PHARMACOLOGY IN MEDICINE:
PRINCIPLES AND PRACTICE

Sachin N. Pradhan, M.D., Ph.D.
Editor

Distinguished Professor
Department of Pharmacology
Howard University College of Medicine
Washington, DC

Roger P. Maickel, Ph.D.
Associate Editor

Professor
Department of Pharmacology and Toxicology
School of Pharmacy and Pharmacal Sciences
Purdue University
West Lafayette, IN

Samar N. Dutta, M.D.,Ph.D.
Associate Editor

Medical Officer
Division of Metabolism and Endocrine Drug Products
National Center for Drugs and Biologics
Food and Drug Administration
Rockville, MD

SP PRESS INTERNATIONAL INC.

Printed in the United States of America

SP Press International Inc.
7806 Honeybee Court
Bethesda, Maryland 20817

International Standard Book Number: 0-9617129-0-2
Library of Congress Catalog Card Number: 86-90514

PREFACE

Information about drugs that is so essential for their therapeutic application in medical practice makes the role of Pharmcology in Medicine extremely important. Medical students heavily burdened with their curriculum in multiferious nonclinical and clinical subjects need a source of drug information which should neither be too voluminous and extensive nor be too light and inadequate. Furthermore, such source should provide not only new and up-to-date information about drugs, but also focus on the new vistas of pharmacology, which are developing and expanding rapidly. These were the objectives which initiated our conceptualization of this textbook and attracted the interest and participation of 106 contributors from more than 60 institutions from USA and abroad.

This textbook is meant for the students of the health profession in general, and medical and pharmacy students in particular. This is a midsize book that contains, in most cases, selective, balanced and up-to-date information and should be helpful for students and teachers for the classroom. The book is organized primarily on the basis of drugs as modifiers of physiological functions rather than on the basis of chemical or pharmacological classifications. This book also goes beyond the traditional practice of the current textbooks of Pharmacology, and provides some new vistas by introducing chapters on much needed topics such as Pharmacogenetics, Pediatric Pharmacology, Geriatric Pharmacology, Immunopharmacology, Peptides, Radiation and Drugs, and also by reorganizing and/or adding chapters on Systemic Pharmacology (such as, Pharmacology of Respiratory and Gastrointestinal Systems, Skin Pharmacology, Ocular Pharmacology, Auditory and Vestibular Pharmacology and Drug Effects on Taste and Smell), Environmental Pharmacology, Diagnosting Agents and Over-the-Counter Drugs.

Each chapter has some salient features: a short table of contents, a brief introductory section; generous tables, schematics, and figures to help make the presentation of the subject more effective and easy to understand; and up-to-date, but less exhaustive bibliography.

A multiauthor book has many positive aspects. Most of our authors have been involved in teaching pharmacology to medical or other health professional students and research in their areas of contribution. Thus each author has the perspective of classroom instruction and is very much aware of students' needs in a course in Pharmacology and/or Toxicology. However, editors are very much aware of some potential problems of a multiauthor book, such as heterogeneity in style and extent of coverage, that would upset the balance among different chapters. To overcome such problems, each chapter has been repeatedly reviewed by editors and consultants and revised as needed. Nevertheless, some residual problems are bound to exist. Although the organization of this project started more than 10 years ago, its publication has been delayed due to some unforeseen problems causing additional shortcomings. The present publisher, SP Press International that was established for publication of this book only, has attempted to rectify some of these and other shortcomings related to publication. Editors realize that it is almost an impossible task to produce a balanced flawless multiauthor book of this size first time around. We hope that comments, criticisms and suggestions from the faculty and students who use this textbook, will help to develop more mature and balanced future editions of the book, the basis of which has now been laid.

It is difficult to thank scores of individuals, too numerous to mention by name, friends, colleagues and consultants who advised and helped in organization, reviewed chapters and provided comments, and participated in preparation and production in various phases of this project. Our special thanks are due to our contributors for their participation in this project, their cooperation in revising and up-dating their chapters as and when needed, and above all, their support and sympathy during the prolonged period of preparation and publication of the book. We are grateful to the Department of Pharmacology and the Office of the Dean, Howard University College of Medicine for their constant whole-hearted support and encouragement in various ways from the very inception to the end of the project, without which the work would never come to a successful completion; in this regard, we are specially appreciative of helps from Dr. Marian Mann, the former Dean of the College of Medicine. Our personal and deep appreciations are to Robert L. Copeland, Jr., Ph.D., Tushar K. Ghosh, Ph.D. and Suwat Wimolwattanapun, M.D. for their reviewing the manuscript in various phases of preparations and their editorial comments. Our sincere thanks are also due to Mrs. Chelvakanie V. Isaac and Mrs. Sandy Willis for their technical assistance in production phase of the book. Finally, our special thanks are due to Dr. Sikta Pradhan who, in addition to her contribution of a chapter, offered her moral, personal and all-out support for publication of this book.

Sachin N. Pradhan
Roger P. Maickel
Samar N. Dutta

CONTRIBUTORS

Armstrong, George D., R.Ph., M.P.H., Chief, Surveillance and Data Processing Branch, Division of Drugs and Biological Product Experience, Office of Epidemiology and Biostatistics, Food and Drug Administration, Rockville, MD

Arvanitakis, Constantine, M.D., F.A.C.P., Associate Professor of Medicine, University of Thessaloniki, Thessaloniki, Greece

Badola, Raghubar, F.F.A.R.C.S., Associate Attending Anesthesiologist, Montefiore Hospital and Medical Center; Assistant Professor of Anesthesiology, Albert Einstein College of Medicine, Bronx, NY

Barnes, Charles D., Ph.D., Professor and Chairman, Department of Veterinary and Comparative Anatomy, Pharmacology and Physiology, Washington State University, College of Veterinary Medicine, Pullman, WA

Berger, Paul, M.D., Chief of Radiotherapy, Bridgeport Hospital, Bridgeport, CT

Berndt, William O., Ph.D., Vice Chancellor for Academic Affairs, Dean for Graduate Studies and Research, University of Nebraska Medical Center, Omaha, NE

Bogaert, M., M.D., Associate Professor, J.F. en C. Heymans Instituut, voor Farmakodynamie en Terapie, der Rijksuniversiteit, de Pintelan 135, B-9000 Ghent, Belgium

Borison, Herbert L., Ph.D., Professor of Pharmacology, Department of Pharmacology and Toxicology, Dartmouth Medical School, Hanover, NH

Bright, Thomas, M.D., Assistant Clinical Professor of Medicine, Assistant Professor of Pharmacology and Toxicology, Indiana University Medical Center, Indianapolis, IN

Brown, R. Don, Ph.D., Professor, Department of Pharmacology and Therapeutics, Louisiana State University Medical Center, Shreveport, LA

Chang, Freddy W., O.D., Ph.D., School of Optometry, Indiana University, Bloomington, IN

Chaudhuri, Gautam, M.D., Ph.D., Assistant Professor, Department of Obstetrics and Gynecology, School of Medicine, Center for the Health Sciences, University of California, Los Angeles, CA

De Schaepdryver, A.F., M.D., Ph.D., Professor of Pharmacology, J.F. en C. Heymans Instituut, voor Farmakodynamie en Terapie, der Rijksuniversiteit, De Pintelan 135, B-9000 Ghent, Belgium

Dettbarn, Wolf-D., M.D., Professor of Pharmacology, Vanderbilt University Medical Center South, Nashville, TN

Dresel, Peter E., Ph.D. Professor and Head, Department of Pharmacology, Dalhousie University, Halifax, Canada

Duncalf, Deryck, M.D., F.F.A.R.C.S., Chairman, Department of Anesthesiology, Montefiore Hospital and Medical Center; Professor of Anesthesiology, Albert Einstein College of Medicine, Bronx, NY

Dutta, Samar N., M.D., Ph.D., Medical Officer, Division of Metabolism and Endocrine Drug Products, National Center for Drugs and Biologics, Food and Drug Administration, Rockville, MD

Dutta, Saradindu, G.V.Sc., Ph.D., Professor of Pharmacology, Wayne State University, College of Medicine, Detroit, MI

Evans, Michael A., Ph.D., Associate Professor of Pharmacology, College of Medicine, University of Illinois Medical Center, Chicago, IL

Garvey, H. Lloyd, Ph.D., Associate Professor, Department of Pharmacology, Howard University College of Medicine, Washington, DC

Goodman, Frank R., Ph.D., Ciba- Geigy Corporation, Summit, NJ

Gordon, David, Ph.D., M.D., M.P.H., Lipid Metabolism - Atherogenesis Branch, Division of Heart and Vascular Diseases, National Heart, Lung and Blood Institute, Bethesda, MD

Green, Sidney, Ph.D., Division of Toxicology, Food and Drug Administration, Washington, DC

Halder, Rebat M., M.D., Assistant Professor, Department of Dermatology, Howard University Hospital, Washington, DC

Hastings, Robert C., M.D., Ph.D., Chief, Laboratory Research Branch, Department of Health and Human Services, U.S. Public Health Service, National Hansen's Disease Center, Carnville, LA

Henkin, Robert I., M.D., Director, Center for Molecular Nutrition and Sensory Disorders, Georgetown University Medical Center, Washington, DC

Hollister, Leo E., M.D., Professor of Medicine, Psychiatry and Pharmacology, VA Medical Center, Palo Alto, CA

Holloway, James A., Ph.D., Professor of Physiology and Neurology, Howard University College of Medicine, Washington, DC

Hook, Jerry B., Ph.D. Vice President, Preclinical R&D, Smith Kline and French Labs, Philadelphia, PA

Hughes, Maysie J., Ph.D., (Formerly of Department of Physiology, Texas Tech University Health Sciences Center, Lubbock, TX), Route #1, Box 137, Elvins, MD

Hunninghake, Donald B., M.D., Co-Director, Lipid Research Clinic, University of Minnesota, Minneapolis, MN

Hurwitz, Aryeh, M.D., Professor of Medicine and Pharmacology, Division of Clinical Pharmacology, Kansas University Medical Center, Kansas City, KS

Jackson, Rudolph E., M.D., Professor and Acting Chairman, Department of Pediatrics, Morehouse School of Medicine; Medical Consultant, Centers for Disease Control, Atlanta, GA

Johnson, Gordon E., Ph.D., Professor and Head, Department of Pharmacology, University of Saskatchewan, Saskatchewan, Canada

Kaliner, Michael A., M.D., Head, Allergic Diseases Section, NIADDKD, National Institutes of Health, Bethesda, MD

Kaul, Lalita, Ph.D., Associate Professor, Community Health and Family Practice, Howard University College of Medicine, Washington, DC

Kenny, Alexander D., Ph.D., D.Sc., Professor and Chairman, Department of Pharmacology, Texas Technical University Health Science Center, Lubbock, TX

Kirkpatrick, Charles H., M.D., Head, Division of Clinical Immunology, National Jewish Hospital and Research Center; Professor of Medicine, University of Colorado School of Medicine, Denver, CO

Knych, Edward T., Ph.D., Associate Professor, Department of Pharmacology, University of Minnesota School of Medicine, Duluth, MN

Kvorning, Sven Ancher, M.D., Chief Physician Emeritus, Sankt Annae Pl. 10, OK1250-Copenhagen, Denmark

Laddu, Atul R., M.D., F.A.C.C., Director of Clinical Research, American Critical Care, McGaw Park, IL

Lal, Harbans, Ph.D., Professor and Chairman, Department of Pharmacology, Texas College of Osteopathic Medicine, Fort Worth, TX

Lathers, Claire M., Ph.D., Associate Professor, Department of Pharmacology, Medical College of Pennsylvania, Philadelphia, PA

Lavappa, K.S., Ph.D., Research Biologist, Division of Toxicology, Genetic Toxicology, Food and Drug Administration, Washington, DC

Leaders, Floyd E., Jr., Ph.D., Technical Evaluation and Management Systems, Inc., 1110 Prestonwood Tower, Dallas, TX

Levine, Donald P., M.D., Assistant Professor of Medicine, Department of Medicine, Wayne State University School of Medicine; Chief, Division of Infectious Diseases, Detroit Receiving Hospital, Detroit, MI

Long, John P., Ph.D., Professor, Department of Pharmacology, University of Iowa College of Medicine, Iowa City, IA

Maickel, Roger P., Ph.D., Professor, Department of Pharmacology and Toxicology, School of Pharmacy and Pharmacal Sciences, Purdue University, West Lafayette, IN

Maines, Mahin D., Ph.D., Dean's Professor of Toxicology, Department of Radiation Biology and Biophysics, University of Rochester School of Medicine and Dentistry, Rochester, NY

Mäkilä, Ulla-Maija, M.D., Ph.D., Visiting Scientist, Department of Physiology and Biophysics, Georgetown University Medical Center, Washington, DC

Maranogos, Paul J., Ph.D., Chief, Unit of Neurochemistry, Biological Psychiatry Branch, National Institute of Mental Health, Bethesda, MD

Mazel, Paul, Ph.D., Professor of Pharmacology and Anesthesiology, George Washington University Medical Center, Washington, DC

McCarthy, Lawrence E., Ph.D., Assistant Professor, Department of Pharmacology and Toxicology, Dartmouth Medical School, Hanover, NH

McNeill, John H., Ph.D., Dean and Professor, Faculty of Pharmaceutical Sciences, Office of the Dean, The University of British Columbia, Vancouver, B.C., Canada

McPhee, Mark, M.D., Assistant Professor of Medicine, University of Kansas Medical Center, Kansas City, KS

Meltzer, Herbert Y., M.D., Douglas Bond Professor of Psychiatry, Department of Psychiatry, School of Medicine, Case Western Reserve University, Cleveland, OH

Merali, Zulfiquar, Ph.D., School of Psychology, University of Ottawa, Ottowa, Ontario

Moore, Kenneth E., Ph.D., Professor of Pharmacology, Michigan State University, East Lansing, MI

Myers, Adam K., Ph.D., Assistant Professor, Department of Physiology and Biophysics, Georgetown University Medical Center, Washington, DC

Neu, Harold C., M.D., Professor of Medicine and Pharmacology, Department of Medicine, College of Physicians and Surgeons of Columbia University, New York, NY

Papac, Rose J., M.D., Chief, Hematology/Oncology, VA Medical Center, West Haven, CT

Paul, Steven M., M.D., Clinical Neuroscience Branch, National Institute of Mental Health, Bethesda, MD

Plaa, Gabriel L., Ph.D., Professor of Pharmacology, Faculte de medecine, Universite de Montreal, Montreal, Quebec, Canada

Popovich, Nicholas G., Ph.D., Associate Professor, Department of Pharmacy Practice, School of Pharmacy and Pharmacal Sciences, Purdue University, West Lafayette, IN

Pradhan, Sachin N., M.D., Ph.D., Distinguished Professor, Department of Pharmacology, Howard University College of Medicine, Washington, DC

Pradhan, Sikta, Ph.D., Pharmacologist, Division of Bioequivalence, Food and Drug Administration, Rockville, MD

Radnay, Paul A., M.D., Attending Anesthesiologist Emeritus, Montefiore Hospital and Medical Center; Professor Emeritus of Anesthesiology, Albert Einstein Collge of Medicine,Bronx, NY

Raines, Arthur, Ph.D., Professor of Pharmacology, School of Medicine and Dentistry, Georgetown University, Washington, DC

Ramwell, Peter W., Ph.D., Professor of Pharmacology, Department of Physiology and Biophysics, Georgetown Medical Center, Washington, DC

Rastogi, Ram B., D.V.M., Ph.D., Associate Director, Clinical Investigation, Medical Research Division, Lederle Laboratories, American Cynamide Co., Pearl River, NY

Rech, Richard H., Ph.D., Professor, Department of Pharmacology and Toxicology, Michigan State University, East Lansing, MI

Rifkind, Basil M., M.D., Chief, Lipid Metabolism - Atherogenesis Branch, Division of Heart and Vascular Disease, NHLBI, National Institutes of Health, Bethesda, MD

Ritschel, W.A., Ph.D., Dr. Univ., Professor of Pharmacokinetics and Biopharmaceutics, College of Pharmacy; Professor of Pharmacology and Cell Biophysics, College of Medicine, University of Cincinnati Medical Center, Cincinnati, OH

Roberts, Jay, Ph.D., Professor and Chairman, Department of Pharmacology, Medical College of Pennsylvania, Philadelphia, PA

Rollinson, Russell D., M.D., (Formerly of Department of Neurology, Vanderbilt University School of Medicine, Nashville, TN). 42 The Avenue. Windsor, Victoria 3181, Australia

Sanders-Bush, Elaine, Ph.D., Professor of Pharmacology, Vanderbilt University School of Medicine, Nashville, TN

Sastry, Annette K., R.N., M.S.N., Assistant Professor, Department of Adult Health, Vanderbilt University School of Nursing, Nashville, TN

Sastry, B.V. Rama, Sc.D., Ph.D., Professor of Pharmacology, Vanderbilt University School of Medicine, Nashville, TN

Schou, Jens, M.D., Ph.D., Professor of Pharmacology, University of Copenhagen, Copenhagen, Denmark

Schyve, Paul M., M.D., Department of Psychiatry, University of Chicago, Pritzker School of Medicine, Chicago, IL

Severs, Walter, B., Ph.D., Professor of Pharmacology, Pennsylvania State University, The Milton S. Hershey Medical Center, Hershey, PA

Silverman, Ira, M.D., Clinical Assistant Professor, Department of Obstetrics and Gynecology, University of California, Los Angeles, CA

Singhal, Radhey L., Ph.D., (Formerly Chairman, Department of Pharmacology, University of Ottawa College of Medicine, Ottawa, Canada). 22 Royal Hung Court, Ottawa, Ontario, Canada

Skolnick, Phil, Ph.D., Chief, Section on Neurobiology, Lab. of Bioorganic Chemistry, NIADDK, National Institutes of Health, Bethesda, MD

Smith, Carol Grace, Ph.D., Visiting Professor, Department of Obstetrics and Gynecology, University of Texas Health Center, San Antonio, TX

Smith, Michael T., M.D., Chairman, Department of Pathology, Wilford Hall USAF Medical Center, Lackland AFB, San Antonio, TX

Sokol, Gerald H., M.D., Director, Radiation Oncology Department, Tampa General Hospital, Davis Island, Tampa, FL

Spector, Sidney, Ph.D., Head, Department of Physiology, Chemistry and Pharmacology, Roche Institute of Molecular Biology, Nutley, NJ

Spratto, George R., Ph.D., Professor of Pharmacology, School of Pharmacy and Pharmacal Sciences, Purdue University, West Lafayette, IN

Spyker, Daniel A., Ph.D., M.D., Medical Center, University of Virginia, School of Medicine, Charlottesville, VA

Steck, Edgar A., Ph.D., (Formerly of Division of Experimental Therapeutics, Walter Reed Army Institute of Research, Washington, DC). 1913 Edgewater Parkway, Silver Spring, MD

Strickland, G. Thomas, M.D., Ph.D., Professor and Director, International Health Program; Professor of Microbiology and Medicine, University of Maryland School of Medicine, Baltimore, MD

Sulser, Fridolin, M.D., Professor of Pharmacology, Tennessee Neuropsychiatric Institute, Nashville, TN

Summy-Long, Joan Y., Ph.D., Department of Pharmacology, Pennsylvania State University, The Milton S. Hershey Medical Center, Hershey, PA

Tamir, Israel, M.D., Department of Pediatrics, Tel Aviv Medical Center, University of Tel Aviv, Tel Aviv, Israel

Thomas, John A., Ph.D., Vice President, Corporate Research, Travenol Labs., Inc., Route 120 & Wilson Road, Round Lake, IL

Tizabi, Yousef, Ph.D., Associate Professor, Department of Pharmacology, Howard University College of Medicine, Washington, DC

Trautman, John R., M.D., Director of Leprosorium, USPHS Hospital, Carnville, LA

Turlapaty, Prasad D.M.V., Ph.D., Associate Director of clinical Research, American Critical Care, McGaw Park, IL

Utz, John P., M.D., Professor of Medicine, Georgetown University School of Medicine, Washington, DC

Vesell, Elliot S., M.D., Professor and Chairman, Department of Pharmacology, Pennsylvania State University, The Milton S. Hershey Medical Center, Hershey, PA

Weisburger, Elizabeth K., Ph.D., Division of Cancer Etiology, NCI, National Institutes of Health, Bethesda, MD

West, William L., Ph.D., Professor and Chairman, Department of Pharmacology, Howard University College of Medicine, Washington, DC

Wilson, John T., M.D., Professor, Department of Pharmacology and Pediatrics; Chief, Section on Clinical Pharmacology, Louisiana State University Medical Center, School of Medicine in Shreveport, Shreveport, LA

Wood, Charles D., Ph.D., Professor of Pharmacology, Department of Pharmacology and Therapeutics, Louisiana State University Medical Center, Shreveport, LA

Yim, George K.W., Ph.D., Professor and Head, Department of Pharmacology, School of Pharmacy and Pharmacal Sciences, Purdue University, West Lafayette, IN

CONTENTS

Section I
GENERAL PRINCIPLES

CHAPTER
1

INTRODUCTION AND HISTORICAL BACKGROUND

John P. Long, Floyd E. Leaders, Jr. and Sachin N. Pradhan

DEFINITION AND SCOPE OF PHARMACOLOGY

Pharmacology (from the Greek *pharmacon*, medicine or drug, and *logos*, a discourse or study) is concerned with the study of drugs. It has been defined as the experimental science that deals with changes induced in living organisms by chemically active substances (with the exception of foods), whether used for therapeutic purposes or not. In a broad sense, pharmacology encompasses all aspects of our knowledge about chemicals that have actions on living systems — their history, source, chemistry, absorption, distribution, biotransformation and fate, biochemical and physiologic effects, mechanism of action, toxic and side effects, therapeutic uses, and interaction with other drugs.

The study of pharmacology necessitates an integrated knowledge of many scientific disciplines to understand how a drug acts and how it can be appropriately used. An in-depth knowledge of biochemistry and physiology is essential, and background knowledge in chemistry, statistics, anatomy, histology, microbiology, and pathology is helpful.

HISTORY OF PHARMACOLOGY

Ever since man's advent on earth, alleviation of pain and suffering and change of mood have been among the main concerns of humankind. To these ends, humans have been involved throughout the history of our species in the ingestion of chemical agents, particularly plant products. Early humans noted that selected plants and herbs seem to produce either harmful or beneficial effects. Out of this misty past every culture, Egyptian, Greek, Roman, Indian, and others, developed a long list of medical folklore with suggested formulations for various diseases.

Eber's *Papyrus*, an Egyptian book of records dating from 1550 B.C., lists numerous recipes of plant products including castor oil (a purgative), colchicum (an antigout drug), and opium (dried exudation from poppy capsule containing narcotic alkaloids) that are still in use. In the Egyptian and even in the early Greek period, medicine was also an integral part of religion and philosophy.

The concept of disease as a pathological process developing in the body, rather than as a visitation from the spirits, was formulated for the first time by Hippocrates (460-377 B.C.). He also made extensive use of medicinal plants (including hyoscyamus, opium, veratrum, and acacia), about 300 of which are mentioned in the Hippocratic writings.

Theophrastus (373-287 B.C.) compiled an herbal guide in which about 450 plants of supposed medicinal value were described. Pedanius Dioscorides, a physician to Roman armies in Asia during the reign of Nero (ca. A.D. 54), described therapeutic uses of 500 medicinal herbs and coined the term *materia medica* for such a compilation.

With the decline of Greek culture, the quest for fresh knowledge slackened. Notable during this period was Claudius Galen (A.D. 130-200), a successful physician in Rome, who compiled an herbal guide describing medical use of about 400 herbs. Crude mixtures of drugs, usually of plant origin, have been named after him as *galenicals.* Under his influence, medicine degenerated into a dogmatic system of polypharmacy throughout the late Roman period and the Middle Ages. Discourse of Apuleius, a prominent Roman herbalist (ca. A.D. 450), on medicinal agents was perpetuated and published in Anglo-Saxon for the first time about A.D. 1000.

During the fourteenth and fifteenth centuries great interest in medicine and pharmacy was aroused throughout Europe. Epidemic diseases, especially leprosy, ergotism, and the black death (bubonic plague), were very prevalent during this time. In the fifteenth century, alchemy brought in by the Arabs rapidly spread over Europe. In search of the philosopher's stone and elixir of life alchemists made important inventions and discoveries that laid the foundations of the modern science, chemistry. In 1438 printing was invented; some earliest printed works provide illustration of a fifteenth century pharmacy.

During the sixteenth century there was further development in pharmacy. In 1546 Valerius Cordus, son of a professor of medicine at Marburg, has his first pharmacopeia printed for use in the community. Its materials were procured from Greek, Roman, and Arabian sources, and it also quoted freely from Galen, Dioscorides, and Avicenna. It contained comparatively few types of preparation. With the Renaissance the Hippocratic spirit was revived.

Paracelsus (1493-1541), the son of a German physician and chemist, with his vast background of knowledge and experience, was appointed professor of physics and surgery at the University of Basel in 1526. Free thought and critical inquiry led him to denounce the prevailing absolute authority of ancient texts, to burn Apuleian herbal in public, and to reject the teachings of Galen. He introduced simple prescription writing and recommended use of chemical substances rather than mixed vegetable galenicals. Because of his background in alchemy, he advocated use of metals in the treatment of disease and introduced mercury in the treatment of syphilis.

In the seventeenth century, Thuillier (1630), a French physician, ascertained that grains infected with ergot fungus were responsible for a form of gangrene of the extremities that was ascribed earlier to a mystical phenomenon known as *ignis sacer*, or holy fire. Robert Boyle and his associate Timothy Clark (1660) showed the therapeutic effectiveness of certain drugs (e.g., opium, antimony, tobacco oil) by the intravenous route, leading to the concept that drugs are transported from the site of administration to the site of action by way of the bloodstream. Johann Wepfer (1679) presented experimental evidence for the convulsive nature of the water hemlock, *Cicuta aquatica*, and that of *Strychnos nux-vomica*, and thus provide a basis for their toxicity.

In the latter half of the eighteenth century, Menghini (1755) showed actions of camphor on animals, and Peter Daries (1776) established that the juices of belladonna leaves, if locally instilled into the eye of an animal, would produce typical dilatation of pupils. William Withering (1785) explained how digitalis relieves edema in cardiac decompensation in a report of his pharmacological investigations in fowls and humans entitled *The Foxglove and An Account of its Medical Properties with Practical Remarks on Dropsy.*

The early part of the nineteenth century saw a surge of interest in the isolation of active principles from plant products. In 1803, Sertürner, a German scientist, isolated morphine from opium. Pelletier and Caventou, French chemists, isolated quinine and cinchonine from cinchona (1820) and strychnine from *Strychnos nux-vomica* used as a Javanese arrow poison; Pelletier and Magendie isolated emetine from ipecac. François Magendie (1783-1855) localized the convulsive action of strychnine in the spinal cord by experimenting on animals with the spinal cord transected or destroyed.

Claude Bernard (1813-1878), a famous pupil of Magendie, reflected on the methods of "experimental medicine," as the undifferentiated field of physiology-pharmacology-biochemistry was then called. Investigating carbon monoxide poisoning, he explained the mechanism of its action. Bernard also conducted a simple but ingenious experiment on frogs that led to localization of the site of action of curare (a South American arrow poison and a muscle-paralyzing agent) at the myoneural junction.

In the second half of the nineteenth century, the center of activity for experimental medicine gradually shifted from France to Germany, with its two important schools of physiology, Johannes Müller's (1801-1858) at Berlin and Ernst Weber's (1795-1878) at Leipzig. Karl Binz (1832-1913), a student of Müller, did fundamental work on cyanide poisoning and quinine. Rudolf Buchheim (1820-1879), a pupil of Weber, established in the basement of his home the first laboratory of experimental pharmacology, where he contributed to the knowledge of atropine and ergot. Buchheim was invited to establish the first chair of pharmacology at the University of Dorpat (Tartu, Estonia) in 1849.

Oswald Schmiedeberg (1838-1921), one of the most famous names in pharmacology and regarded as the founder of modern pharmacology, was a pupil of both Buchheim and the well-known physiologist, Carl Ludwig. He pioneered in the study of drug actions on isolated organs, an avenue of research that has contributed much to the knowledge of how drugs act in the body, and also initiated studies on the fate of drugs in the body. His greatest role, however, was that of a teacher of medical students and future pharmacologists. One of 40 pupils who filled chairs of pharmacology throughout the world was John Jacob Abel, regarded as the father of American pharmacology.

Abel (1857-1938) became the first professor of pharmacology at the University of Michigan (1883) and later at Johns Hopkins University (1893). He introduced Schmiedeberg's teaching methods by lectures, demonstrations, and discussions in pharmacology. Besides devoting considerable time to research and contributing to the isolation of epinephrine and insulin, Abel also founded the *Journal of Pharmacology and Experimental Therapeutics* and the *Journal of Biological Chemistry.*

SUBDIVISIONS OF PHARMACOLOGY

In earlier times, as indicated in the history, pharmacology was little more than a compilation of plant materials used for therapeutic purpose. For proper handling of the *materia medica* or medicinal plant materials, and preparation of his own crude drugs, it was essential for a physician to have a broad botanical knowledge of the crude natural drugs. This led to the development of *pharmacognosy*, a field that deals with the biological, biochemical, and economic aspects of drugs of natural origin and their constituents.

With the development of new drugs and products, the art of preparing, compounding, and dispensing medicine (comprising the field of *pharmacy*), which was at one time in the hands of physicians, has now been delegated almost completely to pharmacists.

Modern pharmacology is usually subdivided into the following major and intimately related subdivisions: pharmacokinetics, pharmacodynamics, therapeutics, and toxicology.

Pharmacokinetics is concerned with the time-course of the concentration of a drug in the blood and at its site of action, and deals with absorption, distribution, metabolism, and excretion of the drug and its metabolites in the intact organism.

Pharmacodynamics is the study of the biochemical and physiological effects of a drug and its mechanism of action. *Immunopharmacology* is the study of immunological aspects of drug action, including effects of drugs on immune response and development of antibodies in response to drugs. The study of the variation of drug effects in relation to their chemical structure (*structure-activity relationship*, or SAR) leads to the development of better drugs. Studies on the pharmacodynamics and pharmacokinetics of a new drug are performed on normal animals and are usually compared in more than one studies of the drug's effects on humans (*clinical trials*) are required before regular therapeutic use is started.

Clinical pharmacology and *therapeutics* deals with application of drugs to the treatment or prevention of diseases; it may be further differentiated into pharmacotherapy and chemotherapy. *Pharmacotherapy* is treatment with drugs directed toward preventing a disease or restoring altered body functions in an existing disease state, as in using digitalis preparation in the treatment of cardiac failure. *Chemotherapy*, as first proposed by Paul Ehrlich, is treatment with drugs to destroy or eliminate pathogenic organisms or cells without (or minimally) affecting the host, as in the treatment of tuberculosis with isoniazid.

Toxicology, or the science (*logos*) of poisons (*toxicon*), deals with the adverse effects of drugs used in therapy, as well as with the effects of many other household, environmental, occupational, and industrial chemicals. These groups of nondrug chemicals may be taken accidentally in high doses or may be absorbed by chronic exposure during their occupational and industrial use. They include heavy metal compounds, industrial solvents, insecticides, pesticides, herbicides, and many others.

For certain drugs, individual variability in therapeutic (or toxic) response is markedly influenced by heredity. *Pharmacogenetics* is the branch of pharmacology that studies the effects of heredity upon drug response. For example, the rate of inactivation of the antitubercular drug isoniazid by acetylation is dependent upon ethnic group: fast acetylation occurs in Eskimos and Japanese, and slow acetylation in Jews, Scandinavians, and North African Caucasians. Hemolysis caused by the antimalarial agent primaquine (and by other drugs) has been shown to be due to a hereditary deficiency of the enzyme glucose-6-phosphate dehydrogenase found in erythrocytes; this occurs in about 10% of black males in the United States and also in some dark-colored Caucasian ethnic groups, including Sephardic Jews, Greeks, Sardinians, and Iranians.

Investigation of drug effects as a function of biological timing, as well as their effects upon rhythm characteristics, has been the concern of a developing discipline called *chronopharmacology* (15). Effects of various chemical agents have shown circadian changes; for example, the peak effects of histamine-induced skin reaction (erythema and wheal) to intradermal injection, or airway reactivity, was shown at close to midnight, whereas the peak acetylcholine-induced bronchial reaction was observed at about noon or early afternoon. Another type of effect includes drug-induced changes in circadian rhythm in human beings, such as alteration of body temperature circadian rhythm by reserpine or alteration of plasma glucose, nonesterified fatty acid (NEFA), and growth hormone circadian rhythms by insulin.

SOURCES OF DRUGS

For many years pharmacologists and chemists, in developing agents for the treatment of disease, used a wide spectrum of chemical entities found in plants and animals. The major sources were plants that, during normal growth, produced a broad spectrum of chemical agents: alkaloids, glycosides, and others. Many of these agents have significant biological actions; determination of the chemical structures of these agents led synthetic chemists to produce many structural analogs. In many cases, marked improvement in therapeutic benefit resulted; on occasion, new areas of pharmacology emerged. Many active biological agents are also produced in animals, even from such lowly creatures as frogs, toads, and marine life. For example, the extraction of hormones from animal endocrine glands for replacement therapy in humans has been of tremendous benefit.

Most drugs recently introduced into medicine had their beginning with modern synthetic chemistry. The chemist, working with biologists, attempts to increase the desired therapeutic action and to diminish toxicity and unwanted activities. This approach was placed on a firm basis at the beginning of the twentieth century with the synthesis of barbiturates for depression of the central nervous system and local anesthetics for inhibition of neural conduction. During the next three decades, although isolated discoveries led to the introduction of new therapeutic agents, advances in drug therapy seemed to falter. In 1935 the American Society for Pharmacology and Experimental Therapeutics even appointed a committee to evaluate whether the society should be continued because there did not seem to be many worthy discoveries. Fortunately for the society (and perhaps the committee), sulfa drugs were introduced, giving pharmacologists something new to study. Marked expansion in applying research to modern medicine via synthetic chemistry occurred following World War II, when several new types of drugs were introduced, including effective drugs for the treatment of mental disease, hypertension, cancer, and a host of additional therapies. These advances in pharmacology have continued. Many valuable synthetic drugs have been added to the treasure house of modern medicine; development of these drugs has been possible due to the joint efforts of chemists and pharmacologists. As presented later in this chapter, however, the path to new drugs is a lengthy and expensive one.

MECHANISM AND SITES OF DRUG ACTION

Most drugs stimulate or inhibit ongoing biological processes. Some compounds serve as substrates for enzyme systems; others attach to enzyme receptors and inhibit enzyme-substrate interactions. Many compounds act on cell membranes to alter the function and/or biological processes within the cell. Such actions of drugs may alter the balance of essential ions such as Na^+, K^+, and Ca^{2+}. A large number of active transport systems have been identified in various cell membranes; drugs may facilitate or inhibit these processes. The biophysical and biochemical alterations induced by drugs are reflected in such physiological effects as changes in blood pressure, heart rate and respiration.

In order to interpret the mechanism of action of most of the drugs (such as autonomic agents, hormones, etc.) in a biological system, it is helpful to conceive of an active site known as *receptor* with which the drug must interact. However, it may be added that such conception is not applicable to certain other drugs like gaseous anesthetics, osmotic diuretics, antiseptics, and chelating agents. Attempts are being made to isolate receptors considered to be active macromolecular components of biological systems, and to identify these entities by modern analytical techniques. The difficulty in analyzing an isolated receptor is great because the process of isolation and purification may cause alterations in morphology and function. As indicated below and discussed in Chapter 3, receptors that belong to some molecular system are usually part of a large molecule and involve a functionally integrated interdependent unit.

Evidence for Receptors. Concepts concerning receptors were consolidated at the end of the nineteenth century by Ehrlich and Hara (5) who used the concept of "lock and key" in their research and drug design: the lock is the receptor, and the key is the drug or chemical that opens the lock and causes alteration of biological function. Ehrlich believed that structural alterations in his active arsenical compounds would be expected to increase still further the interaction with the lock, hopefully resulting in more effective agents for the treatment of syphilis. More sophisticated concepts concerning receptors were evolved by A.J. Clark (3), who by 1933 placed drug-receptor interactions on a mathematical basis and provided for the application of statistics and mathematics to experimental pharmacology. His original idea came from the earlier studies of I. Langmuir, a physical chemist at General Electric, who had described the adsorption of gases onto activated charcoal in 1913. Clark noted that the dose-response curves that he obtained with his chemicals were described by the same mathematical equations (adsorption isotherms) that Langmuir had reported.

During the past 50 years, the concept of the receptor as a functional entity in biological systems has been widely adopted. The components of this basic hypothesis may be outlined as follows:

1. Extremely small doses of chemicals are active. As A.J. Clark demonstrated, adsorption onto a major portion of a cell surface cannot explain biological activity because of the large surface area of cells versus the extremely small surface that could be occupied by the reacting chemical. Biological activity of drugs is observed in the submicromolar range; thus, only a very small part of a cell surface can be occupied by the reacting chemical.

2. It has been observed with all series of active compounds that minor alterations in chemical structure often result in wide variation in biological activity. This is especially true for stimulant compounds; such agents that are termed *agonists*, when bound to the receptor, increase biological function, suggesting rigorous structure and charge requirements for both drug and receptor that must match and be complementary to allow a drug-receptor interaction.

3. For most agonists there has been the discovery of *antagonists*, agents that inhibit or block a receptor. Hypothetically, such agents bind to the receptor but do not produce activation. Antagonists are believed to shield the target receptor and interfere with the approach of an agonist. These agents normally compete with an agonist and follow mass-action relationships; that is, with increasing agonist concentration, the antagonist will be removed from the receptor and biological action reestablished. Likewise, biological action can be terminated by increasing the concentration of the antagonist and removing the agonist from the receptor. This type of interaction between an agonist and antagonist is termed *competitive inhibition*. There are also numerous examples of *noncompetitive antagonists*. With these agents, high-energy bonds are formed with some part of the receptor; the agents cannot be removed from the receptor site merely by increasing the concentration of agonists.

4. *Stereoisomers* are present in many active drugs; generally, only one of the isomers will exhibit high biological activity. This is best explained by a receptor concept that involves three or more binding sites. With this concept, the active isomer would be able to present three points in correct position to the receptor, and the inactive isomer at best would be able to interact at only two points.

LEVELS OF INTEGRATION FOR DRUG ACTION

Drugs interact with the biological systems at various levels, as discussed by Schueler (16) and summarized in Table 1-1. The sites for drug action will invariably be with receptors that are part of the molecular level of integration. Alteration of function at the molecular level results in modification of function at all higher levels and thus results in altered biological activity. For example, drug-receptor interaction brings about changes in the molecular level and this in turn alters the polymolecular system, which then alters cell function. Change in function at the higher levels leads to alterations such as changes in heart rate and blood pressure, relaxation or contraction of smooth muscle, and stimulation or depression of the central nervous system. As illustrated in Table 1-1, involvement of the molecular level and altered interactions at other levels occur in both health and disease. For example, an alteration in the function of an organ or in the state of mental health is preceded by changes at the molecular level of integration. Thus, disease alters the molecular level, and it is the attempts to restore normalcy that comprise the research interest of pharmacologists and the goal of therapy with drugs.

PLACEBO

The effect of a drug administered to a conscious patient often involves more than the effect of the chemical on the body; added to this are the "psychological, physiological, and psychophysiological effects of the medication or procedure given with therapeutic intent, which is independent of or minimally related to the pharmacologic effect of the medication or to the specific effects of the procedure" (17). The reactions to drug administration that are unrelated to the drug's pharmacological effect and that arise from, or are related to, drug administration are known as *placebo effects*. The Latin word *placebo*, meaning "I shall please," referred originally to substances given merely to "please" or appease the patient when no specific medication was available. The placebo effect depends a great deal on the total relationship between physician and patient. An important role is played by the physician, whose prestige, appearance, attitude, sympathetic interest, and other emotional responsiveness form the bases for effectiveness of placebo therapy, including the placebo effect.

Table 1-1
Levels of Integration

Level of Integration	Physical Unit of Level	Remarks
0	Electron, proton, positron, neutron	Has been called the zero level of integration; the zero is purely relative to our state of knowledge.
1	Atom	With the zero level, embraces the active interests of atomic and nuclear physicists with their appropriate techniques.
2	Molecule	Molecule in the ordinary chemical sense, including both micro- and macromolecules. Level of interest for "pure" chemists.
3	Molecular system	Any individual isolated enzyme system with its associated coenzymes, ions, substrates, etc. Receptor is a macromolecular component. Levels 2-4 are of greatest interest to biochemists and enzymologists.
4	Polymolecular system	Embodies the idea of a metabolic pool containing many enzyme systems held in an integrated functional relationship; of particular interest to cytologists and enzymologists.
5	Cellular system	Level of interest for cytologists and cytochemists.
6	Polycellular or tissue system	Of particular interest for histologists, cytologists, and pathologists.
7	Polytissue or organ	Of particular interest in classical organology and physiology (e.g., isolated hearts, smooth-muscle preparations, etc.)
8	Organism	In the sense of a multiorgan organism, such as mammal.
9	Society	According to some, includes only human societies; it is argued that the differentiated aspect of mind is too undeveloped in lower species for this degree of integration.

Source: Ref. 16. (Published by permission of McGraw-Hill, New York)

The effects and roles of placebos in therapy have been discussed by Wolf (19) and Melmon and Morelli (13) and will be briefly summarized here.

Examples and Types of Placebos. Placebos are most commonly represented by the dosage form or the vehicle — pills, capsules, injections, or ingredients — through which the active drug is given, but which itself does not usually possess any medicinal property. Some drugs not actually indicated for the particular disease condition in question may also produce some beneficial placebo effects. The physician in whom the patient has confidence may "please" and do much benefit to the patient simply by being present and performing various procedures (e.g., taking a medical history, performing a physical examination or diagnostic and therapeutic procedures). A variety of diagnostic practices (e.g., drawing blood for laboratory tests, cardiac catheterization) and therapeutic procedures (putting dietary restrictions in peptic ulcer, which may even produce harmful effects; setting up of fluid infusion apparatus even without giving any infusion; performing exploratory surgical operations) may also serve as placebos.

A substance or a procedure serving as a placebo may be called *pure* if it does not have any known physiological or pharmacological effects, or *impure* if it has some effects, but not on the disease process for which it is prescribed. Placebos used for their beneficial or positive effects may also have negative or toxic effects. They are often beneficial even if the physician is aware of their harmful aspects. On the other hand, a drug administered for other reasons may also produce a toxic placebo effect. For example, if the physician is aware of a toxic effect of a drug and warns the patient about it, or if the patient had heard about this toxic effect, the patient may anticipate such an effect in addition to desired effect(s) of the drug. This creates difficulty in interpreting drug response in humans and in distinguishing between the pharmacological and placebo effects of a drug (19). Double-blind studies in which both the patient and physician are unaware of the identity of the drug concerned are therefore of great important in experimental clinical pharmacology.

Placebo "Reactor". Beecher (1) showed that placebo therapy in 1082 patients with conditions including postoperative pain, cough, mood changes, headache, seasickness, anxiety and tension, angina pectoris, and the common cold produced satisfactory relief in 35% of the cases. In a well-designed study involving postoperative pain in 162 patients, Lasagna et al. (9) showed that following placebo (saline) injection, 14% of the patients experienced consistent analgesia, 31% consistently failed to experience any releif of pain, and the remaining 55% were inconsistent. Certain characteristics for both of these groups have been suggested. The patients of the reactor group were more outgoing, more favorably disposed to hospitalization, more concerned with visceral or pelvic complaints, sometimes anxious, more dependent on outside emotional satisfaction, and perhaps less mature compared with the nonreactors. It was difficult, however, to predict the reaction of the patients to placebos on the basis of earlier conversation or examination. Other studies have shown that the frequency of placebo responses varies widely in different studies, and even in the same individual studied at different times, and that all people react to placebos under appropriate circumstances. It is therefore impractical to identify or exclude placebo reactors (7).

Requirements and Possible Mechanisms of Placebo Effect. For a placebo to be effective, the following conditions should be fulfilled: the disease process itself or its symptoms should be amenable to modification in intensity that may vary with time and individuals. Furthermore, the patient may possess resilience and defensive mechanisms that may reduce the intensity of symptoms and even cure the disease. There must also exist a dynamic physician-patient relationship that would strengthen the effect of the placebo in amelioration of the disease process.

The mechanism of placebo effect is not known. The roles of psychological processes such as transference (transfer of emotion from the past environment to new objects) or conditioned response have been proposed to be responsible, at least to some extent. A potential neurochemical substrate has also been suggested for placebo effects in patients suffering from pain. Levine et al. (11, 12) suggested that placebo analgesia may involve opiate receptors the same way as does morphine analgesia. They showed that on pain after extraction of a wisdom tooth placebo would produce analgesia which could be reduced by an opiate antagonist, naloxone. However, such conclusion on mediation of placebo analgesia through the opiate receptors has been disputed by other investigators (4).

Toxicity and Undesired Effects. An impure placebo may produce the usual toxic effect of the active ingredient. An effective placebo may have abuse potential, and its repeated use may cause habit formation.

Failure to diagnose a patient's condition for which a more specific treatment is indicated, and treatment of such a patient with a placebo, would cause much harm to the patient.

Even though use of placebos may be justified in appropriate cases for the sake of relieving the patient's suffering, the patient may also blame the physician for "being tricked;" if the patient finds out, this may worsen the physician-patient relationships and increase the patient's suffering.

Use of Placebo: Indications and Objections. Evidence of the effectiveness of placebos in well-controlled trials (e.g., patients with mild depression), and situations in which no drug is indicated, but the patient requires or demands some "treatment," are some of the justifications for administration of a placebo.

There are, however, some ethical objections to the use of a placebo. Individuals may not be placed in a trial with a placebo if the investigator knows that its potential risk to the patient outweighs potential benefit. Furthermore, use of placebos has been considered as deceitful (8). Placebos have been criticized because they are deceptive, yet defended on the grounds that a physician's beneficial intentions justify the deception. However, deception need not play any essential role in eliciting this powerful therapeutic modality. A positive placebo response can be elicited by physicians in their patients by nondeceptive means. One excellent example of non-deceptive use of placebo occurs in properly designed double-blind research with informed consent. In such research both the subject and the experimenter are unaware of the placebo or the drug, but the patient has been fully informed of the experimental design, about use of placebo in the study, and about the risks and benefits associated with design, and have given free consent (2).

MODERN DRUG DEVELOPMENT

Pharmacologists, chemists, and other scientists in drug research and development work jointly in evaluating new chemical entities and gaining better understanding of known active agents. At the present time, the development of new drugs is limited almost entirely to pharmaceutical companies, although the historic location for drug development has been the academic sector. In general, drug research and development are areas of high risk, high monetary investment, and delayed rewards for successful research. Synthesis and evaluation of thousands of chemical agents are usually necessary for one new drug to be introduced on the market. The cost of developing a new drug to-day in America will therefore range from $35 to $50 million.

This high cost has unfortunately resulted in some negative factors. For example, it is no longer economically feasible to develop drugs for more than 30-50 of the more common diseases that afflict humans. Who will develop the drugs to treat other, less prevalent, diseases? Likewise, the marked monetary increase for drug research and development discourages the introduction of drugs for the treatment of diseases that occur in less affluent areas of the world. In total numbers of afflicted humans, the diseases found in tropical areas are many times more common than disease found in our society.

Government regulations controlling each step of drug research and development have greatly increased over the past two decades (18). The following section will demonstrate the complexities of drug development and also illustrate the tremendous demands that must be met before a new drug may be introduced into therapeutics.

GROWTH OF DRUG REGULATION IN THE UNITED STATES

The dramatic advances in pharmacology together with the accompanying improvement in medical treatment that took place during the first three-quarters of this century have largely overshadowed a parallel development that may be expected to have an impact on further scientific development in the foreseeable future. This development, an increase in regulatory involvement in the drug development process, has not attracted a great deal of attention from scientists outside the pharmaceutical industry. As usual, in retrospect this growth of regulatory interest could have been anticipated within the framework of drug development and medical practice in the United States.

As compounds with increased pharmacological activity and hence more pronounced effectiveness were made available to the medical community, clinical treatment became more and more an extension of applied clinical pharmacology. It is not surprising that this phenomenon was accompanied by the potential for increased side effects and toxicity. Moreover, as the anticipated toxic effects became manifest, sometimes quite dramatically, it might also be expected that an aware and anxious laity would attempt to ensure their safety through legislative means.

Issues of safety and efficacy go back beyond the turn of the century, when they centered on therapeutic use of overtly toxic substances and false and misleading claims for patent medicines and nostrums. The entry of the U.S. government into control of such substances was initiated through the Pure Food and Drugs Acts of 1906, which defined *drug* broadly and regulated labeling, but not advertising, associated with any substance used therapeutically.

More than 30 years passed before any major new legislation was enacted. Then, toxicity resulting from a newly introduced formulation, "Elixir of Sulfanilamide," prompted Congress to act. In June 1938, the Food, Drug and Cosmetic Act extended the government's control over advertising and labeling, and required new drugs to obtain approval (based on safety criteria) from the Food and Drug Administration (FDA) before being allowed in interstate commerce. This act called for submission of a New Drug Application (NDA), containing the results of safety and clinical efficacy investigations. These NDAs were automatically approved if the FDA failed to respond within 60 days.

The 1938 act did not provide for government involvement with investigational plans prior to submission of New Drug Application; the FDA did not enter the picture until a manufacturer actually sought marketing approval. Selection of drugs for clinical trial was completely dependent upon the scientific expertise and ethical conscience of sponsoring firms and their clinical investigators. Although they were not required by law to do so at that time drug manufacturers began to institute premarketing safety tests as a means of self-protection. Extensive toxicity testing was not likely to be demanded by most potential clinical investigators, so this testing was often deferred until after demonstration of clinical utility.

Twenty-four more years went by before enactment of the next major legislative package affecting development of new drugs. This legislation was also in response to the manifestation of drug-induced toxicity during the thalidomide tragedy. Reaction to the birth of deformed babies in Europe following use of thalidomide during pregnancy prompted passage of the Drug Industry Act of 1962, the Kefauver-Harris Amendments to the Food, Drug, and Cosmetic Act of 1938. These amendments produced a new set of guidelines for drug development. One of the major changes brought about by the 1962 legislation related to preclinical safety evaluation. The legislation required the sponsor to submit a Notice of Claimed Investigational Exemption for a New Drug (IND) to the FDA before instituting human testing. Guidelines concerning acceptable criteria for this testing evolved with time. The four phases of clinical investigation are as follows (6):

Phase I. *Clinical Pharmacology*, is intended to include the initial introduction of a drug into the human organism. It may be administered to the usual "normal" volunteer subjects to determine levels of toxicity, and be followed by early dose-ranging studies in patients for safety and, in some cases, early efficacy.

Alternatively, for ethical or scientific considerations, with some new drugs the initial introduction into humans is more properly done in selected patients. When normal volunteers are the initial recipients of a drug, the very early patient trials that follow are also considered part of phase I.

The number of subjects and patients in phase I will, of course, vary with the drug but will generally range between 20 and 80.

Drug dynamic and metabolic studies, in whichever stage of investigation they are performed, are considered to be phase I clinical pharmacological studies. Whereas some, such as absorption studies, are performed in the early stages, others, such as efforts to identify metabolites, may not be performed until later in the investigations.

Phase II. *Clinical Investigation,* is intended to include early controlled clinical trials designed to demonstrate efficacy and relative safety. Normally, these are performed on a limited number or closely monitored patients. This phase will seldom go beyond 100-200 patients on drug, all under rigidly controlled protocols.

Phase III. *Clinical Trials*, are expanded controlled and uncontrolled trials performed after efficacy has been basically established, at least to a certain degree, and are intended to gather additional evidence of efficacy, plus further evidence of safety, tolerance, and definition of adverse effects.

Phase IV. *Postmarketing Clinical Trials,* are of several types:

1. Additional studies to elucidate the incidence of adverse reactions, to explore a specific pharmacological effect, or to obtain more information of a circumscribed nature.
2. Large-scale, long-term studies to determine the effect of a drug on morbidity and mortality.
3. Additional clinical trials, similar to those in phase III, to supplement premarketing data where it has been deemed in the public interest to release a drug for more widespread use before acquisition of all data that would ordinarily be obtained before marketing.

The definition of phase IV is not intended to include studies on new indications.

The 1962 amendments eliminated the automatic approval of any NDA and substituted a 6-month (180-day) review period. Under this act, the 180-day review period is restarted if deficiencies are found in the initial submission. Substantial additional evidence for efficacy as well as safety was now required in the NDA.

In 1970, an additional administrative check was instituted. Through publication in the *Federal Register*, the FDA requested that a period of 30 days elapse between acknowledgment of receipt of an IND by the FDA and initiation of human testing. This became required procedure.

Only 14 years elapsed between 1962 and the next wave of legislation. Historically, selection of the procedures to be used in collection, processing, and reporting of research data had been accepted as the purview of the investigator. Evaluation of whether the procedures used were appropriate and/or adequate was the responsibility of the peer review process that accompanied scientific presentation or publication. This practice was nearly universally accepted in the majority of disciplines of scientific investigation, including biomedical research to support new drug development.

In fulfilling their responsibility to ensure the highest degree of consumer protection possible, the FDA over time had been requiring even more extensive animal testing and supportive evaluations before approving products for marketing. As a matter of policy, these studies were conducted by the person or company desiring to market the product or by contract laboratories at the person's or company's direction. The results of these studies were then submitted to the FDA to become part of the information based upon which the judgment was made to permit or deny introduction of the product into the market place.

REGULATION OF RESEARCH

Before 1976, the FDA shared the concept of research accepted by the scientific community at large and assumed that nonclinical laboratory studies submitted in support of regulated product resulted from the application of appropriate experimental procedures by the investigators. Then, however, the FDA identified a number of problems in the manner in which some ongoing studies were being performed. Based on a concern that significant deviations might exist in the quality and integrity of these types of data generally, the FDA published *Proposed Regulations for Good Laboratory Practice: Nonclinical Laboratory Studies* in November 1976. These regulations were issued in final form as *Nonclinical Laboratory Studies: Good Laboratory Practice Regulation* (GLP regulations) (14) late in 1978 to become effective in June 1979. The period between publication of the proposed and final GLP regulations was one of considerable change in the precepts governing handling of medical research data.

Although the GLP regulations legally applied only to nonclinical laboratory studies in support of research or marketing permits for products regulated by the FDA, their ramifications extended broadly beyond this sector. The Environmental Protection Agency (EPA) published similar proposed GLP regulations within a short time after publication of the FDA version, and other regulatory agencies are expected to follow suit. A concensus is developing within the biomedical research community that because codified procedures now exist for conducting specific types of biomedical research, these procedures will ultimately become either official or unofficial standards for conduct of nearly all animal experimentation.

Similar regulations have been proposed that will apply to clinical investigations and investigators. Examples of early proposals include *Proposed Establishment of Regulations of Obligations of Sponsors and Monitors* (1977), *Standards for Institutional Review Boards for Clinical Investigations: Proposed Establishment of Regulations* (1978), and *Obligations of Clinical Investigators of Regulated Articles: Proposed Establishment of Regulations* (1978).

GLP regulations were not intended to dictate the scientific design of nonclinical investigations. They were, however, intended to define in considerable detail the procedures by which the studies are to be performed. These procedural requirements, the volume of information now required, and the precision with which information must be acquired, processed, and reported have exponentially increased the complexity of handling biomedical data. They have also increased the potential for development of a research administration bureaucracy. This state of affairs will increase drug development research costs and could conceivably discourage commercialization of some potentially useful drugs by making it impossible for small organizations to comply with the requirements.

REFERENCES

1. Beecher, H.K. The powerful placebo. *JAMA* 159:1602, 1955.
2. Brody, H. The lie that heals: The ethics of giving placebos. *Ann. Intern. Med.* 97:112, 1982.
3. Clark, A.J. *The Mode of Action of Drugs on Cells.* Baltimore: Williams & Wilkins, 1933.
4. Editorial. Shall I Please? *Lancet,* December 24/31:1465,1983.
5. Ehrlich, P., and Hara, S. *Die Experimentelle Chemotherapie der Spirillosen.* Berlin: Springer Verlag, 1910.
6. *FDA Introduction to Total Drug Quality.* DHEW publication no. 74-3006, Washington, D.C.: U.S. Government Printing Office, 1973, p. 55.

7. Honigfeld, G. Non-specific factors in treatment. I. Review of placebo reactions and placebo reactors. *Dis. Nerv. Sys.* 25:145, 1964.
8 Joyce, C.R.B. Placebos and other comparative treatments. *Br. J. Clin. Pharmacol.* 13:313, 1982.
9. Lasagna, L., Mosteller, F., von Felsinger, J.M., and Beecher, H.K. A study of the placebo response. *Am. J. Med.* 16:770, 1954.
10. Leaders, F.E., Van Hoose, M.C., and O'Kane, K.C. Computer-based systems for acquisition, management, and reporting of animal data — The biomedical scientist perspective. *Drug Inform. J.* 14:15, 1980.
11. Levine, J.D., Gordon, NC., and Fields, H.L. The mechanism of placebo analgesia. *Lancet* 2:656, 1978.
12. Levine, J.D., Gordon, N.C., Jones, R.T., and Fields, H.L. The narcotic antagonist naloxone enhances clinical pain. *Nature* 272:826, 1978.
13. Melmon, K.L., and Morelli, H.F. *Clin. Pharmacol.* New York: Macmillan, 1972, p. 558.
14. Noel, P.R.B. The data audit. In: *Good Laboratory Practice* (Paget, G.E., ed.) Baltimore: University Park Press, 1979, p. 73.
15. Reinberg, A. New aspects of human chronopharmacology. *Arch. Toxicol.* 36:327, 1976.
16. Schueler, F.W. *Chemobiodynamics and Drug Design.* New York: McGraw-Hill, 1960.
17. Shapiro, A.K. The placebo effect in the history of medical treatment: Implications for psychiatry. *A. J. Psychiatry* 116:298, 1960.
18. Wardell, W.M., and Lasgna, L. *Regulation and Drug Development.* Washington, D.C.: American Enterprise Institute for Public Policy Research, 1975.
19. Wolf, S. The pharmacology of placebo. *Pharmacol. Rev.* 11:689, 1959.

CHAPTER
2

PHARMACOKINETIC BASIS OF DRUG ACTION

Elliot S. Vesell

Pharmacological effects are considered to be produced by the interaction of drug molecules with their specific receptor sites. The intensity and duration of drug action depend upon the number of drug molecules present at any time at such sites. The concentration of a drug at its receptor site(s) as well as in the bloodstream depends upon the absorption, distribution, metabolism, and excretion of the drug. Studying the time course of concentration of a drug in the blood and tissues of an organism is the scope of pharmacokinetics.

The concentration of a drug at its receptor site(s) can rarely be determined directly in human subjects. Ethical reasons prohibit the removal, from living human beings, of pieces of brain, heart, liver, kidney, and other tissues that would be necessary to achieve this goal. Because such tissues change their composition and metabolic activity after death, measurement of drug concentration(s) in postmortem specimens may not accurately reflect the pharmacokinetic properties of drugs in those tissues during life. However, the concentrations of many drugs at their site(s) of action in tissues are in equilibrium with the concentrations of those drugs in the plasma, or in other biological fluids such as saliva. Thus, by measurement of the concentration of drugs at various time points after dosage, in biological fluids such as plasma, saliva, or even urine, it may be possible to describe the time course of the drug in the tissue of interest. Such information provides the cornerstone of the subject of pharmacokinetics, which may be defined as the quantitative description of the rates of movement of drug molecules into, within, and out of the body.

Furthermore, measurement of drug concentrations in blood can provide, for certain drugs, under certain clinical circumstances, an excellent way to determine the appropriate dose of a drug to administer to a patient during chronic therapy, once the initial dose has been given. This procedure, called *individualization* of therapy, is often necessary for two reasons: (1) the margin of safety of many potent drugs is small; thus, the dose of a drug that produces a therapeutic effect is very close to the dose that produces unacceptable, adverse effects; and (2) patients vary greatly, from 4-40-fold, depending on the drug, in the rate at which they can eliminate a drug from their body. Table 2-1 lists the therapeutic concentrations of some commonly used drugs; the values are presented in terms of therapeutic *windows*, that is, the range of values that has been generally found to be efficacious.

Table 2-1
Therapeutic Concentrations of Various Drugs in the Blood

Compound	Therapeutic Blood Level (%)
Acetaminophen	1-3 mg
Aminophylline	1-2 mg
Aminopterin	0.02-0.1 mg
Barbiturates	
Short-acting	0.2-0.4 mg
Intermediate-acting	0.2-0.5 mg
Long-acting	1-2.5 mg
Bishydroxycoumarin	1.8-2.6 mg
Chlordiazepoxide	0.1-0.3 mg
Chlorpheniramine	0.8-1.6 mg
Chlorpropamide	3-14 mg
Diazepam	0.1-0.25 mg
Digoxin	0.07-0.2 μg
Ethchlorvynol	0.2-1.5 mg
Ethyl ether	90-100 mg
Glutethimide	0.02-0.75mg
Halophenate	15-25 mg
Imipramine	0.005-0.016 mg
Lidocaine	0.15-0.4 mg
Lithium	0.5-1.3 mEq[a]
Nortriptyline	5-14 μg
Paraldehyde	3-15 mg
Phenytoin	0.6-1.7 mg for anti-convulsant effect 0.4-2.4 mg for anti-arrhythmic effect
Probenecid	10-20 mg
Procainamide	0.4-0.8 mg
Propranolol	2-5 μg
Quinidine	0.2-0.5 mg
Salicylate	2-10 mg analgesia (therapeutic) 35-40 mg antiarthritic >25 mg rheumatic fever therapy

[a] per liter.

Values below these levels are generally therapeutically ineffective; those above these levels generally produce toxic effects. This concept is presented schematically in Fig. 2-1. Obviously, because of the individual variability between humans in terms of pharmacokinetic phenomena, the same dose of a given drug, administered to three different humans by the same route of administration can produce toxicity in one patient, therapeutic benefit in another, and no effects whatsoever in a third.

Traditionally, the topic of pharmacokinetics is divided into four sets of processes:

1. *Absorption* of drug molecules into the circulation from site(s) of administration.
2. *Distribution* of drug molecules to different tissues after absorption.
3. *Metabolism* or *biotransformation* of drug molecules within the body.
4. *Excretion* of the drug and its metabolite(s).

These four processes are often distinctive in many ways, such as tissue localization and factors that modify their action. Nevertheless, separate treatment of the processes must not be misconstrued as indicating that they are completely independent or proceed at completely different times. On the contrary, in practice they often take place concurrently or simultaneously, and they are often closely interdependent. It should also be strongly emphasized that not only do individual drugs and classes of drugs exhibit different pharmacokinetic properties, but even the same drug can exhibit differing pharmacokinetic behavior in different patients, depending on the course and severity of the disease state involved, the age, diet, and genetic constitution of the patient, the exposure to other drugs, the dose of drug, and the route of administration.

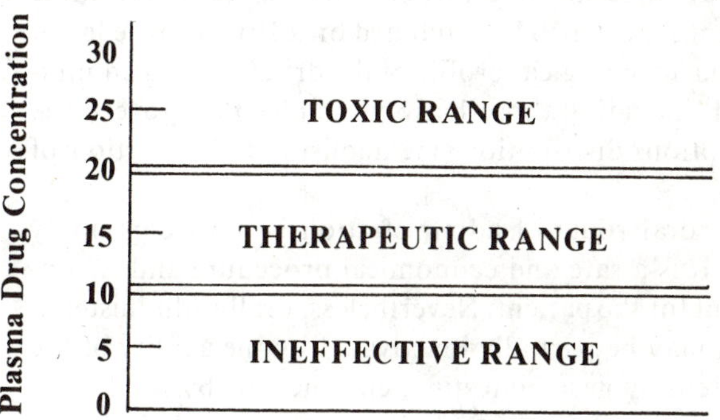

Fig. 2-1 *Relationship between the concentration of drug in serum and its pharmacological effects.*

ABSORPTION

ROUTES OF ADMINISTRATION

There are many different routes by which a drug can be administered: oral (p.o.), rectal, subcutaneous (s.c.), intramuscular (i.m.), intravenous (i.v.), topical, pulmonary, and others. For certain drugs, or in certain therapeutic indications, one route may be used rather than another. For example, the fact that ether is a readily volatile liquid or that nitrous oxide is a gas at room temperature permits these agents to be administered by inhalation.Insulin must be given by s.c. or i.m. injection, since it is broken down and poorly absorbed if given by the oral route. Depending on the locus of an infection, a given antibiotic may be administered p.o., i.v., or topically.

Where a medical emergency exists, such as acute carditis or rheumatic fever, the intravenous route is often selected, since large doses can be administered more rapidly. Access to receptor sites is also more direct when the i.v. route is used, since the time delay involved in gastrointestinal absorption is avoided, as well as a significant amount of inactivation of the drug. By virtue of these same considerations, the i.v. route is more difficult to control and more dangerous to use; it is also more apt to produce toxicity than the oral route.

This introduces a fundamental principle of therapeutics and that is the need for the physician to balance the risks inherent in the prescribing of any drug against the benefits to be derived by the patient from taking that drug. The physician must weigh many factors carefully in making the decision to use one drug at a particular dose and by a specified route of administration. The most potent and often the most useful drug in a given therapeutic situation may have a low *therapeutic index*, indicating a low safety factor; such a drug may have a great capacity to correct physiological derangements but can also produce much harm. Unfortunately a drug that is safe for all is likely to be effective for none. The physician's decision concerning which drug to use, what route of administration to select, and how much to give will depend, in part, on many individual characteristics of the patient, including the course and severity of the disease. However, these decisions must also be grounded on a firm knowledge of the pharmacological profile of the drug(s) being administered, including those basic principles that govern the absorption, distribution, metabolism, and excretion of drugs.

The oral route of administration is most commonly used. It is a safe and economical procedure and is convenient for the patient. Nevertheless, orally administered drugs may be partially inactivated by the acidity of the stomach, by gastrointestinal enzymes, or by food; they may irritate the lining of the GI tract; and they may exhibit large variations among patients, and even in the same patient, because of factors such as differences in gastric emptying time, GI motility, and mixing. Of course, the oral route can only be used in conscious and cooperative patients.

In this regard, it should be noted that failure of patients to take drugs exactly as prescribed by their physician has been termed *noncompliance*; rates of such behavior vary from 40-90%, depending on the socioeconomic conditions of the group studied, the disease, and the physician. The term *noncompliance* tends to place the onus of blame on the patient, whereas the physician who prescribes a drug that the patient cannot afford, does not fully comprehend the importance of taking, or finds too unpleasant in taste or side effects to ingest regularly, must also accept significant responsibility for the subsequent noncompliance.

Because the oral route of administration is the one most commonly used for drugs in general medical practice (accounting for more than 80% of all prescriptions written), it seems appropriate to consider the general principles that govern drug absorption after p.o. administration. It should be recalled that drug absorption is pharmacokinetically significant and closely associated with drug response because the rate of drug absorption determines in large part not only the rate at which a drug reaches its site(s) of action but also the peak drug concentration attained at these site(s) and the time during which such drug concentrations are maintained there. For these reasons, slow or incomplete absorption can be a cause of ineffective therapy.

With respect to the *factors affecting the rate of passage of drug molecules* from the lumen of the gut across the lipid barrier composed of cells lining the gastrointestinal wall, and from these cells into the circulation, the most important consideration from a quantitative point of view is the total surface area available for the absorptive process. Absorption occurs more rapidly when a larger area of the GI tract is available as an absorbing surface. Thus, regardless of the acidity of the stomach, or the acidity or basicity of the drug, comparatively little drug absorption takes place in the stomach; many drugs are significantly absorbed from the upper portion of the small intestine, since that location offers a much greater surface area for absorption to take place than does the stomach.

The absorption rate of drug is greatly influenced by the form in which the drug is administered. Drugs are more rapidly absorbed when given as solutions than as tablets or capsules. Drugs are absorbed more rapidly and more completely from solutions containing higher concentrations than those of lower concentrations. Absorption of a drug from tablets depends upon the disintegration rate of the tablet into small particles, since small particles tend to dissolve more rapidly in the fluids of the GI tract; thus, the smaller the particles into which the tablet disintegrates, the faster the absorption of the drug. In the preparation of a commercial tablet, when the active ingredient(s) are combined with inert binders and excipient(s), the nature of these inert ingredients, the particle size distribution, the compression force used, and the type(s) of granulation, lubricant, filler, and coating — all contribute to the rate of tablet dissolution and hence, the time required for drug action. Therapeutic failure or toxicity may occur because of difference in *bioavilability* (the relative rate and extent at which the administered dose of a given drug reaches the general circulation). In a number of cases — digoxin, prednisone, phenytoin, and many antibiotics — differences in relative bioavailability of the same drug, in the same dose, and given by the same route greatly influence the clinical effects of the therapeutic agent in patients, often with disastrous results.

Once a tablet has disintegrated into small particles, the drug contained in these particles must dissolve into the fluid phase of the contents of the GI tract prior to actual absorption. In this regard, water-soluble drugs dissolve more rapidly into the fluid of the GI tract than do lipid-soluble drugs; in contrast, lipid-soluble drugs move across the mucosal cells of the GI tract and into the circulation faster than do water-soluble drugs. Fig. 2-2 presents a schematic idea of the factors involved in drug absorption, including: gastric emptying time, intestinal transit time, and mesenteric blood flow. Slowing gastric emptying time generally delays drug absorption, since most absorption occurs in the upper portion of the intestine, rather than in the stomach. For the same reason, acceleration of gastric emptying tends to hasten drug absorption. Table 2-2 lists some of the major factors associated with increased or decreased gastric emptying times.

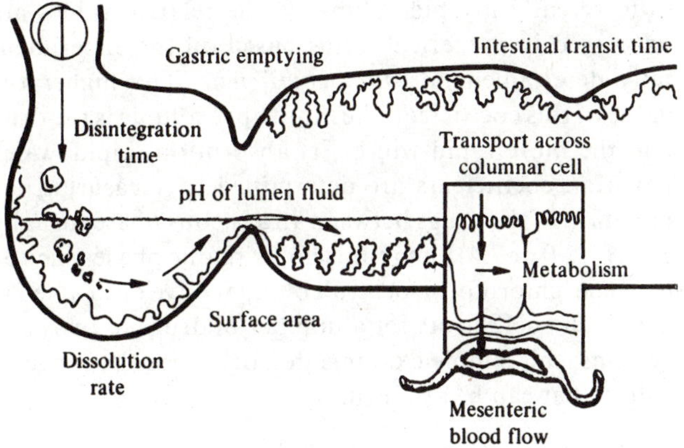

Fig. 2-2. *Factors influencing the rate and extent of drug absorption after ingestion of tablet.* (From Ref. 20)

Depending on the drug, the *presence of food* in the GI tract can either accelerate, delay, reduce, or fail to change the rate of drug absorption (Table 2-3). The presence of food exerts effects on drug absorption by some combination of: influencing blood flow to the GI tract, altering gastric emptying, or modifying intestinal motility. Drug absorption involves the movement of drug molecules by passive diffusion from locations of high drug concentration in the gastrointestinal lumen, across the mucosal cells lining the gut, into adjacent capillaries where the drug is present in much lower concentrations. The faster blood flows through these capillaries, the greater will be the concentration gradient of drug from lumen to capillary, and hence, the faster the drug will move from lumen to blood vessel. Different foods have differing effects on splanchnic blood flow; for example, a high-protein liquid meal will increase but a liquid carbohydrate meal will decrease the rate of splanchnic blood flow.

Certain compounds find a therapeutic use by virtue of their failure to be absorbed from their site(s) of administration. For example, antacids remain in the GI tract to neutralize the high acidity present in the stomach. Neomycin, poorly absorbed from the GI tract, is an effective therapeutic agent against infections of the intestine. Nonabsorbability from the GI tract makes barium sulfate eminently useful as a contrast medium for radiological identification of lesions in that area; soluble barium salts could never be used for this purpose because of their extreme toxicity.

Table 2-2
Factors Influencing or Associated with Changes in the Rate of Gastric Emptying

Decreased Emptying Rate	Increased Emptying Rate
Physiological	*Physiological*
Solids	Liquids
Acids	Gastric distention
Fat	Posture (lying on right side)
Increased osmotic pressure	
Pathological	*Pathological*
"Acute abdomen"	Chronic calcular cholecystitis
Trauma and pain	Gastroenterostomy
Gastric ulcer	
Myocardial infarction	
Hepatic coma	
Migraine	
Myxedema	
Intestinal obstruction	
Paralytic ileus	
Pharmacological	*Pharmacological*
Anticholinergics	Metoclopramide
Ganglionic blockers	Reserpine
Narcotic analgesics	Anticholinesterases
Isoniazid	Sodium bicarbonate
Aluminum hydroxide	
Drugs with anticholinergic side effects	

PASSAGE OF DRUGS ACROSS MEMBRANES

The rate of drug absorption from the GI tract is intimately associated with the rate of passage of drug molecules across the lipid membranes of the mucosal cells that line the gut then into the circulation by crossing the lipid membrane of the splanchnic capillaries. Most drugs traverse this path by the process of *simple diffusion* down a concentration gradient from places of higher drug concentration to places of lower (or zero) drug concentration.

In addition to simple diffusion, some drugs move across lipid membranes by processes of *active transport*. These processes require energy input often in the form of adenosine triphosphate (ATP) and the presence of a carrier system to move the drug across the membrane(s). Active transport allows such compounds as glucose, ionized amino acids, quaternary ammonium cations, and sulfonic acid anions to be absorbed, even *against* a concentration gradient. Thus, these molecules can cross a

Table 2-3
Effects of Food on Drug Absorption

Reduced absorption	*Delayed absorption*
Ampicillin	Acetaminophen
Aspirin	Amoxicillin
Doxycycline	Cephalexin
Isoniazid	Digoxin
Levodopa	Furosemide
Oxytetracycline	Potassium ion
Penicillin G	Sulfadiazine
Tetracycline	Sulfisoxazole
Increased absorption	*Unaffected absorption*
Carbamazepine	Digoxin elixir
Griseofulvin	Penicillin V
Hetacillin	Prednisone
Hydralazine	Theophylline
Lithium citrate	
Metoprolol	
Nitrofurantoin	
Propoxyphene	
Propranolol	
Riboflavin	
Spironolactone	

lipid membrane from a place of lower drug concentration to a place of much higher concentration.

Another mechanism for drug absorption is *pinocytosis*, a process in which the drug is engulfed by an infolding process of a small portion of the cell membrane. Pinocytosis involves a local invagination of the cell membrane; this invagination then buds off to form a sac within the cell. Pinocytosis resembles active transport in that it requires the expenditure of energy; it is used in primitive organisms as a mechanism for ingesting food. It is an interesting phenomenon of importance in host resistance to infection, but is of only minimal significance as a mechanism for drug absorption. In addition to the major processes for drug absorption (simple diffusion and active transport), specialized absorption phenomena such as diffusion through pores and facilitated transport also exist; however, these also are of only very minor significance.

After the first requirement for drug absorption from the gut has been met, namely, that the drug is in solution in the aqueous phase of the GI contents and in contact with the lipid membrane of the cells lining the GI tract, several additional characteristics are involved in the passage of the drug through this membrane. These characteristics constitute significantly important pharmacological principles; they apply to all types of drug absorption and relate as well to other pharmacokinetic processes — distribution, metabolism, and excretion.

Lipid Solubility of Drugs. The rate of passage of a drug across a lipid membrane depends upon the lipid solubility of the drug. This does not mean the amount of drug that can be dissolved in a given amount of lipid, but refers to the relative ability of the drug to preferentially partition into *nonpolar* or lipid phase of a two-phase system in which the other phase is a *polar* or aqueous one. Lipid-soluble drugs are more rapidly absorbed because they can reach the circulation more quickly, traversing more easily the lipid membranes of both the mucosal cells and the cells lining the splanchnic capillary. Thus, the more lipid soluble the drug, the faster it will dissolve in and move across the lipid barriers constituted by the membranes of the cells separating the drug from the circulation. Drugs differ greatly in lipid solubility: the relative values are expressed in numerical terms based on the experimentally determined *partition coefficient.* The higher the value of this coefficient, the more lipid soluble is the drug and the more rapid will be its absorption. Lipid/water partition coefficients are determined by measuring the partition of the drugs between an aqueous phase (usually at pH = 7.0 or 7.4) and immiscible organic phases such as benzene, chloroform, octyl alcohol, or olive oil. Table 2-4 lists such coefficients for a number of drugs in two such systems; this simple example demonstrates the range of values that can be attained.

Table 2-4
Partitioning of Drugs in Lipid/Water and Chloroform/Water Systems (Aqueous Phase at pH 7.4)

Olive Oil/Water		Chloroform/Water	
Drug	Partition Coefficient	Drug	Partition Coefficient
Sucrose	0.00003	Hexamethonium	0
Urea	0.00015	Salicylic Acid	0.2
5-HT	0.06	Barbital	1
Ethanol	0.1	Acetanilide	3
Antipyrine	0.3	Amiphenazole	15
Morphine	0.4	Aniline	17
Codeine	0.8	Quinalbarbitone	23
Tryptamine	0.9	Antipyrine	28
Aminopyrine	1.3	Aminopyrine	73
Barbital	1.4	Thiopental	102
Allobarbital	2.4		
Salicylamide	5.9		
Phenobarbital	5.9		

The Role of Ionization. To predict how rapidly a drug might pass across lipid barriers, one must know the pH values involved as well as the partition coefficients of the drug. Most drugs are either weak acids or weak bases; as such, they exist in aqueous solutions as a mixture of dissociated and undissociated forms. Although the undissociated (unionized) form of a drug molecule can move rapidly across lipid membranes in proportion to lipid solubility and concentration gradient, the dissociated (ionized) form of a drug is relatively lipid insoluble and will not readily cross lipid membranes. Thus, ionized drug forms are absorbed relatively slowly.

To calculate the proportion of drug molecules in the undissociated and dissociated forms, one must know the pH of the solution and the pK_a of the drug. The pK_a is the negative logarithm of the acidic dissociation constant of the drug. When the pH of the solution is equal to the pK_a of the drug, exactly 50% of the total number of drug molecules will be dissociated, and 50% will be undissociated. At pH values other than that equal to the pK_a the relative proportions of dissociated and undissociated drug will vary, as shown in Fig. 2-3. For an acidic drug, HA, the ionization equation may be written:

$$HA \rightleftarrows H^+ + A^-$$

where:

$$K_a = \frac{[H^+][A^-]}{[HA]}$$

As stated above, $pK_a = -\log K_a$.

For a basic drug, B, the ionization equation can be written:

$$B + H_2O \rightleftarrows BH^+ + OH^-$$

where:

$$K_b = \frac{[BH^+][OH^-]}{[B]}$$

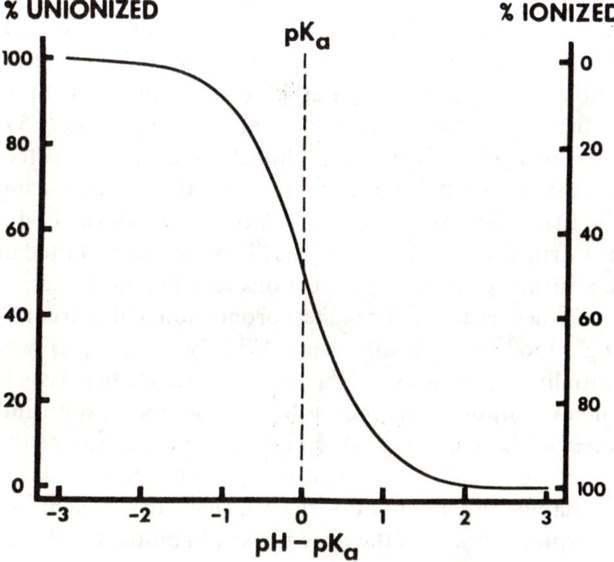

Fig. 2-3. *The effect of pH on the ionization of a weak acid.* The acid is 50% ionized at a pH = pK_a. *At higher pH values, it becomes increasingly more ionized; at lower pH values, it becomes increasingly more unionized. The rate of change of ionization is greatest at pH values near the pK_a.*

For basic drugs, $pK_a = [14 - pK_b]$. The pK_a values of a variety of common drugs are presented in Fig. 2-4. The Henderson-Hasselbalch equation may be used to calculate the fraction of drug in the dissociated and undissociated forms. These values, in turn, will give some estimate of whether the drug will be relatively lipid soluble (and consequently relatively rapidly absorbed) or relatively water soluble (and consequently relatively slowly absorbed).

For an acidic drug:

$$pK_a = pH + \log \frac{[\text{unionized acid}]}{[\text{ionized acid}]}$$

For a basic drug:

$$pK_a = pH + \log \frac{[\text{ionized base}]}{[\text{unionized base}]}$$

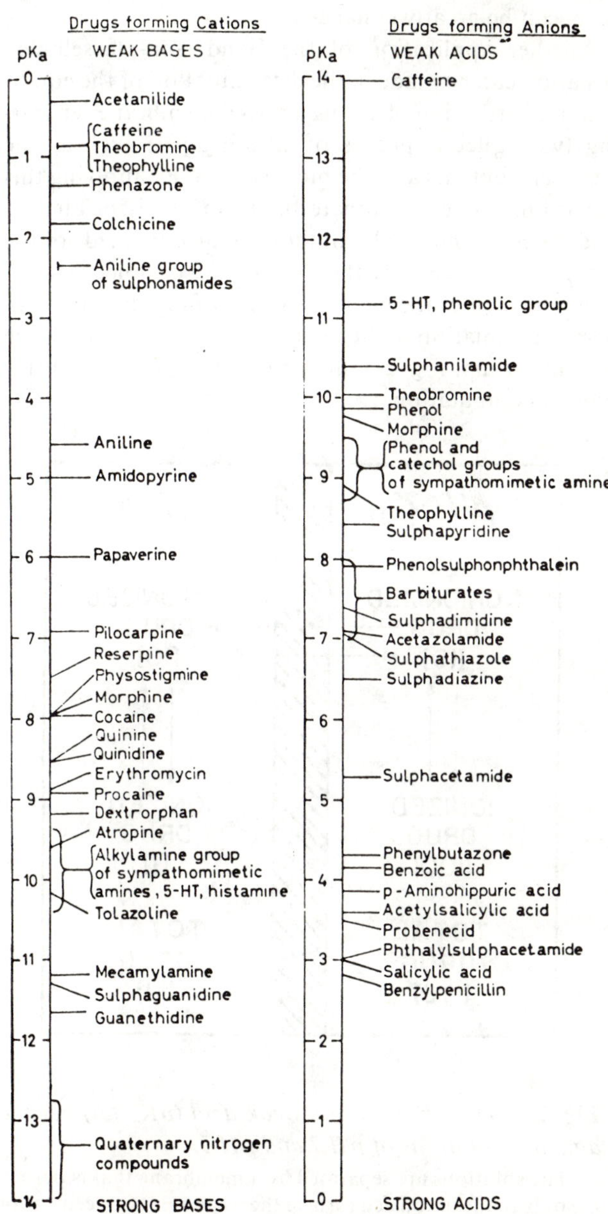

Fig. 2-4. *The pk_a values of some drugs.*

These equations express the ionization of drugs in terms of their pK_a values, rather than in terms of their ionization constants. As stated earlier, at a pH equal to the pK_a, the number of dissociated molecules equals the number of undissociated molecules. If the pH rises above the pK_a, more than half of the total number of drug molecules become ionized (for acidic drugs); conversely, fewer than half the number of drug molecules will be ionized (for basic drugs). If the pH decreases below the pK_a, the opposite effects on ionization take place for acidic and basic drugs, respectively.

Application of the Henderson-Hasselbalch equation to specific drugs and conditions reveals that quinine, a basic drug with a pK_a = 8.4 is ionized approximately 91% at pH = 7.4, 50% at pH = 8.4, and 9% at pH = 9.4. Thus, by raising the pH of the solution by 2 units, the ionization lipid solubility, and hence the rate of absorption of quinine, can be greatly enhanced.

Further application of the Henderson-Hasselbalch equation can be made in the determination of the equilibrium distribution of a drug across a membrane separating two aqueous phases of differing pH, such as the stomach contents and the bloodstream. By applying this equation, one can estimate the ratio of dissociated to undissociated molecules of the drug on either side of the membrane; since only the undissociated molecules can cross the membrane with any degree of rapidity, this can permit calculation of the relative distribution of the drug at equilibrium. Fig. 2-5 illustrates the application of this type of computation.

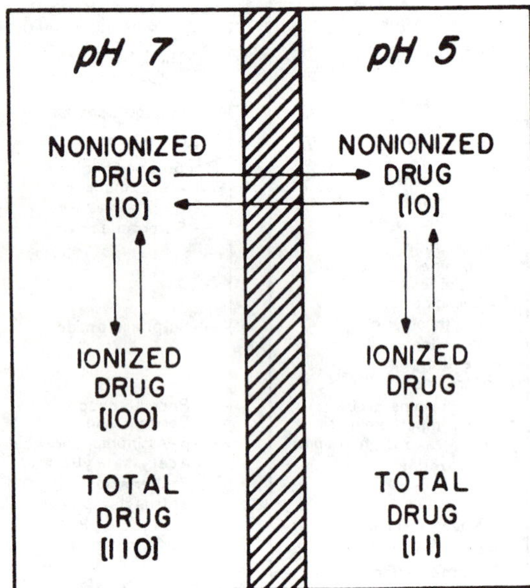

Fig. 2-5. *Distribution of a weak acid (pK_a = 6) between aqueous solutions of pH 7 and pH 5.*

The solutions are separated by a membrane that is permeable only to the unionized form of the weak acid. Concentrations at the steady state are shown in brackets.

EFFECTS OF DRUG INTERACTIONS

Drugs are often given to patients in combination. One drug can interact with another to alter its rate of absorption. Such interactions can also affect drug distribution, biotransformation, or excretion. Although a drug interaction in the GI tract could theoretically result in increased as well as decreased drug absorption, in practice, the latter situation is more common, leading to therapeutic failure. Mechanisms by which such interactions alter the rate or degree of absorption include: formation of complexes or chelates, changes in rates of gastric emptying or GI motility, effects on dissolution or ionization, inhibition of active transport processes, changes in membrane permeability, toxic effects on gastrointestinal mucosa, or combinations of these and other, as yet undefined mechanisms. Examples of drug interactions that can be of clinical significance include: p-aminosalicylic acid causing a decreased GI absorption of rifampin or isoniazid; compounds containing cations such as calcium, magnesium, aluminum, or iron reducing the absorption of tetracyclines; and cholestyramine, which delays the absorption of thyroxine, warfarin, and other acidic drugs.

DISTRIBUTION

The absorption process is complete when all drug molecules reach the circulation; this may take hours or even days. Once in the circulation, drug molecules continue their journey throughout the body, eventually reaching their site(s) of action. In the body, drugs distribute differently, since they have different properties and different affinities for the various tissues of the body. In addition to divergent affinities of drugs for the various tissues of the body, drug distribution also depends upon the relative rate(s) of blood flow to different tissues. Table 2-5 illustrates the markedly differing proportions of the total circulating blood volume (approximately 5.0 liters in a 70 kg normal adult human) that flow to different tissues. As might be expected from these data, during the first few passes of the circulation through the body, any drug present in the blood is likely to be distributed in significantly different proportions to different tissues.

Tissues receiving the highest proportion of the circulating blood (e.g., brain, heart, kidney, and liver) will initially receive most of the drug, whereas other tissues, such as adipose tissue, connective tissue, and smooth and skeletal muscle, receive a much lower proportion of the blood flow, and, consequently, a lower proportion of the available drug. Eventually, the drug in all tissues achieves an equilibrium with the drug present in blood; for this to occur, there must be a redistribution from tissues that had gotten a high initial perfusion to all organs. Although this would theoretically permit all tissues to achieve an equal concentration of the drug, a process which might take many hours, it seldom occurs, since individual drugs will partition between different tissues and the bloodstream in much the same manner as partitioning occurs between the GI contents and the bloodstream in the process of absorption.

A classical example of the important role of redistribution in drug action is that of the ultrashort-acting barbiturate, thiopental. By virtue of its close structural resemblance to the short to intermediate-acting barbiturate, pentobarbital, it was predicted that thiopental would also be relatively long-acting. When thiopental was given to humans, however, its duration of action was found to be surprisingly ultrashort. This situation was later explained by animal studies showing a significant redistribution from the brain to other tissues of the body. Thiopental went initially from the blood to the brain because of the high proportion of blood flow to the brain, coupled with the great affinity of the drug fo fatty tissues (a high lipid solubility). Because of this high lipid solubility, an accumulation of thiopental gradually developed in the adipose tissue of the body, causing blood concentrations to fall, and thiopental to move out of the brain, first into the blood, and eventually into body fat and even into skeletal muscle. This redistribution of thiopental out of the brain occurs because of the very high lipid solubility of the drug and the differences in distribution of blood to various tissues; it explains the short duration of thiopental as a hypnotic on the basis of known pharmacokinetic phenomena.

The story of thiopental also shows that, even after the time required for full equilibrium to be achieved from the point of view of initial circulatory differences among tissues, great differences can still exist among tissues. Such differences in drug accumulation result from the different affinities of drugs for various tissues. For example, highly lipid-soluble compounds, such as DDT, may remain in the adipose tissue of the body for months or years after a single exposure, whereas poorly lipid-soluble drugs, such as penicillin, are largely eliminated from the body within several hours after administration. Penicillin, ionized at plasma pH and poorly able to penetrate lipid barriers, enters the CNS slowly, if at all, after oral or even i.v. administration; thus, it cannot be relied upon to treat CNS infections unless administered directly into the spinal subarachnoid space. Quinine and quinacrine have such avidity for the liver that after several doses of either antimalarial, liver/blood concentration ratios of >4000 can be attained; even though blood levels may drop to virtually undetectable concentrations, liver concentrations may remain high for long periods of time.

Differences among tissues in the initial distribution of a drug as well as in long-term accumulation resulting from differences in lipid solubility or tissue binding among drugs are not the only problems that must be considered when one administers drugs. Partitioning of the drug between the cells of the circulating blood, the plasma water, and the plasma proteins occurs as soon as the molecules of the drug reach the bloodstream. A fundamental principle of pharmacology states that only the *free* form of a drug is available for drug action since only the free form has ready access to the receptor site(s). By virtue of being *bound*, those molecules attached to albumin or other macromolecules are also sequestered from the receptor. This process may provide a safety factor for the body by protecting the organism from a sudden exposure to the full effects of a drug that might prove toxic. The bound form of the drug constitutes a *storage depot* from which the drug can eventually be released; this change from bound to free form occurs when a sufficient number of free drug molecules are removed from the circulation by metabolism, binding to receptors, elimination from the body, or some combination of these. It must also be recognized that binding of drugs to albumin or other macromolecules serves to retain such drug molecules in the body, since they are neither filterable at the glomerulus nor available for metabolic degradation while bound. Thus, binding to albumin or other macromolecules prolongs the presence of drug molecules in the body.

Table 2-5
Blood Flow to Human Tissues

Tissue	Percent Body Weight	Percent Cardiac Output	Blood Flow (ml/100 g tissue per minute)
Adrenals	0.02	1	550
Kidneys	0.4	24	450
Thyroid	0.04	2	400
Liver, Hepatic	2	5	20
Portal		20	75
Portal-drained viscera	2	20	75
Heart (basal)	0.4	4	70
Brain	2	15	55
Skin	7	5	5
Muscle (basal)	10	15	3
Connective tissue	7	1	1
Fat	15	2	1

PROTEIN BINDING

Albumin is capable of binding many drugs and is present mainly in two places; approximately 50% of the albumin molecules in the body are in the plasma protein fraction of the blood, and the other 50% are in the liver. At therapeutic concentration, the extent of binding to plasma proteins varies from as low as 3% for antipyrine to 99% for warfarin. Once the absolute binding capacity of albumin is exceeded, such as after a very large single dose of a drug, or after repetitive dosage with somewhat smaller dosages, any additional drug molecules administered will be present 100% in the free form. These molecules move directly into the pool of free drug molecules and, as such, are immediately available for binding at their receptor site(s) to produce pharmacological effects; thereby, both the therapeutic activity of the drug and the potential for adverse drug reactions are increased. The proportion of the total drug molecules present in the bloodstream that will be bound to albumin will vary depending on the total concentration of drug in the plasma and on how many of the possible binding sites on albumin are occupied.

Another basic pharmacological principle illustrated by the examples of the differences in degree of binding of antipyrine and warfarin concerns the clinical consequences of changes in the degree of binding of a drug. When coadministered, many drugs have the capacity to displace one another from their binding sites. In disease states such as cirrhosis of the liver, or nephrosis, the number of albumin molecules in the body are reduced, and the qualitative capacity of the remaining albumin molecules may be altered. A basic principle of therapeutics states that the clinical consequences of a change in the percent binding of drug to albumin depends upon the value for binding under normal conditions. For drugs that under normal conditions are bound to albumin to the extent of $<90\%$, moderate changes in the percent of drug bound because of coadministered drugs that compete for the binding sites will probably not evoke a dramatic or clinically significant effect. By contrast, for drugs normally bound to albumin $>90\%$, a slight change in drug binding may result in a dramatic alteration in drug effect, since the important factor is not the percent of drug that is bound, but the percent of drug that is free and has access to receptor site(s). Thus, for a drug such as warfarin (which is 99% bound to albumin at usual therapeutic doses) the free fraction of drug can be doubled (from 1 to 2%) by merely decreasing the bound percentage from 99 to 98%, a small change indeed. In contrast, for a drug such as digoxin, which at usual therapeutic doses is bound to albumin only to approximately 25%, a reduction in the bound fraction of 20% (i.e., from 25 to 20%) would result in only a small change (i.e., from 75 to 80%) in the fraction of free digoxin molecules.

APPARENT VOLUME OF DISTRIBUTION

The percent of drug bound to albumin does not tell the whole story; the avidity of drug binding is also an important consideration. For example, a compound such as the x-ray contrast media iophenoxic acid is so avidly bound that, even in low concentrations, it disappears from the body with a half-life of 2.5 years. Since the distribution of drug in the body is such an important characteristic, estimated values of the distribution volume of a drug enable comparisons with other drugs and effective dosages.

The *apparent volume of distribution* of a drug is a term that refers to the volume into which the total amount of a drug in the body would have to be uniformly distributed to provide the concentration of that drug actually measured in the plasma. The formula for calculating the apparent volume of distribution (V_d) of a drug is as follows:

$$V_d = Q/c$$

where Q is the total amount of the drug in the body (in mg) and c is the concentration of drug in the plasma (in mg/l). The value obtained for the apparent volume of distribution of any drug may or may not have physiological significance. For example, drugs such as warfarin and phenytoin are bound almost completely to plasma albumin; such drugs have volumes of distribution equivalent to that of plasma water (i.e., about 4% of body weight or approximately 2.8 l in the average 70-kg man). In contrast, if a drug distributes in the total body water as do antipyrine or ethanol, the value for the apparent volume of distribution will be approximately 42 l, since total body water constitutes approximately 60% of body weight. For compounds such as quinine, quinacrine, or DDT, which localize extensively in certain tissues, the values for V_d may reach several hundred liters; such values are obviously without physiological significance, but they do provide supporting evidence for an extensive accumulation of the drug in one or more tissues.

BIOTRANSFORMATION/DRUG METABOLISM

TISSUE LOCALIZATION OF DRUG-METABOLIZING ENZYMES

Because marked differences often exist between parent drugs and their metabolites, in terms of physicochemical properties and therapeutic effects, biotransformation is perhaps the most significant process that can occur to a drug during its passage through the body. The enzymes that catalyze the biotransformation reactions can be found in a multiplicity of sites throughout the body: blood, GI tract, lungs, brain, kidneys, adrenals, skin. However, from a quantitative point of view, the most important organ for drug-metabolizing activity is the liver. From a quantitative point of view, this reflects that: (1) the concentration of drug-metabolizing enzymes is higher in the hepatocyte than in any other, and (2) the liver contains many more cells with drug-metabolizing enzymes than do other tissues.

BIOLOGICAL SIGNIFICANCE OF THE DRUG-METABOLIZING ENZYME SYSTEMS

Metabolic conversion of a drug to one or more different products has a number of biologically significant aspects.

1. Many drug metabolites are therapeutically inactive; for such drugs, the process of metabolism serves to

terminate their duration of action, thereby also reducing potential toxicity that might otherwise accompany an extended duration of action. In some cases, such as that of PRONTOSIL, which is converted to sulfanilamide *in vivo*, the parent compound is actually inactive; biotransformation in the liver is required to produce the therapeutically active agent. A third type of drug exists, exemplified by allopurinol and diazepam, in which both the parent drug and one or more metabolic products are active. In this most complicated situation (at least from a pharmacokinetic point of view), the intensity and duration of therapeutic activity depend not only on the rate(s) of metabolism of the parent drug and the active metabolite(s), but also on the relative amount(s) of *all* active forms of the drug (i.e., parent drug + active metabolites) in the body and at the active site at any point in time. To evaluate the overall therapeutic activity one requires knowledge of the rate of elimination of each active form from the body, as well as the relative therapeutic activities of the different active forms.

2. Most drugs that are metabolized by the drug-metabolizing enzyme systems are lipid soluble, and hence, would remain in the body for a long duration. The drug-metabolizing enzymes are embedded in the lipid envelope of the smooth endoplasmic reticulum (SER); only lipid-soluble drugs can penetrate the lipid membranes separating them from the SER in the hepatocytes. The lipid-soluble drugs that reach the drug-metabolizing enzyme systems are converted to more polar, less lipid-soluble metabolites that are more readily eliminated from the body (via the urine) than are the parent drugs. Thus, from a homeostatic point of view, one of the major functions of the drug-metabolizing enzyme systems is to convert lipid-soluble drugs, which might remain indefinitely in the body because of their physicochemical properties, into more polar, and hence, more readily excretable meta-bolites. In this concept, the enzyme systems may have developed as an evolutionary protective mechanism to enable terrestrial animals to consume plants containing alkaloids (of high lipid solubility and significant pharmacological activity) and reduce the potential toxicity by converting these compounds to more readily excretable products.

3. For many years, the drug-metabolizing enzyme systems were regarded as detoxification mechanisms. According to this view, the potential toxicity of many organic compounds could be reduced by conversion to less toxic substances. However, this would demand that the enzyme systems for drug metabolism have a capability of sensing whether a precursor or product is of greater toxicity. Some metabolites produced by the drug-metabolizing enzymes are extremely reactive, with the ability to bind covalently to various macromolecules such as proteins and nucleic acids. These chemically reactive intermediates have been associated with subsequent tissue necrosis or cancer. Thus, metabolic conversion of some compounds that are themselves relatively harmless, such as benzo [a]pyrene, may result in producing potent carcinogens. Furthermore, acetaminophen administered in a large dose may cause hepatic necrosis. In this light, the drug-metabolizing enzymes in the hepatic SER are far from being benign detoxification systems.

Finally, it must be mentioned that the so-called drug-metabolizing enzyme systems of the hepatic SER are also involved in a number of other metabolic pathways that are crucial to the metabolism of endogenous compounds such as steroid hormones. It would seem that the only constraint placed upon these systems is the requirement for lipid solubility of their substrates.

MECHANISMS OF DRUG METABOLISM

Most drugs are metabolized by at least several different reactions; some (such as the phenothiazine antipsychotic agents) will have as many as 30 distinct metabolic products. Some drugs, such as barbital, will be metabolized to only negligible amounts, while others, such as succinylcholine, will be hydrolyzed so rapidly that the duration of action of a single dose of the drug is only a few minutes.

Virtually all of the enzymatic chemical reactions that take place in drug matabolism in mammals can be categorized in one of four groups.

1. Hydrolysis
2. Reduction
3. Synthesis
4. Oxidation

The reactions that can be categorized as hydrolysis, reduction,and oxidation are often further grouped together as phase I reactions, whereas the synthesis reactions are often referred to as phase II reactions.

Hydrolysis. Hydrolysis reactions refer to the enzymatic cleavage of esters or amides. These enzymes are located in the liver, as well as in other tissues; the reactions are quite straightforward, involving a cleavage of the ester or amide bond and an addition of water to produce the final products as illustrated in the following examples.

Ester hydrolysis

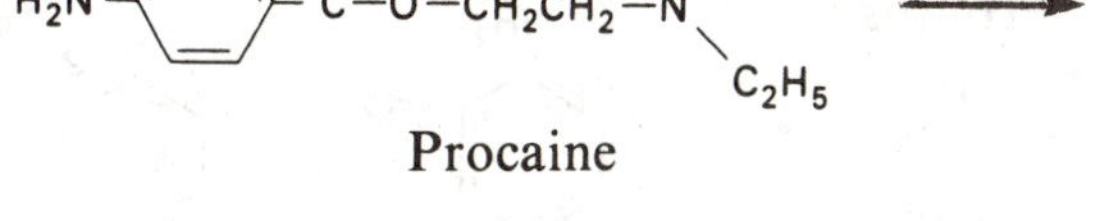

$$H_2N-C_6H_4-\overset{O}{\overset{\|}{C}}-O-CH_2CH_2-N(C_2H_5)_2 \longrightarrow$$

Procaine

$$H_2N-C_6H_4-\overset{O}{\overset{\|}{C}}-OH \;+\; HO-CH_2CH_2-N(C_2H_5)_2$$

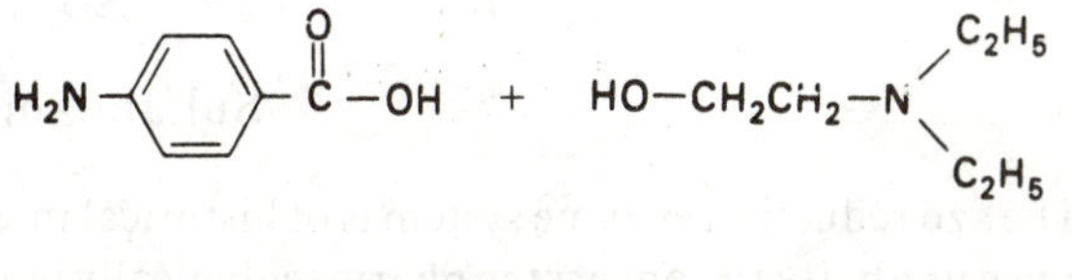

Amide hydrolysis

$H_2N-C_6H_4-CO-NH-CH_2CH_2-N(C_2H_5)_2$ →

Procaine amide

$H_2N-C_6H_4-COOH + NH_2-CH_2CH_2-N(C_2H_5)_2$

Succinylcholine is hydrolyzed extremely rapidly by the pseudocholinesterase(s) of plasma, giving it very short half-life in the body. The differential rates of metabolism (i.e., hydrolysis) of procaine and procainamide are a significant part of the reasons why the former has minimal uses other than as a local anesthetic, whereas the latter has a significant therapeutic application as an anti-arrhythmic agent.

Reduction. Reduction reactions involve the addition of a hydrogen atom to the molecule with the consequent reduction of a structural group such as nitro, azo, or carbonyl. The enzyme systems that perform these reactions are also located primarily in the liver, although some other tissues may contain significant levels of activity. Some of the enzymatic processes involved may best be illustrated by the follwing examples.

Nitro reduction

NO_2 / CHOH / CH-NH-CO-$CHCl_2$ / CH_2OH → NH_2 / CHOH / CH-NH-CO-$CHCl_2$ / CH_2OH

Chloramphenicol

Azo reduction

N=N, NH_2, SO_2NH_2, NH_2 →

Prontosil

NH_2, NH_2, NH_2 + NH_2, SO_2NH_2

Sulfanilamide

The azo reduction enzyme system is of historical interest, since its ability to convert the pharmacologically inactive chemical, PRONTOSIL, into the active antibacterial agent, sulfanilamide, is the first recognized example of the metabolic activation of a drug.

Conjugation (or Synthesis). Conjugation (or synthesis) reactions involve the addition of a significantly large additional chemical structure to the drug molecule by the process of one or more biosynthetic reactions. The most commonly seen examples of drug metabolism via conjugation reactions are pathways involving the addition of acetyl, glucuronyl, or sulfate groups to the drug, or the pathway known as mercapturic acid formation in which the initial step is the conjugation of the drug molecule with a molecule of glutathione. These processes are also predominantly found in the mammalian liver, although there are significant quantities of various conjugating system activities found in other tissues such as kidney and intestines. Some examples of drug metabolism via the pathways of conjugation are as follows.

Acetylation

CO—NH—NH_2 (pyridine ring, N) → CO—NH—NH—$COCH_3$ (pyridine ring, N)

Isoniazid

Glucuronide conjugation

OH (benzene ring) → COOH, H, O, H, OH, H, HO, H, H, OH, O (glucuronide–phenyl)

Phenol

Sulfate conjugation

OH (benzene ring) → OSO_3H (benzene ring)

Phenol

Mercapturic acid formation

Br (benzene ring) → Br (benzene ring), S-CH_2-COOH, NH-CO-CH_3

Bromobenzene

Oxidation. A number of oxidative functions are localized in the enzymatic activities present in the SER. These functions are named by the chemical reactions that they perform: epoxide formation, aromatic hydroxylation, aliphatic hydroxylation, N-dealkylation, O-dealkylation, oxidative deamination, sulfoxidation, N-oxidation, and N-hydroxylation. Several of the more prominent reactions can be described as follows:

N-dealkylation

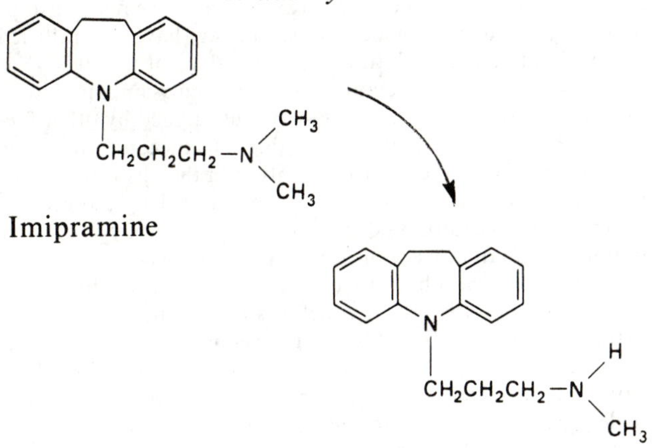

$CH_2CH_2CH_2-N(CH_3)_2$

Imipramine

$CH_2CH_2CH_2-N(H)(CH_3)$

O-dealkylation

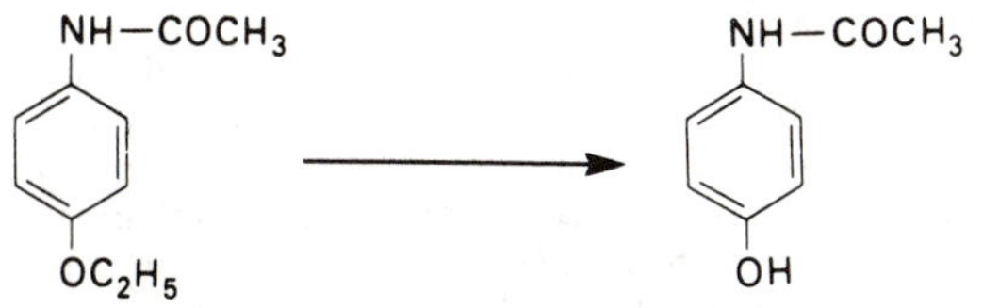

$NH-COCH_3$

OC_2H_5

Phenacetin

$NH-COCH_3$

OH

Sulfoxidation

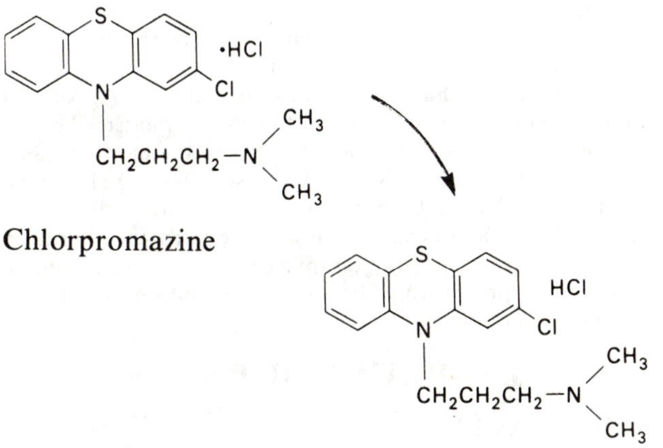

S

•HCl

N

Cl

$CH_2CH_2CH_2-N(CH_3)_2$

Chlorpromazine

S

HCl

N

Cl

$CH_2CH_2CH_2-N(CH_3)_2$

Aromatic hydroxylation

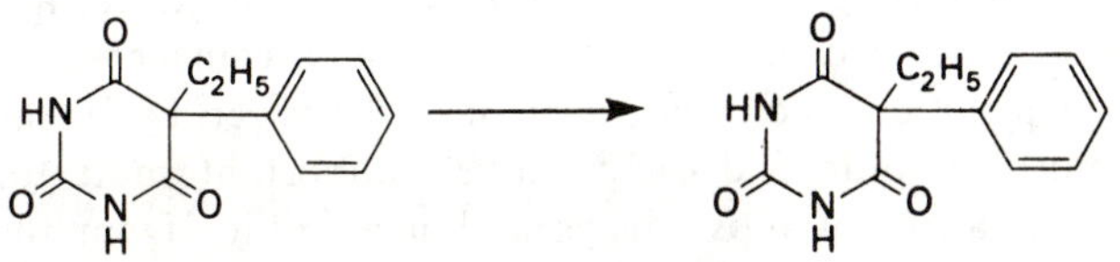

O

C_2H_5

HN

O N O

H

Phenobarbital

O

C_2H_5

HN

O N O

H

Aliphatic hydroxylation

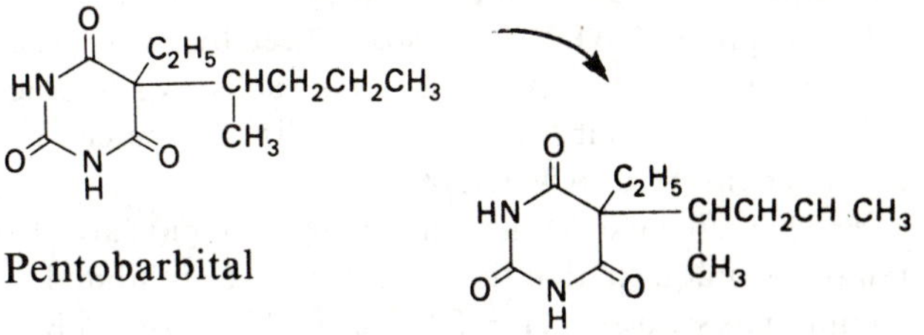

O

C_2H_5

HN $CHCH_2CH_2CH_3$

CH_3

O N O

H

Pentobarbital

O

C_2H_5

HN $CHCH_2CH\ CH_3$

CH_3

O N O

H

The enzyme system(s) located in the smooth endoplasmic reticulum (SER) of the liver, and responsible for these oxidative pathways of metabolism, are often called by one of a variety of names: hepatic mixed-function oxidase system, hepatic microsomal enzyme system, liver oxidative drug-metabolizing enzymes. The requirements for activity include: molecular oxygen, nicotinamide-adenine dinucleotide phosphate (NADPH), and an iron-containing heme that is designated cytochrome P-450. This cytochrome is so named because it exhibits, in its reduced form, an absorption maxima at 450 nm in the presence of carbon monoxide; the P stands for porphyrin. A number of recent studies have shown that multiple molecular forms of this cytochrome (isoenzymes) exist in the SER; these forms apparently bear the responsibility for conferring on the system the extremely broad substrate specificity. For example, a single compound such as the antipsychotic drug, chlorpromazine, can be metabolized by the hepatic mixed-function oxidase system to a number of derivatives representing at least four pathways: sulfoxidation, N-dealkylation, aromatic hydroxylation, and N-oxidation. Indeed, more than one of these reactions can take place on the same molecule, thereby leading to combinations of metabolites.

Another unique facet of these enzymes is their ability to undergo the process known as *induction.* This process may simply be described as an increased protein synthesis in the liver, with resulting increased total liver weight and specific proliferation of the liver SER with enhanced drug-metabolizing activity. A number of drugs and chemicals can produce this effect; depending on the drug administered and the condition of the animal (sex, age, diet, genetic constitution), induction may increase the level of drug-metabolizing activity by as much as 10-fold.

From a structural point of view, the hepatic drug-metabolizing enzyme system(s) consist of three parts: a *phospholipid matrix*, containing a *number of cytochrome P-450s,* and an *NADPH-dependent cytochrome reductase*. The oxidative reactions take place following the general chemical reaction:

$$RH + O_2 + NADP{\cdot}H \xrightarrow[\text{P-450}]{\text{cytochrome}} ROH + H_2O + NADP$$

As can be seen, not only the drug molecule undergoes oxidation; the reduced nicotinamide adenine dinucleotide phosphate (NADPH) is also oxidized by the molecular oxygen. Presumably, one atom of each oxygen molecule goes to the substrate to be oxidized, whereas the other is converted to water.

The hepatic mixed-function oxidase system(s) are also relatively unique in that their activity can be inhibited by compounds such as SKF 525A or by carbon monoxide or a number of environmental toxicants.

OTHER ENZYME SYSTEMS INVOLVED IN DRUG METABOLISM

In addition to the systems localized primarily in the liver and discussed earlier, a variety of additional enzyme systems, localized throughout the body, may also be responsible for the conversion of drugs to chemically changed metabolic products. Indeed, any body enzyme is capable of metabolizing a drug, if the structural characteristics of the drug molecule are suitable for the enzyme. Thus, nonspecific esterases in the blood plasma can degrade drugs such as succinylcholine, monoamine oxidase(s) in brain or liver can oxidize amphetamine, alcohol dehydrogenase can convert a variety of primary alcohol functions to aldehydes, and a number of dehydrogenase systems can attack drugs. However, one facet of drug metabolism remains constant. If a drug structure does not rather closely resemble any of the endogenous body substrates, and if the drug molecule has a significant lipid solubility, the primary route(s) of metabolism will be those of the drug-metabolizing enzymes of the liver.

FACTORS CAUSING VARIATION IN DRUG METABOLISM

The hepatic mixed-function oxidases are particularly susceptible to alteration in activity by a number of factors, some of which are listed in Table 2-6.

Species Difference. Species differences in the pathway(s) of hepatic metabolism of a given drug (qualitative differences) are quite common, as are differential rates of metabolism along the same chemical pathway in differing animal species (quantitative differences). Such species differences make extrapolation from one species to another quite difficult; this can be an especially tricky problem when one attempts to extrapolate from laboratory animals to humans in the course of development of a new drug.

Interindividual Variations. Furthermore, even in a single species, extremely large interindividual variations may occur because of genetic factors involved in the determination of the basal activity of the drug-metabolizing enzyme systems. Such interindividual variability, often referred to as *biological variation*, can create a real problem for the clinician, since the genetic background of the human patient is considerably more heterogeneous than that of the inbred laboratory rat. Thus, when combined with the factors listed in Table 2-6, one can see why interindividual variations in the duration of a drug's action or in its lifetime in the blood of individual humans can easily vary by as much as 50-fold. Nevertheless, regardless of the cause, such individual variations in rates of drug metabolism require that each patient receive differing doses of a drug to achieve maximum therapeutic benefit and to avoid toxicity. This practice, often called *individualization of therapy*, was employed by wise and capable physicians long before the specific causes for such variations between individuals were identified and investigated. Recent studies indicate the cytochrome P-450 genes code for a family of isoenzymes with different yet in many instances overlapping substrate specificities; the absolute number of these isoenzymes is not known and estimates go from 20 (11 being isolated from the rat and the rabbit) to over 1000. These isoenzymes differ in their immunological properties and in spectral and other physical characteristics. These variants of the isoenzymes contribute to the differences in drug metabolism in different persons and individualization of drug action.

Age. The influence of age on drug metabolism must also be considered, since it represents an additional complexity to the understanding of the science of pharmacokinetics. There is no question that individuals of different ages are likely to metabolize the same drug at somewhat different rates. However, attempts to develop specific or precise correlative relationships between the rate of drug metabolism and age have generally led to nonsignificant correlations (i.e., to values of $p > 0.5$). For some drugs, hepatic metabolism is markedly impaired with increasing age, although this may be outweighed by other factors such as those presented in Table 2-6. In addition, in the geriatric patient, other factors involved in the absorption, distribution, protein binding, and excretion of drugs, as well as differences in receptor binding and interactions, may be of more importance than any actions of drug metabolism.

A significant number of situations also exist in which drug metabolism is impaired or functions at a reduced rate in the extremely young patient (i.e., in the neonate). And, of course, the fetal subject represents a special situation. In all of these situations in which a patients presents an extreme of the age scale, it behooves the physician to carefully assess the age factor, and to either arbitrarily reduce the initial level of drug dosage or to observe the patient with extreme care while administering a normal dosage regimen. The particular topics of pediatric and geriatric pharmacology will be discussed in Chapters 29 and 30, respectively.

Diet. Dietary changes have been shown to modify the metabolism of certain drugs. Thus, antipyrine and theophylline half-lives and clearance are prolonged by switching from high to low protein with a reverse change in carbohydrate content of the diet (23). Charcoal broiling of beef, which produces polycyclic hydrocarbons (e.g., benzo [a]pyrene) on the meat surface enhances gastrointestinal and hepatic drug-metabolizing enzyme activity and shortens plasma antipyrine and theophylline half-lives in humans (22). A diet containing certain vegetables such as brussels sprouts, cabbage, turnips, broccoli, cauliflower, or spinach has been shown to accelerate rates of metabolism of antipyrine and phenacetin, probably by inducing some drug-metabolizing enzymes in humans (29).

Environmental Factors. Environmental factors, such as additional drugs, exposure to pesticides and industrial chemicals, nutritional factors (e.g., starvation or quality of diet), alcohol intake, vaccinations, and disease states (e.g., hepatic or renal diseases) have been demonstrated to affect drug metabolism. These factors have been shown to alter the pharmacokinetics of test drugs like antipyrine in volunteers. Some of these factors presumably affect drug metabolism by induction or inhibition of cytochrome P-450 isozymes.

EXCRETION OF DRUGS

RENAL EXCRETION

Drugs can be excreted from the body by many different routes: through the skin in sweat, the lung in expired air, the kidney in urine, the gastrointestinal tract in feces, and the parotid gland in saliva. Urine is, however, by far the most common and quantitatively important route for elimination of most drugs and metabolites from the body. In the functional units of the kidney (the nephrons), processes of glomerular filtration, tubular secre-

Table 2-6
A Partial List of Variables Affecting Drug Disposition in Experimental Animals

Variables in External Environment	Variables in Internal Environment	Pharmacological Variables
Aggregation	Adjuvant arthritis	Drugs
Air exchange and composition	Age	Short vs. long-term administration, bioavailability, dose, withdrawal, presence of other drugs or food, routes of administration, volume of material injected, tolerance, vehicle, etc.
Barometric pressure	Alloxan diabetes	
Cage design, materials	Cardiovascular function	
Cedar and other softwood bedding	Castration and hormone replacement	
Cleanliness	Circadian and seasonal variations	
Coprophagia	Dehydration	
Diet (food and water)	Disease — hepatic, renal, malignant, endocrine (thyroid, adrenal, pituitary)	
Exercise	Estrous cycle	
Gravity	Fever	
Hepatic microsomal enzyme induction or inibition by insecticides, piperonyl butoxide, heavy metals, detergents, organic solvents, ammonia, vinyl chloride, aerosols containing eucalyptol, etc.	Gastrointestinal function, patency, and flora	
Handling	Genetic constitution (strain and species differences)	
Humidity	Hepatic blood flow	
Light cycle	Hibernation	
Migration	Infection	
Noise level	Malnutrition, starvation	
Temperature	Pregnancy	
	Sex	
	Shock (hemorrhagic or endotoxic)	
	Stress	

tion, and tubular reabsorption combine to produce urine and eliminate drugs. *Filtration*, a physical process that partitions blood according to the molecular weight of its constituents, occurs in the glomerulus, which may be considered a network of renal capillaries. The filtration process permits unbound drugs having a molecular weight less than 800 to pass from blood to urine: drugs having a molecular weight > 800 or bound to plasma proteins cannot be filtered. The significance of this filtration process by the kidney can be appreciated when one considers that, in a healthy adult human, about 1200 ml of blood (about 650 ml of plasma) per minute is presented to the two kidneys for filtration. From this total volume, approximately 130 ml/min is transformed into an ultrafiltrate of plasma by the glomerular system; this amounts to the production of a total of about 180 l of ultrafiltrate in a 24-hour day.

As the ultrafiltrate of plasma reaches the loop of Henle in the renal tubule, water and sodium ions are removed, making the urine more concentrated with regard to the remaining constituents. Since approximately 99% of the water that has been filtered at the glomerulus is reabsorbed in the tubules, a drug filtered in the glomerulus may become concentrated as much as 90 to 99-fold during its passage down the renal tubules. If a drug (or drug metabolite) retains a sufficient degree of lipid solubility, the concentration gradient (now in the direction from tubular ultrafiltrate to plasma) directs reabsorption from the renal tubular cell back into the circulation. This reabsorption of a drug or its metabolite(s) across the renal tubular cells has the effect of retaining these compounds in the body, thereby prolonging their therapeutic, as well as toxic, actions. Here again, considerations of the pk_a of the drug and the pH of the urine play significant roles in determining how much of the total concentration of the drug will exist in the dissociated, water-soluble form or in the undissociated, lipid-soluble form that will be reabsorbed through the lipid membranes of the tubular cell and back into the circulation. The net rate of drug elimination in the urine will depend upon a summation of the processes of glomerular filtration and tubular secretion balanced against the tubular reabsorption.

In various forms of renal disease, these processes of drug elimination become impaired or disrupted; as a result, rates of drug elimination may be retarded. Consequently, drugs eliminated in urine tend to be retained in the body for much longer periods than in patients with normal renal function. Such retention is particularly marked for drugs whose elimination occurs mainly via the kidney, such as digoxin, penicillin, and sulfisoxazole. Consequently, in patients with renal disease, doses of such drugs must be reduced, depending on the extent to which renal functions are impaired; the degree of impairment may be estimated by measurements of glomerular filtration rates by determination of creatinine clearance.

BILIARY EXCRETION

Although biliary excretion of drugs generally plays a less important role in humans than in laboratory animals, some drugs (such as the cardiac glycosides and ampicillin) are secreted by the liver into the bile, following which they are partly reabsorbed into the circulation from the gastrointestinal tract when the bile empties into the duodenum. Although some of the drug molecules secreted in the bile are not reabsorbed from the duodenum, but are subsequently excreted into the feces, reabsorption of even a small proportion of the total can lead to a recycling of the drug with a consequent prolongation of the lifetime of the agent in the body. This overall process is called the *enterohepatic circulation*. Approximately 1 liter of bile is secreted each day by the liver, through the common bile duct into the duodenum, where the bile salts aid in the digestion and absorption of fats. The secreted bile salts themselves are almost completely reabsorbed from the intestine, some after hydrolysis by bacterial enzymes in the gut, thus completing their own enterohepatic cycle.

Drugs and drug metabolites, particularly glucuronides, are subject to excretion in the bile if they are polar and their molecular weight exceeds 350. Such drugs, often containing large hydrocarbon structures and polar functional groups, may reach concentration levels in the bile that are several orders of magnitude greater than those in plasma. The polar functional groups are a requirement for the drug molecules to be retained in the bile in high concentrations; if the lipid solubility were not modified, the drugs would merely diffuse across the lipid barriers back into the circulation. However, in the case of the glucuronide conjugates of drugs, once in the duodenum, they are subjected to the actions of bacterial glucuronidase enzymes; the regenerated aglycones are readily reabsorbed across the intestinal mucosa. Thus, for such compounds, the sequence of events in the enterohepatic circulation becomes: DRUG (in blood)→ DRUG-GLUCURONIDE (in liver)→DRUG-GLUCURONIDE (in bile)→DRUG-GLUCURONIDE (in duodenum)→ DRUG (in duodenum)→DRUG (in blood), and so the enterohepatic cycle continues.

Highly polar organic acids and bases are concentrated in bile by active transport processes, similar to those that secrete similar compounds across the renal tubular cells into the urine. Different carrier systems appear to exist in the liver for anions, cations, and cardiac glycosides. Unlike the bile acids and less polar drugs, these very polar acidic and basic drugs do not enter an enterohepatic circulation because no active transport system(s) are available for them in the intestine, and their polarity prevents passive reabsorption. Thus, for compounds such as quaternary ammonium salts, biliary excretion accomplished by the active transport system appears to be an effective means of elimination from the body.

PHARMACOKINETIC PRINCIPLES

For many drugs, a close correlation exists between the concentration of the drug in the blood and the pharmacological or therapeutic effects; the existence of such a relationship allows the measurement of the concentration of a drug in the blood to be used as a determination of its concentration at a distant, inaccessible receptor site. However, this relationship does not hold for all drugs. For example, some drugs are bound so avidly by certain tissues that they may be virtually undetectable in the blood, or present at such low concentrations that their true concentrations in body organs are not relatable. Drugs of this type, as well as drugs that form irreversible covalent bonds with certain macromolecules, may continue to exert their effects long after their concentrations in blood are no longer measurable.

The therapeutic and toxic properties of most pharmacological agents are determined by the characteristics that define the process of absorption, and by those that define the combined, simultaneously occurring processes of distribution, metabolism, and excretion. The final intensity of pharmacological effect(s) depends upon the amount of pharmacologically active substance that actually gets to the site of drug action (the receptor site).

Pharmacokinetics deals with the time course of absorption, distribution, metabolism, and excretion of drugs and their metabolites in the intact organism. The amounts of a drug and its metabolite(s) in readily available body fluids (blood, saliva, urine) are determined as functions of time and dosage; mathematical models are established to quantitatively describe the dynamic processes involved and to permit prediction of subsequent time-concentration relationships. Knowledge of a drug's pharmacological profile within a given individual permits the physician to construct an adequate dosage regimen/schedule that will rapidly and safely produce and maintain the desired therapeutic effect.

For any pharmacokinetic analysis to be useful, the assays upon which the analyses of the drug are based must separate the parent drug from any metabolite(s); this can be a difficult problem, and some currently used methodology fails this requirement of specificity. Nevertheless, most pharmacokinetic principles have been confirmed by investigating the concentration of a drug in blood or plasma as a function of time. An enormous body of literature is available; the following discussion is meant to develop and display certain fundamental pharmacokinetic principles.

PHARMACOKINETIC MODELS OF DRUG DISPOSITION

Numerous observations of drug absorption, distribution, and excretion *in vivo* led to the concept that any biological system can be treated as if there were actual boundaries separating the system into parts (compartments); drugs are transferred from one compartment to another in conformance with first-order kinetics. Although the assumption of first-order kinetics and rate coefficients that are constants is a gross approximation of complex biological phenomena, when utilized with discretion and a clear understanding of the limitations, this approach often proves rewarding; the kinetic assumptions are often validated by studies subsequently performed *in vivo*.

THE ONE-COMPARTMENT PHARMACOKINETIC MODEL

The simplest pharmacokinetic model assumes that, after administration (or after absorption for those drugs administered by routes other than i.v. injection), drugs are instantaneously and homogeneously distributed throughout the fluids and tissues of the body (Fig.2-6). This assumption does not necessarily mean that the concentration of drug in plasma and other body fluids is the same at the same point(s) in time. What the one-compartment model does assume, however, is that changes in plasma drug concentration quantitatively reflect changes occurring in the concentration of that drug in other body tissues and fluids.

For drugs whose distribution in the body follows first-order, one-compartment pharmacokinetics, a plot of the logarithm of the concentration of drug in the plasma against time will be a straight line. The equation describing the plasma decay curve is

$$C = A_e^{-(k_e)t} \quad (1)$$

where K_e is the first-order rate constant for the overall elimination of drug from the body, C is the concentration of drug at time = t, and A is the concentration of drug at time = 0, when all of the drug administered has been absorbed but none has been removed from the body through metabolism or excretion. The apparent first-order constant K_e is usually the sum of the rate constants of a number of individual processes such as renal excretion, biliary excretion, and metabolism. The apparent first-order rate constant for elimination of a drug from the body is related to the biological half-life ($t_{1/2}$) by the equation

$$t_{1/2} = 0.693/k_e \quad (2)$$

Unfortunately, this simple model does not account accurately for the observed time course of most drugs in the body, since most drugs will fit a system containing two, three, or even more compartments, rather than one. A variety of errors, the magnitude of which depend on the nature of a particular drug's distribution, may be introduced into a pharmacokinetic analysis by the assumption that a drug distributes according to the one-compartment model (35,41).

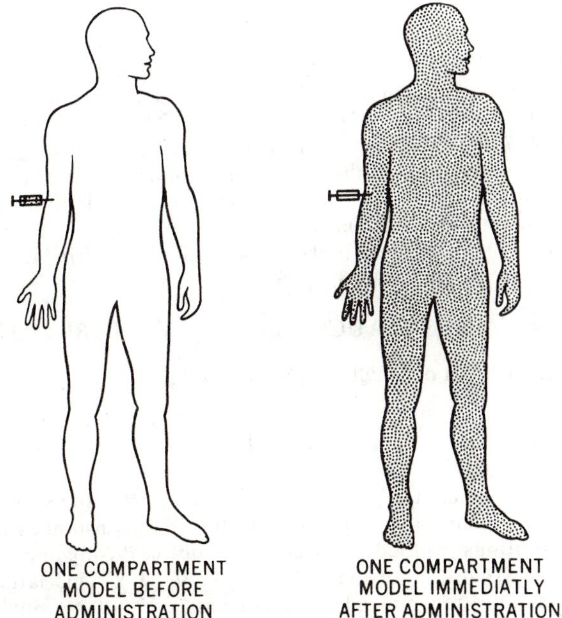

Fig. 2-6. *The one-compartment model.*

THE TWO-COMPARTMENT PHARMACOKINETIC MODEL

For most pharmacokinetic purposes, the mammalian body may be considered as a multicompartment system, with all compartments directly or indirectly in contact with the blood. The rate(s) at which a drug interchanges between the blood and various tissues depends on the rate(s) of blood flow through the tissues, the volume of the tissues, and the relative partitioning of the drug between the blood and the individual tissues. On the basis of similarities in blood flow and partitioning between the blood and tissues, various tissues (organs) may be grouped together so that the body may be regarded as a two- or three-compartment model (35). Because of differential vascularization among tissues, a drug may rapidly exchange between the blood and some tissues; thus together with the blood, these tissues may be considered as one compartment, commonly referred to as the *central compartment*. It should be obvious that this central compartment has no real physiological meaning, but varies with the particular drug being studied. The other tissues may be considered as one or more *peripheral compartments*, the number depending upon the properties of the drug. At some point in time, a state of *distribution equilibrium* between the central and peripheral compartments is reached, whereupon loss of the drug from the blood is described by a nonexponential process indicative of kinetic homogeneity with respect to drug concentrations in all fluids and tissues of the body. The central compartment and one peripheral compartment suffice to describe the pharmacokinetic properties of most drugs (Fig. 2-7).

When for purposes of pharmacokinetic analysis the body has to be subdivided into a central compartment and one or more peripheral compartments, the semilogarithmic plot of blood concentration versus time is not linear, but multiphasic (1, 13, 21, 42). In the case of the two-compartment model represented schematically in Fig. 2-8, where elimination occurs from the central compartment, a semilogarithmic plot of the concentration of the drug in blood against time (Fig. 2-9) can be separated into two distinct linear segments, described by the following equation:

$$C = Ae^{-\alpha t} = Be^{-\beta t} \quad (3)$$

The initial rapid decrease in drug concentration with time is due to the simultaneously occurring processes of drug distribution and drug elimination. The slope of the first, or distributional phase (α) is obtained by subtracting the extrapolated portion of the terminal linear (β) phase from the experimental data, as shown in Fig. 2-9 (17, 38). The half-life for the distributional process is determined from equation 2, where α replaces k_e.

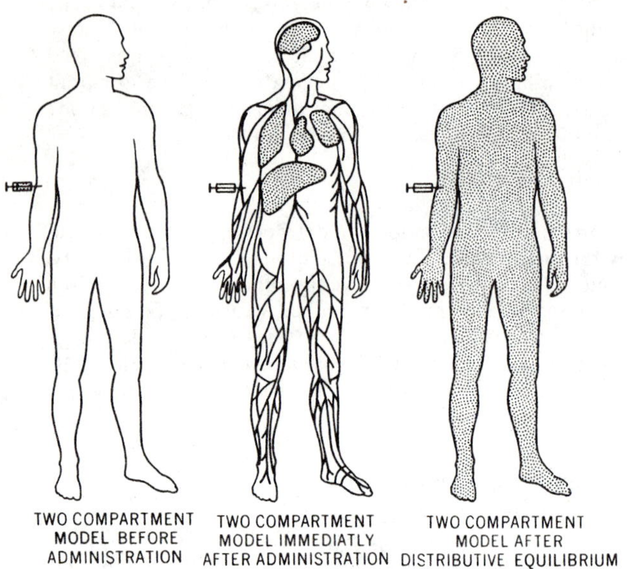

Fig. 2-7. *The two-compartment model.*

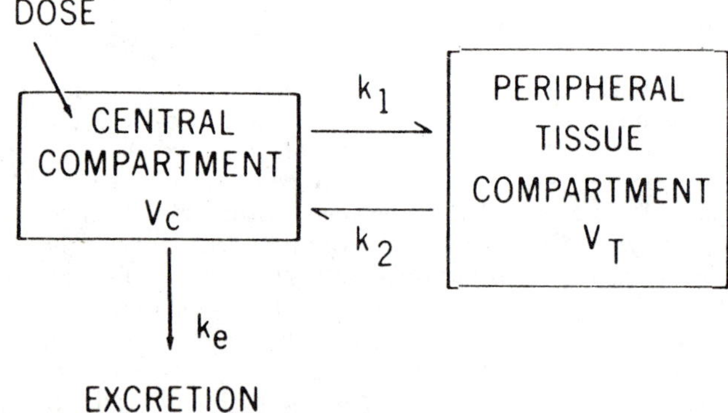

Fig 2-8. *Two-compartment model with elimination occurring from the central compartment.*

The terminal linear phase (β) describes irreversible loss of a drug from the body, usually considered to be the combination of the processes of metabolism and renal excretion, although enterohepatic circulation may be a confounding variable for some drugs. The first-order half-life of this phase is commonly called the *biological half-life* of the drug in the body, and can be calculated from equation 2, where β replaces k_e. The slope of the terminal linear portion of the curve relating the log of the drug concentration to time does not equal the first-order elimination rate constant, k_e (from equations 1 and 2), but is a function of k_e, k_1, and k_2 (6, 27),

$$\beta = k_e \Big/ 1 + \frac{k_1}{k_2} \quad (4)$$

The coefficients A and B in equation 3 are obtained from the intercepts of α and β, respectively. The sum of A + B is taken as the drug concentration at t = 0, on the assumption that the drug has been completely absorbed from its site of administration. Once the four terms in equation 1 are determined, individual rate constants may be calculated. Equations used to calculate the individual pharmacokinetic parameters are published elsewhere (17, 27, 51).

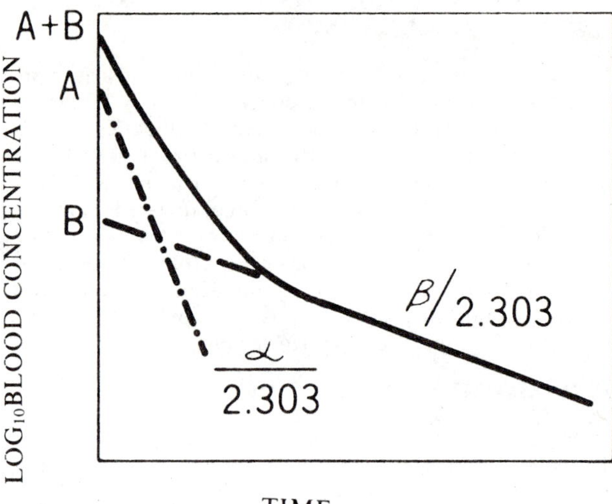

Fig. 2-9. *The logarithm of the drug concentration in blood plotted against time (solid line) after intravenous administration of a drug whose disposition can be described by a two-compartment model.*

The dashed line (— —) represents extrapolation of the terminal (β) phase. The other line (— . —) was obtained by the method of residuals. (From Refs. 17 and 27.)

The apparent volume of the central compartment (Vc), expressed in liters, or in kilogram of body weight, can be determined from the following:

$$Vc = \text{dose administered}/(A + B) \quad (5)$$

Calculation of the apparent volume of any tissue compartment, V_T requires knowledge of the total apparent volume of distribution (V_d), since

$$V_d = V_c + V_T \quad (6)$$

V_d may be calculated by any one of several methods (3, 9, 15, 17, 27, 31, 36, 37). The one in which the area under the blood concentration-time curve (AUC) is used provides the most useful estimate of V_d after single doses of drugs. The AUC is one of the most useful parameters in pharmacokinetics, since it is directly proportional to the total amount of drug that reaches the central compartment. The apparent volume of distribution determined by this method relates the amount of drug in the body to its concentration in the blood at all times during the β phase of the decay curve (3, 9, 15, 17, 27, 31)

$$(V_d)_\beta + \text{dose}/(\beta \times AUC) = \text{dose}/[A/\alpha + B/\beta] \quad (7)$$

Another method of calculating V_d is as follows:

$$(V_d)_{ss} = V_c \left[1 + \frac{k_1}{k_2} \right] \quad (8)$$

where $(V_d)_{ss}$ refers to the volume of distribution at the steady state. This method is useful when dealing with constant drug concentrations in blood, attained after multiple dosing or constant intravenous infusion (17, 27, 31, 36, 37). This latter method is not recommended for calculating V_d after a single dose of a drug, since the conditions under which it was derived apply only for that time at which the net transfer of drug between compartments is zero (3, 15, 36).

CLEARANCE

TOTAL BODY CLEARANCE

As stated earlier, for most drugs the biological half-life ($t_{1/2}$) is a complex function encompassing several discrete pharmacological processes: drug disposition, biotransformation, and urinary elimination. Clearance, on the other hand, permits the expression of rates of drug removal from the body independent of these processes (30, 32, 37, 39). The total body clearance of a drug, resulting from the summation of all processes of elimination, may be determined from the expression

$$\text{Clearance} = (V_c)(K_e) = B\,(V_d)_\beta = \text{dose}/\text{AUC} \quad (9)$$

Perrier and Gibaldi demonstrated that clearance, and not β_1, is a direct measure of the intrinsic metabolic activity of the liver, assuming the liver to be an integral part of the central compartment. Thus, for drugs whose disposition can be described by a two-compartment model (with elimination occurring from the central compartment), clearance is a more meaningful measurement of drug elimination than the disposition rate constant, β. However, for drugs subject to first-pass metabolism, in which the liver is considered to be a compartment peripheral to the central compartment, the use of clearance as an index of drug elimination is limited.

ORGAN CLEARANCE

Clearance may also be used to estimate the efficiency of any organ in removing a drug irreversibly from the blood perfusing that organ (the first-pass effect). The question that arises is whether clearance from plasma or blood is the parameter for physiological interpretation of clearance (38, 39, 53, 54). The rate at which a drug is delivered to the clearing organ(s) is also involved, since clearance reflects both removal of drug (as expressed by the term *extraction ratio*) and blood flow to the organ(s) (38). Rowland et al. (39) and Perrier and Gibaldi (33) used different models to show that the interrelationships of clearance can be described by the equation.

$$\text{Organ clearance} = Q\,\frac{Cl_{intrinsic}}{Q + Cl_{intrinsic}} \quad (10)$$

where Q is the blood flow to the organ, and $Cl_{intrinsic}$ is the maximal capacity of the organ to remove the drug by all pathways in the absence of any flow limitations (i.e., intrinsic organ clearance). The fractional term in equation 10 is equivalent to the extraction ratio. Fig. 2-10 shows the relationship between flow and hepatic drug extraction, and Fig. 2-11 shows the relationship between liver blood flow and total hepatic clearance, for drugs having different extraction ratios.

The pharmacokinetic behavior of a particular drug depends upon the relative values of $Cl_{intrinsic}$ and Q. When $Cl_{intrinsic} >>> Q$ (extraction ratio > 0.8), clearance becomes dependent upon blood flow to the eliminating organ. When $Q >>> Cl_{intrinsic}$ (extraction ratio < 0.2), clearance becomes independent of organ blood flow and is approximately equal to $Cl_{intrinsic}$. For intermediate conditions ($0.2 <$ extraction ratio < 0.8), clearance is partly flow dependent (38, 39, 53, 54).

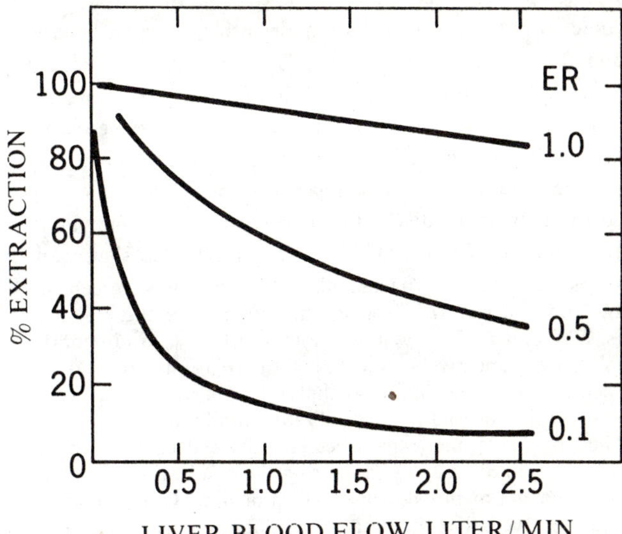

Fig. 2-10. *Relationship between hepatic blood flow and hepatic extraction for drugs with various extraction ratios (ER).* (Revised from Ref. 54.)

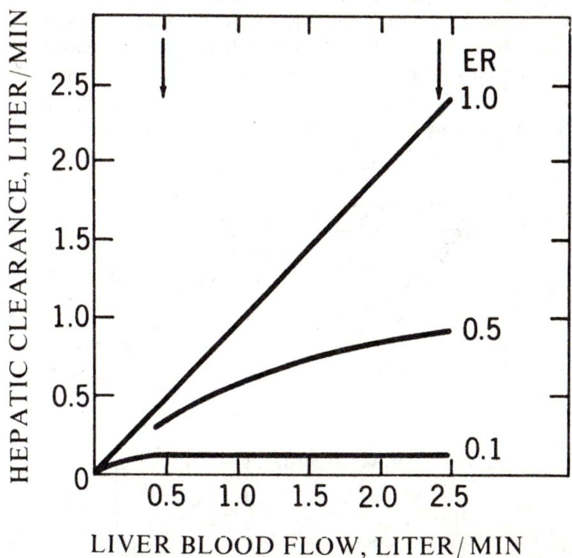

Fig. 2-11. *Relationship between hepatic blood flow and total hepatic clearance for drugs with various extraction ratios (ER).*

Arrows indicate normal physiological range of liver blood flow; extraction values refer to a normal flow of 1.5 l/min. (Revised from Ref. 54.)

One cannot easily measure the organ clearance of drug *in vivo*. However, the total body clearance (TBC) of a drug can be determined from equation 9. If the drug is eliminated both by metabolism and excretion of unchanged drug and if the fraction of drug excreted unchanged (f_e) is known, renal clearance of the drug [Cl_{renal} (f_e)(TBC)] can be calculated. The difference [TBC $-Cl_{renal}$] equals the metabolic clearance of the drug. If the liver is the only organ involved in the metabolism of the drug, then this value equals the hepatic clearance of the drug.

Several physiological or pathological conditions that alter cardiac output, blood distribution, or both can change hepatic blood flow (53). One drug may also exert an effect on the elimination of another drug through a hemodynamic interaction or by altering intrinsic clearance (e.g., by enzyme induction). Alterations in acid-base balance can also affect pharmacokinetic parameters. When pharmacokinetic principles are used to describe the disposition of any drug in an individual patient, one should be aware of the possibility that significant changes may occur in pharmacokinetic parameters for certain drugs and hence in the dosage requirements for these drugs. Figs. 2-12 and 2-13 show how changes in $Cl_{intrinsic}$ and hepatic blood flow, respectively, can change the relationships of drug concentration in the blood to time after intravenous or oral administration of totally metabolized compounds.

The pharmacokinetic parameters described earlier can be estimated for any drug by measuring the concentration of the drug in plasma or blood as a function of time. One should be aware, however, that the parameters obtained always refer to the particular fluid used to determine the drug concentration. Thus, if blood is used, the pharmacokinetic parameters refer to whole blood. Since only the nonprotein-bound drug is pharmacologically active, it would be preferable to refer all pharmacokinetic parameters, regardless of whether obtained from whole blood or plasma, to this free fraction of the totally determined drug concentration, although clearance may be an exception. If the drug concentration is determined from whole blood, one needs to calculate the plasma/erythrocyte partition and the fraction of drug bound to plasma proteins. If plasma drug concentration is measured, only the fraction of drug bound to the proteins needs to be determined. Knowledge of these factors will permit any pharmacokinetic parameter to be obtained in terms of the nonprotein-bound drug concentration, the total concentration in plasma, or the total concentration in blood (7).

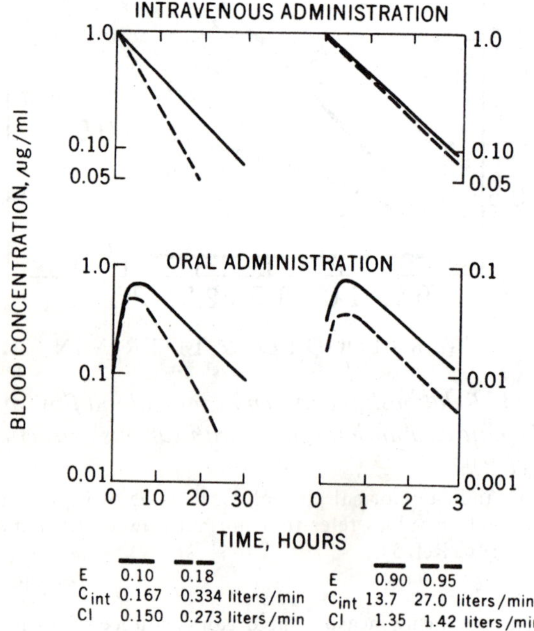

Fig. 2-12. *Effect of increasing hepatic total intrinsic clearance ($Cl_{intrinsic}$) on the curves for total drug concentration in blood vs. time, after i.v. and p.o. administration of equal doses of two totally metabolized drugs.*

Left: a drug with an initial extraction ratio of 0.9. The AUCs after oral administration are inversely proportional to $Cl_{intrinsic}$. (From Ref. 54, reprinted with permission of the publisher.)

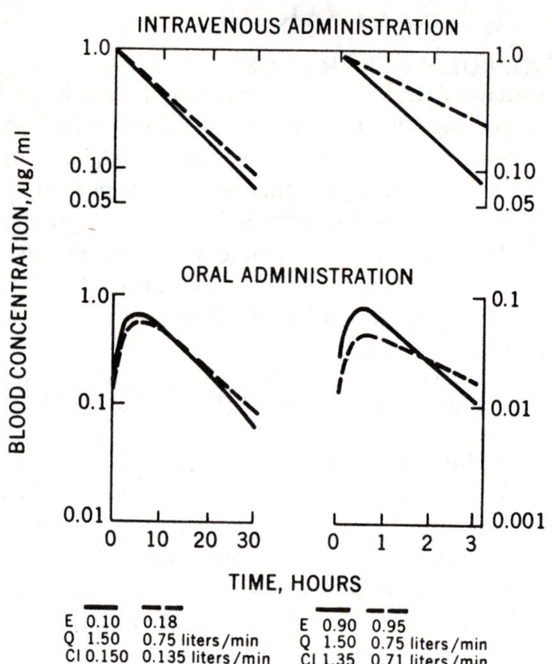

Fig. 2-13. *Effects of decreasing hepatic blood flow on the total blood concentration-time curves after intravenous and oral administration of equal doses of two totally metabolized drugs.*

Left: a drug with a total intrinsic clearance equivalent to an extraction ratio of 0.1 when blood flow equals 1.5 l/min. Right: a drug with an intrinsic clearance equivalent to an extraction ratio of 0.9. (From Ref. 54, reprinted with permission of the publisher.)

The physician rarely takes a sufficient number of samples from a given patient to perform a complete pharmacokinetic analysis. Nevertheless, the physician should be aware of these pharmacokinetic principles, to ensure the half-life determinations of a drug are based solely on samples obtained during the β phase.

Thus far, the pharmacokinetics of drugs administered only by a single intravenous administration have been discussed. However, most drugs are administered by other routes; the following sections describe certain aspects of pharmacokinetics after administration of drugs by routes other than i.v., or with multiple dosages. More comprehensive discussions are available in the literature (6, 10-12, 16, 17, 20, 27, 38, 43, 51).

BIOAVAILABILITY

After oral administration of a drug, the AUC reflects the amount of drug that reaches the systematic sampling site. The ratio of the values $AUC_{p.o.}/AUC_{i.v.}$ has been taken to be an estimate of the relative bioavailability of the drug after oral administration. All drugs, when administered orally, must pass through the gut wall and, when absorbed by the hepatic portal system, must traverse the liver before reaching the systemic sampling site. On the assumption of complete gastrointestinal absorption, it is possible that, for some compounds, a fraction of the dose absorbed may never reach the sampling site because of metabolism within the gut or liver. This first-pass effect, especially with regard to the liver, has received increasing recognition (4, 10-12, 16, 18, 20, 30, 38, 40, 53, 54). Thus far, only a few drugs have been shown to exhibit a large amount of first-pass destruction; most notable examples include imipramine, lidocaine, pethidine, nortriptyline, phenacetin, and propranolol.

A hospitalized patient might initially receive a drug intravenously rather than orally. As mentioned earlier, changes in the patient's physiological and pathological state may be reflected in altered body clearance of these drugs, with resulting alterations of therapeutic impact or effect. Pharmacokinetic considerations reveal that, even if no discernible changes occur in the curve relating drug concentration in the blood to time (and thus, total body drug clearance) when the patient is on intravenous drug therapy, a change in the route of administration from i.v. to p.o., which commonly occurs when the patient is discharged, can alter the pharmacokinetic profile and consequently the dosage requirements (Fig. 2-12 and 2-13, bottom).

For example, consider a drug that induces the hepatic drug-metabolizing enzymes. If the hepatic clearance of this drug, or of a simultaneously administered drug, approaches hepatic flow (i.e., an extraction ratio >0.9), then even though the hepatic enzymes are stimulated changes in the clearance of the drug may not be observable, even if the drug is given i.v. If the drug is administered orally, a decrease in bioavailability (as judged by the AUC) will be evident (Fig 2-12, bottom right). Thus, even though the clearance of the drug remains unchanged, the patient could be receiving as little as 50% of the desired dose.

CHRONIC OR REPETITIVE DOSING

Although some drugs, particularly analgesics, hypnotics, bronchodilators, and neuromuscular-blocking agents, may be used effectively in a single dose, numerous therapeutic agents are given chronically or in repetitive doses. In many instances, doses of chronically administered drugs are taken with sufficient frequency that measurable and often pharmacologically significant concentrations of the drug persist in the body at the time that a subsequent dose is taken. Thus, the drug tends to accumulate at a decreasing rate with increasing numbers of dosage until a steady-state level of the drug is achieved in the blood (Fig. 2-14). For drugs whose disposition follows first-order kinetics, the average steady-state blood concentration is a function of the dose (D), the fraction of dose absorbed (f), the dosing interval (γ), the biological half-life ($t_{1/2} = 0.693/\beta$), and the apparent volume of distribution (V_d), (24). The relationships between the average steady-state blood concentration (C) and these factors is given by the equations (44)

$$C = 1.44\ (t_{1/2})\ x\ (fD)/V_d\ x\ \tau \qquad (11)$$

and

$$\text{Clearance} = (f)\ x\ (D)/C_{ss}\ x\ t_{1/2} \qquad (12)$$

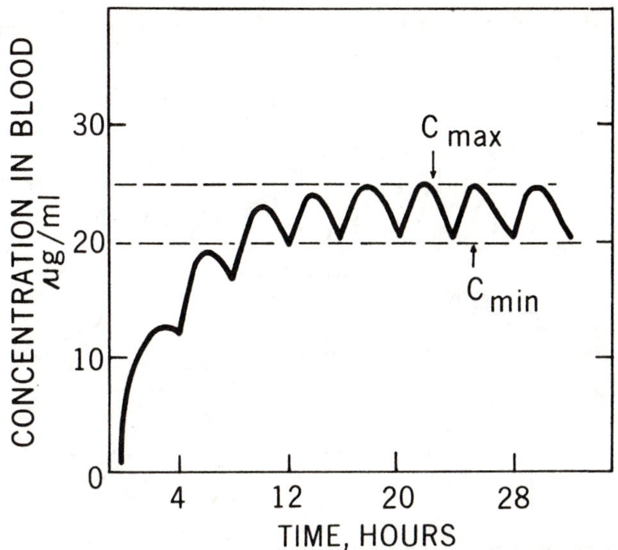

Fig. 2-14. *Typical plot of the concentration of a drug in blood after repetitive oral administration of equal doses at equal time intervals.*

In some cases, the terminal exponential phase of elimination is difficult, if not impossible, to observe, since it occurs only after drug concentrations have decreased by two or more orders of magnitude from those occurring immediately after administration of a single dose. It is possible to reach an apparent steady-state concentration in blood while the drug concentration in an organ or tissue that acts as a "deep" compartment continues to rise. If the site of drug action is in this deep compartment, the discrepancy in pharmacokinetic behavior between blood or plasma and the deep compartment can account for a delayed onset of therapeutic activity, increases in pharmacological effects at times when plasma drug concentrations appear to be at steady-state, or occurrence of pharmacological effects despite negligible drug concentrations in the plasma (Fig. 2-15). When a drug is administered repetitively in a sufficiently high dose, and at a dosage interval equivalent to its half-life, then after one drug half-life following the first dose, the plasma drug concentration will be 50% of the final steady-state concentration. By the end of one drug half-life following the second dose, 75% of the steady-state level will be attained. After one drug half-life following the third dose, 88% of the ultimate steady-state concentration will be attained; 94% of that concentration will be achieved after the fourth dose, and 97, 98, and 99% of steady-state plasma concentration of the drug will be reached after the fifth, sixth, and seventh doses, respectively, as can be derived from equation 11.

USE OF URINE OR SALIVA FOR OBTAINING PHARMACOKINETIC PARAMETERS

The pharmacokinetic parameters in the foregoing discussion can usually be obtained by following the concentration of drug or metabolite(s) in the blood as a function of time (14, 26, 27, 51). The necessary blood samples, drawn by skilled personnel in a clinic or hospital, may be difficult to obtain in old or young patients, or when many serial samples are needed. More accessible body fluids, such as urine or saliva, are more convenient and less discomforting or risky to obtain than blood. Furthermore, such noninvasive methods may offer information on drug disposition that can be either unavailable or difficult to acquire from blood samples.

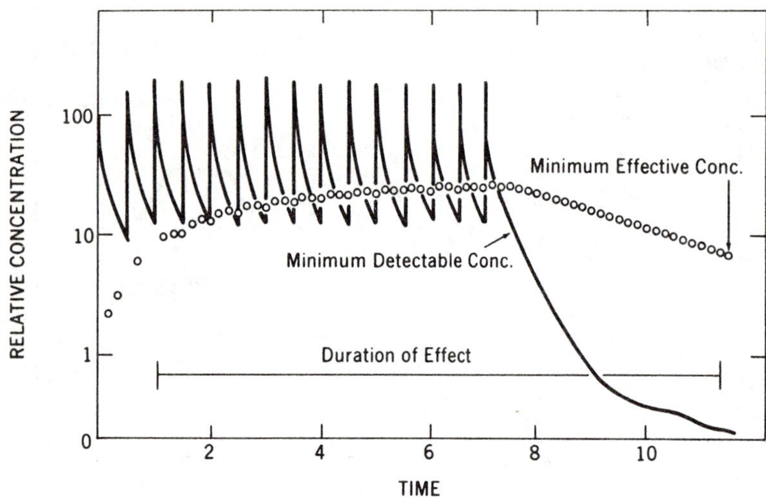

Fig. 2-15. *Relative concentrations of a drug in the central and deep peripheral compartments of a three-compartment system during repetitive administration of equal doses at equal time intervals.*

The curve and the circles represent the central and the deep peripheral compartments, respectively. (From Ref. 14, reprinted with permission of the publisher).

Many potent therapeutic agents, especially those with large volumes of distribution, present problems for pharmacokinetic analysis because even at their peak pharmacological effect the drug concentrations in the blood are very low. Thus, depending on the selectivity and sensitivity of the analytical procedure, determination of the concentration of the drug in blood may not be sufficiently accurate (52).

Because a substantial fraction of the administered dose, either as the unchanged drug or as metabolite(s), is usually excreted in the urine, it would be very useful if such urinary excretion data could be used to obtain an estimate of certain pharmacokinetic parameters. For drugs whose disposition can be described by a one-compartment model, and whose metabolite(s) are rapidly excreted

$$\text{Log (excretion rate of drug or metabolites)} = \log (\text{constant}) - \left[\frac{k_e}{2{\cdot}303}\right]t \quad (13)$$

This same relationships holds for drugs whose disposition conforms to a two-compartment model and whose metabolites are rapidly excreted, except that β replaces K_e (47). Thus, measurement of the rate of elimination of a drug, or any of its metabolites, permits estimation of the drug's biological half-life.

In practice, the logarithm of the amount of drug excreted in a series of equal intervals is plotted versus the midpoint of each time interval. This method requires no knowledge of the total amount of drug or metabolite excreted at infinity, so loss of a single urine specimen does not invalidate the data. Furthermore, collection of urine can be discontinuous; it can be abandoned overnight and started again on the following day. Thus, this method is particularly applicable to investigation of progressive changes in the rate of drug elimination that may occur during the course of drug therapy; it has been successfully used to analyze data on urinary salicylamide excretion in adults (24a) and phenytoin elimination in overdosed children (8). However, fluctuations in the rate of drug elimination do cause appreciable departures from linearity (25, 47).

Another method that can be used is called the *Sigma-minus method* (5, 25, 47). Derived from classic chemical kinetics, this methods discloses the amount of drug in the body from knowledge of the amount of drug or metabolite excreted at any time (U) and the total amount excreted (U $\int$). When elimination is first order

$$\log (U_\infty - U) = \log U_\infty - \left[\frac{\beta}{2{\cdot}303}\right]t \quad (14)$$

Furthermore

$$U_\infty = \frac{K_i \times A_o}{\beta} \quad (15)$$

where K_i is the first-order rate constant for either (1) elimination of metabolite (when elimination is slower than production (2), production of metabolite (when production is slower than elimination), or (3) elimination of unchanged drug (47). A_o represents that fraction of the administered dose reaching the central compartment; when absorption is complete, A_o is equal to the administered dose.

The Sigma-minus method requires knowledge of U and so, in theory, requires the total collection of urine until such time as drug excretion is essentially complete. It has been suggested that urine be collected for a time period equal to 10 times the drug's half-life if one is concerned with defining the complete pharmacokinetic profile of a drug (48). For useful approximation studies, one needs only carry urine collections through three to five drug half-lives, since 87 to 96%, respectively, of a drug is eliminated from the body during these periods.

The fraction of the dose of a drug excreted in the urine depends on the ratio of renal clearance to total body clearance. Thus, any factor affecting total body clearance can affect the ultimate fraction of the dose eliminated in the urine. Furthermore, because renal clearance is a complex function of glomerular filtration, tubular secretion, and tubular reabsorption (34), with the precise combination varying from drug to drug, any factor affecting one or more of the components of renal clearance will also affect the pharmacokinetic parameters. For example, alterations in protein binding and urinary pH can affect the urinary excretion and metabolism of certain drugs (17, 27, 43, 49, 50).

In summary, urinary excretion data permit determination of (1) the overall disposition constant, β, for loss of drug from the body, and (2) the rate constants for urinary elimination of unchanged drug, for production of metabolities, or both (5, 6, 17,25-28, 47, 48, 51). The use of urine is particularly promising for pediatric and geriatric patients.

REFERENCES

1. Balasubramaniam, K., Lucas, S.B., Mawer, G.E. and Simons, P.J. The kinetics of amylobarbitone metabolism in healthy men and women. *Br. J. Pharmacol.* 39:564, 1970.
2. Barr, W.H. Principles of pharmaceutics. *Am. J. Pharm. Educa.* 52:958, 1968.

3. Benet, L.Z. and Ronfeld, R.A. Volume terms in pharmacokinetics. *J. Pharm. Sci.* 58:639, 1969.
4. Cleaveland, C.R. and Shand, D.G. Effect of route of administration on the relationship between β-adrenergic blockade and plasma propranolol level. *Clin. Pharmacol. Ther.* 13:181, 1972.
5. Cummings, A.J., Martin, B.K. and Park, G.S. Kinetic considerations relating to the accrual and elimination of drug metabolites. *Br. J. Pharmacol. Chemother.* 29:136, 1967.
6. Garrett, E.R. Theoretical pharmacokinetics. In: *Klinische Pharmakologie und Pharmakotherapie* (Kuemmerle, H.P., ed.) Munich: Urban and Schwarzenberg, 1971.
7. Garrett, E.R. and Lambert, H.J. Pharmacokinetics of trichloroethanol and metabolites and interconversions among variously referenced pharmacokinetic parameters. *J. Pharm. Sci.*62:550, 1973.
8. Garrettson, L.K. and Jusko, W.J. Diphenylhydantoin elimination kinetics in overdosed children. *Clin. Pharmacol. Ther.* 17:481, 1975.
9. Gilbaldi, M. Effect of mode of administration on drug distribution in a two-compartment open system. *J. Pharm. Sci.* 58:327, 1969.
10. Gibaldi, M., Boyes, R.N. and Feldman, S. Influences of first-pass effect on availability of drugs on oral administration. *J. Pharm. Sci.* 60:1338, 1971.
11. Gilbaldi, M. and Feldman, S. Pharmacokinetic basis for the influence of route of administration on the area under the plasma concentration-time curve. *J. Pharm. Sci.* 58:1477, 1969.
12. Gibaldi, M. and Feldman, S. Route of administration and drug metabolism. *Eur. J. Pharmacol.* 19:323, 1972.
13. Gilbaldi, M., Levy, G. and Hayton, W. Kinetics of the elimination and neuromuscular blocking effect of d-tubocurarine in man. *Anesthesiology.* 36:213, 1972.
14. Gibaldi, M. Levy, G. and Weinraub, H. Drug distribution and pharmacological effects. *Clin. Pharmacol. Ther.* 12:734, 1971.
15. Gibaldi, M., Nagashima, R. and Levy, G. Relationship between drug concentration in plasma or serum and amount of drug in the body. *J. Pharm. Sci.* 58:193, 1969.
16. Gibaldi, M. and Perrier, D. Route of administration and drug disposition. *Drug. Metab. Rev.* 3:185, 1974.
17. Gibaldi, M. and Perrier, D. *Pharmacokinetics.* New York: Marcel Dekker, 1975.
18. Gram, L.F. and Christiansen, J. First-pass metabolism of imipramine in man. *Clin. Pharmacol. Ther.* 17:555, 1975.
19. Gram, L.F. and Overo, K.F. First-pass metabolism of nortriptyline in man. *Clin. Pharmacol. Ther.* 18:305, 1975.
20. Harris, P.A. and Riegelman, S. Influence of the route of administration on the area under the plasma concentration-time curve. *J. Pharm. Sci.* 58:71, 1969.
21. Kaplan, S.A., Weinfeld, R.E., Abruzzo, C.W. and Lewis, M. Pharmacokinetic profile of sulfisoxazole following intravenous, intramuscular, and oral administration in man. *J. Pharm. Sci.* 61:773, 1972.
22. Kappas, A., Alvres, A.P., Anderson, K.E. et al. Effect of charcoal-broiled beef on antipyrine and theophylline metabolism. *Clin. Pharmacol. Ther.* 23:445, 1978.
23. Kappas, A., Anderson, K.E., Conney, A.H. and Alvares, A.P. Influence of dietary protein and carbohydrate on antipyrine and theophylline metabolism in man. *Clin. Pharmacol. Ther.* 20:643, 1976.
24. Levy, G. Pharmacokinetic control and clinical interpretation of steady-state blood levels of drugs. *Clin. Pharmacol. Ther.* 16:130, 1974.
24a. Levy, G. and Matsuzawa, T. Pharmacokinetics of salicylamide elimination in man. *J. Pharmacol. Exp. Ther.* 156:285, 1967.
25. Martin, B.K. Drug urinary excretion data: some aspects concerning the interpretation. *Br. J. Pharmacol. Chemother.* 29:181, 1967.
26. Nelson, E. Kinetics of drug absorption, distribution, metabolism and excretion. *J. Pharm. Sci.* 50:181, 1961.
27. Notari, R.E. *Biopharmaceutics and Pharmacokinetics*, 2nd ed. New York: Marcel Dekker, 1975.
28. O'Reilly, W.J. Pharmacokinetics in drug metabolism and toxicology. *Can. J. Pharm. Sci.* 7:66, 1972.
29. Pantuck, E.J., Pantuck, C.B., Garland, W.A. et al. Stimulatory effect of brussels sprouts and cabbage on human drug metabolism. *Clin. Pharmacol. Ther.* 25:88, 1979.
30. Perrier, D. and Gibaldi, M. Influence of first-pass effect on the systemic availability of propoxyphene. *J. Clin. Pharmacol.* 12:449, 1972.
31. Perrier, D. and Gibaldi, M. Relationship between plasma or serum drug concentration and amount of drug in the body at steady state upon multiple dosing. *J. Pharmacokinet. Biopharm.* 1:17, 1973.
32. Perrier, D. and Gibaldi, M. Clearance and biologic half-life as indices of intrinsic hepatic metabolism. *J. Pharmacol. Exp. Ther.* 191:17, 1974.
33. Perrier, D. and Gibaldi, M. Drug clearance in multicompartment systems. *Can. J. Pharm. Sci.* 9:11, 1974.
34. Pitts, R.F. *Physiology of the Kidney and Body Fluids*, 2nd ed. Chicago: Year Book Medical Publishers, 1968.
35. Riegelman, S., Loo, J.C.K. and Rowland, M. Shortcomings in pharmacokinetic analysis by conceiving the body to exhibit properties of a single compartment. *J. Pharm. Sci.* 57:117, 1968.
36. Riegelman, S. Loo, J.C.K. and Rowland, M. Concept of a volume of distribution and possible errors in evaluation of this parameter. *J. Pham. Sci.* 57:128, 1968.
37. Riggs, D.S. *The Mathematical Approach to Physiological Problems.* Baltimore: Williams & Wilkins, 1963.
38. Rowland, M. Influence of route of administration of drug availability. *J. Pharm. Sci.* 61:70, 1972.
39. Rowland, M., Benet, L.Z. and Graham, G.G. Clearance concepts in pharmacokinetics. *J. Pharmacokinet. Biopharm.* 1:123, 1973.
40. Saidman, L.J. and Eger, E.I. Uptake and distribution of thiopental after oral, rectal, and intramuscular administration: Effect of hepatic metabolism and injection site blood flow. *Clin. Pharmacol. Ther.* 14:12, 1973.
41. Sedman, A.J. and Wagner, J.G. Importance of the use of the appropriate pharmacokinetic model to analyze *in vivo* enzyme constants. *J. Pharmacokinet Biopharm.* 2:161, 1974.
42. Shen, D., Gibaldi, M., Throne, M. et al. Pharmacokinetics of bethanidine in hypertensive patients. *Clin. Pharmacol. Ther.* 17:363, 1975.
43. van Rossum, J.M. Significance of pharmacokinetics for drug design and the planning of dosage regimens, (Ariens, E.T., ed.) In: *Drug Design.* Vol. 11. New York: Academic Press, 1971.
44. van Rossum, J.M. and Tomey, A.H.M. Rate of accumulation and plateau plasma concentration of drugs after chronic medication. *J. Pharm. Pharmacol.* 20:390, 1968.
45. Vesell, E.S. Relationship between drug distribution and therapeutic effects in man. *Ann. Rev. Pharmacol.* 14:249, 1974.
46. Vesell, E.S. and Passananti, G.T. Utility of clinical chemical determinations of drug concentrations in biological fluids. *Clin. Chem.* 17:851, 1971.
47. Vesell, E.S., Passananti, G.T., Glenwright, P.A. and Dvorchik, B.H. Studies on the disposition of antipyrine, aminopyrine, and phenacetin using plasma, saliva, and urine. *Clin. Pharmacol. Ther.* 18:259, 1975.
48. Wagner, J.G. Some possible errors in the plotting and interpretation of semilogarithmic plots of blood level and urinary excretion data. *J. Pharm. Sci.* 52:1097, 1963.
49. Wagner, J.G. Equations for excretion rate and renal clearances of exogenous substances not actively reabsorbed. *J. Clin. Pharmacol.* 7:89, 1967.

50. Wagner, J.G. Pharmacokinetics. *Ann. Rev. Pharmacol.* 8:67, 1968.

51. Wagner, J.G. *Biopharmaceutics and Relevant Pharmacokinetics*. Hamilton, N.Y.: The Hamilton Press, 1971.

52. Werner, M., Sutherland, E.W., III and Abramson, F.P. Concepts for the rational selection of assays to be used in monitoring therapeutic drugs. *Clin. Chem.* 21:1368, 1975.

53. Wilkinson, G.R. Pharmacokinetics of drug disposition: Hemodynamic considerations. *Ann. Rev. Pharmacol.* 15:11, 1975.

54. Wilkinson, G.R. and Shand, D.G. A physiological approach to hepatic drug clearance. *Clin. Pharmacol. Ther.* 18:377, 1975.

ADDITIONAL READING

Books

Avery, G.S. *Drug Treatment, Principles, and Practice of Clinical Pharmacology and Therapeutics*, 2nd ed. Sydney: ADIS Press, 1980.

Goldstein, A., Aronow, L. and Kalman, S.M. *Principles of Drug Action: The Basis of Pharmacology*, 2nd ed. New York: John Wiley, 1974.

LaDu, B.N., Mandel, H.G. and Way, E.L. *Fundamentals of Drug Metabolism and Drug Disposition*. Baltimore: Williams & Wilkins, 1971.

Melmon, K.L. and Morrelli, H.F. *Clinical Pharmacology: Basic Principles in Therapeutics*. New York: MacMillan, 1972.

Hathaway, D.E. (ed.) *Foreign Compound Metabolism in Mammals*, Vol. 6. London: 1981. The Royal Society of Chemistry.

Monographs and Reviews

Albert, A. Ionization, pH, and biological activity. *Pharmacol. Rev.* 4:136, 1952.

Brodie, B.B. and Hogben, C.A.M. Some Physicochemical Factors in Drug Action. *J. Pharm. Pharmacol.* 9:345, 1957.

Conney, A.H. Pharmacological Implications of Microsomal Enzyme Induction. *Pharmacol. Rev.* 19:317, 1967.

Davson, H. The Blood-brain Barrier. In: *The Structure and Function of Nervous Tissue*. Vol. 4 (Bourne, G.H., ed.) New York: Academic Press, 1972, p. 321.

Hartiala, K. Metabolism of Hormones, Drugs, and Other Substances by the Gut. *Physiol. Rev.* 53:496, 1973.

Kulkarni, A.P. and Hodgson, E. The Metabolism of Insecticides: The Role of Monooxygenase Enzymes. *Ann. Rev. Pharmacol.* 24:19, 1984.

Meyer, U.A. The Clinical Pharmacology of Cytochrome P-450. In: *Proceedings of the Second World Conference on Clinical Pharmacology and Therapeutics*. (Lemberger, L. and Reidenberg, M.M., eds.). Washington, D.C.: American Society for Pharmacology and Experimental Therapeutics, 1984, p. 331.

Vesell, E.S. New Directions in Pharmacogenetics. *Fed. Proc.* 43:2319, 1984.

Weinshilboum, R.M. Human Pharmacogenetics. *Fed. Proc.* 43:2295, 1984.

CHAPTER
3

PHARMACODYNAMIC ASPECTS OF DRUG ACTION

Walter B. Severs and Joan Y. Summy-Long

Pharmacodynamics can be defined as the study of drug effects at biochemical and physiological levels together with their mechanisms of actions. The goal of this chapter is to convey general principles of drug-receptor theory, sites and mechanisms of drug action, and quantitative aspects relating drug-receptor interaction, drug dose, and time.

DRUG-RECEPTOR THEORY

DEFINITIONS AND PRINCIPLES

For a drug to produce an effect in a biological system, it must interact, directly or indirectly, with an endogenous molecule of functional importance. Most drugs interact with a macromolecular species defined here as a *receptor*. The result of drug-receptor interaction (i.e., drug action) is a change in a biochemical and/or physiological function of the living organism. An *agonist* is defined as a drug that, when bound to the receptor, increases receptor function. An *antagonist,* although forming a drug-receptor complex, reduces the action associated with the receptor. Agonists and antagonists both have *affinity* (i.e., binding capability) for receptors; agonists have a second property, *intrinsic activity* or *efficacy*. This means that once bound, the agonist-receptor complex initiates the biological function related to the receptor. These important concepts are described later in a quantitative manner. It is necessary at this juncture to point out that the words "agonist" and "antagonist" do not specify whether the biochemistry/physiology related to the receptor is increased or decreased. The receptor may be coupled to either excitatory or inhibitory control mechanisms. An agonist may activate either an excitatory or inhibitory mechanism controlling bodily processes. Similarly, an antagonist may remove either an excitatory or inhibitory mechanism controlling bodily processes.

Drug receptors, as defined, are not necessarily cell components. Plasma macromolecules (lipids, proteins, hormones, enzymes, etc.) may bind drugs and cause a change in the activity of these endogenous substances. For example, heparin binds to active factor IX in plasma, which contributes to the drug's anticoagulant effect. Some macromolecules bind drugs but do not result in a drug action; these are defined as *silent receptors.* Drugs bound to silent receptors act as a reservoir in equilibrium with *free drug* in the biophase. All endogenous molecules that bind drugs are not receptors. Inorganic body components, rather than macromolecules, that bind drugs are not receptors as defined. Agents such as dimercaprol that chelate heavy metals or antacid drugs such as calcium carbonate that neutralize gastric acid exert pharmacological actions independent of macromolecular receptors.

For most drugs the receptor is poorly identified. The following example illustrates the complexity involved with receptor identification. A cell-surface membrane component (receptor) that reacts with a drug may be spatially arranged in an organized, refined manner because of adjacent membrane and subcellular structure. In turn, all structure is related to precise regulation of the extracellular and intracellular fluids. The slightest distortion of this environment by experimental intervention may cause the endogenous receptor to disappear or create an *artifact receptor*. Examples in the literature can be found where "membrane-bound drug receptors" were isolated after homogenizing tissue and applying extensive biochemical manipulations. In some cases it is more likely that a membrane component capable of binding drugs was isolated, rather than a *specific* receptor. Whether the isolated "receptor" existed *in vivo* is uncertain. Even if it were the endogenous receptor, the *coupling* of the biological response with drug-receptor interaction cannot be achieved with a disrupted cell preparation. Nevertheless, multiple approaches to receptor pharmacology have contributed not only to the understanding of drug mechanisms, but also to better comprehension of normal biochemical and physiological processes.

SITES AND MECHANISMS OF DRUG ACTION

Drugs are often classified and identified in terms of specific receptor action and therapeutic use. However, drugs may interact with *several* receptors which may be at *multiple* sites; or, drug interaction may be with one type of receptor which is present in many tissues. Interactions with all receptor types at all sites comprise the potential therapeutic use and toxicology of an individual drug. Atropine and diphenhydramine (BENADRYL) illustrate these principles.

Atropine blocks acetylcholine (ACh) receptors at postganglionic parasympathetic terminals and in some brain pathways. It is said to be *specific* because it interacts with one receptor even though atropine can be considered *nonselective*, although the mechanism of action is specific. In this context, *nonselectivity* means the drug will produce side effects in many patients at a dose necessary for therapeutic benefit. For example, ACh receptor blockade in the bladder may be the therapeutic intent of a urologist treating a patient with cystitis. But the patient may experience a side effect of motor disturbances because atropine also blocks ACh receptors in the basal ganglia in the brain. Conversely, a neurologist may prescribe atropine to block ACh receptors in the basal ganglia as therapy for a Parkinson's disease patient. This individual may suffer from urinary retention because the drug also blocks ACh receptors in the bladder. This illustrates that, with a specific but nonselective drug, a therapeutic effect for one patient can be a side effect for another. However, nonselectivity can be reduced by modifying drug distribution to therapeutic sites. For example, the patient with cystitis could be given methylatropine, a quaternary analog that penetrates the brain only slightly.

Diphenhydramine inhibits both histamine and ACh receptors. Since it has more than one mechanism of action, it is *nonspecific*. Blockade of either ACh or histamine receptors can be the therapeutic goal. Side effects are produced by blockade of the unintended receptor or the therapeutic receptor at undesired sites. Thus, diphenhydramine is nonspecific and nonselective. It is common to classify such drugs based on the receptor affected at the lowest dose. Although diphenhydramine is classified as an antihistamine, the dose differential required to cause anticholinergic action is not great. Specific and nonspecific are relative terms. At some dose level even atropine (a specific drug) probably affects endogenous macromolecules besides ACh receptors. Figure 3-1 illustrates potential drug action on multiple receptors at many sites.

Drugs may produce a particular biological response on a single cell by multiple mechanisms. A cell in the body may receive information from several neurons. Its external surface membranes have specific receptors that interact with locally released neurotransmitter(s); this interaction, in turn, initiates all subsequent events culminating in the physiological function of the nervous system. The same cell may also receive information from blood-borne hormones that interact with other membrane-bound or intracellular receptors. These hormones may influence the same cellular function as the neurons, but they interract with the cell machinery via different receptors. Drugs can simulate the reactions of neurotransmitters and hormones with receptors (i.e., act as agonists). They can also inhibit the reaction of neurotransmitters and hormones with their receptors (i.e., act as antagonists). In this context, drugs modify *endogenous* reactions that determine cells function.

A drug does not necessarily compete with an endogenous substance for a receptor. It may interact with a macromolecule of a cell in a specific manner that never occurs endogenously. Continuing the example of the typical cell, it can be envisioned that a drug binds to a cell-surface or intracellular receptor according to its physico-chemical properties. This type of interaction may never occur endogenously because the body lacks a substance equivalent to the drug. Nevertheless, the drug-receptor interaction can affect a chemical reaction that is coupled to a biological function regulated endogenously by nerves and hormones. The result of drug-receptor interaction may be a conformational change of a surface membrane or intercellular molecule causing changes in ion flux, enzyme activity, etc. Figure 3-2 illustrates some of these principles for a vascular smooth muscle cell whose function is control of peripheral vascular resistance. A careful review of this figure and its legend will provide an overview of the multiple mechanisms that can affect the function of a single cell.

CHARACTERIZATION OF RECEPTORS

Structure-Activity Relationships (SARs). Study of SARs has contributed greatly to the understanding of drug-receptor properties. In this procedure, a structurally identified compound, either endogenous or exogenous to the body, is used to determine molecular characteristics of the receptor. The dose-response (dose-

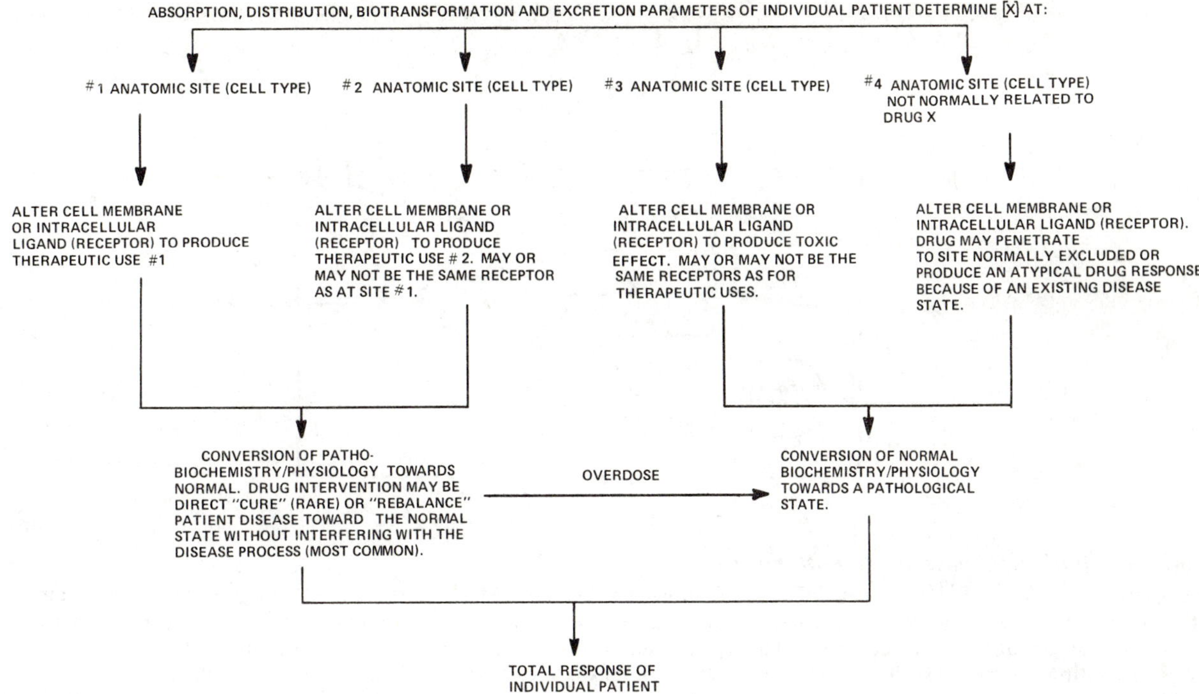

Fig. 3-1. *Representation of a drug with many actions.*

If a drug reacts with the same receptor at different sites, it is *specific* in its mechanism but *nonselective* in its site of action. It would be relatively nonspecific if it reacts with different receptors.

receptor) relationship of this compound is determined with and without a standard antagonist. Many analogs are made in which the molecular shape and reactive groups of the parent compound are modified. These are *quantitatively* tested, alone, and for interaction with the parent drug and antagonist. The goal of this enduring procedure is to define which parts of the parent molecule are essential and nonessential for *affinity* and *intrinsic activity*. By inference from the SAR data, the receptor should have a complementary structure in terms of: stereospecificity, molecular configuration, appropriate reactive groups for bond formation, and *intrareceptor* distance between groups.

Based on knowledge of the receptor size, shape, stereospecificity, and arrangements of reactive groups, a drug can be redesigned to improve specificity and selectivity (reduced side effects, see Fig. 3-1). Redesign of the parent compound can also alter pharmacokinetic properties of the drug, producing more desirable distribution, onset, and/or duration of action. In addition, previously unknown receptors may be discovered. A classic example of the importance of SAR studies comes from the work of Ahlquist (1), who studied five drugs that mimic sympathetic nervous responses, using various tissues in several animal species. Two types of tissue response occurred. In some tissues the five drugs acted as agonists in a *specific* rank order, whereas other tissues responded to the sympathetic agonists in the *reverse* order. Ahlquist concluded that cells innervated by the sympathetic nervous system had two different kinds of receptors: α and β. Prior to this, many physiologists believed that sympathetic neurons released two kinds of transmitters: one *excitatory*, and one *inhibitory*. The concept of α- and β-receptors still provides an important framework for defining drug action.

Continuing SAR work based on exogenous agonists and antagonists suggests two β-adrenergic receptor subtypes: β_1 and β_2 (22, 23). Heart tissue has mostly β_1-receptors that increase rate and contractility, whereas bronchial smooth muscle has mostly β_2-receptors that cause relaxation. Similarly, SAR studies suggest the existence of α_1- and α_2-receptors subtypes (22, 23).

Theoretically, if the complete structure of a receptor were known, drugs could be specifically designed to interact with it, and no extraneous parts of the molecule would exist to combine with other body components and produce side effects. This molecular tailoring would be constrained, however, if the resultant *pharmacokinetic* properties did not allow an adequate drug concentration to reach the *pharmacodynamic* site. In this case, additional molecular modification would be needed to create desirable pharmacokinetic properties; but these additions would increase the potential for reduced specificity of drug action.

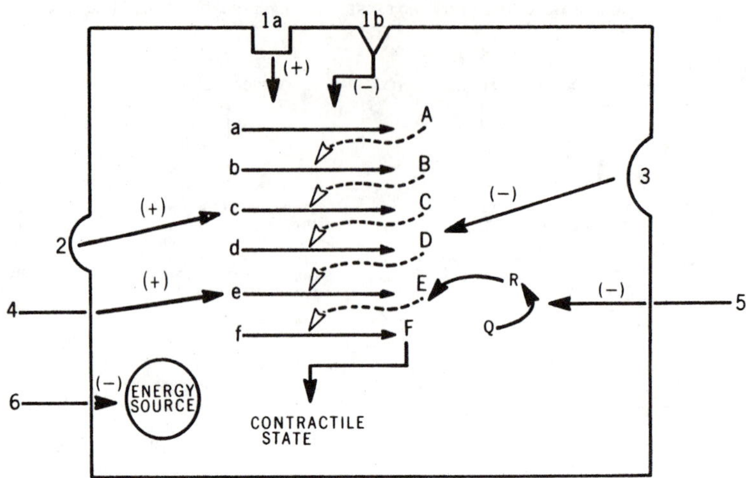

Fig. 3-2. *A hypothetical vascular smooth muscle cell.*

The reactions a → A, b → B, etc., represent an orderly cascade where F is the last determinant of the contractile state. Commonly, the number of reactions, their exact sequence, and molecular nature are unknown. The reactions may be a change in protein conformation, enzyme reaction rate, ion flux, etc. The cell has many membrane-bound receptors that convey information from neurotransmitters and circulating hormones such as norepinephrine, angiotensin, etc. These substances provide excitatory (+) or inhibitory (-) information; the net input determines the degree of muscle contraction. Hypothetical mechanisms of drug action are numbered (1a, b = 6) and illustrated as drug-receptor interactions on the cell surface or at intracellular sites.

1a, b represent an excitatory α (1a) and inhibitory β (1b) adrenergic receptor. These cell membrane-bound receptors convey information from locally released neurotransmitter and blood-borne catecholamines to alter contractility. Drugs may *mimic* endogenous information transfer if they have affinity and intrinsic activity; or *interfere* with *endogenous* information transfer if they bind to the receptor without intrinsic activity. In both cases, the drug *competes* with endogenous catecholamines for the receptors.

2 is an example of a receptor on the cell membrane conveying excitatory information from a circulating hormone (e.g., angiotensin). Activation is arbitrarily shown as affecting c → C to emphasize two concepts. First, it is not necessary (indeed, unknown) that all excitatory membrane receptors couple to the reaction cascade at the same point. Second, if one receptor (such as 1a) is blocked, the contraction scheme can be entered at other sites. α Receptor blockade does not render the cell incapable of functioning in response to other stimuli (angiotensin).

3 represents a cell membrane receptor transmitting *inhibitory*, information from a circulating hormone (perhaps a prostaglandin). Inhibition is arbitrarily shown at D to emphasize again that the same event (state of contraction) can be altered by drugs at multiple reaction sites. Note that if inhibition at D becomes rate limiting, information transfer from all preceding steps fails.

4 shows an excitatory drug *not* mimicking endogenous information transfer from cell membrane receptors. The agonist penetrates the cell according to the concentration of free, un-ionized drug in extracellular fluid. It reacts with an endogenous intracellular ligand and, like D, increases the e → E reaction.

5 shows an inhibitory drug with an intracellular site of action. In this case, the reaction R → Q is inhibited. The drug does not *directly* affect contractile reactions; rather, it reduces E by affecting *another* series of reactions and vasodilation results. A similar drug indirectly increasing E availability can be envisioned.

6 represents drug interference with the cell's energy source. The unavailability of energy, necessary for many cellular processes, nonspecifically reduces contraction.

Radioligand Binding. In recent years the field of *in vitro* receptor purification and *quantification* of drug-receptor interactions has led to numerous applications of these procedures. The technology (for example, see Ref. 9) depends on a starting radioactive drug (radioligand) that binds to a specific receptor of interest with very high affinity; thus, very low doses of ligand are presumed to bind mainly to the specific receptor of interest. Nonspecific binding usually (but not always) is of comparatively low affinity and is minimal at low doses. Since the major amount of radioactivity is bound to a specific receptor, a starting ligand with high specific radioactivity (Curies/mole) is desirable because extremely small doses can be given that minimize nonspecific binding without reducing the amount of radioactivity bound to the specific receptors.

Morphine is an example of a drug whose receptor has been studied by ligand binding (19, 31). *In vitro* radioligand assays show that the partially isolated morphine receptor displays high-affinity binding, saturability, and stereospecificity. Between 70 and 90% of the radioligand binding is specific. In addition, kinetic analysis of various morphine-receptor agonists correlates well with several biological responses. Morphine receptors have endogenous agonists: the enkephalin and endorphin polypeptides. Thus, morphine modifies what is presumed to be an endogenous reaction. High-affinity specific radioligand binding has also been reported for diazepam (VALIUM). Data are available that indicate a correlation between displacement of radioligand binding with clinical antianxiety actions for this series of drugs (28). The body may produce an *endogenous* substance interacting with these receptors. This point is uncertain, but not impossible (5).

Histochemical Procedures. Many methods involve the use of a drug or endogenous substance with an identifiable marker such as a fluorescent or a radioactive species. Fluorescein-coupled substances bound to tissue receptors can be visualized using fluorescent microscopy; tissue-bound radioactive drugs can be located by autoradiography. The unlabeled antibody (peroxidase-antiperoxidase) method utilizes specific antibodies to substances such as peptides (vasopressin, angiotensin) and enzymes (tyrosine and tryptophan hydroxylases). The antibody is reacted with tissue antigen; antiimmune globulin is then added to bind the antibody, followed by peroxidase-antiperoxidase reagent and staining. This provides a powerful tool for receptor localization since it uses *immunologically* specific antisera, and multiple markers can be coupled to each tissue antigen.

One example of histochemical contributions is the autoradiographic localization of nicotinic acetylcholine receptors (NA-R) in the brain (20). The principles are similar to the *in vitro* use of radioligands for purification of receptors. α-Bungarotoxin, from snake venom, specifically and irreversibly binds to NA-R. Pure toxin was labeled with ^{125}I and injected into rat cerebral ventricles. A day later, the animals were killed and brain sections processed. Microscopy and autoradiography showed presumptive NA-R in the stratum oriens of the hippocampal formation, associated with synaptic complexes. If further work shows a biological response to locally applied nicotinic agonists and specific blockade by antagonist, the receptor *function* will be clarified in this brain region. If tissue malfunction is suspected in a disease process, then pharmacological control of the NA-R could be attempted as therapy. Thus, various methods of studying receptors have the potential to define both sites and actions.

QUANTIFICATION OF DRUG-RECEPTOR INTERACTION

HISTORY

Ehrlich and Hata (12) avidly synthesized organic compounds as potential medicinals to treat infectious diseases. They conceptualized that specific chemical receptors exist in parasites but not in humans; thus a drug reacting with these receptors might cure a disease without harming the host. Compound number 606, synthesized by Ehrlich, was an organic arsenical, SALVARSAN. Although the drug was not without side effects in humans, its introduction in 1907 formed the mainstay of therapy for syphilis until the penicillin era.

The first quarter of this century produced a remarkable surge of research in autonomic nervous system pharmacology, culminating in the discovery of chemical transmission at autonomic nerve endings. Much of this work was based on careful observation that the actions of some botanical drugs on tissues closely *simulated*, whereas others specifically *blocked*, the effects of sympathetic or parasympathetic nerve stimulation. Extracts from endogenous tissues (such as the adrenal medulla) also could mimic sympathetic nerve actions. Such work led to the hypothesis that autonomic nerves liberate chemicals that interact with *receptors* on innervated cells. Resolution of the issue of whether neurotransmission was electrical or chemical was provided by Otto Loewi (25), who collected effluent fluid from perfused frog hearts after autonomic nerve stimulation. Transfer of this effluent to the heart of a second frog reproduced the autonomic response of the first heart. The physiology of postganglionic autonomic transmitter release onto a specialized portion of the effector cell became accepted. At the same time, drug mechanisms were described in terms of mimicking or inhibiting transmitter action on specific receptors.

Other important studies provided a scientific basis for older empiricisms that: (a) an individual's response to a particular dose of drug is variable, and (b) there is a relationship between the drug dose and biological response. By extension, if drug response depends on drug-receptor interaction, then drug-receptor interaction must also be dependent on dose. These principles have been well established.

J. H. Burn (6), an eminent Oxford pharmacologist, concluded in 1922 that studying lethality of digitalis in cats was not useful for determining potency of different batches of the drug, an important problem at the time. The lethal dose in three cats, using the same batch of digitalis, was 75, 92, and 125 mg of plant leaf per cat. Such unreliable data, even with the same batch of the drug, suggested an unreliable method. deLind van Wijngaarden (35) pursued the matter further. He determined the *exact* lethal dose of intravenous digitalis in 573 cats; the data generated a classic bell-shaped, Gaussian frequency distribution curve (Fig. 3-3). These experiments showed that the dose of the drug (digitalis) to produce a specified effect (lethality) in one animal had little significance. The true dose to produce a specified effect is the mean (average) dose determined in a large population; individuals vary about that mean. Similar studies by Trevan (34) with digitalis lethality showed that if many frogs were given one of several doses of the drug, the mean (average) lethality (response) was, indeed, related to dose; a quantal dose-response curve was produced. Behrans (4) independently

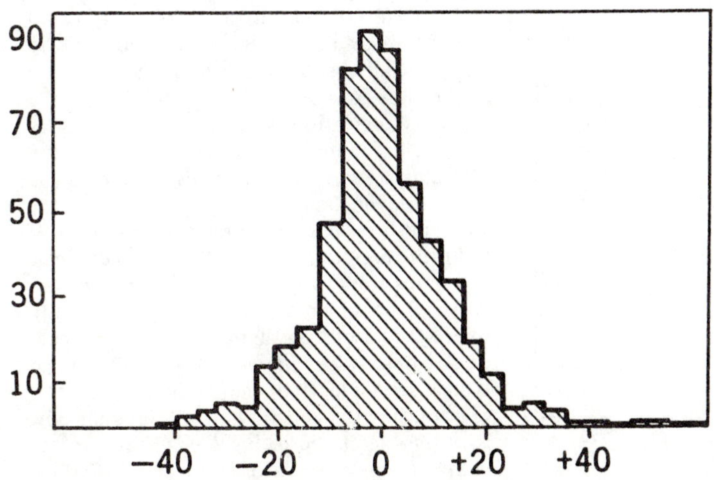

Fig. 3-3. *Digitalis lethality in cats.*
The mean (average) lethal dose of digitalis is shown as zero on the "X" axis; percent deviation (+ or -) from the mean dose is illustrated. The "Y" axis shows the number of acts that died at a particular dose. Almost all individual cats died at doses between 40% above or below the mean. This gaussian or bell-shaped curve is a typical example relating frequency of response to drug dose. (From Ref. 35, with permission of Springer Verlag).

studied another digitalis glycoside (strophanthin) for lethality in frogs by determining the exact i.v. dose required to kill each animal. His data could be plotted as a Gaussian curve and a frequency curve. Moreover, a plot of both Trevan's and Behran's data (normalized for the 50% response dose) yields the same curve (Fig. 3-4). Two independent studies with a drug acting on the same receptors to produce the same effect in the same species yielded identical results. Such early work put quantitative aspects of drug response on a firm basis.

QUANTITATIVE ASPECTS OF DRUG DOSE-RESPONSE

A fundamental principle of pharmacology states that the magnitude of drug effect is a function of the amount of the drug administered to the concentration of free drug available for interaction in the biophase adjacent to the receptor.

Occupation Theory. A quantitative theory applying the laws of mass action to the interaction of drugs with specific receptor groups was first postulated by Clark (7, 8) and later developed by Gaddum (15). These authors provided evidence suggesting that the drug-receptor interaction was similar to the adsorption isotherm relationship described by Langmuir (21). This theory describing the quantitative relationship of drug-receptor interaction has been called the *occupation theory* and has the following theoretical assumptions:

1. Drug action is proportional to the number (or percentage) of receptors occupied.
2. The occupation of receptors by drug molecules follows the law of mass action.
3. Receptors are identical and equally accessible; one drug molecule reacts with one receptor.
4. The amount of the drug bound to receptors is negligible compared with the total amount of drug in the biophase.
5. The maximal drug response occurs when all receptors are occupied.

The equations for *quantification* of drug-receptor interactions are similar to the Michaelis-Menten analysis of enzyme-substrate reactions (17, 27). The example to be presented illustrates a simple case applicable to several drugs. The following equations (see Table 3-1), based on the assumptions specified, explain the relationship of effect and dose according to the law of mass action.

Table 3-1
Abbreviations and Definitions for Quantitative Terms Describing Drug Action

Term	Definition
D	Drug molecule
R	Drug receptor
DR	Drug-receptor complex
DR*	Activated drug-receptor complex
R_t	Total number of drug receptors
k_1	Association rate constant for DR
k_2	Dissociation rate constant for DR
k_3	Dissociation rate constant for DR*
$K_{A,\ B,\ C,\ \text{OR}\ D} = k_2/k_1$	Equilibrium[a] dissociation constant for A (agonist), B, C (antagonists), or D (drug)
$1/K_{A,\ B,\ C,\ \text{OR}\ D}$	Association constant (index of affinity)
E	Effect
E_{max}	Maximum effect (efficacy)
[ ]	Concentration

[a] Equilibrium constants can be indicated by dissociation (k_2/k_1) or association (k_1/k_2) expressions.

According to the law of mass action, a reversible reaction occurs between the drug and receptor.

$$[D] + [R] \underset{k_2}{\overset{k_1}{\rightleftarrows}} [DR] \rightarrow \text{effect} \qquad (1)$$

At equilibrium, the rate of association of [DR] equals the rate of dissociation, thus

$$[D]\ [R]\ k_1 = [DR]\ k_2 \qquad (2)$$

Rearranging yields

$$K_D = \frac{k_2}{k_1} = \frac{[D]\ [R]}{[DR]} \qquad (3)$$

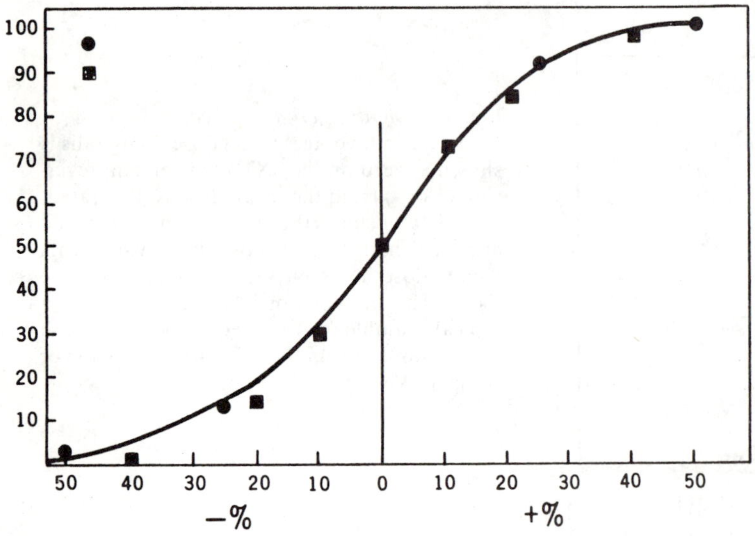

Fig. 3-4. *Digitalis lethality in frogs.* The results of Behrans (1929) (4) and Trevan (1927) (34), as described in the text, are shown. The dose killing 50% of the animals in the two studies was considered equivalent (zero on the "X" axis); deviation (+ or -%) from this dose is indicated. The frequency of response (% on the "Y" axis) is shown in an *integrated* manner. This form of data presentation accounts for 100% of the animals (like the Gaussian curve), but the *assumption* is made that frogs dying at low doses would have died at all higher doses. As the dose is increased from -50 to +50%, the total number of frogs dying *at* or *below* a particular dose is *cumulated*. This results in the typical sigmoidal frequency response plot. The relationship between this and the Gaussian plot is further described in Fig. 3-8. (From Ref. 6, with permission of Oxford University Press).

The total number of receptors is given by

$$[R_t] = [R] + [DR] \qquad (4)$$

Thus. $$[R] = [R_t] - [DR] \qquad (5)$$

Substitution of equation (5) into equation (3) and rearranging yields

$$\frac{[DR]}{[R_t]} = \frac{[D]}{K_D + [D]} \qquad (6)$$

where $\frac{[DR]}{[R_t]}$ is equal to the proportion of drug-receptor complexes at equilibrium.

Assuming the proportion of receptors occupied determines drug effect (E), the maximal response (E_{max}) of the drug occurs when all the receptors (100%) are occupied. If 50% of R_t is occupied, 50% of the maximal response is obtained.

Thus, $$\frac{E}{E_{max}} = \frac{[DR]}{[R_t]} \qquad (7)$$

Substitution of equation (7) in equation (6) and subsequent rearrangements yields

$$E = \frac{E_{max}\,[D]}{K_D + [D]} \qquad (8)$$

or

$$E = \frac{E_{max}}{K_D/[D] + 1} \qquad (9)$$

This equation defines a hyperbola such that when the concentration of the drug is great, the maximal effect is approached; and when [D] = 0, E = 0. Thus, a drug combines with its receptor in relation to the concentration of free drug at the receptor site and the affinity of the drug for that receptor. Simple occupancy, however, cannot explain all drug actions. Two drugs may bind to 50% of the receptors, but one is an *agonist* and the other an *antagonist*. Other aspects must, therefore, be considered.

Different agonists may yield different E_{max} values even at very high drug concentrations. A receptor agonist evoking the maximal tissue response can be considered a full agonist. Other agonists may exert a lesser maximal response. These are called *partial agonists.* The concepts of *intrinsic activity* (3), or *efficacy* (32), were invoked to explain further the relationship between drug-receptor binding and drug action. Ariens (3) introduced the term intrinsic activity to explain the pharmacodynamics of partial agonists; it assumes complete (100%) receptor occupancy is required for the maximal drug response. Stephenson (32) used the term efficacy, which is conceptually similar to, but quantitatively different from, intrinsic activity. The difference is that 100% occupation of receptors is not required for maximal efficacy. Both terms imply that the drug-receptor complex of different agonists may differ in their ability to elicit the drug response (26).

To explain differences in the ability of a drug-receptor complex to elicit the drug response, two forms of the drug-receptor complex are hypothesized: one activated [DR*], the other not [DR]. The ratio [DR*]/[DR] is an expression of efficacy. Equation (1) must be rewritten as

$$[D] + [R] \overset{k_1}{\rightleftarrows} [DR] \overset{k_2}{\rightleftarrows} [DR^*] \overset{k_3}{\rightarrow} \text{drug effect} \qquad (10)$$

where k_1 and k_2 = dissociation constants for the respective reactions. The activated DR* complex directly mediates the drug action. This action can be conceptualized as a change in membrane pore size or ion flux produced by changes in membrane macromolecules initiated by drug-receptor activation. Thus, according to the occupation theory, the effect of a certain agonist increases with time as the proportion of occupied, and activated, receptors increases until equilibrium is obtained as characterized by equation (9).

Efficacy is measured as a ratio between the maximal effect of the individual drug and the maximal effect possible in the tissue studied. It has no dimensions. The association constant ($1/K_D$) can be obtained from the dose-response relationship. According to the assumptions of Clark (7), the drug response is proportional to the fraction of receptors occupied.

In equation (7) the proportion of receptors occupied is given by

$$\frac{E}{E_{max}} = \frac{[DR]}{[R_t]} \qquad (11)$$

when

$$E = 1/2\ E_{max} \qquad (12)$$

Then $$\frac{[DR]}{[R_t]} = \frac{1}{2} \qquad (13)$$

Or from equation (9)

$$E_{50\%} = E_{max/2} = \frac{E_{max}}{K_D/[D_{50\%}] + 1} \qquad (14)$$

Thus,

$$\frac{K_D}{[D_{50\%}]} + 1 = 2 \qquad (15)$$

and $$K_D = [D_{50\%}] \qquad (16)$$

The association constant ($1/K_D$) is, therefore, derived as the reciprocal of the concentration of agonist necessary to produce one-half (50%) of the maximal drug response. This is an index of affinity of the drug for its receptor.

Rate Theory. The *rate theory,* proposed by Paton (30), has also been postulated to quantitatively explain drug-receptor interaction. This theory assumes that drug action is proportional to the rate of drug-receptor combination rather than to the proportion of receptors occupied. Quantitatively, k_2/k_1 or K_D determines the potency, and k_2 the antagonist or agonist properties of the drug. If the rate constant for dissociation (k_2) of the drug from the receptor is high, the drug is a powerful agonist; if the rate is moderate, the drug will be a partial agonist; and if low, the drug is an antagonist. Instead of using efficacy or intrinsic activity to explain partial agonists, Paton (30) explained drug action by the rate of dissociation of the drug from the receptor site. Some experimental support for the rate theory has been obtained and can qualitatively account for several pharmacological observations such as: the long duration of antagonist action on tissue; drugs that have both agonist and antagonist properties; certain forms of tachyphylaxis; and the initial stimulant properties of many antagonists.

Spare Receptors. One of the major assumptions of the occupation theory of drug-receptor interaction is that the maximal response of the tissue is obtained only when all the receptors are occupied. This assumption was questioned as a result of the work of Furchgott (13) and Nickerson (29), who postulated that pretreatment of tissue with irreversible antagonists should decrease the number of receptors available for occupancy and thus reduce the maximal response. In fact, Nickerson (29) demonstrated that after pretreatment of the isolated guinea pig ileum with GD 121 (irreversible antagonist), the dose-response curve of histamine was shifted to the right without changing either the slope or maximal response.

A similar result was obtained by Furchgott (13, 14) and MacKay (26) using dibenamine (antagonist) and epinephrine (agonist) on the isolated rabbit aortic strip. Based on these experiments, the presence of spare receptors was postulated. The maximal effect that can be produced by the tissue is regarded as occurring after the appropriate, but not necessarily maximum, number of receptors have produced their stimulus in the effector organ. Drug concentration and affinity of the agonist still determine receptor occupation. The tissue response, however, is only proportional to the number of receptors occupied until the maximum response is obtained. This theory no longer requires occupation of all receptors to elicit the maximal effect.

It is important to realize that the theories discussed are based on assumptions. They are useful to predict hypothetical curves for comparison with those experimentally derived. These models can explain some, but not all, aspects of drug-receptor interaction. No quantitative system has been developed that can predict the action of all drugs in all test systems. The dose-response relationship must be obtained after biochemical equilibrium when the steady state has been reached. The steady state is best approximated by *in vitro* methods. Frequently, however, the dose-response curve is obtained *in vivo* using peak responses after a single dose of drug. Under *in vivo* conditions, the shape of the curve may vary and could be multiphasic, indicating the presence of compensatory biological responses.

ALLOSTERIC MODELS OF RECEPTORS

Allosteric enzymes are usually rate limiting and strategically located at an early step in a series of reactions. End product often binds to the allosteric enzyme at a site distant from the catalytic site, resulting in a conformational change that affects the rate of enzyme action at the catalytic site, and thereby controls an entire series of reactions.

The receptors located on cell membranes may be under similar control (13). According to this concept, the membrane receptor exists in two forms, active and inactive, which are in equilibrium. Agonists and antagonists are presumed to distort this equilibrium by binding to one form of the receptor more than the other. For example, agonists would bind with greater affinity to the active, rather than the inactive form.

DOSE-RESPONSE CURVE

Equations describing the quantitative aspects of drug actions are represented in graphic form as the dose-response curve. The abscissa shows an increasing concentration of the drug (arithmetic scale) and the ordinate shows the percent of the maximal effect. A hyperbola, as defined from equation (4), is obtained and is illustrated in Fig. 3-5.

A more convenient method of expressing the dose-response relationship is to use the logarithms of the drug concentration rather than arithmetic values on the abscissa. This semilogarithmic plot allows (1) a larger concentration range to be presented, and (2) an optimal illustration of large responses produced by small dosage increments. This form of the dose-response curve, illustrated in Fig. 3-6, is especially useful for evaluating pharmacological antagonism. Characteristics of the dose-response relationship can be easily identified from a log dose-response curve. These characteristics include: affinity, efficacy, slope, potency, and biological variability.

Affinity. Affinity describes the ability of a drug to bind to a receptor. When the affinity is great, only a small concentration of the drug is required to occupy a specified proportion of receptors. The converse is also true. Affinity is thus one index of the effectiveness of a drug

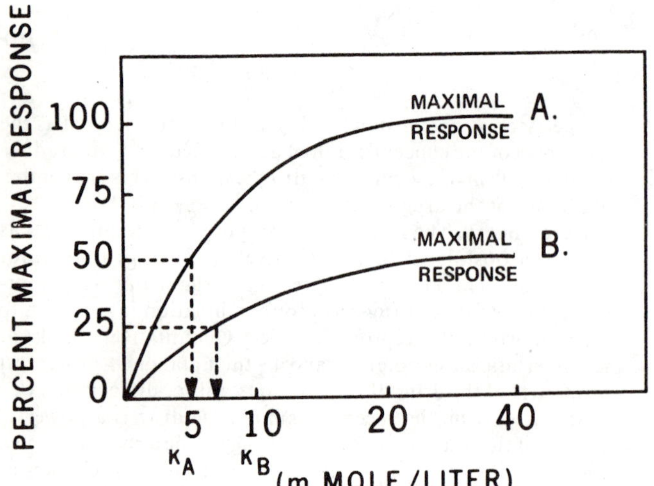

Fig. 3-5. *Dose-response curves for two hypothetical agonists.*

Determination of the equilibrium dissociation constants and maximal response of two agonists, A and B. The equilibrium constants (K_A, K_B) are equal to the drug concentration producing 50% of the maximal drug response. The reciprocal of the equilibrium constant ($1/K_A$, $1/K_B$) is the association constant, a measure of affinity. Agonist A has an efficacy of 1 (maximum effect of A equals maximum effect of the tissue); the efficacy of B is 0.5.

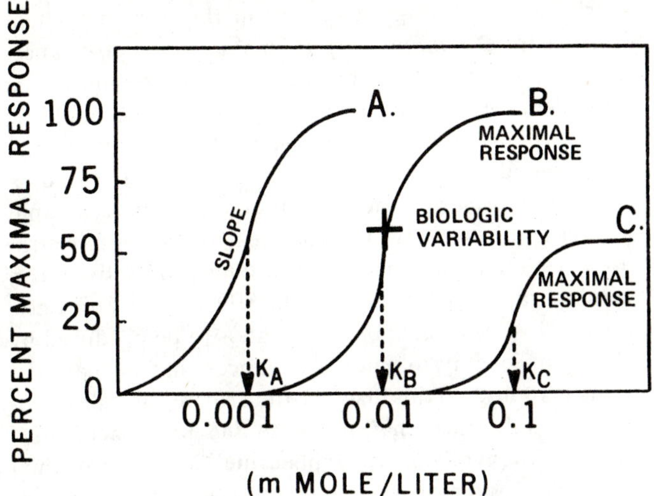

Fig. 3-6. *Semilogarithmic plot of the dose-response curve.*

The curve illustrates the relationship of two agonists (A, B) having different equilibrium-dissociation constants (K_A, K_B) and potencies but with a similar maximal response or efficacy (1.0). The partial agonist C has an equilibrium-dissociation constant of K_C and efficacy of 0.5. The slopes of A, B, and C are similar. Biological variability (+) illustrates the range of doses eliciting the same response and the differences in response produced by one dose.

interaction with its receptor. Affinity is measured as the reciprocal of the dissociation constant (K_D) which is obtained from the dose-response curve as the concentration of the drug required to produce 50% of the maximal response (33) (Figs. 3-5 and 3-6).

Efficacy. Efficacy is defined as the maximal effect produced by the drug. It is estimated from the dose-response curve as the response at which a plateau is asymptomatically reached. For comparative purposes, efficacy is expressed as a ratio of the maximal response produced by the drug and that which can be elicited from the tissue. For comparison of a series of drugs, the relative efficacy of each drug is determined by comparison with the compound producing the greatest response. The opium-derived narcotics and aspirin provide a striking example of differences in drug efficacy. Morphine provides relief of pain of all intensities, whereas aspirin, at any dose, is an effective analgesic for only mild-to-moderte pain.

Potency. Potency defines the dose of a drug necessary to produce a specified response (50%, 75% of the maximal response, etc.). Potency varies inversely with the amount of the drug necessary for drug action (i.e., if large doses are needed to produce the specified effect, the drug has low potency). For comparison of drugs having a similar mechanism of action, relative potency is defined as the ratio of equi-effective doses of compounds. Conceptually, for drugs stimulating similar receptors, potency is influenced by the drug-receptor binding (affinity). The position of the dose-response curve on the abscissa indicates relative potency. For example, in Fig. 3-6, agonist A is 10 times more potent than agonist B; to elicit 50% of the maximal response, 0.01 mmol/ l of B is necessary, whereas a similar response can be obtained with only 0.001 mmol/ l of A. It is appropriate to compare these agonists because their slopes and maximal responses are not different, indicating a similar mechanism of action (33). The data illustrated in Fig. 3-6 were obtained under equilibrium conditions *in vitro.* These conditions minimize the pharmacokinetic differences between drugs; thus, in this example, differences in affinity determine the relative potency.

It is important to distinguish between efficacy and potency. Potency is relatively unimportant in therapeutics, since whether a patient takes 10 μg or 300 mg to achieve the desired effect is of minor importance. Potency may be important in pharmaceutical formulation of drugs. The size of the tablet or capsule may be quite large for a drug with low potency and may consequently reduce patient compliance. Efficacy, however, is an important characteristic of drug action and must be considered if therapy is to be successful.

Slope. The slope of the dose-response curve is an expression of the rate of change in drug response with increasing dose. The slope is best estimated from the central or linear portion of the dose-response curve by least-squares regression analysis. Theoretical explanations of the significance of the slope of dose-response curves in relation to drug action have been reviewed. It can be stated generally, however, that drugs acting by similar mechanisms (e.g., stimulating the same population of receptors) have parallel slopes and attain the same maximal response or efficacy. The semilogarithmic plot of the dose-response curve most conveniently illustrates these characteristics of drug action. It is important to note that because of the sigmoid shape of the dose-response curve, tripling the dose will not necessarily triple the drug effect. Although primarily useful in the theoretical analysis of drug action, the slope of the dose-response curve can be of practical utility. A steep slope suggests the dose range between therapeutic and toxic effects may be narrow. The therapeutic index, is, however, a more appropriate measure of a drug's margin of safety.

Biological Variation. Biological variation is defined as the difference in drug response measured among different people or in the same individual from time to time; it can be illustrated on the dose-response curve as a variation in both (1) the responses produced by one dose, and (2) the doses required for eliciting the same effect. Both genetic and environmental factors influence biological variation in drug response. For example, an exaggerated response (hypersusceptibility) to a "typical" dose of drug may result from a genetically determined deficit in an enzyme necessary for drug metabolism or from differences in bioavailability due to environmental factors or preexisting disease states. Thus, interindividual and intraindividual differences in drug response or drug action are related to alterations in pharmacokinetic and pharmacodynamic processes. Biological factors influencing the response include: age, weight, sex, presence of preexisting pathology, variations in physiology, and psychological factors such as the placebo effect. An abnormal or peculiar drug response has been called *idiosyncrasy,* that is more precisely defined "as a genetically determined abnormal reactivity to a drug" (16). This aspect of biological variation is discussed under pharmacogenetics. Factors related to drug administration also modify drug response in individuals. Repeated administration of the same drug, the route of administration, and drug interactions from combination therapy may also affect biological variability.

With repeated administration of some drugs, a decreased responsiveness or *tolerance* can occur. This decrease in drug effect, often indicative of a change in drug-receptor interaction, can usually be overcome by increasing the dose. Tolerance is not a characteristic of all drugs, nor does it develop to all actions of the same drug. It is reversible, disappearing after drug withdrawal, although cross-tolerance to structurally and/or pharmacologically related drugs is frequent. Tolerance develops by changes in: (a) pharmacokinetic processes that effectively lower the concentration of active drug at the receptor site (e.g., drug disposition or pharmacokinetic tolerance), or by (b) a change in receptor reactivity (cellular or pharmacodynamic tolerance) after repeated drug administration. Drug-disposition tolerance occurs when a drug causes a change in its rate of absorption, distribution, metabolism, and/or excretion such that a decreased concentration of free drug occurs at the receptor site. This form of tolerance can be measured as a change in either the duration of action or the magnitude of peak drug response. Route of administration can alter drug-disposition tolerance. Intravenous administration circumvents absorption and first-pass biotransformation, permitting maximal drug concentrations at the receptor site. However, coexisting increases in drug elimination can decrease duration of action (tolerance) without changing the peak response. Phenobarbital is a well-known example of drug-disposition-induced tolerance. Repeated administration of this compound results in increased phenobarbital metabolism by stimulation of the hepatic microsomal mixed-function oxygenase enzyme system. Although many compounds can affect their own biological disposition, the majority of compounds, including barbiturates, having an action on the nervous system demonstrate *cellular* or *pharmacodynamic* tolerance. This change in receptor responsiveness is best illustrated by tolerance developed to the analgesic and euphoric actions of morphine. The biochemical changes mediating pharmacodynamic tolerance are not well understood.

Tachyphylaxis is the term used to describe a rapid decrease in responsiveness to repeated drug administration. Cellular tolerance or receptor hyporeactivity can explain tachyphylaxis to certain drugs such as nitroglycerin. However, tachyphylaxis can also be produced by depletion of physiological substances that mediate the drug response. In this instance the drug releases an endogenous substance that mediates the pharmacological action. Tachyphylaxis to ephedrine-induced bronchial relaxation and morphine-induced vasodilation is probably caused by depletion of endogenous norepinephrine and histamine, respectively.

ASSESSMENT OF DRUG TOXICITY

No drug is completely safe. For every drug there is a dose that is toxic; thus, the physician must assess the relative risk for each patient undergoing pharmacological treatment. Each drug has at least two frequency or dose-response curves: one for the therapeutic and one for the toxic and/or lethal effects. The safety of the drug depends upon the difference in doses producing therapeutic and toxic responses. The therapeutic index is an expression of the margin of drug safety and is expressed as the ratio of the median lethal dose (LD_{50}) to the median therapeutic dose (ED_{50}). These values are calculated from quantal dose-response curves obtained by plotting number or percent of animals responding against increasing dose (Fig. 3-7). This is contrasted with the typical dose-response curve illustrating graded responses produced by increases in drug concentration. The graded dose-response can be regarded as the frequency distribution of the number of individual units responding. The relationship of the log dose-response curve (quantal or graded response) with the Gaussian frequency distribution is illustrated in Fig. 3-8. A ratio of $LD_{50}/ED_{50} = 2$ tells us that two times more drug is necessary to kill 50% of the animals than is necessary to provide the therapeutic benefit in 50%. Another way of expressing the margin of safety for a drug is the ratio LD_1/ED_{99}. This ratio is an approximation of the relationship between the therapeutic dose effective in nearly all of the animal population with a lethal or toxic effect in virtually none. This expression of relative safety in animals may be a more realistic comparison since it is closer to the goals of the physician (e.g., therapeutic action with minimal side effects). In human subjects limiting side effects are evaluated instead of lethality. Another advantage to the LD_1/ED_{99} ratio is apparent when the slopes of the dose-response curves for efficacy and toxicity differ.

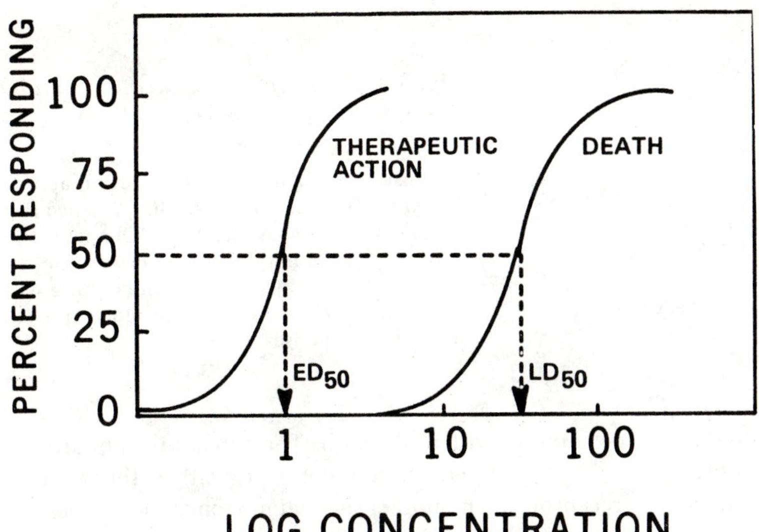

Fig. 3-7. *Quantal log dose-response curves.*
The curves represent the cumulative number of animals responding to either the therapeutic of lethal actions of a drug. The median effective dose (ED_{50}) is the amount of a drug producing a therapeutic response in 50% of the population. The median lethal dose (LD_{50}) is the dose resulting in death in 50% of the animals.

If the drug toxicity is an extension of the therapeutic effect, the slopes for both will be similar (Fig. 3-7). However, if these two actions of the drug are produced by different mechanisms, the slopes would be dissimilar. Collectively, the therapeutic indices and the slopes of the dose-response curves provide a relative assessment of the margin of safety.

DRUG ANTAGONISM

Chemical-Physiological Antagonism. Administration of one drug can quantitatively or qualitatively affect the drug-receptor interaction or pharmacological effects of another drug. Conceptually, one drug can modify the action of other drugs at a variety of sites. Figure 3-9 illustrates three types of antagonism that can occur in biological systems: chemical, pharmacological and physiological. Clinical and pharmacological antagonism involve an interaction of an agonist and an antagonist. Chemical antagonism occurs in independent of a biological receptor. For example, pencillamine chelates mercury to remove the toxic metal from interaction with body proteins and enzyme systems. Physiological antagonism occurs by the action of two agonists producing opposite effects on a physiological system. For example, norepinephrine contracts vascular smooth muscle to increase blood pressure, whereas histamine produces vasodilation that decreases blood pressure.

Pharmacological Antagonism. An agonist is a drug that has both affinity for the receptor and efficacy. The result of the agonist-receptor interaction is a drug effect or response. Antagonists are drugs that have affinity for

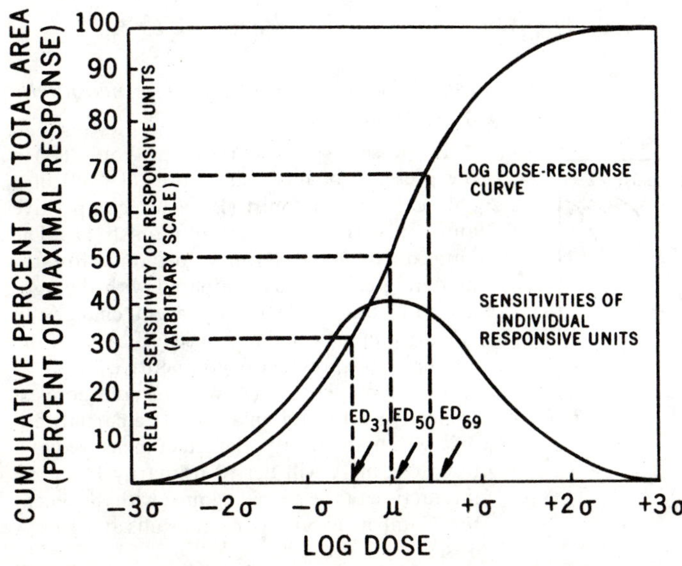

Fig. 3-8. The relationship between a log dose-response curve and a normal frequency distribution (Gaussian) curve.

The "X" axis shows the log dose of the drug where μ (mean) is the dose producing 50% of the maximal response. The standard deviation from this dose is shown at + or - σ. The log dose-response curve is plotted as a function of either the percent maximal response, the cumulative percent of the total area under the Guassian curve, or as the *relative* sensitivity of responsive units on the "Y" axis. The log dose-response curve can be visualized as the summation of responding units from most sensitive (low doses) to least sensitive (high doses). The sensitivities of these individual responsive units are distributed normally, as illustrated by the superimposed Gaussian curve. Since 38% of the total area of the normal curve lies within $\mu + \sigma/2$ (19% on either side), the log dose-response relationship between ED_{31}, ED_{50}, and ED_{69} can be readily estimated. Compare with Figs. 3-3 and 3-4. (From Goldstein, A. *Biostatistics*, 1964, with permission of Macmillan).

AGONIST [A] + RECEPTOR [R] ⇄ AGONIST–RECEPTOR COMPLEX [A][R] → AGONIST EFFECTS

CHEMICAL ANTAGONISM

[A] + ANTAGONIST [B] + [R] ⇄ [A][B] + [R] → NO AGONIST EFFECT

PHARMACOLOGICAL ANTAGONISM

[A] + ANTAGONIST [C] + [R] ⇄ [A] + [C][R] → NO AGONIST EFFECT

PHYSIOLOGICAL ANTAGONISM

[A] + [R] ⇄ [A][R] → AGONIST EFFECT →
AGONIST [X] + $[R_2]$ → $[X][R_2]$ → AGONIST EFFECT
} NO AGONIST EFFECT

Fig. 3-9. *Chemical, pharmacological, and physiological antagonism results in inhibition of agonist effect.*

Illustration of the interaction of an agonist (A) with its receptor (R) in the presence of a chemical (B) or pharmacologic (C) antagonist. Physiological antagonism describes the *net effect* of two agonists (A, X) interacting with different receptors (R, R_2) to produce opposite biological responses.

the receptor but are incapable of producing the biological response; they lack efficacy. Antagonists can interact directly at the same receptor site as the agonist, or affect other reactions necessary for the drug response (Fig. 3-2). If the inhibitory action of an antagonist can be overcome by increasing the concentration of agonist, thereby achieving the same maximal response, the inhibition is termed *competitive*. A competitive antagonist can: (a) reversibly bind to the same receptor site as the agonist, or (b) reversibly or irreversibly bind at a remote receptor site that influences the affinity of the agonist for its receptor. Allosteric modulation of drug-receptor interactions may occur as described for enzyme-substrate regulation. Since the maximal response of the agonist is attainable in the presence of competitive antagonist, the dose-response curve remains parallel but is shifted to the right. This illustrates the decrease in affinity of the agonist for the receptor (Fig. 3-10).

Noncompetitive pharmacological antagonism results when the effects of the antagonist *cannot* be overcome by increasing the concentration of agonist. The affinity of the agonist for the receptor is unchanged but the maximal response (efficacy) is reduced (Fig. 3-10). The noncompetitive antagonist decreases the capacity of the agonist to combine with its receptor. This can occur by binding of the noncompetitive antagonist to either the agonist-receptor site or another site that influences the *capacity* of agonist that combines to its receptor. The agonist can interact with the receptors uninfluenced by the antagonist in a normal manner (similar K_D).

Partial agonists are compounds with affinity but with low or moderate efficacy. A partial agonist with high affinity can competitively inhibit the action of full agonists. Partial agonists thus have both agonist and antagonist properties. The effects of partial agonists, competitive antagonists, and noncompetitive antagonists on the dose-response curve of an agonist are illustrated in Fig. 3-10.

Pharmacological antagonism can be illustrated by applying the Lineweaver-Burk plot used in enzyme kinetics to drug-receptor interactions. Lineweaver and Burk (24) linearly transformed the Michaelis-Menten equation for a more convenient and precise evaluation of enzyme-substrate kinetics. The log dose-response curve is derived mathematically by equations similar to Michaelis-Menten quantification of the enzyme-substrate reaction. For agonist A equation (8) becomes

$$E = \frac{E_{max}[A]}{K_A + [A]} \qquad (17)$$

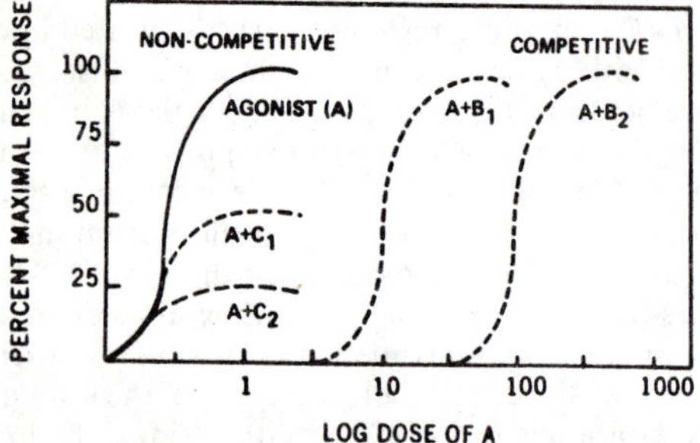

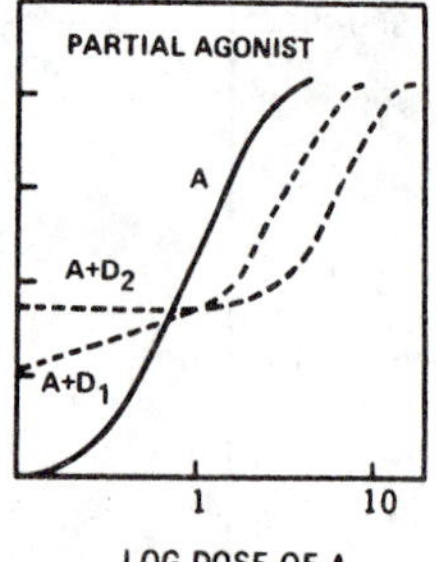

Fig. 3-10. *Competitive and noncompetitive antagonism.*

Log dose-response curve of an agonist (A) in the presence of increasing doses ($1 < 2$) of a competitive antagonist (B), a noncompetitive antagonist (C), or a partial agonist (D). The antagonists have affinity but only low-to-moderate efficacy, as compared with the agonist. Illustrated are the apparent changes in affinity and maximal response (efficacy) of the agonist in the presence of competitive ($A + B_{1+2}$) and noncompetitive ($A + C_{1+2}$) antagonists, respectively. In combination with a partial agonist with high affinity, the effect measured at a low dose of A will derive primarily from the interaction of the partial agonist with the receptor. Competitive antagonism results at higher A doses.

where [A] is the agonist concentration and K_A is the equilibrium-dissociation constant for the agonist (A).

This equation for the dose-response curve can be transformed to linear form by taking the reciprocal of each side of the equation according to Lineweaver and Burk.

$$\frac{1}{E} = \frac{K_A + [A]}{E_{max}[A]} + \frac{1}{E_{max}} = \frac{K_A}{E_{max}} \bullet \frac{1}{[A]} + \frac{1}{E_{max}} \qquad (18)$$

Plotting this equation with 1/E on the ordinate and 1/A on the abscissa results in a straight line, as illustrated in Fig. 3-11. Effects of the competitive (B) and noncompetitive (C) antagonists on the log dose-response curve of agonist A (Fig. 3-11) are linearly transformed in Fig. 3-12. This form of the dose-response curve illustrates the major kinetic differences of competitive (increase $1/K_A$; no change E_{max}) and noncompetitive (no change $1/K_A$; decrease E_{max}) antagonism.

Another useful linear transformation of the Michaelis-Menten equation is the Eadie-Hofstee plot (11, 18). By multiplying both sides of equation (18) by E_{max}, the following equation is obtained:

$$E = -K_A \left(\frac{E}{[A]}\right) + E_{max} \qquad (19)$$

Competitive and noncompetitive inhibition are illustrated by plotting E on the ordinate and E/[A] on the abscissa, according to the Eadie-Hofstee equation (Fig. 3-13). Both the Lineweaver-Burk and Eadie-Hofstee plots allow affinity ($1/K_A$) and maximal efficacy (E_{max}) to be conveniently obtained. However, the Eadie-Hofstee plot is more reliable and will magnify deviations from linearity in the experimental data (10). In contrast, the Lineweaver-Burk (24) transformation minimizes differences between experimentally obtained and theoretically predicted linear points.

TIME-RESPONSE RELATIONSHIP

Drug response is a function of time as well as of dose. The relationship between time and drug response is influenced by dose, route of administration, and pharmacokinetic and pharmacodynamic processes. Following a single dose of drug, time influences all pharmacokinetic and pharmacodynamic processes illustrated in Fig. 3-14 resulting in a drug effect. The time-action curve is obtained by plotting the magnitude of drug response (ordinate) measured at various times after drug administration (abscissa). The following terms are used to express the time course of drug action: *Latency* is the time interval between drug administration and onset of drug action; *duration of action* is the time interval during which a drug response can be measured; and *time of peak response* describes the time at which the maximal drug effect occurs. These basic concepts of time-action are influenced primarily by drug dose and rates of absorption, distribution, bio-transformation, and excretion processes that influence the time at which (a) an adequate drug concentration can be reached at the receptor site, or (b) the least responsive cell can be stimulated. Since latency and duration are defined at the minimal measurable response, the time-action relationship reflects not only pharmacokinetic and pharmacodynamic processes, but limitations of the methods used to evaluate drug action.

Figure 3-14 illustrates these characteristics of the time-action response and how they change with increasing dose. As dosage increases, the latency is shortened and the duration of action is prolonged. The time of peak effect, however, is relatively similar at different doses. As discussed in Chapter 2, the plasma drug concentration correlates with the magnitude of responses in many instances and plasma levels often reflect the concentration of the drug available for receptor interaction. The concentration of the drug in the plasma can then be correlated with the amplitude of drug effect to study the time course of drug action.

MISCELLANEOUS PHARMACODYNAMIC PRINCIPLES

NONSPECIFIC DRUGS: FERGUSON'S PRINCIPLE

Some drugs exert biological effects without involving a chemical reaction. These are almost always depressant and/or toxic actions. Anesthetics are a classic example. Overton and Meyer independently noted that diverse

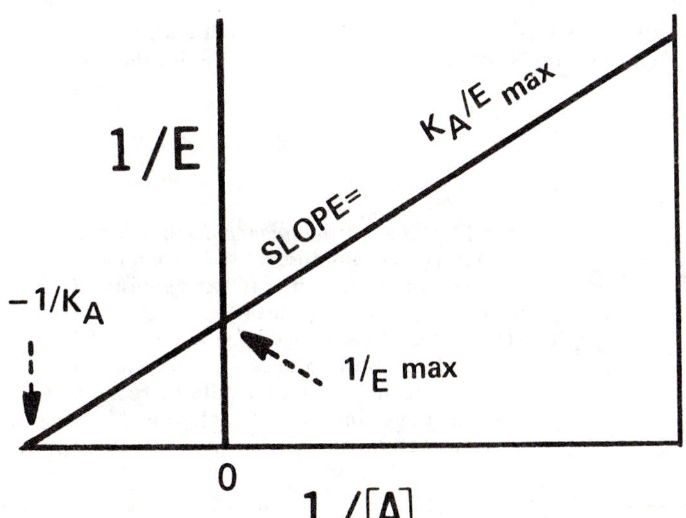

Fig. 3-11. *Lineweaver-Burk linear plot of the dose-response curve.*

The reciprocal of drug effect (1) is expressed as a function of the reciprocal of agonist concentration (1/[C]). The following kinetic parameters can be easily obtained from the line: $1/E_{max}$ at the y intercept, $-1/K_A$ at the x intercept, and K_A/E_{max} is the slope.

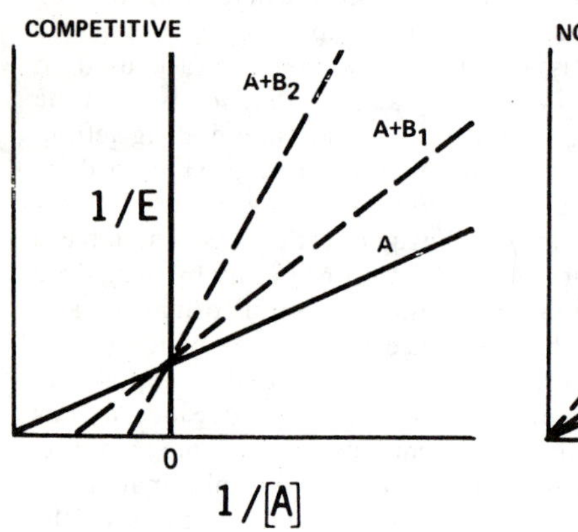

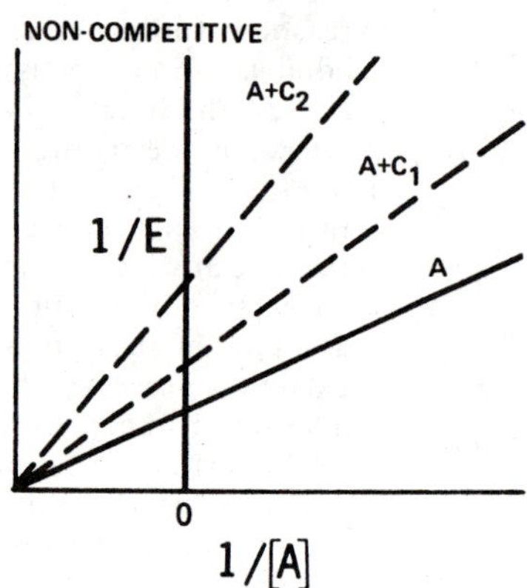

Fig. 3-12. *Lineweaver-Burk linear plots* illustrating the effects of various doses ($1 < 2$) of competitive (B) and noncompetitive (C) antagonists on the dose-response of an agonist (A).

The apparent decrease in the affinity of A ($1/K_A$, x intercept) during competitive inhibition (A vs. A + B_1 or B_2) and the decrease in maximal response (E_{max}, y intercept) associated with noncompetitive antagonism (A vs. A + C_1 or C_2) are illustrated. The log dose-response curves for these linear plots are illustrated in Fig. 3-10.

chemicals capable of producing anesthesia could be ranked on the basis of their lipid/water partition coefficient; increasing lipid solubility increased the depressant action of the drug. Ferguson considered this physical phenomenon (lipid solubility), correlating drug action with a thermodynamic principle, chemical potential (CP), as follows:

$$CP = RT \ln \frac{C}{Cs} \qquad (20)$$

where R is the gas constant, T the absolute temperature, and C/Cs the ratio of actual concentration over the maximum possible concentration of the substance of interest (see Ref. 2 for review). The expression can be constructed for *ideal* gases or solutions.

C/Cs, the *relative saturation,* is of importance, since at equilibrium, CP is the same in all phases. Thus, if C/Cs is known in plasma, it must be the same at unknown cells or parts of cells where the biological action occurs. Many examples of Ferguson's principle (dependence of drug action on chemical potential) illustrate its significance. Multiple volatile substances of diverse structure produce anesthesia at inspired concentrations differing by 200-fold. Comparison of the CP of these substances showed only a seven-fold variability. Another common example of depression is the nitrogen narcosis encountered by divers. The increased solubility of nitrogen in blood under pressure (increased CP) clouds the sensorium and impedes rational thinking. Substituting the lighter helium for nitrogen reduces the CP, enabling divers to think more clearly at greater depths. A further example illustrates the use of this principle in toxicology. Organic solvents kill wireworms at air concentrations varying 4000-fold. Variability was only ninefold when CP was compared (2). CP of these chemicals approximated 0.5 (50% relative saturation in air). The CP for ammonia in the test system was 0.00009; it killed the worms at a CP far less than other chemicals. It is clear that ammonia lethality was related to factors other than its nonspecific presence (CP) alone. Screening new chemicals for toxicity in such systems quickly determines if their relative risk

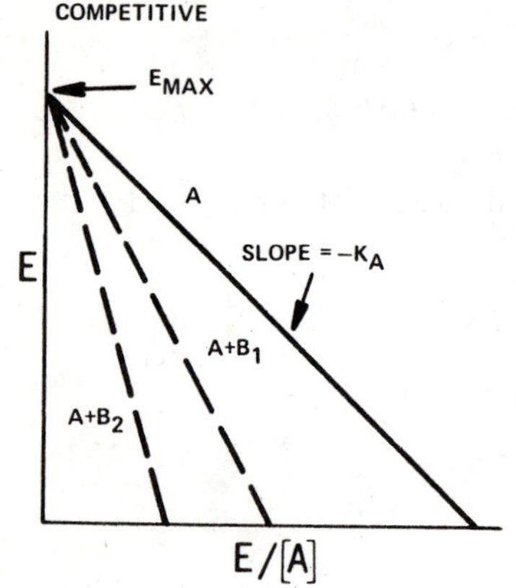

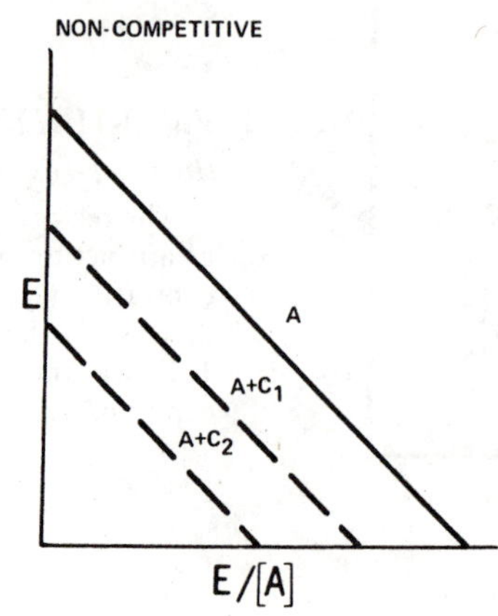

Fig. 3-13. *Eadie-Hofstee linear plots* illustrating the effects of various doses ($1 < 2$) of competitive (B) and noncompetitive (C) antagonists on the dose-response of agonist (A).

Drug effect (E) is plotted as a function of the ratio of drug effect to agonist concentration (E/[A]). The maximal drug effect (E_{max}) is obtained at the y intercept. The slope is $-K_A$.

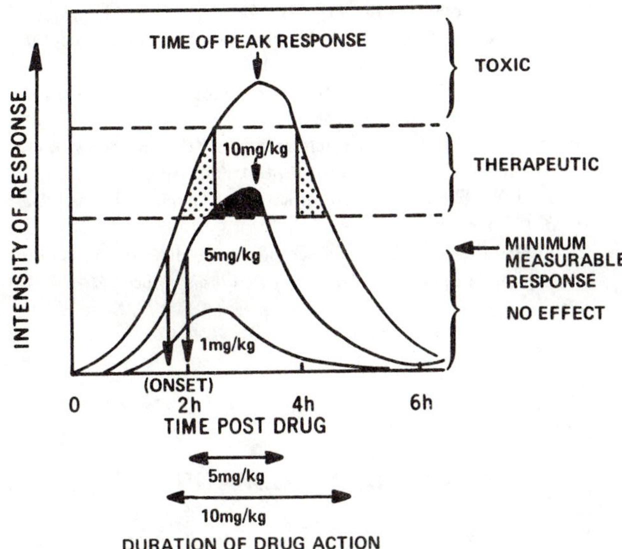

Fig. 3-14. *The time-response curve* illustrates the intensity of drug effect as a function of time.

Drug response intensity ranges from no effect to toxic actions. Various doses (1, 5, 10 mg) of the same drug were administered at time zero. The time interval from drug administration to the first measurable drug response defines onset or latency. The time required to obtain the maximal effect identifies the time of peak response (↓). Duration of drug action (←→) defines the time interval during which the drug produces a measurable response. Shaded areas indicate the duration of therapeutic effects after 5 to 10 mg doses. Note the minimal measurable response is not therapeutic in this instance.

is structurally nonspecific (CP = 0.5) or very great (like ammonia, 0.00009). The residual response variability of the CP may be due to one or more of the following: (a) the drug-biological system deviates from the ideal gas or solution; (b) the biological system is not in equilibrium; (c) a particular drug may have some degree of specific activity as well as sufficient CP for effects. The mechanisms of drugs acting according to Ferguson's principle are undefined. It may be a swelling of cell membranes resulting in uncoupling of enzyme activities, altered ion transport mechanisms, or other nonspecific phenomena.

ENDOGENOUS SUBSTANCES AS DRUGS

Various *endogenous* substances are administered *exogenously* as drugs. Hormones are one example. They are given as replacements or supplements when underproduced or underutilized by the body. It is noteworthy that when endogenous hormones are administered as drugs, their actions are not initiated or regulated by physiological mechanisms, such as insulin release by postprandial hyperglycemia. Therefore, clear rationale is needed to ensure that administration at an arbitrary time is warranted. Even though such substances are endogenous and act on endogenous receptors, exogenous administration only approximates the dose-response and time-action parameters that occur physiologically. Many insulin preparations exist with different dose-response and time-action characteristics. These cannot reproduce the degree of control of blood glucose achieved by normal pancreatic function. Insulin replacement controls diabetes; it is not a cure. Hormones given orally are subject to pharmacokinetic phenomena never encountered endogenously. Thus, orally administered thyroid hormone or cortisone is subject to the variables governing absorption, whereas endogenous hormones secreted into the bloodstream are not subject to these influences.

BIOLOGICAL TESTING

Advances in analytical chemistry have occurred at a rapid rate. Drugs are analyzed by sophisticated techniques such as high-pressure liquid chromatography, mass spectrometry plus gas chromatography, nuclear magnetic resonance, etc. It is perhaps worthwhile to emphasize that chemical analysis is an indirect assessment of drug activity since the intent of therapy is to achieve a biological result. Biological testing is still required in many instances. A partial list of biological tests includes the following: (a) proof of sterility and absence of pyrogens; (b) determination of biologically active isomeric products when chemical analysis cannot distinguish enantiomers (one lot of drug may differ from another); (c) biological testing of natural materials when drug products are not purified to homogeneity such as thyroid extract, vitamin D, etc; (d) identification of biological activity of complex molecules where slight changes in structure destroys drug activity. For example, many polypeptide hormones are routinely radioimmunoassayed but are easily inactivated. Therefore, cross-reactivity of antibody with inactive peptide fragments can invalidate radioimmunoassay methods used to assay active hormones. Thus, careful observation of biological response remains most important.

REFERENCES

1. Ahlquist, R. P. A study of the adrenotropic receptors. *Am. J. Physiol.* 153:586, 1948.
2. Albert, A. Biological activity unrelated to structure: Ferguson's principle. In: *Selective Toxicity*, 4th ed. London: Methuen & Co., 1968.
3. Ariens, E. J. Affinity and intrinsic activity in the theory of competitive inhibition. Part I. *Arch. Int. Pharmacodyn. Ther.* 99:32, 1954.
4. Behrans, B. Zur Auswertung der Digitalisblatter. *Arch. Exp. Pathol. Pharmak.* 140:237, 1929.
5. Biggio, G., and Costa, E. (eds.). *Benzodiazepine Recognition Site Ligands: Biochemistry and Pharmacology*. New York: Raven Press, 1983.

6. Burn, J. H. *Biological Standardization.* New York: Oxford University Press, 1950.
7. Clark, A. J. *The Mode of Action of Drugs on Cells.* London: Arnold, 1933.
8. Clark, A. J. *The Mode of Action of Drugs on Cells.* Baltimore: Williams and Wilkins, 1937.
9. Creese, I., Sibley, D. R., Hamblin, M. W., and Leff, S. E. The classification of dopamine receptors: Relationship to radioligand binding. *Ann. Rev. Neurosci.* 6:43, 1983.
10. Dowd, J. E., and Riggs, D. S. Comparison of estimates of Michaelis-Menten kinetic constants from various linear transformations. *J. Biol. Chem.* 240:863, 1965.
11. Eadie, G. S. The inhibition of cholinesterase by physostigmine and prostigmine. *J. Biol. Chem.* 146:85, 1942.
12. Ehrlich, P., and Hata, S. *Die Experimentelle Chemotherapie der Spirillosen.* Berlin: Springer-Verlag, 1910.
13. Furchgott, R. F. Pharmacological characterization of receptors: Its relation to radioligand-binding studies. *Fed. Proc.* 37:115, 1978.
14. Furchgott, R. F. Receptor mechanism. *Ann. Rev. Pharmacol.* 4:21, 1964.
15. Gaddum, J. H. The quantitative effects of antagonistic drugs. *J. Physiol.* (Lond.) 89:7P, 1937.
16. Goldstein, A., Aronow, L., and Kalman, S. M. *Principles of Drug Action: The Basis of Pharmacology.* New York: Wiley, 1974.
17. Haldane, J. B. S. *Enzymes.* London: Longmans, Green, 1930.
18. Hofstee, B. H. J. Graphical analysis of single enzyme systems. *Enzymologia* 17:273, 1956.
19. Höllt, V., and Herz, A. In vivo receptor occupation by opiates and correlation to the pharmacological effect. *Fed. Proc.* 37:158, 1978.
20. Hunt, S. P., and Schmidt, J. The electron microscopic autoradiographic localization of α-bungarotoxin binding sites within the central nervous system of the rat. Brain Res. 142:152, 1978.
21. Langmuir, I. The adsorption of gases on plane surfaces of glass, mica and platinum. *J. Am. Chem. Soc.* 40:1361, 1918.
22. Lefkowitz, R. J., and Hoffman, B. B. New directions in adrenergic receptor research (Part 1). *Trends Pharmacol. Sci.* 1:314, 1980.
23. Lefkowitz, R. J., and Hoffman, B. B. New directions in adrenergic receptor research (Part 2). *Trends Pharmacol. Sci.* 1:369, 1980.
24. Lineweaver, H., and Burk, D. The determination of enzyme dissociation constants. *J. Am. Chem. Soc.* 56:658, 1934.
25. Loewi, O. Uber humorale ubertragbarkeit der Herznervenwirkung. *Pfluger's Arch.* 189:239, 1921.
26. MacKay, D. The mathematics of drug-receptor interactions. *J. Pharm. Pharmacol.* 18:201, 1966.
27. Michaelis, L., and Menten, M. L. Die Kinetik der Invertinwirkung. *Biochem. Z.* 49:333, 1913.
28. Mohler, H., and Okada, T. Biochemical identification of the site of action of benzodiazepines in human brain by ^{3}H diazepam binding. *Life Sci.* 22:985, 1978.
29. Nickerson, M. Nonequilibrium drug antagonism. *Pharmacol. Rev.* 9:246, 1957.
30. Paton, W. D. M. Theory of drug action based on the rate of drug-receptor combination. *Proc. R. Soc. Ser. B.* 154:21, 1961.
31. Simon, E. J., and Miller, J. M. *In vitro* studies on opiate receptors and their ligands. *Fed. Proc.* 37:141, 1978.
32. Stephenson, R. P. A modification of receptor theory. *Br. J. Pharmacol. Chemother.* 11:379, 1956.
33. Tallarida, R. J. The use of drug-receptor affinity measures in the differentiation of receptors. *Fed. Proc.* 41:2323, 1982.
34. Trevan, J. W. The error of determination of toxicity. *Proc. R. Soc. Ser. B.* 101:483, 1927.
35. van Wijngaarden C. deL. Untersuchungen uber die Wirkungsstarke von Digitalispreparaten. *Arch. Exp. Pathol. Pharmak.* 113:40, 1926.

ADDITIONAL READING

Textbook References

1. Albert, A. *Selective Toxicity,* 4th ed. London: Methuen & Co., 1968.
2. Ariens, E. J. (ed.). *Molecular Pharmacology.* New York: Academic Press, 1964.
3. Bacq, Z. M. (ed.). *Fundamentals of Biochemical Pharmacology.* New York: Pergamon Press, 1971.
4. Goldstein, A. *Biostatistics.* New York: Macmillan, 1964.
5. Levine, R. R. *Pharmacology: Drug Actions and Reactions,* 2nd ed. Boston: Little, Brown, 1978.
6. Tallarida, R. J., and Jacobs, L. S. *Dose Response Relation in Pharmacology.* New York: Springer-Verlag, 1979.

Monographs and Reviews

1. Furchgott, R. F. Receptors: Introduction to symposium. *Fed. Proc.* 37:113, 1978.
2. MacKay, D. The mathematics of drug-receptor interactions. *J. Pharm. Pharmacol.* 18:201, 1966.
3. Paton, W. D. M. The theory of drug action based on the rate of drug-receptor combination. *Proc. R. Soc. Ser. B* 154:21, 1961.
4. Roth, J., and Taylor, S. Receptors for peptide hormones: Alterations in diseases of humans. *Ann. Rev. Physiol.* 44:639, 1982.
5. Seeman, P. Brain dopamine receptors. *Pharmacol. Rev.* 32:229, 1980.
6. Symposium. Neurotransmitter release, receptor regulation and drug interactions. *Fed. Proc.* 40:135, 1980.

CHAPTER
4

BASIC PRINCIPLES OF TOXICITY AND TOXICOLOGY

Gabriel L. Plaa

Toxicology, in its broadest sense, is the scientific discipline concerned with the injurious effects of chemical and physical agents on living systems. It is both a qualitative and a quantitative discipline. The qualitative phase includes the description of the effect, the mechanism(s) of action, the pathogenesis of the response, and the sequelae; the quantitative phase deals with the amounts of agent needed in the biosphere to elicit the effect. The qualitative phase describes the end result of the exposure; the quantitative phase defines the limits of the exposure that lead to such a result. Both aspects are essential in the safety evaluation process — the process by which one determines the safe use of chemical substances by society. It is the quantitative component, however, that permits the establishment of use patterns that will avoid the emergence of an undesirable response. Quantitative considerations are also essential for a better comprehension of the nature of the toxic response.

In the context of this chapter, the scope of the discipline called toxicology will be restricted. The living system of concern will be humans, and only chemical agents will be considered. Furthermore, the term *drug* will be employed only when reference is made to a chemical substance used as a therapeutic agent. Obviously, to understand, predict, prevent, or treat toxic effects of chemical agents in humans, the results of toxicological studies performed in animals are utilized.

The basic principles of toxicology are well described in the works authored by Boyd (4), Doull et al. (9), Hayes (16), Loomis (21), and Zbinden (33, 34). The reader is encouraged to consult these texts for more detailed presentations.

NATURE OF THE TOXIC RESPONSE

ACUTE VERSUS CHRONIC TOXICITY

Toxic effects can be divided into two categories: (1) effects that occur very quickly after a brief exposure to a chemical agent and (2) those that appear only after repetitive exposure to the substance. By tradition, the former are referred to as *acute* and the latter as *chronic* toxic properties. An acute toxic effect is usually one that is observed within the first several days after exposure to the agent. In most instances, all of these reactions are usually discernible within 1-2 weeks after administration. On the other hand, the chronic toxic properties of a substance may not be demonstrable until several months of continuous repetitive exposure.

It is important to realize that the qualitative nature of the toxic reaction may be different depending upon the duration of the exposure. A drug reaction that demonstrates this difference is that associated with chloramphenicol. In the human neonate, the acute drug reaction (grey syndrome) is characterized by cardiovascular collapse, coma and cyanosis. The chronic toxic effects of chloramphenicol, however, are on the bone marrow, resulting in agranulocytosis or aplastic anemia. A similar type of qualitative difference in toxicity profile is seen following exposure to benzene by inhalation. The primary acute toxic manifestation of exposure to this chemical is central nervous system depression. When individuals are exposed repetitively to benzene vapors, however, the dosages may be insufficient to produce central nervous system depression but sufficient to cause bone marrow damage, resulting in aplastic anemia.

LOCAL VERSUS SYSTEMIC TOXICITY

Chemical substances can produce toxic effects at their site of application (*local* toxicity) or after they are absorbed into the circulatory system and distributed to other target organs (*systemic* toxicity). Examples of local toxic reactions include the caustic corrosive effects of strong alkalies, and acids, particularly in the oral cavity and in the esophagus. The gastric irritation caused by salicylates is a manifestation of a local response. On the other hand, the metabolic acid-base imbalance associated with acute salicylate intoxication is a systemic manifestation associated with the effects of salicylates on the central nervous system, pulmonary function, and metabolism. Local toxic effects at the site of injection can be produced by the intravenous administration of thiopental, an ultrashort-acting barbiturate; extravasation of the thiopental solution can result in local vasoconstriction and tissue damage at the site of injection. Respiratory arrest after this drug, however, is a systemic effect. Sulfobromophthalein, when administered intravenously to assess hepatic excretory function, can cause local tissue damage and a necrotizing lesion due to extravasation of this substance. The systemic toxicity of this diagnostic agent, however, is virtually nonexistent at the dosages employed, with the exception of those individuals who are allergic to the agent.

REVERSIBLE VERSUS IRREVERSIBLE TOXICITY

The relative reversibility of a toxic effect depends upon the recuperative properties of the organ affected. An example of this is the hepatic damage produced by ethanol (35). Frequent and repetitive ingestion of intoxicating doses of ethanol over a period of weeks can lead to the development of a fatty liver that is reversible shortly after cessation of the ingestion. Continued exposure to excessive amounts of ethanol for a longer period of time (months or years) can result in alcoholic hepatitis; this lesion is also reversible. The prolonged administration (years) of excessive amounts of ethanol, however, can lead to the production of hepatic fibrosis and the development of cirrhosis. Unfortunately, this lesion is not reversible, although its evolution can be modified upon discontinuation of ethanol ingestion.

DELAYED TOXICITY

Some reactions associated with the chronic administration of drugs take some time to appear. In these situations, the individual is often still being exposed to the agent when the toxicity is manifested. There are other situations in which chemical exposure or drug treatment may actually have ceased, yet sufficient injury has occurred so that the toxic signs do not become evident for some time after termination of the exposure. The delayed neurotoxicity, leading to paralysis, that is associated with triorthocresyl phosphate (TOCP) intoxication is one such example. Mass outbreaks of human poisoning with TOCP have occurred due to the contamination of cooking oils with lubricating oil containing TOCP. The lung fibrosis characteristic of chronic inhalation of asbestos dust or silica dust in certain occupational environments is another example of delayed toxicity. This kind of time-exposure pattern is also observed with chemically induced carcinogenesis. The organism is exposed for a given period of time to the noxious substance, the exposure is terminated, yet at some later date, the production of the neoplasm evolves from the chemical exposure. Such reactions can be observed with laboratory animals under controlled experimental conditions.

Recently, a delayed carcinogenic reaction (hepatic angiosarcoma) has been observed in humans exposed to vinyl chloride in the occupational environment. Furthermore, the therapeutic use of diethylstilbestrol (DES) to maintain pregnancy has been shown to produce vaginal neoplasms in the female progeny of the treated mothers. DES did not affect the mothers, but exposure of the fetus *in utero* was sufficient to produce the neoplasms in the daughters many years later. The phenomenon of delayed toxicity can complicate risk assessment because it may be extremely difficult to establish a cause-and-effect relationship.

ALLERGIC REACTIONS

Immunological reactions to drugs have been established as being responsible for certain adverse effects in humans (2, 21, 23). The drug (or a metabolite) is antigenic or acts as a haptene to stimulate antibody production; the antibody-haptene conjugate or antibody-antigen interaction occurs in a setting leading to tissue injury; an inflammatory process then proceeds and expresses the reaction. In humans, sensitization reactions of this type appear to account for only about 6 - 10% of all drug reactions, and relatively few drugs cause such reactions (23). There has been some discussion among toxicologists as to whether the allergic type of reaction described should be classified as a true toxic reaction (9). Others (4, 9, 16, 21) accept immunological reactions as a part of the toxicity profile of a chemical agent but point out that the response depends upon the host's reaction to the chemical.

TOXICITY VERSUS HAZARD

A distinction must be made between the toxic potential of a chemical substance and its eventual importance when the agent is employed. This is the distinction between *toxicity* and *hazard.* All chemical substances possess toxic properties. When compared quantitatively, some substances are essentially nontoxic because extremely large doses or exposures are required to produce toxic effects; other substances cause toxic reactions when present in very minimal quantities. As first expressed by Paracelsus (16), all chemicals are potentially toxic, depending upon the dose. In the case of hazard, however, one must consider the amount of the chemical the individual is exposed to in a specific environmental setting (therapeutic, occupational, and so on) and the manner in which the chemical is to be utilized. Potentially lethal substances can be used safely (without hazard) in the occupational environment, provided the environment is controlled to prevent ingestion or absorption of sufficient quantities of the material to produce toxicity. In such a situation, although the chemical in question is potentially toxic, it is not hazardous in the manner in which it is being used. *Hazard* has the important component of *use* incorporated in its definition.

With pharmaceutical agents, the difference between the amount of the drug needed to exert its desired biological effect and the amount that produces toxic effects can vary from one drug to another. This margin provides some idea of the relative hazard involved in the use of a particular drug. Thus, the physician is interested in the pattern of use of a drug as well as its toxic properties. He must know whether the toxic effects of the drug occur at dosages that far exceed the therapeutic range, or whether they occur at dosages that are relatively near to those employed therapeutically.

ADVERSE DRUG REACTIONS

Drugs can often produce a number of different effects depending on their pharmacological properties. Several of these may occur in the same patient when the drug is administered in the dosage range normally recommended to obtain the desired therapeutic action. The other effects (the unwanted effects) are commonly termed *side effects.* This term can be confusing, since the classification depends upon the therapeutic indication. For example, several antihistaminic agents possess sedative properties in addition to their major property of blocking the effects of histamine. When these drugs are used in the treatment of allergies, the desired therapeutic action is the antihistaminic response, and the drowsiness that may also occur is called a side effect. Some of these antihistaminic agents, however, can be employed therapeutically to produce sedation; in this instance, sedation is not considered a side effect, because it is the desired therapeutic response. The term side effect should be used when describing an undesirable pharmacological action that accompanies the therapeutic action being sought. An unwanted side effect may be troublesome to the patient (an untoward effect), but this is not always the case.

When the unwanted effect is clearly detrimental (an adverse effect), it seems much more appropriate to call the response an *adverse drug reaction.* Karch and Lasagna (19) defined an adverse drug reaction as one that is noxious and unintended and that occurs at dosages of a drug used appropriately in humans for prophylaxis, diagnosis, or therapy, excluding therapeutic failures. In the last 15 years, there has been a considerable amount of interest in adverse drug reactions. The problem is discussed more extensively by Davies (8), Avery (2), Melmon and Morelli (23), and by the American Medical Association (1). Unfortunately, many of the reports in the literature suffer from inadequate descriptions of the cause-and-effect relationship between the drug and the reaction reported. The physician interested in establishing whether the adverse reaction is attributable to the drug should verify if the methods employed in the reporting of the reaction are sufficient to determine cause-and-effect relationships as defined in Table 4-1. In most studies, there is a notable lack of data concerning controls. Relatively minor symptoms that have been attributed to some drugs given to patients can occur frequently in other groups of patients who are not taking these drugs (29).

It is difficult to assess, in quantitative terms, the incidence and impact of adverse drug reactions. The following estimates, however, have been calculated by Karch and Lasagna (19): (a) In hospitalized patients on acute medical wards, the incidence ranged from 6 to 15%; (b) in other hospital services, the incidence ranged from 1 to 6%. Studies reported by Davies (8) indicated that the incidence ranged from 1 to 28%, although in most cases the figure was between 10 and 20%. In 1963, Zbinden (32) reported an incidence of adverse reactions in 7.3% of 20,000 patients with therapeutic dosages of over 100 drugs. The precise incidence of such reactions is still unknown.

From the point of view of the toxicologist, it is of interest to determine whether these reactions are of the type that would normally be associated with the known properties of the drugs in question or whether they represent aberrant, undetectable types of responses. In quantitative terms, these data are also imprecise. Estimates derived from the published literature do shed some light on this question. Davies (8) reports that the type of reaction that occurs most frequently is a previously known intended action of the drug; the next most com-

Table 4-1
Cause-and-Effect Relationship for Reporting of Adverse Drug Reactions

Definite	A reaction that follows a reasonable temporal sequence from administration of the drug or in which the drug level has been established in body fluids or tissues; that follows a known response pattern to the suspected drug; and that is confirmed by improvement on stopping the drug (*dechallenge*) and reappearance of the reaction on repeated exposure (*rechallenge*).
Probable	A reaction that follows a reasonable temporal sequence from administration of the drug; that follows a known response pattern to the suspected drug; that is confirmed by dechallenge; and that could not be reasonably explained by the known characteristics of the patient's clinical state.
Possible	A reaction that follows a reasonable temporal sequence from administration of the drug; that follows a known response pattern to the suspected drug; but that could have been produced by the patient's clinical state or other modes of therapy administered to the patient.
Conditional	A reaction that follows a reasonable temporal sequence from administration of the drug; that does not follow a known response pattern to the suspected drug; but that could not be reasonably explained by the known characteristics of the patient's clinical state.
Doubtful	Any reaction that does not meet the criteria above.

Source: From Ref. 19.

mon is an exaggeration of the intended pharmacological action of therapeutic doses of the drug; and the third is an allergic reaction. Several independent studies reported in the literature have found that about 80% of the reactions responsible for patient admissions to the hospital were considered to be due to known pharmacological mechanisms. Less than 20% were allergic in character. In other estimates, sensitization reactions involving an antigen-antibody component seem to account for only 6 to 10% of all drug reactions, and relatively few drugs seem to cause these reactions (23). Less than 5% could be attributed to the so-called *idiosyncratic reaction.* Because unpredictable adverse responses appear to be less than 20 to 30% of the total reported adverse drug reactions, it must be concluded that the remaining 70 to 80% are at least understandable and predictable.

There is a certain amount of confusion in the literature concerning the term idiosyncratic reaction. Some authors tend to define these reactions merely in terms of incidence (4, 23). When the reaction occurs only in a small number of individuals and includes both predictable, but unexpected, pharmacological effects and unusual effects of the drug, they may call the reaction idiosyncratic. Goldstein et al. (12), however, deplore the use of the term *idiosyncrasy* as a catch-all classification for unexpected drug reactions. They point out that the characteristic feature in drug idiosyncrasy is a discontinuity from the ordinary distribution of dosage reactivity and feel that such aberrant responses indicate that the drug reaction has a genetic basis. Therefore, they prefer to define *drug idiosyncrasy* as a genetically determined abnormal reactivity to a drug. Most authors would agree that mere frequency of a reaction should not be the basis for such a classification. Some toxicologists, however, might have reservations about restricting the term drug idiosyncrasy to only those situations in which the reaction is based on genetics. Such a restriction would necessitate the inclusion of another classification, the *unexplained drug reaction,* to refer to those reactions that cannot be accounted for by the known toxic properties of the chemical, or by the immunological response or the genetic makeup of the individual. It is not the purpose here to propose the "correct" definition of drug idiosyncrasy, but rather to point out that unfortunately this term is employed differently by different authors. The reader should be aware of this fact when the term is encountered.

DOSE-RESPONSE RELATIONSHIPS

The quantitative aspects of toxicology are extremely important because they are fundamental to the safety evaluation process. This process determines first of all the qualitative toxicological profile of the substance and then determines how the chemical can be employed safely to prevent injury. In the sixteenth century, Paracelsus first expressed the important principle; dosage alone determines poisoning. This principle is the foundation of the quantitative phase of toxicology. It states that all chemical substances are capable of producing injurious effects in living systems. Whether these injurious effects manifest themselves or not, however, depends upon the amount of the chemical present in the biological system. A dose exists below which the injurious properties will not appear. This is the basis of the dose-response relationship that has become the major tenet of the modern toxicologist. In the field of therapeutics, the dose-response relationship is employed to determine whether the desirable therapeutic properties of the drug can be usefully employed in patients without incurring injurious or undesirable effects.

In the twentieth century, there have been marked efforts in the mathematical derivation of reliable quantitative data that can be used for safety evaluation. Most of these procedures have dealt with the acute toxic properties of chemicals, because these properties are more easily controlled and defined. The various procedures and approaches employed are well described by Hayes (16).

SINGLE-DOSE MEDIAN EFFECTIVE DOSAGE

The *median effective dosage* (ED_{50}) is a statistical estimate of the amount of a chemical that produces a defined effect in 50% of a very large population of the test species under specified conditions. This parameter can be estimated in small groups of animals (about 10 per dosage group). The first group receives the smallest amount possible that will produce the intended effect in only a small proportion of the group, whereas the subsequent groups will receive a series of geometrically increasing amounts such that the last group receives a dosage producing the same effect in most of the animals. When only the number of responders in each group is of interest, the results are expressed as the percentage of animals showing the effect being studied. The response measured is an all-or-none response. The classic example of such an analysis is the determination of the *median lethal dosage* (LD_{50}), where the effect being measured is mortality. The toxicologist is interested not only in the ED_{50} value, but also in the relative accuracy of the estimate. A reflection of the relative accuracy of the estimate can be found when the 95% confidence limits of the ED_{50} obtained is determined. These confidence limits indicate the range within which the universal ED_{50} may be expected to fall in 19 of 20 samples taken at random from the same population.

The slope of the dose-response curve is also of interest to the toxicologist. The slope describes how greatly the response will be modified when the dosage is changed. When a compound is said to exhibit a *shallow* dose-response curve, a large change in dosage is required before a significant change in response will be observed. When a compound exhibits a *steep* dose-response curve, however, a relatively small change in dosage will cause a large change in the response.

With a dose-response curve, values other than the ED_{50} can be estimated; the ED_{10} (the dosage affecting 10% of the population) and the ED_{90} (the dosage affecting 90% of the population) can be calculated, as well as their confidence limits. Mathematically, it can be demonstrated that the range of values encompassed by the confidence limits is narrowest at the midpoint (the ED_{50}) and widest at both extremes (ED_{10} and ED_{90}) of the dose-response curve. This merely means that the ED_{50} may be estimated more accurately than the ED_{10} or the ED_{90}. This is the reason why, for quantitative comparisons, toxicologists usually employ the midpoint of the curve (ED_{50}) rather than the extreme ends of the dose-response line.

MULTIPLE-DOSE MEDIAN EFFECTIVE DOSAGE DETERMINATIONS

The quantitative comparisons already described are used universally to determine acute toxic properties of chemicals. Fewer attempts have been initiated to quantitate toxic responses that are observed after multiple treatments, particularly subchronic or chronic exposures. Two groups of investigators have described procedures in which ED_{50} values could be determined in experiments where multiple treatments were employed. Boyd and Boyd (3) described a method in which the compound under study was administered for 100 days, and Hayes (15) described a procedure where the substance was given for a total of 90 doses. The statistical calculation of a 90-dose ED_{50} is comparable with that used for a single-dose ED_{50}. The dosages in the 90-day test are expressed in milligrams/kilogram/day. The ratio between the single-dose and multiple-dose ED_{50} values (the *chronicity index*) can be useful for assessing the cumulative effects of a chemical (3,4, 15, 16). Theoretically, if no cumulative effect occurs over the 90 doses, the ratio (1-dose ED_{50} /90-dose ED_{50}) would be 1.0.

Hayes (16) has determined the chronicity index of several substances in the rat. Sodium chloride, caffeine and benzylpenicillin yielded values of 1.3 to 1.6, indicating a lack of cumulative effect. However, the values for warfarin (a rodenticide) and mirex (a pesticide) were 20.8 and 60.8, respectively; these agents exhibited marked cumulative effect during the 90-dose exposure because the 90-dose ED_{50} values were much smaller than the 1-dose ED_{50} estimates. The utility of this approach has not been exploited by toxicologists, although it appears to deserve considerably more attention than it has received to date.

TIME RELATIONSHIPS

Time relationships can furnish information of practical utility. A rapid onset of toxic effects following treatment of animals at suitable dosages indicates that the chemical under study is absorbed rapidly and acts quickly, whereas a slow onset suggests that the substance may be absorbed slowly or may require biotransformation before it can exert its action. A delay in the appearance of the response may also suggest that the substance produces some anatomical or biochemical lesion that recovers slowly and is the underlying cause of the response. There are statistical procedures that permit this time relationship to be determined in quantitative terms. The *median time to effect* (ET_{50}) devised by Litchfield (20) is such an approach. In this situation, the dosage is not varied; the animals are treated with a near-maximal dosage, and the frequency of response is noted at predetermined time intervals. Thus, the curve that will be generated from such an analysis will depend upon the dosage employed. In general, a progressive increase in dosage beyond that necessary to affect all animals will cause progressively less and less change in the ED_{50} (16).

ESTIMATION OF EFFECTIVE DOSAGES

In the safety evaluation process, toxicologists are interested in establishing the *no observable effect level* (NOEL). By definition, this is the maximal or near-maximal dosage at which no treatment-related effect will be demonstrated. It is a term normally encountered in studies conducted to determine the long-term effects of chemicals. For drugs, this parameter must be further qualified. By definition, a drug is given to a patient to elicit a desirable biological effect. Consequently, the term *no observable adverse effect* is used when dealing with this class of chemical agents. This defines the dosage that will result in no detectable, injurious effect. There is a great imprecision when one actually attempts to determine the no observable adverse effect level because it is the absence of a response that is being measured. In practice, it is easier to deal with the *lowest observable effect* level rather than with the no observable adverse effect level. The determination of such a level is employed to establish safety factors for the use of potentially toxic chemicals by individuals in a defined environment.

The single-dose LD_{50} obtained in animals is employed for predicting possible lethal responses that might occur acutely in the accidental ingestion of chemicals. This is particularly useful in the case of accidental intoxications resulting from commercial products found in the home or work place (13). Table 4-2 summarizes the classification of test materials based on acute oral LD_{50} values. Some examples of commercial products and drugs are included. These values suggest the urgency that is required in the treatment of such intoxications when they occur. Classifications have also been devised for chemicals that might be absorbed through the skin or by inhalation (11).

LOW-INCIDENCE RESPONSES

Despite all the toxicological information required (tests in animals; phase I, II, and III clinical trials) of a new drug before it is permitted to go on the market, it is possible that new therapeutic agents may exhibit their toxic potential only after they have been given to a very large number of patients. The question arises why animal tests apparently fail to detect such effects and why they are disclosed only after large numbers of human are subjected to drugs. Four explanations are possible: (1) the toxic reaction may be a rare event; (2) the reaction may appear only after a long period of administration; (3) the reaction may manifest itself only in the presence of disease; and, (4) the toxic reaction may be one that is not reproducible in animals and is unique to humans.

An all too natural tendency has been to use the last explanation as the one that covers many of those toxic reactions that

Table 4-2
Classification of Toxic Substances and Probable Human Lethal Dosages After Acute Oral Ingestion

Toxicity Rating	Classification	Probable Human Lethal Dosage (70 kg body weight)	Examples
6	Supertoxic	<5 mg/kg (<7 drops)	Atropine, azides, cardiotonic glycosides, cyanides, digoxin, fluoroacetate, heroin, LSD, morphine, nitroglycerin, nitroprussides, paraoxon, phosphorus, selenates
5	Extremely toxic	5-50 mg/kg (<1 teaspoon)	Amitriptyline, amobarbital, amphetamine, antihistaminics, cocaine, codeine, iodine, meperidine, mercuric chloride, nitrites, pentobarbital
4	Very toxic	50-500 mg/kg (<1 ounce)	Allyl alcohol, aspirin, benzene, boric acid, caffeine, carbon tetrachloride, chlorpromazine, DDT, dichromates, fluorides, methaqualone, oxalates, phenobarbital
3	Moderately toxic	0.5-5 g/kg (<1 pint)	Bromides, chloroform, diazepam, diethyl ether, formalin, gasoline, iron salts, lithium salts, magnesium salts, methanol, nitrates, sodium chloride, sulfites
2	Slightly toxic	5-15 g/kg (<1 quart)	Ethanol, lysol, penicillins, soaps, tetracyclines, witch hazel
1	Practically nontoxic	>15 g/kg (<1 quart)	Aluminum hydroxide, calcium carbonate, lanolin, mineral oil, pyrethrum, stearic acid, sucrose

Source: From Ref. 13.

have been reported in humans. An alternative reason, however, can be formulated to explain why it is difficult to produce certain types of toxic reactions in animals. When it is said that an abnormal reaction cannot be reproduced in laboratory animals, it is actually more correct to say that the conditions under which the animals are being tested do not permit the elucidation of the toxic reaction. The evidence is now clear that, at least for several toxic reactions, the conditions of exposure of the animals may markedly affect the appearance of the reaction.

Halothane-induced liver injury (5) and acetaminophen-induced liver injury (25) are two such examples. These toxic reactions came to light because of their occurrence in humans; the experimental counterparts were questionable in laboratory animals. It is now clear, however, that the parent substances themselves do not induce hepatic injury and that the lesion is a result of the formation of reactive metabolites that are considerably more toxic than the parent substances. In animals, the kinetics of metabolism play an extremely important role in the response. With acetaminophen, the formation of the toxic metabolites can be enhanced by pretreating the animals with substances that increase bioactivation by the mixed-function oxidase system of the liver. It is now possible to reproduce human acetaminophen lesions by pretreating rats with phenobarbital prior to the exposure to acetaminophen. Under these conditions, the hepatotoxic properties of acetaminophen become very evident.

In the case of halothane, the substance can undergo biotransformation along several different pathways; tissue oxygen tension can alter the final pathway of metabolism (30). The toxic metabolite of halothane appears to be the result of a reductive activation by the mixed-function oxidase system. In addition, in some subjects, an allergic reaction may occur, resulting in hepatotoxicity. When laboratory animals are pretreated with an inducing agent and are also rendered hypoxic, the reductive pathway becomes more important in quantitative terms and a more toxic metabolite is produced. Under these conditions it is possible to produce hepatic lesions in laboratory animals that resemble those observed in certain cases of intoxication reported in humans.

Two other lesions found in humans that are difficult to reproduce in laboratory animals seem to be due to strain differences within animal species. The kidney injury associated with methoxyflurane does occur in the Fisher 344 rat, but not in the Buffalo or the Sprague-Dawley rat (22). Whether this strain difference is due entirely to a difference in the metabolic activation of methoxyflurane or whether it is due to an increased susceptibility of the kidney in certain strains of rats is not clear. This information, however, has led to experimental conditions in which the pathology of the lesion can now be studied. Anabolic steroids can produce cholestasis and jaundice in humans; this toxic reaction is not reproduced in routine animal testing procedures (28). Certain uncommon strains of inbred mice, however, will exhibit the morphological and biochemical signs of cholestasis after short-term treatment with anabolic steriods, although the lesion cannot be produced in rats (18). Although the explanations for these strain and species differences are yet unknown, the data indicate again that the lesion itself can be reproduced in laboratory animals, and that the conditions of exposure (species or strains selected) regulate the type of lesion observed.

Another explanation for the occurrence of untoward reactions in humans, uncovered only after extended exposure of subjects to drug therapy, is that the toxic reaction may be a rare event. These have been described as *low-incidence toxic reactions*. Frequencies of 0.1, 0.01, and 0.001% are examples of such reactions. Some have raised the question as to why these low-incidence reactions are not detected in laboratory animals. For quantal data, Hayes (16) published values that denote the differences that have to exist between groups in order to demonstrate a treatment-related effect. As one would expect, the differences in response required are dependent upon the size of the group being observed; thus, the background response of the control animals affects the magnitude of the difference required for establishing statistical significance. If the incidence of the response being measured is found to be 0 in the control animals, the effect will have to be observed in 12, 30, or 50% of the treated animals if the groups contain 50, 20, or 10 animals, respectively. If such differences (0 versus 12, 30, or 50%) were observed, one could propose that the effect was related to the treatment and that the difference was statistically significant at $p<0.05$. Thus, in a group of 50 animals a minimum of 6 responders (12% of the group) is needed.

Toxicologists feel much more comfortable when the toxic effect is dosage related; that is, the incidence of the reaction actually increases in the experimental groups as the dosage of the substance given is increased. There is a tendency to deemphasize abnormal responses in treatment groups if a clear dose-response relationship is not observed. This is particularly true when the abnormal response is observed in a low-dosage group but not in a high-dosage group. In the experimental situation, it is assumed that the laboratory animals selected for the test represent a homogenous population. Yet differences in susceptibility do exist in such populations. Dahl et al. (7) carried out a study on hypertensive rats that illustrates this point. They selectively bred from an outbred stock of Sprague-Dawley rats, a subpopulation of rats that was hypersusceptible to the hypertensive effects of sodium chloride. Thus, the original "homogenous" population contained a small group of rats that was susceptible to the hypertensive effects of sodium chloride, but the subpopulation could only be demonstrated when they were selected out of the original population and bred separately in a manner in which their hypersusceptibility could be demonstrated. Newberne (26) has described strain differences in the development of chronic nephritis in rats. Imai and Hayashi (18) showed qualitative and quantitative differences in inbred strains of mice in the response to intrahepatic cholestasis induced by anabolic steroids.

Thus, it is clear that a supposedly homogenous population can contain one or more subpopulations. These observations have important implications on the application of the dose-response principle to treatment-related toxic responses in animal populations. A low-incidence abnormal response is the possible reflection of a particular, susceptible subpopulation; such observations should not be dismissed without considerable thought. When it is said that no dose-response relationship occurs, it is more correct to say that the dose-response relationship that might exist is not evident. Perhaps the effects observed in the small subpopulation of responders may be diluted out by the larger subpopulation of nonresponders.

If it is assumed that undetected susceptible subpopulations exist in laboratory animal populations just as they exist in human populations, it is possible to calculate how many animals would be required to uncover such a response in the animal population, as shown in Table 4-3. Several assumptions have been made in the preparation and the interpretation of these values. The first assumption is that the incidence of the effect in the laboratory animal population is identical to the incidence of the effect in the human population. The second assumption is that the dose-response relationship does not play a role in these reactions (the incidence does not increase as the dosage increases). The number of animals that will have to be tested to uncover an adverse reaction depends upon the expected incidence in the animal population. If the incidence of the reaction in humans and in animals is of the order of 1%

(1:100), approximately 300 animals would have to be tested to have a 95% probability of at least one animal exhibiting the adverse reaction. If the frequency in the human and animal populations is 0.1% (1:1000), about 3,000 animals would have to be tested to have a 95% probability of obtaining at least one animal with the adverse reaction. If the incidence in the two populations is 0.01% (1:10,000), about 30,000 animals would have to be tested in order to have a 95% probability of observing at least one adverse reaction. These calculations demonstrate why it is virtually impossible to expect current animal toxicological tests to uncover low-incidence adverse reactions if a dose-response relationship cannot be demonstrated.

Table 4-3
Minimum Number of Animals Required in a Test Group to Detect an Effect Occurring with the Stated Expected Incidence

Expected Incidence (%)	Number of Animals Required (p = 0.95)
100	1
80	2
60	4
50	5
40	6
20	14
10	29
5	59
2	149
1	299
0.1	2,995
0.01	29,956
0.001	299,572

Source: From Ref. 33.

FACTORS INFLUENCING TOXICITY

CHEMICAL AND PHYSICAL PROPERTIES

The toxicity of a chemical can be influenced by the products used in its formulations as these can affect the solubility and absorption of the chemical. The presence of vehicles, adjuvants, binding agents, and the use of enteric coatings need to be considered when assessing the toxic properties of a chemical formulation. Stability characteristics also need to be known as these can influence the toxic properties of the substance. With pharmaceuticals, the influence of these various factors are assessed before the drug is made available for use.

For industrial chemicals or agricultural chemicals, it is also important to assess the degree of impurities present in the chemical compound as a finished product available for use. The formulation may contain impurities or contaminants that are considerably more toxic than the test agent or that can actually modify the response of the test agent. Such a situation has been demonstrated in the toxicological assessment of the herbicide 2,4,5-trichlorophenoxyacetic acid (2,4,5-T); the presence of an extremely toxic contaminant, 2,3,7,8-tetrachlorodibenzo-p-dioxin (dioxin), is said to be responsible, in part, for the alleged teratogenic effects of 2,4,5-T in animals (9, 17). The problem of impurities is of particular importance in the assessment of the long-term carcinogenic potential of such chemicals.

In the food industry, the various ingredients that may be employed in the processing of a final food product must also be considered. These consist of suspending agents, preservatives, surfactants, lubricants, stabilizers, and so on. Because of years of widespread use in food processing, the bulk of these substances are considered "Generally Recognized As Safe" (GRAS) in the United States. Their GRAS status, however, is currently being reevaluated by the Food and Drug Administration. Siu et al. (31) described the composition of the so-called GRAS list and the problems associated with the assessment of the safety of these substances. Nearly 400 substances are included on the GRAS list, and approximately 1200 more are found on the Flavor and Extract Manufacturers' Association (FEMA) list of flavoring substances.

More recently, there has been concern regarding the various metabolic transformations that a chemical can undergo in mammalian systems. Reactive metabolites, although produced in relatively small quantities, can react with macromolecules to produce organ damage. A number of drugs are biotransformed to reactive metabolites and thus cause toxicity; acetaminophen, furosemide, isoniazid, chloroform, and halothane are examples of such drugs. The concepts involved in this type of reaction were described by Mitchell et al. (24). Their work with acetaminophen is an excellent example of the phenomenon. Normally, only a small portion of the acetaminophen is actually biotransformed into a reactive metabolite. This metabolite then reacts with glutathione, which is present in the liver, and thus is no longer available to react with key macromolecules. However, if the amount of reactive metabolite formed exceeds the amount of normally available glutathione, or if the amount of glutathione present in the liver is reduced, the excess metabolite can react covalently with tissue macromolecules. This irreversible binding is associated with the production of hepatic necrosis.

The experimental work performed to gain a better understanding of this phenomenon has led to some new fundamental concepts regarding toxic reactions. First, it is apparent that very small amounts of highly reactive metabolites can induce toxic responses. Second, endogenous substances such as glutathione can react with these reactive metabolites to render them nontoxic; thus, glutathione appears to function in part as a detoxification pathway. Third, these studies have shown that the existence of a threshold is very important for defining toxicity because acetaminophen does not exert its hepatotoxic effect unless a sufficient amount of reactive metabolite is produced and the normal detoxifying resources of the cells are exhausted. This demonstration of the validity of a threshold concept, an extremely important finding, has implications in the current controversy concerning potentially carcinogenic substances, because at least for a good number of these agents, the carcinogenic properties seem to be due to the production of metabolites that can react with macromolecules.

ROUTES OF EXPOSURE

The route of administration can modify toxicity. In human medicine, the most important route of administration is the oral route. The second most important route is parenteral injection. When this route is employed, absorption is enhanced, and high concentrations of the drug within a given tissue may occur much more rapidly than those that occur after oral administration. Oral administration, however, can favor hepatic biotransformation before distribution to organs.

When chemicals are administered orally, the conditions and manner of administration can influence their toxicity. The presence of food in the stomach can markedly affect absorption. The toxicity of an orally administered drug is generally greatest when it is given on an empty stomach and least when it is incorporated in food. Fractionation of the daily dose generally also reduces toxicity as both the rate of absorption and the rate of biotransformation influence toxicity. The reduction in toxicity that occurs when drugs are given by slow intravenous infusion rather than by a rapid single injection can also be attributed to more efficient distribution, biotransformation, and excretion. It is evident that changes in the rate of administration of a toxic agent can be expected to produce changes in the toxic response. It is important to note, however, that the magnitude of the change or even the direction of the change may be unpredictable.

In the industrial environment, other routes of exposure, the percutaneous route and the inhalation route, are particularly important. For humans, the most common exposure to agricultural chemicals is through contact with the skin. The physical and chemical properties of the substance are the principal determining factors in percutaneous absorption of the compound.

SUBJECT SUSCEPTIBILITY

The physiological characteristics of the individual receiving a drug or being exposed to a chemical in the environment must be taken into consideration when assessing the relative possibility of a toxic reaction. Many such associations have been suspected, but only the recent interest in the assessment of adverse drug reactions has confirmed the phenomenon. They are discussed in greater detail in the following texts: Doull et al. (9), Davies (8), Goldstein et al. (12), and Melmon and Morelli (23).

Racial and ethnic differences in response to drugs are well established; these appear to be due to the genetic makeup of the individuals. Some drugs depend upon acetylation as a major means of biotransformation, and human populations have been characterized into two categories, *rapid acetylators* and *slow acetylators*. Eskimos and Japanese contain a greater proportion of rapid acetylators than other racial stocks, whereas slow acetylators are more prominent among Mediterranean Jews. Slow acetylators have been associated with the development of peripheral neuropathy caused by isoniazid and the lupus type of reaction prevalent with hydralazine. A toxic interaction associated with the combination of phenytoin and isoniazid appears to be more prominent in individuals who are slow acetylators; this interaction is due to an abnormally longer presence of circulating isoniazid in these individuals and the subsequent inhibition by isoniazid of the biotransformation of phenytoin.

Individuals who exhibit a deficiency in glucose-6-phosphate dehydrogenase appear to be more susceptible to hemolytic anemia caused by a number of drugs. This type of genetic deficiency is more commonly found among black Africans, Kurdish and Iraqi Jews, some Mediterraneans, and Filipinos. Racial differences have also been observed among women using oral contraceptives in the production of thromboembolic disease and intrahepatic cholestasis associated with these agents. Women in Scandinavia and Chile appear to be more susceptible to oral contraceptives than other racial, ethnic, or geographical stocks. Acute intermittent porphyria, which can be aggravated by drugs, is more frequent in people of Scandinavian, Anglo-Saxon, or German origin. Genetic alterations resulting in diminished plasma pseudocholinesterase can lead to unusually prolonged muscular paralysis and apnea following the administration of succinylcholine during anesthesia. Malignant hyperthermia also can occur in genetically susceptible individuals following the use of certain anesthetics (usually halothane).

Surveys of adverse drug reactions also indicate that in some instances the toxic response may be related to sex. These associations are less clear than those that have been described for genetically based reactions. In laboratory animals, it is not uncommon to see sex-related differences in toxic responses. A number of these is attributable to the effect of sex hormones on the pharmacokinetics of the chemical in question. Other examples, however, indicate that the differences in susceptibility may be in terms of the organ response. The nephrotoxic properties of chloroform is one such example. Male mice are particularly susceptible to this property of chloroform, whereas females are resistant. The variations are so frequent that it is impossible to make generalizations regarding the relative susceptibility of each sex. It is important to note that such differences in toxicity do exist, however.

Age can also influence susceptibility to toxic properties of chemical substances. In the neonate, who is devoid or deficient in the enzymes involved in drug metabolism, the risk of adverse reactions is increased. Examples of this situation consist of chloramphenicol, sulfonamides, novobiocin, barbiturates, morphine and vitamin K. In addition, in the neonate or very young infant, one can anticipate decreased drug elimination and the presence of an inefficient blood-brain barrier, leading to increased susceptibility to toxic reactions.

It is also now becoming more evident that individuals over 65 years of age are more liable to suffer adverse drug reactions than those under this age. Patients in the 66-75 years of age group appear to be slightly more prone to adverse drug reactions than those in other categories, and individuals older than 75 appear to be even more susceptible. The type of drugs associated with increased problems in elderly individuals include digoxin, coumarin anticoagulants, meperidine, some barbiturates, and some benzodiazepines. Whereas a number of these instances can be related to relative deficiencies in drug metabolism and alterations in the pharmacokinetics of the drugs in question, the data are insufficient to indicate that all of these can be explained merely in these terms.

It should also be recognized that the presence of renal and hepatic disease can predispose certain individuals to adverse drug reactions. Although in these situations impaired renal elimination and impaired hepatic degradation of the drugs in question are involved, the mere presence of renal or hepatic disease does not mean that drug pharmacokinetics will be affected. For example, in the case of hepatic disease, a number of studies indicate that the diseased organ may have sufficient remaining functional capacity to permit normal degradation of drugs when the substances are given in therapeutic dosages.

ANIMAL TESTING PROCEDURES

Only brief descriptions of the various testing procedures employed for safety evaluation will be described in this chapter. The reader should consult the following for more detailed information: Drill and Lazar (10), Ellison (11), Hayes (14), Hayes (16), Loomis (21) and Zbinden (33, 34). The test procedures described here are listed in Table 4-4.

ACUTE TOXICITY STUDIES

One purpose of acute toxicity studies is to determine the toxic signs that occur following the administration of the chemical when it is administered only once. A second purpose is to obtain some idea of the quantitative relationships involved. Initially, the chemical is given to a single species; mice and rats are usually selected for these initial studies. Similar tests may be carried out later in other species. The route of administration selected depends upon the intended use of the compound. Because most drugs are given orally, it is more common to use the oral route in laboratory animals. Such studies, however, are also carried out following parenteral administration or even topical application. When the topical route is employed, both local effects and systemic effects following absorption are of interest. If the likely route of exposure in humans is by inhalation,this route is employed in the animal studies.

Table 4-4
Types of Animal Toxicological Tests

I. *Acute tests (single dose)*
   A. LD_{50} determination (24-hour test and survivors followed by 7 days)
      1. Two species (usually rats and mice)
      2. Two routes of administration (one by intended route of use)
   B. Topical effects on rabbits skin (if intended route of use is topical; evaluated at 24 hour and at 7 days)

II. *Subchronic tests (daily doses)*
   A. Duration, 3 months
   B. Two species (usually rats and dogs)
   C. Three dosage levels
   D. Route of administration according to intended route of use
   E. Evaluation of state of health
      1. All animals weighed weekly
      2. Complete physical examination weekly
      3. Blood chemistry, urinalysis, hematology, and function tests performed on all ill animals
   F. All animals subjected to complete autopsy, including histology of all organ systems

III. *Chronic tests (daily doses)*
   A. Duration, 2 to 7 years depending on species
   B. Species, selected from results of prior prolonged tests, pharmacodynamic studies on several species of animals, possible single-dose human trial studies; otherwise use two species
   C. Minimum of two dosage levels
   D. Route of administration according to intended route of use
   E. Evaluation of state of health
      1. All animals weighed weekly
      2. Complete physical examination weekly
      3. Blood chemistry, urinalysis, hematological examination, and function tests on all animals at 3 to 6-month intervals and on all ill or abnormal animals
   F. All animals subjected to complete autopsy, including histological examination of all organ systems

IV. *Special tests for*
   A. Potentiation with other chemicals
   B. Effects on reproduction
   C. Teratogenicity
   D. Carcinogenicity
   E. Mutagenicity
   F. Skin and eye effects
   G. Behavioral effects

Source: From Ref. 21.

After the administration of a chemical, the animals are observed closely for at least 24 hrs, with a period of follow-up from several days up to 2-3 weeks. The second phase of observation is of particular interest because, if death is delayed, a metabolic product may be involved in causing the toxic response or organ injury that subsequently leads to the death of the animal. Although acute toxicity studies are primarily employed to determine the dosage that produces death, additional information of toxicological importance can be obtained by close observation and physical examination of the animal undergoing this test. These observations can be of use in determining the mechanisms of action leading to toxicity.

When such tests are performed to obtain quantitative measures of toxicity, different groups of animals are given increasing dosages of the compound so that a frequency dose-response curve can be established. From such data, the LD_{50} of the compound can be estimated. These quantitative measurements are important for comparing compounds within a series of studies and also for establishing dosages that will be utilized in subsequent safety evaluation studies.

SUBCHRONIC TOXICITY STUDIES

Most drugs are administered to humans for a prolonged period. It is not unusual for a patient to receive medication for several weeks, months, or even years. Therefore, it is of extreme importance to know what happens to the toxicological profile of a new drug when it is given repetitively over long periods of time. The route of administration employed in such studies is the same as the one used when the compound will be administered to humans. The duration of such studies is a matter of controversy. Generally, most subchronic studies last about 90 days. Because species are known to vary in their response to chemicals, at least two species are utilized in subchronic tests, one of which should be a nonrodent. In practice, rats and dogs are commonly employed, and both males and females are used. At least three dosage levels of the compound, selected so that the highest one will produce some toxic effect, are administered to different groups of animals. Frequent physical examination of the animals to detect the presence of overt behavioral patterns as well as the general well-being of the animals is required. During the 3-month study, when feasible, blood cell counts and blood chemistry studies should be performed. At the end of the study all animals are sacrificed and subjected to a complete autopsy, with histological sections of organs and tissues prepared for microscopic evaluation. All animals that die during the study or are sacrificed because they are moribund are also subjected to a complete postmortem examination.

CHRONIC TOXICITY STUDIES

Chronic toxicity studies are performed for periods longer than 90 days; the chemical tested is either incorporated in the diet or given at least once a day. The oral route of administration is usually employed. Chronic toxicity studies for pharmaceutical preparations are usually run for at least 1 year but may last as long as 2 years. More than one species, both males and females, and at least two dosage levels are used. The high dosage is one that is near the maximally tolerated level. At regular intervals, the animals are subjected to a complete physical examination, and samples are obtained for blood chemistry and urinary analyses. All animals are subjected to a complete autopsy at the end of the study, including histological examination of all organ systems. Animals that die during the course of the study or animals that are moribund are also subjected to a complete autopsy and histological examination.

There have been changes in the terminology employed for the various tests that have been described. At one time, the repetitive dose tests that are carried out for less than 90 days were called subacute; the term *subchronic* is now preferred. In chronic testing procedures, the terms *short-term* and *long-term* are also employed. A test is considered to be long-term if the duration of the test is longer than one-half the average lifetime of the animal species employed. If the duration is shorter than one-half the lifetime, this type of toxicity test is considered short-term.

The object of this battery of acute, subchronic, and chronic tests is to determine the profile of toxicological activity of the chemical in question. The toxicologist will be in a better position to advise the physician as to the possible toxic manifestations that might be expected to occur when a medication is given in large dosages. A second objective is to get a quantitative measure of the dosage at which toxicity begins to appear when the substance is given repetitively. This is of particular importance for establishing the relative safety of drugs.

SPECIAL TESTS

In addition to the battery of tests described, routine special tests are also carried out to determine possible teratogenic manifestations, effects on reproduction, possible mutagenic effects, and finally, assessment of the potential carcinogenic properties of the chemical in question.

Interest in teratogenicity arose only when such a drug-induced phenomenon was discovered in humans from use of the sedative thalidomide. Since that tragedy, methods have been developed for the detection of possible teratogenic effects of chemicals in laboratory animals. Fertilization is produced in rats, mice, or rabbits under controlled laboratory conditions. The drug is then administered to the pregnant animals during the period of fetal organ development for that particular species. Finally, the fetuses are removed by cesarean section prior to delivery, and malformations in the fetuses are detected by direct systematic observation and subsequently by dissection and histological examination of organs. When such a study is carried out, it is also of interest to note whether the chemical can interrupt pregnancy or can even be embryotoxic. Suitable methods are available for determining these parameters (14, 27).

Tests for reproductive performance are also carried out. Both males and females must be examined. Fertilization, maintenance of pregnancy, litter size, fetal development and viability, and lactation are observed. The tests may be repeated through second and third generations of chronically treated animals.

Carcinogenicity testing has become a major preoccupation of toxicologists involved in the safety evaluation process. It is an extremely complex problem, one that has created considerable emotional reactions because of the possible impact on society. Carcinogenicity testing is usually carried out in rodents or dogs maintained over their total life span. Current testing procedures recommend that the chemical be given by a suitable route of administration (the intended route of exposure in humans) and be administered at least at two dosage levels; the dosages utilized are selected in conjunction with the results observed in the chronic toxicity studies.

Large group sizes are required because many potentially carcinogenic substances do not actually induce the development of new types of neoplasms but enhance the appearance of spontaneous tumors known to occur in the test species selected. The incidence of spontaneous tumors in the control group of rats is an important consideration for establishing the validity of the findings. Unfortunately, there is a wide range of incidence for such tumors among different strains of rats, and the selection of the proper strain for specific test purposes is a matter of controversy. Animals that die or are moribund during the study are autopsied, and histological sections are prepared. At the end of the treatment period (usually 24 months for rats), all animals are sacrificed and subjected to a complete autopsy and histological examination.

In recent years, there has been considerable interest in the testing of mutagenicity by short-term testing procedures (6, 11, 14, 16, 21). Both *in vitro* and *in vivo* assays have been developed. Although this field is evolving very rapidly, there is considerable controversy concerning the extrapolation of such data to possible toxic manifestations in humans. Among the *in vitro* tests, there are the Ames *Salmonella* microsomal assay system and variations of this procedure, which consist of incubating the suspected mutagen with a mutant strain of *Salmonella* requiring histidine for growth. In the presence of a mutagen, some of the organisms revert to the prototype form that no longer requires histidine for growth; the number of such colonies are counted. Rat or human liver homogenate can be added to the medium to permit biotransformation of the suspected mutagen.

For *in vivo* tests, there are the dominant-lethal assay, the host-mediated assay, and various cytogenetic methods. In the dominant-lethal procedure, male mice or rats are treated with the test substance and mated with females; the latter are sacrificed and scored for corpora lutea, early fetal deaths, late fetal deaths and total implantations. The assay detects chromosomal aberrations that are incompatible with fetal development. The host-mediated assay uses micro-organisms (*Salmonella*, *Neurospora*, *Escherichia coli*, *Saccharomyces*) grown in the peritoneal cavity of a host (rat, mouse, hamster) as the indicator of genetic damage. The test agent is given to the host, and the mutation frequency in the organisms is subsequently measured. This procedure detects point mutations. For *in vivo* cytogenetic procedures, use is made of various tissues from treated animals or humans: bone marrow, lymphocyte, skin fibroblasts, gametocytes, and amniotic fluid cell cultures. A battery of tests is employed because no single method is adequate for determining the possible risk to humans.

Animal tests are also available to detect possible effects of chemical substances on the skin or on the eye (10, 14). These tests are employed when the projected use pattern of the chemical indicates that contact with the skin or the eye is an important consideration (soaps, detergents, cosmetics, solvents, emulsifiers, ophthalmological preparations, and so on). The tests employed are usually acute in nature, but exposures of longer duration are possible. The effects looked for include primary irritation, corrosion, cutaneous sensitization, phototoxicity, and photoallergy. Rabbits, guinea pigs, and mice are the usual species selected for such tests.

REFERENCES

1. American Medical Association. *AMA Drug Evaluations*, 5th ed. Philadelphia: W.B. Saunders, 1983.
2. Avery, G.S. *Drug Treatment*, 2nd ed. Sidney: Adis Press, 1980.
3. Boyd, C.F. and Boyd, E.M. The chronic toxicity of atropine administered intramuscularly to rabbits *Toxicol. Appl. Pharmacol.* 4:457, 1962
4. Boyd, E.M. *Predictive Toxicometrics* Bristol: Scientechnica, 1972.
5. Brown, B.R. and Sipes, I. Biotransformation and hepatotoxicity of halothane *Anesthesiology* 41:554, 1974.
6. Brusick, D. *Principles of Genetic Toxicology* New York: Plenum Press, 1980.
7. Dahl, L.K., Heine, M. and Tassinari, L. Effects of chronic excess salt ingestion: Evidence that genetic factors play an important role in susceptibility to experimental hypertension. *J. Exp. Med.* 115:1173, 1962.
8. Davies, D.M. *Textbook of Adverse Drug Reactions* Oxford: Oxford University Press, 1977.
9. Doull, J., Klaassen C.D. and Amdur, M.O. (eds.). *Casarett and Doull's Toxicology. The Basic Science of Poisons*, 2nd ed. New York: Macmillan, 1980.
10. Drill, V.A. and Lazar, P. *Cutaneous Toxicity* New York, Raven Press, 1984.
11. Ellison, T. Toxicological effects testing. In: *Guide book: Toxic Substances Control Act* (Dominguez, G., ed.). Cleveland: CRC Press, 1977, pp. 8-11.
12. Goldstein, A., Aronow, L. and Kalman, S.M. *Principles of Drug Action: The Basis of Pharmacology*, 2nd ed. New York: John Wiley, 1974.
13. Gosselin, R.E., Hodge, H.C., Smith, R.P. and Gleason M.N. *Clinical Toxicology of Commercial Products: Acute Poisonings* Baltimore: Williams and Wilkins, 1976.
14. Hayes, A.W. *Principles and Methods of Toxicology* New York: Raven Press, 1982.
15. Hayes, W.J. Jr. The 90-dose LD_{50} and a chronicity factor as measures of toxicity. *Toxicol. Appl. Pharmacol.* 11:327, 1967.
16. Hayes, W.J. Jr. *Toxicology of Pesticides.* Baltimore: Williams and Wilkins, 1975.
17. Hayes, W.J. Jr. *Pesticides Studied in Man.* Baltimore: Williams and Wilkins, 1982.
18. Imai, K. and Hayashi, Y. Steroid-induced intrahepatic cholestasis in mice. *Jap. J. Pharmacol.* 20:473, 1970.
19. Karch, F.E. and Lasagna, L. Adverse drug reactions. A critical review. *JAMA* 234:1236, 1975.
20. Litchfield, J.T. Jr. A method for rapid graphic solution of time-percent effect curves. *J. Pharmacol. Exp. Ther.* 97:399, 1949.
21. Loomis, T.A. *Essentials of Toxicology*, 3rd ed. Philadelphia: Lea and Febiger, 1978.
22. Mazze, R.I. Methoxyflurane nephropathy. In: *Toxicology of the Kidney* (Hook, J.B., ed.) New York: Raven Press, 1981, p. 135.
23. Melmon, K.L. and Morelli, H.F. *Clinical Pharmacology: Basic Principles in Therapeutics*, 2nd ed. New York: Macmillan, 1978.
24. Mitchell, J.R., Jollow, D.J., Gillette, J.R. and Brodie, B.B. Drug metabolism as a cause of drug toxicity. *Drug Metab. Disposit.* 1:418, 1973.
25. Mitchell, J.R., Potter, W.Z., Hinson, J.A., Snodgrass, W.R., Timbrell, J.A. and Gillette, J.R. Toxic drug reactions *Handbook Exp. Pharmacol.* 28:383, 1975.
26. Newberne, P.M. Pathology: Studies of chronic toxicity and carcinogenicity. *JOAC* 58:650, 1975.
27. Palmer, A.K. Regulatory requirements for reproductive toxicology: Theory and practice. In: *Developmental Toxicology* (Kimmel C.A. and Buelke-Sam, J., eds.) New York: Raven Press, 1981, p. 259.
28. Plaa, G.L. and Priestly, B.G. Intrahepatic cholestasis induced by drugs and chemicals. *Pharmacol. Rev.* 28:207, 1976.
29. Reidenberg, M.M. and Lowenthal, D.T. Adverse nondrug reactions. *N. Engl. J. Med.* 279:678, 1968.
30. Sipes, I.G. and Gandolfi, A.J. Bioactivation of aliphatic organohalogens: Formation, detection and relevance. In: *Toxicology of the Liver.* (Plaa, G.L. and Hewitt, W.R., eds.). New York: Raven Press, 1982, p. 181.
31. Siu, R.G.H., Borzelleca, J.F., Carr, C.J. *et al.* Evaluation of health aspects of GRAS food ingredients: Lessons learned and questions unanswered *Fed. Proc.* 36:2519, 1977.
32. Zbinden, G. Experimental and clinical aspects of drug toxicity. *Adv. Pharmacol.* 2:1, 1963.
33. Zbinden, G. *Progress in Toxicology*, Vol. 1 New York: Springer-Verlag, 1973.
34. Zbinden, G. *Progress in Toxicology*, Vol. 2 New York: Springer-Verlag, 1973.
35. Zimmerman, H.J. *Hepatotoxicity* New York: Appleton-Century-Crofts, 1978.

CHAPTER
4.1

PHARMACOGENETICS AND TOXICOGENETICS

Sikta Pradhan and William L. West

Pharmacogenetics refers to a special area of biochemical genetics that relates variation in the responsiveness to drugs to genetic variability (15, 16, 18). It is a relatively new discipline in that the study of human inheritance which includes among its pioneers Francis Galton and Archibald E. Garrod began only 125 years ago (11). Lines of inquiry studied by Galton included characteristics such as intelligence, stature, and fingerprints, but such traits were difficult to analyze quantitatively. The quantitative methods were later introduced by K. Pearson, and improved by R.A. Fisher (11). From these metrical procedures in genetics emerged a somewhat standard approach based on the assumption that the effects of an indeterminate number of genes at different loci, with several alleles at each, combine with environmental factors to produce a phenotype. For example, a large number of enzymes (proteins) are made in the human body, and the amino acid sequence in each polypeptide chain is coded by deoxyribonucleic acid (DNA) in a separate gene locus. From this vast array of structural gene loci, it has been shown that, at certain loci, many different alleles determine structurally distinct versions of an enzyme. Whereas most of these structurally distinct versions are quite rare, in some cases certain alleles at a particular locus may be more frequent. When an inherited trait is controlled by a single genetic locus with two alleles, and if the rarer allele has a frequency of a least 0.01, so that the heterozygote frequency is at least 0.02, the locus is considered to be polymorphic and the phenomenon is often called genetically determined polymorphism. The latter is characterized by individual members of a population that can be categorized into two or more separate types, each containing a unique distribution of isozymes or proteins that differ in their physical and chemical characteristics.

Thus pharmacogenetic research seemingly emerged as a discipline that attempts to understand the hereditary basis for differences in responsiveness to therapeutic effects of a drug between individuals, often called interindividual variation. Whenever a drug is prescribed for a patient, a physician should keep in mind that the patient is genetically unique. Variations in drug effect may be 2-fold, 10-fold, or 100-fold, even among members of the same family. Similar interindividual variations are also observed in respect to adverse effects of a drug or a chemical; such variation can be designated as toxicogenetic.

The major pharmacogenetic studies are involved either in directly measuring the drug-metabolizing capability through enzymatic activities or in detection of genetic variations producing differential drug responses. The bases of variations in response to drugs can be classified into two major categories, (1) pharmacokinetic (i.e., some inherited variations in biotransformation of drugs due to the differences in the activities of the drug-metabolizing enzymes); (2) pharmacodynamics (genetic variation of a major effect producing unique tissue responsiveness). However, each of these categories may represent only the predominant type of reaction and does not rule out partial overlap by the other type.

POLYMORPHISM IN PHARMACOKINETICS

Pharmacokinetic polymorphism has been demonstrated by various researchers (33) using different pharmacogenetic models, such as (1) inherited variations in hepatic N-acetyltransferase, that cause a wide variation in the metabolism of drugs (e.g., isoniazid, hydralazine, etc.); (2) inherited differences in the activity of the hepatic mixed-function oxidase system containing multiple forms of cytochrome P-450 that cause genetic polymorphisms in the oxidative metabolism of debrisoquin, sparteine, etc.

Polymorphic drug metabolism can be classified into groups on the basis of their mode of biotransformation: (1) oxidation, (2) reduction, (3) hydrolysis and (4) conjugation.

OXIDATION

Most of the oxidative drug metabolisms are catalyzed by the hepatic mixed-function oxidase system that contains multiple forms of cytochrome P-450 isozymes. These isozymes differ in their molecular weight, spectral properties, and substrate specificity (12). It was first reported by Kutt et al (20) that the same dose of phenytoin (diphenylhydantoin) can produce toxic effects in an individual who has inherited deficiency in an enzyme that is required for the oxidative drug metabolism. Shahidi (27) also observed that a large dose of phenacetin (acetophenetidin) can cause methemoglobin formation in some individuals due to unusual oxidation of the drug producing methemoglobin-forming metabolites. Vesell (30) observed wide individual variability in the drug-metabolizing capability in different individuals using a so-called model drug, antipyrine (phenazone) metabolized by hydroxylation. In the above studies, it was concluded that most of the drugs having similar characteristics can produce differential effects in different individuals due to the variations in oxidative metabolism. The variations in drug oxidation are partly due to the complex nature of the hepatic mixed-function oxidase system containing varying amounts of isozymes of cytochrome P-450 in individuals with different genetic inheritance.

Over the years, the genetic polymorphisms in the metabolism of many drugs (e.g., debrisoquin, mephenytoin, phenformin, sparteine, tolbutamide, and so on) have been described (Table 4.1-1). With the extensive studies on the polymorphic oxidation of debrisoquin and sparteine, it has been possible to detect two phenotypes, the extensive or fast metabolizer (FM) and poor or slow metabolizer (SM) in all populations investigated (12).

The drugs presented in Table 4.1-1 are metabolized by oxidative enzymatic reactions of different types in the liver smooth endoplasmic reticulum (microsomes).

Table 4.1-1
Drugs Affected by Polymorphic Oxidation

Hepatic mixed function oxidase system containing multiple forms of cytochrome P-450 isozyme is involved in this metabolic process.

Drugs[a]	Metabolic Reaction	Consequence	Mode of Inherit-ance[b]	Frequency of Poor Metabolizer (12)
Debrisoquine	Slow 4-hydroxylation and aromatic hydroxylation	Appreciable orthostatic hypotension	A R	8-9% of the Caucasian British population; 1-9% different ethnic groups
Mephenytoin	Slow 4-hydroxylation	Increased toxicity	A R	6%
Phenacetin	Defective O-deethylation	Methemoglobin formation	U	
Phenformin	Slow 4-hydroxylation	Increased toxicity	A R	
Phenytoin	Moderately slow 4-hydroxylation	Increased toxicity	A D	
Sparteine	Slow oxidation	Increased toxicity	A R	5% of the German population and 2-9% of different ethnic groups[c]
Tolbutamide	Slow aliphatic hydroxylation	Increased toxicity	A R	25%

[a]In addition, other drugs (e.g., dicumarol, phenylbutazone, antipyrine, nortriptyline) are also affected by slow or defective hydroxylation.
[b]A, autosomal; R, recessive; D, dominant; U, unknown
[c]Egyptians, Saudi Arabians, Nigerians, Ghanians, and others (17).

Table 4.1-2
Drugs Affected by Polymorphic Reduction and Hydrolysis

Drugs	Enzyme and Source	Abnormal Metabolic Reaction	Consequent Abnormal Response	Inheritance[b]	Frequency of Poor Metabolizers
Hydrogen peroxide	Catalase in erythrocytes	Slow reduction	Acatalasia	A R	Mainly in Japan (about 1% in certain areas) and also in Switzerland (31)
Succinylcholine[a]	Pseudocholinesterase in plasma	Slow hydrolysis (deesterification)	Prolonged apnea	A R	Approximately 0.05% in Canadian population (29)
Paraoxon	Serum paraoxonase	Slow hydrolysis (deesterification)	Increased toxicity	A R	60-70% in a sample of Caucasian population (21)

[a] This drug can also cause the genetically determined pharmacodynamic reaction.
[b] A, autosomal; R, recessive.

REDUCTION

A pharmacogenetic condition such as acatalasia arises due to the deficiency of the enzyme catalase (EC 1.11.1.6) that facilitates the reduction of hydrogen peroxide to water and free oxygen. A clinical characteristic associated with the genetically inherited deficiency is the absence of frothing when peroxide is applied to a wound (Table 4.1-2). Gross deficiency of catalase is observed in all tissues. In some persons, the ulceration of the mucosa of the nose and mouth occurs and severe oral gangrene may develop; but other individuals with less than 1% of the normal level of catalase remain quite healthy and suffer apparently from no bad effects.

HYDROLYSIS

An important advance was made when it was first discovered by Kalow and Genest (19) that the serum cholinesterase present in suxamethonium-sensitive individuals is atypical in certain of its properties (Table 4.1-2). Serum cholinesterase hydrolyzes a number of drugs of which succinylcholine (suxamethonium) is clinically most important. The drug succinylcholine is widely used as a muscle relaxant in anesthesia and in connection with electroconvulsive therapy. The rapidity of its hydrolysis effectively decreases the amount of succinylcholine that reaches the motor end plates. However, a patient with an atypical form of enzyme (with less hydrolytic activity) develops prolonged apnea lasting from one to several hours after administration of a normal dose of succinylcholine. Clark et al (7) reported that succinylcholine-sensitive people have different genetical inheritance from normal individuals. The enzyme is inhibited by dibucaine. The inhibition studies using dibucaine led to the development of a rather simple test for detecting the atypical form of serum cholinesterase.

CONJUGATION

Conjugate formation is an important pathway in the biotransformation of many drugs (34). Conjugation reactions in humans or with demonstrated clinical significance can be classified into three subgroups: (a) acetylation, (b) methylation and (c) glucuronide formation.

Acetylation. The fundamental aspects of polymorphism in acetylation in humans, first recognized as an abnormal response, was demonstrated in the case of isoniazid (INH) inactivation during the treatment of tuberculosis (14). Individuals with different genetic inheritance were identified as slow or fast acetylators. Later, many other drugs were found to utilize similar enzymatic pathways (Table 4.1-3). This polymorphic acetylation was studied by various investigators (32) in mouse, rat and rabbit models. Although some of the consequent abnormal responses presented in Table 4.1-2 are speculative, there is a close similarity between polymorphic acetylation in humans and that in rat or rabbit models; the results that were observed in animal models could probably be applicable in humans. Individuals with inherited capacity of slow acetylation often suffer from drug toxicity after receiving normal doses of different drugs such as isoniazid, hydralazine etc. that are acetylated because the serum concentrations of these drugs, are usually high.

In addition to those drugs presented in Table 4.1-2, the enzyme acetyltransferase (acetylase) also catalyzes the acetylation of sulfadimidine, sulfapyridine and other sulfonamides, aminoglutethimide and some laboratory chemicals containing an amine or a hydrazine group. It also affects the metabolism of drugs such as clonazepam, nitrazepam, sulfasalazine and caffeine even though they do not contain an amine or a hydrazine group, which is essential for enzyme reactions; perhaps these essential groups are introduced during metabolism (32).

Table 4.1-3
Drugs Affected by Polymorphic Acetylation
(Mediated by acetylase in liver)

Drugs	Abnormal Metabolic Reaction	Consequent Abnormal Response[a]	Inherit-ance[b]	Frequency of Poor Metabolizers (17)
Isoniazid	Fast	Hepatitis	A D	Approximately 45% of Caucasian and 80% of Japanese population
	Slow	Peripheral neuropathy; inhibition of hepatic mixed-function oxidase; increased phenytoin toxicity when INH is given along with phenytoin	A R	52-68% of Caucasian population
Hydralazine	Slow	Lupoid reaction	A R	
Procainamide	Slow	Lupus develops earlier and more frequently	A R	
Phenelzine	Slow	Nausea, drowsiness, etc. are more common	A R	
Sulphasalazine	Slow	Severe reaction, more likely when large doses used	A R	
Dapsone	Slow	Some hematological effects	A R	

[a] Some of these responses are speculative.
[b] A, autosomal; R, recessive; D, dominant.

Methylation. In human biochemical genetic studies, methyl conjugation plays an important role in catecholamine metabolism and in biotransformation of many drugs (2). Research in the field of methyl conjugation was neglected until recently because of a lack of sensitive methods for assaying the enzymes involved. At present with the advancement of sensitive radioactive assay procedures, it has been possible to establish the fact that the activities of these methyltransferase enzymes are regulated by inheritance (34). On the basis of the currently available biochemical genetic data, three different human methyltransferase enzymes are known to exist (34): (a) catechol-O-methyltransferase (COMT) (EC 2.2.2.6), (b) thiopurine methyltransferase (TPMT) (EC 2.1.1.67) and (c) thiol methyltransferase (TMT) (EC 2.2.2.9).

Methylation by COMT. COMT causes O-methylation of catecholamines and some catechol-containing drugs during metabolism (34). This is one of the two major catecholamine-metabolizing enzymes (1). It has been suggested that COMT activity in human erythrocytes might reflect the activity of the enzyme in other tissues (34). It has also been shown that both biochemically and immunologically, red blood cell (RBC) COMT is similar to that in other tissues (34). Weinshilboum et al (36) were the first to indicate in 1974 that inheritance may play an important role in the regulation of the enzyme activity in humans by correlating the RBC COMT activity between siblings. A year later, Gershon and Jonas (13) reported that a change in erythrocyte-soluble COMT activity might cause primary affective disorders. It was further identified that the activity of COMT in erythrocytes is regulated by monogenic (mendelian) inheritance (34).

The major variations in erythrocyte COMT activity are due to the existence of two alleles, one with high activity ($COMT^H$) and the other with low activity ($COMT^L$), at a single locus. The gene frequency of $COMT^L$ and $COMT^H$ were roughly equal in a randomly selected sample of a white population of northern European origin as reported by Weinshilboum and Raymond (35). A recent report indicates that the overall level of COMT is inherited as an autosomal codominant trait (28).

The genetic polymorphism regulating erythrocyte COMT activity is a common polymorphism without any involvement of a rare genetic variant. A close relationship is observed between the metabolism of drugs, such as levodopa (26), methyldopa, isoprenaline (9) and so on, and the overall level of COMT in an individual. The metabolism of these drugs is enhanced in individuals with high activity of COMT enzyme. Therefore, more drug will be needed to elicit the proper therapeutic effect. On the other hand, some toxic effect could be observed after administration of a normal dose of a drug in some individuals having inherited a low level of COMT.

Methylation by TPMT. TPMT catalyzes the S-methylation of thiopurines in the presence of S-adenosyl-L-methionine, which is the methyl donor in the reaction. It is a cytoplasmic enzyme present in RBCs and in different tissues. For a long time no information on the characteristics of the enzyme was available due to the lack of a sensitive assay procedure, as was the case with COMT. Recent experimental evidence on erythrocyte TPMT indicated that the enzyme might be genetically controlled (34) and regulated by a single genetic locus with two alleles of low ($TPMT^L$) and high ($TPMT^H$) enzyme activity. The enzyme activity was inherited as an autosomal codominant trait. The gene frequencies of $TPMT^H$ and $TPMT^L$ were estimated to be 94% and 6%, respectively, in a sample of white population investigated.

The polymorphism for TPMT was the common type as was the case with COMT. This enzyme can metabolize any drug containing thiopurines such as, 6-mercaptopurine, 6-thioguanine, and azathioprine (34). However, the possible significance of action of polymorphic TPMT in clinical response and in drug toxicity has not yet been elucidated.

Methylation by TMT. Like TPMT, TMT enzyme also catalyzes the S-methylation, but in xenobiotic aliphatic sulfhydryl compounds. S-Adenosyl-L-methionine acts as a methyl donor in the reaction (34). TMT catalyzes the S-methylation of sulfhydryl drugs such as captopril and D-penicillamine. This enzyme is present in many tissues including human erythrocytes. However, still at present it remains undetermined whether the genetically regulated level of TMT activity in the erythrocyte also reflects the relative level of TMT activity in other tissues as in the case of COMT and TPMT. From the limited biochemical genetic information on erythrocyte TMT enzyme available at present, experiments of Bremer and Greenberg (4) and Weinshilboum et al (37) show that TMT activity is controlled by inheritance. It has also been indicated that there is a good possibility that genetical inheritance plays an important role in the metabolism of drugs such as captopril and D-penicillamine.

Glucuronide Formation. Certain agents belonging to drug classes, such as antibacterial agents, sedative-hypnotics and antipyretic-analgesics, are disposed through glucuronide conjugate formation by the action of the hepatic glycuronyl transferase. Substances of physiological importance such as bilirubin, vitamins, hormones and so on are also disposed through glucuronide conjugate formation by the action of the hepatic enzyme. Individuals with inherited deficiency of glucuronyl transferase enzyme are affected with a congenital form of nonhemolytic jaundice that is known as Crigler-Najjar Syndrome. This disorder, which is transmitted as an autosomal recessive trait, is also called congenital hyperbilirubinemia because of the presence of excessive amounts of unconjugated bilirubin in the blood.

POLYMORPHISM IN PHARMACODYNAMICS

Adverse reactions may be either normal responses that occur to a greater or lesser degree than a desired response (quantitatively adverse) or an unusual (unique) response (qualitatively abnormal) seemingly involving new receptors (targets) within the organism. A few examples are selected here because they exhibit genetic polymorphism and are clinically relevant (Table 4.1-4).

QUANTITATIVELY ABNORMAL REACTIONS

A genetically determined resistance to the action of oral anticoagulants has been reported (25). In this and subsequent studies two large pedigrees were described in which an autosomal dominant trait for coumarin resistance was recognized (23). In these patients the requirement for vitamin K was greatly increased (24). Even more striking, the required dose for an anticoagulant effect in one patient was observed to be 5-20 times greater than that for his siblings (23). In patients with coumarin resistance, the "normal" dose of an oral anticoagulant is ineffective and most of the evidence suggests defective receptors since the metabolism of these drugs seem to be unchanged.

QUALITATIVELY ABNORMAL REACTIONS

The structure of glucose-6-phosphate dehydrogenase (G-6-PD) is coded at a gene locus on the X chromosome. There are more than 80 different variant forms, each determined by a different allele at this locus (22). They differ from the "normal" enzyme and from each other in electrophoretic mobility, Michaelis constants and pH optima. It seems probable that most, if not all, differ in their structure by single amino acid substitutions in the enzyme. Most important is that the structural differences result in marked changes in the level of activity of the enzyme. G-6-PD in sufficient amounts functions in maintenance of the integrity of red blood cells, particularly in the presence of oxidant drugs such as certain antimalarials, sulfonamides and nitrofurans.

Summarily, the alleles of G-6-PD are rare, but in certain populations they have an unusually high incidence and give rise to a characteristic genetic polymorphism. Some population and their diaspora who have a frequency of more than 1% of the G-6-PD deficiency include Africans, Arabs, Philippinos, Greeks, Indians (Asian), Indonesians, Jews, Kurds, Malaysian, Persian, Romanians, Sardinians, southern Chinese and Thais. The African type (Gd^{a-}) and Mediterranean type (Gd^{b-}) variants have been studied in the greatest detail. Although there

Table 4.1-4
Selected Genetically Determined Adverse Reactions of Pharmacodynamic Origin

Genetic Etiology	Drugs	Adverse Response
Quantitatively adverse		
Defective receptor		
Coumarin resistance	Oral anticoagulants	Resistance to anticoagulation
Qualitatively adverse		
Enzymatic deficiency		
Glucose-6-phosphate dehydrogenase (G-6-PD)	Oxidants	Hemolytic anemia
Methemoglobin reductase	Oxidants	Hemolytic anemia
Hemoglobin variants		
Hemoglobin H	Oxidants	Cyanosis and hemolytic anemia
Hemoglobin Zurich	Sulfonamides	
Disorders precipitated via enzyme-inducing agents		
Hepatic porphyrias	Barbiturates, Griseofulvin	Abdominal pain and paralysis
Unknown etiology		
Malignant hyperthermia	Halothane plus succinylcholine	Increased body temperature

exists a great degree of heterogeneity among the G-6-PD deficiencies, Gd^{b-} may be more severe and result in hemoglobinuria and death (6). In patients with the Gd^{a-} type variant, hemolytic episodes may be arrested at some intermediate level, or it is self-limiting even in the presence of continuous drug administration. The initial hemolysis seems to destroy the older red blood cells, whereas the younger cells seem less vulnerable. In patients with the Gd^{b-} type variant, red blood cells of all ages are destroyed and the hemolytic episodes are not self-limiting. In Gd^{a-} and Gd^{b-} variants the offending drug should be discontinued in the presence of hemolysis, but the Gd^{b-} variant may also require blood transfusion.

Patients with a deficiency of the enzyme methemoglobin reductase may develop methemoglobinemia and cyanosis when given antimalarial drugs such as primaquine, chloroquine, or dapsone (8) and hemolysis may ensue. A genetically determined polymorphism is also responsible for certain red blood cell abnormalities, hemoglobin mutants that are susceptible to hemolysis by certain drugs (3). For example, hemolysis is induced by oxidant drugs in patients with hemoglobin H or Zurich.

Overall, nonimmune hemolysis by oxidant drugs is a relatively rare condition except in populations where erythrocyte abnormalities such as G-6-PD deficiencies or unstable hemoglobins (hemoglobin H or Zurich) exist in high frequency. These abnormalities in some way increase the sensitivity of cells predisposing them to hemolysis by certain drugs.

DISORDERS EXACERBATED BY CERTAIN ENZYME INDUCING AGENTS

The syndrome of acute porphyria is characterized by emotional disturbances, abdominal and muscular pain, and progressively a generalized neuritis and paralysis. The syndrome may be inadvertently precipitated in intermittent acute porphyria, porphyria variegata and coproporphyria by certain drugs such as sedative-hypnotics, antifungals, sulfonylureas, hypoglycemics, anti-anxiety agents, anticonvulsants, and oral contraceptives. These hepatic porphyrias represent several genetically unique disorders that have in common the overproduction of the rate-limiting enzyme, δ-aminolevulinic acid (ALA) synthetase, in the metabolic pathway to porphyrin formation (10). The mechanism for this overproduction may involve an operator gene that is less sensitive to its normal repressor.

In an acute attack, whether it has been precipitated in porphyria variegata, intermittent acute porphyria, or coproporphyria, the patient's life is in danger. In patients with porphyria cutanea tarda, there is photodermatosis that may be precipitated by drugs.

UNKNOWN ETIOLOGY

Malignant hyperpyrexia, a rare complication occurring during general anesthesia, is precipitated by the combination of a general anesthetic (halothane) and a muscle relaxant (succinylcholine). The complication is characterized by hyperthermia, muscular rigidity and acidosis, and represents a serious emergency demanding expert attention. The genetic basis for the condition seems established; however, this does not rule out the possibility that some patients have the complication without a genetic predisposition (5).

REFERENCES

1. Axelrod, J. and Tomchick, R. Enzymatic O-methylation of epinephrine and other catechols. *J. Biol. Chem.* 233:702, 1958.
2. Axelrod, J. and Weinshilboum, R. Catecholamines. *N. Engl. J. Med.* 287:237, 1972.
3. Beutler, E. Drug-induced anemia. *Fed. Proc.* 31:141, 1972.
4. Bremer, J. and Greenberg, D.M. Enzymatic methylation of foreign sulfhydryl compounds. *Biochim. Biophys. Acta* 46:217, 1961.
5. Britt, B.A. Malignant hyperthermia. *Clin. Anesth.* 11:61, 1975.
6. Chan, T.K., Todd, D. and Tso, S.C. Drug-induced hemolysis in glucose-6-phosphate dehydrogenase deficiency. *Br. Med. J.* 2:1227, 1976.
7. Clark, S.W., Glaukbiger, G.A. and La Du, B.N. Properties of plasma cholinesterase variants. *Ann. N.Y. Acad. Sci.* 151:710, 1968.
8. Cohen, R.J., Sachs, J.R., Wicher, D.J. and Conrad, M.E. Methemoglobinemia provoked by malarial chemoprophylaxis in Vietnam. *N. Engl. J. Med.* 279:1127, 1968.
9. Conolly, M.E., Davies, D.S., Dollery, C.T. et al. Metabolism of isoprenaline in dog and man. *Br. J. Pharmacol.* 46:458, 1972.
10. Eales, L. Acute porphyria: The precipitating and aggravating factors. *South African J. Lab. Clin. Med.* 17:120, 1971.
11. Edwards, J.H. Familial predisposition in man. *Br. Med. Bull.* 25:58, 1969.
12. Eichelbaum, M. Polymorphic drug oxidation in humans. *Fed. Proc.* 43:2298, 1984.
13. Gershon, E.S. and Jonas, W.Z. Erythrocyte soluble catechol-O-methyltransferase activity in primary affective disorder. *Arch. Gen. Psychiatry*32:1351, 1975.
14. Hughes, H.B., Biehl, J.P., Jones, A.P. and Schmidt, L.H. Metabolism of isoniazid in man as related to the occurrence of peripheral isoniazid neuritis. *Am. Rev. Respir. Dis.* 70:266, 1954.
15. Kalow, W. *Pharmacogenetics: Heredity and the Response to Drugs.* Philadelphia: Saunders, 1962.
16. Kalow, W. The metabolism of Xenobiotics in different populations. *Can. J. Physiol. Pharmacol.* 60:1, 1982a.
17. Kalow, W. Ethnic differences in drug metabolism. *Clin. Pharmacokinet.* 7:373, 1982b.
18. Kalow, W. Pharmacogenetics and anthropology. In: *Proceedings of the Second World Conference on Clinical Pharmacology and Therapeutics* (Lemberger, L. and Reidenberg, M.M., eds.). Washington, D.C.: American Society for Pharmacology and Experimental Therapeutics, 1984, p. 264.
19. Kalow, W. and Genest, K. A method for the detection of atypical forms of human serum cholinesterase. Determination of dibucaine numbers. *Can. J. Biochem. Physiol.* 35:339, 1957.
20. Kutt, H., Wolk, M. and McDowell, F. Insufficient parahydroxylation as a cause of diphenylhydantoin toxicity. *Neurology* 14:542, 1964.
21. La Du, B.N. and Eckerson, H.W. The polymorphic paraoxonases/arylesterase isozymes of human serum. *Fed. Proc.* 43:2338, 1984.
22. Motulsky, A.G., Yoshida, A. and Stamatoyannopoulos, G. Variants of glucose-6-phosphate dehydrogenase. *Ann. N.Y. Acad. Sci.* 179:636, 1971.
23. O'Reilly, R.A. The second reported kindred with hereditary resistance to oral anticoagulant drugs. *N. Engl. J. Med.* 282:1448, 1970.
24. O'Reilly, R.A. Vitamin K in hereditary resistance to oral anticoagulant drugs. *Am. J. Physiol.* 221:1327, 1971.
25. O'Reilly, R.A. and Aggler, P.M. Determinants of the response to oral anticoagulant drugs in man. *Pharmacol. Rev.* 22:35, 1970.
26. Reilly, D.K., Rivera-Calimlin, L. and Van Dyke, D. Catechol-O-methyltransferase activity: a determinant of levodopa response. *Clin. Pharmacol. Ther.* 28:278, 1980.
27. Shahidi, N.T. Acetophenetidin-induced methemoglobinemia. *Ann. N.Y. Acad. Sci.* 181:822, 1968.
28. Spielman, R.S. and Weinshilboum, R.M. Genetics of red cell COMT activity: analysis of thermal stability and family data. *Am. J. Med. Genet.* 10:279, 1981.
29. Thompson, J.S. and Thompson, M.W. *Genetics in Medicine*, 3rd Ed. Philadelphia: Saunders, 1980, p. 134.
30. Vesell, E. The antipyrine test in clinical pharmacology: conceptions and misconceptions. *Clin. Pharmacol. Ther.* 26:275, 1979a.
31. Vesell, E.S. Pharmacogenetics: Multiple interactions between genes and environment as determinants of drugs response *Am. J. Med.* 66:183, 1979.
32. Weber, W.W. Acetylation pharmacogenetics: experimental models for human toxicity. *Fed. Proc.* 43:2332, 1984.
33. Weinshilboum, R.M. Human pharmacogenetics. *Fed. Proc.* 43:2295, 1984.
34. Weinshilboum, R.M. Human pharmacogenetics of methyl conjugation. *Fed. Proc.* 43:2303, 1984.
35. Weinshilboum, R.M. and Raymond, F.A. Inheritance of low erythrocyte catechol-O-methyltransferase activity in man. *Am. J. Hum. Genet.* 29:125, 1977.
36. Weinshilboum, R.M., Raymond, F.A., Elveback, L.R. and Weidman, W.H. Correlation of erythrocyte catechol-O-methyltransferase activity between siblings. *Nature* (London) 252:490, 1974.
37. Weinshilboum, R.M., Sladek, S. and Klumpp, S. Human erythrocyte thiol methyltransferase: radiochemical microassay and biochemical properties. *Clin. Chim. Acta* 97:59, 1979.

CHAPTER
5

FORENSIC PHARMACOLOGY

Roger P. Maickel

A number of interfaces exist between drugs, medical practice, and the law. It is essential in modern society that every individual involved in the health care system have at least a cursory exposure to those aspects of the law that are intimately involved with the practice of medical therapeutics.

Some facets of forensic pharmacology will be covered elsewhere in this text: illicit drug use (drug abuse), poisoning and toxicology, and the relevant aspects of prescription writing. The topics to be presented in this chapter may be grouped into four categories:

1. Drugs and public safety: An overview of the ways in which therapeutic agents may actively influence the well-being of individuals in the course of their interactions with other individuals or with society as a whole.
2. Federal food, drug and cosmetic laws: A generalized treatment of the interactions of federal laws controlling the use of therapeutic agents in general.
3. Federal drug abuse control laws: A presentation and treatment of the federal statutes and processes regarding those chemicals and therapeutic agents deemed to have significant potential for 'abuse.
4. Drugs and medical malpractice: A brief and selective examination of relevant decisions in judicial cases bearing on the proper and improper use of therapeutic agents in the practice of the healing arts.

The material presented in this chapter is meant for informational, educational and exemplary use. It is not possible to present detailed material on statutes unique to a specific state or locality, nor is it practical to detail every aspect as it relates to each member of the health maintenance team. Rather, attempts have been made to present generalized concepts that may form a basis for more specific learning and judgments by the individual in a unique locale or situation. In addition, some historical perspectives will be given to facilitate a comprehension of the legal and societal aspects of medical therapeutics as the beginning of the twenty-first century approaches.

DRUGS AND PUBLIC SAFETY

Modern society clearly recognizes that its well-being depends on the satisfactory interactions of millions of individuals with other individuals (or groups of individuals) in a diversity of situations. We are also developing an awareness that many chemicals, in addition to those obtained in a pharmacy, possess pharmacological activity (perhaps *biological activity* would be a more precise term) capable of altering the interactions of society's members with each other. Five situations in which an active chemical agent can enter into play and subsequently alter human behavior and performance may be clearly identified. Examples of these situations are:

Agents administered to hospitalized patients
Agents prescribed for and used by outpatients
Agents used for self-medication [over-the-counter (OTC) drugs]
Agents used for "recreational" purposes
Agents present in the environment

In addition to the exposure to a single agent in one or more of these ways, cognizance must also be taken of the possibility of multiple combinations and permutations (polydrug usage); such situations are extremely commonplace. One dramatic example may be noted in the ever-present possibility of the accidental combination of ethanol with a host of agents, ranging from OTC antihistamines to prescription tranquilizers, leading to excessive depression of the central nervous system and even death. In this regard, though the possibility of drug-drug interactions having an adverse effect on the hospitalized patient can theoretically be controlled by the medical care staff, no such control exists for the nonhospitalized subject. When one considers the pharmacologically active agents present in OTC preparations; the widespread use of beverages containing ethanol or caffeine, or tobacco products containing nicotine;

and the exposure incidence of members of society to anesthetic-like volatile solvents (hydrocarbons), toxic gases (carbon monoxide), and plants containing biologically active materials, it seems amazing that drug-drug interactions with adverse effects on the individual are not more numerous than they seem to be.

The role that the modern medical professional must play, in terms of drugs and public safety, is primarily in the dissemination of proper information and the encouragement of a sensible attitudinal development in the patient. Physicians and pharmacists should exercise special care to inform patients of possible hazardous or untoward effects of prescription drugs per se, and should carefully delineate the potential adverse interactions with other drugs — especially OTC agents, caffeine, ethanol and nicotine. Extreme care should be taken to warn patients of the possible adverse effects of drugs that may cause drowsiness (antihistamines, anxiolytics, tranquilizers, etc.) on behavior that requires coordinated psychomotor skills (e.g., driving a motor vehicle or operating machinery). Attention should be paid to warning patients of aspects of drug action that may not be readily apparent to the layperson, such as the morning-after drowsiness following use of sleeping pills, the long duration of action of the desmethyl metabolite of diazepam, or the possible sudden onset of bouts of orthostatic hypotension early in antihypertensive treatment.

From even this brief treatment, it should be obvious to the reader that the members of the health maintenance team bear a heavy burden in the area of public safety in terms of making the patient aware that the pharmacology of therapeutic agents may well include aspects that can be deleterious to the well-being of the individual as well as to other members of society. Though it should not be necessary to apply the concepts and principles of the public health "quarantine," it is most certainly beneficial to society as a whole that the patient who is legitimately using a drug be made fully cognizant of any possible adverse effects that agent may have on his or her ability to perform the usual tasks of daily life.

FEDERAL FOOD, DRUG, AND COSMETIC LAWS

The health care system comes into contact with federal statutes in a number of ways. The present code, known as the Federal Food, Drug and Cosmetic Act, as amended, appears in the U.S. Code under Title 21. A brief review of the historical development of the major federal laws and court decisions in this area is presented in Table 5-1. It must be recognized that most of these federal statutes were passed in response to demands made by the public in response to abuses perceived as being nationwide.

The term *drug* is defined in Sec. 201(g) as

> (A) articles recognized in the official United States Pharmacopeia, official Homeopathic Pharmacopeia of the United States, or official National Formulary, or any supplement to any of them; and (B) articles intended for use in the diagnosis, cure, mitigation, treatment, or prevention of disease in man or other animals; and (C) articles (other than food) intended to affect the structure or any function of the body of man or other animals; and (D) articles intended for use as a component of any articles specified in clause (A), (B), or (C); but does not include devices or their components, parts, or accessories.

The basic constraints of the federal laws with regard to those chemical agents used in human therapeutics are three-fold:

1. *A drug must be pure and accurately labeled* (the 1906 Pure Food and Drugs Act).
2. *A drug must be safe* (the 1938 amendments).
3. *A drug must be effective* (the 1962 amendments).

From this brief review, the obvious conclusions are that the primary burden of compliance with the Federal Food, Drug and Cosmetic Act rests on the shoulders of the pharmaceutical manufacturers. The two areas of most concern to the medical practitioner are in regard to studies of new drugs covered by a Notice of Claimed Investigational Exemption for a New Drug

Table 5-1
Historical Development of Federal Food, Drug, and Cosmetic Legislation

Year	Act	Content/Purpose
1848	National Drug-Import Law	To control quality and purity of imported drugs
1906	Pure Food and Drugs Act	To prohibit interstate commerce of adulterated or misbranded foods and drugs
1912	Sherley amendment	To forbid therapeutic claims that were both false and fraudulent
1938	Food, Drug, and Cosmetic Act amendments	To ensure that manufacturers demonstrate safety, quality and purity of a new drug
1951	Humphrey-Durham amendment	To set up specific definitions for, and classes of, prescription drugs and over-the-counter (OTC) agents
1962	Drug Amendments Act (Kefauver)	To ensure that manufacturers demonstrate efficacy of a new drug

(IND). Any physician participating in clinical studies with such agents must: (1) obtain appropriate informed consent statements from each subject to whom the drug is administered, and (2) keep detailed records of the studies for transmission to the manufacturer.

One other area in which a physician may interact with the Food and Drug Administration (FDA) is that of OTC agents. The FDA does not have jurisdiction over advertised claims for nonprescription drugs. This is the purview of the Federal Trade Commission; the relationship between the two agencies has been solidified by agreements reached in 1954 and updated in 1968. In virtually all situations, the modern physician will interact more directly with state laws regarding the practice of medicine rather than with federal statutes regarding the preparation or advertising of medicines.

FEDERAL DRUG ABUSE CONTROL LAWS

In the area of drugs or other agents that have a significant abuse potential, the health care system is more severely constrained by federal regulations. At the present time, these regulations are contained in the comprehensive Drug Abuse Prevention and Control Act of 1970; the historical development of this legislative area is briefly reviewed in Table 5-2. In contrast to the federal statutes under the Food, Drug and Cosmetic Act, which are primarily concerned with drug safety and purity, the laws dealing with drug abuse control are concerned with everyone from the pharmaceutical manufacturer through the entire health care chain to the drug user.

One of the major aspects of the 1970 law (sometimes referred to as PL 91-513) was the establishment of five "schedules" of controlled substances, as defined and exemplified in Table 5-3. This concept of schedules permits differential treatment of offenses and varying penalties, depending on the schedule in which the drug in question is placed. Basically, as can be seen in Table 5-3, those agents in Schedules I and II would be the most hazardous and have the greatest abuse potential; classification in Schedule I, however, is reserved for those agents having no currently accepted medical use in the United States. Placement of a previously unscheduled agent on

Table 5-2
Historical Development of Federal Drug Abuse Legislation

Year	Act	Content/Purpose
1842	Opium Tax Act	To place a tax on importation of opium for any purpose
1909	Opium Exclusion Act	To prohibit the importing of opium except for medical purposes
1914	Harrison Narcotic Act	To require dealers and dispensers of opium, cocaine, and their derivatives to register annually
1922	Jones-Miller Act	To increase penalties for violation of Harrison Act; limited importation of crude opium and coca leaves for medical purpose *only*
1924	Opium Importing Act	To prohibit importing opium for the manufacture of heroin for *any* use
1928	Revenue Act	To establish social definition of an addict
1937	Marihuana Tax Act	To require payment of tax on all marihuana transactions
1942	Opium Poppy Control Act	To require that domestic growers of opium poppies be licensed by the secretary of the Treasury
1951	Boggs amendment	To establish minimum mandatory sentences for all narcotic and marihuana offenses
1956	Narcotic Drug Control Act	To raise mandatory minimum sentences for conviction of violation of narcotic laws
1965	Drug Abuse Control amendments	To bring amphetamines, barbiturates, and hallucinogens under federal control
1970	Comprehensive Drug Abuse Prevention and Control Act	To establish concept of five drug schedules

one of these schedules, or shifting of an agent from one schedule to another, is done by the U.S. Attorney General with the input and recommendations of the Secretary of the Department of Health and Human Services (DHHS). In fact, the recommendations of the Secretary of DHHS to the Attorney General are binding on the latter official in terms of scientific and medical matters; if the Secretary recommends that an agent not be controlled, that recommendation is binding.

Table 5-3
Definitions and Examples of Scheduled Drugs

Schedule Definition	Examples
Schedule I	
A. The drug or other substance has a high potential for abuse.	Alphacetylmethadol Heroin
B. The drug or other substance has no currently accepted medical use in treatment in the United States.	LSD Marihuana
C. There is a lack of accepted safety for use of the drug or the substance under medical supervision.	Peyote Tetrahydrocannabinols
Schedule II	
A. The drug or other substance has a high potential for abuse.	Amphetamine Codeine
B. The drug or other substance has a currently accepted medical use in treatment in the United States or a currently accepted medical use with severe restrictions.	Hydrocodone Levorphanol Methadone Methylphenidate
C. Abuse of the drug or other substance may lead to severe psychological or physical dependence.	Morphine Opium Oxymorphone Secobarbital Phencyclidine
Schedule III	
A. The drug or other substance has a potential for abuse less than the drugs or other substances in Schedules I and II.	Benzphetamine Glutethimide Methyprylon
B. The drug or other substance has a currently accepted medical use in treatment in the United States.	Nalorphine Phendimetrazine
C. Abuse of the drug or other substance may lead to moderate or low physical dependence or high psychological dependence.	
Schedule IV	
A. The drug or other substance has a low potential for abuse relative to the drugs or other substances in Schedule III.	Chlordiazepoxide Dextropropoxyphene
B. The drug or other substance has a currently accepted medical use in treatment in the United States.	Diazepam Diethylpropion
C. Abuse of the drug or other substance may lead to limited physical dependence or psychological dependence relative to the drugs or other substances in Schedule III.	Fenfluramine Mazindol Pentazocine Phentermine
Schedule V	
A. The drug or other substance has a low potential for abuse relative to the drugs or other substances in Schedule IV.	Loperamide <0.2% Codeine[a] <0.1% Dihydrocodeine[a]
B. The drug or other substance has a currently accepted medical use in treatment in the United States.	<0.1% Ethylmorphine[a] <0.1% Opium[a]
C. Abuse of the drug or other substance may lead to limited physical or psychological dependence relative to the drugs or other substances in Schedule IV.	<2.5 mg Diphenoxylate[b] <0.5 mg Difenoxin[b]

[a] Mixtures of nonnarcotic and narcotic drugs.
[b] Per dosage unit.

Particular aspects of this federal statute that are most relevant to physicians, dentists, nurses and pharmacists are those requiring registration, distribution and dispensing procedures (including aspects of prescription), and storage and record keeping. The responsibility for enforcement lies with the Drug Enforcement Administration (DEA), a unit of the Department of Justice. In addition, state laws may supplement the federal regulations but may not contravene the scheduling principles and characteristics.

DRUGS AND MEDICAL MALPRACTICE

Perhaps no other area is as terrifying to the modern health practitioner as that of medical malpractice and the laws relating thereto. With regard to therapeutic agents, there are seven areas in which specific legal structures may be discussed:

1. A drug may be given that is not the one prescribed.
2. The proper drug may be given in a negligent manner.
3. The patient may become addicted to a narcotic.
4. The drug given may be the wrong one for the patient's illness.
5. The dosage or dosage regimen may be excessive.
6. A serious side effect may occur.
7. A drug allergy may exist.

When the wrong drug is administered by mistake, whether the result is a direct injury to the patient or, because of being deprived of the proper medication, a patient suffers damage, the finding of liability is virtually automatic. The assignment of liability may be to any member of the health care system or some combination of members, depending on the placement of the actual negligent act. For example, a medical technician or nurse administering the wrong solution for test or treatment, a pharmacist dispensing the wrong drug, or a physician administering the wrong agent can each be assigned primary or exclusive responsibility for a negligent act.

Similarly, when a drug dosage is administered in the wrong manner (because of negligence), one or more of the persons involved in the incident may be assigned liability. Thus, in the case of intravenous injection of an agent meant for intramuscular use, the liability rests with the person who made the error and the employer (such as a hospital), but not with the prescribing physician. In general, when a drug is in common use, the physician can rely on nursing personnel to know the correct route of administration; even if the physician does not specify the route, liability is not borne by him. One other possible area of dosage negligence is when an injected dose causes tissue necrosis or other damage because of the nature of the agent or due to poor injection technique. In such cases the person making the injection is generally held responsible, although confounding variables may exist, such as an emergency situation or the need for heroic treatment.

The problems with regard to potential drug addiction of a patient are rather straightforward. For any patient who clearly is terminally ill, extremely aged, or in great pain, the prescription of addictive narcotic analgesics by a physician is clearly justified, even if subsequent addiction does occur. In the case of patients that do not fit any of these classifications, however, there is definite potential liability for the physician. For example, unless one or more nonaddictive analgesic agents are tried first and found to be unsatisfactory, the use of an addictive narcotic is rarely justifiable. When an addictive narcotic is required, the physician's responsibility is twofold. Do not extend treatment beyond the period of absolute necessity, and take proper steps to deal with the addiction problem as soon as medical conditions permit.

The correct drug to be prescribed for a patient's illness is, of course, a question of medical judgment. Such judgment, even if it is upheld only by a modest minority of the medical profession, will clearly remove liability for adverse reactions or for failure of the patient to improve. Should a drug be clearly inappropriate, however, such as the prescription of an antibiotic for a definitively viral disease state, the physician may be liable for either adverse reactions or failure to produce health improvement.

Overdosage of any drug can be the cause of injury and thus can create a liability situation. Proper dosage magnitude and dosage regimens are, of course, matters of medical judgment. A patient's condition may necessitate administration of an agent at a dosage larger than that commonly prescribed or suggested by the manufacturer. The courts will presume that the physician knows the correct dosage and will exercise appropriate care if it is exceeded. The primary burden of proof lies in the plaintiff's demonstrating that the dosage deviated significantly from the manufacturer's recommendations and that this deviation could not be justified on the basis of good medical judgment. Should the overdosage occur by mistake, the physician is clearly liable.

The most common case of drug-related malpractice situations is that of serious side effects of an agent. For example, many cases involving chloramphenicol (a drug that can cause aplastic anemia) have been recorded. Once this serious side effect was identified, warnings were sent to physicians and published in medical journals. Subsequently, liability judgments were assigned to physicians in virtually all cases where the side effect occurred; the only exceptions were in those situations where the illness was shown to be very severe. Even when the drug was shown to be clearly the only effective agent, physicians were held liable for failure to monitor patients' conditions by appropriate laboratory tests.

In all cases of unavoidable side effects, the physician is expected to be cognizant of the predicted adverse effects of the agent. The physician is held responsible for warnings issued by a manufacturer or published in commonly read medical journals; he or she is also bound by other knowledge, such as personal experience. Where the condition of the patient requires administration of a drug known to cause adverse side effects, the situation becomes one of a calculated risk. In general, a twofold burden is placed upon the physician. Use the most effective and least hazardous agent in any given situation, and clearly communicate any necessary warnings to the patient. An example of such a situation would be the case of some more potent nonsteroidal antiinflammatory agents where the physician is presumed to be aware of the potential for gastrointestinal (GI) ulcerogenesis. In such cases clear instructions for drug ingestion with food and warnings to immediately report GI distress and bloody or tarry stools are imperative.

A final area is that of drug-induced allergic reactions, such as anaphylactic shock in penicillin-sensitive individuals. Should such a drug allergy be known to the patient or readily discovered by laboratory tests, it is incumbent upon the physician to be aware of the hazards of medication. The physician is responsible for eliciting such knowledge from the patient and/or confirming it by sensitivity testing; any clear case of administration of an agent to a patient where a known allergy exists is an almost automatic point of liability.

ADDITIONAL READING

Waltz, J.R. and Inbau, F.E. Medical Jurisprudence. New York: Macmillan, 1971.

United States Code, 21 U.S.C. 801-966. Comprehensive Drug Abuse Prevention and Control Act of 1970 Public Law 91-513. October 27, 1970, as amended.

United States Code, 21 U.S.C. 301-392. Federal Food, Drug and Cosmetic Act — Public Law, as amended.

Holder, A.R. Medical Malpractice Law, 2nd ed. New York: John Wiley, 1978.

Section II
DRUGS AFFECTING NEURAL REGULATION OF FUNCTION

CHAPTER
6

PRINCIPLES OF PERIPHERAL AND CENTRAL NEUROTRANSMISSION

Sachin N. Pradhan

GENERAL CONSIDERATION

NEURON AND SYNAPSE

The nervous system which is highly complex in its organization and function, mostly comprises of a specialized cell type called the neuron. A neuron consists of a cell body (soma), a process which carries information from the cell of origin to other cells (axon), and several other processes which receive information from other cells (dendrites). The cell and its processes are covered by a axoplasmic membrane. In some nerves, this membrane is further covered by an insulating sheath of complex lipid mixture (myelin) interrupted at intervals by nodes (node of Ranvier).

Important characteristics of neurons are their electrical excitability and ability to conduct electrical signals over their long axons. During the process of development the nerve cells specialized for conduction and have lost their ability to reproduce. They have very simple processes of metabolism and are extremely sensitive to oxygen lack.

The neuronal processes carry signals from one neuron to another through their points of contact known as the synapse . Depending on the points of contact, various types of synaptic arrangements may occur; thus most commonly the axon of the cell of origin makes functional contact with the dendrites (axodendritic) or the cell body (axosomatic) of the target neuron. Contact may also occur between adjacent cell bodies (somasomatic) or between dendrites (dendrodendritic). Typical axodendritic, somasomatic and dendrodendritic contacts are found within autonomic ganglia. The axon of an interneuron may make contact with an axon terminal of a distant cell (serial axoaxonic), while the latter axon terminal contacts a dendrite, as seen in the dorsal horn of the spinal cord.

Cytological characteristics of neurons resemble those of active secretory cells. They contain (a) large nuclei; (b) mitochondria, organelles scattered in the cytoplasm especially surrounding the nucleus and specialized for oxidative phosphorylation and respiration; (c) microtubules (elongated tubules) present in the axon and dendrites, that provide structural support because of their fibrous protein content and are responsible for transport of macromolecules between the cell body and distal processes; (d) smooth and rough endoplasmic reticulum with clusters of specialized smooth endoplasmic reticulum (Golgi apparatus); and (e) vesicles, large ones in the cell body and small ones near the nerve terminals (synaptic vesicles).

Small vesicles serve as stores for neurotransmitters, and their shape, size and cytochemical properties vary with the neurotransmitter. They accumulate near the presynaptic region from where neurotransmitter are released by process of exocytosis (see below). Presynaptic and postsynaptic membranes show specialized attachment sites which have been called synaptolemma (8). However, autonomic terminals innervating smooth muscles and exocrine glands do not exhibit such synaptolemma. Moreover, many presynaptic terminals show enlargements containing collections of synaptic vesicles often without a synaptolemma.

The neuronal membrane is electrically polarizable. At rest, the potential difference between the inside and the outside of the membrane (i.e. the resting potential) is of the order of -65 to -90 mv, the inside being relatively negative. This resting potential is mostly due to higher (30-50 fold) K^+ concentration inside the neuron compared to that in the extracellular fluid and high permeability of axonal membrane to K^+. Roles of Na^+ and Cl^- which are present in high concentrations in the extracellular fluid are relatively less in this regard because of the less permeability of the membrane at rest to these ions, and lower concentration gradients of these ions across the membrane. Energy-dependent active transport (or pump mechanism) is needed to maintain concentration gradients of the ions.

In response to a stimulus above the threshold level, the membrane permeability to sodium ions increases suddenly and selectively. Sodium ions flow inwards causing rapid deflection of the internal resting potential from its negative to zero and then to a positive value. Thus a local depolarization of the membrane is generated and a nerve action potential (AP) or nerve impulse is initiated. This change is then rapidly compensated by increased permeability to potassium ions which flow outwards, thus resulting in immediate repolarization of the membrane. The region of the axon membrane undergoing these changes remain refractory for a short period. However the ionic channels which are involved in these changes become activated in the adjacent excitable regions causing their excitation and propagation of the AP.

The AP shows 'all-or-none' properties and is constant in form and velocity of conduction for a particular nerve. The speed of conduction depends on the diameter of the nerve fiber. The larger the diameter, the faster is the conduction of the AP. The process of conduction is influenced by myelination of the nerve. In unmyelinated nerves, there is a progressive depolarization along the fibers. However, in myelinated nerves, permeability changes occur only at unmyelinated nodes of Ranvier, and AP is conducted rapidly by jumping from one node to the other (saltatory conduction). Thus the speed of conduction of AP through large diameter (approx. 15 μm) motor fibers is in the order of 100 m/sec, whereas that in the unmyelinated C fibers (diameter approx. 0.5 μm) that conduct the pain sensation, the speed is around 1 m/sec. Conduction of AP is affected by several drugs and toxins that are discussed elsewhere, e.g., local anesthetics (Chapter 10.4), antiarrhythmic agents (Chapter 15.2), tetrodotoxin, saxitoxin and others (Chapter 9).

SYNAPTIC TRANSMISSION

Function of the nervous system, especially the CNS, is dependent upon the interaction between the neurons. During the latter part of the 19th century and early 20th century controversy arose whether there is a continuity between one neuron and the next forming a network (i.e., reticular theory) or the neurons remain separate and independent, but interact across their point of contact or juncture (i.e., 'neuron theory'). The neuron theory was eventually accepted mostly through the histolocial studies of Ramón y Cajal (12).The point of contact or close juncture between neurons was termed the 'synapse' by Sherrington (67) who further suggested that transmission of nerve impulses across synapses would differ from conduction along nerve fibers in several ways; synaptic transmission is one-way and involves certain amount of delay. This delay is known to range from 0.5 to 2 msec (11). Following repetitive presynaptic stimulation at a rapid rate, fatigue of synaptic transmission is manifested (i.e., the number of discharges by postsynaptic neurons first increases and then progressively decreases); however, rapidly repetitive (tetanizing) stimulus applied to presynaptic terminals for a shorter period (than needed to produce fatigue) would usually make neurons more responsive to impulses. This is known as posttetanic facilitation . A number of drugs is known to act selectively at the synapses by modifying neurotransmission.

A controversy further arose between the electrical versus chemical hypothesis pertaining to neurotransmission across the synapse. The electrical field generated due to depolarization of the axonal membrane during conduction of an impulse along the nerve fibre is severely attenuated in the extracellular space in the synaptic region. Synaptic transmission by direct spread of current may occur only in circumstances where large areas of opposing synaptic membrane are in close proximity. Such electrical synapses or ephapses across which electrical current flows permitting transmission of signals are present in invertebrates and some lower vertebrates. Electronic transmission of information has been demonstrated across 'gap junctions' in the CNS (65)

It is now generally accepted that synaptic neurotransmission in the mammals usually occurs through release of specific chemical substances (i.e., neurotransmitters).

NEUROHUMORAL TRANSMISSION

History. Langley (1901) observed that effects of injection of the adrenal gland extract resembled those of the sympathetic stimulation (48). Elliott (1905) suggested that sympathetic nerve impulses acted on smooth muscles by liberating an epinephrine-like substance at the junctional region; he also observed that long after the lesion and degeneration of sympathetic nerves, the effector tissues still showed characteristic responses to the adrenal medullary hormone (24). Dixon (1906) proposed that the vagus nerve released a muscarine-like chemical transmitter (22). Dale (1914) noted a very close similarity between pharmacological effects of acetylcholine (ACh) and responses to stimulation of the parasympathetic nerves and termed the drug effect as parasympathomimetic (21). Loewi (1921) demonstrated that stimulation of the vagus nerve of a perfused frog heart released in the perfusate a substance that could slow the rate of a second heart. He called the substance as 'vagusstoff' (vagus substance: parasympathin) which was later identified as ACh (51).

Loewi (1921) demonstrated an epinephrine-like accelerator substance in the perfusate from the frog's stimulated vagus nerve (a mixed nerve) during the summer when frog's vagus shows a predominance of the sympathetic activity (51). At the same time Cannon and Uridil (1921) reported the release of a similar epinephrine-like substance during stimulation of the sympathetic hepatic nerve; the mediator was termed 'sympathin' by Cannon (13).

This sympathin differed from epinephrine in that epinephrine would produce both excitatory and inhibitory effects, whereas sympathin would produce mainly excitatory effects. Much earlier Berger and Dale (1910) showed that responses to sympathetic nerve stimulation resemble effects of primary sympathomimetic amines more closely than those of epinephrine or other secondary amines (6). Ultimately in 1946 von Euler who observed a close resemblance between norepinephrine and the potent sympathomimetic substance in the highly purified extract of the sympathetic nerve proposed norepinephrine to be the sympathetic neurotransmitter (72).

Sites of Neurotransmission. ACh and NE were accepted as the transmitters released at the postganglionic parasympathetic and sympathetic nerve terminals, respectively. However, neurotransmission at the autonomic ganglia and skeletal neuromuscular junction remained undecided for a long period. Ultimately through the use of newer techniques of intracellular recording and microiontophoretic application of drugs it was established that ACh is the neurotransmitter for all motor nerves at the neuromuscular junction as well as for all preganglionic nerves at both sympathetic and parasympathetic ganglia. ACh is also released at the nerve endings supplying the adrenal medulla. Furthermore, the neurotransmitter role in the CNS has now been established for ACh and NE and so also for dopamine, the precursor of NE. Epinephrine is also being recognized as a central neurotransmitter.

Neurotransmitter: Criteria. Once the evidence that ACh and NE serve as neurotransmitters at various sites in the peripheral nervous system and the neurohumoral transmission across the synapses was conceptually accepted, a large number of substances including amines, amino acids and peptides was indicated for their possible roles as neurotransmitters particularly in the CNS. It became then necessary to formulate the criteria for accepting a chemical as a neurotransmitter. They are as follows: First, the substance must be present in the presynaptic terminals along with its precursor, and the synthesizing enzyme(s) together with any cofactor or ions necessary for its action. Second, the substance should be stored in the presynaptic terminals and must be released from the terminals during the presynaptic nerve activity. The substance can be recovered from the perfusate of an innervated structure during nerve stimulation, but very little, if at all, at rest. Third, the substance must produce its action on the postsynaptic neuron at a specialized site, the postsynaptic receptor, and the effects must be indentical to those of stimulation of the presynaptic pathway. Fourth, the substance should be usually deactivated by the catabolizing enzyme(s) or by re-uptake into the presynaptic terminals or both.

It is difficult for a neurochemical to fulfill all the criteria particularly in the CNS (see latter). However, development of newer techniques have facilitated research on these substances. There are now more than forty such substances and their number is still increasing. It has now been possible to establish several of these substances as neurotransmitters both in the peripheral as well as the central nervous systems. In addition to ACh and NE, other substances such as dopamine, 5-hydroxytryptamine (serotonin), gamma-aminobutyric acid (GABA), substance P and glutamate may be included in this category. However, there are still others which possess many characteristics of a neurotransmitter, but do not fulfill all the criteria. Their role as a neurotransmitter is at present considered as putative. These include histamine, several amino acids, and many neuropeptides.

Multitransmitter Neurons. It was once believed that each neuron, whether peripheral or central, contains one neurotransmitter. There are now many evidences to suggest that more than one neurotransmitter may be present in the same neuron. Thus, enkephalins are found in preganglionic cholinergic neruons (containing ACh), postganglionic sympathetic neurons (containing NE) and adrenal medullary chromaffin cells (containing catecholamines) (27). Vasoactive intestinal polypeptide (VIP) is present in the peripheral cholinergic nerve to exocrine glands (53). Both substance P and ACh are released on stimulation of preganglionic cholinergic nerve to the adrenal medulla (50). The majority of neurons in the rostral ventrolateral medulla projecting to the spinal cord show the presence of substance P-like and phenylethanolamine-N-methyltransferase-like (related to epinephrine) immunoreactivity (52). Part of central serotonin neurons store peptides like substance P, TRF (thyrotropin-releasing factor) and enkephalins (5). Thus these instances appear to show an association of one of the neuropeptides with a traditional amine neurotransmitter.

STEPS IN NEUROTRANSMITTER MECHANISM

Since many drugs serve as an agonist or an antagonist to a neurotransmitter by acting at the various steps of its life cycle, these steps, e.g., synthesis, storage, release, receptor action and disposal of neurotransmitters will be briefly discussesd in general here, and in particular with respect to individual transmitters latter on.

Synthesis. The synthesis of a neurotransmitter occurs within the neuron particularly in the terminal. The precursor of the transmitter which may be present in the diet and is often a common constituent of the body (e.g., an amino acid), enters the neuronal membrane by an active transport system. The enzyme(s) needed for the synthesis are formed in the cell body containing the nucleus that holds the necessary genetic information and may be associated with mitochondrial membrane or freely presented in the neuronal cytoplasm. Macromolecules and organelles can then be transported through microtubules or axoplasmic flow to the nerve terminal where the synthesis occurs. Colchicine, an antigout drug that inhibits mitosis, interferes with the axonal transport by binding to the microtubular protein and disorganizing the microtubular structure.

Storage and Release. The synthesized neurotransmitter is stored in vesicles which remain in the region of the nerve terminal and protect the transmitter from its destruction by cytoplasmic enzymes. During the resting state, the transmitter is released slowly and continually in small amounts that are insufficient to initiate a propagated impulse, but can produce electrical responses on the postsynaptic membrane (miniature end-plate potentials, MEPP) thus indicating physiologic responsiveness of the effector organ.

During nerve stimulation when the AP arrives at the nerve terminal, it causes synchronous release of several hundred quanta. This is initiated by the influx of Ca^{2+} ion into the axonal cytoplasm in response to the AP. Ca^{2+} ions are believed to promote the process of exocytosis causing release of the neurotransmitter. Removal of Ca^{2+} ions from the vicinity of the synapse blocks the neurotransmission.

Presynaptic Receptors. The release of NE or ACh can be inhibited by the action of various chemicals on certain receptor sites in the presynaptic nerve terminals (presynaptic receptors). Presence of NE in the synaptic cleft can inhibit its own release from the nerve terminal by acting on a presynaptic α_2-adrenergic receptor which is hence called 'autoreceptor'. Release of NE can be decreased by α_2-adrenergic agonists and increased by α_2-adrenergic antagonists through their actions on these receptors and also increased by stimulation of presynaptic β_2-adrenergic receptors. α_2-Adrenergic agonists can also inhibit neurally mediated release of ACh from cholinergic neurons. Moreover, release of NE can be inhibited by dopamine, methacholine, adenosine, prostaglandins and enkephalins through their actions on specific presynaptic receptors (47, 54, 69). Binding studies have also confirmed the existence of presynaptic muscarinic receptors on the terminals of catecholamine neurons (33). Decrease of NE release due to α_2-adrenoceptor activation in the central noradrenergic neurons is due to a primary effect at a K^+ channel or at an intracellular Ca^{2+} channel (34).

A similar presynaptic autoreceptor mechanisms inhibiting release of 5-HT appears to exist. These autoreceptors may be somatodendritic, stimulation of which leads to inhibition of firing rate, or may be presynaptic, which on *in vitro* stimulation inhibit impulse-induced 5-HT release (40).

Presynaptic muscarinic receptors have been detected in the cholinergic (parasympathetic) nerves supplying the heart and eye and in the ganglia of the myenteric plexus, which possess postsynaptic muscarinic receptors. Release of ACh which is regulated by these presynaptic receptors, can be blocked by anticholinesterase agents and enhanced by antimuscarinic drugs (41).

Existence of presynaptic cholinoceptive receptors (cholinoceptors) have been proposed in the skeletal myoneural junction. Injection of ACh or an anticholinesterase drug (e.g., physostigmine) into the arterial supply of a skeletal muscle produces fasciculation of muscle fibers of the entire motor unit as well as antidromic action potentials conducted from motor nerve terminals to ventral spinal roots. Both effects are inhibited by curare. These and related observations have led to the suggestion that ACh and some agonists and antagonists act at presynaptic as well as postsynaptic cholinoceptive sites (63).

Action: Postsynaptic Receptors. The released neurotransmitter diffuses across the synaptic cleft and acts on a specialized site, the postsynaptic macromolecular receptor by producing a localized increase in channel permeability to small ions. Depending on the nature of ions, effects of such changes may be of two types: (a) an increased permeability to cations (particularly Na^+) would cause localized depolarization of the membrane resulting in an excitatory effect, i.e., an excitatory postsynaptic potential (EPSP); (b) a selective increase in permeability to only smaller ions such as K^+ and Cl^- which would produce stabilization or hyperpolarization of the membrane, which has an inhibitory effect, i.e., an inhibitory postsynaptic potential (IPSP). These processes involve respective ion-conducting channels or ionophores. The changes in the ionic channel permeability is regulated by the specialized postsynaptic receptor for the neurotransmitter. Depending on whether the receptor responds to ACh or NE, it is termed as cholinergic (or cholinoceptor) or adrenergic (or adrenoceptor) receptor respectively. Each of these receptors are further differentiated into various types and subtypes depending on the site and nature of their action (see latter).

If the postsynaptic potential exceeds a threshold level, an AP is initiated in the postsynaptic neuron or the effector tissue resulting in specific effects, e.g., contraction of a muscle or secretion of a gland. An IPSP would inhibit the effects and oppose the effects of an EPSP initiated by other neurons at the same time and site.

Neurotransmitters can elicit postsynaptic responses through mediation of certain substances serving as second messengers, such as cyclic adenosine 3′,5′-monophosphate (cyclic AMP) and cyclic guanosine 3′,5′-monophosphate (cyclic GMP). Thus the metabolic effect of catecholamines are known to be mediated through cyclic AMP. These substances have been referred to as neuromediators.

Disposal. After the neurotransmitter has produced its effect on the postsynaptic receptor, it is acted on by an enzyme to form an inactive metabolite e.g., inactivation of ACh by AChE to acetate and choline, or removed from the synaptic site by its re-uptake into the presynaptic terminal as in the case of NE. For some neurotransmitters (as for NE), both re-uptake mechanism and inactivation by enzymes (monoamine oxidase, MAO or catechol-o-methyltransferase, (COMT) may be operative (see later).

MISCELLANEOUS NEUROCHEMICALS

In addition to neurotransmitters and neuromediators already discussed, several other types of neurochemicals also play important roles in the CNS. In the brain, there are secretory cells that receive synaptic information from other central neurons and release their secretion directly into the circulation. Examples are posterior pituitary hormones (oxytocin, antidiuretic hormone) secreted by peptide-containing cells of the hypothalamicohypophyseal circuits. These neurosecretory cells have been considered as a form of neuron and the secretions are called neurohormones. However, these hypothalamic neurons may also synapse with neurons in the brainstem and spinal cord, and transmission at these sites may also be mediated by the same substances, but they may not be called neurohormones. Furthermore, while neurotransmitters are usually localized in the nerve terminals, widely distributed, and very rapidly destroyed, and disposed off, neurohormones are localized in discrete areas and have longer duration of action. In addition, several substances (like prostaglandins, substance P, opioid peptides and certain other neuropeptides) have been called as neuromodulators. These substances are capable of influencing neuronal excitability in a less direct manner than the traditionally accepted neurotransmitters. They are of larger molecules than the usually smaller neurotransmitters. They can exert their effects presynaptically by modifying synthesis or release of transmitters from the same or separate nerve terminals, or postsynaptically possibly at the receptor level. The latter agents can also produce their responses through the participation of neuromediators.

NEUROTRANSMISSION IN THE PERIPHERAL NERVOUS SYSTEM

AUTONOMIC NERVOUS SYSTEM

Anatomy. The autonomic nervous system innervates heart, blood vessels, exocrine glands and smooth muscles of various viscera (e.g., gastrointestinal, respiratory and genitourinary tracts) and other structures (e.g., iris and ciliary muscles of the eye and pilomotor muscle of the skin) and regulates various autonomic functions of the body. In contrast to voluntary somatomotor system which innervates the skeletal muscles, function of this system are executed without the conscious control. Hence this system has also been termed as visceral, vegetative or involuntary nervous system.

The autonomic nervous system consists of central and peripheral components. It is evident from investigations in spinal animals including man that elicitation of autonomic reflexes (e.g., involving blood pressure changes, vasomotor responses to alteration of body temperature, sweating, contraction of urinary bladder) can occur at the level of the spinal cord. However, integration of many autonomic functions occurs at supraspinal levels. Thus, regulation of respiration and blood pressure is integrated in the medulla. The hypothalamus plays a prominent role in integration of various autonomic functions e.g., regulation of blood pressure, respiration, body temperature, water balance, sleep, emotions, sexual reflexes, and carbohydrate and fat metabolism. Posterior and lateral hypothalamic nuclei are connected with the sympatho-adrenal system, and anterior and midline nuclei are concerned with parasympathetic functions. The posteromedial hypothalamus is involved in the modulation of the baroreceptor reflex. The other higher centers involved in the integration of various autonomic functions include the neostriatum, limbic system and cerebral cortex. Influence of higher brain centers (e.g., cerebral cortex) on autonomic activity is supported by observations that nervous tension or emotional stress is often associated with autonomic changes (e.g., sweating, increased blood pressure and heart rate, mydriasis, etc.).

Afferent Autonomic Fibers. Autonomic afferent fibers from various viscera pass through the vagus, splanchnic and other autonomic nerves to the CNS. Some autonomic afferents arise from blood vessels of voluntary muscles and certain skin structures and pass through the somatic nerves. Cell bodies of afferent nerves are located in the dorsal root ganglia of spinal nerves and in the corresponding sensory ganglia of certain cranial nerves (e.g., the nodose ganglion of the vagus); their fibers are mostly nonmyelinated.

The afferent fibers mediate visceral sensations (including pain) and participate in various vasomotor, respiratory and viscerosomatic reflexes. Chemoreceptor and baroreceptor reflexes are the examples. Based on the criteria for neurotransmitters (see later) identification of these substances in primary afferents is incomplete in all cases and at present in some cases only circumstantial. L-Glutamate and substance P are the most extensively studied candidates for primary afferent neurotransmitters. L-Glutamate has been implicated as a possible transmitter of large myelinated non-nociceptive (mechanoreceptor) primary afferent fibers. Substance P which is present in the afferent sensory fibers of the dorsal root ganglia and in the dorsal horn of the spinal cord and produces algesic effect is involved in nociceptive afferent neurotransmission. Several other neuropeptides such as vasoactive intestinal polypeptide

(VIP), cholecystokinin (CCK), somatostatin, bombesin which are present in afferent neurons and many of which co-exist with 'traditional' neurotransmitters may also play some role in afferent neurotransmission (64).

Efferent Nerves of the Peripheral Nervous System. Peripheral efferent nerves may belong either to the voluntary (or somatomotor) or involuntary (or autonomic) nervous system. There are certain differences between the efferent nerves of the two systems. The efferent nerves of the somatomotor system originating in the anterior horn cells of the spinal cord or the nuclei of the cranial motor nerves and directly proceed to the skeletal muscles without any interim synapse or terminal plexus. On the other hand, efferent neurons of the autonomic nervous system, emerging out of the brainstem or spinal region, form synapses around cell bodies which remain in clusters (called ganglia) and whose neurons then proceed to innervate the target tissues where effects are produced (effector tissues). Efferent neurons from the brainstem and spinal cord synapsing in the ganglia are called preganglionic fibers, while the ganglionic cell bodies with their axons innervating effector tissues are called postganglionic fibers . Before innervating the effector tissues many autonomic nerves form networks or plexuses. Whereas motor nerves to skeletal muscles and preganglionic fibers of autonomic nerves (which are usually of smaller diameter than motor nerves) are myelinated, postganglionic fibers are generally nonmyelinated. Finally, following lesions or blockade of efferent nerves, skeletal muscles are paralyzed, whereas autonomically innervated smooth muscles and glands generally show some spontaneous activity.

The peripheral component of the autonomic nervous system consists of two divisions: (a) the sympathetic or thoracolumbar outflow, and (b) the parasympathetic or craniosacral outflow (Fig. 6-1).

Sympathetic Nervous System. The sympathetic nerves originate from the cell bodies in the intermediolateral column from the first thoracic to the second or third lumbar segments of the spinal cord. The axons of these cells that form the preganglionic fibers leave the spinal cord along the anterior root, and follow the segmental spinal nerve. They then leave the spinal nerve as myelinated trunk (white rami) and synapse with neurons lying in the sympathetic ganglia located in one of the following areas:

(a) Many fibers terminate in ganglia lying on either side of the vertebral column (paravertebral ganglia) . These ganglia, 22 pairs, are connected to each other by nerve trunks to form two lateral chains. Axons from ganglionic cells (postganglionic fibers) that are nonmyelinated form the gray rami, then pass back to the spinal nerve and are distributed to the effector structures. (b) Located outside the vertebral chain, there are some small intermediate ganglia. They are variable in number and locations and often escape removal during conventional sympathectomy. (c) Some preganglionic fibers pass through the paravertebral ganglionic chain without interruption and synapse with postganglionic neurons in the ganglia lying in the abdomen near the ventral surface of the vertebral column (prevertebral ganglia). These ganglia which are unpaired consist mainly of the celiac (solar) and the superior and the inferior mesenteric ganglia. They are mainly concerned with intestinal movements. (d) A few preganglionic fibers, synapse in ganglia near the organs they innervate (e.g., urinary bladder and rectum); these are called the terminal ganglia.

Parasympathetic Nervous System. This system originates from two sources: cranial outflow consisting of the third, seventh, ninth and tenth cranial nerves, and the sacral outflow. From the Edinger-Westfall nucleus in the tectum of the midbrain emerges the third cranial (oculomotor) nerve which passes via the ciliary ganglia and innervates concentric muscles of the iris and ciliary muscles in the eye. From the medulla, the seventh, ninth and tenth cranial nerves emerge. The seventh cranial or facial nerve forms the chorda tympani which runs into the ganglia lying on and innervating the submaxillary and sublingual glands. The ninth cranial or glossopharyngeal nerve whose parasympathetic fibers originate in the inferior salivatory nucleus pass via otic ganglia to the parotid gland. The tenth cranial or vagus nerve has very wide distribution and innervates the smooth muscles and secretory glands of the viscera of the thorax and abdomen. Its preganglionic fibers are very long and synapse in many small ganglia lying directly on or within the viscera. In the intestine they terminate in the plexuses of Auerbach and Meissner before they synapse with very short postganglionic neruons.

The sacral outflow consists of nerves from second, third and fourth sacral segments of the spinal cord. Preganglionic fibers from these segments proceed to form the pelvic nerves (nervi erigentes) which synapse in terminal ganglia existing near or within the pelvic organs and provide motor and secretary fibers to the terminal portion of the colon, rectum, bladder, uterus, and external genitalia.

Comparison Between Sympathetic and Parasympathetic Nervous Systems. ***Innervation.*** The sympathetic nervous system has a very wide and diffuse distribution; its fibers ramify to a great extent and make synapses with a large number of postganglionic neurons (ratio of pre- to postganglionic neurons being 1:20 or more). Sometimes there is an overlapping of innervation, so that several preganglionic neurons may innervate one ganglion. In contrast, in the parasympathetic system the postganglionic neurons are very short and has 1:1 ratio with the preganglionic neurons (except in Auerbach's plexus the ratio may as high as 1:8000). Distribution of parasympathetic nerve fibers are usually very limited and discrete.

Function. Although the sympathetic nervous system is not essential to life, it protects the organism under stress conditions by regulating circulation, respiration, body temperature and metabolism. Working along with the adrenal medulla as a unit, it prepares the organism for emergency situations e.g., 'flight or fight'. On the other hand, the parasympathetic nervous system which has discrete and localized distribution is concerned with conservation of energy and maintenance of organ function during normal activity.

In most functional systems in the body, these two autonomic nervous systems demonstrate opposite effects and are considered to be physiological antagonists. If a certain function is inhibited by one system, it is usually stimulated by the other. Most viscera are innervated by both autonomic systems and at any time integration of their effects on the viscera determines the level of its activity. However, many autonomic effectors may not have dual innervations. Thus, there is no parasympathetic innnervation of blood vessels. In the eye, while radial muscles of the iris are only supplied by sympathetic nerves, concentric fibers of the iris and ciliary muscles are only supplied by the parasymapthetic third cranial nerve. Actions of the two autonomic systems, instead of being antagonistic, may be complimentary, as observed in male sexual organs in which actions of the two systems are integrated to promote sexual function. Furthermore, there may be a preponderance of influence of one system on some viscera. Thus, there is sympathetic (adrenergic) preponderance on blood vessels, while there is parasympathetic (cholinergic) preponderence on heart, eye, bronchioles, gastrointestinal tract, bladder, and salivary and sweat glands.

Respective effects of adrenergic and cholinergic nerve impulses on effector organs with types of their adrenergic receptors are summerized in Table 6-1.

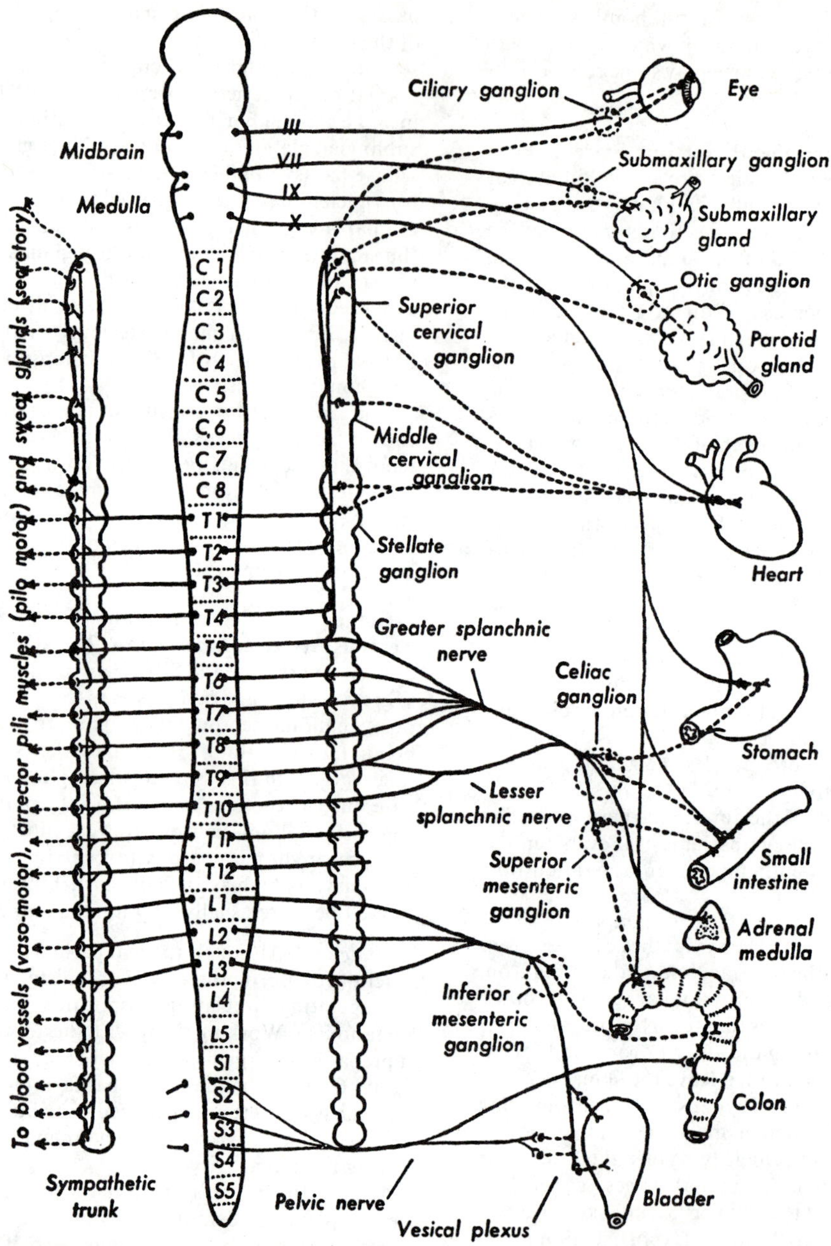

Fig. 6-1. *Connections of autonomic nervous system.*

Courses of preganglionic and postganglionic fibers are shown by intact and broken lines respectively. (From Carpenter, M.B. *Human Neuroanatomy, 7th ed.* Williams and Wilkins, Baltimore, 1976, p. 192, by permission).

ADRENERGIC NEUROTRANSMISSION

History. Adrenergic agents possessing neurohumoral effects generally include three catecholamines: norepinephrine, epinephrine and dopamine. Of these, norepinephrine (NE) is the neurotransmitter for most of the sympathetic postganglionic fibers and certain tracts in the CNS. This substance corresponds to 'Accelerenstoff' of Loewi (1921) which was shown to cause acceleration of the heart when sympathetic nerves were stimulated (51). Earlier, it was considered that epinephrine (but not NE) or both substances were the neurotransmitter(s) at different sites at the postganglionic sympathetic nerve terminals. This concept arose from the observation that sympathetic nerve stimulation caused excitation at some sites and inhibition at others. However, the difference in the responses to these adrenergic agents was later attributed to the existence of two types of adrenergic receptors (or adrenoceptors), as proposed by Ahlquist (2). According to this concept, excitatory responses were mediated by α-receptors, and inhibitory responses were mediated by β-receptors. Furthermore, NE was shown to be the predominant catecholamine in the sympathetic nerves and peripheral tissues by von Euler (72).

Sites. It is now generally accepted that NE which shows predominantly excitatory effects is the neurotransmitter at the postganglionic sympathetic nerve terminals,

Table 6-1
Effects of Autonomic Nerve Impulses on Effector Organs/Tissues

		Adrenergic		Cholinergic
Effector Organ/Tissue	Response[a]	Receptor	Effect[a]	Effect[a]
Eye				
Iris, radial muscle	Contr. (+) (mydriasis)	α_1	++	—
Iris, sphincter muscle	Contr. (+) (miosis)		—	+++
Ciliary muscle	Accommodation[b]	β	-	+++
Heart				
S-A node	Heart rate	β_1	↑ (++)	↓, vagal arrest (- - -)
Atria	Contr., conduc.	β_1	↑ (++)	↓ (- -)
A-V node	Automat., conduc.	β_1	↑ (++)	↓, block (- - -)
His-Purkinje system	Automat., conduc.	β_1	↑ (+++)	little
Ventricles	Contr., conduc., automat.	β_1	↑ (+++)	↓ (?)
Arterioles	Cons. (+), dil. (-)			
Skin and mucosa		α	+++	-
Coronary		α, β_2	+; - -	- (?)
Skeletal muscle		α, β_2	++; - -	-
Cerebral		α	+ (slight)	-
Pulmonary		α, β_2	+ ; -	-
Abdominal viscera		α_1, β_2	+++ ; -	—
Renal		α_1, β_1, β_2	+++ ; -	—
Veins	Cons. (+), dil. (-)	α_1, β_2	++ ; - -	—
Lung				
Bronchial muscle	Contr. (+), relax. (-)	β_2	-	++
Bronchial glands	Secretion	α_1, β_2	↓ ; ↑	↑ (+++)
Stomach (S) and Intestine (I)				
Wall	Motility and tone	α_2, β_2 (S) α_1, β_1, β_2 (I)	↓	↑ (+++)
Sphincters	Contr. (+), relax. (-)	α	+	—
Secretion			↓	↑ (++)
Gallbladder and ducts	Contr. (+); relax. (-)	β_2	-	+
Kidney	Renin secretion	β_1	↑ (++)	—
Urinary bladder				
Detrusor	Contr. (+), relax. (-)	β	-	+++
Trigone and sphincter	Contr. (+), relax. (-)	α	++	- -
Ureter	Motility and tone	α	↑	↑ (?)
Uterus	Contr. (+), relax. (-)	α, β_2	+ (α); - (β_2)[c]	Variable
Sex organs, male		α	Ejaculation (+++)	Erection (+++)
Sweat glands	Secretion	α	Localized (+)	Generalized (+++)
Pilomotor muscles	Contr. (+)	α	++	—
Spleen capsule	Contr. (+), relax. (-)	α, β_2	+++ ; -	—
Adrenal medulla				Epi. & NE secretion
Liver		α, β_2	Glycogenolysis (+++)	Glycogen synthesis (+)
Pancreas acini	Secretion	α	-	++
Fat cells		α, β_1	Lipolysis (+++)	—
Lacrimal gland	Secretion		—	+++
Nasopharyngeal gland	Secretion		—	++
Salivary gland	Secretion (K & water)	α_1	+ (thick)	+++ (watery)
Posterior pituitary	ADH secretion	β_1	+	—

[a] ↑, increase; ↓, decrease; + or -, increase or decrease respectively , number of + or - approximately indicating the intensity of the effect; automat., automaticity; conduc., conduction; cons., constriction; contr. contraction; dil., dilation; relax, relaxation; ADH, antidiuretic hormone; Epi., epinephrine; NE, norepinephrine.

[b] Ciliary muscle relaxation (-) for near vision and contraction (+) for far vision.

[c] Contraction(α) of pregnant uterus, and relaxation (β_2) of pregnant and nonpregnant uterus.

whereas epinephrine which possesses both excitatory and inhibitory effects remains as the major hormone of the adrenal medulla. Dopamine which is mainly present as a precursor to NE, has a minimal independent role in the peripheral nervous system. In the sympathetic ganglia, it is present in the SIF (small, intensely fluorescent) cells and causes inhibition of neurotransmission. It also causes fall of blood pressure by producing dilatation of renal vasculature; this effect is not blocked by α- or β-adrenergic blocking agents. These peripheral effects of dopamine may be due to a local hormone action. However, in the CNS dopamine plays the role of a prominent neurotransmitter in the nigrostriatal (for motor control) as well as mesolimbic and mesocortical (for control of emotional behavior) pathways.

Life Cycle of Catecholamines. Since many drugs used in the treatment of hypertension, psychiatric disorders and other conditions produce their effects by modifying various steps in the life cycle of these catecholamines, their synthesis, storage, release, action, re-uptake and metabolism will be discussed below.

Synthesis. Catecholamines are synthesized from the amino acid precursor, tyrosine. Steps of their synthesis are shown in Figure 6-2 as proposed by Blaschko (7). Tyrosine is available in diet, or in mammals, can be derived from phenylalanine which is also a constituent of diet, by the action of an enzyme phenylalanine hydroxylase present in the liver. Tyrosine is present in the blood from which it is taken up into adrenergic neurons by an active transport stystem. L-Tyrosine which serves as the starting substance for catecholamine synthesis within the adrenergic neurons is converted to dihydroxyphenylalanine (DOPA) by the enzyme tyrosine hydroxylase. This enzyme is stereospecific and converts only naturally occurring L-tyrosine, but not D-tyrosine, tyramine or L-tryptophan. This enzyme is uniquely present in the axoplasm of the adrenergic nerve terminal and also in chromaffin cells of the adrenal medulla and is activated by stimulation of adrenergic nerves and the adrenal medulla. The action of the enzyme is facilitated by the cofactor, tetrahydropteridine and presence of Fe^{2+}, and regulated by the concentration of the end product so that high concentration of NE in the adrenergic nerve terminals inhibits the enzyme. The enzyme is thus subject to end product feedback inhibition (76) and therefore hydroxylation of tyrosine is generally considered as the rate-limiting step in catecholamine biosynthesis (75). Therefore, at this step of biosynthesis pharmacological intervention (such as by metyrosine, an inhibitor of tyrosine hydroxylase) is effective in modifying the NE content of adrenergic neurons.

Phenylalanine

Tyrosine

Tyrosine hydroxylase

Dihydroxyphenylalanine (DOPA)

DOPA decarboxylase

Dopamine

Dopamine β-hydroxylase

Norepinephrine

Phenylethanolamine N-methyltransferase

Epinephrine

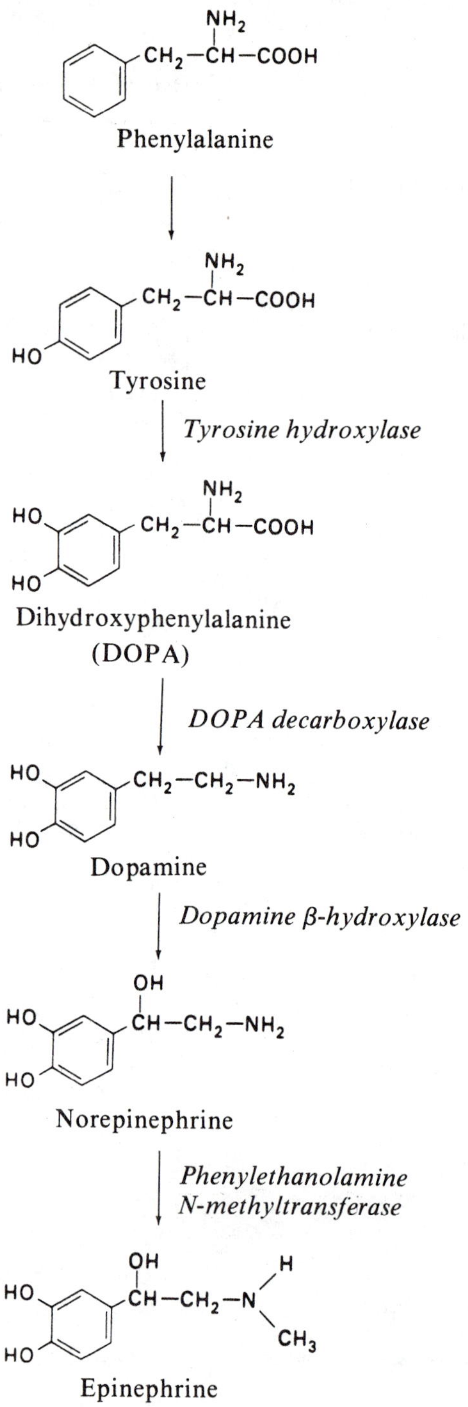

Fig. 6-2. *Synthesis of catecholamine neurotransmitters.*

The next step in the catecholamine biosynthesis involves decarboxylation of L-DOPA to dopamine by mediation of the enzyme DOPA-decarboxylase. Compared to tyrosine hydroxylase, this enzyme is more widely distributed, occurs in the axoplasm of adrenergic nerve terminals as well as in non-nervous tissues like liver, stomach and kidney, and has much higher activity. It requires pyridoxal phosphate (active form of vitamin B_6 as a cofactor. This enzyme is not specific for L-DOPA and also acts on other catecholamine precursors (e.g., tyrosine) as well as other L-amino acids (e.g., 5-hydroxytryptophan, etc.). It can also decarboxylase the drug methyldopa to methyldopamine.

Dopamine is then converted to NE through mediation of the enzyme dopamine-β-hydroxylase (DBH). In contrast to the enzymes tyrosine hydroxylase and DOPA-decarboxylase which are present in the cytoplasm of adrenergic neurons, DBH exists in the vesicles or granules which are localized near the nerve terminals. Synthesis of NE which requires ascorbic acid and fumeric acid as cofactors, occurs within the vesicles. The action of DBH on dopamine is not specific; DBH can act on structurally analogous compounds, such as α-methyldopamine converting it to α-methylnorepinephrine that acts as a 'false transmitter'.

Storage. The synthesized NE remains stored in the vesicles until its release. The vesicles, 0.05-0.2 μm in diameter, are noted as electron-dense granules in electron micrograph, small ones being seen in adrenergic nerve terminals and larger ones in the cell body and axon. They are similar to those at the cholinergic nerve terminals, but can be distinguished by their histochemical staining properties and electron-dense appearence. They contain very high concentration of catecholamines, DBH, ATP, ascorbic acid, some specific proteins (chromogranins) and peptides (e.g., enkephalin precursors). Vesicles not only store catecholamines, but also protect them from being destroyed by intraneuronal monoamine oxidase (MAO).

Release. The sequence of events leading to release of NE following arrival of nerve impulses in adrenergic neurons is not fully known. It would probably resemble that in the adrenal medulla where the release is triggered by liberation of ACh in preganglionic fibers; ACh then interacts with nicotinic receptors in chromaffin cells and produces localized depolarization. This leads to an influx of Ca^{2+} into these cells resulting in liberation of granular contents by the process of exocytosis. The released contents include catecholamines, ATP, some vasoactive peptides or their precursors, chromogranins and DBH (16, 42, 71, 74, 77). Similar role of Ca^{2+} in the process of exocytosis and transmitter release has been demonstrated in case of ACh and appears to occur for NE at the adrenergic nerve terminals. Increased concentrations of DBH and chromogranins in the circulation during increased sympathetic nerve activity also indicate occurrence of exocytosis during NE release. In addition to Ca^{2+}, other factors may influence release of the transmitter from adrenergic nerve terminals (and also possibly other nerve terminals). Several cytoplasmic proteins (e.g., tubulin, calmodulin, neurin, stenin, synexin, chromobindins) have been shown to influence the process of exocytosis by inducing fusion of granular membrane with the plasma membrane (18, 19, 74).

Release of NE can be regulated by the presence of the neurotransmitter in the synaptic cleft (feed-back inhibition). As mentioned earlier, this has been thought to be due to the existence of 'presynaptic receptors' on which the neurotransmitter act to modulate its own release from presynaptic terminals. Some agonists (e.g., clonidine) has been shown to reduce the stimulus-induced release by acting on these presynaptic receptors. There may be more than one presynaptic receptor on adrenergic nerve terminals.

It has been observed that recently stored NE is released preferentially by nerve stimulation or by action of some drugs (e.g., amphetamine, ephedrine, etc.). On this basis the store of NE has been differentiated into two 'pools' -readily releasable and bound (see Chapter 7).

Action. NE released from sympathetic nerve terminals produces effects on various target tissues e.g., smooth muscles, heart, blood vessels and glands. On the smooth muscles, NE as well as other catecholamines can cause either excitation or inhibition of contraction depending on the catecholamine, dose, and site of action. Thus NE possesses predominantly excitatory actions, whereas isoproterenol shows potent inhibitory actions; epinephrine produces both excitatory and inhibitory effects. Depending on the nature of actions, different receptors have been proposed for catecholamines.

Adrenergic Receptors and Subtypes. Ahlquist (2) in 1948 attributed these actions to two different types of receptors and termed them α (excitatory) and β (inhibitory) adrenergic receptors (adrenoceptors). This classification was further corroborated by the capability of the then available certain agents (e.g., phenoxybenzamine) to block the actions related to α-adrenoceptors, but not those related to β-adrenoreceptors, inhibitors for which are now available. On the basis of this classification, α-receptor actions includes excitatory effects (e.g., smooth muscle contraction, blood vessel constrictions), whereas β-receptor actions comprise inhibitory effects (e.g., smooth muscle relaxation, vasodilatation) and cardiac effects [e.g., chronotropic (increase in rate) and inotropic (increase in force of contraction)]. Such receptor actions were also identified in metabolic and CNS effects. Further details are discussed in Chapters 7, 7.1 and 7.2.

Both α and β adrenoceptors have been further differentiated into subtypes (57). Thus β receptors have two subtypes: β_1 has a high affinity for both NE and epinephrine and is found in heart, brain and adipose tissue; and β_2 has a low affinity for NE and is involved in mediation of relaxation of smooth muscles in blood vessels, bronchioles and uterus, and in many metabolic effects. In case of α-adrenoceptors, α_1 subtype is related to excitatory effects (e.g., contraction of smooth muscles, vasoconstriction, etc.) and has a predominant postsynaptic location. On the other hand, the α_2 subtype is mainly localized on presynaptic autonomic nerve terminals. In the adrenergic nerve terminals α_2 receptors appear to produce feedback inhibition of NE release, and serve as autoreceptors involved in regulation of NE release. In the cholinergic nerve terminals in the GI tract such receptors probably mediate inhibitory effects of α-adrenergic agonists. α_2-Receptors also appear to be present postsynaptically in the extrasynaptic sites in blood vessels and in the CNS. Selective agonists and antagonists for α and β receptor subtypes are available (Chapter 7.1 and 7.2), some of which are of therapeutic importance.

Contraction of smooth muscle (e.g., guinea pig vas deference) due to adrenergic nerve stimulation resembles the excitatory effect of ACh and results from localized partial depolarization of the muscle membrane and subsequent increased Na^+ conductance. On the other hand, mechanism of smooth muscle relaxation (e.g. in the GI tract) induced by adrenergic nerve stimulation appears to be complex. α-Receptor stimulation of the smooth muscle causes activation of Ca^{2+}-dependent potassium channels resulting in hyperpolarization. However, actions of adrenergic agonists on presynaptic α_2 receptors in cholinergic nerve terminals which stimulate smooth muscles appear to be important; these agents hyperpolarize the neuron and inhibit the firing rate causing muscle relaxation. These agents may also act on β-adrenoceptors by increasing cyclic AMP (see below).

Mechanism of Metabolic Action. Epinephrine and its congeners produce a number of metabolic effects such as an increase of blood glucose, lactic acid and free fatty acid, transient increase of plasma potassium and increased oxygen consumption. Many of these metabolic effects of catecholamines are produced by activation through β-adrenoceptor action of a membrane-bound protein, adenylate cyclase. The interaction of β-adrenoceptors with adenylate cyclase requires a guanine nucleotide-binding regulatory protein that activates the catalytic component of adenylate cyclase. This enzyme mediates the conversion of ATP to cyclic AMP which is responsible for the metabolic effects of catecholamines. For example, hyperglycemia induced by catecholamines and by glucagon is produced through the action of cyclic AMP which causes (a) activation of hepatic glycogen phosphorylase, the enzyme which converts glycogen to glucose-1-phosphate, and (b) inactivation of glycogen synthetase, the enzyme that promotes synthesis of glycogen by catalyzing the transfer of glycoxyl units from UDP-glucose. Through these dual actions cyclic AMP increases conversion of hepatic glycogen to blood glucose. In the muscle which does not contain glucose-6-phosphatase, lactate becomes the end product of glycogenolysis leading to hyperlactacidemia. In the adipose tissue, activation of triglyceride lipase through similar type of reactions results in hyperlipemia (Fig. 7.1-1 in Chapter 7.1). Thus these metabolic effects of catecholamines appear to be mediated through cyclic AMP. These substances like cyclic AMP and cyclic GMP which mediate the postsynaptic responses of neurotransmitters serve as second messengers and are referred to as neuromediators.

Termination of Action. Termination of actions of NE and epinephrine occurs in two ways: (a) by re-uptake into nerve terminals or also at extraneuronal sites following its diffusion away from the synaptic cleft; (b) by metabolic disposal.

Re-uptake. Uptake of NE into adrenergic nerve terminals involves at least two carrier-mediated active transport systems: one, from the extracellular fluid to the cytoplasm across the axoplasmic membrane; and the other, from the cytoplasm into storage vesicles (granules) across the vesicular membrane. The transport system across the granular membrane, particularly in the adrenal medulla requires ATP and Mg^{2+} ion. The adrenergic neuronal uptake system which has been termed as uptake-1 has high affinity for NE, lower affinity for epinephrine and no affinity for isoproterenol. In contrast, an extraneuronal amine transport system which is present in glia, heart, liver and other non-neuronal tissues and termed uptake-2, shows a reverse order of affinity, being lowest for NE and highest for isoproterenol. Uptake-2 is inhibited by metanephrine and corticosteroid, but not by imipramine like uptake-1. Uptake-2 system may not be of much physiological importance other than for disposal of circulating catecholamines.

Metabolism. Metabolic transformation plays a secondary role in the termination of actions of catecholamines, the reuptake mechanism being the primary one. Two enzymes - monoamine oxidase (MAO) and catechol-O-methyltransferase (COMT) are involved in the initial steps of their metabolism. The enzymatic mechanism to dispose catecholamines in the adrenergic nervous system is less effective than acetylcholinesterase (AChE) in the cholinergic nervous system.

MAO is widely distributed in the body, highest concentration occurring in liver and kidney; it is also present in brain, intestine and all parts of sympathetic nervous system. This enzyme is mostly localized to the outer surface of mitochondria including those within the adrenergic nerve terminals. It causes oxidative deamination of catecholamines (e.g., NE, epinephrine, dopamine) as well as indolamines (e.g., 5-hydroxytryptamine). Because of the predominant intraneuronal distribution of this enzyme, oxidative deamination by MAO does not probably play an important role for removal of NE from the synaptic cleft. It is more likely to be concerned with regulating the content of the cytoplasmic NE pool. It has no effect on the stored NE in the vesicles. Inhibition of MAO does not markedly potentiate the effects of sympathetic stimulation. However, they can cause an increase in levels of biogenic NE, dopamine and serotonin in the brain and can produce significant central and peripheral effects (Chapter 11.5.2).

The enzyme COMT which inactivates NE, epinephrine and other catechols, catalyzes the transfer of methyl groups from S-adenosyl methionine to form metahydroxy compounds (e.g. normetanephrine or metanephrine from NE or epinephrine respectively). Like MAO, this enzyme is also widely distributed in various tissues in the body including the brain, the highest concentrtion occurring in the liver and kidney. Unlike MAO, it is present largely in the cytoplasm and to a smaller extent in the membranes. Most of the catecholamines that are released from the adrenal medulla or sympathetic nerve terminals and enter into circulation are metabolized by COMT. However, inhibition of this enzyme has little potentiating effect on sympathetic stimulation.

Most circulating NE or epinephrine is first O-methylated by COMT to normetanephrine or metanephrine respectively, whereas intraneuronally released NE is initially deaminated by MAO to 3,4-dihydroxyphenylglycolaldehyde (DOPGAL) (as under reserpine action). This aldehyde is either reduced to the glycol, 3,4-dihydroxyphenyl ethylene glycol (DOPEG) by aldehyde reductase (usually in the CNS) or oxidized to 3,4-dihydroxymandelic acid (DOMA) (usually in extraneuronal sites such as liver or intestine). Most of the metabolites formed by either COMT or MAO are then converted by the other enzyme (MAO and related enzymes, or COMT respectively) to the common product either 3-methoxy-4-hydroxyphenylethylene glycol (MOPEG or MHPG) or 3-methoxy-4-hydroxymandelic acid ('vanillyl mandelic acid', VMA as it has been called). Formation of these and other metabolites are shown in a schematic (Fig. 6-3). Similar metabolic degradation of dopamine (the precursor of NE without β-OH group) to homovanillic acid (HVA) and dihydroxyphenyl acetic acid (DOPAC) is described latter in this chapter and also in Chapter 7.4. In a normal adult, 24-hr urine sample may contain VMA (2-4 mg), MHPG (1.2-1.8 mg; about one-fourth of the content is central in origin), normetanephrine (0.1-0.3 mg), metanephrine (0.1-0.2 mg) and some free NE (20-50 μg) and epinephrine (2-5 μg) (31).

CHOLINERGIC NEUROTRANSMISSION

Site. It is now established that in the peripheral nervous system, acetylcholine (ACh) is released and serves as a neurotransmitter at postganglionic parasympathetic (innervating heart, blood vessels, smooth muscles and exocrine glands) and a few sympathetic nerve terminals (e.g. those at the sweat glands and smooth muscle walls of blood vessels in the skeletal muscle), autonomic ganglia, skeletal myoneural junctions and adrenal medulla. It also plays a significant functional role in many areas of the CNS (see latter).

Life Cycle of Acetylcholine. As in the case of catecholamines, many drugs produce their effects by modifying various steps in the life cycle of ACh; these steps in its life cycle will be discussed here.

Synthesis. ACh is synthesized by interaction of choline and acetyl-coenzyme A (acetyl-CoA) catalyzed by the enzyme choline acetyltransferase (choline acetylase). Choline is an essential constituent of diet and found in most tissues of the body. It is taken up from the extracellular fluid into the neural tissue by the active transport. Such uptake which appears to be the rate-limiting step in ACh biosynthesis is mediated by distinct high- and low-affinity sytems. The high-affinity system is found to be responsible for transport of choline to the cholinergic nerve ending. This system is sodium-dependent and inhibited by hemicholinium.

Acetyl-CoA is derived by transacetylation of CoA from a compound acyladenylate (acetyl-AMP) which is formed by reaction of acetate with adenosine triphosphate (ATP) catalyzed by the enzyme acetate thiokinase. Acetyl-CoA is synthesized in the mitochondria present in a large number in the axonal terminal.

The enzyme choline acetyltransferase which is unique to cholinergic neurons is synthesized within the neuronal cell body, like other protein constituents, and then transported to the axonal terminal. The final step in ACh synthesis occur in the cytoplasm mostly in the axonal terminal. Inhibition of choline acetyltransferase has not proved to be therapeutically effective, because neither this enzyme action is not a rate-limiting step, nor are highly potent selective inhibitors available. Synthesis and degradation of ACh are summarized in Fig. 6-4.

Storage and Release. Following its synthesis, ACh is stored in synaptic vesicles present in the presynaptic nerve terminal. These vesicles are 300-600 Å in diameter. Principles of storage and release of ACh, which have been mostly learned from experiments on motor end-plates, probably apply to other sites of cholinergic transmission as well (44, 62).

When action potentials generated by nerve stimulation arrive at the motor nerve terminal, ACh is discharged from the vesicles into the synaptic cleft by a process of exocytosis, as also described for catecholamines. ACh content per synaptic vesicle has been estimated to range from 1000 to over 50,000 molecules. A single motor nerve terminal may contain 300,000 or more molecules of ACh. Release of ACh which is Ca-dependent is facilitated by excess of Ca^{2+} ions and inhibited by excess of Mg^{2+}.

Action. Released ACh molecules then act on the receptor located in the postsynaptic membrane, probably inducing a conformational change in the receptor; as a result the membrane becomes suddenly permeable to cations, especially Na^+, causing its depolarization. This activity is localized only in the synaptic region and of brief duration, because released ACh that is responsible for such action is rapidly hydrolyzed by the enzyme AChE (see below).

At resting state, recording from the motor end plate of skeletal muscle show small (approximately 0.1 to 3.0 mV), spontaneous (about 1/sec) depolarizations (called miniature end-plate potentials, MEPP). These are too much below the threshold level to cause muscle action potential. These potentials can be enhanced by physostigmine and blocked by *d*-tubocurarine indicating that they are ACh-induced. These show that ACh is released from motor nerve endings in constant amounts or quanta. When nerve impulses reach presynaptic terminals, a large number of vesicles discharge ACh into the synaptic cleft causing depolarization of the postsynaptic membrane; if the threshold level is reached, this results in a propagated action potential in the muscle leading to its

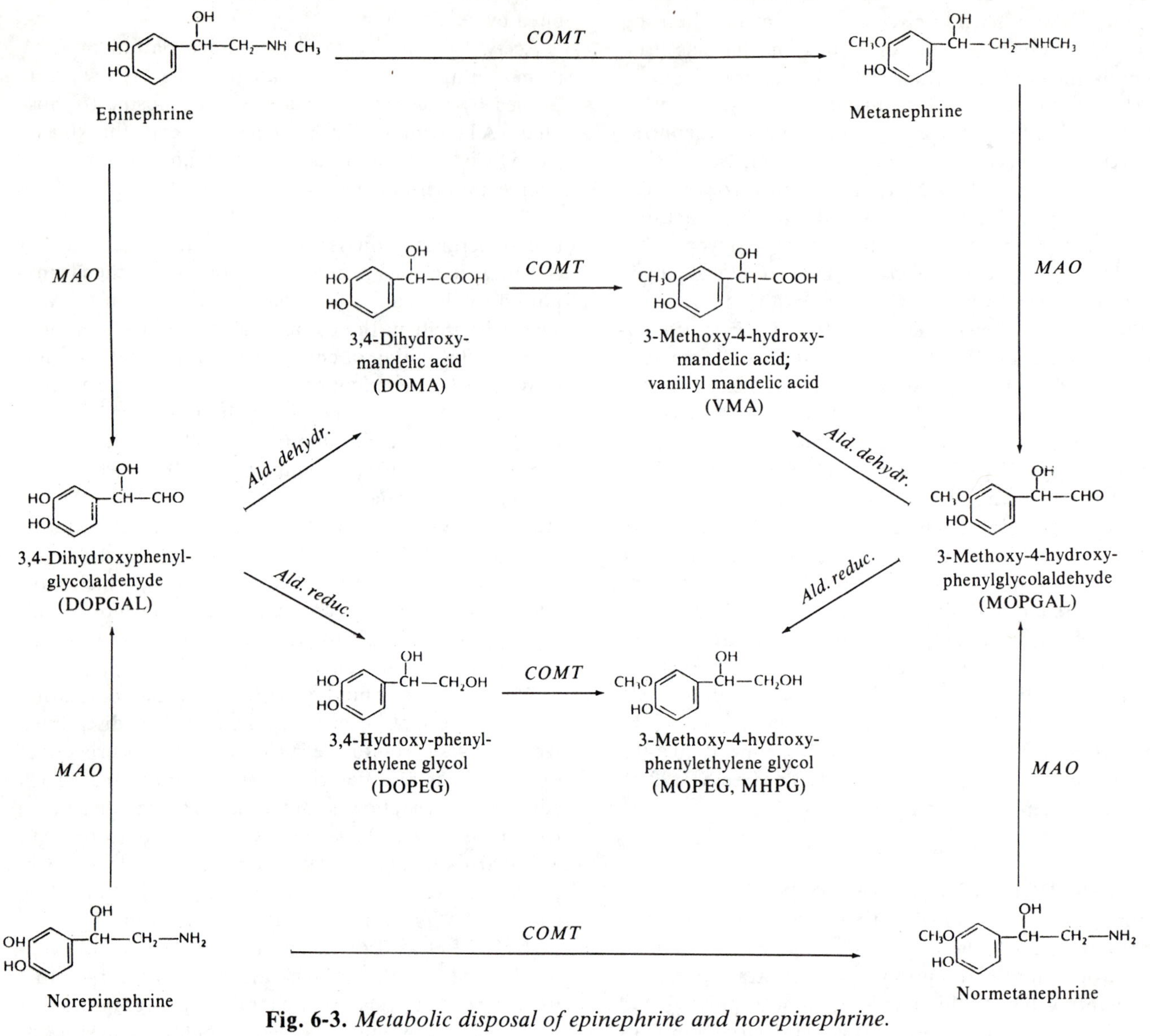

Epinephrine — COMT → Metanephrine

MAO

3,4-Dihydroxy-mandelic acid (DOMA) — COMT → 3-Methoxy-4-hydroxy-mandelic acid; vanillyl mandelic acid (VMA)

Ald. dehydr.

3,4-Dihydroxyphenyl-glycolaldehyde (DOPGAL)

3-Methoxy-4-hydroxy-phenylglycolaldehyde (MOPGAL)

Ald. reduc.

3,4-Hydroxy-phenyl-ethylene glycol (DOPEG) — COMT → 3-Methoxy-4-hydroxy-phenylethylene glycol (MOPEG, MHPG)

MAO

Norepinephrine — COMT → Normetanephrine

Fig. 6-3. *Metabolic disposal of epinephrine and norepinephrine.*

contraction. Further details of the mechanism of muscle contraction has been discussed in Chapter 9.

ACh released from postganglionic autonomic nerves acts on various effectors sites e.g., heart, blood vessels, smooth muscles and exocrine glands. Actions of ACh at these sites resemble those of the alkaloid muscarine and are termed *muscarinic*; they are inhibited by anticholinergic alkaloids (e.g., atropine, scopolamine) and synthetic drugs (Chapter 8.3). On the other hand, actions of ACh released at autonomic ganglia and neuromuscular junctions resemble those of the alkaloid nicotine and hence termed as *nicotinic*. These actions are blocked by respective antagonists such as ganglion blocking agents (Chapter 8.4) and neuromuscular blocking agents (Chapter 9.1). Muscarinic and nicotinic actions of ACh which are mediated by muscarinic (M) and nicotinic (N) receptors respectively are further discussed in Chapter 8.

ACh produces dilatation of isolated blood vessels with intact endothelium. Such vasodilatation induced by an administered choline ester may involve several sites of action including prejunctional inhibitory synapses on the sympathetic nerve fibers and inhibitory cholinergic receptors in the vasculature that are not innervated. Activation of muscarinic receptor apparently causes release of a vasodilator substance (endothelium-dependent relaxing factor) that relaxes the smooth muscle (26).

Disposal. Acetylcholine is rapidly hydrolyzed into acetate and choline by the enzyme AChE. The hydrolysis product choline has only 10^{-5} vasodepressor potency of ACh. Recent biophysical methods have demonstrated that such inactivation of ACh by hydrolysis occurs in less than a millisecond. Enzymes that hydrolyze ACh have been distinguished into two classes depending on their substrates. Thus, AChE that acts specifically on ACh has

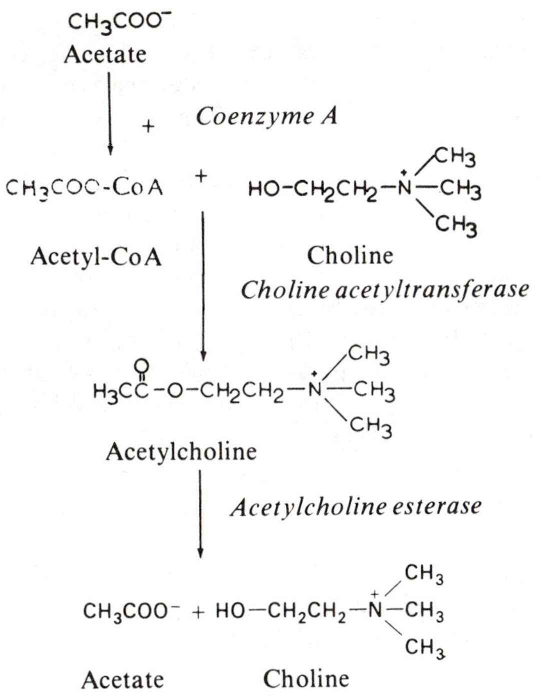

CH_3COO^-
Acetate
↓ + *Coenzyme A*
$CH_3COC\text{-}CoA$ + $HO\text{-}CH_2CH_2\text{-}\overset{+}{N}(CH_3)_3$
Acetyl-CoA Choline
↓ *Choline acetyltransferase*
$H_3C\overset{O}{\overset{\|}{C}}\text{-}O\text{-}CH_2CH_2\text{-}\overset{+}{N}(CH_3)_3$
Acetylcholine
↓ *Acetylcholine esterase*
$CH_3COO^- + HO\text{-}CH_2CH_2\text{-}\overset{+}{N}(CH_3)_3$
Acetate Choline

Fig. 6-4. *Synthesis and degradation of acetylcholine.*

been termed true or specific cholinesterase. It is present in neurons, neuromuscular junctions, and also in certain noncholinergic nerves and other tissues (e.g., erythrocytes). It hydrolyzes ACh in the close vicinity of the nerve ending immediately following its release. On the other hand, another esterase that specifically hydrolyzes butyrylcholine also hydrolyzes ACh. It is present in glial cells, serum, liver, but only slightly in the central and peripheral neuronal tissues. This enzyme is called as butyrylcholinesterase, and also cholinesterase, psuedocholinesterase and serum cholinesterase. While the specific substrate for true AChE is acetyl-β-methylcholine and that for pseudocholinesterase is butyrylcholine, ACh is hydrolyzed by both types of enzymes. Both the enzymes are inhibited by agents known as anticholinesterases such as physostigmine, isoflurophate and others. Further details about these enzymes, their actions, and their inhibition by drugs are discussed in Chapter 8.2.

NEUROTRANSMISSION IN THE CENTRAL NERVOUS SYSTEM

BRAIN REGIONS AND DRUG ACTIONS

A number of brain areas which are responsible for many important physiological functions serves as sites of action of centrally acting drugs.

Cerebral cortices contain not only the areas controlling the motor, sensory and special sensory functions, but also the association areas which are involved with attention, memory, consciousness and abstract thought. These areas may also influence autonomic functions involving cardiovascular and gastrointestinal systems through conscious feedback controls. General anesthetics and other CNS depressant drugs act on these areas.

The *limbic system* which is considered to be mainly involved with emotional control, consists of cortical areas (e.g., olfactory and pyriform lobes, hippocampal gyrus) and subcortical structures (e.g., amygdala and septum). The hypothalamus, anterior thalamic nuclei, the epithalamus, and parts of the basal ganglia are also included in the limbic system by some authors, because of the connections of these structures with other areas and their functional implications. Areas of the neocortex may also be involved in emotional behavior.

The *hippocampus* has been considered to be of importance in the formation of recent memory and in memory loss in Alzheimer's disease. The *hypothalamus*, in addition to regulation of emotion, integrates a number of autonomic functions involving cardiovascular and neuroendocrine systems, and temperature regulation among many others. Visceral functions are also regulated by the thalamic nuclei and the basal ganglia.

The limbic structures through their connections with the extrapyramidal areas (basal ganglia) and the hypothalamus integrate emotional states with motor and visceral activities. Antipsychotic, antianxiety, antidepressant and antimanic drugs are considered to act on these and related areas.

The *brainstem* consisting of the medulla, pons, midbrain and a portion of diencephalon accommodates a very important functional system, the *reticular activating system (RAS)*. The RAS which consists of the reticular formation and the nonspecific thalamocortical projections to the cerebral cortex is involved with central integration for coordination of essential reflexive acts (such as vomiting) and of cardiovascular and respiratory functions. However, RAS is primarily responsible for regulation of sleep and wakefulness. Lesions in the RAS at the midbrain or low diencephalic levels produce permanent sleep and synchronization of EEG (showing low frequency, high voltage waves). On the other hand, electrical stimulation of the RAS produces arousal manifested by behavioral signs of wakefulness with EEG desynchronization (showing low voltage, high frequency waves). Barbiturates and other general anesthetics can produce EEG synchronization and block EEG desynchronization produced by reticular stimulation, thus indicating the RAS as a major site of action of these drugs. Conversely, the CNS stimulants such as amphetamine produce behavioral stimulation and EEG desynchronization presumably also acting through the RAS. However, the CNS depressants and stimulants act at several sites in the CNS, although some site(s) may be predominantly affected.

The *cerebellum* which plays an important role in maintenance of posture may be affected by drugs producing ataxia.

The *spinal cord* with its afferent and efferent peripheral and autonomic nerves plays important roles in many motor, sensory and autonomic functions and somatic and autonomic reflexes. CNS stimulants (e.g., strychnine), general anesthetics, narcotic analgesics are some examples of the drugs acting on the spinal cord.

CENTRAL NEUROTRANSMITTERS

In the CNS several neurotransmitters are involved in mediation of actions of some drugs e.g., reserpine, cocaine, amphetamine, etc. Some neurotransmitters have also been implicated in certain diseases, e.g., dopamine in Parkinson's disease and schizophrenia, biogenic amines in depression and mania. With the discovery of opioid peptides, there has been a great surge of research on central neurochemicals. More than forty neurochemicals have now been indicated or proposed to play the role of a central neurotransmitter. It is however necessary that they should fulfill the criteria of a neurotransmitter before they are designated such a role.

Fulfillment of Criteria of a Central Neurotransmitter. Compared to ACh and NE as neurotransmitters in the peripheral autonomic nervous system, neurochemicals at synapses in the CNS face extreme difficulty in fulfilling the criteria required to be qualified as neurotransmitters. However, in recent years development of sophisticated newer techniques have solved some but not all of the problems. Thus, the first criterion that the transmitter and the mechanism for its production (e.g., synthesizing enzyme, etc.) should be present in the presynaptic neurons has been fulfilled by using microscopic cytochemical methods. These techniques have been combined with production of surgical or chemical lesions of the presynaptic neurons or their tracts to cause disappearance of the alleged neurochemical in those sites. Subcellular fractionation technique has helped further to localize the site of distribution.

The criterion that the transmitter must be released upon physiological stimulation of the presynaptic neuron has yet to be fulfilled for single synapses in the CNS. Electrical stimulation of the nerve pathway *in vivo* and collection of perfusion fluid by push-pull cannula to measure the neurotransmitter content, as is usually done at present, concerns with release of the transmitter from an area hundreds of time larger than a synapse, and over a period thousands of times longer than that of a synpatic potential. However, the recently developed methods such as differential pulse voltammetry (10), and microvoltammetric electrode technic (25) may be more sensitive to permit collection of synaptic neurochemicals *in vivo*. *In vitro* methods of ionic or electrical activation of thin brain slices or subcellular fractions enriched in nerve terminals have also been used to study neurotransmitter release. Such release is dependent on voltage and also calcium content in the medium. Tetrodotoxin which blocks transmembrane movement of Na^+, blocks such release, although not very sensitive.

The criterion that exogenously applied transmitter candidates and the release of the endogenous transmitter should have the same effect on the postsynaptic neuron and both should be blocked by the same pharmacological antagonist can only be loosely fulfilled by qualitative comparison. Such test would require intracellular recording of synaptic potential for a prolonged period *in vivo*, which is difficult to do particularly in case of deep-seated neurons.

Finally, for the criterion that there should be an inactivation or disposal mechanism for the putative neurotransmitter, the microscopic cytochemical methods particularly for detection of the enzyme(s) concerned, as mentioned for the first criterion, have been helpful.

It is difficult for majority of the neurochemicals to fulfill all the criteria rigorously. Although some of the substances such as ACh, NE, DA, 5-HT, GABA for which most of the criteria are fulfilled, are readily accepted as central neurotransmitters, for many others such designation is still putative.

ACETYLCHOLINE

Acetylcholine (ACh) became readily accepted as a central neurotransmitter, after it was established as a neurotransmitter in the postganglionic parasympathetic neuroeffector and neuromuscular junctions as well as in the autonomic ganglia; such role was further supported by marked behavioral effects produced by peripheral cholinergic agonists that pass through the blood-brain barrier or by these agonists after their central administration. It also fulfilled most of the criteria for a central neurotransmitter. In general, the procedures for synthesis, storage, release and disposal of ACh in the CNS appear to resemble those described for peripheral cholinergic synapses.

Distribution. ACh and the enzymes for its synthesis (e.g., choline acetyltransferase or acetylase) and disposal (e.g., AChE) are distributed in many parts of the brain and also in the spinal cord. ACh concentrations in different CNS areas vary, being highest in the striatum, lowest in the cerebellum, and intermediate in pons, medulla, midbrain, hypothalamus, cerebral cortex and other regions. Distribution of ACh resembles that of choline acetyltransferase, but not that of AChE. For instance, in the cerebellum AChE concentration is high, although ACh concentration is low and evidence for cholinergic transmission is weak. Furthermore, AChE is associated with postsynaptic receptor site in the CNS, and is also present in the glial cells which do not contain ACh.

Pathways. Use of a histochemical staining technique for localization of AChE along with selective lesioning of tracts demonstrated a diffuse ascending tegmental-mesencephalic-cortical cholinergic system consisting of several pathways interconnected via ramifications (38, 46). From these, three main cholinergic systems have been identified: (i) a dorsal tegmental pathway with cell bodies in the cuneiform nucleus in the mesencephalic reticular formation projecting to the tectum, pretectal area and thalamus; (ii) a ventral tegmental pathway originating from the substantia nigra and ventral tegmental area and projecting to subthalamus, hypothalamus and basal forebrain areas; (iii) a septal pathway projecting from the septum to all areas of the cerebral cortex, hippocampus and mesencephalon. However, as already mentioned, distribution of AChE does not necessarily correspond to that for ACh.

Recent immunohistochemical studies based on specific monoclonal antibodies against the cholinergic marker choline acetyltransferase have demonstrated that the cortical mantle, amygdala, hippocampus, olfactory bulb and thalamic nuclei receive their cholinergic innervation principally from the basal forebrain and upper brainstem. The source of major cholinergic projections and their area of innervation in the rat and the macaque are as follows: from the medial septal nucleus and the vertical limb nucleus of the diagonal band to the hippocampus; from the lateral portion of the horizontal limb nucleus of the diagonal band to the olfactory bulb; from the nucleus basalis of Meynert and also parts of the diagonal band nuclei to the corticle mantle and the amygdala; from the pedunculopontine nucleus of the pontomesencephalic reticular formation and the laterodorsal tegmental gray of the periventricular area to the thalamus (56).

Effects and Physiological Roles. Eccles and his colleagues (23) using the microintophoretic technique in 1956 demonstrated a prolonged discharge of Renshaw cells in the spinal cord by intra-arterial injection of nicotine and to a less extent also by ACh. Anticholinesterases increased the effect of ACh and the nicotinic cholinergic antagonists, dihydro-β-erythroidine blocked the effects of nicotine and ACh. This indicated the presence of a cholinergic synapse in the pathway of the system. The synapse was possibly formed by motor axon collaterals at the Renshaw cells.

Use of similar technique along with agonists and antagonists has demonstrated the presence of cholinoceptive neurons in many brain areas including the cerebral cortex, thalamus, caudate nucleus, hippocampus, brainstem and others. Action of ACh has been shown to be predominently excitatory, although its inhibitory action has also been demonstrated on some neurons, (e.g., in the brainstem). Furthermore, excitatory action can be either nicotinic or muscarinic, whereas inhibitory action is usually muscarinic. Spinal Renshaw neurons remain as best examples of the central cholinergic nicotinic site.

Involvement of the central cholinergic mechanism in the motor function is further demonstrated by the effects of various cholinergic agonists and antagonists. Thus, the locomotor activity can be increased by nicotine as well as by muscarinic antagonists. Moreover, tremor can be produced by muscarinic agonists (e.g. oxotremorine) and large doses of nicotine, whereas tremor in Parksinson's disease can be reduced by antimuscarinic agents that can penetrate the blood-brain barrier (e.g., atropine, trihexyphenidyl). The striatum is considered to be the site of the drug action in tremor modulation.

Centrally acting cholinergic agonists and antagonists are known to alter states of consciousness or arousal probably mediating through the ventral tegmental pathway.

Involvement of the central cholinergic mechanism has been demonstrated (mostly by using agonists and antagonists) on certain physiological functions including behavior, e.g. food and water intake, motivation, learning and memory. Derrangement of the central cholinergic mechanism has also been implicated in addition to Parkinsonism, in other diseases of the basal ganglia, e.g. Huntington's chorea [decreased choline acetyltransferase (CAT) activity and M receptors], certain degenerative states e.g. Alzheimer's disease (decrease CAT and AChE activity) and also in psychiatric conditions e.g. schizophrenia increased CAT activity, mania (decreased cholinergic activity) and depression (increased cholinergic activity).

CATECHOLAMINES

Although in the peripheral nervous system only norepinephrine plays the predominant role as a catecholamine neurotransmitter, in the CNS three catecholamines, dopamine (DA), norepinephrine (NE) and epinephrine possess separate neuronal systems and play distinct independent roles. Histochemical methods [(formaldehyde or glyoxylic acid-induced fluorescence) (20)] or immunohistochemical methods (32) for synthesizing enzymes specifically needed for each catecholamines have provided the facilities to identify and localize individual catecholaminergic systems.

Dopamine

Although DA is present in the brain as a precursor of NE, it also exists in certain brain areas as a distinct independent entity in neurons that cannot convert DA to NE due to lack of DA-β-hydroxylase. More than half of catecholamine contents in the CNS is dopamine. It occurs in very high concentrations in the basal ganglia (particularly the caudate nucleus), nucleus accumbens, olfactory tubercle, amygdala, median eminence, and some areas of the frontal cortex.

Pathways. Histochemical and immunological technics have demonstrated three major morphological classes of DA neurons: (a) Long projections extending from major DA-containing cells in the mesencephalon (cell groups A8, A9, and A10). From cell groups A8 and A9 located in the substantia nigra, axons ascend in the medial forebrain bundle (MFB) along with NE fibers, some terminating in the caudate nucleus and globus pallidus (nigrostriatal pathway), and others in the limbic system and frontal cortex. From cell group A10 (primarily surrounding the interpeduncular nucleus in the ventral tegmental area) axons project to the nucleus accumbens, amygdala and olfactory tubercle. The latter two groups constitute mesolimbic and mesocortical pathways. (b) Short projections from the cell group A12 within tuberobasal ventral hypothalamus (arcuate nucleus of periventricular nucleus) in mediobasal hypothalamus innervate median eminence and intermediate lobe of pituitary (tuberoinfundibular-hypophyseal and incertohypothalamic systems); (c) Ultrashort neurons having very short or no axon, e.g., amacrine cells of retina and periglomerular cells of the olfactory bulb.

Receptor Subtypes. DA receptors have been suggested to have a number of different subpopulations. Generally considered are two subtypes, D-1 and D-2 on the basis of their association with adenylate cyclase (D-1) or lack of, or more probably negative association with this enzyme (D-2) as well as on the basis of other differences. In addition, analysis of DA agonist/antagonist actions on vascular responses has suggested two subpopulations which do not correspond entirely with the D-1, D-2 subtypes; these pharmacologically differentiated peripheral receptors have been termed DA_1 which subserves smooth muscle relaxation and vasodilatation in renal, mesenteric, coronary and cerebral vascular beds, and DA_2 which upon stimulation inhibits the release of norepinephrine from sympathetic nerve endings (28, 37).

Disposal. Like other catecholamines, DA undergoes metabolic degradation through the actions of COMT and MAO. Formation of DOPAC, HVA and other metabolites are schematically shown in Fig. 6-5.

Functional Role. Microiontophoretic application of DA onto single neurons plays a mainly inhibitory role in the CNS. DA in the nigrostriatal pathway is clearly involved in the motor function. Its role is indicated by the beneficial effects of L-DOPA, the immediate precursor of DA, in the treatment of Parkinson's disease which shows a deficiency of DA in the basal ganglia. Production of extrapyramidal side effects by the antipsychotic (neuroleptic) agents which act as DA receptor antagonists further corroborates this role. DA in the mesolimbic system has been implicated in emotional behavior and is thought to be involved in schizophrenia because of the DA antagonistic actions of antipsychotic drugs; furthermore, clinical efficiency of these drugs parallels their DA antagonistic actions.

In addition, a drug like amphetamine which causes release of DA from presynaptic terminals produces at high doses symptoms resembling those of paranoid psychosis which can be ameliorated by antipsychotic drugs. In addition, DA systems have been thought to provide neural basis for perception, arousal, motivation, memory and learning (37) reward behavior and endocrine secretion (particularly prolactin).

Norepinephrine

NE is distributed in varying concentrations in different areas of the brain being highest in the hypothalamus and certain limbic areas e.g., central nucleus of the amygdala and dentate gyrus of hippocampus.

Its synthesis, storage, release and metabolism are very similar to those of peripheral NE. Development of specific fluorescence histochemical technique has made it possible to identify several NE pathways. The noradrenergic tracts consist of two main ascending pathways and one descending pathway. The ventral noradrenergic (ascending) pathway arises from the cell bodies of A1, A5 and A7 areas in the medulla and pons and innervates mainly the medulla, pons, midbrain and hypothalamus. The dorsal ascending pathway and a descending tract arise from the cell bodies of the locus ceruleus (A6), from which multiple branch axons form plexiform networks and innervate various specific target areas. The dorsal ascending pathway pass through the median forebrain bundle and through the zona incerta to innervate neocortex, hippocampus, amygdala, thalamus, some hypothalamic nuclei and olfactory bulb. Some fibers from the locus ceruleus also innervate Purkinje cells in the cerebellum. Another tract arising from the locus ceruleus descends into the spinal cord.

Microiontophoretic application of NE as well as stimulation of the locus ceruleus produces predominently inhibitory effects on cortical neurons, although some diencephalic and mesencephalic neurons may show excitatory effects. Such inhibition is due to hyperpolarization along with an increase in the passive resistance of the postsynaptic membrane and is mediated by β-adrenergic receptors. These inhibitory effects are slower in onset and longer in duration than those of inhibitory amino acids and stimulate those of cyclic AMP on certain cerebellar and cerebral neurons, which may involve both α and β adrenoceptors.

Adrenoceptors in the CNS show similar subtypes as in the periphery. While α_1-adrenoceptors correspond to the postsynaptic NE neurons, α_2 receptors presumably located on the presynaptic terminals have inhibitory function of regulating NE release. Such inhibitory role of α_2 receptor action has been considered to be the basis of action of some centrally acting antihypertensive drugs (e.g. clonidine). Stimulation of α_2 adrenoceptors on noradrenergic neurons leads to marked inhibition of firing. Postsynaptic α_2-adrenoceptors have also been shown to exist in both CNS and the periphery (57). β_1-Adrenergic receptors may be mainly associated with neurons, whereas β_2-receptors may be related to glial and vascular elements.

Physiological Role. Use of lesion technique and of agonists and antagonists have indicated roles of NE in a number of physiological functions e.g. food intake, sleep, learning and memory, and attentions.

Pharmacological Implication. Since exogenously applied NE very poorly penetrates the blood-brain barrier, drugs modifying neurotransmission have been used to explore the funcitonal role of NE. The dorsal ascending NE pathways which probably mediates the ascending facilitatory influence from the brainstem to the cortex are responsible for phasic arousal responses. This has been indirectly shown by amphetamine that releases presynaptic catecholamines producing an increase in alertness. Conversely, drugs such as antipsychotic neuroleptics are considered to produce sedative action due to their α-adrenoceptor blocking effect.

Other psychotropic drugs such as tricyclic antidepressants and MAO inhibitors are also considered to produce their alleviating effects on depression by elevating levels of NE either by inhibiting its uptake by neurons (e.g., by tricyclics) or by preventing their metabolism (e.g., by MAO inhibitors). These actions are not however selective to NE alone, since other amines such as 5-hydroxytryptamine (5-HT) are also involved particularly in case of depression. Conversely, the Rauwolfia alkaloid, reserpine, which depletes catecholamines (as well as 5-HT) in the central and peripheral nervous systems,produces effects which closely resemble the manifestatioins of depressive states. Thus because of such role of NE and other biogenic amines in induction of a depression-like

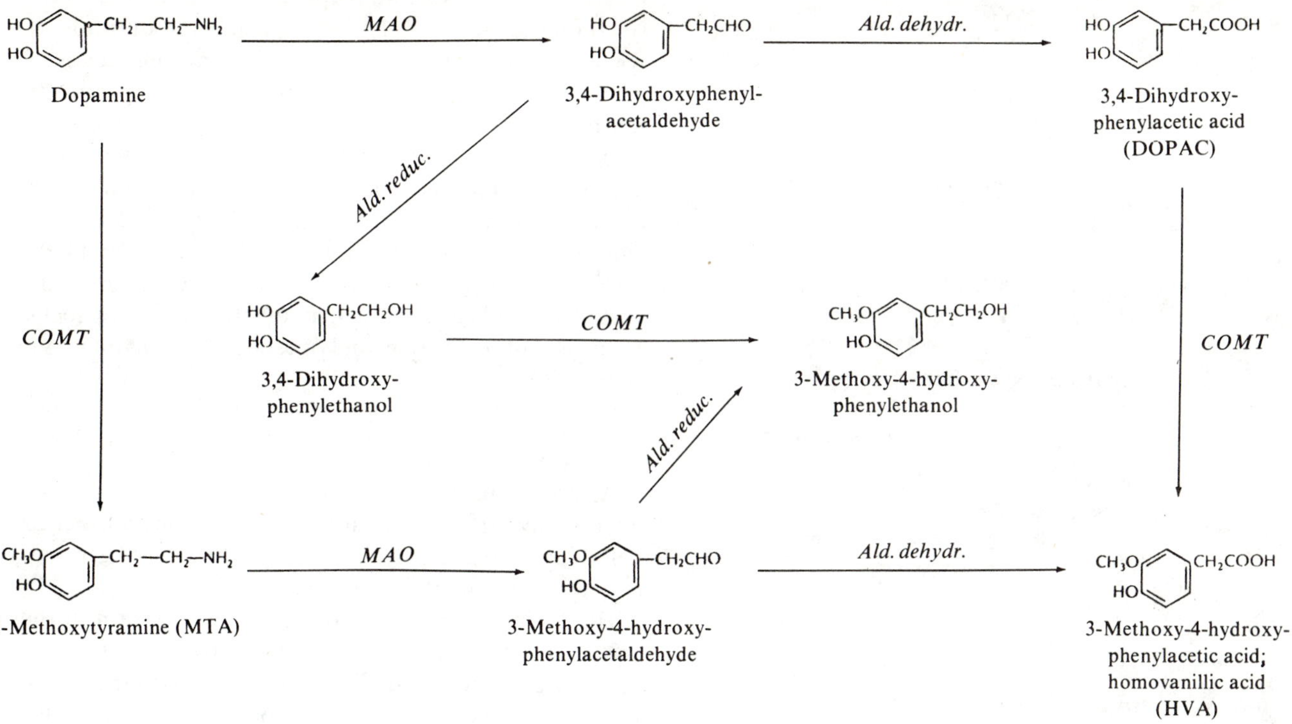

Fig.6-5. *Metabolic disposal of dopamine.*

condition, biogenic amine theory of depresion has been developed.

Epinephrine

By using immunohistochemical technic for assay of phenylethanolamine-N-methyl transferase (PNMT, the enzyme involved in conversion of norepinephrine to epinephrine), PNMT-containig cell bodies have been localized in C1 and C2 cell groups of the reticular formation in the medulla. The PNMT-positive terminals are mainly found in the ventral periventricular gray of the lower brainstem and certain nuclei of the hypothalamus. Complete neural pathways are not clearly known. Amount of epinephrine in the CNS is much smaller than that of NE. The role of adrenergic neurotransmission in the CNS is not well established,but it has been implicated in temperature regulation,food and water intake,regulation of sleep and wakefulness, control of blood pressure and respiration, and secretion of oxytocin and gonadotropin (29).

5-Hydroxytryptamine (5-HT, serotonin)

The indoleamine, 5-hydroxytryptamine (5-HT) that was earlier isolated and identified as "serotonin" in the serum and as "enteramine" in the enterochromaffin cells of the intestine was later found to be present also in the brain (9). Since then, interest in 5-HT has been greatly stimulated to explore its role in the actions of several neuropharmacological agents as well as in various CNS functions and dysfunctions.

5-HT is synthesized from tryptophan, an essential amino acid present in the diet (Fig. 6-6). The amino acid is taken up into neurons by an active process and then converted to 5-hydroxytryptophan (5-HTP) by tryptophan hydroxylase, an enzyme associated with mitochondria. Following this hydroxylation that is a rate-limiting step in 5-HT synthesis, 5-HTP is decarboxylated to 5-HT by L-amino acid decarboxylase. The latter enzyme appears to be somewhat different from DOPA decarboxylase in its characteristics and distribution. 5-HT is metabolized mainly by MAO to form 5-hydroxyindoleacetic acid (5-HIAA). In the pineal gland, 5-HT serves as a precursor in the synthesis of its hormone, melatonin.

Iontophoretic application of 5-HT shows invariably inhibition of firing. Although in some experiments both inhibitory and excitatory responses of the raphe cells to 5-HT have been reported, excitatory responses have been suggested to be due to nonserotonergic cells (1).

Uses of fluoresence histochemistry (20) and orthograde and retrograde tracing techniques (4) have demonstrated most of the 5-HT containing cell bodies in the midline (raphe) regions of the pons and the upper brainstem. While neurons of the caudal raphe cell groups project mainly within the brainstem and spinal cord, more rostral raphe nuclei send ascending fibers passing through the MFB to the forebrain regions. Among the latter groups the dorsal raphe nucleus innervates the cortical regions and the neostriatum, and the median raphe nucleus innervates mainly the limbic structures. There are also projections into the cerebellum and pontomesencephalic reticular formation. A serotonergic pathway from the area postrema to the parabrachial nucleus has been recently described (49).

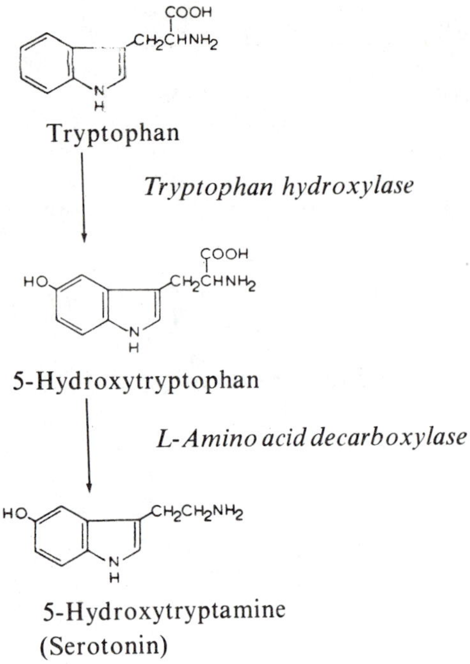

Tryptophan

Tryptophan hydroxylase

5-Hydroxytryptophan

L-Amino acid decarboxylase

5-Hydroxytryptamine
(Serotonin)

Fig. 6-6. *Synthesis of 5-hydroxytryptamine.*

Microintrophoretic application of 5-HT directly inhibits the activity of 5-HT neurons of the dorsal raphe nucleus indicating thereby the presence of receptor within the neuron itself, that mediates a response to its own transmitter ("autoreceptor"). These autoreceptors could reflect the presence of 5-HT collaterals within or between the various raphe nuclei or of 5-HT sensitive presynaptic membrane. Thus as mentioned earlier, these receptors can be somatodendritic or presynaptic. Such receptors have been considered to be involved in the local feedback regulation of 5-HT release (1). In addition to autoreceptors, a neuronal feedback mediated by postsynaptic 5-HT receptors appears to be involved in regulation of serotonergic neurotransmission. Binding studies have revealed at least two subtypes of 5-HT receptors, 5-HT_1 and 5-HT_2 receptors (40).

Pharmacological Importance. 5-HT has been involved in the mechanism of action of many drugs which modify its synthesis (p-chlorophenylalanine), storage (reserpine), release (amphetamine, chloramphetamine, morphine), uptake (tricyclic antidepressants), and catabolism (MAO inhibitors). Chronic administration of lithium has been suggested to induce 5- HT agonistic effects in the brain in humans and animals (58). A number of antidepressant drugs have potent, direct action on 5-HT_2 receptors which may be of clinical importantance (60). 5-HT has been implicated in the mechanism of action of the hallucinogen, lysergic acid diethylamide (LSD) (see Chapter 11.6 for discussion).

Physiological Role. 5-HT is involved in modulation of certain behavior e.g., sleep and wakefulness, sexual behavior and aggression. It appears to play an important role in modulating the latency, spacing and duration of REM episodes within the sleep cycle. Serotonin tends to protect the organism against damage by dampening of sensory stimuli, by reducing aggression potential and by stabilizing mood. Serotonin neurons of midbrain raphe appear to mediate a central clock for regulating circadian oscillatory secretory profiles of several hypothalamic and hypophysial hormones (CRF/ACTH; LRF/LH: TRF/TSH) by acting at the preoptic area. These functions are partly accomplished through modulatory effects on locus ceruleus noradrenergic and mesolimbic dopaminergic neurons (5).

HISTAMINE

Although histamine has been long known for its peripheral effects and some antihistaminics known for their behavioral effects, only recently histamine has been suggested to be a putative central neurotransmitter.

Histamine is present in the mammalian brain in the concentration of about 0.5 nmole (50 to 70 ng)/g of wet tissue, highest concentration being in the hypothalamus. Its presence in the pituitary is associated with mast cells. It is also present in raphe nucleus, central gray, substantia nigra, basal ganglia, septal nuclei, thalamus and periventricular gray as in the case of dopamine and serotonin (30).

Histamine is formed from histidine by decarboxylation mediated by the enzyme histidine decarboxylase. This enzyme is also present in the brain with highest concentration in the hypothalamus. Histamine is inactivated by methylation and necessary enzyme is also present in the brain. Histamine does not pass through the blood-brain barrier, but administration of histidine can raise the level of brain histamine. Subcellular fractionation technic has demonstrated the presence of histamine in nerve terminals. Most of the histamine content in the brain is associated with its mast cells. Unilateral lesions of the lateral hypothalamus result in a repletion of histidine decarboxylase on the same side of lesion. Active reuptake and release *in vitro* or *in vivo* for this amine have not been demonstrated. CNS shows both H_1 and H_2 subtypes of histamine receptors, although H_2 receptor action appears to be more prominent.

Histamine stimulates adenylate cyclase in a particulate preparation of the hippocampus; this effect is synergistically enhanced by GTP and competitively blocked by H_2-antagonists (e.g., metiamide and cimetidine)(30). Histamine-induced accumulation of cyclic AMP is potentiated by adenosine; this effect involves both H_1 and H_2 receptors (39). Iontophoretic application of histamine depresses neuronal firing in the cerebral cortex and also in the hypothalamus and reticular formation. Many hypothalamic neurons are however excited by histamine. Depression of cortical neurons in rats has been blocked by H_2-antagonists, but not specifically.

Pharmacological Importance. Drugs such as compound 48/80 or polymyxin B cause release of histamine in the CNS mostly by liberating the amine from the mast cells granules. Also morphine causes release of histamine in the CNS and decreases the level of histamine in the hypothalamus, brainstem and cortex after 9-21 days of treatment. Many centrally acting drugs (e.g., phenothiazine neuroleptics) show antihistaminic properties, whereas the antihistamine agents show some central effects, especially sedation.

AMINO ACIDS

Certain amino acids e.g., γ-aminobutyric acid (GABA) and glycine have been considered to play roles of central neurotransmitters, although several problems have been faced in accepting such role of these amino acids. It is difficult to discriminate the role of these amino acids as neurotransmitters from that as precursors for protein synthesis. Their presence in abundance throughout the CNS makes it difficult to identify their release during discharge of a single neuronal circuit. After their microiontophoretic application, they produce prompt, powerful and readily reversible, but redundant effects indicating a nonspecific action on neuronal discharge. A lack of selective antagonists in some cases, and also lack of technic for their cytochemical identification prevent their effective investigation. However, at present results of many investigations support their role as central neurotransmitters. Usually the monocarboxylic ω-amino acids (e.g., GABA, glycine, β-alanine, taurine) are inhibitory, and the dicarboxylic acids (e.g., glutamate and aspartate) are excitatory. Some of these will be discussed here.

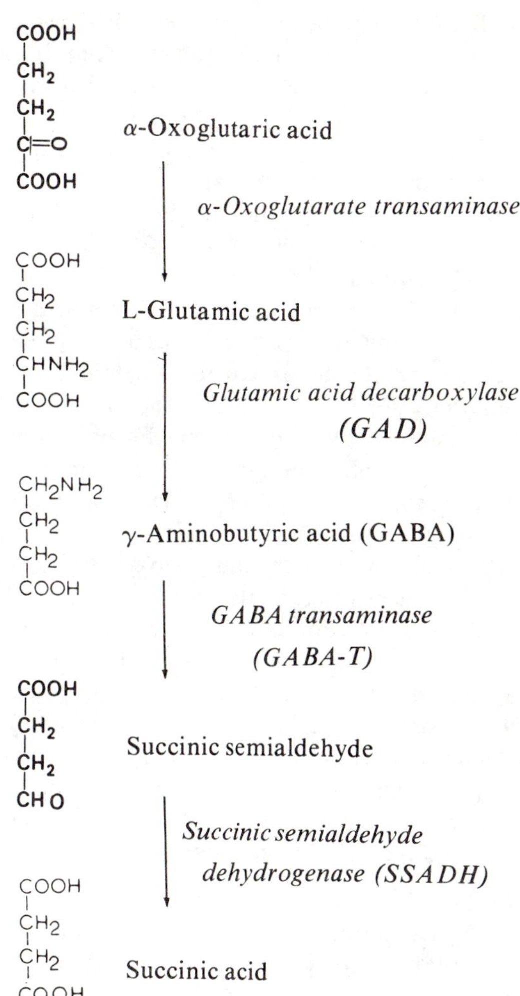

Fig. 6-7. *Synthesis and biotransformation of γ-aminobutyric acid.*

GABA

GABA is a unique chemical constituent of the mammalian brain, not being found in any other tissues. It is probably the principle inhibitory neurotransmitter in the brain. It is distributed unevenly in the CNS (both in the brain and spinal cord), its concentration being highest in the substantia nigra, followed by pallidium, hypothalamus, and superior colliculi and smallest in the cerebral cortex.

GABA is formed by decarboxylation of L-glutamic acid, which is catalized by the enzyme glutamic acid decarboxylase (GAD) requiring the presence of pyridoxal phosphate as a cofactor. GAD is unique to the mammalian CNS and is mainly associated with neurons, although it is also present in the glial cells and other tissues. GABA is metabolized to succinic semialdehyde by the action of the enzyme GABA transaminase (GABA-T) which also requires pyridoxal phosphatase as a cofactor. Both GAD and GABA occur in presynaptic terminals and GABA-T is associated with mitochondria. Succinic semialdehyde is then rapidly metabolized to succinic acid by the enzyme succinic semialdehyde dehydrogenase (Fig. 6-7).

The distribution of GABA follows that of GAD, both being demonstrated in the nerve terminals. GAD is localized in the nervous system where inhibitory nerve endings are recognized, thus indicating that GABA is an inhibitory neurotransmitter at least in some parts of the brain (35). GABA has been shown to be released from presynaptic nerve terminals and to produce hyperpolarization of the postsynaptic neurons probably by increasing chloride ion conductance which is disposed from the synaptic cleft probably via sodium-dependent uptake mechanism rather than by GABA-T effect.

Pathway. Use of immunocytochemical method has enabled visualization of GAD and localization of presumptive GABA-ergic neurons and nerve-terminals. By such method a GABA-ergic pathway from the caudate nucleus to the substantia nigra has been demonstrated.

GABA-ergic inhibitory synapses have been similarly shown clearly between cerebellar Purkinji neurons and their targets in Deiter's nucleus and also in cerebellar cortex, olfactory bulb, cuneate nucleus and hippocampus. Use of other methods have also demonstrated some presumptive GABA-ergic pathways from the substantia nigra, zona reticulata, the zona incerta and the reticular formation of the mesencephalon (3).

GABA Receptor. Depending on their binding to agonists, GABA receptors can be differentiated into high- and low-affinity forms. These sites may represent recognition templates for modulatory peptides like GABA-modulin. Properties of these receptors are also mutually regulated by activation of coupled benzodiazepine/barbiturate/ionophase binding sites. This supports the presently accepted view that benzodiazepines potentiate the effects of GABA which are implicated in their anticonvulsant and anxiolytic agents. Two types of GABA receptors have been differentiated depending on their agonists and antagonists. For the classical $GABA_A$ receptor, muscimol is a potent agonist, and bicuculline and picrotoxin are competitive and noncompetitive antagonists respectively; baclofen is inactive. The other receptor $GABA_B$ which appears to be predominently localized presynaptically and many of which appear to be associated with noradrenergic terminals, is insensitive to bicuculline and picrotoxin, but is activated by baclofen (66).

Glycine

Glycine appears to be an inhibitory amino acid transmitter abundantly present in the ventral quadrant of the spinal cord and also in the reticular formation (excluding cuneate nucleus). It has been localized in spinal interneurons by electron microscopy autoradiography. It produces inhibitory effects on motoneurons due to hyperpolarization caused by increase in chloride ion conductance. It appears to mediate the action of recurrent inhibitory neurons in the spinal cord. Its action is antagonized by strychnine which also inhibits the hyperpolarizing responses to β-alanine, but not to GABA.

Glutamate and Aspartate

The dicarboxylic acids such as glutamic acid and aspartic acid occur in high concentrations in the brain, and also in the spinal cord and retina. They exert potent excitatory effects on neurons in CNS areas. Such excitation has a rapid onset and termination of action, and is produced by a depolarizing action. Because of their wide spread distribution in the CNS and involvement in the intermediary metabolism it has been difficult to analyze experimental data in terms of evidence for or against their excitatory neurotransmitter role in the CNS. However, certain evidences e.g. (a) presence of excess of L-glutamate in the dorsal root compared to the ventral root, (b) its presence in the synaptosome (nerve-ending fraction) of brain homogenates, (c) selective high-affinity uptake system for L-glutamate and other similar aminoacids in the spinal cord and medulla, (d) reduction of uptake of L-glutamate (thought to be into nerve terminals) in the dorsal column nuclei after dorsal column lesions, (e) release of preloaded labelled glutamate as well as endogenous L-glutamate from the rat dorsal column stimulation (64), are highly suggestive of a transmitter role for L-glutamate (and L-aspartate) in the CNS. Kainic acid, an analog of glutamic acid, has been used as a neurotoxin to produce selective lesions in neuronal cell bodies, while sparing adjacent axons (17). Using various pharmacological agonists and antagonists as well as from binding studies, the existence of three receptors for excitatory amino-acids has been proposed; these are activated by the specific agonists, N-methyl-D-aspartic acid (NMDA), kainic acid (KA) and quisqualic acid (QA) (66). L-Aspartate appears to act preferentially on the NMDA receptor and L-glutamate at the quisqualate (and possibly on kainate) receptor. It seems likely that L-glutamate is a possible transmitter of large myelinated non-nociceptive mechanoreceptor primary afferent fibers and is released onto a postsynaptic receptor of kainate or quisqualate type in the dorsal horn (64).

NEUROPEPTIDES

Although many peptides have long been known for their various functions in different systems, discovery of encephalins and endorphins in the brain has stimulated discovery of multiferious neuroactive peptides in the brain. As a result, a large number of peptides have already been identified in the mammalian CNS and their number is continually increasing.

These peptides appear to produce their effects at least in three different ways in the CNS: (a) as local hormones that are released into the blood stream to act at target area away from their site of release; (b) as local neurohormones that are released into local portal systems; and (c) as local neurotransmitters that act on close neuroeffector structures.

Many of these CNS peptides are distributed also in different tissues where they carry on their specific functions (e.g. in cholecystokinin and gastrin in the GI tract, glucagon and vasoactive intestinal polypeptide, VIP in the pancreatic islets, etc.). Since many of these peptides occur as well in the gut, they have been called "peptides of the brain and gut". Because of their diffuse distribution and location of many of them in both neutral and endocrine systems, they have been termed "peptide of the diffuse neuroendocrine system" (Chapter 13.1.1).

Neuropeptide transmitters differ from the biogenic amine and amino acid transmitters in many ways. The latter neurotransmitters are synthesized from dietary constitutents through the mediation of one or more enzymes within the neuron; the synthesized neurotransmitter is then stored in the nerve terminal and then released. The neuropeptide on the other hand, is synthesized in the endoplasmic reticulum into a larger precursor molecule (propeptide) coded by mRNA. The propeptide is then cleaved to form the secretory vesicles that are transported to the nerve terminal prior to release. Furthermore, for neuropeptides there is no active re-uptake mechanism, that makes the availability of the peptide at the nerve terminal entirely dependent on the distant site of synthesis. Also for most of the neuropeptides (except for opioids) there is a lack of specific receptors and appropriate antagonists, which make their investigation difficult.

Substance P

Substance P (SP) is a well known peptide containing 11 amino acids discovered more than 55 years ago by von Euler and Gaddum (73). SP is found in high concentrations in the dorsal root of the spinal cord. It is also present in the basal ganglia and hypothalamus and in low concentrations in the frontal cortex, hippocampus and cerebellum. SP is synthesized in the cell bodies of primary afferents and from there transported both to the peripheral and central endings of the sensory axon. it is stored in large dense-core vesicles in nerve terminals in the dorsal horn and can be localized in brain synaptosomal fractions. It can be released from spinal cord and medullary slices by elevated extracellular potassium levels in a calcium-dependant manner and also from the spinal cord *in vitro* and *in vivo* experiments by electrical stimulation of peripheral nerves. Such release can be inhibited by opioid analgesics.

Microiontophoretic experiments show that SP depolarizes spinal neurons and has predominantly excitatory effects. These effects have slow onset and long duration suggesting that the peptide may have a long-term regulatory or modulatory function rather than a traditional neurotransmitter role (64). Use of radioimmunoassay and immunocytochemical techniques have demonstrated dense SP-immunoreactive staining in laminae I and II of the dorsal horn. SP has been found in a proportion of small diameter primary afferent neurons (likely to be C fibers) projecting to the dorsal horn of the spinal cord and medulla. The peptide is greatly depleted from the dorsal horn upon dorsal rhizotomy or peripheral nerve injury. It can be hypothesized that SP is an important neurochemical mediator for certain kinds of noxious peripheral stimuli. SP is further discussed in Chapter 13.1.1

OPIOID PEPTIDES

The discovery of opiate receptors in 1973 was followed by discovery (in 1975) of opioid peptides, enkephalins which possess morphine-like activities and serve as endogenous ligands to these receptors. These and related peptides acting on the opiate receptors have been suggested to play the role of neurotransmitters.

There are two naturally occurring enkephalins, methionine-enkephalin (Met-enkephalin) and leucine-enkephalin (Leu-enkephalin); both are pentapeptides. In addition, larger peptides possessing opiate-like properties also exist in the CNS. Examples include β-endorphin which has 30 amino acids, and dynorphin which has 17 amino-acids.

Three endogenous opioid precursors (e.g., pro-opiocortin, proenkephalin and prodynorphin) have been identified (43). In a peptide-containing neuron a peptide is synthesized in the rough endoplasmic reticulum in which the propeptide is cleaved to the form in which it is secreted and is stored in the secretory vesicle. The latter is then transported from the perinuclear cytoplasm to the nerve terminals. Release of enkephalins occurs in response to depolarizing stimuli and is calcium-dependent. No active re-uptake system for the peptides has been described.

The enkephalins and β-endorphin interact with μ and δ receptors, while dynorphin has high affinity for κ-receptors. However, there is a lack of selectivity of the endogenous ligands. Unlike endorphins and dynorphin, enkephalines are very susceptible to the degrading action of peptidases.

From the functional standpoint, the enkephalins, endorphin and dynorphin appear to belong to two distinct systems. Because of wide distribution, very rapid destruction, localization in nerve terminals, calcium-dependent release, the enkephalins are considered to act as short acting neurotransmitters. β-Endorphin with its localized distribution in the hypothalamus and pituitary, and with its longer duration of action may serve as a neurohormone. Both systems are apparently involved in modulation of pain. Dynorphin appears to serve both ways.

Further discussions on opiate receptors and opioid peptides, particularly distribution and types of the receptors and distribution and functional roles of the peptides are provided in Chapter 10.1

INTERACTION OF NEUROTRANSMITTERS

Neurotransmitters play important roles in mediation of many physiological functions, but their actions appear to be complicated. The simple concept of one neuron, one neurotransmitter and one action does not appear to be plausible. One and the same neuron may contain more than one transmitter and sometimes neurotransmitters with apparent opposing actions (52).

The presynaptic action of a neurotransmitter would exert an inhibitory influence on the postsynaptic release of the same or another neurotransmitter. Furthermore, there are considerable evidences for interaction and interdependence among several neurotransmitters including ACh, NE, DA, 5-HT, histamine and GABA at various (e.g., neuroanatomical, neurochemical, functional and behavioral) levels in the CNS (for review see 61; also 14, 45, 55, 68). Interactions between NE or DA and amino acid transmitters (15, 59) and between DA and neuropeptides (36, 70) have also been demonstrated.

Finally, it may be stated that execution and maintenance of a certain physiological function would involve the actions of several neurotransmitters each with a facilitatory or an inhibitory effect. Balance of their effects would determine the existing (normal) state of the function. Pathological conditions or pharmacological manipulation may affect one or more of these components leading to imbalance of the multitransmitter system. Therapeutic use of a drug would be concerned with the correction of a neurotransmitter disorder produced by a pathological condition. For example, the extrapyramidal motor function is maintained by balance of the facilitatory dopaminergic system and the inhibitory cholinergic system. In Parkinson's disease, pathological damage to the nigrostriatal DA neurons results in dopaminergic deficiency and cholinergic hyperactivity causing neurotransmitter imbalance and manifestation of extrapyramidal disorders; amelioration of the disorder can be produced by compensating the DA deficiency by administration of L-DOPA or DA agonists and/or inhibiting the cholinergic hyperactivity by anticholinergic agents (Chapter 9.4).

REFERENCES

1. Aghajanian, G.K. and Wang, R.Y. Physiology and pharmacology of central serotonergic neurons. In: *Psychopharmacology -A Generation of Progress* (Lipton, M.A., DiMascio, A. and Kilam, A.F., eds.). New York: Raven Press, 1978, p. 171.
2. Ahlquist, R.P. A study of adrenotropic receptors. *Am. J. Physiol.,* 153:586, 1948.
3. Araki, M., McGeer, P.L. and McGeer, E.C. Presumptive γ-aminobutyric acid pathways from the midbrain to the superior colliculus studied by a combined horse-radish peroxidase-γ-aminobutyric acid transaminase pharmacohistochemical method. *Neuroscience* 13:433, 1984.
4. Azmitia, E.C. The serotonin-producing neurons of the midbrain median and dorsal raphe nuclei. In: *Handbook of Psychopharmacology,* Section II, Vol. 9 (Iversen, L.L., Iversen, S.D. and Snyder, S.H., eds.). New York: Plenum Press, 1978, p. 233.
5. Baumgarten, H.G. and Lachenmayer, L. Anatomical features and physiological properties of central serotonin neurons. *Pharmacopsychiatry* 18:180, 1985.
6. Berger, G. and Dale, H.H. Chemical structure and sympathomimetic action of amines. *J. Physiol.(Lond.)* 41:19, 1910.
7. Blaschko, H. The specific action of L-dopa decarboxylase. *J. Physiol. (Lond.)* 96:50P, 1939.
8. Bodian, D. Neuron junctions: a revolutionary decade. *Anat. Rec.* 174:73, 1972.
9. Brodie, B.B. and Shore, P.A. A concept for a role of serotonin and norepinephrine as chemical mediators in the brain. *Ann. N.Y. Acad. Sci.* 66:631, 1957.
10. Buda, M., De Simoni, G., Gonon, F. and Pujol, J.-F. Catecholamine metabolism in rat locus coeruleus as studied by *in vivo* differential pulse voltammetry. I. Nature and origin of contributors to the oxidation current at +0.1 V. *Brain Res.* 273:197, 1983.
11. Bullock, T.H. and Hagiwara, S. Intracellular recording from the giant synapse of the squid. *J. Gen. Physiol.* 40:565, 1957.
12. Cajal, S. Ramón y. Les preuves objectives de l'unité anatomique des cellules nerveuses. *Trab. Lab. Invest. Biol. Univ. Madr.* 29:1, 1934.
13. Cannon, W.B. and Uridil, J.E. Studies on the conditions of activity in endocrine glands. VIII. Some effects on the denervated heart of stimulating the nerves of the liver. *Am. J. Physiol.* 58:353, 1921.
14. Capuzzo, A., Borasio, P.G., Fabbri, E. et al. Alpha-adrenoceptor-mediated inhibition of acetylcholine release in guinea-pig superior cervical ganglion. *Neurosci. Lett.* 43:215, 1983.
15. Collins, G.G., Probett, G.A., Anson, J., and McLaughlin, N.J. Excitatory and inhibitory effects of noradrenaline on synaptic transmission in the rat olfactory cortex slice. *Brain Res.* 294:211, 1984.
16. Costa, E. Guidotti, A., Hanbauer, I. et al. Adrenal medulla: regulation of biosynthesis and secretion of catecholamines and enkephalins. In: *Neurology and Neurobiology* (Usdin, E., Carlsson, A., Dahlström, A. and Engel, J., eds.) *Catecholamines: Basic and Peripheral Mechanisms,* Vol. 8A. New York: Alan R. Liss Inc., 1984, p. 153.
17. Coyle, J.T., Schwarcz, R., Bennet, J.P. and Campochiaro,P. Clinical neuropathologic and pharmacologic aspects of Huntington's disease: correlates with a new animal model. *Prog. Neuropsychopharmacol.* 1:13, 1977.
18. Creutz, C.E. Cis-unsaturated fatty acids induce the fusion of chromaffin granules aggregated by synexin. *J. Cell Biol.* 91:247, 1981.
19. Creutz, C.E., Dowling, L.G., Sando, J.J. et al. Characterization of the chromobindins: soluble proteins that bind to the chromaffin granule membrane in the presence of Ca^{2+}. *J.Biol. Chem.* 258:14664, 1983.
20. Dahlström, A. and Fuxe, K. Evidence for the existence of monoamine-containing neurons in the central nervous system. I. Demonstration of monoamines in the cell bodies of brainstem neurons. *Acta Physiol. Scand.* 232:1, 1964.
21. Dale, H.H. The action of certain esters and ethers of choline, and their relation to muscarine. *J. Pharmacol. Exp. Ther.* 6:147, 1914.
22. Dixon, W.E. Vagus inhibiton. *Br. Med. J.* 2:1807, 1906.
23. Eccles, J.C., Eccles, R.M. and Fatt, P. Pharmacological investigations on a central synapse operated by acetylcholine. *J. Physiol. (Lond.)* 131:154, 1956.
24. Elliott, T.R. The action of adrenaline. *J. Physiol. (Lond.)* 32:401, 1905.
25. Ewing, A.G., Bigelow, J.C., and Wightman, R.M. Direct *in vivo* monitoring of dopamine released from two striatal compartments in the rat. *Science* 221:169, 1983.
26. Furchgott, R.F. The role of endothelium in the responses of vascular smooth muscle to drugs. *Annu. Rev. Pharmacol. Toxicol.* 24:175, 1984.
27. Gilbert, R.F.T. and Emson, P.C. Neuronal coexistence of peptides with other putative transmitters. In: *Handbook of Psychopharmacology. Vol. 16, Neuropeptides* (Iversen, L.L., Iversen, S.D. and Synder, S.H., eds.). New York: Plenum Press, 1983, p. 519.
28. Goldberg, L.I. Dopamine: Receptors and clinical applications. *Clin. Physiol. Biochem.* 3:120, 1985.
29. Goldstein, M., Lew, J.Y., Matsumoto, Y. et al. Localization and function of PNMT in the centeral nervous system. In: *Psychopharmacology - A Generation of Progress* (Lipton, M.A., DiMascio, A. and Kilam, A.F., eds.). New York: Raven Press, 1978, p. 261.
30. Green, J.P., Johnson, C.L., and Weinstein, H. Histamine as a neurotransmitter. In: *Psychopharmacology - A Generation of Progress* (Lipton, M.A., DiMascio, A. and Kilam, A.F., eds.). New York: Raven Press, 1978, p. 319.
31. Henry, J.B. (ed.). *Clinical Diagnosis and Management by Laboaratory Methods 17th ed.* Philadelphia: Saunders, 1984, p. 316.
32. Hökfelt, T. et al. Aminergic and peptidergic pathways in the nervous system with special reference to the hypothalamus. In: *The Hypothalamus* (Reichlin, S., Baldessarini, R.J. and Martin, J.B., eds.). New York: Raven Press, 1978, p. 69.

33. Hoss, W., and Ellis, J. Muscarinic receptor subtypes in the central nervous system. *Int. Rev. Neurobiol.* 26:151, 1985.
34. Illes, P., and Dörge, L. Mechanism of α_2-adrenergic inhibition of neuroeffector transmission in the mouse vas deferens. *Naunyn-Schmiedeberg's Arch. Pharmacol.* 328:241, 1985.
35. Ishikawa, K., Watabe, S., and Goto, N. Laminal distribution of γ-aminobutyric acid (GABA) in the occipital cortex of rats: evidence as a neurotransmitter. *Brain Res.* 277:361, 1983.
36. Jolicoeur, F.B., De Michele, G., Barbeau, A., and St-Pierre, S. Neurotensin affects hyperactivity but not stereotypy induced by pre and post synaptic dopaminergic stimulation. *Neurosci. Biobehav. Rev.* 7:385, 1983.
37. Kaiser, C., and Jain, T. Dopamine receptors: Functions, subtypes and emerging concepts. *Medicinal Res. Rev.* 5:145, 1985.
38. Karczmar, A.G. and Dun, N.J. Cholinergic synapses: physiological, pharmacological and behavioral consideration. In: *Psychopharmacology - A Generation of Progress* (Lipton, M.A., DiMascio, A. and Killam, A.F., eds.). New York: Raven Press, 1978, p. 293.
39. Kebabian, J.W. and Nathanson, J.A. (eds.). *Cyclic Nucleotides. Handbook of Experimental Pharmacology,* Vol. 58. Berlin: Springer-Verlag, 1982.
40. Kehr, W. Receptor-mediated regulation of 5-hydroxytryptamine metabolism: current knowledge and open questions. *Pharmacopsychiatry* 18:193, 1985.
41. Kilbinger, H. Presynaptic muscarine receptors modulating acetylcholine release. *Trends Pharmacol. Sci.* 5:103, 1984.
42. Kirshner, N. Function and organization of chromaffin vesicles. *Life Sci.* 14:1153, 1974.
43. Kosterlitz, H.W. Opioid peptides and their receptors. *Proc. R. Soc. Lond. B* 225:27, 1985.
44. Krnjević, K. Chemical nature of synaptic transmission in vertebrates. *Physiol. Rev.* 54:418, 1974.
45. Kubo, T., and Su, C. Effects of serotonin and some other neurohumoral agents on adrenergic neurotransmission in spontaneously hypertensive rat vasculature. *Clin. Exp. Hypertens. [A]* 5:1501, 1983.
46. Kuhar, M.J. Central cholinergic pathways: physiologic and pharmacologic aspects. In: *Psychopharmacology - A Generation of Progress* (Lipton, M.A., DiMascio, A. and Killam, A.F., eds.). New York: Raven Press, 1978, p. 199.
47. Langer, S.Z. Presynaptic regulation of the release of catecholamines. *Pharmacol. Rev.* 32:337, 1980.
48. Langley, J.N. Observations on the physiological action of extracts of the supra-renal bodies. *J. Physiol. (Lond.)* 27:237, 1901.
49. Lansa, A.J. and Van Der Kooy, D. A serotonin containing pathway from the area postrema to the parabranchial nucleus in the rat. *Neuroscience* 14:1117, 1985.
50. Livett, B.G., Boksa, P., Dean, D.M. et al. Use of isolated chromaffin cells to study basic release mechanisms. *J. Autonom. Nerv. Syst.* 7:59, 1983.
51. Loewi, O. Über humorale Übertragbarkeit der Herznervenwirkung. *Pflügers Arch. Gesamte Physiol.* 189:239, 1921.
52. Lorenz, R.G., Saper, C.B., Wong, D.L. et al. Co-localization of substance P- and phenylethanolamine-N-methyltransferase-like immunoreactivity in neurons of ventrolateral medulla that project to the spinal cord: potential role in control of vasomotor tone. *Neurosci. Lett.* 55:255, 1985.
53. Lundberg, J.M., Anggard, A., and Fahrenkrug, J. Complementary role of vasoactive intestinal polypeptide (VIP) and acetylcholine for cat submandibular gland blood flow and secretion. I. VIP release. *Acta Physiol. Scand.* 113:317, 1981.
54. Majewski, H. and Starke, K. Prejunctional effects of catecholamines. *Biblthca Cardiol.* 38:53, 1984.
55. McCall, R.B. Serotonergic excitation of sympathetic preganglionic neurons: a microiontophoretic study. *Brain Res.* 289:121, 1983.
56. Mesulam, M-M, Mufson, E.J., Wainer, B.H. and Levey, A.I. Central cholinergic pathways in the rat: an overview based on an alternative nomenclature (Ch1-Ch6). *Neuroscience* 10:1185, 1983.
57. Molinoff, P.B. α- and β-Adrenergic receptor subtypes properties, distribution and regulation. *Drugs* 28(suppl. 2):1, 1984.
58. Müller-Oerlinghausen, B. Lithium long-term treatment. Does it act via serotonin? *Pharmacopsychiatry* 18:214, 1985.
59. Nieoullon, A., Kerkerian, L., and Dusticier, N. Presynaptic dopaminergic control of high affinity glutamate uptake in the striatum. *Neurosci. Lett.* 43:191, 1983.
60. Örgen, S.O., Fuxe, K. and Agnati, L. The importance of brain serotonergic receptor mechanisms for the action of antidepressant drugs. *Pharmacopsychiatry* 18:209, 1985.
61. Pradhan, S.N., and Bose, S. Interactions among central neurotransmitters. In: *Psychopharmacology: A Generation of Progress* (Lipton, M.A., DiMascio, A., and Killam, K.F., eds.) New York: Raven Press, 1978, p. 271.
62. Reichardt, L.F. and Kelly, R.B. A molecular description of nerve terminal function. *Annu. Rev. Biochem.* 52:871, 1983.
63. Riker, W.F., Jr. and Okamoto, M. Pharmacology of motor nerve terminals. *Annu. Rev. Pharmacol.* 9:173, 1969.
64. Salt, T.E. and Hill, R.G. Neurotransmitter candidates of somatosensory primary afferent fibres. *Neuroscience* 10:1083, 1983.
65. Schmitt, F.O., Dev, P. and Smith, B.H. Electrogenic processing of information by brain cells. *Science* 193:114, 1976.
66. Sharif, N.A. Multiple synaptic receptors for neuroactive amino acid transmitters new vistas. *Int. Rev. Neurobiol.* 26:851, 1985.
67. Sherrington, C.S. The central nervous system. In: *A Textbook of Physiology,* Vol. 3, 7th ed. (Foster, M. ed.). London: Macmillan, 1897.
68. Spampinato, U., Nowakowska, E., and Samanin, R. Increased release of striatal dopamine after long-term treatment with methadone in rats: inhibition by agents which increase central 5-hydroxytryptamine transmission. *J. Pharm. Pharmacol.* 35:831, 1983.
69. Starke, K. Presynaptic receptors. *Ann. Rev. Pharmacol. Toxicol.* 21:7, 1981.
70. van Heuven-Nolsen, D., De Kloet, E.R., De Wied, D., and Versteeg, D.H. Microinjection of vasopressin and two related peptides into the amygdala: enhancing effect on local dopamine neurotransmission. *Brain Res.* 293:191, 1984.
71. Viveros, O.H. and Wilson, S.P. The adrenal chromaffin cell as a model to study cosecretion of enkephalins and catecholamines. *J. Autonom. Nerv. Syst.* 7:41, 1983.
72. von Euler, U.S. A specific sympathomimetic ergone in adrenergic nerve fibres (sympathin) and its relations to adrenaline and noradrenaline. *Acata Physiol. Scand.* 12:73, 1946.
73. von Euler, U.S., and Gaddum, J.H. An unidentified depressor substance in certain tissue extracts. *J. Physiol. (Lond.)* 72:74, 1931.
74. Weiner, N. Multiple factors regulating the release of norepinephrine consequent to nerve stimulation. *Fed. Proc.* 38:2193, 1979a.
75. Weiner, N. Tyrosine-3-monooxygenase (tryosine hydroxylase). In: *Aromatic Amino Acid Hydroxylases: Biochemical and Physiological Aspects* (Youdim, M.B.H. ed.). New York: John Wiley & Sons, Inc., 1979b, p. 141.
76. Weiner, N., Cloutier, G., Bjur, R. and Pfeffer, R.I. Modification of norepinephrine synthesis in intact tissue by drugs and during short-term adrenergic nerve stimulation. *Pharmacol. Rev.* 24:203, 1972.
77. Winkler, H., Fischer-Colbrie, F. and Weber, A. Molecular organization of vesicles storing transmitter: chromaffin vesicles as a model. In: *Chemical Neurotransmission-75 Years* (Stjärne, L., Hedqvist, P., Lagercrantz, H. and Wennmalm, A., eds.). London: Academic Press, 1981, p. 57.

CHAPTER
7

DRUGS AFFECTING CATECHOLAMINERGIC NEUROTRANSMISSION

Sidney Spector and Sachin N. Pradhan

SITES OF CATECHOLAMINE RELEASE

Of three physiologically important catecholamines, norepinephrine and dopamine are mainly involved in the neurotransmission in the central as well as sympathetic nervous systems. Epinephrine, a hormone from the adrenal medulla, is also involved in regulation of target organs with sympathetic innervation. Although present in the CNS, epinephrine's role is not very definite (Chapter 6).

Norepinephrine (NE) is released from most of the postganglionic sympathetic nerve terminals, adrenal medulla, and other chromaffin tissue, and certain tracts within the CNS (Chapter 6). *Epinephrine* is the major hormone of the adrenal medulla. Approximately 80% of medullary catecholamines are epinephrine, the rest being made up of NE. It is also present in other chromaffin cells. Some tracts are also demonstrable in the CNS. *Dopamine* is a predominant central neurotransmitter (e.g., in nigrostriatal, mesolimbic, tuberoinfundibular and tuberohypophyseal pathways). Small dopaminergic interneurons (SIF cells) are demonstrable in sympathetic ganglia, and dopamine receptors are present in renal and mesenteric vascular beds (Chapter 6).

FUNCTIONAL USES OF CATECHOLAMINES

From these locations the catecholamines perform and modulate many important functions. In the CNS they are involved in various functions: (a) NE in the regulation of mood and emotions, reward, behavior, motivation and autonomic control; (b) dopamine in the regulation of motor activity, emotions and endocrine functions; and (c) epinephrine in the regulation of temperature, food and water intake, sleep and wakefulness, and control of blood pressure and respiration (Chapter 6). In the periphery, epinephrine and NE are mainly concerned with the autonomic regulation of target tissues like heart, blood vessels, and smooth muscles and exocrine glands in eye and in respiratory, gastrointestinal and genitourinary systems (Table 7-1). In these aspects dopamine is comparatively much less potent.

MODIFICATION OF CATECHOLAMINERGIC TRANSMISSION BY DRUGS OR CHEMICALS

Drugs can interact with the biosynthesis, release, uptake and disposition of the various catecholamines (2, 8), as well as at the receptor to modify neurotransmission (Figure 7-1), as described in Chapter 6.

Synthesis Briefly, synthesis of catecholamines inside the sympathetic neurons involves the uptake of the amino acid tyrosine into the neuron where it is then converted to DOPA (dihydroxyphenylalanine), which in turn is converted to dopamine and then to NE. Several agents can depress overall catecholamine synthesis by inhibiting the specific enzymatic steps involved in their biosynthesis. Thus, metyrosine (α-methyl-*p*-tyrosine) and catechols

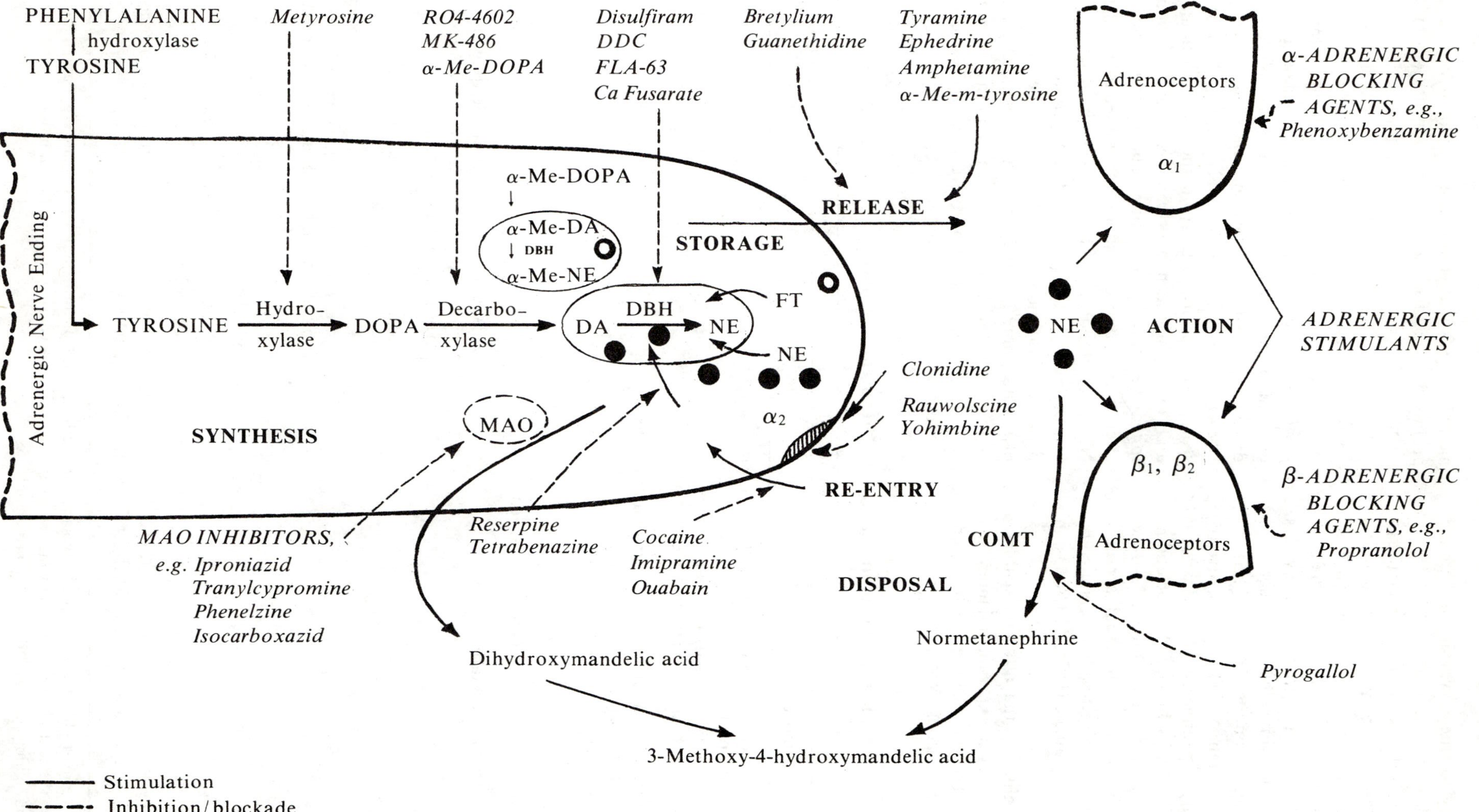

Fig. 7-1. *Pharmacology of adrenergic neurotransmission.*
(Abbrv. FT, False transmitter; DA, Dopamine; NE, Norepinephrine; MAO, Monoamine oxidase; DBH, DA-β-hydroxylase; DDC, Diethyldithiocarbamate; FLA-63, *bis*-(1-methyl-4-homopiperazinyl-thiocarbonyl) disulfide.)

inhibit tyrosine hydroxylase, the enzyme involved in the rate-limiting step of this synthesis.

DOPA decarboxylase (also known as aromatic L-amino acid decarboxylase) is responsible for the conversion of DOPA to dopamine. This enzyme is not specific. Many other endogenous metabolites and exogenous chemicals and drugs are similarly acted upon by this enzyme. Thus, this enzyme is involved in production of tyramine from tyrosine, histamine from histidine, 5-hydroxytryptamine (serotonin, 5-HT) from 5-hydroxytryptophan, and α-methyldopamine from α-methyldopa. Several compounds (namely, R04-4602, MK-486 and α-methyldopa) can inhibit this step. Dopamine-β-hydroxylase, the enzyme that hydroxylates the β carbon of dopamine and converts dopamine to NE, is inhibited by disulfiram, diethyldithiocarbamate (DDC), FLA-63 and calcium fusarate.

Most of the enzyme inhibitors that affect the synthesis of catecholamines are mainly of experimental interest at present and not much of therapeutic benefit in hypertension and other clinical conditions except for drugs like methyldopa (β-methyldopa), since their effects are compromised by feedback and other compensatory mechanisms.

Storage and Release. Synthesized catecholamine molecules are stored in granulated vesicles at the nerve terminals where they are thought to exist in more than one *pool*. The concept of *pools* originated because of differences in the pattern of release of NE induced by different drugs and procedures. Thus, from one pool (*free*, *mobile*, or *easily releasable* pool, or pool I) release of NE from the storage vesicles occurs by sympathetic nerve stimulation and by agents such as tyramine, phenylethylamine, ephedrine and amphetamine. The sympathomimetic effect of the latter compounds is attributed to the released NE, and is not observed following sympathetic denervation of the tissue, or depletion of its NE content following preadministration of reserpine. Hence, these agents (all of which are noncatecholamines) have been called indirect-acting sympathomimetic agents in contrast to norepinephrine, epinephrine, isoproterenol and phenylephrine that act directly on the adrenoceptors.

Table 7-1
Classification of the Effects of Adrenoceptor Agonists

Type of Effects	Type of Adrenoceptors	
	α-Adrenoceptor Action[a]	β-Adrenoceptor Action[b]
Peripheral excitatory	Contraction of smooth muscles [e.g., iris dilator, pilomotor, splenic capsule, sphincters (gastrointestinal), pregnant uterus (rabbit, dog, human), nictitating membrane (cat)]	
	Constriction of arterioles as in skin, mucous membrane; also in kidney, abdominal viscera, skeletal muscle, etc.	
	Increased salivary secretion	
	Increased sweat secretion (localized)	
Peripheral inhibitory	Intestinal relaxation	β_2, Relaxation of smooth muscles [e.g., in gastrointestinal tract, bronchus, bladder, uterus (rat, pregnant cat, human)]
		β_2, Vasodilation (e.g., in heart, skeletal muscle, lung, abdominal viscera)
Cardiac excitatory		β_1, Increase in heart rate (positive chronotropic effect) and force of contraction (positive inotropic effect)
Metabolic		β_1, Increase in lipolysis
		β_2, Increase in glycogenolysis and gluconeogenesis
CNS excitatory	Respiratory stimulation (analeptic effect), decrease of appetite (anorectic effect), increase in wakefulness (arousal effect), receptor sites not definite	

[a] Mostly involving α_1-receptors to be blocked by phenoxybenzamine, dibenamine, phentolamine, tolazoline, ergot alkaloids, etc., except for clonidine in the central nervous system which stimulates α_2-receptors causing presynaptic inhibition.
[b] Blocked by propranolol, sotalol, practolol, dichloroisoproterenol, etc.

The amount of NE that remains in the storage granule after release from pool I can be completely depleted by reserpine. This tightly bound pool of NE is called the *bound pool*, or pool II. The NE in pool I is the newly synthesized NE and has a very rapid turnover with a half-life of 2 hr. In contrast, pool II has a half-life of 24 hr. Equilibrium exists between these two pools.

The release of NE is prevented by the drugs bretylium and guanethidine which are called adrenergic neuronal-blocking agents. Guanethidine can also cause a release of catecholamines prior to its blocking action.

Receptor Action. As mentioned in Chapter 6, released NE acts on two different types of adrenergic receptors, or adrenoceptors referred to as α and β, depending on the nature of their actions (1, 17). Table 7-1 lists the α and β adrenoceptor actions under five broad categories: peripheral excitatory, peripheral inhibitory, cardiac excitatory, metabolic and central excitatory. β-Receptor actions are further subdivided into β_1 (cardiac actions and lipolysis) and β_2 (smooth muscle and other metabolic actions) (15, 16, 24).

α-Adrenoceptors also appear to be of more than one type (4, 9, 15). The α-receptors at the postsynaptic sites located in the smooth muscle and exocrine gland cells are responsible for producing excitatory actions and are designated as α_1. On the other hand, there are adrenoceptor sites on the presynaptic nerve terminals; activation of these receptors (α_2) mediates presynaptic feedback inhibition of release of norepinephrine and perhaps acetylcholine (7, 14, 20). Activation of such receptors on cholinergic nerve terminals in the gastrointestinal tract by α-adrenergic agonists probably causes inhibitory effects at this site. α_2-Receptors may be present in some central sites such as cerebral cortex and lower brainstem (possibly in nucleus tractus solitarius), as well as in peripheral tissues such as uterus and parotid gland. These α_2-receptors are stimulated by clonidine and blocked by piperoxan and yohimbine.

The agents stimulating these adrenergic receptors have been variously termed sympathomimetic agents (as their effects resemble stimulation of sympathetic nervous system), adrenergic stimulants or agents, adrenergic agonists, adrenergic receptor or adrenoceptor agonists. Similarly, terms used to identify agents that block these receptors have also been diverse: sympatholytic or adrenolytic agents; adrenergic-, adrenergic receptor-, or adrenoreceptor-blocking agents or antagonists.

As already indicated, adrenergic stimulants can be classified as direct-acting (on the adrenoceptors) or indirect-acting, the effects of the latter being mediated through release of NE from storage sites. Furthermore, both adrenoceptor agonists and antagonists can be classified depending on the receptor they exert their action upon (α or β).

False Transmitters Methyldopa causes inhibition of DOPA decarboxylase; since the enzyme exists far in excess of the amount required for catecholamine synthesis, this action is not enough to explain the effect of this drug, causing progressive reduction in blood pressure and heart rate. Moreover, the inhibition of the enzyme occurs for a relatively short period, while the effect on blood pressure lasts longer. Methyldopa is decarboxylated by the aromatic L-amino acid decarboxylase to α-methyldopamine and then on to α-methylnorepinephrine. α-Methyl-NE then occupies the same storage sites as NE in the adrenergic nerve terminals, displacing the stored NE and thereby reducing the stored amount of the active neurotransmitter. During nerve stimulation, both NE and α-methyl-NE are released; however, the amount of NE released is much less, and consequently postsynaptic adrenoceptors would manifest less effects. Such diminished receptor action can be attributed to the transmitter-like substances that share the same storage site and the same release process as the true neurotransmitter, but possess comparatively less potency. Such substances have been termed *false transmitters* (12, 18). In addition to α-methyl-NE, other false transmitters include metaraminol and octopamine; their formation is shown in Fig. 7-2.

Termination of Action As discussed in Chapter 6, released NE is rapidly (a) removed from the synaptic cleft, mostly by a process of re-uptake or re-entry into the nerve terminal to be stored in the vesicles, or (b) disposed of by dilution through diffusion out of the synaptic cleft, and by metabolic transformation initiated by two enzymes, catechol-O-methyl-transferase (COMT) and monoamine oxidase (MAO) (3). Of these, the re-uptake process plays a major role in terminating the action of released catecholamines. With respect to enzymatic disposition of NE action, MAO metabolizes the transmitter mainly within the nerve terminal, whereas COMT in the liver is of importance to metabolize and inactivate the circulating endogenous and exogenous catecholamines.

Re-uptake. NE is subject to a re-uptake process from the synaptic cleft into the neuron (uptake-1) by at least two active transport systems—one across the axoplasmic membrane from the extraneuronal fluid into the neuronal cytoplasm and the other from the cytoplasm into the storage vesicles. Such active transport processes across the neuronal and vesicular membranes may result in concentrating NE 10,000-fold within the vesicles. Uptake by extraneuronal tissue has been termed as uptake-2, which has higher affinity for epinephrine, whereas uptake-1 by the neural tissue has higher affinity for NE (11, 25).

The evidence of the transport system across the axoplasmic membrane is indirect and is based on selective blockade by several drugs. Thus cocaine, antidepressants (e.g., imipramine) and ouabain can selectively block the plasma membrane re-uptake and thereby increase and prolong the action of catecholamines at the postsynaptic receptor sites.

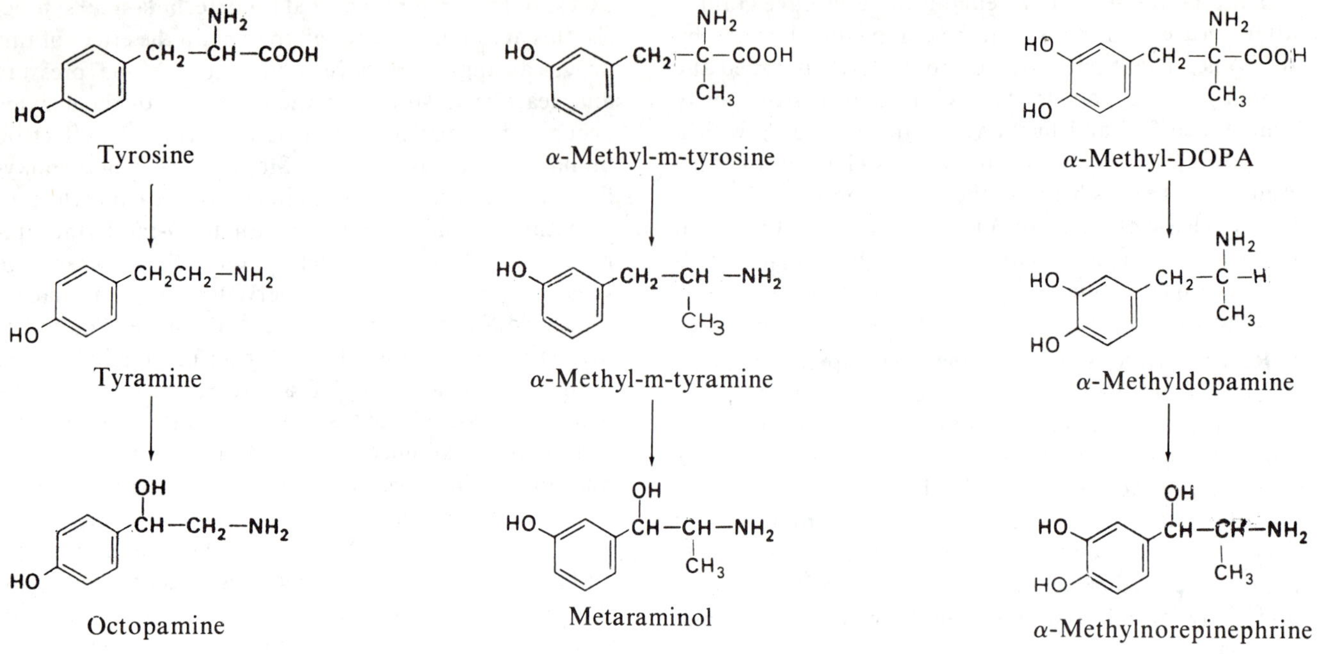

Tyrosine → Tyramine → Octopamine

α-Methyl-m-tyrosine → α-Methyl-m-tyramine → Metaraminol

α-Methyl-DOPA → α-Methyldopamine → α-Methylnorepinephrine

Fig. 7-2. *False transmitters.*

The transport system across the vesicular membrane has been studied more completely. This system requires adenosine triphosphate (ATP) and Mg^{++} and is inhibited by very low concentrations (40 nM) of reserpine. Reserpine can also block uptake of dopamine into storage vesicles where NE is synthesized from dopamine by the enzyme dopamine-β-hydroxylase. Thus NE synthesis is decreased by reserpine. Increased concentrations of free catecholamines within the neuron can inhibit tyrosine hydroxylase and thereby regulate its rate of synthesis by end-product inhibition. Free catecholamine in the cytoplasm is inactivated by mitochondrial MAO. Acting through these mechanisms, reserpine depletes the stores of catecholamines (and also 5-HT) in the brain, adrenal medulla, and other organs with catecholaminergic innervation.

Disposition. COMT plays a greater role than MAO in enzymatic inactivation of circulating catecholamines. Despite the importance of COMT, compounds (e.g., pyrogallol) that inhibit COMT does not have any therapeutic importance. MAO inhibitors (e.g., pargyline, tranylcypromine, nialamide), on the other hand, can cause an increase in the level of NE in the brain and other tissues, resulting in several pharmacological effects (as antidepressant and antihypertensive). Some of these effects may be due to other than MAO inhibition. However, their uses as antidepressants and antihypertensive agents are not encouraged currently because of their adverse effects.

It now appears that MAO exists in two forms with different substrate specifications (10, 22). MAO-A is predominantly in the liver and intestinal mucosa, and MAO-B in certain regions of the brain e.g., basal ganglia. Although controversial, selective inhibition of these two isozymes by drugs has been claimed (19) (Chapter 7.4).

INHIBITION OF ADRENERGIC NERVE ACTIVITY BY DRUGS

Activity of the adrenergic nerve can be inhibited by several mechanisms as discussed earlier (Fig. 7-3).

1. Preventing release of NE from the adrenergic nerve terminal (e.g., by guanethidine, bretylium)
2. Depleting the store of NE in the adrenergic neurons (e.g., by reserpine)
3. Replacing NE by less potent false transmitters (e.g., α-methyldopa)
4. Preventing released NE from acting on the adrenoceptors (e.g., by α- and β-adrenoceptor-blocking agents)
5. Decreasing release of NE through feedback inhibition induced by presynaptic α_2-adrenoceptor stimulation [e.g., by clonidine (α_2-adrenoceptor agonists)].

CATECHOLAMINE NEUROTOXIN

6-HYDROXYDOPAMINE

6-Hydroxydopamine (6-OHDA) acts as a relatively selective neurotoxin to catecholaminergic nerve terminals (13, 21). Effects of 6-OHDA on the peripheral noradrenergic neurons may be due to uptake-1 and accumulation in the nerve membrane amine pump that can be inhibited by the uptake blockers such as desipramine. However, since its action is not affected by reserpine, its uptake into the storage granules does not appear

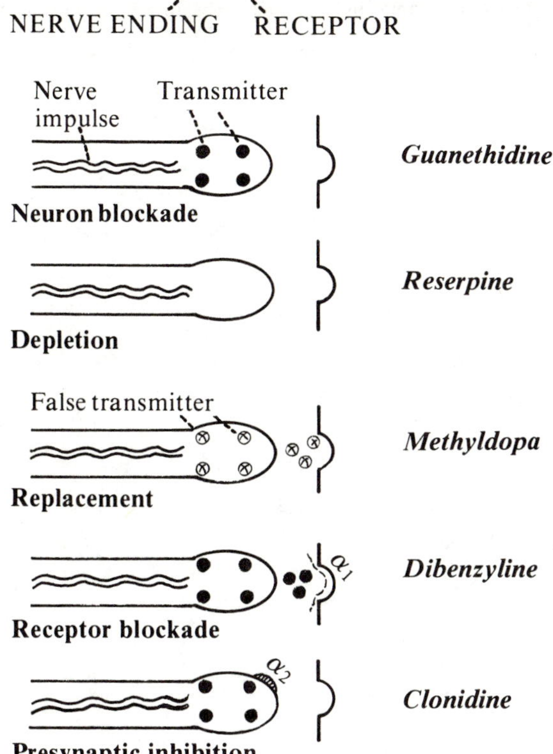

Fig. 7-3. *Different approaches of inhibition of adrenergic neurotransmission.*

to be a necessary step for nerve damage. While inside the neuron, 6-OHDA is bound in a granular storage pool and can be released by nerve stimulation, thus acting as a false neurotransmitter. It may displace and cause release of norepinephrine from the storage site, showing an initial sympathomimetic effect. In sufficiently high concentration, presumably in the cytoplasmic pool, 6-OHDA generates highly reactive products (suggested to be peroxides, superoxides, hydroxyindoles and quinones). These products react nonspecifically with neuronal structures and cause destruction of sympathetic nerve endings, which resembles the effect of surgical sympathectomy. In adult animals peripheral noradrenergic nerve cell bodies and the proximal axons are not affected, and complete regeneration of the nerve terminals usually occurs. In newborn animals destruction of the entire noradrenergic neuron may occur and may be permanent. Such process of chemical sympathectomy, as it may be called, is more complete than that produced by nerve growth factor antisera (immunosympathectomy). 6-OHDA does not cross the blood-brain barrier, and the central catecholaminergic neurons are not affected. However, after intraventricular or local administration, both noradrenergic and dopaminergic neurons in the CNS are affected, the former being more susceptible.

Attempts to use 6-OHDA in the therapy of glaucoma have been unsatisfactory. Following its subconjunctival injection, sympathetic innervation of the anterior portion of the eye is destroyed and intraocular pressure decreases. However, with regeneration of the nerves in 3-4 months the beneficial effect ceases. Its repeated injections cause inflammation and fibrosis.

REFERENCES AND ADDITIONAL READING

1. Ahlquist, R.P. A study of the adrenotropic receptors. *Am. J. Physiol.* 153:586, 1948.
2. Axelrod, J. The formation, metabolism, uptake and release of noradrenaline and adrenaline. In: *The Clinical Chemistry of Monoamines* (Varley, H. and Gowenlock, A.H., eds.). Amsterdam: Elsevier, 1963, p. 5.
3. Axelrod, J. The fate of noradrenaline in the sympathetic neurone. *Harvey Lect.* 67:175, 1973.
4. Berthelsen, S. and Pettinger, W.A. A functional basis for classification of α-adrenergic receptors. *Life Sci.* 21:595, 1977.
5. Burn, J.H. and Rand, M.J. The action of sympathomimetic amines in animals treated with reserpine. *J. Physiol.* (London) 144:314, 1958.
6. Cooper, J.R., Bloom, F.E. and Roth, R.H. *The Biochemical Basis of Neuropharmacology*, 3rd ed. New York: Oxford University Press, 1978.
7. Dixon, W.R., Mosimann, W.F. and Weiner, N. The role of presynaptic feedback mechanisms in regulation of norepinephrine release by nerve stimulation. *J. Pharmacol. Exp. Ther.* 209:196, 1979.
8. Euler, U.S. von. Regulation of catecholamine metabolism in the sympathetic nervous system. *Pharmacol. Rev.* 24:365, 1972.
9. Hoffman, B.B. and Lefkowitz, R.J. Alpha-adrenergic receptor subtypes. *N. Engl. J. Med.* 302:1390, 1980.
10. Houslay, M.D. and Tipton, K.F. Multiple forms of monoamine oxidase: Fact and artifact. *Life Sci.* 19:467, 1976.
11. Iversen, L.L. Uptake processes for biogenic amines. In: *Handbook of Psychopharmacology* Vol.3 (Iversen, L.L., Iversen, S.D. and Snyder, S., eds.). New York: Plenum Press, 1975, p. 381.
12. Kopin, I.J. False adrenergic transmitters. *Ann. Rev. Pharmacol.* 8:377, 1968.
13. Kostrzewa, R.M. and Jacobowitz, D.M. Pharmacological actions of 6-hydroxydopamine. *Pharmacol. Rev.* 26:199, 1974.
14. Langer, S.Z. Presynaptic receptors and their role in the regulation of transmitter release. *Br. J. Pharmacol.* 60:481, 1977.
15. Lee, G.M. A hitch-hikers's guide to the galaxy of adrenoceptors. *Br. Med. J.* 283:173, 1981.
16. Minneman, K.P., Hegstrand, L.R. and Molinoff, P.B. Simultaneous determination of beta-1 and beta-2 adrenergic receptors in tissues containing both receptor subtypes. *Mol. Pharmacol.* 15:286, 1979.
17. Moran, N.C. Adrenergic receptors. In: *Adrenal Gland Vol. 6, Sect. 7, Endocrinology. Handbook of Physiology* (Blaschko, H., Sayers, G. and Smith, A.D., eds.). Washington, D.C.: American Physiology Society, 1975, p. 447.
18. Muscholl, E. Adrenergic false transmitters. In: *Catecholamines. Handbuch der Experimentellen Pharmakologie* Vol. 33, (Blaschko, H. and Muscholl, E., eds.). Berlin: Springer-Verlag, 1972, p. 618.
19. Riederer, P., Youdim, M.B.H., Birkmayer, W. and Jellinger, K. Monoamine oxidase activity during (-)-deprenyl therapy: Human brain postmortem studies. *Adv. Biochem. Psychopharmacol.* 19:377, 1978.
20. Starke, K. Regulation of noradrenaline release by presynaptic receptor systems. *Rev. Physiol. Biochem. Pharmacol.* 77:1, 1977.
21. Thoenen, H. Surgical, immunological, and chemical sympathectomy. In: *Catecholamines. Handbuch der Experimentellen Pharmakologie*, Vol. 33 (Blaschko, H. and Muscholl, E., eds.). Berlin: Springer-Verlag, 1972, p. 813.
22. Usdin, E., Weiner, N. and Youdim, M.B.H. (eds.). *Structure and Function of Monoamine Enzymes.* New York: Marcel Dekker, 1977.
23. Westfall, T.C. Local regulation of adrenergic neurotransmission. *Physiol. Rev.* 57:659, 1977.

24. Wolfe, B.B., Harden, T.K. and Molinoff, P.B. *In vitro* studies of β-adrenergic receptors. *Ann. Rev. Pharmacol. Toxicol.* 17:575, 1977.

25. Yamaguchi, N., DeChamplain, J. and Nadeau, R.A. Regulation of norepinephrine release from cardiac sympathetic fibers in the dog by presynaptic alpha and beta receptors. *Circ. Res.* 41:108, 1977.

CHAPTER
7.1

ADRENERGIC AGENTS

Sachin N. Pradhan and Sidney Spector

Adrenergic agonists, which are also called adrenoceptor agonists or adrenoceptor agents, can be classified into catecholamines and noncatecholamines. Catecholamines, such as epinephrine, norepinephrine, isoproterenol and others, directly act on the adrenergic receptors or adrenoceptors. Noncatecholamines, such as amphetamines, ephedrine, tyramine, and others, act by releasing norepinephrine from the storage sites in the adrenergic neurons, which in turn acts on the adrenoceptors. Hence they are called indirectly acting adrenergic agents. However, some noncatecholamines, such as phenylephrine, act directly on adrenoceptors. Other noncatecholamines, such as ephedrine, have both direct and indirect effects because ephedrine, which shows marked bronchodilator action, is dependent upon released norepinephrine for its action, although norepinephrine itself does not have much effect on the bronchus. Adrenergic agents of both types will be discussed in this chapter. Dopamine, although a catecholamine, has somewhat different site and type of action compared with other catecholamines; its pharmacology is discussed in Chapter 7.4. Agents discussed here act on various adrenoceptors (e.g., α_1, β_1, and β_2). Clonidine acts on α_2-adrenoceptors and is discussed in Chapter 15.3. Certain selective β_2-adrenoceptor agonists with less untoward effects, such as metaproterenol, are of therapeutic importance for their bronchodilator effect. Although most of the β_2-adrenoceptor agonists are noncatecholamines, some contain the catechol nucleus. Some of these agents are also discussed here.

CHEMISTRY

Most of the adrenergic agonists possess a parent structure, β-phenylethylamine, that consists of a benzene ring and an ethylamine side chain. Substitutions are made in the benzene ring as well as in the α- and β-carbons and the terminal amine groups of the side chain (Table 7.1-1).

Substitution on the Benzene Ring. Substitution of OH groups in the 3 and 4 positions of the benzene ring produces O-dihydroxybenzenes, or catechols. Amines derived from catechols are catecholamines that include

Table 7.1-1
Chemical Structures and Major Therapeutic Uses of Adrenergic Agonists

					Major Therapeutic Uses and Adrenoceptors Involved				
	Ring (positions 1–6)	β CH —	α CH —	NH	Nasal Deconges- tant (N)	Pressor (P), Vaso- constrictor (V)	Antialler- gic (A), Broncho- dilator (B)	Cardiac Stimulant (C)	CNS Stim- ulant (S), Anorectic (A)
					α	α	β_2	β_1	
Phenylethylamine		H	H	H					
Catecholamines									
Epinephrine	3-OH, 4-OH	OH	H	CH_3		P,V	A,B	C	
Norepinephrine	3-OH, 4-OH	OH	H	H		P,V			
Dopamine	3-OH, 4-OH	H	H	H		P			
Dobutamine	3-OH, 4-OH	H	H	a				C	
Isoproterenol	3-OH, 4-OH	OH	H	$CH(CH_3)_2$			B	C	
Isoetharine	3-OH, 4-OH	OH	CH_2CH_3	$CH(CH_3)_2$			B		
Noncatecholamines									
Tyramine	4-OH	H	H	H					
Amphetamine		H	CH_3	H					S,A
Methamphetamine		H	CH_3	CH_3		P			S,A
Hydroxyamphetamine	4-OH	H	CH_3	H	N	P		C	
Fenfluramine	3-CF_3	H	CH_3	C_2H_5					A
Ephedrine		OH	CH_3	CH_3	N	P	B	C	
Mephentermine		OH	CH_3	H	N	P			
Metaraminol	3-OH	OH	CH_3	H		P			
Phenylephrine	3-OH	OH	H	CH_3	N	P			
Methoxamine	2-OCH_3, 5-OCH_3	OH	CH_3	H		P			
Methoxyphenamine	2-OCH_3	H	CH_3	CH_3			B		
Metaproterenol	3-OH, 5-OH	OH	H	$CH(CH_3)_2$			B		
Terbutaline	3-OH, 5-OH	OH	H	$C(CH_3)_3$			B		
Albuterol	3-CH_2OH, 4-OH	OH	H	$C(CH_3)_3$			B		

[a] $-CH(CH_3)-(CH_2)_2-C_6H_4-OH$

dopamine, norepinephrine, epinephrine, and isoproterenol.

Most direct-acting adrenergic agonists possess both α-and β-adrenoceptor activity. The maximal α and β activity depends on the presence of OH groups in the 3 and 4 positions. The ratio of the α and β activity varies from drug to drug.

Hydroxy groups in the 3 and 5 positions, as in metaproterenol and terbutaline, produce selective β-receptor actions [e.g., bronchodilation (in asthma)] without causing significant cardiac effects. Absence of one or both OH groups in the 3 and 4 positions reduces overall potency, as in the case of phenylephrine, which, compared with epinephrine, has less α- and no β-receptor activity. Absence of one or both OH groups, especially the 3-OH group, increases oral effectiveness and duration of action of compounds, particularly with an α-methyl group. Absence of polar hydroxy group in the phenylethylamine structure makes the compounds (such as ephedrine and amphetamine) lose direct peripheral sympathomimetic activity; furthermore, such compounds become more lipophilic and capable of crossing the blood-brain barrier and show more central activity.

Substitution on the α-Carbon Atom. Substitution of a CH_3 group on the α-carbon atom in the noncatecholamines such as ephedrine or amphetamine blocks their oxidation by monoamine oxidase (MAO) and prolongs their duration of action, since catechol-O-methyltransferase (COMT) can affect their metabolism. The duration of action of a similarly substituted catecholamine (e.g., α-methylnorepinephrine or nordefrin) is not prolonged. For the same reason, metaraminol has a more prolonged action compared with norepinephrine.

Substitution on the β-Carbon Atom. Substitution of OH group on the β-carbon atom greatly enhances the agonistic activity, both at α- and β-adrenoceptors, but lowers lipid-solubility and reduces CNS-stimulant activity. Thus, compared with methamphetamine, ephedrine possesses more bronchodilator and pressor effects and less central stimulant effects.

Optical Isomerism. Optical isomers are produced either by α- or β-carbon substitutions. Naturally occurring compounds such as *l*-epinephrine or *l*-norepinephrine with levorotatory substitutions in the β-carbon are 10 or more times as potent as the unnatural dextroisomers with respect to their peripheral adrenergic activity. On the other hand, *d*-amphetamine, which has dextrorotatory substitution on the α-carbon atom, is more potent than *l*-amphetamine in its central activity.

Substitution on the Amino Group. Increase in the size of the alkyl substitution on the amino group increases the β-receptor activity: isoproterenol (isopropyl substitution) > epinephrine (methyl substitution) > norepinephrine (none). Less substitution increases the selectivity of α-receptor activity, although N-methylation increases the activity: epinephrine > norepinephrine > isoproterenol.

CATECHOLAMINES

EPINEPHRINE

Pharmacological Effects.

Cardiovascular System. *Heart.* Epinephrine increases the rate (positive chronotropic effect), and the force of contraction (positive inotropic effect) of the heart by acting on the β_1-receptor in the cells of the pacemaker, conducting tissues, and myocardium, respectively. These effects are due to a direct cardiac stimulation and are independent of changes in cardiac function resulting from increased venous return and other vascular effects.

Epinephrine increases positive inotropic action, resulting in shortening of the systole and increases in the stroke volume. This effect, along with increase in heart rate, enhances the cardiac output. The work of the heart and its oxygen consumption are increased, but disproportionately, so that the work done relative to oxygen consumption (i.e., cardiac efficiency) is lessened. During induced tachycardia, depolarization of SA node cells is accelerated; the conduction velocity in the bundle of His, Purkinje fibers, and ventricles is increased; and the refractory period of the atrial and ventricular muscles is shortened.

In normal human ECG, epinephrine decreases the amplitude of the T wave. The downward deviation in the ST segment has also been shown in patients with angina pectoris during spontaneous or epinephrine-induced attacks of pain as well as in animal experiments with relatively high doses of epinephrine.

In isolated cardiac preparations or in the cat papillary muscle, epinephrine increases excitability, rate of spontaneous beating, and contractile force, and induces automaticity in quiescent muscles.

Blood vessels. Epinephrine produces its effects mainly on the small arterioles and precapillary sphincters, and to a lesser extent on the veins and large arteries. Its effect varies in different vascular beds. Epinephrine constricts the blood vessels in the skin, mucosa, kidney, and salivary glands by acting on their α_1-adrenoceptors. However, the effects of epinephrine on the vascular bed vary with the doses used. At low doses, it dilates the blood vessels to the skeletal muscles by its action on the β_2-receptors; at higher doses, these blood vessels are constricted through its action on the α_1-adrenoceptors, which are also present in the skeletal muscles and which partially balance the effects on the β_2-adrenoceptors.

Epinephrine as well as sympathetic stimulation enhances the coronary blood flow. This increased coronary flow is due to the net effect of several factors; the flow is slightly reduced because of mechanical compression from forcible contraction of the surrounding myocardium, but due to an increase in duration of the diastole and increased aortic blood pressure, the overall flow is enhanced. Epinephrine also directly acts on the adrenoceptors present in the coronary arteries, which have both α_1- and β_2-receptors. However, in humans, the α_1-adrenoceptor is predominant and so its overall effect is vasoconstriction. A metabolite (e.g., adenosine) that may be produced in the heart during myocardial hypoxia may elicit a dilator effect on the coronary vessels.

Blood Pressure. Rapid intravenous injection of epinephrine causes a characteristic biphasic effect on the blood pressure. It causes an increase and then a decrease of both systolic and diastolic blood pressure. As the systolic pressure increases more than the diastolic pressure, the pulse pressure also increases. The mean blood pressure quickly rises to a peak, then falls below the normal before returning to the control level. The pressor effect is proportional to the dose and fails to show tachyphylaxis with repeated doses. Epinephrine-induced pressor effect is due to (1) increased inotropic and chronotropic effects on the heart that enhance the systolic pressure, and (2) increased peripheral resistance due to constrictor effects on several vascular beds including those in the skin, mucosa and kidney that would increase the diastolic blood pressure.

This effect is, however, counterbalanced by vasodilator effects of epinephrine on β_2-receptors in other vascular beds such as the splanchnic and skeletal muscles, particularly at lower concentrations. Such vasodilation is responsible for the depressor effect of a small i.v. dose (0.1 μg/kg), slow i.v. infusion (10-30 μg/min), or s.c. injection (0.5-1 mg) of epinephrine, and also for the delayed hypotensive effect of a high dose of epinephrine when its blood concentration is decreased.

The initial increase of the pulse rate may be slowed markedly at the peak of the pressor effect by a compensatory vagal discharge arising via the baroreceptor mechanism. Such reflex bradycardia can be blocked by atropine.

Respiratory System. Intravenous injection of epinephrine in humans or animals may cause brief apnea, partly due to a direct effect and partly due to reflex inhibition (through the baroreceptor mechanism) of the brainstem respiratory center. This apnea may be followed by mild brief respiratory stimulation, causing increase in the rate and the tidal volume.

Epinephrine produces significant bronchodilation through stimulation of β_2-adrenoceptors in the bronchial smooth muscle. It can effectively counteract bronchoconstriction occurring in bronchial asthma and other anaphylactic conditions, or induced by histamine, bradykinin, cholinoceptor agonists, and other autacoids or drugs. This effect is due to nonspecific physiological antagonism and has to be differentiated from competitive antagonism elicited by antihistamines in histamine-induced bronchoconstriction. Epinephrine also produces vasoconstriction in the bronchial mucosa by acting at the α_1-adrenoceptor and can relieve bronchial congestion and increase the vital capacity. In addition, it prevents antigen-induced histamine release, similar to β-adrenoceptor agonists such as isoproterenol and salbutamol. These effects of epinephrine are of therapeutic importance in bronchial asthma.

Gastrointestinal System and Urinary Bladder. In general, epinephrine causes relaxation of the smooth muscles in the walls of the hollow viscera, especially those in the stomach, intestine and bladder via the β_2-receptor action; on the other hand, the pyloric, ileocecal, trigone and bladder sphincters contract due to α-receptor action. Inhibitory responses mediated by β_2-receptors are probably due to an increase in K^+ conductance, causing hyperpolarization. Epinephrine also inhibits gastric secretion in the resting condition and increases secretion induced by food, histamine and bethanechol (13, 14).

Eye. Sympathetic stimulation or i.v. administration of epinephrine or norepinephrine (but not their conjunctival instillation into the normal eye) causes mydriasis (due to contraction of the radial muscle of the iris), widening of the palpebral fissure (due to contraction of the smooth muscle of the levator palpebrae superioris), and protrusion of the eyeball (due to contraction of the unstriped muscle of the orbit). Epinephrine usually decreases intraocular pressure in normal and glaucomatous (wide-angle) eyes; this may be the effects of both a decrease in production of the aqueous humor due to local vasoconstriction and an increased outflow.

Other Smooth Muscles. Epinephrine produces contraction of the smooth muscle in some tissues, in addition to that of the blood vessels in the skin and mucous membrane, due to α-adrenoceptor stimulation. It contracts the splenic capsule and reduces the size of the spleen in some species, but not in humans. Pilomotor activity can be observed after an intradermal injection of very dilute solutions of epinephrine and norepinephrine, but not following their systemic administration.

The effect of epinephrine on the uterus varies with the dose of the drug, species, state of gestation and phase of sexual cycle. *In vitro*, it contracts strips of the human pregnant and nonpregnant uterus, however, it produces brief relaxation of human uterus *in situ* during the last month of pregnancy and at parturition. On the basis of this latter observation, more effective β_2-adrenoceptor stimulants such as albuterol (salbutamol) and terbutaline are used to delay premature labor.

Metabolism. Catecholamines elevate the blood glucose level by increasing glycogenolysis in the liver through β_2-adrenoceptor stimulation, gluconeogenesis, and decreased glucose clearance from the circulation (3). Insulin secretion is inhibited through α-receptor stimulation and enhanced through β_2-receptor stimulation; however, the predominant effect of epinephrine is an inhibition of insulin secretion. The uptake and utilization of glucose by peripheral tissues are also inhibited, at least partly because of its action on insulin secretion. Through β_2-receptor stimulation of adenylate cyclase (11, 15, 22) epinephrine also increases glycogenolysis in the skeletal muscle but elevates concentration of lactic acid due to a lack of glucose-6-phosphatase in this tissue (Fig. 7.1-1). Abolition of glucose mobilization requires simultaneous blockade of α-adrenoceptors in the liver and of β_2-adrenoceptors in the skeletal muscle.

Catecholamines also elevate levels of free fatty acid in the blood by activation of lipase (in the adipose tissue), which accelerates the breakdown of triglycerides to glycerol and free fatty acid. Such lipolytic action is mediated by cyclic adenosine monophosphate (cAMP) via β_1-receptor stimulation (Fig. 7.1-1). The lipolytic action may provide an oxidizable substrate and enhance metabolism (calorigenic action); norepinephrine has a similar action.

Catecholamines may also stimulate ketogenesis directly or indirectly (hormone mediated) in the liver. Epinephrine produces transient hyperkalemia followed by prolonged hypokalemia. Infusion of norepinephrine (NE) has been shown to decrease the plasma level of alanine in normal subjects, and prolonged infusion of epinephrine results in a decrease in plasma levels of branched-chain amino acids.

The direct metabolic effects of epinephrine are greater (about 10 times) than those of norepinephrine. Compared with epinephrine, isoproterenol has a less glycogenolytic effect, but an equal lipolytic effect.

Pharmacokinetics. Given orally, epinephrine is rapidly conjugated and oxidized in the gastrointestinal mucosa and liver and does not reach effective blood concentrations. Its subcutaneous injection produces local vasocon-

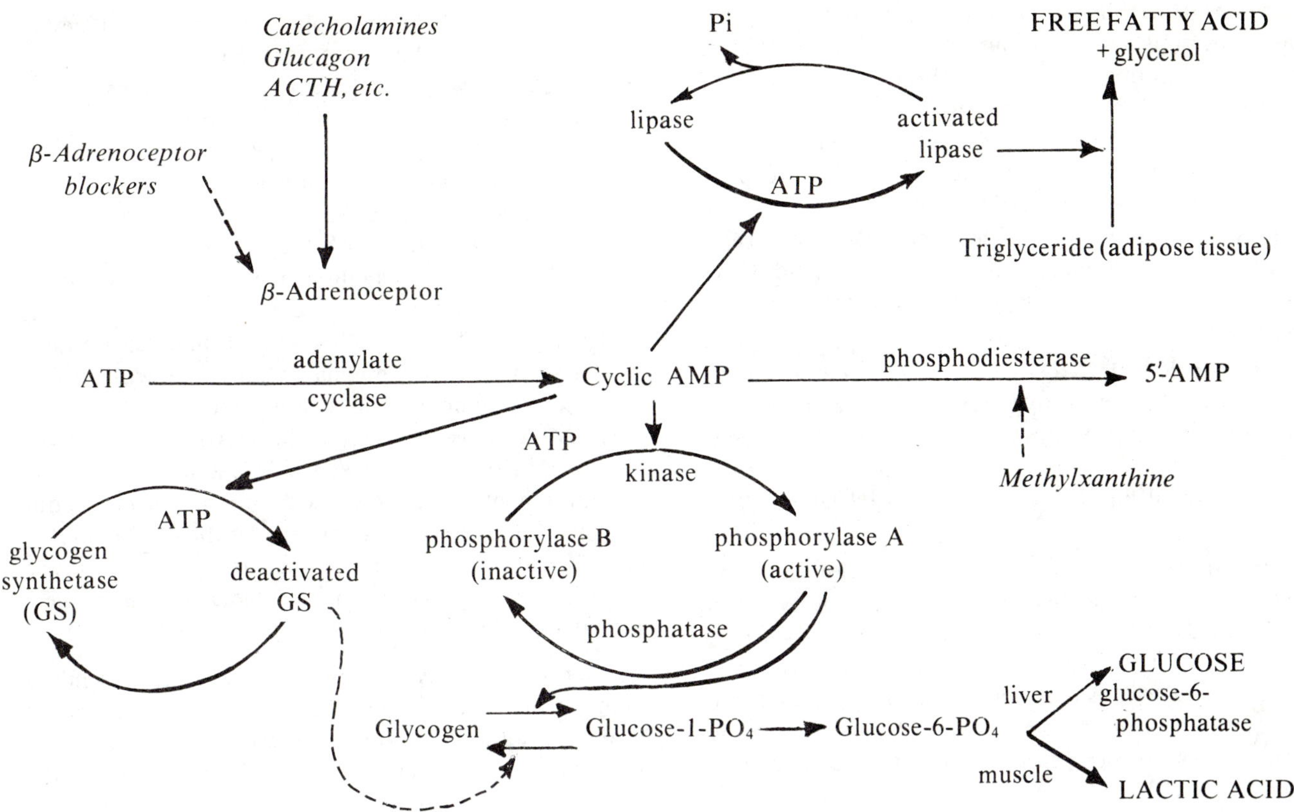

Fig. 7.1-1. *Regulation of carbohydrate and fat metabolism through β-adrenoceptor and effects of epinephrine.*

striction, slowing down its absorption, which can be hastened by massage and heat. Absorption after intramuscular administration is more rapid than after a subcutaneous injection. When inhaled in a concentrated solution (1%), the effect is mainly localized to the respiratory tract, although some systemic effects may be produced.

The plasma clearance rate of NE and epinephrine has been calculated at various steady-state concentrations following their graded infusions. In young humans, the plasma clearance rate of epinephrine was reported to be about 52 ml/kg/min at a steady state of plasma epinephrine concentration of 24-74 pg/ml. At a high steady-state plasma epinephrine concentration (e.g., 90-1020 pg/ml), the mean clearance rate is about 70% higher (approximately 90 ml/kg/min). The mean plasma clearance rate for NE was shown to be 25 ml/kg/min at a steady-state plasma NE level of 229-345 pg/ml. It appears that both epinephrine and NE stimulate their own plasma clearance rate, probably due to increased enzymatic degradation.

Catecholamines are cleared from the extracellular fluid by re-uptake into adrenergic postganglionic nerve endings, where they are mainly stored, or into extraneuronal cells, where they are metabolized. The former has a higher affinity for NE than epinephrine, and the latter has a higher affinity for epinephrine. The uptake into postganglionic nerve terminals has no affinity for isoproterenol. Recent studies have shown that the catecholamine clearance rate in the plasma is modulated by β-adrenoceptors only, and β-adrenergic blockade can markedly reduce the clearance rate of epinephrine and of both exogenously and endogenously released NE.

Epinephrine, like norepinephrine, is rapidly inactivated by both reuptake into the adrenergic nerve terminals and metabolic transformation by two enzymes, COMT and MAO. The greater part of a dose of epinephrine is excreted as metabolites in the urine; only a small amount may appear as epinephrine in the urine of normal persons, but it may be present in large amounts in the urine of pheochromocytoma patients.

COMT methylates OH group at the meta position of the catechol nucleus. Thus, congeners of epinephrine lacking in the 3-OH group are unaffected by COMT; they depend on MAO or other enzymes for their metabolism. The acid and glycol metabolites of catecholamines are produced by the enzyme MAO which have a number of inhibitors; it is now being shown that there are two MAO enzymes, each with a specific substrate. If the amines have an α-methyl group, they do not serve as substrates for the MAO enzyme.

Adverse Effects. Epinephrine may produce fear, anxiety, restlessness, tremor, throbbing headache, dizziness, palpitation and respiratory difficulty. These reactions often subside rapidly with rest. Hyperthyroid and hypertensive persons are often susceptible to these effects. More serious effects include cerebral hemorrhage and cardiac arrhythmias, particularly after large or rapid i.v. doses. A marked pressor effect may be counteracted by nitrites, sodium nitroprusside, or α-adrenoceptor blockers. Ventricular arrhythmia may occur when the drug is given along with a halogenated hydrocarbon anesthetic or in patients with an organic heart disease. Epinephrine induces anginal pain in patients with angina pectoris.

Therapeutic Uses. Most common uses of epinephrine are in bronchospasm, hypersensitivity reactions, and cardiac arrest, for prolongation of infiltration anesthesia, and as a topical hemostatic. These and other therapeutic uses of epinephrine are further discussed later in this chapter.

Comparison with Other Adrenergic Agonists. The effects of epinephrine discussed here as a prototype can be classified into five categories: peripheral excitatory, peripheral inhibitory, cardiac excitatory, metabolic and central excitatory, as described in Chapter 7 and Table 7-1. The effects of various adrenergic agonists can be compared with those of epinephrine with respect to these action categories; they are summarized in Table 7.1-2.

NOREPINEPHRINE

Pharmacological Effects. Norepinephrine [1,β-(3,4-dihydroxyphenyl)-α-aminoethanol, *l*-noradrenaline, levarterenol] resembles epinephrine in its cardiac (β_1-adrenoceptor) and excitatory (α-adrenoceptor) effects; it is somewhat less effective on α-receptors of most organs but is approximately equipotent on β_1-adrenoceptors. However, it is much less potent in its inhibitory and metabolic (β_2-adrenoceptor) effects. As with epinephrine, the *l*-isomer is much more potent than the *d*-isomer.

Cardiovascular Effects. Norepinephrine produces overall vasoconstriction and very little vasodilation, thus increasing the peripheral resistance and the diastolic blood pressure. As a result, the pressor effect of norepinephrine is greater and lasts longer than that of epinephrine, and secondary hypotension is very little or absent. Norepinephrine resembles epinephrine in its potency in stimulating β_1 (cardiac) receptors. However, due to the compensatory vagal reflex activity in response to its marked pressor effect, bradycardia is produced and the cardiac output may be unchanged or even decreased, although the stroke volume may be increased.

Other Effects. Compared with epinephrine, norepinephrine is less active with respect to its β_2-receptor effects. It causes only a slight increase in the tidal volume of respiration and a slight decrease in gastrointestinal motility. The effects on other smooth muscles are minimal except for the pregnant human uterus, which responds by an increase in the frequency of contraction. The CNS response to norepinephrine is minimal, as in the case of epinephrine: the drug may cause some restlesness and apprehension. In large doses, norepinephrine produces metabolic effects approximating those of epinephrine, which include glycogenolysis (in liver and muscle resulting in hyperglycemia and lactacidemia, respectively) as well as lipolysis.

Pharmacokinetics. Norepinephrine closely resembles epinephrine in its pharmacokinetics. It is not absorbed after oral administration because of its destruction by gastric secretions and rapid enzymatic inactivation in the liver (first-pass effect) and intestinal wall. It is also poorly absorbed following its s.c. injection because of local vasoconstriction. The drug is usually given by the i.v. route. Its pressor effect is brief due to its rapid inactivation by uptake into adrenergic nerve terminals,conjugation in liver, and deamination by MAO. It is excreted in the urine as metabolites with only a small fraction excreted unchanged.

Adverse Effects. Therapeutic doses of norepinephrine can produce adverse effects analogous to those produced by epinephrine, although they are less marked. They are characterized by anxiety, headache, palpitations and respiratory difficulty; however, these effects are transient and not usually dangerous. Its overdosage can produce extreme hypertension resulting in severe headache, sharp retrosternal and pharyngeal pain, intolerance to light, pallor, sweating and vomiting.

Table 7.1-2
Pharmacological Effects of Various Adrenergic Agents[a]

	Peripheral Excitatory α_1	Peripheral Inhibitory β_2	Cardiac Excitatory β_1	Metabolic Endocrine	CNS Excitatory
Epinephrine	++++	++++	++++	+++	+
Norepinephrine	++++	0/±	+++/++	0/+	+
Isoproterenol	0	++++	++++	+	±
Phenylephrine	+++	0/±	+	0	±
Ephedrine	++	++	+	0/+	++
Amphetamine	++	–	+	0	+++

[a] + to ++++ signify graded intensity of effect; ±, slight but variable effect; 0, lack of any effect.

During the i.v. infusion, extravasation at the site of injection produces cutaneous vasoconstriction that may result in necrosis and sloughing of the tissue. Careful infusion techniques or the local infiltration of an α-adrenoceptor-blocking agent will decrease the incidence of necrosis.

Therapeutic Uses. Norepinephrine may be useful in the treatment of cardiogenic shock to maintain adequate blood pressure by peripheral vasoconstriction. However an excessive increase in the blood pressure must be avoided so as not to overburden the heart or compromise circulation to the kidneys and other organs.

ISOPROTERENOL

Isoproterenol acts almost exclusively on β-adrenoceptors and has virtually no actions in the α-adrenoceptors. Its major effects are exerted on the cardiovascular system, the smooth muscles of the respiratory and gastrointestinal tracts, and the vasculature in skeletal muscle.

Isoproterenol's positive chronotropic and inotropic cardiac actions combined with its vasodilator effects (particularly in the skeletal muscle) and an increase in the venous return tend to increase the cardiac output and lower the peripheral vascular resistance. Usually there is an increase in the systolic pressure and a decrease in the diastolic pressure that together result in a reduction in mean arterial pressure. Higher doses cause a more dramatic fall in the mean arterial pressure.

The smooth muscle of the bronchi is relaxed by isoproterenol. However, only in the presence of bronchial constriction due to asthma or certain bronchoconstrictor drugs there is an observable increase in the tidal volume during the induced relaxation. Tolerance can develop to this effect with chronic use of the drug.

Isoproterenol is inhibitory to both tone and motility of the gastrointestinal tract. The drug can also decrease the uterine activity even in the presence of epinephrine.

Other effects of isoproterenol are not prominent. Isoproterenol is known to speed up the rate of contraction and relaxation of slow skeletal muscle fibers (slow motor units) leading to finger tremor (1). The latter effect is mediated through extrafusal β_2-receptors. It is equipotent to epinephrine in activating lipolysis, but less effective in producing hyperglycemia. CNS stimulation can occur but is negligible at therapeutic doses.

When administered as an aerosol (2) or parenterally, isoproterenol is quickly absorbed. Oral administration, however, results in an unpredictable absorption. It is enzymatically metabolized by COMT in the liver and excreted in the urine. It is not taken up in the adrenergic nerve terminals nor is it metabolized by MAO.

The adverse effects are associated with its actions on the cardiovascular system, but are much less marked than those produced by epinephrine. Common effects include palpitation, tachycardia, and possibly angina and various arrhythmias.

Isoproterenol is therapeutically used in the treatment of moderate-to-severe bronchial asthma and is a potent cardiac stimulant in the emergency treatment of heart block.

DOPAMINE

Dopamine, a metabolic precursor of NE and epinephrine, produces effects on α- and β-adrenoceptors. It can also release NE from the adrenergic nerve terminals. In addition, it activates specific dopaminergic receptors. It is also a central neurotransmitter. Dopamine causes dilation of renal and mesenteric blood vessels through activation of the dopaminergic receptors following infusion of low concentrations ($< 10\ \mu g/kg/min$) (7). At higher doses, it increases cardiac contractility due to its β_1-receptor action and through release of NE from the sympathetic nerve terminals. At still higher doses ($> 20 \mu g/kg/min$), blood pressure is increased due to generalized vasoconstriction resulting from its α-receptor action. Further details of dopamine pharmacology are discussed in Chapter 7.4, and its central actions are discussed in Chapters 9.4 and 11.6.1.

DOBUTAMINE

Dobutamine resembles dopamine except for an aromatic substitution on its amino group, and it has selectivity for the β_1-receptors (6, 16). It exerts a more effective inotropic than chronotropic action and enhances AV conduction (18). Increased cardiac contractility and cardiac output can be prevented by β-adrenoceptor blockers; the β-blockers, however, can increase total peripheral resistance to some extent, suggesting an α-receptor action of dobutamine on blood vessels. In contrast to dopamine, it has no effect on the dopaminergic receptors in the renal vasculature. Adverse effects include cardiac arrhythmias, although their incidence is lower than that with other catecholamines.

NONCATECHOLAMINES

AMPHETAMINE

Amphetamine structurally resembles ephedrine and generally produces similar effects to other adrenoceptor agonists. It has potent stimulant effects on the cerebrospinal axis, and these actions overshadow its peripheral effects. Depending on the dose, the stimulant effects result in feelings of mental alertness, anxiety, insomnia, tremor, and toxic psychosis. Peripherally, amphetamine causes mydriasis, inhibition of gastrointestinal motility, and a precursor response due to vasoconstriction. In addition, it usually causes reflex bradycardia and relaxation of the bronchial muscles, but these effects are not prominent in therapeutic doses.

The drug acts indirectly on both α- and β-adrenoceptors by releasing endogenous NE from the adrenergic nerve terminals. Acute overdosage with amphetamine results in an accentuation of the usual pharmacological effects, and withdrawing the drug from abusers may produce symptoms of chronic fatigue and depression.

Therapeutically, amphetamine is useful in the management of narcolepsy and children with minimal brain dysfunction. It can also be used adjunctively in the treatment of obesity in combination with a program to restrict caloric intake.

The CNS stimulant action of the drug is further discussed in Chapter 11.3, and its abuse liability, in Chapter 11.6.

METHAMPHETAMINE

Methamphetamine may be regarded as a derivative of either amphetamine or ephedrine. The drug is used mainly as a CNS stimulant. Methamphetamine is nearly equipotent to *d*-amphetamine as a CNS stimulant and is more potent than ephedrine as a pressor agent, seldom requiring more than one dose. Its abuse potential is identical to that of amphetamine.

HYDROXYAMPHETAMINE

Chemically, hydroxyamphetamine differs from amphetamine by the addition of a 4-OH group. The actions of hydroxyamphetamine are similar to those of ephedrine except that the drug lacks CNS-stimulant activity. It is used as a mydriatic for ophthalmoscopy and for localization of the lesion in Horner's syndrome. It is a weaker mydriatic than phenylephrine, producing maximal mydriasis in 45 to 60 minutes, with recovery in about 6 hours.

EPHEDRINE

Ephedrine, an alkaloid that was formerly obtained from a Chinese plant *ma huang (Ephedra vulgaris)* and used in ancient Chinese medicine for centuries. It is now commercially prepared by organic synthesis. It is a mixed-acting adrenomimetic amine that stimulates both α- and β-receptors directly and can also release NE from adrenergic nerve terminals. In contrast to epinephrine, its pressor response occurs much slower and lasts much longer; it is effective orally, is a potent CNS stimulant, and exhibits tachyphylaxis.

Ephedrine, following i.v. injection, produces an increase in blood pressure partly due to vasoconstriction and mainly due to increase in myocardial contractility and cardiac output.

Ephedrine produces effects on smooth muscle similar to those caused by epinephrine. The drug relaxes the bronchial musculature, but is slower in onset and less potent than epinephrine. When applied locally to the conjunctiva, it causes mydriasis, being most effective in individuals with lightly pigmented irises. It is also effective as a nasal decongestant by causing vasoconstriction in the nasal mucous membrane.

Ephedrine produces CNS stimulation like amphetamine, and most of the adverse effects seen are due to its action on the CNS. These include nausea, vomiting, vertigo, nervousness, and apprehension. Ephedrine is effective when administered by almost all routes. It is completely absorbed and distributed throughout the body. It is resistant to MAO but is deaminated to some extent in the liver, and up to 40% of ephedrine is excreted unchanged in the urine.

Ephedrine is therapeutically used in the treatment of asthma, as a nasal decongestant, and as a mydriatic agent in ophthalmology.

MEPHENTERMINE

Mephentermine acts both directly on the adrenoceptors and indirectly by liberation of norepinephrine from the nerve terminals. Its actions are similar to those of methamphetamine except that the CNS effects are weak. It produces a pressor effect due to an increase in the peripheral vascular resistance and cardiac output. It causes a positive inotropic effect on the heart, but the chronotropic effect is variable, depending on reflex bradycardia. Mephentermine is administered by parenteral injection, and the duration of action depends on the route of administration. The pressor effects may last up to 1 hour following s.c. injection and 4 hours after its i.m. injection. In large doses, mephentermine can depress cardiac function and affect the CNS, as manifested by drowsiness, incoherence, and convulsions.

METARAMINOL

Metaraminol is similar in effects to norepinephrine but is a mixed-acting adrenoceptor agonist with its direct actions on the adrenoceptors and indirect actions through the release of endogenous norepinephrine. However, it is less potent, and the duration of its action is more prolonged. The drug is essentially a pure α-adrenoceptor stimulant and causes peripheral vasoconstriction that results in a marked increase in blood pressure followed by reflex bradycardia. In addition, it increases the force of contraction and cardiac output in hypotensive conditions. It is administered by oral and parenteral routes. Its subcutaneous administration causes tissue necrosis. Metaraminol is principally used as a pressor agent in hypotensive states. It is also used to treat paroxysmal atrial tachycardia.

PHENYLEPHRINE

The actions of phenylephrine are similar to those of norepinephrine, but it is less potent and has a longer duration of action. It produces peripheral vasoconstriction, increased blood pressure, and reflex bradycardia. It does not produce CNS stimulation nor does it induce ventricular arrhythmias. Phenylephrine is used as a pressor agent, decongestant, and mydriatic, and is also used to treat paroxysmal atrial tachycardia.

METHOXAMINE

Methoxamine acts directly and almost exclusively on the α-adrenoceptors, causing vasoconstriction and increasing blood pressure. It is not a cardiac stimulant but produces reflex bradycardia. No significant CNS stimulation is caused by this drug. It is used as a pressor agent in hypotensive conditions to abort attacks of paroxysmal atrial tachycardia.

METHOXYPHENAMINE

Methoxyphenamine is structurally similar to methamphetamine but differs in pharmacological properties, with significant CNS and α-adrenoceptor stimulant actions. Its major effects are on the β-adrenoceptors in the smooth muscle, causing relaxation, particularly in the bronchi. It has weak cardiovascular effects.

α-ADRENOCEPTOR AGONIST

CLONIDINE

Clonidine, an imidazole derivative (closely related to tolazoline), is considered to act as an α-adrenoceptor agonist by stimulating both central and peripheral α_1-and α_2-adrenoceptors. Following its parenteral administration, it produces an initial pressor action followed by prolonged hypotension. The pressor action appears to be due to its effect on the peripheral α_1-adrenoceptors, and hypotension is considered to be due to its agonistic effect on the central α_2-adrenoceptors such as in the lower brain-stem vasomotor area (possibly in the nucleus tractus solitarius). Its action on presynaptic α_2-receptors appears to decrease the central adrenergic outflow by inhibiting neural release of norepinephrine (8, 9). The effect of clonidine on blood pressure can be antagonized by yohimbine, which is primarily an α_2-antagonist. Clonidine is mainly used as an antihypertensive agent and is discussed in detail in Chapter 15.3.

SELECTIVE β_2-ADRENOCEPTOR AGONISTS

The following agents selectively act on the β_2-adrenoceptors, causing relaxation of smooth muscles of bronchi, uterus, and blood vessels of the skeletal muscles, but they usually have much less cardiac stimulant actions compared with isoproterenol.

METAPROTERENOL

Metaproterenol is analogous to isoproterenol except that its actions are mainly on β_2-adrenoceptors in the bronchial musculature, with little effect on the β_1-adrenoceptors in the myocardium. It is resistant to metabolism by COMT and as a result has a prolonged action and may be administered by inhalation, orally, or subcutaneously. Metaproterenol causes an increase in the peak expiratory flow and a decrease in the bronchial resistance. The adverse effects are generally those described for adrenoceptor agonists, characterized by tachycardia, palpitations, and hypertension. It is useful as a bronchodilator in the treatment of bronchial asthma. Administered by inhalation, it is approximately as effective as isoproterenol but has a longer duration.

TERBUTALINE

The pharmacological effects of terbutaline are nearly the same as those of metaproterenol. The drug is a selective β_2-adrenoceptor agonist and is used mainly as a bronchodilator in asthma (19, 24). The drug is not methylated by COMT and has a longer duration of action (4 to 7 hours). It can be administered orally or by subcutaneous injection. Because of their muscle-relaxant action on the uterus, terbutaline, metaproterenol, and albuterol have been used successfully to delay delivery in premature labor. For this purpose they are given by i.v. infusion. The side effects include nervousness, muscle tremor, headache, drowsiness, nausea and vomiting, sweating, and maternal and fetal tachycardia.

ALBUTEROL AND ISOETHARINE

Albuterol (salbutamol) and isoetharine, β_2-adrenoceptor agonists, are also strong, specific bronchodilators (2) with only weak effects on the myocardium. They resemble terbutaline in their therapeutic uses and side effects.

FENOTEROL

Fenoterol (BEROTEC) is a selective β_2-adrenoceptor agonist available in the aerosol form in Canada and Europe. Its bronchodilator action is equivalent to albuterol, but superior to isoproterenol (17). The drug has a long duration of action up to 8 hours. Mild tremor and shaking have been reported in a few patients as side effects (20) with minimal cardiovascular effects. It is used for the management of asthma as an oral and a nasal spray preparation. It has also been used to arrest premature labor. The drug is not available in the United States.

MISCELLANEOUS β-ADRENOCEPTOR AGONISTS

PRENALTEROL

Prenalterol is a phenol derivative resembling isoproterenol in its chemical structure and is a relatively selective β_1-adrenoceptor agonist. It increases myocardial contractility and cardiac output (10). Its effects on heart rate, peripheral resistance, and blood pressure are variable.

In humans, the bioavailability of prenalterol following oral administration is about 25%, and its elimination half-life is of about 1 to 2 hours. Intravenous and oral administration of the drug has been reported to cause an increase in heart rate, systolic blood pressure, and pulse pressure in normal human volunteers (23), with little effect on renal plasma flow and glomerular filtration rate (12).

The drug has been tried in patients with postischemic heart failure, and in patients with severe refractory chronic congestive heart failure. Prolonged use of prenalterol may cause desensitization, thus limiting its therapeutic usefulness in the treatment of acute heart failure (4). Side effects of prenalterol include nausea, ventricular ectopic beats, and tachycardia. It is available as a solution (1 mg/ml) and as 10-, 20-, and 50-mg tablets for investigational use.

PIRBUTEROL

Pirbuterol is an orally active nonselective β-adrenoceptor agonist. In unanesthetized instrumented dog, pirbuterol has been reported to cause increase in heart rate and ventricular contractile force (5). It resembles isoproterenol with regard to its chronotropic effect. In humans it increases cardiac contractility and output, reduces peripheral vascular resistance and blood pressure, and may cause a mild tachycardia. In clinical trials tremor and nervousness were reported to occur as side effects, and marked decrease in its hemodynamic effects were reported after several weeks of therapy, probably resulting from down-regulation of β-adrenoceptors. The drug is available currently for investigational use only for patients with refractory congestive heart failure.

THERAPEUTIC USES

ALLERGIC DISORDERS

Bronchial Asthma. Bronchial asthma is characterized by smooth muscle spasm, edema of the bronchial mucosa, and increased mucus secretion. Epinephrine, isoproterenol, and the newer selective β_2-adrenoceptor stimulants are effective in relieving respiratory distress in asthma by their potent bronchodilator action (21). In addition, epinephrine causes vasoconstriction in the mucosa by its α_1-receptor action. Acute attacks are usually relieved within 3 to 5 minutes after an s.c. injection of epinephrine (0.2 to 0.5 mg) or after oral inhalation of epinephrine (1% solution), isoproterenol (0.5 or 1% solution), or administration of other β_2-stimulants.

Other Allergic Conditions. An s.c. injection of epinephrine promptly relieves itching, urticaria, serum sickness, serum reaction, hay fever, angioneurotic edema, and other acute allergic disorders. Epinephrine (1:1000, 0.5 ml, s.c.) is the drug of choice for treating hypersensitivity reactions to penicillin. Angioneurotic edema in the larynx, causing suffocation, can be promptly relieved by epinephrine inhalation.

USES OF VASCULAR EFFECTS

Because of their vasoconstrictor effects in the skin and mucosa and pressor effects, adrenergic agents have been useful in the following situations.

Topical Hemostatic. In case of hemorrhage from the skin and mucosa, epinephrine applied topically can produce its hemostatic effect by acting on the arterioles and capillaries. It is still occasionally used for this purpose in dental practice as well as in professional sports.

With Local Anesthetics. Epinephrine is usually mixed with local anesthetics to retard their absorption and prolong their duration of action and decrease their systemic toxicity.

Nasal Decongestion. Vasoconstrictor effects of the sympathomimetic amines in the mucous membrane caused through their α-adrenoceptor action have been useful in the treatment of nasal congestion in hay fever, allergic rhinitis, sinusitis, and other upper respiratory conditions. Amines with such nasal decongestant actions are marked in Table 7.1-1. However, such effects of these drugs are followed by rebound congestion, and their prolonged use may cause chronic rhinitis.

Hypotension. Sympathomimetic amines with pressor effects may be used to relieve hypotension associated with spinal anesthesia or due to overdosage of antihypertensive agents. They may be given as an emergency measure in acute hemorrhage. However, before such treatment is initiated there should be sufficient evidence for adequate perfusion of the vital organs during hypotension. Attention should initially be given to other appropriate measures such as restoration of the blood volume.

Following surgical removal of a pheochromocytoma, the blood pressure may drop markedly. Norepinephrine has been infused to maintain blood pressure. However, replacement of the fluid volume would be more appropriate.

Shock is a clinical syndrome associated with circulatory insufficiency and protracted underperfusion of the vital tissues. Management varies with its pathogenesis. In cardiogenic shock, in addition to fluid-volume replacement, α-adrenoceptor agonists have been used to restore the blood pressure. The goal of therapy is to restore and maintain adequate arterial pressure in order to restore perfusion of the vital tissues such as brain, heart, kidney, liver, and intestine. However, the patient should be monitored carefully so as to avoid overloading of the heart, as well as excessive vasoconstriction in the vital organs. In this regard, dopamine appears to be an appropriate agent because of its ability to produce peripheral vasoconstriction with vasodilation in the renal and mesenteric vascular beds. Dobutamine and isoproterenol are also used to improve perfusion of tissues. Infusion of norepinephrine, mephentermine, and metaraminol has been used to maintain adequate blood pressure. Use of these drugs in shock is discussed in detail in Chapter 15.3.

Cardiac Uses. Epinephrine and isoproterenol have been useful in restoring rhythm during cardiac arrest and heart block with syncopal attacks. Epinephrine should not be used and may even worsen the situation during ventricular fibrillation; isoproterenol may be less harmful in such a case. Ephedrine and hydroxyamphetamine are both orally effective and long acting. However, in these situations drug therapy should be used as a temporary measure; wherever possible, appropriate physical measures such as cardiac pacemaker, defibrillation, or external cardiac compression should be used.

Ophthalmic Uses. Sympathomimetic amines, particularly ephedrine (0.1%), hydroxyamphetamine (1%), and phenylephrine (1-2%), are used to produce mydriasis that, in contrast to the anticholinergic agents, is not associated with cycloplegia or increase of intraocular pressure. Epinephrine and phenylephrine are used in wide-angle glaucoma to decrease production of the aqueous humor (Chapter 21.1).

Central Uses. Ephedrine, amphetamine, methamphetamine, and dextroamphetamine are used to treat narcolepsy; tolerance does not appear to develop. Amphetamine and its analogs are used as anorectic agents, but abuse liability and central stimulant effects are problems; they have been given in combination with some sedatives to overcome the stimulant effects. In contrast, fenfluramine and similar compounds (Table 7.1-1), which also have anorectic effects do not show CNS-stimulant effects nor do they disturb REM sleep.

Dextroamphetamine has some beneficial effect in parkinsonism, but levodopa is superior. Amphetamines have a calming effect in hyperkinetic children. Side effects include insomnia, irritability, headache, periods of excessive crying, and depression. Their continued use can cause anorexia, leading to depressed growth. An equally effective drug, methylphenidate, may have less growth-reducing effect. Dextroamphetamine is used as an adjunct to drugs used in grand mal and absence seizure epilepsy to counteract their side effects, such as sedation and ataxia, and to allow their administration in effective amounts. In absence seizure, it may be given alone or along with trimethadione or other drugs to prevent attacks.

PREPARATIONS

As Nasal Decongestants

Solution for Topical Application

Epinephrine HCl: 0.1%.

Naphazoline HCl: 0.05 and 0.1%.

Oxymetazoline HCl: (AFRIN) 0.025% (for children) and 0.05% (for adults).

Phenylephrine HCl: 0.25 and 1%.

Tetrahydrozoline HCl: 0.05%.

Tuaminoheptane sulfate: 1%.

Xylometazoline HCl: 0.05 and 0.1%.

Tablets and Capsules

Phenylpropanolamine HCl: tablets (25, 35, and 50 mg) *capsules* (25 mg); and 1% solution. For adults, 25 mg q. 4 hourly, p.o., and solution for topical.

Pseudoephedrine HCl: tablets (30 and 60 mg); *capsules* (time release, 120 mg).

Pseudoephedrine sulfate: tablets (time release, 120 mg). For adults, 60 mg t.i.d.; for children, 4 mg/kg/day.

As Bronchodilator

Epinephrine suspension (in oil) 1:1000 or *Epinephrine HCl* (solution) 1:1000. For adults, 0.2-0.5 ml of 1:1000 solution q 2 hr s.c.; for children, 0.01 ml/kg q 4 hr for oral inhalation, 0.1-1.0% of solution or suspension.

Ephedrine sulfate: capsules (25 and 50 mg), syrup (11 and 20 mg/5 ml). For adults, 20 to 50 mg q 4 hrs; for children, 3 mg/kg/day.

Isoproterenol HCl: solution (1:100, 1:200 and 1:400) for oral inhalation; tablets (10 and 15 mg) for sublingual administration.

Isoproterenol sulfate: suspension of 2 mg/ml for oral inhalation.

Metaproterenol sulfate (ALUPENT, METAPREL): tablets (10 and 20 mg); syrup (10 mg/5 ml). For adults, 10-20 mg t.i.d.

Terbutaline sulfate (BRETHINE, BRICANYL) tablets (2.5 and 5 mg); solution (1 mg/ml). For adults, tablets 2.5 mg t.i.d. or 0.25 mg, s.c.; for children, tablets 1.25-2.5 mg t.i.d. or 0.01 mg/kg in solution.

For Shock

Dopamine HCl (INTROPIN): aqueous solution 40 mg (=32.3 mg of base)/ml, i.v. infusion at a rate of 2-5 μg/kg/min may be increased to 50 μg/kg/min in seriously ill patients.

Dobutamine HCl (DOBUTREX): available in powder form 250 mg; reconstituted solution is infused i.v. at a usual rate of 2.5-10 μg/kg/min.

Epinephrine HCl: solution (1:1,000 and 1:10,000 for s.c., i.m., or i.v. injections). For adults, 0.5 ml of 1:1,000, i.m. or s.c., and 0.25-0.5 of 1:10,000 i.v.; for children, 0.3 ml of 1:1,000, i.m.

Norepinephrine bitartrate: aqueous solution equivalent to 1 mg of base/ml. For adults, 2-8 ml of solution added to 500 ml of 15% dextrose solution: for i.v. injection; for children, 1 ml of solution added to 250 ml of 5% dextrose for continuous i.v. infusion.

Isoproterenol HCl: aqueous solution (1:5,000). For adults, 5-10 ml of solution added to 500-1,000 ml of 5% dextrose continuous i.v. infusion at a rate of 0.5-5 μg/min.

Metaraminol bitartrate: available as 1% solution. For adults, single i.v. dose 2-5 mg or 0.2-0.5 g/l of 5% dextrose for continuous i.v. infusion; for children, 0.01 mg/kg, i.v., single dose or 1 mg/25 ml of 5% dextrose for i.v. infusion. For adults, i.m. dose 5-10 mg; for children, 0.1 mg/kg.

Methoxamine HCl (VASOXYL): solution (10 or 20 mg/ml) for i.m. injection and for i.v. injection (3-5 mg). Dose 10-20 mg.

REFERENCES AND ADDITIONAL READING

1. Bowman, W.C. Adrenergic activators and inhibitors. In: *Handbook of Experimental Pharmacology*, Vol. 54/II (Szekers, L., ed.). New York: Springer-Verlag, 1980, p. 47.
2. Choo-Kang, Y.F.J., Parker, S.S. and Grant, I.W.B. Response of asthmatics to isoprenaline and salbutamol aerosols administered by intermittent positive-pressure ventilation. *Br. Med. J.* 4:465, 1970.
3. Exton, J.H. Mechanisms involved in effects of catecholamines on liver carbohydrate metabolism. *Biochem. Pharmacol.* 28:2237, 1979.
4. Farah, A.E., Alousi, A.A. and Schwarz, R.P. Positive inotropic agents. *Ann. Rev. Pharmacol. Toxicol.* 24:275, 1984.
5. Gold, F.L. and Horowitz, L.D. Hemodynamic effects of pirbuterol in conscious dog. *Am. Heart J.* 102:591, 1981.
6. Goldberg, L.I., Hsieh, Y.-Y. and Resnekov, L. Newer catecholamines for treatment of heart failure and shock: An update on dopamine and a first look at dobutamine. *Progr. Cardiovasc. Dis.* 19:327, 1977.
7. Goldberg, L.I., Volkman, P.H. and Kohli, J.D. A comparison of the vascular dopamine receptor with other dopamine receptors. *Ann. Rev. Pharmacol. Toxicol.* 18:57, 1978.
8. Haeusler, G. Further similarities between the action of clonidine and a central activation of the depressor baroreceptor reflex. *Naunyn-Schmiedebergs Arch. Pharmacol.* 285:1, 1973.
9. Haeusler, G. Clonidine-induced inhibition of sympathetic nerve activity: No indication for a central presynaptic or an indirect sympathomimetic mode of action. *Naunyn-Schmiedebergs Arch. Pharmacol.* 286:97, 1974.
10. Kirlin, P.C. and Pitt, B. Hemodynamic effects of intravenous prenalterol in severe heart failure. *Am. J. Cardiol.* 47:670, 1981.
11. Lefkowitz, R.J. and Williams, L.T. Molecular mechanisms of activation and desensitization of adenylate cyclase coupled β-adrenergic receptors. *Adv. Cyclic Nucleotide Res.* 9:1, 1978.
12. Meurer, K.A., Long, R., Hombach, V. et al. Effect of β_1-selective adrenergic agonist in normal human volunteers. *Klin. Wochenschr.* 53:425, 1980.
13. Pradhan, S.N. and Wingate, H.W. Effects of adrenergic agents on gastric secretion in dogs. *Arch. Int. Pharmacodyn.* 140:399, 1962.

14. Pradhan, S.N. and Wingate, H. Effects of some adrenergic blocking agents on gastric secretion in dogs. *Arch. Int. Pharmacodyn.* 162:303, 1966.
15. Rall, T.W. Role of adenosine 3′,5′-monophosphate (cyclic AMP) in actions of catecholamines. *Pharmacol. Rev.* 24:399, 1972
16. Sonnenblick, E.H., Frishman, W.H. and LeJemtel, T.H. Dobutamine: A new synthetic cardioactive sympathetic amine. *N. Engl. J. Med.* 300:17, 1979.
17. Steil, I.G. and Rivington, R.N. Adrenergic agents in acute asthma: Valuable new alternatives. *Ann. Emerg. Med.* 12:493, 1983.
18. Tuttle, R.R. and Mills, J. Dobutamine: Development of a new catecholamine to selectively increase cardiac contractility. *Circ. Res.* 36:185, 1975.
19. Wallace, R.L., Caldwell, D.L., Ansbacher, R. and Otterson, W.N. Inhibition of premature labor by terbutaline. *Obstet. Gynecol.* 51:387, 1978.
20. Watanabe, S., Turner, W., Renzetti, A. *et al.* Bronchodilator effects of nebulized fenoterol. *Chest* 80:292, 1981.
21. Webb-Johnson, D.C. and Andrews, J.L. Bronchodilator therapy. *N. Engl. J. Med.* 297:476, 1977.
22. Weiner, N. The role of cyclic nucleotides in the regulation of neurotransmitter release from adrenergic neurons by neuromodulators. In: *Essays in Neurochemistry and Neuropharmacology*, Vol. 4 (Youdim, M.B.H., Lovenberg, W., Sharma, P.F., and Lagnado, J.R., eds.). New York: John Wiley, 1980, p. 69.
23. Weiss, A., Pfister, B., Imhof, P. *et al.* Haemodynamic effects, plasma concentrations and tolerance of orally administered prenalterol in man. *Eur. J. Clin. Pharmacol.* 18:383, 1980.
24. Wolfe, J.D., Tashkin, D.P., Calvarese, B. and Simmons, M. Bronclhodilator effects of terbutaline and aminophylline alone and in combination in asthmatic patients. *N. Engl. J. Med.* 298:363, 1978.

ADDITIONAL READING

Sanders, V.M., and Munson, A.E. Norepinephrine and the antibody response. *Pharmacol. Rev.* 37:229, 1985.

CHAPTER

7.2

ADRENERGIC BLOCKING AGENTS

Charles D. Barnes and Maysie J. Hughes

The first evidence of compounds that could specifically alter the response to sympathetic activity was presented in 1906 by Dale (12). He demonstrated, by use of the ergot alkaloids, the conversion of adrenaline's (epinephrine) vasopressor effect to a depressor effect. After extensive studies, Ahlquist (1) proposed that two types of adrenergic receptors or adrenoceptors existed and that the receptor for which blocking agents were available should be called the α-adrenoceptor, whereas the receptors that were not inhibited by these compounds should be called β-adrenoceptors. Ten years elapsed before dichloroisoproterenol, a β-specific partial antagonists, was synthesized and tested (44). Since that time, a progressively increasing number of β-adrenoceptor antagonists have been synthesized, and the most successful, propranolol, has been studied extensively and used in clinical treatment. Pharmacological evidence now suggests that at least two types of β-receptors exist (23, 27). The type of β-adrenoceptor that stimulates lipolysis and is found in cardiac muscle has been designated β_1, whereas adrenoceptors found in smooth muscle appear to be largely of the β_2 type. There is now evidence that more than one type of α-adrenoceptor exists as well (5, 15, 40). These have been termed α_1 (formerly α or postsynaptic) and α_2 (initially called presynaptic).

Labetalol, an interesting new compound under clinical investigation, has both α- and β-blocking properties, and its combined activity appears to have considerable potential. This type of compound may lend support to the concept that there is only one adrenoceptor with a variety of stereo configurations (22, 24) and that its pharmacological activity may be dependent on the metabolic state of the cell.

A number of other categories of drugs affect adrenergic activity by mechanisms unrelated to a direct blockade of the receptor site. Thus, alterations in sympathetic activity can result from modification of central activity, inhibition of catecholamine synthesis, depletion of catecholamine storage in the nerve terminals, prevention of norepinephrine release from nerve terminals, and replacement of norepinephrine in the storage granules with less active compounds known as *false transmitters*.

α-ADRENOCEPTOR BLOCKING AGENTS

Epinephrine has an affinity for both α- and β-adrenoceptors, and the normal vascular response to this hormone is a net vasoconstriction and increased blood pressure caused by α-adrenoceptor stimulation. However, *epinephrine reversal*, which results in vasodilation and a drop in blood pressure, can be produced in experimental animals after α-adrenoceptor blockade exposes the β-adrenoceptor effect.

α-Blockade decreases peripheral resistance by reducing the number of vascular α-adrenoceptors capable of reacting with catecholamines released by the sympathetic nerve terminals and the adrenal medulla. This vasodilation is augmented by the response of β-adrenoceptors to circulating epinephrine. Cardiac output is usually increased, and tachycardia may be observed, because the β-receptors in the heart are unaffected and can respond to reflex increases in sympathetic activity resulting from decreased blood pressure. Although there is evidence that cardiac tissue contains a small component of α-receptors, these receptors do not normally make a significant contribution to sympathetic regulation of the heart. Those vascular areas that are predominantly under the control of α-receptor activity may actually receive increased blood flow (i.e., kidney and splanchnic regions).

Besides affecting the cardiovascular system, some of these compounds cross the blood-brain barrier and are associated with a number of CNS-mediated changes. Although no definitive data relate these effects directly to α-blockade, an apparently dose-related central depression or excitation does occur, and high drug concentrations cause stimulation, even to the point of convulsion. The direct effect of α-blockade on gastrointestinal activity appears to be negligible, possibly because the α-receptors cause relaxation of the smooth muscle (50). Nausea and vomiting, which may occur with such drugs, are related to central nervous system stimulation.

Most metabolic activity of catecholamines is mediated by β-receptors, but α-receptors also appear to be involved in the inhibition of insulin and glucagon release. Following α-blockade, β-receptors manifest stimulatory activity, causing an increase in circulating insulin.

The bronchoconstricting properties of α-receptors suggest that α-blocking agents may be of some value in controlling asthma (47), and the α-blocking agents have been shown in clinical trials to be moderately effective in producing bronchodilatation in asthmatics (38). Moxisylate thymoxamine, an experimental α-blocker, has been shown to be approximately 60% effective in inhibiting exercise-induced bronchospasm (39).

The designation of α_2-adrenoceptors was necessitated by the discovery that the synaptic endings of noradrenergic neurons have a negative feedback system for reducing transmitter release and that the system involves an α-receptor whose properties differ from the postsynaptic receptor's. This α_2-receptor has now also been identified on the soma of noradrenergic neurons where it produces inhibition (autoinhibition) (1). A study on the action of presynaptic α-adrenoceptor blockade on transmitter release and effector response casts some doubt on the functional relevance of negative feedback regulation of

Table 7.2-1
A Partial List of α-Adrenoceptor Blocking Agents

Generic Name	Trade Name	Receptor Blocking Action	Available Dose
Azapetine	ILIDAR	α_1, α_2	Tablet: 25 mg
Dibenamine		α_1, α_2	Not used clinically
Dihydroergotoxine	HYDERGINE	α_1, α_2	Tablet: 0.5 mg Ampuls: 0.3 mg/ml
Moxisylate		α	Investigational
Phenoxybenzamine	DIBENZYLINE	α_1, α_2	Tablet: 10 mg Ampuls: 100 mg/2 ml
Phentolamine	REGITINE	α_1, α_2	Hydrochloride tablet: 50 mg Mesylate powder for injection: 5 mg
Piperoxane	BENODAINE	α_2	Not used clinically
Prazosin	MINIPRESS	α_1	Capsule: 1, 2, 5 mg
Tolazoline	PRISCOLINE	$\alpha_1 < \alpha_2$	Tablet: 25 mg Time release tablet: 80 mg Injection: 25 mg/ml
Yohimbine		α_2	Not used clinically

transmitter release, however (20). Recent ligand binding studies indicate that there are inhibitory α_2-adrenoceptors in the smooth muscle of the gut (50).

Several α-adrenoceptor blocking agents, classified as short acting and long acting, are listed in Table 7.2-1; their structures are given in Fig. 7.2-1.

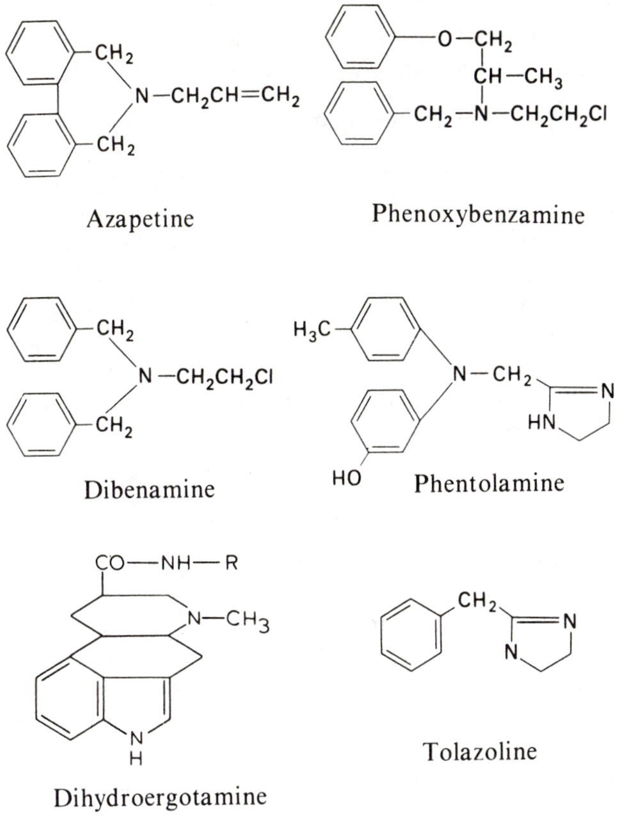

Azapetine

Phenoxybenzamine

Dibenamine

Phentolamine

Dihydroergotamine

Tolazoline

Fig. 7.2-1. *Structures of some α-adrenoceptor antagonists.*

SHORT-ACTING AGENTS

All agents in this class are relatively short acting and comprise several subgroups, including the ergot alkaloids and 2-substituted imidazolines.

ERGOT ALKALOIDS

In the Middle Ages naturally occurring ergot alkaloids of fungal origin caused epidemic poisoning by contaminating grain foods, particularly rye bread. These alkaloids have complex and varied effects besides α-adrenergic blockade. These effects include gastrointestinal hyperactivity, increased uterine motility, peripheral vasoconstriction resulting in severe ischemia of the extremities, and various CNS manifestations. Dihydrogenation of these compounds increases α-blocking activity and decreases direct vasoconstrictor activity, as in the case of dihydroergotamine (Fig. 7.2-1).

Dihydroergotoxine mesylate (HYDERGINE) is a mixture of three dihydrogenated compounds: dihydroergocornine, dihydroergocristine, and dihydroergocryptine (also see Chapter 19).

Therapeutic Uses. Dihydroergotoxine mesylate has been used to a limited extent in treating elderly patients, ostensibly to increase cerebral blood flow and correct mental problems; there is no evidence that it has been effective, however. Some ergot preparations are used in obstetrics; these uses will be discussed in Chapter 19.

2-SUBSTITUTED IMIDAZOLINES

Tolazoline and phentolamine are two short-acting α-adrenoceptor blocking agents of the class 2-substituted imidazolines (Fig. 7.2-1).

Tolazoline is absorbed from the gastrointestinal tract rapidly and fairly completely and, in turn, quickly excreted, unchanged by the kidney. One-half of the absorbed agent appears in the urine within approximately 2 hours. In comparison, phentolamine is poorly absorbed from the gastrointestinal tract, with only one-fifth reaching the circulation by this route.

Tolazoline and phentolamine are used clinically as moderate, short-acting α-blocking agents. Phentolamine has been found to be approximately five times as effective as tolazoline in blocking the vasoconstrictor effect of injected epinephrine. Nickerson and Gump (33) suggested that both agents have histaminelike action, and more recent evidence suggests that tolazoline releases histamine (19, 28). Histamine release would explain tolazoline's stimulatory actions on the heart, gastrointestinal motility, and secretions as well as its exacerbation of peptic ulcers. The fact is that tolazoline is much more effective in blocking α_2 than α_1 receptors; thus disinhibiting noradrenergic neurons must also be kept in mind. Some of the gastrointestinal responses are blocked by atropine, suggesting that acetylcholine may also be involved. Furthermore, both tolazoline and phentolamine have antiserotonin properties.

Therapeutic Uses. Phentolamine was used as a pharmacological tool to test for pheochromocytoma in hypertensive patients as it is short acting and lacks major side effects at the test dose used in the office procedure. Sensitive laboratory methods of directly determining catecholamines and their metabolites in urine have since become available, and these techniques are now replacing pharmacological challenge in the diagnosis of pheochromocytoma. However, in both pheochromocytoma surgery and postoperative management, phentolamine is used to prevent acute hypertensive episodes.

Both phentolamine and tolazoline have been used in treating shock: to increase blood flow to abdominal viscera for better metabolic and fluid regulation and to improve circulation when fluid replacement causes elevated venous pressure. They are also used in treating

Raynaud's disease, pulmonary edema, and various occlusive peripheral arterial diseases. In most of these cases, however, the clinically useful doses are generally smaller than those necessary to cause α-blockade, and the release of endogenous histamine could explain the observed effects.

Adverse effects. Adverse effects include orthostatic hypotension, cardiac arrhythmias, anginal pain and tachycardia, gastrointestinal stimulation, abdominal pain, nausea, vomiting, diarrhea, and exacerbation of peptic ulcers.

LONG-ACTING AGENTS

Long-acting agents have α-antagonist actions that are produced slowly and are very prolonged. The delayed onset results from the slow formation of reactive intermediate compounds that combine irreversibly with the α-adrenoceptors.

HALOALKYLAMINES

These drugs are related structurally to nitrogen mustard. The best-known members of this group are dibenamine and phenoxybenzamine (Fig. 7.2-1).

The tertiary amines in these compounds cyclize to form a reactive ethylenimonium intermediate. This three-membered ring then breaks, and the resulting highly reactive carbonium ion is probably what reacts with the α-adrenoceptor.

Because of its toxic effect on tissue, dibenamine is not used clinically. Phenoxybenzamine is used clinically and can be taken by mouth, but it is usually given parenterally. Even when phenoxybenzamine is given intravenously, there is a slow onset of blockade that may be due in part to the time required for ethylenimonium ions to form and irreversible binding to occur.

Adverse Effects. When taken orally, phenoxybenzamine causes marked gastric irritation, nausea, and vomiting, and its absorption is variable; therefore, treatment is usually parenteral. Common complaints with either parenteral or oral treatment are orthostatic hypotension, tachycardia, swelling of the nasal mucosa, and miosis.

Therapeutic Use. Phenoxybenzamine has been used during surgery to decrease peripheral vasoconstriction and coronary arterial spasm and to improve renal blood flow. Although it has been used widely in the treatment of hypertension and peripheral vascular disease, its effectiveness has not been established.

SELECTIVE α_1-ADRENOCEPTOR ANTAGONIST

PRAZOSIN

Prazosin is a quinazoline derivative with the following chemical formula:

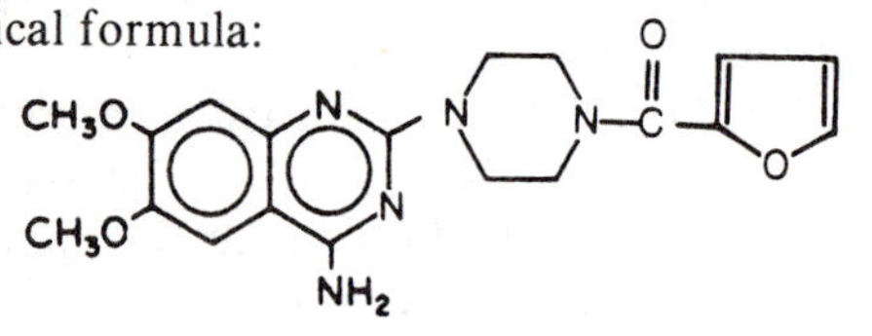

Prazosin was the first of a new chemical class of adrenoceptor antagonists with a high selectivity for the α_1-adrenoceptor. Such selectivity of this compound, which is orally active, has been useful in treatment of patients with hypertension and congestive heart failure. Since prazosin does not block presynaptic α_2-adrenoceptors, it causes little or no increase in heart rate, plasma renin, or plasma norepinephrine (10), in contrast to nonselective adrenoceptor blockers like phentolamine.

Further details of its pharmacology, therapeutic use, and adverse effects are given in Chapter 15.3.

β-ADRENOCEPTOR BLOCKING AGENTS

The first partial β-adrenoceptor antagonist to be synthesized and tested was dichloroisoproterenol, which was quickly followed by a succession of other β-blocking agents. Pronethalol was the first compound tested clinically, but was withdrawn because animal studies implicated it in tumor formation in mice (36). Later, tolamolol was also withdrawn from clinical trials for the same reason. In both cases, the doses that induced tumors were greater than those normally used for patient treatment, and there was some question of whether endogenous viral activation was involved. There has been no evidence that any of the other β-antagonists are carcinogenic.

Propranolol, which was also tested during the 1960s, has been used extensively for more than 15 years in treating a variety of cardiovascular diseases. There has been a proliferation of β-blocking drugs since then, and a number of them have appeared on the market for clinical use, whereas others are still undergoing clinical trials (11, 14, 30).

It was soon recognized that there were at least two types of β-adrenoceptors; therefore, β-adrenoceptor antagonists were divided into several categories, according to degree of selectivity (24). Those compounds that were more effective in preventing cardiac stimulation (cardioselective) were designated β_1-antagonists, whereas those that were more effective in blocking vasodilation were designated β_2-antagonists. However, the majority of the β-blocking compounds are nonselective and/or relatively effective at both types of β-sites (Table 7.2-2). A different type of selectivity has been suggested regarding a β_1-receptor blocker mepindolol, which blocks chronotropic β_1-receptors to a greater degree than β_1-inotropic receptors (8). It must be noted that even cardioselective is a relative term and applies only to low drug dosages; the selectivity disappears at higher dose levels. As yet, there is no clinically useful selective β_2-blocking agent, but butoxamine (structurally dissimilar to the other β-antagonists) is being studied experimentally as a compound of this type (26).

All the β-blocking compounds currently in use or having clinical potential are structural variations of the original partial β-antagonist dichloroisoproterenol. Like dichloroisoproterenol, some of the new compounds have

Table 7.2-2
A Partial List of β-Blocking Agents

Generic Name	Trade Name	Receptor Blocking Action	Agonistic Activity[b]	Available Doses
Acebutolol[a]	SECTRAL	β_1	P	Tablet: 100, 200 mg Injection: 5 mg/ml
Alprenolol[a]	APTINE	β_1, β_2	P	Tablet: 50 mg Injection: 1 mg/ml
Atenolol	TENORMIN	β_1	N	Tablet: 100 mg
Butoxamine		β_2	N	Experimental
Bunitrolol[a]		β_1, β_2	P	Experimental
Metoprolol	LOPRESSOR	β_1	N	Tablet: 50, 100 mg
Nadolol	CORGARD	β_1, β_2	N	Tablet: 40, 80, or 120 mg
Niteralol		β_1, β_2	N	Experimental
Oxprenolol[a]	TRASICOR	β_1, β_2	P	Tablet: 20 - 160 mg
Para-oxprenolol		β_1, β_2	N	Experimental
Penbutolol[a]		β_1, β_2	P	Experimental
Pindolol[a]	VISKEN	β_1, β_2	P	Tablet: 5 mg
Practolol	ERALDIN	β_1	P	Injection: 2 mg/ml
Propranolol	INDERAL	β_1, β_2	N	Tablet: 10 - 80 mg Injection: 1 mg/ml
Sotalol	SOTACOR	β_1, β_2	N	Tablet: 80 mg Injection: 2 mg/ml
Sulfinalol[c]		β_1	N	Experimental
Timolol[a]	BLOCADREN	β_1, β_2		Tablet: 5, 10 mg Ophthalmic solutions: 0.1 -1.0%

[a] Compounds having membrane-stabilizing properties similar to propranolol's.
[b] P, partial agonistic activity; N, no agonistic activity.
[c] "Direct" vasodilation.

some agonistic as well as antagonistic activity; thus, their clinical usefulness could be significantly limited. In addition to considering β-blockers as a group, this chapter will discuss in some detail a representative β-blocking agent of each type.

STRUCTURAL COMPARISON OF SOME β-ADRENOCEPTOR AGONISTS AND ANTAGONISTS (FIG. 7.2-2)

The β-receptor activity of epinephrine is increased by alkyl substitution on the amino group in the side chain, with an isopropyl substitution causing maximum activity (isoproterenol). Substitutions on the ring determine the β-blocking action (dichloroisoproterenol). There is evidence that the addition of amidic substituents to the alkylamino moiety can confer cardioselectivity (25). Potency is determined primarily by the asymmetric β-carbon on the side chain, with the (-) levo-form 20 to 100 times more active than the (+) dextro-isomer. The clinically used β-antagonists are racemic mixtures of the two forms.

GENERAL CONSIDERATIONS

Pharmacological effects of β-blocking compounds fall into two general categories: (a) those effects that are the result of β-adrenoceptor blockade, and (b) those actions that are independent of adrenoceptor interactions. β-Receptor inhibition affects cardiac and smooth muscle activity, metabolism, hormones, and, in the case of the lipid-soluble compounds, the CNS. Nonreceptor-mediated effects include the membrane-stabilizing (local anesthetic) properties of many of the β-agonists, a serious oculocutaneous syndrome (practolol), and some minor allergic reactions. The membrane-stabilizing

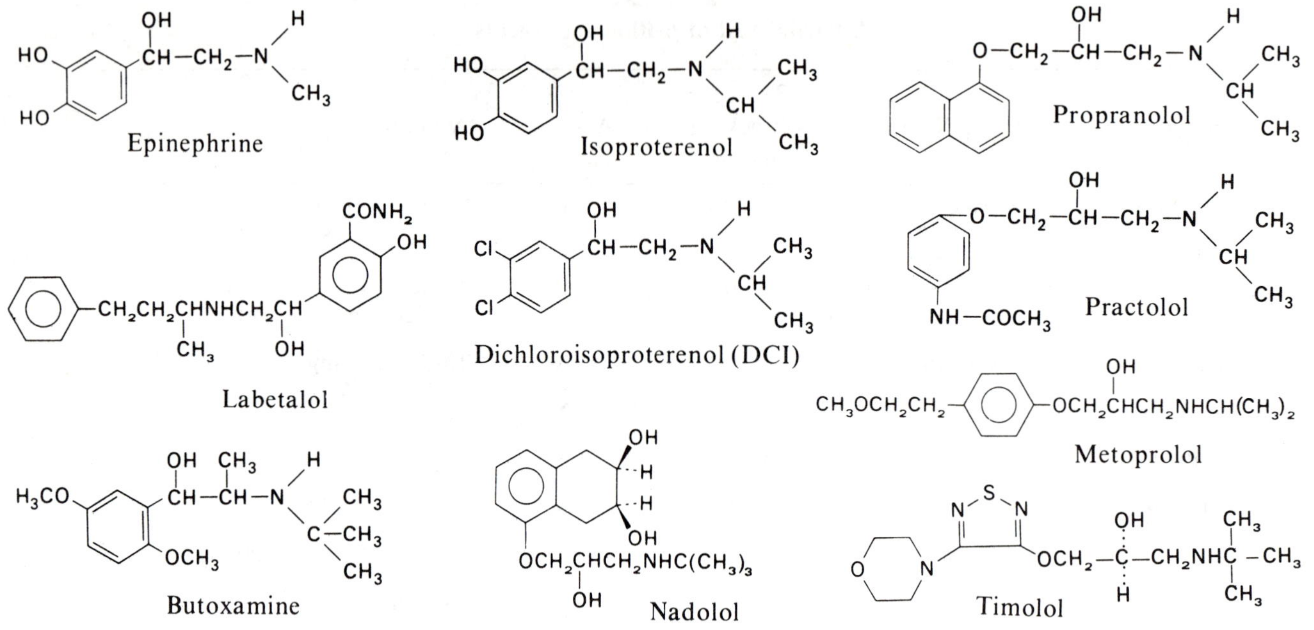

Fig. 7.2-2. *A structural comparison of some β-adrenoceptor agonists and antagonists.*

action of β-blockers seems to be highly correlated with their lipid solubility. Lipophilic β-blockers cross the blood-brain and placental barriers.

Effects Related to β-Adrenoceptor Blockade

Serious Bradycardia and Heart Failure. β-Blocking drugs may aggravate the condition of patients with partial or complete conduction blocks or severe congestive failure; therefore, careful consideration should be given to each individual case before treatment. The membrane-stabilizing properties of some of these drugs, which cause a reduction in contractility, may contribute to the detrimental effects of β-blockade.

Bronchoconstriction. β-Receptors mediate relaxation of bronchial smooth muscle. Blockade of these receptors (β_2) can cause constriction and serious complications in the asthmatic patient. In general, β-antagonists are not recommended for patients with pulmonary problems; however, some β-agents (nonselective) are much less likely to cause ventilatory complications.

Metabolic Changes. Hyperglycemic and diabetic patients who take insulin may have prolonged hypoglycemia when treated with β-antagonists. To a large extent, this probably results from the decreased mobilization of skeletal muscle glycogen and a reduction in mobilization of free fatty acids from fat stores, both of which are mediated by β_1-receptors. Because α-adrenergic receptors inhibit whereas β-receptors stimulate insulin release, increased insulin secretion is not involved.

β-Blockade is also responsible for inhibition of hepatic phosphorylase activity, facilitation of glucose uptake in peripheral tissues, increased secretion of growth hormone, and inhibition of glucagon secretion.

Renin-Angiotensin System. The effect of β-blockade on plasma renin activity has not been completely resolved, but the current evidence suggests that, if renin plasma levels are high or normal in a standing position, a reduction is obtained by β-blockade. However, if levels are low or normal in a supine position, no measurable changes are observed. Other studies have shown that some of the same drugs (timolol, atenolol and practolol) lower renin levels in both the standing and supine positions. Propranolol and atenolol have been reported to be both effective and ineffective in altering renin plasma levels; however, these reported responses were both dose and drug dependent. It has been proposed that one of the major mechanisms by which β-blocking agents moderate hypertension is a reduction of plasma renin activity, but the data are less than conclusive.

Central Nervous System. Most of the β-antagonists (with the exception of practolol) are lipid-soluble to some extent and enter the central nervous system (13). The slow onset of antihypertensive activity has been attributed by some to a central β-blocking action of these drugs (20). But a central β-blocking action cannot explain the antihypertensive actions of practolol, which is not lipid-soluble and does not enter the central nervous system. Practolol's d-isomer has little β-blocking effect, but is hypotensive when administered intracerebroventricularly. β-Blocking compounds are used experimentally in treating various abnormal mental states, and propranolol appears to be useful in treating some schizophrenics. Some of the unpleasant but generally not serious side effects of these compounds occur in the CNS and appear as hallucinations, sleep disturbances, lethargy, depression, dizziness, nausea and vomiting. It has been noted that chronic treatment with β-blocking agents increases dopamine, norepinephrine and epinephrine contents of some brain sites, particularly the norepinephrine-rich nucleus locus ceruleus (18) without changing amounts at peripheral sites.

Presynaptic Effects. Propranolol has been shown to reduce norepinephrine release from sympathetic nerves. This has led to the hypothesis that sympathetic presynaptic β-receptors, activated by low concentrations of catecholamine, lead to an increased release of the transmitter (48). These receptors appear to be of the β_2-subgroup because they are stimulated primarily by β_2- and not β_1-agonists and are blocked by butoxamine (43, 45, 49, 51). Rather than acting as a positive feedback in response to norepinephrine, this mechanism probably responds to the increased circulating levels of epinephrine released from the adrenal medulla during times of stress. Clinically, this mechanism may contribute to the beneficial effects of β-blockade in the treatment of hypertension by preventing increased sympathetic neurotransmitter secretion during emotionally stressful situations. Additionally, the chronic administration of propranolol or one of the β_1-blocking agents (acebutolol, metoprolol, or practolol) has been shown to reduce tyrosine hydroxylase and dopamine-β-hydroxylase activities (43). Such inhibition would reduce the availability of norepinephrine for release at sympathetic nerve endings. It is not known whether the decrease in activity of these enzymes is the result of a direct inhibitory action of the β-blocking drugs or a consequence of reduced preganglionic nerve activity caused by CNS β-blockade. In any event, mechanisms exist through which both β_1- and β_2-blocking drugs can reduce the release of norepinephrine presynaptically.

Effects Unrelated to Receptor Activity. An important effect of some of these drugs (acebutolol, alprenolol, oxprenolol, pindolol and propranolol) is membrane stabilization similar to that seen with the local anesthetics. This property becomes manifest at higher plasma levels of the drugs and can cause myocardial depression. Chronotropic activity is reduced by β-blockade, independent of this quinidine-like effect. This is manifested by a reduction in contractility that is greater than that resulting from catecholamine blockade alone.

Practolol has caused serious immunological problems. It is responsible, in some cases, for an oculocutaneous syndrome and/or a sclerosing peritonitis; both of these very serious side effects have reduced its long-term use in patient treatment. The oculocutaneous syndrome can involve eyes, ears, and skin and may include conjunctivitis, keratitis, serious otitis media, and a psoriasis-like plaque of the skin.

OTHER CONSIDERATIONS

Some of these agents (alprenolol, oxprenolol, pindolol and practolol) also have partial agonist activity (intrinsic sympathomimetic activity) similar to dichloroisoproterenol, the first antagonist synthesized. In the case of pindolol, the agonist properties are of sufficient magnitude to limit its usefulness for some types of treatment (see Table 7.2-2).

NONSELECTIVE β-ADRENOCEPTOR ANTAGONISTS

PROPRANOLOL

Propranolol, in addition to its β-blocking action, also has a stabilizing effect (similar to that produced by local anesthetics) on cell membranes. It is very lipid-soluble and has a generalized distribution; in the CNS, it can attain a high concentration (15 times that found in plasma). Like most β-antagonists, propranolol is readily absorbed from the gastrointestinal tract with an oral bioavailability of about 90%. Plasma levels vary widely among individuals receiving the same dosage because much of the drug is altered in first-pass metabolism by the liver. If the dose is very low, almost none appears in the systemic circulation; however, the percentage that reaches the general circulation increases with the dose. At higher dosages, hepatic catabolism appears to become saturated because the percentage increase in plasma levels exceeds the percent increase in the dose of the drug administered.

Propranolol is more than 95% metabolize, and its metabolites are largely excreted by the kidney. The metabolic products of liver catabolism include 4-hydroxypropranolol and other active compounds that appear to have shorter half-lives than propranolol. Although propranolol is largely (90-95%) bound to plasma proteins and has a plasma half-life of 3 to 6 hours, its effect on the β-receptor lasts from 10 to 12 hours (probably because of tissue binding); therefore, oral doses are usually given twice daily. Care should be taken when administering the drug intravenously because disproportionately smaller doses achieve higher plasma concentrations.

Adverse Effects. Adverse effects are of two types: those caused by generalized β-blockade and those caused by other properties of the drug. Those resulting from a generalized β-blockade include heart failure, cardiac arrest, severe bradycardia, and AV block. In some cases, side effects include arterial insufficiency, marked vasoconstriction in the extremities, increased peripheral resistance, increased airway resistance, and gastrointestinal hyperactivity (53). If the patient has received prolonged treatment with propranolol, it is advisable to reduce the dosage slowly because abrupt withdrawal of this medication has been reported to precipitate arrhythmias and infarctions. Propranolol is inactivated primarily by conjugation in the liver; therefore, the status of hepatic function needs to be considered when propranolol is being administered.

Effects of propranolol that are not related directly to peripheral β-blockade include CNS manifestations such as insomnia, vivid dreams, nightmares, hallucinations, dizziness and depression. These effects may result from β-adrenoceptor blocking action or, as evidence suggests, from blockade of $serotonin_2$ ($5\text{-}HT_2$) receptors as well (16).

Propranolol treatment alters carbohydrate and fat metabolism as well as adenylate cyclase activity that is normally initiated by β-receptor activation. It inhibits a rise in plasma free fatty acids and may induce hypoglycemia in some patients. Increased fatigue, alterations in sodium excretion, and decreased red cell affinity for oxygen have also been reported.

Therapeutic Uses

Treatment of Hypertension. The effects of propranolol are complex and involve a number of mechanisms, of which none alone accounts adequately for propranolol's beneficial effects. The direct β-blocking action on the vasculature would tend to produce an increased peripheral resistance (blockade of dilatation, which does occur occasionally as an unwanted side effect). Normally, however, the contribution of β-adrenergic vascular dilatation is minimal and, therefore, does not generally make much of a contribution to the total peripheral resistance. The drop in blood pressure achieved by treatment with propranolol alone is usually not very significant, and no postural hypotension is seen. It has been suggested that a CNS action may be responsible for beneficial effects on hypertension (similar to those that follow clonidine treatment).

It has been suggested that propranolol's β-blocking action on the heart decreases cardiac output and lowers blood pressure by reducing both the chronotropic and inotropic responses to catecholamines. Propranolol has been reported to inhibit renin release as well as the chain of events that is initiated by renin activation of angiotensin and that culminates in the release of aldosterone by angiotension II. The prevention of this series of events causes a reduction in angiotension-induced vasoconstriction as well as the circulating volume that results from aldosterone-induced sodium retention. The prevention of these actions is believed to contribute to a reduction in blood pressure. This clinical evidence is not completely clear because these effects appear to be restricted to those individuals who have high initial renin-angiotensin levels. Treatment with propranolol does not appear to have any significant effect on low or normal renin levels unless relatively high doses are used. Mechanism of antihypertensive action of propranolol is also discussed in Chapter 15.3.

Treatment of Other Disease States. Propranolol has also been used successfully in the treatment of cardiac arrhythmias, tachycardia of both atrial and ventricular origin, digitalis-induced anginal pain, and after acute myocardial infarction. It is used in hypertrophic obstructive cardiomyopathy, aortic dissection, thyrotoxicosis, pheochromocytoma, essential tremor, and migraine attacks. The beneficial effects of propranolol in treating these conditions are probably the result of its quinidine-like action as well as its β-blocking effects. Propranolol appears to be promising in the treatment of schizophrenia (45).

NADOLOL

Nadolol is a nonselective β-adrenoceptor antagonist (Fig. 7.2-2) and lacks both intrinsic sympathomimetic and membrane-stabilizing properties. Its β-blocking potency in animals is about two to four times that of propranolol, but in humans it is equipotent to propranolol when given orally.

About 30% of an oral dose of nadolol is absorbed from the gastrointestinal tract, and its absorption is not influenced by the presence of food or diuretics (e.g., furosemide, hydrochlorothiazide). Peak plasma concentrations of the drug are reached within 3 to 4 hours after administration. About 30% of the drug circulates bound to plasma proteins. The drug has a low lipid solubility and, as such, its penetration into the CNS is very low, which may explain its few CNS side effects. It has a long half-life of 14 to 24 hours in individuals with normal renal function. The drug is metabolized to a small extent; about 75% of the drug is excreted unchanged in the urine, and to a lesser extent in the feces. Elimination of nadolol is affected markedly in patients with severe impairment of renal function. Side effects of nadolol are attributed to β-blocking activity and similar to propranolol. Because of nadolol's low brain penetration, its CNS side effects are fewer than those of the more lipophilic β-blocking agents. It is contraindicated in bradycardia, AV block, congestive heart failure, and cardiogenic shock. Patients with bronchial asthma or chronic obstructive pulmonary disease should be treated with a β-blocker with relative β_1-selectivity (e.g., metoprolol) instead of nadolol.

The drug is effective in the treatment of angina pectoris and hypertension. Because of its long half-life, it is given once daily. For hypertension, the recommended initial daily dose of nadolol is 40 mg, gradually increased by 40-80 mg at intervals of 3-7 days to its usual maintenance dose of 80-320 mg (rarely up to 640 mg). For angina pectoris, the initial and premaintenance dosages are similar to those for hypertension, and the usual daily maintenance dose is 240 mg. Patients with renal impairments require dose adjustments.

TIMOLOL

Timolol is a nonselective β-adrenoceptor antagonist (Fig. 7.2-2) without membrane-stabilizing or sympathomimetic properties. On a weight basis, it is about 8-10 times as potent as propranolol. The drug is well absorbed from the gastrointestinal tract, and its plasma half-life is about 5 hours. Timolol has been shown to prolong the duration of exercise that can be tolerated before angina occurs, and to decrease the resting heart rate and both systolic and diastolic blood pressure. Timolol has been demonstrated to reduce mortality and reinfarction in patients surviving acute myocardial infarction. The protective mechanism and the pharmacological properties of the drug that are responsible for the effect on mortality and reinfarction have not been clarified. Side effects of timolol are attributable to β-adrenoceptor blockade.

SELECTIVE β_1-ADRENOCEPTOR ANTAGONISTS

PRACTOLOL

The structure of practolol is given in Fig. 7.2-2.

Adverse Effects. Serious adverse effects that result from treatment with practolol are referred to as the oculocutaneous syndrome, which involves a practolol complex with immunoglobulins. The syndrome can result in severe eye, ear and skin rashes and sclerosing peritonitis (52). These symptoms usually appear only after several years of treatment, but their occurrence has limited the use of practolol. Other β_1-blocking compounds do not appear to cause similar difficulties.

Therapeutic Uses. Practolol is a relatively selective β_1-antagonist that has its major effect on cardiac β-receptors and is minimally active on β_2-receptors except at high dosages. The direct effect of blockade is a decrease in heart rate, myocardial contractility, and cardiac output. Practolol, sotalol and atenolol do not have the quinidine or local anesthetic-like effects of propranolol and a number of other β-blocking compounds; however, practolol does have a partial agonistic activity similar to that seen with some other β-blockers.

Practolol is the least lipid-soluble of the β-blocking agents and does not cross the blood-brain barrier in measurable amounts. It is not metabolized to any extent, and 95% is excreted unchanged in the urine; this is also the case with sotalol. This property results in each of these compounds having a plasma half-life of two to three times that of propranolol.

Practolol is effective in the treatment of cardiac arrhythmia and angina but does not reduce cardiac output or produce bronchospasm to the extent that nonspecific β-blockers might (29).

METOPROLOL

Metoprolol is a relatively selective β_1-adrenoceptor antagonist devoid of agonistic activity. Compared with propranolol, its potency to inhibit the inotropic and chronotropic responses to isoproterenol is similar, but its potency to inhibit the vasodilator responses to isoproterenol is 50 to 100 times less. Metoprolol is well absorbed after oral administration. Its half-life is about 3 hours. It is excreted by the kidney, largely as inactive metabolites; 10% or less is excreted unchanged. Metoprolol resembles propranolol in its efficacy in treatment of mild-to-moderate hypertension. As with other antihypertensive agents, it should be given with a diuretic. The adverse effects of metoprolol that are secondary to cardiac β-blockade are similar to those of propranolol and the same precautions apply. Clinically effective doses of metoprolol may increase airway resistance in asthmatic patients, although to a lesser extent than propranolol.

SELECTIVE β_2-ADRENOCEPTOR ANTAGONIST

BUTOXAMINE

The structure of butoxamine is given in Fig. 7.2-2.

Therapeutic Uses. Butoxamine is the only β-blocking compound that is not a modification of the basic isoproterenol structure but is instead an N-tert-butyl methoxamine, at the present time it is the only β_2-selective agent (26). It blocks the metabolic effects of epinephrine, including increasing blood levels of glucose and free fatty acids. It also blocks the inhibitory effects of catecholamines on uterine and vascular smooth muscle without altering cardiac responses. This drug is still experimental and has not been clinically tested.

β-ANTAGONISTS WITH INTRINSIC SYMPATHOMIMETIC ACTIVITY

Bunitrolol and penbutolol are two new β-blocking agents with intrinsic sympathomimetic activity and vasodilator action (6). Bunitrolol (7) reduces peripheral vascular resistance (32) and does not decrease cardiac output in patients with coronary artery disease (4, 44). Penbutolol has also been shown to be active as an antihypertensive agent (16), but its vasodilator activity probably does not result from sympathomimetic stimulation. Because both of these agents are potent β-blocking agents that do not cause significant myocardial depression but have the ability to reduce peripheral resistance, they may find their use in the management of patients with both angina pectoris and impaired left ventricular function or hypertension.

COMBINED β- AND α-ADRENOCEPTOR ANTAGONIST

LABETALOL

The structure of labetalol is given in Fig. 7.2-2.

Pharmacokinetics. Labetalol can be administered orally, is rapidly absorbed, and causes plasma levels to peak within 1 or 2 hours with a low bioavailability ($\simeq$40%). Its plasma half-life is between 3.5 and 4.5 hours with $\simeq$50% protein bound. Evidence from animal experiments indicates that the highest tissue concentrations are found in the lung, liver and kidney. There does not appear to be measurable brain uptake, probably because labetalol is not as lipophilic as some of the other β-activity compounds (i.e., propranolol). Much of the oral dose is metabolized in the intestinal lumen and wall; $\simeq$5% of the drug is excreted unchanged. The conjugated metabolites appear in both urine and feces over a period of several days.

Therapeutic Uses. Labetalol is being studied extensively in clinical trials as an antihypertensive agent and, to a lesser extent, in pheochromocytoma surgery and clonidine withdrawal. This new compound has both α- and β-activity (9). Its action on β-receptors is nonspecific and similar to that of propranolol, whereas its action on α-receptors is like that of phenoxybenzamine. However, it is much more effective as a β- than an α-blocking agent. The β-blockade is approximately three times more potent than the α-blocking effect and should therefore have the clinical advantage of reducing static blood pressure without completely blocking the dynamic aspects of reflex control. Postural hypotension does occur in some individuals, but usually only at high-dose levels and/or during the first weeks of treatment. Labetalol can significantly reduce blood pressure, peripheral resistance, and heart rate; however, it has a lesser effect on stroke volume and cardiac output.

Labetalol (0.5 to 2 mg/day, i.v.) will cause a rapid (1-3 min) decrease in blood pressure in both normal and hypertensive subjects. The hypotensive response is similar to that obtained when propranolol and hydralazine are used in combination.

Labetalol appears to have little effect on the CNS. Its effect on plasma renin-angiotensin levels is independent of route of administration, dose and duration of treatment. High doses ($\simeq$ 1.2 g/day) given orally for a few days do not appear to alter plasma renin levels; however, either several months' treatment with doses in this range or intravenous treatment can reduce renin-angiotension plasma concentrations.

Labetalol does not appear to have any significant effect on ventilatory functions in control of asthmatic patients, even though many other β-receptor antagonists (i.e., propranolol) can cause severe bronchoconstriction.

WITHDRAWAL OF β-ADRENOCEPTOR ANTAGONISTS

In about 1 to 5% of patients with coronary artery disease, abrupt cessation of treatment with a β-adrenoceptor blocker leads to severe angina, mycocardial infarction, arrhythmias, or sudden death. Ambulatory patients are more likely to manifest these effects than hospitalized patients in bed rest. The precise mechanism for these withdrawal side effects of β-blockers is not clearly understood. It has been suggested that following withdrawal of β-adrenoceptor blockade there is sudden disappearance of beneficial therapeutic effects of these drugs such as decreases in plasma renin activity, platelet aggregation, heart rate-blood pressure response to stress. Deregulation of β-adrenoceptors and hyperresponsiveness to β-sympathomimetics have also been suggested as possible mechanisms for withdrawal side effects.

DRUG INTERACTIONS

With such agents as alprenolol and propranolol, liver metabolism is considerable, and consideration must be given to this first-pass effect if the patient is taking any other agents that decrease the hepatic blood flow, reduce the efficacy of the microsomal enzyme system, or cause other changes in the liver's capacity to metabolize drugs.

The interactive effects of adrenergic-blocking agents and agents such as tyramine, ephedrine, amphetamine, reserpine, or guanethidine, which release catecholamines, are obvious. Less commonly anticipated interactions are those occurring with the administration of such drugs as butyrophenones, phenothiazines, and tricyclic antidepressants, which have secondary autonomic effects. These agents all act as α-adrenoceptor antagonists and enhance activity of concomitantly administered α-blockers.

On the other hand, if two agents have a greater effect when coadministered than either has when given alone, there may be good cause for using them together in a therapeutic regime. For example, when alprenolol and the diuretic chlorthalidone were coadministered for their hypotensive effect, only one-fourth of the dose level required for administering either alone was necessary (3). Similar effects have been seen when other diuretics are administered with atenolol (41) and propranolol (31, 35). A smaller dose of two agents in combination, although attaining the desired action, may also reduce unwanted side effects that might occur when a higher dose of either agent is administered alone.

Table 7.2-3
Adrenoceptor Antagonists and Their Actions

Receptor	Action[a]	Blocking Agents	
		Specific	Nonspecific
α_1	Vasoconstriction (s)		
	Heart (s)	Azapetine	Dibenamine
	Iris, radial muscle (c)	Clozapine	Dihydroergotamine
	Bladder sphincter (c)	Corynanthine	Mianserin
	Vas deferens (c)	Phenoxybenzamine	Phentolamine
	GI sphincter (c)	Prazosin	
	Bronchial smooth muscle (c)	Urapidil[b]	
α_2	Adrenergic neurons (i)	Piperoxone	
	Norepinephrine release (i)	Rauwolscine	
	Renin release (i)	Tolazoline	
	Intestinal smooth muscle (r)	Yohimbine	
β_1	Heart (s)	Atenolol	
	Norepinephrine release (s)	Metoprolol	
	Adipose tissue lipolysis (s)	Para-oxprenolol	
	Liver glycogenolysis (s)	Practolol	Alprenolol
		Sotalol	Nadolol
β_2	Bronchial smooth muscle (r)		Oxprenolol
	GI smooth muscle (r)		Pindolol
	Bladder detrusor (r)	Butoxamine	Propranolol
	Ciliary muscle (r)		

[a] c = contract; r = relax; s = stimulate; i = inhibit.
[b] has α_2 agonist properties.

A combination of a β-blocker [alprenolol (37) or propranolol] with the vasodilator hydralazine has been administered to minimize the tachycardia and palpitations that could result from using the vasodilator alone. Furthermore, combining a β-blocker with a vasodilator prevents the rise in plasma renin caused by the latter.

Propranolol and hydralazine cause an increase in the systemic bioavailability of propranolol.

SUMMARY

Table 7.2-3 summarizes actions of the various adrenoceptor antagonists.

REFERENCES

1. Ahlquist, R. P. A study of the adrenoceptor receptors. *Am. J. Physiol.* 153:586, 1948.
2. Aghajanian, G. K., and Cedarbaum, J. M. Central noradrenergic neurons: Interaction of autoregulatory mechanisms with extrinsic influences. In: *Catecholamines: Basic and Clinical Frontiers* (Usdin, E., Koplin, G. J., and Barches, J., eds.). New York: Pergamon Press, 1978, p. 619.
3. Angervall, G., and Bystedt, U. The effect of alprenolol and alprenolol in combination with saluretics in hypertension. *Acta Med. Scand.* 554:39, 1974.
4. Banim, S. O., da Silva, A., and Balcon, R. Haemodynamic observations with KO. 1366 (bunitrolol): A new beta-adrenergic blocking agent. *Curr. Med. Res. Opinion* 4:630, 1977.
5. Barker, K. A., Harper, B., and Hughes, I. E. Possible subdivisions among α-adrenoceptors in various isolated tissues. *J. Pharm. Pharmacol.* 29:129, 1977.
6. Baum, T., Rowles, G,. Shropshire, A. T., and Gluckman, M. I. Beta-adrenergic blocking and cardiovascular properties of two new substances, Ko 1313 and Ko 1366. *J. Pharmacol. Exp. Ther.* 176:339, 1971.
7. Boissier, J. R., Coutte, R., Advenier, C., and Giudicel, J. R. Beta-adrenolytic and hemodynamic effects of penbutolol. *Therapie* 28:1251, 1973.
8. Bonelli, J. Comparative haemodynamic studies with mepindolol-sulphage (SHF 222) and propranolol (Inderal, Docition) in the isoproterenol test. *J. Int. Med. Res.* 6:317, 1978.
9. Brogden, R. N., Heel, R. D., Speight, T. M., and Avery, G. S. Labetalol: A review of its pharmacology and therapeutic use in hypertension. *Drugs* 15:251, 1978.
10. Colucci, W. S. Alpha-adrenergic receptor blockade with prazosin. *Ann. Intern. Med.* 97:67, 1982.
11. Conally, M. E., Kersting, F., and Dollery, C. T. The clinical pharmacology of beta-adrenoceptor-blocking drugs. *Prog. Cardiovasc. Dis.* 19:203, 1976.
12. Dale, H. H. On some physiological actions of ergot. *J. Physiol.* (Lond.) 34:163, 1906.
13. Dollery, C. T., and Lewis, P. J. Central hypotensive effect of propranolol. *Postgrad. Med. J.* 52:116, 1976.
14. Fitzgerald, J. D. Beta-blockade and mechanisms of disease. *Postgrad. Med. J.* 52:184, 1976.
15. Furchgott, R. F. The classification of adrenoceptors (adrenergic receptors). An evaluation from the stand point receptor theory. In: *Handbook of Experimental Pharmacology,* Vol. 33, Catecholamines (Blaschko, H., and Muschall, E., eds.). Berlin: Springer-Verlag, 1972, p. 283.
16. Green, A. R., Johnson, P., and Nimgaonkar, V. L. Interactions β-adrenoceptor agonists and antagonists with the 5-hydroxytryptamine$_2$ (5-HT$_2$) receptor. *Neuropharmacology* 22:657, 1983.
17. Hansson, L., Olander, R., Aberg, H., Malmcrona, R., and Westerlund, A. Treatment of hypertension with propranolol and hydralazine. *Acta Med. Scand.* 190:531, 1971.
18. Heimburger, M., Denoroy, L. Renaud, B., Sassard, J., Cohen, Y., and Wepierre, J. Effects of chronic β-blocker treatment on catecholamine levels in spontaneously hypertensive rats. *Biochem. Pharmacol.* 32:2739, 1983.
19. Hughes, M. J., and O'Brien, L. J. Liberation of endogenous compounds by tolazoline. *Agents and Actions* 7:225, 1977.
20. Ishimore, T., Shiratsuchi, K., Izumi, A., and Himori, N. No evidence for involvement of the peripheral sympathetic nervous system in the antihypertensive action of β-adrenoceptor blocking agents in spontaneously hypertensive rats. *Folia Pharmacol.* Jap. 80:463, 1982.
21. Kalsner, S. The effects of yohimbine on presynaptic and postsynaptic events during sympathetic nerve activation in cattle iris: A critique of presynaptic receptor theory. *Br. J. Pharmacol.* 78:247, 1983.
22. Kunos, G., Mucci, L., and Jaeger, V. Interconversion of myocardial adrenoceptors: Its relationship to adenylate cyclase activation. *Life Sci.* 19:1597, 1976.
23. Lands, A. M., Arnold, A., McAuliff, J. P., Luduena, F. P., and Brown, T. G. Differentiation of receptor systems activated by sympathomimetic amines. *Nature* 214:597, 1967.
24. Lands, A. M., Luduena, E. D., and Buzzo, H. J. Differentiation of receptors responsive to isoproterenol. *Life Sci.* 6:2241, 1967.
25. Large, M. S., and Smith, L. H. β-Adrenergic blocking agents. 22. 1-Phenoxy-3 [[(substituted-amino) alkyl]amino]-2-propanols. *J. Med. Chem.* 25:1286, 1982.
26. Levy, B. The adrenergic blocking activity of N-tert-butylmethoxamine (butoxamine). *J. Pharmacol. Exp. Ther.* 151:413, 1966.
27. Levy, B., and Wilkenfeld, B. E. Selective interactions with beta-adrenergic receptors. *Fed. Proc.* 29:1362, 1970.
28. Light, K. E., and Hughes, M. J. Liberation of histamine by compound 48/80, tolazoline, betahistine, and burimamide from isolated spontaneously beating guinea pig and rabbit atrial pairs. *Agents Actions* 9:141, 1979.
29. MacDonald, A. G., and McNeill, R. S. A comparison of the effect on airway resistance of a new beta-blocking drug, ICI 50, and propranolol. *Br. J. Anaesth.* 40:508, 1968.
30. McDevitt, D. G. The assessment of β-adrenoceptor blocking drugs in man. *Br. J. Clin. Pharmacol.* 4:413, 1977.
31. Mitchell, I., Lodge, R,. and Lawson, A. A. Adjuvant effect of bendrofluazide on propranolol in hypertension. *Scott. Med. J.* 17:326, 1972.
32. Naylor, W. G., and Tay, J. Effect of O-2-hydroxy-3-(tert.-butylamino) propoxybenzonitrile HCl (KO 1366) on beta-adrenergic receptors in the cardiovascular system. *J. Pharmacol. Exp. Ther.* 180:302, 1972.
33. Nickerson, M., and Gump, W. S. The chemical basis for adrenergic blocking activity in compounds related to dibenamine. *J. Pharmacol. Exp. Ther.* 97:25, 1949.
34. Nickerson, M., and Kunos, G. Discussion of evidence regarding induced changes in adrenoceptors. *Fed. Proc.* 36:2580, 1977.
35. O'Brien, E. T., and MacKinnon, J. Propranolol and polythiazide in treatment of hypertension. *Br. Heart J.* 34:1042, 1972.
36. Paget, G. E. Carcinogenic action of promethalol. *Br. Med. J.* 2:1266, 1963.
37. Pape, J. The effect of alprenolol in combination with hydralazine in essential hypertension. *Acta Med. Scand.* 554:55, 1974.
38. Patel, K. R., and Kerr, J. W. Alpha-receptor-blocking drugs in bronchial asthma. *Lancet* 1:348, 1975.
39. Patel, K. R., Kerr, J. W., MacDonald, E. B., and MacKenzie, A. M. The effect of thymoxamine and cromolyn sodium on postexercise bronchoconstriction in asthma. *J. Allergy Clin. Immunol.* 57:285, 1976.
40. Patil, K. R., Miller, D. D., and Trendelenburg, U. Molecular geometry and adrenergic drug activity. *Pharmacol. Rev.* 57:285, 1976.
41. Petrie, J. C., Galloway, D. B., Webster, J., Simpson, W. T., and Lewis, J. A. Atenolol and bendrofluazide in hypertension. *Br. Med. J.* 4:133, 1975.

42. Powell, C. E., and Slater, I. H. Blocking of inhibitory adrenergic receptors by a dichloro analog of isoproterenol. *J. Pharmacol. Exp. Ther.* 122:480, 1958.

43. Raine, A. E. G., and Chubb, I. W. Long term β-adrenergic blockade reduces tyrosine hydroxylase and dopamine β-hydroxylase activities in sympathetic ganglia. *Nature* 267:265, 1977.

44. Reale, A., Nigri, A., and Gioffre, A. Evidence for improved cardiac performance after beta-blockade in patients with coronary artery disease. *J. Int. Med. Res.* 4:338, 1976.

45. Roberts, E., and Amadren, P. (eds.). *Propranolol and Schizophrenia* Kroe Foundation Series, Vol. 10. New York: Alan R. Liss, 1978

46. Sainani, G. S., Shah, G. M., Nandi, J. S., and Gulati, R. B. A pilot study of once-daily penbutolol in hypertension. *Pharmatherapeutical* 1:493, 1977.

47. Simonsson, G.B., Svedmyr, N., Skoogh, B.E., Andersson, R., and Bergh, N. P. In vivo and in vitro studies on alpha-receptors in human airways: Potentiation with bacterial endotoxin. *Scand. J. Resp. Dis.* 53:227, 1972.

48. Stjarne, L., and Brundin, J. Dual adrenoceptor-mediated control of noredrenaline secretion from human vasoconstrictor nerves: Facilitation by β-receptors and inhibition by α-receptors. *Acta Physiol. Scand.* 94:139, 1975.

49. Stjarne, L., and Brundin, J. β-Adrenoceptors facilitating noradrenaline secretion from human vasoconstrictor nerves. *Acta Physiol. Scand.* 97:88, 1976.

50. U'Prichard, D. C., and Snyder, S. H. Distinct α-noradrenergic receptors differentiated by binding and physiological relationships. *Life Sci.* 24:79, 1979.

51. Weinstock, M., Thoa, N. B., and Kopin, I. J. β-Adrenoceptors modulate noradrenaline release from axonal sprouts in cultured rat superior cervical ganglia. *Eur. J. Pharmacol.* 47:297, 1978.

52. Wright, P. Untoward effects associated with practolol administration: Oculomucocutaneous syndrome. *Br. Med. J.* 1:595, 1975.

53. Zacharias, F. J. Patient acceptability of propranolol and the occurrence of side effects. *Postgrad. Med. J.* 52:87, 1976.

ADDITIONAL READINGS

Cavero, I., and Roach, A. G. The pharmacology of prazosin, a novel antihypertensive agent. *Life Sci.* 27:1525, 1980.

El-Etr, A. A., and Glisson, S. N. Alpha-adrenergic blocking agents. *Int. Anesthesiol. Clin.* 16:239, 1978.

Gross, F. (ed.). *The cardioprotective Action of Beta-Blockers.* Baltimore: University Park Press, 1976.

Hansson, L. Effects of beta adrenoceptor blocking agents on haemodynamic parameters. *Acta Med. Scand.* (suppl.) 606:49, 1977.

Lydtin, H. Side effects and contraindications of beta-receptor blocking agents. *Klin. Wochenschr.* 55:415, 1977.

Lowenthall, D.T. et al. Mechanism of action and clinical pharmacology of β-adrenergic blocking drugs. *Am. J. Med.* 77:119, 1984.

Petrie, J. C., Galloway, D. B., Jeffers, T. A., and Webster, J. Adverse reactions to beta-blocking drugs: A review. *Postgrad. Med. J.* 52:63, 1976.

Saxena, P. R., and Forsyth, R. P. (eds.). Beta-adrenoceptor blocking agents. In: *The Pharmacological Basis of Clinical Use.* New York: Elsevier, 1976.

Scriabine, A. β-Adrenoceptor blocking drugs in hypertension. *Ann. Rev. Pharmacol. Toxicol.* 19:269, 1979.

Zimmerman, T. J., Kass, M. A., Yablonski, M. E., and Becker, B. Timolol maleate. *Arch. Ophthalmol.* 97:656, 1979.

CHAPTER
7.3

ADRENERGIC NEURON BLOCKING DRUGS

H. Lloyd Garvey

Drugs classified as adrenergic neuron blocking agents depress impulse transmission at the postganglionic adrenergic nerve terminals. This depression may be accomplished by the prevention of normal release of norepinephrine (NE) after nerve stimulation. Members of this class of drugs (guanethidine, bretylium, bethanidine, and debrisoquin) have been reported to act as substrates for the neuronal membrane amine pump, which is normally involved in the reuptake of NE after its release. Uptake of these drugs by the adrenergic neurons results in dissociation of electrical activity and impaired transmission of impulse across the junction between the adrenergic nerve terminals and the effector cells. Although the exact mechanism for dissociation of electrical activity is not clearly known, it has been suggested that interference with Ca^{2+}-mediated release mechanism or local anesthetic action of these drugs may be responsible. The initial entry of these drugs into the adrenergic neurons may result in transient release of NE, evidenced by a rise in blood pressure and cardiac stimulation. In humans, although all neuron blocking agents except for bretylium cause NE depletion after prolonged administration, this event plays no major role in the pharmacological activity of these drugs. Bretylium produces effects on the electrical properties of cardiac muscle, which led to its principal therapeutic use as an antiarrhythmic drug (2, 12). Because of the rapid development of tolerance, its use as an antihypertensive drug has been abandoned.

GUANETHIDINE

Guanethidine, [2-(octahydro-1-azocinyl) ethyl] guanidine, is a synthetic adrenergic neuron blocking agent (Fig. 7.3-1). It is most often used in the treatment of severe hypertension that is resistant to other antihypertensive agents (8).

Pharmacological Actions. The important pharmacological actions of guanethidine are the result of its ability to inhibit the vascular smooth muscle tone induced by sympathetic stimulation due to decreased liberation of norepinephrine. Following its administration, there is a progressive fall in systemic and pulmonary arterial pressure associated with decrease in heart rate and cardiac output. The hypotensive effect of the drug is most marked in the erect posture or during exercise (5, 6, 14). The antihypertensive action is also associated with impairment of cardiovascular reflexes.

Pharmacokinetics. Guanethidine is poorly (3-50%) absorbed from the gastrointestinal tract when given orally, and the absorbed drug undergoes first-pass metabolism. Patients vary in their response to the drug due to its erratic absorption, variable rate of biotransformation, and renal elimination. At least three phases of drug elimination have been described: an initial rapid phase, a second phase with a half-life of about 20 hours, and a third phase of 5 to 14 days (11). Elimination of its principal metabolites is mainly by the bile and kidney.

BETHANIDINE AND DEBRISOQUIN

Several compounds structurally related to guanethidine and bretylium have been synthesized and tested for adrenergic neuron blocking action. Two of these compounds, bethanidine (1-benzyl-2,3-dimethylguanidine) and debrisoquin (3,4-dihydro-2-[1H] isoquinolinecarboxamidine) are currently undergoing clinical trials as potential antihypertensive agents (Fig. 7.3-1).

Both bethanidine and debrisoquin are similar to guanethidine in action. Both drugs gain access to the adrenergic neuron by active transport but cause less depletion of catecholamines than guanethidine. Debrisoquin possesses monoamine oxidase-inhibiting activity. The actions of bethanidine and debrisoquin have more rapid onset but shorter duration (4, 7). Thus, it is possible to attain a maintenance dose of these drugs more quickly. There is also less danger of prolonged hypotension with these agents than with guanethidine. Compared with guanethidine, bethanidine is more reliably absorbed (50-70%) from the gastrointestinal tract.

It is not metabolized in the body and is excreted unchanged in the urine. Thus, a reduction of dosage is necessary in the presence of renal failure. The half-life of bethanidine is 2 to 2.5 hours. Debrisoquin is also well absorbed and is partly metabolized. Some individuals have a genetic inability to metabolize debrisoquin. Thus, dosage requirements for this drug vary considerably. Approximately 95% of the drug is excreted in the urine, mainly as metabolites within 24 hours and about 12% is excreted unchanged in the feces. The major metabolite, 4OH-bethanidine, is inactive.

Like guanethidine, bethanidine and debrisoquin are effective and reliable drugs in the management of hypertension. Diarrhea is not observed with these two drugs. Otherwise, they show minor differences from guanethidine in their effectiveness and side effects. Drug interactions and contraindications are similar to those of guanethidine described in Chapter 15.3, although there is less tendency to produce hypertensive crises in patients with pheochromocytoma. Neither drug is approved for use in hypertension in the United States.

GUANADREL

Guanadrel (HYLOREL) is a new adrenergic neuron blocking drug with a chemical structure similar to that of guanethidine (1) (Fig. 7.3-1). It is rapidly absorbed from the gastrointestinal tract after oral administration, and the maximum hypotensive effect occurs within 4 to 6 hours. The drug is largely (85% of a dose) excreted unchanged in the urine. The frequency of major drug-related side effects such as morning orthostatic faintness, orthostatic symptoms during the day, and diarrhea is less with guanadrel than that encountered with guanethidine. It is generally recommended for use in step 2 therapy for moderate hypertension as an alternative to methyldopa.

BRETYLIUM

TM 10 (choline 2,6-xylylether) was the first strongly basic compound demonstrated to have adrenergic neuron-blocking actions. However, because of its pronounced cholinergic side effects such as salivation and intestinal spasm, this agent was not used clinically but was responsible for initiating the search for other useful congeners.

Bretylium [O-bromo benzyl] ethyl-dimethyl ammonium-p-toluenesulfonate was the first congener of TM 10 to be used in humans (3) (Fig. 7.3-1). Bretylium blocks the activation of sympathetic nerves without causing depletion of catecholamines. Agents that block amine transport mechanisms will antagonize the effects of bretylium. High concentrations of bretylium accumulate in adrenergic nerves, and it has been suggested that its pharmacological properties may be in part related to a local anesthetic action. Like guanethidine, bretylium does not interfere with adrenomedullary catecholamines. It increases the sensitivity of target tissues to circulating or exogenously administered catecholamines. Poor oral absorption and side effects such as postural hypotension and parotid swelling, as well as the development of tolerance, have made bretylium an undesirable agent in the management of hypertension. It is currently employed as an antiarrhythmic agent for the management of recurrent ventricular arrhythmias that are resistant to conventional treatment and in arrhythmias associated with an increased sympathetic activity (Chapter 15.2). However, the frequent occurrence of potentially serious side effects prevents its use as a first-line drug in the management of cardiac arrhythmias.

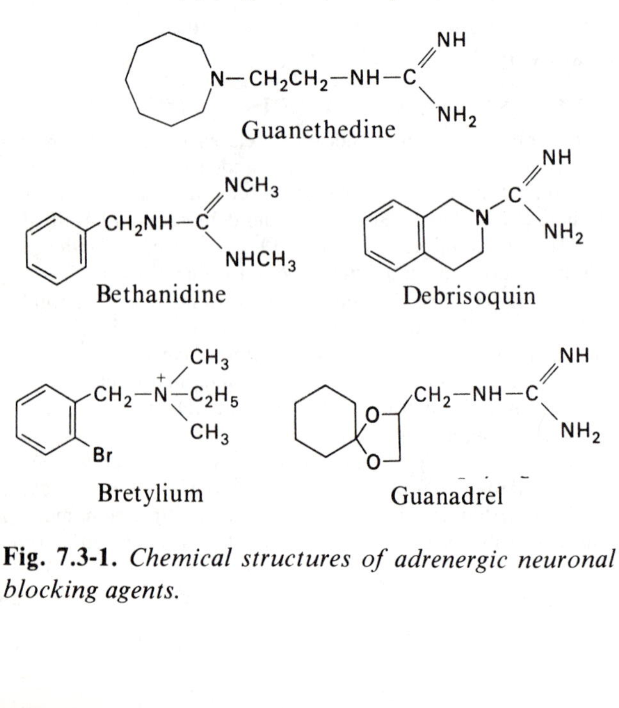

Guanethedine

Bethanidine

Debrisoquin

Bretylium

Guanadrel

Fig. 7.3-1. *Chemical structures of adrenergic neuronal blocking agents.*

Adverse Effects. Debrisoquin and bethanidine are associated with fewer side effects than guanethidine, and the severity of these effects may decrease with continued use of the drug or by reduction in their dosages. All adrenergic neuron-blocking drugs produce orthostatic hypotension that is marked in the early morning, in hot weather, after exercise, after heavy meals, and during fever. The timing of occurrence of hypotension seems to be related to the pharmacokinetics of the individual drug. With bethanidine, due to its shorter half-life, the hypotension generally occurs within 1 to 2 hours of postmedication. Debrisoquin and guanethidine have greater negative chronotropic action on the heart than bethanidine. About 25% of patients taking guanethidine show postural hypotension, compared with about 18-19% in those taking bethanidine or debrisoquin. The most common side effect of guanethidine is diarrhea. This is much less common with debrisoquin and bethanidine. Other side effects of these drugs include failure of ejaculation, impotence, dizziness, nasal stuffiness, syncope and weakness. The frequency of the major side effects is less with guanadrel than with guanethidine. Transient hypertension and increased frequency of premature ventricular contractions may occur early in the treatment with bretylium due to release of NE from adrenergic postganglionic nerve endings. Concomitant use of bretylium and digitalis may precipitate toxicity of the latter.

Therapeutic Uses. Adrenergic neuron blocking drugs such as bethanidine, debrisoquin, guanadrel and guanethidine are used in the management of moderate-to-severe hypertension and reported to be equally effective by most investigators. They are also employed in the management of renal hypertension, including hypertension due to renal amyloidosis and renal artery stenosis (9).

Efficacy of guanethidine may be demonstrated at dose levels as low as 5 mg, but larger doses are usually required in patients with severe hypertension. Because the drug is only partially absorbed, it is not possible to predict dosage requirements for individual patients. The erratic absorption does not fully account for the dosage variability observed, because resistant patients are unresponsive even to parenteral doses at which it is effective in sensitive patients (13). The initial dose of bethanidine is 5-10 mg three times a day, which may be increased by 5 mg or more. The usual doses of debrisoquin are 20-60 mg/day for either mild or severe hypertension. Several clinical studies have confirmed the equivalent efficacy of guanadrel and guanethidine in respect to the onset or extent of blood pressure control in patients with essential hypertension (10). The initial dose is 10 mg/day, gradually increased until blood pressure level is achieved. The usual maintenance dose is 25 to 75 mg/day. It is available as 10- and 25-mg tablets. Concurrent therapy with diuretic and/or adrenergic-blocking drugs will improve the hypotensive effect and lower the dosage requirement of neuron blocking agent.

In life-threatening ventricular arrhythmias (ventricular fibrillation not responding to lidocaine), bretylium tosylate is given i.v. at a dose of 5 mg/kg initially; if ventricular fibrillation persists, a second injection at a dose of 10 mg/kg may be repeated. In other forms of ventricular arrhythmias, it is administered i.m. or i.v. (slow infusion) at a dose of 5-10 mg/kg; the dose may be repeated, if needed (see Chapter 15.2).

Preparations. Preparations and doses of adrenergic neuron-blocking drugs are given in Chapter 15.3.

REFERENCES

1. *AMA Drug Evaluation*, 5th ed. American Medical Association, 1983, p. 717.
2. Amsterdam, E.A., Massumi, R.A., Zelis, R. and Mason, D.T. Use of bretylium tosylate in the management of cardiac arrhythmias. *Heart Lung* 1:269, 1972.
3. Aviado, D.M. and Dil, A.H. The effects of a new sympathetic blocking drug (bretylium) on cardiovascular control. *J. Pharmacol. Exp. Ther.* 129:328, 1960.
4. Chrysant, S.G., Nishiyama, K. Adampoulos, P.N. et al. Systemic hemodynamic effects of bethanidine in essential hypertensive man. *Circulation* 52:137, 1975.
5. Clezy, T.M. Oral contraceptives and hypertension: The effects of guanethidine. *Med. J. Aust.* 1:638, 1970.
6. Dollery, C.T., Emslie-Smith, D. and Milne, M.D. Clinical and pharmacological studies with guanethidine. *Lancet* 2:381, 1960.
7. Gifford, R.W., Jr. Bethanidine suflate: A new antihypertensive agent. *JAMA* 193:901, 1965.
8. Goldberg, L.I. and Zimmerman, A.M. Guanethidine and methyldopa as therapeutic agents in hypertension. A comparative review. *Postgrad. Med.* 33:548, 1963.
9. Kastrup, E.K. and Boyd, J.R. Antihypertensives. In: *Facts and Comparisons*. St. Louis: Facts and Comparisons, 1979, p. 454.
10. Malinow, S.H. Comparison of guanadrel and guanethidine efficacy and side effects. *Clin. Ther.* 5:284, 1983.
11. Oates, J.A., Mitchell, J.R. Feagin, O.J. et al. Distribution of guanidinium antihypertensives: Mechanism of their selective actions. *Ann. N.Y. Acad. Sci.* 179:302, 1972.
12. Patterson, E. and Lucchesi, B.R. Bretylium: A prototype for future development of antidysrhythmic agents. *Am. Heart J.* 106:426, 1983.
13. Rahn, K.H. and Goldberg, L.I. Comparison of antihypertensive efficacy and intestinal absorption and excretion of guanethidine in hypertensive patients. *Clin. Pharmacol. Ther.* 10:858, 1969.
14. Richardson, D.W., Wyso, E.U., McGee, J.H. et al. Circulatory effects of guanethidine. Clinical, renal and cardiac responses to treatment with a novel antihypertensive drug. *Circulation* 22:184, 1960.

CHAPTER
7.4

DOPAMINERGIC AGONISTS AND ANTAGONISTS

Kenneth E. Moore

Dopaminergic receptors are located in the brain, the anterior pituitary, and the mesenteric and renal vasculature. Dopaminergic agonists and antagonists are drugs that mimic and block, respectively, the actions of dopamine at these receptor sites. These drugs have a variety of pharmacological actions and therapeutic uses. This chapter will focus on the basic and clinical pharmacology of dopaminergic agonists. The basic pharmacology of dopaminergic antagonists and the therapeutic use of these drugs as antipsychotic agents are discussed in Chapter 11.5.1.

DISTRIBUTION OF DOPAMINERGIC NEURONS IN THE BRAIN

Dopamine was originally believed to function primarily as a precursor for the synthesis of norepinephrine and epinephrine. It was not until the late 1950s that the development of sensitive fluorometric assays permitted the quantification of the microgram quantities of dopamine that exist in the brain. Because dopamine is a precursor of norepinephrine, it was expected that the regional distribution of dopamine and norepinephrine would be the same; this was found not to be the case. Whereas norepinephrine is distributed throughout the brain, with the highest concentrations in the hypothalamus, dopamine is concentrated in the striatum (caudate nucleus and putamen). This region, which is almost devoid of norepinephrine, contains neurons that make up part of the extrapyramidal system; this system is involved with the initiation of motor movement and with postural reflexes. It was postulated, therefore, that in addition to serving as precursor for norepinephrine, dopamine may play a neurotransmitter role in the central regulation of motor functions.

This proposal was strengthened by the finding that brains of patients suffering from Parkinson's disease were discovered at autopsy to have a low content of dopamine in the striatum. It is now known that brains of patients with Parkinson's disease are characterized by a loss of nigrostriatal dopaminergic neurons (1). These neurons have cell bodies in substantia nigra and terminals in the striatum (Fig. 7.4-1). Ascending dopaminergic neurons that constitute the mesolimbic-mesocortical systems have cell bodies in the medial ventral tegmentum and terminals in various limbic (e.g., olfactory tubercle, nucleus accumbens, septum) and cortical (e.g., frontal, entorhinal, cingulate) regions (2, 8). Collectively, the ascending dopaminergic neurons have been referred to as the mesotelencephalic system (11).

A small number of dopamine-containing neurons, comprising the tuberoinfundibular-hypophysial and incertohypothalamic systems, are located in the hypothalamus. Cell bodies of the tuberoinfundibular and tuberohypophysial dopaminergic neurons are located in the arcuate and periventricular nuclei in the mediobasal hypothalamus. Short axons of tuberohypophysial neurons project from these cells to the pituitary (neurointermediate lobe); other axons, constituting the tuberoinfundibular system, project to the external layer of the median eminence. The former neurons have been postulated to play a role in the release of hormones from the posterior pituitary (e.g., α-melanocyte-stimulating hormone, β-endorphin). Tuberoinfundibular dopaminergic neurons are believed to influence the release of luteinizing hormone, growth hormone, and prolactin from the anterior pituitary (9, 12). Dopamine-containing cells have also been identified in autonomic ganglia (SIF cells) of some species, in the retina, spinal cord, and in the kidney (4, 6, 11).

EVENTS OCCURRING AT A DOPAMINERGIC SYNAPSE

The neurochemical events occurring at the terminals of dopaminergic neurons are similar to those at noradrenergic neurons (Fig. 7.4-2). Tyrosine is transported into the nerve terminal, where it is converted to L-dihydroxyphenylalanine (DOPA) by the rate-limiting enzyme, tyrosine hydroxylase. DOPA, in turn, is decarboxylated to dopamine by aromatic L-amino acid decarboxylase. Whereas tyrosine hydroxylase is distributed only to catecholamine-containing neurons or cells, the decarboxylase is ubiquitous, being identified in other neurons, glia, and blood vessels in the brain, and in a variety of peripheral tissues, especially the liver. Newly synthesized dopamine can be stored in synaptic vesicles or it can be released in response to nerve action potentials or drugs. Tyrosine hydroxylase appears to be regulated, in part, by end-product inhibition so that concentrations of dopamine in the nerve terminal remain fairly constant despite alterations in the amount of transmitter released. Once released, dopamine can activate receptors on the postsynaptic membrane (postsynaptic receptors) or on the dopaminergic nerve terminal itself (presynaptic or autoreceptors). Activation of these latter receptors inhibits the release and synthesis of dopamine. Thus, synaptic concentrations of dopamine appear to modulate the amount of amine that is synthesized and released through this short-loop feedback mechanism.

Dopamine is removed from the synaptic cleft by an active uptake mechanism that transports the amine back into the presynaptic nerve terminal. Once inside the neuron, dopamine can be stored and subsequently released, or it can be converted by mitochondrial monoamine oxidase (MAO) to dihydroxyphenylacetic acid (DOPAC) and lost from the nerve as this inactive metabolite. DOPAC, in turn, can be O-methylated by catechol-O-methyltransferase (COMT), an enzyme located in glial cells, to form homovanillic acid (HVA). A small amount of released dopamine is converted to 3-methoxytyramine (3MT) by COMT and then to HVA by extraneuronal MAO. These metabolites of dopamine can be measured in the brain or CSF; their concentrations can provide a biochemical index of the activity of dopaminergic neurons in the brain, an increased concentration of metabolites generally reflecting increased activity.

Some of the events occurring at terminals of tuberoinfundibular dopaminergic neurons, which appear to have evolved characteristics suited to release dopamine into blood, are slightly different from those described earlier. First, instead of forming synapses, many dopaminergic neurons in the median eminence end in close approximation to the perivascular spaces of the hypothalamic-hypophyseal portal system (Fig. 7.4-1). Dopamine released from these neurons is transported in the blood to the anterior pituitary, where it activates receptors on prolactin-secreting cells, thereby inhibiting the release of this hormone. Tuberoinfundibular neurons also differ from other dopaminergic neurons in that they lack a high-affinity uptake system and presynaptic receptors (10).

Dopaminergic receptors have been characterized *in vitro* by determining the binding characteristics of radioactive agonists or antagonists to cell membrane fragments, and by monitoring the activity of dopamine-sensitive adenylate cyclase, which is believed to be linked to some receptors. These two techniques do not measure the same putative receptor sites, and there is some evidence for the existence of a family of dopaminergic receptors just as there is for multiple noradrenergic receptors (e.g., α_1, α_2, β_1, β_2). Selected dopaminergic agonists have different relative affinities for receptors located at different sites (e.g., the profile of activities of dopaminergic agonists in the brain is different from that in the renal vascular bed) (5).

Dopaminergic receptors have been identified at a variety of sites other than those at terminals of dopaminergic neurons (Table 7.4-1). Some of these are tonically activated (e.g., those on prolactin-secreting cells in anterior pituitary), as evidenced by the effects that dopaminergic antagonists have on functions regulated by these receptors. Other dopaminergic receptors appear to be activated only by exogenously administered dopaminergic agonists (e.g., in the area postrema). Because it is a flexible molecule, dopamine can assume a variety of positions; thus, it is not surprising that in addition to activating different putative dopaminergic receptors, this amine can, at high doses, also activate α- and β-adrenergic receptors.

Table 7.4-1
Activation of Different Dopaminergic Receptors

Location of Receptors	Results of Stimulation
Striatum	Initiation of motor function; excessive stimulation results in stereotyped behaviors
Limbic and cortical regions	Arousal, increased activity; excessive stimulation may result in mania, hyperactivity (schizophrenia?)
Median eminence	Release of growth hormone-releasing hormone and of luteinizing hormone-releasing hormone
Area postrema	Emesis
Anterior pituitary	Inhibition of prolactin release
Posterior pituitary	Inhibition of α-melanocyte-stimulating hormone, β-endorphin
Smooth muscle in renal, mesenteric, coronary, and cerebral vascular beds	Vasodilation
Sympathetic ganglia	Inhibition of transmission (?)

DRUG-INDUCED ALTERATIONS OF DOPAMINERGIC TRANSMISSION PROCESSES

Drugs can mimic or disrupt dopaminergic transmission in a variety of ways; some of these are depicted schematically in Fig. 7.4-2.

Drugs That Mimic or Enhance Dopaminergic Transmission

Drugs that Act Directly on Dopaminergic Receptors. Compounds with markedly different chemical structures (e.g., apomorphine, bromocriptine) are capable of activating both pre- and postsynaptic dopaminergic receptors. There is no drug currently available for clinical investigation that selectively activates presynaptic dopa-

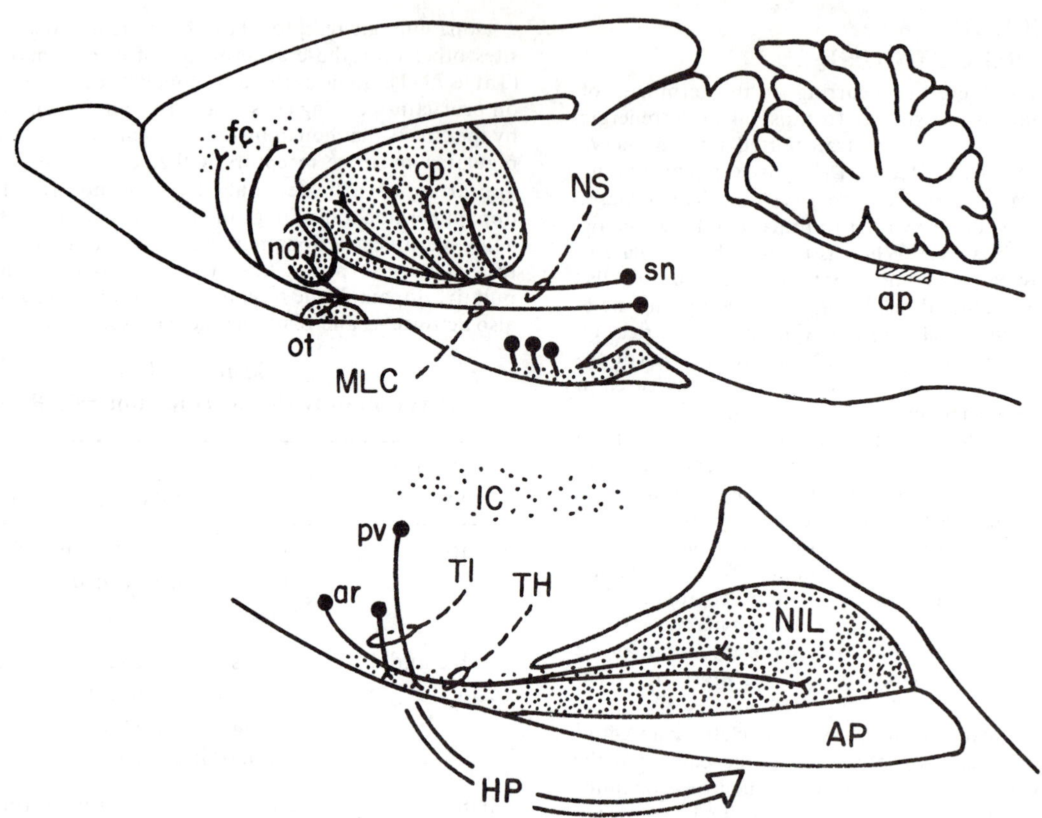

Fig. 7.4-1. *Distribution of dopaminergic neuronal systems in the rat brain.*

The lower figure is an enlargement of the mediobasal hypothalamus and the pituitary. Abbreviations: ap, area postrema; ar, arcuate nucleus; cp, caudate-putamen (striatum); fc, frontal cortex; me, median eminence; na, nucleus accumbens; ot, olfactory tubercle; pv, periventricular nucleus; AP, anterior pituitary; NIL, posterior pituitary (neurointermediate lobe); HP, hypothalamic-hypophysial portal system. Dopaminergic neuronal systems: IC, incertohypothalamic; MLC, mesolimbic-cortical; NS, nigrostriatal; TH, tuberohypophyseal; TI, tuberoinfundibular.

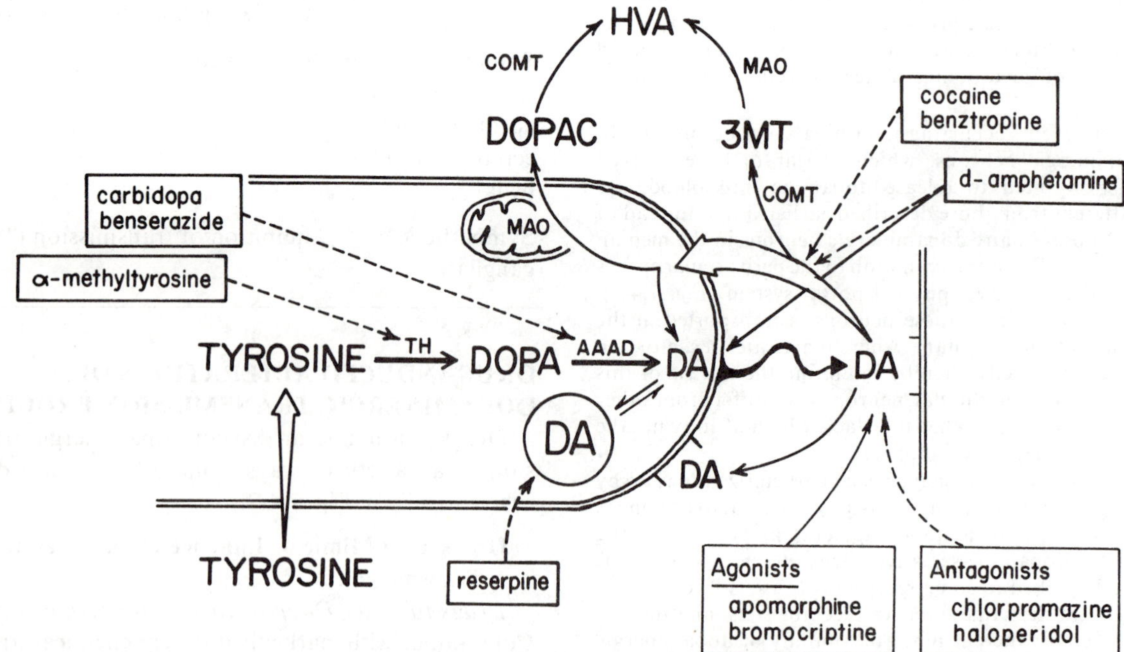

Fig. 7.4-2. *Schematic diagram of a dopaminergic synapse depicting sites at which drugs have been postulated to act.*

Abbreviations: AAAD, aromatic L-amino acid decarboxylase; COMT, catechol-o-methyltransferase; DA, dopamine; DOPAC, dihydroxyphenylacetic acid; MAO, monoamine oxidase; 3MT, 3-methoxytyramine; TH, tyrosine hydroxylase; stimulation ——▸; inhibition ----▸

minergic receptors, although several experimental compounds (e.g., 3PPP, TL99) have been reported to activate selectively these receptors in animal tests (7). Presynaptic dopaminergic agonists, by inhibiting synthesis and release of dopamine, might be expected to block dopaminergic transmission and thereby have some clinical utility.

Drugs that Release or Block the Reuptake of Dopamine. There are no drugs currently available that specifically and selectively block the neuronal uptake of dopamine. Cocaine and d-amphetamine will block the uptake of dopamine, but they also block the uptake of norepinephrine; d-amphetamine also directly releases dopamine. Benztropine blocks the uptake of dopamine and not norepinephrine, but this drug has powerful antimuscarinic properties.

Drugs that Block Dopaminergic Transmission

Drugs that Deplete Dopamine in the Nerve Terminal. Reserpine depletes dopamine from neurons in the brain, but it also depletes neurons of other neurotransmitters as well (e.g., norepinephrine, 5-hydroxytryptamine). Furthermore, it would appear that newly synthesized dopamine can maintain dopaminergic transmission despite the depletion of dopamine stores by reserpine treatment.

Drugs that Block Dopamine Synthesis. α-Methyltyrosine inhibits tyrosine hydroxylase and thereby inhibits the synthesis of dopamine. The drug does not specifically inhibit dopamine synthesis as tyrosine hydroxylase also catalyzes the rate-limiting step in the synthesis of norepinephrine and epinephrine. Because aromatic L-amino acid decarboxylase is not rate limiting, it is difficult to disrupt endogenous synthesis of dopamine with inhibitors of this enzyme. Furthermore, this enzyme is also involved with the synthesis of norepinephrine and 5-hydroxytryptamine. Inhibitors of aromatic L-amino acid decarboxylase (e.g., carbidopa, benserazide) are useful in blocking the peripheral formation of dopamine following the administration of L-DOPA.

Drugs that Block Dopaminergic Receptors. There are several chemical classes of drugs (e.g., derivatives of phenothiazine and butyrophenone) that block dopaminergic receptors; the pharmacological properties and clinical uses of these drugs are discussed in Chapter 11.5-1.

DOPAMINERGIC AGONISTS

Most efforts to find new dopaminergic agonists with unique chemical structures have resulted from a desire to find drugs that might have some advantage over L-DOPA for the treatment of Parkinson's disease. Some of the side effects of L-DOPA represent major therapeutic uses of other dopaminergic agonists. For example, the vomiting and endocrine upsets caused by L-DOPA are shared by other dopaminergic agonists; these effects have been utilized therapeutically (e.g., apomorphine to induce vomiting; bromocriptine to treat hyperprolactinemia-induced galactorrhea).

DOPAMINE

Because dopamine has poor lipid-solubility and carries a charge at physiological pH, it does not readily pass through cellular membranes. Accordingly, the drug is not absorbed following oral administration, and its pharmacological effects after parenteral administration are limited to actions in the periphery. In addition to activating specific dopaminergic receptors, dopamine can be thought of as a sympathomimetic amine, since at higher concentrations it also activates both α- and β_1-adrenergic receptors. Intravenous infusions of low doses of dopamine (<10 μg/kg/min) selectively activate dopaminergic receptors to cause vasodilation in renal, mesenteric, coronary, and cerebral vascular beds, and to decrease systemic blood pressure. At doses greater than 20 μg/kg/min, dopamine increases blood pressure due to generalized vasoconstriction resulting from α-adrenergic receptor activation. At intermediate doses, dopamine increases cardiac contractility due to a direct action on β_1-receptors and to an ability to release norepinephrine from sympathetic nerve terminals. The inotropic action on the myocardium is generally not accompanied by an increase in heart rate or the development of arrhythmias. Thus, dopamine is a beneficial cardiac stimulant in patients with ischemic heart disease.

Dopamine is a useful drug for the treatment of hemodynamic imbalances caused by shock resulting from myocardial infarctions, trauma, renal failure, endotoxins, etc. In this condition there is a reduced blood pressure and a reduced blood flow to vital organs. The administration of dopamine increases cardiac output and systolic but not diastolic pressure. Because dopamine increases renal blood flow, glomerular filtration, sodium and potassium excretion, and urine flow, it offers a distinct advantage for the treatment of shock over other sympathomimetics, which reduce blood flow in renal and mesenteric vascular beds.

Dopamine has a short duration of action, as it is rapidly metabolized by MAO and COMT (Fig. 7.4-2). Effects of overdosage (e.g., hypertension) are reversed quickly after stopping the infusion of the drug. Other side effects include nausea and vomiting, angina pectoris, and cardiac arrhythmias.

L-DOPA

Dopamine per se cannot be used to activate receptors in the CNS, since it does not pass the blood-brain barrier. However, its immediate synthetic precursor, L-DOPA, is transported into the brain, where it can be decarboxylated to form dopamine. Thus, in order to produce dopaminergic agonistic effects at a site within the CNS, L-DOPA or a lipid-soluble, nonpolar dopaminergic agonist must be administered.

There are also a number of compounds that can directly or indirectly stimulate the dopamine receptors; some of these dopamine agonists are described here.

APOMORPHINE

Apomorphine is obtained by treating morphine with strong acid. It has the following chemical structure:

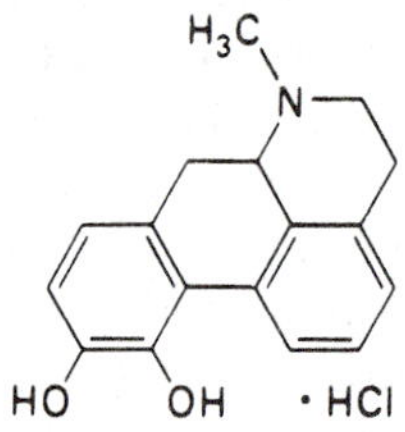

H_3C N HO OH · HCl

This drug is without analgesic properties but is a very short-acting agonist of central and peripheral dopaminergic receptors. Following intravenous administration, apomorphine does ameliorate the symptoms of Parkinson's disease, but its short duration of action and side effects make it unsuitable for treating this condition. Apomorphine is used clinically to treat poisoning resulting from the oral administration of various compounds because of its ability to stimulate dopaminergic receptors in the area postrema and thus cause vomiting.

BROMOCRIPTINE

Bromocriptine is an ergot derivative that has dopaminergic agonist properties (Table 19-1). It is a potent, long-lasting, and orally effective dopaminergic agonist. Bromocriptine is effective in ameliorating the symptoms of Parkinson's disease (3), and for the treatment of endocrine disorders. Like all dopaminergic agonists, bromocriptine inhibits the release of prolactin and can thereby disrupt lactation. In patients with galactorrhea and amenorrhea associated with elevated serum concentrations of prolactin, bromocriptine can suppress the galactorrhea and reinstate normal ovulatory menstrual cycles.

Dopaminergic agonists increase serum concentrations of growth hormone in normal individuals, but acromegalics respond in just the opposite way to these drugs. Thus, bromocriptine has some utility in treating acromegaly by decreasing serum concentrations of growth hormone. Bromocriptine mesylate (PARLODEL) is available as 2.5-mg tablets and 5-mg capsules for oral administration.

AMANTADINE

Amantadine, an antiviral drug used for prophylaxis of A_2 influenza (Chapter 25.1), has been observed to release dopamine from peripheral neuronal storage sites in animals receiving infusions of this neurotransmitter. This drug also causes dopamine release from nigrostriatal neurons and other central sites. Amantadine might exert a similar action on the residual, intact dopaminergic terminals in the striatum of patients with Parkinson's disease. Amantadine acts by augmenting the release of dopamine and other catecholamines from neuronal storage sites and delaying their reuptake into the storage sites.

Preparations. Dopamine hydrochloride (INOTROPIN) is available in 5-ml ampules containing 40, 80 or 160 mg/ml that must be diluted before use. It is used only by intravenous infusion (2 to 50 μg/kg/min) for treatment of shock.

L-DOPA or levodopa (DOPAR, LARODOPA) is available in 100-, 250-, or 500-mg tablets or capsules for oral administration. The optimal dosage is determined for each patient by gradually increasing the amount given, generally in three daily doses, ranging from 0.5 to 1 g/day initially up to 3 to 8 g/day. The dose of L-DOPA can be markedly reduced if the drug is administered concurrently with a decarboxylase inhibitor. Preparations containing fixed combinations of L-DOPA and carbidopa (SINEMET) are currently available. Although carbidopa is available as a single-entity drug (LODOSYN) reserved for investigational use, it is effective only when administered with levodopa. The combination product, SINEMET (which contains levodopa and carbidopa in a ratio of 10:1), is recommended for general use. In these combinations, treatment of parkinsonian patients is initiated with approximately 300 mg L-DOPA/day, increasing gradually up to a dose of 2000 mg/day.

Apomorphine hydrochloride is available in 6-mg hypodermic tablets. Subcutaneous injection of 2 to 10 mg apomorphine is used to induce vomiting in cases of oral ingestion of noncorrosive toxic substances. Vomiting generally occurs within 10 to 15 min. The injection must *not* be repeated because the drug can cause respiratory depression.

Bromocriptine mesylate (PARLODEL) is available in 2.5-mg tablets for oral administration.

Amantadine hydrochloride (SYMMETREL) is available in 100-mg capsules, 50-mg/5-ml syrup.

DOPAMINERGIC ANTAGONISTS

Dopaminergic antagonists displace the specific binding of radioactive dopamine or direct-acting dopamine agonists from cell membrane fragments prepared from dopamine-rich regions of the brain (e.g., striatum), and they also block dopamine-stimulated adenylate cyclase in these same cell membrane fragments. These drugs also inhibit various dopamine-related functions (Table 7.4-1).

These dopamine antagonists belong to several different chemical classes (phenothiazines, thioxanthines, butyrophenones, dihydroindolones, dibenzodiazepines, dibenzoxazepines); they are used as preanesthetic medication and as antiemetics, and to treat mental disorders such as schizophrenia. Because the main therapeutic use is as antipsychotic or neuroleptic agents, they are discussed in Chapter 11.5-1.

REFERENCES

1. Bernheimer, H., Birkmayer, W., Hornykiewicz, O., Jellinger, K., and Seitelberger, F. Brain dopamine and the syndromes of Parkinson and Huntington. *J. Neural Sci.* 20:415, 1973.
2. Bunney, B. S., and Aghajanian, G. K. Mesolimbic and mesocortical dopaminergic systems: Physiology and pharmacology. In: *Psychopharmacology: A Generation of Progress* (Lipton, M. A., Dimascio, A., and Killam, K. F., eds.). New York: Raven Press, 1978, p. 159.
3. Calne, D. B. Role of ergot derivatives in the treatment of parkinsonism. *Fed. Proc.* 37:2207, 1978.

4. Dinnerstein, R. J., Vannice, J., Henderson, R. C., Roth, L. J., Goldberg, L. I., and Hoffmann, P. C. Histofluorescence techniques provide evidence for dopamine-containing neuronal elements in canine kidney. *Science* 205:497, 1979.
5. Goldberg, L. I. The vascular dopamine receptor as a model for other dopamine receptors. *Adv. Biochem. Psychopharmacol.* 19:119, 1978.
6. Koslow, S. H. Dopamine and other catecholamine containing SIF cells. *Adv. Biochem. Psychopharmacol.* 16:553, 1977.
7 Martin, G. E., Haubrich, D. R., and Williams, M. Pharmacological profiles of the putative dopamine autoreceptor agonists, 3-PPP and TL-99. *Eur. J. Pharmacol.* 76:15, 1981.
8. Moore, K. E., and Kelly, P. H. Biochemical pharmacology of mesolimbic and mesocortical dopaminergic neurons. In: *Psychopharmacology: A Generation of Progress* (Lipton, M. A., Dimascio, A., and Killam, K. F., eds.). New York: Raven Press, 1978, p. 221.
9. Moore, K. E., and Wuerthele, S. M. Regulation of nigrostriatal and tuberoinfundibular-hypophyseal dopaminergic neurons. *Prog. Neurobiol.* 13:325, 1979.
10. Moore, K. E., Demarest, K. T., Johnston, C. A., and Alper, R. H. Pharmacological and endocrinological manipulations of tuberoinfundibular and tuberohypophyseal dopaminergic neurons. In: *Neuroactive Drugs in Endocrinology* (Müller, E. E., ed.). Amsterdam: Elsevier/North Holland, 1980, p. 109.
11. Moore, R. Y., and Bloom, F. E. Central catecholamine neuron systems: Anatomy and physiology of the dopamine systems. *Ann. Rev. Neurosci.* 1:129, 1978.
12. Weiner, R. I., and Ganong, W. F. Role of brain monoamines and histamine in regulation of anterior pituitary secretion. *Physiol. Rev.* 58:905, 1978.

ADDITIONAL READING

Calne, D., Chase, T. N., and Barbeau, A. Dopaminergic Mechanisms. *Advances in Neurology,* Vol. 9, New York: Raven Press, 1975.

Costa, E., and Gessa, G. L. Nonstriatal Dopaminergic Neurons. *Advances in Biochemical Psychopharmacology,* Vol. 16, New York: Raven Press, 1977.

Horn, A. S., Korf, J,. and Westerink, B. H. C. *The Neurobiology of Dopamine.* New York: Academic Press, 1979.

Roberts, P. J., Woodruff, G. N., and Iversen, L. L. Dopamine. *Advances in Biochemical Psychopharmacology,* Vol. 19, New York: Raven Press, 1978.

Usdin, E., Carlsson, A., Dahlström, A., and Engel, J. Catecholamines, Part A, B and C. In: *Neurology and Neurobiology,* Vol. 8A, 8B and 8C, New York: Alan R. Liss, 1984.

CHAPTER
8

DRUGS AFFECTING CHOLINERGIC NEUROTRANSMISSION

Sachin N. Pradhan

SITES OF ACETYLCHOLINE RELEASE

Acetylcholine (ACh) plays an important role in neurotransmission in both the peripheral (autonomic and somatic) and central nervous systems (11). As discussed in Chapter 6, it is secreted at: (a) the postganglionic parasympathetic as well as some sympathetic nerve endings [e.g., in sweat glands (13) and in blood vessels in skeletal muscles]; (b) sympathetic and parasympathetic ganglia, and the adrenal medulla, which is innervated by preganglionic autonomic fibers; (c) motor end-plates at the neuromuscular junction of skeletal muscles (14, 15); and (d) certain synapses in the CNS.

MODIFICATION OF CHOLINERGIC NEUROTRANSMISSION BY DRUGS OR CHEMICALS

Because of its wide distribution throughout the peripheral and central nervous systems, ACh is involved in a multitude of functions. These functions are modified by drugs affecting various phases of the life cycle of the cholinergic neurotransmitter e.g., synthesis, storage, release, receptor action and disposition of ACh [all of which have been discussed in many reviews (10, 14, 17, 18)]. These phases with their modification by various drugs will be briefly described here.

Synthesis. ACh is synthesized from choline and acetyl coenzyme A by choline acetylase (choline acetyltransferase) (13, 19). The rate of its synthesis can be reduced by an experimental chemical, hemicholinium (HC-3), which prevents uptake of choline into the cholinergic neurons.

Storage and Release. ACh is stored in synaptic vesicles and released from presynaptic terminals into synaptic clefts by exocytosis. This release, mediated by nerve stimulation, is facilitated by the presence of Ca^{2+} (20), and inhibited by the lack of Ca^{2+} or the presence of Mg^{2+}. Release is stimulated by carbachol (23) and blocked by botulinum toxin, local anesthetics, and α-bungarotoxin (16, 24).

Receptor Action. The pharmacological actions of ACh can be described in terms of the actions of two naturally occurring plant alkaloids: muscarine and nicotine. Historically, these two sets of actions have been designated as muscarinic by Schmiedeberg (21) and nicotinic by Langley (12), respectively.

The chemical structures as well as brief discussions on pharmacology of these two alkaloids are presented as follows:

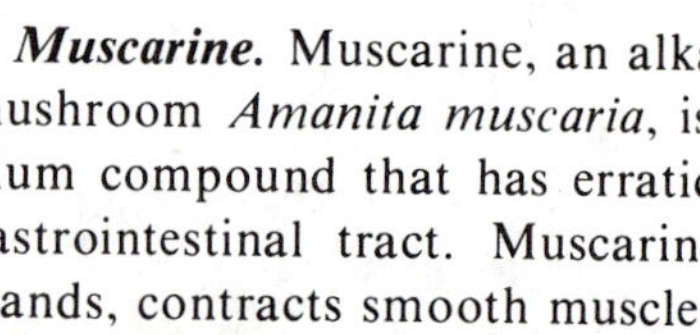

Muscarine

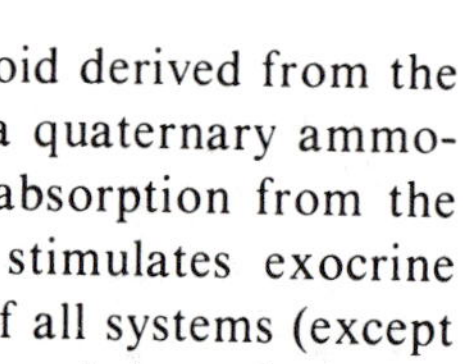

Nicotine

Muscarine. Muscarine, an alkaloid derived from the mushroom *Amanita muscaria*, is a quaternary ammonium compound that has erratic absorption from the gastrointestinal tract. Muscarine stimulates exocrine glands, contracts smooth muscle of all systems (except those of blood vessels which dilate), and slows the heart. It has very little effect on the CNS due to lack of passage across the blood-brain barrier. Onset of effects begins about 0.5 hour after ingestion of muscarine-containing mushroom with sweating, salivation, lacrimation, abdominal cramps, diarrhea, urination, and visual disturbances. There also may be bradycardia, hypotension, nausea, vomiting, malaise and headache. All of these muscarinic effects are reversible by the administration of an adequate dose of a cholinoceptor antagonist, such as atropine. (For effects of other types of mushroom, see Chapter 8.1).

Nicotine. Nicotine is an alkaloid isolated from leaves of tobacco, *Nicotiana tabacum*. Its pharmacology is discussed in detail in Chapter 11.3. Briefly summarized, it causes excitation of autonomic ganglia, producing a mixture of sympathetic and parasympathetic responses. It causes stimulation of catecholamine release mediated through the sympathetic nervous system, as well as from the adrenal medulla and chromaffin cells. It evokes a variety of cardiovascular and pulmonary reflexes; heart rate and blood pressure may increase or decrease. Gastrointestinal tone and motility are generally increased due to combined activation of parasympathetic ganglia and cholinergic nerve endings. Nicotine causes depolarization of motor end-plate of skeletal muscles and produces fasciculations. It readily enters the CNS to produce muscle twitches, tremors and convulsions. Furthermore, nicotine causes initial excitatory actions that are followed by depression of functions of the central and autonomic nervous systems, and the neuromuscular junction. Death from respiratory paralysis may occur quickly.

Cholinoceptors. Receptors for ACh (cholinoceptors) differ, depending on their site of action. Cholinoceptors at postganglionic nerve terminals of all parasympathetic target tissues or organs (including heart, blood vessels, smooth muscles and exocrine glands) and some sympathetic target tissues (e.g., sweat glands) have been described as muscarinic, since ACh actions at these sites resemble actions of muscarine. Such receptors are also present in the autonomic ganglia and CNS (1, 2) (see Fig. 8.4-1). Choline esters (such as methacholine, bethanechol and carbachol) that cannot pass through the blood-brain barrier act only on the peripheral receptors, whereas cholinomimetic alkaloids (e.g., pilocarpine and arecoline) act directly on both peripheral as well as central receptors. They are blocked by muscarinic cholinoceptor antagonists (anticholinergic agents) including alkaloids such as atropine, scopolamine, and their analogs, and some synthetic chemicals.

Cholinoceptors at the preganglionic nerve terminals in the autonomic ganglia and at the terminals of first-order neurons (nerves to skeletal muscles and the adrenal medulla) have been described as nicotinic, since ACh action at these sites resembles that of nicotine. These sites are stimulated at low doses and depressed at high doses. Furthermore, these receptors are heterogenous in nature so that they are not blocked by the same chemical agents. Effects of nicotine at the autonomic ganglia and neuromuscular junctions are blocked by ganglion blocking and neuromuscular blocking agents, respectively, with some amount of overlap in their actions. The adrenal medulla is little affected by these compounds.

The muscarinic receptor has been characterized and quantified by specific ligand-binding studies in various tissues in the periphery as well as CNS (2, 22). Extensive studies have been done in nicotinic cholinergic receptors that have been isolated from the electric organs of the aquatic species of *Electrophorus* and characterized, as described in Chapter 9.

The muscarinic and nicotinic actions of acetylcholine are presented in Table 8-1.

Like α- and β-adrenergic receptors, the nicotinic and more recently the muscarinic receptors have been proposed to be classified into respective subtypes on the basis of studies with their selective agonists and antagonists. Nicotinic (N) receptors in autonomic ganglia with dimethylphenylpiperazinium (DMPP) as a selective agonist and hexamethonium as a comparatively more selective antagonist have been designated as N_1 subtype. Likewise, receptors in skeletal muscle with phenyltrimethylammonium as a selective nicotinic agonist and decamethonium as a selective nicotinic antagonist have been called N_2 subtypes. However, in the autonomic ganglia certain actions of acetylcholine are blocked by atropine, but not by hexamethonium or decamethonium, suggesting the presence of muscarinic receptors also in the autonomic ganglia (Chapter 8.4).

Two subtypes of muscarinic (M) receptors have also been proposed (8, 9). In experiments using lower esophageal sphincter (LES) of the opossum (5, 6), it was observed that muscarinic agonists McN-A-343 [4-(m-chorophenyl carbamoyloxy)-2-butyltrimethyl-ammonium chloride] caused relaxation of LES that could be blocked by atropine as well as by tetrodotoxin, a neuronal poison; on the other hand, contraction of the LES induced by another muscarinic agonist, bethanechol, could also be blocked by atropine, but not by tetrodotoxin. It was concluded (5, 6) that McN-A-343-induced relaxation of the LES was the result of stimulation of an M_1 receptor located on an inhibitor ganglionic neuron, and bethanechol-induced contraction of the LES was due to stimulation of an M_2 receptor located on the sphincter smooth muscle rather than on a neuron. Pirenzepine, an antimuscarinic agent (Chapter 8.3) selectively blocks McN-A-343-induced LES relaxation, but not the bethanechol-induced LES contraction (7).

Selective action of pirenzepine on M_1 subtype was further corroborated in experiments in pithed rats (8) in which the dose of this drug necessary to antagonize McN-A-343-induced hypertension (thought to be due to stimulation of M_1 receptors) was less than one-fortieth the dose necessary to antagonize vagally mediated bradycardia (thought to be due to M_2-receptor stimulation). The locations, agonists, and antagonists of cholinoceptor subtypes are summarized in Table 8-2 (4).

Table 8-1
Muscarinic and Nicotinic Actions of Acetylcholine

	Muscarinic Action	Nicotinic Action
Effector site or function		
Cardiovascular system		
Blood vessels	Dilation	Constriction[a] at high doses after atropine
Heart (rate and force of contraction)	Decreased	Increased at high doses after atropine
Blood pressure	Decreased	Increased at high doses after atropine
Smooth muscles (bronchi, gastrointestinal, bladder, concentric iris, and ciliary muscles, etc.)	Contraction	Contraction[a]
Exocrine glands (secretion) (salivary, gastrointestinal, lacrimal, sweat, etc.)	Increased	Variable
Skeletal muscle	—	Stimulated
Autonomic ganglia	—	Stimulated
Adrenal medulla	—	Catecholamines released
Relation to dose	Sensitive to low concentration of ACh; effects increase with the dose	Low dose stimulates and high dose depresses
Blocking agent	Atropine	Multiple blockers[b]

[a] Net effect after balancing the opposing actions of sympathetic and parasympathetic ganglion stimulation.
[b] Nature of blockers varies depending on the effector sites (ganglia, neuromuscular junction, or adrenal medulla).

Disposition. Acetylcholine is rapidly hydrolyzed to acetic acid and choline by acetylcholinesterase that is distributed in the vicinity of the sites of its release. Choline is taken up by the neuron for resynthesis of ACh; this is in contrast to adrenergic neurons where reuptake of the intact neurotransmitter molecule occurs. Rapid enzymatic destruction makes ACh actions at the receptor very transient. The action of this catabolic enzyme can be inhibited by compounds of varied chemical nature (anticholinesterase or cholinesterase inhibitors), thereby preserving concentration and prolonging the action of ACh both at muscarinic and nicotinic receptor sites.

Sites and mechanisms of these drugs that affect different stages in the metabolism of ACh and modify its effects at different receptor sites are summarized in a schematic diagram (Fig. 8-1). These drugs will be discussed in detail in the following chapters.

Table 8-2
Tentative Classification of Cholinoceptors

Receptor Type/ Subtype	Location(s)	Agonist	Antagonist
Nicotinic (N)	Autonomic ganglia, skeletal muscle	Nicotine	d-Tubocurarine
N_1	Autonomic ganglia	Dimethylphenyl-piperazinium (DMPP)	Hexamethonium
N_2	Skeletal muscle	Phenyltrimethyl-ammonium	Decamethonium
Muscarinic (M)	Glands, smooth and cardiac muscles, autonomic ganglia	Muscarine	Atropine
M_1	Autonomic ganglia	McN-A-343	Pirenzepine
M_2	Glands, smooth and cardiac muscles	Bethanechol	?

Source: Modified from Ref. 4.

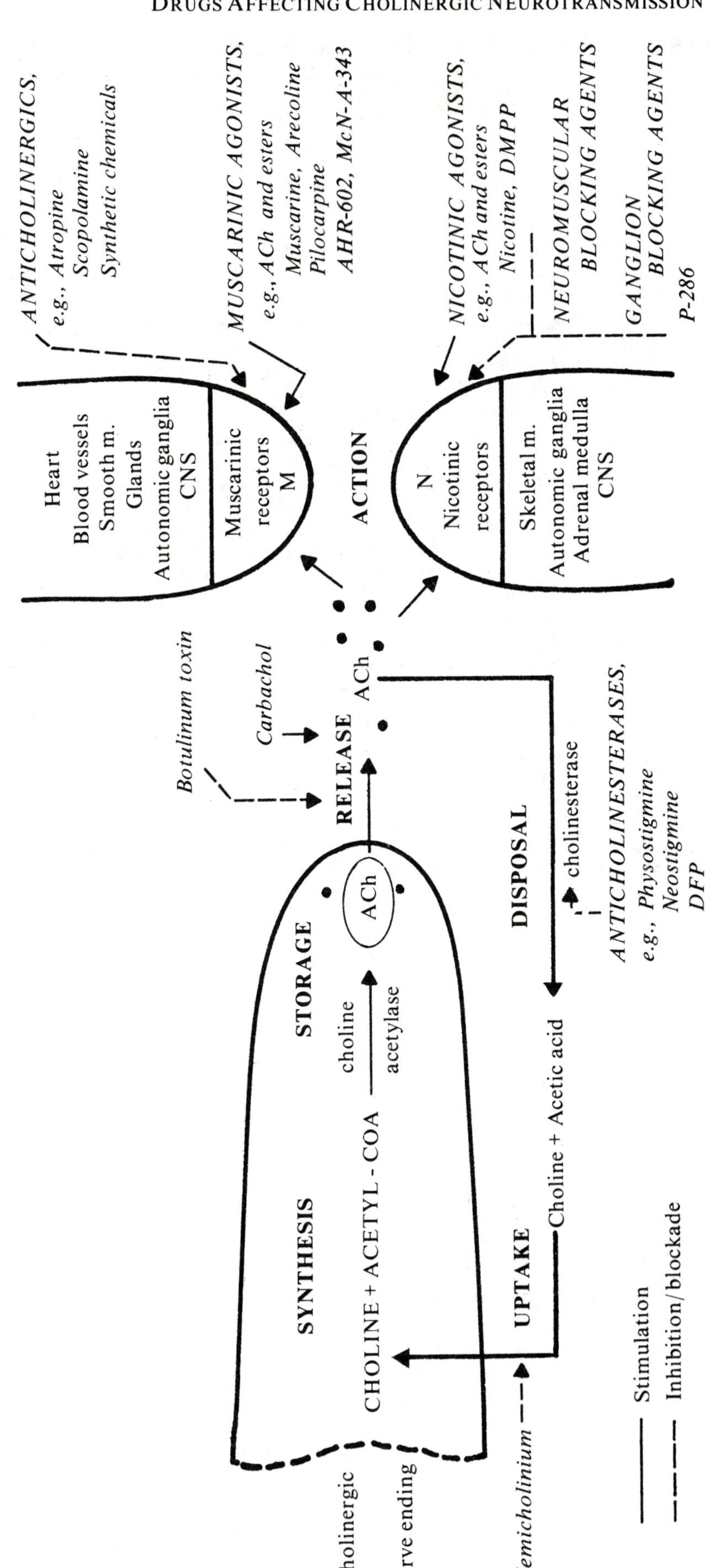

Fig. 8-1. *Pharmacology of cholinergic neurotransmission.*

REFERENCES

1. Bebbington, A., and Brimblecombe, R. W. Muscarinic receptors in the peripheral and central nervous systems. *Adv. Drug Res.* 2:143, 1965.
2. Birdsall, N. J. M., Burgen, A. S. V., and Hulme, E. C. The binding of agonists to brain muscarinic receptors. *Mol. Pharmacol.* 14:737, 1978.
3. Bolton, T. B. The permeability change produced by acetylcholine in smooth muscle. In: *Drug Receptors* (Rang, H. P., ed.). Baltimore: University Park Press, 1973, p. 87.
4. Feldman, M. Inhibition of gastric acid secretion by selective and nonselective anticholinergics. *Gastroenterology* 86:361, 1984.
5. Goyal, R. K., and Rattan, S. Nature of vagal inhibitory innervation to lower esophageal sphincter. *J. Clin. Invest.* 55:1119, 1975.
6. Goyal, R. K., and Rattan, S. Neurohumoral, hormonal, and drug receptors for the lower esophageal sphincter. *Gastroenterology* 74:598, 1978.
7. Gilbert, R., Rattan, S., and Goyal, R. K. Pharmacologic identification of muscarinic M_1 and M_2 receptor subtypes (abstr). *Gastroenterology* 84:1166, 1983.
8. Hammer, R., Giachetti, A. Muscarinic receptor subtypes: M_1 and M_2 biochemical and functional characterization. *Life Sci.* 31:2991, 1982.
9. Hammer, R., Giraldo, E., and Giachetti, A. Pirenzepine, the first M_1-receptor antagonist. In: *Receptor Update*, Asia Pacific Congress Series No. 13. Amsterdam Excerpta Medica, 1982, p. 90.
10. Hebb, C. O. Biosynthesis of acetylcholine in nervous tissue. *Physiol. Rev.* 52:918, 1972.
11. Krnjevic, K. Chemical nature of synaptic transmission in vertebrates. *Physiol. Rev.* 54:418, 1974.
12. Langley, J. N., and Dickinson, W. L. On the local paralysis of peripheral ganglia, and on the connection of different classes of nerve fibers with them. *Proc. R. Soc. Lond.* [*Biol.*], 46:423, 1889.
13. Lloyd, D. P. C. Cholinergy and adrenergy in the neural control of sweat glands. In: *Studies in Physiology* (Curtis, D. R., and McIntyre, A. K., eds.). New York: Springer-Verlag, 1965, p. 169.
14. Michelson, M. J., and Zeimal, E. V. *Acetylcholine: An Approach to the Molecular Mechanism of Action.* Oxford: Pergamon Press, 1973.
15. Nachmansohn, D. The neuromuscular junction: The role of acetylcholine in excitable membranes. In: *The Structure and Function of Muscle*, 2nd ed., Vol. 3 (Bourne, G. H., ed.). New York: Academic Press, 1973, p. 31.
16. Patrick, J., and Stallcup, B. α-Bungarotoxin binding and cholinergic receptor function on a rat sympathetic nerve line. *J. Biol. Chem.* 252:8629, 1977.
17. Potter, L. T. Synthesis, storage, and release of acetylcholine from nerve terminals. In: *The Structure and Function of Nervous Tissue*, Vol. 4 (Bourne, G. H., ed.). New York: Academic Press, 1972, p. 105.
18. Rang, H. P. Acetylcholine receptors. *Q. Rev. Biophys.* 7:283, 1975.
19. Rossier, J. Choline acetyltranesterase: A review with special reference to its cellular and subcellular localization. *Int. Rev. Neurobiol.* 20:283, 1977.
20. Rubin, R. P. *Calcium and the Secretory Process.* New York: Plenum Press, 1974.
21. Schmiedeberg, O., and Koppe, R. *Das Muscarin, das giftige Alkaloid des Fliegenpilzes.* Leipzig: F.C.W. Vogel, 1869.
22. Snyder, S. H., Chang, K. J., Kuhar, M. J., and Yamamura, H. I. Biochemical identification of the mammalian muscarinic cholinergic receptor. *Fed. Proc.* 34:1915, 1974.
23. Volle, R. L., and Koelle, G. B. The physiological role of acetylcholinesterase (AChE) in sympathetic ganglia. *J. Pharmacol. Exp. Therp.* 133:223, 1961.
24. Wang, G., Molinaro, S., and Schmidt, J. O. Ligand responses of the α-bungarotoxin binding sites from skeletal muscle and the optic lobe of the chick. *J. Biol. Chem.* 253:8507, 1978.

ADDITIONAL READING

Waser, P.G. Morphology and molecular function of the cholinergic synapse. *Eur. J. Anaesthesiol.* 2:105, 1985.

CHAPTER
8.1

CHOLINOCEPTOR AGONISTS

Roger P. Maickel and Sachin N. Pradhan

TERMINOLOGY AND CLASSIFICATION

Cholinergic agonists that resemble acetylcholine (ACh) in their effects (hence called cholinomimetic agents) act on the autonomic effector cells innervated by the postganglionic parasympathetic nerve endings, and their effects closely simulate stimulation of the parasympathetic nervous system. As such, they are called parasympathomimetic agents. These agonists act on the cholinergic receptors and can be called cholinoceptor agonists or cholinoceptive agents.

The cholinoceptor agonists that act *directly* on the cholinergic receptors can be divided into two groups: (1) ACh and synthetic choline esters (e.g., methacholine, bethanechol, and carbachol) and (2) cholinomimetic alkaloids [e.g., muscarine, nicotine (discussed in Chapter 8), pilocarpine, and arecoline]. In addition, another group of cholinomimetic compounds that *indirectly* act by inhibiting acetylcholinesterase, and thereby increasing the concentration of ACh at the receptor site, is known as anticholinesterase (anti-AChE) agents; they are discussed in Chapter 8.2.

PHARMACOLOGICAL EFFECTS

The metabolism of ACh and sites of its release have been discussed in Chapters 6 and 8. It has also been mentioned (Chapter 8) that the pharmacology of ACh is a combination of its muscarinic and nicotinic effects. In this chapter, the pharmacology of cholinoceptor agonists will be briefly discussed using ACh as the prototype agent with reference to its muscarinic and nicotinic components; this will be followed by a discussion of the pharmacology of different choline esters while comparing them with ACh.

ACETYLCHOLINE

Muscarinic Effects. The primary actions of ACh are exerted at the muscarinic cholinoceptors located in tissues supplied by all parasympathetic and some sympathetic (e.g., to sweat gland) postganglionic nerve terminals; these actions include slowing of heart, vasodilation, contraction of smooth muscles of the gastrointestinal, urinary, and respiratory tracts as well as the eye, and increase in secretions of various exocrine glands. In addition, such receptors are located in the ganglia and CNS; pharmacological actions due to activation of these receptors are complex.

Cardiovascular System. ACh decreases the rate and force of contraction of the heart and reduces cardiac output and systolic blood pressure. Although blood vessels lack parasympathetic innervation, they contain cholinoceptors; action of ACh on these receptors causes vasodilation, leading to reduction of peripheral resistance and diastolic blood pressure.

Administration of a small i.v. dose of ACh results in a marked decrease in blood pressure and compensatory reflex tachycardia. It appears to produce dilation of resistance vessels, more so than the capacitance vessels. As the dose is increased, the effect on the heart resembles that of vagal stimulation (i.e., bradycardia, decrease in atrial and ventricular contractile force, and prolongation of atrial and AV conduction). Complete blockade of conduction through the AV node occurs at still larger doses.

Gastrointestinal Tract. ACh increases tone, amplitude of contraction, and peristaltic movement as well as secretory activity of stomach and intestine. In addition, relaxation of the anal sphincter coupled with increased intestinal peristalsis leads to defecation. Higher doses lead to belching, nausea. vomiting, and intestinal cramps. ACh also causes an increase in the tone and motility of the gallbladder, and biliary ducts.

Urinary Tract. Choline esters increase ureteral peristalsis and contract detrusor muscle of the bladder, but the trigone and external sphincters relax, resulting in micturition. In addition, there is an increase in the maximal voiding pressure, and the bladder capacity is decreased.

Respiratory Tract. ACh causes bronchoconstriction and an increase in bronchial secretion. The outpouring of secretions from the bronchial gland together with the constriction of the smooth muscles of the bronchioles cause cough, choking, and wheezing, particularly in persons with a history of bronchial asthma. The chemoreceptors in aortic and carotid bodies are stimulated by a decrease in pO_2, resulting from the precipitous hypotension produced by ACh administration.

Eye. Choline esters when applied topically to the eye cause contraction of concentric muscle of the iris (miosis) and spasms of the ciliary muscle, thereby facilitating drainage of aqueous humor through Schlemm's canal and producing intraocular hypotension (Chapter 21.1). ACh and related quaternary ammonium agents are without effect when instilled directly into the eye because of poor penetration.

Glands. ACh stimulates secretion from the exocrine glands (e.g., bronchial, salivary, and sweat) in addition to the gastrointestinal glands, as mentioned earlier. The sialagogic action of choline esters results in copious flow of saliva from the submaxillary glands. In addition, these agents increase the blood flow through the gland and enhance the formation of saliva. The composition of the saliva approaches that of the ultrafiltrate of plasma, whereas normal saliva is hypotonic and high in potassium. The gastric glands are stimulated to produce a large volume of secretion that is highly acidic and rich in mucin and pepsin.

Nicotinic Effects. ACh depolarizes the respective effector sites in the skeletal muscles and autonomic ganglia, but at a dose much higher than that it produces prominent muscarinic effects. Nicotinic receptors are also present in the CNS.

OTHER CHOLINE ESTERS

Three choline esters, methacholine, carbachol and bethanechol (Fig. 8.1-1), are briefly discussed with a view of comparing their pharmacological properties with those of acetylcholine (Table 8.1-1). The pharmacological actions of choline esters have been reviewed (7, 8).

METHACHOLINE

Methacholine differs from ACh only by the addition of a methyl group at the β-carbon position of choline. This structural change modifies the pharmacological properties of the molecule in several ways. It considerably slows the rate of hydrolysis of the compound by acetylcholinesterase and prolongs its duration of action (compared with ACh), and it also makes methacholine act more selectively on the muscarinic receptors without any nicotinic action. Compared with ACh, the actions of methacholine on the cardiovascular system are qualitatively similar, but its effective dose is only about 0.5% as large. Its only clinical use is for the treatment of atrial tachycardia; in this, however, it has been replaced by other therapeutic regimens.

CARBACHOL (CARBAMYLCHOLINE)

In contrast to ACh and methacholine, the acid component of carbachol is carbamic rather than acetic acid. The carbamic acid-ester link is totally resistant to hydrolysis by either acetylcholinesterase or plasma cholinesterase. Carbachol has muscarinic and prominent nicotinic effects. It has weak cardiovascular effects (vasodilation,

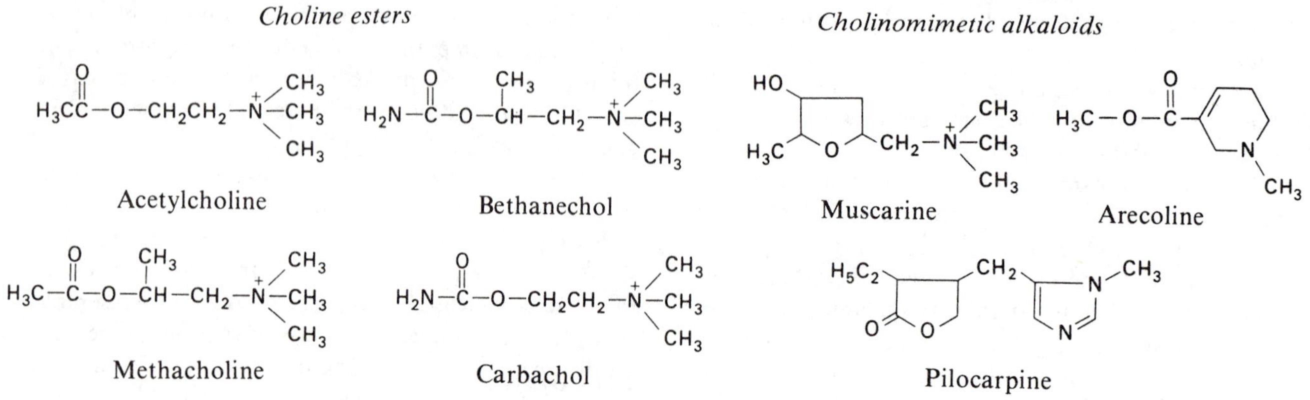

Choline esters

Acetylcholine: $H_3C-C(=O)-O-CH_2CH_2-N^+(CH_3)_3$

Bethanechol: $H_2N-C(=O)-O-CH(CH_3)-CH_2-N^+(CH_3)_3$

Methacholine: $H_3C-C(=O)-O-CH(CH_3)-CH_2-N^+(CH_3)_3$

Carbachol: $H_2N-C(=O)-O-CH_2CH_2-N^+(CH_3)_3$

Cholinomimetic alkaloids

Muscarine

Arecoline

Pilocarpine

Fig. 8.1-1. *Chemical structures of cholinoceptor agonists.*

Table 8.1-1
Comparative Pharmacological Properties of Some Cholinoceptor Agonists

		Effects					
		Muscarinic					Nicotinic[a]
	Susceptible to AChE	Cardio-vascular	Gastrointes-tinal, Bladder	Eye	Sweating	Antagonism by Atropine	
Acetylcholine	+++	++	++	+	+	+++	++
Methacholine	+	+++	++	+	+	+++	+
Carbachol	–	+	+++	++	+	+	+++
Bethanechol	–	±	+++	++	+	+++	–
Pilocarpine	–	±	++	+++	++	++	+
Arecoline	–	±	±	++	±	++	–

[a]For details on nicotinic actions, see Chapters 8 and 8.4.

cardiac slowing) and marked effects on eye, gastrointestinal tract, and urinary bladder. Compared with other choline esters, it is antagonized to a less extent by atropine. In addition, it stimulates the autonomic ganglia and skeletal muscle. Its chemical stability and marked activity at ganglia and neuromuscular junctions make it useful as a pharmacological tool. Its therapeutic use is limited to ophthalmic use as a miotic agent (see Chapter 21.1).

BETHANECHOL

Bethanechol is a choline ester with structural features common to those of both methacholine and carbachol, with β-methyl group and carbamic acid substitutions. Because of these features, bethanechol has the pharmacological properties of methacholine combined with the chemical characteristics of carbachol. Bethanechol is not hydrolyzed by either true or pseudocholinesterases, and it does not stimulate autonomic ganglia or skeletal muscle. Bethanechol appears to have a more selective action on the gastrointestinal tract and urinary bladder than ACh and methacholine. It exhibits mainly muscarinic activity and is used for the management of postoperative urinary retention or neurogenic atony of the bladder.

SUCCINYLCHOLINE

Succinylcholine is another ester of choline having two choline molecules connected to a succinic acid molecule. This ester acts as a depolarizing muscle relaxant and is further discussed in Chapter 9.1.

CHOLINOMIMETIC ALKALOIDS

PILOCARPINE

Pilocarpine, the principal alkaloid from leaves of the Brazilian shrub *Pilocarpus jaborandi,* is a tertiary amine (Fig. 8.1-1) that has marked muscarinic actions, particularly on sweat and other exocrine glands and smooth muscles.

Glands. Pilocarpine causes marked secretion of sweat, saliva, tears, mucus, and of the gastric, pancreatic, and intestinal glands. In contrast to normal saliva, which is hypotonic and contains a larger amount of potassium than the extracellular fluid, saliva secreted after pilocarpine administration resembles more closely an ultrafiltrate of plasma (3). Induced gastric secretion is rich in acid, pepsin, and mucin, and resembles that produced by vagal stimulation.

Smooth Muscles. Local application of pilocarpine to the eye causes marked miosis, spasm of accommodation, and transitory increase of intraocular pressure followed by its fall (Chapter 21.1). Pilocarpine also contracts smooth muscles of intestine, bronchus, ureter, bladder, and others. In high doses, it may cause intestinal colic; in asthmatic patients, it may precipitate an attack.

Cardiovascular System. Pilocarpine actions on the cardiovascular system are complex. In small doses (0.1 mg/kg i.v.), it produces a slight fall of blood pressure; with larger doses, this is followed by considerable rise of pressure that is increased by nicotine and abolished by atropine. With clinical doses (7.5 to 10 mg), the slight pressor effect and tachycardia observed have been attributed to epinephrine output from the adrenal medulla. Pilocarpine also stimulates autonomic ganglia.

CNS. Pilocarpine produces a characteristic arousal response, as does muscarine, arecoline, and anti-AChE agents; this response can be blocked by atropine.

Effects of pilocarpine are compared with those of choline esters in Table 8.1-1.

Therapeutic Uses. Pilocarpine has important ophthalmic use as a miotic in glaucoma (Chapter 21.1).

ARECOLINE

Arecoline, an alkaloid from areca or betel nut, the seeds of *Areca catechu,* is a tertiary amine with an ester linkage (Fig.

8.1-1) that has parasympathomimetic actions (closely related to pilocarpine) that can be reversed by atropine. In addition, it has a mild CNS stimulant effect and produces a sense of well-being. It is a familiar psychotropic agent in Southeast Asia, Indonesia, and East Africa, where millions of people chew and ingest it regularly in the form of betel, a preparation made up of slices of nuts mixed with lime and flavoring ingredients, such as herbs or spices, wrapped in leaves from the betel pepper, *Piper betle*. An initial intense increase in salivation is followed by a genial euphoria and sense of well-being. Arecoline has no known therapeutic use in humans.

THERAPEUTIC USES

The cholinoceptor agents are useful for ophthalmic, gastrointestinal, and genitourinary disorders. The ophthalmic use of these agents is extensively discussed in Chapter 21.1. Bethanechol is effective in relief or prevention of postoperative abdominal distention and gastric atony following bilateral vagotomy, as well as in management of megacolon and constipation induced by ganglion-blocking agents. It is given orally with meals because it increases both acidity and volume of gastric secretions. In cases of gastric atony without complete retention, bethanechol is given orally with meals; when there is complete gastric retention without any passage of food into the duodenum, the drug given orally is not adequately absorbed from the stomach and should be given subcutaneously.

Bethanechol is useful in restoring normal micturition in some patients with acute urinary retention following surgery or parturition (2, 4, 6). Subcutaneous administration of the drug would cause urination and possibly defecation. During the injection of the drug the stomach should be empty to avoid vomiting.

Methacholine and bethanechol are also useful in the diagnosis of pancreatic enzymatic function, and in atropine poisoning; a failure to elicit the characteristic parasympathetic stimulation is indicative of belladonna intoxication.

ADVERSE EFFECTS

The adverse effects of cholinoceptor agonists are extensions of their pharmacological actions and include salivation, headache, nausea, vomiting, diarrhea, and difficulty in accommodation. They may lower blood pressure and should be avoided in patients with hypotension. Because they cause bronchospasm, they are contraindicated in patients with bronchial asthma, and because they stimulate gastric motility and secretion, they are also contraindicated in patients with peptic ulcer. Bethanechol should never be administered intravenously, as it may cause severe muscarinic effects such as acute circulatory failure and/or cardiac arrest.

MUSHROOM POISONING

Named after the fungus *Amanita muscaria*, muscarine is present in small, usually toxicologically insignificant amounts in this species. Ingestion of *Amanita muscaria* usually provokes strong psychotomimetic effects and behavioral changes (probably due to muscimol, a GABA agonist), but it causes little or no parasympathomimetic effects (1). On the other hand, fungi of the species *Inocybe* and *Clitocybe* contain clinically significant amounts of muscarine. Onset of illness begins about one-half hour after ingestion; the symptoms indicating muscarinic toxicity include sweating, salivation, lacrimation, abdominal cramps, diarrhea, nausea, vomiting, malaise, headache, urination, visual disturbance, bradycardia, hypotension and shock. These effects are reversible by an adequate dose of a muscarinic antagonist, such as atropine (see also Chapter 29).

Intoxication with other fungi are much more difficult to treat, since they contain unrelated chemical compounds. Mushroom poisoning should not be considered to be due to muscarine unless the classic signs of muscarinic overactivity are present. More severe forms of mushroom poisoning are caused by the members of the genus *Amanita* (1, 9, 10), which contain thermostable toxins termed *amatoxins*. The principal toxins include: (1) phallotoxins (from *A. phalloides*), bicyclic heptapeptides, fast-acting, but not lethal after ingestion; they combine with F-actin, stabilizing this protein against several destabilizing influences; (2) virotoxins (from *A. virosa*), monocyclic heptapeptides, like phallotoxins, fasting-acting, probably not lethal; and, (3) amatoxins (toxic components of *Amanita* species), bicyclic octapeptides, that can lead to death within several days by inhibiting nuclear RNA polymerase II (10). They cause cellular destruction mostly in gastrointestinal tract mucosal cells, hepatocytes, and renal tubular cells. The symptoms of poisoning are late, appearing usually 6-24 hr following ingestion, and are characterized by abdominal pain, diarrhea and hematuria. Death results from renal or hepatic failure.

Thioctic acid, a Krebs cycle coenzyme, has been claimed to reduce the mortality in a number of reports, although not confirmed. Intravenous pencillin has been used in combination with thioctic acid and steroids; it competes with amanitin for binding sites on serum proteins and causes more toxin free to renal excretion. Steroids may have a similar action, but their role is less clear. Different types of mushroom toxins, their effects, and treatment are summarized in Table 8.1-2 (5).

Preparations. *Acetylcholine Chloride for Ophthalmic Solution* (MIOCHOL): 1% solution in 5% mannitol.

Bethanechol Chloride, USP (URECHOLINE, etc.): 5-, 10-, 25- or 50-mg tablets; 5-mg/ml solution for injection.

Carbachol Ophthalmic Solution, USP: in concentrations of 0.75, 1.5, 2.25 and 3% for local instillation; or 0.01% solution for instillation into the anterior chamber during surgery.

Pilocarpine Hydrochloride and Pilocarpine Nitrate, USP: Ophthalmic solutions, hydrochloride (0.25-10%), nitrate (0.5-6%). A drug-delivery system (OCUSERT, a pilocarpine-containing reservoir bounded by two layers of polymer to control delivery of the drug) is availlable for producing sustained drug release (20 or 40 μg/hour).

Table 8.1-2
Mushroom Toxins, Effects, and Treatment

Principal Mushrooms	Toxin	Incubation Period (hr)	Mechanism/ Site of Action[a]	Symptoms	Treatment; Expected Recovery
Clitocybe dealbata, C. cerussata, C. illudens, Inocybe species	Muscarine & muscarinic compounds	0.5-2	Affects ANS	Sweating, salivation, lacrimation, blurred vision, abdominal cramps, watery diarrhea, hypotension, and bradycardia	Atropine sulfate, 1-2 mg; i.v. for severe poisonings; symptoms subside in 6-24 hr
Coprinus atramentarius, Clitocybe clavipes	Coprine	0.5[b]	Disulfiram-like effect; affects ANS	Flushing, paresthesias, metallic taste, tachycardia, cardiac arrhythmias, hypotension, nausea, vomiting, and sweating	Avoid alcohol; recovery usually 2-4 hr
Amanita muscaria, A. pantherina	Ibotenic acid and other isoxazoles	0.5-2	Affects CNS	Dizziness, incoordination, ataxia, muscular jerking, hyperkinetic activity, stupor, and hallucinations	Avoid sedatives that may exacerbate symptoms; avoid atropine unless severe cholinergic symptoms occur; recovery 4-24 hr
Psilocybe cubensis, P. baeocystis, and others	Psilocybin and other indoles	0.5-1	Affects CNS	Mood elevation, apprehension, hyperkinetic activity, muscle weakness, drowsiness, and hallucinations	Reassurance; benzodiazepine for severe symptoms; recovery within 6-10 hr
Many different genera and species	Diverse, mostly unknown	0.5-2	Affects GI	Nausea, vomiting, abdominal cramps, and diarrhea	Hydration, support; recovery several hours to days
Gyromitra esculenta and other species	Monomethylhydrazine, gyromitrin	6-12	Cellular destruction	Nausea, vomiting, watery or bloody diarrhea, abdominal pain, muscle cramps, loss of coordination; convulsions, coma, and death in severe cases	Pyridoxine hydrochloride, 25 mg/kg i.v. for neurological symptoms; titrate dose to symptoms, up to 15-20 g/day; intensive support; recovery in days; death in 5-7 days in severe poisonings
Amanita phalloides, A. bisporigera, A. ocreata, A. verna, A. virosa, Galerina autumnalis, G. marginata, G. venenata, Lepiota species	Cyclopeptides, amanitin	6-24	Cellular destruction, hepatic, renal, and GI necrosis	Nausea, vomiting, abdominal pain, profuse diarrhea; short remission, then jaundice, liver and renal failure, convulsions, coma and death	Thioctic acid, 75 mg i.v. every 6 hr, to start, then 25-150 mg every 6 hr, titrated to symptoms and transaminase level; penicillin G sodium, 250 mg/kg/day i.v., vitamin B complex, vitamin K, 40 mg daily; ?high-dose corticosteroids; ?plasma exchange, charcoal hemoperfusion; intensive monitoring; recovery days to weeks; death in 4-7 days in severe poisonings

[a] ANS, autonomic nervous system; CNS, central nervous system; GI, gastrointestinal tract.
[b] Half an hour after alcohol intake, as long as 5 days after eating mushroom.
Source: Modified from Ref. 5, by permission.

REFERENCES

1. Becker, C.E., Tong, T.G., Boerner, U. *et al.* Diagnosis and treatment of *Amanita phalloides*-type mushroom poisoning. *West. J. Med.* 125:100, 1976.
2. Diokno, AC and Korrenhoefer, R. Bethanechol chloride in neurogenic bladder dysfunction. *Urology* 8:455, 1976.
3. Dreisbach, R.H. Effect of parasympathetic stimulants on Ca^{45} transfer in rat parotid glands *in vitro*. *Am. J. Physiol.* 204:497, 1963.
4. Finkbeiner, A.E., Bissada, N.K. and Welch, L.T. Uropharmacology: choline esters and other parasympathomimetic drugs. *Urology*, 10:83, 1977.
5. Hanrahan, J.P. and Gordon, M.A. Mushroom poisoning. Case reports and a review of therapy *JAMA* 251:1057, 1984.
6. Khanna, O.P. Disorders of micturition: Neuropharmacologic basis and results of drug therapy. *Urology* 8:316, 1976.
7. Kosterlitz, H.W. Effects of choline esters on smooth muscle and secretions. In: *Physiological Pharmacology*, Vol. 3, *The Nervous System, Part C: Autonomic Nervous System Drugs* (Root, W.S. and Hofmann, F.G., eds.). New York: Academic Press, 1967, p. 97.
8. Rand, M.J. and Stafford, A. Cardiovascular effects of choline esters. In: *Physiological Pharmacology*, Vol. 3, *The Nervous System, Part C: Autonomic Nervous System Drugs* (Root, W.S. and Hofmann, F.G., eds.). New York: Academic Press, 1967, p. 1.
9. Weiland, T. and Faulstich, H. Amatoxins, phallotoxins, phallolysin and antamanide: The biologically active components of poisonous *Amanita* mushrooms. *CRC Crit. Rev. Biochem.*5:185, 1978.
10. Wieland, T. The toxic peptides from Amanita mushrooms. *Int. J. Peptide Protein Res.* 22:257, 1983.

CHAPTER
8.2

CHOLINESTERASE INHIBITORS

B.V. Rama Sastry and Annette K. Sastry

CHOLINESTERASES

Enzymes that hydrolyze choline esters are cholinesterases. They are usually subdivided into acetyl-, propionyl-, butyryl-, or benzoyl-cholinesterases depending upon the choline ester that is hydrolyzed at the highest rate (5, 16, 19). Cholinesterases hydrolyze acetylcholine into choline and acetic acid; they also hydrolyze esters other than choline esters at very low rates. There are two major cholinesterases: acetylcholinesterase (acetylcholine hydrolase, EC 3.1.1.7), also named true cholinesterase, and butyrylcholinesterase (acylcholine acyl-hydrolase, EC 3.1.1.8), or pseudocholinesterase. It is customary to refer to butyrylcholinesterase as cholinesterase to distinguish it from acetylcholinesterase. Acetylcholinesterase occurs in nervous tissue, erythrocytes, snake venoms, and the tissue from electric eels. Butyrylcholinesterase occurs in serum. The two types of enzymes differ greatly with regard to substrate specificity, substrate concentration patterns, sensitivity toward inhibitors, and molecular properties.

Acetylcholine is hydrolyzed rapidly by both cholinesterases. Acetyl-β-methylcholine is a specific substrate for acetylcholinesterase; its hydrolysis by butyrylcholinesterase is not significant. Butyrylcholine is a specific substrate for butyrylcholinesterase; it is very slowly hydrolyzed by acetylcholinesterase. There are also selective inhibitors by which both enzymes can be distinguished. For an inhibitor to be considered selective, the concentration that causes complete inhibition of one enzyme (I_{100}) should have no measurable inhibitory effect on any other enzyme. Ambenonium is a selective inhibitor of acetylcholinesterase, and pancuronium is a selective inhibitor of butyrylcholinesterase.

DISTRIBUTION AND LOCATION

Acetylcholinesterase is present in all conducting fibers of nerve and muscle, in the presynaptic and postsynaptic membranes of junctional sites in the nervous system, in red blood cells, and in variable concentrations in several other tissues (17). The enzyme is found in high concentrations at all sites at which acetylcholine serves as a transmitter, including the skeletal-neuromuscular junction, autonomic ganglia, postganglionic parasympathetic neuroeffector sites, and certain synapses in the central nervous system (CNS).

Acetylcholinesterase, in contrast to butyrylcholinesterase, is a membrane-bound enzyme and is localized in close proximity to the sites of action of acetylcholine but separated from acetylcholine stores within the membranes. This arrangement allows acetylcholinesterase to fulfill its regulatory role on the functions of released acetylcholine without interfering with the accumulation of adequate reserves of acetylcholine.

At cholinergic neuroeffector sites, most of the acetylcholinesterase activity is localized in the ganglia, which usually are in close proximity to the effector cells, and in the axonal terminations of the short postganglionic fibers (12). In those ganglia where the postganglionic fiber is adrenergic (e.g., stellate), most acetylcholinesterase is localized on the outer surface of the terminal presynaptic fibers. When the postganglionic fiber is cholinergic (e.g., ciliary ganglion), there is high acetylcholinesterase activity in both the presynaptic and postsynaptic fibers. Acetylcholinesterase activity is also high within the postganglionic fibers of parasympathetic ganglia. Most of the acetylcholinesterase at the neuromuscular junction is postsynaptic. The presynaptic membrane contains significantly less acetylcholinesterase. In humans and other mammals, the highest butyrylcholinesterase activity is present in the plasma and in the liver, and its moderate activity is also demonstrated in the brain, retina, cerebrospinal fluid, muscle, and several other tissues.

FUNCTION

Acetylcholinesterase is the main enzyme responsible for the disposition of acetylcholine following its liberation from nerve terminals. Acetylcholinesterase is also active presynaptically and plays a role in regulating acetylcholine levels in cholinergic nerve terminals.

The function of butyrylcholinesterase is not well understood (13). Several types of evidence indicate that many cells have the capacity for the synthesis of acetylcholine. Butyrylcholinesterase may prevent accumulation of acetylcholine in the blood. It has been suggested that butyrylcholinesterase may serve as a precursor of acetylcholinesterase.

The muscle relaxant, succinylcholine, and several local anesthetics that are esters (e.g., procaine or tetracaine; Chapter 10.4) are metabolized by butyrylcholinesterase. Inherited abnormalities of this enzyme may adversely affect the course of anesthesia.

MECHANISM OF ACTION

Acetylcholinesterase contains two active sites, an anionic site and an esteratic site, in its active center. Acetylcholine binds to the enzyme surface through its quaternary nitrogen and the carbonyl carbon. The positively charged quaternary nitrogen of acetylcholine is attracted by coulombic forces, probably to strongly negative phosphate groups at the anionic site or to a negative ester group, and the carbonyl carbon to a positively charged nucleophilic group consisting of histidine and serine at the esteratic site of the active center of acetylcholinesterase (Fig. 8.2-1). In addition, covalent bond formation between the ester group and esteratic site and dipolar forces in the ester oxygen atom may also be involved in the binding.

The hydrolysis of acetylcholine occurs in at least three steps. At first, a high-energy unstable complex of the enzyme and unchanged substrate is formed (step 1). This complex goes on to form a more stable acetylated enzyme and yields choline (step 2). The acetylated enzyme reacts with water and dissociates into free enzyme and acetic acid (step 3). The reactions between acetylcholinesterase and acetylcholine, and this enzyme with its inhibitors, are illustrated in Fig. 8.2-1.

The hydrolysis of acetylcholine by acetylcholinesterase occurs at a very fast rate. The turnover time (i.e., the time necessary for one active center to break down one molecule of substrate) of this enzyme for acetylcholine is about 30-60 μsec or even less. The mechanism for the hydrolysis of acetylcholine by butyrylcholinesterase is similar to that of acetylcholinesterase. The high reactivity of the esteratic site is probably due to the interaction of the hydroxyl group of serine with the imidazole group of histidine.

CHOLINESTERASE INHIBITORS

TYPES

Cholinesterase inhibitors prevent the hydrolysis of acetylcholine by interfering with one of the steps in its hydrolysis (15,21). They prevent the formation of the enzme-acetylcholine complex by interacting with: (1) the anionic site, and forming a reversible enzyme inhibitor complex (e.g., edrophonium); (2) both anionic and esteratic sites in the same manner as acetylcholine (physostigmine and neostigmine); (3) the esteratic site, and forming a stable acylated enzyme (e.g., organophosphorus inhibitors); and (4) the anionic site of the acetylated enzyme, and preventing its hydrolysis by water (e.g., several alkylammonium ions). Fluoride ions become attached to sites different from the active center of cholinesterase to both free and acetylated enzymes and interfere with both acetylation and deacetylation of cholinesterase.

Several clinically useful cholinesterase inhibitors act by mechanisms 1 and 2, and organophosphorus and organosulfonates inhibit cholinesterase by mechanism 3. All mechanisms of cholinesterase inhibitors are schematically shown in Fig. 8.2-1.

The cholinesterase inhibitors may be reversible or irreversible. The reversible inhibitors dissociate readily from the enzyme and can be easily removed by dialysis with full restoration of enzyme activity. The binding of enzymes and irreversible inhibitors can only be broken up by the use of reactivators (e.g., pralidoxime) causing the return of enzyme activity.

The reversible inhibitors may be competitive or noncompetitive. Clinically useful cholinesterase inhibitors are reversible and competitive. Cholinesterase inhibitors used as insecticides and pesticides are noncompetitive and irreversible. Several examples of those inhibitors are listed in Tables 8.2-1 and 8.2-2.

PHARMACOLOGICAL ACTIONS

The systemic administration of cholinesterase inhibitors causes generalized cholinergic responses. The majority of their effects are due to the sparing effects upon acetylcholine released as a transmitter at various sites in the nervous system. The prominence and intensity of effects are dependent upon the dose. The most prominent effects at low doses are those originating due to activation of muscarinic receptors. These include (1) decreased heart rate, vasodilation, and decreased arterial pressure; (2) increased gastrointestinal activity, abdominal cramps, and involuntary defecation; (3) increased bronchial constriction and spasm; (4) pupillary constriction (pinpoint pupils); (5) increase in the secretions of salivary, lacrimal, sweat, gastric, and mucosal glands; and (6) involuntary micturition. At these doses, cholinesterase inhibitors have little effect at the skeletal-neuromuscular junction.

Higher doses of cholinesterase inhibitors cause muscle fasciculations associated with augmentation of miniature end-plate and excitatory postsynaptic potentials, and conversion of twitch to tetanus; ultimately, depolarization block may be seen. In this situation, nondepolarizing agents (e.g., d-tubocurarine) may cause significant improvement.

Ganglionic stimulant and subsequent blocking effects can be observed after very high doses of cholinesterase inhibitors. Pallor and elevation of blood pressure may be seen in an occasional case as an effect of accumulated acetylcholine at sympathetic ganglia.

A variety of central effects may be produced after high or toxic doses of those cholinesterase inhibitors that cross the blood-brain barrier. These include drugs that contain a tertiary nitrogen (e.g., physostigmine) but not a quaternary nitrogen (e.g., neostigmine).These effects are characterized by stimulation followed by depression, and include giddiness, tension, anxiety, jitteriness, restless-

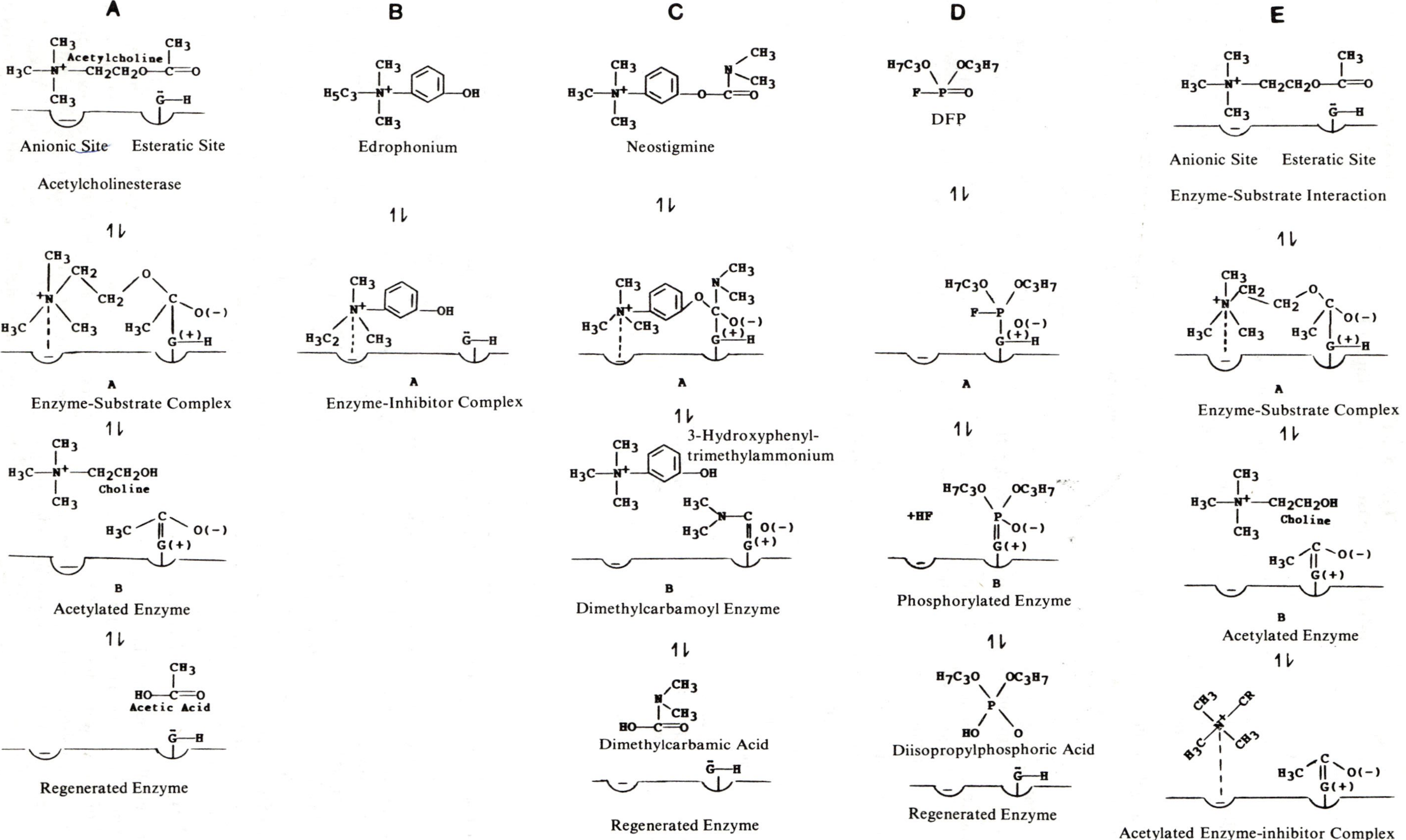

Fig. 8.2-1. *Steps involved in the hydrolysis of acetylcholine by acetylcholinesterase (A), and the inhibition of acetylcholinesterase by reversible inhibitors (e.g., edrophonium) (B), carbamate inhibitors (neostigmine) (C), organophosphorus inhibitors (e.g., DFP) (D), and alkylammonium ions (E).* In all cases, the reactions can be represented by three steps except in the case of inhibitors that are completely reversible, where the reaction is represented by a single step.

Table 8.2-1
Anticholinesterase Agents in Clinical Use

Generic Name (Proprietary Name)	Chemical Classification	I50 (M) AChE (BChE)	Kinetic Classification	Clinical Uses	Preparations[a]
Physostigmine sulfate, USP (ESERINE)	alkaloid heterocyclic carbamate	2.2×10^{-7} (3.2×10^{-8})	slowly reversible, competitive	to produce miosis; awakening from anesthesia	S, 0.25%, 0.5% I, 2mg/2 ml O, 0.25%
Neostigmine methyl sulfate, USP (PROSTIGMIN)	aromatic carbamate	1.7×10^{-7} (8×10^{-8})	slowly reversible, noncompetitive	treatment of myasthenia gravis (MG); reversal of residual neuromuscular block	T, 15 mg I, 0.25-1mg/ml
Pyridostigmine bromide, USP (MESTINON)	heterocyclic carbamate	6.8×10^{-9} (1.9×10^{-7})	reversible, competitive	same as those of neostigmine	T, 60 mg Sy, 12mg/ml
Edrophonium chloride, USP (TENSILON)	phenolic quaternary ammonium	1.1×10^{-5} (1.4×10^{-3})	reversible, competitive	diagnosis of MG; residual neuromuscular block	I, 10 mg/ml
Ambenonium chloride, NF (MYTELASE)	aromatic bisquaternary ammonium	7.5×10^{-10} (2.6×10^{-6})	reversible, competitive	treatment of MG	T, 10,25 mg
Demecarium bromide, USP (HUMORSOL)	aromatic bisquaternary ammonium		reversible, competitive	to produce miosis	S, 0.125%,0.25%
Hexafluorenium bromide (MYLAXEN)	aromatic bisquaternary ammonium	2.2×10^{-6} (1.5×10^{-7})	reversible, competitive	prolongation of the neuromuscular effect of succinylcholine	I, 20 mg/ml
Isoflurophate, USP, DFP (FLOROPRYL)	organophosphate	10^{-9} (10^{-10})	irreversible	miosis	S, 0.1% (in vegetable oil) O, 0.025%
Echothiophate iodide, USP (PHOSPHOLINE)	organophosphate	1.5×10^{-8} (1.0×10^{-9})	irreversible	treatment of glaucoma and MG	S, in special diluent

[a] I, injection (in ampuls); O, ointment (ophthalmic); S, solution (ophthalmic); Sy, syrup; T, tablet.

ness, emotional lability, excessive dreaming, insomnia, nightmares, headache, tremor, apathy, withdrawal and depression, bursts of slow waves of elevated voltage in EEG especially on overventilation, drowsiness, difficulty in concentrating, slowness of recall, confusion, slurred speech, ataxia, generalized weakness, coma with absence of reflexes, Cheyne-Stokes respiration, convulsions, and depression of respiratory and circulatory centers with dyspnea, cyanosis, and fall in blood pressure.

PRINCIPAL CHOLINESTERASE INHIBITORS

Although several cholinesterase inhibitors are available, only some are used clinically. They will be discussed in this section. All of these cholinesterase inhibitors are effective against both types of cholinesterases. Most widely used cholinesterase inhibitors are reversible (Table 8.2-1).

PHYSOSTIGMINE

Physostigmine was the first specific cholinesterase inhibitor. The properties of the drug were studied as early as 1855, and its structure was determined in 1925. It served as a prototypic drug for the development of other reversible cholinesterase inhibitors. Neostigmine, pyridostigmine, and edrophonium have some structural similarities to physostigmine.

Physostigmine is a tertiary amine alkaloid extracted from the Calabar bean, the dried ripe seed of a woody vine, *Physostigma venenosum*, which grows in tropical West Africa. It is also synthesized chemically.

Physostigmine is well absorbed from the gastrointestinal tract and crosses the blood-brain barrier. It appears about equally effective against acetylcholinesterase and/or butyrylcholinesterase. It forms a carbamyl enzyme as an intermediate, and its effects may be readily

Table 8.2-2
Organophosphorus Compounds of Pharmacological and Toxicological Interest

Common Name	Mammalian Toxicity or LD_{50} in Rat (mg/kg, p.o.)	Uses
A. *Substituted cyanide or halogen phosphates*		
DFP, diisopropyl phosphorofluoridate	highly toxic	potent, irreversible inactivator, with ophthalmological use
Mipafox	highly toxic	early insecticide; selective inhibitor of butyrylcholinesterase
Tabun	highly toxic	toxic "nerve gas"
Sarin	highly toxic	toxic "nerve gas"
Soman	highly toxic	toxic "nerve gas"
Dimefox	3	strong systemic pesticide; highly persistent
B. *Orthophosphates*		
Dichlorvos	25	nonpersistent insecticide
Chlorfenvinphos	10-39	insecticide, quasisystemic, not very persistent
Mevinphos	7	pesticide with low contact selectivity and negligible persistence
C. *Orthothionphosphates*		
Parathion	3-10	insecticidal spray for foliages, quasisystemic insecticides
Diazinon	235	quasisystemic pesticide, not persistent
D. *Dithiophosphates or phosphorodithioates*		
Malathion	1400	agricultural insecticide; low mammalian toxicity
Dimethoate	200-500	strong systemic pesticide; persistent
Menazon	1200-1980	strong systemic pesticide; fairly persistent
Azinphosmethyl	16	pesticide with low contact selectivity; not persistent, phytotoxic
E. *Thionphosphonates*		
Ethyl p-nitrophenyl benzene thionphosphonate, "EPN"		pesticide, widely used; also inhibits carboxyesterases
F. *Pyrophosphates*		
Tetraethyl pyrophosphate (TEPP)	0.5	pesticide of low contact selectivity; negligible persistence
G. *Pyrophosphoramides*		
Schradan	5	pesticide of strong systemic properties; moderately persistent
H. *Phosphinylthiocholines*		
Echothiophate (PHOSPHOLINE, 217 MI)		potent choline derivative; used in treatment of glaucoma; relatively stable in aqueous solution

or slowly reversible depending upon the dose. Its half-life is relatively short, in humans about 1-2 hr.

The principal use of physostigmine is as a miotic, and it is used to treat narrow-angle glaucoma and to reverse the mydriasis caused by atropine. Physostigmine is also the antidote of choice to treat poisoning with belladonna alkaloids.

NEOSTIGMINE

Neostigmine is a synthetic reversible cholinesterase inhibitor. It is a quaternary ammonium nitrogen compound that is poorly and irregularly absorbed from the gastrointestinal tract, and it does not cross the blood-brain barrier. The presence of the quaternary nitrogen enables the drug to have a direct action on both nicotinic and muscarinic receptors that makes it particularly useful for its effect at the neuromuscular junction.

Neostigmine is a very powerful anticurare agent. It increases the amount of acetylcholine liberated from

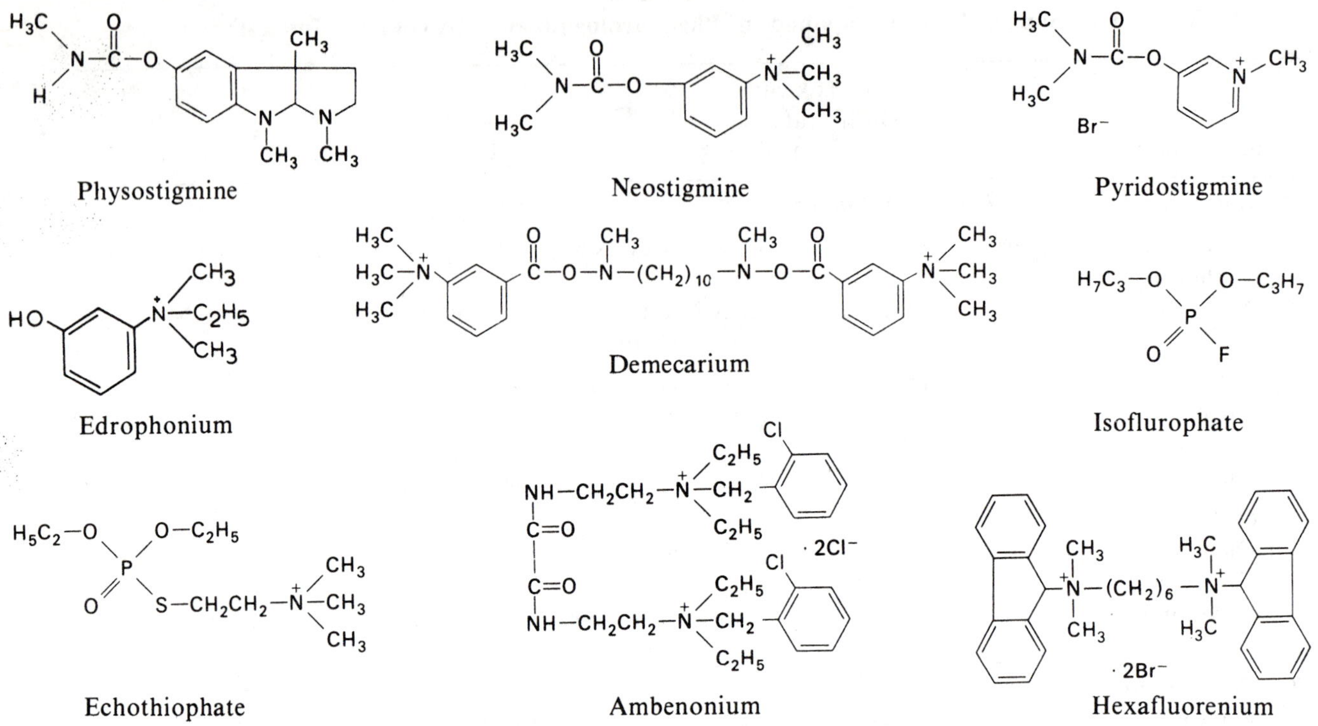

Fig. 8.2-2. *Chemical structures of anticholinesterase agents.*

nerve terminals, preserves the liberated acetylcholine by inhibiting acetylcholinesterase, and has a direct action on the skeletal-neuromuscular end-plate. The neuromuscular effects of neostigmine have made it very beneficial in the management and diagnosis of myasthenia gravis. It is also useful as a miotic and in treating postoperative atony of the intestine and urinary bladder.

PYRIDOSTIGMINE

Pyridostigmine is a reversible cholinesterase inhibitor with pharmacological properties similar to those of neostigmine. It is about 100 times less potent for inhibiting cholinesterases but has a long duration of action. After intravenous administration, it is eliminated by glomerular filtration and secretion. After intramuscular administration in humans, the half-life of pyridostigmine is about 2 hr; it increases to 4-5 hr after oral administration. Pyridostigmine induces less severe, although typical, side effects.

EDROPHONIUM

Edrophonium is a synthetic cholinesterase inhibitor with a shorter onset and duration of action than neostigmine. The absence of the carbamate group in its chemical structure results in a marked reduction in its potency to inhibit acetylcholinesterase compared with physostigmine or neostigmine. It interacts with the anionic site to form a reversible enzyme substrate complex (Fig. 8.2-1B). It also stimulates cholinergic receptors on the motor end-plate by direct action. It is more effective at the skeletal-neuromuscular junction than at postganglionic parasympathetic neuroeffector sites.

Edrophonium is useful in establishing the diagnosis of myasthenia gravis and in differentiating between myasthenia weakness (or "crises") and cholinergic crises.

Edrophonium exhibits powerful anticurare action and is used to reverse curare-induced paralysis of skeletal muscle. This effect is prolonged and does not appear to be related to the inhibition of acetylcholinesterase but rather to the facilitation of transmitter release and the direct displacement of curare from the motor end-plate.

Edrophonium has a short duration of action, and therefore its side effects are not as severe as those of other cholinesterase inhibitors. Most of its muscarinic symptoms are seen after intravenous administration and are readily reversed with atropine.

AMBENONIUM

Ambenonium is a bisquaternary compound with anticholinesterase activity about six times higher than that of neostigmine. It facilitates transmission at the neuromuscular junction, has anticurare actions and, at high doses, exhibits neuromuscular blocking activity. The drug is generally given orally (initial dose 5 mg; maintenance dose, 10-30 mg/kg) when treating myasthenia gravis and has fewer side effects and a longer duration of action than neostigmine. It has a greater tendency to accumulate than neostigmine. It is useful in treating patients who cannot tolerate bromide ions in neostigmine bromide or pyridostigmine bromide.

ORGANOPHOSPHORUS INHIBITORS OF CHOLINESTERASE

The organophosphorus compounds were discovered by a German team concerned primarily with the development of nerve gases. Most organophosphorus insecticides are based upon the following general molecular pattern, where X and Y are alkoxy or substituted amino groups, and Z is often, but not always, a group derived from an acid HZ.

$$\begin{matrix} X & & O \text{ or } S \\ & P & \\ Y & & Z \end{matrix}$$

Table 8.2-2 lists some of these compounds with their toxicity and uses.

ORGANOPHOSPHORUS INHIBITORS USED IN THERAPEUTICS

DIISOPROPYL PHOSPHOROFLUORIDATE (ISOFLUROPHATE)

Diisopropyl phosphorofluoridate [diisopropyl fluorophosphate (DFP)] produces an irreversible inactivation of the cholinesterases (Fig. 8.2-1D). The difference between DFP and agents such as physostigmine lies in the persistency of action. Diisopropylphosphoryl-enzyme complex forms as an intermediate. No spontaneous hydrolytic reactivation occurs with this intermediate. Both acetylcholinesterase and butyrylcholinesterase are inactivated by DFP; DFP, however, has a greater affinity for the latter enzyme. The complete inhibition by DFP of the butyrylcholinesterase activity of an organ is not accompanied by functional alterations. It is only when the dose of DFP used is sufficient to produce a decrease in acetylcholinesterase in excess of 50% that such changes are observed. Therefore butyrylcholinesterase plays a minor role, if any, in the junctional events of cholinergic transmission.

DFP is a volatile, colorless oily liquid having a characteristic peppermintlike odor. Its solubility in water is limited, but it is readily soluble in oil. In aqueous solution, it undergoes hydrolysis to form hydrofluoric acid and is rendered biologically inert. DFP is stable in peanut or sesame oil or in the form of water-free ointment for as long as 3 months.

DFP is useful for the treatment of certain types of glaucoma and strabismus, and as an antidote against the harmful effects of atropine on preglaucomatous and glaucomatous eyes (Chapter 21.1).

ECHOTHIOPHATE IODIDE

Echothiophate iodide is a long-acting cholinesterase inhibitor with pharmacological actions on the peripheral nervous system similar to those of DFP. Spontaneous reactivation of the phosphorylated enzyme occurs more rapidly with echothiophate than with DFP. Echothiophate is soluble in water, and it is relatively stable in refrigerated solutions for months.

The presence of a quaternary ammonium group in the molecule limits the actions of echothiophate to the peripheral nervous system. The poor penetration of the blood-brain barrier by echothiophate is probably related to its low solubility in lipids. The peripheral signs of intoxication are similar to those seen following the administration of other cholinesterase inhibitors. Death results due to paralysis of the muscles of respiration, bronchoconstriction, and the accumulation of bronchial secretions.

Echothiophate is used for the treatment of glaucoma. It is used in 0.1-0.25% solution in physiological saline with 0.5% chlorobutanol as preservative. Echothiophate is supplied in the form of a powder, and solutions can be prepared fresh to desired strength.

ORGANOPHOSPHORUS COMPOUNDS USED AS NERVE GASES, INSECTICIDES, AND PESTICIDES

Compounds that are nerve gases and those used for their insecticidal activity are listed in Table 8.2-2. They are divided into eight groups based upon the modifications in chemical structure. Based upon their field use, they can be divided into three main subgroups (8):

> *Subgroup* 1. These are compounds of low chemical stability. They are soluble in water and usually somewhat less soluble in oil. The sprayed substance is usually also the effective substance at the site of action in insects [e.g., tetraethylpyrophosphate (TEPP), mevinphos, dichlorvos].
>
> *Subgroup* 2. These are compounds of moderate or high chemical stability. They are of low solubility in water but usually soluble in oil. The sprayed substance is activated before it reaches its site of action in insects (e.g., parathion, chlorfenvinphos, azinphos-methyl, diazinon, malathion).

SUBGROUP 1

Because of the low hydrolytic stability of compounds in the first group, they persist for only a few hours after spraying. Tetraethylpyrophosphate (TEPP), one of the first organophosphates to be employed as an insecticide, belongs to this group. It has a half-life of about 8 hr *in vitro*. Under field conditions, its half-life should be much less than that found *in vitro*. Its instability and its high acute toxicity to higher animals has rendered its use obsolete.

Mevinphos has superseded TEPP and has an acute toxic dose about four times higher than that of TEPP. It is somewhat more stable than TEPP. It is used for spraying fruit and vegetable plants just before harvesting.

Unlike many of the substances in the remaining two groups, compounds such as TEPP and mevinphos appear to be the actual toxicants at the site of action; they do not seem to be altered or "activated" to more potent cholinesterase inhibitors.

Dichlorvos is a substance that lies intermediate between subgroups 1 and 2. Its solubility in water (1%) is much lower than that of TEPP and mevinphos. It is rapidly hydrolyzed and is therefore nonpersistent. Its complex with cholinesterase in erythrocytes and plasma is not very stable, and consequently the cholinesterase activity returns to normal levels more quickly than it does after the enzyme has been attached by most other organophosphorus compounds. This is of importance in relation to possible harmful effects arising from exposure to successive small doses of the compound.

SUBGROUP 2

The substances in subgroup 2 are soluble in oil but of very limited solubility in water. Parathion, malathion, azinphos-methyl, and diazinon are representatives of this group. In contrast to substances such as TEPP, most substances in this second group undergo activation before they reach their site of action in the insect.

Parathion and certain other quasisystemic compounds exhibit high toxicity to animals, limited selectivity to insects, and moderate persistence. Malathion and diazinon have lower mammalian toxicity than parathion. Some of the early members of this group were sufficiently persistent and caused a serious residue problem, especially when applied to edible crops too close to the time of harvesting; the introduction of such materials as malathion has dramatically altered this situation. In view of the relative instability and low mammalian toxicity of malathion, it can be used on edible crops up to 1 day before harvesting. The corresponding requirement for parathion is 4 weeks, whereas azinphos-methyl and diazinon have the intermediate requirements of 3 weeks and (usually) 2 weeks, respectively.

SUBGROUP 3

The third group comprises the systemic poisons. They are materials that are able to enter the plant through its leaves and roots. They possess marked chemical stability to hydrolysis. Some systemic compounds have only a weak contact toxicity, with the result that beneficial organisms in the vicinity at the time of application may not be seriously affected by the poison. Their limited contact toxicity is due to the fact that the sprayed substance itself is usually only a weak cholinesterase inhibitor, the actual toxicant at the site of action being a more potent inhibitor formed from it by metabolism.

Schradan and dimefox, in common with other early organophosphorus insecticides, are of high toxicity to vertebrates, but some later compounds — dimethoate and menazon — are less toxic. Not only are organophosphorus compounds employed extensively as systemic compounds in plants, but certain of them have been found suitable for both systemic and superficial application to animals for the control of endo- and ectoparasites. They are, for example, employed in veterinary hygiene for the control of grubs of blowfly and warble fly. Clearly, the mammalian toxicity of certain organophosphorus compounds of suitable structure can be very low in comparison with the toxicity they show toward insects and to some other invertebrates.

SELECTIVITY, ACTIVATION, AND DEGRADATION

Both activation by the enzyme systems of insects and decomposition accelerated by enzymes in higher animals can contribute significantly to the selective action of organophosphorus insecticides. TEPP probably undergoes no activating change either in insects or in higher animals prior to reaction with cholinesterase. Both spontaneous and enzymatic hydrolysis destroy it rapidly in all organisms. Mevinphos is probably degraded in a similar manner by hydrolytic cleavage of the O-C bond that attaches the 5-carbon portion of the molecule to the phosphorus atom. In both cases, nontoxic metabolites are formed. No selective activation or destruction occurs with these compounds.

Many phosphorothionates, including parathion and malathion (subgroup 2), undergo enzymatic oxidation in insects and mammals. When this occurs, their cholinesterase activity is sometimes greatly enhanced. The reaction involves the substitution of oxygen for sulfur on the dative bond of the molecule. Thus, parathion is oxidized to the more potent and more water-soluble paraoxon.

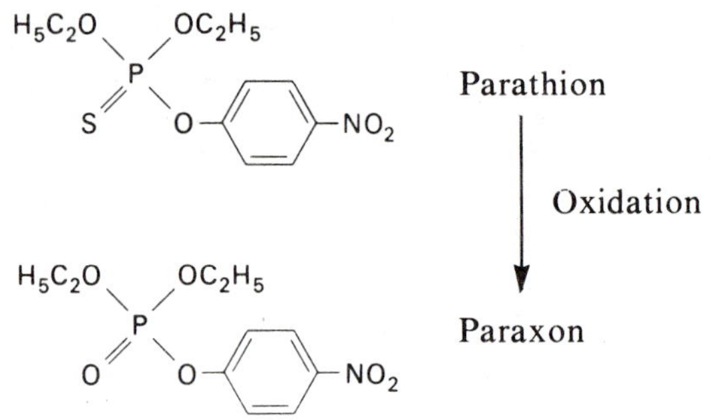

H_5C_2O, OC_2H_5, P, S, O, NO_2 — Parathion

↓ Oxidation

H_5C_2O, OC_2H_5, P, O, O, NO_2 — Paraxon

It is known that insect fat bodies and preparations from insect gut also activate thionates. Similar activation has been noted for malathion, diazinon, and other common insecticidal phosphorothionates. For some of these, such as malathion, both hydrolytic and oxidative systems may play a part in their metabolism. Such metabolism may result in activation or in destruction. There are differences in the hydrolytic and oxidative actions in different organisms, and this variability is said to account for the remarkable selectivity of malathion. In mammals, the hydrolytic process in the presence of carboxyesterase leads to inactivation. This normally occurs quite rapidly, whereas oxidation leading to activation is slow. In insects, the opposite is usually the case.

When insects develop resistance to malathion, this is often due to an increase in the quantity or activity of a carboxyesterase operating in the same way as the carboxyesterase present in mammals. The activated form of schradan is likely to be the hydroxymethyl derivative.

N(CH_2 OH)(CH_3) ⟶ N-methoxide

The latter may rapidly isomerize *in vivo* to a less active N-methoxide (N-O-CH_3).

THERAPEUTIC USES

Among the cholinesterase inhibitors, the reversible inhibitors and the carbamate inhibitors are widely used.

Myasthenia Gravis. The main symptom of myasthenia gravis (MG) is severe weakness and rapid fatigability of skeletal muscle. The complete etiology of the disease is not known. Several observations indicate that failure of neuromuscular transmission is the main cause of the disease (14). It is indicated that both presynaptic and postsynaptic cholinergic mechanisms are involved in the etiology of myasthenia gravis. An autoimmune response involving the thymus gland has also been implicated. Regardless of the underlying mechanism, there is an insufficiency of acetylcholine required for neuromuscular transmission, and the rational treatment of the disease is to increase the amount of available acetylcholine or improve the neuromuscular transmission (10, 11, 22).

Reversible cholinesterase inhibitors and carbamates are used for both the diagnosis and treatment of myasthenia gravis. For diagnosis, both edrophonium and neostigmine are convenient to use. In the majority of cases, dramatic improvement in muscle strength can be observed shortly after the administration of either of these two drugs. Effective quaternary ammonium compounds, neostigmine, ambenonium, and pyridostigmine, which do not exhibit central nervous system side effects, are used. These drugs are given orally, but in severe cases neostigmine can be given parenterally. The maximal muscle strength attained following optimal doses of these agents is about the same, but the effectiveness of therapy varies among individual patients. With insufficient drug, a myasthenia crisis may result. If there is too much drug, a cholinergic crisis may be precipitated (4).

Glaucoma. Glaucoma is a disease characterized chiefly by an increase in intraocular pressure. There are three types of glaucoma: primary, secondary (e.g., aphasic glaucoma after cataract extraction), and congenital. Primary glaucoma is further classified into narrow-angle (acute congestive) and wide-angle (chronic simple) types. Pathophysiology of different types of glaucoma and use of cholinesterase inhibitors and other drugs are discussed in Chapter 21.1. To describe briefly, the purpose of the therapy is to reduce the intraocular pressure to the normal level. In narrow-angle glaucoma, this is done by instilling into the conjunctival sac a combination of a cholinesterase inhibitor (e.g., physostigmine salicylate, 1% solution) with a cholinomimetic agent (e.g., pilocarpine nitrate, 4%). Administration of acetazolamide, a carbonic anhydrase inhibitor, to reduce the secretion of aqueous humor is used as adjunctive therapy.

Physostigmine and pilocarpine are also used in chronic simple glaucoma, although in varying concentrations. Long-acting cholinesterase inhibitors (e.g., echothiophate, demecarium) have been used in the past with the risk of the development of lenticular opacities and a specific type of cataract.

Atony of the Urinary Bladder. Reversible cholinesterase inhibitors stimulate the smooth muscle of the urinary bladder and are used for the treatment of postoperative acute nonobstructive urinary retention and atony of the urinary bladder. Among cholinesterase inhibitors, neostigmine is useful for this purpose. It facilitates contraction of the detrusor muscle of the urinary bladder; postoperative dysuria is relieved, and the time interval between operation and spontaneous urination is shortened.

Atony of the Intestinal Tract. Reversible cholinesterase inhibitors are used for relief of abdominal distention from a variety of medical and surgical causes. Neostigmine is the most common cholinesterase inhibitor used. The subcutaneous dose of neostigmine methylsulfate for postoperative paralytic ileus is about 0.5-1.0 mg, and the oral dose of neostigmine bromide is about 15 mg. Peristaltic activity begins in 10-30 min after parenteral administration, and 2-4 hr after oral administration. Neostigmine and other drugs are to be viewed mainly as adjuvant agents in the treatment of distention, for which other appropriate measures (e.g., removal of mechanical obstruction, if any, or suction through rectal tube, etc.) may be necessary.

Postanesthetic Delirium. Functional integrity of the reticular-activating system is intimately concerned with the maintenance of an alert and wakeful state. Acetylcholine plays an important role in the functioning of this system. Inhalation anesthetics that depress this system also interfere with the turnover rate of acetylcholine in the rat brain. Therefore, it is reasonable to assume that anticholinergic premedication drugs, and possibly inhalation anesthetics, do suppress acetylcholine activity in the brain of the anesthetized patient. This reasoning forms the basis for the use of a cholinesterase inhibitor for awakening patients from postanesthetic somnolence and for preventing delirium (1,3, 9). For this purpose, physostigmine salicylate (0.014 mg/kg, i.m.) can be given in one dose 20 min after surgery (18,20). Physostigmine has been effective, especially in shortening the arousal time in postoperative patients who have received anticholinergic drugs, antihistamines, benzodiazepines, and droperidol and in reducing the disorientation and agitation occasionally caused by these agents. Its routine use, however, is not recommended (1).

Acute Anticholinergic Syndrome. Several centrally acting drugs produce acute toxic psychosis characterized by agitation, confusion, and peripheral signs of cholinergic blockade. These drugs include several plant toxins (e.g., *Atropa belladonna, Datura stramonium,* which contain atropinelike principles), antispasmodics that cross the blood-brain barrier, antidepressants (e.g., imipramine), H_1 receptor antagonists with central effects (e.g., diphenhydramine, promethazine), and several antiparkinsonian drugs (benztropine), and antipsychotic drugs (e.g., thioridazine).

Cholinesterase inhibitors that cross the blood-brain barrier are suitable to reverse the central anticholinergic syndrome. Physostigmine is the drug of choice. It can reverse the central and peripheral effects of high doses of atropine (212 mg) (6). Physostigmine can also be of great diagnostic help in evaluating an acute toxic reaction superimposed on an underlying psychosis.

CHOLINESTERASE REACTIVATORS

The phosphorylated esteratic site of cholinesterase undergoes hydrolytic regeneration at a slow or negligible rate. Nucleophilic agents such as hydroxylamine (H_2NOH), however, can reactivate the enzyme much more rapidly. Highly effective reactivation may be produced by a molecule containing both a quaternary N-atom and an oxime group, spaced at an appropriate distance, such as pyridine-2-aldoxime methylchloride (PAM, 2-formyl-1-methylpyridinium chloride oxime, pralidoxime, PROTOPAM). Reactivation with this compound occurs at about a million times the rate of that with hydroxylamine. Certain bisquaternary oximes are even more potent as reactivators. An example is obidoxime chloride [1,1-(oxydimethylene) bis (4-formylpyridinium) dichloride dioxime].

Chemical structures of some cholinesterase reactivators are as follows:

Pralidoxime chloride (PAM; Protopam chloride)

Obidoxime chloride

1,3-Bis(pyridine-4-aldoxime) propane dibromide (TMB-4)

PRINCIPLES OF THE ACTION

When the quaternary ammonium group of pralidoxime is attracted electrostatically to the anionic site, the oxime group of the former is oriented optimally to exert nucleophilic attack on the electrophilic phosphorus atom of the phosphorylated esteratic site; the oximephosphonate is then split off, leaving the regenerated enzyme (Fig. 8.2-3) (21, 23). The phosphorylated cholinesterase formed by some inhibitors such as the active metabolite of octamethyl pyrophosphoramide (OMPA) is not reactivated by the oximes and hydroxamic acids.

AGING OF PHOSPHORYLATED CHOLINESTERASES AND REACTIVATION

Cholinesterases inhibited by organophosphates, depending on the duration of the interaction between the enzymes and the inhibitors, become gradually refractory to reactivation by nucleophilic compounds. This phenomenon is termed *aging*. Aging is caused by the transformation of the enzyme by a chemical reaction, probably dealkylation, between the phosphoryl (or other similar) group and the enzyme, to an inactive

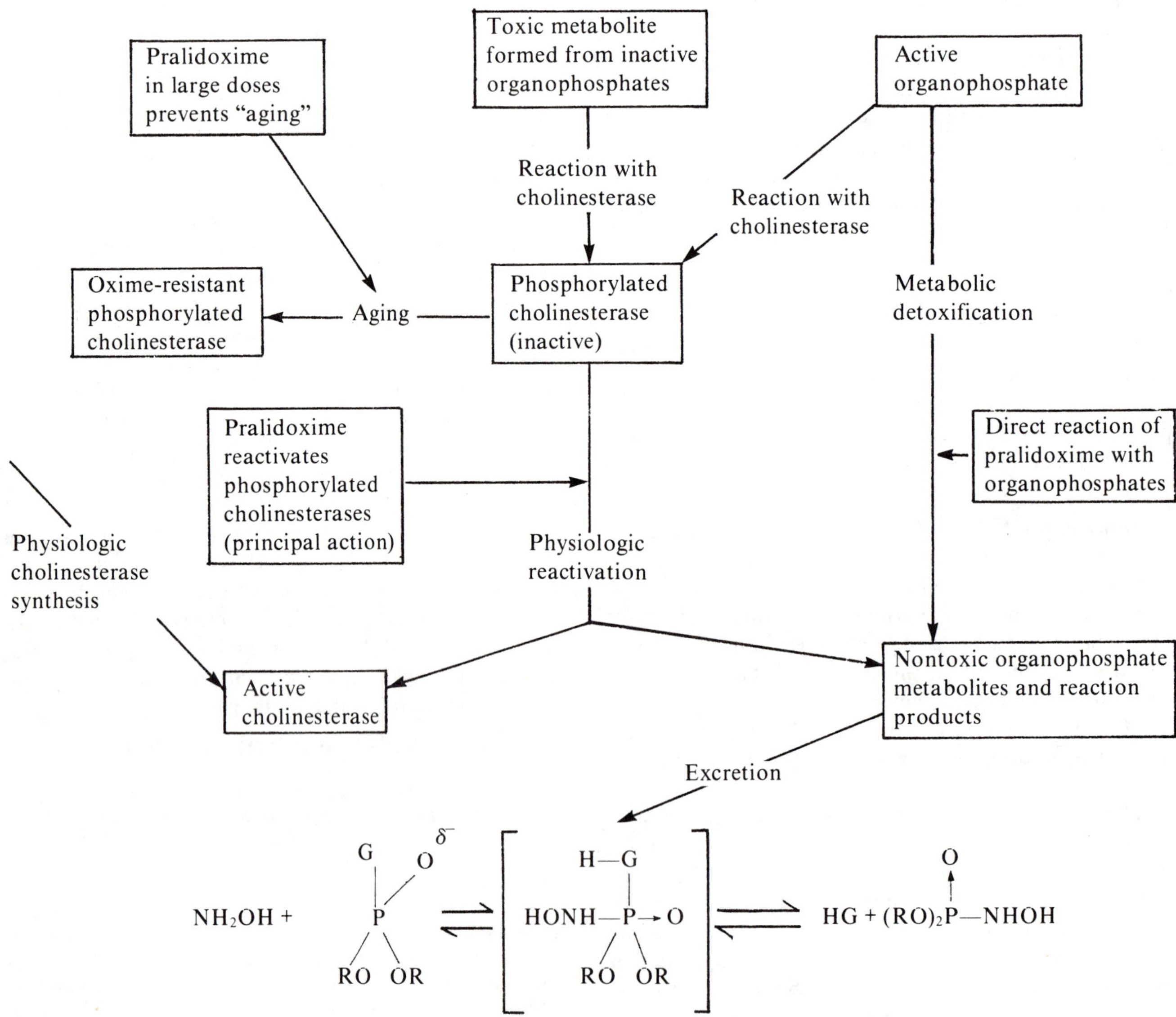

Fig.8.2-3. *Mechanisms of action of PAM.*

form. In addition to the chemical structure of the inhibitory group and the time elapsed before the application of the reactivator, the type of enzyme, the temperature, and the pH also have considerable influence on aging. Aging can occur not only *in vitro* but also *in vivo*.

Aging occurs very rapidly with soman with a half-life of less than 90 sec (i.e., 50% of the phosphorylated enzyme can be reactivated at this time) and much more slowly with tabun or sarin. Organophosphates containing a quaternary ammonium group (e.g., PHOSPHOLINE) cannot be reactivated by oximes, and they seem to age instantaneously. Butyrylcholinesterase tends to age more rapidly than acetylcholinesterase.

PHARMACOLOGY OF REACTIVATORS

The reactivating efficacy of oximes and hydroxamic acids *in vivo* is most marked at the skeletal-neuromuscular junction. The total blockade of transmission produced by a dose of an organophosphorus compound can be reversed by the intravenous injection of an oxime within a few minutes. Antidotal effects are less striking at autonomic effector sites and insignificant in the CNS [except with the nonquaternary compounds, such as diacetyl monoxime (DAM)].

High doses of pralidoxime and related compounds can in themselves cause neuromuscular blockade and other effects. Such actions are minimal at clinical doses. If pralidoxime is injected intravenously more rapidly than the recommended rate of 500 mg/min, it can produce mild weakness, blurred vision, diplopia, dizziness, headache, nausea, and tachycardia (5).

The oximes are largely metabolized by the liver, and the metabolic products are excreted by the kidney.

ACUTE INTOXICATION FROM CHOLINESTERASE INHIBITORS

Intoxication from cholinesterase inhibitors may occur as a complication of the therapy of myasthenia gravis and is referred to as *cholinergic crisis*. This effect may also result from accidental or intentional intoxication with organophosphates.

The signs and symptoms of intoxication from cholinesterase inhibitors and its treatment are described in detail in Chapter 28.2.

REFERENCES

1. *AMA Drug Evaluations*, 5th ed. Chicago: American Medical Association, 1983, p. 368.
2. Calvey, T.N. and Chan, K. Plasma pyridostigmine levels in patients with myasthenia gravis. *Clin. Pharmacol. Ther.* 21:187, 1976.
3. Chapin, J.W. and Wingard, D.W. Physostigmine reversal of benzquinamide-induced delirium. *Anesthesiology* 46:364, 1977.
4. Foldes, F.F. The management of anticholinesterase intoxication in myasthenia gravis patients. In: *Cholinergic Mechanisms* (Waser, P.G., ed.). New York: Raven Press, 1976, p. 399.
5. Foldes, F.F. Enzymes of acetylcholine metabolism. In: *Enzymes in Anesthesiology* (Foldes, F.F., ed.). New York: Springer-Verlag, 1978, p. 89.
6. Forrer, G.R. and Miller, J.J. Atropine coma: A somatic therapy in psychiatry. *Am. J. Psychiatry* 115:455, 1958.
7. Granacher, R.P. and Baldessarini, R.J. Physostigmine: Its use in acute antidepressant and antiparkinson drugs. *Arch. Gen. Psychiatry* 32:375, 1975.
8. Hassall, K.A. Organophosphorus insecticides. In: *World Crop Protection*, Vol. 2, *Pesticides*. Cleveland: CRC Press, 1969, p. 102.
9. Hill, G.E., Stanley, T.H. and Sentker, C.R. Physostigmine reversal of postoperative somnolence. *Canad. Anaesth. Soc. J.* 24:707, 1977.
10. Hobbiger, F. Pharmacology of anticholinesterase drugs. In: *Neuromuscular Junction* (Zaimis, E., ed.), *Handbook of Experimental Pharmacology*, Vol. 42. Berlin: Springer-Verlag, 1976, p.487.
11. Karczmar, A.G. Introduction: History of research with anticholinesterase agents. In: *Anticholinesterase Agents* (Karczmar, A.G., ed.), *International Encyclopedia of Pharmacology and Therapeutics*, Section 13, Vol. 1. London: Pergamon Press, 1970, p. 1.
12. Koelle, G.B. Current concepts of synaptic structure and function. *Ann. N.Y. Acad. Sci.* 183:5, 1971.
13. Koelle, G.B., Koelle, W.A., Smyrl, E.G., Davis, R. and Nagle, A.F. Histochemical and pharmacological evidence of the function of butyrylcholinesterase. In: *Cholinergic Mechanisms and Psychopharmacology*. New York: Plenum Press, 1977, p. 125.
14. Lindstrom, J.M. Nicotinic acetylcholine receptors in myasthenia gravis. In: *Cell Receptor Disorders* (Melnechuk,T., ed). La Jolla, Calif.: Western Behavioral Sciences Institute, 1978, p. 10.
15. Main, A.R. Structure and inhibitors of cholinesterase. In: *Biology of Cholinergic Function* (Goldberg, A.M. and Hanin, I., eds.) New York: Raven Press, 1976, p. 269.
16. Oosterbann, R.A. and Jansz, H.S. Cholinesterases, esterases, and lipases. In: *Comprehensive Biochemistry* (Florkin, M. and Stotz, E.H., eds.), Vol. 16, New York: Elsevier, 1965, p. 1.
17. Sastry, B.V.R. and Sadavongvivad, C. Cholinergic systems in non-nervous tissues. *Pharmacol. Rev.* 30:65, 1979.
18. Savage, G.J. and Metzger, J.T. The prevention of postanesthetic delirium. *Plast. Reconstr. Surg.* 62:81, 1978.
19. Silver, A. *The Biology of Cholinesterases*. New York: North Holland Publ. Co., 1974.
20. Smith, D.B., Clark, R.B., Stephens, S.R., Sherman, R.L. and Hyde, M. Physostigmine reversal of sedation in parturients. *Anesth. Analg.* (Cleve.) 55:478, 1976.
21. Usdin, E. Reactions of cholinesterases with substrates, inhibitors, and reactivators. In: *Anticholinesterase Agents* (Karczmar, A.G., ed.), *International Encyclopedia of Pharmacology and Therapeutics*, Section 13, Vol. 1, London: Pergamon Press, p. 47.
22. Van Woert, M.H. Myasthenia gravis, Eaton Lambert syndrome, and familial dysautonomia. In: *Biology of Cholinergic Function* (Goldberg, A.M. and Hanin, I., eds.). New York: Raven Press, 1976, p. 567.
23. Wills, J.H. Toxicity of anticholinesterase and its treatment. In: *Anticholinesterase Agents* (Karczmar, A.G., ed.). *International Encyclopedia of Pharmacology and Therapeutics*, Section 13, Vol. 1, London: Pergamon Press, 1970, p. 357.

CHAPTER
8.3

MUSCARINIC CHOLINOCEPTOR ANTAGONISTS

Roger P. Maickel and Sachin N. Pradhan

As discussed earlier, the cholinoceptors or cholinergic receptors are of two types: muscarinic and nicotinic. The drugs that act by blocking the cholinoceptors of either type are termed cholinoceptor antagonists. Of these, the drugs-blocking or inhibiting actions of acetylcholine at the nicotinic cholinergic receptors are called *nicotinic cholinoceptor* (or *N-cholinoceptor) antagonists* or *antinicotinic agents.* Their examples are: ganglion blocking agents (Chapter 8.4) and neuromuscular blocking agents or peripheral muscle relaxants (Chapter 9.1). The drugs that block or inhibit the action of acetylcholine at the muscarinic receptors are called *muscarinic cholinoceptor* (or *M-cholinoceptor) antagonists* and are to be discussed in this chapter. They can also be called *antimuscarinic, muscarinic cholinergic blocking agents* (or *M-cholinergic antagonists).* They have also been termed *cholinolytic, anticholinergic, cholinoceptor,* or *cholinergic antagonists or blocking agents,* although such terms cannot strictly exclude nicotinic components. Because the muscarinic receptors are located at the postganglionic parasympathetic nerve endings, these drugs are also called *parasympatholytic* agents. The main actions of the drugs belonging to this group qualitatively resemble those of the well-known member, atropine; hence, they have also been termed *atropine* or *atropine-like.*

CLASSIFICATION AND CHEMISTRY

Cholinoceptor antagonists may be classified as (a) natural alkaloids (atropine and scopolamine), (b) semisynthetic compounds (homatropine, methylscopolamine), and (c) synthetic compounds (methantheline and propantheline). The structures of several natural and semisynthetic cholinoceptor antagonists are presented in Fig. 8.3-1.

The natural alkaloids atropine (dl-hyoscyamine) and scopolamine (l-hyoscine), obtained from plants of the order Solanaceae (such as *Atropa belladonna, Datura stramonium, Hyoscyamus niger),* are organic esters of

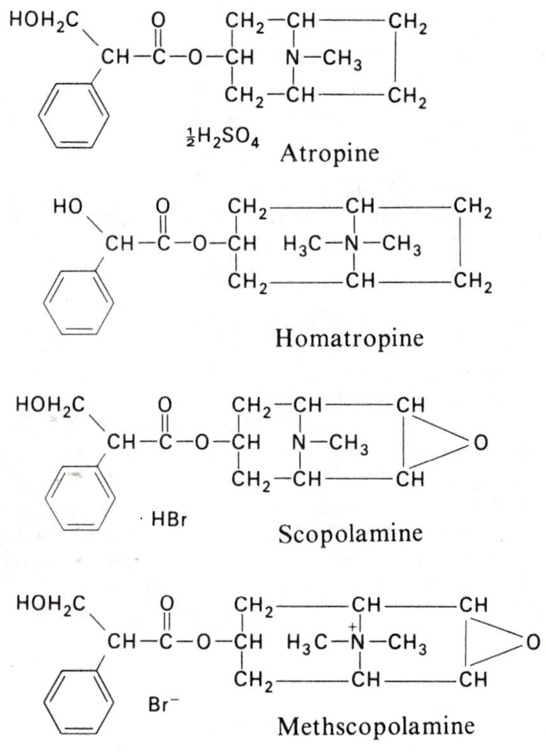

$\frac{1}{2}H_2SO_4$ Atropine

Homatropine

· HBr Scopolamine

Br^- Methscopolamine

Fig. 8.3-1: *Chemical structures of anticholinergic alkaloids and their analogs.*

tropic acid and an organic base such as tropine (atropine) or scopine (scopolamine), differing structurally by the presence of an oxygen bridge between carbons of the organic base (Fig. 8.3-1). The plant synthesizes only the levorotatory isomers, which are much more active than the dextro forms. To ensure a consistent, stable product, l-hyoscyamine is racemized to the dl mixture before it is marketed as atropine.

The semisynthetic compounds are structurally similar to the natural alkaloids. Homatropine is a tertiary amine formed from tropine and mandelic acid, whereas methylatropine and methylscopolamine are quaternary ammonium derivatives of atropine and scopolamine, respectively, produced by the addition of a second methyl group to nitrogen of the tropine nucleus.

A search for anticholinergic drugs that would be selectively more effective on either the gastrointestinal tract or the CNS, with reduced undesired side effects, has led to the development of several classes of synthetic anticholinergic agents (Fig. 8.3-2). Some of these compounds are discussed extensively in Chapter 9.4, since their primary use is in treating parkinsonism.

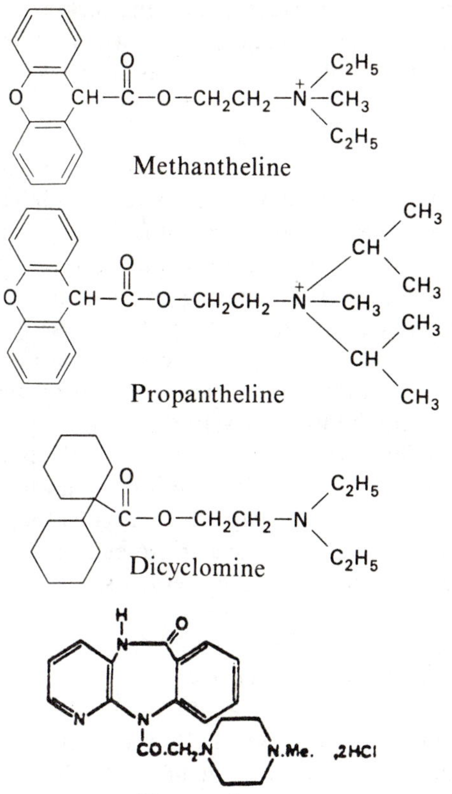

Methantheline

Propantheline

Dicyclomine

Pirenzepine

Fig. 8.3-2: *Chemical structures of some synthetic anticholinergic agents.*

BELLADONNA ALKALOIDS

Pharmacological Effects. Many of the organs innervated by the parasympathetic nervous system are only partially controlled by it. Many also receive sympathetic innervation not inhibited by cholinoceptor antagonists. Moreover, the function of many organs is only modulated, not controlled, by the parasympathetic nervous system. For example, the heart and gut have intrinsic pacemakers that can function independently of the nervous system. The gut is also poorly innervated; only a few cells receive direct innervation, with the rest responding to signals passed from one cell to another in the syncytial net. On the other hand, most of the blood vessels do not have parasympathetic nerve supply, although they are cholinoceptive and dilate in the presence of ACh and related cholinergic agents.

Antimuscarinic agents are not equally effective on different parasympathetically innervated organs. Thus, gradually increasing doses of these agents are needed to decrease the following muscarinic functions: secretion of exocrine (salivary, bronchial, and sweat) glands $<$ iris circular muscle contraction (miosis), ciliary muscle action (accommodation), vagal effect on heart rate (bradycardia) $<$ bladder contraction (micturition), and intestinal tone and motility $<$ gastric secretion and motility. Thus, a dose of an antimuscarinic agent that will reduce gastric secretion and motility will also affect intestine and bladder contraction and will cause tachycardia, cycloplegia, mydriasis, and decrease of secretions.

These agents have little effect on ACh action at nicotinic receptors. Thus, atropine produces only partial block of ganglionic neurotransmission at a relatively high dose, and causes slight block at the neuromuscular junction at extremely high doses. On the other hand, quaternary ammonium analogs of atropine and scopolamine interfere more readily with ganglionic and neuromuscular transmission in doses that produce muscarinic blockade. In the CNS, cholinergic transmission appears to be both muscarinic and nicotinic at various sites in the brain and predominantly nicotinic in the spinal cord. Atropine and related tertiary amines penetrate the blood-brain barrier and act on the central muscarinic receptors. Quaternary compounds do not cross the blood-brain barrier and have very few CNS effects.

The cholinoceptor antagonists act by reversibly combining with muscarinic receptors on the effector cells. They cause competitive blockade of ACh at the receptors. Muscarinic cholinergic blockade is highly selective and can be overcome by increasing the concentration of ACh at the receptor site. Muscarinic cholinergic antagonists have little affinity for histaminergic, serotonergic, or noradrenergic receptors.

The basic effect of atropine is antagonism at cholinergic receptors, regardless of their innervation. Thus, both the sweat glands (which are cholinergic even though they are innervated by the sympathetic nervous system) and the small blood vessels (which are dilated by acetylcholine even though they are not innervated by the parasympathetic nervous system) are inhibited by atropine.

Atropine is considered to combine reversibly with muscarinic receptors and compete with acetylcholine for attachment to the receptor. It does not prevent the liberation of acetylcholine at nerve endings nor does it combine chemically with acetylcholine. It prevents acetylcholine from exerting its action due to receptor blockade. It is generally accepted as a competitive antagonist of acetylcholine at the muscarinic receptor. However, in a quantitative investigation using isolated guinea pig ileum, a noncompetitive antagonism of atropine to acetylcholine action was demonstrated (5).

Antagonism of acetylcholine at muscarinic sites can also be produced by a number of nonspecific drugs (including phenothiazines, tricyclic antidepressants, and antihistamines) that have some structural relationship to cholinoceptor antagonists. Such drugs may produce clinically significant blockage of parasympathetic nervous function when given in usual therapeutic doses, and cause severe CNS effects in toxic overdoses.

Atropine has the capacity to prevent or antagonize all the muscarinic effects of acetylcholine and will be discussed as the prototype agent.

Cardiovascular System. In usual therapeutic doses (0.4-1 mg), atropine may cause a transient bradycardia as a result of central vagal stimulation. At high doses (2 mg), atropine produces an inhibitory effect on vagal influences, thereby allowing spontaneous expression of the pacemaker activity of the SA node and maximum conduction through the atrium and the AV node, causing tachycardia with shortening of the PR interval. This effect is most marked in healthy young adults with high vagal tone. In the very young and in the elderly, atropine, even at large doses, produces only little acceleration of the heart.

Because the parasympathetic nervous system has little direct influence on blood vessels, atropine has no significant effect on blood pressure or circulation. Even at high doses, blood pressure and cardiac output are not altered because of compensatory hemodynamic mechanisms. When atropine is administered by rapid intravenous injection, it may transiently block transmission in sympathetic ganglia and thereby cause a sudden drop in blood pressure. Moreover, at a very high dose (10 mg) atropine can cause dilation of cutaneous blood vessels, particularly in the blush area in the cheeks or face (atropine flush). The exact mechanism of this action, which appears to be unrelated to the antimuscarinic effect, is unclear but may involve some compensatory response to provide heat loss to counteract the temperature rise induced by atropine. The vasodilation produced by cholinergic agonists or cholinesterase inhibitors can be prevented by atropine.

Eye. The effects of atropine on the eye are discrete and predictable. If the drug is applied to the conjunctiva, the circular muscle of the iris and the ciliary muscles are paralyzed, resulting in pupillary dilation (mydriasis) and loss of accommodation (cycloplegia), respectively. The mydriasis is due to the unopposed activity of the radial muscle. This effect subsides slowly in 7 to 12 days. Mydriasis caused by sympathetic stimulation is not accompanied by cycloplegia, due to lack of sympathetic innervation in the ciliary muscle. However, in persons with narrow-angle glaucoma the cholinoceptive antagonist should not be used. The paralysis of the concentric muscle, causing dilation of the pupil and the relaxation of ciliary muscle, allows the iris to block the angular space of the anterior chamber, thus preventing the drainage of aqueous humor through Schlemm's canal and causing an increase in intraocular pressure.

Gastrointestinal Tract. Belladonna alkaloids can completely abolish the effects of cholinoceptor agonists on the gastrointestinal tract, but they only incompletely reduce the effects of vagal impulses on motility and secretion. On the tone and peristaltic activity of the stomach and intestine these alkaloids produce marked and prolonged inhibitory effects. Enhanced motility and tone produced by parasympathomimetic drugs, insulin hypoglycemia, and certain emotional stimuli are inhibited by atropine. Responses to drugs acting through the complex system of intramural nerve plexuses, such as those produced by nicotine, morphine, and serotonin, are also inhibited. Intestine may also manifest atropine-resistant tone and motility. The alkaloids in moderate doses do not block the effects of histamine and vasopressin.

The alkaloids can completely abolish salivary secretion but only partially reduce gastric secretion. At a dose of 1 mg, atropine can usually reduce the volume of gastric secretion, but not the concentration of acid. Copious secretion of gastric juice, rich in the both acid and pepsin produced by injection of cholinoceptor agonists (e.g., methacholine, carbachol, or pilocarpine) is completely blocked by atropine. Secretion produced by histamine, alcohol or caffeine is reduced but not abolished by atropine in usual doses.

Respiratory Tract. The smooth muscles of the bronchi and bronchioles are relaxed by atropine, resulting in widening of the airway. The reduction of parasympathetic influence on bronchioles produced by atropine may help to relieve bronchoconstriction caused by irritants in the lung, cholinoceptive agonists, anticholinesterase agents, and/or psychogenic factors. Atropine is a more potent bronchodilator than scopolamine but less potent than epinephrine or isoproterenol against bronchoconstriction induced by electrical stimulation of the vagus. Belladonna alkaloids inhibit secretions of the upper and lower respiratory tract and produce dryness of mucous membranes; hence, they are used in preanesthetic medication. They can also reduce reflex laryngospasm that may occur due to respiratory tract secretion during general anesthesia.

Other Smooth Muscle. Atropine causes some relaxation of smooth muscles of the bile ducts and gallbladder, but it has little effect on bile secretion. The relaxation of the biliary sphincter is incomplete, so these drugs are of little value in relieving biliary spasm. Therapeutic doses of atropine cause relaxation of smooth muscles of the urinary tract. The tone and contractions of the ureter are diminished, and the detrusor muscle of the bladder is relaxed by atropine. The cholinoceptor antagonists have little or no effect on uterine tone or motility.

Exocrine Glands. Cholinergic stimulation of glandular secretions may be prevented by the administration of atropine. Secretion may be blocked in glands that are totally or principally cholinergic, such as salivary and sweat glands, resulting in dry mouth and hot, dry skin. In organs that receive both sympathetic and parasympathetic innervation, such as the lower respiratory tract and pancreas, the secretions are less voluminous and more viscid.

Central Nervous System. Atropine interferes with muscarinic cholinergic transmission in the brain, resulting in mild sedation, dysphoria, or severe toxic psychoses depending on the dose. In usual therapeutic doses (0.5-1 mg) atropine causes mild CNS stimulation manifested by increased vagal impulses resulting in mild bradycardia, and slight increase in the rate and depth of respiration, partly due to central influences and partly due to increased dead space produced by bronchial dilation. Atropine at slightly higher doses (beginning with 0.75 mg, gradually increasing to 15 or even 20 mg/day) can suppress muscular rigidity in parkinsonism. Atropine in large doses (10 mg or more) produces marked central effects characterized by restlessness, disorientation, irritability, hallucinations, and delirium. The initial stimulation is followed by depression and respiratory paralysis that eventually leads to coma and death.

Other Effects. The inhibition of sweating may cause hyperthermia noted after large doses of atropine, particularly in children.

Pharmacokinetics. Atropine and scopolamine are readily absorbed from the gastrointestinal tract following oral administration and may also be absorbed from mucous membranes. They disappear rapidly from the blood and distribute into extracellular spaces. Although these compounds are esters, they are not hydrolyzed by cholinesterases. About 50% of a dose of atropine is excreted unchanged in the urine, with the rest metabolized in the liver and eliminated slowly as metabolites. The half-life of atropine is between 12 and 36 hours. The metabolic fate of scopolamine is less well understood.

Adverse Effects. The cholinoceptive antagonists are generally safe and their adverse effects, primarily extensions of their pharmacological effects, are usually not life-threatening. Dry mouth, blurred vision, tachycardia, urinary hesitancy, dizziness, and fatigue are common troublesome effects. More serious adverse effects include interference with the fluid dynamics of the anterior chamber of the eye, which aggravates glaucoma, and pronounced urinary retention if the urethra is partly obstructed such as by a hypertrophied prostate.

Acute Poisoning. Poisoning by cholinoceptor antagonists can occur accidently by ingestion of certain plants of the order Solanaceae or from an overdose of anticholinergic drugs. It can also occur after an overdose of phenothiazines, tricyclic antidepressants, antihistamines, or any other drugs with anticholinergic properties.

Intoxication by these drugs occurs quickly and is manifested by hot, dry, scarlet skin, dry mouth, very blurred vision, tachycardia, and hyperthermia. The CNS effects are characterized by excitation, ataxia, confusion, delirium, hallucinations, and with very high doses, convulsions, respiratory collapse, and coma. The signs of acute toxicity may persist for a few hours to several days.

Treatment of acute toxicity includes gastric lavage to limit further absorption and physostigmine to counter the peripheral and CNS effects; diazepam causes sedation and is useful for the control of seizures (see Chapter 32).

SUBSTITUTES FOR BELLADONNA ALKALOIDS

Atropinelike drugs are of great therapeutic importance, and therefore attempts have been made to develop agents with selective effects at various cholinergic sites.

SUBSTITUTE FOR OPHTHALMIC USE

As already mentioned, *homatropine,* a semisynthetic agent, is used solely as a topical mydriatic and cycloplegic. It differs from atropine in being one-tenth as potent, more rapid in onset, and shorter in duration of action (Chapter 21.1).

QUATERNARY AMMONIUM COMPOUNDS DESIGNED FOR GASTROINTESTINAL EFFECTS

Methantheline and propantheline (Fig. 8.3-2) are potent antimuscarinic compounds with more selective gastrointestinal actions. Their absorption after oral administration is poor and unreliable. Penetration of conjunctiva is also poor, and hence they are not used in ophthalmology. Their transport through the blood-brain barrier is also poor, and thus their CNS effects are minimal.

The ratio of ganglion blocking activity to antimuscarinic activity is higher than that for belladonna alkaloids. Compared with atropine, the quaternary ammonium anticholinergic compounds appear to produce relatively greater gastrointestinal effects and less antimuscarinic side effects. This additional potency may be due to ganglion blocking action that may also account for some of their side effects, such as impotence and postural hypotension. At high and toxic doses, these derivatives may cause neuromuscular blockade resulting in respiratory and other skeletal muscle paraylsis.

Propantheline is two to five times more potent than methantheline in this respect. Other compounds are listed under preparations.

PIRENZEPINE

Pirenzepine is a selective antimuscarinic anticholinergic agent (1, 3). Its chemical structure is in Fig. 8.3-2. This agent reduces gastric acid secretion and also heals ulcers without producing serious side effects, probably by preferential blocking of a certain subtype (M_1) of muscarinic cholinoceptors (see Chapter 8). The site of action of this drug on acid secretion may be at an M_1 site away from the parietal cell and has been postulated to be in the parasympathetic or enteric ganglia, which needs further confirmation.

Like the conventional anticholinergic drugs, in therapeutic doses, pirenzepine inhibits basal as well as pentagastrin-stimulated gastric acid secretion to about 50% and 30%, respectively. However, it inhibits insulin-stimulated gastric secretion to a greater degree, indicating its greater effect on a cholinergic stimulus. Similar effect was shown in sham-feeding experiments. Pirenzepine thus appears to act as an antimuscarinic drug (4).

In contrast to the conventional antimuscarinic drugs, in acid peptic disorders it inhibits gastric secretion at a much lower dose than required to inhibit salivation and contraction of smooth muscles of the eye, stomach, and esophagus, and to produce tachycardia (1). It is also effective on Zollinger-Ellison syndrome, but no typical antimuscarinic side effects have been observed (2). Although there are M_1 receptors in the brain, pirenzepine does not enter the brain to any appreciable extent (4) and lacks central effects.

SYNTHETIC TERTIARY AMINE ANTIMUSCARINIC AGENTS

Tertiary amine compounds such as cyclopentolate and tropicamide are used in ophthalmic practice, and dicyclomine (Fig. 8.3-2) is used as an antispasmodic in gastrointestinal, biliary, and urinary tracts.

SYNTHETIC ANTIPARKINSONIAN DRUGS

Several tertiary amine antimuscarinic agents (Fig. 9.4-1) have more selective actions on the CNS and less peripheral side effects; as such, they are used in the treatment of idiopathic and iatrogenic parkinsonism. These compounds are discussed in Chapter 9.4.

THERAPEUTIC USES

The major therapeutic uses of cholinoceptor blocking agents lie in five areas: as antispasmodics in the adjunctive treatment of peptic ulcer; in the treatment of cardiac bradyarrhythmias; as preanesthetic medication; in the treatment of idiopathic and iatrogenic parkinsonism (see Chapter 9.4); and as cycloplegic/mydriatic agents in ophthalmic practice (see Chapter 21.1).

Although the inability to act selectively on specific organs is usually an impediment to the use of cholinoceptor antagonists, the wide range of their actions is beneficial to those poisoned by cholinoceptor agonists or cholinesterase inhibitors. Although large doses may be required, atropine can reverse all of the muscarinic effects but not the neuromuscular paralysis and ganglionic effects of cholinesterase inhibitors.

Gastrointestinal Uses. The use of anticholinoceptor drugs in the management of peptic ulcer has decreased with the introduction of cimetidine, an H_2-receptors antagonist. Atropine and related compounds reduce peristaltic and secretory activities of the gastrointestinal tract. The original (and still used) preparations were extracts or tinctures of belladonna. The synthetic and semisynthetic compounds, especially quaternary amines that do not cross the blood-brain barrier, lessen undesirable side effects. These agents relieve pain in peptic ulcer by inhibiting gastric motility and secretions (although the actual concentration of hydrochloric acid and the amounts of pepsin and mucus are only slightly reduced). They are usually administered before meals and at bedtime; dosage regimens and requirements vary markedly among patients, so that therapy generally begins with a minimal dose and is increased until clinical efficacy is achieved with minimal adverse effects.

Cardiac Uses. The capacity to inhibit the cardiac vagus nerve permits reduction of reflexly induced bradycardia or cardiac dysrhythmias, such as some of those that may occur after strokes or head injuries or as a result of manipulation of viscera during surgery. It can also prevent bradyarrhythmias produced by cholinergic agonists such as succinylcholine. In patients with myasthenia gravis, atropine should be given intravenously if a severe muscarinic reaction occurs during its diagnosis using edrophonium; atropine is also given during its therapy with anti-AChE agents to control muscarinic side effects. Atropine may reduce the degree of AV block in conduction defect due to increased vagal tone. It may be occasionally useful in the diagnosis of accelerated AV conduction (Wolff-Parkinson-White syndrome) by normalizing the QRS complex duration. Some of the dysrhythmias that follow myocardial infarction have a vagal component, and the use of atropine in this situation has been advocated, particularly in situations where there is a pronounced sinus bradycardia. Careful selection of cases is necessary to avoid unmasking lethally abnormal sympathetic activity. Atropine is more active in accelerating heart rate (thereby preventing bradycardia), whereas scopolamine (which may slow heart rate) is preferred when tachycardia must be avoided as in patients with mitral stenosis.

Use in Anesthesia. Atropine, scopolamine, and glycopyrrolate are preferred as preanesthetic medications. These agents reduce the stimulation of salivary and respiratory system secretions often caused by some inhalation anesthetics and by succinylcholine. In addition, they prevent bradycardia, hypotension, and even cardiac arrest that may result from anesthesia or surgical procedures. For women in labor, scopolamine can produce tranquilization and amnesia; combined with an opioid, it produces a soporific state known as twilight sleep. Scopolamine has a significant sedative effect and may reduce the problems of postoperative nausea and vomiting; unfortunately, it has a greater probability of evoking CNS symptoms such as dizziness, hallucinations, and delayed awakening from general anesthesia, especially in the elderly. Both atropine and scopolamine readily cross the blood-brain barrier and may evoke the syndrome of emergence delirium in postoperative patients. For this reason, the quaternary compound, glycopyrrolate, which has minimal central cholinergic blocking effects, may be more useful in the elderly or in patients with considerable postoperative pain.

Other Uses. A few of the CNS actions of muscarinic antagonists are useful. Scopolamine (l-hyoscine) is one of the best preventatives of motion sickness (Chapter 21.2). Scopolamine produces more sedation, relative to its peripheral effects, than atropine, and it has been used in some over-the-counter preparations intended to induce sleep.

DRUG INTERACTIONS

Antimuscarinic drugs interact with antihistamines, antidepressants (tricyclic antidepressants as well as MAO inhibitors), and antipsychotic drugs by increasing their anticholinergic side effects. They act additively with levodopa or amantadine in the treatment of parkinsonism and with antacids in the treatment of peptic ulcers.

Preparations. *Belladonna extract:* tablets (15 mg; contains 0.2 mg of atropine), 15 mg t.i.d. *Belladonna tincture:* contains approximately 0.3 mg/ml of alkaloids (mainly atropine); for adults, 0.6-1 ml t.i.d.; for children, 0.03 ml/kg t.i.d.

Hyoscyamine hydrobromide: compounding needed for prescription; 0.25 mg t.i.d., p.o., s.c., i.m., or i.v.

Atropine sulfate: tablets (0.3, 0.4, and 0.6 mg); solution (0.3-1.2 mg/ml for s.c. injection); also tablets (hypodermic; 0.3, 0.4, and 0.6 mg).

Homatropine methylbromide: tablets (5 and 10 mg, p.o.); 2.5-10 mg four times a day; for children, 3-6 mg four times a day.

Methylscopolamine bromide: tablets (2.5 mg); for adults, 2.5-5 mg four times a day; for children, 0.2 mg/kg four times a day. Solution (1 mg/ml for s.c. or i.m. injection) at a dose of 0.25-1 mg q.6 hr.

Methylatropine nitrate (METROPINE); tablets (1 mg); for adults 1-2 mg.

Anisotropine methylbromide (VALPIN): tablets (10 mg); elixir (10 mg/5 ml); for adults 10 mg t.i.d., p.o.

Diphemanil methylsulfate (PRANTAL METHYLSULFATE): tablets (100 mg); 100-200 mg q.4 to 6 hr. for adults.

Glycopyrrolate (ROBINUL): tablets (1 and 2 mg); 1-2 mg t.i.d. initially, then 1 mg b.i.d. Solution (0.2 mg/ml for s.c., i.m., or i.v.); 0.1 or 0.2 mg t.i.d. for adults.

Methantheline bromide (BANTHINE): tablets (50 mg); for adults, 50-100 mg q.6 hr. (initial), then one-half the initial dose. Solution for i.m. injection at a dose of 50 mg q.6 hr.

Oxyphenonium bromide (ANTRENYL BROMIDE): tablets (5 mg); 10 mg t.i.d. for adults; for children, 0.8 mg/kg in divided doses.

Adephenine HCl: tablets (75 mg); 75-100 mg t.i.d. for adults.

Dicyclomine HCl (BENTYL): tablets (20 mg); capsules (10 mg); syrup (10 mg/5 ml); solution (10 mg/ml). For adults, 10-20 mg t.i.d., p.o. or i.m.; for children, 10 mg t.i.d.; for infants, 5 mg t.i.d. not to be given i.v.

Isometheptene HCl: solution (for i.m. injection 100 mg/ml); for adults, 100 mg q.6 hr.

REFERENCES

1. Baron, J. H., and Londong, W. (eds). Advances in basic and clinical pharmacology of pirenzepine: Proceedings of Second International Symposium on Pirenzepine. *Scand J. Gastroenterol.* 15:1, 1980.
2. Collen, M. J., S. J. Pandol, and J. P. Raufman, et al. Beneficial effects of pirenzepine, selective anticholinergic agent, in patients with Zollinger-Ellison syndrome, (abst.). *Gastroenterology* 82:1035, 1982.
3. Feldman, M. Inhibition of gastric acid secretion by selective and nonselective anticholinergics. *Gastroenterology* 86:361, 1984.
4. Jaup, B. H. Studies on the mode of action of pirenzepine in man with special reference to its anticholinergic muscarinic properties. *Scand. J. Gastroenterol.* (suppl. 68), 16:1, 1981.
5. Marshall, P. B. Antagonism of acetylcholine by hyoscyamine. *Br. J. Pharmacol.* 10:345, 1955.

CHAPTER
8.4

GANGLIONIC STIMULANTS AND BLOCKING AGENTS

Samar N. Dutta and Sachin N. Pradhan

Both sympathetic and parasympathetic ganglia contain nicotinic receptors that are acted up on by nicotinic cholinergic agonists and antagonists. There are also muscarinic receptors, particularly in the sympathetic ganglia that are also acted up on by muscarinic cholinergic agonists and antagonists. The classic ganglion blocking agents block the action of acetylcholine at the nicotinic receptors of both sympathetic and parasympathetic ganglia and inhibit the function of both autonomic systems. They are potent in their action and have been used earlier for the treatment of hypertension. They are also used in physiological and pharmacological research. However, because of lack of selectivity, resulting in a broad range of adverse effects and development of tolerance, their therapeutic uses are extremely limited.

Therefore, discussion on ganglion blocking agents in this chapter will be very brief. This discussion will be initiated by a brief presentation on receptors in the ganglia.

RECEPTORS IN GANGLIA

Acetylcholine (ACh) is the principal neurotransmitter at the autonomic ganglionic synapse. However, intracellular recording of autonomic ganglion cells shows multiple receptor systems for ganglionic neurotransmission. Stimulation of preganglionic nerve or microiontophoretic application of ACh to the postganglionic neurons (e.g., in a mammalian superior cervical ganglion) generates triphasic postsynaptic action potentials consisting, in sequence, of (1) an initial excitatory postsynaptic potential (EPSP with a latency of 1 msec and duration of 10-20 msec), (2) an inhibitory postsynaptic potential (IPSP) with an approximate latency of 35 msec., and (3) a late EPSP (with latency and duration of several hundred milliseconds). Figure 8.4-1 illustrates these action potentials with drugs enhancing and suppressing them. On the basis of the nature of agonists and antagonists acting on the different components of the action potentials, existence of at least three different receptors has been considered as shown in this figure. It shows that the initial EPSP that represents the primary pathway for ganglionic neurotransmission involves nicotinic receptors and is sensitive to classic nondepolarizing blocking agents like hexamethonium.

IPSP and late EPSP represent secondary pathways and involve muscarinic receptors; they are sensitive to atropine but not to classic ganglion blockers. In addition, dopamine and

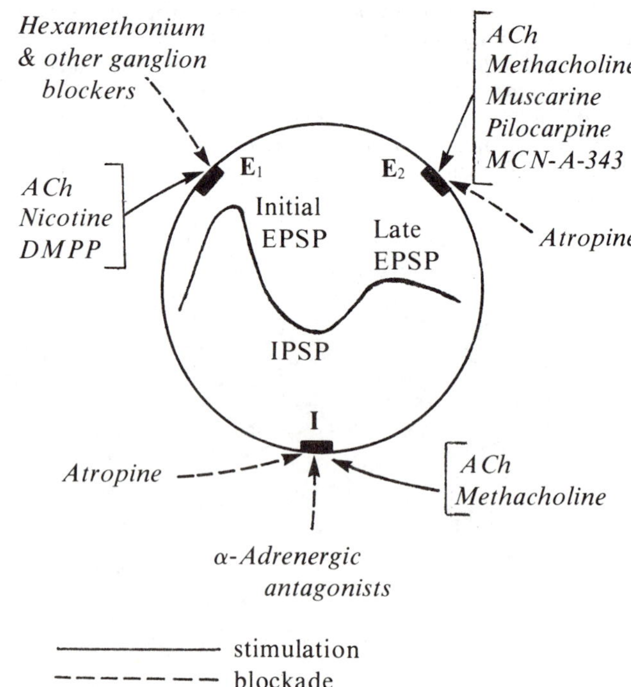

Fig. 8.4-1. *Drugs affecting different cholinergic receptors in (mammalian superior cervical) ganglia.*

norepinephrine have been shown to cause hyperpolarization. IPSP and catecholamine-induced hyperpolarization can be blocked by α-adrenergic antagonists. Because both atropine and α-adrenergic antagonists block IPSP, ACh released at preganglionic nerve terminals may act on a catecholamine-containing interneuron, causing release of dopamine or norepinephrine that in turn hyperpolarizes the ganglion cells. Presence of such interneurons has been demonstrated by dopamine- or norepinephrine-containing small, intensely fluorescent (SIF) cells and adrenergic nerve terminals in sympathetic ganglia.

CLASSIFICATION OF GANGLION STIMULANTS AND BLOCKING AGENTS

Drugs that stimulate cholinoceptors in autonomic ganglia are of two types:

1. Drugs that cause rapid stimulation and are blocked by nondepolarizing ganglion blocking agents. Their effects mimic initial EPSP; nicotine and dimethylphenylpiperazinium (DMPP) are examples.
2. Drugs that cause stimulation with delayed onset and are blocked by atropine. Their effects mimic the late EPSP; muscarinic and methacholine are examples.

Drugs that block cholinoceptors in the autonomic ganglia can also be classified into two groups:

1. Drugs that cause initial stimulation of ganglia by ACh-like action and then maintain persistent depolarization producing blockade (e.g., nicotine).
2. Drugs that impair transmission by competing with ACh for ganglionic cholinoceptors and do not produce initial depolarization and stimulation. They prevent initial EPSP; hexamethonium and other conventional ganglion blockers are examples. Only this group of drugs is clinically important and will be further discussed.

These ganglion blocking agents, as they will henceforth be called, are further classified into two groups based on their chemical structure, the quaternary and tertiary amines, as shown in Fig. 8.4-2.

GANGLION STIMULANTS

Stimulants of autonomic ganglia have no therapeutic importance, but are used as experimental tools. The natural alkaloids, such as nicotine, lobeline, muscarine, and several synthetic compounds, DMPP, McN-A-343, are examples (Chapter 8). Of these, nicotine is of much toxicological importance; it is discussed in Chapters 8 and 11.3. Lobeline (α-lobeline), an alkaloid of *Lobelia inflata* (Indian tobacco) has similar action as nicotine, but is less potent. Muscarine action is discussed in Chapter 8.

GANGLION BLOCKING AGENTS

Pharmacological Effects. The quaternary ammonium compounds such as hexamethonium are known to act by competing with acetylcholine for receptor sites at ganglionic synapses. Mecamylamine and pempidine have been shown to alter the sensitivity of receptors in addition to a competitive blocking action similar to that of quaternary ammonium compounds.

Most of the autonomic effector organs or sites have dual autonomic innervations having opposing actions. However, the sum total of these effects on an individual site, instead of completely balancing each other, shows predominance of one autonomic component; thus sympathetic (adrenergic) predominance is found in heart, smooth muscles of eye, gastrointestinal tract and bladder, and salivary glands; and, sympathetic (cholinergic) predominance in sweat glands. Accordingly, as a result of action of the ganglion blocking drugs, which block both sympathetic and parasympathetic ganglia to a similar degree, the predominant component at a particular site appears to be depressed. Thus, these agents appear to act as adrenergic-blocking agents in their effects on blood vessels and as cholinergic blocking agents on heart, smooth muscles, and exocrine glands.

The primary pharmacological effects attributed to blockade of sympathetic ganglion outflow include hypotension, particularly postural hypotension, and increased cutaneous blood flow. Parasympathetic interference may cause dilatation of pupils, cycloplegia, dry mouth, and inhibition of intestinal movement. The tertiary amines, mecamylamine or pempidine, are able to cross the blood-brain barrier and can cause CNS stimulation characterized by involuntary movements, acute mania, and seizures. Tolerance develops to both quaternary and tertiary compounds, but there is no evidence for the development of cross-tolerance among them.

Pharmacokinetics. Gastrointestinal absorption of quaternary ammonium compounds is generally both erratic

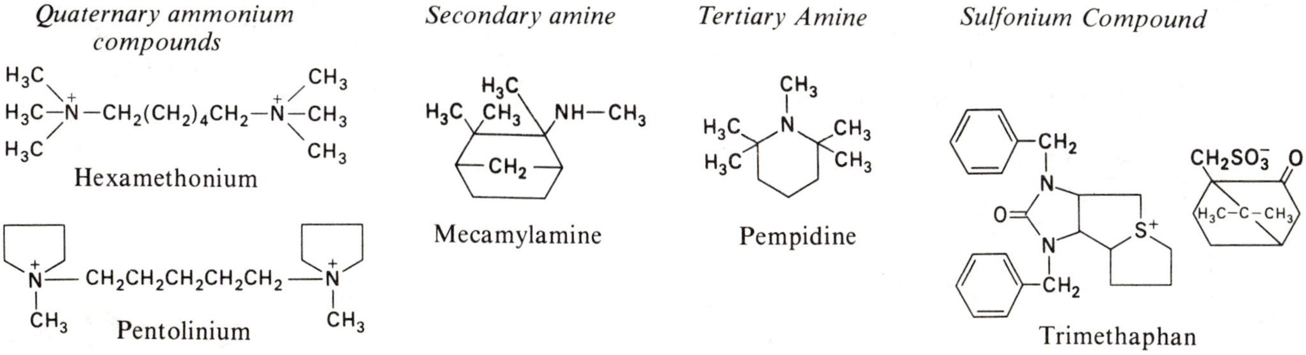

Quaternary ammonium compounds

$(H_3C)_3\overset{+}{N}-CH_2(CH_2)_4CH_2-\overset{+}{N}(CH_3)_3$

Hexamethonium

Pentolinium (CH_3-pyrrolidinium$-CH_2CH_2CH_2CH_2CH_2-$pyrrolidinium-CH_3)

Secondary amine

Mecamylamine

Tertiary Amine

Pempidine

Sulfonium Compound

Trimethaphan

Fig. 8.4-2. *Chemical structures of ganglion blocking agents.*

and incomplete due to the inhibitory effect on peristalsis in the gastrointestinal tract as well as poor penetration of quaternary ions across cellular membranes. Further distribution is limited to the extracellular space, and the unchanged compound is eliminated via the kidney. Both mecamylamine and pempidine are readily and completely absorbed from the small intestine. These agents are distributed throughout the body, including the CNS, and may accumulate in kidney and liver. Mecamylamine is slowly eliminated unchanged through the kidney and hence has a longer duration of action than most other ganglion blocking agents. Trimethaphan, an agent that contains a triethylsulfonium ion, has a very brief duration of action and is usually administered by i.v. drip, whereas the duration of action of other compounds varies between 6 and 12 hours.

Side Effects and Contraindications. The principal side effect of ganglion blocking drugs is marked hypotension, which may lead to impaired cerebral circulation and impaired glomerular filtration. Other side effects include anticholinergic effects, such as pupillary dilation, dry mouth, urinary retention, constipation, paralytic ileus, and failure of erection and ejaculation. Tremors, confusion, and hallucination may occur with mecamylamine due to central actions, but these reactions are not shared by quaternary compounds. Some degree of tolerance develops to the side effects with continued administration. Ganglion blocking drugs are contraindicated in patients with severe coronary artery disease, cerebrovascular insufficiency, diabetes mellitus on oral hypoglycemic drugs, glaucoma, or enlarged prostate.

Therapeutic Uses. Because of various potential adverse effects of ganglion blocking drugs, particularly orthostatic hypotension, urinary retention, and paralytic ileus, their clinical use is limited to the treatment of severe or malignant forms of hypertension and hypertensive emergencies only. Trimethaphan is considered as a drug of choice in the treatment of hypertension associated with acute dissecting aortic aneurysm and has also been used for production of controlled hypotension during neurosurgery and some cardiovascular operations. Therapy with ganglion blocking agents is further discussed in Chapter 15.3.

Drug Interactions. Ganglion blocking drugs potentiate the pressor effects of norepinephrine, phenylephrine, and other indirectly acting sympathomimetic agents, and also the depressor effects of acetylcholine, histamine, and other hypotensive drugs. This can be explained by the fact that ganglion blocking agents interfere with the reflex adjustment of the circulation. When blood pressure is increased or decreased, normally baroreceptor homeostatic mechanism attempts to normalize the pressure by adjusting the sympathetic and parasympathetic outflows. In presence of ganglion blocking agents, these autonomic outflows are inhibited at the ganglion level, thereby interfering and delaying the homeostatic mechanism. Concomitant use of alcohol and ganglion blocking drugs results in enhanced hypotensive effect due to synergism.

Preparations. *Trimethaphan camsylate* (ARFONAD): 10-ml ampules (50 mg/ml).

Mecamylamine hydrochloride, USP (INVERSINE): tablets (2.5 and 10 mg). Dose 2.5 mg twice daily.

GENERAL READING

Birmingham, A. T. A comparsion of the skeletal neuromuscular autonomic ganglion-blocking potencies of five non-depolarizing relaxants. *Br. J. Pharmacol.* 70:501, 1980.

Doyle, A. E. The introduction of ganglion-blocking drugs for the treatment of hypertension. *Br. J. Clin. Pharmacol.* 13:63, 1982.

Eranko, O., Small intensely fluorescent (SIF) cells and nervous transmission in sympathetic ganglia. *Ann. Rev. Pharmacol. Toxicol.* 18:417, 1978.

Gardier, R.W. et al. A mechanism of tolerance to the antihypertensive effect of ganglionic blocking agents in rats. *Arch. Int. Pharmacodyn. Ther.* 267:35, 1984.

Gurney, A.M. and Rang, H.P. The channel blocking action of methonium compounds on rat submandibular ganglion cells. *Br. J. Pharmacol.* 82:623, 1984.

Leigh, J. M. The history of controlled hypotension. *Br. J. Anaesth.* 47:745, 1975.

Libet, B. Generation of slow inhibitory and excitatory postsynaptic potentials. *Fed. Proc.* 29:1945, 1970.

Libet, B. The role SIF cells play in ganglionic transmission. *Adv. Biochem. Psychopharmacol.* 16:541, 1977.

Purves, D., and Lichtman, J. W. Formation and maintenance of synaptic connections in autonomic ganglia. *Physiol. Rev.* 58:821, 1978.

Salem, M. R. Therapeutic uses of ganglionic blocking drugs. *Int. Anesthesiol. Clin.* 16:171, 1978.

Volle, R. L. Ganglionic transmission. *Ann. Rev. Pharmacol.* 9:135, 1969.

Weight, F. F., Schulman, J. A., Smith, P. A., and Busis, N. A. Long-lasting synaptic potentials and the modulation of synaptic transmission. *Fed. Proc.* 38:2084, 1979.

Moe, G. K., Rennick, B. R., Capo, L. R., and Marshall, M. R. Tetraethylammonium as an aid in the study of cardiovascular reflexes. *Am. J. Physiol.* 157:158, 1949.

CHAPTER
9

DRUGS AFFECTING MUSCLE TONE AND CONTRACTION

Sachin N. Pradhan

SKELETAL MUSCLE TONE AND ITS REGULATION

Skeletal muscles receive their motor nerve supply from the anterior horn cells of the spinal cord and the analogous nuclei of the brain stem. A nerve supplying a muscle contains both motor (efferent) and sensory (afferent) fibers. A single motor nerve fiber (an axon) is responsible for the innervation of a definite group of muscle fibers, sending a filament to each muscle fiber of the group. All efferent nerves to voluntary muscle stimulate the muscle to contract. Relaxation is achieved by reducing or terminating the neuromotor stimuli. The activity of the motor unit system may be responsible to a certain extent for tension or tone always present in muscle even when it is at rest.

Tapping the tendon, or belly, of a muscle to elicit the tendon jerk, stretches the muscle between its points of origin and insertion only very briefly. Such stretching stimulates the muscle to twitch. Stretch, or myotatic reflex, is responsible for maintenance of tone of the muscle, which may be viewed as the resistance of a muscle to passive elongation or stretch. A schematic diagram of such a reflex arc is given in Fig. 9-1.

The efferent neurons are of two types: (1) skeletomotor neurons (or α-motoneurons) consisting of large cell bodies and innervating skeletal (extrafusal) muscles and (2) fusimotor neurons (or γ-motoneurons) with smaller cell bodies connecting the intrafusal muscle fibers. Activation of fusimotor neurons (primarily from supraspinal centers) would result in contraction of intrafusal muscle fibers and an increase in discharge from that particular muscle via the group-Ia afferent fibers to skeletomotor neurons (i.e., the γ-loop) that in turn would contract the skeletal (extrafusal) muscle fibers. γ-motoneurons chiefly contribute to the postural tone.

The brain stem reticular formation, which exerts a powerful influence on α- and γ-motoneurons, has a large facilitatory zone (extending from the middle of the medulla to the subthalamus) and a smaller inhibitory zone (in the caudal portion of the medulla). The facilitatory reticular formation receives strong excitatory input from ascending sensory pathways as well as from the eighth cranial nerve through the vestibular nuclei. The motor cortex, basal ganglia, and the cerebellum also control and harness the reticular activity. The facilitatory reticular formation exerts descending influence via the reticulospinal and vestibulospinal pathways, and has its action heavily biased toward extensor reflexes. The

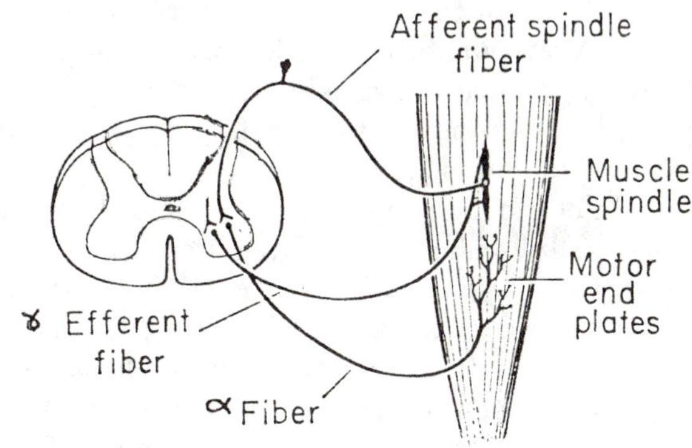

Fig.9-1. *A simple reflex arc showing the spinal center with afferent and efferent pathways.*

motor functions of the reticular formation are chiefly directed toward control of muscle tone and posture. These functions have been mainly studied in decerebrate cats, in which the increased extensor tone has been shown to be mediated by two mechanisms that can act separately or together. One mechanism involves direct action of the descending pathways upon α- or skeletomotor neurons either through monosynaptic connection or via spinal interneurons. The second mechanism is via γ- or fusimotor neurons and γ-loop. In this way descending impulses from the brain stem can activate extensor motoneurons and thereby reflexly increase extensor skeletomotor neuron discharges causing extensor hypertonia. Thus, although the final common path for control of muscle tone is the motor unit consisting of the skeletomotor neuron and the muscle fibers it innervates, both α- and γ-motor mechanisms can modulate the activity of the motor unit acting through monosynaptic and polysynaptic pathways. Drugs can modify muscle tone by acting specifically on α- or γ-motor mechanisms or nonspecifically blocking the polysynaptic pathways or affecting neuronal excitability.

NEUROMUSCULAR JUNCTION

Motor nerve fibers to the skeletal muscle are myelinated up to the point of their entry into the muscle. Near the muscle each branch of the myelinated motor axon is divided into as many as 200 divergent unmyelinated terminal filaments. Usually one branch terminal forms a single end-plate region on a single muscle fiber. Each unmyelinated axon terminal remains embedded in an indentation in the surfaces of the muscle fiber. The cell membranes of nerves (axonal membrane) and muscles (sarcolemma), each of which are continuous and distinct, remain separated by a (primary) synaptic cleft approximately 50 nm wide. The outer surface of the nerve terminal, which is away from the muscle cell, remains covered with a Schwann cell sheath that also covers preterminal axon; thus, the unmyelinated nerve fiber remains completely insulated from the surrounding connective tissue.

Synaptic Trough. The motor nerve terminal is embedded in a region ofthe muscle fiber (synaptic trough) where the muscle cell membrane is thrown into folds (palisades or secondary synaptic clefts) that open into the primary synaptic clefts (Fig. 9-2).

The motor nerve terminals contain mitochondria and many small globular bodies having structureless interiors called synaptic vesicles. The nerve terminals along their courses show a series of nodulelike enlargements, where the density of the vesicles is much greater than that in the intermediate regions. These vesicles that contain the neurotransmitter, acetylcholine, are frequently seen to be congregated within the axoplasm just opposite each postjunctional fold of the muscle membrane. At this position the axon membrane shows thickened local regions called *active regions.*

Nicotinic Cholinergic Receptor. Nicotinic cholinergic receptor with which acetylcholine (ACh) combines to initiate the end-plate potential (EPP) has been isolated from the electric organs of the aquatic species of *Electrophorus* and, especially, *Torpedo* (2, 9). The electric organ is derived embryologically from the myoid tissue, but unlike the skeletal muscle, a significant fraction of the surface of its membrane contains cholinergic receptors and is excitable. The receptor is capable of binding with snake venom α-bungarotoxin (13), which has high affinity and selectivity for the receptor and which has been initially used to facilitate its isolation (3).

The ACh receptor is a glycoprotein made up of five subunits, chains of about 500 amino acids. It comprises four types of polypeptide chains of apparent molecular weights [determined by SDS gel electrophoresis of 39,000 (α), 48,000 (β), 58,000 (γ), and 64,000 (δ) in the stoichiometry $\alpha_2\beta\ \gamma\ \delta$ (6)]. The estimate of molecular weights thus determined may be about 10% low compared with those determined by sedimentation equilibrium. The complete amino acid sequences of each of these four subunits have been determined.

The two of the subunits (α) that are identical contain binding sites for both ACh and α-bungarotoxin (4). The toxin competes with the cholinergic agonists and antagonists for the same binding sites in the receptor. The other three chains (β, γ, δ) are unique and may have additional ACh binding sites, perhaps involved in desensitization of

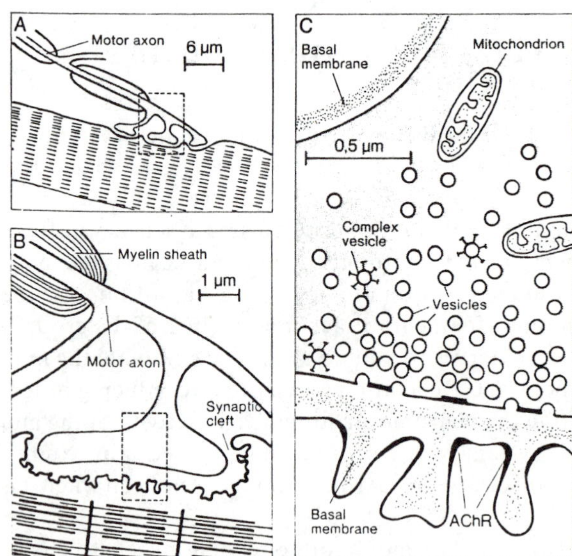

Fig.9-2. *A-C: Elements of a cholinergic synapse in a neuromuscular junctiion.*

Sections through the end-plate region of a skeletal muscle fiber; B and C are enlarged sections of A and B, respectively. These are schematized from electron micrographs of many authors. The synaptic cleft is disproportionately wide in each drawing. AChR denotes subsynaptic localization of the ACh receptors; the basal membrane may be the site for localization of the cholinesterase. (From Ref. 11 by permission).

the receptor in the presence of high ACh concentration (7). Most likely subunit arrangement (proposed by Karlin) is α-γ-α-δ-β (6). However, Stroud has proposed a different order of the subunits: α-β-α-γ-δ, as shown in the three-dimensional model for ACh receptor in Fig. 9-3, which also marks the neurotoxin binding sites (12). Other chemicals acting at different location in the receptor molecule include local anesthetics, psychotropic drugs, antiviral agents, plant poisons, detergents, and alcohols.

The central region of the receptor is traversed by a cylindrical pore perpendicular to the membrane, about 7.2 Å in diameter. The pore is presumably the ion channel gated by cholinergic ligands (like ACh).

According to previous theory, when two ACh molecules attach to a receptor on the muscle cell the channel rapidly opens, allowing free flow of ions such as sodium and potassium across the membrane. The channel remains open for a few milliseconds, then closes; the ACh molecule dissociates, leaving the receptor free to bind another ACh molecule and to begin the cycle. The new *patch clamp* technique reveals further details to this process of ionic permeability changes (7). It is now known that at least two open states of the channel exist of which the shorter open time represents binding to a single ACh molecule and the longer open time represents a more stable state after binding with two ACh molecules. The channel open times are interrupted by very brief closed times, averaging 50 msec; sometimes ACh receptors enter a state where only one-third of the normal amount of open-state current flows; and variations in the ion flow across the membrane increases when the channel is open.

NEUROMUSCULAR TRANSMISSION

Stimulation of a motor nerve generates a nerve action potential (NAP) that travels along the nerve to the branch

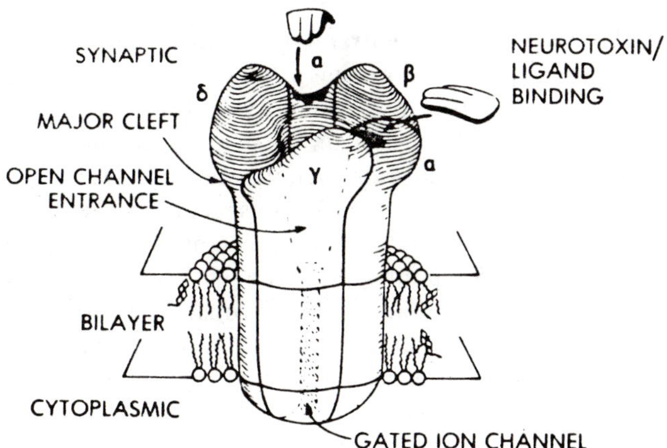

Fig.9-3. *Three dimensional structure of the ACh receptor with the neurotoxin-binding sites as deduced from x-ray scattering and electron microscopy. Positions around the receptor crest are tentative.* (From Ref. 12 by permission).

terminals, where it causes a small influx of Ca^{2+} ions. The entering Ca^{2+} causes the ACh vesicles to approach the prejunctional (presynaptic) membrane that, as well as the vesicle membrane, becomes negatively charged. The ACh vesicles then fuse with the presynaptic membrane and release their ACh content into the synaptic cleft by a process known as exocytosis. Such mechanism might be expected to produce a steady increase in the total area of the presynaptic membrane. However, this does not happen because new synaptic vesicles are constantly being formed at the edges of the synaptic region by pinocytosis (Chapter 2). By the latter process, the membrane of the emptied vesicle incorporated with the synaptic membrane is pulled back into the cytoplasm by contractile filaments, forming a basket that is later converted to a cistern. The cistern is then filled with resynthesized ACh forming a new ACh vesicle that migrates toward the center of the nerve terminal, and the cycle is repeated.

Released ACh diffuses across the synaptic cleft (200 Å) within approximately 0.1 msec, and combines to the ACh receptors located on the outside of the sarcolemma (postjunctional muscle membrane); ACh injected inside the muscle is ineffective. ACh acting on the postjunctional membrane receptor simultaneously opens up channels for Na^+ and K^+ in the sarcolemma, resulting in depolarization of the end-plate and generation of an end-plate potential (EPP).

After its release, ACh normally acts on the postsynaptic membrane for only a very short time (1-2 msec), since some of it diffuses away and some is hydrolyzed by the enzyme acetylcholinesterase (AChE); it is split into the ineffective components choline and acetic acid. Special staining methods have shown that AChE is present at the end-plate in large amounts (specific or true cholinesterase), but cholinesterase is also present in the plasma (pseudocholinesterase). Thus, the ACh that diffuses from the end-plate into the surrounding extracellular space and into the bloodstream is also broken down into choline and acetic acid. Most of the choline product of ACh hydrolysis is reuptaken into the presynaptic terminal by active transport and is reutilized for ACh synthesis.

A vesicle spontaneously releases a quantum (10^3-10^4 molecules) of ACh that produces a miniature end-plate potential (MEPP), as occurs at the rate of 2/sec. When a nerve impulse is elicited, about 200 vesicles release ACh simultaneously, producing a normal EPP of 10-15 mv. If the EPP exceeds 15 mv, an action potential is produced on the muscle membrane. The muscle action potential (MAP) travels along the muscle membrane and is carried into the central portion of the myofibril by the transverse tubular system (Fig. 9-4). The transverse tubules (or T tubules) are formed apparently by invagination of the plasma membrane. They form part of the internal membrane system (also referred to as triad). Each transverse tubule is in intimate contact on either side with the dilated ends (cisternae) of the sarcoplasmic reticulum (thus form-

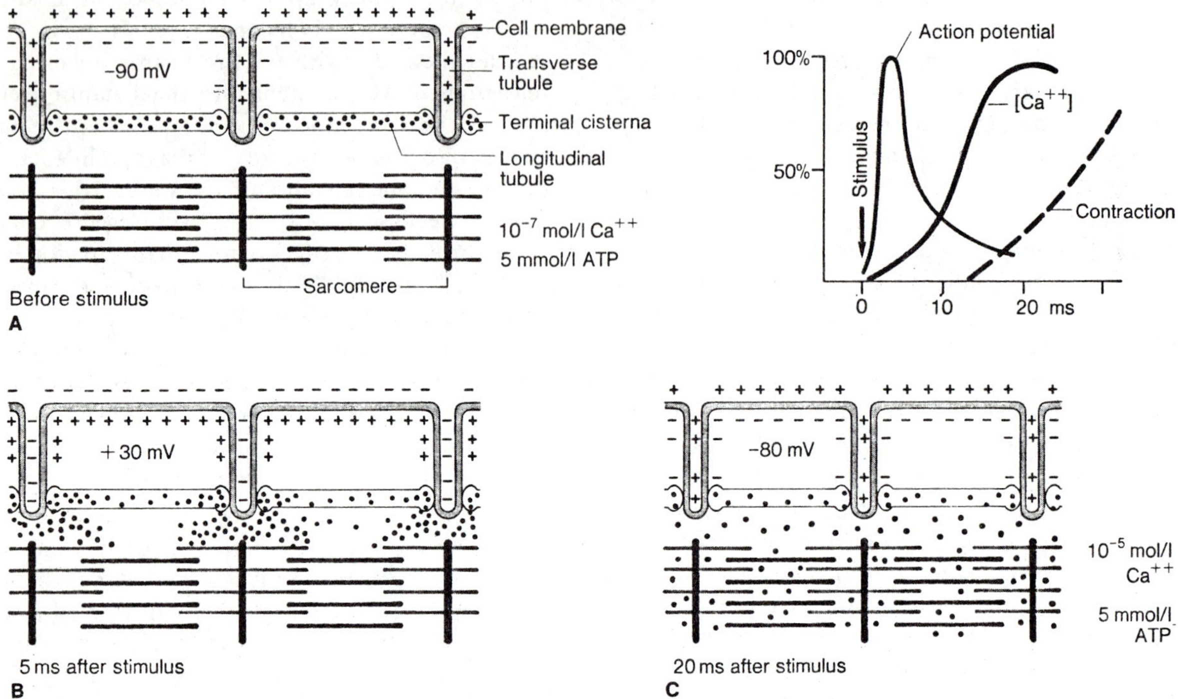

Fig.9-4. *Diagram of the excitation-contraction coupling.*
A: A relaxed muscle fiber with the polarized cell membrane. The intracellular Ca^{2+} concentration is below 10^{-7} M. B: During the action potential the polarization of the cell membrane and the transverse-tubule membrane is reversed; Ca^{2+}ions begin to flow out of the terminal cisternae. C: The intracellular Ca^{2+} concentration has reached approxmately 10^{-5} M at the end of the action potential; the sarcomeres of the myofibrils contract. Inset: the temporal sequence of events in the excitation-contraction coupling during the latency and at the beginning of contraction in the frog sartorius (0^0C) . (From Ref. 10 by permission).

ing a group of three tubules or triads). A continuity between the membrane of the T tubules and that of the lateral cisternae has been revealed by electron microscopic studies; this has led to the suggestion that just as an action potential can travel from plasma membrane to T tubules, it can also pass across the junction between T tubules and lateral cisternae, thus depolarizing the membrane of the sarcoplasmic reticulum. When the MAP invades the sarcoplasmic reticulum, it produces a release of Ca^{2+} from the reticulum. The released Ca^{2+} may bring the level of cytosol Ca^{2+} from a normal of $\sim 10^{-7}$M-$\sim 10^{-6}$M, which would trigger interactions of troponin, actin, and myosin, resulting in muscle contraction. A few milliseconds after the Ca^{2+} is released, the reticulum reabsorbes the Ca^{2+} causing muscle relaxation. The events between arrival of the nerve impulse at the nerve ending and the initiation of an impulse in the muscle are referred to as *neuromuscular transmission;* the events between muscle fiber impulse and contraction are referred to as excitation-contraction coupling to distinguish them from the contraction process itself. The events beginning from the stimulation of a motor nerve to the contraction of a skeletal muscle along with their sites and mechanism are summarized in Table 9-1.

MODIFICATION OF MUSCLE TONE BY VARIOUS AGENTS

Muscle tone can be affected by agents that modify muscle contraction by acting at various steps in the process of neuromuscular transmission.

Agents Acting on Central Regulation of Muscle Tone. Certain centrally acting drugs produce muscle relaxation by their more selective action on γ-motoneuron system (e.g., benzodiazepines) or on the α-motoneuron system (e.g., phenothiazine antipsychotic agents). Drugs like mephensin appear to block nonspecific polysynaptic responses (Chapter 9.2). CNS depressants like inhalation anesthetics and hypnotic-sedative agents also cause muscle relaxation by stabilizing the neuronal membrane so as to decrease transmitter release in response to nerve stimulation and also by depressing postsynaptic responsiveness.

Agents Acting on Nerve Impulse. Propagation of nerve action potential is inhibited by local and general anesthetics and tetrodotoxin. Local anesthetics (and also general anesthetics like barbiturates) block conduction of the nerve impulse by decreasing or preventing large transient

Table 9-1
Sites and Mechanisms of Events Leading to Skeletal Muscle Contraction and Drug Actions

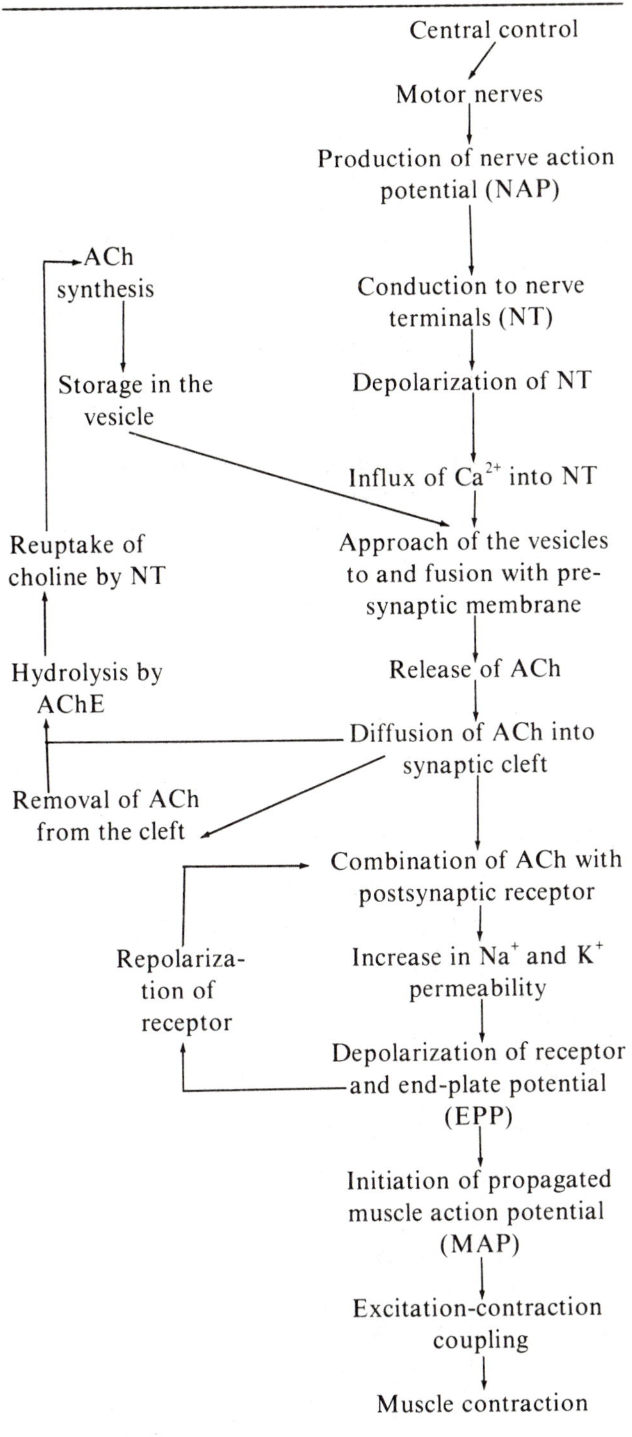

increase in the permeability of the membrane to Na^+ ions associated with membrane depolarization. Tetrodotoxin (from Japanese puffer fish) and saxitoxin (from shell fish feeding on dinoflagellates, *Gonyaulax*) block sodium channels in the excitable membrane (5). On the other hand, batrachotoxin, a steroidal alkaloid secreted by a South American frog, produces muscle paralysis by causing persistent depolarization through a selective increase in sodium permeability (1).

Agents Acting on ACh Synthesis and Release. Hemicholinium reduces ACh release by inhibiting choline reuptake into the cholinergic nerve terminal and ACh synthesis. Botulinus toxin binds irreversibly to the site of action in the prejunctional membrane and prevents release of ACh by exocytosis. Release by exocytosis is facilitated by low concentration of ethanol and excess of Ca^{2+} (8). Black widow spider venom causes complete release of ACh from all vesicles, causing muscle cramps.

Agents Acting on End-plate Depolarization. An α-toxin (α-bungarotoxin) from venom of krait, *Bungarus multicintus,* or varieties of cobra, *Naja naja,* binds irreversibly to cholinergic receptors and blocks neuromuscular transmission (13). d-Tubocurarine competitively blocks the action of ACh at the cholinergic receptor site at the postjunctional membrane, thus reducing the MEPP and EPP. This block can be reversed by increasing the concentration of ACh, such as following administration of anticholinesterases. Hence, these agents are called *competitive neuromuscular-blocking* agents. Since they do not depolarize or otherwise disturb the receptor, they are also termed *nondepolarizing* or *stabilizing* agents.

Succinylcholine and decamethonium produce an initial depolarization like ACh, but unlike ACh they persist at the neuromuscular junction, thereby prolonging the depolarization. During this period of persistent depolarization, the muscle is unable to respond to ACh or nerve stimulation. Drug effect is manifested as initial transient muscular fasciculations followed by muscle relaxation. These agents have been termed *depolarizing* agents. Their effects are similar to those of high, paralyzing doses of ACh in the presence of an antiacetylcholinesterase (anti-AChE) agent. Their effect is not antagonized by anti-AChE agents.

Quinine decreases the excitability of the motor end-plate region of skeletal muscle, and following a single maximal stimulus increases the refractory period of muscle, although the tension response is increased; as a result, responses to repetitive nerve stimulation and to acetylcholine are reduced. Thus, it produces a curarelike effect and can antagonize the action of physostigmine like curare. Quinine can symptomatically relieve myotonia congentina and aggravate symptoms of myasthenia gravis.

Agents Acting Directly on the Muscle. Dantrolene causes reduction of skeletal muscle contraction by acting directly on the skeletal muscle through uncoupling of excitation from contraction probably by impairing release of calcium from the sarcoplasmic reticulum.

The effects of drugs on various processes involving muscle tone and contraction are summarized in Table 9-2.

Table 9-2
Effects of Drugs on Processes Involving Muscle Tone and Contraction

Process/Site	Stimulated By	Inhibited By
Central[a]		
α-Motoneuron system	—	Major (antipsychotic) tranquilizers
γ-Motoneuron system	—	Minor (antianxiety) tranquilizers
Polysynaptic neurotransmission	—	Mephenesin and other central muscle relaxants
Peripheral		
Nerve action potential	—	Tetrodotoxin, saxitoxin, batrachotoxin, local anesthetics
Acetylcholine		
Synthesis	—	Hemicholinium
Release	Excess of Ca^{2+}, black widow spider venom	Lack of Ca^{2+}, Mg^{2+}, botulinum toxin, procaine
End-plate		
Depolarization	Neostigmine, DFP, K^+	Competitive neuromuscular blocking agents (e.g., curare alkaloids)
Repolarization	—	Depolarizing agents (e.g., succinylcholine)
Muscle action potential	Ca^{2+}, veratrine	Quinine
Muscle contraction	—	Lack of Ca^{2+}, dantrolene

[a] CNS stimulants and depressants also affect the muscle tone and contraction by acting on various central mechanisms and sites.

REFERENCES

1. Alburquerque, E. X., Seyama, I., and Narahashi, T. Characterization of batrachotoxin-induced depolarization of the squid giant axons. *J. Pharmacol. Exp. Ther.* 184:308, 1973.
2. Colquhoun, D. Mechanisms of action at the voluntary muscle end-plate. *Ann. Rev. Pharmacol.* 15:307, 1975.
3. Fambrough, D. Control of acetylcholine receptors in skeletal muscle. *Physiol. Rev.* 59:165, 1979.
4. Heidmann, T., and Changeux, J. P. Structural and functional properties of the acetylcholine receptor protein in its purified and membrane bound states. *Ann. Rev. Biochem.* 47:317, 1978.
5. Kao, C. Y. Tetrodotoxin, saxitoxin, and their significance in the study of excitation phenomena. *Pharmacol. Rev.* 18:997, 1966.
6. Karlin, A. The anatomy of a receptor. *Neurosci. Commentaries* 1:111, 1983.
7. Miller, J. A. Molecular hardware of cell communication: Describing the acetylcholine receptor, a nontechnical summary of the reviews in this issue. *Neurosci. Commentaries* 1:93, 1983.
8. Miyamoto, M. D. The actions of cholinergic drugs on motor nerve terminals. *Pharmacol. Rev.* 29:226, 1978.
9. Rang, H. P. Acetylcholine receptors. *Q. Rev. Biophys.* 7:283, 1975.
10. Rüegg, J. C. Muscle. In: *Human Physiology* (Schmidt, R. F., and Thews, G., eds.). New York: Springer-Verlag, 1983, p. 32.
11. Schmidt, R. F. The transmission of excitation from cell to cell. In: *Human Physiology* (Schmidt, R. F., and Thews, G., eds.). New York: Springer-Verlag, 1983, p. 51.
12. Stroud, R. M. Acetylcholine receptor structure. *Neurosci. Commentaries* 1:124, 1983.
13. Wang, G., Molinaro, S., and Schmidt, J. O. Ligand responses of the α-bungarotoxin binding sites from skeletal muscle and the optic lobe of the chick. *J. Biol. Chem.* 253:8507, 1978.

ADDITIONAL READING

Viby-Mogensen, J. Clinical assessment of neuromuscular transmission. *Br. J. Anaesth.* 54:209, 1982.

CHAPTER
9.1

PERIPHERAL MUSCLE RELAXANTS

Sachin N. Pradhan

HISTORY

The European conquerors of the Amazon basin found natives using poison-tipped darts shot from blowguns to hunt birds and monkeys. The poison acted rapidly, causing the game to die quickly and fall from the treetops to the forest floor, where it could be picked up easily by the hunters. Despite the lethal action of the poison on the prey, people ate the flesh with impunity. The poison, prepared ritually from plants, intrigued the Europeans who sought information on its nature and mechanism. Crude material was brought to Europe and in the late 1850s a French scientist, Claude Bernard, began studies that are classics of experimental biology (5). Bernard learned that curare caused paralysis of skeletal muscle by acting at the precise point where nerves meet muscles, the area now known as the neuromuscular junction. These experiments not only identified the neuromuscular junction, but also showed that a specific agent could be used to study neuromuscular transmission, thereby opening the way to the study of synaptic function and neurohumoral transmission. Curare and its synthetic derivatives still play an essential role in the investigation of synaptic physiology.

In 1935 King published the structure of d-tubocurarine (19), the active principle in curare; 6 years later Griffith and Johnson described its use to produce muscle relaxation during surgery (16). These events opened the era of modern anesthesiology. Formerly, a surgeon had to use force to move powerful abdominal or limb muscles out of the way, or the anesthetist had to give dangerously high concentrations of diethyl ether to induce relaxation. Tubocurarine permits complete muscle relaxation at safe concentrations of anesthetics and allows anesthesiologists to adjust anesthesia to the needs of each patient.

CLASSIFICATION

Various types of agents affecting muscle tone and contraction were discussed in Chapter 9. Among them, the clinically effective agents that cause peripheral muscle relaxation are known as neuromuscular blocking agents. They affect end-plate depolarization and, as indicated in Chapter 9, can be classified into two groups: (1) competitive (nondepolarizing) agents such as d-tubocurarine, gallamine, and so on, and (2) depolarizing agents such as succinylcholine and decamethonium. The agents of the first group competitively block the depolarizing action of acetylcholine (ACh) on the receptor (in the end-plate), and this block can be reversed by increasing the concentration of ACh. They themselves do not depolarize the receptor. On the other hand, the depolarizing agents cause initial depolarization of the end-plate like ACh, but unlike ACh they persist at the neuromuscular junction and prolong depolarization, during which the end-plate is unable to respond to ACh or nerve stimulation. Because repolarization of the end-plate and its repetitive firing by vollies of ACh are needed to produce miniature muscle contractions in order to maintain muscle tone, flaccid paralysis is manifested during persistent depolarization of the end-plate. Anticholinesterase agents do not reverse such blockade, rather they may potentiate it.

However, under clinical circumstances involving depolarizing agents blockade has been observed. In the case of succinylcholine, by increasing its concentration, in time the blockade changes from a depolarizing type (called phase I) to a nondepolarizing type (phase II). The type of blockade may depend on the general anesthetic used. Thus fluorinated hydrocarbons may predispose the system to nondepolarization blockade (31). The pharmacology of the competitive and depolarizing neuromuscular blocking agents has been described in several recent reviews (13, 21, 27, 28, 31, 32). In addition to discussion on the two types of neuromuscular blocking agents, this chapter will include a drug, dantrolene, which unlike neuromuscular blocking agents or centrally acting muscle relaxants, reduces skeletal muscle contraction by uncoupling excitation from contraction.

CHEMISTRY

A few generalizations (with some exceptions) can be made in connection with the structure-activity relationship regarding the neuromuscular blocking agents. Quaternary ammonium groups appear to be an important part of these compounds. Most of the therapeutically used compounds have two quaternary ammonium groups; gallamine has three groups. Such a structure suggests that electrostatic or coulombic association exists between the cationic groups of the drug and certain anionic centers in their receptor. Quaternization of nitrogen in many drugs like atropine, strychnine, quinine, and so on, increases their neuromuscular blocking effect. However, tertiary amine β-erythroidine and β-hydroerythroidine possess potent neuromuscular blocking effects; quaternization of nitrogen in these compounds abolishes their blocking effect.

The competitive agents (e.g., d-tubocurarine, β-erythroidine, gallamine, pancuronium) have relatively bulky rigid molecules compared with the more flexible structure of the depolarizing compounds (e.g., succinylcholine, decamethonium).

The distance between the quaternary nitrogens in the depolarizing agents may vary up to the limit of the maximum bond distance (e.g., 1.45 nm for decamethonium), but is usually less for the rigid competitive blockers (1 ± 0.1 nm). The internitrogen distance for d-tubocurarine is 1.03 nm. In d-tubocurarine all the polar groups reside on one of its surfaces, whereas in l-tubocurarine, which is 20- to 60-fold less potent than its d-isomer and has similar internitrogen distance, the polar group does not reside on one surface.

MECHANISM OF ACTION

It was mentioned earlier that ACh released from the nerve terminal at the neuromuscular junction acts on postsynaptic receptors outside the sarcolemma by opening up the ionic channels, which results in end-plate potential (EPP). Recent sophisticated electrophysiological techniques such as direct recording from a single-receptor channel with a suction electrode on denervated skeletal muscle have been used to further analyze the electrical events associated with EPP. Such techniques (22, 23) have demonstrated that the fundamental event elicited by an agonist is an all-or-none opening and closing of individual ionic channels in the receptor, resulting in a square wave pulse with an average open channel conductance of ~ 30 pico siemens and duration of about 1 msec. EPP is the summation of such pulses resulting from all the receptor channels opening at the time. An antagonist like d-tubocurarine (3) competes with ACh for combining with the receptor and reduces the frequency of channel opening, but not the conductance or duration of opening for a single channel. This results in decrease in amplitude and duration of the EPP, which is dose dependent (10).

Depolarizing agents like decamethonium produce channel opening during their binding with the receptor, but probability of opening is less than that caused by ACh or carbachol. Hence, decamethonium may be designated as a partial agonist; it can also block the channel directly at high concentrations (1).

NEUROMUSCULAR BLOCKING AGENTS

COMPETITIVE BLOCKING AGENTS

d-TUBOCURARINE

Pharmacological Effects

Skeletal Muscles. With an intravenous dose (10-15 mg) of d-tubocurarine in humans, flaccid paralysis occurs rapidly without any initial muscular fasciculation (as seen with the depolarizing agents). The muscles of eye and jaw are affected first, followed by those of other small muscles of head and neck, as manifested by difficulty in speech, ptosis, strabismus, diplopia, and dysphagia. Limbs that are next affected feel heavy and are difficult to move. Then intercostal muscles and finally diaphragm are affected, showing signs of paralysis. Relaxation of abdominal muscles occurs after substantial paralysis of ventilatory muscles. During the stage of complete muscle paralysis, sensations and consciousness remain unaffected.

A single intravenous dose produces maximum paralysis in 3-5 min. The action begins to wear off in about 20 min and may persist for more than an hour in some individuals. Some residual effect may remain for a longer period. When a second dose is repeated within 24 hours, usually less dose is needed to produce equilvalent effect.

Histamine Release. d-Tubocurarine causes histamine release. Bronchospasm, hypotension, and excessive bronchial and salivary secretion observed after its administration are suggested to be due to histamine. d-Tubocurarine also produces typical histaminelike wheals when injected intracutaneously or intraarterially in humans. Antihistamines can prevent these effects.

Cardiovascular Effects. Rapid intravenous injection of large doses of d-tubocurarine causes rapid severe hypotension. The latter may result from peripheral vasodilation due to induced histamine release and ganglion blockade in addition to increased venous pooling in relaxed muscles.

Other Effects. In addition to hypotension, induced blockade of autonomic ganglia may cause decrease of tone and motility of the gastrointestinal tract.

Pharmacokinetics. Tubocurarine is inactive when given orally, unless huge doses are ingested. The drug is ionized and does not easily cross lipid membranes; hence, its absorption is erratic and incomplete. That is why, despite the lethality of the poison on prey, the flesh could be eaten with impunity; this was known to the South American Indians. The drug is always administered intravenously, and because the neuromuscular junctions are well supplied with capillaries it acts quickly. The distribution is limited to the extracellular space, and the drug appears to concentrate in the neuromuscular junction. However, the action at the neuromuscular junction begins to decline in 20 min due to redistribution of the drug. About 40% of the drug is excreted unchanged in urine over several hours, with some amounts being excreted in the bile or metabolized. Tubocurarine does not readily penetrate the blood-brain barrier nor does it cross the placenta.

Drug Interactions. The muscle relaxant effect of d-tubocurarine is potentiated or prolonged by a number of drugs. Of the inhalation anesthetics, potentiation is most marked with enflurane (14) and isoflurane, less with ether and methoxyflurane, and least with halothane and cyclopropane. Potentiation or prolongation of tubocurarine effect is also observed with many antibiotics (24) [e.g., aminoglycosides (streptomycin, neomycin, viomycin, kanamycin, gentamicin, amikacin), tetracyclines, polypeptides (polymyxins A and B, colistin), clindamycin, and lincomycin]. Streptomycin resembles Mg^{2+} ions in producing neuromuscular blockade by inhibiting release of ACh from preganglionic nerve terminals through competition with Ca^{2+} ions and to a less extent also by stabilizing the postjunctional membrane. Other aminoglycosides also show a similar mechanism to varying degrees. Such blockade is reversed by Ca salts and only inconsistently by anti-AChE agents (e.g., neostigmine). On the other hand, tetracyclines produce the blockade possibly by Ca^{2+} ion chelation, and Ca salts also reverse such block. Local anesthetics, quinidine, β-adrenoceptor-blocking agents, magnesium sulfate, and trimethaphan have also been reported to potentiate tubocurarine effect.

Neuromuscular blockade by tubocurarine can be reversed by anti-AChE agents like neostigmine and edrophonium that prevent destruction of endogenous ACh and also act directly at the neuromuscular junction. These agents can be used to treat respiratory depression due to overdose of d-tubocurarine and other competitive neuromuscular blocking agents. Epinephrine and norepinephrine show weak anticurare action.

METOCURINE

Metocurine (dimethyl tubocurarine iodide), a semisynthetic derivative, is similar to tubocurarine except that it is approximately twice as potent, shorter in duration, and has less effect on circulatory system.

GALLAMINE

Compared with tubocurarine, gallamine, a synthetic compound, has slightly shorter duration of action, and a slightly larger dose of neostigmine may be needed to reverse its effect. It has an atropinelike effect, blocks cardiac vagus, and may cause sinus tachycardia and occasionally increased cardiac output and hypertension. Its blocking effect is diminished by respiratory acidosis and enhanced by alkalosis. It is excreted solely by the kidney.

PANCURONIUM

Pancuronium has a steroid structure with two quaternary ammonium group (Fig. 9.1-1). Compared with tubocurarine, it is about five times more potent. At equipotent dosage, it has a comparable onset and shorter duration of action. This drug does not cause ganglion blockade, and rarely, if at all, histamine release. Hence, bronchospasm and hypotension are not observed. In addition, it may increase heart rate, cardiac output, and arterial pressure primarily due to its vagolytic action and secondarily by blocking the neuronal uptake of norepinephrine. Atrioventricular conduction is accelerated, but cardiac contractility and peripheral resistance remain unaffected. It can inhibit plasma cholinesterase and prolong the action of succinylcholine.

Pancuronium is also administered intravenously and is distributed similarly as tubocurarine. However, it is hydrolyzed slowly in the liver to form the 3-hydroxy and 17-hydroxy derivatives with a potency of 0.5 and 0.01, respectively, of the precursor. About 80% of a dose of pancuronium is eliminated in urine (mostly as metabolites) when renal function is normal. The drug enters the fetal circulation in an insignificant amount, and hence it may be used safely in obstetrical anesthesia.

Adult dose for intubation is 0.1 mg/kg i.v. and for surgery, initially 0.04-0.1 mg/kg, followed by 0.01-0.02 mg/kg repeated as required. These doses are for use with nitrous oxide and must be reduced when used with more potent inhalation agents.

VECURONIUM

Vecuronium (NORCURON; Org NC 45), a monoquaternary analog of pancuronium, is a nondepolarizing muscle relaxant (6) (Fig. 9.1-1). Compared with pancuronium, it is about 1.5 times more potent, has a similar onset time, and about one-third to one-half duration of action (12). Unlike pancuronium, it causes minimal cumulative effects on repeated administration. The drug does not cause histamine release or significant ganglionic or vagal blockade, nor does it interfere with norepinephrine uptake (15). Consequently, it has little or no cardiovascular effects.

Its relative short duration of action and lack of cumulative effects can be explained by its rapid plasma clearance. In patients with chronic renal failure, clearance is

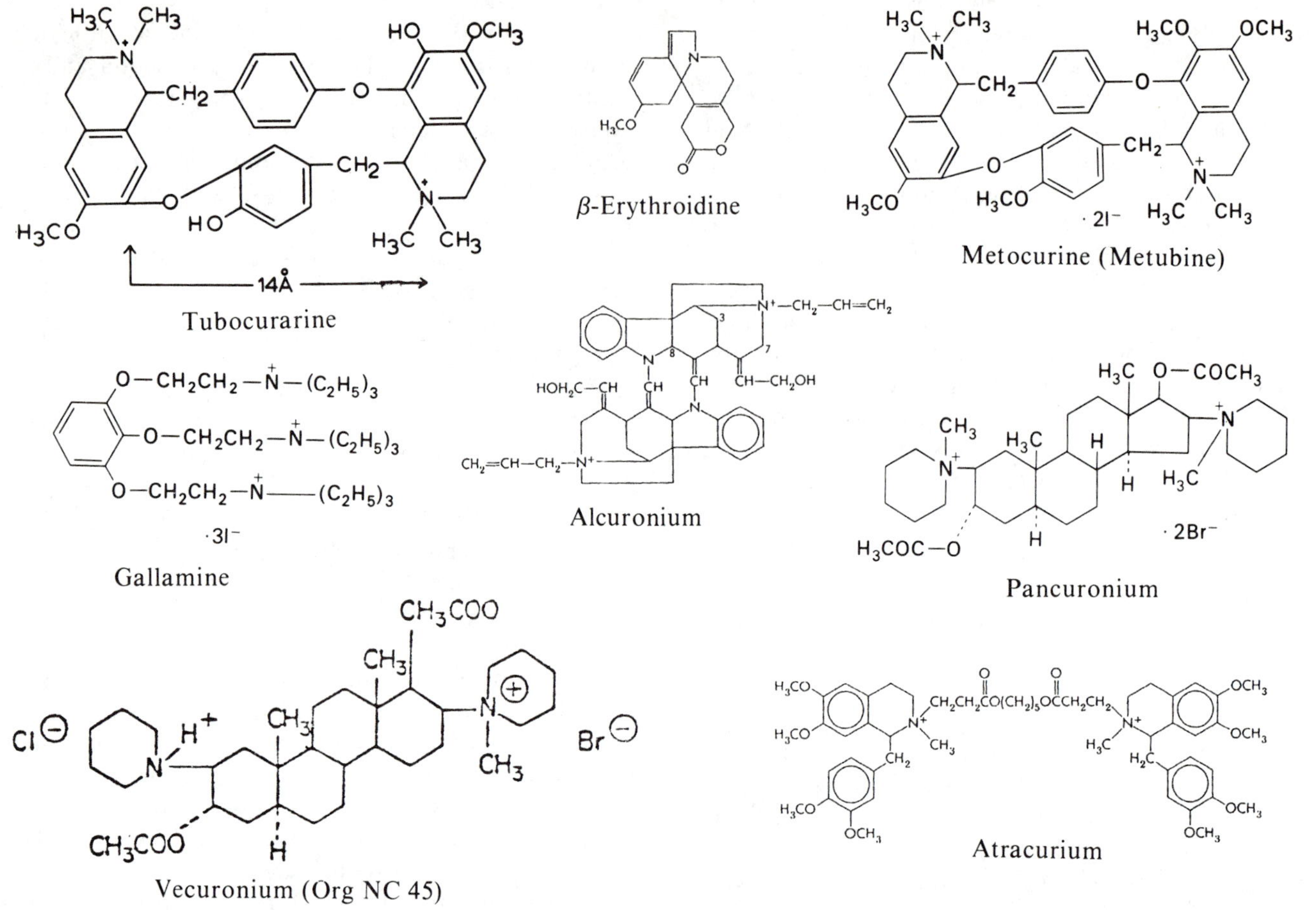

Tubocurarine

β-Erythroidine

Metocurine (Metubine)

Gallamine

Alcuronium

Pancuronium

Vecuronium (Org NC 45)

Atracurium

Fig. 9.1-1. *Competitive blocking agents.*

reduced by 12% with only a 32% prolongation of action compared with patients with normal renal functions. Animal studies also demonstrate increases in intensity and duration of neuromuscular blockade following temporary or permanent hepatic exclusion.

The drug is used to provide muscle relaxation during surgery and for endotracheal intubation. Its effect is readily reversible by neostigmine, pyridostigmine, or other anticholinesterase agents.

Adult dose i.v. for intubation is 0.07-0.14 mg/kg, and for surgery 0.04-0.1 mg/kg initially, followed by 0.015-0.02 mg/kg, repeated as needed.

ATRACURIUM

Atracurium, a symmetrical bis-quaternary ester (Fig. 9.1-1) is an investigational nondepolarizing muscle relaxant.

It is approximately as potent as d-tubocurarine, but with a shorter duration of action. A dose of 0.3 mg/kg produces adequate relaxation for 15-20 min (24). Muscle paralysis is readily antagonized by neostigmine. It appears from animal studies that plasma cholinesterase inhibition or renal or hepatic impairment does not significantly affect the duration of action. Such doses do not appear to produce any cardiovascular side effects (4, 17). Higher doses given in animal studies produce hypotension that could be partially antagonized by antihistamines.

The drug is inactivated by ester hydrolysis or by an alkaline-catalyzed Hofmann elimination of the bridging chain from one of the quaternary nitrogen atoms (4).

Intravenous dose is initially 0.3-0.6 mg/kg; subsequent doses are 0.05-0.1 mg/kg.

DEPOLARIZING BLOCKING AGENTS

SUCCINYLCHOLINE

Succinylcholine is the only neuromuscular blocking agent that is commonly used at present. Succinylcholine appears very closely as if two molecules of ACh have been joined together in mirror image as shown in Fig. 9.1-2.

Neuromuscular Blocking Effects. Succinylcholine produces neuromuscular blockade by persistent depolarization (phase I) followed by sensitization (phase II) of the muscle end-plate. Failure of the muscle end-plate to repolarize and lack of its repetitive firing that maintains the muscle tone result in a flaccid paralysis. Succinylcholine has a rapid onset (1 min) and short duration (5-10 min following 1-mg/kg doses). Tachyphylaxis may occur after rapid administration. The flaccid paralysis is pre-

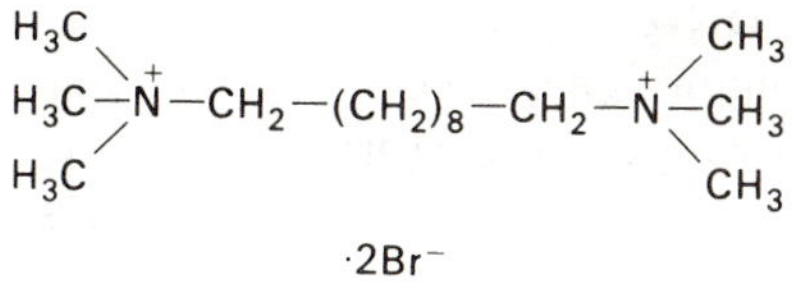

$(H_3C)_3\overset{+}{N}-CH_2-(CH_2)_8-CH_2-\overset{+}{N}(CH_3)_3 \cdot 2Br^-$

Decamethonium

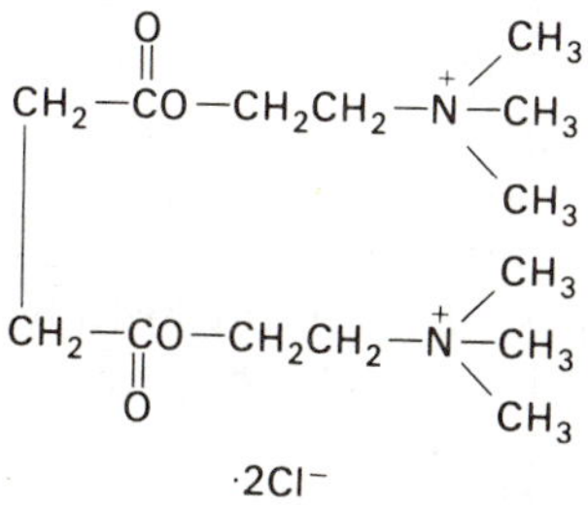

$\cdot 2Cl^-$

Succinylcholine

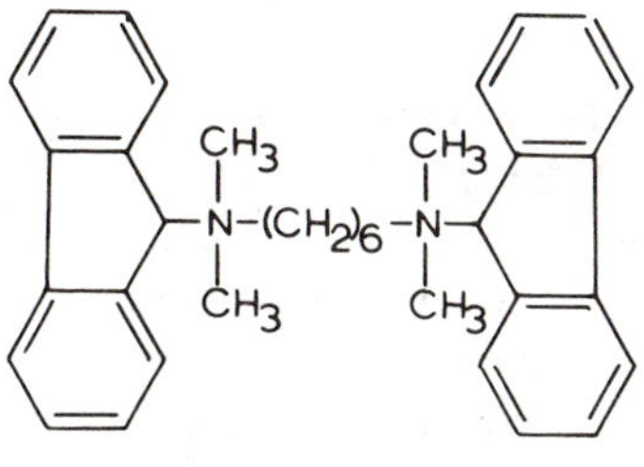

Hexafluorenium

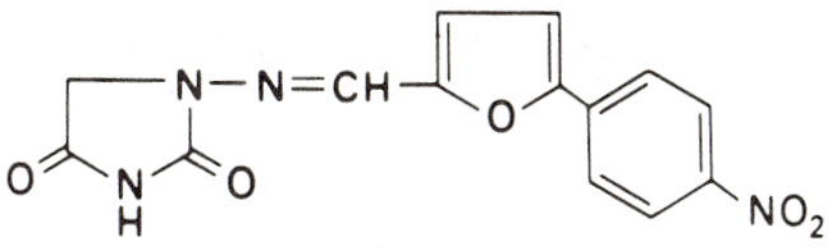

Dantrolene

Fig. 9.1-2. *Depolarizing muscle relaxants, related agents and dantrolene.*

ceded by transient muscle fasciculations, especially visible over cheeks and abdomen; paralysis then develops over arm, neck, and leg muscles with slight weakness of the facial and pharyngeal muscles. Weakness of respiratory muscles follows.

Duration of paralysis by succinylcholine is brief because it is almost completely hydrolyzed by pseudocholinesterase. However, in patients with a genetically determined abnormal variant of plasma pseudocholinesterase succinylcholine-induced paralysis (such as in postoperative apnea) may be prolonged. Such patients can be identified by testing their ability to metabolize succinylcholine. Under standardized test condition, dibucaine, a local anesthetic, inhibits the normal enzyme about 80% and the abnormal enzyme about 20%. The "dibucaine number" indicates the extent of the existence of the abnormal enzyme. Although several genetic variants of the enzyme have been identified, those related to dibucaine are the most important.

In contrast to the effect of the competitive neuromuscular blocking agents, succinylcholine-induced phase I paralysis cannot be antagonized; rather it may be potentiated and prolonged by anticholinesterases such as neostigmine. The plasma cholinesterase level can also be lowered, and postoperative apnea can be prolonged by exposure to long-acting anticholinesterase agents such as organophosphorus pesticides or topical use of agents like echothiophate for open-angle glaucoma or accommodative esotropia. The response to a peripheral nerve stimulator following a small dose can be tested to detect such complications.

Following a single large dose, repeated administration, or prolonged infusion of succinylcholine, decreased receptor sensitivity may occur, causing a desensitization block (dual, antidepolarizing or phase II block). For succinylcholine, whereas 1-3 mg/kg can produce phase I block, 3-5 mg/kg dose would cause phase II block. Hypokalemia may also prolong the response to succinylcholine. Postoperative apnea can be prolonged through phase II block. Such apnea during phase II block can best be managed by controlled ventilation. Anticholinesterases may act as antagonists during phase II block as in the case of nondepolarizing agents.

Phase II block produced by succinylcholine is not always observed clinically, is sometimes slow to develop, and does not always assume all the characteristics of nondepolarizing block. For these reasons, phase II block has not been clearly defined or understood. Considerable controversy exists as to the characteristics, time course, and mechanism of phase II block (11).

Hexafluorenium, primarily a plasma cholinesterase inhibitor with capability of mild competitive neuromuscular blockade, can enhance its duration of action and abolish initial muscular fasciculations; however, occasional bronchospasm is observed due to combined use of these drugs.

The distribution of succinylcholine is similar to tubocurarine. In therapeutic doses, it does not cross the blood-brain barrier or enter placental circulation in appreciable quantities. It owes its short duration of action to the rapid metabolism by pseudocholinesterase found in plasma and liver. It is excreted mainly as metabolites.

Adverse Effects. Succinylcholine can cause both *nodal and ventricular arrhythmias,* increased arterial pressure, and decrease or increase in heart rate partly due to stimulation of nicotinic receptors in both sympathetic and parasympathetic ganglia and muscarinic receptors in the sinus node of the heart. Prior administration of atropine can prevent some of the effects such as nodal arrhythmias, bradycardia, and sinus arrest.

Administration of succinylcholine to patients with severe burns, major crush injuries, spinal cord injuries, multiple sclerosis of recent onset, tetanus, and diseases of upper motor or diffuse lower motor neurons has cause severe *ventricular arrhythmias and cardiac arrest.* The latter effects have been related to exaggerated release of potassium into the blood following depolarization of the supersensitive denervated muscle. The duration of sensitivity varies from a week to a year or more depending on the disease. In the case of burns, such sensitivity may develop between 5 and 120 days when succinylcholine should be avoided.

The *intraocular pressure can be increased* following succinylcholine injection. The increase occurs 1 min after injection, is maximum between 2 and 4 min, and lasts for 5-10 min. It occurs during the stage of generalized muscle fasciculations. Despite the increase of intraocular pressure, succinylcholine is safe for use in intraocular surgery, if it is administered at least 6 min prior to surgery.

In some patients succinylcholine-induced abdominal muscle fasciculations can *increase intragastric pressure.* A dose of 1 mg/kg may increase the pressure up to 40 cm of water, which would exceed the normal pressure of 28 cm of water needed to open the cardioesophageal sphincter. This may make vomiting or regurgitation more likely with the potential hazard for aspiration of the gastric contents. Pretreatment with nondepolarizing relaxants may prevent this adverse effect.

Succinylcholine can produce *muscle contracture* of varying degrees in patients with myotonia congenita or myotonia dystrophica. Contracture is also an early sign of *malignant hyperthermia* induced by succinylcholine given as an adjuvant to a volatile general anesthetic. Further details regarding this complication with its management are discussed later in this chapter.

Pain and stiffness often occur in the neck, shoulder, and subcostal muscles after surgery in which succinylcholine is used. The effects appear 12-24 hours postdrug and last for several hours to days. They usually occur in patients aged 20-50 years, and their incidence is more in ambulatory than in bedridden patients. They do not appear to be related to muscle fasciculations. Pretreatment with competitive muscle relaxants prior to succinylcholine and postoperative diazepam may reduce the incidence of pain.

Myoglobinuria is observed in 40% of prepubertal children and only rarely in adults following use of succinylcholine. This effect does not appear to be related to severity of fasciculations.

Therapeutic Uses. Because of its rapid and short action, the drug is primarily indicated for brief procedures such as endotracheal intubation, endoscopy, relief of laryngospasm, orthopedic manipulation, and electroconvulsive therapy.

DECAMETHONIUM

Decamethonium (Fig. 9.1-2) is a depolarizing neuromuscular blocking agent that has the same mechanism of action as succinylcholine, has a longer duration of action than the latter. Complete recovery occurs in about 20 min. It is excreted unchanged by the kidneys. This drug is now rarely used.

BENZOQUINONIUM

Benzoquinonium is a synthetic neuromuscular blocking agent possessing certain features of both the competitive and depolarizing agents. It also possesses marked anticholinesterase activity.

HEXAFLUORENIUM

Hexafluorenium [hexamethylene-bis (9-fluorenyldimethyl ammonium)] has the structure shown in Fig. 9.1-2. It is primarily a plasma cholinesterase inhibitor with mild nondepolarizing (competitive) neuromuscular blocking potency. It delays the enzymatic hydrolysis of succinylcholine and thus increases the duration and intensity of its action. It may diminish or prevent the muscle fasciculations and pain often associated with succinylcholine; however, the combined use of the two drugs may occasionally cause bronchospasm.

COMPARISON OF COMPETITIVE AND DEPOLARIZING BLOCKING AGENTS

Pharmacological effects of succinylcholine are compared with those of d-tubocurarine in Table 9.1-1. These two compounds are being taken as representatives from depolarizing and competitive neuromuscular blocking agent groups, respectively. Autonomic and cardiovascular effects of several competitive neuromuscular blocking agents are also compared with those of succinylcholine in Table 9.1-2.

THERAPEUTIC USES

In clinical usage as adjuncts to anesthesia, a number of factors will directly influence the choice of agent. Succinylcholine is generally the agent of choice for short procedures, since it is rapidly metabolized and therefore has a short and easily controlled duration of action. One problem with the use of this agent is the genetic variant in serum cholinesterase that makes some subjects experience an abnormal, prolonged response to the drug. This pharmacogenetic phenomenon has been discussed extensively by Kalow (18). Percentage of inhibition of serum cholinesterase by dibucaine is usually expressed as a number—the dibucaine number. The use of a preoperative dibucaine number test can successfully predict the likelihood of a given subject having the abnormally low serum enzyme activity (7).

Gallamine and decamethonium are largely excreted as unchanged molecules via the kidney and should therefore not be used in patients with impaired renal function. Tubocurarine and pancuronium may be less effective in patients with liver disease who have high plasma globulin levels. Even though these drugs are extensively metabolized, their use in patients with renal disease should be carefully undertaken, since renal excretion of both unchanged drug and metabolites is still required.

ADVERSE EFFECTS

The major problems from use of the neuromuscular blocking agents are associated with respiratory depres-

Table 9.1-1
Comparative Neuromuscular Blocking Effects of a Typical Nondepolarizing (e.g., Tubocurarine) and a Depolarizing (e.g., Succinylcholine) Muscle Relaxant

		Succinylcholine	
	d-Tubocurarine	Phase I	Phase II
Effect on motor end-plate	Blockade of ACh-induced depolarization	Persistent depolarization	Repolarization and desensitization to ACh
Initial muscle contraction	None	Transient fasciculation	None
Response to tetanic stimulation (50-100 Hz)	Unsustained	Well-sustained	Poorly sustained tetanus; decrease of action potential
Posttetanic facilitation of twitch height	Occurs	None	Occurs
A train-of-four ratio (T4/T1)[a]	< 0.25	> 0.7	< 0.3
Effect of anticholinesterases on neuromuscular blockade	Reversal	Addition/ synergism	Reversal

[a]Ratio of the amplitude of the last twitch of a train-of-four (T4) at 2 Hz to amplitude of the first twitch (T1)
Source: Data are based on Refs. 11 and 20.

Table 9.1-2
Autonomic and Cardiovascular Effects of Peripheral Muscle Relaxants

	Effects on[a]					
Drugs	Autonomic Ganglia	Muscarinic Receptor (Cardiac)	NE Release	NE Uptake	Histamine Release	Resultant Cardiovascular Effects
Tubocurarine	– –	0		0	+ + +	Hypotension, tachycardia
Metocurine	–	0		0	+ +	Same, but less than tubocurarine
Gallamine	0	– – –	+	0	0	Sinus tachycardia, occasionally hypertension
Pancuronium	0	– –	+	– –	0	Tachycardia, hypertension
Vecuronium	0	0		–	0	Little or no effect
Atracurium	0	0			+	Little or no effect
Succinylcholine	+	+	+		+	Heart rate increased or decreased, hypertension

[a]+, Stimulation or increase; –, inhibition, blockade, or decrease; 0, no effect. Number of + or – approximately indicate degree (e.g., mild, moderate, or marked).
Source: From Ref. 6.

sion leading to inadequate postoperative ventilation. Normally, a period of controlled positive ventilation is sufficient to reverse the effects of the agents; if inadequate respiration occurs, it may be due to overdosage, the presence of complicating pathological conditions, or interactions with other drugs (some inhalation anesthetics and some antibiotics) (14, 25).

Succinylcholine has been reported to produce severe arrhythmias in some subjects, and because it tends to have an intraocular hypertensive effect, should not be used in patients with deep, penetrating ocular wounds. Tubocurarine causes histamine release and ganglion blockade and thereby can produce circulatory and respiratory adverse effects.

Attempts have been made to develop nondepolarizing competitive blockers devoid of autonomic effects. Although great progress has been made in this direction, pancuronium, one of the most commonly used drugs, does produce tachycardia and occasional bronchospasm. Its analog norcuron with its shorter duration of action and lack of autonomic effects appears to be a promising new drug (30).

PREPARATIONS

All of these agents are available only in solution, since intravenous administration is the only route utilized, with the exception of children, where succinylcholine may be given i.m.

Tubocurarine chloride, USP (d-tubocurarine chloride, TUBARINE)—sterile solution (3 or 15 mg/ml). *Metocurine iodide,* USP (dimethyl tubocurarine, METUBINE IODIDE) solution (2 mg/ml).

Gallamine triethiodide, USP (FLAXEDIL)—solution (20 or 100 mg/ml).

Pancuronium bromide (PAVULON)—solution (1 or 2 mg/ml).

Succinylcholine chloride, USP (ANECTINE, etc.)—sterile powder (0.5 and 1 g); sterile solution (20, 50, or 100 mg/ml).

Hexafluorenium, USP (MYLAXEN)—solution (20 mg/ml in 10-ml vial).

Decamethonium bromide, USP (SYNCURINE)—sterile solution (1 mg/ml in 10-ml vial).

DANTROLENE

Dantrolene (Fig. 9.1-2) unlike any other muscle relaxant, is thought to exert its major actions within the muscles. The drug, as shown, uncouples excitation from contraction seemingly by impairing the release of calcium from the sarcoplasmic reticulum (29). Thus, the electrical activity of muscle is unaffected but the contractile activity is compromised. Unlike neuromuscular blocking agents such as curare in animal studies, dantrolene has an upper limit of efficacy in diminishing muscle contractile strength, with degrees of depression rarely exceeding 60% of the initial strength, after even maximally tolerated doses. The drug is approximately equally effective in directly or indirectly stimulated muscles and seemingly is without effect on neuromuscular transmission. Dantrolene seems relatively specific for skeletal as opposed to cardiac or smooth muscle. The drug, by virtue of its actions on muscle, weakens contraction strength of normal muscles as well as those experiencing spasticity. If on-balance residual function is enhanced by the alleviation of an overlying incapacitating hypertonus, the drug may be useful. Dantrolene does exhibit some CNS-depressant actions that may indirectly contribute to a reduction in muscle tone, but it does not impair polysynaptic reflexes preferentially like the centrally acting muscle relaxants.

Dantrolene is hepatotoxic in a significant proportion of individuals and has proved fatal in several instances. The drug should not be used unless clear evidence of a beneficial effect on function develops within a month. Liver function tests are essential; patients at higher dose levels are at higher hepatic risk. Other adverse reactions include drowsiness, dizziness, weakness, general malaise, fatigue, and diarrhea. The drug has recently been reviewed (25).

Dantrolene (DANTRIUM) is available in 50- and 100-mg tablets as well as a suspension containing 5 mg/ml for oral use. An intravenous preparation has recently been made available containing 20 mg of dantrolene sodium for administration in 60 ml of diluent.

Dantrolene relieves spasticity and improves functional capacity for a majority of hemiplegic and paraplegic patients, but it produces weakness that may handicap the patient (9). Dantrolene is recommended for use as an adjunct to supportive therapy in malignant hyperthermia, a hyperpyrexia that occurs rarely during surgery as a reaction to anesthetics or neuromuscular blocking drugs. Excessive release of calcium from the sarcoplasmic reticulum may be responsible for skeletal muscle contraction causing hyperpyrexia that may prove fatal.

MALIGNANT HYPERTHERMIA AND ITS MANAGEMENT

Malignant hyperthermia (2) is a potentially fatal disorder that can be triggered by a variety of stimuli including general anesthetics and neuromuscular blocking agents. It can be induced by any volatile anesthetic, but its onset is usually more abrupt with the use of succinylcholine. Its incidence is increased by premedication with belladonna alkaloids.

This complication develops rarely (1:14,000) in genetically susceptible individuals. Such patients have hereditary deficiency on the part of the sarcoplasmic reticulum to sequester calcium. Therefore, a trigger can cause a sudden and prolonged release of calcium with muscle contraction, lactic acid production, and increase in body temperature.

Signs. In a susceptible person, administration of succinylcholine can cause rigidity that may be first noticed in jaw muscles. Continued use of this or other depolarizing muscle relaxant may intensify rigidity. Tachycardia or tachyarrhythmia may be the earliest sign in susceptible patients without succinylcholine. Other early signs include tachypnea, hypertension, and flushing. Acidosis and elevation of serum potassium levels occur. Hyperthermia is a late sign that results from heat production in the skeletal muscle and liver. Disseminated intravascular clotting and oozing of blood at the surgical site may occur.

Treatment. Sequential steps of treatment include the following: (1) immediate discontinuation of anesthesia; (2) hyperventilation with 100% oxygen; (3) intravenous administration of dantrolene, starting with a 1 mg/kg dose and repeating as necessary to a maximum of 10 mg/kg; (4) correction of acidosis with sodium bicarbonate; (5) control of hyperkalemia, if present, by injection of regular insulin (10 units); (6) cooling (surface cooling in children and intravenous iced saline in adults);

and (7) maintenance of urinary output above 2 ml/kg/hr to prevent renal damage due to myoglobinuria.

Necessary supportive and symptomatic treatment should be done. For anesthesia in susceptible patients, neuroleptic analgesia is preferred. In addition to dantrolene, a barbiturate or a benzodiazepine may be used for premedication with or without a narcotic. A nondepolarizing muscle relaxant may be used. General anesthetics (except for nitrous oxide), succinylcholine, or other depolarizing muscle relaxants, or belladonna alkaloids should be avoided.

REFERENCES

1. Adams, P. R., and Sakmann, B. Decamethonium both blocks and opens end-plate channels. *Proc. Natl. Acad. Sci. US* 75:2994, 1978.
2. *AMA Drug Evaluations,* 5th ed. Chicago: American Medical Association, 1983, p. 438.
3. Armstrong, D. L., and Lester, H. A. The kinetics of tubocurarine action and restricted diffusion within the synaptic cleft. *J. Physiol.* (London): 294:365, 1979.
4. Basta, S. J., Ali, H. H., Savarese, J. J. et al. Clinical pharmacology of atracurium besylate (BW 33A): A new non-depolarizing muscle relaxant. *Anesth. Analg.* 61:723, 1982.
5. Bernard, C. *Leçons sur les Effects des Substances Toxiques et Medicamenteuses.* Paris: J. B. Baillière et Fils, 1857.
6. Bowman, W. C. Non-relaxant properties of neuromuscular blocking drugs. *Br. J. Anesth.* 54:147, 1982.
7. Churchill-Davidson, H. C. (ed.). 1978. Neuromuscular blocking agents. In: *Practice of Anesthesia,* 4th ed. Philadelphia: W. B. Saunders, 1978, pp. 879.
8. Cronnelly, R., and Morris, R. B. Antagonism of neuromuscular blockade. *Br. J. Anaesth.* 54:183, 1982.
9. Davidoff, R. A. Pharmacology of spasticity. *Neurology* (Minneapolis) 28:46, 1978.
10. Dionne, V. E., Steinbach, J. H., and Stevens, C. F. An analysis of the dose-response relationship at voltage-clamped frog neuromuscular junctions. *J. Physiol.* (London) 281:421, 1978.
11. Durant, N. N., and Katz, R. L. Suxamethonium. *Br. J. Anaesth.* 54:195, 1982.
12. Fahey, M. R., Morris, R. B., Miller, R. D. et al. Clinical pharmacology of ORG NC45 (Norcuron): A new nondepolarizing muscle relaxant. *Anesthesiology* 55:6, 1981.
13. Feldman, S. Neuromuscular blocking drugs. In: *Practice of Anaesthesia,* 4th ed. (Churchill-Davidson, H. C., and Wylie, W. D., eds.). Philadelphia: W. B. Saunders, 1978, p. 865.
14. Fogdall, R. P., and Miller, R. D. Neuromuscular effects of enflurane, alone and combined with d-tubocurarine, pancuronium, and succinylcholine in man. *Anesthesiology* 42:173, 1975.
15. Gregoretti, S. M. et al. Heart rate and blood pressure changes after ORG NC45 (vercuronium) and pancuronium during halothane and enflurane anesthesia. *Anesthesiology* 56:392, 1982.
16. Griffith, H. R., and Johnson, G. E. The use of curare in general anesthesia. *Anesthesiology* 3:418, 1942.
17. Hunter, J. M., and Jones, R. S., and Utting, J. E. Use of atracurium in patients with no renal function. *Br. J. Anaesth.* 54:1251, 1982.
18. Kalow, W. Genetic factors in relation to drugs. *Ann. Rev. Pharmacol.* 5:9, 1965.
19. King, H. Curare alkaloids. I. Tubocurarine. *J. Chem. Soc.* (London): 1381, 1935.
20. Lee, C. M. Train-of-4 quantitation of competitive neuromuscular block. *Anesth. Analg.* 54:649, 1975.
21. MacLagan, J. Competitive neuromuscular blocking drugs. In: *Neuromuscular Junction* (Zaimis, E., ed.). Berlin: Springer-Verlag, 1976, p. 421.
22. Naharashi, T. Neurotoxins: Pharmacological dissection of ionic channels of nerve membranes. In: *The Nervous System* Vol. 2 (Tower, D. B., ed.). New York: Raven Press, 1975, p. 101.
23. Neher, E., and Sakmann, B. Single channel currents recorded from the membrane of denervated frog muscle fibres. *Nature* 260:799, 1976.
24. Payne, J. P., and Hughes, R. Evaluation of atracurium in anaesthetized man. *Br. J. Anaeth. 53:45, 1981.*
25. Pinder, R. M., Brogden, R. N., Speight, T. M., and Avery, G. S. Dantrolene sodium: A review of its pharmacological properties and therapeutic efficacy in spasticity. *Drugs* 13:3, 1977.
26. Pittinger, C., and Adamson, R. Antibiotic blockade of neuromuscular function. *Ann. Rev. Pharmacol.* 12:169, 1972.
27. Riker, W. F. Prejunctional effects of neuromuscular blocking and facilitatory drugs. In: *Muscle Relaxants* (Katz, R., ed.). Amsterdam:L Excerpta Medica, 1975, p. 59.
28. Smith, S. C. Neuromuscular blocking drugs in man. In: *Neuromuscular Junction* (Zaimis, E., ed.). Berlin: Springer-Verlag, 1976, p. 593.
29. Van Winkle, W. B. Calcium release from skeletal muscle sarcoplasmic reticulum: Site of action of dantrolene sodium? *Science* 193:1130, 1976.
30. Walts, L. F. Neuromuscular blocking drugs. *Otolaryngol. Clin. North Am.* 14:501, 1981.
31. Zaimis, E. The neuromuscular junction: Area of uncertainty. In: *Neuromuscular Junction* (Zaimis, E., ed.). Berlin: Springer-Verlag, 1976, p. 1.
32. Zaimis, E., and Head, S. Depolarizing neuromuscular blocking drugs. In: *Neuromuscular Junction* (Zaimis, E., ed.). Berlin: Springer-Verlag, 1976, p. 365.

CHAPTER
9.2

CENTRALLY ACTING MUSCLE RELAXANTS

Arthur Raines

In contrast to the peripheral muscle relaxants (discussed in Chapter 9.1) that act directly on the skeletal muscles or at the myoneural junctions, there are drugs that cause muscle relaxation by affecting certain central mechanisms regulating muscle tone. As such, these drugs are referred to as the *centrally acting muscle relaxants.*

This group of drugs is mainly used for treatment of skeletal muscle hypertonus leading to pain, discomfort, and limitation of motion. The conditions in which the centrally acting muscle relaxants are used can be classified into two groups differing as regards etiology and mode of therapy: spasm and spasticity.

Skeletal muscle *spasm* is an acute muscle stiffness associated with musculoskeletal pain leading to lack of mobility. The etiology is usually (not always) of skeletal muscle origin and associated with trauma, contusion, muscle strain, or sprain. Sometimes it is caused by an inflammatory process. The etiology can occasionally be neurogenic, as in a spinal disk protrusion creating pressure on nerve roots; such instances require more specific interventions. Often spasm results from excessive use of muscles by otherwise sedentary individuals; this condition is often referred to as the common *charley horse.* Individuals whose muscles are weak and who may be overweight occasionally experience *low back syndrome,* characterized by muscle contraction, pain, and immobility in the lumbosacral spinal area that can be triggered by a strain to this musculature and can be incapacitating. Similarly, the neck musculature can be a source of twisting of the neck in a contracture *(torticollis).*

Muscle spasm can be episodic in susceptible individuals, with more severe bouts lasting as long as 2-3 weeks. In most cases where strain, sprain, trauma, or inflammation are causal, the condition is self-limiting and usually resolves itself in 4-7 days without the need for therapeutic interventions. In these conditions, rest and heat are usually beneficial and muscle relaxant drugs are only adjunctive as they are of only limited value.

The second group of hypertonic muscle disorders, referred to as *spasticity,* are the consequence of chronic neurological disorders produced by upper motor neuron lesions as obtained in stroke, spinal cord injury, multiple sclerosis, cerebral palsy, amyotrophic lateral sclerosis, and several less prevalent neurological disorders. The symptoms observed are muscle contracture, clasped knife responses, weakness and clonus. These symptoms usually persist throughout life with occasional exacerbations and remissions.

Spasticity appears to be due to a net loss of inhibitory influences on spinal motoneurons and can be of the γ, α, or mixed type, depending upon the motoneuron population which is primary in producing muscle contractures. In the γ type, the release of these small motoneurons leads to stretching of the polar regions of muscle spindles and consequent discharge of the spindle afferent fibers and reflex activation of α motoneurons. In α spasticity, excitation of these motoneurons appears to be direct and does not involve appreciable reflex excitement. It is likely that most cases of spasticity involve a variable combination of α and γ contributions to spasticity. Additionally, evidence exists that indicates that presynaptic inhibition is diminished in patients with longstanding upper motor neuron lesions (4). Accordingly, drugs that enhance presynaptic inhibition may be of value in spasticity for this reason. Clearly, spasticity is not a single motor disturbance but is a term somewhat loosely applied to several disorders of motor control of varying etiology and local origin (21).

Spasticity comprises the major disabling neurological disorder, being much greater in scope than epilepsy and parkinsonism combined in both number of people affected and cost of rehabilitative care.

The goal of treatment is to maximize utilization of residual neuromuscular function. This requires physical and often drug therapy. It is important to recognize that patients often use spastic limbs for support or other purposes, and the manner in which spasticity may be useful must be taken into account before administering drugs that are intended to diminish spasticity. It should be pointed out here that, as with those drugs used for muscle spasm, available agents provide only modest benefit.

DRUGS USED IN THE THERAPY OF MUSCLE SPASM

The centrally acting muscle relaxants used for treatment of spasm do not show any high order of efficacy. Because the most prominent sign of the spasm is pain (a subjective response), placebos are often as effective as these drugs. They do not appear to exert any specific action on the musculoskeletal systems as opposed to depressing other centrally controlled functions.

Intravenous administration, whenever possible (as with mephenesin and methocarbamol), leads to more readily demonstrable muscle relaxation. It requires about 5-10 times as much of the drug administered orally to produce the equivalent of intravenous dosing (19). Oral dosing is usually not up to such levels.

MECHANISM OF ACTION

The mechanism of muscle relaxant action of this group of drugs is thought to occur by depressing internuncial cells and thereby diminishing the facilitatory background activity on spinal motoneurons. The polysynaptic reflexes are more readily depressed than monosynaptic reflexes. These drugs also inhibit supraspinal influences (both facilitatory and inhibitory), impinging on spinal motoneurons affecting muscle stretch reflexes, primarily in the lateral reticular area of the brain stem. These drugs produce sedation and drowsiness as their common side effects, which may reflect depressed neuronal activity essential for wakefulness in the medial reticular ascending system. These drugs also exhibit anticonvulsant activity in several animal models. These actions to inhibit polysynaptic as compared with monosynaptic systems and depression of descending influences as well as anticonvulsant actions are widely observed for other nonspecific CNS depressants.

Some centrally acting muscle relaxants used in the therapy of spasm are listed with their proprietary name, daily dose, and dosage form in Table 9.2-1; their chemical structures are given in Fig. 9.2-1.

MEPHENESIN

Mephenesin, introduced in the late 1940s (5), is usually regarded as the prototype centrally acting muscle relaxant. It was the first to enjoy widespread use and may be credited with creating the drug class. Mephenesin diminishes muscle tone in experimentally induced rigid states (e.g., decerebrate, decerebellate rigidity) without measurable effect on neuromuscular transmission. Ironically, although it has received the most investigative attention and probably exhibits the most favorable separation between doses needed to produce a reduction in motor tone and sedative effects than the others of this class, the drug is no longer marketed. This situation derives from the facts that National Academy of Science-National Research Council's (NAS-NRC) evaluation rated the drug less than "effective," that patent protection had long elapsed, and that potential sponsors lacked interest in conducting the requisite controlled clinical trials.

Although with large doses of mephenesin (particularly by the intravenous route) a reduction in motor tone could often be produced in humans, this effect tended to be short lived; the alcoholic hydroxy group was readily conjugated with glucuronic acid, causing the drug's rapid inactivation. This short-lived course of action was successfully remedied by masking this alcoholic hydroxy

Table 9.2-1
Centrally Acting Muscle Relaxants Used in Therapy of Skeletal Muscle Spasm and Spasticity

Name	Trade Name	Dosage Forms[a]	Daily Dose[b]
Mephenesin	TOLSEROL[c]	T: 500 mg	1-2 g
Methocarbamol, USP	ROBAXIN	T: 500, 750 mg	1-2 g, p.o.
		I: 100 mg/ml	1-3 g, i.v.
Chlorphenesin	MAOLATE	T: 400 mg	800 mg
Chlorzoxazone	PARAFLEX	T: 250 mg	250-750 mg
Metaxalone	SKELAXIN	T: 400 mg	800 mg
Carisoprodol	RELA, SOMA	T: 350 mg	350 mg
Orphenadrine citrate, USP	NORFLEX	T: 100 mg	100 mg, p.o.
		I: 30 mg/ml	60 mg, i.m. or i.v.
Cyclobenzaprine hydrochloride, USP	FLEXERIL	T: 10 mg	10 mg
Diazepam	VALIUM	T: 2, 5, 10 mg	2-10 mg
		I: 5 mg/ml	2-10 mg
Baclofen	LIORESAL	T: 10 mg	5-20 mg

[a] T = tablet; I = injection.
[b] Dose to be taken 2 to 3 times a day and to be increased gradually if needed.
[c] No longer available.

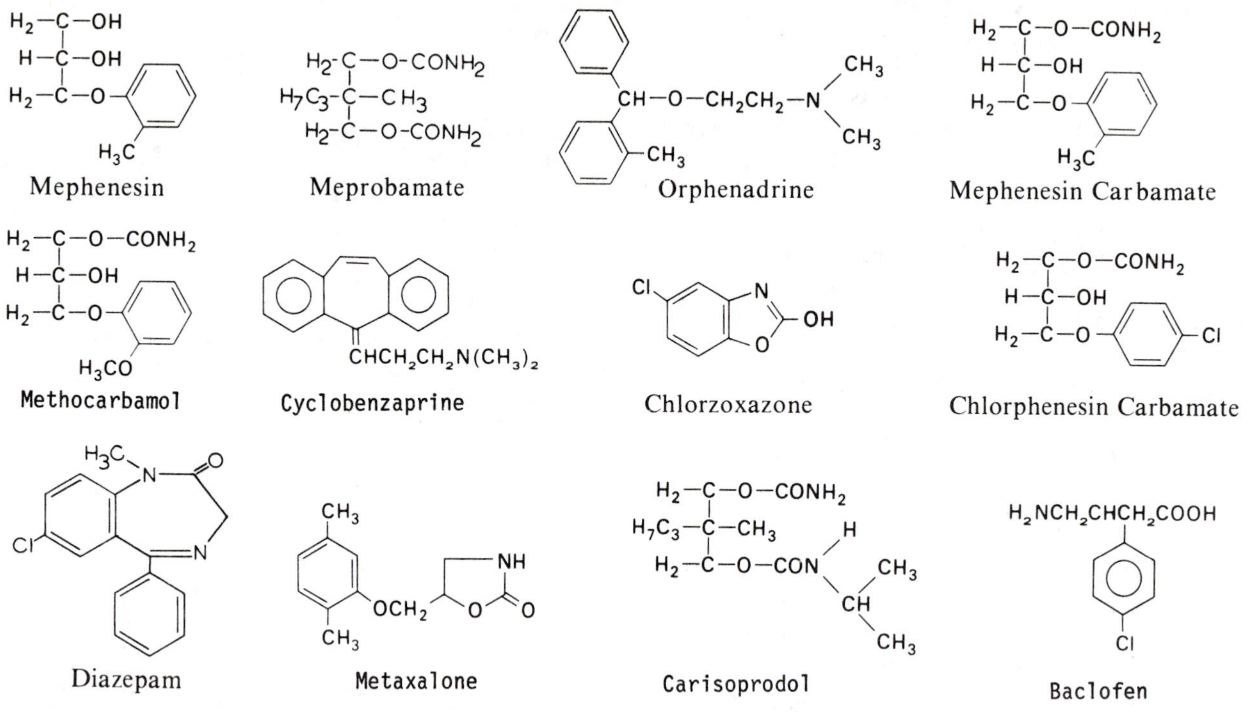

Mephenesin Meprobamate Orphenadrine Mephenesin Carbamate

Methocarbamol Cyclobenzaprine Chlorzoxazone Chlorphenesin Carbamate

Diazepam Metaxalone Carisoprodol Baclofen

Fig. 9.2-1. *Chemical structures of centrally acting muscle relaxants.*

group by esterification with carbamic acid. Unfortunately, the carbamylation appears to have enhanced the drug's capacity for nonspecific CNS depression, as is the case with mephenesin carbamate, which is no longer marketed.

OTHER MUSCLE RELAXANTS

Several centrally acting muscle relaxants resemble mephenesin in their pharmacological actions. These include *methocarbamol* and *chlorphenesin carbamate* (two carbamylated derivatives of mephenesin), *chlorzoxazone* and *metaxalone* (oxazole derivatives), *carisoprodol* (N-isopropyl derivative of meprobamate), *orphenadrine* (a methyl derivative of diphenhydramine), and *cyclobenzaprine* (Table 9.2-1 and Fig. 9.2-1). Diazepam also relieves spasm through central action.

As shown in Table 9.2-1, in addition to their oral use as tablets methocarbamol, orphenadrine, and diazepam are also available for intravenous administration to relieve severe, acute muscle spasm of local origin caused by inflammation or trauma. Intravenous methocarbamol also is effective in reducing spasticity in selected patients. The parenteral form of methocarbamol contains 1 g of the drug in 10 ml of 50% polyethylene glycol 300. The latter diluent in large doses has been shown to be nephrotoxic and should not be administered to patients with suspected or known renal impairment. Its intravenous administration should be slow (not to exceed 300 mg/min), and the total daily dose by this route should not exceed 3 g daily.

ORPHENADRINE

Orphenadrine, a methyl derivative of diphenhydramine, is alleged to be less soporific than diphenhydramine but shares with this agent appreciable anticholinergic properties that account for the most prevalent adverse effects of the drug. It appears to have analgesic properties. Orphenadrine is available as either the hydrochloride salt advocated for use in parkinsonism or as the citrate salt for musculoskeletal discomfort.

CYCLOBENZAPRINE

Cyclobenzaprine is the most recently marketed drug for the amelioration of muscle spasm of local origin. Chemically the drug bears a similarity to tricyclic antidepressants and the antiepileptic drug carbamazepine. Cyclobenzaprine shares with the former drugs the capacity to potentiate norepinephrine, antagonize reserpine, exert anticholinergic actions, and produce sedation. It has been shown to depress experimentally induced rigid states, whether produced by midcollicular decerebration (γ rigidity), anemic decerebration (α rigidity), or ischemia of the spinal cord (18). The drug has some efficacy as an adjunct to rest and physical therapy, and appears about equal to diazepam in this regard.

Cyclobenzaprine is well absorbed after oral administration, with peak plasma levels occurring after 2 to 4 hours (13). The drug has an appreciable half-life ranging from 1-3 days and is highly bound (about 93%) to plasma proteins when present in the usual therapeutic range of 10-30 ng/ml (13).

Due to its cocaine-like effect on norepinephrine reuptake, the drug is contraindicated in patients receiving monoamine oxidase inhibitors or who have cardiac disease or hyperthyroidism. The atropine-like actions suggest that individuals with glaucoma or benign prostatic hypertrophy should likewise not receive the drug.

DIAZEPAM

Diazepam, the most widely used of the benzodiazepines, possesses anticonvulsant, sedative, hypnotic, and muscle relaxant properties (Chapter 11.4). Diazepam enhances spinal presynaptic inhibition in experimental animals (12, 16). The drug appears to enhance the efficacy of γ-aminobutyric acid (GABA) by an action on GABA receptors (12). GABA is thought to be the depolarizing transmitter for presynaptic inhibition, and it has thus been argued that diazepam, by enhancing presynaptic inhibitions, diminishes motor tone (18, 20). The parenteral preparation may be used but carries with it greater risk, as mentioned for intravenous diazepam in Chapter 11.4.

DRUGS USED IN THE THERAPY OF SPASTICITY

DIAZEPAM

Diazepam (discussed earlier in this chapter and also in Chapters 11.4) enjoys rather wide use in the treatment of spasticity. Dose levels are established by gradually increasing the dose until either a satisfactory response is produced or a degree of lethargy which is unacceptable develops. The latter is the usual limiting factor in the dosage.

BACLOFEN

Baclofen is p-chloro-phenyl-γ-aminobutyric acid, a lipid soluble analog of GABA. The drug was prepared on the assumption that it would penetrate the blood-brain barrier and activate GABA receptors, whereas GABA itself was too polar to enter the CNS (14). Although the drug does enter the CNS and exert depressant actions, it is unclear whether these effects are the result of GABA-mimetic actions (7); data from different systems indicate that baclofen can mimic or antagonize GABA or have no influence on GABAergic function. It has been proposed that baclofen antagonizes substance P on spinal motoneurons (11, 17). Baclofen does not have any direct neuromuscular blocking effect. It diminishes the transmission of monosynaptic extensor and polysynaptic flexor reflexes in the spinal cord, probably by presynaptic hyperpolarization leading to inhibition of release of putative excitatory neurotransmitters, glutamic and aspartic acids from primary afferent fibers (1). The drug does exert an overall CNS depressant action, which is frequently observed as an adverse effect but which may be a significant factor in motor tone reduction. Other adverse effects associated with baclofen are drowsiness, weakness, fatigue, confusion, headache, insomnia, hypotension and nausea, vomiting, and leg edema.

Recommended dose is initially 15 mg daily (in three divided doses), gradually increasing the daily dose every 3 days until the desired therapeutic effect is achieved or toxicity limits further dosing. Usual daily doses are in the order of 40-80 mg (Table 9.2-1). Patients who do not experience benefit within a month should have the drug gradually discontinued, as abrupt withdrawal has been associated with hallucinations.

PHENOTHIAZINES

Phenothiazines (discussed in Chapter 11.5.1) have shown efficacy (6, 8) in the treatment of spasticity, although they are not officially approved for such use in this country. Phenothiazines (with chlorpromazine as the prototype) are known to block γ-motoneuron discharges and hence cause desensitization of the muscle spindles. This depression of γ-motoneurons may be the consequence of central α-adrenergic blockade of descending noradrenergic influences (15). Phenothiazines are strikingly effective in abolishing the extensor rigidity of the midcollicularly decerebrated cat. This classic preparation demonstrates γ-motoneuron hyperactivity leading to spindle discharges that produce a reflex hypertonus. Undue sedation and peripheral α-adrenergic blockade leading to orthostatic hypotension are the limiting factors for the use of this group of drugs.

PHENYTOIN

Phenytoin, an antiepileptic drug (see Chapter 11.4) depresses muscle spindles (2) directly, and markedly potentiates chlorpromazine's capacity to diminish the extensor tone of the midcollicularly decerebrated cat (3). Early clinical results indicate that phenytoin is useful in the treatment of spasticity, especially when given with chlorpromazine (8). These results need further confirmation, however.

DANTROLENE

In addition to the centrally acting muscle relaxants discussed earlier, dantrolene is effective in treatment of spasticity. Unlike the centrally acting relaxants, this drug reduces skeletal muscle contraction by uncoupling excitation from contraction perhaps by decreasing the amount of calcium released from the sarcoplasmic reticulum (9, 10). Dantrolene is discussed in Chapter 9.1.

REFERENCES

1. American Medical Association. In: *AMA Drug Evaluation*, 5th ed. Chicago, 1983, p. 355.
2. Anderson, R. J., and Raines, A. Suppression by diphenylhydantoin of afferent discharges arising in muscle spindles of the triceps surae of the cat. *J. Pharmacol. Exp. Ther.*, 191:290, 1974.
3. Anderson, R. J., and Raines, A. Suppression of decerebrate rigidity by phenytoin and chlorpromazine. *Neurology*, 26:858, 1976.
4. Ashby, P., and Verrier, M. Neurophysiologic changes in hemiplegia. *Neurology*, 26:1145, 1976.

5. Berger, F. M. Spinal cord depressant drugs. *Pharmacol. Rev.*, 1:243, 1949.
6. Burke, D., Hammond, C., Skuse, N., and Jones, R. A phenothiazine derivative in the treatment of spasticity. *J. Neurol. Neurosurg. Psychiatr.*, 38:469, 1979.
7. Calne, D. B. The pharmacology of spasticity. In: *Clinical Neurophysiology*, Vol. 1. (Klawans, H. L., ed.). New York: Raven Press, 1976, p. 137.
8. Cohan, S. L., Raines, A., Panagakos, J., and Armitage, P. Phenytoin and chlorpromazine in the treatment of spasticity. *Arch. Neurol.*, 37:360, 1980.
9. Ellis, K. O., and Carpenter, J. F. Studies on the mechanism of action of dantrolene sodium. *Naunyn-Schmiedebergs Arch. Pharmacol.*, 275:83, 1972.
10. Ellis, K. O., and Carpenter, J. F. Mechanisms of control of skeletal muscle contraction by dantrolene sodium. *Arch. Phys. Med. Rehab.*, 55:362, 1974.
11. Fotherby, K. J., Morrish, N. J., and Ryall, R. W. Is lioresal (baclofen) an antagonist of substance P? *Brain Res.*, 113:210, 1976.
12. Haefely, W. E. Synaptic pharmacology of barbiturates and benzodiazepines. *Agents Actions*, 7:353, 1977.
13. Hucker, H. B., Stauffer, S. C., Albert, K. S. et al. Plasma levels and bioavailability of cyclobenzaprine in human subjects. *J. Clin. Pharmacol.*, 117:719, 1977.
14. Koella, W. P. Baclofen: Its general pharmacology and neuropharmacology. In: *Spasticity: Disordered Motor Control* (Feldman, R. G., Young, R. R., and Koella, W. P., eds.). Yearbook, Chicago, 1980, p. 383.
15. Maxwell, D. R., and Sumpter, E. A. A comparison of the action of some drugs on decerebrate rigidity muscle spindle activity and alpha-adrenoceptors. *Br. J. Pharmacol.*, 50:355, 1974.
16. Polc, P., Mohler, H., and Haefely, W. The effect of diazepam on spinal cord activities: Possible sites and mechanisms of action. *Naunyn-Schmiedebergs Arch. Pharmacol.*, 284:319, 1974.
17. Saito, K., Konishi, S., and Otsuka, M. Antagonism between lioresal and substance P in rat spinal cord. *Brain Res.*, 97:177, 1975.
18. Share, N. N., and McFarlane, C. S. Cyclobenzaprine: A novel centrally acting muscle relaxant. *Neuropharmacology*, 14:675, 1975.
19. Smith, C. M. Relaxants of skeletal muscle. In: *Physiological Pharmacology* (Root, W. S., and Hofmann, F. G., eds.). New York: Academic Press, 1965, p. 1.
20. Verrier, M., MacLeod, S., and Ashby, P. The effect of diazepam on presynaptic inhibition in patients with complete and incomplete spinal cord lesions. *Can. Sci. Neurol.*, 2:179, 1975.
21. Young, R. R., and Delwaide, P. J. Drug therapy: Spasticity. *N. Engl. J. Med.*, 1:28, 96, 1981.

CHAPTER
9.3

THERAPY OF NEUROMUSCULAR DISEASE

Russell D. Rollinson and Wolf-D. Dettbarn

The *motor unit* consists of anterior horn cell, peripheral nerve, neuromuscular junction and muscle. Diseases that affect the motor unit are collectively considered the *neuromuscular diseases*. Therapy of the neuromuscular diseases aims at arresting progress, improving function, alleviating symptoms, and ultimately curing the underlying process. However, our present understanding of the pathophysiological mechanisms operant in these disorders is incomplete; hence, for example, in muscular dystrophy, at present, the cause is unknown and therefore treatment is empirical or symptomatic. In myasthenia gravis, on the other hand, our present understanding of the mechanism is such that arrest and cure of this disorder is now possible.

Therapy encompasses not only pharmacological agents, but also physical therapy and occasionally surgical procedures. The emphasis of this chapter will be on the pharmacological management of these disorders.

CLASSIFICATION OF NEUROMUSCULAR DISORDERS

1. Anterior horn cell: motor system disorders, amyotrophic lateral sclerosis, hereditary spinal muscular atrophies (4)
2. Peripheral nerve: peripheral neuropathies (11)
3. Neuromuscular junction: myasthenia gravis, myasthenic syndrome (Eaton-Lambert syndrome), botulism, and tick paralysis (9)
4. Myopathies (18)

ANTERIOR HORN CELL DISEASES

Anterior horn cell diseases include amyotrophic lateral sclerosis and the various subcategories of the spinal muscular atrophies. They are of unknown etiology and lead to progressive weakness, wasting, fasciculation, and variable spasticity. These diseases are due to dysfunction of the cells of the motor system, both upper and lower motor neurons, at brain stem and spinal levels with sparing of ocular motility, sensation and mentation.

There are at present no drug therapies that can be applied on a rational basis; rather, they have been directed toward symptomatic relief. Various therapies have been tried on an empirical basis; these include guanidine hydrochloride and snake antivenom. However, there is no conclusive evidence as yet that these agents are effective. Symptomatically, the problem of most difficulty for patients with amyotrophic lateral sclerosis is weakness; this is not usually amenable to therapy, although conditions such as foot drop may be treated with splinting. Difficulty in swallowing is a major late complaint of this disease. It may be due either to lower motor neuron weakness or to spasticity of the muscles of swallowing. If due to spasticity, relief can be obtained with a minor surgical procedure involving sectioning of the cricopharyngeus muscle. Terminally, the major problem is swallowing difficulty, which produces aspiration of gastric contents into the respiratory tree. This can be overcome temporarily with the use of a nasogastric tube or feeding through gastrostomy.

Several new drugs have been introduced specifically for the treatment of spasticity. Spasticity is manifested by increased tone and involuntary spasms of muscles. This usually involves the lower extremities in amyotrophic lateral sclerosis.

BACLOFEN

Baclofen (LIORESAL), a lipophilic analog of γ-aminobutyric acid (GABA), crosses the blood-brain barrier more readily than GABA itself. Administered orally, it inhibits both monosynaptic and polysynaptic reflexes at the spinal level, possibly by hyperpolarization of the presynaptic nerve terminals, and thus increases the threshold for producing flexor reflexes. Weakness, clonus and reflexes are not significantly altered (10). Further details about its mechanism of action, dosage and side effects are given in Chapter 9.2 and Table 9.2-1.

DANTROLENE SODIUM

Dantrolene Sodium (DANTRIUM) is another useful agent in spasticity. A muscle relaxant, it exerts its action directly on skeletal muscle. Capsules are available in 25- and 100-mg sizes. Oral administration should begin at 25 mg b.i.d. and increase to 100 mg q.i.d. For children, a starting dose of 1 mg/kg b.i.d. is gradually increased to a maximum of 3 mg/kg q.i.d., not to exceed 400 mg/day. Side effects include weakness, euphoria, light-headedness, dizziness, drowsiness and fatigue, diarrhea, liver enzyme elevation and depression of white cells. Relative contraindications include coexistent heart and lung disease (6), as well as active hepatic disease (for further details, see Chapter 9.1).

PERIPHERAL NEUROPATHIES

The majority of polyneuropathies are amenable to classification with the use of biochemical studies, clinical neurophysiological tests, and nerve biopsy (see Table 9.3-1) (12, 13). The most ubiquitous conditions occurring throughout the world include leprosy, vitamin deficiency (including alcoholism), and diabetes mellitus. However, among the patients requiring admission for investigation of peripheral nerve disease, an etiological diagnosis is reached in only about half the cases.

Therapy is therefore directed toward the underlying cause, although often our knowledge of the pathogenesis is insufficient to reverse the basic disorder, such as diabetic polyneuropathy. However, removal of toxins, treatment of infections (diphenylsulfone for leprosy), vitamin deficiency replacement (B_1, B_6, B_{12}), and release of entrapment neuropathies are often indicated and usually constitute satisfactory treatment. Uremic neurophathy responds well to dialysis and renal transplantation. Attacks of porphyric neuropathy cease when all causative drugs are avoided (e.g., barbiturates, sulfonamides nd griseofulvin).

The place of corticosteroids in the treatment of polyneuropathy is controversial. In postinfectious polyneuropathy (Guillain-Barré syndrome) where there is a rapidly ascending flaccid

Table 9.3-1
Peripheral Neuropathy

Category	Example	Treatment
Inherited	Charcot-Marie-Tooth	Supportive
	Dejerine-Sottas	
	Refsum's	
Toxic	Arsenic, antimony, bismuth, gold, lead, thallium, phosphorus, mercury	Identification, elimination, and use of chelating agents
Drugs	Vincristine, isoniazid, disulfiram, emetine, nitrofurantoin, phenytoin, alcohol	Recognition, and use of pyridoxine with isoniazid
Infectious	Leprosy	Dapsone, rifampin
	Brucellosis	Tetracyclines
	Diphtheria	Penicillin
	Infectious mononucleosis	Supportive
	Tick paralysis	Supportive
Postinfectious	Guillain-Barré syndrome	Supportive Consider steroids for severe cases
Collagen vascular disorders	Systemic lupus erythematosus, rheumatoid arthritis, polyarteritis nodosa	Appropriate immunosuppressive therapy
Deficiency states	Thiamine, niacin, Vitamin B_{12}, folic acid, pyridoxine	Replacement
Metabolic disease	Renal failure	Diet, dialysis, transplant
	Liver disease	Treat underlying cause
	Diabetes mellitus	Good control
	Porphyria	Avoid drugs that precipitate attacks such as griseofulvin, barbiturates, sulfonamides
Unknown	Hypothyroidism	Thyroxine
	Multiple myeloma	Chemotherapy
	Associated with malignancy	Symptomatic
	Amyloidosis	Symptomatic
	Recurrent idiopathic	Steroids

motor neuropathy often leading to respiratory failure and autonomic dysfunction, there is little evidence to support their continued use. However, it must also be noted that in practice they are commonly administered. Chronic recurrent polyneuropathy may be remarkably steroid responsive, and a trial of prednisone at 60-80 mg/day for a 2- to 3-week period should identify the steroid-responsive cases.

Instruction in the care of anesthetic feet and hands is mandatory. Episodes of repeated unrecognized trauma can destroy fingers and toes. Pain associated with neuropathy is fortunately uncommon. When encountered, treatment should begin with simple analgesics such as buffered acetylsalicylic acid. Sometimes long-acting narcotics cannot be withheld. However, before these drugs are used, other measures such as the administration of carbamazepine, phenytoin, and antidepressants should be tried. Counterstimulation with cutaneous electrodes may give relief when applied to an isolated peripheral nerve or painful area.

NEUROMUSCULAR JUNCTION DISORDERS

Neuromuscular junction disorders include myasthenia gravis, Eaton-Lambert syndrome, botulism and tick paralysis.

MYASTHENIA GRAVIS

Myasthenia gravis is a disease, probably of immunological origin, characterized by weakness and abnormal fatigability of striated muscle. The weakness is commonly of the bulbar musculature (ptosis, diplopia, dysarthria, dysphagia and respiratory difficulties) and less often the skeletal muscles. Weakness is partially or completely reversed by cholinesterase inhibitors. The demonstration of an acetylcholine receptor antibody in the serum of 85-95% of patients with myasthenia gravis supports the view that the mechanism is immunological and the site of attack is postsynaptic (9). Myasthenia gravis is associated with thymic pathology, hyperplasia and thymoma, and other diseases of immunological origin, such as thyroid disease, systemic lupus erythematosus, pemphigus, pernicious anemia and rheumatoid arthritis.

Diagnosis. The diagnosis of myasthenia gravis is based not only on the clinical and neurophysiological findings (use of repetitive stimulation, demonstrating a decrementing response), but also on the use of pharmacological agents active at the synapse that either improve or aggravate the weakness.

Edrophonium chloride (TENSILON) is used intravenously as a diagnostic test. As an anticholinesterase agent, it is a short-lasting, reversible inhibitor of acetylcholinesterase. It may be used subcutaneously or intramuscularly. However, the clinical response is transient. One should be following one or two parameters of strength: abnormalities of eye movements (ptosis, ophthalmoplegia), facial weakness, weakness of neck flexors, difficulty with grip strength, inability to maintain straight-arm or straight-leg raising. To add sensitivity, the test can be done in a double-blind fashion.

Improvement of muscle strength can be expected to occur within 30-45 sec after intravenous injection and will be maintained for 3-4 min. Dosage varies with age and weight of the patient. For infants, 0.15 mg/kg; for children, 0.2 mg/kg; and for adults, 10 mg is suggested. Initially, one-fifth of the total dosage is given. This is to detect sensitivity and the rare syncopal reaction that can occur with use of full dosage. If there is no response after 60 sec, the remainder is injected.

The effect of edrophonium chloride is transient and may sometimes be overlooked. Some, therefore, have recommended the use of *neostigmine methylsulfate* (PROSTIGMINE) because of its longer action, and this may be preferable in children and questionable placebo responders. This can be used orally, intravenously, subcutaneously, or intramuscularly. Intramuscularly, the dose is 1.5-2 mg for adults; 0.1-0.25 mg for neonates; 0.1 mg/10 lb of body weight for children. Onset of improvement with neostigmine is delayed 10-30 min, but the clinical improvement is maintained for about 2 hr. Various pharmacological agents will increase muscle weakness in myasthenia gravis, chiefly tubocurarine, decamethonium, quinidine and quinine. Rarely nowadays are these employed as diagnostic tests because of the hazards and other diagnostic tests available, such as repetitive stimulation and antiacetylcholine receptor antibody assay (21).

Therapy. Therapy includes the use of drugs directly improving neuromuscular transmission, drugs that modify the immune mechanism, procedures that modify the immune mechanisms, and at least one surgical procedure.

The *anticholinesterases* (Chapter 8.2) have been the mainstay of treatment in myasthenia gravis. (These drugs prolong the action of released acetylcholine by inhibiting acetylcholinesterase. Acetylcholine accumulates, and its actions are potentiated and prolonged at nicotinic as well as muscarinic sites.) Three reversible anticholinesterases, neostigmine, pyridostigmine (MESTINON), and ambenonium (MYTELASE), have been used in prolonged oral therapy. In general, inhibition lasts for 2-4 hr. None of these drugs is superior when compared with the other in giving the desired effect. Pyridostigmine is preferred because it causes less muscarinic side effects, such as diarrhea, abdominal cramps, and salivation.

The oral dose and frequency of medication has to be determined for each individual patient. In general, one or two tablets (neostigmine 15 mg/tablet or pyridostigmine 60 mg/tablet) 3 to 4 times daily is sufficient. In more severe cases the dosage can be increased to 3 to 4 tablets at 2-4 hr. During the course of treatment, the dose will have to be adjusted to that which will give maximal benefit. To check the effectiveness of the dosage of edrophonium, a very short-lasting inhibitor can be given i.v. 1-2 hr after an oral dose. If the patient improves, then the oral dose has been too small; no improvement after edrophonium indicates that the oral dose is optimal. Should further weakness occur, then the oral dosage is probably too large.

To avoid major fluctuations in the patient's strength, the intervals between doses should be carefully considered. A slowly released (8-12 hr), sustained-action form of pyridostigmine may be taken at bedtime. Medication should be timed in patients with swallowing difficulties 1-2 hr before meals. The patient requires sufficient anticholinesterase medication to produce optimal improvement in muscle strength without producing unwanted side effects.

A variety of drugs in addition to those discussed earlier have been employed to supplement the action of the anticholinesterase medications. Ephedrine, potassium chloride, triamterene, spironolactone and calcium have been used. These agents have some beneficial effects, but none has modified the management of myasthenia gravis. Their mode of action is not clear, but each is active at the neuromuscular junction and probably increases release of acetylcholine presynaptically.

The unwanted muscarinic side effects may be controlled by oral doses of atropine (0.4-0.6 mg/tablet) when given with each dose of cholinesterase inhibitor.

Immunosuppressants have been used in the therapy of myasthenia gravis. Adrenocorticosteroids have a long and varied history in the treatment of this disease. However, it is now accepted that prednisone and adrenocorticotropic hormone (ACTH) do have a place in the treatment of generalized myasthenia gravis (22, 23). The rationale for their use was initially on an empirical basis. Presently, with the recent advances in the understanding of the pathophysiology of myasthenia gravis, their main therapeutic effect is attributed to their immunosuppressive action. However, corticosteroids also have a positive action at the neuromuscular junction, enhancing transmission;

they have also been of benefit in cases of refractory ocular myasthenia gravis. However, high doses of these agents can produce an initial deterioration in the strength of the myasthenic patient. This seems more likely to occur when the individual patient is also on cholinesterase inhibitors. Therefore, patients should have anticholinesterase therapy reduced with the institution of prednisone or followed carefully for the signs of cholinergic weakness.

Oral prednisone is the drug of choice, beginning with 25 mg every other day, with increments of 25 mg every second or third dose. The patient's muscle strength is charted and vital capacity measured twice daily. If vital capacity falls below 500 ml (or 15 ml/kg), ventilatory assistance is usually required. One gradually increases to 100 mg every other day. Once remission is achieved (return to near-normal strength and functional capacity), the dosage can be reduced slowly, no more than 5 mg every 2 weeks. If deterioration occurs with reduction of dosage, the former dosage is reinstituted.

Others have recommended a rapid induction with prednisone or ACTH. Prednisone is begun 60-80 mg daily or ACTH, 100 IU. When improvement begins, usually within the first 2 weeks, medication is changed to alternate days — for example, prednisone 100 mg. Less steroid side effects are encountered with alternate-day therapy. If a patient fails to respond to steroid treatment within 4-6 weeks, it is unlikely that he ever will, and consequently alternate therapy should be sought. Steroid therapy should be continued for 12-24 months to avoid relapse in the steroid-responsive cases.

Azathioprine (IMURAN) is an analog of 6-mercaptopurine with antimetabolite and immunosuppressive activities (Chapter 13.5.3). The mechanisms of action are not clearly established. It is administered orally as 50-mg tablets. The major side effect in humans is bone marrow depression. Regular leukocyte counts are essential — weekly at outset, then every 2 weeks; after 3 months, every 3-4 weeks. The usual recommended dosage is 1-2 mg/kg/day. However, some physicians recommend 2-3 mg/kg/day. If the leukocyte count falls below 3000/ml, the dosage of azathioprine should be reduced by 50 mg/day with a repeat count in 5 days; if the count is less than 2000/ml, medication should be discontinued until the count rises again. Azathioprine should then be reintroduced at a lower dose (16).

Hepatotoxicity, in the form of liver function test elevations and cholestatic jaundice, has been reported, but these symptoms are generally completely reversible when the drug is withheld. Nausea, anorexia and vomiting may be encountered at the initiation of azathioprine. Females of reproductive age should avoid pregnancy while taking azathioprine because of the risk of teratogenicity. Once again, azathioprine can be combined with steroid medication as with inflammatory muscle disease.

Cyclophosphamide (CYTOXAN), a nitrogen mustard, is an alkylating agent. It is administered orally as 25- and 50-mg tablets and is used for its immunosuppressive properties. Side effects include alopecia, which is usually reversible even without interruption of therapy. Nausea and vomiting are common. Mucosal ulceration, skin pigmentation, hepatoxicity, interstitial pulmonary fibrosis, hemorrhagic cystitis, inappropriate antidiuretic hormone (ADH) secretion, sterility, teratogenic effects, mutations and cancer have been reported. Dosage is usually 2.5 mg/kg/day. It, too, can be used alone or in combination with other agents such as prednisone (21).

A procedure for modifying the immune response is plasmapheresis. Plasma exchange may be followed by a short-term remission, and clinical improvement is associated with a decrease in the serum acetylcholine receptor antibody. The procedure is time consuming and expensive and is usually reserved for patients who have failed to respond to chemotherapy and thymectomy. Most patients treated with plasmapheresis are also on high doses of steroids and/or other immunosuppressives, such as azathioprine or cyclophosphamide (8).

Thoracic duct lymph drainage as an immunosuppressive procedure in myasthenia gravis has been employed since 1970. This procedure has been used during myasthenic crises, following thymectomy in patients with severe weakness, and in cases of severe chronic myasthenia where all other therapy has failed. Drainage is performed for 7-14 days, with about one-third to one-half of plasma volume drained each day. This volume is replaced by albumin and electrolyte solutions only. IgG, complement, and titers of antiacetylcholine receptor antibodies are reduced during this therapy (2).

A *surgical procedure* may also be indicated. All patients who are examined for myasthenia gravis should be screened for the presence of a thymoma. A thymoma may be present on a routine chest x-ray. Its overall incidence is about 10% of all myasthenic patients. Thymoma is most commonly found in elderly males; young females rarely have it. High titers of anti-striated muscle antibody and the presence of HLA-2 may be markers for the presence of thymoma as well. Nowadays computerized body tomography would be the investigation of choice for the presence of a thymoma. Overall, the group of patients with thymoma carry a worse prognosis when compared with the group without thymoma. Patients with generalized myasthenia gravis who have either severe disease or disease refractory to chemotherapy should be considered for thymectomy. In some medical centers, thymectomy is used as the treatment of choice for generalized myasthenia gravis because it may induce a remission of myasthenia gravis. The time of onset of the remission from the time of surgery is variable and can range from a very short period to many years after the thymectomy (19).

Contraindications. The neuromuscular blocking drugs of the depolarizing type, such as succinylcholine and decamethonium, are contraindicated. Furthermore, drugs such as procainamide, quinidine, quinine and chlorpromazine have been associated with increasing the muscular weakness in patients with myasthenia gravis. Some antibiotics, notably streptomycin, neomycin, polymyxin, kanamycin and colistimethate, have neuromuscular blocking properties. When a myasthenic patient with respiratory and bulbar weakness suddenly has symptoms of anxiety, sedatives and major tranquilizers should be avoided. These symptoms may reflect cerebral hypoxia, and blood gas analysis and vital capacity should be performed rather than resorting to sedation of the patient.

EATON-LAMBERT SYNDROME

Eaton-Lambert syndrome (myasthenic syndrome) is a disorder of neuromuscular transmission first described in association with malignancy. This group of patients is characterized by increasing proximal weakness without major bulbar signs. EMG and repetitive stimulation demonstrate an incremental rather than a decremental response, the latter being seen in myasthenia gravis. The defect is probably presynaptic, due to a defect in the basic inhibition of the release of acetylcholine from the nerve terminals. Treatment with cholinesterase inhibitors and other standard treatments for myasthenia gravis is unrewarding. Guanidine hydrochloride is thought to increase acetylcholine release from the nerve terminal and is administered orally as 25-mg tablets. The usual therapeutic range is 10-30 mg/kg/day. Side effects including nausea and vomiting, paresthesias, dry mouth, ataxia, confusion, mood changes, dryness and scaling of skin, atrial fibrillation, hypotension, bone marrow depression, renal tubular necrosis, and chronic interstitial nephritis all have been reported (20).

BOTULISM

Acute poisoning caused by the exotoxin of *Clostridium botulinum* occurs generally through the ingestion of contaminated food, primarily occurring in home-canned fruits and vegetables. This exotoxin acts on the presynaptic side of the neuromuscular junction and other cholinergic synapses, causing blockade of transmission by preventing the release of acetylcholine. All cranial nerves with the exception of the first and second are affected. Diplopia, blurred vision, and difficulty in swallowing and speaking are present. Associated with this is limb weakness and respiratory impairment. Once clinical evidence of this disease is present, the patient's stomach should be lavaged and a cathartic administered; 10,000 U of polyvalent antitoxin should be administered i.v. along with 50,000 U i.m. every 18-24 hr. Guanidine hydrochloride has recently been shown to be beneficial in a dosage of 35-50 mg/kg (5).

TICK POISONING

Tick poisoning causing neuromuscular blockade has been demonstrated to be similar to that of botulism. However, no detailed analysis of neuromuscular transmission has been described in humans. Guanidine has not been used for treatment.

MYOPATHIES

Muscular dystrophy is usually a genetically determined progressive primary disease of muscle. The therapy is aimed at (1) genetic counseling and detection of the carrier state in asymptomatic relatives, (2) symptomatic treatment, prevention of contractures, physical therapy and (3) vigorous treatment of infections and other complications.

Various therapeutic modalities have been tried in Duchenne muscular dystrophy, the most severe form encountered, among them steroids and megavitamin therapy, immunosuppression, and drugs such as penicillamine without success. Continued research into the basic pathophysiological mechanisms may provide hope for the sufferers of these diseases in the future.

Almost any endocrine disease, both hyperfunction and hypofunction, can produce a proximal myopathy. Therefore, any patient with evidence of muscle disease should be carefully screened for some underlying endocrine abnormality, as the treatment of these usually leads to a gratifying return of strength. Proximal weakness is common in thyroid disease and, if looked for, is found in the majority of cases. Long-term steroid therapy with corticosteroids can produce proximal muscle weakness in itself. The steroids most likely to cause severe proximal weakness when used for prolonged periods include dexamethasone and triamcinolone.

Inflammatory myopathies comprise a number of conditions of probable autoimmune origin. The muscle bears the brunt of the pathology, but skin and other organ systems may be involved. The latter group usually comprises patients with obvious evidence of underlying collagen vascular disease, such as systemic lupus erythematosus, rheumatoid arthritis, or scleroderma. There appears to be an increased incidence of dermatomyositis and underlying malignancy in the over 45 age group, but a direct relationship has not been established (3). All of the treatment regimens involve the use of immunosuppressive agents, such as corticosteroids, methotrexate, and azathioprine (1, 7).

The childhood variety of *dermatomyositis* is a fairly stereotyped condition and the pathology is a vasculitis. Treatment should be begun early with a single daily high dose of prednisone (60-80 mg). It was first administered on an empirical basis for these diseases and is now believed to work by its immunosuppressive properties. Prednisone is effective when given orally. Side effects associated with long-term usage include fluid retention and weight gain, hypertension, susceptibility to infections, carbohydrate intolerance, osteoporosis, peptic ulceration, posterior subcapsular cataracts, personality changes and psychotic episodes, skin changes (such as easy bruising) and acne. With the exception of cataract formation, these side effects are seen less often when alternate-day therapy is used. The clinician is guided by the clinical improvement of muscle weakness and the return to normal of the elevated muscle enzymes, such as the creatine phosphokinase levels. Usually, the enzyme activity declines in the first 2 weeks, followed by improvement in the muscle strength thereafter. As the enzymes approach normal levels, steroid therapy can be changed to alternate-day dosage at the same level. The dosage is then guided by the foregoing parameters to obtain the lowest possible dose that will maintain the patient at normal or near-normal strength. Therapy should be continued for at least 2 years from the first symptoms. As in all cases of inflammatory myopathy, poor results are usually related to: (1) late diagnosis, (2) inadequate dosage of steroids at the outset, (3) failure to maintain steroids for at least a 2-year period.

The approach in the adult cases of polymyositis and dermatomyositis is along similar lines. However, because diagnosis is not usually made early in these conditions, the therapy is delayed and therefore the prognosis is poorer. There are some patients who do not seem to respond to prednisone alone; that is, they continue to have significant muscle weakness and muscle enzyme elevation with adequate steroid therapy. A trial of at least 6-8 weeks of prednisone in high doses is needed before a case should be labeled steroid resistant.

The next drug that is most commonly used is the folic acid analog and dihydrofolate reductase inhibitor, methotrexate (1). Intravenous administration is preferred as being less toxic than the oral route. Methotrexate also has powerful immunosuppressive activity. A test dose of 5 mg is administered initially and hematological and liver functions are monitored to detect hypersensitivity. The drug is then administered weekly in a dosage of 10-40 mg, gradually increasing to maximum tolerable levels within this range.

Prior to each injection, blood counts and liver function tests should be checked along with a general physical examination of the patient to detect side effects. These include nausea and vomiting (usually transient following the injection), ulceration of the gastrointestinal tract, hepatitis, skin rashes, bone marrow suppression, and occasionally nonbacterial pneumonitis (need for regular chest x-rays). Should any of these be evident, the medication should be withheld.

Methotrexate is usually combined with prednisone. In patients who require high maintenance doses of prednisone, methotrexate can be used for its steroid-sparing effect. Azathioprine has also been used with some success in this condition and is given orally at a dosage 1-2 mg/kg/day; this was discussed earlier.

Overall, with these therapeutic regimens, mortality has been reduced to 10-20% from 50%. However, some argue that this improvement can be attributed to, for example, better respiratory care and antibiotics rather than to prednisone.

MISCELLANEOUS CONDITIONS

MYOTONIA

Myotonia is a slow relaxation after voluntary effort or after direct percussion of the muscle. It can occur without weakness, as in myotonia congenita, or with weakness, as in myotonic dystrophy, or with periodic paralysis. Treatment of this condition depends on the degree of disability caused by the myotonia. In the past, agents such as quinine, procainamide and diphenylhydantoin have been tried with variable success. Acetazolamide (DIAMOX), a carbonic anhydrase inhibitor, is thought to stabilize the muscle membrane in this condition (15). It is administered orally in a dosage 125-750 mg, beginning with 125 mg b.i.d. Side effects include paresthesias, anorexia, weight loss, renal calculi, renal failure, osteoporosis, and hematological and hepatic dysfunction.

PERIODIC PARALYSIS

Periodic paralysis is a group of conditions in which periodic muscle weakness has been associated with hypokalemia, hyperkalemia, and, rarely, normokalemia. Acute treatment of hypokalemic periodic paralysis has been the oral use of potassium salts, 20-100 meq. Intravenous potassium is particularly difficult to administer because concentrated potassium therapy is hazardous. Chronic treatment with acetazolamide, as mentioned earlier, appears to be the therapy of choice in hypokalemic periodic paralysis (14). The prophylactic administration of potassium does not prevent recurrent attacks of weakness. In the hyperkalemic variety, immediate treatment with high-carbohydrate foods or fluids is usually effective. Rarely, in severe attacks, intravenous glucose, insulin, calcium, or bicarbonate may be indicated. The electrocardiogram must be monitored throughout this therapy. Although acetazolamide has been noted to be of benefit in this condition, thiazide diuretic may be preferable for chronic treatment because it is at least as effective and may be associated with fewer side effects. Dietary management with high-carbohydrate and low-sodium intake has also been reported to be effective.

MUSCLE CRAMPS

Muscle cramps are caused by several conditions. Ordinary muscle cramps (charley horse) manifest themselves by a painful hard contraction of a single muscle that can last up to a few minutes. This condition may be precipitated by a trivial movement or by a forceful contraction of the shortened muscle, and it is ended by stretching the muscle. Treatment for recurrent idiopathic cramps is usually not successful. However, agents such as diphenylhydantoin, carbamazepine and quinine have been tried. Pathological cramps may be associated with disorders of carbohydrate and lipid metabolism. The former is typified by McArdle's syndrome and the latter by deficiencies of carnitine palmityl transferase. Abnormalities of the glycolytic pathway are manifested by cramps that appear early during exercise. Those in fatty acid metabolism are accompanied by cramps that occur late in exercise. Cramps can also be caused by abnormalities of the lower motor neuron, such as neuropathy and radiculopathy, anterior horn cell disease, myxedema, salt depletion or diuretic therapy, pregnancy, uremia, and renal dialysis.

MUSCLE STIFFNESS

Muscle stiffness is caused by several disorders of the neuromuscular system. Isaac's syndrome is a nonhereditary condition with onset in childhood or adult life. Distal muscle stiffness with slow relaxation without myotonia is present. Symptoms slowly spread proximally and may involve trunk and cranial nerves. Diagnosis is made by the EMG findings of persistent motor unit activity at rest. Symptomatic treatment with carbamazepine or diphenylhydantoin can produce excellent relief (17). The condition of stiff-man syndrome is probably related to a disorder of the central nervous system function, which responds well to diazepam therapy.

SPASTICITY

Spasticity is manifested by increased deep tendon reflexes, extensor plantar responses, and involuntary flexor spasms. These spasms are often accompanied by severe pain and sometimes involuntary bowel and bladder movements. Despite physical therapy, the patient's limbs usually become deformed and fixed by contractures or pseudocontractures that position them in either flexion or extension. Drugs such as meprobamate, chlordiazepoxide and diazepam have been of limited use because they tend to cause significant sedation at therapeutic doses. However, baclofen and dantrolene are useful (see Chapters 9.1 and 9.2).

REFERENCES

1. Arnett, F.C., Whelton, J.C., Zizic, T.M. and Stevens, M.B. Methotrexate therapy in polymyositis. *Ann. Rheum. Dis.* 32:536, 1973.
2. Bergstrom, K., Franksson, C., Matell, G. *et al.* The effect of thoracic duct lymph drainage in myasthenia gravis. *Neurolology* 9:157, 1973.
3. Bohan, A. and Peter, J.B. Polymyositis and dermatomyositis. *N. Engl. J. Med.* 292:344, 1975.
4. Brooke, M.H. *A Clinician's View of Neuromuscular Diseases.* Baltimore: Williams & Wilkins, 1977, p. 34.
5. Cherrington, M. Botulism: Ten year experience. *Arch. Neurol.* 30:432, 1974.
6. Chiatte, S.B. and Basmajian, J. Dantrolene sodium: Long term effects in severe spasticity. *Arch. Phys. Med. Rehab.* 54:311, 1973.
7. Currie, S. and Walton, J.N. Immunosuppressive treatment in polymyositis. *J. Neurol. Neurosurg. Psychiatry.* 34:447, 1971.
8. Dau, P.C., Lindstrom, J.M. and Cassel, C.K. (eds.). Plasmapheresis and immunosuppressive drug therapy in myasthenia gravis. *N. Engl. J. Med.* 297:1136, 1977.
9. Drachman, D.B. Myasthenia gravis. *N. Engl. J. Med.* 298:136, 186, 1878.
10. Duncan, G.W., Shanani, B.T. and Young, R.R. An evaluation of baclofen treatment for certain symptoms in patients with spinal cord lesions. *Neurology* (Minneapolis) 26:441, 1976.
11. Dyck, P.J., Thomas, P.K. and Lambert, E.H. (eds.). *Peripheral Neuropathy*, Vols. 1 and 2, Philadelphia: W.B. Saunders, Co. 1975.
12. Evans, O.B. Polyneuropathy in childhood. *Pediatrics* 64:96, 1979.
13. Freemon, F.R. Causes of polyneuropathy. *Acta Neurol. Scand.* (suppl.) 59:1, 1975.
14. Griggs, R.C., Engel, W.K. and Resnick, J.S. Acetazolamide treatment of hypokalemic periodic paralysis. *Ann. Intern. Med.* 73:39, 1970.
15. Griggs, R.C., Moxley, R.T., Riggs, J.F. and Engel, W.K. Effects of acetazolamide on myotonia. *Ann. Neurol.* 3:531, 1978.
16. Hertel, G., Mertens, H.G., Reuther, P. and Ricker, K. The treatment of myasthenia gravis with azathioprine. In: *Plasmapheresis and the Immunobiology of Myasthenia Gravis* (Dau. P.C., ed.), Boston: Houghton Mifflin, 1979, p. 315.
17. Isaacs, H. and Heffron, J.J.A. The syndrome of "continuous muscle fibre activity" cured: Further studies. *J. Neurol. Neurosurg. Psychiatry* 37:1231, 1974.
18. Moxley, R.T. III. In: *Current Neurology* Vol. I (Tyler, H.R. and Dawson, D.M., eds.). Boston: Houghton Mifflin, 1978, p. 1.
19. Mulder, D.G., Hersmann, C. and Buckberg, G.D. Effect of thymectomy in patients with myasthenia gravis. *Am. J. Surg.* 128:202, 1974.
20. Oh, S.T. and Kim, K.W. Guanidine hydrochloride in Eaton-Lambert syndrome. *Neurology* (Minneapolis) 23:1084, 1973.
21. Patten, B.M. Myasthenia gravis: Review of diagnosis and management. *Muscle and Nerve* 1:190, 1978.
22. Seybold, M.E. and Drachman, D.B. Gradually increasing doses of prednisone in myasthenia gravis. *N. Engl. J. Med.* 290:81, 1974.
23. Warmolts, J.R. and Engl, W.K. Benefit from alternate day prednisone in myasthenia gravis. *N. Engl. J. Med.* 286:17, 1972.

CHAPTER 9.4

THERAPY OF PARKINSONISM AND OTHER DYSKINETIC DISORDERS

Sachin N. Pradhan

PARKINSONISM

Parkinson's disease is a chronic, progressive movement disorder that is characterized by: (1) akinesia or bradykinesia (slowness in the initiation and execution of voluntary movements), (2) tremor at rest (involuntary, rhythmic oscillatory movements of parts of the body resulting from alternating contractions of opposing muscles), (3) rigidity (an increased resistance to passive movements), and (4) loss of postural reflexes (abnormal fixation of posture, equilibrium, and righting reflex). The majority of cases are idiopathic whereas a small number result from viral infections (postencephalitic), vascular accidents, tumors, trauma, or toxic chemicals (exposure to carbon monoxide or manganese). Drugs that disrupt dopaminergic transmission processes (e.g., phenothiazines, reserpine) can cause extrapyramidal side effects that resemble those of Parkinson's disease (see Chapter 11.6.1).

Neuropathological examination of the brains of patients suffering from idiopathic parkinsonism reveals loss of pigmentation and cell bodies in substantia nigra. There is no obvious histological damage to the caudate or putamen, but dopamine concentration in these regions is severely reduced, indicating loss of nigrostriatal dopaminergic neurons (2).

It is generally believed that dopaminergic neurons originating in the substantia nigra exert an inhibitory effect on neurons, including cholinergic neurons, in the striatum. A decrease of dopaminergic transmission in the striatum results in a concomitant increase in the turnover of acetylcholine, which is believed to be an index of cholinergic nerve activity. Prior to the advent of dopaminergic agonists, the symptoms of Parkinson's disease were treated with anticholinergic (antimuscarinic) drugs. It would appear, therefore, that there is an increased cholinergic tone in the extrapyramidal system of parkinsonian patients that results from the lack of inhibitory dopaminergic input.

Cholinergic hyperactivity in parkinsonism can be further substantiated by using certain cholinergic agents as tools to produce some manifestations of this condition. Thus oxytremorine, a synthetic compound that acts as a muscarinic agonist in the periphery as well as in some central areas like basal ganglia, can produce parkinsonismlike effects such as tremor, rigidity, and ataxia. This imbalance can be partially counteracted by blocking the effects of acetylcholine at muscarinic receptors. Similarly, the extrapyramidal side effects of dopamine receptor-blocking drugs (neuroleptics) can be reversed by the administration of antimuscarinic drugs.

A more direct approach to reversing the consequences of the loss of nigrostriatal dopaminergic nerves is to restore dopaminergic functional activity in the striatum by administering dopaminergic agonists. Dopamine per se is not effective because it does not pass the blood-brain barrier, but its immediate synthetic precursor, L-dopa, is transported into the brain and decarboxylated locally to form dopamine. Dopa is pharmacologically inactive, so that the therapeutic and side effects of this compound are primarily due to the actions of its decarboxylated products.

Thus, two types of drugs are used in the therapy of Parkinson's disease: (1) dopamine agonists including levodopa and other agents that would enhance dopaminergic activity directly or indirectly in the brain, and (2) anticholinergic agents. Fig. 9.4-1 provides the chemical structures of some of these agents.

L-DOPA (LEVODOPA)

Pharmacological Effects. Administered in gradually increased doses for an adequate period of time, levodopa

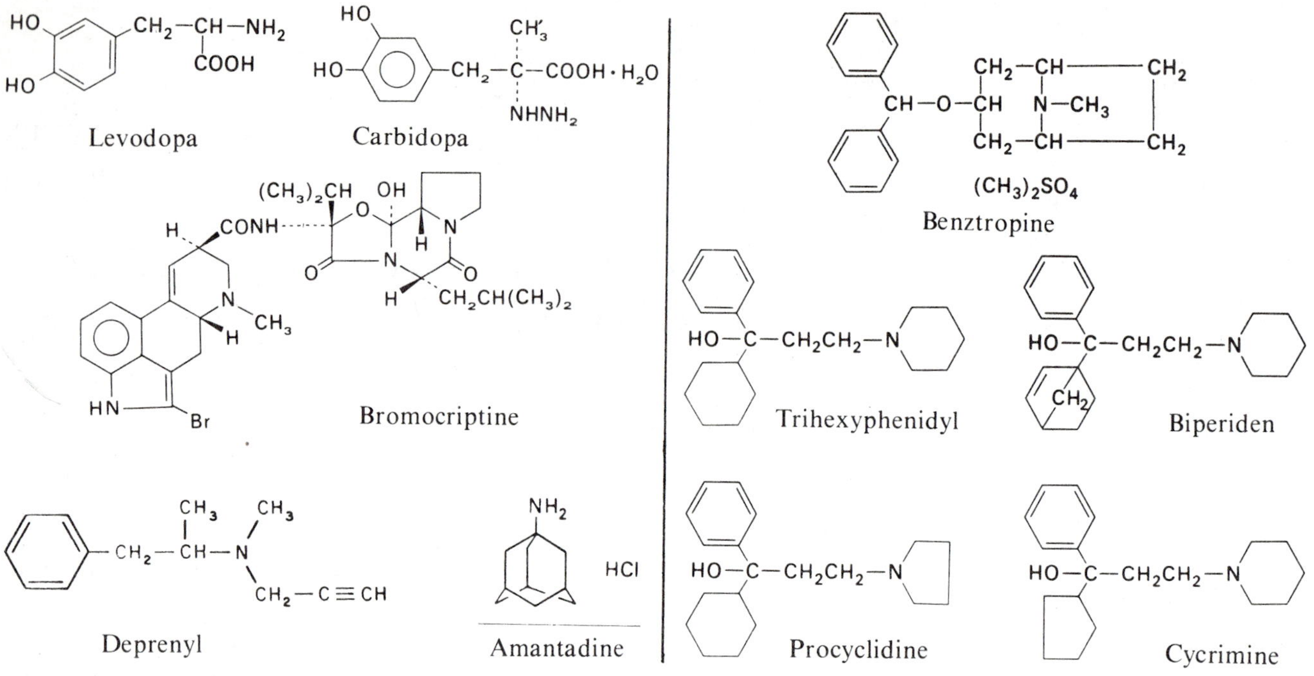

Levodopa Carbidopa

Bromocriptine

Deprenyl Amantadine

Drugs affecting brain dopamine

Benztropine

Trihexyphenidyl Biperiden

Procyclidine Cycrimine

Anticholinergic agents

Fig. 9.4-1. *Chemical structures of some drugs used in therapy of Parkinson's disease.*

relieves symptoms and improves functional capacity in approximately 75% of the patients with parkinsonism. Bradykinesia, rigidity, and, to a lesser extent, tremor are ameliorated. Balance, posture, gait, handwriting, swallowing, and facial expression are improved to a variable degree, and mood is often elevated. Feelings of apathy are replaced by increased vigor and a sense of well-being. Levodopa generally does not reverse parkinsonian symptoms induced by antipsychotic drugs, presumably because this syndrome results not from dopamine deficiency but from dopamine receptor blockade that cannot be overcome by an additional quantity of dopamine.

It is generally believed that dopamine formed from dopa acts on receptors in the striatum to restore the "dopaminergic tone" that has been lost as a result of nigrostriatal nerve degeneration.

Adverse Reactions and Precautions. The majority of patients with parkinsonism who are treated with levodopa experience side effects resulting from actions of dopamine in the periphery (outside the blood-brain barrier in the CNS). These effects are generally dose dependent and reversible, but they can be severe enough to limit use of the drug.

Gastrointestinal. Nausea, vomiting, and anorexia occur in most patients, if the initial dose is high, if the dose is increased rapidly, or if the drug is taken without food. They are partially due to the action of dopamine on receptors in the area postrema (chemoreceptor trigger zone) that initiates the vomiting reflex. Nausea and vomiting frequently limit the dose of levodopa, although some tolerance may develop to these actions. These symptoms may be controlled by titrating the dose, giving the drug along with food, or in conjunction with a peripheral dopa decarboxylase inhibitor. Nonphenothiazine antiemetics may be given, but dopamine antagonists (phenothiazines, butyrophenones, and others) would counteract the therapeutic actions and should be avoided. Other gastrointestinal disturbances include abdominal pain, diarrhea, constipation, and activation of peptic ulcer.

Neurological. The neurological effects are dose related and frequently occur during long-term use. Mild, intermittent dyskinesias involving mouth, tongue, face, and neck are common after a few months; some tolerance may develop to these dyskinesias. These are followed by involuntary choreiform movements of limbs and still later by severe generalized choreoathetoid movements. Respiratory abnormalities (irregular gasping or hyperventilation) may occur. Tolerance does not develop to these side effects; rather, symptoms tend to increase if the dose is not reduced. These abnormal movements can be reduced by lowering the dose or by pyridoxine, which would also reduce therapeutic efficacy of levodopa.

In patients treated with levodopa for 1 year or more, episodic emergence of symptoms of parkinsonism (akinesia, tremor, and rigidity) lasting for a few minutes to several hours is common. Such episodes may be of three forms: (a) end-of-dose akinesia (wearing of effect) that occurs between the doses and appears at increasingly shorter intervals, as the therapy is continued for longer period, onset decreasing from 4 hours to 2 to 3 hours; (b) the "on-off" phenomena—patients swing from on and off periods, representing a marked change from mobility to relative immobility, which may occur unexpectedly and bears no relation to the time of the last dose; (c) akinesia paradoxica that may develop suddenly during a dyskinetic episode, and is often precipitated by stress. All three forms have also been regarded as examples of on-off phenomena by some physicians (1).

Psychiatric. Psychic disturbances occur commonly in the elderly, particularly those receiving anticholinergics in combination with levodopa. These are more likely to occur in patients with prior history of mental illness. These may be mild reactions such as nervousness, anxiety, and sleep disturbances. They may be serious in some patients showing confusion, delirium, depression, hypomania, paranoia, and hallucinations. These indicate central stimulant action of levodopa. Action of levodopa on the hypothalamus may produce renewed sexual interest.

Cardiovascular. Orthostatic hypotension may occur early in therapy. Some tolerance develops to this effect. Transient flushing of skin and palpitation may occur. Cardiac arrhythmias develop only occasionally due to activation of β_1-adrenergic receptors and can usually be controlled by propranolol.

Endocrine Effects. Acting through the dopamine receptor in tuberoinfundibular-hypophyseal system, levodopa decreases the secretion of prolactin. On the other hand, release of growth hormone that is increased in responses to levodopa in normal subjects is minimal or absent in parkinsonian patients.

Abnormalities of Laboratory Tests. Changes of color of urine (red when voided and black when exposed to air) have been reported. Urinary metabolites of levodopa cause false-positive tests for ketoacidosis by dip-stick test.

Drug Interactions. *Pyridoxine* enhances extracerebral decarboxylation of levodopa by the pyridoxine-dependent enzyme dopa decarboxylase. Therefore the patient should avoid pyridoxine or multivitamins containing pyridoxine. *Antipsychotic drugs* such as phenothiazines and butyrophenones can produce parkinsonism-like syndrome and reduce the action of levodopa. Phenothiazines should not be used to prevent emetic effects of levodopa. *Reserpine,* which depletes the stores of central dopamine, can also block the action of levodopa. *Anticholinergic drugs* act synergistically with levodopa to alleviate the symptoms of parkinsonism. *Nonspecific monoamine oxidase (MAO) inhibitors* such as phenelzine and isocarboxazid enhance central effects of levodopa, other catecholamines, and their metabolites; hypertensive crisis and hyperpyrexia are consequences.

LEVODOPA AND DOPA-DECARBOXYLASE INHIBITORS

Approximately 95% of orally administered levodopa is metabolized in the periphery and thus is unavailable for actions in the CNS. Accordingly, large doses (3-6 g/day) of this amino acid must be administered, and occasionally 2-3 months of treatment is necessary before its beneficial effects are available. These large doses frequently cause nausea and vomiting, presumably due to dopamine effect on chemoreceptor trigger zone which is located outside the blood-brain barrier. The administration of a peripheral decarboxylase inhibitor permits the dose of levodopa to be markedly reduced (1-2 g/day).

Carbidopa. Carbidopa is a dopa decarboxylase inhibitor that does not readily enter the CNS when given in small doses. By blocking conversion of levodopa to dopamine in the periphery, carbidopa increases the brain concentration of levodopa to be decarboxylated to dopamine, thereby increasing the therapeutic efficacy of levodopa and reducing its peripheral side effects such as nausea, vomiting, and cardiac effects. However, the central side effects of levodopa such as orthostatic hypotension, involuntary motor movements, and psychic effects are not altered by carbidopa. In fact, these central reactions may appear earlier and be more severe than with levodopa alone. Nausea and vomiting may still occur in approximately 15% of patients; as with levodopa alone, these effects can be minimized by giving the drug with food. A combination of carbidopa with levodopa in the ratio of 1:4 has been found to be better than the previous combination used (1:10) (3).

Benserazide. Benserazide is a similar dopa decarboxylase inhibitor to carbidopa, but it is marketed in Europe and Canada.

DOPAMINE AGONISTS

Levodopa clearly relieves symptoms of parkinsonism, but does not alter the progressive course of the disease. Many patients show a good response to L-dopa, but fail to maintain this response over a period of several years. Several compounds, to be described here, that act directly or indirectly as dopamine agonists have been tested for ameliorating the symptoms of Parkinson's disease.

PIRIBEDIL

Piribedil, a dopamine receptor agonist, has been shown to produce improvement in parkinsonism patients. It is less effective than levodopa and is occasionally a useful adjuvant to levodopa therapy (7). Dose can be started at 20-40 mg three times a day and increased not to exceed 300 mg daily. Side effects include dyskinesia and mental confusion.

AMANTADINE

Amantadine (1) an antiviral agent (Chapter 25.1) that augments release and delays uptake of dopamine and thereby enhances dopaminergic action in the striatum (Chapter 7.4), moderately reduces the signs and symptoms and improves functional activity in some parkinsonian patients. It is clearly less efficacious than levodopa but produces a more rapid response (2-5 days) and fewer side effects; its doses are easier to adjust. It is slightly more efficacious than the anticholinergic agents. However, its efficacy deteriorates in 3-6 months. Therefore it is used by some physicians episodically for short intervals to provide additional therapeutic support when needed.

The drug may be used alone for initial therapy, but is more efficacious when given with levodopa or anticholinergics. It is particularly beneficial in patients who cannot tolerate the maximum effective dose of levodopa. Pharmacokinetics and adverse effects of amantadine are discussed in Chapter 25.1.

ERGOT DERIVATIVES

Ergot derivatives, which demonstrate dopaminergic activity in animal models of parkinsonism, have been tried in parkinsonian patients (4-6). These compounds include lergotrile, lisuride, and bromocriptine, the last one being the most studied and promising. Lergotrile showed similar effects to bromocriptine but was barred because of hepatotoxicity.

BROMOCRIPTINE

Bromocriptine (1) is more effective than anticholinergic agents and amantadine and less effective than levodopa in the management of parkinsonism. Approximately 50-70% of patients respond favorably to adequate doses of bromocriptine. In general, neurological improvement occurs at daily dose levels of 80-100 mg.

Adverse Reactions. Adverse effects at mean daily doses of 10-50 mg include, in order of frequency, transient dizziness, nausea and vomiting, postural hypotension, colicky abdominal pain, constipation, blurred vision, frequent extrasystoles and digital vasospasm in response to cold, and jaundice. With higher daily doses (50-100 mg or more) erythromelalgia, mental disturbances, and dyskinesia may occur.

DEPRENYL

Deprenyl (1) an inhibitor of MAO-B, which occurs predominantly in the brain, prevents degradation and preserves dopamine in the basal ganglia and produces significant, although limited, role in therapy of Parkinson's disease. The drug itself does not have any effect on parkinsonism in doses up to 15 mg/day. Given with levodopa alone or levodopa plus carbidopa, deprenyl increases the duration of action of levodopa and is beneficial in overcoming early morning stiffness and immobility; it has also been shown to be quite effective in diminishing the incidence of on-off phenomena.

Adverse Effects. Increased incidence of dyskinesia occurs in 33% of patients. Incidence of nausea, dryness of mouth, confusion, and dizziness is 10-20% and that of orthostatic hypotension, syncope, circumoral paresthesia, hallucinations, and unpleasant taste is 5% or less. This agent is not apt to produce "beer, cheese, and wine" type of hypertensive crisis as is seen with MAO-A inhibitors. However, 1 patient in a group of 32 patients was reported to develop hypertension.

This drug is not currently available in the United States, and its place in treating Parkinson's disease has not been established.

ANTICHOLINERGIC AGENTS

Anticholinergic agents were the drugs of choice for treatment of parkinsonism before introduction of levodopa and are still useful in patients with minimal symptoms, in those in whom levodopa is contraindicated (e.g., presence of cardiac arrhythmias, cardiac failure, or recent cardiac infarction), or in those unable to tolerate levodopa because of side effects. Given in combination, they act synergistically to improve the therapeutic efficacy of levodopa alone or with carbidopa. They are also useful in management of extrapyramidal syndrome induced by antipsychotic drugs.

These drugs reduce the excitatory effect of the cholinergic system in the striatum resulting from dopamine deficiency in pathological or drug-induced parkinsonism and thereby maintain the balance between the two neurotransmitter systems regulating motor function in the basal ganglia.

The anticholinergic drugs that cross the blood-brain barrier are efficacious in therapy of Parkinson's disease, indicating that their effect is central. Quaternary ammonium compounds do not have effect on Parkinson's disease. Belladonna alkaloids, atropine, and scopolamine were the first centrally acting anticholinergic agents used in Parkinson's disease, but because of their peripheral side effects, they have been largely replaced by synthetic central anticholinergic agents which produce fewer peripheral side effects. These are listed in Table 9.4-1.

Of these compounds, trihexyphenidyl or benztropine is preferred for initiating therapy or may be added to levodopa to achieve maximum improvement. Ethopropazine and antihistamines are used primarily as adjunct. Because of their sedative effects, antihistamines can also help counteract the insomnia that may follow use of levodopa and anticholinergic drugs.

The adverse effects are related to the peripheral or central cholinergic-blocking activity of these drugs. The most common adverse effects include dryness of mouth, mydriasis, cycloplegia, tachycardia, constipation, urinary retention, and psychic disturbances. Sudden withdrawal of these drugs can cause a rebound worsening of parkinsonism, and therefore they should be withdrawn slowly.

THERAPY OF PARKINSONISM

The goals in therapy of parkinsonism (1) are to provide maximum relief of the major symptoms (e.g., bradykinesia, rigidity, tremor) and to maintain some freedom of movement and activity. Drug therapy is palliative and not curative. A total program of therapy should also include physiotherapy, exercise, and psychological support.

The choice of drugs depends principally on the severity of the disease. Relatively inactive patients with minimal disorder may not need any drug therapy. When the disease progresses, central anticholinergic agents may be used initially. In patients in whom anticholinergics are contraindicated, amantadine may be used. A combination of amantadine with anticholinergics has an additive effect.

In moderate or severe disease conditions levodopa with decarboxylase inhibitor (e.g., carbidopa) is most effective. Combination of carbidopa with levodopa (preferably in 1:4 ratio) offers the best relief for rigidity and akinesia. It improves quality of life and reduces mortality by 50%. The greatest benefit occurs in the first 3 years. Combination therapy also eliminates complications such as nausea, vomiting, and cardiac and respiratory arrhythmias; pyridoxine need not be avoided during such treatment. However, the abnormal involuntary movements, hallucinations, occasional psychosis, and a dopa-resistant state may appear earlier and limit the treatment

Table 9.4-1
Centrally Active Anticholinergic Drugs

Drugs	Dosage Form[a]	Initial Dose (mg)	Usual Daily Dose (mg)
Piperidyl compounds			
Biperiden (AKINETON)	T 2 mg; I 5 mg/ml	2, t.i.d.	5-20
Cycrimine (PAGITANE)	T 1.25, 2.5 mg	1.25, t.i.d.	12.5-20
Procyclidine (KEMADRIN)	T 2,5 mg	5, b.i.d.	20-30
Trihexyphenidyl (ARTANE, TREMIN)	T 2,5 mg C 5 mg E 2 mg/5 ml	2, b.i.d./t.i.d.	15-20 or >
Tropano derivatives			
Benztropine (COGENTIN)	T 0.5, 1,2 mg; I 1 mg/ml	0.5 to 1 mg at bedtime	4-6
Antihistamines			
Chlorphenoxamine (PHENOXENE)	T 50 mg	50, t.i.d.	150-400
Diphenhydramine (BENADRYL)	C 25, 50 mg E 12.5 mg/5 ml I 10 or 50 mg/ml	25, t.i.d.	100-200
Orphenadrine (DISIPAL)	T 50 mg	50, t.i.d.	50-250
Phenothiazine			
Ethopropazine (PARSIDOL)	T 10,50,100 mg	50, once or b.i.d.	100-600

[a] T, tablet; I, injection; C, capsule; E, elixir.

efficacy (3). Since dopaminergic drugs (with or without decarboxylase inhibitors) are limited in their duration of effectiveness, the drugs should be reserved for severe stage of the disease.

When levodopa is contraindicated in a patient, or a patient shows tolerance or significant fluctuation in therapeutic response to levodopa or its combination with carbidopa, a dopamine agonist like bromocriptine can be used.

After 2-5 years, responsiveness to levodopa gradually diminishes and end-of-dose akinesia, on-off phenomena, and /or psychic disturbances are commonly observed. Bromocriptine or amantadine has been added to the regimen of such patients. However, neither drug is uniformly effective in reducing the incidence or severity of such adverse effects or preventing the reduction of responsiveness to levodopa. Currently, investigated drugs like deprenyl, a MAO-B inhibitor which prolongs dopamine action, may be helpful in reducing difficulties of levodopa therapy.

Preparations. Preparations and doses for some dopamine agonists are given in Chapter 7.4. Those for anticholinergic agents are given in Table 9.4-1.

MISCELLANEOUS DYSKINETIC DISORDERS

Different types of extrapyramidal movement disorders have been clinically distinguished as dyskinesias or involuntary abnormal movements. Some of these disorders that respond to pharmacological treatment to varying extents (1) are discussed here.

MYOCLONUS

Myoclonus is characterized by brief muscular contraction of sudden onset and closely related to epileptic seizures. They respond to antiepileptic drugs and are discussed in Chapter 11.5.

TICS

Tics (habit spasms) like myoclonus are characterized by isolated muscle twitches or jerks that are often repetitive and stereotyped. They are commonly associated with anxiety and can be controlled by will indicating that they are not strictly involuntary. The antianxiety drugs may relieve some simple disorders, but chronic multiple tics (Gilles de la Tourette's syndrome) that may need effective treatment respond to antipsychotic drugs, particularly haloperidol. If the latter fails, fluphenazine, clonazepam, clonidine, or carbamazepine should be tried.

TREMOR

Tremor is a rhythmic oscillatory movement resulting from involuntary alternating contraction of opposing muscle groups. It may be static (present at rest, as in parkinsonism), postural or action (present throughout the course of a movement, as in senility), or intention (enhanced toward the end of movement, as in cerebellar disease, multiple sclerosis, and delirium tremor). Physiological postural tremor is enhanced in amplitude by anxiety, stress, fatigue, thyrotoxicosis, or induced by epinephrine, isoproterenol, amphetamine, bronchodilators, tricyclic antidepressants, and lithium. Propranolol has been useful in reducing amplitude of postural tremor. Drug-induced tremors are readily stopped by discontinuation of drugs.

Essential tremor is a postural or action tremor that is clinically similar to physiological tremor. Its frequency is in the range of 4-12 Hz and primarily involves the upper extremities. It is sometimes familial and develops in adults without any demonstrable neurological abnormalities (benign hereditary tremor).

β-Adrenergic blocking agents diminish tremor in amplitude. Propranolol has been used extensively, but whether the response depends on a central or peripheral action is unclear. Metoprolol, a relatively selective β_1-blocker has been sometimes useful, particularly when propranolol is contraindicated as in patients with concomitant pulmonary disease. Thus, dysfunction of β_1-adrenoceptors has been implicated in some cases of tremor, since they respond to both propranolol as well as metoprolol. However, tremor produced by a sympathomimetic bronchodilator such as terbutaline is blocked by propranolol, which is both β_1 and β_2-adrenoceptor antagonist, but not by metoprolol, a β_1-antagonist, suggesting that such tremor is mediated mainly by the β_2-adrenoceptors. Small quantities of alcohol may also suppress essential tremor, but only for a brief period.

HUNTINGTON'S DISEASE

Huntington's disease is a progressive hereditary disorder due to degeneration of the basal ganglia and cerebral cortex and characterized by choreiform movements and mental deterioration. It usually begins in adult life, and its inheritance is based on a single autosomal gene. Juvenile-onset Huntington's disease begins in the first or second decade of life and is characterized by bradykinesia and muscular rigidity resembling parkinsonism more than chorea.

Development of chorea appears to be the result of imbalance between several neurotransmitters in the basal ganglia [e.g., dopamine, acetylcholine, γ-aminobutyric acid (GABA), and perhaps others]. Thus in Huntington's disease, as a result of widespread degenerative changes in the basal ganglia, levels of acetylcholine and choline acetylase as well as GABA and the enzyme glutamic acid decarboxylase (GAD), concerned with its synthesis, are markedly reduced. On the other hand, functional overactivity is manifested in dopaminergic nigrostriatal pathways as demonstrated by pharmacological studies (see later). Accordingly, therapy is directed toward correcting the neurotransmitter imbalance. However, drug therapy is only a small part of the overall management of adults with this disease. The goal of therapy is to antagonize the brain dopaminergic overactivity or enhance cholinergic activity.

Drugs that impair dopaminergic activity either by depleting central monoamines (e.g., reserpine, tetrabenazine) or by blocking dopamine receptors (e.g., antipsychotic agents) are often beneficial in reducing chorea, whereas levodopa that enhances dopaminergic activity aggravates the abnormalities. However, levodopa may be of short-term benefit in juvenile-onset Huntington's disease. Antipsychotic drugs (phenothiazines, butyrophenones) antagonize dopamine overactivity and lessen chorea in adult-onset disease. Drugs with minimal anticholinergic activity may be preferred.

Reserpine, which depletes cerebral dopamine by preventing intraneuronal storage, is often effective in suppressing chorea in a daily dose of 2-5 mg, but side effects such as hypotension, sedation, depression, diarrhea, and nasal stuffiness may be troublesome. Tetrabenazine (NITOMAN), also a dopamine-depleting agent, has been effective in reducing chorea of Huntington's disease. Since this drug is not expected to produce serious side effects, such as receptor supersensitivity (as in tardive dyskinesia related to antipsychotic drugs) or severe depression and hypotension (as in the case of reserpine), tetrabenazine is considered a drug of choice by some physicians in Europe. This drug is available in the United States only as an investigational agent.

Attempts have been made to enhance cholinergic activity by administering precursors of acetylcholine, such as choline and deanol. However, deanol may interfere with choline transport into the brain despite elevation of plasma choline levels and hence may not be clinically effective in chorea. Choline has been shown to be effective in some patients.

In view of the concomitant deficiency of GABA in the basal ganglia of patients with Huntington's disease, drugs have been used to increase GABA activity. Baclofen, an analog of GABA, has not been effective in chorea. Isoniazid, an antitubercular drug, which inhibits GABA aminotransferase and thereby increases GABA levels in animals, has been shown to produce clinical improvement in patients with Huntington's disease, but its dose was three to five times the antitubercular dose and may have serious adverse effects.

TARDIVE DYSKINESIA

Tardive dyskinesia is characterized by a variety of abnormal movements that develop after long-term neuroleptic treatment and is discussed in Chapter 11.6.1.

Pathogenesis of neuroleptic-induced tardive dyskinesia has been ascribed to development of supersensitivity of postsynaptic dopamine receptors. Central noradrenergic hyperactivity and presynaptic dopaminergic overactivity may also be involved (8). Available therapy aims at restoring the neurotransmitter balance by increasing cholinergic activity and/or decreasing dopaminergic overactivity. As mentioned in Chapter 11.6.1, attempts to increase cholinergic activity by using deanol, choline, or lecithin have been beneficial in some cases but not in others; they also produce side effects.

Dopaminergic activity can be interfered with either by receptor blockade or by dopamine depletion. Unfortunately, the receptor-blocking drugs are the ones that cause this dyskinesia as a late effect. If tardive dyskinesia develops during or after antipsychotic drug therapy, larger doses or restitution of therapy usually terminates the choreiform activity. Although neuroleptics are significantly superior to most other therapy, if possible, such therapy best be avoided to prevent a spiral phenomenon of continued use of higher doses of such drugs to cause temporary suppression of dyskinesia. If antipsychotic therapy has to be continued despite tardive dyskinesia, use of a weak dopamine antagonist like thioridazine may produce less adverse effects; however, there are no clinical data to support this recommendation. Clozapine (LEPONEX), a new drug which is not yet approved for use in the United States, has not been reported to cause tardive dyskinesia. However, this drug can cause agranulocytosis.

A dopamine-depleting agent, tetrabenazine (an investigational drug), would not produce supersensitivity like antipsychotic agents, or serious adverse effects like the other amine-depleting agent, reserpine, and is considered a drug of choice by some physicians in Europe. A combination of reserpine and haloperidol has been used with benefit in some patients. Several GABA-mimetic agents such as baclofen, muscimol, γ-acetylenic-GABA, benzodiazepines, and sodium valproate have also been tried with varying amounts of good results. Among the nonneuroleptic drugs, catecholamine-depleting agents and GABA-mimetic agents appear to be promising (9, 10). Several other drugs such as lithium, methyldopa, amantadine, clonidine, and propranolol have been investigated with limited benefit and /or marked adverse effects (1).

BALLISMUS

Ballismus is a violent dyskinesia consisting of continual, usually unilateral, purposeless flinging movement of the limbs. The muscles involved are in the shoulder and pelvic girdle. It is most often produced by acute vascular infarction of the subthalamic nucleus. It responds quite well to antipsychotic drugs such as haloperidol, perphenazine, and others.

DYSTONIAS

Dystonias are abnormal, sustained, often bizarre posturing movements of neck, jaw, eyes, and trunk (e.g., torticolis, masse-ter spasm, grimacing, perioral spasms, protrusion of tongue, dysphagia, blepharospasm, oculogyric crisis, and opisthotonus). It may be idiopathic, hereditary, caused by perinatal cerebral injury and encephalitis, or induced by drugs (e.g., antipsychotics and other antidopaminergic agents such as antiemetics like metoclopramide and prochlorperazine). Drug-induced dystonias can be treated by antihistaminics (e.g., diphenhydramine) or centrally acting anticholinergic agents (e.g., benztropine, biperiden).

WILSON'S DISEASE

Wilson's disease is a rare autosomal recessively inherited disorder of copper metabolism; it is characterized by degenerative changes in the brain, particularly in the basal ganglia, and cirrhosis of liver, and marked by increased concentration of copper in the brain and viscera. A brownish pigmented ring at the corneal margin is pathognomonic of the disease.

Treatment involves the removal of excess copper by a chelating agent, penicillamine, followed by maintenance of copper balance. Mechanism of action and pharmacological and adverse effects of this drug are discussed in Chapter 28.1.

REFERENCES

1. *AMA Drug Evaluation*, 5th ed. Chicago: American Medical Association, 1983, p. 329.
2. Bernheimer, H., Birkmayer, W., Hornykiewicz, O., Jellinger, K., and Seitelberger, F. Brain dopamine and the syndromes of Parkinson and Huntington. *J. Neural. Sci.* 20:415, 1973.
3. Boshes, B., Sinemet and the treatment of parkinsonism. *Ann. Intern. Med.* 94:364, 1981.
4. Calne, D. B. Developments in the pharmacology and therapeutics of parkinsonism. *Ann. Neurol.* 1:111, 1977.
5. Calne, D. B. Parkinsonism: Clinical and neuropharmacologic aspects. *Postgrad. Med.* 64:82, 1978.
6. Calne, D. B. Role of ergot derivatives in the treatment of parkinsonism. *Fed. Proc.* 37:2207, 1978.
7. Feigenson, J. S., Sweet, R. D., and McDowell, F. H. Piribedil: Its synergistic effect in multidrug regimens of parkinsonism. *Neurology* 26:430, 1976.
8. Jeste, D. V., and Wyatt, R. J. Dogma disputed: Is tardive dyskinesia due to postsynaptic dopamine receptor supersensitivity. *J. Clin. Psychiatry* 42:455, 1981.
9. Jeste, D. V., and Wyatt, R. J. Therapeutic strategies against tardive dyskinesia: Two decades of experience. *Arch. Gen. Psychiatry* 39:803, 1982.
10. Simpson, G. M. et al. Management of tardive dyskinesia: Current update. *Drugs* 23:381, 1982.
11. Weiner, M. Update on antiparkinsonian agents. *Geriatrics* 37:81, 1982.

CHAPTER
10

DRUGS AFFECTING PERCEPTION OF PAIN

Sachin N. Pradhan and James A. Holloway

MEANING OF PAIN

Pain is a complex experience that includes not only the sensation provoked by noxious or tissue-damaging stimulation produced by injury or disease but also emotional reactions and certain associated autonomic, psychological, and behavioral responses. Reactions to pain may vary from one person to another and from time to time in the same person. They arouse the subject and demand immediate attention. Reflexive, complex autonomic and somatic motor responses are initiated to promote escape or avoidance. Cultural background, past experience, and emotional level preceding the exposure to noxious stimulation influence the response. The most important factor, however, is perhaps the personality of the sufferer. Thus, the perception of pain is immensely modified by reactions induced by multidimensional factors including attentional, cognitive, motivational and emotional variables.

NEURAL PATHWAYS OF PAIN

Pain acts as a signal warning about possible damage to a tissue. Pathways that transmit pain messages serve as a pain-signaling system required to protect the body. Pain is produced by excitation of functionally distinct types of pain receptors or nociceptors. Sensation is carried by afferent fibers of the dorsal root ganglia to the substantia gelatinosa of the spinal cord or by cranial nerve V to the brain stem trigeminal nuclear complex. From these sites, the spinothalamic neurons carry sensory impulses to the thalamus and then to the sensory cortex. Although these systems carry specific sensory-discriminative impulses to higher centers of pain perception, another system is concerned with the unpleasant and aversive aspects of pain sensations and involves the ascending reticular-activating system that projects to the cortex via medial thalamic nuclei and to the limbic areas. This system thus participates in the attentional and emotional aspects of pain and is concerned with the suffering aspect arousing the desire to escape the pain. Whereas the sensory aspect of pain may remain similar among different individuals and at different times in the same individual, the suffering aspect shows variations depending on personality and situational and cultural factors. Thus, a headache may be ignored or treated with a mild analgesic, but when it becomes known to be due to a brain tumor, the pain appears to become intolerable.

The trigeminothalamic neurons (projecting from the nucleus caudalis in the medulla to the thalamus) consist of: (1) nociceptive-specific neurons that respond only to intense mechanical and thermal stimuli and appear to receive input only from small myelinated (Aδ) and unmyelinated (C) afferent fibers; (2) wide, dynamic-range neurons that are activated by hair movement and mechanical forces less than 1 g [many respond to noxious heat, and appear to receive input from Aδ and C primary afferents and also from myelinated (Aβ) afferents]; and (3) low-threshold mechanoreceptives neurons that respond to light touch, pressure, or hair movements and appear to receive input from large Aβ afferents. They can inhibit or suppress the responses of nociceptive-specific and wide, dynamic-range neurons (2).

CHEMICAL MEDIATORS OF PAIN

A number of substances have been shown to produce pain when applied on a blister base or injected in different layers of or under the skin or injected parenterally. These include acetylcholine, potassium ions, acids (lactic or hydrochloric), histamine, 5-hydroxytryptamine (5-HT), bradykinin, and prostaglandins.

Of these agents, histamine, 5-HT, and bradykinin appear to be more probable candidates as mediators at the nociceptor level. They are released soon after injury and can cause pain if given in small quantities, probably within the range of physiological concentrations. They also produce hyperemia and swelling as in inflammation, and thus induce inflammatory pain. Prostaglandins themselves do not induce pain except in very high doses, but they can potentiate pain induced by other algesic agents (e.g., bradykinin). They are thought to sensitize the nociceptors. Once released, prostaglandins can cause inflammation, releasing algesic agents like bradykinin and histamine whose actions on the already sensitized nerve endings are then facilitated. Hence, prostaglandins are considered as neuromodulators of nociceptor mechanisms.

The chemical neurotransmitters in the first-order afferent nociceptive neurons may include substance P and glutamate. Substance P is present predominantly in the neurons composing the dorsal horn of the spinal cord. Glutamate, although found in many areas of the CNS, is concentrated primarily in the dorsal afferent root of the spinal cord, and particularly in the central branches of the primary afferent neurons. Hence, they are considered as neurotransmitters within the primary sensory neurons. These agents are briefly described subsequently.

Histamine and 5-HT produce pain when applied on a blister base in humans or injected intraarterially in dog spleen. These amines are widely distributed in all tissues, particularly in platelets, basophils, and tissue mast cells. They are released during tissue damage, inflammation, and other conditions. Histamine has been implicated in producing headache. A role of 5-HT is postulated in migraine headache during which a subject is markedly supersensitive to this amine. An antagonist to 5-HT (e.g., methysergide) has been used as prophylactic to such headache.

Bradykinin, a nonapeptide kinin, formation of which requires a complex cascade of reactions (Chapter 13.1.3), is a potent algesic agent. It is particularly relevant in inflammatory pain. Its repeated application causes tachyphylaxis. Bradykinin is known to release prostaglandins, which potentiate the algesic action of bradykinin.

Prostaglandins are a complex group of derivatives of a polyunsaturated fatty acid, arachidonic acid (Chapter 13.2). They are formed and released in response to noxious stimuli and play an important role as pain mediators. Prostaglandins are not stored within the cells but are produced from phospholipid precursors in the cell membrane during pain; bradykinin may act as a releaser. Certain steps in their formation are known to be blocked by some substances that serve as effective therapeutic agents in relief of pain. Thus, the glucocorticoid steroids block the activity of phospholipase A_2, the enzyme responsible for the formation of arachidonic acid, via synthesis of a protein or a peptide. The ability of the steroids to block the formation of prostaglandins parallels their antiinflammatory activity. In the next step of prostaglandin synthesis, arachidonic acid is converted to cyclic endoperoxides by the enzyme cyclooxygenase, which is inhibited by aspirin and other minor analgesics (Fig. 13.2-1). Thus, the effects of both aspirin-like drugs and the steroids are probably peripheral and at the nociceptor level; the steroids produce a more general blockade of all proinflammatory mediators.

Substance P (SP), an undecapeptide (Chapter 13.1.1), is present in the primary sensory neurons. This peptide is found in association with pain fibers as in the skin or dental pulp. The central branch of the sensory fibers containing SP terminates mainly in the dorsal horn of spinal cord. Strong afferent stimulation releases SP from the perfused cord, indicating that SP is an excitatory transmitter of the first afferent synapse of the pain pathway. However, since excitation produced by SP is markedly slower than that induced by natural stimulation, SP has been proposed instead to act as a neuromodulator that modifies neuronal excitability. SP is also widely distributed in the CNS and has been shown to produce algesic and analgesic actions, depending on the species, the dose, and the route of administration.

PAIN-MODULATION SYSTEMS

When the message from the nociceptors is transmitted along the primary afferent fibers (small myelinated and unmyelinated neurons) to the spinal cord, it is subjected to two important modifications at this level: (a) through involvement of the sympathetic nervous system and (b) by action of large myelinated afferent fibers. The sympathetic nervous system can induce pain that can be illustrated by occurrence of causalgia, the severe burning pain that is sometimes produced after nerve injury. Such pain is completely relieved by sympathetic block. On the other hand, as already mentioned earlier, the transmission of a pain message carried along the nociceptive specific and wide, dynamic-range neurons at the spinal cord can be suppressed by the large myelinated afferent fibers. This phenomena is probably the basis of certain local therapeutic procedures such as massage, acupuncture, and transcutaneous electric nerve stimulation (TENS) (1, 3).

In addition to these, a descending pain-modulating network with links in the midbrain, medulla, and spinal cord has recently been discovered. Existence of such a system is based on several lines of evidence: (a) analgesia produced by electrical stimulation of discrete brain areas, (b) discovery of opiate receptors in brain areas, (c) isolation of opioid peptides and their localization in the brain, and (d) effects of microinjection of opiate and lesioning of specific brain areas.

It has been demonstrated in rats as well as in patients with intractable pain that electrical stimulation of the midbrain periaqueductal gray matter (dorsal raphe nucleus) and diencephalic periventricular region can inhibit nociceptive neurons in the trigeminal nucleus caudalis and the spinal cord dorsal horn. Repetitive (10-30 Hz) electrical stimulation of these midbrain and diencephalic regions can suppress for minutes the heat-induced responses of nociceptive-specific and wide, dynamic-range trigeminothalamic neurons.

Modulation of pain within the CNS by chemical mediators has also been revealed in recent years. Specific opioid receptors are ubiquitous. They have been identified at several levels of the pain pathways such as the dorsal horn of the spinal cord, spinal trigeminal nucleus, the medullary raphe nuclei, and periaqueductal gray matter; such receptors also exist in other CNS areas regulating mood and behavior and neuroendocrine functions (e.g., locus ceruleus, striatum, and hypothalamus) and in small intestine; opiates and opioids would act on these receptors to produce their analgesic, euphoric (or dysphoric), constipating, and other effects. Presence of opioid receptors in mood- and behavior-regulating areas may indirectly imply emotional aspects of pain.

The opioid receptors are also acted on by the endogenous opioid peptides such as endorphins and enkephalins that show morphinelike effects. Endorphins, whose distributions are similar to those of opioid receptors, have longer-lasting action and are viewed as neurohormones, whereas enkephalins (Met-enkephalin and Leu-enkephalin), which have wider distributions and shorter actions, are suggested to function as neurotransmitters or modulators of synaptic function. Short enkephalin-releasing interneurons have been suggested to exist in the substantia gelatinosa; when activated by noxious stimuli or by glutamate, these neurons release enkephalins that act exclusively at postsynaptic sites producing tonic inhibitory inputs that can be blocked or antagonized by naloxone.

The endogenous descending pain-modulation or analgesia-producing system can be described at midbrain, medullary, and spinal cord levels (1, 3). At the midbrain level, this system involves the periaqueductal gray (PAG), an area rich in endorphins and opiate receptors and an important site for induction of analgesia produced by electrical stimulation as well as microinjection of opiates. Excitatory inputs are sent from PAG to serotonin-containing cells of the nucleus raphe magnus (NRM) and the adjacent magnocellular nucleus of the reticular formation (Rmc) of the medulla, which in turn send efferent fibers to the spinal cord. At the spinal level, efferent fibers from the NRM and Rmc descend in the dorsal lateral fasciculus to terminate among pain transmission cells concentrated in laminae I and V of the dorsal horn. The NRM exerts an inhibitory effect, via enkephalinergic neurons, specifically on nociceptive (substance P-containing) primary afferent fibers. The pain transmission (second order) neurons, which may be activated by substance P-containing small-diameter primary afferents, project to supraspinal sites and indirectly, via the nucleus gigantocellularis of the reticular formation, excite the cells of the descending analgesia system in the PAG and NRM, thus establishing a negative feedback loop.

In summary, the endogenous analgesia-producing system has the following major characteristics: it is at least partially endorphin mediated; it involves serotonergic mechanisms; it depends on activation of descending efferent pathways that inhibit pain-transmission neurons; and, it is effectively activated by noxious stimulation. Although the description of this endogenous system is far from complete, an outline of the mechanisms of pain suppression has emerged.

For its functioning the pain-modulation system depends mostly on the release of endorphin, although other neurotransmitters may be involved. This system is set in motion by noxious stimuli and stress and limits perception of pain by interfering with the afferent input at the level of the spinal cord. This system is also affected by psychological factors that may be responsible for causing variations in pain perception. Analgesic effect of placebo has been demonstrated in patients with postoperative dental pain, and the pain-modulation system may involve release of endorphins. Naloxone, an opioid antagonist, produces significant hyperalgesia in patients responding to placebo, but has little effect in nonresponsive patients (1, 3).

The observations on the pain-signaling as well as the pain-modulation systems discussed previously led to the formalization of a *gate-control theory* (4) at several CNS levels, regulated by afferent inputs of both large (Aβ) and small (Aδ and C) fibers reaching the spinal cord or by activation of descending regulatory pathways. Neural mechanisms in the substantia gelatinosa of the spinal cord dorsal horn act like a gate that increases or decreases the flow of nerve impulses from the peripheral afferent fibers to the CNS. In this way, an increase in large fiber input would result in dampening of transmission by negative feedback and, hence, close the gate, whereas increased small fiber input would exacerbate the pain state by a positive feedback effect thereby opening the gate. A similar gating mechanism may exist in the trigeminal system.

THERAPEUTIC INTERVENTION

On the basis of previous discussion relating to the existence of a pain-transmission and pain-modulation system, there are at least two general classes of approaches to pain management: one is to block the pain-transmission system and the other is to turn on or stimulate the pain-suppression system. Table 10-1 summarizes the sites and mechanisms of action of various analgesic agents acting on these two systems. Thus, the pain transmission is affected by steroids and aspirin-like drugs that would relieve pain at the nociceptor level by inhibiting synthesis of prostaglandins. Local anesthetics act by blocking afferent nerves transmitting the impulses generated by nociceptive stimuli. On the other hand, narcotic analgesics like morphine or codeine activate the pain-suppression system by acting at the specific site in the

Table 10-1
Morphological and Biochemical Basis of Therapy of Pain

Morphological Sites	Chemical Mediators	Therapeutic Agents or Procedures
Chemosensitive nociceptors (peripheral)	Algesic agents (e.g., histamine, 5-hydroxytryptamine, bradykinin, prostaglandins)	Steroids[a] Aspirin[a], indomethacin[a]
Afferent fibers		
Fine fibers (A, C) from nociceptors	Substance P	Local anesthetics
Large fibers (Aβ) from mechanoreceptors	—	Counterirritants
Spinal and higher central modulatory systems	Endorphin[b], enkephalins[b]	Morphine, codeine, and other narcotics
	5-Hydroxytryptamine[b]	Antidepressants
Sensory cortex, reticular formation, spinal cord, etc.	—	General anesthetics
Limbic system, hypothalamus and cortex	—	Tranquilizers (i.e., diazepam)

[a]Inhibit prostaglandin synthesis.
[b]Analgesic.

brain. They bind to the opiate receptors and activate the descending inhibitory neurons that release 5-HT at their spinal endings as an inhibitory neurotransmitter or neuromodulator and thus suppress nociceptive impulses at the level of the spinal cord. Because both endorphins and opiate receptors are present in the spinal cord, local application of morphine or other narcotics is expected to produce analgesia. In fact, their epidural or intrathecal administration has produce powerful and long-lasting analgesia that can be reversed with opiate antagonists. Antidepressants (tricyclic antidepressants or monoamine oxidase inhibitors) may exaggerate and prolong the effects of some opioid analgesics, probably by modifying the metabolism of 5-HT and other neurotransmitters involved.

General anesthetics (such as halothane, ether, nitrous oxide, barbiturates) have been shown to depress both spontaneous and evoked activity of neurons in laminae IV-VI of the spinal cord dorsal horn (of some vertebrates) where first-order nociceptive afferent neurons make their synapses. They also act at the level of the reticular-activating system. Pain perception (at the sensory cortex) is inhibited by the general anesthetics in stage I of anesthesia, which is called stage of analgesia. Cognitive, affective, and attentional components of the pain can be inhibited by tranquilizers such as diazepam that reduce apprehension and anxiety associated with the cause of pain (such as surgical procedure).

Counterirritant methods (e.g., application of pressure or mustard plaster on a painful site, scratching to relieve itch) have been used for centuries. Vibration, pressure, or tactile stimuli have also been used recently to alter response to pain under experimental situations. These techniques suggest selective enhancement of large fiber input that in turn suppresses transmission of noxious input. Relief of pain by transcutaneous electrical stimulation of large fibers is also based on a similar mechanism. Stimulation of the dorsal columns with implanted electrodes, which has been less successful as a pain reliever, also selectively activates large fibers. Success of intense auditory stimuli (audioanalgesia) to suppress pain produced by dental procedures under some conditions can be related to central control mechanism and psychological processes such as suggestions. Methods such as hypnosis, behavioral modification, and placebo drugs are based on such pain control measures.

Acupuncture, which has been practiced for centuries in China with much success, is effective in selective patients and involves many of the pain control mechanisms previously discussed. In laboratory experimental studies, the acupuncture needling technique has been shown to cause a slight increase in pain thresholds and reduce pain sensitivity and the willingness of the subject to report pain. Elevation of tooth-pulp thresholds produced by acupuncture has been shown to be reversed by naloxone. Thus, the mechanism of acupuncture-produced analgesia may partially be related to endogenous opioid peptides and descending brain stem pathways that are also activated by opiate drugs.

REFERENCES

1. Basbaum, A. I., and Fields, H. L. Endogenous pain control mechanisms: Review and Hypothesis. *Ann. Neurol.* 4:451, 1978.
2. Dubner, R. Neurophysiology of pain. *Dent. Clin. North Am.* 22:11, 1978.

3. Fields, H. L. Neurophysiology of pain and pain modulation. *Am. J. Med.* 77 (3A):1, 1984.

4. Yaksh, T. L., and Hammond, D. L. Peripheral and central substrates involved in the rostrad transmission of nociceptive information. *Pain* 13:1, 1982.

ADDITIONAL READING

Albe-Fessard, D. et al. Diencephalic mechanism of pain sensation. *Brain Res.* 356:217, 1985.

Beers, R.F., Jr., and Bassett, E.G. (eds.). *Mechanisms of Pain and Analgesic Compounds.* New York: Raven Press, 1979.

Hirst, M. The changing nature of pain control. Clinical aspects of endorphins and enkephalins. *Canad. Dent. Assoc. J.* 51:493, 1985.

Mayer, D. J., and Price, D. D. Central nervous system mechanisms of analgesia. *Pain* 2:379, 1976.

Melzack, R., and Dennis, S. G. Pain mechanisms: Theoretical approaches. In: *Mechanisms of Pain and Analgesic Compounds.* New York: Raven Press, 1979, p. 185.

Terenius, L. Biochemical mediators in pain. *Triangle* 20:19, 1981.

CHAPTER
10.1

NARCOTIC AGONISTS AND ANTAGONISTS

Sachin N. Pradhan and Samar N. Dutta

NARCOTIC ANALGESICS

The word *opium* is derived from the Greek word for "juice," the alkaloid being extracted from the juice of unripe poppy capsules. The alkaloid was isolated in 1803 by a German pharmacist who named it *morphine* after Morpheus, the Greek god of dreams. In succeeding years, other opium alkaloids (e.g., codeine and papaverine) were isolated and by the middle of the nineteenth century these alkaloids found their way into clinical practice in preference to crude opium preparations.

With the introduction of the hypodermic needle, parenteral use of morphine led to increased frequency of its compulsive abuse. Recognition of the serious dependence liability of morphine stimulated the search for nonaddictive analgesics, and as a result various semisynthetic and synthetic analgesic compounds were developed.

The term *opiate* refers to components of the opium plant that have narcotic properties similar to morphine, and the term opioid generally refers to synthetic and endogenous opiate-like compounds that are directly acting agents and whose effects are stereospecifically blocked by pure narcotic antagonists like naloxone.

CLASSIFICATION

There are two main classes of narcotic analgesics used in humans: (1) opium alkaloids and derivatives, and (2) synthetic analogs. Compounds under each class are further subdivided into smaller groups based on their chemical structures, as shown in Table 10.1-1.

CHEMISTRY OF OPIUM ALKALOIDS

Opium is an air-dried product of the milky exudate of the unripe seed capsules of the poppy plant, *Papaver somniferum*, indigenous to Asia Minor. This brownish gummy mass contains more than 20 alkaloids that constitute about 25% of its weight. Alkaloids contained in opium belong to distinct chemical classes: (1) phenanthrene (e.g., morphine, 10% of opium; codeine, 0.5%, thebaine, 0.2%), and (2) benzylisoquinoline (e.g., papaverine, 1%, noscapine, 6%). Of these, only morphine and codeine cause analgesia, and they are abused as narcotics.

Morphine is a pentacyclic alkaloid regarded as a derivative of phenanthrene bridged across the 4,5-positions by oxygen and across the 9,13-positions by an ethanamine chain that creates a six-membered piperidine ring with a methylated nitrogen. The ring A is fully aromatic and carries a phenolic OH group at position 3. The ring C carries a nonphenolic secondary OH group at position 6, and an isolated double bond between C7 and C8. The structure of morphine originally proposed by Gullard and Robinson in 1925 and confirmed by synthesis in 1950 (shown in Table 10.1-2) possesses asymmetric centers at positions 5, 6, 9, 13, and 14. The naturally occurring alkaloid is levo-enantiomorph; its dextro-enantiomorph available by synthesis is almost inactive as an analgesic (9).

Thebaine differs from morphine in having little analgesic action and producing seizures at relatively low dosages, possessing both OH groups methylated, and having two double bonds in the rings ($\Delta_{6,8}$, $\Delta_{9,15}$). Substitutions at certain positions in the morphine or thebaine structure led to development of a number of narcotic analgesics and antagonists, and these are shown in Table 10.1-2. A number of semisynthetic compounds have been prepared from morphine and thebaine. Chemical transformation of ring C of morphine has produced several useful drugs like hydromorphone, oxymorphone, metopon, and others. Acetylation of the 3- and 6-OH groups of morphine produces diacetylmorphine (heroin) which, although more potent than the parent compound, is more toxic and has a higher addiction liability (9). Removal of the N-methyl group of morphine gives normorphine, which is probably a metabolite and which when compared with morphine shows less potency when given paren-

Table 10.1-1
Narcotic Analgesics with Their Dosage, Duration of Analgesia, and Characteristic Features

Drugs and Classes	Analgesic Effect: Parenteral Dose[a] (s.c./i.m.) (mg)	Duration of Analgesia (hr)	Oral Dose[a] (mg)	O/P Potency Ratio[b]	Abstinence Symptom (Compared with Morphine)	Characteristic Features[c]
OPIUM ALKALOIDS AND DERIVATIVES						
Morphine and Derivatives						
Morphine	10	4-5	60	L (1/6)		
Heroin (diacetylmorphine)	3	3-4	U	L	Similar	
Hydromorphone (dihydromorphinone, DILAUDID)	1.5	4-5	6.5	L (1/5)	Similar	F
Oxymorphone (dihydrohydroxymorphinone, NUMORPHAN)	1-1.5	4-5	6.6	L (1/6)	Similar	F
Metopon (methyldihydromorphinone)	3.5	4-5			Similar	
Codeine and Derivatives						
Codeine	120	3-4 (4-6)	200 (10-30)	H (3/5)	Less	A
Hydrocodone (dihydrocodeinone, HYCODAN)		(4-8)	200 (5-10)		Less	A
Dihydrocodeine (PARACODIN)	60	4-5			Less	A
Oxycodone (dihydrohydroxycodeinone, PERCODAN)	10-15	4-5 (4-5)	15-20 (3-20)	H (2/3-1)	Less	A
SYNTHETIC ANALOGS						
Diphenylpropylamine Derivatives						
Methadone (DOLOPHINE)	7.5-10	3-5	20	H (1/2)	Less	E
Acetylmethadol (L-α-acetylmethadol, LAAM)					Less	E
Propoxyphene (dextropropoxyphene, DARVON)	240	4-5			Less	D
Phenylpiperidine derivatives						
Meperidine (pethidine, DEMEROL)	80-100	2-4	50-100	M (1/3)	Similar	C, D
Alphaprodine (NISENTIL)	40-60	1-2			Similar	C
Anileridine (LERITINE, APODOL)	25-30	2-4			Similar	C
Morphinan derivatives						
Levorphanol (LEVO-DROMORAN)	2-3	4-5	4	H (3/5)	Similar	
Butorphanol (STADOL)	1.5-2.5	4-5		L	Less	B
Benzomorphan derivative						
Pentazocine (TALWIN)	60	3-4		M (1/3)	Less	B

[a] Dose equianalgesic of 10 mg of i.m. morphine.
[b] Oral/parenteral potency ratio; H, high; M, moderate; L, low.
[c] A, used as an antitussive (figures in parentheses are oral antitussive doses and their duration of action); B, mixed agonist-antagonist; C, causes little or no constipation; D, causes marked irritation at injection site; E, may show cumulative effects on repeated dosage; F, available as suppository.

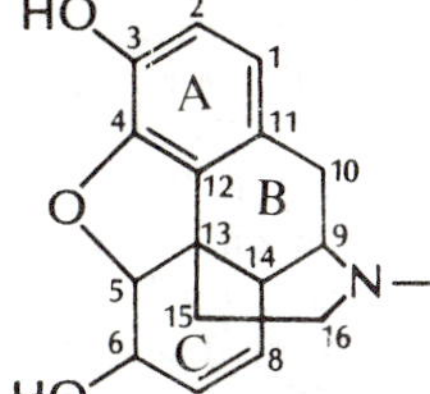

Table 10.1-2
Structure of Narcotic Agonists and Antagonists Chemically Related to Morphine

Morphine Derivatives	Substitutions of Radicals or Groups at Different Positions[a] in Morphine Structure				
	3-OH	6-OH	N-CH_3	7C = 8C	Others
Heroin	-$OCOCH_3$	-$OCOCH_3$	-	-	-
Hydromorphone	-	=O	-	C-C	-
Metopon	-	=O	-	C-C	5-CH_3
Oxymorphone	-	=O	-	C-C	14-OH
Levorphanol	-	-H	-	C-C	b
Codeine	-OCH_3	-	-	-	-
Hydrocodone	-OCH_3	=O	-	C-C	-
Oxycodone	-OCH_3	=O	-	C-C	14-OH
Nalorphine	-	-	-$CH_2CH{=}CH_2$	-	-
Naloxone	-	=O	-CH_2-$CH{=}CH_2$	C-C	14-OH
Naltrexone	-	=O	-CH (cyclopropyl)	C-C	14-OH
Nalbuphine	-	-	-CH_2 (cyclobutyl)	C-C	14-OH
Butorphanol	-	-H	-CH_2 (cyclobutyl)	-	14-OH[b]

[a]Indicated by numerals prefixed to an atom or a radical.
[b]No oxygen between C4 and C5.

terally but equal potency when given intracisternally in mice. N-allyl derivative of normorphine provides nalorphine, which antagonizes a wide spectrum of morphine actions (9).

Thebaine is a precursor of some important 14-OH compounds such as oxycodone and naloxone. Etorphine, a derivative of thebaine, is more than 1000 times as potent as morphine. Etherification of the phenolic OH group reduces its analgesic potency as seen in codeine (methyl ether), dionine (ethyl ether), and others.

OPIATE RECEPTORS

A variety of experimental evidence led to the postulation of the existence of opiate receptors related to analgesia in the mammalian nervous system. A methodological procedure for study of receptors was developed by Goldstein and coworkers (18). The direct demonstration of the presence of stereospecific and saturable binding sites or receptors for opiate agonists and antagonists in the nervous tissue was demonstrated simultaneously by Simon, Terenius, and Pert and Snyder in 1973. These developments have been described in several reviews (33, 44, 54, 55, 57). The receptors with high affinity that bind with antagonists are probably protein in nature, because various protein reagents, including sulfhydryl compounds, markedly inhibit their binding with opiates (29). Because of high selectivity, the stereoisomers of opiate such as levorphanol and dextrorphan have practically no binding affinity.

Distribution. Opiate receptors with high binding affinity are present in cerebral cortex (temporal and frontal lobes, supraorbital gyrus), amygdala, septum, thalamus (medial nuclei), hypothalamus (supra- and preoptic nuclei), and brain stem (periventricular gray). Opiate receptors with moderate to low or poor binding affinity have been reported to be distributed in various other regions of brainstem, caudate-putamen, hypothalamus, neocortex, olfactory bulb, hippocampus, and thalamus (29). The type and magnitude of response of various areas to the brain to opiates are probably related to the differences in the distribution of specific receptors. Opiate receptors are also found in some endocrine glands such as the pituitary and adrenal gland, and the innervation of certain smooth muscle systems (e.g., myenteric plexus of the guinea pig ileum and mouse vas deferens). It has been shown that these binding sites are concentrated in the synaptosomal cell fraction, suggesting a loction in the vicinity of synapses (52).

Types of Receptors. On the basis of experiments in spinal dog preparations, Martin (39) has postulated that there are three stereochemically related opiate receptors: μ (mu), κ (kappa), and σ (sigma). The μ receptor on which morphine acts predominantly as an agonist, is associated with analgesia, respiratory depression, euphoria, and physical dependence; the κ receptor, which is acted on mainly by ketocyclazocine and only slightly by morphine as agonists, involves analgesia, miosis, and sedation; the σ receptor, on which SKF 10,047 (N-allylnorcyclazocine) acts as an agonist is linked to psychotomimetic effects, mydriasis, and vasomotor and respiratory stimulation. Nalorphine and pentazocine are antagonists with high affinity (and no agonist activity) for μ receptors; they have agonist activity for κ and σ receptors (39). The σ site binds specifically N-allylnorcyclazocine in the presence of cyclazocine and can be displaced by phencyclidine (63, 64).

After the discovery of the enkephalins, Kosterlitz's group observed that opiates were more potent than enkephalins in inhibiting electrically induced contractions in the guinea pig ileum, whereas enkephalins were more potent in the isolated mouse vas deferens (36). They suggested the existence of two different receptor types in two tissues: a receptor in the guinea pig ileum that prefers morphine and congeners, which they called μ (analogous to Martin's μ receptor), and the other in mouse vas deferens that prefers enkephalin, which they called δ (delta for vas deferens). The same group found the evidence of similar receptor heterogeneity in the CNS. Radiolabeled enkephalin binding is displaced more easily by enkephalins than by opiates and vice versa, suggesting existence of morphine-selective μ and enkephalin-selective (δ) sites. These putative subclasses of opiate receptors have differential distributions in the CNS (ratio of μ and σ sites being highest in the thalamus) and can be selectively inhibited (enkephalin-selective site by ethanol and other aliphatic alcohols) (52).

On further analysis of the opiate receptors by using naloxone as an irreversible ligand for the high-affinity active site, the μ receptors have been separated into two subclasses. The μ_1 receptor corresponds to the high-affinity binding sites for opiates and appears to be responsible for analgesia under normal circumstances. The subclass μ_2 corresponds to the low-affinity binding site for the opiates after naloxone treatment and binds morphine far better than enkephalin. The low-affinity enkephalin receptor site corresponds to previously described receptor and binds enkephalin more potently than morphine (62).

OPIOID PEPTIDES

In 1975, Hughes, Kosterlitz and associates (24, 25) isolated and characterized two related pentapeptides from pig brain that exhibited morphinelike inhibitor action on electrically induced contraction of guinea pig ileum, which could be antagonized by naloxone. They named these peptides *enkephalins* (from the Greek, meaning "in the head"): methionine-enkephalin (Met-enkephalin) and leucine-enkephalin (Leu-enkephalin). This group also reported that the amino acid sequence in Met-enkephalin was the same as in the residue (61-65) in the pituitary hormone, β-lipotropin (β-LPH), that was isolated by C.H. Li in 1965 and found to possess weak lipolytic activity. In the same year (1975), Goldstein and coworkers reported the presence of peptidelike substance in the bovine pituitary gland that acts like morphine (58). From this substance, two polypeptides were isolated and sequenced; they were found to have structures identical to sequences 61-76 and 61-77 of β-LPH. In the meantime the so-called C-terminal fragment (with amino acid sequences 61-91) of β-LPH was shown to have potent opioid activity, although the intact β-LPH molecule was devoid of such activity. These opioid polypeptides were termed *endorphins* (endogenous morphins), the C-terminal fraction being renamed β-endorphin, and β-LPH 61-76 and β-LPH 61-77 as α- and γ-endorphins, respectively (52). α- and γ-endorphins are now thought by most investigators to be breakdown products of β-endorphin (54). The amino acid sequence of human porcine and bovine β-endorphins show variations in positions 23, 27, and 31. The amino acid sequences of these and other opioid peptides are shown in Table 10.1-3. A large-molecular polypeptide (MW 31,000) has been suggested to be the precursor of both adrenocorticotropic hormone (ACTH) and β-endorphin (37).

Human β-endorphin has been synthesized, and the opioid activity of the synthetic product is comparable with that of the natural peptide assayed on the guinea pig ileum. In the ileum assay, human β-endorphin has been shown to be 55% more active than normorphine and four times more potent than Met-enkephalin.

Recently, a peptide called α-neoendorphin has been isolated from pig hypothalmus; it contains 15 amino acids, of which the first 8 have been sequenced (28). Another peptide has been isolated and sequenced by Goldstein, et al (19, 20) and is named dynorphin because of its greater potency. It has 17 amino acids (dynorphin 1-17). This peptide also has two short forms (dynorphin 1-8 and dynorphin 1-9) (Table 10.1-3).

Distribution. Unlike opiate receptors, which are localized in the synaptosomal fractions, the enkephalins are distributed in the neurons and their processes; enkephalin immunoreactivity in the cell bodies has also been observed in certain cell groups. Enkephalin-containing neurons are primarily short interneurons located in specific regions in the CNS.

The distribution of opiate receptors and enkephalins correlates fairly closely and involves brain structures whose functions are linked to opiate actions. Thus, small enkephalin-containing interneurons and opioid receptors are found in the areas of the CNS related to perception of pain (dorsal horn of spinal cord, particularly substantia gelatinosa, spinal trigeminal nucleus, thalamus, periaqueductal and periventricular

Table 10.1-3
Amino Acid Sequence of Opioid Peptides

Met-enkephalin (5)[a]	Tyr-Gly-Gly-Phe-Met-NH_2
Leu-enkephalin (5)	Tyr-Gly-Gly-Phe-Leu-NH_2
β-Endorphin (31)[a]	
	5 10
Human	H-Tyr-Gly-Gly-Phe-Met-Thr-Ser-Glu-Lys-Ser-
	15 20
	Gln-Thr-Pro-Leu-Val-Thr-Leu-Phe-Lys-Asn-
	25 31
	Ala-Ile-Ile-Lys-Asn-Ala-Tyr-Lys-Lys-Gly-Gln-OH
	23 27 31
Porcine	Val His Gln-OH
Bovine	Ile His Gln-OH
Dynorphin (17)	Tyr-Gly-Gly-Phe-Leu-Arg-Arg-Ile-Arg-Pro-Lys-Leu-Trp-Asp-Asn-Gln

[a] Amino acid sequences of the following peptides in terms of that of β-lipotropin (β-LPH) are: β-endorphin, 61-91; α-endorphin, 61-76; γ-endorphin, 61-77; Met-enkephalin, 61-65.

gray), emotional behavior (limbic system), neural regulation of endocrine functions (median eminence), and respiratory depression (solitary nucleus of the brain stem which regulates visceral reflexes including respiration). However, distribution of opiate receptors does not correlate with that of the opioid peptides in certain areas. Thus, the globus pallidus has the highest enkephalin content, whereas it is relatively low in opiate receptors. Certain cortical areas rich in opiate receptors have low levels of enkephalins (52). Unlike other limbic areas, the hippocampus is low in opiate receptors, but high enkephalin immunoreactivity has been shown in certain hippocampal areas; responsiveness to electrophoretically applied dynorphin has also been demonstrated in a majority of hippocampal neurons. Dynorphin has been shown to be the major opioid peptide in the hippocampus (21). At least three possible opioid peptide systems have been suggested to exist in hippocampus: (1) dynorphin-containing dentate granule cell-mossy fiber system; (2) dynorphin-containing cells in CA 1 and CA 3-4 cellular fields; and (3) a third peptide system showing enkephalin immunoreactivity and extending from the lateral entorhinal/perirhinal cortex to dentate granule cells. These pathways into this limbic structure may indicate a role of these peptides in neuropsychiatry (21). The enkephalins are also present in the sympathetic ganglia, myenteric plexus of the gastrointestinal tract (mostly in the upper parts), plasma, and cerebrospinal fluid. Immunoreactivity has also been detected in adrenal medulla, pheochromocytoma, and abdominal ganglioneuroblastoma (8). Met-enkephalin and Leu-enkephalin have been shown to occur in completely separate neurons in the brain and intestine (15).

β-Endorphin occurs mainly in the hypothalamus and in the pars intermedia and pars distalis of the pituitary gland. Some β-endorphin-containing axon terminals have been found in the central gray matter, which is concerned with modulation of pain, and endorphin immunoreactivity in the plasma, cerebrospinal fluid, placenta, semen, pancreas, and thyroid. Dynorphin has been shown to be present in hippocampus, hypothalamus, posterior pituitary, and submucous plexus of the gastrointestinal tract.

Some Functional Roles. There are at least three receptors, mu (μ), kappa (κ), and delta (δ), that are closely related to the opioid peptides. The enkephalins act as short-acting agonists or neurotransmitters at δ receptors. Dynorphin 1-17 is a long-acting agonist or modulator at κ receptors, whereas short forms (dynorphin 1-8 or dynorphin 1-9) are short-acting agonists at κ receptors. From a functional standpoint, the enkephalins, dynorphins and β-endorphin appear to belong to two distinct and separate systems. Because of wide distribution, very rapid destruction, localization in the nerve terminal, and calcium-dependent release with depolarization of intestine, the enkephalins are considered to serve as short-acting neurotransmitters. β-Endorphin with its location in the hypothalamus and pituitary and with longer duration of action may function as a neurohormone. Leu- and Met-enkephalins and related small peptides are released from the adrenal medulla into the blood, thus acting as neurohormones in this situation (35). β-Endorphin may also act as a neurotransmitter in a discrete pathway in the brain (7). Both the systems are apparently involved in modulation of pain. Dynorphin appears to serve both ways. β-Endorphin is a long-acting agonist at μ receptors, whereas the short-length opioid peptides of enkephalin and dynorphin families participate in neurotransmission; the longer-length peptides of all three families (e.g., peptide E, dynorphin, β-neoendorphin, β-endorphin) contribute in neuronal or hormonal modulation (59).

Biochemically, opiates and enkephalin decrease adenylate cyclase activity and reduce cyclic adenosine monophosphate (cAMP) levels in neuroblastoma clones which possess specific opiate receptors. This effect is antagonized by naloxone. Adenylate cyclase activity and cAMP levels return to control level when cells are exposed to morphine for several days and become tolerant, they are increased when morphine is removed (27). Thus, cAMP also seems to be a second messenger for enkephalin.

In general, the opioid peptides form chemical messengers (neurotransmitters, neuromodulators, hormones, or neurohormones) of a widespread inhibitory system (59). At the cellular level, they cause depression of transmitter release or membrane hyperpolarization due to opening of potassium channels (59). Although both types of peptides have similar affinities for opiate receptors, β-endorphin is much more active than the enkephalins. Some of the characteristic actions of enkephalins and β-endorphin are summarized in Table 10.1-4. In addition, β-endorphin administered intraventricularly causes hypothermia, hyperglycemia, and in some species respiratory depression. In humans, i.v. injection of β-endorphin causes dry mouth, orthostatic hypotension, and mild cognitive impairment (30).

Although many clinical studies on opioid peptides have been conducted, no novel therapeutic applications have yet been established. Clinical areas in which opioid peptides appear to be involved include analgesia, opiate-induced coma, postmenopausal flushing, opiate dependence, and as yet undefined sub types of schizophrenia (13). They can be significantly inhibited by naloxone. The opioid inhibition of pain needs a preexisting noxius stimulus to activate the inhibitory system involving the opioid peptides (31). This explains the mechanism of action of acupuncture and transcutaneous nerve stimulation. Enkephalins are rapidly metabolized and are unlikely to provide adequate analgesia with parenteral administration. Synthetic β-endorphin on intrathecal injection can produce analgesia of a mean duration over 33 hr. To date, endorphins, enkephalins, and their analogs have shown tolerance and dependence after prolonged administration and produce cross-tolerance with morphine (59).

Opioid peptides are also involved in various stress situations such as anesthesia, hypoxia, shock, etc. (43). Plasma levels of β-endorphin were found to be elevated following surgery and amphetamine administration when plasma cortisol levels were also increased, indicating thereby a stresslike situation. These suggest a linkage between endogenous opioid system and hypothalamic-pituitary axis (12). Opioid peptides exert tonic inhibitory control over corticotropin and gonadotropins via inhibition of corticotropin-releasing factor (CRF) and gonadotropin-releasing hormone (GRH), respectively, although they are probably concerned with release of CRF in conditions of stress (59). A role of the peptides in postmenopausal flushing is suggested by significant reduction of such flushing by naloxone (13). Involvement of these peptides in opiate dependence is indicated by high endorphin levels in the cerebrospinal fluid samples in opioid-dependent subjects; elevated endorphin level persists even during methadone treatment (46).

MORPHINE

Pharmacological Effects. The pharmacology of morphine is discussed here in detail as a prototype of narcotic analgesics. The remaining drugs will be briefly described

Table 10.1-4
Characteristics of Opioid Peptides

Properties	β-Endorphin	Enkephalins
Analgesia[a]	+ (longer duration)	+
Wet-dog shakes	+	+
Release of vasopressin, growth hormone, and prolactin	+	+
Motility and muscle tone	Akinesia and muscular rigidity	Hypermotility
Effects on CNS neurotransmitters	Inhibit drug-induced DA release; ↑ midbrain 5-HT; ↓ ACh turnover	Inhibit release of ACh, NE
Release of the peptide during stress	+	
Rate of metabolism	Resistant to degradation in plasma and CSF	Very rapid in serum and tissue homogenates
Antidiarrheal action		+ (Potent), reversed by naloxone
Action on brain adenylate cyclase	Uncertain	Stimulation
Addiction potential and withdrawal behaviors	+	+

[a]Tolerance develops to analgesia.
+, characteristic property of the peptides.

with reference to their inherent characteristics and differences.

Central Nervous System (CNS). The effects of morphine on the CNS are complex and comprise both depressant and stimulant actions depending on the dose, the site of action, species of animal, and individual variations. The depressant actions on the CNS are predominant and manifested by its sedative, hypnotic, and analgesic properties, respiratory inhibition, and hypothermic and delayed antiemetic effects. Morphine also exerts a direct depressive action at the spinal cord level (dorsal horn interneurons), mainly concerned with motor reflexes (6).

Morphine also produces stimulant effects at certain central sites. Thus it causes nausea and emesis through its stimulatory action on the chemoreceptor trigger zone (CTZ) in the area postrema of the medulla, miosis through its action on the oculomotor nucleus, and bradycardia and intestinal spasticity through its action on the vagal nuclei. In some species of animals, as in cats, horses, pigs, cows, tigers, and other species, relatively low doses of morphine cause excitation. Although such doses produce analgesia in these animals, they show restlessness, hyperactivity, fright, mydriasis, and hyperthermia. High doses of morphine and its analogs may produce convulsions, patterns of which are more supraspinal than spinal in nature. These effects can be reversed by naloxone. Some neurons seem to be excited (or disinhibited) by opiates. Morphine has been shown to increase discharge rates of Renshaw cells in the spinal cord that cannot be antagonized by naloxone (29).

Behavioral Effects. Morphine and several other narcotic analgesics have been shown to affect a number of unlearned (spontaneous) and learned behaviors in animals.

Spontaneous behavior. Small doses of morphine produce stimulation of locomotion, rearing, grooming, eating, and drinking behaviors in rats. Spontaneous motor activity in rats is increased by small doses and decreased by high doses of morphine. Decreased activity by high doses of morphine is inversely related to brain concentrations of morphine (26). Morphine-induced increase of motor activity is antagonized by narcotic antagonists (47).

Aggressive behavior has been induced by apomorphine (41) (10-30 mg/kg, s.c.) but not by morphine itself. However, during morphine withdrawal dependent rats may manifest hyperirritability or hyperalgesia to noxious stimuli or even intermale fighting behavior. Another type of aggression within morphine-withdrawn pairs (intermale) has also been described (56).

Conditioned behavior. Morphine causes a dose-related decrease in responding under a multiple fixed-interval, fixed-ratio schedule of food presentation in monkeys and pigeons (17). Narcotic antagonists have been shown to block those responses of morphine. Morphine also attenuates a quickly learned conditioned emotional response; however this effect does not appear to be a consequence of an influence upon the initial performance (4).

The effects of morphine have been tested in self-stimulation experiments on positively reinforcing brain areas (e.g., posterior or lateral hypothalamus), electrical stimulation of which produces rewarding or reinforcing effects. In such experiments, morphine causes an initial decrease in response for 1 to 2 hours postinjection, followed by subsequent enhancement of responses that is mostly dose dependent. With repeated administration, tolerance develops to the initial depression but not to its facilitatory effect. In studies on threshold measurements, the facilitatory effect has been correlated with lowering of threshold of rewarding brain stimulation, which does not develop tolerance and can be reversed by naloxone. In addition, morphine has been shown also to raise the threshold for stimulation of negatively reinforcing brain areas (e.g., midbrain reticular formation), electrical stimulation of which would cause aversive effects (32). In humans, continued drug-seeking behavior with respect to narcotics may be ascribed to such facilitation of rewarding (pleasing) brain stimulation as well as attenuation of aversive (pain) perceptions.

Drug-seeking behavior. A number of narcotic analgesics such as morphine, codeine, methadone, pentazocine, and propoxyphene have been shown to act as positive reinforcers in self-administering trained animals (e.g., monkeys and rats) implanted with intravenous catheters, and they can induce a drug-seeking behavior. After development of physical dependence, when withdrawal signs are manifested because of cessation of narcotic administration or when a narcotic antagonist is injected, the rate of responding under certain operant schedules maintained by drug injection is enhanced. In morphine-dependent animals, responding may be maintained so as to result in termination of the injection of narcotic antagonists. The rate and pattern of responding controlled by the schedule of termination of drug injection are comparable with the schedules of electric shock avoidance; such schedules produce negative reinforcement (16). Thus, increased responding may lead to morphine injection (positive reinforcement) during withdrawal. As a result, withdrawal would be terminated or postponed in narcotic-dependent animals. Self-administration behavior of animals has been shown to be influenced by various factors such as (1) dosage of drug and its interaction to other drugs, (2) organismic variables (e.g., genetic factors, age, sex of the subject), and (3) environmental variables. The role of conditioning in narcotic drug addiction is discussed further in Chapter 11.6.

EEG. At therapeutic dose levels, morphine produces synchronization of EEG characterized by high-voltage, low-frequency waves similar to that produced in natural sleep or after a low dose of a barbiturate. Morphine significantly decreases REM (rapid eye movement) sleep, increases non-REM light sleep (stages 1 and 2), and reduces non-REM deep sleep (stages 3 and 4).

Heroin produces a biphasic response on EEG: initial high-amplitude, low-frequency α-rhythm associated with increased θ and δ rhythms (60). Repeated administration of methadone leads to EEG changes characterized by a decrease in the mean α- and β- activities and increased θ- activity. When a maintenance dose level is established, EEG activities return to premethadone patern, indicating the development of tolerance. Methadone also partially blocks the EEG changes induced by heroin. EEG changes elicited by heroin are also blocked by cyclazocine and naloxone.

Analgesia. Analgesia is a reliable characteristic of morphine in different species of animals. It occurs without impairment of consciousness, sensitivity to touch, hearing, vision, or motor, or intellectual function. Continuous dull pain is more effectively relieved than sharp intermittent pain. In addition to relief of pain and discomfort, some patients may feel euphoric. A normal pain-free subject, however, may exhibit dysphoria to morphine consisting of mild anxiety and fear instead of analgesia.

The *site and mechanism* of narcotic analgesia have been briefly discussed in Chapter 10. Morphine is believed to act on several sites in the CNS for producing analgesia. The electrical stimulation of various brain areas (e.g., the periaqueductal gray, the dorsal raphe nuclei, and the periventricular gray) or microinjection of opioid and opioid peptides produces a profound analgesia that could largely be reversed by naloxone. Cross-tolerance develops between analgesia produced by these procedures. Stimulation of periaqueductal gray that appears to cause release of endogenous peptides or microinjection of opioids in this area influence the ascending and descending fibers concerned with modulation of pain. The descending fibers exert an inhibitory influence on the spinal interneurons in the dorsal horn. Opioid-induced analgesia involves several neurotransmitter systems. 5-Hydroxytryptamine (5-HT) appears to be particularly involved; since analgesia produced by stimulation of the periaqueductal gray or the dorsal raphe nuclei could be abolished by depletion of 5-HT or by interruption of tryptaminergic pathways, it is likely that the descending pathways to spinal dorsal horn could be tryptaminergic (4, 61).

Exogenous administration of cAMP has also been demonstrated to antagonize morphine analgesia. Manipulation of endogenous cAMP by pharmacological agents also influences analgesic actions of morphine. A single injection of morphine has been shown to increase significantly the cAMP levels in the rat cerebral cortex (15). Chronic administration of opiate alkaloid results in prolonged increase in adenylate cyclase.

Sedation. Morphine and related drugs at therapeutic analgesic doses produce drowsiness, lethargy, apathy, or mental confusion in patients with pain and in normal healthy volunteers. Sedation and hypnosis may result after relief of pain and due to its accompanying psychological and physical exhaustion. Former addicts, however, show tolerance to these effects. Morphine-induced sedation is not accompanied by slurring of speech or marked motor incoordination. When the opioids are used as preanesthetic medication in combination with other sedatives, generally additive effects are observed. The site of depressant action of opioids (producing sedtion and hypnosis) appears to lie in the sensory area of the cerebral cortex.

Neuroendocrines. Both alkaloid narcotics and opiatelike peptides influence hypothalamic-pituitary hormonal functions. Conversely, hormones of the anterior pituitary such as ACTH, thyroid-stimulating hormone (TSH), prolactin, luteinizing hormone (LH), follicle-stimulating hormone (FSH), growth hormone (GH), β-lipotropin (β-LPH), and β-melanocyte-stimulating hormone (β-MSH) affect the expression of opiate-induced spectrum of actions.

The acute effects of these compounds on pituitary hormones show considerable variations because of species differences, dosages employed, duration of administration, stress effect, and other uncertain variables. Generally, both alkaloid and peptide opiates seem to increase ACTH, GH, prolactin (PRI), and antidiuretic hormone (ADH) and decrease TSH, LH, and FSH secretions of the anterior pituitary (14). Morphine has been reported to increase β-MSH secretion also. As regards site and mechanism of action of these opiates on the neuroendocrine system, it has been postulated that they act through a specific CNS site and probably change hypoothalamic releasing and/or inhibitory hormonal effects on the pituitary. Increased ACTH secretion due to morphine has been shown to stimulate adrenocortical steroid secretion and to decrease plasma testosterone as a result of depressed LH release from the anterior pituitary. Although morphine is known to stimulate ADH release from the posterior pituitary in dogs and rats, it has been shown to stimulate diuresis in humans (14).

Hypothalamic hormones such as TRH and somatostatin (growth hormone-inhibiting factor) have been shown to antagonize morphine-induced GH release, and TRH alone antagonizes β-EP-induced inhibition of motor activity (22).

Pupil reaction. Morphine and many of its surrogates cause pupillary constriction (miosis), which is a characteristic sign in humans. In overdose with an opiate drug, miosis is greatly accentuated so that a pinpoint pupil is produced. The exact mechanism of this effect is not clear, but it is believed to be mediated through stimulation of the third cranial nerve nucleus (Edinger-Westphal). The diagnosis of opiate poisoning may be confused in the advanced stages because of mydriasis associated with hypoxia. Some variations among species have been noted in the pupillary response to opiates; cats, pigs, cows, etc. may show mydriasis. In the latter species, morphine causes an excitation of the CNS. Miotic action of morphine is blocked by atropine and related compounds. Tolerance does not develop to the miotic actions of opiates.

Respiration. Respiratory centers in the brain stem are very sensitive to morphine and are depressed by a very small dose. Morphine affects all the components of respiration such as rate, minute volume, and tidal exchange, and may induce irregular periodic breathing. The respiratory depressant effect generally precedes the onset of analgesia. Morphine and related compounds also depress the response of brain stem respiratory centers to elevated blood carbon dioxide tension. Pontine and medullary centers that regulate respiratory rhythmicity are also believed to be depressed under the influence of opiates. Voluntary control of respiration is also affected by morphine, and this is considered therapeutically beneficial in the management of pulmonary edema. In the latter condition the patient's effort to breath, may aggravate the underlying pathology. In equianalgesic doses, all opioids cause respiratory depression. Death due to overdose of opiate in humans usually occurs following respiratory arrest. Morphine also causes depression of the cough center in the medulla; the antitussive action, however, is not attributed to the same part of the molecule that is responsible for analgesia.

Vomiting. Morphine and its derivatives at a therapeutic dose often cause nausea and vomiting in ambulatory patients as a result of stimulation of the chemoreceptor trigger zone (CTZ) of emesis in the area postrema of the medulla. These drugs have also been reported to increase the sensitivity of the vestibular apparatus. After initial stimulation of CTZ, depression of the vomiting center occurs, thereby rendering it nonresponsive to emetics (e.g., apomorphine). The emetic action of morphine and related drugs is antagonized by narcotic antagonists and certain phenothiazines with dopamine-blocking action.

Cardiovascular System. Morphine and its derivatives in therapeutic doses cause very little or no effect on cardiovascular functions. However, these drugs cause orthostatic hypotension associated with marked peripheral vasodilation, resulting in fainting. Vasodilation is partly due to the release of histamine and is blocked by antihistamines. Medullary depression may also play a role in vasodilation. Cardiac response to morphine in patients with myocardial infarction is inconsistent and often produces marked hypotension and bradycardia. Hypovolemic patients are more susceptible to vasodepressor action of morphine and other narcotics.

Phenothiazines produce a marked potentiation of the hypotensive action of morphine. Morphine indirectly causes dilatation of the cerebral vascular bed by raising the carbon dioxide tension in the blood.

Gastrointestial System. Morphine and its derivatives decrease gastric motility and increase the tone of the antral portion of the stomach, which delays the passage of gastric content through the duodenum. On the smooth muscle of small and large intestines, opiates increase the resting tone almost to the point of spasm and decrease propulsive peristaltic movements. The tone of the ileocecal valve and that of the anal sphincter is greatly increased. The actions on the stomach and small and large intestine contribute to the constipating effects. Atropine can partially antagonize the spasmogenic actions of morphine. Gastric, biliary, and pancreatic secretions are all inhibited by the drugs.

Miscellaneous Effects. The tone of the detrusor muscle of the urinary bladder, bronchiolar smooth muscle, and biliary tract is stimulated by morphine. Carbohydrate metabolism is also affected by these drugs in humans and in other species of animals. Morphine may cause transient hyperglycemia in humans, which results from mobilization of liver glycogen through release of epinephrine from the adrenals. Morphine given centrally or peripherally has been shown to cause hyperthermia in the cat (10) but lowers temperature in the dog, rabbit, and primate.

Pharmacokinetics. Morphine is absorbed readily from the gastrointestinal tract, nasal mucous membrane (when it is used as snuff), and lung (smoking of opium). Following oral administration, however, only 20% of a given dose reaches the systemic circulation, and about 80% of the dose is lost during the passage from the intestine to systemic circulation (first-pass effect). Oral administration of morphine provides very low plasma levels of free morphine because of its rapid conjugation in the mucosal cells of small intestine and in the liver (8). Maximum plasma level of morphine is noted 10-20 minutes after i.m.and s.c. administrations (8). Approximately 35% of circulating morphine is protein (albumin) bound. The half-life of morphine is about 2-2.5 hours. Morphine is distributed in high concentrations in the kidneys, liver, lung, spleen, adrenals, and thyroid gland. Much lower concentrations are found in the brain because of the blood-brain barrier. Morphine and related drugs cross the placenta and can cause respiratory depression, miosis, and withdrawal symptoms in neonates born to addicted mothers.

Morphine is extensively metabolized in the body. Glucuronide conjugation is the major (about 70%) pathway for metabolism of morphine, and this results in formation of highly polar glucuronides. Glucuronide conjugation occurs in the intestine, liver, kidney and placenta. Sulfate conjugation is a minor pathway for morphine metabolism, and about 5-10% of a dose is eliminated as morphine-3-sulfate (8). About 5% of morphine undergoes oxidative N-dealkylation of N-methyl to form the active metabolite, normorphine; N-oxidation and hydro xylation of morphine at position 2 have also been shown to occur. Renal and biliary excretion are prime pathways for morphine and its metabolites. About 3-10% of the drug is excreted unchanged in the urine by glomerular filtration. Morphine also undergoes enterohepatic circulation (51) and about 10% is excreted in the feces as glucuronide-conjugated metabolite.

Elderly patients are sensitive to injected morphine and have higher blood levels of the drug, presumably due to its altered rate of metabolism and excretion. Presence of microsomal oxidative enzymes and UDP glucuronyl transferase activity has been reported in human fetus (45). Chronic use of enzyme inducers such as cigarette smoking, barbiturates, and alcohol may result in stimulation of microsomal enzymes in the fetus and newborn and increased oxidative N-demethylation of morphine.

Adverse Effects. Besides analgesia, morphine produces other pharmacological actions that could be considered adverse effects. These include drowsiness, mood changes, mental clouding, nausea, vomiting, dizziness, epigastric discomfort, respiratory depression, constipation, and biliary colic. Patients with previous history of asthma may develop bronchoconstriction. Morphine may occasionally cause orthostatic hypotension, syncope, peripheral vasodilation, and circulatory collapse.

Contraindications and Precautions. Morphine and other related drugs are contraindicated in certain acute disease states (e.g., acute abdomen, suspected acute head injuries). Narcotic analgesics will interfere with the accurate clinical assessment of the patients. Narcotics should be used with extreme caution in patients with hypopituitary hypothyroidism, Addison's disease, anemia, and severe malnutrition.

Drug Interactions. Additive effects may be produced when morphine and related drugs are used concurrently with phenothiazines, MAO inhibitors, and tricylic antidepressants.

Tolerance and Physical Dependence. Both tolerance and physical dependence occur following repeated use of narcotic analgesics, and these are adequately covered in Chapter 11.6.

MORPHINE CONGENERS

Hydromorphone (dihydromorphinone, 7,8-dihydromorphinone) is a semisynthetic derivative of morphine (Tables 10.1-1 and 10.1-2). It is about 5 times more potent than morphine in producing analgesia. At equianalgesic doses, it produces less sedation than morphine. It is less constipating and infrequently causes nausea and vomiting. It does not produce miosis. Its adverse reactions are similar to morphine, and tolerance and physical dependence seem to appear more rapidly.

Oxymorphone (7,8-dihydro-14-hydroxydihydromorphinone) is another semisynthetic morphine derivative (Tables 10.1-1 and 10.1-2). It is about 7 to 10 times as potent as morphine in producing analgesia, but it has no significant antitussive activity. Its absorption from the gastrointestinal tract is unreliable, and parenteral routes are preferred for its therapeutic use. Its adverse effects, tolerance, and addiction liability are similar to those of morphine.

METOPON

The analgesic potency of metopon (methyldihydromorphinone) is twice that of morphine; its full effect can be manifested after its oral administration. It is devoid of emetic and respiratory-depressant effects in therapeutic dose. Its side effects are less than those of morphine, but addiction liability and withdrawal syndrome are similar to those of morphine.

CODEINE

Codeine is a naturally occurring alkaloid of opium (0.5%) and is produced synthetically by substituting a methyl group for the phenolic-hydroxyl radical in morphine (Tables 10.1-1 and 10.1-2). Its analgesic potency is about one-twelfth to one-tenth that of morphine. It produces fewer gastrointestinal effects than morphine, and it is about one-third as effective as morphine in suppressing cough. It can suppress morphine withdrawal symptoms only in doses 5 to 6 times as great as morphine itself. Codeine is more effective when given parenterally than when administered orally in equivalent doses. As an analgesic, about 120-130 mg of codeine administered subcutaneously is equivalent to 10 mg of morphine sulfate by the same route, but at these doses codeine seems to produce more adverse effects.

Codeine is absorbed readily from the gastrointestinal tract, and peak plasma levels occur within 1 to 2 hours. Its plasma half-life is bout 3 to 4 hours (6 hours after overdosage) (23). Codeine is mainly metabolized in the liver through N-demethylation, O-demethylation (approximately 10% to form morphine), and conjugation reactions. It is mainly excreted in the urine, 37% as glucuronide and 10% unchanged. Adverse reactions to codeine are similar to those produced by morphine. Respiratory arrest is associated with a plasma codeine level of about 5 μg/ml. Tolerance and dependence can occur with codeine, but dependence develops rarely to its oral use. The codeine withdrawal syndrome is milder than that of morphine but easily detectable. Codeine may be abused in the form of elixir (e.g., terpin hydrate), with possible complications developing from simultaneous physical dependence on both codeine and alcohol.

Depressant effect of codeine may be intensified and prolonged with simultaneous administrations of phenothiazines, MAO inhibitors, and tricyclic antidepressants.

HEROIN

Heroin is the 3,6-diacetyl derivative of morphine (Tables 10.1-1 and 10.1-2). As an analgesic, it is about 2 to 3 times more potent than morphine, with a more rapid onset of action. Pharmacological actions of heroin are attributed to morphine. In equivalent doses the subjective effects, effects on psychomotor performance, rate of development of tolerance, and qualitative and quantitative aspects of withdrawal symptoms of heroin and morphine are quite comparable (50). Psychomotor performance of a tolerant subject may still remain normal, but generally more time is spent in bed with curtailed social activity.

Heroin is readily absorbed from the gastrointestinal tract and through nasal mucous membrane. It is abused through the intravenous route most commonly. Heroin is rapidly hydrolyzed by esterases in blood or liver to monoacetylmorphine (MAM), which is further hydrolyzed to morphine. Both heroin and MAM are more lipid soluble than morphine and pass through the blood-brain barrier in the adult more easily and rapidly than morphine. Heroin is excreted in the urine largely as free and conjugated morphine.

HYDROCODONE

Hydrocodone (7,8-dihydrocodeinone) is closely related to oxycodone, in which the 14-hydroxyl group is replaced by hydrogen (Tables 10.1-1 and 10.1-2). It is available in the United States with a trade name of HYCODAN that also contains homatropine methylbromide. It is orally active, and its analgesic potency is equal or slightly more than that of morphine and has a longer duration of action than that of codeine. Its addiction liability is greater than that of codeine. Withdrawal symptoms with hydrocodone are less severe than with morphine but have greater intensity than with codeine.

OXYCODONE

Oxycodone is a modified codeine compound with a chemical formula 7,8-dihydro-14-hydroxycodeinone (Tables 10.1-1 and 10.1-2). It is effective when given orally. Analgesic potency of oxycodone is slightly less than that of morphine, but with similar duration of action (i.e., 4 to 5 hours). Addiction liability and withdrawal symptoms are similar to those of morphine.

METHADONE AND CONGENERS

Bockmühl and Ehrhart synthesized methadone (6-dimethylamino-4,4-diphenyl-3-haptanone) (Table 10.1-1 and Fig. 10.1-1), which is distinctly different chemically from morphine (5). The pseudopiperidine ring structure has been found to be essential for its opioid action. Qualitatively, pharmacological actions of methadone are similar to those of morphine. Analgesic potency and duration of action following i.m. injection of methadone are similar to morphine. Methadone is relatively more effective orally than morphine, since it has a longer duration of action with respect to its peak effect. The cardiovascular action of methadone, however, is less prominent than that of morphine, and compensatory cardiovascular responses are not affected by it.

Methadone is almost completely absorbed from the gastrointestinal tract and from sites of subcutaneous administration. After oral administration, the peak concentration of methadone in blood occurs in about 4 hours (1 to 2 hours after s.c. or i.m. injection). It is highly (84-87%) bound to plasma protein, about 70% to albumin and the remainder to globulin. Concentrations of methadone in liver, lung, and kidneys are higher than in blood. Methadone crosses placental barrier.

Following a single dose, the half-life of methadone is about 5 hours and it is reduced to about 2 to 5 hours after repeated administrations. Patients with severe liver disease manifest prolonged half-life of methadone.

The liver is the principal site for metabolism of methadone, and through N-demethylation, mono-N-demethylmethadone (pyrrolidine), a major metabolite, and pyrroline are formed. There are also minor hydroxylated and

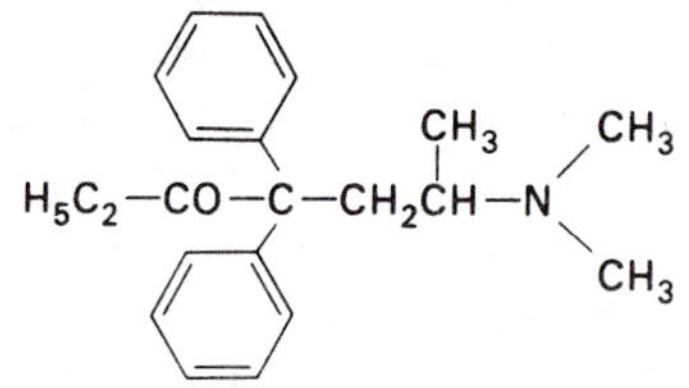

Methadone

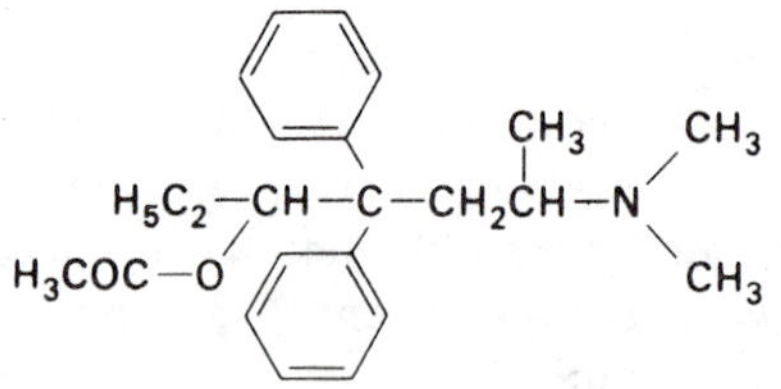

Methadyl acetate
Levomethadyl acetate

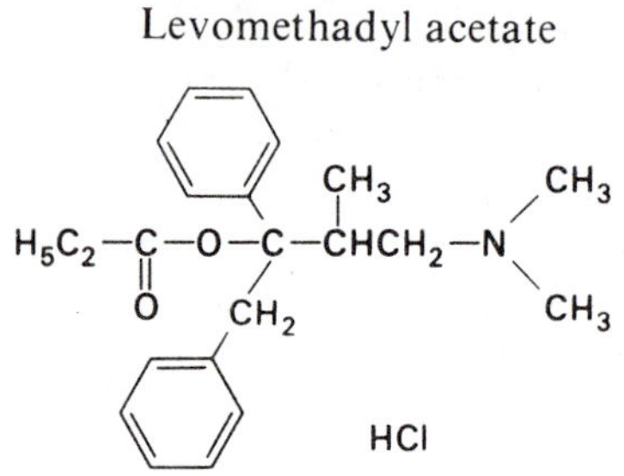

Propoxyphene

Fig. 10.1-1. *Synthetic analgesics of the diphenylpropylamine series.*

conjugated metabolites of the drug. The principal route of excretion of its metabolites appears to be through kidney, although an enterohepatic circulation possibly exists. Acidification of urine enhances renal excretion of methadone. Narcotic addicts maintained on methadone (orally or subcutaneously) are known to develop partial tolerance to its emetic, anorectic, sedative, miotic, respiratory-depressant, and cardiovascular effects. Tolerance to the depressant effects develops more slowly with methadone than with morphine in some individuals. Overt behavioral effects similar to those caused by morphine are more common with parenteral administration of methadone than when it is given orally. Rifampin has been reported to induce withdrawal syndrome in patients maintained on methadone. The precise mechanism for such interaction has not been clearly established. Desipramine and diazepam have also been reported to alter metabolism of methadone when these drugs are used concurrently. The overall addiction potential of methadone is comparable with that of morphine. Intravenous abuse of methadone is similar to i.v. heroin abuse.

METHADYL ACETATE

Methadyl acetate is a methadone congener introduced as α-dl-and α-l-acetylmethadol (LAAM) in the treatment of heroin physical dependence (Table 10.1-1 and Fig. 10.1-1). It has a slower onset of action than methadone, and the duration of action is much longer (more than 72 hours). Therefore, it can surpass opioid withdrawal symptoms for as long as 96 hours with a single oral dose. An oral dose of 80 mg three times a week has been suggested as a substitute for 100 mg of methadone per day. Studies have shown that several of its pharmacological properties and prolonged duration of action are probably due to its biotransformation to acetylnormethadol and acetylbisnormethadol. Fecal excretion seems to be a major route for elimination of methadyl acetate and its metabolites. Chronic administration of methadyl acetate has been reported to result in enhanced metabolism of the drug and the elimination of its metabolites.

PROPOXYPHENE

Propoxyphene is structurally related to methadone (Fig. 10.1-1), and there are 4 stereoisomers, of which only dextropropoxyphene elicits analgesic action. The levo-isomer is not an analgesic but has an antitussive action. Its pharmacological actions are similar to those of codeine, but probably less potent than the latter in producing analgesia. Orally, approximately 65 mg of d-propoxyphene are about as effective as 30-45 mg of codeine for analgesia. Hydrochloride salt of propoxyphene is more readily absorbed from the gastrointestinal tract than the less water-soluble napsylate preparation. After a single oral dose, the half-life of propoxyphene has been reported to be 4 to 6 hours. It is extensively metabolized in the liver and there are a number of metabolites (norpropoxyphene, dinorpropoxyphene, propoxyphene-carbinol, and dinorpropoxyphene-carbinol, etc.) of which norpropoxyphene and dinorpropoxyphene continue to be excreted in the urine for several days in humans.

The common adverse reactions to propoxyphene include dizziness, drowsiness, nausea, and vomiting; these occur more frequently in ambulatory patients. Acute intoxication with this drug is manifested by severe respiratory and circulatory depression, miosis, and coma (reversible by nalorphine). Focal or generalized convulsions, toxic psychosis, cardiac arrhythmias, and pulmonary edema have also been reported in overdosage. The addiction liability of d-propoxyphene is somewhat less than that of codeine.

MEPERIDINE AND CONGENERS

MEPERIDINE

Meperidine (Fig. 10.1-2) is a synthetic analgesic of the phenylpiperidine series. Although chemically dissimilar,

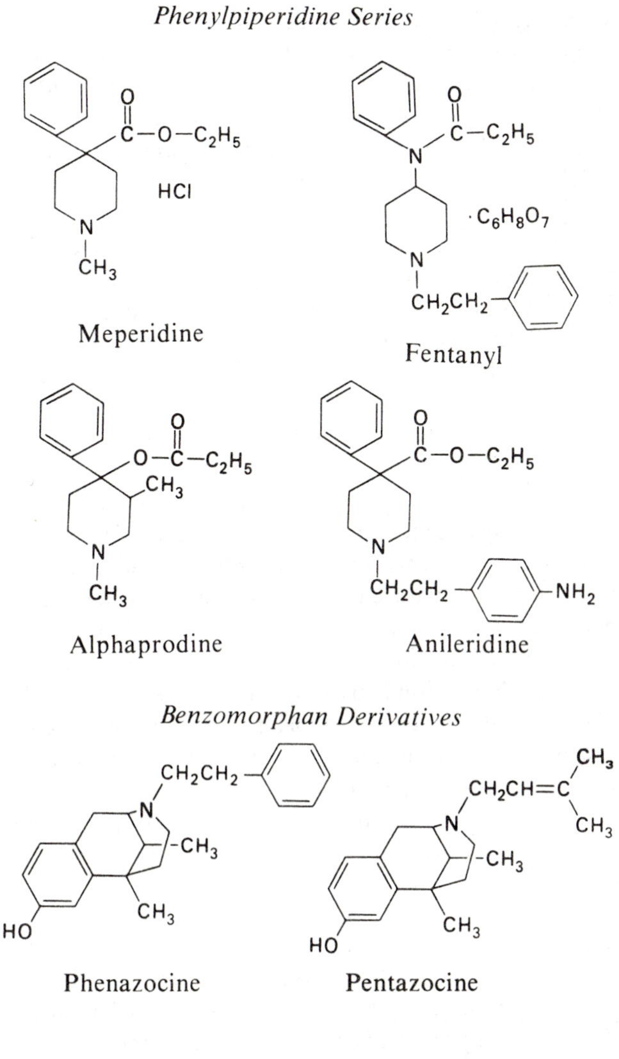

Phenylpiperidine Series

Meperidine (HCl) — Fentanyl ($\cdot C_6H_8O_7$)

Alphaprodine — Anileridine

Benzomorphan Derivatives

Phenazocine — Pentazocine

Fig. 10.1-2. *Synthetic analgesics of the phenylpiperidine and benzomorphan series.*

the molecule of meperidine seems to conform to the steric configuration of the opiate receptors. Its analgesic potency is one-tenth to one-eighth that of morphine, and the duration of action extends from 2 to 4 hours. The onset of action is somewhat rapid (less than 10 minutes) compared with morphine.

Pharmacological properties of meperidine are similar to those of morphine, but it has little or no effect on the pupil size in humans. Respiratory-depressant action of the drug can be antagonized by narcotic antagonists (e.g., nalorphine, naloxone, levallorphan). A single administration of meperidine does not have any appreciable effects on the EEG in humans. However, if large doses are administered at short intervals, the EEG shows characteristic low-frequency, high-amplitude waves, and abnormal slow wave activity persists even after the development of tolerance.

Following oral administration, about 50-60% of a dose is absorbed, and peak blood levels occur in about 1 to 2 hours. About 65-75% of it is protein bound in the circulation, which decreases with age and is increased by alcohol intake. The half-life of meperidine is about 7 to 8 hours, and increases in patients with cirrhosis and hepatitis. It crosses placenta and its concentration in fetal circulation is equal to maternal blood levels. Meperidine is metabolized into inactive compounds, meperidinic and normeperidinic acids, normeperidine, and meperidine-N-oxide. Conjugated products of these metabolites are excreted in the urine. About 6% of a dose is excreted unchanged in the urine, and it is increased to about 28% in acid urine.

In general, adverse reactions, addiction liability, and clinical features of tolerance and physical dependence of meperidine are similar to those of morphine. Tolerance to excitatory effects of meperidine does not seem to develop even after prolonged use of large doses.

In meperidine addicts, hallucinations, muscular twitchings, and convulsions may occur at high doses. The threshold dose level for the convulsant effects of meperidine is much lower than that of morphine in humans, so that when the daily dose reaches 3 g, myoclonic jerks or generalized seizures may develop. Convulsions may also occur when nalorphine is administered to antagonize respiratory depression caused by meperidine.

All sedative-hypnotics, MAO-inhibitors, tricyclic antidepressants, and the phenothiazines cause additive CNS depression when used concurrently.

Alphaprodine and anileridine have similar pharmacological properties to meperidine, but they are twice as potent.

FENTANYL

Chemically, fentanyl is related to the synthetic phenylpiperidine derivatives. On a weight basis, it is 80 to 100 times more potent an analgesic than morphine. It has a very short duration of analgesic action but causes prolonged and recurrent respiratory depression in humans. Its analgesic and euphoric actions are effectively blocked by narcotic antagonists (e.g., nalorphine, naloxone). It is used for neuroleptic analgesia, in combination with droperidol, a neuroleptic agent. At larger doses, it produces muscular rigidity and apnea, which can be antagonized by narcotic antagonists. A single i.v. injection causes marked ventilatory depression within 2 to 3 minutes after injection, and there is gradual recovery in about 60 minutes. About 7% of the drug is excreted in urine unchanged and 69% as metabolites. About 9% of the administered dose is excreted in the feces, mainly as metabolites.

MORPHINAN DERIVATIVE

LEVORPHANOL

Levorphanol is levo-3-hydroxy-N-methylmorphinan. N-methylmorphinan can be considered as a molecule of morphine without the allylic alcohol moiety, the oxygen bridge, and the phenolic hydroxyl group (Table 10.1-2). It retains all of the analgesic activity of racemorphan (dl-3-hydroxy-N-methylmorphinan). It is about 3 to 5 times as potent as morphine for producing analgesia. Consequently, it is also more potent than morphine with respect to respiratory depression, stimulation of smooth muscle, and physical dependence. Orally, it is less effective than when it is given subcutaneously. The adverse reactions to the drug and withdrawal symptoms are similar to morphine. Overdosage with levorphanol is antagonized by narcotic antagonists.

BENZOMORPHAN DERIVATIVES

PHENAZOCINE

Phenazocine is a synthetic 6,7-benzomorphan derivative (α-2-hydroxy-5,9-dimethyl-2-phenethyl-6,7-benzomorphan) (Fig. 10.1-2). Both orally and parenterally, its analgesic potency is about three times that of morphine. Side effects are fewer than with morphine, and there is less circulatory depression at higher doses. In comparison with morphine, tolerance to phenazocine develops at a slower rate, and the withdrawal syndrome that follows its abrupt discontinuation is milder but more prolonged. Its abuse potential in humans is very high, and this drug is no longer available in the United States.

PENTAZOCINE

Pentazocine [dl-α-5,9-dimethyl-2-(3,3-dimethylallyl)-2-hydroxy-6,7-benzomorphan] is an analgesic of the benzomorphan series (Fig. 10.1-2), but it also has a weak antagonistic action.

Pentazocine is usually classified as a nonnarcotic analgesic. Given parenterally, pentazocine is one-sixth to one-fourth as potent an analgesic as morphine. In terms of total analgesic effect, pentazocine is one-third as potent orally as parenterally. Its pharmacological properties encompass those of agonists of the morphine type and of antagonists of the nalorphine type. Respiratory depression caused by pentazocine can be reversed only by naloxone; antagonists of the nalorphine type are not effective against pentazocine.

Pentazocine does not produce hypotension as seen with morphine; however, it increases the pulmonary arterial pressure and a rise in central venous pressure, and thereby tends to increase the cardiac work.

This drug is well absorbed from the gastrointestinal tract; its peak blood levels occur in 1 to 3 hours after oral ingestion and in 15 to 60 minutes after i.m. injection. Following its i.m. administration, the analgesic effect reaches its peak after 30 to 60 minutes and lasts for 2 to 3 hours. After oral ingestion, the peak effect is delayed and lasts somewhat longer than after i.m. injection. With its rapid onset and short duration of action the time-course of pentazocine resembles that of meperidine. About 60-70% of it is protein bound, and it crosses both blood-brain and placental barriers. The drug is extensively metabolized in the liver, and its metabolites, glucuronide conjugates, and unchanged (10%) portion are excreted in the urine. About 60% of an administered dose is eliminated within 24 hours.

Nausea, vomiting, and dizziness occur most frequently with this drug. Drowsiness and respiratory depression are also observed. Cardiovascular side effects (such as tachycardia, palpitation, and transient hypertension), hyperhydrosis, urinary retention, constipation, and euphoria are occasionally observed after administration of pentazocine. It can produce psychotomimetic reactions such as visual hallucinations, dysphoria, nightmares, and feelings of depersonalization. After a large i.v. dose, epileptiform convulsions may occur. Sterile abscess formation can result following it repeated injection into a single area.

Following chronic use, tolerance can develop to pentazocine. Its overall dependence liability is low, but, psychological and physical dependence have been observed primarily after parenteral administration, especially in persons with a history of dependence on other drugs. Pentazocine has less abuse potential than nalorphine or cyclazocine. It is rarely the first drug of abuse; most patients concurrently abuse pentazocine (parenterally) and sedative-hypnotics, alcohol, or heroin. Pentazocine and tripelennamine in combination have been reported to produce an euphoric state similar to that of a heroin-cocaine combination (34). On abrupt withdrawal of the drug, an atypical abstinence syndrome of mild intensity (nausea, vomiting, abdominal cramps, restlessness, dizziness, chills, and fever) ensues. Some patients may not show withdrawal symptoms. Because it is a mild narcotic antagonist, pentazocine precipitates withdrawal manifestation in subjects on a methadone maintenance program. Methadone maintenance, however, is often used to alleviate withdrawal symptoms in pentazocine-dependent subjects, particularly in treating "complicated withdrawal" where a less addictive drug such as diazepam has failed (40).

Pentazocine is effective in relief of moderate pain and as a preoperative medication. It is less effective than morphine in severe pain. It may be useful in obstetrics, but causes respiratory depression in the fetus comparable with that produced by meperidine. Because its dependence liability is less than that of morphine, pentazocine can relieve chronic pain when given before development of appreciable dependence on opiates.

MIXED AGONISTS-ANTAGONISTS

A varying degree of antagonist property has been observed in analgesics like nalbuphine and butorphanol in addition to pentazocine, discussed earlier. The antagonist property is more marked in nalorphine, which also possesses a weak agonist activity.

NALBUPHINE

Nalbuphine (n-cyclobutylmethyl-7,8-dihydro-14-hydroxymorphine) is chemically related to oxymorphone and naloxone (Tables 10.1-2 and 10.1-5) and has both analgesic and antagonist properties.

Nalbuphine has about the same analgesic potency as that of morphine, but it is approximately three times more potent than pentazocine. Its antagonist activity is about 10 times more potent than that of pentazocine. In general, pharmacological properties of nalbuphine are comparable with those of morphine. Its addiction liability is similar to that of pentazocine, and sudden withdrawal of its administration results in the manifestation of an opiatelike withdrawal syndrome milder than that produced by morphine, but more intense than that produced by pentazocine. Like pentazocine, because of its antagonist activity nalbuphine also precipitates withdrawal symptoms in patients who are receiving narcotic analgesics.

Systemic arterial pressure may increase somewhat in doses up to 3 mg/kg. Cardiac index, heart rate, systemic vascular resistance, pulmonary capillary wedge pressure, and pulmonary vascular resistance remain unchanged.

Respiratory depression is equal to that produced by morphine at equianalgesic doses. Nalbuphine may precipitate bronchial asthma.

The drug is metabolized in the liver and excreted by the kidneys. It should therefore be used with caution in patients with liver or kidney disease.

Adverse effects of nalbuphine are essentially similar to those of morphine. Sedation is most common with nalbuphine. Unlike morphine, respiratory depression that occurs with an analgesic dose of the drug is not increased with its larger doses. Its psychotomimetic effects are less than those of pentazocine.

This drug is indicated as a preoperative medication and as a supplement to general anesthesia, and for postoperative pain. It is effective in relieving moderate-to-severe pain from a variety of causes (e.g., cancer, trauma). As an obstetric analgesic, 10 to 15 mg of the drug is comparable

Table 10.1-5
Narcotic Antagonists of Various Chemical Groups

Antagonists	Analgesic Potency (Morphine = 1)	Antagonist Potency (relative to nalorphine) Rat[a]	Monkey	Humans[b]	Addiction Liability	Psychotomimetic Effect[c]
Morphine analogs						
Nalorphine	0.25-0.17	1	1	1	+	30
Naloxone	0	7	7	7		
Naltrexone	0	14	6-13	17		
Nalbuphine		0.5-0.17	0.11	0.25		72
Morphinans						
Levallorphan	50	2-5	4	2-5		12
Benzomorphans						
Pentazocine	0.33	0.014	0.03	0.02	+	60
Cyclazocine	0.33	4-6	4-5	6	+	1

[a]Prevention of analgesia or narcosis.
[b]Precipitation of morphine withdrawal.
[c]Dose (mg, s.c.) showing LSD-like effect.
Source: Adopted from Ref. 50.

with 75 to 100 mg of meperidine, both having similar effects on mother and neonate. It is contraindicated in narcotic addicts and also in patients with increased intracranial pressure.

BUTORPHANOL

Butorphanol is related chemically to levorphanol (Tables 10.1-2 and 10.1-5) and pharmacologically belongs to the same classes as pentazocine and nalbuphine, which have both analgesic and weak antagonist properties.

Butorphanol's analgesic activity is about 4 to 7 times more potent than morphine on weight basis. Pharmacological action of butorphanol are basically similar to those of morphine. Incidence of nausea and vomiting is less than that of morphine. Its antagonist activity is about 10 to 30 times that of pentazocine and 2.5% of that of nalozone. Butorphanol has low addiction liability.

Respiratory depression caused by 2 mg butorphanol equals that of 10 mg morphine; and does not increase with the dose. Changes in pCO_2 are small. The duration of respiratory depression is dose related.

Butorphanol increases pulmonary artery pressure, pulmonary wedge pressure, left ventricular end-diastolic pressure, systemic arterial pressure, and pulmonary vascular resistance. It increases the work of the right heart.

Following i.m. injection, peak plasma level is reached in about 30 to 60 minutes. The half-life of butorphanol is about 2.5 to 3.5 hours. It is mainly metabolized in liver to inactive hydroxybutorphanol, which is excreted in the urine.

The most common adverse reactions to butorphanol are sedation, nausea, and sweating. Other reactions are similar to those caused by other potent narcotic analgesics.

Butorphanol is a potent analgesic, the duration of which is 3 to 4 hours. The onset of action following i.m. administration is in 10 minutes. The drug may be used to relieve gallbladder colic, as it does not increase intrabiliary pressure. It may be used as a preoperative medication and as a supplement to nitrous oxide-oxygen anesthesia. It is contraindicated in narcotic addicts and in patients suffering from liver or kidney disease.

THERAPEUTIC USES OF NARCOTIC ANALGESICS

Narcotic analgesics are principally indicated in the treatment of constant dull or sharp pain (e.g., of visceral origin), postoperative pain, as well as pain caused by coronary, pulmonary, or peripheral vascular thrombosis, neoplasm, fractures, burns, and biliary or renal colic. They are also used as preanesthetic medication, as sedative-hypnotics in special circumstances (e.g., cardiac asthma), as cough suppressants, and as antidiarrheal agents.

In general, parenteral dose of morphine is about 0.1 to 0.15 mg/kg. The oral equianalgesic dose is about 4 to 5 times the parenteral dose.

Codeine at a dose of 20 to 45 mg every 3 hours is fairly effective in relieving superficial pain originating from integumentary structures. Meperidine, methadone, and dihydromorphine are generally preferred to combat moderate-to-severe acute deep pain where sedation is not required and to avoid constipation. Propoxyphene, oxycodone, and pentazocine are usually used in the treatment of chronic painful conditions. In the management of cancer pain, the analgesia need should not be equated with psychic or physical dependence. In the treatment of cancer pain, tolerance is a more important problem than physical dependence. Meperidine and pentazocine produce tissue irritation and pain at the site of injections and as such they are not suitable for the management of chronic pain in cancer patients.

In changing the route of administration of narcotic analgesics (e.g., from parenteral to oral), one should take into consideration the oral/parenteral potency ratio. Oral administration of these drugs result in slower onset, a lower peak effect, and longer duration of analgesic action than when administered parenterally (5).

In acute pulmonary edema, morphine reduces anxiety, which tends to cause exacerbation of the condition, and thereby helps in alleviation of the condition. Morphine is given s.c., i.m., or i.v. at doses of 10 to 20 mg, depending on the severity of the condition. In paroxysmal atrial tachycardia, when all other measures fail to correct arrhythmia, morphine 10 to 15 mg, s.c., may be given.

In myocardial infarction, morphine is traditionally given for the relief of pain. It may reduce blood pressure and cardiac output. There is great variation in the individual patient's analgesic and hemodynamic response to morphine. Morphine, even though it is spasmogenic, is commonly used for relief of pain in biliary colic, in combination with atropine.

For obstetric analgesia, meperidine is generally used and as a result the neonate may have a low Apgar score: but this does not affect the newborn detrimentally. Morphine, when given 3 to 4 hours before parturition, may cause respiratory depression in the neonate.

Acute narcotic withdrawal syndrome is generally treated initially by administering the drug of abuse followed by gradual detoxification with methadone. This is discussed in more detail in Chapter 11.6. The use of narcotic analgesics in preanesthetic medication, for suppression of cough, and for diarrhea is discussed in Chapter 17.1.

NARCOTIC ANTAGONISTS

Antagonism of morphine and heroin-induced respiratory depression by nalorphine (N-allylnormorphine) was reported by Pohl as early as 1915, but not until 1951 was the clinical significance of this antagonism critically exploited. The search for better narcotic antagonists led to the introduction of several congeners of morphine and other narcotics [e.g., naloxone (1-N-allyl-7,8,dihyro-14-hydroxynormophinone), naltrexone (N-cyclopropylmethyl-14-hydroxydihydromorphinone), pentazocine, and cyclazocine]. The chemistry and structure-activity relationships of narcotic antagonists have been reviewed by Harris (17) and Archer and coworkers (1). Tables 10.1-2 and 10.1-5 list several important narcotic antagonists from different chemical groups, with some of their characteristics.

Pharmacological Effects. These drugs compete with morphine (or other opioids) at the receptor sites and antagonize most of their pharmacological actions. However, some of these compounds, such as nalorphine, may exert their action on certain receptor sites to produce morphinelike (agonistic) and other (e.g., psychotomimetic) effects that may vary in potency; these agents are termed agonist-antagonists or partial antagonists. Drugs such as naloxone and naltrexone, which appear to have little, if any, agonistic action, are called pure antagonists. It is now generally considered that narcotic agonists and antagonists act on different conformations of the same receptor site (53).

In the absence of physical dependence nalorphine-type antagonists may add their morphinelike action to those elicited by morphine (e.g., intensifying respiratory depression and miosis), if the dose of the latter is relatively low. On the other hand, if the dose of morphine is high, the same dose of nalorphine or levallorphan will antagonize morphine action by displacing it from the receptor site. Pretreatment with nalorphine has been shown to prevent or reverse the initial temperature response to narcotics and antagonize the development of tolerance to these effects (3). In a physically dependent organism, precipitation of withdrawal symptoms is believed to be produced by "unmasking" the counteradaptive processes responsible for physical dependence.

Naloxone is a pure antagonist, and it is 10 to 20 times more potent than nalorphine and 5 to 7 times more potent than levallorphan. The "pure" antagonist naloxone at a dose of 0.4 mg given i.v. at short intervals may effectively reverse the respiratory and CNS depression caused by narcotics. Relative potency of narcotic antagonists is shown in Table 10.1-5. A very small dose (< 5) $\mu g/kg$) of naloxone is required to precipitate withdrawal from exogenous opiates (48). After high doses (2 and 4 mg/kg) naloxone causes somatic effects in normal volunteers. These effects include "buzz", tingling, numbness of the extremities, dizziness, a heavy head, lethargy, nausea, and vomiting lasting for about 15-30 min. Behavioral changes induced by increasing doses of naloxone include irritability, anxiety, tension, difficulty in concentrating, and lack of appetite lasting for about 24-48 hours (11). At about 10 mg dose, naloxone has been reported to release catecholamines in a patient with pheochromocytoma presumably from chromaffin cells, suggesting an opioid modulation of sympathetic output (38).

Naloxone can antagonize the psychotomimetic and dysphoric actions of nalorphine and cyclazocine at higher doses (10-15 mg). These antagonists also compete with morphinelike drugs for enkephalin receptor sites.

Naltrexone, because of its low incidence of side effects, oral effectiveness, and prolonged duration of action, has therapeutic advantages over other antagonists. It is about eight times as potent and has three times longer duration of action than naloxone in rats. In humans, it is 17 times more potent than naloxone in producing acute withdrawal symptoms in narcotic physical dependence.

Pharmacokinetics. About 20% of a dose of naloxone given orally reaches the systemic circulation, and peak blood levels occur in about 30-60 min. A fast first-pass effect probably exists with naloxone. The half-life of naloxone is about 60 min. Naloxone is metabolized by glucuronide conjugation, N-dealkylation, and reduction. Naltrexone is absorbed from the gastrointestinal tract, and a first-pass hepatic biotransformation results in rapid appearance of metabolites in the blood. The peak plasma concentrations occur in about 1 hour following oral administration. The half-life of naltrexone is about 10 hours. Naltrexone is metabolized to 6-β-naltrexol and 2-hydroxy-3-methoxy naltrexol. The metabolites are excreted mostly (38-70% of a dose) through the kidney and slightly (about 2-3% of a dose) through feces.

Therapeutic Uses. Narcotic antagonists are used in the treatment of acute intoxication, particularly for respiratory depression caused by morphine and related drugs (e.g., hydromorphone, oxymorphine, methadone, anileridine, alphaprodine, levorphanol, meperidine, piminodine, fentanyl, d-propoxyphene, and pentazocine). Because naloxone is free of any respiratory-depressant action, it is the drug of choice to antagonize narcotic-induced respiratory depression; the usual dose of the drug in adults is 0.4 mg (i.v.), repeated every 2-3 min if no immediate improvement is seen. In children and in newborn infants, it is administered at a dose of 0.01 mg/kg initially, repeated after 5-6 min if no improvement occurs, and may be repeated in 30-90 min. Due to the relatively short half-life of naloxone, patients who respond to the drug should be observed for 24 hours for possible recurrence of depression. Agonist-antagonists (e.g., cyclazocine) can be used as analgesics. They are also used in the diagnosis of physical dependence on narcotic drugs. Nalorphine does not precipitate withdrawal symptoms in the case of dependence on meperidine with a daily intake of less than 3 g. Naloxone can also antagonize overdose due to dextromethorphan. Opioid antagonists have been used in a variety of other conditions such as cardiovascular shock, hypercapnia, schizophrenia, and manic depression (42). Naltrexone has been recommended in the treatment of narcotic dependence in order to reduce or block the reinforcing effect of the narcotic (see Chapter 11.6).

REFERENCES

1. Archer, S., Albertson, N. F., and Pierson, A. K. Structure-activity relationships in the opioid antagonists. In: *Agonist and Antagonist Actions of Narcotic Analgesic Drugs* (Kosterlitz, H. W., Collier, H. O. J., and Villareal, J. E., eds.). Baltimore: University Press, 1973, p. 25.
2. Ary, M., and Lomax, P. Influence of narcotic agents on temperature regulation. In: *Neurochemical Mechanism of Opiates and Endorphins.* Advanced Biochemistry Psychopharmacology, Vol. 20 (Loh, H. H., and Ross, D. H., eds.). New York: Raven Press, 1979, p. 429.
3. Babbini, M., Gaiardi, M., and Bartoletti, M. Effects of morphine on a quickly learned conditioned suppression in rats. *Psychopharmacologia,* 33:329, 1973.
4. Beaumont, A., and Hughes, J. Biology of opioid peptides. *Ann. Rev. Pharmacol. Toxicol.,* 19:245, 1979.
5. Beaver, W. T. Management of cancer pain with parenteral medication. *JAMA,* 244:2653, 1980.
6. Besson, J. M., and Le Bars, D. Effect of morphine on the transmission of painful messages at the spinal level. In: *Factors Affecting the Actions of Narcotics* (Adler, M. L., Manara, L., and Samanin, R., eds.). New York: Raven Press, 1978, p. 103.
7. Bloom, F., Battenberg, E., Rossier, J., Ling, N., and Guillemin, R. Neurons containing β-endorphin in rat brain exist separately from those containing enkephalin: Immunocytochemical studies. *Proc. Natl. Acad. Sci. USA,* 75:1591, 1978.
8. Brunk, S. F., and Delle, M. Morphine metabolism in man. *Clin. Pharmacol. Ther.,* 16:51, 1974.
9. Casy, A. F. The structure of narcotic analgesic drugs. In: *Narcotic Drugs Biochemical Pharmacology* (Clouet, D. H., ed.). New York: Pergamon Press, 1971, p. 1.
10. Clark, W. G., and Cumby, H. R. Hyperthermic responses to central and peripheral injections of morphine sulphate in the cat. *Br. J. Pharmacol.,* 63:65, 1978.
11. Cohen, M. R., Cohen, R. M., Pickar, D. et al. Behavioral effects after high dose naloxone administration to normal volunteers. *Lancet,* 2:1110, 1981.
12. Cohen, M. R., Pickar, D., Dubois, M. et al. Clinical and experimental studies of stress and the endogenous opioid system. *N. Y. Acad. Sci.,* 398:424, 1982.
13. Copolov, D. L., and Helme, R. D. Enkephalins and endorphins clinical, pharmacological and therapeutic implications. *Drugs,* 26:503, 1983.
14. DeWied, D., Van Ree, J. M., and de Jong, W. Narcotic analgesia and the neuroendocrine control of anterior pituitary function. In: *Narcotics and the Hypothalamus* (Zimmerman, E., and George, R., eds.). New York: Raven Press, 1974.
15. Donovan, M. P., Thomas, J. A., and Ling, G. M. Morphine analgesia and tolerance: A possible role of cyclic AMP. *Bull. Narcotics,* 29:9, 1977.
16. Goldberg, S. R., Hoffmeister, T., Schlichting, V., and Wultke, W. Aversive properties of nalorphine and naloxone on morphine-dependent rhesus monkeys. *J. Pharmacol. Exp. Ther.,* 179:269, 1971.
17. Goldberg, S. R., and Morse, W. H. Some behavioral effects of morphine, naloxone and nalorphine, alone and in combination, compared in the squirrel monkey and the pigeon. *Fed. Proc.,* 33:550, 1974.
18. Goldstein, A. Opioid peptides (endorphins) in pituitary and brain. *Science,* 193:1081, 1976.
19. Goldstein, A., Tachibana, S., Lowney, L. I. et al. Dynorphin-(1-13), an extraordinarily potent opioid peptide. *Proc. Natl. Acad. Sci. USA,* 76:6666, 1979.
20. Goldstein, A., Fischli, W., Lowney, L. I. et al. Porcine pituitary dynorphin: complete amino acid sequences of the biologically active heptadecapeptide. *Proc. Natl. Acad. Sci. USA,* 78:7219, 1981.
21. Henriksen, S. J., Chouvet, G., McGinty, J., and Bloom, F. E. Opioid peptides in the hippocampus: anatomical and physiological considerations. *N. Y. Acad. Sci.,* 398:207, 1982.
22. Holaday, J. W., and Loh, H. H. Endorphin-opiate interactions with neuroendocrine systems. In: *Neurochemical Mechanisms of Opiates and Endorphins.* Advanced Biochemistry Psychopharmacology, Vol. 20 (Loh, H. H., and Ross, D. H., eds.). New York: Raven Press, 1979, p. 227.
23. Huffman, D. H., and Ferguson, R. L. Acute codeine overdose: correspondence between clinical course and codeine metabolism. *Johns Hopkins Med. J.,* 136:183, 1975.
24. Hughes, J. Isolation of an endogenous compound from the brain with pharmacological properties similar to morphine. *Brain Res.,* 88:295, 1975.
25. Hughes, J. W., Smith, T., Kosterlitz, H. et al. Identification of

two related pentapeptides from the brain with potent opiate agonist activity. *Nature*, 255:577, 1975.

26. Iida, N., Tetsuo, O., and Eikichi, H. Relationship between the morphine-induced spontaneous locomotor activity and the concentration of morphine in brain or in plasma of rats (Report 2). *Jap. J. Pharmacol.*, 24:88, 1974.
27. Iwamoto, E., and Way, E. L. Opiate actions and catecholamines. In: *Neurochemical Mechanisms of Opiates and Endorphins.* Advanced Biochemistry Psychopharmacology, Vol. 20 (Loh, H. H., and Ross, D. H., eds.). New York: Raven Press, 1979, p. 357.
28. Kangawa, K., Matsuo, H., and Igarashi, M. α-Neo-endorphin: a "big" Leu-enkephalin with potent opiate activity from porcine hypothalami. *Biochem. Biophys. Res. Commu.*, 86:153, 1979.
29. Klemm, W. R. Opiate mechanisms: evaluation of research involving neuronal action potentials. *Progr. Neuropsychopharmacol.*, 5:1, 1981.
30. Kline, N. S., Li, C. H., Lehmann, H. E. et al. β-Endorphin induced changes in schizophrenic and depressed patients. *Arch. Gen. Psychiatry*, 34:1111, 1977.
31. Koob, G. F., and Bloom, F. E. Behavioral effects of opioid peptides. *Br. Med. Bull.*, 39:89, 1983.
32. Kornetsky, C., and Bain, G. Biobehavioral bases of the reinforcing properties of opiate drugs. *N. Y. Acad. Sci.*, 398:241, 1982.
33. Kosterlitz, H. W., and Hughes, J. Development of the concepts of opiate receptors and their ligands. *Adv. Biochem. Psychopharmacol.*, 18:31, 1978.
34. Lahmeyer, H. W., and Steingold, R. G. Medical and psychiatric complications of pentazocine and tripelennamine abuse. *J. Clin. Psychiatry*, 41:275, 1980.
35. Livett, B. G., Dean, D. M., Whelan, L. G. et al. Co-release of enkephalin and catecholamines from cultured adrenal chromaffin cells. *Nature*, 289:317, 1981.
36. Lord, J. A. H., Waterfield, A. A., Hughes, J., and Kosterlitz, H. W. Endogenous opioid peptides: multiple agonists and receptors. *Nature*, 267:495, 1977.
37. Mains, R. E., Eipper, B. A., and Ling, N. Structure of a common precursor to corticotropin and endorphin. *Proc. Natl. Acad. Sci. USA*, 74:3014, 1977.
38. Mannelli, M., Maggi, M., Defeco, M. L. et al. Naloxone administration releases catecholamines. *N. Engl. J. Med.*, 308:654, 1983.
39. Martin, W. R. The effects of morphine- and nalorphine-like drugs in the nondependent and morphine-dependent chronic spinal dog. *J. Pharmacol. Exp. Ther.*, 197:517, 1976.
40. Maxmen, J. S. Methadone treatment of pentazocine abuse. *Ann. N. Y. Acad. Sci.*, 398:87, 1982.
41. Mckenzie, G. M. Apomorphine-induced aggression: Characteristics, pharmacological intervention, and site of action. *Psychopharmacol. Bull.*, 9:19, 1973.
42. McNicholas, L. F., and Martin, W. R. New and experimental therapeutic roles for naloxone and related opioid antagonists. *Drugs*, 27:81, 1984.
43. McQueen, D. S. Opioid peptide interactions with respiratory and circulatory systems. *Br. Med. Bull.*, 39:77, 1983.
44. Miller, R. J., and Cuatrecasas, P. Neurobiology and neuropharmacology of the enkephalins. In: *Neurochemical Mechanisms of Opiates and Endorphins*, Advanced Biochemistry Psychopharmacology, Vol. 20 (Loh, H. H., and Ross, D. H., eds.). New York: Raven Press, 1979, p. 187.
45. Misra. A. L. Metabolism of opiates. In: *Factors Affecting the Actions of Narcotics* (Adler, M. L., Manara, L., and Samanin, R., eds.). New York: Raven Press, 1978, p. 297.
46. O'Brien, C. P., Terenius, L., Wahlstrom, A. et al. Endorphin levels in opioid-dependent human subjects: A longitudinal study. *N. Y. Acad. Sci.*, 398:377, 1982.
47. Parker, R. B. Effect of morphine, narcotic antagonists, and the interaction of morphine and narcotic antagonists on mouse locomotor activity. *Pharmacologist*, 15:203, 1973.
48. Pert, C., and Garland, B. L. The mechanism of opiate agonist and antagonist action. In: *Receptors and Hormone Action*, Vol. 3 (Birnbaumer, L., and O'Malley, B. V. W., eds.). New York: Academic Press, 1978, p. 535.
49. Pickworth, W. B., and Sharpe, L. G. EEG-behavioral dissociation after morphine-like drugs in the dog: Further evidence for two opiate receptors. *Neuropharmacology*, 18:617, 1979.
50. Pradhan, S. N., and Dutta, S. N. Narcotic analgesics. In: *Drug Abuse: Clinical and Basic Aspects* (Pradhan, S. N., and Dutta, S. N., eds.). St. Louis: C. V. Mosby, 1977, p. 49.
51. Säwe, J., Dahlström, B., Paalzow, L., and Rane, A. Morphine kinetics in cancer patients. *Clin. Pharmacol. Ther.*, 30:629, 1981.
52. Simon, E. J. Opiate receptors and opioid peptides: an overview. *N. Y. Acad. Sci.*, 398:327, 1982.
53. Simon, E. J., and Groth, J. Kinetics of opiate receptor inactivation by sulfhydryl reagents: Evidence for conformational change in presence of sodium ions. *Proc. Natl. Acad. Sci. USA*, 72:2404, 1975.
54. Simon, E. J., and Hiller, J. M. The opiate receptors. *Ann. Rev. Pharmacol. Toxicol.*, 18:371, 1978.
55. Snyder, S. H. The opiate receptor and morphine-like peptides in the brain. *Am. J. Psychiatry*, 135:645, 1978.
56. Sparber, S. B., Gellert, V. F., Lichtblau, L., and Eisenberg, R. The use of operant behavior methods to study aggression and effects of acute and chronic morphine administration in rats. In: *Factors Affecting the Action of Narcotics* (Adler, M. L., Manara, L., and Samanin, R., eds.). New York: Raven Press, 1978.
57. Terenius, L. Endogenous peptides and analgesia. *Ann. Rev. Pharmacol. Toxicol.*, 18:189, 1978.
58. Teschemacher, H., Opheim, K. E., Cox, B. M., and Goldstein, A. A peptide-like substance from pituitary that acts like morphine. *Life Sci.*, 16:1771, 1975.
59. Thompson, J. W. Opioid peptides. *Br. Med. J.*, 288:259, 1984.
60. Volavka, J., Zaks, A., Roubicek, J., and Fink, M. Electrophysiologic effects of diacetylmorphine (heroin) and naloxone in man. *Neuropharmacology*, 9:587, 1970.
61. Way, E. L., and Glasgow, C. Recent development in morphine analgesia: Tolerance and dependence. In: *Psychopharmacology: A Generation of Progress* (Lipton, M. A., DiMascio, A., and Killam, K. F., eds.). New York: Raven Press, 1978, p. 1535.
62. Wolozin, B. L., and Pasternak, G. W. Classification of multiple morphine and enkephalin binding sites in the central nervous system. *Proc. Natl. Acad. Sci. USA*, 78:6181, 1981.
63. Zukin, R. S., and Zukin, S. R. Demonstration of [^{3}H] cyclazocin binding to multiple opiate receptor sites. *Mol. Pharmacol.*, 20:246, 1981.
64. Zukin, S. R., and Zukin, R. S. Specific [^{3}H] phencyclidine binding in rat central nervous system. *Proc. Natl. Acad. Sci. USA*, 76:5372, 1979.

ADDITIONAL READING

Kosterlits, H.W. The Wellcome Foundation lecture, 1982. Opioid peptides and their receptors. *Proc. R. Soc. Lond. (Biol.)* 225:27, 1985.

CHAPTER 10.2

ANALGESIC-ANTIPYRETICS

Paul Mazel

The analgesic-antipyretics are drugs that relieve pain, inflammation, and lower body temperature, but do not have any sedative or hypnotic effects; nor do they produce significant tolerance, physical dependence, and abuse liability. These drugs relieve pain of low-to-moderate intensity (e.g., headache, arthralgia, myalgia, dysmenorrhea,and others).

Two of the world's most widely used drugs, aspirin (acetylsalicylic acid) and acetaminophen (N-acetyl-para-aminophenol), were introduced into medicine well over 80 years ago and are used in the treatment of mild-to-moderate pain and as antipyretics. Although differing substantially in structure, both compounds exert their antipyretic and analgesic actions by similar mechanisms. It has been estimated that Americans consume 20 billion aspirin tablets annually (40 tons each day) (16). Both aspirin and acetaminophen are present in more than 200 proprietary preparations (22), widely advertised and sold over the counter for self-medicating purposes.

In an excellent recent symposium all aspects of analgesics-antipyretics were discussed (60).

SALICYLATES

History. The word "salicylate" is derived from *Salicaceae*, the botanical name for the willow family. The therapeutic properties of an extract of the willow bark were reported as early as 1763 by Rev. Edward Stone (58). The bark contains a glycoside (salicin) that yields salicylic acid plus glucose on hydrolysis. With time, salicylic acid (orthohydroxybenzoic acid) had been accepted for rheumatic conditions, but it is quite irritating. To overcome this problem, various derivatives were synthesized that would be better tolerated. Substitution in the phenolic group (Fig. 10.2-1) led to the development of aspirin, which is the acetylated derivative; another widely used salicylate, found in nature in oil of wintergreen, is the methyl ester of salicylic acid (Fig. 10.2-1).

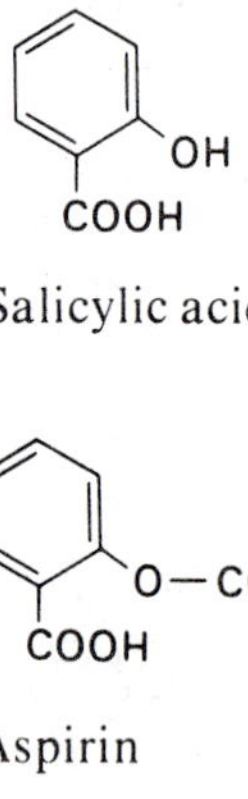

OH
COOH

Salicylic acid

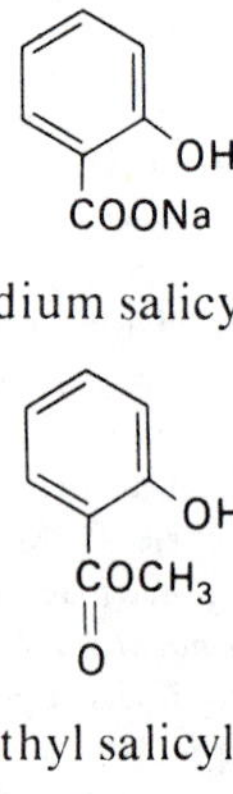

OH
COONa

Sodium salicylate

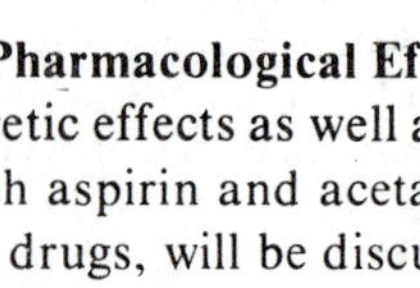

O—$COCH_3$
COOH

Aspirin

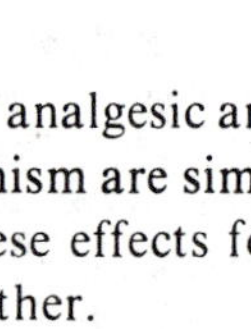

OH
$COCH_3$
‖
O

Methyl salicylate

Fig.10.2-1. *Structural formulas of salicylates.*

Pharmacological Effects. Since the analgesic and antipyretic effects as well as their mechanism are similar for both aspirin and acetaminophen, these effects for both the drugs, will be discussed here together.

Analgesia. Both aspirin and acetaminophen relieve pain of slight-to-moderate intensity and are effective in pain associated with headache, myalgia, arthralgia, neuralgia, bursitis, arthritis, dysmenorrhea, neuritis, fibrositis, post-tooth extraction, vascular headache, and musculoskeletal pain. Neither aspirin nor acetaminophen induce tolerance, addiction, or euphoria, nor do they produce sedation. The effective dose for analgesia is 0.6 g; increasing the dose will not increase the intensity of effect. If an additional effect is desired, it is better to repeat the dose every 4 hr. For children, a dose of 65 mg/year of age is recommended.

Antipyresis. Both acetaminophen and aspirin decrease temperature in fever by heat loss through promotion of peripheral vasodilation and sweating. Thus, there is a normalization of temperature-regulating system. Aspirin and acetaminophen have been shown to inhibit the temperature-elevating effect of leukocytic pyrogen (6). The antipyretics decrease body temperature in febrile patients but have no effect on normal body temperature. Clark has recently reviewed the mechanism of antipyretic action of salicylates and related compounds (6).

Mechanism of Action. Although aspirin-like drugs have been used for over 80 years, their mechanism(s) of action have included: (a) uncoupling of oxidative phosphorylation (4); (b) the release of an endogenous antiinflammatory peptide from plasma proteins; and, (c) interference with the migration of leukocytes. None of the proposed mechanisms have satisfactorily explained the observed actions of aspirinlike compounds (57).

A substantial body of evidence has accumulated demonstrating that aspirinlike compounds and acetaminophen exert their analgesic and antipyretic effects by affecting the synthesis of prostaglandins (55, 58), namely, the formation of prostaglandin E_2 (PGE_2) and prostaglandin $F_2\alpha$ ($PGF_2\alpha$) by inhibiting the action of prostaglandin synthetase (cyclooxygenase) as shown in Fig. 10.2-2.

In humans, injection of prostaglandins causes pain along the veins into which they are infused, as well as headache. Furthermore, PGE_1, when injected either into the cerebral ventricles or anterior hypothalamus, has been reported to be the most powerful pyretic agent known. Evidence has accumulated that when cell membranes are distorted or damaged by physical trauma or other injurious processes, prostaglandins are released; pain and fever are produced. In addition, the prostaglandins enhance the pain induced by such substances as bradykinin, substance P, serotonin, and histamine (57). Thus, by preventing prostaglandin release, aspirinlike compounds also prevent sensitization of the pain receptors (free nerve endings) to mechanical stimulation or to chemical mediators.

Supporting evidence relating the effect of aspirinlike compounds, including acetaminophen, to prostaglandins includes the following:

1. Aspirin as an analgesic is effective only on those tissues in which prostaglandin formation has been demonstrated. Thus, aspirin is ineffective in uninflamed tissues.

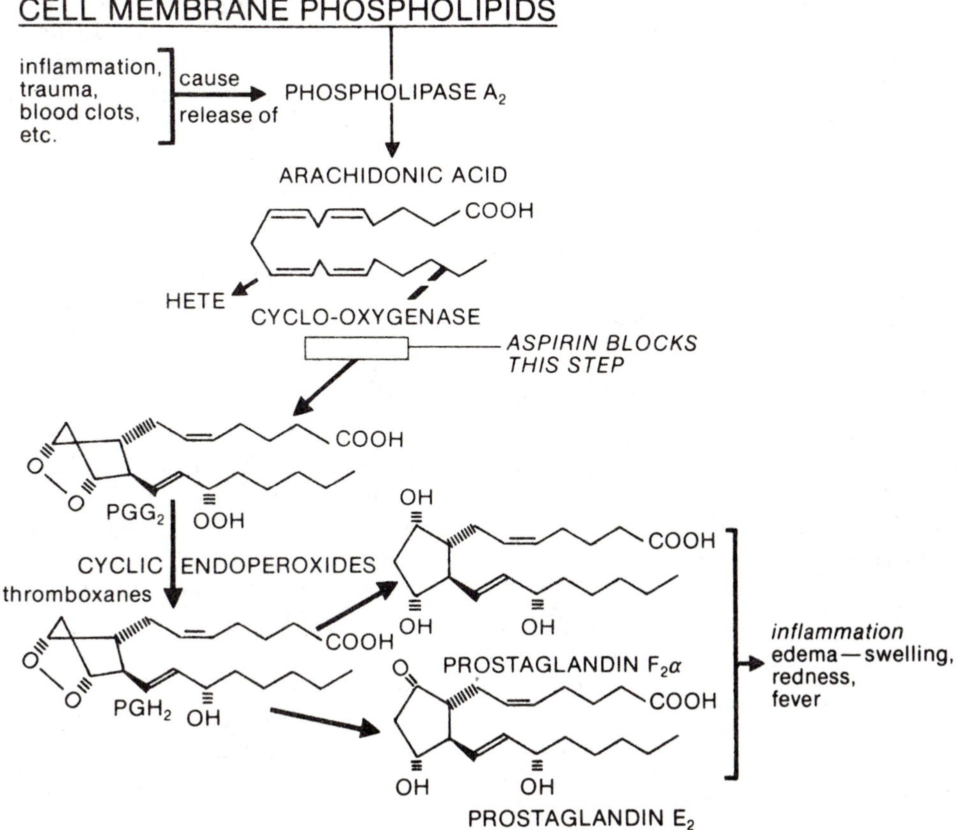

Fig.10.2-2. *Inhibition of prostaglandin synthesis by aspirin (from Ref. 55).*

2. Administration of aspirinlike compounds has been shown to decrease prostaglandin metabolites by 77-98%.

3. Aspirinlike compounds decrease the prostaglandin content of synovial fluid from arthritic patients.

4. Aspirin decreases prostaglandin generation from isolated, incubated platelets.

5. The hyperthermic effect of centrally injected arachidonate, a prostaglandin precursor, is blocked by aspirin and acetaminophen. Prostaglandins have also been shown to be required for pyrogen-induced fever.

6. The antipyretics (aspirin/acetaminophen) are competitive with leukocytic pyrogens, shown by a shift in the log dose-response curve, which exert their effects through prostaglandins.

7. Aspirin has been shown not to block the inflammatory effect of injected prostaglandins, demonstrating that its action is related to preventing synthesis and release.

8. The effect of aspirinlike compounds on prostaglandin synthesis has been found to be true in all animal species studied thus far.

Miscellaneous Effects

Uricosuric Effects. Salicylic acid has been found to affect renal tubular reabsorption and secretion of uric acid. With low doses (1-2 g/day), uric acid secretion is inhibited, as reflected in increased uric acid concentrations. Tubular reabsorption of uric acid is also inhibited, resulting in an enhanced excretion of uric acid and decreased uric acid concentrations. With large doses of salicylates (greater than 5 g/day), there is evidence of uricosuria, and plasma urate levels decrease. Wherever possible, one should avoid giving small doses of salicylate with uricosuric agents.

Platelet Aggregation. Following blood vessel injury, circulating platelets adhere to exposed collagen and release adenosine diphosphate (ADP), producing aggregation of the platelets, followed by release of epinephrine, serotonin, and platelet factor III. All of the released substances produce local vasoconstriction and inhibit bleeding. The release of endogenous ADP by platelets is most important in initiating this reaction. Salicylates inhibit the platelet release of ADP and hence serotonin, epinephrine, and platelet factor III (35). The mechanism by which aspirin acts has not been completely elucidated, but it has been demonstrated that aspirin inhibits prostaglandin synthesis in the platelet, which in turn modulates the levels of adenyl cyclase and hence cyclic adenosine monophosphate (cAMP) (45, 51).

Small doses (300 mg) of aspirin can produce effects on aggregation in normal individuals, which may last from 4 to 7 days. The clinical implications of these effects are reflected in an increased prolongation of the bleeding time. The effects of aspirin could be significant in postsurgical cases (tonsillectomy) by producing severe hemorrhage (50). Furthermore, aspirin has been shown to affect fetal platelets and could produce neonatal hemorrhage (36).

In view of aspirin's effect on platelets and bleeding time, the drug should be avoided in patients with severe hepatic damage, hypoprothrombinemia, vitamin K deficiency, or hemophilia.

Coagulation. Large doses of aspirin have been shown to prolong plasma prothrombin time (28). Administration of vitamin K will prevent the hypoprothrombinemia produced by aspirin. It is believed that aspirin competes with vitamin K in the enzymatic mechanisms involved in the synthesis of the coagulant protein. Mechanism of action of aspirin on platelets has been recently reviewed (20).

Metabolic Effects. Salicylates affect intermediary metabolism. Large doses uncouple oxidative phosphorylation (4, 33). The uncoupling of a number of adenosine triphosphate (ATP)-dependent reactions results in increasd heat production and oxygen consumption. Carbohydrate metabolism is also affected. With increasing doses, hyperglycemia, glycosuria, and a depletion of liver and muscle glycogen may be observed. In the diabetic, large doses may actually decrease blood sugar levels.

Large doses of aspirin can also affect nitrogen metabolism; there is an increase in nitrogen excretion because of increased protein breakdown, and a negative nitrogen balance may result. Fat metabolism is also affected, with decreased lipogenesis, increased oxidation of fatty acids in muscle and liver, and decreased concentration of plasma free fatty acids.

Salicylates have been shown to affect the binding of thyroxine to plasma proteins by competitive displacement. Release of free thyroxine causes a decrease in thyrotropin secretion and a decrease in thyroid activity. The results of the protein-bound iodine test can be altered; this should be considered in patients chronically taking salicylates.

Local Effects. Salicylic acid is keratolytic and is used in the treatment of warts, corns, and fungal infections. Methyl salicylate is used as an external preparation only, as a liniment and counterirritant.

Pharmacokinetics

Absorption. Salicylates are acidic compounds with a pk_a of 3.5 and exist in the stomach and intestine largely as the undissociated acid. The lipid-soluble unionized form is well absorbed orally, particularly in aqueous solution (41). The dissolution rate of the tablet form of aspirin limits its rate of absorption; this is probably affected by various pharmaceutical formulations (25). Buffered aspirin tablets may be absorbed faster because the addition of the antacid would increase the dissolution rate by increasing the pH near the aspirin particles (25), although there are no meaningful differences in the rate of absorption of buffered preparations compared with nonbuffered. Administration of aspirin with a glass of warm water may be as effective in enhancing absorption as the buffered preparation. With the effervescent tablet form of aspirin, the problem of dissolution rate is eliminated; absorption may be significantly enhanced. If large amounts of alkali are administered with aspirin, the elimination rate of salicylic acid through the kidneys could be increased, which would decrease the duration of action of the drug. With the ingestion of large doses of aspirin, the rate of absorption may be decreased due to decreased gastric emptying time and a decrease in absorption from the upper part of the small intestine.

Distribution. Peak plasma levels of salicylate, administered as aspirin, are reached in about 2 hours, then gradually decline. Levy has reported the biological half-life of aspirin in the systemic circulation to be 15-20 minutes (25). Orally administered aspirin is partly hydrolyzed in the intestine and on its first pass through the liver to salicylic acid (25). Thus, the pharmacological effects of aspirin are probably attributable to salicylic acid. The half-life of salicylates lengthens with the dose: 3.1-3.2 hours at 300 to 650-mg dose, 5 hours at 1 g, and 9 hours at 2-g dose. In addition, as the half-life increases, urinary excretion decreases. Thus, increasing doses without increasing the interval between them may lead to accumulation and toxic effects (26). In blood, salicylate is bound to plasma albumin (50-90%), depending on the concentration; this may have significant clinical implications, particularly concerning drug interactions with other compounds (e.g., anticoagulants), which can lead to significant side effects. In patients with hypoalbuminemia, from whatever cause, the protein binding of salicylates would be decreased, leading to side effects as a result of the increased levels of free drug. There are a number of compounds that compete with salicylates for plasma protein binding sites. These include: thyroxine, triiodothyronine, penicillin, thiopental, phenytoin, sulfinpyrazone, bilirubin, corticosteroids, and uric acid. Therapeutic blood levels for salicylates usually range from 2 to 10 mg/dl. Antiinflammatory effects are associated with 15-to 30-mg/dl blood levels. However, toxic manifestations (as tinnitus, CNS stimulation or depression, hyperventilation, etc.) begin to appear at 15- to 30-mg/dl and higher blood levels.

Once absorbed, salicylates are distributed to all body tissues and extracellular fluids. At therapeutic concentrations, the volume of distribution has been reported to be 150-200 ml/kg, which corresponds to the extracellular space (25). Salicylates can be found in synovial, spinal, and peritoneal fluids and saliva. Salicylates readily cross the placental barrier and can be found in the milk of nursing mothers (8).

Metabolism. Once absorbed and distributed, the duration of action of salicylates is determined by metabolism (hepatic microsomal and mitochondrial enzymes) and the rate of excretion of the unchanged salicylic acid. The metabolic fate of salicylic acid is shown in Fig. 10.2-3. The several pathways include: (a) conjugation of salicylic acid with glycine, yielding salicyluric acid, which accounts for approximately 25% of the total metabolites; (b) conjugation with glucuronic acid, yielding salicyl phenol glucuronide and salicyl acyl glucuronide, accounting for another 25% of the metabolites; (c) hydroxylation to gentisic acid (2, 5-dihydroxybenzoic acid), which represents a small amount (about 1%) of the total metabolites; and, (d) excretion of unchanged salicylic acid by glomerular filtration and tubular secretion, which accounts for approximately 50% of the administered compound (21, 25, 27).

Kinetics of Elimination. It has been well documented that two of the important pathways for salicylate elimination can be readily saturated at relatively low plasma levels of salicylate concentration; the time necessary to eliminate a given fraction of a dose will increase as the dose of drug is increased. With increasing doses, the formulation of salicylurate and salicyl phenolic glucuronide takes a much longer time to excrete, and because the two pathways are saturable, an increase in the serum concentration of free salicylate may be observed; a 50% increase in the daily dose of aspirin produces a 300% rise in the concentration of salicylate (25).

The clinical significance of the kinetics of elimination is that a small increase in dose may yield a sharp increase in blood levels. In doses of less than 10 mg/kg, the drug is eliminated in the percentages described for the five metabolites. With increasing doses, the percentage of salicyluric and salicyl phenolic glucuronide will decrease, thus increasing the levels of salicylic acid. This will not only enhance the therapeutic response but will also increase the contribution of the renal excretory pathway to the elimination of salicylates.

Excretion. The excretion of salicylates involves glomerular filtration, active renal tubular secretion, and passive renal tubular back-diffusion. The undissociated, lipid-soluble form is passively reabsorbed. Thus, the renal clearance of salicylate is quite sensitive to changes in urine pH. As the urine pH is increased above 6, there will be a large increase in the ionized form of the drug and

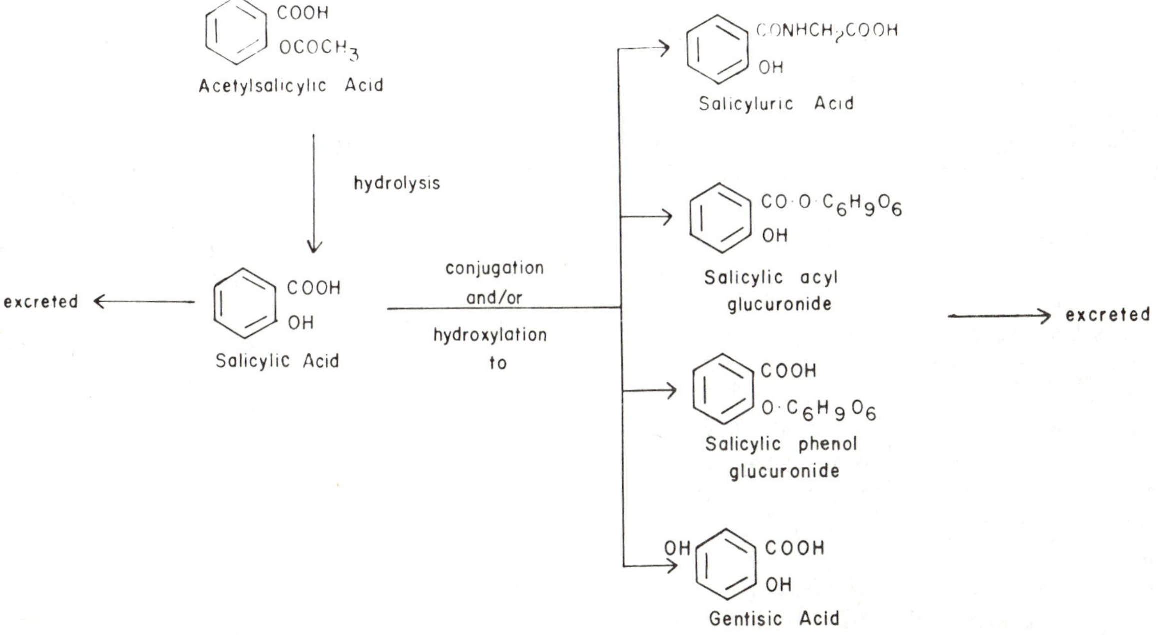

Fig.10.2-3. *Biotransformation and excretion of aspirin (from Ref.21).*

thus a marked increase in the renal clearance of salicylate (27). This is an important factor in the treatment of salicylate overdosage.

Adverse Effects

Gastrointestinal Effects. Aspirin has been shown to produce a number of gastrointestinal problems including epigastric distress, nausea, vomiting, heartburn, dyspepsia, gastritis, ulceration, and bleeding. The most serious of these is gastric mucosal damage and the resulting blood loss from the gastrointestinal tract. This subject has been recently reviewed by Fromm (13). It has been demonstrated that acidic conditions are required for salicylate to produce damage. The low pH keeps the salicylate in the un-ionized lipid-soluble diffusible form. As the salicylate penetrates the cells facing the lumen, it produces alterations in the mucosa, allowing for an increased diffusion of acid and producing cellular damage. Along with this back-diffusion into the mucosa, there is also a release of histamine from mast cells, which further stimulates acid secretion and resulting tissue damage. There is also an effect on adenosine triphosphate (ATP) and oxidative phosphorylation which, in turn, would interfere with active ion transport processes. Light and electron microscopic studies demonstrate that salicylate causes structural alterations of the gastric mucosa. Thus, salicylates would be expected to aggravate the symptoms of peptic ulcer, and their use would be contraindicated (13).

Hepatic Toxicity. Reversible liver toxicity, manifested as hepatitis, has been seen in patients susceptible to systemic lupus erythematosus even at therapeutic plasma salicylate concentrations (47). The liver toxicity is very unusual and disappears when the drug is withdrawn.

Hypersensitivity. In view of the large amounts of salicylate used in our society, the incidence of allergic reactions can be considered rare. Reactions to aspirin include angioneurotic edema, urticaria, skin rash, asthma, and hypotension.

Aspirin has a great potential for causing acute airway obstruction in patients with the following triad: asthma (nonallergic), nasal polyps, and sinusitis (46). Other analgesics and tartrazine (FD & C yellow # 5), a dye used in providing a yellow color for foods and medication, may cause airway obstruction in aspirin-sensitive patients. It has been speculated that aspirin may affect prostaglandin synthesis increasing formation of $PGF_2\alpha$ and the levels of cyclic nucleotides, which in turn could affect histamine release from mast cells in lung tissue (59). Aspirin should be used with caution in patients with severe chronic asthma. Weinberger has recently reviewed the problem of analgesic sensitivity in adults and children with asthma (59).

Atropine inhibits the bronchoconstrictor effect of aspirin. There may also be a relationship to slow-reacting substance of anaphylaxis (SRS-A) because $PGF_2\alpha$ and SRS-A are both formed from arachidonic acid. Settipane (52) has recently reviewed the problem of aspirin intolerance.

Pregnancy. Corby (8) has recently reviewed the role of aspirin in pregnancy and concluded that "conclusive evidence of adverse effects in humans is lacking." Based on animal data, however, a potential hazard does exist and "the indiscriminant use of aspirin during pregnancy is contraindicated." Animal studies have shown that the administration of aspirin in high doses results in an increased incidence of congenital anomalies. Administration of aspirin late in pregnancy has been associated with a decrease in birth weight of infants, and an increase in the incidence of stillbirths and neonatal deaths. There is a possibility of an increase in the length of pregnancy and labor as well as an increase in antepartum and postpartum bleeding.

Drug Interactions. Aspirin (salicylate) is associated with a significant number of drug interactions (Table 10.2-1), many of which occur by aspirin's affecting the

Table 10.2-1
Aspirin-Drug Interactions

Mechanism of Interaction	Potential Result
1. *Competing for plasma protein binding sites*	
Aspirin + oral anticoagulants (coumarins)	Increased risk of bleeding by affecting platelet function and decreasing protein binding of anticoagulant
Aspirin + chlorpropamide	Potentiation of hypoglycemic effect
Aspirin + methotrexate	Increased levels of free methotrexate
2. *Effects on excretion*	
Aspirin + probenecid	Decreased uricosuric effect of probenecid by affecting secretory mechanism
Aspirin + methotrexate	Increased blood levels of methotrexate as aspirin competes for active tubular secretion mechanism; may get methotrexate accumulation and toxicity
Aspirin + antacids	Increased rate of aspirin absorption followed by decreased plasma levels due to increased rate of excretion; efficacy could be decreased in arthritic patient
3. *Effects on metabolism*	
Aspirin + corticosteroids	Steroid stimulation of hepatic metabolism of salicylates will decrease salicylate below therapeutic levels

Source: Adopted from Ref. 33.

physiological disposition of other drugs and vice versa. Aspirin competes for plasma protein binding sites and will displace a previously bound drug, resulting in an increased blood level of the displaced drug and possibly an exaggerated pharmacological effect. For example, by displacing oral anticoagulants (coumarins), there may be an increased risk of bleeding. The combination of anticoagulants and aspirin should be used cautiously because, in addition to displacement, aspirin has an effect on platelets that will increase the risk of bleeding. In such patients acetaminophen may be a proper substitute. Aspirin also decreases plasma prothrombin levels. The hypoglycemic effect of chlorpropamide and the anticancer effect of methotrexate may be exaggerated by the same mechanism (plasma protein displacement).

A second mechanism for aspirin interaction is at the level of the kidney. By competing for active renal tubular secretion, aspirin can decrease methotrexate excretion. The effect on renal tubules and plasma proteins can increase methotrexate levels, leading to accumulation and toxicity. Aspirin in low doses will decrease the uricosuric effect of probenecid and of sulfinpyrazone by affecting the secretory mechanism. Salicylate excretion itself will be affected by concomitant ingestion of large amounts of antacids. Antacids will help increase the rate of excretion and hence the efficacy of the drug. The resulting decrease in plasma level may be significant in an arthritic patient.

Administration of aspirin in conjunction with corticosteroids may decrease plasma salicylate levels below therapeutic because steroids have been shown to increase hepatic metabolism of salicylates (15, 22). Salicylate dosage should be adjusted when steroid dosage is reduced, so as to avoid salicylate accumulation and the risk of toxicity.

Ingestion of ethyl alcohol with aspirin may enhance the aspirin-induced fecal blood loss. It would be prudent to eliminate alcohol in patients with a tendency for gastrointestinal bleeding.

In view of the described interactions of aspirin, acetaminophen would be considered a reasonable alternative when analgesic and/or an antipyretic effect is desired. Because acetaminophen does not have antiinflammatory properties, this drug is not an alternative when aspirin is used for its antiinflammatory properties. The therapeutic implications of drug interactions with aspirin and acetaminophen are discussed in a recent article by Hayes (17).

Aspirin Overdosage (48, 49, 53, 54). The most common drug in childhood accidental poisoning is aspirin, as this drug is readily available in the home. Serious intoxication in a child may result if the amount ingested exceeds 150-170 mg/kg. In the adult, the fatal dose of salicylate has been estimated to be 20-30 g. Plasma salicylate levels are essential in diagnosis and management. Serum levels of 70-90 mg/dl would be associated with severe toxicity in the first 6 to 12 hours. A nomogram relating blood levels to toxicity has been published by Done (11, 12). The mild form of salicylate toxicity (salicylism) will present itself as nausea, vomiting, gastrointestinal irritation, dizziness, tinnitus, headache, and mental confusion (19, 36), effects that are usually reversible on withdrawal of the drug.

Done has classified the degree of salicylate intoxication as follows: mild (some hyperpnea and lethargy; vomiting, hyperthermia, hypocapnea without frank acidosis); moderate (severe hyperpnea, marked lethargy and /or excitability, no coma or convulsions, compensated metabolic acidosis in the child); severe (coma, possibly convulsions, uncompensated metabolic acidosis in the child after 12 hours) (11).

Thus, the initial event in salicylate toxicity is stimulation of the respiratory center of the brain, resulting in hyperpnea and tachypnea. Increased carbon dioxide exhalation will result in a decrease in plasma carbon dioxide and a rise in plasma pH, leading to an initial respiratory alkalosis. To compensate for this, there will then be an increase in renal excretion of bicarbonate. The second major event in salicylate toxicity is the uncoupling of oxidative phosphorylation, leading to increase in oxygen utilization, glucose demand, gluconeogenesis,and heat production,resulting in the hyperpyrexia characteristic of salicylate intoxication. Hyperglycemia may be seen early in intoxication as glucose stores are depleted. Coupled with all of these events, there is an alteration in glucose metabolism (indirectly since salicylates inhibit Krebs cycle dehydrogenases), which leads to accumulation of lactic and pyruvic acids (diminished aerobic glycolysis). Furthermore, the metabolism of lipids is increased with the formation of ketone bodies (β-hydroxybutyric acid, acetoacetic acid, and acetone). The effects of salicylate on metabolism result in a decreased plasma pH and metabolic acidosis. There is also water and electrolyte loss leading to dehydration. The loss of sodium and potassium results in poor buffering capacity. Decreased fluid intake and emesis further aggravate the existing dehydration, and water losses may be substantial. In essence, the greater the time from ingestion until treatment, the greater the possibility of the development of acidosis. The prothrombin time is also increased.

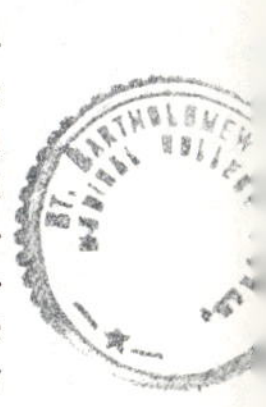

Treatment of Aspirin Overdosage. Treatment of salicylate toxicity should be directed at:

Minimizing absorption of the salicylate. If the patient is seen soon enough and is conscious, administer syrup of ipecac to induce vomiting.

Attempting to reduce the temperature. The use of tepid water, alcohol sponges, and ice packs are indicated.

Initiating procedures to hasten salicylate elimination. Urine alkalinization will enhance salicylate excretion by threefold to fivefold. It is desirable to increase the urine pH above 7.5 by administering tromethamine (THAM) or sodium bicarbonate. Isotonic sodium bicarbonate (7.5 g%) may be administered in lactated Ringers's solution. At this high pH (7.5), virtually all of the salicylate will be in the charged, water-soluble, nonreabsorbable form and therefore readily excreted. In cases of severe acidosis, sodium bicarbonate may not change urine pH significantly.

Other measures. (a) When adequate urine flow has been established, potassium in concentrations of 20-40 mEq/l should be administered, as it is difficult to achieve urine alkalinization in the face of severe potassium depletion. Furthermore, without potassium and bicarbonate, hypernatremia is risked. (b) Be certain enough fluids are given to correct dehydration. (c) Administer parenteral vitamin K to counteract aspirin's effect on prothrombin. (d) Correct any existing hypoglycemia by giving i.v. glucose.

Aspirin overdose and its treatment are also discussed in Chapter 32.

Causes of Morbidity. Salicylate intoxication may produce central nervous system dysfunction, which may be seen as seizures, coma, or cerebral edema. The acidosis produced by high levels of salicylate will favor the transport of salicylate into the brain. There may be impaired cardiac function due to decreased myocardial metabolism, which will lead to decreased cardiac output, congestive heart failure, and possibly cardiac arrhythmias. A late finding in salicylate toxicity is pulmonary edema. The overall effects of salicylate intoxication, at its worst, are tissue hypoxia and brain death.

A statistical association between the use of medicines containing salicylates and an increase in the risk of Reye's syndrome has been reported. Reye's syndrome is a childhood disease that usually follows flu or chickenpox. The syndrome is a rare but life-threatening encephalopathy characterized by vomiting and lethargy that may progress to delirium, coma, and death. It has been estimated that 600-1200 cases occur each year in the United States, and it is fatal in 20-30% of the cases. In view of this association, the FDA requires that aspirin be labeled to indicate that the drug not be used by anyone under 16 years of age with influenza, chickenpox, or influenzalike illnesses unless it is prescribed by a physician (14).

From the foregoing discussion, it is clear that aspirin should also not be used in patients with bleeding disorders (hemophilia), patients deficient in platelets (thrombocytopenia), and patients on anticoagulants.

Aspirin is also used to treat a rare childhood disease (800 cases in the United States since 1976) called Kawasaki disease (mucocutaneous lymph node syndrome). Aspirin is used to lower high fever and to prevent blood platelets from clumping.

Preparations. *Sodium salicylate,* USP: tablets (300, 600 mg). *Aspirin,* USP: tablets (65-650 mg); enteric-coated tablets (ECOTRIN) (300 and 600 mg); capsules (300 mg); suppositories (65-1300 mg). There are a number of buffered aspirin preparations available (BUFFERIN, ASCRIPTIN) and an effervescent preparation (ALKA-SELTZER). For relief of mild pain and fever, the dosages used are 0.3-0.6 g every 3 to 4 hours.

PARA-AMINOPHENOL DERIVATIVES

Acetaminophen (N-acetyl-para-aminophenol) (Fig. 10.2-4) is a widely used analgesic and antipyretic. Although actually developed 80 years ago, it did not become widely used until Brodie and Axelrod in 1949 demonstrated that phenacetin (Fig. 10.2-4) was metabolically converted to acetaminophen, which was later shown to be an effective analgesic and antipyretic (1, 23). In contrast to aspirin, acetaminophen has no antiinflammatory properties. Extensive promotion has made acetaminophen a widely used analgesic and antipyretic both in the United States and Britain. It is marketed in this country under many brand names and is sold in almost 200 proprietary combinations.

Pharmacokinetics. Acetaminophen is a weak acid (pK_a 9.5) due to its aromatic hydroxyl group. It is rapidly and well absorbed from the gastrointestinal tract with peak plasma levels seen in about 70 minutes (range 60-120 minutes) (1, 23); peak plasma levels are attained faster when liquid preparations are used. The compound is widely distributed throughout most body tissues and fluids; with therapeutic doses, serum concentrations range between 5 and 20 mg/l. The drug has a half-life of 1.5-3 hours and volume of distribution of 1-1.2 l/kg. There is little significant plasma protein binding at therapeutic plasma levels, although at toxic levels there is marked increase in the amount of protein bound (1, 23).

In contrast to aspirin, acetaminophen does not follow saturable kinetics. On oral administration, approximately 25% of the dose undergoes first-pass metabolism by the liver (1). Only a small percentage (approximately 1%) of the dose is excreted unchanged; most is conjugated with glucuronide (approximately 63%), sulfate (approximately 34%), cysteine (3%), and mercapturic acid. Andrews et al. (2) identified eight acetaminophen excretion products: unchanged acetaminophen, acetaminophen sulfate, 3-hydroxy-acetaminophen-3-sulfate, 3-methoxy-acetaminophen-sulfate, acetaminophen-glucuronide, 3-methoxy-acetaminophen-glucuronide, acetaminophen-3-cysteine, and acetaminophen-3-mercapturate (2).

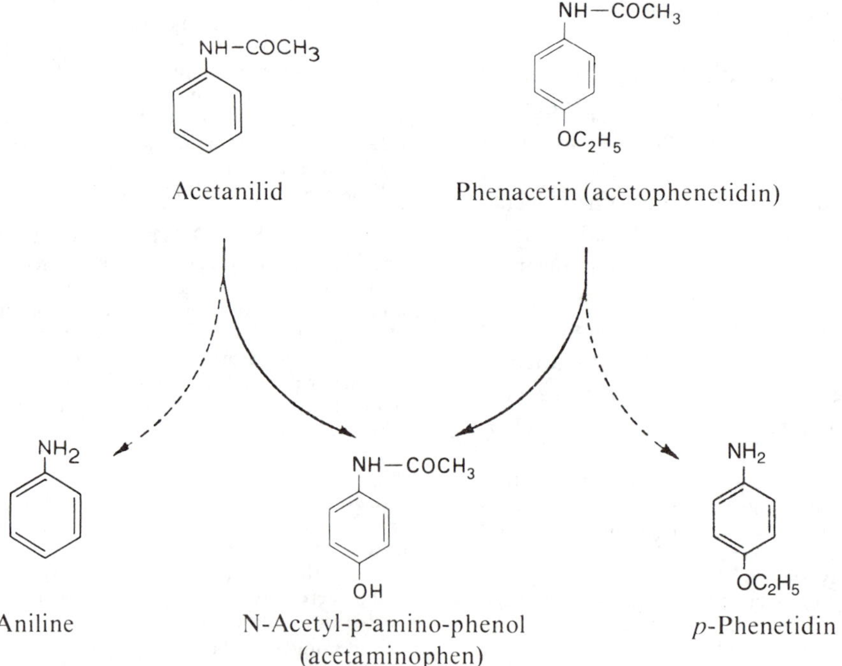

Fig. 10.2-4. *Structural formulas of para-aminophenol compounds.*

Acute Overdosage. Approximately 4% of acetaminophen is inactivated through a hepatic cytochrome P-450 pathway (Fig. 10.2-5). With large doses of acetaminophen (140 mg/kg for the therapeutic range), the conjugating mechanism utilizing hepatic glutathione becomes depleted (1, 23). Thus, metabolism now forms a toxic intermediate that binds covalently to hepatocellular macromolecules and thereby causes hepatic necrosis. The formulation of the arylating metabolite by microsomal enzymes may be increased through enzyme induction by pretreatment with phenobarbital (30, 32). Corocran and coworkers (9, 10) have provided strong circumstantial evidence on the sequence of events in the formation of the reactive intermediate. They postulate the formation of N-hydroxy-acetaminophen that is then rapidly dehydrated to the reactive N-acetyl-p-benzoquinonimine, the ultimate toxic species. Further evidence for the role of glutathione has been demonstrated by Mitchell and coworkers (30, 32), who have shown that when glutathione levels are decreased (pretreatment with diethyl maleate) there is increased formation of the toxic intermediate and thus increased formation of covalently bound metabolite, which in turn leads to centrilobular hepatic necrosis. The plasma half-life is significant in estimating prognosis; a number of studies have demonstrated that if the serum half-life is in excess of 4 hours, one can expect to develop hepatic damage (23, 40). Plasma levels of 300 μg/ml at 4 hours have been associated with hepatic damage, whereas blood levels of less than 120 μg/ml are unlikely to be followed by liver damage (23).

Treatment of severe acetaminophen overdosage includes administration of substances that will slow the formation of toxic metabolite or combine with the metabolite, thus protecting hepatic macromolecules from arylation (37, 39, 43, 44). On admission, if it has been less than 24 hours since the overdose, the stomach should be washed out or ipecac syrup administered (within less than 12 hours). A loading dose of acetylcysteine (MUCOMYST), 140 /kg, should be administered, as a 5% solution in cola, grapefruit juice, or orange juice. Plasma acetaminophen assays should be performed 4 hours after ingestion to assure that peak acetaminophen levels have been achieved. If plasma levels are below 150 μg/ml, then the acetylcysteine can be discontinued. If the plasma levels are above 200 μg/ml at the 4 hours period, then it is recommended that acetylcysteine be administered in doses of 70 mg/kg of body weight every 4 hours for 17 doses.

Three phases have been described for the clinical course of events associated with acetaminophen overdose (42). In the first phase (within hours), there is anorexia, nausea, vomiting and diaphoresis. The patient is pale and feels very sick. In the second phase, these symptoms decrease in intensity but persist for as long as 48 hr. Hepatic bilirubin and prothrombin time are markedly increased, and the liver becomes enlarged and tender. In the third phase (3-5 days later), there is evidence of jaundice, coagulation defects, hypoglycemia, encephalopathy, renal failure and myocardiopathy. Death is due to hepatic failure.

It should be remembered that although acetaminophen has significant toxic effects in large overdosage, in normal therapeutic use it has few adverse reactions. The mortality rates from accidental or suicidal overdosage with acetaminophen probably differ very little from aspirin. Aspirin overdose, however, is probably much easier to treat and manage than is acetaminophen overdosage.

Anticholinergic agents (propantheline), by decreasing gastric emptying time, may decrease the rate of acetaminophen absorption but not the total amount of drug absorbed. This may be significant in the rate of onset of the analgesic effect but is less significant when the drug is used on a long-term basis. Drugs that increase gastric emptying (e.g., metoclopramide) enhance the rate, but not the total amount, of acetaminophen absorbed (17).

Acetaminophen overdose and its treatment are also discussed in Chapter 32.

Preparations. Acetaminophen is available in tablets of 325 and 500 mg, capsules containing 500 mg, elixir containing 120 mg/5 ml (teaspoonful), drops containing 60 mg/0.6 ml, and chewable tablets containing 80 mg in each tablet.

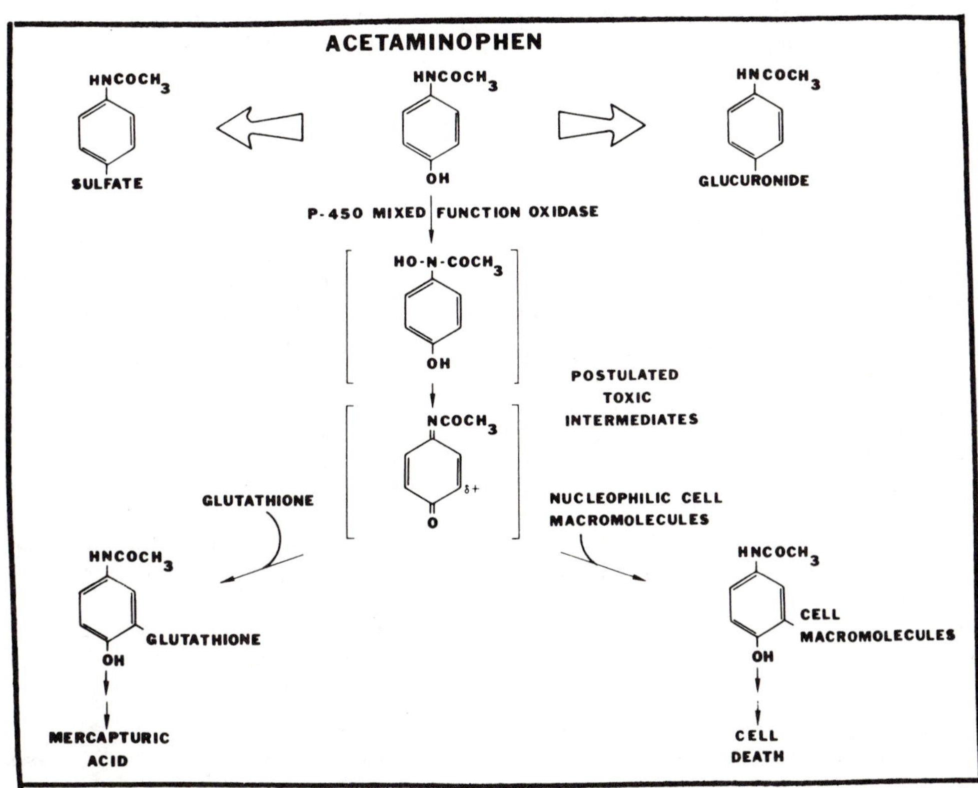

Fig. 10.2-5. *Pathways of acetaminophen metabolism (from Ref. 29).*

THERAPEUTIC USES

Acetaminophen and aspirin have the same general indications for use, that is, analgesic-antipyretic. Acetaminophen does not possess the antiinflammatory properties of aspirin but has become very popular in recent years because it has few of the adverse effects associated with aspirin. Unlike salicylates, with acetaminophen there is no occult bleeding, few drug interactions and little hypersensitivity or stomach upset. When compared with phenacetin (no longer recommended), there is no methemoglobinemia, nephrotoxicity, tolerance, or habituation.

The nonnarcotic analgesics, in view of their proven efficacy and low toxicity, are widely used on a worldwide basis. Their usefulness has been demonstrated in all types of pain (except deep visceral), from the discomforts of the common cold to the pain associated with malignancy. Both aspirin and acetaminophen can be found as part of the formulation of cold remedies, in combination with antihistamines, sedatives, sympathomimetic amines, muscle relaxants, nasal decongestants and narcotic analgesics.

The combination of a nonnarcotic analgesic with codeine is a rational one (7). Codeine acts in the central nervous system on the opiate receptor, where the nonnarcotics exert their main effects at a peripheral level. Thus, the use of such a combination will provide additive effects in the treatment of pain.

Although aspirin is contraindicated in certain clinical conditions (peptic ulcer, gastrointestinal bleeding problems), the nonnarcotic analgesics should be considered the initial agents to be used in treating various painful syndromes. Narcotics should be added when the painful conditions cannot be controlled with either aspirin or acetaminophen.

REFERENCES

1. Ameer, B. and Greenblatt, D.J. Acetaminophen. *Ann. Intern. Med.* 87:202, 1977.
2. Andrews, R.S., Bown, D.C., Brunett, J., Saunders, A. and Watson, K. Isolation and identification of paracetamol metabolites. *J. Int. Med. Res.* 4 (suppl. 4):34, 1976.
3. Avery, G.S. (ed.). *Drug Treatment. Principles and Practice of Clinical Pharmacology and Therapeutics.* New York: Adis Press, 1980.
4. Bosund, I. The effect of salicylic acid, benzoic acid, and some of their derivatives on oxidative phosphorylation. *Acta Chem. Scand.* 11:541, 1957.
5. Brodie, B.B. and Axelrod, J. The fate of acetophenetidin (phenacetin) in man and methods for the estimation of acetophenetidin and its metabolites in biological material. *J. Pharmacol. Exp. Ther.* 97:58, 1949.
6. Clark, W.G. Mechanisms of antipyretic action. *Gen. Pharmacol.* 10:71, 1979.
7. Cooper, S.A. and Beaver, W.T. A model to evaluate mild analgesics in oral surgery outpatients. *Clin. Pharmacol. Ther.* 20:241, 1976.
8. Corby, D.G. Aspirin in pregnancy: Maternal and fetal effects. *Pediatrics* 62 (suppl. 2):930, 1978.
9. Corcoran, G.B., Mitchell, J.R., Vaishnav, Y.N. and Horning, E.C. Sulfhydryl adduct and acetaminophen formation from N-hydroxyacetaminophen: Mechanistic implications. *Pharmacologist* 21:220, 1979.
10. Corcoran, G.B., Mitchell, J.R., Vaishnav, Y.N. and Horning, E.C. Evidence that acetaminophen and N-hydroxyacetaminophen form a common arylating intermediate, N-acetyl-p-benzoquinonimine. *Mol. Pharmacol.* 18:536, 1980.
11. Done, A.K. Aspirin overdosage: Incidence, diagnosis and management. *Pediatrics* 62 (suppl.):890, 1978.
12. Done, A.K. and Temple, A.R. Treatment of salicylate poisoning. *Mod. Treat.* 8:528, 1971.
13. Fromm, D. Salicylate and gastric mucosal damage. *Pediatrics* 62 (suppl.):938, 1978.
14. U.S. Food and Drug Administration. Salicylate labeling may change because of Reye syndrome. In: *FDA Bulletin*, Vol. 12(2), August, 1982.
15. Graham, G.G., Champion, G.D., Day, R.D. and Paull, P.D. Patterns of plasma concentrations and urinary excretion of salicylate in rheumatoid arthritis. *Clin. Pharmacol. Ther.* 22:410, 1977.
16. Gwill, J.R., Robertson, A. and McChesney, E.W. Determination of blood and other tissue concentrations of paracetamol in the dog and man. *J. Pharm. Pharmacol.* 15:440, 1963.
17. Hayes, A.H., Jr. Therapeutic implications of drug interactions with acetaminophen and aspirin. *Arch. Intern. Med.* 141:301, 1981.
18. Hammond, A.L. Aspirin: New perspective on everyman's medicine. *Science* 174:48, 1971.
19. Hill, J.B. Salicylate intoxication. *N. Engl. J. Med.* 228:1110, 1973.
20. Hook, J.C. Mechanism of action: Aspirin. *Thromb. Res.* 4 (suppl.):47, 1983.
21. Kimmel, C.A., Wilson, J.G. and Schumacher, H.J. Studies on metabolism and identification of the causative agent in aspirin teratogenesis in rats. *Teratology* 4:15, 1971.
22. Klineberg, J.R. and Miller, R. Effect of corticosteroids on blood salicylate concentrations. *JAMA* 194:601, 1965.
23. Koch-Weser, J. Acetaminophen. *N. Engl. J. Med.* 295:1297, 1976.
24. Leist, E.R. and Banwell, J.G. Products containing aspirin. *N. Engl. J. Med.* 291:710, 1974.
25. Levy, G. Clinical pharmacokinetics of aspirin. *Pediatrics* 62 (suppl.):867, 1978.
26. Levy, G. Comparative pharmacokinetics of aspirin and acetaminophen. *Arch. Intern. Med.* 141:279, 1981.
27. Levy, G. Pharmacokinetics of salicylate in man. *Drug Metab. Rev.* 9(1):3, 1979.
28. Meyer, O. and Howard, B. Production of hypoprothrombinemia and hypocoagulability of the blood with salicylates. *Proc. Soc. Exp. Biol. Med.* 53:234, 1943.
29. Mitchell, J.R., McMurtry, R.J., Statham, C.N. and Nelson, S.D. Molecular basis for several drug-induced nephropathies. *Am. J. Med.* 62:518, 1977.
30. Mitchell, J.R., Jollow, D.J., Potter, V.Z., Davis, D.C., Gillette, J.R. and Brodie, B.B. Acetaminophen-induced hepatic necrosis. I. Role of drug metabolism. *J. Pharmacol. Exp. Ther.* 187:185, 1973.
31. Mitchell, J.R., Jollow, D.J., Potter, W.Z., Gillette, J.R. and Brodie, B.B. Acetaminophen-induced hepatic necrosis. IV. Protective role of glutathione. *J. Pharmacol. Exp. Ther.* 187:211, 1973.
32. Mitcheli, J.R. and Jollow, D.J. Metabolic activation of drugs to toxic substances. *Prog. Hepatol. Gastroenterol.* 68:392, 1975.
33. Miyahara, J.T. and Karler, R. Effect of salicylate on oxidative phosphorylation and respiration of mitochondrial fragments. *Biochem. J.* 97:194, 1965.

34. Murphy, D.E. (ed.). Symposium on paracetamol and the liver: Overdosage and its management. *J. Int. Med. Res.* 4 (suppl. 4): 1, 1976.
35. O'Brien, J.R. Aspirin haemostasis and thrombosis. *Br. J. Haematol.* 29:523, 1975.
36. Pearson, H.A. Comparative effects of aspirin and acetaminophen on hemostasis. *Pediatrics* 62 (suppl.):926, 1978.
37. Peterson, R.G. and Rumack, B.H. Treating acute acetaminophen poisoning with acetylcysteine. *JAMA* 237:2496, 1977.
38. Pierce, A.W., Jr. Salicylate intoxication. *Postgrad. Med.* 48:243, 1970.
39. Piperno, E. and Bersenbruegge, D.A. Reversal of experimental paracetamol toxicosis with N-acetylcysteine. *Lancet* 2:738, 1976.
40. Prescott, L.F., Wright, N., Roscoe, P. and Brown, S.S. Plasma paracetamol half-life and hepatic necrosis in patients with paracetamol overdosage. *Lancet* 1:519, 1971.
41. Rowland, M., Riegelman, S., Harris, P.A. *et al.* Absorption kinetics of aspirin in man following oral administration of an aqueous solution. *J. Pharm. Sci.* 61:379, 1972.
42. Rumack, B.H. and Matthew, H. Acetaminophen poisoning and toxicity. *Pediatrics* 55(6):871, 1975.
43. Rumack, B.H. and Peterson, R.G. Acetaminophen overdose: Incidence, diagnosis, and management in 416 patients. *Pediatrics* 62 (suppl.):898, 1978.
44. Rumack, B.H., Peterson, R.C., Koch, G.G. and Amara, I.A. Acetaminophen overdose. *Arch. Intern. Med.* 141:380-385, 1981.
45. Salzman, E.W. Cyclic AMP and platelet function. *N. Engl. J. Med.* 286:358, 1972.
46. Samter, M. Intolerance to aspirin. *Hosp. Practice* 8:85, 1973.
47. Seaman, W.E., Ishak, K.G. and Plotz, P.H. Aspirin-induced hepatotoxicity in patients with systemic lupus erythematosus. *Ann. Intern. Med.* 80:1, 1974.
48. Segar, W.E. The critically ill child: Salicylate intoxication. *Pediatrics* 44:440, 1969.
49. Segar, W.E. and Holliday, M.A. Physiologic abnormalities of salicylate intoxication. *N. Engl. J. Med.* 259:1191, 1958.
50. Singer, R. Aspirin: A probable cause for secondary posttonsillectomy hemorrhage. *Arch. Otolaryngol.* 42:19, 1945.
51. Smith, J.B. and Willis A.L. Aspirin selectively inhibits prostaglandin production in human platelets. *Nature* 231:235, 1971.
52. Settipane, G.A. Adverse reactions to aspirin and related drugs. *Arch. Intern. Med.* 141:328, 1981.
53. Temple, A.R. Pathophysiology of aspirin overdosage toxicity with implications for management. *Pediatrics* 62 (suppl.):873, 1978.
54. Temple, A.R. Acute and chronic effects of aspirin toxicity and their treatment. *Arch. Intern. Med.* 141:364, 1981.
55. Vane, J.R. Inhibition of prostaglandin synthesis as a mechanism of action for aspirin-like drugs. *Nature (New Biol.)* 231:232, 1971.
56. Vane, J.R. The mode of action of aspirin and similar compounds. *J. Allergy Clin. Immunol.* 58:691, 1976.
57. Vane, J.R. The mode of action of aspirin and similar compounds. *Hosp. Formulary* 10:618, 1976.
58. Vane, J.R. Inhibitors of prostaglandin, prostacyclin and thromboxane synthesis. In: *Advances in Prostaglandin and Thromboxane Research*, Vol. 4 (Coceani, F. and Olley, P.M., eds.). New York: Raven Press, 1978, p. 27.
59. Weinberger, M. Analgesic sensitivity in children with asthma. *Pediatrics* 62 (suppl.):910, 1978.
60. Zimmerman, M. and Long, D.M. (eds.). Antipyretic analgesic current worldwide therapy status. *Am. J. Med.* 75:1, 1983.

ADDITIONAL READING

Graham, D.Y., and Smith, J.L. Aspirin and the stomach. *Ann. Intern. Med.* 104:390, 1986.

Seeff, L.B., Cuccherini, B.A., Zimmerman, H.J. et al. Acetaminophen hepatotoxicity in alcoholic. *Ann. Intern. Med.* 104:399, 1986.

Wallenburg, H.C.S. et al. Low-dose aspirin prevents pregnancy-induced hypertension and pre-eclampsia in angiotensin-sensitive primigravida. *Lancet* 1:2, 1986.

CHAPTER
10.3

ANTIARTHRITIC DRUGS

Samar N. Dutta

RHEUMATOID ARTHRITIS

Rheumatoid arthritis is a constitutional disease of unknown etiology in which inflammatory changes occur throughout the connective tissues of the body. Its most characteristic symptom is the polyarthritis, particularly involving the small joints of hands and feet. Articular inflammation and joint destruction are the results of complex interaction between inflammatory cells, immunologically competent cells, synovial lining cells, and their soluble products (39). Arthritis is manifested by pain on use, stiffness, and swelling of joints.

DRUGS FOR RHEUMATOID ARTHRITIS

Drug therapy of rheumatoid arthritis is mainly aimed at suppression of the inflammatory process and relief of symptoms to alter the outcome of the pathological process. Drugs for rheumatoid arthritis are listed with dosage form and daily doses in Table 10.3-1; structures of some of these drugs are given in Fig. 10.3-1.

NONSTEROIDAL ANTIINFLAMMATORY DRUGS (NSAIDs)

SALICYLATES

The pharmacology of salicylates has been described in detail in Chapter 10.2. Only their use in rheumatoid arthritis will be discussed here.

Aspirin is the most commonly used salicylate preparation in treatment of rheumatoid arthritis, and unless a specific contraindication exists it should be tried first in all patients. Aspirin possesses analgesic, antipyretic, and antiinflammatory actions. The latter is evident at maximally tolerated doses. Gastrointestinal disturbances (nausea, vomiting, and gastric distress), which occur in about 10-30% of patients receiving high doses of aspirin, can be minimized by taking the drug with food or with antacids. Other salicylate preparations, for example, magnesium salicylate, choline salicylate, choline magnesium trisalicylate, and salsalate (salicylsalicylic acid) have been reported to cause less gastric irritation. Elderly patients manifest less tolerance to aspirin and other salicylates.

The usual daily oral or rectal (suppository) dose of aspirin in adult patients with rheumatoid arthritis is about 2.6-5.2 g. Children with a body weight of less than 50 lbs are treated at a daily dose of 100 mg/kg for juvenile

Table 10.3-1
Drugs Used in Therapy of Rheumatoid Arthritis

Drugs	Dosage Form[a]	Average Daily Dose
Nonsteroidal antiinflammatory		
Aspirin	T, 75, 300, 325, 600, 650 mg	3.6-5.4 g
Magnesium salicylate	T, 300 mg	1.8-4.8 g
Choline salicylate	S, 5 ml equivalent to 600 mg of aspirin	3.6 g
Choline magnesium trisalicylate	T, each provides 500 mg of salicylate	3.0 g
Salsalate	T, 325, 500 mg	3.0 g
Indomethacin (INDOCIN)	C, 25,50 mg	100-200 mg
Ibuprofen (MOTRIN, RUFEN)	T, 300, 400, 600 mg	1.6-2.4 g
Fenoprofen (NALFON)	T, 600 mg, C, 300 mg	2.4 g
Naproxen (NAPROSYN)	T, 250 mg	500-700 mg
Benoxaprofen (ORAFLEX)	T, 600 mg	600 mg
Phenylbutazone	T, 100 mg	300-400 mg
Oxyphenbutazone (AZOLID, BUTAZOLIDIN)	T, 100 mg	300-400 mg
Tolmetin (TOLECTIN)	T, 200 mg	0.6-1.8 g
Sulindac (CLINORIL)	T, 150, 200 mg	300 mg
Mefenamic acid (PONSTEL)	C, 250 mg	0.75-1.0 g
Piroxicam (FELDENE)	C, 10, 20 mg	20 mg
Specific antiarthritic (slow-acting antirheumatic)		
Gold		
Aurothioglucose (SOLGANAL)	Susp, 50 mg/ml in oil	25-50 mg weekly
Gold sodium thiomalate (MYOCHRYSINE)	S, 10, 25, 100 mg/ml	—
Auranofin	T, investigational drug in United States	6 mg
D-Penicillamine (CUPRIMINE, DEPEN)	C, 125, 250 mg, T, 250 mg	125-500 mg
Hydroxychloroquine (PLAQUENIL)	T, 200 mg	200-400 mg
Levamisole	Investigational drug in United States	150 mg weekly
Corticosteroids		
Prednisone	T, 1, 2.5, 5, 10, 20 mg	5-10 mg
Prednisolone	T, 1, 2.5, 5 mg	5-10 mg
Immunosuppressants		
Cyclophosphamide (CYTOXAN)	T, 25, 50 mg	75-100 mg
Azathioprine (IMURAN)	T, 50 mg	100-150 mg

[a] T, tablet; C, capsule; S, solution; Susp, suspension.

rheumatoid arthritis. Effective therapeutic serum concentration of salicylate lies between 15 and 25 mg/100 ml and higher blood levels result in manifestation of toxicity. Concomitant use of salicylate and nonsteroidal antiinflammatory drugs is not recommended because the former reduce the serum levels of nonsteroidal antiinflammatory drugs and thereby interfere with their therapeutic efficacy.

INDOMETHACIN

Chemistry. Indomethacin is 1-(p-chlorobenzoyl)-5-methoxy-2-methylindole-3-acetic acid (Fig. 10.3-1).

Pharmacological Effects. Indomethacin is both antiinflammatory and antipyretic. Its antiinflammatory action has been attributed to its ability to inhibit a step in the biosynthesis of prostaglandins (see Fig. 10.2-2).

Indomethacin has been shown to interact *in vitro* with the adenylate cyclase system and to inhibit phosphodiesterase. The resultant increase in intracellular cyclic adenosine monophosphate (cAMP) stabilizes membranes of polymorphonuclear leukocytes, thus interfering with the release of enzymes involved in the inflammatory response (34). Leukocyte infiltration into the inflammatory sites is also inhibited by indomethacin in rats. Like aspirin, indomethacin also uncouples oxidative phosphorylation. It is a more potent antipyretic than aspirin, aminopyrine, or phenylbutazone in pyrogen-induced fever in rabbits and rats, but it has no significant effect on the normal body temperature.

Pharmacokinetics. Indomethacin is well absorbed after oral administration and when given rectally as a supposi-

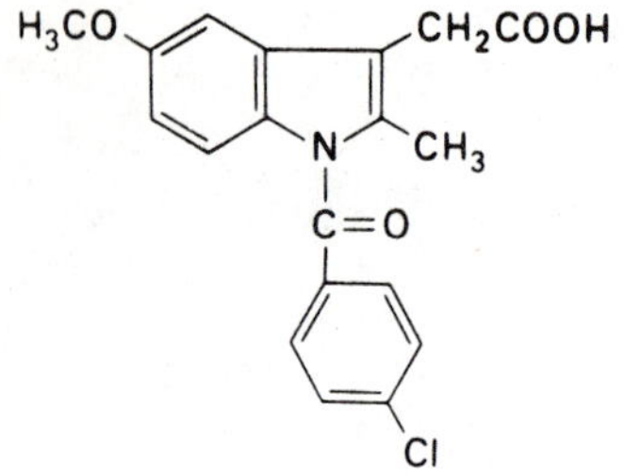

Indomethacin 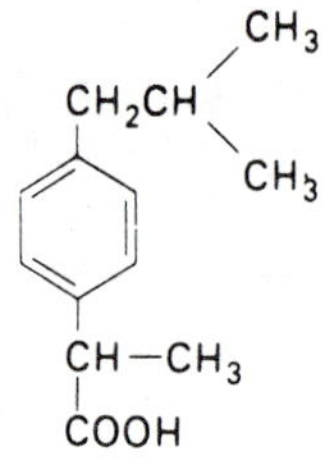 | Ibuprofen 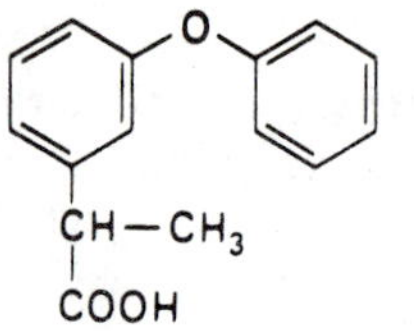 | Fenoprofen 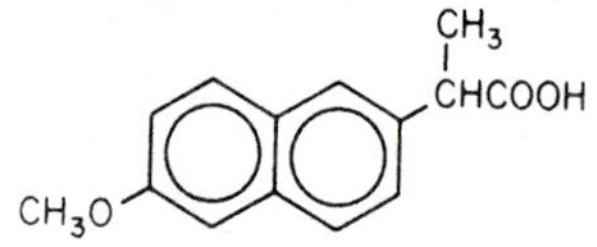 | Naproxen

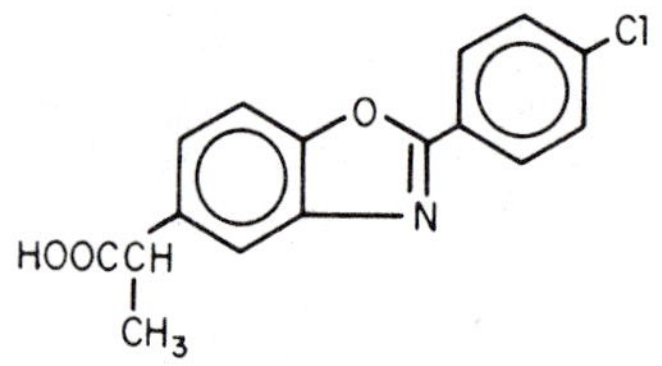

Benoxaprofen 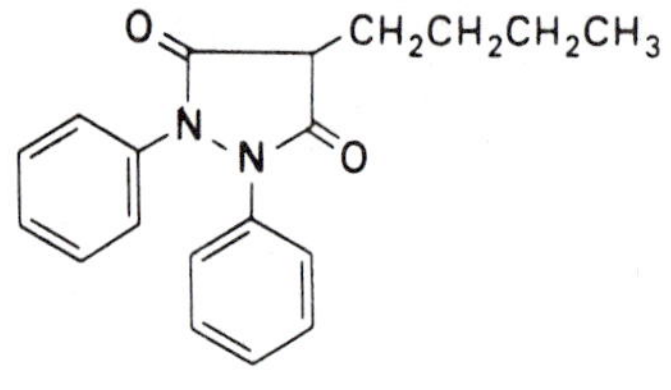 | Phenylbutazone 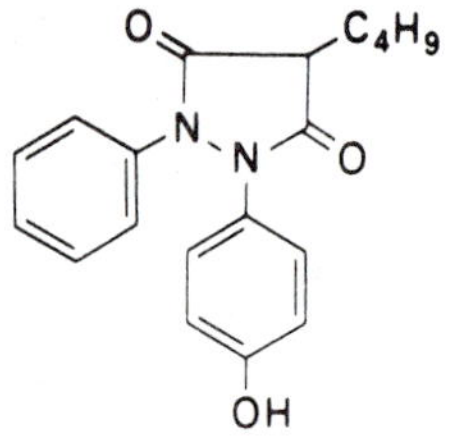 | Oxyphenbutazone 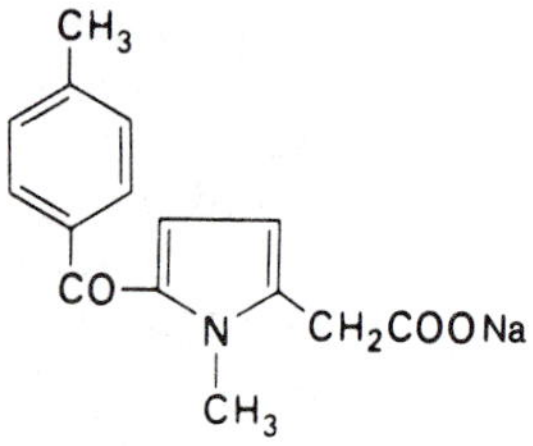 | Tolmetin sodium

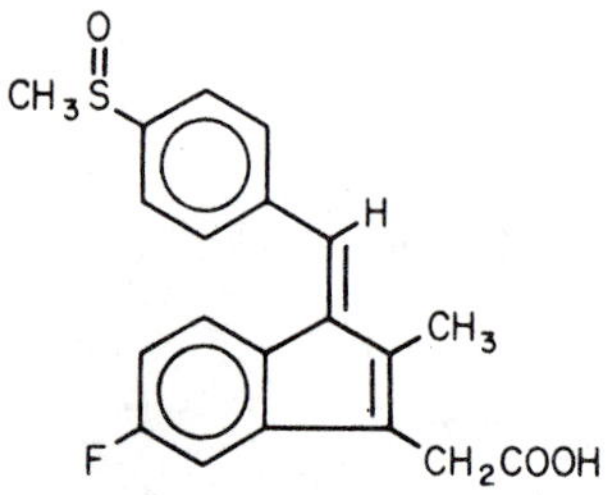

Sulindac 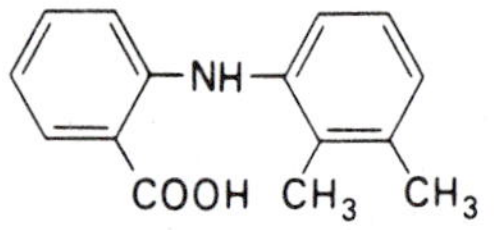 | Mefenamic acid 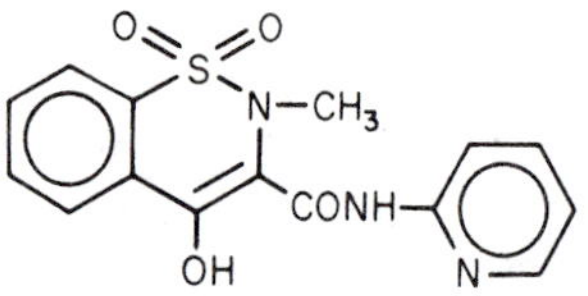 | Piroxicam 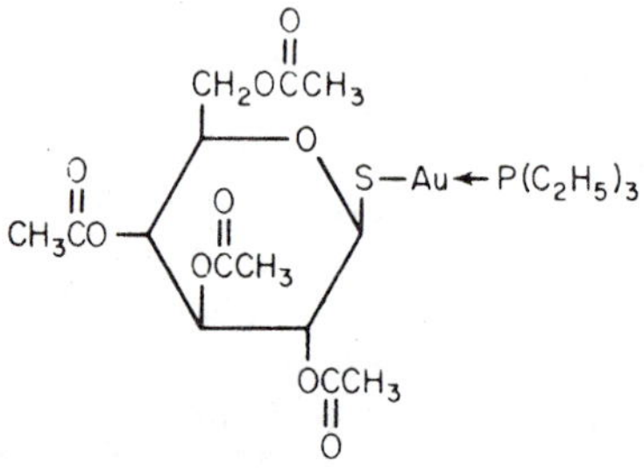 | Auranofin

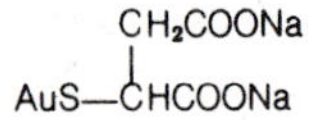

Gold sodium thiomalate 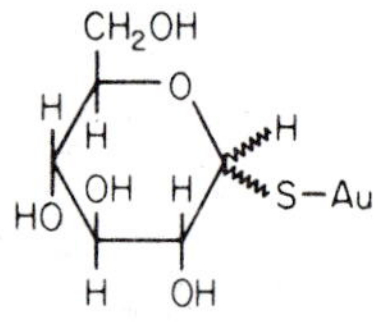 | Aurothioglucose 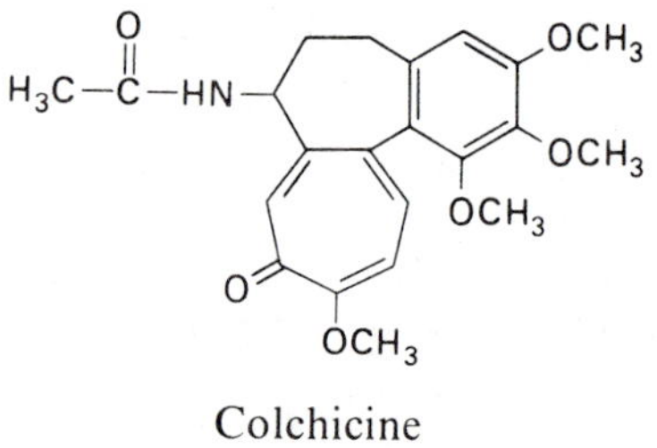 | Colchicine 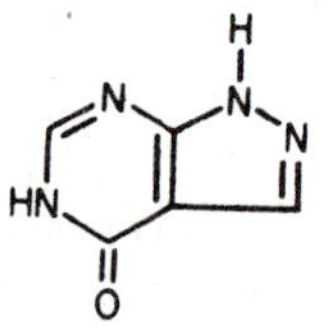 | Allopurinol

Fig. 10.3-1. *Chemical structures of drugs in the therapy of rheumato*

tory. Plasma half-life has been reported to be highly variable (4 to 11 hours), possibly as a result of enterohepatic recycling (18, 24). It is believed to undergo extensive O-methylation and N-deacylation in humans. Generally, peak synovial fluid concentration results about an hour later than the peak serum level, and after about 4 to 5 hours the levels are almost equal. Biliary excretion of indomethacin has been demonstrated in several species of animals.

Side Effects. Gastrointestinal complications in the form of dyspepsia, nausea, and diarrhea are commonly observed within the first few weeks of treatment. Headache is also a common side effect of indomethacin, and it may be associated with dizziness, depression, and malaise. Some cases of gastrointestinal bleeding and toxic hepatitis associated with indomethacin treatment have been reported (17, 21). Other side effects include tinnitus, bone marrow depression, pruritus, rash, edema, hypertension, and various bleeding episodes. In elderly patients with diminished glomerular filtration rate, even azotemia may develop. Indomethacin has also been shown to cause transient rise in blood urea nitrogen and creatinine.

Many of these side effects are possibly due to inhibition of prostaglandin synthetase.

Drug Interaction (2, 10, 12). Aspirin decreases intestinal absorption of indomethacin; furosemide decreases plasma concentration of indomethacin. Probenecid decreases renal excretion of unchanged indomethacin and thus increases its plasma level. Indomethacin inhibits renin-aldosterone response to furosemide, thereby decreasing natriuretic and antihypertensive effect of furosemide. Severe hypertension was observed after ingestion of an appetite suppressant, phenylpropanolamine, with indomethacin (19).

Therapeutic Uses. Indomethacin is effective in active stages of moderate-to-severe rheumatoid arthritis, severe ankylosing spondylitis, severe osteoarthritis, and acute gouty arthritis. In rheumatoid arthritis, some of the common gastrointestinal and central nervous systems (CNS) side effects of indomethacin can be avoided by gradually increasing the dose. It has been found to be effective in relieving night pain and morning stiffness. As such, it is recommended for administration at night. In ankylosing spondylitis, indomethacin is considered as the drug of choice by many. There appears to be no difference in therapeutic efficacy between indomethacin and other newer nonsteroidal agents. Patients with osteoarthritis of the hip are reported to have benefited by relief of pain, stiffness, and increased range of abduction of the hip as a result of treatment.

Indomethacin is widely used in the management of acute gout. The initial daily dose varies from 200 to 500 mg on the first day, followed by reduction of the dose to 100-150 mg/day. If there is no response within 2 weeks, the therapeutic trial of indomethacin should be terminated.

Contraindications. Indomethacin is contraindicated in children, in pregnant or lactating women, in patients who are hypersensitive to aspirin, and in patients with a history of hypersensitivity to chemically related drugs.

IBUPROFEN

Chemistry. Ibuprofen, 2-(4-isobutylphenyl) propionic acid (Fig. 10.3-1), was introduced in therapy in 1969.

Pharmacological Effects. Ibuprofen is about 16-32 times more potent an antiinflammatory agent than aspirin against ultraviolet light-induced erythema in guinea pigs, and 3-4 times more potent than aspirin against adjuvant-induced arthritis (a chronic polyarthritic condition) in rats. In the animal model, its analgesic activity has been shown to be about 8-16 times greater than aspirin, and it exhibits mainly a peripheral action (1). Both in adjuvant-induced arthritis in rats and in clinical trials, it has been reported to potentiate the action of corticosteroids.

The mechanism of action of ibuprofen is believed to be the suppression of prostaglandin biosynthesis. Prostaglandins tend to sensitize tissues to mediators of inflammation. Several other mechanisms have also been proposed such as stabilization of cell membrane permeability and inhibition of leukocyte adherence and chemotaxis.

Pharmacokinetics. Ibuprofen is well absorbed after oral administration, and peak plasma level is reached within 1 to 2 hours after administration. Its absorption is somewhat slower, and peak plasma levels are less when administered postprandial. Its half-life is about 2 hours. The drug is avidly (99%) bound to serum albumin, but at peak serum concentrations less than 20% of its albumin-binding capacity is utilized. Ibuprofen can be displaced by other chemically related drugs *in vitro,* but the clinical significance of such interaction is not clearly established. The drug is extensively metabolized in the liver; within 24 hours after an oral dose, ibuprofen and its metabolites are excreted in the urine almost totally. Two of its principal inactive metabolites are 2-4-(2-hydroxy-2-methyl-propyl) phenylpropionic acid and 2-4-(2-carboxypropyl) phenylpropionic acid.

Side Effects. Side effects of ibuprofen include gastrointestinal symptoms (nausea, dyspepsia and, rarely bleeding). It has also been reported to exacerbate bronchospasm like aspirin, presumably through suppression of prostaglandin biosynthesis. Reversible toxic amblyopia, inhibition of platelet aggregation, rise in blood urea nitrogen (BUN) and serum creatinine, and meningeal syndrome in patients with systemic lupus erythematosus have been reported to occur infrequently when treated with ibuprofen.

Drug Interactions. Ibuprofen may interact with anticoagulants and oral hypoglycemic agents, which are also protein bound in circulation. A steroid-sparing effect of ibuprofen has been reported, and as such it complements corticosteroid therapy.

Therapeutic Uses. Ibuprofen is most useful in rheumatoid and osteoarthritis. For greater antiinflammatory actions, a higher dose of the drug (> 1200 mg/day) is required. At a lower dose, its actions are mostly analgesic. Some studies have reported its use in gout at a very high dose. In osteoarthritis of the spine, at a dose of 900 mg daily it has been shown to be equally effective as indomethacin (75 mg daily) or phenylbutazone (300 mg daily), with fewer side effects. Recent studies have shown its usefulness in the management of dysmenorrhea.

FENOPROFEN

Chemistry. Chemically, fenoprofen [DL-2(3-phenoxyphenyl) propionic acid] is related to indomethacin and tolmetin (Fig. 10.3-1). Its calcium salt is a racemic mixture.

Pharmacological Effects. The antiinflammatory, analgesic, and antipyretic actions of fenoprofen have been shown in various animal models. Its mechanism interferes with formation or release of PGE_1 and PGE_2 from various tissue components and thereby reduces the concentration of one of the mediators of inflammation at the affected site(s). It also inhibits the formation of prostacyclins and thromboxanes.

Pharmacokinetics. Fenoprofen is rapidly and well absorbed from the gastrointestinal tract. The pK_a (4.5) of fenoprofen calcium favors its gastric absorption. Concurrent administration of aspirin may interfere with its gastric absorption. Peak plasma level (20-30 μg/ml) is reached in about 60-120 min following a single dose. The average half-life is about 2 to 3 hours. More than 95% of fenoprofen is bound to plasma albumin. Its metabolic product, fenoprofen glucuronide, is readily excreted in urine. If fenoprofen is given to a patient with impaired renal function, care should be exercised and the patient's renal function frequently checked.

Side Effects. Compared with aspirin, fenoprofen is relatively well tolerated (less occult gastrointestinal bleeding). Gastric irritation is the common side effect.

Therapeutic Uses. Fenoprofen is useful in the treatment of patients with rheumatoid arthritis and osteoarthritis. The recommended dose is 2.4 g/day. Some investigations have shown that it has no advantage over high doses of aspirin in rheumatoid arthritis (12). In acute gouty arthritis, it has also been shown to be useful.

NAPROXEN

Chemistry. Naproxen is an aromatic acid derivative of propionic acid (Fig. 10.3-1). The sodium salt has high dissolution characteristic.

Pharmacological Effects. Like other drugs of this group, naproxen's antiinflammatory action is believed to be due to inhibition of prostaglandin biosynthesis, although some minor mechanism(s) may also be involved in this respect (35). On a number of animal models, naproxen has been shown to possess marked antiinflammatory, analgesic, and antipyretic activity.

Pharmacokinetics. Naproxen is well absorbed after oral administration as well as in suppository dosage form. Peak plasma concentration is usually achieved within 1 to 2 hours after its oral administration. It is highly (99%) bound to plasma protein. Its absorption from upper gastrointestinal tract is interfered with by food and alkali such as magnesium oxide and aluminum hydroxide. Naproxen's half-life is about 13 hours. About 95% of a given dose of naproxen is excreted in the urine, mostly conjugated with glucuronic acid. About 25% of the drug is oxidized to 6-desmethyl-naproxen and excreted in the urine as such or as the conjugated product. It is contraindicated in pregnant women and women who are breast-feeding, because it crosses the placental barrier and it is secreted in breast milk.

Adverse Effects. Gastrointestinal irritation is the common side effect of naproxen. However, such irritation is less than that caused by aspirin. Other reported side effects include gastrointestinal bleeding, headache, lightheadedness, stomatitis, nausea, skin rash, and neonatal jaundice (competitive albumin binding resulting in increased free bilirubin).

Drug Interaction. Plasma level of naproxen can be elevated by simultaneous administration of probenecid; such elevation results from greater affinity of probenecid for glucuronyl transferase. Potential interactions between naproxen and protein-bound drugs (e.g., aspirin, warfarin, tolbutamide) may occur, but thus far they are not considered clinically significant.

Therapeutic Uses. Naproxen has been shown to be effective in rheumatoid arthritis, osteoarthritis of hip and knee, ankylosing spondylitis, and acute gout. It is also useful in a variety of painful conditions associated with inflammation. In the majority of controlled clinical trials, it has been reported to be well tolerated and as effective as aspirin (28). The average daily dose of naproxen is about 500 mg, and because of its relatively long half-life, it may be given twice daily.

BENOXAPROFEN

Chemistry. Benoxaprofen chemically is 2-(4-chlorophenyl)-α-methyl-5-benzoxazole acetic acid. It is a nonsteroidal, antiinflammatory drug derived from propionic acid.

Pharmacological Effects. Pharmacological effects of the drug are similar to those of naproxen and ibuprofen, but it is a relatively weak inhibitor of prostaglandin synthesis (7). The exact mode of its antiinflammatory action is not yet clear.

Pharmacokinetics. Benoxaprofen (Fig. 10.3-1) is readily absorbed after oral administration, and has long half-life of 29 to 35 hours. In elderly patients a much longer half-life has been reported after a daily dose of 600 mg (16).

Side Effects. About 65% of patients were reported to develop side effects of benoxaprofen (15). Patients with rheumatoid arthritis seem to develop side effects more frequently than patients with osteoarthritis. The most frequent side effects of benoxaprofen are skin rash, photosensitivity, and onycholysis. Elderly patients may be more susceptible to major gastrointestinal bleeding (29). Fetal cholestatic jaundice has been reported in several elderly patients receiving this drug.

The drug has been recently withdrawn from the market in the United States because of increased incidence of hepatotoxicity.

PHENYLBUTAZONE AND OXYPHENBUTAZONE

Phenylbutazone and its analog oxyphenbutazone (Fig. 10.3-1) have antiinflammatory, analgesic, and antipyretic effects. They are usually more effective in acute gouty arthritis and ankylosing spondylitis than in rheumatoid arthritis. They have serious adverse effects, however, and are used only for brief periods. The most serious adverse effect is bone marrow depression. Rashes, water retention, and edema, and gastrointestinal disorders (ranging from mild irritation to ulceration) are commonly observed. Jaundice, hepatitis, purpura, and hematuria also occur. They may prolong the prothrombin time in patients receiving coumarin anticoagulants. These drugs are contraindicated in children 14 years of age or under and in elderly patients.

TOLMETIN

Chemistry. Tolmetin is a pyrrole acetic acid derivative that has a structural resemblance to indomethacin (Fig. 10.3-1).

Pharmacological Effects. Tolmetin's antiinflammatory, antipyretic, and analgesic activities have been demonstrated in experimental animal models (37, 38). Inhibition of prostaglandin biosynthesis has been mentioned as the possible mechanisms for its antiinflammatory action. Tolmetin has been shown to possess a mild antiplatelet effect like that of aspirin and tends to prolong bleeding time.

Phamacokinetics. Tolmetin is almost entirely absorbed after oral administration, and the peak serum level is achieved within 40 min after administration. It has a half-life of 60 min and is 99% bound to plasma albumin. It is almost totally excreted in the urine within 24 hours, as an inactive dicarboxylic acid derivative that constitutes 70% of the recovered dose, and the rest is either unchanged or conjugated.

Therapeutic Uses. In view of its potent antiinflammatory and desirable analgesic activity, tolmetin is used in the treatment of rheumatoid arthritis, osteoarthritis, ankylosing spondylitis, and nonarticular rheumatism. It has a prompt onset of therapeutic action, and generally 600-1800 mg/day is given in three equally divided doses. No clinically significant drug interactions have been reported with tolmetin.

Side Effects. Epigastric pain, nausea, and vomiting are usual side effects. Peptic ulcer has been reported to occur in patients with a history of such disease. Headache, dizziness, skin rash, edema (with retention of sodium), and hypertension have been observed occasionally.

SULINDAC

Chemistry. Sulindac is an indene analog of indomethacin (Fig. 10.3-1). The fluoro substitute at C-5 seems to influence its analgesic activity. The drug's biological activity is largely attributable to its sulfide metabolite.

Pharmacological Effects. The pharmacological profile of sulindac is similar to that of indomethacin, and in several species of animal models it has been shown to have analgesic, antiinflammatory, and antipyretic properties. The only sulfide derivative has demonstrated inhibition of prostaglandin biosynthesis.

Pharmacokinetics: Sulindac is rapidly absorbed (about 88%) from the stomach and upper intestine. The peak plasma levels of sulindac and its sulfide, after a single oral dose, are reached at 1 and 2 hours postmedication, respectively. The average half-life of sulindac and its sulfide has been reported to be 8 and 16 hours, respectively. Two principal metabolites of sulindac are formed in the liver, with the possibility of its additional bacterial reduction in the large bowel to a very small extent. It is oxidized to the sulfone and then reversibly reduced to the sulfide. Sulindac and its two metabolites undergo enterohepatic circulation. Sulfone derivatives and its conjugates are eliminated mainly through urine. The sulfide is eliminated from plasma after reoxidation to sulindac and through fecal excretion of the nonabsorbed portion.

Therapeutic Uses. In rheumatoid arthritis and osteoarthritis, sulindac is as effective as indomethacin and aspirin. The average daily dose is about 300 mg. It is also used in gout. In ankylosing spondylitis, sulindac is less effective than indomethacin and phenylbutazone (17).

Side Effects. About 25% of patients on the drug develop gastrointestinal complaints, of which constipation is the most common. Its CNS-related side effects are much less compared with those of indomethacin. There are reports of an aseptic meningitis syndrome developing in patients with connective tissue diseases after the administration of sulindac (13).

MEFENAMIC ACID

Chemistry and Pharmacological Effects. Mefenamic acid is an anthranilic acid derivative (Fig. 10.3-1). Its analgesic, antiinflammatory, and antipyretic properties have been shown in animal studies. In addition to its inhibitory effects on prostaglandin biosynthesis, mefenamic acid possibly also blocks peripheral action of prostaglandin on receptors (30).

Pharmacokinetics. Mefenamic acid is well absorbed following oral administration, and peak plasma level of the drug is achieved in about 2 hours. The half-life of the drug is about 4 to 6 hours. The drug is metabolized in the liver, and most of it is excreted in the urine as a conjugated metabolite. Roughly 20% of mefenamic acid is excreted in the feces.

Side Effects. The most common side effect of mefenamic acid is diarrhea. However, occult gastrointestinal bleeding, indigestion, nausea, vomiting, abdominal pain, vertigo, dizziness, skin rash, hemolytic anemia, bone marrow hypoplasia, and agranulocytosis have been reported to a lesser degree. The drug may potentiate the anticoagulant effect of warfarin, and in asthmatics it may exacerbate the condition. The drug is contraindicated in patients with peptic ulcer or impaired renal function.

Therapeutic Uses. Mefenamic acid is used in rheumatoid arthritis. The drug is given initially at a dose of 500 mg, and then the dose is reduced by 250 mg every 6 to 8 hours; therapy should not last more than 1 week.

PIROXICAM

Piroxicam belongs to the oxicam (enolic acid derivatives) family of nonsteroidal antiinflammatory drugs (NSAIDs) and is chemically different from the majority of the latter group of drugs, which fall into the category of carboxylic acids (Fig. 10.3-1).

Pharmacological Effects. Piroxicam is a very potent NSAID tested in various animal models of pain and inflammation (36). The drug has also been shown to exert antiinflammatory, antiedema, and inhibitory activity in animal (dog) models of human gout. It inhibits chemotaxis, platelet aggregation, and prostaglandin biosynthesis, all of which are involved in the various steps of inflammation cascade. The drug does not interfere with the spasmogenic action of histamine, acetylcholine, serotonin, and prostaglandins. Like other NSAIDs, piroxicam also delays expulsion of the full-term fetus in pregnant rats, and this is attributed to drug-induced reduced availability of prostanoids. In various species of animals, the LD_{50} (oral) of piroxicam ranges between 270 and 700 mg/kg. Long-term administration of the drug has been reported to cause gastrointestinal lesions and renal papillary necrosis in rats, mice, and dogs. The drug has not been shown to be teratogenic or carcinogenic (36)

Pharmacokinetics. Piroxicam is rapidly absorbed following oral administration, and its peak plasma concentration is achieved within 1 hour after administration. The drug reaches the synovial fluid promptly. It has a long half-life of about 45 hours in humans. Hydroxylation is the principal pathway for its metabolism in humans. The hydroxylated metabolite is either excreted as such or further undergoes glucuronic acid conjugation. About 2-5% of a single dose is excreted unchanged in the urine. The metabolites of piroxicam lack any inhibitory activity on prostaglandin biosynthetase. Several other metabolites of the drug have been identified in laboratory animals, but their importance in humans has not been determined. The plasma concentration of piroxicam at a dose of 20 mg/day reaches a plateau in about 5-7 days. The drug is bound to plasma proteins to the extent of 99% or more, and such binding is not affected by concurrent administration of aspirin or anticoagulants.

Side Effects. Gastrointestinal side effects in the form of epigastric and abdominal discomfort, constipation, flatulence, diarrhea, and nausea are the most common problems observed in about 19% of patients. Other infrequent side effects of the drug include headache, dizziness, skin rash, pruritus, tinnitus, palpitation, erythema, and edema. Side effects are slightly more common in older patients over 70 years of age.

Therapeutic Uses. Piroxicam is indicated for acute and long-term use in the relief of signs and symptoms of rheumatoid and osteoarthritis. The recommended single daily dose of piroxicam for these conditions is 20 mg. The drug has also been reported to be effective in ankylosing spondylitis and acute gout. The drug has been reported to be slightly more effective in gout at a dose of 40 mg/day than at a dose of 20 mg/day. Preliminary studies have reported that piroxicam-induced analgesia is comparable with aspirin in postpartum pain, postfracture pain, episiotomy pain, postoperative pain, and dental pain (25).

The drug is available as 10- and 20-mg capsules.

SLOW-ACTING ANTIRHEUMATIC AGENTS

GOLD

Chemistry and Pharmacology. At present, only water-soluble compounds of gold are used; colloidal gold preparations are no longer employed. The two most common preparations, gold sodium thiomalate and aurothioglucose (Fig.-10.3-1), both contain approximately 50% of gold by weight. The mechanism of action of gold in rheumatoid arthritis has not been clearly defined. Several potential mechanisms have been advanced, such as inhibition of lysozomal enzyme system, lysozomal membrane stabilization, inhibition of phagocytic activity of macrophages and polymorphonuclear leukocytes in the synovial fluid, inhibition of capillary permeability, and stabilization of collagen tissue (27).

Pharmacokinetics. Following intramuscular injection of either gold salts, the peak plasma level is reached within a few hours; the half-life of gold is about 5 to 6 hours. The drug is widely distributed throughout the body and concentrated mainly in the reticuloendothelial system (liver and spleen), renal tubules, and synovial fluid. It binds principally to plasma albumin and fibrinogen. About 30% of an administered dose is excreted in urine and 10% in feces over a 7-day period. There is no correlation between serum concentration of gold and either its therapeutic effects or its toxicity.

Side Effects. Side effects are usually not seen at doses less than 300-500 mg of gold salts. Approximately 30% of patients treated with gold salts manifest adverse reactions (10). The most common toxic manifestations are dermatitis (preceded by pruritus and eosinophilia) and stomatitis preceded by metallic taste. Nephrotoxicity manifested by proteinuria and/or microscopic hematuria has been reported to occur in 3-17% of patients. In rare instances these manifestations progress to the nephrotic syndrome or acute tubular necrosis. The most severe toxic effects of gold salts include thrombocytopenia, agranulocytosis, leukopenia, and aplastic anemia. Anaphylactoid or "nitritoid reactions" characterized by flushing, sweating, dizziness, and syncope may occur with myochrysine but can be avoided by using an oil-based preparation (SOLGANAL).

Because of high risk of toxicity, each patient receiving gold salts should be carefully evaluated initially by clinical history, urinalysis, and blood tests prior to each injection of gold. If no evidence of toxicity appears within 3-4 months, laboratory tests may be done at intervals of 2-4 weeks and subsequently at intervals of 6-8 weeks. Therapy should be discontinued at the earliest appearance of adverse reactions.

Gold salts are contraindicated in severely undernourished patients, in pregnancy, in presence of systemic lupus erythematosus, and in patients with history of gold hypersensitivity, active hepatitis, serious renal disease, or blood dyscrasia.

Therapeutic Uses. Gold therapy is considered in adult and juvenile patients with active rheumatoid arthritis who have failed to respond to a conservative regimen of salicylate, rest, and physical therapy. Some patients with psoriatic arthritis have also been reported to be benefited by gold therapy. The initial dose of either preparation for adults is 10-25 mg/week to test idiosyncrasy to the drug. Thereafter, it is 25-30 mg each week in the second and third weeks followed by 50 mg weekly until a total dose of 800-1000 mg has been administered. Therapy is discontinued if no therapeutic response occurs after about 1 g has been given. A good responder may be maintained at a weekly dose of 25 mg. In juvenile rheumatoid arthritis, the usual weekly dose is 1 mg/kg (not to exceed 25 mg except for large-bodied adolescents) for 20 weeks or longer if the patient continues to show therapeutic progress without toxicity.

AURANOFIN

Auranofin is a synthetic gold compound with a molecular weight of 678.5 (Fig. 10.3-1). It is lipid-soluble and is about 29% gold by weight. The precise mechanism of action by which auranofin exerts its effect in patients with rheumatoid arthritis has not been clearly established. It inhibits antibody production in adjuvant arthritis in rats (32). Other suggested mechanisms include inhibition of tissue-damaging events, such as lysozomal enzyme release, biological action of prostaglandin E, oxygen radical production, and antibody-dependent cell-mediated cytotoxicity (33). Unlike parenteral gold, auranofin is orally active, and in patients with rheumatoid arthritis about 25% of an oral dose may be absorbed (3). It significantly binds to erythrocytes (40-60%), and exhibits a long half-life of 16-25 days, depending on the duration of treatment (4). The drug is mostly excreted in feces. Currently available evidence indicates that auranofin at a dose of 3 mg twice a day is equally effective as gold sodium thiomalate in rheumatoid arthritis (5). When auranofin is added to baseline antiinflammatory medication, patients with rheumatoid arthritis may experience greater clinical and laboratory improvement. Diarrhea is the most frequent side effect of the drug. Mild and episodic skin rash may also occur with equal frequency.

PENICILLAMINE

Chemistry and Pharmacology. Penicillamine is D-β, β-dimethylcysteine prepared by hydrolysis of penicillins. It is a chelating agent particularly useful in removing excess of copper in patients with Wilson's disease (see Chapter 28.1 and Fig. 28.1-2). The mechanism of action of penicillamine in rheumatoid arthritis is not clear. The drug has been shown to improve grip strength, relief of pain, erythrocyte sedimentation rate, and hemoglobin levels (9). It is rapidly absorbed following oral administration and excreted mainly through the kidney.

Adverse Effects and Contraindications. The most common side effects are pruritus, skin rash, and alterations in taste. The skin rash may resemble pemphigus and disappears after withdrawal of the drug. Serious side effects include hematological reactions (thrombocytopenia, leukopenia, agranulocytosis, and aplastic anemia) and nephrotoxicity (proteinuria and hematuria). Therapy is discontinued if toxicity appears. The drug is contraindicated in patients allergic to penicillins. A number of autoimmune syndromes such as myasthenia gravis, Goodpasture's syndrome, stenosing alveolitis, polymyositis, and lupus have been reported to be associated with penicillamine therapy.

Therapeutic Uses. The use of penicillamine in rheumatoid arthritis is considered investigational, and it should be reserved for patients who have progressive disease not responding to the conventional therapeutic regimen. Routine urinalysis and blood tests should be performed at intervals of 2 weeks during the first 6 months of treatment and thereafter once a month. Marked decrease in serum albumin level and/or appearance of nephrotoxicity necessitates immediate withdrawal of penicillamine therapy. An individualized dosage schedule should be established based on clinical response and side effects. The initial dose is 125-250 mg every day for 4-8 weeks; the dose may then be increased by an increment of 125 mg daily at 2- to 3-month intervals. If no therapeutic response occurs at a daily dose of 750 mg for 2-3 months, further increase in dose may increase the incidence of adverse effects. A patient with good therapeutic response may be maintained at an average daily dose of 500-750 mg daily. Gold and penicillamine are not used concurrently because adequate data on possible adverse interactions are lacking at present. Other drugs (except gold, chloroquine, cytotoxics, and phenylbutazone) may be used along with penicillamine, but their doses should be tapered when the latter induces good therapeutic response. During therapy, a complete blood count with a direct platelet count and urinalysis should be performed at 2-week intervals for the first 6 months and thereafter monthly.

CHLOROQUINE AND HYDROXYCHLOROQUINE

The 4-aminoquinoline compounds have been used in the treatment of rheumatoid arthritis. Hydroxychloroquine is an approved drug for this indication, but chloroquine is no longer approved. Details of chemistry and pharmacology of 4-aminoquinolines are discussed in Chapter 26.3.

Hydroxychloroquine has a moderate antiinflammatory effect in rheumatoid arthritis attributable to its actions such as stabilization of lysozomal membranes, inhibition of lymphocyte response, and leukocytic chemotaxis. It is rapidly and almost completely absorbed from the gastrointestinal tract and widely distributed throughout the body, with maximum concentration being in eyes, liver, and spleen. Every melanized tissue of the body contains still more concentrated drug. Melanized tissues retain nearly therapeutic drug concentrations long after 99% excretion of the drug from the rest of the body. Higher amount of the drug in the melanin in the retinal pigmented epithelium may cause ocular toxicity (20). About 50% of the drug is found protein bound in plasma. About 30-50% of hydroxychloroquine is biotransformed in the liver, chiefly by disethylation (21). About 60% of a dose of the drug is excreted in the urine; and the rest through feces, skin, and by other metabolic degradation processes. The half-life of hydoxychloroquine is about 50 hours. Acidification of urine enhances drug excretion and alkalinization decreases it.

Adverse Effects. Common side effects of hydroxychloroquine include accommodation delay, tanning allergic skin rash, nausea and diarrhea, and abdominal cramps. The most serious complication is generally irreversible retinopathy at higher daily doses. The drug may be deposited in the cornea (usually reversible if the medication is stopped without delay), resulting in blurring of vision.

Contraindications. The drug is contraindicated in patients with lysosomal storage disease such as Gaucher's, acute intermittent porphyria, neuromyopathy, or significant renal or hepatic dysfunction. The use of the drug in psoriatic arthritis is controversial. The drug is also contraindicated in children and pregnant women.

Therapeutic Uses. Hydroxychloroquine is indicated in rheumatoid arthritis as a second-line treatment in patients who fail to respond to nonsteroidal antiarthritic drugs and for all cases of progressive disease. The drug may be tried prior to initiation of gold or penicillamine therapy, or in patients unable to take the latter drugs. The usual initial dose of hydroxychloroquine is 200 mg once or twice daily. The daily dose should not exceed 6-6.5 mg/kg. Therapeutic response to this drug is slow (2-6 months). Long-term use at a daily dose exceeding 400 mg is not recommended and should be avoided. Therapy is continued indefinitely.

LEVAMISOLE

Levamisole, an anthelmintic drug with immunostimulant properties (see Chapter 13.5.3), was found to have beneficial effect on patients with rheumatoid arthritis. The drug is still considered investigational in the United States. Chemistry and pharmacological actions are dealt with in Chapter 26.4.

The mechanism of action of levamisole in rheumatoid arthritis is uncertain. The drug does not possess a direct antiinflammatory action. It has been suggested that this drug acts by its effect on T cells and neutrophils (14) (Chapter 13.5.2). Levamisole is rapidly and well absorbed from the gastrointestinal tract. It is principally metabolized in the liver and has a half-life of about 4 hours.

Adverse Effects. In a multicenter study (23), levamisole has been reported to elicit mild side effects in about 41% of patients. The common side effects are gastrointestinal upset and skin rashes. A dose-dependent agranulocytosis has been reported to occur in about 5% of patients (more common in the female).

Therapeutic Uses. Therapeutic efficacy of levamisole in rheumatoid arthritis is still inconclusive. In clinical trials, levamisole has been given at a dose of 150 mg once a week.

CORTICOSTEROIDS

Chemistry and pharmacology of glucocorticoids are discussed in Chapter 12.4. Prednisone, prednisolone, and methylprednisolone are most commonly used in rheumatoid arthritis. These drugs are administered orally and absorbed well from the gastrointestinal tract. In plasma; these drugs are substantially protein bound and predominantly metabolized in the liver to water-soluble compounds that are excreted in the urine within 48 hours. For side effects, see Chapter 12.4.

Therapeutic Uses. Currently, systemic corticosteroids are used in patients with rheumatoid arthritis under the following conditions: (1) patients with polysynovitis who have failed to respond to first- and second-line drugs for rheumatoid arthritis, and (2) patients with marked constitutional symptoms (e.g., fever, weight loss, neuropathy, etc.). The dose of corticosteroids should be individualized and generally started at 4-5 mg daily, gradually increasing up to 10 mg daily. The daily dose should not exceed 10 mg except in severe cases. To minimize the side effects of corticosteroids, an alternate-day therapy (consisting of twice the daily dose given as one morning dose every 48 hours) is recommended.

For temporary relief of pain in joints, an intermediate-acting glucocorticoid such as triamcinolone hexacetonide or triamcinolone acetonide is administered intraarticularly in rheumatoid arthritis with involvement of a few joints. The relief of pain may last for days to months (average duration is about 4 weeks), depending upon the preparation chosen.

IMMUNOSUPPRESSANTS

Although many cytotoxic drugs have been tried in rheumatoid arthritis, the purine antagonist azathioprine and the alkylating agent cyclophosphamide are the most commonly used agents in this class.

Chemistry and Pharmacology. Chemistry and general pharmacological considerations of these two drugs are discussed in Chapter 27. Azathioprine, by alteration in the synthesis and function of DNA or by interfering with purine metabolism, may cause decreased T-cell function and modification of the "autoimmune" disorder. Cyclophosphamide, by interfering mostly with the DNA structure, alters the rate of growth of rapidly dividing cells. Pharmacokinetics of azathioprine and cyclophosphamide are discussed along with other immunosuppressants in Chapter 13.5.3.

Adverse Effects and Contraindications. Toxicity from azathioprine and cyclophosphamide generally falls into four major categories: (1) bone marrow depression, (2) susceptibility to infection, (3) hepatotoxicity, and (4) gastrointestinal complications. Cyclophosphamide in addition causes alopecia, azoospermia, anovulation, and hemorrhagic cystitis. Long-term use of both drugs has been reported to cause malignancy of hematological tissues and solid tumors (8).

Therapeutic Uses. Azathioprine and cyclophosphamide are used in patients with advanced severe rheumatoid arthritis when other available antirheumatoid drugs have failed. Therapy should begin with small doses, 1-3 mg/kg/day. If therapeutic benefits fail to occur by 12-16 weeks, the treatment should be discontinued. When allopurinol is given concurrently, the dose of azathioprine should be reduced by 60-70%, as the former drug inhibits the metabolism of the latter.

GOUT

Clinically, gout is characterized by recurrent acute attacks of severe inflammation of a single peripheral joint followed by a spontaneous remission. There is deposition of microcrystals in and about the joints. The crystals are monosodium urate in gout and calcium pyrophosphate dihydrate in pseudogout. For clinical gout, the primary biochemical abnormality is hyperuricemia. Both genetic and acquired abnormalities of purine metabolism may be responsible for the hyperuricemia (6). Clinical phases of gout consist of acute arthritis from periarticular deposits of urate, a spontaneous remission period, and chronic arthritis resulting from continued deposition of the crystals leading to formation of gouty tophi producing eroded joints.

DRUGS FOR GOUT

The therapeutic objectives are (1) termination of acute attack, (2) prophylaxis of acute arthritis and control of hyperuricemia, and (3) prevention of further progression of pathological process.

1. *Drugs for acute arthritis*
   - Colchicine
   - Nonsteroidal antiinflammatory drugs (e.g., phenylbutazone, indomethacin, ibuprofen, sulindac)
   - Glucocorticoids
2. *Prophylaxis for acute arthritis attacks*
   - Colchicine
   - Allopurinol
   - Uricosuric drugs
     - Probenecid
     - Sulfinpyrazone
3. *Chronic gout*
   - Colchicine
   - Nonsteroidal antiinflammatory drugs
   - Allopurinol

COLCHICINE

Chemistry. Colchicine is an alkaloid (Fig. 10.3-1) obtained from bulbs of the autumn crocus (*Colchicum autumnale).* A semisynthetic product (democoline) is also available.

Pharmacological Effects. Colchicine has a selective antiinflammatory effect in gouty arthritis. Although it is not an analgesic, colchicine provides dramatic relief of acute attacks of gout but not of other types of pain. It also has an antimitotic effect and has been widely used as an experimental tool in studies on cell division. Colchicine has a variety of other pharmacological effects (e.g., inhibition of histamine release from mast cells, and insulin secretion from β cells of pancreatic islets, hypothermia, and others), most of which do not appear to be related to its effects in gout.

Pharmacokinetics. Colchicine is well absorbed following oral administration, and the peak plasma level is achieved within 2 hours. Leukocyte colchicine concentrations are much higher than peak plasma levels and last longer. The metabolism of colchicine in humans is not clearly understood.

Mechanism of Action. Colchicine's mechanism of action in gout is not clear. The drug does not have any effect on the renal excretion of uric acid or its blood concentration. It binds microtubular protein and interferes with the function of mitotic spindles. As a result, fibrillar microtubules in the granulocytes disappear, and the migration of granulocytes into the inflamed area is inhibited. Microurate crystals are phagocytosized by leukocytes and incorporated in a glycoprotein that has been suggested to cause acute gouty arthritis. Colchicine appears to act by inhibiting the production or release of this glycoprotein.

Adverse Effects. Colchicine causes nausea and vomiting as well as abdominal pain and diarrhea in a large percentage of patients. Gastrointestinal intolerance-seems to protect patients from toxicity. These side effects are not seen when the drug is administered intravenously, but this route may be potentially risky, as inflammation and tissue necrosis may result from local extravasation of colchicine. Other infrequent side effects of colchicine include aplastic anemia, bone marrow depression, myopathy, alopecia, and hemorrhagic gastroenteritis. Severe toxicity to colchicine usually results from prolonged use of overdose. There are rare reports of azoospermia (22) and chromosomal abnormalities (11).

Therapeutic Uses. Colchicine is effective in the treatment of acute gout and is used prophylactically to prevent acute attacks or to diminish the intensity of acute attacks. For acute attacks, it is given at a dose of 0.5 or 0.6 mg hourly or 1-1.2 mg initially, followed by 0.5 or 0.6 mg every 2 hours until gastrointestinal side effects appear; or a maximum dose of 7-9.6 mg in a 24-hour period is administered (31). For prophylactic purposes, the usual dose of colchicine is 0.5-1 mg daily. For rapid relief of pain and fewer gastrointestinal side effects, the drug can be administered intravenously at a dose of 1-2 mg initially, then 0.5 mg every 3-6 hours if needed. The total dose of colchicine intravenously for one course should not exceed 4 mg. It is available in ampules (1 and 2 mg) for i.v. injection and as tablets, 0.6 mg for oral administration.

PHENYLBUTAZONE AND OXYPHENBUTAZONE

The effectiveness of phenylbutazone and oxyphenbutazone in treatment of acute gouty arthritis is comparable with that of colchicine or indomethacin. In daily doses of 600 mg or more, they have mild uricosuric action, but their antiinflammatory and analgesic actions are more useful in acute gout. Their adverse effects were described in the previous section.

ALLOPURINOL

Chemistry. Allopurinol is an analog of hypoxanthine (Fig. 10.3-1).

Pharmacology. Allopurinol reduces the production of uric acid by inhibiting the enzyme xanthine oxidase, which converts hypoxanthine to xanthine and then xanthine to uric acid, resulting in lowering of both serum and urine urate levels. Furthermore, allopurinol inhibits *de novo* synthesis of purine. It is well absorbed orally. Only a small portion of allopurinol circulates as protein bound. The drug is metabolized by xanthine oxidase to oxypurinol, which also inhibits xanthine oxidase and has a long half-life of about 18-30 hours. The long half-life of oxypurinol permits once-a-day administration of allopurinol. Allopurinol has been reported to inhibit hepatic microsomal enzyme activity, and this probably accounts for potentiation of warfarin action and for prolongation of half-life of probenecid when used concurrently (27).

Adverse Effects. The common side effects of allopurinol are hypersensitivity reactions characterized by maculopapular skin rash as well as exfoliative, urticarial, or purpuric lesions occurring in about 5% of patients. Gastrointestinal symptoms such as nausea and diarrhea may also occur. Rare side effects include bone marrow depression, neuropathy, abnormal liver enzymes, and xanthine stones. The dose of allopurinol should be individualized. For mild cases, it is used at a daily (single) dose of 200-300 mg and in severe cases at a daily dose of 400-600 mg. The dose of allopurinol should be reduced in patients with renal impairment or hepatic disease. Combined use of allopurinol and cytotoxic agents requires a 60-70% reduction of latter drugs.

PROBENECID

Probenecid is a derivative of benzoic acid [p-(dipropylsulfamyl) benzoic acid]. It interferes with the tubular reabsorption of urate and thereby acts as an effective uricosuric drug. In chronic renal failure with a glomerular filtration rate less than 30 ml/min, however, its uricosuric activity is insignificant. Probenecid decreases renal excretion of penicillin, indomethacin, and sulfonylureas.

The drug is well absorbed from the gastrointestinal tract and has a plasma half-life of 6-12 hours. It is rapidly metabolized, and the metabolites are excreted in the urine.

Probenecid has a few mild side effects such as allergic skin rash, flushing, dizziness, and gastrointestinal complaints such as anorexia, nausea, and vomiting. Hemolytic anemia (in patients with glucose-6-phosphate dehydrogenase deficiency), aplastic anemia, necrosis of liver, and peptic ulceration are rare adverse reactions to probenecid. Probenecid and salicylates are not used in combination because salicylates reduce the therapeutic effect of the former drug.

By lowering serum uric acid levels, probenecid can prevent or inhibit changes in the joints in chronic gout. The dose of probenecid should be individualized with monitoring of urinary uric acid. The initial daily dose of probenecid is 500-750 mg for a week or more; the dose is then increased weekly by an increment of 500 mg until serum uric is normalized. Most patients are controlled at a daily maintenance dose of 1-1.5 g in divided doses. Probenecid is not effective in acute attacks of gout. During early probenecid therapy, acute gouty attacks may occur that require concomitant colchicine therapy for prophylaxis.

SULFINPYRAZONE

Although sulfinpyrazone is a congener of phenylbutazone, it has no antiinflammatory and analgesic actions. The mechanism of uricosuric action of sulfinpyrazone is like that of probenecid, that is inhibition of renal tubular reabsorption of filtered urate. It is a more potent uricosuric drug than probenecid on a weight basis. The drug is rarely used for the treatment of hyperuricemia

Table 10.3-2
Drugs in Therapy of Various Arthritic Conditions

Form of Arthritis	Drugs	Dosage Schedule
Sjögren's syndrome	Glucocorticoids	Same as for rheumatoid arthritis
Felty syndrome	Glucocorticoids	Same as for rheumatoid arthritis
Rheumatoid vasculitis	Glucocorticoids	
	Prednisone	100 mg/day
	D-Penicillamine	1-1.5 g/day
Ankylosing spondylitis	Indomethacin	75-150 mg/day
	Phenylbutazone	200-300 mg/day
Reiter's syndrome	Phenylbutazone	Initially 600-800 mg/day followed by 200-300 mg/day
	Indomethacin	100-150 mg/day
	Cytotoxic drugs	
	Azathioprine	1-3 mg/kg/day
Systemic lupus erythematosus	Hydroxychloroquine	100 mg once or twice daily
	Glucocorticoids	
	Prednisolone	20-25 mg daily
Necrotizing vasculitis	Glucocorticoids	
	Prednisone	60-100 mg/day
	Methylprednisolone	1 g/day, pulse therapy
	Cyclophosphamide	2-3 mg/kg/day
	D-Penicillamine	1-1.5 g/day
Osteoarthritis	Indomethacin	Same as for rheumatoid arthritis
	Triamcinolone	
	Hexacetonide	10 mg (intraarticular injection)
Psoriatic arthritis	Phenylbutazone	Same as for rheumatoid arthritis
	Oxyphenbutazone	
	Indomethacin	

because of its possible serious adverse effects in the form of blood dyscrasias.

OTHER ARTHRITIC DISORDERS

Drugs used in arthritic disorders other than rheumatoid arthritis and gout are listed in Table 10.3-2.

REFERENCES

1. Adams, S. S., and Buckler, J. W. Ibuprofen and flurbiprofen. *Clin. Rheum. Dis.* 5:359, 1979.
2. Barraclough, D. Drug interactions in the management of rheumatoid arthritis. *Aust. N.Z. J. Med.* (Suppl. 1) 8:106, 1978.
3. Blocka, K., Droomgoole, S., Furst, D., and Paulus, H.E. Single dose pharmacokinetics of 195 Au-auranofin using a total radiation counting chamber. *Arthritis Rheu.* 23:654, 1980.
4. Blocka, K., Frust, D. E., Landaw, E., Droomgoole, S., Blomberg, A., and Paulus, H. E. Single dose pharmacokinetics of auranofin in rheumatoid arthritis. *J. Rheumatol.* (Suppl. 8) 9:110, 1982.
5. Blodgett, R. C. Auranofin: Experience to date. *Am. J. Med.* 75 (6A):86, 1983.
6. Boss, G. R., and Seegmiller, J. E. Hyperuricemia and gout: Classification, complications, and management. *N. Engl. J. Med.* 300:1459, 1979.
7. Cashin, C. H., Dawson, W., and Kitchen, E. A. The pharmacology of benoxaprofen. *J. Pharm. Pharacol.* 29:330, 1977.
8. Craig, G. L., and Buchanan, W. W. Antirheumatic drugs: Clinical pharmacology and therapeutic use. *Drugs* 20:453, 1980.
9. Dixon, A. St. J., Davies, J., Dormandy, T. L. et al. Synthetic D(-) penicillamine in rheumatoid arthritis: Double-blind controlled study of a high and low dosage regimen. *Ann. Rheum. Dis.* 34:416, 1975.
10. Editorial: Gold for rheumatoid arthritis. *Br. Med. J.* 1:471, 1971.
11. Ferreira, M. L., and Buoniconti, A. Trisomy after colchicine therapy. *Lancet* 2:1304, 1968.
12. Fries, J. F., and Britton, M. C. Fenoprofen calcium in rheumatoid arthritis: A controlled double-blind crossover evaluation. *Arthritis Rheum.* 19:933, 1976.
13. Gaeton, D., Lorino, M. D., and Hardin, J. G., Jr. Sulindac-induced meningitis in mixed connective tissue disease. *South. Med. J.* 76:1185, 1983.
14. Goldstein, G. Mode of action of levamisole. *J. Rheum. Dis.* (Suppl. 4) 5:143, 1978.
15. Halsey, J. P., and Cardoe, N. Benoxaprofen: Side-effect profile in 300 patients. *Br. Med. J.* 284:1365, 1982.
16. Hamdy, R. C., Murnane, B., Perera, N., Woodcock, K., and Koch, I. M. The pharmacokinetics of benoxaprofen in elderly subjects. *Eur. J. Rheumatol. Inflam.* 5:69, 1982.
17. Huskisson, E. C. Antiinflammatory drugs. *Semin. Arthritis Rheum.* 7:1, 1977.
18. Kwan, K. C., Breault, G. O., Umbenhauer, E. R., McMahon, F. G., and Duggan, D. E. Kinetics of indomethacin absorption, elimination, enterohepatic circulation in man. *J. Pharmacokinet. Biopharmaceut.* 4:255, 1976.
19. Lee, K. Y., Beilin, L. J., and Vandongen, R. Severe hypertension after ingestion of an appetite suppressant (phenylpropanolamine) with indomethacin. *Lancet* 1:1110, 1979.
20. Mackenzie, A. H. Antimalarial drugs for rheumatoid arthritis. *Am. J. Med.* 75 (6A):48, 1983.

21. McChesney, E. W., Banks, W. F., Jr., and McAuliff, J. P. Laboratory studies of the 4-aminoquinoline in man after various oral dosage regimens. *Antibiot. Chemother.* 12:583, 1962.

22. Merlin, H. E. Azoospermia caused by colchicine. *Fertil. Steril* 23:180, 1972.

23. Multicenter Study Group. A multicenter randomized double-blind study comparing two dosages of levamisole in rheumatoid arthritis. *J. Rheum. Dis.* (Suppl. 4) 5:5, 1978.

24. Palmer, L., Bertilsson, L., Alvan, G., Orme, M., Sjoqvist, F., and Holmstedt, B. Indomethacin: Quantitative determination in plasma by mass fragmentography including pilot pharmacokinetics in man. In: *Prostaglandin Synthetase Inhibitors* (Robinson, H. J., and Vane, J. R., eds.). New York: Raven Press, 1974, p. 91.

25. Pitts, N. E. Efficacy and safety of piroxicam. *Am. J. Med.* 72:77, 1982.

26. Rhymer, A. R., and Gengos, D. C. Indomethacin. *Clin. Rheum. Dis.* 5:541, 1979.

27. Roe, R. L. Drug therapy in rheumatoid diseases. *Med. Clin. North Am.* 61:405, 1977.

28. Semon, L. S., and Mills, J. A. Nonsteroidal antiinflammatory drugs. *N. Engl. J. Med.* 302:1179, 1977.

29. Stewart, I. C. Gastrointestinal haemorrhage and benoxaprofen. *Br. Med. J.* 284:163, 1982.

30. Tolman, E. L., and Partridge, R. Multiple sites of interaction between prostaglandins and non-steroidal antiinflammatory agents. *Prostaglandins* 9:349, 1975.

31. Wallace, S. L., and Ertel, N. H. Occupancy approach to colchicine dosage. *Lancet* 2:1250, 1970.

32. Walz, D. T., DiMartino, M. J., Chakrin, L. W., Sutton, B. M., and Misher, A. Antiarthritic properties and unique pharmacologic profile of a potential chrysotherapeutic agent: Sk & F D-39162. *J. Pharmacol. Exp. Ther.* 197:142, 1976.

33. Walz, D. T., DiMartino, M. J., Griswold, D. E., Intoccia, A. P., and Flanagan, T. L. Biologic actions and pharmacokinetic studies of auranofin. *Am. J. Med.* 75 (6A):90, 1983.

34. Weiss, B., and Hait, W. N. Selective cyclic nucleotide phosphodiesterase inhibitors as potential therapeutic agents. *Ann. Rev. Pharmacol. Toxicol.* 17:441, 1977.

35. Willoughby, D. A., and Koh, M. Experimental aspects of nonsteroidal and antirheumatic drugs. *Eur. J. Rheumatol. Inflam.* 2:5, 1979.

36. Wiseman, E. H. Pharmacologic studies with a new class of nonsteroidal antiinflammatory agents—the oxicams—with special reference to piroxicam (Feldene). *Am. J. Med.* 72:2, 1982.

37. Wong, S. Pharmacology of tolmetin: 1-Methyl-5-p-toluoylpyrrole-2-acetic acid. In: *Tolmetin: A New Non-Steroidal Anti-Inflammatory Agent* (Ward, J. R., ed.). Princeton, N.J.: Excerpta Medica, 1975, p. 1.

38. Wong, S., Gardocki, J. F., and Pruss, T. P. Pharmacologic evaluation of Tolectin (Tolmetin, MCN-2559 and MCN-2891): Two anti-inflammatory agents. *J. Pharmacol. Exp. Ther.* 185:127, 1973.

39. Zvaifler, N. J. Pathogenesis of the joint disease of rheumatoid arthritis. *Am. J. Med.* 75 (6A):3, 1983.

ADDITIONAL READING

O'Brien, W.M. et al. Rare adverse reactions to nonsteroidal antiinflammatory drugs. *J. Rheumatol.* 12:347, 1985.

Webster, J. Interactions of NSAIDs with diuretics and β-blockers, mechanisms and clinical implications. *Drugs* 30:32, 1985.

CHAPTER
10.4

LOCAL ANESTHETICS

George K.W. Yim

Local anesthetics are agents that, when applied at specific sites, block sensory afferents, thereby producing pain relief and preventing accompanying reflex responses. In higher concentrations, these agents not only block motor nerves, but are also capable of severely depressing other excitable structures, such as conduction pathways in the heart, and pontomedullary respiratory centers. Thus, proper injection technique and precautions, such as the addition of vasoconstrictors, are necessary to restrict the distribution of these agents so that local anesthesia is indeed obtained.

Not all nerve blockers are local anesthetics. Table 10.4-1 presents some properties that distinguish local anesthetics from other agents (e.g., neurolytics, biotoxins, and membrane labilizers) which also block nerve impulses. The term local anesthetic usually refers to classic agents such as procaine and lidocaine that reversibly block nerve conditions. The names of these agents usually end in the suffix "caine," which stems from the prototypical local anesthetic, cocaine. (For the sake of clarity, the term *local anesthetic action* will be restricted to describe the nerve-blocking actions of the classic local anesthetics, whereas their myocardial depressant and other actions will be referred to as *actions common to local anesthetics*.

MECHANISMS OF ACTION

Local Anesthetics. The local anesthetics act by blocking the activation (opening) of sodium channels induced by depolarization of the nerves. It is the ionized form of the local anesthetic that actually blocks the sodium channels. However, only the unionized form can readily penetrate the myelin sheath and the nerve membrane. The pK_a (7.5-9) leaves 5 - 20% in the nonionized (unprotonated) form at tissue pH. This lipid-soluble, unionized form penetrates through axonal membranes, then ionizes in the neural cytoplasm. This cation then binds at the intracellular openings of the sodium channels, thereby reducing the inward flow of Na^+ ions that usually accompany axonal depolarization. Initially, the smaller and more slowly depolarizing sodium current results in: (a) slowing of the rising phase of the action potential; (b) slowing of the conduction rate of the nerve impulse; and, (c) decreased excitability and prolongation of the refractory period. Greater reduction of the inward sodium current eventually prevents the generation of the nerve action potential (4). At higher concentrations, block of potassium channels also contributes to the decreased excitability and prolongation of the refractory period (Fig. 10.4-1).

In low concentrations, local anesthetics are relatively specific for blocking sodium channels, whereas in high concentrations they also block calcium channels. Thus, low concentrations of local anesthetics or the specific sodium-channel blocker, tetrodotoxin (TTX), can selectively block the fast Na^+ component (initial rising phase) of the cardiac action potential, without affecting the slow Ca^{2+} phase. In contrast, low concentrations of the Ca^{2+} antagonist, verapamil, selectively block the plateau without affecting the fast component. Depression of Ca^{2+}-dependent phenomena by high concentrations of local anesthetics probably accounts for the few manifestations of local anesthetic toxicity that are not due to neuronal blockade (i.e., depression of myocardial contraction and platelet aggregation).

During continuous regional anesthetic procedure, frequent administration of local anesthetics often demonstrates a progressive decrease of anesthetic effect. Changes in the local pH in the vicinity of the nerve seem to be involved in the genesis of tachyphylaxis. The locally

Table 10.4-1
Agents That Block Nerve Impulses

Blocker	Effects on: Resting Membrane Potential	Na^+ Channel	K^+ Channel	Mechanism/Consequence
Local anesthetics (procaine)	No change	Block at internal site	Block	Unionized base penetrates nerve, but cationic form blocks Na^+ channel
Neurolytics (ethanol, phenol)	Depolarization	Block	Block	Disruption of lipid membrane; irreversible block
Biotoxins (TTx)	No change	Block at external site	No block	Polar; poor penetration of lipid neural sheaths
Membrane labilizers (DDT, veratridine)	Depolorization	Prevent channel closing	Block	Initial firing followed by depolarization block

acting buffering mechanism that is responsible for providing adequate quantity of anesthetic base for diffusion through axonal membrane is altered to effect a reduced analgesic response. Tachyphylaxis occurs more rapidly with local anesthetics with a lower pK_a e.g., mepivacaine (pK_a = 7.6 (13).

Neurolytics. When applied locally in sufficient concentrations, neurolytic agents such as ethanol and phenol are believed to penetrate into the lipid neuronal membranes, decrease resting permeability to potassium ions, and thereby cause depolarization. Subsequently, the structural integrity of the neuronal membranes is apparently disrupted, as irreversibility characterizes the nerve block induced by these agents. Phenol (5-10% in glycerol) has been injected into the subarachnoid space for long-lasting pain relief in terminal cancer, or for relief of spasticity in patients with prior CNS damage (16). These agents are not selective for pain afferents, as indicated by a 2-15% incidence of paresthesias, paralysis, and urinary incontinence. Ethanol had been similarly used to destroy specific nuclei in the brain (i.e., for chemical pallidectomy to decrease severity of Parkinson's disease). Prior injection of a reversible local anesthetic such as procaine was usually used to verify the accuracy of the intended stereotaxic injection site.

Biotoxins. Biotoxins, such as tetrodotoxin (TTX, puffer fish toxin) and saxitoxin (STX, paralytic shellfish toxin) are among the most potent toxic substances known. These polar compounds block nerve action potentials by binding to and plugging the extracellular openings of axonal sodium channels (3). They do not affect potassium or calcium channels, nor do they affect synaptic potentials, and thus have been used extensively as pharmacological tools for identifying Na^+-type spike potentials. Most TTX-insensitive spikes involve the flux of ions other than Na^+ (e.g., Ca^{2+} spikes of certain invertebrate neurons). Because of the profound and prolonged anesthesia produced when TTX is injected into the subarachnoid space, the evaluation of these biotoxins in spinal anesthesia has been suggested.

Membrane Labilizers. Local anesthetics and Ca^{2+} (in high concentrations) have been classed as membrane stabilizers, or agents that keep neuronal membranes from being excited, and likewise protect red blood cells from osmotic disruption. In contrast, membrane labilizers (e.g., DDT and veratridine) render red blood cells more sensitive to disruption by hypotonic solutions, and also cause axonal depolarization, repetitive firing, and eventual conduction failure by depolarization block. DDT has since been found to block the K^+ channel, and also to prolong the inward Na^+ influx (i.e., block sodium inactivation).

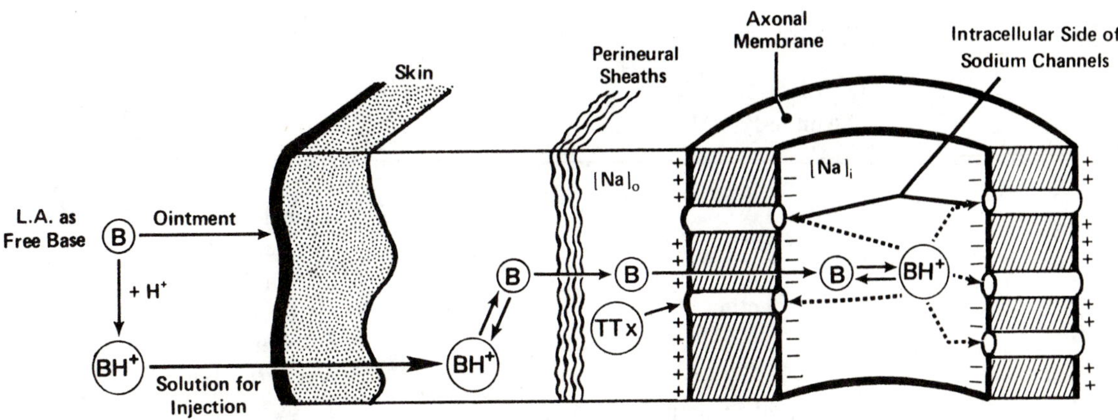

Fig. 10.4-1. *Passage of local anesthetic to site of action.*

STRUCTURE-ACTIVITY RELATIONSHIPS

General Structure. The clinically useful local anesthetics consist of a lipophilic group (usually a substituted phenyl ring) and a hydrophilic group (usually a tertiary amine) connected by an ester- or an amide-linked intermediate chain (Table 10.4-2). Since these structural requirements are common to numerous other drug classes, clinically useful local anesthetics may share some of the actions of these other drug classes (i.e., antiarrhythmics, anticonvulsants, and myocardial depressants).

The solubility characteristics of local anesthetics have important implications in their actions. Thus, the aqueous solubility of the hydrophilic amine salts permits the parenteral injection of aqueous solutions of local anesthetics. The pK_as of these agents range from 7.5 to 9, and consequently, significant amounts of the un-ionized free base are present at normal body pH (Table 10.4-3). The lipophilic group facilitates penetration of the free base through the perineural structures and the nerve membrane. Within the cytoplasm, the free base is again protonated to form the active local anesthetic.

Diminished nerve-blocking potency and reduced central toxicity (i.e., convulsions) are exhibited by more hydrophilic agents, such as procainamide (an antiarrhythmic agent), and quaternary analogs. Thus, quaternary analogs of a lidocaine-like antiarrhythmic agent retain the antiarrhythmic, but not the convulsant actions of the parent compound.

Ester-Type Versus Amide-Type Local Anesthetics. From the clinical viewpoint, an important structural characteristic of current local anesthetics is whether they are esters or amides, because allergic reactions have been observed primarily with the esters, rather than with the amides. The allergies appear to be due to a *p*-aminobenzoic aicd (PABA)-like portion of the ester-type agents. In this regard, an experimental local anesthetic (tetrahydronaphthalene) was developed on the basis that it would not form PABA, a product of procaine hydrolysis and, therefore, would be less apt to elicit cross-allergic reactions in individuals hypersensitive to procaine.

The reduced systemic toxicity of procaine, relative to cocaine, has been attributed to hydrolysis of the ester bond. Many of the other esters are readily hydrolyzed by plasma cholinesterase. Ortho substitutions on the aromatic ring hinder hydrolysis of the esters.

The amides are metabolized mainly by the liver microsomal amide hydrolases. Ortho substitution reduces the generation of aniline-like metabolites of the amides, which have been implicated in methemoglobin formation by certain amide-type local anesthetics.

PHARMACOKINETICS

Factors Affecting the Onset of Local Anesthesia. In a clinical situation, the minimum effective concentration (Cm) of a local anesthetic necessary for blocking the desired nerve can usually be attained only by injecting concentrated solutions of the agent near the nerve. Even then, there is a latent period (3 to 10 minutes), with highly lipid-soluble agents having both slower onset and longer duration of action. Further increases in concentration may shorten the latency to some degree, but only at the possible expense of greater systemic toxicity. Local anes-

Table 10.4-2
Structures of Local Anesthetics

Lipophilic Group - Intermediate Chain - Hydrophilic Chain	Other Examples
$H_2N-C_6H_4-C(=O)-O-CH_2CH_2-N(C_2H_5)_2 \cdot HCl$ Ester-type: Procaine	Chloroprocaine Tetracaine Cocaine
$2,6-(CH_3)_2C_6H_3-NH-CO-CH_2-N(C_2H_5)_2$ HCl Amide-type: Lidocaine	Bupivacaine Mepivacaine
Phenyl — ester / keto / ether / etc. — $(CH_2)_n$ — $N(R_1)(R_2)$ General Structure	Neuroleptics[a] Antidepressants Cholinolytics Antihistamines Calcium antagonists Antiarrhythmics

[a] Other classes of agents that possess basic structural requirements for local anesthetic action.

Table 10.4-3
Properties of Clinically Important Local Anesthetic Agents

Agent and Trade Name[a]	Type	pK_a	Lipid-Solubility (at pH 7.4)	Plasma Protein Binding (%)	EAC[b]	Duration of Action	Primary Site of Metabolism	Principal Clinical Use	Toxicity
Chlorprocaine (NESACAINE)	Ester	8.7	Low	?	2	Short	Plasma	Most block techniques, obstetric block	Least
Procaine (NOVOCAINE)	Ester	8.9	Low	?	2	Short	Plasma	Infiltration	↓
Prilocaine (CITANEST)	Amide	7.9	Medium	55	1	Intermediate	Liver	i.v. regional, single-dose nerve block	
Lidocaine (lignocaine; XYLOCAINE)	Amide	7.9	Medium	64	1	Intermediate	Liver	All block techniques, including topical	
Mepivacaine (CARBOCAINE)	Amide	7.6	Medium	78	1	Intermediate	Liver	As above, except topical	
Etidocaine (DURANEST)	Amide	7.7	High	94	0.5	Long	Liver	Surgical blocks requiring muscle relaxation	
Bupivacaine (MARCAINE)	Amide	8.1	High	95	0.25	Long	Liver	obstetric block, postoperative pain	
Tetracaine (amethocaine; DECICAINE)	Ester	8.5	High	?	0.25	Long	Plasma	Topical	
Dibucaine (cinchocaine; NUPERCAINE)	Amide	?	High	?	0.25	Long	Liver	Spinal	
Cocaine	Ester	?	Medium	?	1.0	Intermediate	Liver	Topical	Most

[a] In capitals within parentheses.
[b] EAC = equivalent anesthetic concentration with cocaine as 1.
Source: Modified Table 4 of Ref. 10.

thetics are less effective in acidic (e.g., inflammed) sites, and in highly vascularized areas that require the use of the most potent agents.

Several neurophysiological studies have shown that axons with smaller diameters are generally more sensitive to local anesthetics. Hence, the smaller pain afferents (C-fibers) are often blocked more quickly and for longer periods than the Ia motor afferents. Location of the sensory fibers in a nerve trunk also influences the onset of anesthesia in the innervated area. In the extremities, proximal sensory innervation is supplied by the axonal bundles (mantle) situated close to the surface of the nerve trunk, and the distal innervation arises from the interior or core bundles. During nerve block of extremities, analgesia first develops proximally, and then spreads to distal parts. During brachial plexus block, motor blockade frequently develops before sensory block, and this is attributed to blockade of motor fibers in the bundles peripheral to core sensory axons. During recovery, activity would return to the outer fibers before the core fibers.

Factors Affecting the Duration of Local Anesthesia. In the usual situation, the Cm of the local anesthetic is much higher than the plasma concentration. Thus, the duration of action is independent of the plasma half-life of these agents. The duration of nerve block increases: (a) with increased lipophilic properties of the local anesthetic, and (b) with decreased blood flow to the site of action. Thus the recovery time after tetracaine (*in vitro*) is 20 times longer than that of the more hydrophilic agent, procaine (Table 10.4-3). Conversely, lidocaine-induced nerve block lasts about 40 minutes as compared with the 400-minutes nerve block induced by the more lipophilic agent, bupivacaine. Dibucaine and chlorpromazine have almost irreversible blocking actions *in vitro*. They are apparently bound to the neuronal membranes by powerful close-range Heitler-London forces.

Increased blood flow resulting from direct vasodilation induced by certain local anesthetics (lidocaine) facilitates their removal from the site of injection. Addition of a vasoconstrictor (e.g., epinephrine HCl in 1:200,000 dilution) slows blood flow sufficiently to prolong the anesthetic action and reduce systemic absorption by about 30%. Such vasconstrictors should not be coadministered with cocaine, as cocaine itself is a vasoconstrictor.

Factors Affecting the Blood Levels. The plasma levels of local anesthetics are determined by the balance of factors that affect other basic compounds. If the rate of absorption is sufficiently slow, metabolism, protein binding, and excretion would prevent the development of toxic blood levels. Thus, the minimum effective concentration and volume of anesthetic solution should be administered. Following topical application to highly vascular mucosal areas such as the trachea and uterus, plasma levels may slowly reach 50% of those obtained with i.v. injections. Careful injection technique is especially important when using small-gauge needles in the neck region. Inadvertent intraarterial injection (i.e., into the lingual or external carotid arteries) may cause the back flow of the highly concentrated solution into the carotid arteries perfusing the brain, thus resulting in convulsions. Such central toxic manifestations may not be observed if the same small dose is injected intravenously, because of consequent dilution before the agent reaches the cerebral circulation.

Metabolism. Little or no metabolism of ester agents takes place at the site of action [e.g., in case of spinal anesthesia there is no cholinesterase (ChE) in the CSF, and the true ChE does not hydrolyze procaine]. In humans, procaine and some ester-type local anesthetics are readily hydrolyzed by plasma ChE, resulting in the excretion of only 2-3% of unchanged compound in the urine. Extensive hydrolysis of cocaine by plasma ChE has recently been reported.

Amide-type agents such as lidocaine undergo N-dealkylations and hydrolysis in the liver by microsomal enzymes. The N-dealkylated, unhydrolyzed lidocaine metabolites retain some anesthetic activity. Plasma concentrations of amide-type agents may be elevated three to four times above control in patients with hepatic tumors, or cirrhosis. Thus, ester-type agents would be preferred for such patients.

Protein Binding. The unionized local anesthetic bases bind to plasma proteins such as albumin and globulins. The binding is reversible and serves as a reservoir from which potentially toxic systemic levels can be released (e.g., by respiratory acidosis). Long-acting, potent, and highly lipophilic drugs (e.g., tetracaine, bupivacaine) are more protein bound than other hydrophilic counterparts (e.g., procaine and lidocaine).

THERAPEUTIC USES

Surface Anesthesia. Prior to tonometry, 1-2 drops of lidocaine (4%) or (1%) are usually sufficient to anesthetize the avascular cornea. However, melanin binding may delay the onset of action in pigmented eyes. Adequate anesthesia can be assumed if a second administration 3 minutes later does not cause smarting. With irritation and inflammation (i.e., of the conjunctiva), increased blood flow and facilitated removal of the agents usually necessitate repeated applications.

Benzocaine (ethyl aminobenzoate, ANESTHESIN) is an anesthetic agent widely used in sunburn and hemorrhoidal preparations. The local anesthetics that are used parenterally (i.e., procaine) usually do not penetrate the unbroken skin. However, epicutaneous application of a new lipophilic agent, ketocaine (10% in dimethylacetamide), can provide cutaneous topical anesthesia.

Infiltration Anesthesia. Infiltration anesthesia often involves the intradermal or subcutaneous injection of procaine or lidocaine into an area to be anesthetized (e.g., the base of a tooth prior to drilling, edges of a wound prior to suturing, or site of entry of a large needle for spinal anesthesia). Benzyl alcohol (0.9%, in saline) can provide intradermal analgesia lasting 3 minutes without causing discomfort. Lidocaine (0.05%) causes burning and stinging, but the analgesia lasts about 20 minutes. With field block of areas such as scalp and abdominal wall, the superficial nerves are effectively blocked by injecting the agent around, rather than directly at the area to be anesthetized. When inducing local anesthesia for opening of an abscess, the risk of bacterial spread is less with an intracutaneous wheal directly over the abscess than with field block.

Nerve Block. The injection of local anesthetics around nerve trunks, whether the site is distal from the spinal cord (e.g., pudendal or brachial nerve block); just outside the spinal cord (epidural, caudal blocks); or within the subarachnoid space (spinal block), results in anesthesia of the innervated areas. The possibility of piercing and permanently damaging nerves or injecting a large, and hence systematically toxic, dose in nearby large veins emphasizes the need for specialized training and experience when using these approaches. There are selected monographs with excellent illustrations of the location of vessels and anatomical landmarks (2, 8).

Regional Anesthesia in Obstetrics. Lumbar, epidural, or saddle-block anesthesia can provide marked maternal pain relief with minimal danger to the fetus and neonate. Low spinal (caudal, sacral, saddle) blocks provide pain relief mainly during the second stage of labor (Table 10.4.-4). High spinal blocks provide excellent pain relief during both stages, but disruption of the pain afferents at the T10-T12 level is accompanied by block of thoracolumbar sympathetic efferents to the peripheral vasculature. The resultant loss in vascular tone is apt to result in maternal hypotension with a disproportionate reduction of fetal circulation. To decrease the incidence and severity of possible fetal distress, maternal hypotension can be prevented or minimized by the prior administration of balanced i.v. fluids, and positioning the mother so her enlarged uterus does not occlude the aorta or inferior vena cava. To reverse maternal hypotension, centrally acting pressor agents such as ephedrine are recommended. Peripherally acting agents such as phenylephrine and methoxamine produce uterine vasoconstriction and thus may be harmful to the fetus.

Paracervical block results in a much higher incidence of fetal distress (approximately 20% with lidocaine) owing to extensive absorption of the agent into the fetal circulation (14). Slowing of labor increases the need for forceps delivery and may be due to: (a) uterine relaxation by epinephrine (when used as a vasoconstrictor additive); (b) depressed release of oxytocin; and, (c) depression of uterine activity secondary to maternal hypotension. Prolonged labor and fetal acidosis may result in significant iontrapping of the local anesthetics by the fetus. Ester-type agents that would be rapidly metabolized by maternal blood might be preferred in such situations.

During regional anesthesia, systemic toxicity may result from inadvertent intravascular injection, rather than from absorption from the epidural or other sites. Headaches following spinal anesthesia are frequently due to accidental puncture of the dura with the large epidural, caudal needle or catheter. Inadvertent subarachnoid injection of the epidural dose (two to three times spinal dose in volume) would result in total spinal anesthesia (characterized by abrupt hypotension and respiratory arrest).

Contraindications for regional anesthesia would include the existence of fetal distress and maternal hypotension (i.e., due to hemorrhage). The risk of aspiration pneumonitis is an important consideration, if the pregnant mother (full term) has a full stomach. With regional anesthesia, the mother would be fully conscious and her swallowing reflexes would not be impaired as under general anesthesia. The overall incidence of anesthetic complications for conduction anesthesia is about twice that observed after inhalation anesthesia. However, high-inspired maternal O_2 levels and vigorous, well oxygenated babies could be delivered during both general anesthesia and lumbar epidural analgesia for elective cesarean section.

TOXICITY AND MANAGEMENT

The untoward reactions associated with the use of local anesthetic agents can be classified according to probable source of the reactions. As summarized in Table 10.4-4, these include: (a) complications due to the techniques by which the agent is administered; (b) manifestations related to additive vasoconstrictor substances, (c) allergic reactions to the agents; and, (d) toxic actions of local anesthetics (Table 10.4-5).

Complications Due to Techniques. Motor paralysis and sensory deficits of varying degrees may persist well

Table 10.4-4
Use of Local Anesthetics in Childbirth

Source of Pain	Entry Level of Pain Afferents	Anesthetic Procedure For Pain Relief	Adverse Effect
First stage labor:			
Contraction of uterus Dilation of cervix	T10-T12	Paracervical	Absorption into fetal circulation: fetal depression
		High spinal	Block sympathetic nerves: maternal hypotension
Second stage labor:			
Distention of vulva and birth canal	S2-S4	High spinal	
		Low spinal	

Anesthetic Procedure	Maternal Status			Fetal Status	
	Satisfactory Analgesia (%)	Hypotension (%)	Forceps Delivery (%)	Fetal Distress (%)	Vigorous Baby at 5 min (%)
Saddle (low spinal)	98	12	—	1	—
Epidural (lumbar)	96	24	16	2	96
Spinal			10	—	97
Paracervical	—		—	10-20	

beyond the usual 6 to 12-hour recovery period following nerve or spinal blocks. In some instances, these deficits may result from mechanical severance of nerve fibers by the needles used to administer the agent. It has been suggested that local anesthetics block axonal transport which raises the question as to whether these agents can block this vital transport long enough to cause distal neuronal degeneration as has been observed with metabolic inhibitors.

Complications Due to Added Vasoconstrictors. Anxiety, tachycardia, palpitations, and hypertension are untoward manifestations that may be due to: (a) anxiety of the patient arising from the scheduled operative procedures; (b) the actions of vasoconstrictor agents that are coadministered to slow systemic absorption of the local anesthetic; or, (c) central excitation due to the local anesthetic. Tissue sloughing at the site of injections is more apt to occur when high concentrations of vasoconstrictor agent are used. Vasoconstrictors should not be coinjected with local anesthetics in anatomical structures with terminal vessels (e.g., digits or penis); the resultant prolonged and intense vasospasm may lead to gangrene. α-Adrenergic blockers such as phentolamine have been recommended for reversing the vasospastic actions of the additives.

Allergic Reactions. True allergy to local anesthetics is generally believed to be relatively rare. Some patients may develop edema, hives, wheezing, and bronchospasm following ester-type local anesthetics. Although cardiovascular and respiratory collapse may develop as manifestations of an anaphylactoid reaction, the possibility of inadvertent intravascular injection of the agent must also be considered. Dentists and others who frequently handle these agents may develop contact dermatitis.

Procaine-sensitive patients are likely to show cross-sensitization with other ester-type agents (i.e., chloroprocaine and tetracaine) and with sulfonamides and methylparabens (p-hydroxybenzoic acid derivatives). The structures of the latter two compounds implicate an important role of the PABA-like portion of the ester-type agents. In contrast, allergic reactions to the amide-type agents appear to be virtually nonexistent. It has been speculated, but not established, that "lidocaine allergy" may be due to the preservative additive, methylparaben, rather than to lidocaine itself.

Once an individual is suspected to be hypersensitive to local anesthetics, the most conservative approach would be to avoid further use of any local anesthetic. Using skin tests to identify an acceptable local anesthetic may subject a patient to an underdetermined risk of evoking an anaphylactoid reaction from the skin test itself.

Toxicity Due to Local Anesthetic Agents. It has been emphasized that the actions of local anesthetics are local only if high concentrations are restricted to the desired site of nerve blockade. Fig. 10.4-2 illustrates the target sites and consequences of not localizing a local anesthetic.

Central Nervous System Toxicity. Toxic systemic levels of local anesthetics often result in initial CNS excitation followed by depression. A depressive or excitatory

Table 10.4-5
Adverse Reactions Encountered with the Use of Local Anesthetics

Adverse Effects	Mechanism	Significance (Management)
Tissue sloughing at site of injection	Due to extravasation of concentrated vasoconstrictor	(α-Adrenergic blocker)
Gangrene of digits	Vasospasm of terminal vessels	(α-Adrenergic blocker)
Anxiety, excitation	Dopaminergic stimulation?	Sign of possible systemic toxicity
Tremors, convulsions	Removal of tonic inhibition	Usually not life-threatening (diazepam)
Coma, respiratory depression	Depression of respiratory center	(Artificial respiration; O_2)
Hypertension	Central sympathetic stimulation	(Diazepam, α-Adrenergic blocker)
Hypotension	Sympathetic inhibition; myocardial depression	Systemic absorption (isoproterenol)
	Direct vasodilator action	(Dopamine)
AV block, cardiac arrest		(Cardiac massage, isoproterenol, electrical pacing)
Ventricular fibrillation		(Cardiac massage, electrical defibrillation; do not use antiarrhythmic agents)

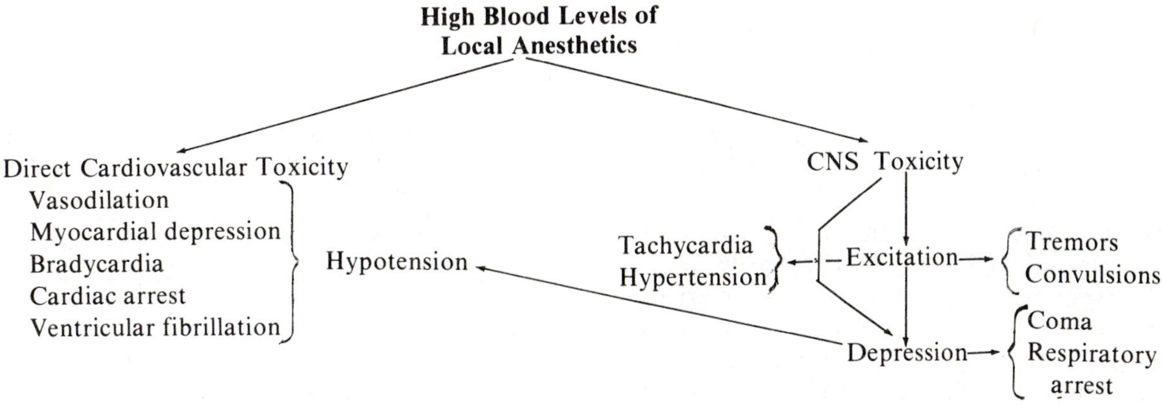

Fig. 10.4-2 *Systemic toxicity of local anesthetics.*

action seems to depend on a balance of effect between inhibitory and excitatory centers in the brain. The CNS excitation can proceed from anxiety, confusion, tremor, and convulsive jerks to generalized seizures. Tachycardia and hypertension are autonomic manifestations of such seizures. Loss of consciousness, coma, and depression of central respiratory and vasomotor centers are manifestations of CNS depression that may not be preceded by seizures (15). These latter depressant actions are likely an extension of the desired therapeutic actions of local anesthetics (i.e., nerve-blocking actions). The local anesthetics reach the central site of action by crossing the blood-brain barrier, because of its lipid nature is similar to that of the nerve sheath. Thus, although more potent local anesthetics have been found, they have also proven to be more toxic. Indeed, an almost perfect correlations (r = 0.9) exists between local anesthetic concentrations and lethal doses (in mice) of a series of local anesthetic agents.

Site and Mechanisms of LA Seizures. Convulsive discharges during local anesthetic seizures seem to originate first in the amygdala. Local anesthetics do not appear to directly excite neurons; rather, when applied directly to spinal, cuneate, cortical, vestibular, and cerebellar neurons by iontophoresis from multibarrel micropipettes (9), they depress firing. The generally held explanation of local anesthetic-induced seizures is that these drugs block inhibitory mechanisms, thereby releasing excitatory mechanisms. Neurons of the amygdala receive a powerful inhibitory input from dorsal raphe nucleus. It appears that local anesthetics diminish the inhibitory influence of raphe inhibition, and thereby induce synchronized firing of neurons in the amygdala, which subsequently spreads to neighboring brain regions, and then to somatic and autonomic efferent pathways.

Local anesthetic seizures themselves are usually not considered life-threatening (7). However, maternal acidosis and hypotension can contribute to fetal distress and depression of the newborn. Local anesthetic seizures can best be antagonized by diazepam. Barbiturates are not commonly used because of their greater respiratory depressant action. Anticonvulsant agents such as phenytoin, trimethadione, and mephenesin that are useful in grand mal, petit mal, and strychinine-induced seizures, respectively, are ineffective against local anestheitc seizures (5).

Cardiovascular Toxicity. Hypertension, due to increased central sympathetic discharge, is likely a manifestation of CNS stimulation at subconvulsive level. The central pressor action may oppose direct peripheral cardiovascular depression, and thereby minimize the net hypotension that is finally observed. Only with a few local anesthetic-type agents [e.g., cocaine and phencyclidine (PCP)] is hypertension enough to be of concern. The hypertension can be reduced centrally by diazepam or peripherally by ganglionic and/or sympathetic blockade.

Diminished central vasomotor outflow (via the sympathetic nerves) and consequent severe hypotension are almost invariably the result of high spinal or epidural administration. Inadvertent intravascular injection can lead to direct depression of vascular or cardiac smooth muscle or cardiac conducting system. Vasoconstrictors such as norepinephrine and dopamine can be used to counter the vasodilation; and epinephrine and isoproterenol have been used for their stimulant actions on the heart. AV block, cardiac arrest, and ventricular fibrillation are serious arrhythmis that are sometimes observed with clinically useful local anesthetics and also with agents with similar chemical structures and pharmacological actions. Following high doses of prilocaine, sufficient o-toluidine is formed to cause symptoms of methemoglobinemia in humans.

DRUG INTERACTIONS

Procaine-Sulfonamide Antagonism. The hydrolysis product of procaine, para-aminobenzoic acid, inhibits the actions of sulfonamides. Thus, during sulfonamide therapy of meningitis, local infections have persisted in areas infiltrated with procaine prior to diagnostic spinal taps. The use of agents that are not derivatives of para-aminobenzoic acid is recommended in this situation.

Prolongation of Neuromuscular Blockade. In high concentrations, local anesthetics can depress neuromuscular transmission. Thus, the duration of apnea produced by succinylcholine or curare may conceivably be prolonged (11).

Local Anesthetic-Antiarrhythmic Agents. Antiarrhythmic agents of the local anesthetic type (e.g., lidocaine and procainamide) themselves cause ventricular fibrillation in toxic doses. Fibrillating dog hearts (electrically induced) have been found to be more resistant to electrical defibrillation following commonly used antiarrhythmic agents such as lidocaine, quinidine, and diphenylhydantoin (1). These findings suggest that agents such as lidocaine and procainamide should not be used in attempts to antagonize ventricular fibrillation due to local anesthetic overdosage. Potassium salts appear to be a promising aid to effective electrical defibrillation of LA-induced ventricular fibrillation.

Preparations

Amides:

Bupivacaine HCl (MARCAINE): 0.25, 0.5, and 0.75% solutions with or without epinephrine 1:200,000.

Lidocaine HCl (XYLOCAINE): 2.5 and 5% ointment (for skin); jelly 2% (in cystoscopy); solution 2 and 4% (topical spray for mouth, nose, nasopharynx).

Mepivacaine HCL (CARBOCAINE): 1 and 2% solutions with methylparaben (preservative) for infiltration and nerve block; 1, 1.5, and 2% solutions without the preservative for epidural anesthesia.

Prilocaine HCl (CITANEST): 1, 2, and 3% solutions with or without methylparaben; 1-2% for infiltration; 0.5% for i.v. regional anesthesia; 1% solution for caudal and epidural anesthesia.

Etiodocaine HCl (DURANEST): 0.5% solution with or without ephinephrine 1:200,000 for infiltration or peripheral nerve block; 1% solution for epidural block with or without epinephrine; 1.5% solution with epinephrine for intraabdominal anesthesia.

Dibucaine HCl (NUPERCAINE): 0.5% cream and 1% ointment; solutions for spinal anesthesia, 0.667 mg/ml (hypobaric), 2.5 mg/ml in 5% glucose (hyperbaric), and 5 mg/ml (hypobaric), 2.5 mg/ml in 5% glucose (hyperbaric), and 5 mg/ml (isobaric).

Esters:

Cocaine HCl: Tablets 135 mg and powder (crystals); 0.25-0.5% solution for corneal anesthesia.

Piperocaine HCl (METYCAINE): Power 120-g container, and 2% solution; 1-4% solution for topical, 5-20% for proctoscopy, and 2% solution for infiltration and nerve block.

Procaine HCl (NOVOCAINE): 1, 2, and 10% solutions; 0.25-0.5% solution for infiltration anesthesia, 1-2% solution for nerve block, and 10% solution plus 10% glucose for subarachnoid anesthesia.

Chlorprocaine HCl (NESACAINE): 1, 2, and 3% solutions; single-dose containers of 2 and 3% are for caudal and epidural anesthesia.

Tetracaine HCl (PONTOCAINE): 1% cream and 0.5% ointment for skin and other topical use; 0.5 and 2% solution; powder 20 mg: 0.2 and 0.3% solutions (for saddle-back, perineal anesthesia) and 1% solution for subarachnoid anesthesia.

Benzocaine (AMERICAINE): Cream 5%; ointment 5 and 20% (for hemorrhoids); spray 20%; otic solution 20%.

REFERENCES

1. Babbs, C.F., Yim, G.K.W., Whistler, S.J., et al. Elevation of ventricular defibrillation threshold in dogs by antiarrhythimic drugs. *Am. Heart J.* 98:345, 1979.
2. Bennett, C.R. *Monheim's Local Anesthesia and Pain Control in Dental Practice,* 7th ed. St. Louis: Mosby, 1984.
3. Catterall, W.A. Neurotoxins that act on voltage-sensitive sodium channels in excitable membranes. *Ann. Rev. Pharmacol.* 20:15, 1980.
4. Covino, B.G. and Vassallo, H.G. *Local Anesthetics: Mechanisms of Action and Clinical Use.* New York: Grune and Stratton, 1976.
5. deJong, R.H. *Physiology and Pharmacology of Local Anesthesia.* Springfield, Ill.: Charles C. Thomas, 1970.
6. deJong, R.H. Toxicity of local anesthetics. *JAMA* 239:1166, 1978.
7. deJong, R.H. and Bonin, J.D. Death from local anesthetic-induced convulsions in mice. *Anesth. Analg.* 59:401, 1980.
8. Eriksson, F. (ed.): *Illustrated Handbook in Local Anesthesia.* Phildelphia: W.B. Saunders, 1980.
9. Garrison, D.S., Sinclair, J.G., Kee, R.D. and Yim, G.K.W. The differential action of intravenous lidocaine on cerebellar inhibition and cerebellar disfacilitation. *Brain Res.* 77:443, 1974.
10. Mather, L.E., and Cousins, M.J. Local anesthetics and their current clinical use. *Drugs* 18:185, 1979.
11. Matsuo, S., Rao, D.B.S., Chandry, I. and Foldes, F.F. Interaction of muscle relaxants and local anesthetics at the neuromuscular junction. *Anesth. Analg.* 57:580, 1978.
12. Ralston, D.H. and Shnider, S.M. The fetal and neonatal effects of regional anesthesia in obstetrics. *Anesthesiology* 48:38, 1978.
13. Savarese, J.J. and Covino, B.G. Pharmacology of local anesthetic drugs. In: *Anesthesia* (Miller, R.D., ed.). New York: Churchill Livingstone, 1981, p. 563.
14. Shnider, S.M. Experience with regional anesthesia for vaginal delivery. In: *Anesthesiologist, Mother, and newborn* (Shnider, S.M. and Moya, F., eds.). Baltimore: Williams & Wilkins, 1974, p. 38.
15. Steen, P.A. and Michenfelder, J.D. Neurotoxicity of anesthetics. *Anesthesiology* 50:437, 1979.
16. Wood, K.M. The use of phenol as a neurolytic agent. A review. *Pain* 5:205, 1978.

CHAPTER
11

DRUGS AFFECTING CONSCIOUSNESS AND MENTAL PROCESSES

Sachin N. Pradhan

In the previous chapters drugs affecting central functions such as central motor control (Chapters 9.2, 9.3 and 9.4) and pain perception (Chapter 10.1) have been dealt with. In the following chapters other drugs acting on the central nervous system (CNS) will be discussed. Although the centrally active agents can affect a variety of CNS functions (such as consciousness, food intake, sex, reward mechanism, motor activity, autonomic controls including cardiovascular functions and respiration, and many others), these chapters will mainly deal with two broad groups of drugs used therapeutically. These include (1) those affecting consciousness and state of excitability, and (2) others affecting mood, emotion, and behavior. The latter group will also include some nontherapeutically used substances such as marijuana and hallucinogens. Before discussing these broad groups, some comments on the mechanisms, and some characteristics of drug actions in the CNS will be made.

MECHANISM OF ACTION

There are many drugs whose molecular mechanisms of action are diverse and sites of action are diffuse and not clearly identifiable. Effects of these drugs may be considered as *nonspecific*. Thus several CNS depressants such as general anesthetics, many sedative-hypnotics, and alcohols depress the excitable brain tissues at many levels by stabilization of neuronal membranes; no definite neurochemical mechanism for these drugs has been elucidated. On the other hand, several centrally acting drugs are known to act at certain target areas and through certain neurochemical or electrophysiological mechanisms. The effect of such drugs can be designated as *specific*. Thus certain neurotransmitters are involved in the mechanism of action of several drugs. As for examples, the CNS stimulants like strychnine and picrotoxin are known to disinhibit the effects of the inhibitory amino acids glycine and γ-aminobutyric acid(GABA),respectively. Reserpine, an antihypertensive alkaloid, produces its effects by depleting various areas of the brain of the biogenic amines such as catecholamines and serotonin. Tricyclic antidepressants (e.g., imipramine) produce their effects by reducing neuronal re-uptake of the biogenic amines (e.g., norepinephrine and serotonin) and thereby enhancing their concentrations as well as by producing anticholinergic effects in the relavant brain areas.

Neurotransmitters acting in the CNS have been discussed in Chapters 6, 9.4, 10, 10.1 and others. In order to facilitate understanding of the mechanism of action of drugs that involve neurotransmitters, as discussed in subsequent chapters, a summary of some physiological, pathological, and pharmacological features of several established central neurotransmitters (e.g., acetylcholine, norepinephrine, dopamine, serotonin, and γ-aminobutyric acid) is presented in Table 11-1.

SOME CHARACTERISTICS OF DRUG ACTIONS IN THE CNS

Because of the restricted permeability through the blood-brain barrier (the lipid-soluble membrane separating the plasma from the interstitial space of the brain), certain systemically administered drugs and substances cannot gain adequate concentration in the brain. Such permeability restriction is much less prominent in the regions of the hypothalamus and several other specialized brain areas (e.g., the median eminence, area postrema, pineal gland, subfornical organ, and subcommissural organ). In addition to macromolecules, selective barrier to permeation exists also for quaternary nitrogen-

Table 11-1
Physiological and Pathological Roles of the Central Neurotransmitters and Their Pharmacological Manipulation

Features	Acetylcholine	Norepinephrine	Dopamine	Serotonin	γ-Aminobutyric acid
Brain areas with high concentration	Striatum, pons, medulla, midbrain, hypothalamus, cortex	Hypothalamus, brainstem	Neostriatum, n. accumbens, olfactory tubercle	Hypothalamus, midbrain, pons, medulla, hippocampus	Substantia nigra, basal ganglia, hypothalamus, midbrain
Pathways in the CNS containing the neurotransmitter	(1) A dorsal tegmental pathway (cuneate n. to tectum, pretectal area, and thalamus); (2) a ventral tegmental pathway (substantia nigra and ventral tegmental area to subthalamus, hypothalamus, and basal forebrain area); (3) a septal pathway (septum to cerebral cortex hippocampus, and midbrain); (4) motoneuron collaterals to Renshaw cells in the spinal cord	(1) A dorsal ascending bundle [locus ceruleus (A6) to hippocampus, cortex, cerebellum]; (2) a ventral ascending bundle [medulla and pons, (A1, A2, and A5) to medulla, pons, in brain, and hypothalamus] (3) a descending pathway [medulla (A1) to lateral column of spinal cord]	(1) A nigrostriatal pathway [substantia nigra (A8 & A9) to caudate n. and globus pallidus]; (2) mesolimbic-mesocortical pathways (A10 area in midbrain) to n. accumbens, amygdala, septum, olfactory tubercle, and frontal entorhinal, cingulate cortex; (3) tuberoinfundibular and tuberohypophyseal pathways (arcuate and periventricular n. of hypothalamus to median eminence and posterior pituitary)	Raphe nuclei to cortex, hippocampus, hypothalamus, and caudate n, also to cerebellum and pontomesencephalic reticular formation	A pathway from globus pallidus to substantia nigra
Physiological function	Control of arousal reaction, motor function, food and water intake, motivated behavior, learning and memory	Control of arousal reaction, mood, reward behavior	Control of motor function, emotion, endocrine secretion, reward behavior, arousal reaction	Control of sleep wakefulness, aggression, sexual behavior	General inhibitory effect in the CNS
Possible pathological implication	Parkinson's disease Huntington's chorea, Alzheimer's disease, Schizophrenia, Depression	Depression	Parkinson's disease, Schizophrenia,	Depression	Epilepsy, Huntington's chorea, Parkinson's disease
Pharmacological manipulation:[a]					
Effect enhanced by	Deanol, choline (P); muscarine, nicotine (RA); physostigmine (CB)	Amphetamine (RE); clonidine (α_2-RA), isoproterenol (β-RA); desipramine (UB); MAO inhibitor (CB)	Levodopa (P); amphetamine (RE); apomorphine, bromocriptine (RA); MAO inhibitor (CB)	Tryptophan, 5-hydroxytryptophan (P); LSD (RA?)[b]; fluoxetine, imipramine (UB)	Musicimol, β-alanine, taurine (RA); amino-oxyacetic acid (CB)
Effect inhibited by	Atropine, scopolamine, trihexyphenidyl (RB)	α-Methyl-p-tyrosine (SB); reserpine (D); phenoxybenzamine (α-RB), propranolol (β-RB)	α-Methyl-p-tyrosine (SB); reserpine (D); γ-hydroxybutyrate (RI)	p-Chlorophenylalanine (SB); reserpine (D); LSD (RB)[b]	Bicuculline, picrotoxin (RD)

[a] Precursor (P); release enhancer (RE); receptor agonist (RA); uptake blocker (UB); catabolism blocker (CB); synthesis blocker (SB); depletor (D); release inhibitor (RI); receptor blocker (RB).

[b] LSD has been shown to act as a receptor blocker as well as a receptor agonist for 5-HT.

containing compounds (e.g., *d*-tubocurarine), penicillin, and even some small charged molecules such as neurotransmitters and their metabolites. Although biogenic amines (like norepinephrine, dopamine, 5-hydroxytryptamine) cannot pass the blood-brain barrier by passive diffusion, their amino acid precursors (e.g., tyrosine, L-DOPA, 5-hydroxytryptophan) can cross the barrier by an active transport system.

Drugs can produce inhibition or stimulation in certain areas of the brain. Stimulation can be achieved either by blockade of an inhibitory process or disinhibition (e.g., convulsions produced by picrotoxin through blockade of action of GABA, an inhibitory amino acid) or by direct stimulation of excitatory neurons (e.g., in the case of pentylenetetrazol). The mechanisms of the neuronal stimulation may differ, depending on the agent, and would include: decreased synaptic recovery time, increased release and duration of action of a neurotransmitter, increased polysynaptic responsiveness, and so forth. An excitatory effect is sometimes observed with low concentrations of certain depressant drugs [e.g., stage of excitation (stage II)] during induction of general anesthesia and "stimulant effects" of ethanol. Increase of their concentration produces uniform gradual depression. Such stimulation is usually considered to be due to depression of inhibitory systems or to a transient increase in the release of excitatory neurotransmitters.

Acute, excessive stimulation of the CNS is usually followed by a depression, as is observed in case of grand mal epilepsy as well as following the administration of high doses of CNS stimulants (e.g., strychnine, pentylenetetrazol). Attempts to inhibit such central stimulation by a general CNS depressant (e.g., pentobarbital) would produce an additive effect on the poststimulation depression; serious adverse effects result from depression of vital medullary centers.

Conversely, although acute drug-induced depression may not result in manifestation of stimulant effects, chronic and repeated administration of CNS depressants (e.g., barbiturates, alcohol) would result in prolonged hyperexcitability on withdrawal of such drugs, thus demonstrating a rebound phenomena (Chapter 11.6).

A centrally acting drug may not act equally at all levels of the CNS. Thus, if the concentration of a general anesthetic (e.g., ether, chloroform) is gradually increased, a progressive, irregularly descending paralysis of the CNS is observed. The cerebral cortex, followed by subcortical centers, is affected first; then the lower part of the spinal cord shows depression; last, the medulla with its vital structures are depressed. Such progressive involvement of different CNS structures is not observed during use of a rapidly acting intravenous anesthetic agent. Furthermore, in the case of convulsant drugs, high doses of different agents are shown to produce different types of convulsions due to their different site of actions. Thus, strychnine produces a tonic type of convulsions by predominantly acting on the spinal cord. Picrotoxin and pentylenetetrazol produce clonic-tonic (predominantly clonic) convulsions by acting mainly on the brainstem. Amphetamine which acts at still higher levels in the CNS (e.g.,cerebral cortex),produces mainly clonic convulsions.

DRUGS AFFECTING CONSCIOUSNESS AND EXCITABILITY

The levels of consciousness and CNS excitability or arousal vary with different physiological states such as drowsiness (in which mental alertness is decreased, but consciousness is not lost) and sleep (in which the subject loses consciousness, but can be aroused by stimuli) and pathological conditions such as coma (i.e., a state of unconsciousness from which the subject cannot be aroused by stimuli). These states can at least superficially be reproduced by drug actions, although their mechanisms may differ. Thus, drugs can act as sedatives (producing sedation), hypnotics (inducing sleep), and anesthetics (producing a state of unconsciousness from which the subject cannot be aroused by stimuli). Sometimes the same drug can produce all these stages depending on the dose.

The changes in the CNS excitability are reflected in two processes, brain electrical activity or electroencephalogram (EEG) and skeletal muscle activity (tone and contraction), which serve as good indicators. Thus, with the decrease in levels of consciousness and excitability, the EEG changes from desynchronization to synchronization; muscle tone usually shows gradual decrease. There are, however, some exceptions to this generalization. The effects of hypnotics are compared only with the slow-wave phase of sleep, since during paradoxical (or rapid eye movement, REM) sleep, EEG desynchronization is observed although there is marked hypotonia of the neck muscle. Furthermore, during induction of general anesthesia, excitability and muscle tone increase during the second stage, followed by their gradual decreases.

On the other hand, the level of CNS excitability may be enhanced from mild excitement and restlessness to manic or hypomanic (mild-to-moderate mania) episodes. CNS stimulants like amphetamine can cause euphoria,restlessness, and excitement. With increase of dose,excitement may be increased, and at still higher doses convulsions and psychosis may occur. At high doses, pentylenetetrazol, picrotoxin, and strychnine may produce convulsions. EEG would show desynchronization and, during convulsions, high-amplitude spikes appear.

The reticular activating system (RAS) is involved in the actions of CNS depressants and stimulants.

DRUGS AFFECTING MOOD, EMOTION, AND BEHAVIOR

Mood, emotion, and behavior are modified by certain substances used for nontherapeutic purposes as well as by therapeutic agents. Thus, cocaine and amphetamine can produce elevation of mood, euphoria and, on prolonged use and repeated and high doses, psychosis. Lysergic acid diethylamide (LSD), phencyclidine (PCP), and mescaline induce various types of hallucinations and other psychotic manifestations. On the other hand, antipsychotic agents (e.g., chlorpromazine, haloperidol, etc.) are used to treat psychotic disorders affecting mood, emotion, and behavior as well as chemically induced psychotic manifestations, if required. Reserpine, historically used as an effective antipsychotic agent, produces serious mental depression,which led to its limited therapeutic use (except as an antihypertensive agent). Elevation of mood in depressed patients is achieved by tricyclic antidepressants (e.g., imipramine, amitriptyline, and others). Excessive excitement (manic or hypomanic condition) can be produced by high doses of amphetamine or cocaine. Lithium salts are used for treatment of manic or hypomanic patients; in acute mania haloperidol or chlorpromazine is used.

Although these drugs may act on various sites in the CNS, the limbic structures appear to be mainly affected in most of the situations. The exact mechanisms of action of the agents producing or inhibiting these psychiatric disorders are not known. However, in many cases, roles of neurochemicals, particularly neurotransmitters, have been implicated through certain direct or indirect evidence. Thus, drugs used in the treatment of depression, such as tricyclic antidepressants and monoamine oxidase (MAO) inhibitors, act by elevating the levels of biogenic amines with or without decreasing the activity of acetylcholine in the CNS. This and other evidences have been the basis for the aminergic hypothesis of depression (Chapter 11.5). Furthermore, the neuroleptic drugs used in the therapy of schizophrenia are known to act mainly by blocking the dopaminergic effects at the receptor sites in the mesolimbic, mesocortical, and other central dopaminergic pathways. This indirect therapeutic evidence has led to the proposition of a dopaminergic theory of schizophrenia, although no clear dopaminergic hyperactivity has been demonstrated in this disorder (Chapter 11.5). It appears that many psychiatric (as also in neurological) disorders may be the result of a derangement of the function of one or more central neurotransmitters resulting in the imbalance of a multitransmitter system participating in maintenance of the physiological function. The effective therapeutic agent(s) attempts to rectify the imbalance and normalize the function.

CHAPTER
11.1

GENERAL ANESTHETICS

Raghubar Badola, Paul A. Radnay and Deryck Duncalf

General anesthesia is a state of drug-induced loss of consciousness whereby surgical procedures can be carried out painlessly. Inhalation anesthetic agents were the first to be used for the production of general anesthesia. Later added to the anesthesiologists' armamentarium were the intravenous agents, which offered the promise of greater specificity and fewer undesirable side effects. Inhalation anesthetics have the advantage of relatively greater controllability; with flammable agents, however, the risk of explosion is considered by many to be an unacceptable hazard and electronic devices frequently preclude their use. The use of flammable anesthetics has thus declined to a vanishing point in the United States (12).

Despite the introduction of many newer agents into the field, an ideal anesthetic agent or a combination of agents is still lacking.

HISTORY

Control of pain during surgical operations has been a pressing problem for humankind; hence, it is remarkable that many chemicals with anesthetic properties were known long before they were tried for surgical anesthesia. It was not until the 1840s, in fact, that ether and nitrous oxide were first used for that purpose.

Some important landmarks in clinical anesthesia include the following:

1803: Morphine isolated by Sertürner.
1844: Wells attempted unsuccessfully to demonstrate the use of nitrous oxide as a surgical anesthetic.
1846: Morton successfully demonstrated in Massachusetts General Hospital the use of ether as a general anesthetic.
1847: Simpson introduced chloroform.
1868: Andrews of Chicago combined oxygen with nitrous oxide.
1872: Clover introduced the nitrous oxide/ether sequence.
1934: Waters introduced cyclopropane.
Waters and Lundy introduced thiopental sodium.
1939: Meperidine synthesized by Schaumann and Eisleb.
1941: Steroid anesthetics described by Selye.
1956: Johnstone introduced halothane.
1959: DeCastro and Mundeleer introduced neurolept analgesia.
1960: Artuso introduced methoxyflurane.
1962: Fentanyl was first introduced by Janssen.
1963: Enflurane synthesized by Terrell.
Droperidol synthesized by Janssen.
1965: Isoflurane synthesized by Terrell.

1966: Ketamine was first used by Corssen and Domino.
1980: Isoflurane approved by U.S. Food and Drug Administration for use in clinical practice.

THEORIES OF MECHANISM OF ACTION

The general anesthetic agents are known to act on the reticular-activating system, cerebral cortex, and spinal cord. Large nerve fibers are resistant to the action of anesthetics; the site of action is therefore likely to be the synaptic region, or the nerve terminals. Anesthetics do not act at a specific receptor site in the cell. This is suggested by the diversity in chemical structure of anesthetics ranging from xenon, nitrous oxide, to halothane and isoflurane.

The exact mechanism of action of the anesthetic agents is not clearly known. However, some generalizations have been made. At the cellular level (33), anesthesia is produced by some physical change or a short-term biochemical event. This is inferred because anesthesia can be induced rapidly and recovery from it can be equally rapid. Because of a lack of precise mechanism of their action, several widely different theories have been proposed from time to time to explain the anesthetic action. Some of them follow:

Lipid Theory. Meyer and Overton proposed that anesthetic action was a function of lipid solubility within the cell (45). The products of maximum alveolar concentration (MAC) and its oil/gas partition coefficient varies less than 2-fold over a 70,000-fold range of anesthetic partial pressures (66).

Because of this strong correlation between anesthetic potency and their solubility in lipids, it has been reasoned that general anesthetics interact with either the lipid bilayer of the cell membrane, or the hydrophobic regions of essential proteins within the cell membrane, or both.

Critical-Volume Theory. The critical-volume theory offers a physical mechanism for the lipid theory in that for induction of anesthesia a critical molar-volume fraction of an inert substance must be attained in membranes (52). This would expand biological membranes causing compression of ionic channels or the proteins binding it; thereby modifying ionic exchange or transmitter release. This theory offers an explanation for pressure reversal of anesthesia. High pressure (100 atmospheres or over) can reverse the action of anesthetics in certain bacteria and animals (47). It is proposed that high pressure reverses the expansion of the membrane caused by anesthetics. The degree of reversal of anesthetic action by pressure varies between anesthetics; this suggests multiple hydrophobic sites where anesthetics produce expansion.

Protein Conformational Change Theory (18). The protein conformational change theory is based on the premise that anesthetics inactivate the lipoproteins of cell membranes. It presupposes that the lipid-soluble anesthetics will have an affinity for the hydrophobic regions of these proteins. Thus, it is a variant of the critical-volume theory.

Lateral-Phase Separation Theory (68). Anesthetics act by dissolving in membrane lipids causing an increase in membrane fluidity and volume and a decrease in compressibility. This restricts the mobility of the protein molecules surrounding ionic pores. The protein molecules are not able to expand, and the ionic pores remain closed. This interferes with the ionic exchange, which in turn affects nerve transmission or the release of a transmitter.

Aqueous-Phase Theories. Pauling, invoking gas hydrate (53), and Miller, et al. basing their assumption on the "iceberg effect" (48) postulated that anesthetic molecules form hydrated microcrystals or clathrates that can interfere with neuronal excitability. However, recent studies have shown very poor correlations between hydrate formation and potency of inhalation anesthetics.

Microtubule Theory (1). The microtubule theory of anesthetic action proposes that reversible depolymerization of microtubules in nerve cells occurs.

STAGES AND PLANES OF ANESTHESIA

Classic Concepts. Anesthetic agents cause dose-related depression of vital functions. Likewise, the incidence of untoward side effects is dose-related. On the other hand, inadequate anesthesia may not provide appropriate surgical conditions, and under these circumstances surgical stimulation can provoke undesirable reflexes.

Certain signs can be identified that serve as landmarks of anesthetic depth. Snow recognized that ether anesthesia has clearly identifiable stages and planes. Guedel (22) deserves credit for much of the currently accepted classification of stages of ether anesthesia, shown in Fig. 11.1-1.

There are four stages of anesthesia discussed next.

I. ***Stage of Analgesia.*** The analgesia stage extends from the beginning of induction to loss of consciousness. Artusio has divided this stage into three planes. In the third plane, the patient is analgesic, amnesic, and cooperative. This stage of analgesia is better demonstrated during recovery from deeper stages of ether anesthesia. The eyelash reflex is abolished with the loss of consciousness.

II. ***Stage of Excitement or Uninhibited Response.*** The stage of excitement or uninhibited response extends from the loss of consciousness to the onset of automatic respiration. The skeletal muscle tone increases. There may be breath holding, struggling, or vomiting. Pupils dilate due to sympathetic stimulation. These undesirable effects can be minimized by preoperative psychological preparation, adequate premedication, and rapid smooth induction. The eyelid reflex is absent.

III. ***Stage of Surgical Anesthesia.*** This stage extends from onset of automatic respiration to respiratory paralysis. With the onset of automatic respiration and loss of the eyelid reflex, the anesthetic stage is set for surgical procedures. This stage, the stage of surgical anesthesia as it is called, has been induced by the processes occurring in stages I and II, which together are therefore called the induction period. The third stage is divided into four planes.

Plane 1. Plane 1 extends from the onset of automatic respiration to cessation of eyeball movement. The eyeballs move from side to side or may be fixed in an up or down position. The pupils are normal in size and react to light. Breathing is deep and regular. The conjunctival reflex is absent.

Plane 2. Plane 2 extends from the cessation of eyeball movement to commencement of intercostal paralysis. The depth of breathing is less than in plane 1, but intercostal and diaphragmatic breathing are synchronous. The corneal reflex is abolished.

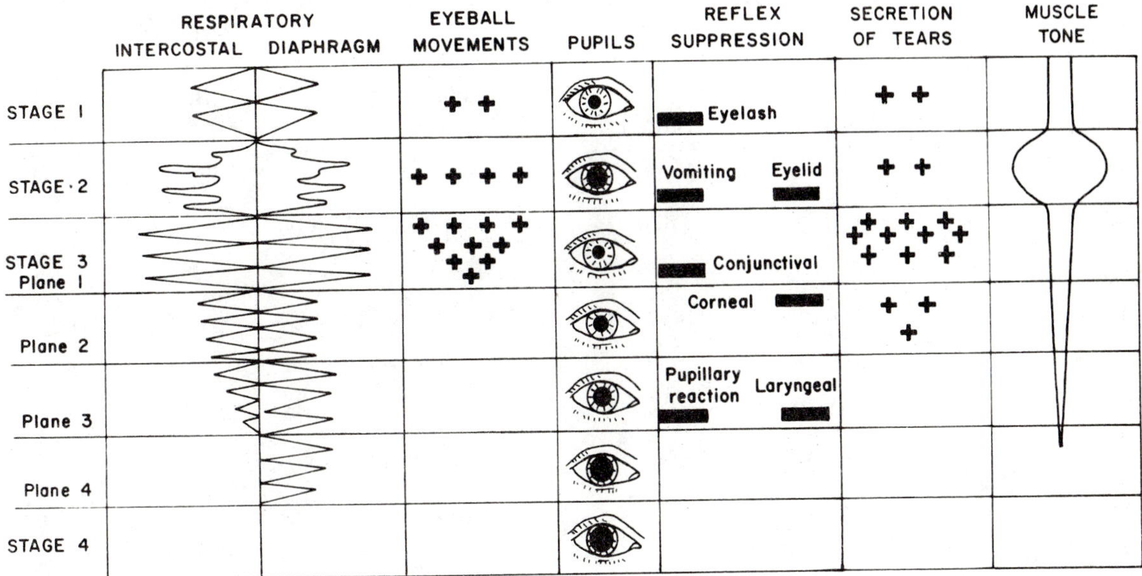

Fig. 11.1-1. *Signs and reflex reactions of the stages and planes of anesthesia.*

The wedge-shaped areas indicate the variability in disappearence of signs and reflexes in several planes of anesthesia depending on the person, anesthetic used, and other factors.

Plane 3. Plane 3 extends from the commencement to completion of intercostal paralysis. The chest lags behind the abdomen during inspiration. Diaphragmatic activity is increased. The tidal volume is reduced. The pupillary reflex for light is abolished, and the pupils are moderately dilated.

Plane 4. Plane 4 extends from complete intercostal paralysis to diaphragmatic paralysis. During inspiration, only the diaphragm moves, pushing the abdominal wall forward, and there is retraction of the chest wall and intercostal spaces. During expiration the diaphragm relaxes, the abdomen descends, and the chest wall resumes its normal position (the chest wall and abdomen move in opposite directions). This type of breathing is called *external paradoxical respiration.* Ventilation is inadequate and requires assistance. The pupils are dilated and do not react to light.

IV. ***Stage of Medullary Paralysis.*** The stage of medullary paralysis extends from the onset of diaphragmatic paralysis to cardiovascular collapse. This is the stage of overdose and should be corrected at once by discontinuing anesthesia and instituting artificial ventilation. With elimination of ether into the expired air, anesthesia will lighten and patient will recover. If cardiac arrest occurs, external cardiac massage and full cardiorespiratory resuscitation must be instituted.

Limitations and Modifications. The signs characteristic of stages of anesthesia with other agents may differ from those caused by ether. For example, halothane fails to enlarge the pupils with increasing depth. With the intravenous agents, the picture is more complex. For example, barbiturates given intravenously may produce respiratory arrest even during light anesthesia, and the patient may move in response to surgical stimulation. Moreover, the concomitant use of muscle relaxants may obscure these signs.

Neurophysiological Basis. The reticular formation in the brain stem is a multineuronal system that is intimately connected with wakefulness. It not only innervates the spinal and bulbar neurons and controls posture and movement, but also modulates the activities of the cerebral cortex. Collaterals from the sensory afferent pathways excite the brain stem reticular formations which in turn activates the cerebral cortex through nerve fibers originating in the nonspecific thalamic (midline, intralaminar, and other) nuclei and spreading diffusely throughout the cerebral cortex (so-called thalamocortical projections). The interaction of cerebral cortex with the reticular-activating system via thalamocortical projections seems to be responsible for wakefulness, alertness, and arousal.

General anesthetics block the electroencephalogram (EEG) arousal response to high-frequency reticular stimulation or to a noxious stimulus, and the subject remains unconscious, although impulses may still be conducted along the lemniscal pathways and excite the neurons in the sensory cortex. This depression of reactive capability of reticular formation by general anesthetics has been considered a neural basis of anesthesia (39).

Depression of the reticular-activating system may not be the sole mechanism of anesthetic state. Some anesthetics such as enflurane and ketamine produce marked enhancement of EEG response in the reticular formation in the presence of deep anesthesia (49).

Anesthetics seem to act on various central nervous system areas including the spinal cord (30). Halothane suppresses response in neurons in Rexed's lamina IV in the dorsal horn. Nitrous oxide depresses lamina V. Ketamine and narcotics suppress spontaneous unit activity in Rexed's laminae I and V,

Table 11.1-1
Physical and Chemical Characteristics of Inhalation Anesthetic Agents

Agent	Molecular Formula	Vapor Pressure at 20°C (mmHg)	Flammability Volume (%)	Partition Coefficients At 37°C Blood/Gas	Oil/Gas	MAC (%) V/V
Nitrous Oxide	N_2O	38,760	Nonflammable	0.47	1.4	105
Cyclopropane	C_3H_6	4,800	Air 2.4-10.4; $O_2$2.5-60	1.4-0.6	11.8	9.2
Ethylene	C_2H_4	—	Air 3.1-32; O_2 3-80	0.41	1.3	67
Diethyl Ether	$(C_2H_5)_2O$	442	Air 1.9-48; O_2 2-82	12.1	65	1.92
Divinyl Ether	$(C_2H_3)_2O$	553	Air 1.7-27; O_2 1.8-85	2.8	58	a
Ethyl Chloride	C_2H_5Cl	988	Air 3.8-15.4; O_2 4-67	3	a	a
Fluroxene	CF_3CH_2-O-C_2H_3	286	Air 3.1-32; $O_2$4.5-80	1.37	47.7	3.4
Chloroform	$CHCl_3$	160	Nonflammable	8.4	394	a
Trichlorethylene	CCl_2=CHCl	65	Air nonflammable O_2 10-65	9.2	960	a
Halothane	$CF_3CHClBr$	243	Nonflammable	2.3	224	0.75
Methoxyflurane	CH_3-O-CF_2CHCl_2	23	Nonflammable	12	970	0.16
Enflurane	CHF_2-O-CF_2CHFCl	175	Nonflammable	1.9	98	1.68
Isoflurane	CHF_2-O-$CHClCF_3$	238	Nonflammable	1.41	98	1.15

[a]Not known in humans.

that are known to respond principally to noxious stimuli. This may explain partly the analgesic action of ketamine.

Barbiturates depress or block monosynaptic reflex response in the cat spinal cord without interfering with the conduction of nerve impulses along sensory or motor nerve fibers. There is depression of excitatory postsynaptic potential. There is also a decrease in the release of transmitter from the afferent nerve terminals.

The precise location of the site of anesthetic action responsible for production of general anesthesia is not determined.

QUANTITATION OF ANESTHETIC POTENCY

Snow determined minimum inspired concentrations of ether and chloroform that produce general anesthesia. Eger and his colleagues later put this approach on a sounder basis by substituting alveolar for inspired concentration (15) and introduced the concept of *minimum alveolar concentration* (MAC), which is defined as the minimum alveolar concentration of an anesthetic at 1 atmosphere pressure that produces immobility in 50% of patients or animals (ED_{50}) exposed to noxious stimuli (see Table 11.1-1). It is a measure of anesthetic potency. (Potency is inversely proportional to the partial pressure of an agent to achieve a given anesthetic effect).

MAC has become established as an index of potency and as a reliable guide to the depth of anesthesia, because the end point of abolition of movement in response to a noxious stimulus is an important landmark in anesthetic depth and is equally applicable to all inhalation anesthetics.

Partial pressure of an inhalation anesthetic in the alveoli, arterial blood, and at its site of action in the CNS reaches the same value if sufficient time is allowed for equilibration. Consequently, at this point MAC equals partial pressure of the anesthetic at its site of action in the CNS.

The value of MAC is unaffected by the intensity of surgical stimuli, duration of administration of anesthesia or variation in patients' sex. Similarly changes in blood acid or base, carbon dioxide, oxygen tension, anemia, and blood pressure over a wide range from normal do not alter MAC.

MAC decreases with age. Hypothermia reduced MAC for all agents. The inhalational agents' effect on MAC is additive (e.g. half MAC of N_2O and half MAC of halothane equals 1 MAC of either halothane or nitrous oxide). Depletion of central catecholamines reduces MAC value, whereas an increase has the opposite effect.

UPTAKE AND DISTRIBUTION OF INHALATION ANESTHETICS

During induction of inhalation anesthesia, the partial pressure in the inspired gases is higher than the alveolar partial pressure. In a relatively short period of time, the partial pressure of the inhalation anesthetic in the alveoli is equal to the partial pressure in the arterial blood, and that in turn comes rapidly in equilibrium to that in the brain because of the high blood flow to the brain.

Alveolar anesthetic partial pressure is therefore assumed to be equal to brain anesthetic partial pressure that determines the depth of anesthesia. Factors that affect alveolar anesthetic partial pressure indirectly affect the partial pressure of anesthetic in the brain. The process of equilibration of the partial pressure of the anesthetic between the inspired air and the brain during induction can be discussed in the following steps: (1) equilibrium of the partial pressure in the inspired air and the alveoli, (2) uptake of the anesthetic in the blood, and (3) uptake in the tissue (including brain).

(1) **Equilibration of the Partial Pressures in the Inspired Air and the Alveoli.** On induction of anesthesia, the partial pressure of the anesthetic in the inspired gas is higher than that of the alveoli. The rate at which the alveolar concentration rises toward the concentration in inspired gases is directly proportional to the alveolar ventilation (Fig. 11.1-2A) and inspired concentration of the anesthetic gas, and inversely to the functional residual capacity of the lung and the uptake of the anesthetic by blood. If no anesthetic were to leave the lungs to enter the blood, the rate of rise of alveolar partial pressure toward the inspired concentration would be very rapid, and in a relatively short period of time the partial pressure of the anesthetic in the alveoli would equal the inspired concentration. However, the rate of rise of anesthetic alveolar partial pressure is slowed by anesthetic uptake into the blood, and the rate of rise of alveolar partial pressure toward the inspired concentration is a balance between the input of ventilation and uptake into the blood.

Input of an anesthetic in the alveoli is also influenced by the following.

(a) Concentration effect. The partial pressure of the anesthetic in the alveoli rises rapidly, if the inspired concentration is high. This is known as the *concentration effect* (14) (Fig. 11.1-2B).

(b) Second gas effect. Uptake of large volumes of first or primary gas (usually nitrous oxide) accelerates the alveolar rise of a second gas given concomitantly. This is called *second gas effect* (17). Two mechanisms are involved:

(i) *Increase in inspired ventilation.* In the first few minutes of anesthesia large volumes of nitrous oxide are taken up from the alveoli by the pulmonary capillary circulation. This results in a net increase in inspired ventilation, thus accelerating the alveolar concentration of all other vapors or gases administered simultaneously (second gas) to rise toward their inspired concentration.

(ii) *Concentrating effect.* Uptake of large volumes of primary gas (nitrous oxide) from the lungs reduces the total volume of gases in the lung (64). This increases the concentration of the remaining gases including that of the second gas. Lung volume is restored by inspiring more gas mixture. Concentrating effect plays a greater role when uptake of second gas is small, while increase in ventilation plays greater role in raising the concentration of a soluble second gas. For the second gas effect to occur, there must be a high concentration of anesthetic in the inspired gas, and in practice, this is seen only with nitrous oxide.

(2) **Uptake of the Anesthetic in the Blood.** The rate of uptake into the blood is determined by: (a) blood solubility of the anesthetic, (b) cardiac output, and (c) anesthetic partial pressure gradient between the alveoli and pulmonary capillaries, that is, the venous blood returning to the lungs.

Blood solubility, or *blood/gas partition coefficient*, may be defined as the ratio of concentration of an anesthetic between the blood and gas phases when the partial pressure between the two phases is equal. The high blood solubility delays the rate of rise of the alveolar partial pressure of the anesthetic (Fig. 11.1-2C), causing slow induction and slow recovery.

An increase in cardiac output has the effect of exposing alveolar gas to a greater amount of blood in a unit time. Anesthetic uptake is accelerated and the rate of rise of anesthetic partial pressure in the alveoli is decreased, thus slowing the induction of anesthesia (Fig. 11.1-2D).

The third factor is the concentration gradient between the alveolus and returning venous blood. The greater the gradient between the two phases, the greater is the uptake into blood and the slower the rate of rise in alveolar concentration.

Anesthetic agent with low blood solubility will have smaller uptake in blood, and its alveolar concentration will rise rapidly. Any change in the cardiac output and minute ventilation will have minimal effect in hastening the onset of anesthesia. On the other hand, when the solubility in the blood is high, a decrease in ventilation or an increase in the cardiac output will considerably prolong the induction of anesthesia and vice versa.

Uptake in the Tissues (including brain). Tissue uptake of an anesthetic is dependent upon the *tissue/blood solubility coefficient* (ratio of concentration of anesthetic between tissue and blood when the partial pressure between the two phases is equal), the tissue size, the blood flow to the tissues, and the arterial blood-to-tissue partial pressure difference.

The higher the tissue solubility, the greater the removal of anesthetic from the blood, hence the lower the partial pressure in returning venous blood and the higher the uptake from alveoli. Tissue capacity is equal to the tissue/blood partition coefficient times the mass of the tissue. The rate of saturation of the tissue is dependent on the ratio of capacity to blood flow.

The vessel-rich group (VRG), the muscle group (MG), and the vessel-poor group (VPG) of tissues have similar tissue/blood partition coefficients, but very different blood flows per unit volume of tissues.

VRG, which includes the brain, heart, kidneys, liver, splanchnic bed, and the endocrine glands, is rapidly saturated with anesthetic because of high blood flow relative to capacity. It ceases removing appreciable volumes of anesthetic in 5 to 15 minutes after induction.

Muscle and skin, which form the MG, equilibrate slower because MG blood flow (liters/kilogram/minute) is about one-twenty-second VRG blood flow.

Although perfusion per unit volume of fat (FG) is very close to MG, saturation of FG never takes place clinically because of the high fat/blood partition coefficient and the far greater capacity of the fats for the anesthetics. VPG includes ligaments, bones, and cartilages, has very poor blood supply, and does not clinically affect the uptake and distribution of anesthetics.

Diffusion of Nitrous Oxide into Air-Containing Spaces in the Body. Nitrous oxide is 34 times more soluble in blood than nitrogen. Thus, nitrous oxide diffuses into closed air (gas) spaces rapidly, even before nitrogen can leave these spaces. This rapid surge of nitrous oxide increases the pressure and/or

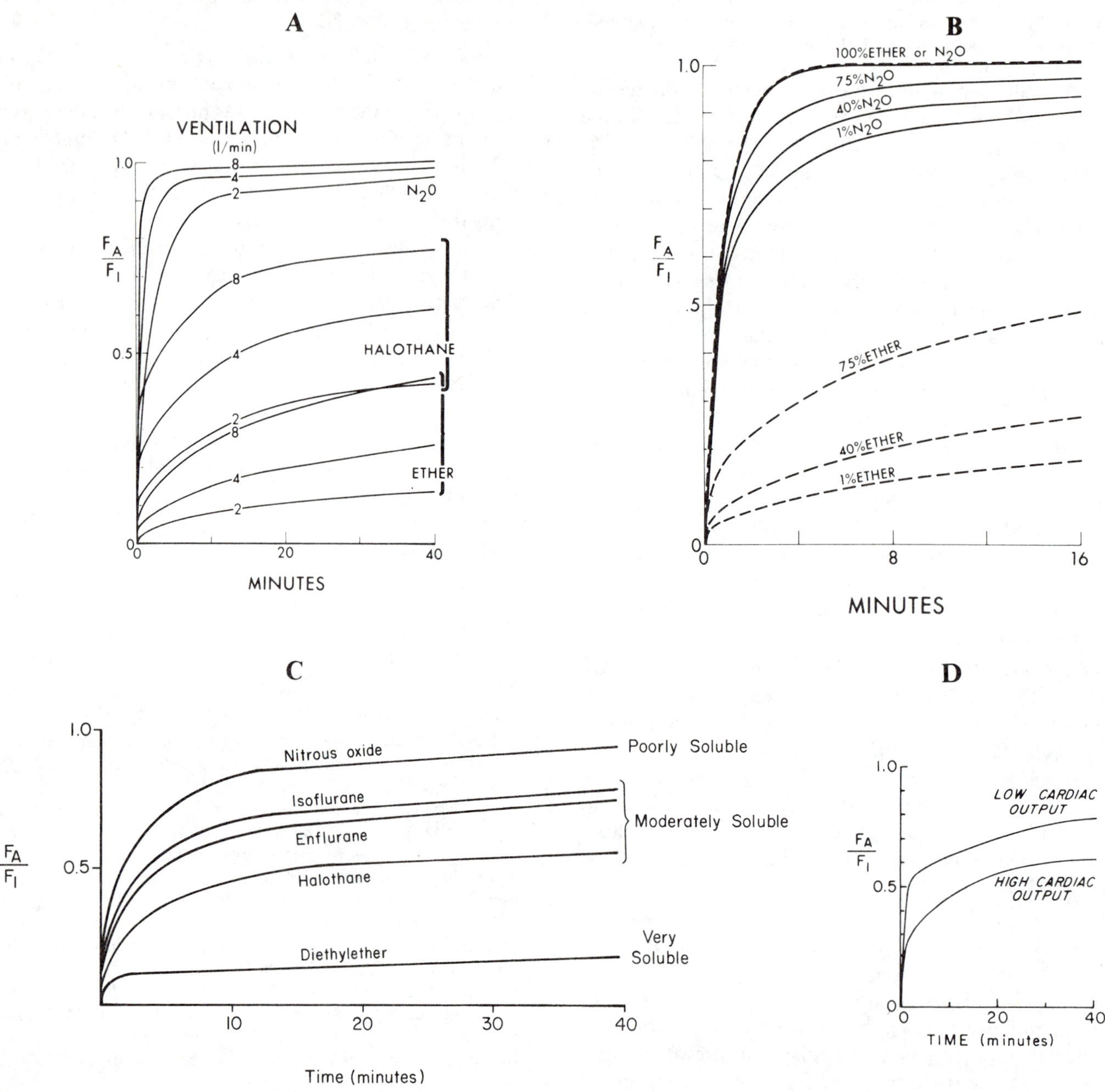

Fig. 11.1-2. *Factors influencing the rate of rise of alveolar concentration of an anesthetic.* F_A/F_I represents alveolar to inspired concentration ratio.

A. Effect of ventilation. Increase in the alveolar ventilation from 2 to 4 to 8 liters/min accelerates the rise in alveolar concentration of the anesthetic.

B. Effect of inspired concentration of the anesthetic. Alveolar concentration rises more rapidly towards inspired concentration, if concentration of the inspired gas is increased. (Both A and B from Ref. 15, by permission).

C. Influence of solubility. The increase of the ratio of the alveolar (F_A) to the inspired (F_I) concentration varies inversely with solubility in the blood. The increase is relatively rapid for insoluble gases compared with those that are more soluble. (Modified from Ref. 73).

D. Effect of cardiac output. Increase in cardiac output slows down the rate of rise of alveolar anesthetic concentration. (From Ref. 73, by permission).

volume of these spaces.

Pneumothorax and noncommunicating emphysematous bullae may rapidly enlarge in size when nitrous oxide is being used, causing respiratory and circulatory embarrassment. Bullae may rupture, producing pneumothorax and air embolism.

In cases of intestinal obstruction, nitrous oxide can increase the distension of bowels containing air.

The sinuses and middle ear have noncompliant walls. Thus, there is a rise in pressure if their outlets are blocked. Tympanic membrane grafts tend to be disrupted by the increase in middle ear pressure when nitrous oxide is used.

Air is usually injected to outline the ventricles during pneumoencephalography. If this procedure is done under nitrous oxide anesthesia, the volume of gases in the ventricles expands with a rise in intracranial pressure.

Diffusion Hypoxia with Nitrous Oxide Anesthesia (19). At the end of anesthesia, nitrous oxide and oxygen are discontinued and the patient is allowed to breathe room air. In 2 to 3 minutes the blood oxygen saturation falls and then returns to normal in the next 2 to 3 minutes. This is explained by the dilution of alveolar oxygen by the outpouring of a large volume of nitrous oxide into the lungs from the circulation. This dilutes not only the oxygen but also the carbon dioxide in the alveoli with a resultant fall in arterial oxygen and carbon dioxide tension. Oxygen percentage in the alveoli may fall as low as 10%. The fall in the carbon dioxide tension potentiates the respiratory depression due to drugs administered during anesthesia. As a result hypoventilation or apnea may occur. It is therefore advisable to administer oxygen for about 5 minutes after discontinuing nitrous oxide.

Elimination. Anesthesia is usually terminated long before the VPG and FG tissues equilibrate with the alveolar partial pressure.

With each breath, anesthetic is eliminated from the lungs, and the alveolar concentration falls; there is a corresponding fall in the arterial blood and brain (VRG) tension. Muscle group tension falls more slowly because of poorer blood supply, and fat and VPG take the longest time to eliminate the anesthetic because of high solubility of the anesthetic in the former (fat) and very poor blood supply in the latter.

Consciousness is regained when anesthetic tension in the brain falls below a critical level. Slow elimination of anesthetic from muscle and fat accounts for the drowsiness and hangover lasting for hours in the postoperative period. Recovery from inhalational anesthesia can be accelerated by an increase in cardiac output and ventilation.

Metabolic Degradation. Inhalation anesthetics have classically been considered inert in their properties, undergoing no chemical change in the body and being excreted unchanged mainly from the lungs. A small amount of unchanged anesthetic appears in sweat, urine, and other secretions. However, using radioactive isotopes of volatile anesthetics (19), it has been demonstrated that halothane, ether, chloroform, and methoxyflurane are biodegraded.

The liver is the principal site of metabolism of anesthetics. The microsomal cytochrome P-450 enzyme system is mainly responsible for the biotransformation reactions. The main pathways involve dehalogenation, ether cleavage, and conjugation.

Biodegradation of anesthetics begins with the uptake of anesthetic into the body and continues until the agent is completely eliminated from the body. Anesthetics are largely exhaled unchanged via the lungs. A small fraction is changed to volatile metabolites that are also eliminated from the lungs. A large proportion of anesthetic metabolism results in the formation of nonvolatile compounds that are excreted in urine, bile, and feces over a period of days to weeks. Anesthetics with high lipid solubility tend to concentrate in the fat depots, from which they are released slowly into the bloodstream to be metabolized and excreted.

TOXICITY OF TRACE ANESTHETIC CONCENTRATION

The epidemiological data provide evidence of a moderate increase in the risk of spontaneous abortion in exposed females, and higher incidence of congenital abnormalities in children of anesthetists working during pregnancy. These conclusions have been questioned because of flaws in design of the studies (11). Until a direct cause and effect relationship for any hazardous effect of anesthetics is obtained through appropriate surveys, concentration of anesthetics in the operating room atmosphere should be kept below a certain minimum (25 parts per million for nitrous oxide and 0.5 parts per million for halothane). However, in order to safeguard against any possible hazard, modern operating rooms have provisions for scavanging waste anesthetic agents.

PREMEDICATION

Drugs are used before the administration of anesthesia with the following objectives: (1) to allay the anxiety of the patient by producing sedation, tranquility, and amnesia, without undue depression, and (2) to decrease hazards associated with the anesthesia and operation.

Premedication is used to help facilitate smooth induction of anesthesia, reduce excessive salivary and bronchial secretions, reduce vagal slowing of the heart, prevent postoperative nausea and vomiting, and help relieve pain, if present in the pre- and postoperative period.

More than one drug is usually required to achieve the desired effects. Anticholinergics are used to block the vagal slowing of the heart and to dry secretions in the respiratory and gastrointestinal tracts. Other objectives are attempted with a wide variety of sedatives, hypnotics, tranquilizers, narcotics, and antiemetics.

Drugs alone are not enough to abolish anxiety. A preoperative visit by the anesthetist to explain the related problems and provide reassurance is more helpful than drugs to relieve anxiety, although a combination of preoperative visit and premedicant drugs is complementary and produces the lowest incidence of anxiety.

The choice of drugs and their dosage for premedication should be decided on an individual basis, although each age group has its own requirements.

Adequate preoperative sedation is particularly important in children, where separation from parents, unfamiliarity of surroundings, and anticipation of pain can produce anxiety that may make anesthesia difficult. Vagal reflexes are brisk in children, and anticholinergics are prescribed to avoid reflex slowing of the heart. Anticholinergics should be avoided if the child has fever. Oral route of premedication is desirable in children when the psychological advantages offered by the premedication will not be offset by the trauma associated with an intramuscular injection (9).

Premedication in adults is used to relieve anxiety in the preanesthetic period. These objectives can be achieved by administering drugs intravenously just prior to or during anesthesia.

Elderly patients have increased sensitivity to sedatives and narcotics. Drug metabolism is reduced in the elderly. Starvation and protein depletion and declining levels of estrogens could account for decreased rate of drug biotransformation. Elderly patients may be receiving a wide variety of therapeutic agents; thus, there are more chances of drug interaction and enzyme induction. The sensitivity of the heart to anticholinergics is diminished in old age. Arterial oxygen tension declines linearly with age, and oxygen supply to the vital organs may be borderline. Sedatives and narcotics should be given with discretion, and smaller doses should be prescribed to avoid respiratory and cardiovascular depression.

DRUGS COMMONLY USED IN PREMEDICATION

Barbiturates. As premedicants, barbiturates in therapeutic doses act mainly as sedatives, with minimal effects on respiration or blood pressure. For this purpose, 50 to 150 mg of pentobarbital may be given in adults by the intramuscular route. In children from 1 to 10 years of age, it is usually prescribed as 2 to 3 mg/kg intramuscular, 90 minutes preoperatively. Barbiturates are painful on injection due to the solvent glycol in the solution.

Benzodiazepines. Benzodiazepines are frequently used for premedication by oral or intramuscular routes. They produce dose-related cerebral depression, and effects vary from tranquility, anterograde amnesia, sedation, or drowsiness to actual anesthesia. They are best given 60 to 90 minutes before operation. Diazepam is the most commonly used drug. Dose is 5 to 10 mg by oral or intramuscular route.

Lorazepam is also used because it has excellent anterograde amnesic effect and long duration of action.

Narcotic Analgesics. Narcotic analgesics are usually prescribed in premedication with barbiturates or nonbarbiturate hypnotics to diminish the requirement of potent anesthetics, reduce rapid shallow breathing produced by halogenated inhalation anesthetics, and provide some analgesia in the recovery phase of anesthesia. The dose of morphine is 0.1 to 0.2 mg/kg i.m; of meperidine 1 to 2 mg/kg i.m. given 60 minutes preoperatively.

All narcotics may depress respiration and, if given in large doses, cause hypoxia and may prolong the uptake of anesthetic gases. Postural hypotension and fainting can follow a head-up tilt. Nausea and vomiting can occur.

Narcotics are unsuitable drugs to use for the outpatient because recovery from anesthesia may be prolonged.

Anticholinergics. Atropine is the drug of choice to prevent or treat reflex slowing of the heart during anesthesia. The usual pediatric dose is 0.02 mg/kg i.m., 30 minutes preoperatively. The adult dose is 0.4 to 0.6 mg i.m.

Scopolamine is a good sedative and produces retrograde amnesia. It is a more effective drying agent for secretions than atropine; but less effective as a vagolytic agent. The dose range from 0.005 to 0.01 mg/kg i.m., 1 hour preoperatively. Scopolamine can cause disorientation and restlessness, especially in the elderly, but this action can be reversed by intravenous administration of physostigmine in 1 mg increments to a total of 3 mg.

Glycopyrrolate is a quaternary ammonium compound and unlike hyoscine and atropine does not cross the blood-brain barrier; hence, it does not produce central sedation or postoperative delirium. Its duration of action is longer than that of atropine. It also reduces gastric secretions and acidity. Tachycardia is less pronounced than with atropine.

Anticholinergics are not prescribed routinely in the preoperative medication, because secretions are no longer a major problem as they were when ether and cyclopropane were in use. It is better to give the drug intravenously as the need arises. Unpleasant dry mouth and tachycardia in the preoperative period are thus avoided.

Anticholinergics should be avoided in thyrotoxicosis and tachycardia and in children with fever or in hot climate. Heat loss is greatly interfered with because of abolition of sweating by anticholinergics, causing a further rise in temperature, metabolism, and tachycardia.

Oral administration of the following combination of drugs in an elixir to children for outpatient anesthesia has been found to be predictable in its action without any apparent side effects (9). It consists of the following mixture: meperidine (1.50 mg/kg), diazepam (0.20 mg/kg), and atropine (0.02 mg/kg). The onset of action is within 10 minutes. Premedicated children exhibited less crying and less secretions, and their gastric pH was >6.

INDIVIDUAL GENERAL ANESTHETICS

Several commonly used general anesthetics with their chemical structures are presented in Fig. 11.1-3.

NITROUS OXIDE

Physical Properties. Nitrous oxide is colorless, sweet-smelling, nonirritating gas. Its specific gravity is 1.5. It is nonflammable but supports combustion of other objects even in the absence of oxygen. Nitrous oxide is stable in the presence of soda lime. It dissolves in plasma, where it is 34 times more soluble than nitrogen. Nitrous oxide is eliminated essentially unchanged, mostly via the lungs.

Central Nervous System. Nitrous oxide is a weak anesthetic, and surgical anesthesia at ambient pressure is not possible in a normal healthy adult using nitrous oxide as a sole anesthetic agent in the presence of adequate oxygen. It is therefore of practical advantage to supply more than 30% oxygen with nitrous oxide and provide additional anesthetic by using intravenous agents or one of the more potent inhalation anesthetics.

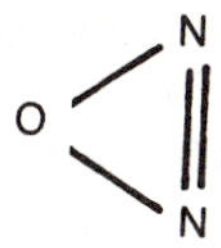

Nitrous Oxide
(dinitrogen monoxide)

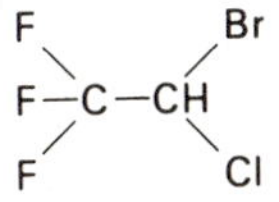

Halothane
(2-bromo-2-chloro-1,1
1-trifluoroethane)

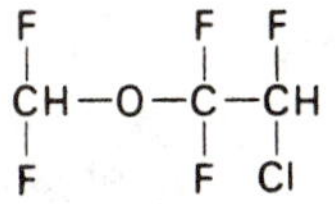

Enflurane
(2-chloro-1,1,2-trifluoroethyl
difluoromethyl ether)

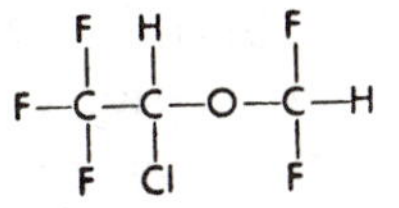

Isoflurane
(1-chloro-2,2,2-trifluoroethyl
difluoromethyl ether)

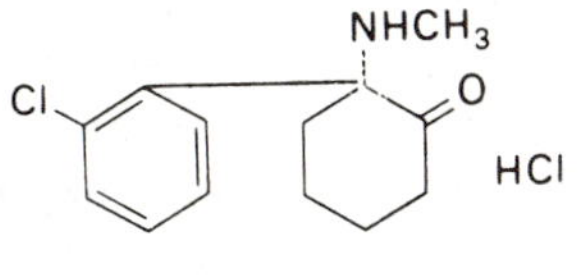

Ketamine

Fig. 11.1-3. *Chemical structure of some commonly used general anesthetics.*

Nitrous oxide has analgesic properties and, at subanesthetic concentrations with oxygen, is used frequently to provide analgesia in obstetrics, dentistry, and relief of pain in acute trauma.

Nitrous oxide increases intracranial pressure by increasing the cerebral blood flow, and enhances cerebral cortical oxygen utilization (54). However, the cerebral effects of nitrous oxide are modified by background anesthesia. At two dose levels of morphine 1 mg/kg and 3 mg/kg, 70% nitrous oxide and 30% oxygen produce no alteration in cerebral blood flow or metabolism in normal humans (27), whereas cerebral metabolic rate for oxygen and cerebral blood flow are both increased when nitrous oxide is added to halothane oxygen anesthesia in dogs. Pretreatment with thiamylal prevents any increase initially.

Respiratory System. Nitrous oxide is a weak respiratory stimulant (13). Ventilation is usually increased under nitrous oxide anesthesia. Respiratory depression produced by enflurane is antagonized by nitrous oxide (35). Alveolar-arterial oxygen tension difference is increased during general anesthesia, and it is recommended to use at least 35% oxygen with nitrous oxide to ensure adequate oxygenation. Nitrous oxide administration causes an increase in pulmonary vascular resistance, more if there is a preexisting pulmonary hypertension (58).

Cardiovascular System. *In vitro*, nitrous oxide causes direct depression of the myocardium, which is substantially less than that caused by halothane. Nitrous oxide resembles halothane and ether in its mechanism of producing myocardial depression, as it inhibits extracellular Ca^{2+} inside the cell to effect contraction. Myocardial depression produced by nitrous oxide can be reversed by the administration of Ca^{2+} or by digitalization. Nitrous oxide also stimulates sympathetic nervous activity by central action, and this tends to antagonize direct myocardial depression.

In clinical practice, cardiovascular effects of nitrous oxide vary with the background anesthetic, duration of administration, type of ventilation (spontaneous or controlled), and depth of anesthesia.

When nitrous oxide is added to halothane anesthesia, its effects at equipotent depth of anesthesia are predominantly those of sympathetic stimulation, such as increase in arterial blood pressure, cardiac output, and total peripheral resistance. Sympathetic stimulation is also observed in combination with ether or fluroxene. Addition of nitrous oxide to enflurane anesthesia causes less cardiovascular stimulation, and there is less cardiac depression with enflurane-nitrous oxide-oxygen mixture than enflurane-oxygen, at equipotent depths.

Cardiac depression is seen even at 10% nitrous oxide when added to morphine-oxygen anesthesia, and each incremental change in nitrous oxide concentration causes further cardiac depression (42). Blood pressure is maintained in the presence of decreased cardiac output by an increase in the total peripheral resistance.

Metabolism. Essentially all nitrous oxide is excreted unchanged via the lung, and a small amount is metabolized in the gut to free nitrogen (69). Activity of methionine synthesis in liver is depressed in patients anesthetized with nitrous oxide. This may impair DNA and protein synthesis (34).

HALOTHANE

Physical Properties. Halothane (FLUOTHANE) is a colorless heavy liquid. Vapor concentrations within anesthetic range are nonflammable, nonirritating, and have a pleasant odor. Halothane is stored in amber-colored bottles to prevent decomposition by light. Thymol 0.01% (w/w) is added to stabilize the compound. Halothane is decomposed when exposed to ultraviolet light or ionizing radiation and therefore should not be used in their presence. The decomposition products are toxic (8).

Halothane is highly soluble in rubber (rubber/gas partition coefficient 121.1 at 760 mmHg and 24°C), and its uptake by rubber may significantly alter its concentration delivered to the patient, especially if using low-flow techniques. In the presence of moisture, halothane corrodes aluminum, brass, tin, solder, and lead. Copper and chromium are not attacked.

Halothane is stable in the presence of soda lime, although it is broken down in traces (0.2%) into a toxic compound $CF_2=CBrCl$ (59). In a semiclosed system, its accumulation to near-toxic concentrations does not occur. Soda lime adsorbs halothane as an inverse function of its water content. Exposure to humidified gas prevents or reverses this adsorption. Fresh soda lime has enough water content and does not adsorb halothane to a significant extent (21).

Central Nervous System. Anesthesia with halothane can be induced rapidly because of its high potency and the fact that it is nonirritating to inhale. Solubility in the blood and brain is low which permits rapid buildup of partial pressure of halothane in the arterial blood and brain and also provides greater flexibility in the control of depth of anesthesia because the alveolar concentration can follow rapidly the inspired concentration. For the same reasons, recovery from anesthesia is also rapid.

Cerebral blood flow is increased, and there is a decrease in cerebral vascular resistance even at normal carbon dioxide tension. The increase in the cerebral blood flow by halothane is unrelated to cerebral metabolic rate. There is a rise in cerebrospinal fluid pressure, but this rise can be prevented if the patient is hyperventilated before the halothane is introduced (43).

Respiratory System. Respiration is depressed early with halothane, and 3 MAC of ether is required to give the same degree of carbon dioxide retention as 1 MAC of halothane. Depression is more at the cost of volume than rate. Halothane causes preferential suppression of intercostal muscle function, with relative sparing of diaphragmatic activity (70), which impairs the stability of the rib cage and predisposes to paradoxical ventilation (28). Assisted or controlled ventilation is easy to perform under halothane anesthesia and becomes necessary to ensure adequate ventilation. Pharyngeal and laryngeal reflexes are depressed early, and salivary and bronchial secretions are inhibited. Halothane produces bronchodilatation and has been shown to reverse the antigen-induced bronchoconstriction. The mechanism of action involves depression of reflex pathways as well as direct effect on airway smooth muscle (25). It is one of the drugs of choice in asthmatics. Metabolism of 5-hydroxytryptamine is inhibited in the lungs during halothane anesthesia (55).

Halothane is a potent depressant of peripheral chemoreceptor-mediated ventilatory reflexes, and in concentrations as low as 0.1 MAC, halothane greatly decreases ventilatory response to hypoxia, whereas ventilatory response to carbon dioxide is unaltered (31). Halothane concentration of 1.1 and 2 MAC abolishes the hypoxic response completely, whereas response to carbon dioxide is fairly brisk. Respiratory stimulant effect of carbon dioxide is progressively depressed with increasing depth of anesthesia. Pulmonary vasoconstrictor response to hypoxia is not impaired at light levels of halothane anesthesia (65).

Cardiovascular System. Halothane causes a fall in blood pressure proportional to the depth of anesthesia. Halothane has a direct inhibitory influence on the smooth muscle of the peripheral vessels and also reduces the vasoconstrictor tone of the peripheral vessels by interfering with the normal action of endogenous norepinephrine. The plasma concentration of this catecholamine is increased during the induction of anesthesia with halothane (29).

The dose-dependent negative inotropic effect of halothane on the heart has been documented in a number of reports (16, 61). This could be due to enzyme inhibition in the myocardium or halothane blocking the action of norepinephrine on the myocardium. Halothane blocks the activation of myocardial adenylate cyclase by catecholamines, which may explain at least in part the myocardial depressant effect of halothane. There is depression of contractile force, stroke volume, and cardiac output. Myocardial metabolism is depressed with a decrease in myocardial oxygen extraction (62). Parasympathetic nerves to the heart are sensitized, causing bradycardia. When anesthesia is prolonged for 5 hours or more, myocardial depression is not seen with deepening of anesthesia; heart rate is increased, and cardiac output and stroke volume return toward or above normal.

Ventricular dysrhythmias under halothane anesthesia bear direct relationship to hypoxia and hypercarbia. Sinoauricular node is depressed, and AV nodal rhythm is frequently seen. The exact mechanism of ventricular arrhythmias during halothane anesthesia is not certain. Earlier, it was proposed that halothane sensitized the myocardium to the effect of epinephrine, causing increased automaticity at a ventricular pacemaker site. Later studies have shown that with halothane ventricular automaticity is suppressed (38). This has led to the suggestion that reentry of excitation mechanism through the AV node may be the mechanism of ventricular arrhythmias during halothane anesthesia (36). Halothane prolongs the AV nodal conduction time and also His-Purkinje and ventricular conduction time and predisposes to reentry (4).

Care should be exercised when epinephrine is to be injected in the presence of halothane anesthesia, and it is safer to limit the dose to 10 ml of 1:100,000 epinephrine over a 10-minute period.

Protection against ventricular arrhythmias due to epinephrine injection to reduce bleeding is increased by using 0.5 or 1.0% lidocaine solution as a vehicle for injection. Fasting renders the heart more prone to premature ventricular contraction under halothane anesthesia (46).

Coronary vascular resistance is decreased. It is probably due to direct action of halothane on the coronary vessels. Coronary vascular reserve is increased (72). Baroreceptor reflex control of heart rate is markedly depressed with a low concentration of 0.7% end tidal halothane concentration, and at moderate depths of anesthesia (1.1% end tidal) the reflex is abolished. Halothane has been found to be a safe anesthetic during severe anemia in dogs (37).

Muscular System. Moderate relaxation can be produced by the depression of the central nervous system. Halothane has minimal action of its own at the neuromuscular junction, but potentiates the myoneural effect of non-depolarizing muscle relaxants and slightly antagonizes the effect of depolarizing agents. Halothane potentiates the ganglion blocking properties of d-tubocurarine, a combination useful to produce deliberate hypotension.

Shivering is commonly seen after halothane anesthesia and seems to be related to heat loss to the environment due to peripheral vasodilation.

Gastrointestinal System. Salivary and gastric secretions are not stimulated, and gastrointestinal motility is reduced. Nausea and vomiting is moderate. Common bile duct pressure in dogs is reduced with halothane, and rises in common bile duct pressure in response to fentanyl are abolished to a great extent by halothane (75).

Kidneys. Halothane decreases renal blood flow, glomerular filtration rate, urinary sodium excretion, and urinary volume. These are secondary to extrarenal influences such as sympathetic stimulation, systemic hemodynamics, and extrarenal hormonal factors.

Elimination of extrarenal factors unmasks the direct renal vasodilation effect on kidneys (7). During halothane anesthesia, autoregulation of renal blood flow is maintained until the normal lower autoregulatory limit of pressure is reached.

Uterus and Fetus. Halothane readily crosses the placental barrier and depresses fetal respiration. It relaxes the uterus and, therefore, is a useful agent to produce external version and to relax the contraction ring of the uterus. Excessive bleeding during cesarean section and postpartum hemorrhage can occur due to interference with retraction and contraction of the uterus.

Metabolism. Most of halothane is exhaled from the lungs unchanged; approximately 20% of halothane absorbed in the body undergoes biodegradation in the liver (56). Included among its urinary metabolites are free bromide, free fluoride ions, trifluoroacetic acid, and two toxic volatile metabolites of reductive pathways, CF_3CH_2Cl and CF_2CHCl (59), which are far below their toxic concentration.

Halothane Hepatitis. Following halothane anesthesia an unexplained jaundice has been observed in rare cases. Hepatitis following halothane anesthesia was thought of as an allergic response to halothane in humans, and it was recommended not to repeat halothane within 3 to 12 months. However, unexplained hepatitis following a single exposure to halothane is unlikely an allergic response. No correlation between repeated administration of halothane and hepatitis has been established.

An active metabolite of halothane rather than the parent molecule was proposed as hepatotoxin. Halothane is normally metabolized via oxidative pathways in humans and animals to a great extent, but the metabolites are nontoxic (71).

In those rare cases that develop hepatitis following halothane anesthesia, it is likely that the metabolism of halothane takes a reductive pathway. Animal studies have shown that in an enzyme-induced liver if hypoxia is superseded, the metabolism of halothane takes a nonoxygen-dependent pathway liberating hepatotoxic intermediates with increased covalent binding with hepatocytes, leading to hepatic necrosis (44).

In a recent study, halothane anesthesia administered to enzyme-induced rats in hypoxic atmosphere consistently produced hepatic necrosis. Neither enflurane nor isoflurane anesthesia produced significant injury in this model (23).

ENFLURANE

Physical Properties. Enflurane (ETHRANE) is a clear, colorless, nonflammable liquid. Enflurane is more stable than halothane, requires no preservative, and is not decomposed by sunlight.

The relatively low blood and tissue solubility of enflurane and its high potency allow rapid induction and recovery from anesthesia. Alveolar concentration approaches inspired concentration quickly and permits flexibility in the control of the level of anesthesia. Rats anesthetized with enflurane have lower anesthetic indices (concentrations producing apnea and cardiac arrest, divided by the anesthetizing concentration) than those anesthetized with methoxyflurane, halothane, or isoflurane.

Central Nervous System. Cerebral blood flow and intracranial pressure are increased due to dilation of cerebral vessels, and hyperventilation reverses this increase. Cerebral irritability is increased under enflurane anesthesia. The electroencephalogram may show convulsive activity with or without muscle movements. Hypercarbia and reduction in enflurane concentration reduce such irritability, whereas hypocapnia and increased enflurane concentration increase it. Enflurane decreases cerebral metabolic rate, and there is an increase in glucose and glycogen reserve.

Epileptic activity associated with enflurane anesthesia increases the cerebral metabolism only to the preanesthetic level. There is no evidence of hypoxic damage to the patient associated with enflurane-induced convulsive activity.

In children, enflurane can cause tonic-clonic twitching of hands and feet when used as the sole anesthetic agent for endotracheal intubation (74). Halothane may be a more suitable agent, without the potential hazard of central nervous system excitation, when endotracheal intubation in children without a muscle relaxant is planned.

Respiratory System. Enflurane produces more respiratory depression at a given MAC level than either halothane or isoflurane (10). Nitrous oxide, when added, antagonizes some of this depressant effect (35).

Enflurane produces a dose-dependent reversible depression of mucociliary flow in the tracheobronchial tree. Enflurane, like halothane, is a bronchodilator (24). Lungs of mice infected with influenza virus while exposed to enflurane anesthesia had a decrease in virus titers, less abnormal lung pathology, and increased survival as compared with those animals receiving halothane, diethyl ether, and pentobarbital anesthesia (32).

Cardiovascular System. Myocardial depression, reduction in cardiac output, and decreased blood pressure are significantly greater with enflurane than with halothane (16, 50). With spontaneous ventilation, cardiac output, stroke volume, and heart rate are increased. Total peripheral resistance and arterial blood pressure are decreased (10). Cardiovascular stimulation is due to sympathetic stimulation by an increase in arterial pCO_2. There is a suggestion that the coronary arteries may be dilated.

If anesthesia is prolonged over 7 hours, with controlled ventilation initial circulatory depression shows reversal, and even an increase above control values is seen. This may be a β-adrenergic stimulant effect of prolonged enflurane anesthesia.

Blood pressure reduction is more pronounced in the absence of surgical stimulation and if the patient has high blood pressure before induction of anesthesia. Hypotension is easily corrected by reduction in the concentration of inspired enflurane, administration of fluids, surgical stimulation, or vasopressors.

Release of norepinephrine at sympathetic nerve endings in the heart is inhibited. Sensitization of heart to epinephrine is very little with enflurane when compared with halothane. Lidocaine 0.5 to 1% when added to epinephrine has a protective effect against epinephrine-induced ventricular irritability during enflurane anesthesia (26).

Neuromuscular Effects. Enflurane produces muscle relaxation by central nervous system depression and its effect at the neuromuscular junction. Both tetanic and twitch response of muscle to indirect nerve stimulation are depressed, and 6% enflurane abolishes the twitch response.

Enflurane potentiates nondepolarizing and depolarizing muscle relaxants and one-half to one-third of the usual relaxant dose is required. The mechanism of action of enflurane at the neuromuscular junction is probably due to alteration of the sensitivity of the end-plate region.

Enflurane, like isoflurane, is twice as potent as halothane in augmenting a neuromuscular block by pancuronium or d-tubocurarine. But enflurane is more potent than isoflurane or halothane in augmenting a vecuronium-induced neuromuscular block (57).

Metabolism. Because of low solubility, about 80% of the administered enflurane is excreted unchanged through the lung. About 2 to 5% is metabolized in the liver, liberating free fluoride ions.

Adverse Reactions. There is no evidence that enflurane is toxic in patients with liver disease. Enflurane does not deplete blood glutathione, a compound involved in body detoxification mechanisms. Although the circulating concentration of fluoride ion derived from enflurane (up to 20 μM) exceeds that from halothane, nephrotoxicity usually does not occur. However, fluoride levels in nephrotoxic range (> 40 μM) of short duration have been reported under enflurane anesthesia in patients enzyme-induced with isoniazid (20). No evidence of renal dysfunction was seen, probably due to rapid pulmonary excretion of enflurane in the postoperative period (41).

Enflurane has no adverse effect on male reproductive organs or on male reproductive processes (6). At present, there is no convincing experimental evidence that enflurane is carcinogenic (5).

ISOFLURANE

Physical Properties. Isoflurane (FORANE) is an isomer of enflurane. It is liquid at room temperature and does not require stabilizer for storage.

Central Nervous System. Because of the low blood solubility of isoflurane, induction of anesthesia and recovery is quicker than with enflurane or halothane. It also makes the depth of anesthesia easier to control.

Isoflurane may be the drug of choice in neuroanesthetic practice (2, 3, 67). Under isoflurane anesthesia, cerebral blood flow is not significantly increased. EEG shows isoelectric pattern, and cerebral metabolic oxygen requirements are markedly reduced; this may have some protective value in situations of ischemia or hypoxia. CSF production and resistance to reabsorption of CSF do not increase. Autoregulation of cerebral blood flow is better maintained. The intracranial pressure is not significantly increased even though the cerebral blood volume is increased. This presumably is a result of a decrease in CSF volume. Halothane on the other hand, causes a rise in intracranial pressure, and the cerebral blood volume. Cerebral blood flow is significantly increased. Autoregulation of the cerebral blood flow is not well maintained, and cerebral metabolic oxygen requirements are decreased, but less than isoflurane. The resistance to reabsorption of CSF and the rate of CSF production are both increased. With enflurane, there is an increase in intracranial pressure, cerebral blood flow is significantly increased, and the EEG shows seizure like bursts of spikes. CSF production and resistance to reabsorption of CSF are both increased.

Isoflurane has a higher margin of safety than enflurane, methoxyflurane, or halothane. Rats anesthetized with isoflurane have the highest anesthetic index (concentration producing apnea or cardiac arrest, divided by anesthetizing concentration).

Respiratory System. There is marked depression of respiration, and ventilatory response to carbon dioxide is depressed most with enflurane and equally with halothane and isoflurane. With increasing depth of anesthesia using isoflurane, tidal volume is decreased but, unlike halothane, there is no compensatory increase in rate. Surgical stimulation counteracts the major part of the respiratory depression. Isoflurane is less depresssant to hypoxic ventilatory response than enflurane. It has a mildly pungent odor that may be a disadvantage during induction of anesthesia by mask in children. Hiccoughs can occur during light anesthesia and emergence.

Cardiovascular System. Isoflurane causes less myocardial depression than halothane or enflurane. Stroke volume is reduced, but cardiac output is maintained by an increase in the heart rate. Cardiovascular stability is maintained even at deeper levels of anesthesia. There is dose-related decrease in peripheral vascular resistance, and vasodilation is greater than that produced by halothane. It maintains stability of cardiac rhythm in patients challenged by administration of catecholamines, and the amount of epinephrine required to produce extrasystoles is almost three times greater than during halothane anesthesia. Nitrous oxide, when added to isoflurane anesthesia, produces some degree of α-adrenergic stimulation, which is more than with enflurane and less than with halothane (60). Isoflurane is shown to inhibit hypoxic pulmonary vasoconstriction.

Muscle. Isoflurane potentiates the effects of depolarizing and nondepolarizing muscle relaxants. This potentiation is similar to enflurane but is two to three times greater than with halothane. Augmentation of caffeine-induced contracture is less with isoflurane than with halothane or enflurane.

Uterus. Isoflurane produces uterine muscle relaxation that is dose related. At low doses, it increases uterine blood flow.

Metabolism and Organ Toxicity. Molecular stability of isoflurane is marked. Less than 0.3% of fluorine in isoflurane is metabolized in the body to inorganic fluoride ion, showing the relative lack of its biotransformation in the body and suggesting lack of hepatic and renal toxicity (40).

Some properties of three commonly used halogenated anesthetics (halothane, enflurane, and isoflurane) are compared in Table 11.1.-2.

ANESTHETIC AGENTS RARELY OR NO LONGER USED

Certain anesthetic agents widely used in the past are no longer or rarely used because of their flammability and/or toxicity. Some of these agents are briefly described here.

DIETHYL ETHER

Ether is a colorless volatile liquid with penetrating smell. It is highly flammable.

Central Nervous System. Induction of anesthesia with ether is slow due to its high blood solubility and pungent character. Its margin of safety is high. Muscular relaxation is good in the presence of adequate respiration and is produced mainly by a central action, and in high concentration, also by neuromuscular blockade due to stabilization of postjunctional membrane.

Respiratory System. Ether is an irritant to the airway and increases bronchial and salivary secretions. It dilates the bronchi. It stimulates respiration by central action (51).

Cardiovascular System. Heart rate is increased and blood pressure is maintained even in deep anesthesia due to increased sympathetic activity. There is a reflex release of catecholamines from the adrenal medulla, increasing the heart rate, cardiac output, and blood pressure. In adrenalectomized animals, cardiac depression is produced. During anesthesia with ether, this cardiac depression is balanced by catecholamine-induced stimulation; in deep anesthesia, cardiac depression is observed. In toxic dose, respiration is stopped before circulatory failure.

About 65 to 90% inhaled ether is excreted unchanged via lung, and about 15% is oxidized to CO_2 and water.

Nausea and vomiting are common after ether anesthesia. Acidosis, dehydration, and fever in children may predispose to convulsions under ether anesthesia.

CYCLOPROPANE

Cyclopropane is a colorless, flammable, and highly explosive gas with a sweet smell.

Central Nervous System. Due to its low blood solubility, induction and emergence are rapid. Recovery is delayed after a prolonged administration due to its high fat solubility. Postoperative excitement may occur and can be avoided by short-acting barbiturates. Muscle relaxation may be adequate at deeper levels of anesthesia. Cyclopropane produces analgesia in subanesthetic concentrations. Nausea and vomiting are common in the postoperative period, probably due to stimulation of the chemoreceptor trigger zone.

Respiratory System. The respiratory center may be directly depressed, but there is a wide margin of safety before occurrence of vasomotor depression.

Table 11.1-2
Comparison of Three Commonly Used Halogenated Anesthetics

Properties	Grades[a] +	++	+++
Stability	H	E	I
Solubility in blood	I	E	H
Pungency	H	I	E
Biodegradation (metabolism)	I	E	H
Increase in heart rate	H	E	I
Arrhythmia	I	E	H
Circulatory depression	I	H	E
Respiratory depression	H	I	E
Muscle relaxation (potentiation of muscle relaxants)	H	I	E
Seizures			E
Cerebral blood flow and intracranial pressure	I	E	H
Renal and hepatic toxicity	I	E	H

[a]Grades indicated by pluses are only qualitative, + signifying mild or least and +++ signifying marked or most. H = halothane; E = enflurane; I = isoflurane.

Cardiovascular System. Blood pressure remains unchanged and may even rise slightly. Cardiac output is increased under light anesthesia and decreased as the anesthesia deepens. Under cyclopropane anesthesia, norepinephrine concentration in the myocardium increases due to sympathetic stimulation, which may account for the initial increase in the cardiac output and may further increase with the increase in carbon dioxide tension resulting in ventricular arrhythmias. Blood flow to skin is increased, causing an increase in bleeding during surgery.

ETHYLENE

Ethylene is a colorless, nonirritating, flammable gas with slightly sweetish and unpleasant odor and taste.

Induction with ethylene is rapid, but anesthesia is not very deep and is adequate only for minor superficial operations. Muscular relaxation is minimal. Respiration and blood pressure are relatively unaffected. Bronchial and salivary secretions are minimal.

CHLOROFORM

Chloroform, $CHCl_3$, was the first halogenated hydrocarbon used in anesthesia and is a potent general anesthetic. It is nonflammable. Chloroform has a low margin of safety, as it depresses cardiac muscle and conducting tissue, and also depresses the heart reflexly via its action on vagal and vasomotor centers. It sensitizes myocardium to catecholamines, producing arrhythmias. Ventricular fibrillation is an ever-present danger. Chloroform causes general vasodilation. It is hepatotoxic and nephrotoxic.

TRICHLORETHYLENE

Trichlorethylene, $CHCl—CCl_2$, is an excellent analgesic.In analgesic and light anesthetic concentration, it is nonflammable and practically nontoxic, but not suitable for deep general anesthesia. It reacts with soda lime in CO_2 absorbers to form dichloroacetylene, which can produce cranial nerve palsy, and hence should not be used in closed or semiclosed circuits. At deeper planes of anesthesia, it produces tachypnea with shallow respiration, sinus bradycardia, and cardiac arrhythmias.

METHOXYFLURANE

Physical Properties. Methoxyflurane (PENTHRANE), is a clear, colorless liquid. Its vapor density is 7.4; saturated vapor pressure at room temperature is 23 mmHg, which is equivalent to approximately 3 volumes percent, and therefore the maximum concentration a vaporizer can deliver. Solubility in rubber is very high, rubber/gas partition coefficient at 25 °C is 635, and 25 to 30% of anesthetic introduced into the circuit is adsorbed by its rubber components.

Central Nervous System. Induction of anesthesia is prolonged due to its low volatility, high solubility in rubber, and high blood solubility. To some extent, these effects are offset by its high potency. At subanesthetic concentrations, it produces good analgesia. Good muscular relaxation is produced. There is negligible effect at the neuromuscular junction, and site of action is central probably in the spinal cord.

Respiratory System. Respiration is depressed more in volume than rate and, at deeper levels, assisted or controlled ventilation is necessary. It is not irritating to respiratory mucosa and is easy to inhale.

Cardiovascular System. There is a fall in blood pressure proportional to the depth of anesthesia, primarily due to a fall in the cardiac output. Catecholamines are not increased, and methoxyflurane is not in itself a contraindication of epinephrine during anesthesia. Peripheral resistance is unchanged and muscle blood flow is not increased.

Metabolism. Association between methoxyflurane and hepatotoxicity has not been established. Of all currently used anesthetics, methoxyflurane is most extensively metabolized in the body. Nearly 50% of the absorbed methoxyflurane is metabolized in the liver, liberating free fluoride ions. This is mainly because cytochrome P-450 can act on the methoxyflurane molecule at two sites, one causing dechlorination and the other ether cleavage. The major metabolic products of methoxyflurane have been identified as methoxydifluracetic acid, oxalic acid, inorganic fluoride, and carbon dioxide.

Free fluoride ions affect the distal renal tubules, rendering them unresponsive to antidiuretic hormone, causing vasopressin-resistant polyurea and azotemia. Renal toxicity is manifest when serum inorganic fluoride level exceeds 50 μM. This level is likely to be reached if methoxyflurane is administered for more than 2 MAC hours.

Use of methoxyflurane has virtually disappeared from clinical practice because of its renal toxicity.

INTRAVENOUS ANESTHETICS

Most sedatives, hypnotics, tranquilizers, neuroleptics, and narcotics, if injected intravenously, are capable of contributing to or causing anesthesia. They may be used for induction of anesthesia, as a sole anesthetic, or as a supplement to inhalation or regional anesthetics. Intravenous anesthesia became popular because of the ease of its administration and its wide acceptance by patients.

The various agents used for induction or supplementation of anesthesia may be divided into the following categories:

(1) Barbiturates (thiopental, methohexital, thiamylal); (2) narcotic analgesics (morphine, meperidine, fentanyl); (3) neuroleptic-narcotic combination (droperidol-fentanyl, INNOVAR); (4) benzodiazepines (diazepam, midazolam, lorazepam); and (5) ketamine.

BARBITURATES

Pharmacology of barbiturates is discussed in Chapter 11.2. Duration of action of most of the sedative-hypnotic barbiturates is usually too long for their safe use as anesthetics. However, the ultrashort-acting barbiturates (e.g., thiopental, thiamylal, methohexital), have very short duration of action and have been used as i.v. anesthetics with safety and better control. They are used extensively for induction of anesthesia. They lack analgesic effect and, as induction agents, should be combined with narcotic or inhalational agents.

Pharmacological Effects. After a single i.v. anesthetic dose of thiopental, consciousness is lost in 10-20 seconds and returns in about 20-30 minutes. This short-lasting anesthetic effect is caused by redistribution of the drug from the brain (which it enters rapidly and where the initial concentration is high) to other tissues of the body (such as adipose and muscle).

Thiopental causes depression of the cerebral cortex and reticular-activating system and is an anticonvulsant. It decreases cerebral blood flow, intracranial tension, and cerebral oxygen consumption. The pain threshold is lowered by its antianalgesic properties.

Respiratory System. Thiopental causes dose-related respiratory depression, affecting the drive to respiration and its rhythmic character. It depresses the respiratory center rapidly. A fast i.v. injection may lead to temporary apnea. It sometimes causes coughing, laryngospasm, and bronchospasm. Insertion of an airway, or presence of saliva, may precipitate one or more of these effects.

Cardiovascular System. Reduction of myocardial contractility leading to decrease of cardiac output and hypotension may occur immediately after rapid i.v. injection. As a compensatory measure, tachycardia and increase of total peripheral resistance may develop.

Pharmacokinetics. The usual induction dose is 3 to 5 mg/kg i.v. Anesthesia is deeper whenever the protein binding is less. The amount of drug administered should be reduced in patients with liver disease.

After a single dose of thiopental, the level in the plasma falls rapidly due to redistribution, and the patient regains consciousness. In 30 minutes, the original concentration in the brain falls to 10%. It is metabolized at a rate of 15%/hour and has been reported to have a body half-life as long as 6 hours.

It may be mentioned that room temperature may change the dose of barbiturates for induction. In low-volume states, myasthenia gravis, severe anemia, and myxedema, it should be given with great care. Porphyria, inadequate airway, and lack of facilities for artificial ventilation, are absolute contraindications to its use.

Complications are perivenous or accidental intraarterial injections. Both require immediate treatment, lidocaine for the former and lidocaine, heparin, stellate ganglion block, papaverine, or phenoxybenzamine to reduce spasm for the latter.

Thiamylal is similar to thiopental, but methohexital is rapid acting and has a short duration of action. Compared with thiopental, it is about 3 times more potent and less irritating. It may cause cough, hiccoughs, and apnea with greater frequency. It may produce involuntary muscle movements.

NARCOTIC ANALGESICS

The pharmacology of narcotic analgesics is described in Chapter 10.1. In addition to their preanesthetic use, narcotic analgesics are used intravenously to provide analgesia during general anesthesia that reduces the dose of general anesthetics. Morphine, and fentanyl are used frequently for this purpose.

Used in large doses, these narcotics can produce general anesthesia, but results in prolonged respiratory depression requiring controlled ventilation.

Morphine may be used as a component of neuroleptic or balanced anesthesia (described next); the first i.v. dose should be about 0.1 to 0.2 mg/kg. It also causes facilitation of mechanical ventilation. Morphine may be used in neuroleptic anesthesia either for cardiac or noncardiac surgery, where the surgery is of long duration. Mechanical ventilation will be needed postoperatively.

Fentanyl is most frequently used as a component of neuroleptic anesthesia. Fentanyl is a synthetic narcotic, related to phenylpiperidines. It produces sedation and anxiolytic effects. Its analgesic effect is 80 to 100 times greater but shorter than that of morphine. After large doses, there appears to be complete amnesia. It reduces cerebral blood flow and cerebral oxygen consumption. It causes nausea and vomiting and may produce miosis and bradycardia due to its parasympathomimetic effects, which can be prevented by atropine. It depresses respiration, but for a much shorter duration than morphine or meperidine. In large doses, it produces chest rigidity, which may be eliminated by use of a muscle relaxant or administration of naloxone. If respiratory depression is marked, mechanical ventilation is instituted.

Fentanyl has been recently advocated in very large doses for neuroleptic anesthesia in aortocoronary bypass or other cardiac surgery with oxygen, mostly in patients with little cardiac reserve. Fentanyl in a 20-μg/kg dose is claimed to increase heart rate and arterial blood pressure, without changing stroke volume, central venous pressure, or peripheral vascular resistance. It is metabolized in the liver, and about 10% is excreted unchanged in the urine.

NEUROLEPTIC-NARCOTIC COMBINATIONS

Neuroleptics (as the antipsychotic drugs were originally called; see Chapter 11.5.1) like droperidol produce a state of calmness with reduced anxiety, emotionality, and motor activity, and indifference to the environment. The patient becomes drowsy and placid, but remains arousable.

Droperidol is a butyrophenone derivative. It potentiates the hypnotic effects of thiopental and other CNS depressants, and the analgesic effects of narcotics and nitrous oxide. It markedly inhibits the chemoreceptor trigger zone of the area postrema in the medulla and antagonizes the emetic effects of narcotics and postoperative vomiting. It is a cerebral vasoconstrictor and reduces cerebral blood flow and cerebrospinal fluid pressure. It has short α-adrenoceptor-blocking, hypotensive, and antiarrhythmic effects. It increases blood levels of glucose and growth hormone. It can be given up to a dose of 150 μg/kg. At a 75 μg/kg dose, it greatly decreases ketamine-induced emergence delirium or hallucination.

When such a drug is combined with a potent narcotic analgesic such as fentanyl, a state of neuroleptic analgesia is produced in which patients with altered consciousness and analgesia remain responsive to command. Combination of these drugs with nitrous oxide and oxygen is termed neurolept anesthesia.

Contraindications. Neuroleptic-narcotic combination is not advised during the first trimester of pregnancy or in patients receiving MAO inhibitors. It should not be used in patients suffering from Parkinson's disease or other extrapyramidal disturbances because droperidol may produce extrapyramidal effects in large doses. It is advisable to use diphenhydramine with narcotics for premedication to prevent extrapyramidal disturbances.

BENZODIAZEPINES

Benzodiazepines are sedative, anticonvulsant, muscle relaxant, anxiolytic and amnestic (Chapter 11.5.3). *Diazepam*, a potent and widely used benzodiazepine, can be given intravenously to induce anesthesia. The usual dose to produce anesthesia is 0.2 to 0.3 mg/kg, and onset of its effect may be delayed by 1 to 2 minutes. Diazepam may be used for induction of anesthesia, and preoperatively to reduce anxiety and facilitate induction.

Midazolam is a water-soluble benzodiazepine. It is less suitable as an induction agent (0.15 mg/kg), but it is more reliable for maintenance of anesthesia and produces better amnesia compared with thiopental. It may cause a drop in blood pressure and cerebrospinal fluid pressure and depression in respiration. The drug is biotransformed in the liver, and there is minimal renal excretion of the active drug.

Lorazepam is not suitable for induction but is an excellent sedative and causes retrograde amnesia. Its dose is between 1 and 4 mg i.m. for premedication. It may, however, be given i.v. Patients may sleep longer after anesthesia when premedicated with lorazepam.

KETAMINE

Certain arylacycloalkylamines such as phencyclidine and ketamine produce CNS depression, analgesia, amnesia, immobility, and a feeling of dissociation from the environment. Phencyclidine was the first such dissociative anesthetic used but was later discontinued due to its frequent production of hallucination and psychological problems.

Ketamine (2-[O-chlorophenyl]-2-[methylamino] cyclohexanone) is a rapidly acting general anesthetic. Ketamine produces a somnolent state in which some patients appear to be awake but dissociated from their environment, unresponsive to pain, and having no recall. Somatic pain appears to be more effectively blocked than visceral pain. It produces no muscle relaxation but may produce generalized extensor spasm during emergence from anesthesia. In a 1 to 2 mg/kg dose given i.v. or 5 mg/kg dose i.m., a feeling of dissociation becomes apparent in about 15 seconds; unconsciousness occurs in about 50 seconds and lasts for 10 to 15 minutes. Analgesia and amnesia outlast the anesthetic effect.

Emergence delirium and hallucinations are ketamine's greatest drawbacks. The incidence in children is less than 5%. Droperidol (75 μg/kg), diazepam (0.3 mg/kg), and lorazepam (1 to 4 mg) have been recommended for their reduction or elimination. A diazepam-ketamine combination is used by many to prevent emergence delirium and bad dreams.

Because ketamine increases salivation, belladonna preparation should be given as part of the premedication. It was found recently that lorazepam eliminates salivation. Ketamine is heat sparing.

Respiratory System. Ketamine causes transient depression of the respiratory center. Pharyngeal and laryngeal reflexes remain active. Bronchodilation is produced. Oxygen inhalation is recommended for at least 5 minutes after an injection.

Cardiovascular System. A dose of 2 mg/kg i.v. or 5 mg/kg i.m. causes an increase of systolic and diastolic blood pressures and heart rate. Supplementary injections do not cause additional increase in either. The cardiovascular-stimulating effect is greater when the drug is given intravenously and is minimized by an intramuscular injection. The stroke work and peripheral resistance remain unchanged, or the latter may decrease. It is antiarrhythmogenic. Ketamine exerts its circulatory changes by central sympathetic stimulation. It is metabolized rapidly into alcohols that are excreted in urine.

Indications. Ketamine is the anesthetic of choice for the burned patient (particularly in children) because of the risk with low blood pressure. It is recommended for asthmatic patients. It is useful for minor surgical or diagnostic (cardiac and radiological) procedures. Its use is not recommended for epileptic patients, or patients with increased intracranial pressure.

Ketamine is not absolutely safe for patients with full stomach where a patent airway cannot be guaranteed.

Preparation. *Ketamine hydrochloride* solution (equivalent to base) 10, 50 and 100 mg/ml for i.m. and i.v. injection.

MUSCLE RELAXANTS

Muscle relaxants (neuromuscular blocking agents) are important adjuvants in modern anesthetic practice. Availability of safe technique for artificial ventilation is a prerequisite for their use. Balanced anesthesia should ensure hypnosis, analgesia, and muscular relaxation. Surgical procedures requiring profound muscular relaxation would need deeper levels of anesthesia causing respiratory and cardiovascular depression. Muscle relaxants used during anesthesia would provide relaxation without the need to deepen the anesthetic level. Effects of these muscle relaxants are discussed in Chapter 9.1.

REFERENCES

1. Allison, A.C. and Nunn, J.F Effects of general anesthesia on microtubules. A possible mechanism of anesthesia. *Lancet* 2:1326, 1968.
2. Artru, A.A. Isoflurane does not increase the rate of CSF production in the dog. *Anesthesiology* 6:193, 1984.
3. Artru, A.A. Relationship between cerebral blood volume and CSF pressure during anesthesia with isoflurane or fentanyl in dogs. *Anesthesiology* 60:575, 1984.
4. Atlee, J.L. and Alexander, S.C. Halothane effects on conductivity of the AV node and His-Purkinje system in the dog. *Anesth. Analg. (Clev.)* 56:378, 1977.
5. Baden, J.M., Egbert, B. and Mazze, R.I. Carcinogen bioassay of enflurane in mice. *Anesthesiology* 56:9, 1982.
6. Baden, J.M., Land, P. C., Egbert B. et al. Lack of toxicity of enflurane on male reproductive organs in mice. *Anesth. Analg. (Clev.)* 61:19, 1982.
7. Bastron, R.D., Pyle, J.L. and Inagaki, M. Halothane induced renal vasodilation. *Anesthesiology* 50:126, 1979.
8. Bosterling, B., Trevor, A. and Trudell, J.R. Binding of halothane-free radicals to fatty acids following ultraviolet irradiation. *Anesthesiology* 56:380, 1982.
9 Brzustowicz, R.M., Nelson, D.A., Betts, E.K. et al. Efficacy of oral premedication for pediatric outpatient surgery. *Anesthesiology* 60:475, 1984.

10. Calverley, R.K., Smith, T.N. et al. Ventilatory and cardiovascular effects of enflurane anesthesia during spontaneous ventilation in man. *Anesth. Analg. (Clev.)* 57:610, 1978.
11. Cohen, E.N. Inhalational anesthetics may cause genetic defects, abortions, and miscarriages in operating room personnel. In: *Controversy in Anesthesiology* (Eckenhoff, J.E., ed.) Philadelphia: W.B. Saunders, 1979, p. 47.
12. Duncalf, D. Flammable anesthetics are nearing extinction. *Anesthesiology* 56:217, 1982.
13. Eckenhoff, J.E. and Helrich, M. The effect of narcotics, thiopental and nitrous oxide upon respiration and respiratory response to hypercapnia. *Anesthesiology* 19:240, 1958.
14. Eger, E.I., II. Effect of inspired anesthetic concentration on the rate of rise of alveolar concentration. *Anesthesiology* 24:153, 1963.
15. Eger, E.I., II. *Anesthetic Uptake and Action*. Baltimore: Williams and Wilkins, 1974, p. 1.
16. Eger, E.I., II, Smith, N.T. and Stoelting, R.K. et al. Cardiovascular effects of halothane in man. *Anesthesiology* 32:396, 1970.
17. Epstein, R.M., Rackow, H. and Salanitre, E. Influence of the concentration effect on the uptake of anesthetic mixtures: The second gas effect. *Anesthesiology* 25:364, 1964.
18. Eyring, H., Woodbury, J.W. and D'Arrigo, J.S. A molecular mechanism of general anesthesia. *Anesthesiology* 38: 415, 1973.
19. Fink, B.R. Diffusion anoxia. *Anesthesiology* 16:511, 1955.
20. Fish, M.P. and Rice, S.A. Isoniazid metabolites and anesthetic metabolism. *Anesthesiology* 51:S256, 1979.
21. Grodin, W.K. and Epstein, R.A. Halothane adsorption by sodalime. *Anesthesiology* 51:317, 1979.
22. Guedel, A. Third stage ether anesthesia: subclassification regarding significance of position and movements of eyeball. *Am. J. Surg.* 34: 53, 1920.
23. Harper, M.H., Collins, P.C., Johnson, B. et al. Hepatic injury following halothane, enflurane, and isoflurane anesthesia in rats. *Anesthesiology* 56;14, 1982.
24. Hirschman, C.A. and Bergman, A. Halothane and enflurane protect against bronchospasm in an asthma dog model. *Anesth. Analg. (Clev.)* 57:629, 1978.
25. Hirshman, C.A., Edelstein, G., Peetz, S. et al. Mechanism of action of inhalational anesthesia on airways. *Anesthesiology* 56:107, 1982.
26. Horrigan, R.W., Eger, E.I., II and Wilson, C. Epinephrine induced arrhythmias during enflurane anesthesia in man: A nonlinear dose-response relationship and dose-dependent protection from lidocaine. *Anesth. Analg. (Clev.)* 57:547, 1978.
27. Jobes, D.R., Kennell, E.M., Bush, G.L. et al. Cerebral blood flow and metabolism during morphine nitrous oxide anesthesia in man. *Anesthesiology* 47:16, 1977.
28. Jones, J.C., Faithful D. and Jordan, C. et al. Rib cage movement during halothane anesthesia in man. *Br. J. Anaesth.* 51:399, 1979.
29. Joyce, J.T., Roizen, M.F., Gerson, J.I. et al. Induction of anesthesia with halothane increases plasma norepinephrine concentrations. *Anesthesiology* 56:286, 1982.
30. Kitihata, L.M., Taub, A. and Sato, I. Lamina-specific suppression of dorsal horn unit activity by nitrous oxide and by hyperventilation. *J. Pharmacol. Exp. Ther.* 176:101, 1971.
31. Knill, R.L. and Gelb, A.W. Ventilatory responses to hypoxia and hypercapnia during halothane sedation and anesthesia in man. *Anesthesiology* 49:224, 1978.
32. Knight, P.R., Bedows, E., Nahrwold, M.L. et al. Alterations in influenza virus pulmonary pathology induced by diethyl ether, halothane, enflurane, and pentobarbital anesthesia in mice. *Anesthesiology* 58:209, 1983.
33. Koblin, D.D. and Eger, E.I., II. Current concepts—Theories of narcosis. *N. Engl. J. Med.* 301:1322, 1979.
34. Koblin, D.D., Waskell, L., Watson, J.E. et al. Nitrous oxide inactivates methionine synthetase in human liver. *Anesth. Analg. (Clev.)* 61:75, 1982.
35. Lam, A.M., Clement, J.L., Chung, D.C. et al. Respiratory effects of nitrous oxide during enflurane anesthesia in humans. *Anesthesiology* 56:298, 1982.
36. Linc, J., Sasyniuk, B.L. and Dresel, P.E. Halothane epinephrine induced cardiac arrhythmias and the role of heart rate. *Anesthesiology* 43:548, 1975.
37. Loarie, D.J., Wilkins, P., Tyberg, J. et al. The hemodynamic effects of halothane on anemic dogs. *Anesth. Analg. (Clev.)* 58:195, 1979.
38. Logic, R.L. and Marrow, D.H. The effect of halothane on ventricular automaticity. *Anesthesiology* 36:107, 1972.
39. Magoun, H.W. *The Waking Brain*. Springfield, Ill.: Charles C. Thomas, 1963.
40. Mazze, R.I., Cousins, M.J. and Barr, G.A. Renal effects and metabolism of isoflurane in man. *Anesthesiology* 40:536, 1974.
41. Mazze, R.I., Woodruff, R.E. and Heerdt, ME. Isoniazid-induced enflurane defluorination in humans. *Anesthesiology* 57:5, 1982.
42. McDermott, R.W. and Stanley, T.H. The cardiovascular effects of low concentrations of nitrous oxide during morphine anesthesia. *Anesthesiology* 41:89, 1974.
43. McDowall, D.G., Barker, J. and Jennett, W.B. Cerebrospinal fluid pressure measurements during anesthesia. *Anaesthesia* 21:189, 1966.
44. McLain, G.E., Sipes, I.G. and Brown, B.R. An animal model of halothane hepatotoxicity: Roles of enzyme induction and hypoxia. *Anesthesiology* 51:321, 1979.
45. Meyer, H.H. *The Theory of Narcosis*. Harvey Lecture, 1905-1906, p. 11.
46. Miletich, D.J., Albrecht, R.F. and Seals, C. Responses to fasting and lipid infusion of epinephrine induced arrhythmias during halothane anesthesia. *Anesthesiology* 48:245, 1978.
47. Miller, S.L. A theory of gaseous anesthetics. *Proc. Natl. Acad. Sci. USA* 47: 1515, 1961.
48. Miller, K.W., Paton, W.D.M., Smith, R.A. et al. The pressure reversal of general anesthesia and the critical volume hypothesis. *Mol. Pharmacol.* 9:131, 1973.
49. Mori, K. and Winters, W.D. Neural background of sleep and anesthesia. *Int. Anesth. Clin.* 13:67, 1975.
50. Mote, P.S., Pruett, J.K. and Gramling, Z.W. Effect of halothane and enflurane on right ventricular performance in hearts of dogs anesthetized with pentobarbital sodium. *Anesthesiology* 58:53, 1983.
51. Muallem, M., Larson, C.P. Eger, E.I., II. The effects of diethyl ether on $PaCO_2$ in dogs with and without vagus, somatic and sympathetic block. *Anesthesiology* 30:185, 1969.
52. Mullins, L.J. Some physical mechanisms in narcosis. *Chem Rev.* 54:289, 1954.
53. Pauling, L. A molecular theory of anesthesia. *Science* 134:15, 1961.
54. Pelligrino, D.A., Hoffman, W.E. et al. Nitrous oxide markedly increases cerebral cortical metabolic rate and blood flow in goat. *Anesthesiology* 60:405, 1984.
55. Rannels, D.E., Watkins, C.A. and Biebuyck, J.F. Effect of halothane on uptake and metabolism of 5-hydroxytryptamine by rat lungs perfused *in vitro*. *Anesthesiology* 51:251, 1979.
56. Rehder, K., Forbes, J., Alter, J. et al. Halothane biotransformation in man: A quantitative study. *Anesthesiology* 28:711, 1967.
57. Rupp, S.M., Miller, R.D. and Gencarelli, P.J. Vecuronium induced neuromuscular blockade during enflurane, isoflurane and halothane anesthesia in humans. *Anesthesiology* 60:102, 1984.
58. Schute, U., Hess, E. and Tarnow, J. Pulmonary vascular responses to nitrous oxide in patients with normal and high pulmonary vascular resistance. *Anesthesiology* 57:9, 1982.

59. Sharp, J.H., Trudell, J.R. and Cohen, E.N. Volatile metabolites and decomposition products of halothane in man. *Anesthesiology* 50:2, 1979.

60. Smith, N.T., Calverley, R.K., Prys-Roberts, C. et al. Impact of nitrous oxide on the circulation during enflurane anesthesia in man. *Anesthesiology* 48:345, 1978.

61. Sonntag, H. Donath, U., Hillebrand, W. et al. Left ventricular function in conscious man and during halothane anesthesia. *Anesthesiology* 48:320, 1978.

62. Sonntag, H., Merin, R.G., Donath, U. et al. Myocardial metabolism and oxygenation in man awake and during halothane anesthesia. *Anesthesiology* 51:204, 1979.

63. Stevens, W.C., Eger, E.I., II, Joas, T.A. et al. Comparative toxicity of isoflurane, halothane, fluroxane and diethyl ether in human volunteers. *Can. Anaesth. Soc. J.* 20:357, 1973.

64. Stoelting, R.K and Eger, E.I., II. An additional explanation for the second gas effect. *Anesthesiology* 30:273, 1969.

65. Sykes, M.K., Gibbs, J.M., Loh, L. et al. Preservation of the pulmonary vasoconstrictor response to alveolar hypoxia during the administration of halothane to dogs. *Br. J. Anesth.* 50:1185, 1978.

66. Tanifugi, Y., Eger, E.I., II and Terrell, R.C. Some characteristics of an exceptionally potent inhaled anesthetic thiomethoxyflurane. *Anesth. Analg. (Clev.)* 56:387, 1977.

67. Todd, M.M. and Drummond, J.C. A comparison of the cerebrovascular and metabolic effect of halothane and isoflurane in the cat. *Anesthesiology* 60:276, 1984.

68. Trudell, J.R. A unitary theory of anesthesia based on lateral phase separations in nerve membranes. *Anesthesiology* 46:5, 1977.

69. Trudell, J.R., Hong, K., O'Neil, J.R. et al. Metabolism of nitrous oxide by human and rat intestinal contents. *Anesthesiology* 51:258, 1978.

70. Tusiewicz, K., Bryan, A.C. and Froese, A.B. Contributions of changing rib cage-diaphragm interactions to the ventilatory depression of halothane anesthesia. *Anesthesiology* 47:327, 1977.

71. Van Dyke, R.A., Chenoweth, M.B. and Van Poznak, A. Metabolism of volatile anesthetics I. Conversion *in vivo* of several anesthetics to $^{14}CO_2$ and chloride. *Biochem. Pharmacol.* 13:1239, 1964.

72. Verrier, E.D., Edelist, G., Consigny, M. et al. Greater coronary vascular reserve with halothane. *Anesthesiology* 51:63, 1979.

73. Wood, M. and Wood, A. *Drugs and Anesthesia: Pharmacology for Anesthesiologists.* Baltimore: Williams and Wilkins, 1982, pp. 253, 255.

74. Yakaitis, R.W., Blitt, C.D. and Angiulo, J.P. End-tidal enflurane concentration of endotracheal intubation. *Anesthesiology* 50:59, 1979.

75. Zylanoff, P.L., Mark-Savage, P., Martucci, R.W. et al. Common bile duct responses to anesthetic agents in dogs. *Anesthesiology* 51:32, 1979.

ADDITIONAL READING

Stock, J.G. Unexplained hepatitis following halothane. *Anesthesiology* 63:424, 1985.

Ueda, I. et al. Molecular mechanisms of anesthesia. *Anesth. Analg.* 63:929, 1984.

CHAPTER
11.2.1

SEDATIVE-HYPNOTICS

Samar N. Dutta and Sachin N. Pradhan

Hypnotics are a class of drugs that have the property of inducing sleep for a reasonable duration, *sedatives* produce a calming effect and drowsiness. Most of these drugs are also *anxiolytics,* as they can induce the calming effect without producing drowsiness. Many of them also have anticonvulsant effects. These drugs do not provide analgesia in therapeutic doses, but do manifest additive toxic effects when combined with each other or with alcohol, and at high doses produce unconsciousness.

HISTORY

One of the deities in the Greek pantheon was Hypnos, god of sleep, to whom people prayed for sleep. Hypnos depicted bearing a poppy stalk, and products of poppy were characterized as sleep-inducing in almost every ancient medical treatise. Bromides were introduced in medicine in 1857 by Sir Charles Locock for treatment of epilepsy; during the late nineteenth and early twentieth centuries, bromides (sodium or potassium) were used as sleeping pills. Chloral hydrate, the oldest hypnotic agent, was synthesized by Liebig in 1832 and came to general use as a sedative-hypnotic agent during the latter part of the nineteenth century.

With the introduction of veronal, a barbituric acid derivative, in 1903 by von Mering and Fischer, a new era of hypnotics began. In the 1920s and 1930s, short- to intermediate-acting hypnotics such as amobarbital, pentobarbital, and secobarbital were added to this class. Interest in a group of chemical compounds having a quinazoline 3-oxide structure led to the development of chlordiazepoxide in 1961, followed by that of diazepam, both being benzodiazepine derivatives, as tranquilizers. In 1970, another benzodiazepine compound, flurazepam, was introduced as a hypnotic agent.

CLASSIFICATION

Sedative-hypnotics can be classified into three groups: (1) barbiturates, (2) benzodiazepines, and (3) miscellaneous drugs. Benzodiazepines are discussed mainly in Chapter 11.5.3 and also in Chapter 11.4.

BARBITURATES

Chemistry. Adolf von Beyer first synthesized barbituric acid in 1863. Barbiturates are derivatives of barbituric acid, which is a cyclic ureide formed by condensation of urea with malonic acid. The reaction is:

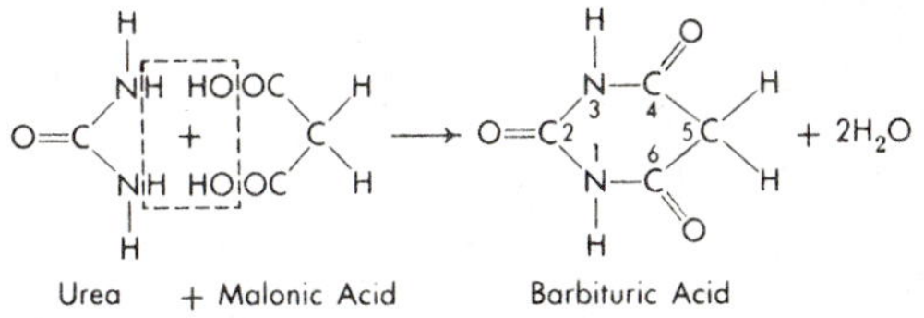

Urea + Malonic Acid → Barbituric Acid + $2H_2O$

The chemical structures of these derivatives with their hypnotic doses and half-lives are given in Table 11.2-1. Substitution of hydrogens attached to C-5 by alkyl or aryl groups results in the development of hypnotic drugs, and a phenyl group substitution to the same carbon atom will produce a compound with anticonvulsant property. A sulfur substitution for oxygen at C-2 results in the formation of thiobarbiturates. If a methyl group is added to the nitrogen at the 3-position, N-methyl barbiturates such as hexobarbital are formed. Thiobarbiturates and methohexital are generally used for intravenous anesthesia.

Barbiturates are poorly soluble in water and are acidic in nature. Sodium salts are more soluble in water, resulting in greater absorption from the intestinal tract.

Classification. Traditionally, barbiturates are classified into groups relative to duration of action based on animal studies carried out by Tatum (20). They belong to three classes: (1) ultrashort-acting, (2) short-to intermediate-acting, and (3) long-acting (Table 11.2.1-1). This classification, however, has little significance in predicting their therapeutic effectiveness as hypnotics in acute

Table 11.2.1-1
General Formula and Classification of Barbiturates

GENERAL FORMULA:

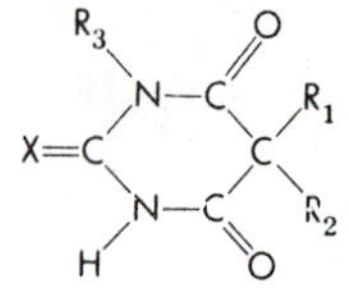

Drug Name	R_1	R_2	R_3	X	Usual Hypnotic Dose (g)
Ultrashort-acting [a] (half-life, 3-8 hours)					
Thiopental (PENTOTHAL)	Ethyl	1-Methylbutyl	H	S	
Thiamylal (SURITAL)	Allyl	1-Methylbutyl	H	S	
Methohexital (BREVITAL)	Allyl	1-Methyl-2-pentynyl	CH_3	O	
Methitural (NERAVAL)	2-Methyl-thioethyl	1-Methylbutyl	H	S	
Short-to-intermediate-acting (half-life, 14-42 hours)[b]					
Secobarbital (SECONAL)	Allyl	1-Methylbutyl	H	O	0.1-0.2
Amobarbital (AMYTAL)	Ethyl	Isopentyl	H	O	0.05-0.2
Heptabarbital (MEDOMIN)	Ethyl	1-Cyclohepten-1-yl	H	O	0.1-0.2
Butabarbital (BUTISOL)	Ethyl	sec-Butyl	H	O	0.1-0.2
Vinbarbital (DELVINAL)	Ethyl	1-Methyl-1-butenyl	H	O	0.1-0.2
Metharbital[c] (GEMONIL)	Ethyl	Ethyl	CH_3	O	0.1-0.2
Probarbital (IPRAL)	Ethyl	Isopropyl	H	O	0.1-0.2
Pentobarbital (NEMBUTAL)	Ethyl	1-Methylbutyl	H	O	0.1
Talbutal (LOTUSATE)	Allyl	sec-Butyl	H	O	0.1-0.2
Butethal (NEONAL)	Ethyl	Butyl	H	O	0.1
Hexethal (ORTAL)	Ethyl	n-Hexyl	H	O	0.1-0.2
Cyclobarbital (PHANODORN)	Ethyl	Cyclohexen-1-yl	H	O	0.1-0.2
Aprobarbital (ALURATE)	Allyl	Isopropyl	H	O	0.1
Allobarbital (DIAL)	Allyl	Allyl	H	O	0.1
Butalbital (SANDOPTAL)	Allyl	Isobutyl	H	O	0.2
Butallylonal (PERNOTON)	sec-Butyl	2-bromoallyl	H	O	0.2
Long-acting (half-life, 24 to 96 hours) [b]					
Barbital (VERONAL)	Ethyl	Ethyl	H	O	0.3-0.5
Phenobarbital [c] (LUMINAL)	Ethyl	Phenyl	H	O	0.1-0.2
Mephobarbital [c] (MEBARAL)	Ethyl	Phenyl	CH_3	O	0.1-0.2

[a] Anesthetic (intravenously).
[b] Hypnotic (orally) unless otherwise indicated.
[c] Anticonvulsant.

use. Several studies have shown that there is little difference in overall therapeutic effects among these three groups of barbiturates (10, 14). Drugs belonging to a particular class, however, may exhibit characteristic pharmacotherapeutic properties. Shorter-acting drugs are more lipid-soluble and their increased lipid-solubility influences their pharmacokinetics.

Pharmacological Effects. Barbiturates reversibly depress the activity of all excitable tissues (nervous system tissues are more sensitive than muscle tissues).

Central Nervous System. The CNS is highly sensitive to barbiturates which, depending on the drug, dose, and route of administration, produce effects ranging from sedation to surgical anesthesia. The anesthetic doses of short- to intermediate-acting and long-acting barbiturates are dangerously close to the lethal dose.

Several studies have shown that with barbiturates (e.g., pentobarbital) the induction of sleep is faster and of longer duration than placebo (21, 23). Barbiturate-induced sleep in normal volunteers differs from normal sleep in causing reduction of rapid eye movement (REM) sleep, which is dose dependent (7, 12). Repeated administration of barbiturates may produce tolerance to the latter effect. Withdrawal after chronic use is attended by a rebound increase in the REM sleep and disturbed dreams. *Paradoxical excitement* can occur in certain individuals following administration of small doses of barbiturates. Individuals awakening from barbiturate-induced sleep often manifest residual daytime effects of hypnotics, characterized by drowsiness, hangover, headache, and decreased performance of cognitive and motor functions. Barbiturates are not primarily analgesics; they may modify a patient's reaction to pain at doses that will impair consciousness. In the presence of severe pain, a small dose of barbiturate alone may cause hyperalgesia and delirium.

Phenobarbital, mephobarbital, and metharbital possess selective anticonvulsant properties independent of their sedative effects. However, all barbiturates reduce seizure activity in anesthetic doses.

Miscellaneous Effects. At sedative-hypnotic doses, barbiturates have no appreciable effects on the autonomic nervous system. However, at anesthetic doses hypothalamic thermoregulatory and medullary vasomotor centers are inhibited.

Barbiturates cause severe respiratory depression by inhibiting neurogenic drive and the responses to hypoxia, increased pCO_2, and low pH. At therapeutic dose levels, barbiturates have only slight effects on cough reflex. Similarly, the cardiovascular system is least affected at hypnotic doses except for mild bradycardia and hypotension. Intravenous administration of barbiturates results in decrease in cardiac output, increased peripheral resistance, and increased heart rate. Urine volume is markedly decreased at anesthetic doses as a result of hemodynamic changes and indirectly due to stimulation of antidiuretic hormone (ADH) release. Barbiturates may inhibit gastric secretion and the tone of intestinal smooth muscle by central as well as peripheral mechanisms.

Repeated administration of barbiturates may stimulate the hepatic microsomal enzyme systems, resulting in an increased rate of metabolism of barbiturates themselves and a variety of other drugs whose efficacy can be decreased. Other sedative-hypnotic drugs, including alcohol, also stimulate hepatic microsomal enzyme systems (resulting in rapid metabolism of barbiturates). This contributes to the development of cross-tolerance.

Nonmicrosomal enzymes e.g., δ-aminolevulinic acid (ALA) synthetase, may also be stimulated by barbiturates. Because ALA synthetase activity is defective in acute intermittent porphyria, barbiturates aggravate the clinical signs and symptoms in such patients.

Mechanism and site of action. Barbiturates selectively inhibit multineuronal conduction of the ascending reticular formation of the brainstem. This system is viewed as maintaining a state of wakefulness under normal conditions. Areas of the cerebral cortex, limbic system, and hypothalamus are also sensitive to barbiturates, but how this can be correlated to their pharmacological actions has not been clearly demonstrated. It has also been suggested that barbiturates interfere with the release of one or more of the central neurotransmitters [e.g., acetylcholine (ACh), γ-aminobutyric acid (GABA) or norepinephrine (NE)] and thereby inhibit central synaptic transmission.

Pharmacokinetics. Major pharmacokinetic indices such as absorption, distribution, protein binding, duration of action, and renal excretion of barbituric acid derivatives are greatly influenced by the high lipid-solubility of their un-ionized moieties. Sodium salts having greater solubility in the intestinal tract are readily absorbed following oral administration. Ultrashort-acting barbiturates (e.g., thiopental) have the highest lipid/water partition coefficient, enter the brain almost instantaneously following intravenous administration, and produce a state of anesthesia. Short- to intermediate-acting and long-acting barbiturates have a considerably smaller partition coefficient, and as such they move in and out of the brain relatively slowly. Compared with thiobarbiturates, higher doses of the latter would be needed to produce anesthesia. Although ultrashort-acting barbiturates, by virtue of their high lipid-solubility, gain rapid entry to the brain, their levels in the brain and blood rapidly decline as a result of distribution to other tissues. The latter phase is then followed by a slower elimination phase. The more water-soluble barbiturates are also distributed in all tissues, but slowly. Polarity of these compounds influence their protein binding (60-80% in the case of thiopental, 44% for secobarbital, and 42% for phenobarbital). Concentration of barbiturates in different tissues other than plasma is also determined by protein binding; somewhat higher amounts accumulate in the liver and kidney. High concentration in fat may occur after repeated administrations.

Barbiturates undergo biotransformation in the liver by one or more of the following pathways: (1) oxidation or removal of substituents at the C-5 position, (2) demethylation at N-3, (3) replacement of S at C-2 of thiobarbiturates by oxygen, and (4) cleavage of the ring structure between N-1 and C-4. Oxygenated metabolites of barbiturates generally exert very little hypnotic action. However, some oxygenated methyl- and thiobarbiturates retain their hypnotic-sedative property. Fetuses and newborn infants only later develop the enzyme system needed for the biotransformation of barbiturates. Thus, barbiturates can cause severe respiratory depression of the baby when given during labor.

The kidney plays a significant role in the excretion of unchanged long-acting barbiturates (e.g., barbital and phenobarbital). Alkalinization of urine promotes renal elimination of long-acting barbiturates (e.g., phenobarbital) rather than the short- to intermediate-acting compounds.

Patients with acute hepatic disease develop rapid sedation to intravenous administration of barbiturates (18) because of prompt increase in blood levels resulting from decreased metabolism, and perhaps from reduction in the distribution space (2). Impaired renal function may lead to accumulation of relatively inactive metabolites of certain barbiturates (e.g., amobarbital), causing manifestation of their pharmacological effect (1). In elderly subjects, hydroxylation of amobarbital has also been shown to be decreased, resulting in higher plasma concentration after a single oral dose (11).

Tolerance and cross-tolerance. Both human and animal studies have demonstrated the development of tolerance to barbiturates. In humans, a limited tolerance develops to the drugs because of slight increase over the tolerant dose could lead to acute overdose. In animal models, tolerance to barbiturates is associated with a progressive decrease in sleeping time, but the lethal dose remains unaffected. Increased rate of metabolism due to induction of microsomal enzyme systems has been suggested as the principal mechanism for development of tolerance. Increased adaptation of the central nervous system to these drugs may also contribute to development of tolerance. Tolerance to barbiturates disappears following abstinence for 1 or 2 weeks. A significant degree of cross-tolerance develops among general anesthetics, alcohol, barbiturates, benzodiazepines, and nonbenzodiazepine hypnotics. Cross-tolerance between barbiturates and narcotics has not been clearly demonstrated.

Psychological and Physical Dependence. The chronic abuse of sedative-hypnotics leads to the development of psychological and physical dependence. Unlike dependence of the narcotic type, physical dependence produced by the barbiturates does not exhibit a typical dose-response relationship. Physical dependence to sedative-hypnotics is discussed in detail in Chapter 11.6.

Side Effects and Contraindications. A wide variety of adverse reactions are produced by barbiturates, including respiratory depression, lethargy, confusion, and disorientation as well as paradoxical excitement in elderly subjects, hangover, nausea, vomiting, hypersensitivity reactions in the form of skin rash, and increased cognitive dysfunction in patients with impairment of renal function. In addition, barbiturates frequently have a potential for inducing dependence and acute overdose. Barbiturates should be administered with caution to pregnant women and nursing mothers because these drugs produce depressant effects on the fetus and the newborn. There is some suggestive evidence for increased incidence of brain tumors in children exposed to barbiturates prenatally or treated with these drugs in early childhood (6). Elderly subjects receiving barbiturates have been reported to manifest low blood calcium concentration (24). The clinical significance of this finding has not been clearly determined. Barbiturates are absolutely contraindicated in patients with acute intermittent porphyria.

Drug Interactions. Central nervous system depressant effects of barbiturates are potentiated by monoamine oxidase inhibitors (e.g., isocarboxazid, phenelzine, tranylcypromine). Because barbiturates enhance the synthesis and activity of hepatic microsomal enzyme systems and thereby stimulate the rate of metabolism of warfarin and dicumarol, tricyclic antidepressants, phenytoin, griseofulvin, and adrenocorticoids, the dosage of the latter drugs needs to be adjusted to achieve the desired level of therapeutic effects. This phenomenon also accelerates the formation of polar vitamin D metabolites, which are biologically inactive, and the net result is a reduced hepatic production of the active metabolite, 25-hydroxyvitamin D_3. This signals a state of vitamin D deficiency. Some children receiving long-term phenobarbital as anticonvulsant may develop biochemical or clinical evidence of vitamin D deficiency.

Acute overdose. Ingestion of about 10 times the hypnotic dose of barbiturates produces severe toxicity. The degree of severity of acute intoxication with barbiturates has been graded from 1 through 4 by several investigators (16). Grade 1 represents mild intoxication characterized by drowsiness, confusion, ataxia, and possibly lateral nystagmus. As the degree of toxicity progressively increases, the clinical manifestations such as sleep (but responding to painful stimuli), decreased deep tendon reflexes, pupillary constriction, loss of corneal reflex, respiratory depression, and hypotension successively occur. Grade 4 is characterized by deep coma not responding to painful stimuli, slow and shallow respiration, unequal or dilated pupils, loss of tendon and gag reflexes, weak and rapid pulse, and pulmonary edema. The patient may go into shock or respiratory arrest leading to death. The lethal dose of barbiturates is often in the range of 1.5-2 g (about 15-20 times the hypnotic dose). Concomitant use of alcohol worsens toxicity of barbiturates. Patients who survive the initial toxicity may develop a number of complications or sequelae such as residual CNS damage (due to hypoxia), renal failure, pulmonary abscess or pneumonia, blisters of the skin, and myoglobinuria (17).

For many years, it was believed that in some individuals acute intoxication with barbiturates resulted from "amnesia" or "automatism," which led to ingestion of several doses in the course of a restless night. However, intensive investigations, have found that such automatism has no pharmacological background and the term is used by patients or their kin to avoid public revelation. (4).

Diagnosis and Treatment of Barbiturate Overdose. The diagnosis of barbiturate poisoning is generally made from history and physical findings. Flaccid coma with reacting pupils, hypothermia, and hypotension are seen on very few conditions other than barbiturate intoxication. Study of blood barbiturate levels offers a reliable means for determining the type of barbiturates (i.e., whether they are long- or short-acting agents). However, due to variation in individual tolerance, and often due to concurrent use of alcohol, the depth of coma and the blood barbiturate level may not show a dependable correlation. The electroencephalogram (EEG) may also be helpful in diagnosis of barbiturate intoxication; a mild case of poisoning shows fast activity of 20-30 cycles/sec particularly in the frontal regions (20).

The management of acute barbiturate poisoning includes emptying the stomach by gastric lavage (in comatose patients) with cuffed endotracheal tube, or by induced vomiting with syrup of ipecac immediately after ingestion. If the patient is unresponsive, adequate ventilation should be maintained by the insertion of endotracheal tube. Tracheostomy and bronchoscopic suction may be necessary if atelectasis becomes evident. Respiratory support by machine may be necessary if ventilatory failure develops. A sufficient i.v. fluid in the form of 5% glucose and forced diuresis hastens the elimination of barbiturates. Alkalinization of urine also enhances excretion of phenobarbital. In patients deeply comatose for a significant duration, the electrolyte imbalances should also be corrected. Pulmonary and urinary infection should be prevented by the use of appropriate antibiotics. Hemodialysis is indicated in patients under deep coma due to long-acting barbiturates and if anuria or uremia develops.

CHLORAL HYDRATE AND RELATED COMPOUNDS

Chloral hydrate has a simple structure (Fig. 11.2.1-1) and is the oldest of the hypnotic agents. It was synthesized by Liebig in 1832, and Oscar Liebrich in 1869 demonstrated its hypnotic effects. Triclofos and chloral betaine are two derivatives of chloral hydrate. Chloral betaine is a chemical complex of chloral and betaine.

Pharmacological Effects. Chloral hydrate has reliable sedative, hypnotic, and anticonvulsant effects. The exact mechanism of its hypnotic action is not clearly known. In the body it is rapidly reduced to trichloroethanol, which has hypnotic properties. Chloral hydrate produces sleep within 30 min of administration. At the therapeutic dosage, it has very little effect on respiration and blood pressure. Deep reflexes are not depressed and a patient can be easily awakened from chloral hydrate induced sleep. The drug has anticonvulsant property and very little or no analgesic activity. Chloral hydrate at low hypnotic doses (0.5-1 g) does not appear to suppress the REM phase of sleep.

Pharmacokinetics. Chloral hydrate is rapidly absorbed from the gastrointestinal tract. It is quickly metabolized in the liver and other tissues to trichloroethanol, so that appreciable amounts of chloral hydrate are difficult to detect in the blood. Trichloroethanol and its glucuronide conjugate (urochloralic acid) achieve peak blood levels within an hour after administration. Trichloroethanol has a half-life of 6-9 hours. A small fraction of chloral hydrate and a larger portion of trichloroethanol are also converted to an inactive metabolite, trichloroacetic acid, which accumulates in the body following long-term use. Trichloroethanol glucuronide is excreted in the urine and constitutes about 15-35% of a dose of chloral hydrate. Only a small amount of trichloroethanol is excreted in the urine unchanged. Small amounts of glucuronide acid-conjugated chloral hydrate are excreted in the bile. Although chloral hydrate is not metabolized by the

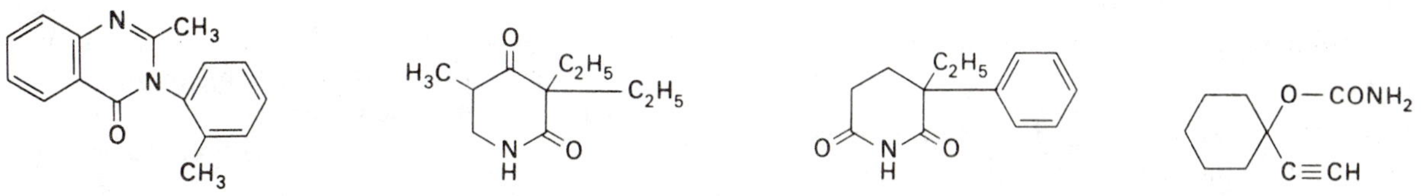

Methaqualone   Methyprylon   Glutethimide   Ethinamate

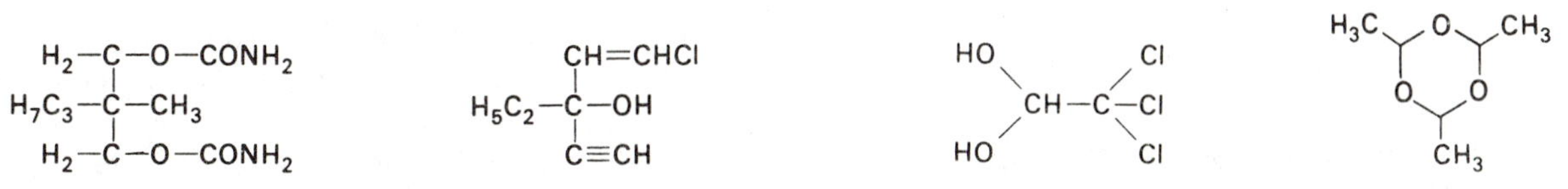

Meprobamate   Ethchlorvynol   Chloralhydrate   Paraldehyde

Fig.11.2.1-1. *Chemical structures of some commonly used and abused sedative-hypnotic agents.*

hepatic microsomal enzyme systems, it stimulates these enzymes and thereby increases the rate of metabolism of compounds such as dicumarol and warfarin.

Tolerance and dependence. Continued use of chloral hydrate results in the development of tolerance in less than 2 weeks. The drug is also capable of producing psychological and physical dependence (Chapter 11.6).

Side effects and overdose. Chloral hydrate may cause gastric irritation. In rare cases, it can cause paradoxical excitation. Acute overdose from chloral hydrate may result at a dose about 4-10 times the hypnotic dose. Clinical manifestations of chloral hydrate overdose are similar to barbiturates, but there is an additional risk of myocardial depression and cardiac arrhythmia. Acute overdose may cause permanent liver and kidney damage. Chloral hydrate is secreted in breast milk and hence may cause lethargy in babies.

Drug interactions. Trichloroacetic acid, one of the minor metabolites of chloral hydrate, may potentiate the actions of anticoagulants (e.g., warfarin) by displacing them from the plasma protein binding sites. Chloral hydrate has been reported to interact with furosemide to cause marked vasomotor instability (15). The combination of chloral hydrate and ethanol may be lethal in overdose. Because alcohol dehydrogenase is involved in the oxidation of alcohol and the reduction of chloral hydrate, combined use of these two agents may result in marked sedation due to inhibition of ethanol metabolism and stimulation of chloral hydrate conversion to trichloroethanol, having hypnotic action. Concurrent use of oral anticoagulants and chloral hydrate requires adjustment of the former drug because their metabolism is stimulated by the enzyme induction process discussed earlier.

CHLORAL DERIVATIVES

Triclofos sodium and chloral betaine have the same pharmacological properties as chloral hydrate, but they do not have unpleasant taste and odor. However, triclofos, produces many adverse reactions such as headache, hangover, gastrointestinal complaints, and nightmares.

PARALDEHYDE

Paraldehyde is a polyether of cyclic structure (Fig. 11.2.1-1) formed by polymerization of three molecules of acetaldehyde. It is a colorless liquid with a strong odor and a burning, unpleasant taste. When exposed to light and air, it readily decomposes, first to acetaldehyde, and then is oxidized to acetic acid.

At therapeutic doses, the pharmacological actions of paraldehyde resemble those of barbiturates. It is rapid acting and at therapeutic doses produces mild respiratory depression and hypotension. It readily passes the placental barrier and produces CNS depression in neonates.

Paraldehyde is rapidly absorbed from the gastrointestinal tract, and the peak level in the brain is reached within 30 min. It is largely metabolized in the liver, contrary to the belief that it is excreted unchanged via the lungs.

In the usual doses, paraldehyde does not cause serious side effects. However, prolonged use of large doses (up to 80 ml/day), may cause acidosis, bleeding gastritis, muscular irritability, azotemia, oliguria, and leukocytosis. Toxic doses of paraldehyde when administered intravenously can lead to pulmonary hemorrhage and edema and right ventricular failure. The lethal dose of paraldehyde in humans varies from 12 to 100 ml. In spite of its strong, disagreeable taste and odor, it is liable to be abused, particularly by chronic alcoholics.

METHAQUALONE

Methaqualone is 2-methyl-3-o-tolyl-4(3H)-quinazolinone (Fig. 11.2.1-1). It is an effective sedative-hypnotic agent with a wide range of other activities, including anticonvulsant, antispasmodic, anxiolytic, local anesthestic, and antihistaminic properties. It is rapid acting; drowsiness appears within 10-20 min after its oral administration.

Methaqualone is rapidly absorbed following oral administration and is 80% protein bound. The drug has a long elimination half-life of about 20 to 40 hours or up to 70 hours (9). Repeated administration leads to accumulation in the body. Methaqualone is largely metabolized in the liver and only a trace of it, about 2% is excreted unchanged in the urine.

Side effects of methaqualone are occasional nausea, headache, hangover, drowsiness, lethargy, and dryness of mouth. Acroparesthesia and peripheral neuropathy have also been reported to occur in some patients. Acute overdosage is characterized by delirium, coma, hyperreflexia, and convulsions. The lethal dose may be as low as 8 g, and fatal blood levels are 0.5-1.5 mg/100 ml. Psychological and physical dependence develops following long-term use of the drug at doses larger than usual therapeutic doses. Withdrawal seizures may occur following its use at a dose of about seven times the usual hypnotic dose for about 1 month (19). Tolerance to methaqualone develops rapidly within 2 weeks of continued use; the mechanism is more likely physiological rather than stimulation of hepatic microsomal enzyme system.

Concomitant use of methaqualone and ethanol has been shown to increase blood and brain levels of the former, contributing to high incidence of toxicity (22). Methaqualone is no longer produced in the U.S.A.

GLUTETHIMIDE AND METHYPRYLON

Both glutethimide and methyprylon are piperidenediones and structurally related to barbiturates (Fig. 11.2.1-1). Although these drugs were introduced to replace barbiturates, they provided no therapeutic advan tage over barbiturates. The onset and duration of their hypnotic action resemble closely that of the short-acting barbiturates.

Because glutethimide is poorly soluble in water, its absorption from the gastrointestinal tract is somewhat erratic. Its half-life is about 5 to 22 hours. The drug is largely metabolized in the liver, and its metabolites enter the enterohepatic circulation. Less than 2% of a dose is excreted unchanged in the urine. It has an active metabolite, 4-hydroxyglutethimide, which has a longer half-life than the parent compound. It is a potent stimulator of the hepatic microsomal enzyme and forms an active metabolite.

Side effects of glutethimide include generalized skin rash, nausea, blurred vision, hypersensitivity reactions, acute intermittent porphyria, thrombocytopenia, and leukopenia. Most of the serious side effects to the drug occur rarely.

Severe intoxication may be produced by the drug at a dose of 10 times the hypnotic dose, and the lethal dose is about 20-40 times the usual hypnotic dose. Acute overdose is characterized by prolonged coma, respiratory depression (less than barbiturates), and marked circulatory depression. The fatal blood level of glutethimide varies from 1.5-3 mg/100 ml. High mortality is associated with acute intoxication due to glutethimide. Long-term use of the drug, even at a daily dose of 2.5 g, may cause psychological and physical dependence.

Methyprylon has a half-life of about 4 hours. The drug is largely metabolized in the liver, and a trace of it is excreted in the urine unchanged. Side effects of methyprylon include occasional mild gastric upset, dizziness, headache, skin rash, and paradoxical excitement. In acute overdose, severe respiratory depression and coma occur. Its lethal dose is highly variable and ranges from 6-20 g. Methyprylon is liable to cause both psychological and physical dependence.

ETHCHLORVYNOL

Ethchlorvynol is an acetylenic carbinol (Fig. 11.2.1-1). It is a rapid-acting hypnotic drug with anticonvulsant and muscle relaxant properties. The drug is rapidly absorbed from the gastrointestinal tract, and the onset of hypnotic effect is generally seen within 15-20 min after administration; the peak blood level is achieved in about 2 hours. It has a half-life of approximately 6 hours and is mostly metabolized in the liver; about 10% of a dose is excreted unchanged in the urine. Ethchlorvynol has been reported to form a long-acting metabolite (13). The drug produces various side effects, including hypotension, nausea, and hangover. Acute overdose with ethchlorvynol is manifested by marked hypotension, respiratory depression, bradycardia, and coma. There is a great individual variation in the lethal dose of ethchlorvynol, which may be as low as 14 times the hypnotic dose, but patients have survived after ingestion of 120 times the usual hypnotic dose. Long-term use of the drug in quantities two to three times the hypnotic dose may result in the development of dependence.

ETHINAMATE

Ethinamate is a carbamate (Fig. 11.2.1-1), a group to which meprobamate belongs. It is generally considered milder than other hypnotics in the recommended doses. The drug is rapidly absorbed from the gastrointestinal tract and is distributed in the body fat, liver, and brain tissue. Peak blood levels are achieved in about 1 hour after administration; it has a half-life of approximately 2.25 hours. It is extensively metabolized (hydroxylated and conjugated) in the liver and possibly elsewhere. Severe toxicity develops following acute overdose, and it is potentially addicting.

MISCELLANEOUS DRUGS

A number of drugs primarily used for various other purposes may also possess hypnotic action. Examples of these drugs are antihistamines (e.g., diphenhydramine and methapyrilene), neuroleptics (e.g., thioridazine), and antidepressants (e.g., amitriptyline).

Diphenhydramine is sometimes given to children and the elderly as a sedative or for hypnotic purposes.

Thioridazine is used to relieve nocturnal agitation of elderly psychotic patients. The drug, however, may produce side effects such as tardive dyskinesia, postural hypotension, and anticholinergic effects.

Amitriptyline and doxepin are two antidepressants that are used to normalize disturbed sleep patterns (hyposomnia or hypersomnia) in clinically depressed individuals. The mechanism of action and side effects are discussed in Chapter 11.5.2 .

Most of the commonly used over-the-counter hypnotics contain an antihistamine and/or an anticholinergic (e.g., scopolamine). There are a number of hazards associated with these compounds, such as potentiation of alcohol or other prescription hypnotic drugs, organic brain syndrome, anticholinergic side effects in the elderly, and possible carcinogenic effect of methapyrilene (5)which has been hence withdrawn from the market. l-Tryptophan, an essential amino acid, has been used as a hypnotic agent (8). Although at low doses it is well tolerated except for nausea and vomiting, the effects of its long-term use need further studies. Tryptophan metabolites may be carcinogenic to the bladder in animals (3).

THERAPEUTIC USES

Insomnia. Short-term use of hypnotics including barbiturates (secobarbital, pentobarbital, and amobarbital, possibly phenobarbital and butabarbital), methyprylon, and the benzodiazepines (flurazepam, nitrazepam, and possibly others) do affect sleep more than placebos do.

Benzodiazepines such as flurazepam, temazepam, and triazolam and barbiturates such as pentobarbital, amobarbital, and secobarbital are used as hypnotics. Ideally, a sedative hypnotic drug should induce sleep with rapid onset, maintain sleep for a reasonable period of time, be without residual hangover after the patient awakens, and have no potential for the development of tolerance and no likelihood for abuse. Most authors agree that the benzodiazepines, when used with other treatment measures for a limited period of time, are the preferred drugs for treating insomnia. Benzodiazepines possess one important advantage over the barbiturates and nonbarbituturates; their therapeutic index is extremely high. When taken alone, large amounts of benzodiazepines can be ingested with little or no hazard of prolonged or severe central nervous system depression. The recurrence of insomnia is rapid following withdrawal of treatment with triazolam because of its short half-life. When a benzodiazepine with a long half-life, such as flurazepam, is discontinued, insomnia recurs gradually over several days. Glutethimide in various comparative efficacy studies has not been shown to possess clear effectiveness. Ethchlorvynol is a weak and short-acting hypnotic. Methyprylon may be a useful hypnotic drug because of its short half-life.

Barbiturates and glutethimide both reduce stage 4 sleep and REM sleep, but flurazepam reduces stage 4 sleep only. If hypnotics have to be used for longer than a week or two, except for flurazepam, almost all require larger doses to produce the initial effect. Hypnotics of all classes increase total sleep time during the initial phase of treatment, but only benzodiazepines have been shown to do so in insomnic patients beyond 3-14 days of treatment. For daytime sedation, butabarbital and phenobarbital are currently preferred.

Other Uses. Phenobarbital is also used for seizure disorders and in the management of withdrawals from other hypnotics, including chloral hydrate, glutethimide, methaqualone, methyprylon, and meprobamate. It is also used by pregnant women as a prophylaxis for neonatal hyperbilirubinemia. Paraldehyde is sometimes used as an alternative to benzodiazepines in the management of alcohol withdrawal.

REFERENCES

1. Breimer, D. D. Clinical pharmacokinetics of hypnotics. *Clin. Pharmacokinet.*, 2:93, 1977.
2. Breimer, D. D., Zilly, W., and Richter, E. Pharmacokinetics of hexobarbital in acute hepatitis and after apparent recovery. *Clin. Pharmacol. Ther.*, 18:443, 1975.
3. Bryan, G. T. The role of urinary tryptophan metabolites in the etiology of bladder cancer. *Am. J. Clin. Nutr.*, 24:841, 1971.
4. Dorpat, T. L. Drug automatism, barbiturate poisoning, and suicide behavior. *Arch. Gen. Psychiatr.*, 31:216, 1974.
5. Food and Drug Administration. *Tentative final orders regarding over-the-counter sedatives and sleeping aids.* U.S. Government Printing Office, Washington, D.C., 1978.
6. Gold, E., Gordis, L., Tonascia, J., and Szklo, M. Increased risk of brain tumors in children exposed to barbiturates. *J. Natl. Cancer Inst.*, 61:1031, 1978.
7. Hartmann, E. The effect of four drugs on sleep patterns in man. *Psychopharmacologia*, 12:346, 1968.
8. Hartmann, E. L-tryptophan: A rationale hypnotic with clinical potential. *Am. J. Psychiatr.*, 134:366, 1977.
9. Heck, H., Maloney, K., and Aubar, M. Long-term urinary excretion of methaqualone in a human subject. *J. Pharmacokinet. Biopharmaceut.*, 6:111, 1978.
10. Hinton, J. M. A. A comparison of the effects of six barbiturates and a placebo on insomnia and motility in psychiatric patients. *Br. J. Pharmacol.*, 20:319, 1963.
11. Irvine, R. E., Grove, J., Toseland, P. A., and Trounce, J. R. The effect of age on the hydroxylation of amylobarbitone sodium in man. *Br. J. Clin. Pharmacol.*, 1:41, 1974.
12. Kay, D. C., Jasinski, D. R., Eisenstein, R. B., and Kelly, O. A. Quantified human sleep after pentobarbital. *Clin. Pharmacol. Ther.*, 13:221, 1972.
13. Kripke, D. F., Lavie, P., and Hernandez, J. Polygraphic evaluation of ethchlorvynol (14 days). *Psychopharmacology*, 56:221, 1978.
14. Lasagna, L. A study of hypnotic, drugs in patients with chronic diseases: Comparative efficacy of placebo, methyprylon (Noludar), meprobamate (Miltown, Equanil), pentobarbital, phenobarbital, secobarbital. *J. Chron. Dis.*, 3:122, 1956.
15. Malach, M., and Berman, N. Furosemide and chloral hydrate: Adverse drug interacton. *JAMA*, 232:638, 1975.
16. Mathew, H., and Lawson, A. A. H. Acute barbiturate poisoning: A review of two years' experience. *J. Med.*, 35:539, 1966.
17. McCarron, M. M., Schulze, B. W., Walberg, C. B., Thompson, G. A., and Ansari, A. Short-acting barbiturate overdosage. *JAMA*, 248::55, 1982.
18. Richter, E., Zilly, W., and Brachtel, D. Zur Frage der Barbituratoleranz bei Patienten mit akuter Hepatitis. *Deutsch. Med. Wochenschr.*, 97:254, 1972.
19. *Sleeping Pills, Insomnia, and Medical Practice.* National Academy of Sciences, Washington, D.C., 1979, p. 17.
20. Tatum, A. L. The present status of the barbiturate problem. *Physiol. Rev.*, 19:472, 1939.
21. Teutsch, G., Mahler, D. L., Brown, C. R. et al. Hypnotic efficacy of diphenhydramine, methapyrilene, and pentobarbital. *Clin. Pharmacol. Ther.*, 17:195, 1975.
22. Whitehouse, L. W., Peterson, G., et al. Effect of ethanol on the pharmacokinetics of 2-^{14}C-methaqualone in the rat. *Life Sci.*, 20:1871, 1977.
23. Wolff, B. B. Evaluation of hypnotics in outpatients with insomnia using a questionnaire and a self-rating technique. *Clin. Pharmacol. Ther.*, 15:130, 1974.
24. Young, R. E., Ramsay, L. E., and Murray, T. S. Barbiturates and serum calcium in the elderly. *Postgrad. Med. J.*, 53:212, 1977.

ADDITIONAL READING

Lane, S.J. Development of tolerance to chronic barbital treatment in the cerebellar cyclic guanosine monophosphate system and its response to subsequent barbital abstinence. *J. Pharmacol. Exp. Therap.* 232:569, 1985.

CHAPTER

11.2.2

ALCOHOLS

Samar N. Dutta and Sachin N. Pradhan

ALCOHOLS

ETHYL ALCOHOL (ETHANOL, C_2H_5OH)

Ethyl alcohol is the active ingredient in various alcoholic beverages such as beer, wine, whiskey, gin, and brandy. It is also a component in medicinal elixirs.

Pharmacological Effects

Central Nervous System. Ethanol is a nonspecific depressant of the central nervous system. Electroencephalograph (EEG) recordings show low frequency and high amplitude of alpha activity under ethanol-induced CNS depression. At high doses, the deep-sleep pattern of delta activity is exhibited, but the sleep component of rapid eye movement (REM) is inhibited (7). Reticular formation has been shown to be more sensitive to the depressant effect of ethanol (37), which exerts greater depressant effect on inhibitory than on excitatory functions in the brain. Ethanol-induced positional nystagmus, dizziness, and nausea are probably due to its effects on the vestibular function in the semicircular canal of the inner ear. Some of the early effects of ethanol (e.g., excessive activity and increased electrical activity of the cerebral cortex) are due to inhibition of certain subcortical structures that modulate the cortical activity. At high doses, ethanol depresses cortical, brainstem, and spinal neurons.

Ethanol affects simple motor functions such as maintenance of standing posture and eye and speech movements, as well as complex motor skills. The taste or odor sensation is impaired even at a low dose of ethanol. Visual motor coordination is usually impaired after ingestion of moderate amounts of ethanol in most social drinkers. Various behavioral functions are also impaired by ethanol. The learning process is slow and less effective under the influence of ethanol. Either at low or high doses ethanol causes impairment of memory, particularly in tests involving the recall of poorly learned information.

Ethanol has been shown to increase sociability, self-esteem, and expressions of an exhilarated mood. Powers of attention and concentration, as well as faculties of judgment and discrimination are impaired under the influence of ethanol. It increases aggressive behavior under certain conditions, and high blood ethanol levels have been reported in a large number of people who have committed homicide (15).

Ethanol at a concentration range of 10-500 mg/dl has been reported to cause graded contractile responses in rat cerebral arterioles and venules *in vivo* and in isolated canine basilar and middle cerebral arteries. At this concentration range, ethanol produces graded effects of euphoria, mental haziness, muscular incoordination, stupor, and coma in humans (1). These observations suggest that ethanol produces hypoxia in the brain by affecting cerebral circulation. This study further showed that calcium antagonists like nimodipine and verapamil completely reversed or prevented alcohol-induced cerebrovasospasm.

Binding sites for ethanol in the brain cell membrane have been described (18), but they do not have the high affinity and selectivity of the receptor sites. It has been suggested that the action of ethanol on the brain is partially due to its effect on γ-aminobutyric acid (GABA) transmission (34). Its acute administration has been reported to decrease synthesis of GABA, and GABA-receptor binding (27). Neurohypophyseal melanophore-stimulating hormone (MSH) and MSH-ACTH have been shown to antagonize some acute effects of ethanol on the CNS (28). Chronic administration of arginine-vasopressin (AVP) was reported to increase duration of tolerance to the sedative and hypothermic actions of ethanol in rats (19).

Cardiovascular System. The acute effects of ethanol on blood pressure are conflicting (39). Cutaneous blood vessels are dilated, whereas splanchnic vessels are constricted. Perivascular, intracarotid, or systemic administration of its graded doses has been reported to cause vasoconstriction of rat cortical arteries (1). A pressor effect of ethanol has been demonstrated in moderate drinkers with hypertension (39). Ethanol has complex effects on cerebral blood flow and autoregulation (8).

Acute exposure to moderate doses of ethanol can predispose to cardiac arrhythmias (atrial flutter, fibrillation, ventricular tachycardia) in alcoholic patients with heart disease (17). High incidence of arrhythmias was reported in patients hospitalized for alcohol withdrawal treatment, and none of the patients had any known cardiac disease (52). Almost all abnormal electrocardiographic changes were corrected after acute withdrawal phase.

Gastrointestinal System. Gastric acid secretion is stimulated by low concentration of ethanol, mediated by release of gastrin from the antral region and possibly by histamine release. Saliva flow and intestinal motility are also stimulated by ethanol at a low dose, but at high doses these functions are depressed. In high concentration (e.g., 10-15%) there is an initial increase in mucus secretion followed by congestion and irritation of gastric mucosa. Tissue damage may occur at a concentration of 20% or above. A sense of well-being and stimulation of end-organs for taste are believed to be the mechanism for the appetite-stimulating property of ethanol.

Moderate ethanol abuse has been reported to be associated with a striking changes in intestinal permeability, resulting in increased absorption of test solution of ^{51}Cr-labeled edetic acid (9). It has been suggested that ethanol-induced increased intestinal permeability could result in the absorption of toxic nonabsorbable compounds of molecular weight less than 5000, which may cause damage to extraintestinal sites.

Metabolic Effects. Chronic alcoholic subjects may have blood sugar levels lower than normal. However, true hypoglycemia ($<$ 50 mg%) may occur in malnourished persons and heavy drinkers. Impairment of hepatic gluconeogenesis is the mechanism for such action of ethanol. Both chronic and acute alcoholism induces hypertriglyceridemia, and that may lead to fatty liver, pancreatitis, and promotion of atherogenesis. Chronic alcoholics may manifest low serum phosphate, magnesium, potassium, and calcium. Mechanisms for these serum changes are probably multifactorial (2).

Kidney and Endocrine System. Acute ingestion of ethanol causes diuresis in normal volunteers, and there is a rapid increase in free water clearance and decrease in urine osmolality, whereas glomerular filtration rate remains unchanged. The principal mechanism for the diuretic action of ethanol is inhibition of release of antidiuretic hormone (ADH). With chronic ingestion, however, the diuretic action does not persist. Ethanol does not change the sensitivity of the renal tubules to either endogenous or exogenous ADH.

Ethanol also interferes with the renal excretion of uric acid, resulting in elevation of serum uric acid level that may lead to precipitation of gout. Alcoholic uricemia can be distinguished from primary uricemia by its return to normal values upon termination of ethanol use. Ethanol decreases the rate of synthesis and plasma level of testosterone following its repeated administration (16) and can increase plasma cortisol level in both alcoholics and nonalcoholics (30).

Acid-base Balance. In nonalcoholic subjects, ethanol causes mixed metabolic and respiratory acidosis. Metabolic acidosis results from increased hepatic ketogenesis and is partly due to increased formation of lactate and β-hydroxybutyrate. Respiratory acidosis results from depression of respiration. Arterial pH may rise during withdrawal syndrome of ethanol, but its mechanism is not clear.

Miscellaneous Effects. Ethanol causes a fall in body temperature due to loss of heat from increased sweating and cutaneous vasodilation. It exerts a direct effect on bone marrow cells, causing increased vacuolation of the red and white cell precursors. Blood platelet counts and serum iron levels are both decreased by ethanol (26). Ethanol impairs sexual functions in either sex; high doses of ethanol cause structural changes in the sperm cells and slow their motility. In women, uterine contractions are inhibited during childbirth and lactation by ethanol administered intravenously.

Alcoholic women often suffer from amenorrhea, infertility, and spontaneous abortions (20). Female monkeys following self-induced ethanol dependence have been reported to manifest amenorrhea, atrophy of the uterus, small ovarian mass, and marked depression of luteinizing hormone levels (29). Intravenous administration of ethanol to pregnant monkeys was reported to cause marked collapse of umbilical vessels promptly and resulted in severe hypoxia and acidosis in the fetus (32).

Pharmacokinetics. Ethanol is rapidly absorbed from the gastrointestinal tract; approximately 25% is absorbed from the stomach and the remainder from the upper small intestine. A number of factors interfere with the gastrointestinal absorption of ethanol; these are concentration of ethanol, presence of food (most pronounced with high-protein foods and least with high-carbohydrate food), low body temperature, and heavy physical exercise. Ethanol is also absorbed through the skin. Ethanol is detected in the blood in less than 5 min after ingestion, and the peak concentration is achieved in about 30-60 min. It is distributed rapidly throughout the body. Its concentration in cerebrospinal fluid, urine, and pulmonary alveolar air bear a steady relationship with blood concentrations.

It is generally accepted that the disappearance of ethanol from the blood of humans and experimental animals follows zero-order kinetics (i.e., linear), until very low values are reached. The possibility of nonlinearity at early times of elimination has been suggested by some investigators (51). However, in contrast to ethanol, most drugs are eliminated by first-order kinetics [i.e., there is a rate constant of elimination (K_e) which is the proportion of the drug concentration being eliminated].

Ethanol is metabolized mainly in the liver. There are three enzyme systems that can independently oxidize ethanol to acetaldehyde. The principal pathway of ethanol oxidation involves alcohol dehydrogenase, which requires nicotinamide adenine dinucleotide (NAD) as a cofactor. The second and the third pathways involve a catalase and the microsomal ethanol oxidizing system (MEOS) for metabolism of ethanol. The latter pathway has been suggested to be responsible for the rapid rate of ethanol metabolism in chronic alcoholics.

The quantitative significance of oxidation of ethanol via MEOS and the action of catalase is controversial, but it has been suggested that these two pathways contribute approximately 10-20% of total metabolism of ethanol (40). It has been suggested that acetaldehyde formed by the oxidation of ethanol could undergo condensation reactions with endogenous amines to form pharmacologically active tetrahydroisoquinoline compounds. One of these compounds, salsolinol (dopamine plus acetaldehyde) has been reported in higher concentration in the urine of alcoholics undergoing detoxification (27).

Acetaldehyde is rapidly oxidized by acetaldehyde dehydrogenase to acetyl-coenzyme A (acetyl CoA) via acetate. Both acetyl CoA and acetate, the end products of ethanol metabolism in the liver, are finally oxidized to carbon dioxide and water. The rate of oxidation of ethanol is constant and is dependent of its concentration in the blood. In humans, a typical rate of oxidation is about 150 mg of ethanol per kilogram of body weight per hour, or roughly 1 oz of 90-proof whiskey per hour. Disulfiram inhibits oxidation of acetaldehyde, and its concomitant use with ethanol leads to elevation of blood acetaldehyde levels. Repeated ingestion of ethanol increases the rate of its own metabolism. In starvation, the rate of ethanol metabolism is inhibited.

Tolerance and Physical Dependence. Tolerance to ethanol develops usually after a short period of exposure. When ethanol concentration in the blood is raised very slowly, few symptoms may appear, even at very high-dosage level. The underlying mechanism(s) for tolerance is (are) not clearly known, but it is generally ascribed to increased rate of ethanol metabolism.

Chronic consumption of ethanol results in increased activity of microsomal ethanol oxidizing system which contributes to the accelerated rate of its metabolism. A concomitant increase in drug-metabolizing enzymes explains increased metabolic tolerance of chronic alcoholics to a variety of other drugs (e.g., aminopyrine, tolbutamide, propranolol, meprobamate, phenobarbital, and rifamycin). The tolerance of the alcoholic to various drugs has also been attributed to the CNS adaptation. Due to the development of metabolic tolerance the half-life of drugs like warfarin, phenytoin, tolbutamide, and isoniazid may be 50% shorter in abstaining alcoholics than nondrinkers. An acute dose of ethanol, however, with some exceptions inhibits the metabolism of other drugs mostly through competition for a shared microsomal metabolic pathway (25).

Adverse Effects. Chronic alcoholism has long been associated with both malnutrition and liver disease. Although malnutrition was previously suggested by many investigators to be an important factor in the development of liver disease in the mid-1960s, evidence began to appear indicating that liver injury in alcoholic patients may be independent of the nutritional status. A recent Veterans Administration Cooperative Study has shown a high prevalence of malnutrition in chronic alcoholics and a progressive increase in frequency and severity of the malnutrition with the severity of the liver disease (31). The presence of such features as ascites, jaundice, or hemorrhage in alcoholics should point to the possibility of the chronic liver disease. The mechanism by which ethanol induces liver damage is still the subject of debate. It is not clear whether alcoholic hepatitis or cirrhosis develops as a result of the direct toxic effect of ethanol or its metabolites (24), or by the way of immunological mechanisms (42).

The concept of ethanol as a myocardial toxin is generally accepted by clinicians. Chronic alcoholics gradually develop subclinical cardiomyopathy which facilitates electrical irritability (5). Several investigators have suggested that excessive ethanol consumption predisposes humans to hemorrhagic stroke and sudden death (4, 49).

There is a possibility of decrease in the risk of myocardial infarction and death from coronary heart disease in individuals who drink low amounts of ethanol (about three drinks per day). The suggested mechanism of this protective effect of ethanol is an increase in the level of high-density lipoprotein in the blood and increased fibrinolytic activity (43). However, a high incidence of hypertensive vascular disease has been reported to occur in alcoholics (3, 6).

At high doses, ethanol changes many information-processing components of learning and memory (11). Zimeldine, a relatively specific blocker of serotonin uptake (35), has been reported to attenuate the disrupting effects of ethanol on memory and learning (50).

Epidemiological studies have demonstrated that ethanol consumption during pregnancy results in increased perinatal mortality and morbidity (46). Excessive ethanol consumption during pregnancy causes developmental anomalies in the fetus referred to as the fetal alcohol syndrome (12). Teratogenic effects of maternal alcoholism are directly attributed to ethanol and vary with the quantities and time of exposure to ethanol during gestation. Developmental anomalies include short palpebral fissures, a hypoplastic upper lip with thinned vermilion, and diminished to absent philtrum, as well as growth inhibition and mental retardation.

Both acute and chronic abuse of ethanol have been reported to be responsible for a wide spectrum of pancreatic disorders (e.g., acute necrotizing, acute edema tous, acute relapsing, and painless pancreatitis) (14). The pathogenesis of ethanol-induced changes in structure and function of pancreas is unclear. It seems to be multifactorial; inappropriate activation of zymogens probably plays a major role (14).There are rare incidences of myopathy in chronic alcoholics (45, 47). The pathophysiological basis for chronic alcoholic myopathy remains obscure.

Deficiencies of vitamins (thiamine, pyridoxine, folate, ascorbic acid, and vitamin A) may arise in alcoholic subjects through a combination of reduced dietary intake, malabsorption, reduced tissue uptake, and increased hepatic metabolism (44). A number of neurological disorders are encountered in chronic alcoholism and these include Wernicke-Korsakoff syndrome, polyneuropathy, cerebellar degeneration, central pontine myelinolysis, and Marchiafava-Bignami disease (33). Wernick's encephalopathy represents the acute phase of Wernicke-Korsakoff syndrome: it is characterized by oculomotor disturbances, cerebellar ataxia, and mental confusion and is caused by thiamine deficiency; Korsakoff's psychosis, the chronic phase, is characterized by amnesia.

Epidemiological studies have suggested positive association between chronic ethanol consumption and increased risk of developing cancer of the mouth, pharynx, larynx, esophagus, colon, rectum, lung, or prostate (10, 38). Ethanol may act as a chemical carcinogen ("initiator"), or function as a cocarcinogen or as a tumor promoter.

Acute Overdose. The clinical findings of ethanol intoxication are exhilaration and excitement, irregular behavior, staggering and slurred speech, incoordination of movement and gait, stupor, convulsions, hypoglycemia, and coma. Blood ethanol levels and clinical manifestations of ethanol are presented in Table 11.2.2-1.

Mild-to-moderate degrees of intoxication with ethanol require no particular therapeutic measures. Alcoholic stupor is often self-limited and in the absence of abnormal vital signs needs no special therapy. In the case of coma due to ethanol intoxication, measures should be taken to counter respiratory depression, hypoglycemia, and ketoacidosis. Hemodialysis should be considered if the blood ethanol concentration is 500 mg/dl or above. Although use of analeptic drugs such as pentylenetetrazol and mixtures of picrotoxin and caffeine antagonize alcohol-induced CNS depression, they may cause powerful cerebrocortical stimulation, leading to convulsions.

Table 11.2.2-1
Clinical Manifestations at Increasing Blood Ethanol Levels

Blood Ethanol (mg/dl)	Signs and Symptoms
30	Mild euphoria
50-150	Incoordination, impaired reaction time, blurred vision
150-300	Ataxia, mental confusion, impaired vision, staggering speech, hypoglycemia
300-500	Stupor, hypoglycemia, convulsions
500 and above	Coma and death

Drug Interactions. A large number of interactions between ethanol and other drugs have been cited. Clinically important interactions are presented in Table 11.2.2-2.

Therapeutic Uses. Ethanol is widely used as a skin disinfectant, and a 70% aqueous solution exerts optimum bactericidal action. Intravenous ethanol has been used to inhibit premature labor because of its direct inhibitory action on uterine contractions.

METHYL ALCOHOL

Methyl alcohol (methanol) is commonly referred to as wood alcohol, and it is present in paint solvent, varnish, antifreeze, and solid canned fuel.

Methanol poisoning could occur from its ingestion, inhalation, or cutaneous absorption. Unlike ethanol, the presence of food materials in the gastrointestinal tract is less likely to interfere with the blood levels of methanol. Ethanol consumption immediately before or with methanol ingestion usually decreases the toxicity of the latter. An 8-hr exposure to methanol vapor at about 3000 ppm may result in methanol intoxication (22). It is rapidly absorbed through the skin, and toxic effects have been reported as a result of prolonged contact with methanol (48). The symptoms of acute methanol poisoning following oral ingestion usually appear 12-48 hr after intake. These symptoms include abdominal pain, nausea, vomiting, weakness, dizziness, shortness of breath, cerebral aberrations, blurring of vision, symptoms of shock, severe metabolic acidosis, blindness, and coma, and death results from respiratory arrest and/or cardiovascular collapse. Lethal dose (oral) of methanol is between 50 and 100 ml (36). Inhalation of methanol vapor results in irritation to the mucous membrane. It may also cause headache, vertigo, tinnitus, visual disturbances, tracheitis, and bronchitis. In addition to systemic toxic effects,

Table 11.2.2-2
Interaction of Ethanol with Other Drugs

Interacting Drugs	Effects	Probable Mechanism
Acetaminophen	Hepatotoxicity	Increased production of toxic metabolites
Anticoagulants (oral)	Decreased anticoagulant action	Increased hepatic metabolism
Antihistamines	CNS depression	Additive action
Barbiturates	Decreased sedation	Increased hepatic metabolism
Disulfiram	Abdominal pain, flushing, vomiting, mental confusion	Inhibition of intermediary metabolism of alcohol
Hypoglycemics (oral, e.g., sulfonylureas)	(1) Reduced effectiveness	Increased metabolism due to enzyme induction
	(2) Increased hypoglycemia	Marked inhibition of gluconeogenesis
	(3) Disulfiram-like effects of alcohol	Inhibition of intermediary metabolism
Metronidazole	Disulfiram-like effect	Inhibition of intermediary metabolism of alcohol
Salicylates	Gastrointestinal	Additive damaging effect on gastric mucosa
Phenytoin	Decreased or increased effectiveness	Increased metabolism due to enzyme induction or decreased metabolism

inflammatory changes to the skin may occur following prolonged dermal contact with methanol.

Accumulation of formic acid, a metabolic product of methanol, has been reported to play a major role in the metabolic acidosis in methanol intoxication in humans (13). Treatment of methanol poisoning includes bicarbonate administration to control acidosis, ethanol infusion to inhibit methanol metabolism and to decrease blood levels of formate, and hemodialysis to decrease the blood levels of formic acid and methanol. Additional supportive measures are taken to provide adequate ventilation.

ISOPROPYL ALCOHOL

Various industrial or home-cleaning products (windshield-washer solvent, jewelery and lens cleaners), antifreeze preparations, and skin lotions contain isopropyl alcolol in varying amounts. Following an oral dose, most of it is absorbed within 30 min absorption being delayed with large doses (23). Cutaneous absorption of isopropyl alcohol is negligible, but significant absorption may occur by inhalation. About 80% of an absorbed dose is excreted as acetone, and the remaining 20% is excreted unchanged by the kidney. Both unchanged alcohol and its metabolite acetone are excreted through the lungs, secreted in saliva and gastric juice. Like ethanol, the elimination of isopropyl alcohol closely follows first-order kinetics.

As little as 20 ml of isopropyl alcohol may cause acute intoxication and symptoms may appear within 30 min of ingestion. In humans the lethal dose of isopropyl alcohol is about 5-8 oz. Symptoms relative to gastrointestinal system occur initially which include abdominal pain, gastritis, vomiting, and hematemesis. It is twice as potent a CNS depressant as ethanol, and it causes dizziness, muscle incoordination, headache, mental confusion, and coma. The latter may be deep and long-lasting because of the slow rate of metabolism (21). Acute intoxication is also associated with nonacidotic acetonemia and acetonuria. Other less frequent symptoms of its intoxication include hypotension, renal tubular necrosis, hypothermia, myopathy, and hemolytic anemia. Prognosis of acute intoxication may be poor in patients with both coma and hypotension and with a serum concentration greater than 400 mg/dl.

Management of acute intoxication with isopropyl alcohol includes induction of emesis by ipecac syrup, if the patient is alert, or gastric emptying by lavage, and supportive measures to maintain adequate ventilation, blood volume and electrolyte balance, and hemodialysis.

REFERENCES

1. Altura, B.M., Altura, B.T. and Gebrewold, A. Alcohol-induced spasms of cerebral blood vessels: Relation to cerebrovascular accidents and sudden death. *Science*, 220:331, 1983.
2. Anderson, R., Cohen, N., Haller, R. *et al.* Skeletal muscle phosphorus and magnesium deficiency in alcoholic myopathy. *Mineral and Electrolyte Metabolism*, 4:106, 1980.
3. Ashley, M.J. and Rankin, J.G. Alcohol consumption and hypertension — The evidence from hazardous drinking and alcoholic populations. *Aust. NZ J. Med.*, 9:201, 1979.
4. Ashley, M.J. and Rankin, J.G. Hazardous alcohol consumption and diseases of the circulatory system. *J. Stud. Alcohol.*, 41:1040, 1980.

5. Ballas, M., Zoneraich, S., Zoneraich, O. and Rosnev, F. Noninvasive cardiac evaluation in chronic alcoholic patients with alcohol withdrawal syndrome. *Chest*, 82:148, 1982.
6. Barboriak, P.N., Anderson, A.J., Hoffmann, R.G. and Barboriak, J.J. Blood pressure and alcohol intake in heart patients. *Alcoholism*, 6:234, 1982.
7. Barry, H., III. Alcohol. In: *Drug Abuse: Clinical and Basic Aspects* (Pradhan, S.N. and Dutta, S.N., eds.). C.V. Mosby, St. Louis, 1977, p. 78.
8. Berglund, M. and Risberg, J. Regional cerebral blood flow during alcohol withdrawal. *Arch. Gen. Psychiatry*, 38:351, 1981.
9. Bjarnason, I., Ward, K. and Peters, T.J. The leaky gut of alcoholism: Possible route of entry for toxic compounds. *Lancet*, 1:179, 1984.
10. Breeden, J.H. Alcohol, alcoholism and cancer. *Med. Clin. North Am.*, 68:163, 1984.
11. Butters, N. and Cermak, L.S. *Alcoholic Korsakoff's Syndrome: An Information Processing Approach to Amnesia.* Academic Press, New York, 1980.
12. Clarren, S.K. and Smith, D.W. The fetal alcohol syndrome. *N. Engl. J. Med.*, 298:1063, 1978.
13. Fulop, M. Methanol intoxication. *Lancet*, 1:338, 1982.
14. Gokas, M.C. Ethanol and the pancreas. *Med. Clin. North Am.*, 68:57, 1984.
15. Goodwin, D.W. Alcohol in suicide and homicide. *J. Stud. Alcohol*, 34:144, 1973.
16. Gordon, G.G. *et al.* Effect of alcohol (ethanol) administration on sex-hormone metabolism in normal man. *N. Engl. J. Med.*, 295:793, 1976.
17. Greenspoon, A. and Schaal, S.F. The "Holiday Heart": Electrophysiologic studies of alcohol in alcoholics. *Ann. Intern. Med.*, 98:135, 1983.
18. Grenell, R.G. The binding of alcohol to brain membranes. In: *Alcohol Intoxication and Withdrawal, Advances in Experimental Medicine and Biology*, Vol. 59 (Gross, M.M., ed.). Plenum Press, New York, 1975.
19. Hoffman, P.L., Ritzmann, R.F., Walter, R. andTabakoff, B.Arginine vasopressin maintains alcohol tolerance. *Nature*, 276:614, 1978.
20. Hugues, J.N., Cofte,T., Perret, G. *et al.* Hypothalamo-pituitary ovarian function in thirty-one women with chronic alcoholism. *Clin. Endocrinol.*, 12:543, 1980.
21. Lacoutre, P.G.,Wason, S., Abrams, A. and Lovejoy, Jr., F.H. Acute isopropyl alcohol intoxication. *Am. J. Med.*, 75:680,1983.
22. Leaf, S. and Zatman, L.J. A study of the conditions under which methanol may exert a toxic hazard in industry. *Br. J. Ind. Med.*, 9:19, 1952.
23. Lehman, A.J., Schwerma, H. and Rickards, E. Isopropyl alcohol: Rate of disappearance from the blood stream of dogs after intravenous and oral administration. *J. Pharmacol. Exp. Ther.*, 82:196, 1942.
24. Lewis, K.O. and Paton, A. Could superoxide cause cirrhosis? *Lancet*, 2:188, 1982.
25. Lieber, C.S. Metabolism and metabolic effects of alcohol. *Med. Clin. North Am.*, 68:3, 1984.
26. Lindenabaum, J. and Lieber, C.S. Hematologic effects of alcohol in man in the absence of nutritional deficiency. *N. Engl. J. Med.* 281:333, 1969.
27. Little, H.J. and Wing, D.R. Alcohol. In: *Preclinical Psychopharmacology* (Grahame-Smith, D.G., ed.). Excerpta Medica, Princeton, 1983, p. 398.
28. McGivern, R.F., Harris, J.M., Yessaian, N. *et al.* Antagonism of ethanol induced sleep-time by α-MSH, MSH/ACTH 4-10 and naloxone. *Subst. Alcohol Actions/Misuse*, 1:335, 1980.
29. Mello, N.K., Bree, M.P., Mendelson, J.H. *et al.* Alcohol self-administration disrupts reproductive function in female Macaque Monkeys. *Science*, 221:677, 1983.
30. Mendelson, J.H., Ogata, M. and Mello, N.K. Adrenal function and alcoholism. *Psychosom. Med.*, 33:145, 1971.
31. Menderhall, C.L., Anderson, S.,Weesner, R.E. *et al.* Protein-calorie malnutrition associated with alcoholic hepatitis. *Am. J. Med.*, 76:211, 1984.
32. Mukherjee, A.B. and Hodgen, G.D. Maternal ethanol exposure induces transient impairment of umbilical circulation and fetal hypoxia in monkeys. *Science*, 218:700, 1982.
33. Nakada,T. and Knight, R.T. Alcohol and the central nervous system. *Med.Clin. North Am.*, 68:121, 1984.
34. Nestoros, J.N. Ethanol selectivity potentiates GABA-mediated inhibition of single feline cortical neurones. *Life Sci.*, 26:519, 1980.
35. Ogren, S.O., Ross, S.B., Hall, H., Holm, A.C. and Renyi, A.L. The pharmacology of zimelidine: A 5-HT selective. *Acta Psychiatr. Scand.*, (Suppl. 290) 63:127, 1981.
36. Paul, J.K. *Methanol Technology and Application in Motor Fuels.* Noyes Data Corp., Park Ridge, N.J., 1978.
37. Perrine, M.W. Alcohol influences on driving-related behavior: A critical review on laboratory studies of neurophysiological, neuromuscular, and sensory activity. *J. Safety Res.*, 5:165, 1973.
38. Pollack, E.S. Nomura, A.M.Y., Heilbrun, L.K. *et al.* Prospective study of alcohol consumption and cancer. *N. Engl. J. Med.*, 310:617, 1984.
39. Potter, J.F. and Beevers, D.G. Pressor effect of alcohol in hypertension. *Lancet*, 1:119, 1984.
40. Rognstad,R. and Grunnet, N. Enzymatic pathways of ethanol metabolism. In: *Biochemistry and Pharmacology of Ethanol*, Vol. I (Majchrowicz, E. and Noble, E.P., eds.). Plenum Press, New York, 1979, p. 65.
41. Sato, C., Matsuda, Y. and Lieber, C.S. Increased hepatotoxicity of acetaminophen after ethanol consumption in the rat. *Gastroenterology,* 80:140, 1981.
42. Saunders, J.B. Alcoholic liver disease. *Br. Med. J.*, 287:1819, 1983.
43. Segel, L.D., Klausner, S.C., Harney Gnadt, J.T. and Amsterdam, E.A. Alcohol and the heart. *Med. Clin. North Am.*, 68:147, 1984.
44. Sherlock, S. Nutrition and the alcoholic. *Lancet*, 1:436, 1984.
45. Salvin, G., Martin, F., Ward, P. *et al.* Chronic alcohol excess is associated with selective but reversible injury to type 2B muscle fibers. *J. Clin. Pathol.*, 36:772, 1983.
46. Streissguth, A.P., Landesman-Dwyer, S., Martin, J.C. and Smith, D.W. Teratogenic effects of alcohol in humans and laboratory animals. *Science,* 209:353, 1980.
47. Sunnasy, D.,Cairns, S.R., Martin, F. *et al.* Chronic alcoholic skeletal muscle myopathy: A clinical histological and biochemical assessment of muscle lipid. *J. Clin. Pathol.*, 36:778, 1983.
48. Tada, O., Nakaaki, K., Fukabori, S. and Yonemoto, J. An experimental study on the cutaneous absorption of methanol in man. *J. Sci. Labor*, 51:143, 1975.
49. Taylor, J.R. Alcohol and strokes. *N. Engl. J. Med.*, 306:1111, 1982.
50. Weingartner, H.,Rudorfer, M.W., Buchsbaum, M.S. and Linnoila, M. Effects of serotonin on memory impairments produced by ethanol. *Science*, 221:472, 1983.
51. Wilkinson, P.K., Reynolds,G., Holmes, O.D., Yang, S. and Wilkin, L.O. Nonlinear pharmacokinetics of ethanol: The disproportionate AUC-dose relationship. *Alcoholism: Clin.Exp. Res.*, 4:384, 1980.
52. Zoneraich, S., Ballas, M., Zoneraich, O. and Rosner, F. Alcohol and the heart. *Ann. Intern. Med.*, 98:671, 1983.

CHAPTER
11.3

CENTRAL NERVOUS SYSTEM STIMULANTS

Richard H. Rech

A great many substances can cause an increase in neuronal activity of the central nervous system (CNS) by a variety of mechanisms. The ultimate cause is a disturbance in the normal balance of excitatory and inhibitory activities of the CNS. This balance fluctuates over narrow limits in the healthy person. Once a gross, generalized disturbance has developed, whether initiated by reduced inhibition (e.g., strychnine) or enhanced excitement (e.g., pentylenetetrazol), the symptoms of excessive output are similar: generalized tonic-clonic convulsions. At threshold doses, however, or as the effects of intoxication with various stimulants, convulsant agents first appear, there are differences in symptom patterns that reflect the different mechanisms and/or sites of action. These include varied influences on consciousness and on cognitive and emotional processes.

This chapter examines the analeptics (picrotoxin, pentylenetetrazol and doxapram type), certain toxic substances of natural origin (strychnine), a few drugs used socially and subject to abuse (nicotine, caffeine), and some aspects of the psychomotor stimulants (amphetamine-like drugs). Some of these agents (e.g., caffeine) produce in overdose mainly clonic seizures, asymmetrical coordinated flailing, or "running" movements of the limbs. Because effective respiration is usually maintained, this syn drome is not likely to be fatal. On the other hand, the tonic convulsant activity of strychnine poisoning is characterized by prolonged phases of uncoordinated contraction of all skeletal muscles, the rigid posture assumed being determined by the more powerful muscle sets. Thus, oxygen debt accumulates from the cramp of the respiratory muscles as well as from the bouts of excessive activity, and death is often the outcome.

Drugs classified as CNS stimulants have few therapeutic applications. In the past, one category of CNS stimulants has been used as *analeptics*, agents intended to reverse marked CNS depression, usually from an overdose of barbiturate or other depressant drug. Unfortunately, the demonstration of effective antagonism of drug-induced depression has been inconsistent, and the difference between the analeptic dose and convulsant dose for most of these agents is very narrow. Furthermore, the stimulant phase is often of short duration and is followed by generalized depression that may then be refractory to further treatment. The current proven therapy of choice for depressant drug overdose is the support of vital functions through artificial respiration and peripherally acting drugs (40). Some agents may have limited value in treating certain pulmonary ailments (e.g., emphysema) or reducing the recovery time from general anesthesia (more common in veterinary than in human medicine) (16).

The current consensus on the use of analeptics is that they do no good in emergency treatment of depressant drug overdose and may do considerable harm. Nevertheless, this stance should not discourage continued research effort to discover an analeptic with sufficient efficacy and specificity in stimulating respiration and other vital functions (40).

CNS stimulants in this class are also important as toxicological (strychnine) or abuse (caffeine) problems, as well as being effective diagnostic (pentylenetetrazol) and research (picrotoxin) tools in the study of synaptic interrelationships in the CNS. These agents qualify as analeptics in that the lowest effective doses demonstrate CNS stimulation as the major pharmacological effect. Examples of drugs in other classes that stimulate the CNS in overdose are the local anesthetics (procaine), antihistamines (pyrilamine), tricyclic antidepressants (imipramine), and atropine, to name a few (see appropriate sections of this text for details).

CLASSIFICATION OF CNS STIMULANTS

CNS stimulants may be classified according to their predominant site of stimulation, as given in Table 11.3-1. The diversity in chemical structures among this class of drugs defies attempts to establish structure-activity relationships and suggests that multiple mechanisms are involved in drug-induced convulsant effects.

The representation of the sites of action for these substances must not be taken too literally. Most of these drugs appear to cause neuronal excitation of any portion of the CNS, providing the drug dosage is adequate. The

Table 11.3-1
Classification of CNS Stimulants by Major Sites of Action

Forebrain	Brainstem	Spinal Cord	Peripheral Receptors
	Picrotoxin	Strychnine	α-Lobeline
Amphetamine group	Bemegride	Tetanospasmin	Nicotine
Caffeine	Doxapram group		Doxapram group
Pentylenetetrazol	Thiosemicarbazide		
	Pentylenetetrazol		

relative selectivity of a lower dose for one portion of the CNS is probably a reflection of a higher density of subcellular components through which the drug exerts its action. Strychnine excites indirectly the spinal motoneurons in threshold doses by blocking the prominent inhibitory control exerted via recurrent collaterals and Renshaw-type interneurons on spinal motoneurons, thus disrupting the normal mechanism that tonically protects against reflex hyperexcitability. Strychnine will, however, excite a neuronally isolated slab of cerebral cortex as the dose level is increased (27), as a reflection of blocking a lower density of recurrent Renshaw-type inhibitory neurons in the circuitry of cortical pyramidal cells. Moreover, given the widespread and complex interconnections of the CNS, one must expect that even subconvulsant doses of these agents may result in heightened excitability in CNS areas remote from a direct local effect of the drug.

Classifications of stimulants have also been based on mechanism (e.g., picrotoxin as a GABA antagonist) and on use or medical consequences of exposure. For example, d-amphetamine is a psychomotor stimulant by virtue of the increased alertness and enhanced motor activity it induces especially in the presence of fatigue. Nicotine may be considered a social drug in reference to tobacco use but is labeled a poison as an ingredient in insecticides. Therefore, any single classification is inadequate to fully characterize the agents in this group.

INDIVIDUAL AGENTS

STRYCHNINE

Strychnine has long been used as a rodenticide, placed in wafers or other bases to whet the appetite. For decades it also had a reputation as a "tonic" for human consumption, being prepared as chocolate-coated tablets. Such use in the past was a source of poisonings of children, pets, and farm animals, but this practice is much less common today. Strychnine is occasionally found as an adulterant with illicit drugs. For this reason, individuals involved in overdose aid for abused drugs should be familiar with symptoms of strychnine poisoning.

Strychnine is the most important alkaloid (Fig. 11.3-1) in the seeds of several species of *Strychnos*, particularly the Indian plant *nux-vomica*. This latter name has led to the erroneous assumption that the substance is emetic. The alkaloid is rapidly and completely absorbed after oral administration and is rapidly degraded by liver microsomal enzymes (40). Thus, protection against convulsant effects usually needs to be maintained for only a few hours.

All mammalian and many other vertebrate nervous systems are affected similarly by strychnine. An initial hyperreflexia rapidly phases into violent spastic jerks and then to more prolonged convulsant activity, predominantly of a tonic nature. Reciprocal interactions between spinal motoneurons become ineffective and all motoneurons are maximally excited. The posture taken during the tonic seizure depends on the relative strength of flexor and extensor muscles. In humans, an arching of the back may cause only the heels and back of head to touch the floor (opisthotonos). Symmetrical extensor thrusts precede and follow (during fatigue) these episodes of tonic extension and are often precipitated by stimuli via any sensory modality. Arms are drawn tightly across the chest, fists clenched, and the facial contortion takes the form of a hideous grimace. Consciousness is usually maintained during initial seizures, so that the victim suffers great stress and pain. Hypoxia ensues due to asphyxia and excessive oxygen utilization, causing fatigue and respiratory embarrassment between tonic bouts and eventual death. The victim seldom survives as many as five seizure episodes. Thus, the preferred treatment is prompt depression of the CNS (i.v. thiopental or diazepam, nitrous oxide by inhalation) before seizures are manifested or early in their course.

McCulloch (see Ref. 40) utilized a technique developed by his mentor, Dusser de Barenne, called *strychnine neuronography* to establish functional connections of cortical sites with other portions of the CNS. Neurons locally stimulated by applied strychnine generated spikes along major axon projections throughout the CNS, but these spikes did not pass synapses. Purpura and Grundfest (24) and Rech and Domino (27) utilized local application of strychnine to the cerebral cortex in the study of cortical inhibitory processes. Thus, strychnine has been and remains an important research tool in neurophysiological studies of mechanisms of postsynaptic inhibition. More recently, strychnine has been shown to block the neurotransmitter glycine from its receptors, which generate one type of inhibitory postsynaptic potential in some of the larger neurons of the CNS (36). The alkaloid does not block inhibitory synaptic potentials generated by γ-aminobutyric acid (GABA), however.

The elaboration of strychnine's mechanism of action has thus been valuable for studying the neurotransmitter properties and central sites of action of glycine (17). Because tetanospasmin (tetanus toxin) causes a similar (but irreversible) pattern to that of strychnine, it is not surprising to learn that this neurotoxin affects the glycine synapse, apparently by suppressing release of this inhibitory neurotransmitter, although other mechanisms may also be involved (15). The mechanism of seizures induced by intracerebroventricular l-kynurenine was suggested as an

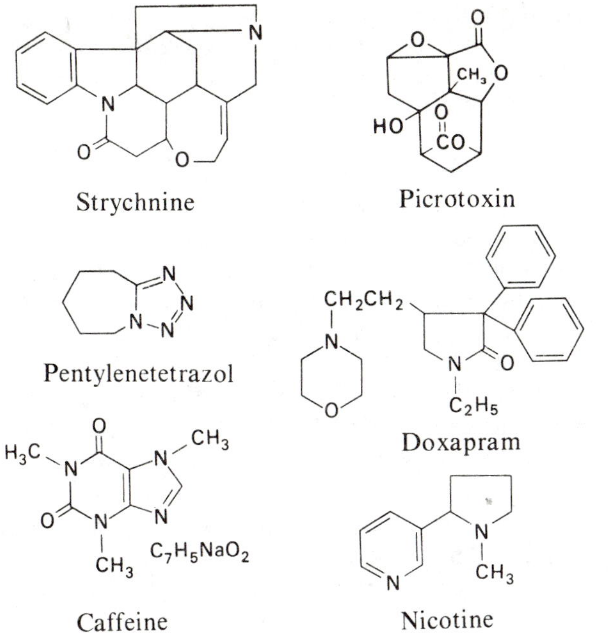

Strychnine

Picrotoxin

Pentylenetetrazol

Doxapram

$C_7H_5NaO_2$

Caffeine

Nicotine

Fig. 11.3-1. *Chemical structures of CNS stimulants.*

impaired release of glycine at inhibitory synapses in the brain, since l-glycine administration was a very effective antagonist (19). Glycine treatment was ineffective against strychnine. Some claims have been made for the facilitation of memory processes by treating laboratory animals with subconvulsant doses of strychnine (5), presumably by enhancing stimulus-response association for certain types of stimuli. The drug has had recent trials for treatment of neonatal nonketotic hyperglycinemia (20). Despite some amelioration of symptoms, the ultimate course of the disease was not altered.

PICROTOXIN

Picrotoxin is a nonnitrogenous neutral compound found in the seeds of *Anamirta cocculus*, a shrub of the East Indies. The natives have used the berries as a neurotoxin by casting them into a pond to catch fish; the fish floated to the top for easy harvest. The natives were not themselves poisoned by eating the fish because the active principle is rapidly and completely degraded by the digestive juices. Picrotoxin (Fig. 11.3-1) is a complex which on partial degradation forms two dilactones, picrotin (inert) and picrotoxinin (active). Perhaps the required breakdown of the complex is responsible for the significant delay in onset of effects even after i.v. administration. The action is rather short-lived, about 1 hr (40), presumably because of rapid metabolic degradation of picrotoxinin.

When picrotoxin is administered to otherwise untreated subjects, little effect is noted until convulsions ensue. These are initially clonic (asymmetrical and uncoordinated), but with more intense effects or larger doses tonic components (flexion followed by extension) are seen. A brainstem origin is suggested by the salivation and emesis observed with stimulant doses. There is little difference between the dose that induces respiratory stimulation and elevated blood pressure and that which initiates convulsions. The molecular mechanism of action has been characterized as the agent causing a decreased probability of opening of chloride channels at inhibitory synaptic sites (2). These effects probably relate to an interference with GABA-mediated inhibition, both presynaptic and postsynaptic. The threshold effects apparently involve brainstem functions because GABA-type inhibitory synapses predominate in that portion of the CNS. Picrotoxin, however, does not interact with GABA at the GABA receptors but via a site closely associated and coupled to the chloride ionophore (35). Bicuculline, a similar convulsant agent, is a more selective GABA antagonist. Thiosemicarbazide toxicity also resembles picrotoxin and results from a depletion of brain GABA by interfering with pyridoxal activation of glutamic acid decarboxylase. GABA applied to portions of the brain can convert depolarizing excitatory potentials into hyperpolarizing ones (28), although larger concentrations of GABA actually provoke repetitive seizure discharge. Furthermore, diazepam, an anticonvulsant that appears to act at least in part by enhancing GABA synaptic activity in the brain, is a most effective antagonist of picrotoxin. Even so, benzodiazepine receptor sites are distinct from picrotoxin sites, as well as from GABA sites (9, 13). The picrotoxin sites appear more closely associated with pentobarbital effects and inhibitory purine analogs (22). Large doses of naloxone are reported to have an analeptic effect, which may relate to a GABA-receptor antagonism rather than a blockade of endogenous opioid activity (10). These are all suggestive of a prominent role for GABA-inhibitory mechanisms in modulating CNS reflex excitability, although these mechanisms are complex and still poorly understood (40).

Since its introduction by Maloney and Tatum in 1932 (38), picrotoxin had gained considerable popularity for a time as an antidote in barbiturate poisoning. But the drug has been obsolete as a clinical analeptic for at least several decades, though still important as a research tool (40).

PENTYLENETETRAZOL

Unlike picrotoxin, pentylenetetrazol (Fig. 11.3-1) is effective by the oral as well as parenteral routes and with very short latency. The drug was synthesized first in 1924 and quickly introduced as an analeptic (40).

This drug appears to act at all levels of the CNS in about the same dose range, with a short duration due to rapid metabolism (half-life = 41.5 min). Onset of seizures with threshold doses is heralded by brief extensor thrusts, followed by clonus. Larger doses lead to prolonged clonic-tonic patterns and terminal flexor, extensor tonus. This agent is often classified as a brainstem stimulant, but the evidence for this claim is not very substantial. Indeed, the cerebral cortex and/or thalamic nuclei seem most sensitive. An acute neuronally isolated slab of cerebral cortex in unanesthetized dogs showed hypersynchrony earlier than the surrounding intact cortex following the i.v. injection of pentylenetetrazol (27). Picrotoxin, on the other hand, induced a high-frequency hypersynchrony in intact cortex sooner than in the isolated region. Bircher *et al.* (see Ref. 40) administered pentylenetetrazol at various levels of the CNS and achieved the highest potency and shortest latency for electrical seizures when applying the agent to the neocortex. Other evidence for a slightly greater sensitivity of telencephalic centers has been reviewed by Wang and Ward (40). Effects of the drug on peripheral structures are secondary to the generalized hyperactivity of the CNS. Thus, earlier marketing as a cardiotonic under the trade name of CARDIAZOL had no rationale.

The excitatory effect of pentylenetetrazol appears to depend upon a reduced neuronal recovery time between action potentials. This may be the result of an increase in permeability to potassium ions (41). The net effect would be an increase in discharge frequency of excitatory neurons, facilitation of the spread and synchronization of excitatory waves, and eventual avalanching into seizure patterns. Inhibitory neurons may also have a decreased recovery time to partially offset the excitation, but the balance is in favor of excitation. This proposal gains credence in considering the interactions between pentylenetetrazol and trimethadione. The latter drug brings about an increase in synaptic recovery time, is an effective antiepileptic in petit mal seizures, and induces sedation and disturbed mentation as common side effects. In a variety of experimental preparations, trimethadione and pentylenetetrazol exhibit a remarkable mutual antagonism (3). Moreover, pentylenetetrazol was found to produce a spike-dome pattern of electrical discharge when applied to neuronally isolated cortex in unanesthetized dogs (27) or to intact cortex of chronically prepared unanesthetized cats (R. H. Rech and E. C. Beck, unpublished observations), and spike-dome electroencephalographic patterns are diagnostic of petit mal epilepsy. These patterns may involve the activation of nerve terminals of thalamic origin impinging upon cortical interneurons. This analeptic may also influence or be influenced by, perhaps indirectly, GABA synaptic activity, benzodiazepine receptor binding (39), α-adrenergic receptor activity, and central cholinergic mechanisms (26). Indeed, multiple mechanisms of seizure causation have generally been proposed (41).

Pentylenetetrazol was used in the past as convulsive therapy in psychiatric illness, but flurothyl has certain advantages (30). In any case, electroconvulsive therapy (ECT) appears to be preferred over chemical methods when convulsant therapy is indicated in actual practice. Pentylenetetrazol has been used for some time, by oral administration, in geriatric patients to combat senility and depression, but its usefulness is still debated. Recent experimental evidence suggests that chronic pentylenetetrazol retards signs of aging in rat hippocampus, as well as improving the capacity of aging rats for reversal learning (18). The stimulant is effectively used by specialists as a diagnostic aid to activate an epileptogenic focus in suspected epilepsy. There is a controversy as to whether or not repeated administration of the drug induces kindling for seizure propensity (6, 38). Bemegride, a glutarimide convulsant with a similar mechanism, has also been employed to activate epileptogenic foci but appears to have no advantage over pentylenetetrazol. Because the respiratory stimulant dose of pentylenetetrazol is very close to the convulsant dose, the agent was particularly dangerous when tried as an analeptic and has not been used for many years for this purpose.

DOXAPRAM, NIKETHAMIDE, ETHAMIVAN

These synthetic agents have all had trial as analeptics in the hope of achieving some relative specificity in stimulating central respiratory neurons. Nikethamide (N,N-diethylpyridine-3-carboxamide), the earliest, is a rather weak stimulant. The implication taken from the trade name (CORAMIN) that the drug stimulates the heart is not true. Early experiments suggested that respiratory stimulation was indirect via an effect on the carotid bodies; later work did not substantiate this (40). Nikethamide has sometimes been used as an analeptic on the basis that it is so weak it will do no harm. However, there are occasional reports of the drug causing depression in its own right. The agent is metabolized to the vitamin nicotinamide.

Ethamivan (3-methoxy-4-hydroxy-N,N-diethylbenzamide) was introduced in 1952 as an analeptic. There appears to be little basis for even relative specificity for stimulation of the respiratory center (40). A portion of the respiratory stimulation may be mediated by activation of pulmonary artery chemoreceptors. When used as an analeptic in treating overdose of a narcotic analgesic, ethamivan has reversed the respiratory depression and even precipitated convulsions without counteracting the coma. As therapy for diseases of respiratory insufficiency, the drug has augmented minute volume, but mainly as an increase in dead-space ventilation.

Doxapram (Fig. 11.3-1) is relatively new on the scene of analeptics. The agent is well absorbed by all routes of administration and has a short latency to onset. After i.v. injection, the stimulation is short-lived (5-12 min), although of longer duration following repeated doses. As with nikethamide and ethamivan, this drug appears to enhance directly the activity of excitatory neurons in the CNS, although the agent also appears to sensitize peripheral receptors. Doxapram is the one analeptic for which there is convincing evidence of a relative specificity to stimulate respiratory, or at least medullary, vital centers (16, 40). The ratio of convulsant dose to respiratory stimulant dose is at least 25 and perhaps as high as 75, according to the circumstances of use. Furthermore, a dose (0.25 mg/kg) that increased the discharge rate of medullary inspiratory neurons did not affect nearby nonrespiratory neurons. Ten times this dose was the threshold for stimulation of the nonrespiratory neurons.

Threshold doses of doxapram affect ventilation by an increase in tidal volume, mainly as a result of activating the carotid bodies. Somewhat larger doses are required to stimulate respiration (both depth and rate) by direct medullary influences, after section of the carotid sinus nerve. A pressor response occurs concurrently, although i.v. doses greater than 2 mg/kg cause transient hypotension. In barbiturate-anesthetized animals, there may be prominent respiratory stimulation without indication of increased arousal or change in skeletal muscle tone. In fact, a recent study indicated that doxapram intensified and prolonged the anesthesia produced by pentobarbital (12). The presence of chlorobutanol in the commercial doxapram preparation accounted for some of the enhanced effect. By way of contrast, this analeptic was effective in reducing the anesthetic level [i.e., pretreatment increased the minimum alveolar concentration (MAC)] of halothane in dogs (33). The increased oxygenation of the blood is claimed to relate, in part, to an improved ventilation-perfusion ratio. Some reports suggest that repeated doses have a diminished effect, but i.v. infusions have maintained an increased ventilation over quite long periods.

Side effects of doxapram used as an analeptic include tachycardia, arrhythmias, coughing, sneezing, vomiting, itching, urinary retention, and hyperpyrexia. Larger doses may cause laryngospasm, muscle rigidity, and bronchospasm. Recommended doses are 0.5-2 mg/kg maximum in single or divided doses for shortening post-anesthetic recovery. Intermittent i.v. infusions as an adjunct in treating drug-induced CNS depression should be limited to 24 mg/kg/day, or a total dose of 3 g. Tremors and convulsions are rare, except in epileptics, for whom the drug is contraindicated. Patients under treatment with sympathomimetics or monoamine oxidase inhibitors are more likely to suffer severe pressor effects or arrhythmias. For respiratory insufficiency, doxapram is best given by infusion along with oxygen therapy. Although the use of doxapram as an analeptic is quite limited in human medicine, it is more commonly used in veterinary practice (16), in particular to hasten recovery from anesthesia. A recent double-blind study indicates that the drug may be efficacious for this purpose in selected human patients (37). As discussed by Wang and Ward (40), if doxapram had been available before the widespread acceptance of the Scandinavian method of treating depressant drug overdose, the adjunctive use of this agent in human medicine might be more common.

AMPHETAMINE, METHYLPHENIDATE, COCAINE

Amphetamine, methylphenidate, and cocaine do not properly belong to the analeptic group on the basis of the criteria set forth earlier. They are psychomotor stimulants and are discussed in that category in Chapters 7.1 and 11.6. Hyperreflexia, tremors, and convulsions are a consequence of overdose. The amphetamines (racemic β-phenylisopropylamine; d-isomer, dextroamphetamine; N-methyl derivative methamphetamine) are sympathomimetic agents with prominent CNS effects and some therapeutic applications dealt with elsewhere. Methylphenidate (methyl-α-phenyl-2-piperidine-acetate hydrochloride) is an amphetaminelike agent in its CNS effects and is the drug of choice in the childhood hyperkinetic syndrome.

These drugs have been employed to lessen the CNS depression caused by barbiturates, alcohol, and similar drugs. Any stimulation of respiration, however, appears to be indirect via an action on brain catecholaminergic modulatory systems. It is controversial whether they can significantly improve respiratory exchange in deep coma resulting from excessive doses of a CNS depressant of the barbiturate type. On the other hand, dextroamphetamine is remarkably effective in reversing marked sedation and behavioral retardation resulting from reserpinelike drugs (29). Cocaine also resembles the amphetamines in terms of its central actions, and all three types of agents are a serious problem in current-day drug abuse (Chapter 11.6). Cocaine has a more narrow range between the psychostimulant and convulsant doses, particularly with intravenous use, probably due to the combined mechanisms of amphetaminelike CNS stimulation and the local anesthetic-type convulsant side effect (Chapter 10.4). The general impression that abuse of this drug only rarely leads to fatalities is not supported by objective evidence. An important consequence of fatal doses is the hyperthermia induced rather than effects on the cardiovascular system (7).

CAFFEINE

Caffeine and other xanthine derivatives (theophylline, theobromine) have had nonmedical uses for centuries as components of coffee, tea, and cocoa (40). Caffeine (Fig. 11.3-1) is the most active as a CNS stimulant. The drug is rapidly assimilated by all routes of administration; it is broken down over several hours and excreted mainly as 1-methylxanthine and 1-methyluric acid.

The effects of caffeine are exerted primarily on the CNS and cardiovascular system. Lower doses orally (100-200 mg, a cup or two of coffee) appear to affect neocortex to enhance intellectual effort, especially in the presence of drowsiness or fatigue. Older reports have indicated that perception is improved, reaction time is decreased, and psychomotor productivity (e.g., typing) is enhanced both in terms of increased output and reduced errors. However, this was not substantiated by a recent double-blind clinical study, which characterized the stimulant effects as distinctly different from those of d-amphetamine, although both drugs improved vigilance (25). Although most users characterize the effects of caffeine as pleasant, there is no distinct euphoria of the type produced by amphetamines or cocaine. Larger doses may produce unpleasant effects, particularly in the nonuser, such as hyperesthesia, restlessness, tremor, insomnia, and palpitation. Some individuals may suffer a rebound lethargy, although this is not definitely established in the case of coffee drinkers. Only very large oral doses bring about overt excitement, delirium, and clonic seizures. Caffeine and sodium benzoate injection i.m. 0.5-1 g can increase ventilation by sensitizing the respiratory center to CO_2, especially if already depressed. Its use as an analeptic is often promulgated on the basis that, although the drug is too weak to do much good, it can probably do no harm. Nevertheless, the excitement due to larger doses is followed by a rebound depression. Furthermore, a recent double-blind study showed no effect of the usual doses of caffeine to counteract the central depression of alcohol in healthy adult males (21), although strong coffee is commonly employed to sober up an inebriated subject. Effects on other organ systems are described in Chapters 16.1 and 17.

Acutely administered caffeine modestly increases blood pressure, plasma catecholamine levels, plasma renin activity, and urine production; however, these effects are not observed on chronic caffeine consumption. On acute administration caffeine also increases serum free fatty acid levels and gastric acid secretion and alters mood and sleep patterns (8).

A number of effects of methylxanthines have been described at the cellular level, including interactions among these effects, and may account for the CNS stimulation produced. Sutherland and coworkers have shown that these drugs inhibit phosphodiesterase to elevate tissue levels of cyclic adenosine-3′,5′-phosphate. Catecholamines also promote an increase in cyclic adenosine monophosphate (AMP) by stimulating synthesis. Methylxanthines appear to release catecholamines from nerve endings or tissues. These effects may increase cellular energy production as well as facilitate some aspects of neuronal transmission. In addition, the drugs influence intracellular calcium distribution in a way that may increase the activity of some excitable tissues. The precise role of these cellular actions of methylxanthines in the CNS stimulant effects of caffeine remains to be elucidated (31).

A mutual antagonism of effects between caffeine and benzodiazepines appears to be more specific than just a physiological interaction. Electrophysiological responses to diazepam in spinal cats were antagonized by caffeine, whereas those to phenobarbital were not (23). Caffeine 50 mg/kg also reversed the increased threshold to rage (by electrical stimulation of the hypothalamus) as achieved by pretreating cats with diazepam. A similar increase in threshold by pretreatment with phenobarbital was not altered by caffeine. Other effects of diazepam were antagonized by caffeine, including the anticonflict activity of the benzodiazepine. The interaction was considered to involve influences at purinergic rather than benzodiazepine receptors. Thus, xanthines and benzodiazepines appear to exert mutually antagonistic effects. These findings, especially with reference to the low doses of caffeine required to reverse the anxiolytic properties of diazepam, may reflect on the therapeutic efficacy of benzodiazepines in the treatment of coffee drinkers for anxiety disorders. Caffeine may be effective as systemic therapy for neonatal apnea and as a topical treatment of atopic dermatitis (8).

Chronic use of caffeine may induce appreciable tolerance in regard to restlessness and insomnia, although the increased mental altertness appears to persist. Chronic ingestion of relatively large daily amounts of caffeine in the form of coffee is an established practice in our society, although the effects in most adults appear to be benign. Children appear to be more sensitive to the stimulant actions even after moderate doses (25), and some authorities suggest that they be denied access to caffeine-containing beverages. Occasional adults drink enough coffee to disturb their behavior or cause significant sleep loss. Limited use of caffeine is also indicated in patients with peptic ulcer, hypertension, and certain cardiac conditions. Caffeine does not appear to be associated in several conditions in which it has been implicated earlier [e.g., myocardial infarction; lower urinary tract, renal, or pancreatic cancer; fibroblastic breast disease; or teratogenicity (8)]. A potential role of its chronic use in causation of cardiac arrhythmias and gastrointestinal ulceration will require further study (8).

NICOTINE

Nicotine, an alkaloid (Fig. 11.3-1) and a volatile liquid, is included as a powerful CNS stimulant of toxicological and sociomedical interest. Nicotine is, however, usually classified under drugs that affect autonomic ganglia, the study of which was greatly facilitated by use of this agent as a tool (Chapter 8). The agent occurs in nature as the most important constituent of tobacco.

The drug is absorbed rapidly even from intact skin, which accounts for some poisonings by insecticides, and is rapidly metabolized in liver, kidney, and lung. The CNS stimulant actions of lower doses account in large measure for the popularity of tobacco products (Chapter 11.6). Large doses of nicotine depress the CNS, compounding the postictal depression that follows tremors and clonic convulsions exhibited earlier (34). Death occurs by respiratory failure, including blockade of the neuromuscular junction after exposure to very large amounts. Nicotine is, in fact, one of the deadliest and most potent poisons known. The stimulation of respiration is particularly prominent, partly by exciting the chemoreceptors of the carotid and aortic bodies. Emesis is caused by both central and peripheral actions. The central effects of the toxin are reported to be blocked in part by diverse agents: antiparkinsonian drugs, anticonvulsants, curariform agents, hypnotics, and adrenergic-blocking drugs, but mainly in an experimental context. In the clinical management of acute poisoning there is no specific antidote, and treatment is largely symptomatic.

The pharmacology of nicotine is exceedingly complex (34), not only due to the biphasic effects at various sites in the brain, but also because of the multiple sites in the periphery at which the drug acts directly. These include effects on autonomic ganglia and skeletal neuromuscular functions; release of catecholamines, 5-hydroxytryptamine, and histamine from body stores; and stimulation of chemoreceptors, mechanoreceptors, thermal receptors, and pain receptors. Thus, the actions attributable to direct stimulant or depressant effects on CNS neurons are difficult to isolate. Many effects are related to activation or blockade of cholinergic receptors of the "nicotinic" type (Chapter 8.1 and 8.4), including those in the CNS. Other effects, however, are probably due to increased permeability of cell membranes. Desynchronization of the electroencephalogram ("EEG arousal") appears to relate to an activation of central cholinergic receptors of the nicotinic type (34). On the other hand, facilitation of conditioned avoidance by nicotine resembles that of d-amphetamine, whereas discriminative properties of nicotine only partly generalize to amphetamine and are antagonized by mecamylamine (1, 11, 32). Low doses in the nonsmoker cause a powerful emesis in large part by stimulating the chemoreceptor trigger zone in the area postrema of the medulla oblongata (34). An antidiuretic action results from the release of antidiuretic hormone. Larger doses affect various brain regions to produce tremors and then clonic convulsions, although a very large overdose may obscure these motor components as the secondary depressant phase develops within a few minutes. Respiratory stimulation is prominent after smaller doses, primarily by excitation of peripheral chemoreceptors.

Cardiovascular changes caused by nicotine derive from actions at many sites in the body. Tachycardia and increased blood pressure are due to a combination of reflex excitation via sensory receptors, stimulation of sympathetic ganglia, and release of catecholamines from the adrenal medulla and sympathetic nerve endings, as well as blockade of vagal autonomic ganglia. Nevertheless, the earliest effect may be a slowing of the pulse as the central vagal nucleus is excited by nicotine, in part indirectly via the carotid body reflex mechanism. Complex changes in blood pressure occur that are not well understood (34). The pupils are also constricted in the early phase and dilated later. In the terminal phases of poisoning, cardiovascular collapse occurs as a consequence of CNS depression, ganglionic blockade, and cardiac arrhythmias. However, lethality is usually the result of respiratory failure as muscles of respiration are paralyzed.

Taking into account the potency and lethal potential of nicotine as a toxin in humans, one may wonder that tobacco users survive chronic exposure long enough to suffer late sequelae such as emphysema and lung cancer. A remarkable tolerance develops to many of the central actions on chronic use, to the extent that a heavy smoker who inhales may achieve brain levels of the drug that would cause marked toxicity in the novice, yet show no signs of discomfort. Consider that the smoke from half a pack of cigarettes contains about one acute lethal dose of nicotine for the average adult. The psychostimulant action appears to show less tolerance and is probably the basis of the addiction seen in some heavy smokers (11). Anorectic effects of nicotine apparently show no tolerance, as opposed to the pattern observed with amphetamine (4). Other aspects of nicotine have been reviewed in a recent symposium proceedings (1, 11, 32).

Many of the effects of acute exposure to nicotine have obvious noxious qualities, and nicotine can in fact be used as a punisher in a typical Geller-Seifter-type operant conflict procedure with monkeys as subjects (14). Yet the very same dose levels will be self-administered as a positive reinforcer when these animals are trained in a different context. Mecamylamine antagonizes both the positively reinforcing and punishing effects of nicotine.

α-Lobeline is an alkaloid from *Lobelia inflata* (Indian tobacco) with effects very much like nicotine. It was once employed as a respiratory stimulant, an effect that was largely peripheral via the chemoreceptors, but has long since been discontinued for that use.

DRUG INTERACTION

Interaction of CNS stimulants with certain drugs are listed in Table 11.3-2.

Preparations The following are some preparations of the CNS stimulants:

Pentylenetetrazol (METRAZOLE, NIORIC, etc.): oral,

Table 11.3-2
Interactions between CNS Stimulants and Other Drugs

CNS Stimulant	Interacting Drug	Effects
Amphetamine	Guanethidine, methyldopa	Interference with (decrease) the hypotensive effects
	MAO inhibitors	Hypertensive crisis
	Epinephrine-sensitizing anesthetics	Cardiac arrhythmias
	Antipsychotic drugs	CNS effects of amphetamine antagonized
Amphetamine or methylphenidate	Tricyclic antidepressants	Increased blood levels of-antidepressants
	Phenytoin, primidone	Potentiation of toxicity of anti-epileptics
	Digitalis	Cardiac arrhythmias

tablets (0.1 g), elixir (100 mg/5 ml); injection, 10% solution (1-ml ampules).

Doxapram hydrochloride, USP (DOPRAM): 20 mg/ml, 20-ml vials, for i.v. injection, 0.5-1.5 mg/kg doses; also by i.v. infusion starting at the rate of 5 mg/min and later reducing by 50% or more.

Ethamivan, USP (EMIVAN): not available commercially in the United States.

Nikethamide (CORAMIN): 25% solution, bulk, oral, or 1.5-ml ampules for i.v., i.m. injection.

Methylphenidate hydrochloride, USP (RITALIN): oral, tablets (5, 10, 20 mg); 10 mg, b.i.d. or t.i.d.; for hyperkinetic children, initially 0.25 mg/kg daily, dose is doubled each week to an optimal daily dose of 2 mg/kg (two equal divided doses given before breakfast and lunch).

Caffeine, USP: white crystalline substance. *Caffeine and sodium benzoate injection*, USP: i.m. injection (500-mg/2-ml ampules containing 250 mg of caffeine).

Amphetamine sulfate, USP (BENZEDRINE): white water-soluble powder, tablets (5, 10 mg), slow-release capsules (15 mg). *Dextroamphetamine sulfate*, USP (DEXEDRINE): tablets (5, 10 mg), elixir (1 mg/ml), slow-release capsules (5, 10, 15 mg). *Dextroamphetamine phosphate*, USP: tablets (5 mg). *Methamphetamine hydrochloride* (DESOXYN, FETAMIN): d-isomer; tablets (2.5, 5 mg), slow-release tablets (5, 10, 15 mg). Amphetamines are schedule II drugs under narcotic regulation.

REFERENCES

1. Abood, L.G., Reynolds, D.T., Booth, H., Bidlack, J.N. and Schawab, L.S. sites and mechanisms for nicotine's action in the brain. *Neurosci. Biobehav. Rev.* 5:479, 1981.
2. Aicken, C.C., Deisz, R.A. and Lux, H.D. On the action of the anticonvulsant 5,5-diphenylhydantoin and the convulsant picrotoxin in crayfish stretch receptor. *J. Physiol.* (London), 315:157, 1981.
3. Angel, A. and Clarke, K.A. The effects of trimethadione on pentetrazol-induced discharges of primary muscle spindle afferents from the hind limb of the rat. *Br. J. Pharmacol.* 72:75, 1981.
4. Baettig, K., Martin, J.R. and Classen, W. Nicotine and amphetamine: Differential tolerance and no cross-tolerance for ingestive effects. *Pharmacol. Biochem. Behav.* 12:107, 1980.
5. Brennan, M.J. and Gordon, W.C. Selective facilitation of memory attributes by strychnine. *Pharmacol. Biochem. Behav.* 7:451, 1977.
6. Cain, D.P. Transfer of pentylenetetrazol sensitization to amygdaloid kindling. *Pharmacol. Biochem. Behav.* 15:533, 1981.
7. Catravas, J.D. and Waters, I.W. Acute cocaine intoxication in the conscious dog: Studies on mechanism of lethality. *J. Pharmacol. Exp. Ther.* 217:350, 1981.
8. Curatolo, P.W. and Robertson, D. The health consequences of caffeine. *Ann. Int. Med.* 98:641, 1983.
9. Davis, W.C. and Ticku, M.K. Picrotoxin and diazepam bind to two distinct proteins: Further evidence that pentobarbital may act at the picrotoxinin site. *J. Neurosci.* 1:1036, 1981.
10. Dingledine, R., Iversen, L.L. and Brenker, E. Naloxone as a GABA antagonist: Evidence from iontophoretic, receptor binding and convulsant studies. *Eur. J. Pharmacol.* 47:19, 1978.
11. Dougherty, J., Miller, D., Todd, G. and Kostenbarder, H.B. Reinforcing and other behavioral effects of nicotine. *Neurosci. Biobehav. Rev.* 5:487, 1981.
12. Flint, B.A., Ho, I.K., Mo, B.P.N. and Rigor, B.M. Enhancement of pharmacological responses of pentobarbital by Dopram. *Clin. Toxicol.* 15:169, 1979.
13. Fujimoto, M. and Okabayashi, T. Effect of picrotoxin on benzodiazepine receptors and GABA receptors with reference to the effect of Cl^- ion. *Life Sci.* 28:895, 1981.
14. Goldberg, S.R. and Spealman, R.D. Maintenance and suppression of behavior by intravenous nicotine injections in squirrel monkeys. *Fed. Proc.* 41:216, 1982.
15. Huck, S., Kirchner, F. and Takano, K. Rhythmic activity in the cerebellum and spinal cord of rabbits receiving tetanus toxin intravenously. *Naunyn-Schmiedeberg's Arch. Pharmacol.* 317:51, 1981.
16. Jones, L.M., Booth, N.H. and McDonald, L.E. (eds.). *Veterinary Pharmacology and Therapeutics.* Ames, Iowa: Iowa State University Press, 1977, pp. 406-408.
17. Kehne, J.H., Gallager, D.W. and Davis, M. Strychnine: Brainstem and spinal mediation of excitatory effects on acoustic startle. *Eur. J. Pharmacol.* 76:177, 1981.
18. Landfield, P.W., Baskin, R.K. and Pitler, T.A. Brain aging correlates: Retardation by hormonal-pharmacological treatments. *Science* 214:581, 1981.
19. Lapin, I.P. Antagonism of L-glycine to seizures induced by L-kynurenine, quinolinic acid and strychnine in mice. *Eur. J. Pharmacol.* 71:495, 1981.
20. MacDermot, K.D., Nelson, W., Reichert, C.M. and Schulman, T.D. Attempts at use of strychnine sulfate in the treatment of nonketotic hyperglycinemia. *Pediatrics* 65:61, 1980.
21. Nuotto, E., Mattila, M.J., Seppala, T. and Konno, K. Coffee and caffeine and alcohol effects on psychomotor function. *Clin. Pharmacol. Ther.* 31:68, 1982.
22. Olsen, R.W. and Leeb-Lundberg, F. Endogenous inhibitors of picrotoxin-convulsant binding sites in rat brain. *Eur. J. Pharmacol.* 65:101, 1980.
23. Polc, P., Bonetti, E.P., Pieri, L., Cumin, R., Angioi, R.M., Mohler, H. and Haefely, W.E. Caffeine antagonizes several central effects of diazepam. *Life Sci.* 28:2265, 1981.
24. Purpura, D.P. and Grundfest, H. Physiological and pharmacological consequences of different synaptic organizations in cerebral and cerebellar cortex of cat. *J. Neurophysiol.* 20:494, 1957.
25. Rapoport, J.L., Jensvold, M., Elkins, R., Buchsbaum, M.S., Weingartner, H., Ludlow, C., Zahn, T.P., Berg, C.J. and Neims, A.H. Behavioral and cognitive effects of caffeine in boys and adult males. *J. Nerv. Ment. Dis.* 169:726, 1981.
26. Rastogi, S.K., Puri, J.N.,Sinha, J.N. and Bhargava, K.P. Involvement of central cholinoceptors in metrazol-induced convulsions. *Psychopharmacology* 65:215, 1979.
27. Rech, R.H. and Domino, E.F. Effects of various drugs on activity of the neuronally isolated cerebral cortex. *Exp. Neurol.* 2:364, 1960.
28. Rech, R.H. and Domino, E.F. Effects of gamma-aminobutyric acid on chemically- and electrically-evoked activity in the isolated cerebral cortex of the dog. *J. Pharmacol. Exp. Ther.* 130:59, 1960.
29. Rech, R.H. and Stolk, J.M. Amphetamine-drug interactions that relate brain catecholamines to behavior. In: *Amphetamines and Related Compounds* (Costa, E. and Garattini, S., eds.). New York: Raven Press, 1970, pp. 385-413.
30. Report of the Council. A convulsant agent for psychiatric use: Flurothyl (Indoklon). *JAMA* 196:29, 1966.
31. Robison, G.A., Butcher, R.W. and Sutherland, E.W. *Cyclic AMP.* New York: Academic Press, 1971.
32. Rosecrans, J.A. and Meltzer, L.T. Central sites and mechanisms of action of nicotine. *Neurosci. Biobehav. Rev.* 5:497, 1981.
33. Roy, R.C. and Stullken, E.H. Electroencephalographic evidence of arousal in dogs from halothane after doxapram, physostigmine, or naloxone. *Anesthesiology* 55:392, 1981.
34 Silvette, H., Hoff, E.C., Larson, P.S. and Haag, H.B. The actions of nicotine on central nervous system functions. *Pharmacol. Rev.* 14:137, 1962.
35. Simmonds, M.A. A site for the potentiation of GABA-mediated responses by benzodiazepines. *Nature* 284:558, 1980.
36. Snyder, S.H. The glycine synaptic receptor in the mammalian nervous system. *Br. J. Pharmacol.* 53:473, 1975.

37. Steele, R.J.C., Walker, W.S., Irvine, M.K.A., Lee, D. and Taylor, T.V. The use of doxapram in the prevention of postoperative pulmonary complications. *Surg. Gynecol. Obstet.* 154:510, 1982.
38. Stripling, J.S. and Hendricks, C. Facilitation of kindling by convulsions induced by cocaine or lidocaine but not by pentylenetetrazol. *Pharmacol. Biochem. Behav.* 15:793, 1981.
39. Syapin, P.J. and Rickman, D.W. Benzodiazepine receptor increase following repeated pentylenetetrazol injections. *Eur. J. Pharmacol.* 72:117, 1981.
40. Wang, S.C. and Ward, J.W. Analeptics. *Pharmacol. Ther.* B3:123, 1977.
41. Woodbury, D.M. Convulsant drugs: Mechanisms of action. In: *Antiepileptic Drugs: Mechanisms of Action* (Glaser, G.H., Penry, J.K. and Woodbury, D.M., eds.). New York: Raven Press, 1980, pp. 249-303.

GENERAL READING

Cooper, J.R., Bloom, F.E. and Roth, R.H. *The Biochemical Basis of Neuropharmacology*, 2nd ed. New York: Oxford University Press, 1974, pp. 217-224.

CHAPTER
11.4

ANTIEPILEPTIC AGENTS

Arthur Raines

The epilepsies are a group of diverse disorders characterized by repeated convulsive (or nonconvulsive) seizures and are generally estimated to occur with an incidence ranging from 1 to 2 in 200 persons. Hughlings Jackson, the great nineteenth century neurologist, defined a seizure as "a state produced by an abnormal excessive neuronal discharge within the gray matter of the brain." The seizures may take any of a variety of forms and be more or less severe, involving motor, sensory, autonomic, and/or behavioral changes. Drugs with utility in prevention and management of the epilepsies are termed *antiepileptic drugs*. The term *anticonvulsant drug* is a more general term that encompasses the antiepileptic drugs but also includes all agents that prevent (or diminish the intensity or duration of) convulsions in experimental circumstances. The management of the epilepsies is a multifaceted problem, with antiepileptic drugs being only one (albeit perhaps the most important) factor.

CLASSIFICATION OF EPILEPSIES

Epileptic seizures are commonly referred to as (a) symptomatic (known etiology; for example, head trauma, hypoxia, circulatory defects, infections, and neoplasms; about 25%), and (b) idiopathic (etiology unknown; about 75%). The International League Against Epilepsy developed the most commonly used classification (21), which is based on the signs and symptoms characteristic of seizure patterns the epileptic patient presents. This classification has been most useful and was recently revised (11). Presently it is based on (a) the clinical seizure type, (b) the ictal (during seizure) electroencephalographic pattern, and (c) the electroencephalographic interictal expression. Although important, issues of anatomic substrate, etiology, and age are not specifically addressed in the current classification of seizures. The major categories recognized are partial seizures, generalized seizures, and unclassified seizures.

Some brief description of the principal characteristics

of the most prominent types of seizures, along with the data of Table 11.4-1, provide a picture of the clinical features usually observed. Further details can be obtained by consulting the Commission on Classification's report (11) or modern textbooks of neurology.

I. PARTIAL SEIZURES

As implied, partial seizures involve only a limited portion of the brain, and because this may be virtually anywhere, symptoms can be most variable and are described based upon motor, sensory, autonomic, or psychic symptoms.

A. Simple Partial Seizures. Simple partial seizures tend to be brief (less than a minute in duration); consciousness is unimpaired. An example of a simple partial seizure with motor signs [Table 11.4-1; I.A.1.(a)] would exist if the initiating lesion was in a portion of the brain controlling hand function. Abrupt twitchings and tonic or clonic (see later discussion) muscle activity in the hand might occur. If the cerebral discharge spreads (travels, marches) in an orderly progression to involve the arm, shoulder girdle, trunk, and/or whole body, it is referred to as a *Jacksonian seizure* [Table 11.4-1; I.A.1.(b)].

B. Complex Partial Seizures. These attacks are characterized by altered or impaired consciousness, often with confusion and subsequent amnesia. During the seizure, fully coordinated behaviors or motor activities (e.g., dressing or undressing, chewing, swallowing, automatic ambulatory activity, grooming, mimicry, aggression) occur that may be appropriate at another time or place. The seizure may occur abruptly or evolve from a simple partial seizure.

These seizures, which usually originate in the temporal lobe, occur primarily in adults and are the most commonly observed pattern. Onset of the seizure may be marked by symptoms that are recalled, called an *aura*. These attacks usually last for 1-5 min.

C. Partial Seizures Evolving to Secondarily Generalized Seizures. All partial seizures can spread and develop into a generalized seizure involving both cerebral hemispheres. When the seizure becomes generalized, consciousness is usually lost.

II. GENERALIZED SEIZURES

During a generalized seizure, neuronal discharge occurs throughout the entire gray matter (or most of it) simultaneously in both hemispheres. Features include: loss of consciousness and for generalized tonic-clonic seizures, en masse autonomic phenomena, and not infrequently, bilateral symmetrical motor signs consisting of either convulsions or hypotonia. There are basically two types of generalized seizures, convulsive and nonconvulsive.

1. Convulsive: tonic-clonic (grand mal); tonic; clonic infantile spasms; and myoclonic and have an appreciable active motor component.
2. Nonconvulsive: absence (petit mal); atonic, and akinetic.

A. Convulsive Generalized Seizures

Convulsive generalized seizures exhibit prominent motor manifestations. Tonic movements consist of sustained contractions, whereas clonic movements consist of alternating contractions and relaxations occuring in rapid succession. Myoclonus refers to a brief, involuntary muscle contraction.

1. Tonic-Clonic (Grand Mal) Seizures. This pattern consists of a tonic phase during which the body assumes an opisthotonic attitude, followed by a clonic phase. During the seizure, the electroencephalogram (EEG) consists of high-voltage, high-frequency activity with sustained electrical activity during the tonic phase and the tendency to bursting in the clonic stages with bursts in phase with clonic movements. There is mobilization of autonomic function from the onset (increased heart rate, blood pressure, increased bladder pressure, usually without urinary incontinence, mydriasis, apnea, cyanosis due to vascular congestion, and glandular hypersecretion). Cessation of the seizure results in a return to normal autonomic functioning as well as relaxation of previously constricted sphincters and subsequent loss of bladder control. The EEG during the postictal stage shows low-voltage, slow-wave activity.

2. Tonic Seizures. Tonic seizures consist of sustained contraction of involved muscles and are divided into three subtypes depending upon topographical area involved (trunk, trunk and limbs, and total body). These are encountered mainly in children.

3. Clonic Seizures. Clonic seizures are associated with a brief, tonic spasm causing falling and a series of bilateral muscle contractions that may be generalized and symmetrical (one side predominating). Autonomic changes are insignificant. The pattern is seen frequently during febrile illness and may also occur during non-REM sleep.

4. Myoclonic Seizures. Myoclonic seizures are brief, usually without loss of consciousness; only occasionally are there autonomic changes. There is usually bilateral flexion leading to jerking movements, spontaneous and isolated myoclonus, and topographical distribution of clonus. An increase in the intensity and involvement of all muscle groups results in massive bilateral myoclonus. These seizures may be spontaneous or precipitated by photic stimulation and movement (action myoclonus), or may occur during or following arousal from slow-wave sleep.

5. Infantile Spasms. These are very brief (1 sec) episodes of spasms experienced by infants; they usually are concomitant with mental retardation. The etiology may be metabolic abnormalities.

B. Nonconvulsive Generalized Seizures. Nonconvulsive generalized seizures are seizures lacking prominent motor activity.

1. Absence (Petit Mal) Seizures. Absence seizures are classified as typical and atypical. The distinction is that the atypical demonstrate a briefer impairment of consciousness and less abrupt onset and termination of the event, as well as the presence of tonic motor activity, than the typical seizures. Atypical seizures are known as petit mal variants or the Lennox-Gastaut syndrome. Typical seizures are subdivided into simple (impaired consciousness only) and complex (impairment of consciousness accompanied by other signs, such as disturbed sensorium). During an absence seizure, the patient appears to be in a trance during which time there is a temporary alteration or suspension of mental functions. In susceptible individuals, this seizure type can be induced by hyperventilation. The EEG during these seizures consists of a characteristic spike-wave (or spike-dome) pattern over the entire surface of the brain. This pattern occurs at a frequency of about 3 cycles/sec.

2. Atonic Seizures. Atonic seizures (drop attacks) occur predominantly during childhood. There is an abrupt loss of postural muscle tone and the patient collapses. No movements are involved.

3. Akinetic Seizures. Akinetic seizures show loss of movement without atonia. Posture is maintained and loss of consciousness is less profound. This is predominantly a type of childhood epilepsy.

III. UNCLASSIFIED SEIZURES

Seizures are designated unclassified when insufficient information exists to clearly categorize or distinguish them from other patterns.

Status Epilepticus. Status epilepticus refers to a prolonged seizure, or frequent recurrences of seizures without recovery in between, and may be associated with any of the seizure varieties. Such a condition may be related to known causes (infec-

Table 11.4-1
Classification of Seizures

I. Partial (Focal, Local) Seizures

Partial seizures are those in which, in general, the first clinical and electroencephalographic changes indicate initial activation of a system of neurons limited to part of one cerebral hemisphere. A partial seizure is classified primarily on the basis of whether or not consciousness is impaired during the attack. When consciousness is not impaired, the seizure is classified as a simple partial seizure. When consciousness is impaired, the seizure is classified as a complex partial seizure. Impairment of consciousness may be the first clinical sign, or simple partial seizures may evolve into complex partial seizures. In patients with impaired consciousness, aberrations of behavior (automatisms) may occur. A partial seizure. may not terminate, but instead progresses to a generalized motor seizure. Impaired consciousness is defined as the inability to respond normally to exogenous stimuli by virtue of altered awareness and/or responsiveness (see Definition of Terms).

There is considerable evidence that simple partial seizures usually have unilateral hemispheric involvement and only rarely have bilateral hemispheric involvement: complex partial seizures, however, frequently have bilateral hemispheric involvement.

Partial seizures can be classified into one of the following three fundamental groups:

A. Simple partial seizures
B. Complex partial seizures
   1. With impairment of consciousness at onset
   2. Simple partial onset followed by impairment of consciousness
C. Partial seizures evolving to generalized tonic-clonic convulsions (GTC)
   1. Simple evolving to GTC
   2. Complex evolving to GTC (including those with simple partial onset)

Clinical Seizure Type	EEG Seizure Type	EEG Interictal Expression
A. *Simple partial seizures*		
(consciousness not impaired)	Local contralateral discharge starting over the corresponding area of cortical representation (not always recorded on the scalp)	Local contralateral discharge
1. *With motor signs*		
(a) Focal motor without march		
(b) Focal motor with march (jacksonian)		
(c) Versive		
(d) Postural		
(e) Phonatory (vocalization or arrest of speech)		
2. *With somatosensory or special sensory symptoms* (simple hallucinations, e.g., tingling, light flashes, buzzing)		
(a) Somatosensory		
(b) Visual		
(c) Auditory		
(d) Olfactory		
(e) Gustatory		
(f) Vertiginous		
3. *With autonomic symptoms or signs* (including epigastric sensation, pallor, sweating, flushing, piloerection and pupillary dilatation).		
4. *With psychic symptoms* (disturbance of higher cerebral function). These symptoms rarely occur without impairment of consciousness and are much more commonly experienced as complex partial seizures.		
(a) Dysphasic		
(b) Dysmnesic (e.g., dé-jà-vu)		
(c) Cognitive (e.g., dreamy states, distortions of time sense)		
(d) Affective (fear, anger, etc.)		
(e) Illusions (e.g., macropsia)		
(f) Structured hallucinations (e.g., music, scenes)		
B. *Complex partial (psychomotor) seizures*		
(with impairment of consciousness, may sometimes begin with simple symptomatology)	Unilateral or frequently bilateral discharge, or diffuse or focal in temporal or frontotemporal regions	Unilateral or bilateral generally asynchronous focus: usually in the temporal or frontal regions

Table 11.4-1
Classification of Seizures (Continued)

Clinical Seizure Type	EEG Seizure Type	EEG Interictal Expression
1. Simple partial onset followed by impairment of consciousness (a) With simple partial features (A.1-A.4) followed by impaired consciousness (b) With automatisms 2. With impairment of consciousness at onset (a) With impairment of consciousness only (b) With automatisms		
C. *Partial seizures evolving to secondarily generalized seizures* (this may be generalized tonic-clonic, tonic, or clonic)	Above discharges become secondarily and rapidly generalized	
1. Simple partial seizures (A) evolving to generalized seizures 2. Complex partial seizures (B) evolving to generalized seizures 3. Simple partial seizures evolving to complex partial seizures evolving to generalized seizures		

II. Generalized Seizures (Convulsive or Nonconvulsive)

Generalized seizures are those in which the first clinical changes indicate initial involvement of both hemispheres. Consciousness may be impaired and this impairment may be the initial manifestation. Motor manifestations are bilateral. The ictal electroencephalographic patterns initially are bilateral, and presumably reflect neuronal discharge which is widespread in both hemispheres.

Clinical Seizure Type	EEG Seizure Type	EEG Interictal Expression
A. 1. *Absence seizures (Petit mal)*	Usually regular and symmetrical 3 Hz but may be 2-4 Hz spike-and-slow wave complexes and may have multiple spike-and-slow wave complexes; abnormalities are bilateral	Background activity usually normal although paroxysmal activity (such as spikes or spike-and-slow-wave complexes) may occur; this activity is usually regular and symmetrical
(a) Impairment of consciousness only (b) With mild clonic components (c) With atonic components (d) With tonic components (e) With automatisms (f) With autonomic components (b through f may be used alone or in combination)		
2. *Atypical absence (Lennox-Gastaut syndrome; Petit mal variant)*	EEG more heterogeneous: may include irregular spike-and-slow-wave complexes, fast activity or other paroxysmal activity; abnormalities are bilateral but often irregular and asymmetrical	Background usually abnormal; paroxysmal activity (such as spikes or spike-and-slow-wave complexes) frequently irregular and asymmetrical
May have (a) Changes in tone that are more pronounced than in A.1		

Table 11.4-1
Classification of Seizures (Continued)

Clinical Seizure Type	EEG Seizure Type	EEG Interictal Expression
(b) Onset and/or cessation that is not abrupt		
B. *Myoclonic seizures* *Myoclonic jerks* (single or multiple)	Polyspike-and-wave, or sometimes spike-and-wave or sharp-and-slow waves	Same as ictal
C. *Clonic seizures*	Fast activity (10 Hz or more) and slow waves: occasional spike-and-wave patterns	Spike-and-wave or polyspike-and-wave discharges
D. *Tonic seizures*	Low voltage, fast activity or a fast rhythm of 9-10 Hz or more, decreasing in frequency and increasing in amplitude	More or less rhythmic discharges of sharp-and-slow waves, sometimes asymmetrical; background is often abnormal for age
E. *Tonic-clonic seizures (Grand mal)*	Rhythm at 10 or more Hz, decreasing in frequency and increasing in amplitude during tonic phase, interrupted by slow waves during clonic phase	Polyspike-and-waves or spike-and-wave, or sometimes sharp-and-slow wave discharges
F. *Atonic seizures (Drop attacks)* (combination of the above may occur, e.g., B and F, B and D).	Polyspikes and wave or flattening of low-voltage fast activity	Polyspike-and-slow-wave

III. Unclassified Epileptic Seizures

Includes all seizures that cannot be classified because of inadequate or incomplete data and some that defy classification in hitherto described categories. This includes some neonatal seizures, e.g., rhythmic eye movements, chewing, and swimming movements.

IV. Addendum

Repeated epileptic seizures occur under a variety of circumstances: (1) As fortuitous attacks, coming unexpectedly and without any apparent provocation; (2) as cyclic attacks, at more or less regular intervals (e.g., in relation to the menstrual cycle, or the sleep-waking cycle); (3) as attacks provoked by: (a) nonsensory factors (fatigue, alcohol, emotion, etc.) or (b) sensory factors, sometimes referred to as "reflex seizures."

Prolonged or repetitive seizures (status epilepticus). The term *status epilepticus* is used whenever a seizure persists for a sufficient length of time or is repeated frequently enough that recovery between attacks does not occur. Status epilepticus may be divided into partial (e.g., Jacksonian), or generalized (e.g., absence status or tonic-clonic status). When very localized motor status occurs, it is referred to as epilepsia partialis continua.

Source: From Ref. 11 (Reproduced with some modification with permission from the Commission on Classification and Terminology of the International League Against Epilepsy).

tions, abrupt withdrawal of anticonvulsant medication) or unknown mechanisms. When generalized tonic-clonic status epilepticus occurs, a state of hypoxia usually ensues and emergency treatment is required.

Epileptogenic focus. The fact that seizures occur intermittently and are often associated with a discrete anatomical lesion has led to the concept of an epileptogenic focus. This may be an area of hyperexcitable nervous tissues adjacent to a neoplasm, scar, vascular abnormality leading to hypoxia, infectious process, foreign body, and the like. Areas such as these can discharge excessively, leading to particular symptoms dependent on the area involved. This discharge can occur at times between seizures (interictally) without triggering obvious seizure manifestations (see Table 11.4-1). The focal area, by virtue of its functional connections and proximity to other CNS areas, occasionally recruits these otherwise normal neural populations as a focal discharge grows and spreads to become more widespread. The triggered focal area may be responsible for the aura (olfactory, tingling, familiar feeling) that is often the immediate warning of an impending seizure that patients often perceive at the onset of an attack. The epileptogenic focus may then be localized by EEG studies and in a small selected number of cases may be surgically removed. The major therapeutic approach to the control of the epilepsies, however, is with antiepileptic drugs. Some drugs are thought to depress all neural tissues, including the focus-preventing seizures, whereas others may prevent seizure spread from the focus and thus abort seizures.

GENERAL CONSIDERATIONS

The objective of therapy is to keep the patient seizure-free (or as seizure-free as possible) without drug-induced impairment of functions. With the drugs presently available, seizures in approximately 55% of epileptic patients can be regarded as adequately controlled (10)

(1) Appropriate selection of drug. Certain agents are of value only in certain seizure varities and may even worsen other forms of epilepsy. Drug selection is based upon a thorough (including EEG) evaluation of the seizure type and the known utility and limitations of the agents under consideration.

(2) Individualization of therapy. Each patient requires care-

ful adjustment of dose of the most effective agent that provides a minimum of adverse effects. The institution of therapy involves the establishment of what may be a lifelong drug-taking process. It is noteworthy that excessive doses of antiepileptic drugs that are useful in a seizure disorder can actually worsen the seizures (42). Often if a drug is introduced at lower dose, tolerance to some of the adverse effects develops and the patient can comfortably tolerate a daily dose that, if given initially, would produce an unacceptable degree of adverse effects. Similarly, if an antiepileptic drug is to be withdrawn for whatever reasons (change of medication, discontinuation), but not due to a serious or life threatening adverse reaction, this must usually be done very gradually so as to preclude the precipitation of seizures. In cases where another medication is being substituted, it must be administered while the patient is being weaned of the drug to be discontinued.

(3) Appreciation of CNS-depressant effects of all antiepileptic drugs. The universal side effects that may be anticipated with all antiepileptic drugs are to some degree dose-related, drug-induced impairments of function that may manifest as a motor or sensory disturbance.

(4) Knowledge of pharmacokinetic factors. Modern treatment of epilepsy demands a working knowledge of the absorption, distribution, and elimination of antiepileptic drugs.This is true for sustained treatment to prevent seizures or emergency treatment to manage seizures.

Although in treating an acute episode, agents that arrest the seizure are administered i.v., in the chronic treatment situation agents with appreciably long half-lives (carbamazepine and valproic acid are exceptions) are the most useful; only with these latter agents can reasonably stable blood levels and therefore brain levels be achieved, and they usually allow for less frequent dosing with a concomitant improvement of compliance with the prescribed drug regimen. Before one begins to assess the utility of a dose regimen, it is extremely important that adequate time (at least four to five half-lives) be permitted to elapse, so that one is dealing with steady-state conditions.

(5) Sensible use of serum level data. Within the past 20 years, determination of the concentrations of antiepileptic drugs in blood serum and other body fluids has shown that the effective and toxic concentration ranges for various drugs can be stated. These data are a useful guide in the same sense that the average dose or dose range for a drug can be stated. Each individual must, however, have therapy tailored to his or her specific needs.

(6) Drug combinations. As a rule, "never use two when one will do." The adddition of a second agent is warranted after the initial agent has been thoroughly explored and has failed to provide adequate control alone in nontoxic doses. Drug combinations are most rational when two or more agents exert different mechanisms of action and their toxicities are divergent. There are, however, added complexities of taking more than one drug with respect to the pharmacokinetics (including protein binding), drug interaction, and other factors for each drug, and the potential for combined toxicities.

It is common for more than one type of epilepsy to exist in a patient. Only when major seizures are brought under control does it occasionally become apparent that some less obvious form of epilepsy is also present. Such an instance could provide a rational basis for multiple-drug therapy.

(7) Long-term monitoring and follow-up. Because the epilepsies are often lifelong disorders that may change over months or years (sometimes disappearing altogether) and the medications used have the capacity on chronic exposure to affect adversely various organ systems of the body, the patient (or the patient's family) and physician develop a longstanding partnership in monitoring the course of therapy. Because many of the agents can influence hematopoiesis and liver function, tests of these systems as well as other clinical laboratory tests must be performed routinely.

(8) Usage in pregnancy. It has been observed that whereas the incidence of birth defects in the nonepileptic population is about 2.5-3%, the incidence in epileptic mothers who have not been using drugs for epilepsy during their pregnancy is about 6%; and the incidence of birth defects in epileptic mothers using antiepileptic drugs is abnout 9%. These data, although they show statistically significant differences between groups, do not permit the conclusion that the drugs are teratogenic or even that they increase risk, since adequate control data are not available. Because of this observation, virtually all antiepileptic drug labeling contains a statement to notify prescribers that a teratogenic risk might exist, but that major seizures constitute a known risk. The labeling further points out that at this time there is little reason to believe that any one antiepileptic drug is safer than the others with regard to risk of birth defects.

(9) New drug development. Today most drugs are developed as a result of lengthy testing procedures. Experimental work peculiar to antiepileptics include (a) the demonstation of anticonvulsant activity in animal models exhibiting convulsions (induced by electrical stimulation, drugs, or chemicals), and (b) the demonstration of utility in epilepsy by controlled clinical trials. The subject of experimental models of epilepsy has been reviewed (31,32,47,55,68). Guidelines for drug testing have been published by the FDA (26,27) and are discussed in a recent symposium (7).

DRUGS USED FOR THE CHRONIC PROPHYLACTIC CONTROL OF SEIZURES

BROMIDE ION

Although rarely used today, the bromide salts introduced by Sir Charles Locock (44), physician to the royal family of England, were the first effective agents for the control of epileptic seizures. The various bromide salts (Na, K, Li, Ca, and Sr) were used in doses of up to several grams daily. The ion, which moves into the body's chloride space, has an exceedingly long half-life in humans (about 12 days). Toxicity (bromism), manifesting as skin rash, gastric distress, lethargy, and mental changes, was very common, since the therapeutic and toxic plasma concentrations are essentially the same (10-20 mEq/1). Soon after the introduction of newer agents, bromides were regarded as obsolete. Their inclusion here is for historical purposes.

BARBITURATES

Although all of the depressant barbiturates (as well as most other CNS depressants) can be shown to exhibit anticonvulsant activity in animals or even treat status epilepticus in humans, only three are marketed for chronic use in epilepsy: phenobarbital, mephobarbital, and metharbital. It is significant that these drugs either have long half-lives or are biotransformed to barbiturates with long half-lives.

PHENOBARBITAL

In 1912, the year that phenobarbital (Fig. 11.4-1) became available, Hauptmann used the drug in a neurological/psychiatric clinic in Freiburg, Germany (25); he reported that epileptic patients either had their seizures markedly ameliorated or totally prevented. Since then, it has been and is still the most extensively studied and clinically used barbiturate for the control of seizures.

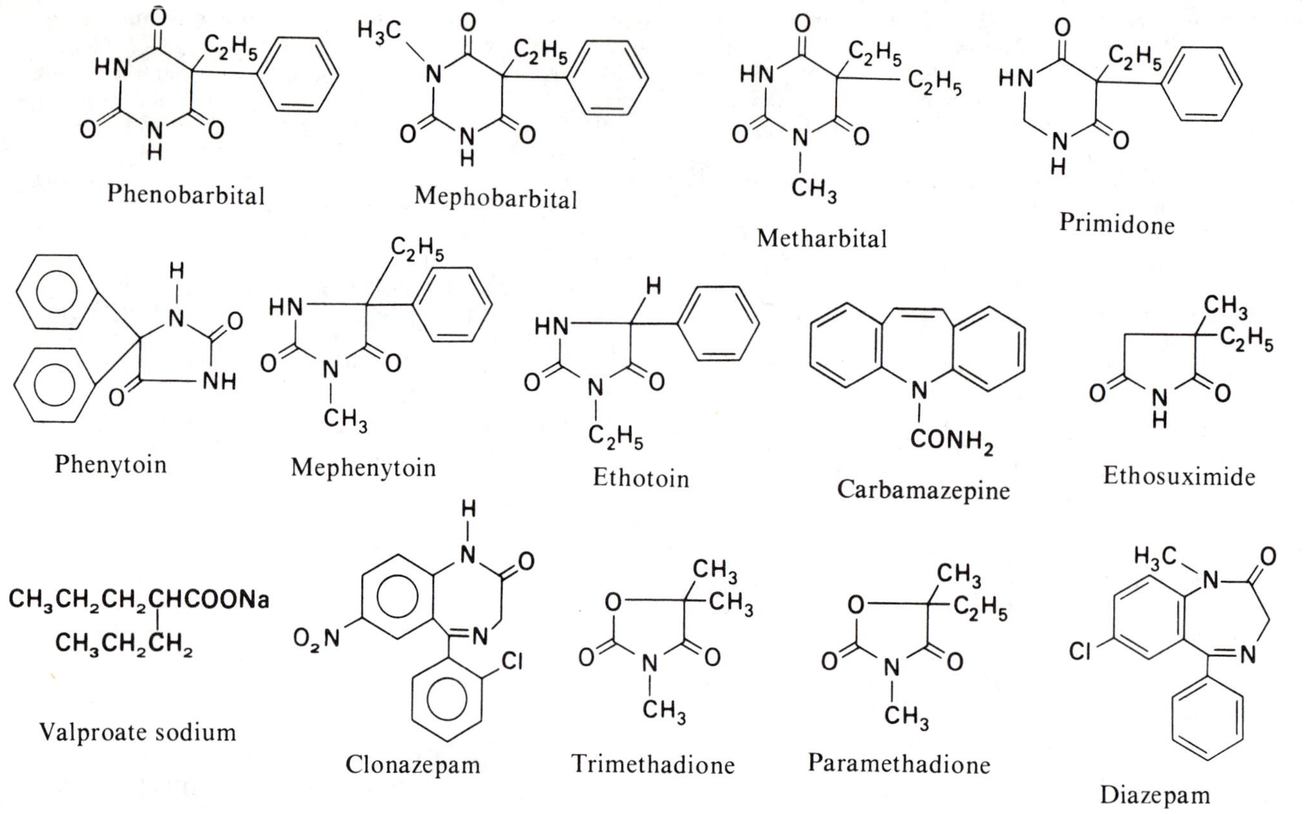

Phenobarbital
Mephobarbital
Metharbital
Primidone

Phenytoin
Mephenytoin
Ethotoin
Carbamazepine
Ethosuximide

$CH_3CH_2CH_2CHCOONa$
$CH_3CH_2CH_2$

Valproate sodium
Clonazepam
Trimethadione
Paramethadione
Diazepam

Fig. 11.4-1. *Chemical structures of antiepileptic drugs.*

The chemistry, pharmacokinetics, and pharmacological actions and interactions of phenobarbital are presented along with other barbiturates in Chapter 11.2.1. However, a few points on pharmacokinetics applicable to humans will be further discussed here. Some pharmacokinetic characteristics of phenobarbital and other antiepileptic drugs are compared in Table 11.4-2.

Table 11.4-2
Summary of Pharmacokinetic Characteristics of Principal Antiepileptic Drugs in Adults[a]

Antiepileptic Drugs	Plasma Half-Life (hr)	Plasma Protein Binding (%)	Dosage (mg/kg/day)	Serum Levels Therapeutic Range for Efficacy (μg/ml)
Phenobarbital	60-144	40-60	1-5	20-40
Primidone	8-12	< 10	7-14	5-15
Phenytoin	7-42	85-90	4-7	10-20
Carbamazepine	12-30	80	10-20	5-10
Ethosuximide	24-72[b]	< 10	20-40	40-100
Valproic acid	8-12	85-95	15-60	50-100
Clonazepam	22-32	80	0.02-0.3	0.02-0.06

[a]Drug package labeling should be consulted for dosing in infants and children.
[b]The $t_{1/2}$ of ethosuximide seems to depend upon age. The mean $t_{1/2}$ for children has been reported to be around 30 hours, whereas that of adults, closer to 60 hours (8, 9).

Absorption in humans after oral administration of phenobarbital appears to be relatively complete, although peak plasma levels after doses of 2-3 mg/kg do not usually occur for 12-18 hr. After larger doses, peak levels seem to be further delayed, suggesting that the rate-limiting step is the dissolution of the poorly soluble drug. Oxidative metabolism of phenobarbital is quite slow and the drug has a half-life in humans of 3-6 days. The drug induces hepatic drug-metabolizing enzymes such that the rates of metabolism of it and many other drugs are accelerated. Because the drug has a long half-life, administering the drug at maintenance doses will require 2-4 weeks for a steady state to be achieved. This latent period can be reduced to about 4 days if the maintenance dose is doubled for the first 4 days (68), while the patient is hospitalized for supervision. The long half-life also makes it possible to administer the dose once a day to most patients, thus simplifying the medication regimen and improving compliance. Inadvertent failure to take a single dose is not likely to precipitate seizures, because the daily dose merely replenishes the daily losses that constitute a small fraction (about one-sixth to one-tenth) of the body's store of the drug. It should be noted that at maintenance dose levels during early weeks of treatment, although it might take a week to increase the plasma concentration by 15% on a reasonable daily dose, discontinuation of the drug can lead to a fall in blood concentration of about 15% in 1 day.

Mechanism of Action. Barbiturates have been shown to depress polysynaptic neural transmission at lower doses than simple (monosynaptic) transmission. Failure of synaptic transmission is associated with presynaptic and postsynaptic membrane stabilization. At the molecular level, barbiturates exhibit actions similar to local anesthetics, blocking action potentials without changing resting membrane conductance (3,33,50).

Adverse Reactions. The commonly observed toxic manifestation is sedation, which often disappears (i.e., tolerance develops) as therapy is continued, even as brain levels are rising (68). However, tolerance to the antiepileptic actions of phenobarbital does not seem to develop, and is not regarded as a clinical problem. Paradoxical excitement is seen in some children and elderly individuals who receive barbiturates. Motor disturbances (nystagmus and ataxia) and visual disturbances have also been observed. Megaloblastic anemia and a hemorrhagic disorder of the newborn that is reversed by vitamin K administration are also associated with barbiturate use. Osteomalacia, apparently produced by a hypermetabolism of vitamin D secondary to induction of the hepatic microsomal oxidizing system, can also develop, particularly in institutionalized individuals who do not receive adequate sunlight.

Therapeutic Uses. Phenobarbital is the most useful barbiturate as an antiepileptic drug. The drug may be viewed as either a broad-spectrum antiepileptic agent or a drug lacking in anticonvulsant selectivity. Although its greatest use is in major tonic-clonic seizures, it is useful in most types of convulsive disorders. It is an inexpensive agent available in a wide variety of dosage forms. Compared with several other depressant barbiturates in terms of anticonvulsant activity and capacity to produce a neurological motor impairment, phenobarbital has a more favorable ratio of anticonvulsant/toxic dose (56).

Preparations. *Phenobarbital,* USP and *phenobarbital sodium,* USP are available in tablets for oral use in strengths in multiples of 15 mg up to 90 mg and as elixir of phenobarbital, a palatable liquid containing about 15 mg per teaspoonful.

MEPHOBARBITAL

Introduced in 1936, mephobarbital is the N-methyl derivative of phenobarbital (Fig. 11.4-1).

The addition of the methyl group enhances the lipid solubility of the drug (but diminishes further the water solubility). Thus, compared with phenobarbital, this drug can move more rapidly into the brain from the blood, but after oral administration its absorption is incomplete, thus requiring somewhat higher doses. The liver efficiently demethylates mephobarbital to form phenobarbital. Thus, the daily administration of mephobarbital leads to the coexistence of both drugs, with a preponderance of phenobarbital that probably accounts for most of the antiepileptic as well as other actions of mephobarbital. In humans, mephobarbital has a half-life substantially shorter than 12 hr and fails to accumulate to any significant degree, whereas phenobarbital with its much longer half-life accumulates in the body to achieve values within its therapeutic range. Like phenobarbital, mephobarbital is used in all forms of epilepsy but has not demonstrated any advantage over phenobarbital.

Mephobarbital, USP (MEBARAL) is available in tablets for oral use in strengths of 32, 50, 100, and 200 mg.

METHARBITAL

Introduced in 1950, metharbital is the N-methyl derivative of barbital (Fig. 11.4-1), a depressant barbiturate with a long half-life and low potency.

The hepatic N-demethylation of metharbital is apparently complete and the derived barbital probably accounts for metharbital's activity. Metharbital is well absorbed after oral administration. It offers no demonstrated advantage over phenobarbital and, like phenobarbital, is used in all forms of epilepsy. Barbital is eliminated primarily unchanged in the urine. Toxicity consists of drowsiness, gastric distress, dizziness, skin rash, and occasionally increased irritability.

Metharbital, USP (GEMONIL) is available as 100 mg tablets for oral use. The usual dose for adults is about 300 mg daily.

DEOXYBARBITURATES

PRIMIDONE

Introduced in 1952, primidone is the product obtained by replacement of the carbonyl group of the urea moiety in phenobarbital with a methylene group (Fig. 11.4-1).

Although the drug has a very low aqueous solubility, it is well absorbed after oral administration, peak plasma levels usually occurring 3 hr after oral administration (5). However, substantial interindividual differences exist (20). Primidone is not bound to plasma proteins in significant amounts; its half-life in humans is about 6 hr. It is biotransformed by (1) oxidation of the methylene group at position 2 to form phenobarbital, and (2) ring opening with loss of the carbon atom at position 2 leading to the formation of phenylethylmaloneamide (PEMA). Experiments in animals indicate that PEMA, although low in potency, exhibits anticonvulsant activity. The degree to which phenobarbital is responsible for primidone's antiepileptic efficacy is unresolved (40). The serum level of phenobarbital derived from primidone rises into its therapeutic range (5) and clearly plays a major part in the efficacy of administered primidone. Primidone finds its most extensive use in generalized tonic-clonic, complex partial (psychomotor), myoclonic, and akinetic seizures.

Adverse Reactions. Primidone has the same adverse effects as observed with phenobarbital; additionally, impotence has been reported.

Preparations. The average adult dose is 0.75-1.5 g daily. *Primidone*, USP (MYSOLINE) is available in tablets containing 50 and 250 mg and in a suspension containing 250 mg per teaspoonful.

HYDANTOINS

PHENYTOIN (DIPHENYLHYDANTOIN)

Phenytoin is a primary antiepileptic drug used in generalized tonic-clonic, and complex partial (psychomotor), akinetic, and myoclonic seizures. In 1938, Merritt and Putnam (48) evaluated scores of phenyl-containing chemicals for their capacity to increase the threshold to electrically induced major motor seizures in cats, and found diphenylhydantoin (now called phenytoin) to elevate seizure thresholds manyfold in nontoxic doses. After some preliminary animal testing, Merritt and Putnam (49) tried the drug in 200 patients with epilepsy and demonstrated that the drug was most useful (46). Recent work in experimental animals (68) indicates that when shorter durations (0.2 sec) of stimulation are used, phenytoin's most prominent effects are to abolish the tonic hindlimb extension that is the outstanding feature of maximal electroshock seizures; the drug does not elevate seizure thresholds under these circumstances.

Chemistry. Hydantoins, like barbiturates, are weak acids and cyclic ureides. This group is formed by the condensation of urea with a glycolic acid derivative to form a five-membered ring (Fig. 11.4-1). Phenytoin, by far the most important and useful member of the group, has a pK_a reported to be in the range of 8.0-9.2. It is usually administered as the sodium salt which is quite soluble at highly alkaline pH values.

Pharmacokinetics. Taken orally as a salt or acid, phenytoin exists as an insoluble acid at the pH values prevailing in the stomach. The solubility is so low in the stomach that absorption from this site is slight. Only when the drug reaches the small intestine, where (a) the pH is higher, so as to solubilize more drug, (b) there is a larger absorbing surface of the tissues, and (c) bile is present, does substantial absorption occur.

Diluents of the active constituent and the capacity of the pharmaceutical preparation to dissolve and its rate of release of drug are important factors for the first step in absorption. As diluents, calcium salts retard the absorption of phenytoin whereas lactose does not. This may be important if a patient uses antacids, particularly to deal with gastric discomfort produced by the drug. The particle size of the acid is important, as the expanded surface area of fine particles provides greater opportunity for dissolution. Additionally, some patients have been identified who are malabsorbers of the drug. At usual therapeutic serum concentrations (10-20 μg/ml), phenytoin is about 90% bound to plasma proteins. Cerebrospinal fluid and saliva, which are in equilibrium with the free drug in plasma, contain (as expected) about one-tenth the plasma concentration. Measurement of drug in saliva is a developing technique that may, if sufficiently sensitive, in some instances replace serum determinations. It appears that phenytoin is bound to albumin and the same two α-globulins that bind thyroxine and T_3, salicylic acid, phenylbutazone, and sulfafurazol and probably other highly plasma protein-bound drugs. Administration of highly protein-bound drugs may lead to an increase in free (active) phenytoin. This can lead to an increased loss from the body, if oxidation is proceeding by first-order kinetics, because it is the free form that is available for biotransformation. On the other hand, if saturation (zero-order) kinetics obtain (see later), drug loss rate will not be accelerated. It should also be noted that phenytoin can displace other highly protein-bound drugs from their binding sites.

In cases of renal failure and azotemia or hypoproteinemia, phenytoin binding with plasma proteins is diminished. This can lead to toxicity with modest total plasma concentrations (59) of the drug.

The amount of drug in the plasma when a steady state is achieved is also a function of metabolism. The drug, like phenobarbital, is primarily biotransformed by parahydroxylation of one of the phenyl rings to form hydroxyphenylphenylhydantoin (HPPH), which is inactive. A small amount of the m-OH derivative is also formed. These oxidation products appear to involve the formation of an epoxide intermediate that may be responsible for some organ toxicities due to its high reactivity. A dihydrodiol intermediate also appears to be formed. The inactive hydroxylated compounds appear in urine largely as the glucuronide conjugates. The half-life of phenytoin in human serum is extremely variable, with values for humans ranging from about 7 to 40 hr with a mean of 22 hr; a subpopulation of genetically determined slow metabolizers has also been identified (37).

The rate of metabolism is influenced by the liver's state of enzyme induction and by the presence of other drugs that may interfere with phenytoin metabolism. The metabolism of phenytoin is a saturable process at concentrations that are occasionally clinically achieved, a situation that makes the half-life dose-dependent. This is further complicated by the fact that therapeutic and toxic concentrations are close. Thus, to obtain therapeutic levels, the rate of administration approaches the maximal rate at which phenytoin can be degraded (45). These factors predispose to the great variability in biotransformation rates reflected in the range of half-lives pointed out earlier. Although there is an increase (on the average) in serum level in some individuals produced by an increase in dose, for any individual this is totally unpredictable. The saturability of the biotransformation process accounts for a frequently observed (but often confusing) abrupt and substantial disproportionate increase in serum levels and toxicity of the drug after a modest increase in dose.

Mechanism of Action. In animal experiments, phenytoin is most effective in abolishing the tonic hind limb extensor phase of maximal electroshock seizures (68). The drug fails to antagonize clonic seizures produced by a variety of chemical convulsants and may exacerbate them (62) but blocks the tonic hind limb extension produced by large doses of convulsant drugs. Because clinically the drug often prevents convulsions without preventing the aura and because epileptogenic foci can often be detected in individuals whose convulsions are controlled by phenytoin, it is thought by many that the seizures are actually aborted rather than prevented and that the drug prevents the spread of the seizure discharge rather than the focal discharge itself. The capacity of phenytoin to curb the spread of excitation leading to recruitment in brain tissue has a parallel in the capacity of the drug under experimental conditions to prevent the spread of excitation within the cat spinal cord that occurs subsequent to high-frequency conditioning of the monosynaptic reflex pathway (posttetanic potentiation, PTP), described by Esplin (16). It has been proposed that suppression of PTP in the brain might be the way the drug acts to control epilepsy (16); this proposed mechanism of action to account for antiepileptic activity has recently been questioned (39) and should not be regarded as proven.

The most intriguing aspect of the drug's actions is its lack of activity on nervous tissues when they are at lower levels of activity, but a marked suppression of neural discharges when they are excessive. This property can be seen in axonal function (30,70), and autonomic reflexes (57).

Phenytoin's fundamental mechanisms of action are still actively sought and debated. The drug is often described as a stabilizer of excitable membranes, because it exerts prominent depressant actions only when the tissues are substantially activated. The focal point of the drug's actions at this time are the cations (that move into neurons and are associated with nerve excitation and neurosecretion), namely, sodium and calcium. Woodbury (73) showed that phenytoin diminished the amount of intracellular sodium in brain cells of animals experiencing electrically induced convulsions, and he and others (63,73) have proposed that phenytoin activates the sodium-potassium adenosine triphosphatase (ATPase) that is associated with active extrusion of sodium from excitable cells (60,69). Thus, it is argued that the enhanced sodium influx associated with excessive depolarization of neurons is compensated for by an increased extrusion of sodium. The valadity of this hypothesis has been questioned (2,15). Other workers have reported a reduction in sodium movements through excitable membranes and have suggested that reducing sodium influx into neurons might explain the drug's membrane-stabilizing properties (19,43,51,54,61). Several workers (24,65,66,75) have reported that calcium influx into excitable membranes is inhibited by phenytoin and that this action explains or contributes to the drug's effects to arrest excessive or neuronal activity. Phenytoin inhibits the increase in cyclic adenosine monophosphate (cAMP) and cyclic guanosine monophosphate (cGMP) that occurs when brain tissues are excited electrically or pharmacologically (18,19,34). These cyclic nucleotides appear intimately involved in excitation-secretion coupling.

Phenytoin has also been reported to inhibit the calcium-dependent phosphorylation of specific proteins isolated from rat brain nerve terminal structures (14). Phenytoin's inhibitory actions are antagonized by calcium. If these phosphorylations participate in neurotransmitter release processes, this may be a mechanism of the drug's actions. Phenytoin apparently exerts several actions, the sum total of which are responsible for its observed clinical effects as an antiepileptic drug.

Adverse Effects. Large doses of phenytoin in animals produce nystagmus and tremor. With still larger doses in animals, postural tone is lost and tremor progresses to clonic muscle movements; unlike barbiturates, phenytoin does not induce sleep. Humans also exhibit a motor disturbance as described here. This constellation of effects is usually alluded to as a *cerebellar syndrome*. The mechanisms probably involve a derangement of the cerebellar-vestibular system and a peripheral proprioceptive deficit produced by depression of muscle spindle function (1). The motor deficits are usually reversible, but after long-term drug use at high doses may persist for indefinite periods after drug removal. It is thought that phenytoin can produce a cerebellar cell loss (64), but this is not totally resolved (12). Increased frequency of seizures, an encephalopathy, and peripheral neuropathy have been observed. Gingival hyperplasia and increased growth of body hair are often concomitants of phenytoin therapy. Other adverse effects seemingly involving immune responses include skin rash, fever, Stevens-

Johnson syndrome, lymphadenopathy and lupus erythematosis. Osteomalacia, hepatitis and some blood dyscrasias (neutropenia, agranulocytosis, and aplastic anemia) are also occasionally observed in patients receiving phenytoin.

Drug Interactions. Phenytoin's gastric absorption is inhibited by calcium and antacid therapy (4,36). Its metabolism is accelerated by inducers (such as phenobarbital) of the microsomal mixed-function oxidase system; this has not proven a serious problem because dose adjustment can compensate for changes in rate of metabolism.

Several agents (e.g., bishydroxycoumarin, phenyramidol, disulfiram, chloramphenicol) have been reported to elevate the plasma levels of phenytoin and increase its half-life, presumably by interfering with phenytoin's biotransformation by competing for hepatic enzyme system components (35). Because phenytoin is bound to plasma proteins extensively, the addition of other drugs highly bound to these proteins can displace the drug and increase the proportion of free drug with resultant enhancement of therapeutic or toxic effects.

Preparations. The usual adult dose of phenytoin is 300-400 mg daily. *Phenytoin sodium* (diphenylhydantoin sodium; DILANTIN) — capsules (30 or 100 mg), flavored tablets (50 mg), suspensions (for pediatric use, containing either 30 or 125 mg per teaspoonful), and vials (2 and 10 ml, containing 50 mg of sodium salt/ml for i.v. injection).

ETHOTOIN

Ethotin is 3-ethyl-5-phenylhydantoin (Fig. 11.4-1). It has not been studied as extensively as, nor does it enjoy the wide use of, phenytoin. Its indications for use and spectrum of toxicity are similar to those for phenytoin. Its potency is, however, lower than that of phenytoin, with effective serum concentrations being about twice those of phenytoin. Additionally, its half-life in humans is only 6-12 hr (76), making for more frequent administration and larger doses than phenytoin.

The drug is dealkylated to form phenylhydantoin, which is then further biotransformed by two routes: (1) parahydroxylation (like phenytoin) and (2) ring opening to form 2-phenylhydantoic acid.

Preparations. *Ethotoin* (PEGANONE) is available as tablets containing 250 or 500 mg. Usual daily doses are of the order of 2-3 g daily given in four to six divided doses.

MEPHENYTOIN

Mephenytoin is 3-methyl-5-phenyl-5-ethylhydantoin (Fig. 11.4-1). The compound thus has the ring structure of phenytoin and the side chains of phenobarbital; in animal experiments it exhibits similarities to both agents. This agent is N-demethylated to form 5-phenyl-5-ethylhydantoin (NIRVANOL), which probably accounts for most of the actions of the drug.

The drug has the same spectrum of anticonvulsant activity as phenytoin and ethotoin but exhibits some serious side effects. Thus, whereas ataxia and gingival hyperplasia may not occur with as great a frequency as seen with phenytoin, agranulocytosis, aplastic anemia, hepatitis, and exfoliative dermatitis have been reported to occur following mephenytoin's use (22). These serious side effects limit this drug's use to patients whose seizures cannot be adequately controlled with safer agents. Blood counts and liver function tests are especially important with this agent.

Mephenytoin is biotransformed via two routes: p-hydroxylation (like other phenylhydantoins) and N-demethylation. These routes are not mutually exclusive. Because this compound has an asymmetric carbon atom at position 5 on the ring, it is possible that the two pathways reflect stereospecific enzymatic processes.

Preparations. *Mephenytoin*, USP (MESANTOIN) is available as 100-mg tablets. Adult maintenance doses are 200-600 mg daily, arrived at by starting with 50-100 mg daily for the first week and increasing gradually each week by 50-100 mg.

CARBAMAZEPINE

Carbamazepine is an iminostilbene, chemically designated 5H-dibenz(b, f)azepine-5-carboxamide (Fig. 11.4-1). It is virtually insoluble in water. The drug was shown to exert an activity profile much like phenytoin in animal models of epilepsy. Like phenytoin, the drug has been useful in treating trigeminal neuralgia.

In 1974, carbamazepine was approved for use as an antiepileptic drug, following by about 8 years its introduction for this purpose in Europe. Carbamazepine exhibits a spectrum of antiepileptic efficacy equivalent to phenytoin, being useful in most types of epilepsy except absence (petit mal) seizures. The drug does not have prominent sedative properties, and its chemical structure (which is not unlike tricyclic antidepressants such as imipramine) led to the presumption that the drug had mood-elevating properties. Presently, the drug is being investigated for use in depression and mania.

Pharmacokinetics. Some pharmacokinetic characteristics of carbamazepine are given in Table 11.4-2. Its half-life generally varies from 12 to 30 hr after acute administration and from 7 to 12 hr after chronic use, apparently due to induction of hepatic enzymes. The drug is oxidized to several hydroxy derivatives that appear in urine. The 10, 11-epoxide is an active metabolite and accounts for about 10% of the administered dose; it is thought by some to be primarily responsible for the toxicities observed after carbamazepine administration.

Adverse Effects. These include depression of blood cell formation (red, white, and platelets), which although of infrequent occurrence can prove disastrous and requires monitoring for hematopoietic changes. Other adverse effects include dizziness, unsteadiness, drowsiness, jaundice, and changes in liver function tests and in kidney function.

Preparation. Usual adult doses are of the range of 600-1200 mg daily. *Carbamazepine*, USP (TEGRETOL) is supplied in tablets containing 200 mg.

DRUGS USED FOR THE TREATMENT OF SIMPLE AND COMPLEX ABSENCE (PETIT MAL) SEIZURES

SUCCINIMIDES

ETHOSUXIMIDE

Introduced in 1960 and chemically α-methyl α-ethylsuccinamide (Fig. 11.4-1), ethosuximide is the most extensively used of the succinimides and vies with valproic acid as the drug of first choice in the treatment of absence seizures. Ethosuximide is useful in reducing the frequency of attacks.

Ethosuximide is soluble in water and is well absorbed after oral administration, reaching peak plasma levels in 1-4 hr. Its other pharmacokinetic characteristics (8,9,53,74) and dose are given in Table 11.4-2.

The mechanism of action of ethosuximide may be related to an enhancement of synaptic refractoriness (6).

Adverse Effects. Nausea, vomiting, anorexia, headache, fatigue, lethargy, dizziness, and hiccups appear to be dose-related, whereas skin rash, blood dyscrasias, allergy, and systemic lupus erythematosus are not. Monitoring of liver and renal function is essential, as abnormalities have been reported.

Preparations. *Ethosuximide*, USP (ZARONTIN) is available in tablets containing 250 mg or as a syrup containing 250 mg per teaspoonful.

OTHER SUCCINIMIDES

Other succinimides are methsuximide, USP (CELONTIN), available as 150- and 300-mg capsules, and phensuximide, USP (MILONTIN), available as 500-mg capsules and as a suspension containing 300 mg per teaspoonful. These have been used when responses to ethosuximide have not been satisfactory. Since the advent of valproic acid as a primary agent, these lesser succinimides have even less justification as alternative agents.

VALPROIC ACID

Valproic acid is a simple fatty acid (dipropyl acetic acid) that is a liquid and is as useful as ethosuximide in absence seizures (Fig. 11.4-1).

The drug is the latest antiepileptic drug to be approved in the United States and, though limited by its official labeling to absence seizures, has a broad spectrum of efficacy in a variety of othert seizure disorders. It is likely that additional controlled clinical trials will lead to an extension of indications.

The drug is rapidly absorbed after oral absorption, reaching peak blood levels within 4 hr. The drug is extensively (about 90%) bound to plasma proteins, leading to interactions with other drugs (e.g., phenytoin) that are also protein bound. A major urinary metabolite is 2-propyl glutaric acid. Its pharmacokinetic characteristics and doses are listed in Table 11.4-2.

Mechanism of Action. The mechanism by which valproic acid favorably influences seizures is not known. The drug inhibits the enzyme γ-aminobutyric acid decarboxylase (GAD), a degradative enzyme for the inhibitory neurotransmitter γ-aminobutyric acid (GABA), thus elevating GABA levels in CNS tissues. It is considered to be the probable reason for valproic acid's efficacy. Interestingly, valproic acid causes enhancement of GABA concentrations that is most marked in brain areas rich in GABAergic nerve terminals (28).

Adverse Effects. Due to the relatively large amounts of drug usually ingested (1-2 g daily), gastric symptoms occur frequently. These consist of nausea, vomiting, and cramps. Sedation and ataxia are observed but may often be the result of elevated phenobarbital levels when the drugs are used concurrently (see earlier). Weight gain and hair loss (reversible) as well as blood clotting disorders have been described as adverse effects of valproic acid.

Drug Interactions. As a consequence of displacing phenytoin from plasma proteins, valproic acid may produce a reduction in total, but an increase in free (i.e., not protein-bound), phenytoin in blood (46). Valproic acid does not appear to induce hepatic microsomal enzyme systems but may substantially elevate phenobarbital levels (60), seemingly by interfering with the latter's biotransformation (29). The drug (which may rarely produce a thrombocytopenia) appears to enhance the actions of warfarin and aspirin in interfering with fibrinogen formation, platelet aggregation, and thus blood clotting.

Preparations. *Valproic acid* (DEPAKENE) is available as a capsule containing 250 mg and a syrup containing 250 mg of valproic acid as sodium salt equivalent per teaspoonful. Enteric coated tablets have recently been made available. Usual doses are 15-60 mg/kg daily.

CLONAZEPAM

Clonazepam is a member of the benzodiazepine group of drugs (Fig. 11.4-1).

These agents possess antianxiety, hypnotic, muscle relaxant, and anticonvulsant properties. Clonazepam distinguishes itself from other members of the group by its high potency. It is most effective as an antagonist of pentylenetetrazol-induced seizures. The drug has some efficacy in absence seizures, as well as akinetic and myoclonic seizures, but it suffers from some serious shortcomings. Tolerance develops to the anticonvulsant efficacy of clonazepam in a substantial proportion of patients. The drug is quite sedating and has the disadvantages of dependence production and abuse liability.

Clonazepam is well absorbed and reaches peak blood levels in 1-2 hr. The activity is sustained, and clonazepam's half-life in serum ranges from 18-50 hr. Five metabolites have been identified in urine resulting from oxidation or reduction of clonazepam. Other pharmacokinetic properties and dose are given in Table 11.4-2.

Adverse Effects. Lethargy, ataxia, and behavioral changes are the more frequently encountered adverse effects, and those with a lesser incidence are cardiovascular, renal, hematopoietic, gastrointestinal, hepatic, and dermatological changes.

Preparations. *Clonazepam*, USP (CLONOPIN) is available in tablets containing 0.5, 1.0, and 2.0 mg. Doses for adults range from 1.5 to 20 mg daily.

OXAZOLIDINEDIONES

TRIMETHADIONE (TMO)

Trimethadione (Fig. 11.4-1) became available clinically in 1945. Its anticonvulsant properties consist of efficacy against pentylenetetrazol as well as electrically induced seizures.

The drug is useful in the treatment of absence seizures and was an important agent before succinimides and valproic acid became available. Presently, it and paramethadione receive little use and only then in patients who have not responded adequately to either ethosuximide or valproic acid.

Mechanistic studies indicate that trimethadione prolongs synaptic recovery periods in cat spinal cord monosynaptic systems (17) and that the drug is a good antagonist to pentylenetetrazol but lacking the potency of benzodiazepines.

In humans, trimethadione is rapidly absorbed after oral administration, with peak plasma levels occurring in 30 min to 2 hr; binding to plasma proteins is negligible. Trimethadione is N-demethylated to form dimethadione (DMO), an active metabolite that accumulates to substantially higher blood levels than the administered agent due to its longer persistence (the half-life of DMO is 6-13 days; that of TMO is 12-24 hr). The accumulation of DMO correlates better with anticonvulsant efficacy than blood levels of TMO. Therapeutic serum concentrations of TMO range from about 6 to 41 μg/ml and from 475 to 1200 μg/ml for DMO (74).

Preparations. *Trimethadione*, USP (TRIDIONE) is available as a 300-mg capsule, a 150-mg tablet, and a liquid containing 200 mg per teaspoonful.

PARAMETHADIONE

Paramethadione differs little from trimethadione; it is also N-demethylated to a longer-acting active metabolite (Fig. 11.4-1).

Preparations. *Paramethadione*, USP (PARADIONE) is available in 150-mg and 300-mg capsules and as a solution containing 300 mg/ml. The latter is in a 65% alcohol solution and must be diluted. The usual dose is 900-2400 mg daily for adults and 300-900 mg daily for children.

DRUGS USED FOR THE TREATMENT OF STATUS EPILEPTICUS OR RECURRENT SEIZURES

Persistent seizure activity is a real medical emergency, and when it is of the major motor variety, represents an immediate threat to life with a fatal outcome in 10-40% of untreated cases; therefore, treatment is always indicated. There is not usually time to identify and specifically treat any of a number of potential causes (e.g., vitamin B_6 deficiency, hypoglycemia, infection, etc.) of a seizure, treatment of which might not in any case cause a rapid disappearance of the seizure. A differential diagnosis to identify cause of the seizure may be carried out and specific therapy initiated after the seizure is brought under control.

The treatment of a convulsing patient usually consists of the intravenous administration of an adequate dose of antiepileptic medication to arrest the seizure. The intravenous route is clearly the most appropriate because the low aqueous solubility of most antiepileptic drugs at physiological pH makes absorption from intramuscular or other depot sites unreliable as regards rate, although extent may eventually be complete. The drug employed must not have an undue latency in penetrating the blood-brain barrier and exerting its pharmacological effects. Because the use of an adequate dose implies a titration of sorts, drugs with unduly long latencies would favor overdosing with resultant excessive CNS depression developing later and having substantial persistence. Because the blood-brain barrier is a two-way street, agents that enter extremely rapidly (such as the ultrashort-acting barbiturates) may prove unsatisfactory because their antiepileptic actions would be fleeting. Ideally, an agent used in the emergency treatment of ongoing seizure activity would: (a) enter the CNS reasonably rapidly so that the effect of a given amount of drug could be assessed before additional drug is administered; (b) have a sufficient duration of action so that after the emergency has been brought under control longer-acting medication could be administered parenterally, or perhaps even orally, and have an opportunity to develop its antiepileptic actions; (c) have minimal actions on organ systems other than the CNS: (d) not produce excessive CNS depression with doses that are antiepileptic. [Patients will experience CNS depression (postictal depression, essentially a postseizure neuronal exhaustion) after a major seizure, and the depth and duration of this depression will be a direct function of seizure severity and duration, ranging from mild and brief disorientation to deep coma. A drug-induced depression will add to this postictal depression and may produce profound respiratory depression requiring mechanical support. In any case of treatment for severe seizure activity, the possible need for respiratory support must always be kept uppermost in mind. Necessary support equipment must be available], and (e) must be convenient to administer, and must not interact with other drugs or parenteral fluids. At the present time there is no available agent that meets all these criteria.

DIAZEPAM

Diazepam is perhaps the best-known and most widely used of the benzodiazepine series of CNS depressants (Fig. 11.4-1).

The important pharmacological actions ascribed to the class are anxiolytic (tranquilizing), sedative-hypnotic, muscle relaxant, and anticonvulsant. Only the latter will be considered here, Details of its other pharmacological actions, pharmacokinetics, mechanism of action, toxicity, tolerance, and drug dependence are discussed in Chapter 11.6.3.

Mechanism of Action. The benzodiazepine group of drugs are extemely potent antagonists of convulsions produced by the convulsant drug pentylenetetrazol. The mechanism of action of agents of the benzodiazepine series is thought to involve an intensification of the actions of the inhibitory neurotransmitter GABA. Benzodiazepines appear to enhance the affinity of GABA for its receptors (Chapter 11.6.3).

Therapeutic Uses. Notwithstanding the rather remarkable capacity of these agents to prevent or abolish pentylenetetrazol-induced seizures and their seeming actions on GABA systems, the utility of the benzodiazepines in the prophylaxis of seizures in epilepsy is poor. Diazepam is generally acknowledged as having little or no value in the chronic management of epilepsy unless anxiety factors are provocative of seizure activity. The use of clonazepam in epilepsy is discussed elsewhere.

Diazepam is generally regarded as the *drug of choice for the emergency treatment of major seizures*; its use is regarded as being successful in 75% of instances in which it is employed. It is effective in a variety of seizure types. The reason for diazepam's position with regard to other agents is its favorable therapeutic index; doses that arrest major seizures tend to produce less respiratory depression that equieffective doses of other CNS depressants. However; diazepam should not be considered as an innocuous agent; by the intravenous route apnea, coma, and death have been observed (23).

Diazepam's actions after i.v. administration develop promptly as blood and brain come into equilibrium in about 5 min, reflecting the drug's high lipid solubility. Thus, the drug may be readministered at 10- to 15-min intervals. The rate of injection as well as dose are important determinants of drug action because the blood concentrations (and hence brain concentrations) fall through the process of redistribution rather than metabolism. Only with several repeated injections would the latter process be a factor in the abatement or termination of drug action. Injection of a dose should not be rapid (particularly in neonates and young children), as effects will be greatly enhanced; alternatively, it is possible to infuse the drug so slowly as never to achieve therapeutic concentrations. Because of the drug's rather rapid emergence from brain as blood concentrations fall, a significant proportion (33-40%) of patients initially brought under control with diazepam experience convulsions within an hour.

It is particularly noteworthy that the doses (in adults, 10-30 mg i.v.) of diazepam employed to treat status epilepticus will often induce sleep if similarly administered to conscious individuals. Thus, it appears difficult to ascribe to diazepam a specific anticonvulsant property in terminating seizures.

Preparations. The usual dose for adults is 5-10 mg i.v. This may be repeated at 10- to 15-min intervals up to a maximum of 30 mg. Diazepam has poor aqueous solubility and for parenteral use is dissolved in a vehicle containing 40% propylene glycol, 10% alcohol, and a benzoate buffer. This solution must not be mixed with other drugs or for convenience injected into a container of intravenous fluid (saline, dextrose in saline, etc.); the drug will precipitate under most conditions. Likewise, whereas just soluble materials may be injected into a vein (given the confluence of venous blood, the presence of proteins, and mixing in the heart) inadvertent intraarterial injections must be scrupulously avoided; the latter has resulted in gangrene and loss of limb.

Diazepam, USP (VALIUM) is available in 2-ml vials containing 5 mg/ml diazepam.

PHENYTOIN

Phenytoin may be given intravenously for the control of seizure types that are susceptible to the drug, but due to its capacity to produce cardiovascular depression, the rate of administration must not exceed 50 mg/min. Therapeutic serum concentrations can be achieved in this manner utilizing doses of the order of 12-18 mg/kg (41,71); thus, a therapeutic dose of 1 g of drug would require at least a 20-min infusion.

The drug penetrates the brain rapidly and CSF contains about one-tenth the plasma concentration, reflecting the proportion of free (nonprotein-bound) drug (74). An advantage of phenytoin in treating status epilepticus is that the levels established by the acute administration of the drug may remain in the therapeutic range up to 12 hr after injection, thus providing prolonged activity and allowing maintenance therapy by oral administration to follow. The drug also has the advantage of not profoundly depressing the sensorium when the latter is being monitored as an index of the degree of brain damage. Under these circumstances, because the infusion is slow and a sustained therapeutic concentration of drug established, biotransformation rather than redistribution accounts for the decline in serum levels.

Individuals with compromised cardiopulmonary function are at greater risk of cardiovascular or respiratory depression than those with normal cardiopulmonary function. Hypotension, cardiac conduction defects, and cardiovascular collapse with fatal outcome have occurred after intravenous phenytoin. The danger is minimized by slow infusion.

The intramuscular route is not recommended because the drug which is injected in a solution containing 40% propylene glycol and 10% ethanol, and at pH 12 precipitates in intramuscular sites. This leads to very low blood levels and perhaps necrotic changes in muscle. One must likewise guard against inadvertent intra-arterial injection, extravasation of the highly alkaline solution and avoid mixing the drug solution with other drugs or i.v. fluids.

PHENOBARBITAL

Phenobarbital may be used to terminate status epilepticus, but its value as a good antiepileptic drug is compromised in this context by its rather slow penetration into the CNS. Peak effects usually develop in about 30 min after injection, making titration difficult. The drug's value is in its persistence of effect; hence, it finds use after seizures have been brought under control by a rapidly acting drug lacking persistence (such as diazepam). Like phenytoin solutions, phenobarbital (containing the soluble sodium salt) solutions are quite alkaline and suffer the same problems as regards extravasation, mixing solutions, or intramuscular uses. Phenobarbital's long half-life (3-6 days) makes it most valuable, because patients may enjoy sustained protection and can maintain therapeutic concentrations with oral medication. As with phenytoin, blood levels decline largely due to loss of drug from the body (via metabolism and renal loss) rather than redistribution. Dangers, as with all depressant barbiturates, consist of excess CNS depression, with the respiratory apparatus at greatest risk. Usual doses of phenobarbital are 150-400 mg administered at rates of 25-50 mg/min. Cumulative doses of up to about 1 g in 24 hr have been suggested.

OTHER DRUGS

Short- and intermediate-acting barbiturates such as pentobarbital and amobarbital, which have redistribution characterstics not unlike those of diazepam, have been successfully used to treat convulsions. Because of the apprent smaller therapeutic index of these agents as compared with diazepam, the former drugs have been used less in recent years. Paraldehyde can be used to treat convulsions, but due to problems with decomposition of the drug, neural damage upon intramuscular injection, and local irritation from intravenous injection, it has been used when diazepam or other more frequently used agents prove inadequate. Last, general anesthesia may be used to terminate seizures when other more conventional therapies have failed.

REFERENCES

1. Anderson, R.J. and Raines, A. Suppression by diphenylhydantoin on afferent discharges arising in muscle spindles of the triceps surae of the cat. *J. Pharmacol. Exp. Ther.* 191:290, 1974.
2. Ayala, G.F. and Johnston, D. The influences of phenytoin on the fundamental electrical properties of simple neural systems. *Epilepsia* 18:3, 1977.
3. Blaustein, M.D. Barbiturates block Na^+ and K^+ conductance increases in voltage-clamped lobster axons. *J. Gen. Physiol.* 51:193, 1968.
4. Bochner, F., Hooper, W.D., Tyrer, J.H. and Eadie, M.J. Factors involved in an outbreak of phenytoin intoxication. *J. Neurol. Sci.* 16:481, 1972.
5. Booker, H.E., Hosokawa, K., Burdette, R.D. and Darcey, B. A clinical study of serum primidone levels. *Epilepsia* 11:395, 1970.
6. Capek, R. and Esplin, B. Effects of ethosuximide on transmission of repetitive impulses and apparent rates of transmitter turnover in the spinal monosynaptic pathway. *J. Pharmacol. Exp. Ther.* 201:320, 1977.
7. Cereghino, J.J. and Penry, J.K. Testing of antiepileptic drugs in humans: clinical considerations. In: *Antiepileptic Drugs: Mechanisms of Action.* (Woodbury, D.M., Penry, J.K. and Pipperger, C.E., eds.). New York: Raven Press, 1982, p. 141.
8. Chang, T., Dill, W.A. and Glazko, A.J. Ethosuximide: Absorption, distribution and excretion. In: *Antiepileptic Drugs: Mechanism of Action.* (Woodbury, D.M., Penry, J.K. and Schmidt, R.P., eds). New York: Raven Press, 1972, p. 417.
9. Chang, T., Burkett, A.R. andGlazko, A.J. Ethosuximide: Biotransformation. In: *Antiepileptic drugs: Mechanisms of Action.* (Woodbury, D.M., Penry, J.K. and Schmidt, R.P., eds.). New York: Raven Press, 1972, p. 425.
10. Coatsworth, J.J. *Studies on the Clinical Efficacy of Marketed Antiepileptic Drugs.* NINDS monograph no. 12, DHEW publication no. (NIH) 73-51. Washington, D.C.: U.S. Government Printing Office, 1971.
11. Commission on Classification. Proposal for revised clinical and electroencephalographic classification of epileptic seizures. *Epilepsia* 22:489, 1981.
12. Dam, M. Neurologic aspects of toxicity. In: *Antiepileptic Drugs* (Woodbury, D.M., Penry, J.K. and Schmidt, R.P., eds.). New York: Raven Press, 1972, p. 227.
13. Delgado, J.M.R. and Mihailovic, L. Use of intracerebral electrodes to evaluate drugs that act on the central nervous system. *Ann. N.Y. Acad. Sci.* 64:644, 1956.
14. De Lorenzo, R.J. and Freedman, S.D. Possible role of calcium-dependent protein phosphorylation in mediating neurotransmitter release and anticonvulsant action. *Epilepsia* 18:3, 1977.
15. Deupree, J.D. The role or non-role of ATPase activation by phenytoin in the stabilization of excitable membranes. *Epilepsia* 18:309, 1977.
16. Esplin, D.W. Effects of diphenylhydantoin on synaptic transmission in cat spinal cord and stellate ganglia. *J. Pharmacol. Exp. Ther.* 120:301, 1957.
17. Esplin, D.W. and Curto, E.M. Effects on trimethadione on synaptic transmission in the spinal cord: Antagonism between trimethadione and pentylenetetrazol. *J. Pharmacol. Exp. Ther.* 121:457, 1957.
18. Ferrendelli, J.A. and Kinscherf, D.A. Phenytoin: Effects on calcium flux and cyclic nucleotides. *Epilepsia* 18:331, 1977.
19. Ferrendelli, J.A. and Kinscherf, D.A. Similar effects of phenytoin and tetrodotoxin on cyclic nucleotide regulation in depolarized brain tissue. *J. Pharmacol. Exp.Ther.* 207:787, 1978.
20. Gallagher, B.B. and Baumel, I.P. Primidone: Absorption, distribution and excretion. In: *Antiepileptic Drugs: Mechanisms of Action.* (Woodbury, D.M., Penry, J.K. and Schmidt, R.P., eds.). New York: Raven Press, 1972, p. 357.
21. Gastaut, H. Clinical and electroencephalographic classification of epileptic seizures. *Epilepsia* 11:102, 1970.
22. Goldensohn, E.D. The epilepsies. In: *Scientific Approaches to Clinical Neurology.* (Goldensohn, E.S. and Appel, S.H., eds.). Philadelphia: Lea and Febiger, 1977, p. 654.
23. Greenblatt, D.J. and Koch-Weser, J. Adverse reactions to intravenous diazepam: A report from the Boston collaborative drug surveillance program. *Am. J. Med.Sci.* 266:261, 1973.
24. Hasbani, M., Pincus, J.H. and Lee, S.H. Diphenylhydantoin and calcium movement in lobster nerves. *Arch. Neurol.* 31:250, 1974.
25. Hauptmann, A. Luminal bei Epilepsie. *Munchen. Med. Wchnschr.* 2:1907, 1912.
26. HEW (FDA) 77-3040. *General Considerations for the Clinical Evaluation of Drugs.* September, 1977.
27. HEW (FDA) 77-3045. *Guidelines for the Clinical Evaluation of Anticonvulsant Drugs* (Adults and Children). September, 1977.
28. Iadarola, M.J., Raines, A. and Gale, K. Differential effects of n-dipropylacetate and aminooxyacetic acid on gamma-aminobutyric acid levels in discrete areas of rat brain. *J. Neurochem.* 33:1119, 1979.
29. Kapetanovic, I., Kupferberg, H.J., Porter, R.J. and Penry, J.K. Valproic acid-phenobarbital interactions: A systematic study using isotopically labled phenobarbital in an epileptic patient. In: *Proc. of Wodadibot @4 Workshop of the Determination of Antiepileptic Drugs in Body Fluids.* Voksenasen, Norway, June 7-9. New York: Raven Press, 1979.
30. Korey, S.R. Effects of dilantin and mesantoin on the giant axon of the squid. *Proc. Soc. Exp. Biol. Med.* 76:297, 1951.
31. Krall, R.L., Penry, J.K., Kupferberg, H.J. and Swinyard, E.A. Antiepileptic drug development: I. History and a program for progress. *Epilepsia* 19:393, 1978.
32. Krall, R.L., Penry, J.K., White, B.G., Kupferberg, J.H. and Swinyard, E.A. Antiepileptic drug development: II. Anticonvulsant drug screening. *Epilepsia* 19:409, 1978.
33. Krupp, P., Bianchi, C.P. and Syarez-Kurtz, G. On the local anesthetic effect of barbiturates. *J. Pharm. Pharmacol.* 21:763, 1969.

34. Kupferberg, H.J., Lust, W.D., Yonekawa, W., Passonneau, J.V. and Penry, J.K. Effect of phenytoin (diphenylhydantoin) on electrically-induced changes in the brain levels of cyclic nucleotides and GABA. *Fed. Proc.* 35:583, 1976.
35. Kutt, H. Biochemical and genetic factors regulating Dilantin metabolism in man. *Ann. N.Y. Acad.Sci.* 179:704, 1971.
36. Kutt, H. Interactions of antiepileptic drugs. *Epilepsia* 16:393, 1975.
37. Kutt, H., Wold, M.,Scherman, R. and McDowell, F. Insufficient parahydroxylation as a cause of diphenylhydantoin toxicity. *Neurology* (Minneapolis) 14:542, 1964.
38. Kutt, H., Winters, W. and McDowell, F. Inhibition of parahydroxylation of diphenylhydantoin by antituberculosis chemotherapy. *Neurology* (Minneapolis) 16:594, 1966.
39. LaManna, J., Lothman, E., Rosenthal, M., Somjen, G. and Younts, W. Phenytoin: Electric, ionic and metabolic responses in cortex and spinal cord. *Epilepsia* 18:3, 1977.
40. Leal, K.W.,Rapport, R.L.,Wilensky, A.J. and Fried, P.N. Single dose pharmacokinetics and anticonvulsant efficacy of primidone in mice. *Ann. Neurol.* 5:470, 1979.
41. Leppik, I.E., Patrick, B.K. and Cranford, R.E. Treatment of acute seizures and status epilepticus with intravenous phenytoin. *Adv. Neurol.* 34:477, 1983.
42. Levy, L.L. and Fenichel, G.M. Diphenylhydantoin activated seizure. *Neurology* 15:716, 1965.
43. Lipicky, R.J., Gilbert, D.L. and Stillman, I.M. Diphenylhydantoin inhibition of sodium conductance in squid giant axon. *Proc. Natl. Acad.Sci.* 69:1758, 1972.
44. Locock, C. Discussion of a paper by Sieveking. *Lancet* 1:527, 1857.
45. Martin, Ernst, Tozer, T.N., Sheiner, L.B. and Riegelman, S. The clinical pharmacokinetics of phenytoin. *J. Pharmacokinet Biopharmaceut.* 5:579, 1977.
46. Mattson, R.H., Cramer, J.A., Williamson, P.D. and Novelly, R.A. Valproic acid in epilepsy: Clinical and pharmacological effects. *Ann. Neurol.* 3:20, 1978.
47. Mercier, J. Anticonvulsant drugs. In: International Encyclopedia of Pharmacology and Therapeutics. Section 19. Vols. 1 and 2. New York: Pergamon Press, 1973.
48. Merritt, H.H. and Putnam, T.J. A new series of anticonvulsant drugs tested by experiments on animals. *Arch. Neurol. Psychiat.* 39:1003, 1938.
49. Merritt, H.H. and Putnam, T.J. Sodium diphenyl hydantoinate in the treatment of convulsive disorders. *JAMA* 11:1068, 1938.
50. Narahashi, T., Frazier, D.T., Deguchi, T., *et al.* The active form of pentobarbital in giant squid axons. *J. Pharmacol. Exp. Ther.* 177:25, 1971.
51. Neuman, R.S. and Frank, G.B. Effects of diphenylhydantoin and phenobarbital on voltage-clamped myelinated nerve. *Can. J. Physiol. Pharmacol.* 55:42, 1977.
52. Penry, J.K. Usefulness of serum anti-epileptic drug levels in the treatment of epilepsy. In: *Drug Interactions* (Morselli, P.L., *et al.*, eds.). New York: Raven Press, 1974, p. 299.
53. Penry, J.K. and Newmark, M.E. The use of antiepileptic drugs. *Ann. Intern. Med.* 90:207, 1979.
54. Perry, J.G., McKinney, L. and DeWeer, P. Cellular mode of action of the antiepileptic 5, 5-diphenylhydantoin. *Nature* (London) 272:271, 1978.
55. Purpura, D.P., Penry, J.K.,Tower, D.B., *et al. Experimental Models of Epilepsy: A Manual for the Laboratory Worker.* New York: Raven Press, 1972.
56. Raines, A., Blake, G.J.,Richardson, B. and Gilbert, M.B. Differential selectivity of several barbiturates on experimental seizures and neurotoxicity in the mouse. *Epilepsia* 20:105, 1979.
57. Raines, A. and Niner, J.M. Blockade of a sympathetic nervous system reflex by diphenylhydantoin. *Neuropharmacology* 14:61, 1975.
64. Snider, R.S. and del Cerro, M. Proliferating membranes in cerebellum resulting from intoxication. In: *Antiepileptic Drugs: Mechanisms of Action.* (Woodbury, D.M., Penry, J.K. and Schmidt, R.P., eds.). New York: Raven Press, 1972, p. 237.
65. Sohn, R.S. and Ferrendelli, J.A. Anticonvulsant drug mechanisms: Phenytoin, phenobarbital, and ethosuximide and calcium flux in isolated presynaptic endings. *Arch. Neurol.* 33:626, 1976.
66. Su, P.C. and Feldmen, D.S. Motor nerve terminal and muscle membrane stabilization by diphenylhydantoin administration. *Arch. Neurol.* 28:376, 1973.
67. Svensmark, O. and Buchthal, F. Accumulation of phenobarbital in man. *Epilepsia* 4:199, 1963.
68. Swinyard, E.A. Electrically induced convulsions. In: *Experimental Models of Epilepsy* (Purpura, D.P., Penry, J.K.,Tower, D.B., Woodbury, D.M. and Walter, R.D., eds.). New York: Raven Press, 1972, p. 433.
69. Toman, J.E.P. The neuropharmacology of antiepileptics. *EEG Clin. Neurophysiol.* 1::33, 1949.
70. Vastola, E.F. and Rosen, A. Suppression by anticonvulsants of focal electrical seizures in the neocortex. *EEG Clin. Neurophysiol.* 12:327, 1960.
71. Wilder, B.J. Efficacy of phenytoin in treatment of status epilepticus. *Adv. Neurol.* 34:441, 1983.
72. Wilder, B.J.,Ramsay, R.E.,Willmore, L.J., *et al.* Efficacy of intravenous phenytoin in the treatment of status epilepticus: Kinetics of central nervous system penetration. *Ann. Neurol.* 1:511, 1977.
73. Woodbury, D.M. Effect of diphenylhydantoin on electrolytes and radiosodium turnover in brain and other tissues of normal, hyponatremic, and postictal rats. *J. Pharmacol. Exp. Ther.* 115:74, 1955.
74 Woodbury, D.M. Pharmacology and mechanisms of action of antiepileptic drugs. In: *Scientific Approaches to Clinical Neurology*, Vol. 1. Philadelphia:Lea and Febiger, 1977, p. 693.
75. Yaari, Y., Pincus, J.H. and Argov, Z. Phenytoin and transmitter release at the neuromuscular junction of the frog. *Brain Res.* 160:497, 1979.
76. Yonekawa, W., Kupferberg, H.J., Cantor, F. and Dudlley, K. Ethotoin distribution in epileptic patients. *Pharmacologist 17:1975 (Abst. 99).*
58. Raines, A. and Standaert, F.G. Pre- and postjunctional effects of diphenylhydantoin at the cat soleus neuromuscular junction. *J. Pharmacol. Ekxp. Ther.* 153:361, 1966.
59. Reidenberg, M.M., Odar-Cederlof, I., von Bahr, C., Borga, O. and Sjogvist, F. Protein binding of diphenylhydantoin and desmethylimipramine in plasma from patients with poor renal function. *N. Engl. J. Med.* 185:164, 1977.
60. Schobben, F.,Van der Kleijn, E. and Gabreels, F.J.M. Pharmacokinetics of di-n-propylacetate in epileptic patients. *Eur. J. Clin. Pharmacol.* 8:97, 1975.
61. Schwartz, J.R. and Vogel, W. Diphenylhydantoin: Excitability reducing action in single myelinated nerve fibers. *Eur. J. Pharmacol.* 44:241, 1977.
62. Shulman, A. and Laycock, G. Action of central nervous system stimulant and depressant drugs in the intact animal. *Eur. J. Pharmacol.* 2:17, 1967.
63. Seigel, G.J. and Goodwin, B.B. Sodium-potassium-activated adenosine triphosphatase of brain microsome: Modification of sodium inhibition by diphenylhydantoin. *J. Clin. Invest.* 51:1164, 1972.

CHAPTER
11.5

PSYCHIATRIC DISORDERS: INTRODUCTION

Herbert Y. Meltzer and Paul M. Schyve

PSYCHIATRIC DISORDERS

Psychiatric disorders have traditionally been divided along the two axes. First, disorders have been classified as organic or nonorganic (functional). *Organic disorders* are those with a known or presumed physical etiology, such as delirium, dementia, and alcohol intoxication or withdrawal. *Functional disorders* are those that traditionally have been thought to have a psychological, rather than biological etiology. Recent advances in biological psychiatry suggest that disorders traditionally considered functional, such as schizophrenia and affective disorders (mania, depression), have biological etiologies (2, 8, 11). Both biological and psychological interventions may be appropriate in organic disorders (e.g., delirium and dementia) and in functional disorders (e.g., schizophrenia and obsessive-compulsive disorder).

The second major axis along which psychiatric disorders have been distributed is that of personality disorder, neurosis, and psychosis. The techniques regularly utilized by an individual to cope with the challenges of living are called *personality traits.* For example, those with a compulsive personality trait tend to approach problems by careful analysis and avoidance of emotionality. When this style fails or is inappropriate, the individual is usually able to shift to alternative methods of problem solving. A *personality disorder* refers to a personality trait in which this flexibility is lost. In the compulsive personality disorder, for example, restricted ability to express emotion, obstinacy, indecisiveness, and perfectionism may pervade almost all aspects of life. Personality traits usually are present throughout life. Personality disorders may develop out of personality traits and are rarely responsive to drug therapy.

The *neuroses* are characterized by the presence of specific psychological symptoms of which the patient is acutely aware and of which he or she complains. Neuroses are usually not lifelong but are characterized by episodes or exacerbations with acute symptomatology. Unlike the inflexible traits found in the personality disorder, neurotic symptoms are painful and useless but irresistible. The patient with an obsessive-compulsive neurosis, for example, may find, to his consternation, that the same thoughts keep repeating themselves in his head, despite their uselessness, their interference with his thinking about other things, and his desire to stop them. The neurotic person, however, does not lose touch with the reality of the world around him. Neurotic disorders include cyclothymic, dysthymic, phobic, anxiety, somatoform, dissociative, and psychosexual disorders.

In *psychosis,* the connection with the real world is impaired. By their very presence, certain symptoms are indicative of a loss of the ability to adequately test reality. Hallucinations in which nonexistent stimuli are perceived as coming from the external world, delusions in which incorrigible false beliefs (not supported by a social or religious subculture) are held, disorders of thought in which clear and logical thinking are significantly impaired, and disorders of movement, such as catatonia, in which the physical activity of the patient demonstrates no relationship to the external world, all either demonstrate a loss of touch with reality or make reality testing impossible. The presence of any of these symptoms justifies the label of psychosis. The adjective *psychotic* may be used with regard to symptoms, people, and disorders.

The utility of somatic treatments for mental disorders is related to their position along this axis of severity. There is little indication for somatic treatments in the personality disorders. Selected neurotic disorders respond, at least in part, to antianxiety and antidepressant drugs. Most psychotic disorders are treated by somatic therapies: antipsychotic, antimanic, and antidepressant drugs or electroconvulsive therapy (ECT).

SYNDROMES OF PSYCHIATRIC DISORDER

The following descriptions of psychiatric disorders utilize the classifications and criteria of the *Diagnostic and Statistical Manual of Mental Disorders,* third edition (DSM-III) (7) developed by the American Psychiatric Association and, in keeping with the purpose of this textbook, emphasize those disorders in which pharmacotherapy has been found to be of use.

DISORDERS USUALLY FIRST EVIDENT IN INFANCY, CHILDHOOD, OR ADOLESCENCE

Disorders usually first evident in infancy, childhood, or adolescence include *mental retardation,* which is characterized by significantly subaverage general intellectual functioning (Wechsler IQ below 70), with an onset prior to age 18, accompanied by deficits in adaptive behavior. About one-quarter of the patients have known biological (e.g., chromosomal) abnormalities, but the specific cause in the other three-quarters of patients is not known. Especially in the severe and profound subtypes, these patients may demonstrate aggressive behavior toward themselves or others that may be reduced by antipsychotic medication.

Attention deficit disorder is characterized by developmentally inappropriate short attention and impulsivity beginning before age 7, and it may be accompanied by hyperactivity. It is sometimes accompanied by "soft" neurological signs, learning disabilities, motor and/or perceptual dysfunction, and EEG abnormalities. Treatment has included the use of antipsychotics, sedatives, and stimulants; the use of methylphenidate, a stimulant, in children with hyperactivity is generally recognized as helpful (13).

Stereotyped movement disorders are conditions in which there are abnormal gross motor movements. *Tic disorders* are characterized by recurrent, involuntary, repetitive, purposeless motor movements, often increased by anxiety. *Tourette's disorder* is characterized by tics and includes multiple vocal *tics* of complicated sounds, words, or obscenities. Tourette's disorder is usually lifelong, three times more common in boys than in girls, and often accompanied by nonspecific EEG abnormalities, hyperactivity, or soft neurological signs (17). Its symptoms often lead to significant social and occupational impairment. Haloperidol has been used successfully in the treatment of tics, particularly some cases of Tourette's disorder (17). Other medications, including low doses of dopamine agonists such as bromocriptine or apomorphine, are under investigation (9).

Pervasive developmental disorders are characterized by abnormalities in psychological functions necessary for the development of social skills and language. The abnormalities are severe and, in contrast to children with specific developmental disorders, are not normal for any stage of development, even an earlier one. *Infantile autism* is a syndrome developing within the first 30 months of life, characterized by a lack of responsiveness to and lack of interest in people, associated with failure to develop normal attachment behavior. Language may be absent and, if present, contains abnormal patterns such as echolalia. The child exhibits bizarre responses to the environment (e.g., ritualistic behavior), abnormality in mood, abnormal responsiveness to stimuli, or abnormal body movements (e.g., rocking).

Childhood-onset pervasive developmental disorder is a syndrome that develops between 30 months and 12 years of age. The patient demonstrates severely impaired emotional speech. In all types of pervasive developmental disorder, antipsychotics may be used to treat primary school-age children and are particularly helpful in reducing anxiety and decreasing disorganized thought processes (4). Enuresis that is abnormal for the age of the individual has frequently been improved by the administration of the tricyclic antidepressant imipramine, whose efficacy is postulated to be related to its effect on the developmental delay of the nervous system believed to be a predisposing factor (1).

ORGANIC MENTAL DISORDERS

The organic mental disorders include the *senile and presenile dementias* (differentiated by age of onset after or before age 65, respectively) and *substance-use disorders* (intoxication, withdrawal delirium, dementia, amnestic disorder, delusional disorder, hallucinosis, affective disorder, personality disorder, or atypical or mixed disorder). The senile and presenile dementias are characterized by gross and microscopic pathological changes in the brain, and the substance-use organic mental disorders are related to the causative agent, such as alcohol, barbiturates, amphetamines, or hallucinogens.

SCHIZOPHRENIC DISORDERS

The schizophrenic disorders are illnesses manifested by delusions and hallucinations in a clear sensorium, and often by incoherent or illogical speech, loosening of associations, marked poverty of content of speech, blunted, flat, or inappropriate affect, and odd (catatonic) or grossly disorganized behavior. Signs of the illness must last continuously for at least 6 months at some time during the person's life; during the active phase of the illness, the symptoms must be associated with significant impairment in two or more areas of routine daily functioning. The illness must have an onset before age 45 and not be attributable to any organic mental disorder or to mental retardation. Schizophrenia occurs in about 1% of the population, is equally common in males and females, and is most frequently found in the lower socioeconomic classes, although this probably results from a downward drift of the individual who develops schizophrenia. The likelihood of hereditary predisposition to schizophrenia is high, although it also appears that environment plays a role in its manifestation.

It is likely that the schizophrenic syndrome has multiple etiologies, i.e., it is a syndrome that is the manifestation of multiple diseases (20). A common pathway in either the pathophysiology or in the psychopathology of many of the diseases may account for the success of biological or psychological interventions, respectively, in more than one disease manifested by the schizophrenic syndrome. For example, antipsychotic drugs, which block dopamine receptors, may be efficacious in a number of diseases in which a step in the pathophysiology is excessive dopaminergic activity in a particular area of the brain. This efficacy would be observed even if different diseases involved different areas of the brain, or involved different etiologies for the dopaminergic overactivity, such as excessive presynaptic production of dopamine, decreased reuptake of dopamine, dopamine postsynaptic receptor supersensitivity, autoreceptor subsensitivity, or other abnormalities in the dopamine system because of decreased or increased trace metals or vitamin deficiencies.

PARANOID DISORDERS

The paranoid disorders are a group characterized primarily by persistent persecutory delusions or delusions of jealousy, in the absence of the characteristic schizophrenic symptoms, such as bizarre delusions, or of a full depressive or manic syndrome. Persecutory delusions may be very simple or complex, but usually involve a single theme or series of connected themes and are often associated with an exaggeration of small slights, anger or resentment, seclusiveness, and eccentric behavior. Because of the absence of disorganization in the patient's mental functioning, daily and occupational activities may be performed rather well, although social and marital relationships are impaired. The paranoid disorders (paranoia and shared, acute, or atypical paranoid disorders) are usually treated with antipsychotic medications.

PSYCHOTIC DISORDERS NOT ELSEWHERE CLASSIFIED

Psychotic disorders not elsewhere classified are characterized by at least one of the following psychotic symptoms: delusions, hallucinations, incoherence, loosening of associations, marked poverty of content of thought, marked illogicality, or behavior that is grossly disorganized or catatonic. In *schizophreniform disorder,* the clinical picture is similar to that of schizophrenia, except that the total duration of illness is less than 6 months. A *brief reactive psychosis* is characterized by a psychotic symptom(s) lasting at least a few hours but no more than 1 week and precipitated by an obviously significant stress, such as death of a loved one or combat. Although there may be subsequent temporary mild depression, a full return to the premorbid level of adjustment is expected. As with other psychotic syndromes, the foregoing are typically treated with antipsychotic medication.

AFFECTIVE DISORDERS

Affective disorders are characterized primarily by an abnormality of mood, which may be elevated, depressed, or alternating between these two poles. One or more episodes of depression with no episodes of elevated mood (mania) is called *unipolar disorder,* and one or more episodes of mania, with or without depressive episodes, is called *bipolar disorder.* An affective disorder that arises in an individual with no previous history of psychiatric disorder other than mania or depression is called *primary,* whereas that which arises in an individual with a preexisting nonaffective psychiatric illness is called *secondary.* No differences in signs and symptoms have been shown between primary and secondary disorders, but the course, prognosis, and family history of these patients may differ (10).

Depression may be a normal state of mood, a symptom that can occur in many illnesses, or a diagnostic category. The latter, called *major depression* in the DSM-III, is characterized by dysphoric mood (depressed, sad, hopeless, irritable, worried) or loss of interest or pleasure in all or most usual activities. Associated symptoms, of which four must be present to make the diagnosis, include: increased or decreased appetite or increased or decreased weight; increased or decreased sleep; loss of energy or tiredness; psychomotor agitation or retardation; loss of interest or pleasure in activities or decreased libido; feelings of self-blame or inappropriate guilt; decreased concentrations; and suicidal ideation or suicidal attempt. A controversial distinction has been made between those depressions thought to stem from environmental and psychological causes, and those depressions thought to arise independently of the environment, usually from a biological etiology. The first group has been called reactive, neurotic, exogenous, or minor, and the second group has been called endogenous, psychotic, biological, and vegetative. The latter group is characterized by a lack of reactivity to environmental changes, severe guilt, often a distinct quality to the depressed mood, and so-called vegetative signs such as decreased libido, diurnal mood variation (mood is regularly worse in the morning than in the evening), early morning awakening, psychomotor retardation or agitation, and anorexia accompanied by weight loss. There is some evidence that depressed patients with endogenous, or especially vegetative, features are more responsive to antidepressant medications than are patients without such features, but this is far from being a universal rule. The risk of suicide must be carefully evaluated in all patients with a depressive illness, and because suicidal risk is usually transient, it is of utmost importance to take whatever steps are necessary, including involuntary hospitalization, to protect the patient from self-harm until the risk of suicide has diminished.

In addition to major depression, the classification of major affective disorders also includes bipolar disorder, which is distinguished by episodes of *mania.* A distinction is made between bipolar patients who have fully developed manic episodes (referred to as *bipolar I*) and patients who only become hypomanic *(bipolar II).* A manic episode is characterized by prominent and persistent elevated, expansive, or irritable mood, often accompanied by increased activity, talkativeness, racing thoughts, grandiosity, distractibility, and decreased need for sleep. *Hypomania* is characterized by mild-to-moderate increases in motoric rate and elevated mood, without delusions or hallucinations. Unlike patients with depression, who frequently complain about their feelings and may believe there is something wrong with their mind, the grandiosity in mania often leads the patient to insist that he is not only well, but better than usual for himself, and better than other people. The patient with manic episodes may also experience episodes of depression, which are similar to the depression of a unipolar major depression, although more likely to be characterized by psychomotor retardation and hypersomnia. Lithium carbonate is efficacious in the treatment of acute mania and may be prophylactic for recurrent manic and depressed episodes in bipolar disorders.

ANXIETY DISORDERS

Anxiety disorders are illnesses in which anxiety is the most prominent symptom, or is experienced if the individual resists giving in to his or her symptoms. Anxiety is a feeling of fear that lacks an appropriate stimulus or is grossly out of proportion to the stimulus. Because anxiety occurs in many other disorders, such other disorders must be ruled out before the diagnosis of anxiety disorder is made. *Phobic disorders* are characterized by repeated avoidance or desire to avoid a specific object or situation because of irrational fears, which the patient recognizes as unreasonable. Agoraphobia (fear of being alone), social phobia (fear of a specific social situation), and simple phobia (fear of a specific object or situation) may lead to serious impairment, depending upon the characteristics of the phobic object or situation. Although phobias have been traditionally treated by psychotherapy or behavioral techniques, recent studies have suggested they may respond to tricyclic antidepressants or monoamine oxidase inhibitors (23, 30).

Panic disorder, a type of anxiety disorder, is characterized by unexplainable attacks of severe anxiety accompanied by autonomic symptoms such as dyspnea, palpitations, chest pain, choking, dizziness, vertigo, sweating, and trembling. Although usually recurrent and episodic, it occasionally becomes chronic and may lead to agoraphobia. Panic disorder has been reported to be responsive to β-adrenergic blockers such as propranolol (27). Recent studies suggest alprazolam may be useful in panic disorder. *Generalized anxiety disorder* is chronic generalized anxiety in the absence of phobic, panic, or obsessive-compulsive disorder. Although rarely incapacitating, it may lead to mild impairment, and self-medication with alcohol or drugs is common. The antianxiety agents, such as the benzodiazepines, are probably the medications of choice in this syndrome. *Obsessive-compulsive disorder* is characterized by obsessions (recurrent, persistent thoughts or impulses not experienced as voluntarily produced) or compulsions (behaviors that the patient feels driven to perform). The patient desires to resist the obsessions or compulsions, and recognizes their irrationality. Attempts to resist a compulsion lead to increasing anxiety that can be relieved by performing the behavior. Chlorimipramine, a new tricyclic antidepressant not available in the United States, has reportedly been effective in some cases of obsessive-compulsive disorder (32). Other drugs which potentiate serotonin via reuptake blockade may also be effective, e.g., zimeldine and fluoxetine.

BIOLOGICAL BASIS OF PSYCHIATRIC DISORDERS

The ability of drugs to induce or diminish psychopathology in humans provides some of the most important clues to the nature of the biological abnormalities that underlie the major psychiatric disorders (schizophrenia, paranoia, and the affective disorders). The major psychiatric disorders are partially genetically determined, as evidenced by a multitude of well-controlled twin and family studies, as well as adoption studies in which infants have been either adopted away from mentally ill parents or into families with one or more such parents (13). Such studies have demonstrated that there is a heritable vulnerability to develop schizophrenia or the affective disorders, but environmental factors are critical in determining the onset and course of the illnesses. There is a strong presumption that polygenic inheritance rather than single genes are involved in the schizophrenic and affective disorders. However, there is some evidence for X-linked inheritance in a small number of cohorts of bipolar affective disorders. Further studies of linkage of known genetic markers to the psychoses with larger, better-defined samples are needed.

The biological factors that contribute to the etiology of schizophrenia and the affective disorders have not been elucidated, although a number of cogent hypotheses have been developed, as shall be reviewed shortly. Only limited progress has been achieved because of the enormous complexity of the brain, the difficulty of studying the brain directly in humans, the empirical basis of available diagnostic systems, the high probability that each of the major mental illnesses is not a single disorder [i.e., there is considerable heterogeneity in schizophrenia and the affective disorders (11)], problems in applying diagnostic criteria in a reliable manner, patient cooperation in clinical research, and contamination of clinical studies by prior drug treatment. There is a wide range of phenotypes within the major mental illnesses, especially schizophrenia. Each phenotype (e.g., for schizophrenia: paranoid undifferentiated, chronic deteriorating, acute recurrent, etc.) may result from unique biological factors, from shared biological factors, or from a mixture of common and unique abnormalities. The same is true for the various forms of affective disorders.

These problems have impeded but not entirely blocked progress in our understanding of the causes of the mental illnesses. The psychotropic drugs whose use is discussed in the ensuing chapters have been enormously valuable tools in the study of the pathophysiology of schizophrenia and the affective and anxiety disorders. Through studies of the mechanism of their effects, important advances have been made in our knowledge of the basic chemistry and physiology of the brain. This chapter will briefly discuss some of the major theories of the etiology of schizophrenia and the affective disorders.

SCHIZOPHRENIA

DOPAMINE HYPOTHESIS

The major current hypothesis of the etiology of schizophrenia is that it is due to increased dopaminergic activity in the mesolimbic or mesocortical dopaminergic pathways (5, 22). However, the direct evidence in support of this hypothesis is quite sparse. Most, but not all, postmortem studies of brains from schizophrenics and controls have shown increased numbers of dopamine (DA) receptors in the caudate nucleus and the nucleus accumbens of chronic schizophrenic patients (16). However, this may be the result of neuroleptic treatment rather than a cause of the illness. Increased receptors in both the nucleus accumbens and the caudate nucleus indicate that both major dopaminergic systems, the limbic and the nigrostriatal, respectively, are involved in schizophrenia or that the increased number of receptor sites is indeed due to prior drug treatment. Increased levels of DA have also been found in the brains of schizophrenics. This could be an indication of increased synthesis or decreased turnover of DA in the brain. Administration of amphetamine to rats on a chronic basis leads to decreased numbers of ^{3}H-spiroperidol binding sites in both the caudate and nucleus accumbens, presumably due to enhanced release of DA by this drug and subsequent down-regulation of receptor sensitivity. There is no suggestion of such a decrease in the postmortem studies of schizophrenic brains, which argues against continued excessive release of DA in schizophrenics. Because postmortem studies have so many potential sources of error, the studies of DA levels and receptor number have not provided strong support for the DA hypothesis of schizophrenia as classically stated.

Studies of the levels or rate of formation of the DA metabolite homovanillic acid (HVA) in the cerebrospinal fluid (CSF) provide no evidence for enhanced DA turnover in schizophrenia (2). Serum prolactin levels provide a measure of the activity of the tuberoinfundibular DA neurons; prolactin levels are normal in most schizophrenics.

Indirect support for the role of DA in schizophrenia comes from the studies of central nervous system stimulants such as amphetamine and phencyclidine (PCP), which are indirect DA agonists. A major component of the action of these drugs is release of DA and blockade of its uptake. Low doses of these agents can exacerbate psychotic symptoms in schizophrenics as well as cause psychoses in vulnerable individuals, and, if given for a prolonged period, at high doses and under stressful conditions, could probably induce psychoses in anyone. Neuroleptic drugs can diminish or block these psychoses.

The ability of neuroleptic drugs to diminish delusions and hallucinations and reduce thought disorder in schizophrenia, as well as in PCP-induced and amphetamine-induced psychoses, is proportional to their ability to inhibit the specific binding of ^{3}H-neuroleptics to DA receptors in the limbic system and striatum (22). These drugs also inhibit a DA-stimulated adenylate cyclase and various receptors of neurotransmitters such as histamine, norepinephrine, and serotonin. However, only the inhibitory effect on ^{3}H-neuroleptic binding correlates with antipsychotic potency.

Chronic administration of neuroleptic agents may lead to supersensitivity of DA receptors as evidenced by shifts in the behavioral, biochemical, and electrophysiological responses to DA agonists in animals treated with such agents. Supersensitivity of striatal DA receptors may be a factor in the development of tardive dyskinesia, a movement disorder involving the tongue, lips and facial musculature, which usually begins after several years of neuroleptic treatment (14). High dosage, female sex, and old age enhance the chances of developing this disorder.

Further support for the importance of DA in psychosis comes from studies of the synergistic antipsychotic action of α-methylparatyrosine (AMPT) and neuroleptics. AMPT is an inhibitor of tyrosine hydroxylase, the rate-limiting enzyme in DA synthesis. Combined inhibition of DA synthesis and DA receptor blockade leads to successful treatment of some schizophrenics who do not respond to neuroleptics alone.

The available pharmacological evidence suggests that reduction of dopaminergic activity is useful in the treatment of acute mania and psychotic (delusional) depression as well as acute exacerbations of schizophrenia. Indeed, the schizophrenic symptomatology sometimes referred to as *process schizophrenia* or the defect state (i.e., anergia, loss of volition, flat affect, impoverished speech and anhedonia) does not appear to respond as well to neuroleptic treatment as do symptoms such as hallucinations, delusions and catatonia. The latter are referred to as positive symptoms. They are also present in some manics and depressed patients. Neuroleptics are as useful in diminishing positive symptoms in these patients as in schizophrenia. Therefore, DA appears to be significant not as a unique feature of schizophrenia but for positive symptoms common to the major psychoses. The fact that reduction of dopaminergic activity is clinically useful does not allow one to conclude that there is an absolute increase in dopaminergic activity in such patients. It may be that reduction of dopaminergic activity restores the balance among neurotransmitters in the brain.

OTHER NEUROTRANSMITTERS OR NEUROMODULATORS IMPLICATED

There is some evidence for primary roles of serotonin (5-HT), norepinephrine (NE), γ-aminobutyric acid (GABA), histamine, prostaglandins, phenethylamine, and β-endorphin in schizophrenia (17). We have reviewed this in detail elsewhere (12). The most salient findings are of elevated levels of the indole hallucinogen N,N-dimethyltryptamine in the urine or blood of schizophrenics, increased NE in the brain and CSF of schizophrenics, increased GABA in CSF, abnormal responses to injected histamine, elevated CSF prostaglandins, increased urinary phenethylamine, increased plasma and CSF β-endorphin, and clinical improvement of chronic auditory hallucinations with naloxone, an antagonist of the endogenous opiates (31). The probable heterogeneity of schizophrenia makes it difficult to test these theories definitively. Assuming that the chemical determinations and clinical reports are reliable, it is possible that some schizophrenic individuals are deviant in their characteristics but that group differences do not exist.

OTHER POTENTIAL BIOLOGICAL BASES

There has been considerable attention given to the possibility that schizophrenia might be a consequence of *viral infections*, either slow viruses or acute viral infections. Herpes simplex infections of the CNS have been associated with schizophreniform psychopathology, and various studies have reported increased levels of viral antibodies in populations of schizophrenic patients (18). Viruslike agents have been reported to be present in the brains of some deceased schizophrenic patients, but the problem of postmortem contamination makes such results in need of further verification.

There is evidence from studies of *brain blood flow* with radioactive xenon and brain metabolic activity using ^{18}F-deoxyglucose and positron emission tomography that the frontal lobes of chronic schizophrenics have decreased blood flow and metabolic activity compared with normal controls and patients with affective disorders (12). These studies are only in their preliminary stages but show promise as examples of techniques that will permit noninvasive studies of small brain regions in schizophrenic patients. Decreased frontal lobe metabolic activity is attractive as a basis for the biology of schizophrenia because of the important role this area has in personality, memory, logical thinking and cognitive processing.

Schizophrenics have been reported to have abnormal ventricles and asymmetries on computed axial tomography (CAT) scans. These reports need independent confirmation with better quantification of the scans. Such abnormalities may also be present in manic-depressive patients as well as schizophrenics. Abnormalities of the cerebellum have been reported in schizophrenic brains in various CAT scan studies and one postmortem study.

There are numerous reports of decreased platelet monoamine oxidase (MAO) activity in schizophrenia (21). However, these studies appear to be contaminated by the effects of chronic neuroleptic treatment, which has now been shown to inhibit MAO activity. Brain MAO activity is not reduced in schizophrenics.

Schizophrenic patients, as well as patients with other affective psychoses, have various neuromuscular abnormalities (19, 20). During a period of acute psychotic symptoms, many psychotic patients have increased serum creatine phosphokinase (CPK), aldolase, and pyruvate kinase activity. Isoenzyme studies have established that the origin of these enzymes is skeletal muscle. These increases do not appear to be due to the effect of drugs, hyperactivity, stress, or trauma but may reflect underlying muscle abnormalities and disruption of the central nervous system regulation of the neuroleptic and endocrine influence on muscle membrane permeability. Morphological studies of skeletal muscle have found increased numbers of atrophic muscle fibers as well as more selective changes in muscle fiber architecture. Paranoid schizophrenic patients also have increased branching of subterminal motor nerves. Electrophysiological studies have demonstrated increased motor unit territory in schizophrenics and an abnormality of the H-reflex recovery curve. The latter, the electrically-evoked monosynaptic spinal cord reflex, is sensitive to CNS dopaminergic influences. The increase in the secondary facilitation component of the H-reflex recovery curve, which is present in some patients irrespective of the type of major psychoses, is compatible with increased dopaminergic activity.

CONCLUSIONS

At present, we cannot precisely identify which regions of the brain are abnormal in schizophrenia or how they become abnormal, reversibly or irreversibly. We do not know whether neuroleptic agents alter the long-term course of the illness. Nevertheless, pharmacological treatment of schizophrenia has proven to be the most effective means of treating this protean disorder, as will be discussed in Chapter 11.5.1.

AFFECTIVE DISORDERS

BIOGENIC AMINE HYPOTHESIS

The *biogenic amine* hypothesis of depression proposes that depression is due to a relative decrease in the amount of NE (26), DA (25), or 5-HT (24), or a relative excess of acetylcholine (ACh) in critical areas of the brain that regulate mood, motor activity, and vegetative functions. Mania is believed to be associated with opposite changes in the activity of these neuronal systems, especially NE and ACh, although one theory proposes that decreased 5-HT activity may be essential but not sufficient for both mania and depression. The original basis for this hypothesis was the pharmacological evidence that reserpine, which depletes central nervous system (CNS) catecholamines and 5-HT, precipitated depressive episodes in about 15% of the patients who received this drug for the treatment of hypertension, whereas monoamine oxidase inhibitors, the first effective antidepressant drugs, increased brain NE, DA and 5-HT. Subsequent studies demonstrated that, at least acutely, the tricyclic antidepressants such as imipramine and amitriptyline could potentiate the activity of brain NE or 5-HT by inhibiting their uptake into presynaptic neurons, the principal means of their inactivation.

The direct evidence to support the monoamine hypothesis is relatively slim. Thus, the levels of the major metabolite of NE, 3-methoxy-4-hydroxyphenylglycol (MHPG), in the urine of bipolar depressed patients have been found to be reduced in a number of studies, although not all data are consistent with this (18). This is believed to reflect reduced central noradrenergic activity, although the proportion of MHPG in urine that is of central origin is still in dispute. Urinary MHPG output may reflect secondary phenomena such as anxiety, decreased blood pressure, and decreased locomotor activity. Patients with decreased urinary MHPG levels are reported to respond better to imipramine than to amitriptyline. Conversely, the response to amitriptyline has been reported to be better in patients with higher urinary MHPG levels. Attempts to treat depression by administration of the NE precursor, L-DOPA, have been unsuccessful, possibly because insufficient increases in brain NE occur after L-DOPA administration.

There are other studies reporting abnormalities related to catecholamines in the peripheral tissues of depressed patients. Dopamine-β-hydroxylase (DBH), the enzyme involved in the conversion of DA to NE, has been found to be decreased in the plasma of patients with psychotic depression and increased in nonpsychotically depressed patients. There is no evidence that these peripheral differences are reflected by central differences. Erythrocyte catechol-o-methyl transferase activity has been reported to be increased in patients with affective disorders and some of their first-degree relatives, but this has not been confirmed. CSF epinephrine has been reported to be decreased in depressed patients and to increase to normal levels after treatment.

The direct evidence for an abnormality of DA in depression is even less compelling than for NE. Thus, there is minimal evidence that homovanillic acid (HVA) or its rate of production is decreased in the CSF of depressed patients or increased in manic patients. Postmortem studies of suicidal depressed patients have found normal activity of tyrosine hydroxylase, the rate-limiting enzyme in the synthesis of dopamine. One of the new antidepressant drugs, bupropion, has been shown to enhance dopamine release, without any effect on 5-HT or NE synthesis, release, uptake, or catabolism, suggesting that increasing dopaminergic activity may have an antidepressant effect in humans. The synergistic action of dopamine receptor blockers, such as chlorpromazine, and tricyclic antidepressants in the treatment of psychotic depression is well established, suggesting that impaired dopaminergic neurotransmission does not preclude an antidepressant action. AMPT, the inhibitor of DA and NE synthesis, has some antimanic effects but does not induce depression in treated depressed patients. Apomorphine, a direct-acting dopamine agonist, can induce depressive symptoms, and the magnitude of the growth hormone (GH) response to apomorphine in psychotic patients has been reported to be correlated with the degree of depressive symptoms. However, bromocriptine, another dopamine agonist, may have some antidepressant effects. Thus, there is no single coherent model that can encompass these findings.

There is more direct evidence for an abnormality of 5-HT in depression than for any other neurotransmitter. Thus, depressed patients, especially those with histories of nearly successful suicide attempts, have been reported to have decreased levels of 5-hydroxyindoleacetic acid (5-HIAA), the major metabolite of 5-HT, in the CSF. Decreased levels of 5-HT and 5-HIAA have also been found in the brains of suicidal depressed patients. The uptake of 5-HT in the blood platelets of depressed patients has been found to be decreased in bipolar and unipolar depressed patients. Some of the newer antidepressant drugs such as fluoxetine and zimelidine have been shown to have relatively specific inhibitory effects on the uptake of 5-HT by neurons. There are numerous studies, some of which have been well controlled, showing that the precursors of 5-HT, tryptophan and 5-hydroxytryptophan, have antidepressant effects in their own right and, when administered together with MAO inhibitors or 5-HT uptake blockers, potentiate the antidepressant effects of these agents. There is some evidence that these treatments are particularly effective in patients who have low 5-HIAA in the CSF. Parachlorophenylalanine (PCPA), an inhibitor of 5-HT synthesis, has been reported to cause a recurrence of depressive symptomatology in recovered depressed patients. Although these studies would suggest decreased 5-HT is a factor in depression, it has also been hypothesized that increased serotonergic activity may be an etiological factor in depression. There is unequivocal evidence that some antidepressant drugs (e.g., amitriptyline, trazadone and mianserin) may block some 5-HT receptors.

There have been some attempts made to divide depressions into those due to catecholamine, principally NE, deficiencies and those due to 5-HT deficiencies. It has been argued that imipramine and its metabolites have a relatively specific capacity to inhibit the uptake of NE, whereas amitriptyline and its metabolites have a relatively specific effect upon 5-HT uptake. There is some clinical evidence that depressed patients who do not respond to imipramine will respond to amitriptyline and vice versa. The major problems with this proposal are that blockade of amine uptake is probably not the mechanism by which these antidepressants work; modification of receptor sensitivity, which both these drugs produce to an equivalent extent, appears to be more important. Second, under physiological conditions both imipramine and amitriptyline appear to block both NE and 5-HT uptake either directly or through their metabolites and so are not selective for either neurotransmitter. Third, drugs such as zimelidine, fluoxetine, and their metabolites, which appear to have no direct effect upon NE uptake compared with their potent, selective 5-HT uptake blockade, are as effective in unselected populations of depressed patients who did not respond to 5-HT uptake blockade. It would be expected that these agents would not be as effective as the standard tricyclics, imipramine and amitriptyline. The argument is based upon the well-founded assumption that all these drugs are effective antidepressants in 70-90% of depressed patients.

There is minimal direct evidence to support the hypothesis of increased cholinergic activity in depression. Erythrocyte acetylcholinesterase (AChE) activity has been reported to be decreased in euthymic manic-depressive patients, but CSF AChE is normal in depressed patients. Administration of physostigmine, an inhibitor of cholinesterase, has been reported to produce depressive symptoms in manic patients and normal controls. Many of the tricyclic antidepressant drugs have potent anticholinergic properties. It has been proposed that the anticholinergic effects of these agents contribute to their antidepressant properties. Amitriptyline and doxepin have particularly potent anticholinergic effects, imipramine and protriptyline are intermediate, and nortriptyline and desipramine have the least anticholinergic effect.

In recent years, there has been extensive investigation of the effects of chronic treatment (2 or more weeks) with tricyclic antidepressants, MAO inhibitors, or repeated electroconvulsive shock treatments on receptor sensitivity in rat brain and peripheral tissues. Thus, decreased β-adrenergic receptor (or β-adrenoceptor) sensitivity, decreased α_2-adrenoceptor sensitivity, subsensitivity of presynaptic DA receptors, and subsensitivity of postsynaptic 5-HT receptors have been reported following chronic administration of the antidepressant treatments. In general, these results have been demonstrated for all classes of antidepressant drugs, even those that do not block reuptake, such as trazodone, mianserin, iprindole, and doxepin. Fluoxetine does not produce β-adrenoceptors sensitivity, but it is not yet entirely clear how effective it is as an antidepressant. Decreased α_2-adrenoceptor sensitivity is believed to lead to increased release of NE and cause the subsensitivity of postsynaptic β-adrenoceptors as a consequence of increased NE release. The time-course of these effects is consistent with the delayed efficacy of the antidepressant treatments, but there is as yet no definitive evidence linking these changes to antidepressant action in humans. Recent studies have explored the possibility of using α_2-adrenoceptors on blood platelets, β-adrenoceptors on lymphocytes, and the neuroendocrine response to the α_2-receptor agonist, clonidine, as a means of demonstrating changes in receptor sensitivity in depressed patients before and after antidepressant treatment.

The study of the metabolites of catecholamines and indolamines in mania has not been as informative as in depression. MHPG levels in urine appear to be higher just prior to a manic episode than during a depression, but the levels in manic patients are not elevated in comparison with normals. CSF MHPG levels are also not elevated in manic patients. CSF 5-HIAA levels have been reported to be normal or decreased in manic patients.

Lithium has significant effects on brain 5-HT, NE, and DA turnover. It also increases 5-HT and blocks the neuroleptic-induced increase in DA receptor sensitivity as indicated by biochemical, behavioral, and electrophysiological measures. The importance of these effects for clinical efficacy in mania is unknown.

There is as yet no consensus on any single monoamine as a key factor in depression. Because the majority of nonpsychotic depressed patients respond to whatever antidepressant is given to them, and indeed, frequently spontaneously remit, it is difficult to utilize the relatively selective NE or 5-HT uptake blockers or DA releasers to determine which neurotransmitters are involved in depression. Drugs with selectivity for down-regulating β-, α_2-, adrenoceptor and 5-HT receptors would be needed to determine which, if any, of these effects might be critical to their antidepressant action.

NEUROENDOCRINE ABNORMALITIES

Numerous studies have been made of cortisol, thyrotropin-releasing hormone (TRH), prolactin, GH, and gonadotropin secretion in depressed patients. There is abundant evidence of increased adrenal corticoid secretion in depressed patients. Increased serum cortisol, 24-hour urinary-free cortisol, and increased numbers of cortisol secretory episodes have been reported. Recently, the dexamethasone suppression test has been reported to be abnormal in 40-50% of patients with major depression (6). The specificity of the test for major depressive illness has been reported to be as high as 97%, but this claim needs independent verification. The cause of the increased adrenal corticoid secretion is not elevated adrenocorticotropic hormone (ACTH) levels, as a number of studies have found ACTH levels are normal in depressed patients.

The thyroid-stimulating hormone (TSH) response to i.v. TRH, 500 μg, is blunted in about 25% of depressed patients. It is also blunted in alcoholics. Some authors propose only bipolar depressed patients have blunted TRH responses. Available evidence indicates that the depressed patients with blunted TRH responses are not the same ones who fail to suppress cortisol after dexamethasone. Basal serum prolactin levels are normal or slightly increased in depressed patients.

Plasma melatonin levels have been reported to be increased in some manic patients and to undergo a phase reversal in some (daytime elevation and nighttime decrease). Elevated melatonin could reflect increased β-adrenergic influence on the pineal during mania. The disturbance of melatonin diurnal rhythm may be another example of the disturbance of circadian cycle regulation in mania.

SLEEP AND DEPRESSION

The sleep of patients with primary depression is characterized by sleep discontinuity, namely, frequent awakenings, sleep reduction, and shortened rapid eye movement (REM) latency (i.e., the time from sleep onset to the first REM period) (15). There is some evidence that this sleep abnormality persists after recovery. These changes are somewhat more prominent in bipolar than unipolar patients.

CIRCADIAN RHYTHMS

Abnormalities in circadian rhythms have been reported in a variety of biological indices of patients with affective disorders. These include cyclical variations in cortisol and prolactin secretion, urinary MHPG, platelet 5-HT levels, serum dopamine-β-hydroxylase activity, CSF melatonin levels, motor activity, and body temperature. It has been proposed that in depression, certain circadian rhythms are phase advanced (shifted earlier). It has also been suggested that mania may be a disorder of synchronization of circadian rhythms, whereby the normal biological clock of slightly more than 24 hours becomes phase advanced at the onset of mania as indicated by shifts to earlier times of sleep parameters and daily temperature peak.

ENDOGENOUS OPIATES

There have been a few studies attempting to demonstrate a relationship between the endogenous opiate system and the affective disorders. Increased levels of opioid peptides have been found in the plasma or CSF of some manic patients. Pain sensitivity appears to be less in patients with affective disorders, suggesting a possible enhancement of opiatelike activity.

CONCLUSIONS

There is as yet no definitive understanding of the biology of the affective disorders. Monoamine hypothesis has had great heuristic value, but there is no consistent body of evidence supporting a relative deficiency of any single neurotransmitter in depression or excess in mania. It may be that a range of neurotransmitter imbalances can all produce the same clinical syndromes and that modification of the neurotransmitter imbalance by a diversity of means can normalize the abnormalities that lead to depression or facilitate the brain's adaptive means of restoring normal function.

REFERENCES

1. Anders, T. F., and Freeman, E. D. Enuresis. In: *Basic Handbook of Child Psychiatry*, Vol. 2 (Noshpitz, J. D. ed.). New York: Basic Books, 1979, pp. 546-555.
2. Bowers, M. B., Jr. Central dopamine turnover in schizophrenic syndrome. *Arch. Gen. Psychiatry*. 31:50. 1974.
3. Bushsbaum, M. S. Neurophysiological aspects of the schizophrenic syndrome. In: *Disorders of the Schizophrenic Syndrome* (Bellak, L. ed.). New York: Basic Books, 1979, pp. 152-180.
4. Campbell, M. Psychopharmacology. In: *Basic Handbook of Child Psychiatry*, Vol. 3 (Noshpitz, J. D. ed.). New York: Basic Books, 1979, pp. 376-409.
5. Carlsson, A. Antipsychotic drugs, neurotransmitters and schizophrenia. *Am. J. Psychiatry*. 135:164, 1978.
6. Carroll, B. J., Feinberg, M., Greden, J. C., Tarika, J., Albala, A. A. et al. A specific laboratory test for the diagnosis of melancholia. *Arch. Gen. Psychiatry*. 38:15, 1981.
7. *Diagnostic and Statistical Manual of Mental Disorders*, 3rd ed. Washington, D.C.: American Psychiatric Association, 1980.
8. Eisenberg, L. Hyperkinetic reactions. In: *Basic Handbook of Child Psychiatry*, Vol. 2 (Noshpitz, J. D. ed.). New York: Basic Book, 1979, pp. 439-453.
9. Feinberg, M., and Carroll, B. J. Effects of dopamine agonists and antagonists in Tourette's disease. *Arch. Gen. Psychiatry*. 36:979, 1979.
10. Goodwin, D. W., and Guze, S. B. *Psychiatric Diagnosis*, 2nd ed. New York: Oxford University Press, 1979.
11. Green, A. R., and Costain, D. W. The biochemistry of depression. In: *Psychopharmacology of Affective Disorders*, (Paykel, E. S., and Coppen, A. eds.). Oxford: Oxford University Press, 1979, pp. 14-40.
12. Ingvar, D. H., and Franzen, G. Abnormalities of cerebral blood flow distribution in patients with chronic schizophrenia. *Acta Psychiar. Scand*. 50:425, 1974.
13. Kety, S. S., Rosenthal, D., Wender, P. H., and Schulsinger, F. The types of prevalence of mental illness in the biological and adoptive families of adopted schizophrenics. In: *The Transmission of Schizophrenia*, (Rosenthal, D., and Kety, S. S. eds.). London: Pergamon, 1968, pp. 345-362.
14. Klawans, H. L. The pharmacology of tardive dyskinesia. *Am. J. Psychiatry* 130:82, 1973.
15. Kupfer, D. J., Broudy, D., Coble, P. A., and Spiker, D. G. EEG sleep and affective psychosis. *J. Aff. Dis*. 2:17, 1980.
16. Lee, T., Seeman, P., Tourtellotte, W. W., Farley, L. J., and Hornykeiwicz, O. Binding of ^{3}H-neuroleptics and ^{3}H-apomorphine in schizophrenic brains. *Nature* 274:897, 1978.
17. Lucas, A. R. Tic: Gilles de la Tourette's syndrome. In: *Basic Handbook of Child Psychiatry*, Vol. 2 (Noshpitz, J. D. ed). New York: Basic Books, 1979, pp. 667-684.
18. Maas, J. W. Biogenic amines and depression: Biochemical and pharmacological separation of two types of depression. *Arch. Gen. Psychiatry* 32:1357, 1975.
19. Meltzer, H. Y. Neurotransmitter dysfunction in schizophrenia. *Schiz. Bull*. 2:106, 1976.
20. Meltzer, H. Y. Biology of schizophrenia subtypes: A review and proposal for method of study. *Schiz. Bull*. 5:460, 1979.
21. Meltzer, H. Y. Biochemical studies in schizophrenia. In: *Disorders of the Schizophrenic Syndrome* (Bellak, L. ed.). New York: Basic Books, 1979, pp. 45-135.
22. Meltzer, H. Y., and Stahl, S. M. The dopamine hypothesis of schizophrenia. *Schiz. Bull*. 2:19, 1976.
23. Mountjoy, C., Roth, M., Garside, R., and Leitch, I. A clinical trial of phenelzine in anxiety, depressive, and phobic neurosis. *Br. J. Psychiatry* 131:486, 1977.
24. Murphy, D. L., Campbell, I., and Costa, J. L. Current studies of the indoleamine hypothesis of the affective disorders. In: *Psychopharmacology: A Generation of Progress* (Lipton, M. A.,

DiMascio, A., and Killam, K. F., eds.). New York: Raven Press, 1978, pp. 1235-1247.

25. Randrup, A., Munkvad, J., Fog, R., Geriacn, J., Molander, L., Kjollberg, B., Scheel-Kruger, J. Mania, depression, and brain dopamine. In: *Current Developments in Psychopharmacology*, Vol. 2. New York: Spectrum, 1975, pp. 206-248.

26. Schildkraut, J. J. The catecholamine hypothesis of affective disorder: A review of supporting evidence. *Am. J. Psychiatry* 122:509, 1965.

27. Shader, R. I., Good, M. I., and Greenblatt, D. J. Anxiety states and beta-adrenergic blockade. In: *Progress in Psychiatric Drug Treatment*, Vol. 2 (Klein, D. F., and Gittelman-Klein, R., eds.). New York: Brunner/Mazel, 1976, pp. 509-528.

28. Sulser, F., and Vetulani, F., and Mobley, P. L. Mode of action of antidepressant drugs. *Biochem. Pharmacol.* 27:257, 1978.

29. Torrey, E. F., and Peterson, M. R. Slow and latent viruses in schizophrenia. *Lancet* 2:22, 1973.

30. Tyrer, P., Candy, J., and Kelly, D. A study of the clinical effects of phenelzine and placebo in the treatment of phobic anxiety. *Psychopharmacologia* 32:237, 1973.

31. Volovka, J., and Davis, L. D., and Ehrlich, Y. H. Endorphins, dopamine, and schizophrenia. *Schiz. Bull.* 5:227, 1979.

32. Yaryura-Tobias, J. A., Neziroglu, F., and Bergman, L. Chlorimipramine for obsessive-compulsive neurosis: An organic approach. *Curr. Therap. Res.* 20:541, 1976.

CHAPTER
11.5.1

DRUGS FOR THERAPY OF PSYCHOSIS

Herbert Y. Meltzer, Paul M. Schyve
and
Kenneth E. Moore

HISTORY

The use of drugs for the treatment of psychotic disorders started approximately in the middle of this century [the history of antipsychotic agents has been summarized by Caldwell (3)]. Lithium was introduced for treatment of mania in 1949. In the 1950s, the extract of a plant indigenous to India, *Rauwolfia serpentina*, and later its pure alkaloid, reserpine, were used for treatment of psychotic disorders with encouraging results, although the hypotensive and sedative properties of the plant product as well as its beneficial effects in the treatment of mental disorders had been known for a long time. However, reserpine and related compounds that deplete monoamines from the central and peripheral neurons sometimes produced serious adverse effects, such as profound hypotension and mental depression, and hence their primary use is now limited to treatment of hypertension, or schizophrenic patients refractory to dopaminergic antagonists (see later).

Initial studies with the compounds now classified as phenothiazine neuroleptics were carried out in France in the early 1950s. Before that time, promethazine, a substituted phenothiazine that blocks histamine but not dopamine receptors, was known to possess sedative properties but was of no benefit in the treatment of agitated mental patients. Because promethazine increased the effects of other central nervous system depressants, it was used to enhance the actions of general anesthetics. A number of chemical modifications of the promethazine molecule were made in an effort to enhance the central "sedative" effects of this drug. As a consequence of this effort, Charpentier in 1949-1950 synthesized chlorpromazine, which was found to have less antihistaminic but more sedative actions than promethazine. Chlorpromazine was first employed by Laborit and his colleagues (9) as a component in a preanesthetic "lytic cocktail" to cause sedation and hypothermia. It was noted, however, that although chlorpromazine did not markedly alter the level of consciousness, it did cause patients to become indifferent to their surroundings and made them less concerned about anxiety-producing situations. In 1952, Delay and Deniker reported on their much-cited early work showing that chlorpromazine exerted a quieting effect on excited, overactive psychiatric patients without clouding consciousness.

The effects of chlorpromazine on mental patients in the United States was first reported by Lehmann and Hanrahan (10) in 1954. The use of chlorpromazine and related neuroleptics produced significant symptomatic improvement in many chronically hospitalized individuals, permitting their discharge to community care programs. The use of these agents facilitates social and rehabilitative treatment programs in and out of the hospital because patients are more accessible to opportunities for learning new social skills and staff are less engaged in purely custodial activities. The number of patients in mental hospitals declined dramatically coincident with the widespread use of chlorpromazine: from a peak of approximately 550,000 patients in 1956 to less than 340,000 in 1970, despite a general increase in the country's population. Public policy changes, however, contributed to this increase in discharge rates as much as drug efficacy.

The efficacy of chlorpromazine has stimulated the search for other types of antipsychotic compounds. Of particular importance in this regard was the development of butyrophenone derivatives, such as haloperidol and its analogs, by Janssen in Belgium in the late 1950s.

Although the neuroleptic drugs are mainly used to treat schizophrenia, they are also useful in the treatment of mania, delusional depression, unspecified functional psychoses, dementia and other organic syndromes where some decrease in CNS arousal is desired. This chapter describes general principles concerning these agents and discusses their use in schizophrenia. Their use for other indications is described in specialty texts and journals.

CHEMISTRY

Drugs currently used in therapy of psychosis in the United States include compounds mainly from five major chemical classes: (a) phenothiazines, which have three subclasses, aliphatic, piperidine and piperazine; (b) structurally similar thioxanthenes; (c) butyrophenones (phenylbutylpiperidines and the newer diphenylbutylpiperidines); (d) dihydroindolones; and (e) the dibenzodiazepines and dibenzoxazepines (Fig. 11.5.1-1). Other types of antipsychotic drugs used elsewhere in the world include substituted benzamides (e.g., sulpiride and sultopride). Rauwolfia alkaloids (which are primarily of historical interest) and related synthetic heterocyclic amine-depleting agents are rarely used

Phenothiazines have a tricyclic structure in which two benzene rings are linked by a sulfur and a nitrogen atom (Fig. 11.5.1-1). Substitution of nitrogen at position 10 by a carbon atom connected to the side chain with a double bond makes a thioxanthene nucleus. Substitutions of phenothiazines and thioxanthenes at positions 2 and 10 are of special interest. The nature of substituents at position 10 in these nuclei influences

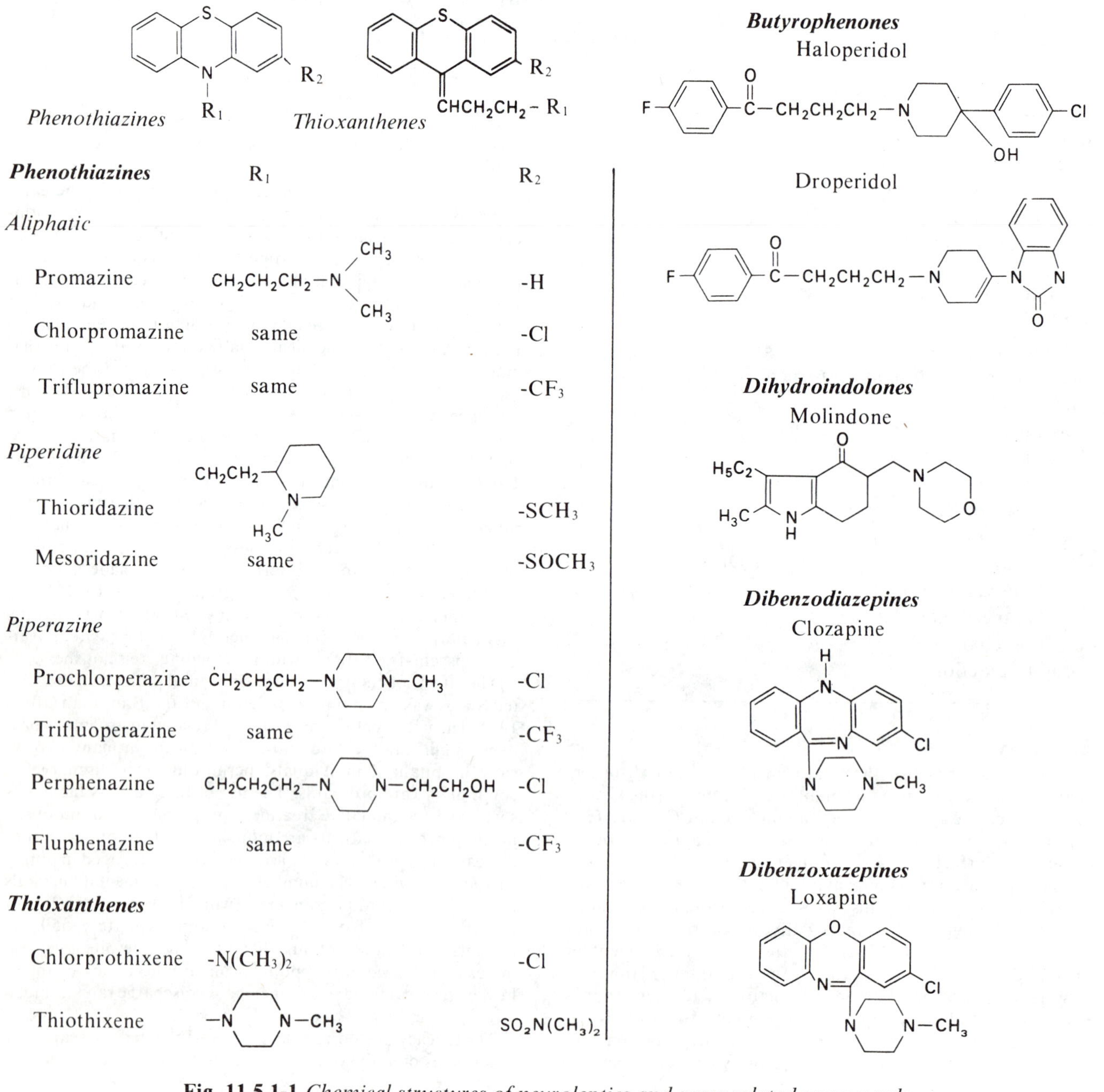

Phenothiazines (ring N bears R_1; ring position 2 bears R_2) — *Thioxanthenes* (ring carbon bears $=CHCH_2CH_2-R_1$; ring position 2 bears R_2)

Phenothiazines	R_1	R_2
Aliphatic		
Promazine	$CH_2CH_2CH_2-N(CH_3)_2$	-H
Chlorpromazine	same	-Cl
Triflupromazine	same	$-CF_3$
Piperidine		
Thioridazine	CH_2CH_2-(N-methyl-2-piperidyl) (H_3C on N)	$-SCH_3$
Mesoridazine	same	$-SOCH_3$
Piperazine		
Prochlorperazine	$CH_2CH_2CH_2-N$(piperazine)$N-CH_3$	-Cl
Trifluoperazine	same	$-CF_3$
Perphenazine	$CH_2CH_2CH_2-N$(piperazine)$N-CH_2CH_2OH$	-Cl
Fluphenazine	same	$-CF_3$
Thioxanthenes		
Chlorprothixene	$-N(CH_3)_2$	-Cl
Thiothixene	$-N$(piperazine)$N-CH_3$	$SO_2N(CH_3)_2$

Butyrophenones

Haloperidol: F–C_6H_4–$\overset{O}{\overset{\|}{C}}-CH_2CH_2CH_2-N$(piperidine, 4-OH, 4-$C_6H_4$–Cl)

Droperidol: F–C_6H_4–$\overset{O}{\overset{\|}{C}}-CH_2CH_2CH_2-N$(tetrahydropyridine)–N(benzimidazolone)

Dihydroindolones

Molindone: H_5C_2, H_3C, N–H, O, N(morpholine)

Dibenzodiazepines

Clozapine: H–N, =N, Cl, N(piperazine)$N-CH_3$

Dibenzoxazepines

Loxapine: O, N=, Cl, N(piperazine)$N-CH_3$

Fig. 11.5.1-1. *Chemical structures of neuroleptics and some related compounds.*

their pharmacological activity. For both groups of compounds, particularly with phenothiazines, drugs with an *aliphatic* side chain (e.g., chlorpromazine and triflupromazine) are relatively low in potency, with marked sedative and autonomic side effects (e.g., hypotension); those with a *piperidine* side chain (e.g., thioridazine) are of similar or somewhat greater potency, with lower incidence of extrapyramidal side effects; those with a *piperazine* side chain (e.g., fluphenazine) are the most potent compounds, with greater extrapyramidal effects and less sedation and autonomic effects.

All the clinically used neuroleptics of phenothiazine and thioxanthene groups have a chain of three carbon atoms between position 10 of the central ring and the nitrogen of the first amine group (which is always tertiary) of the connected side chain. In contrast, there are only two carbon atoms between position 10 and the first amino nitrogen in a similar side chain in antihistamine phenothiazines (e.g., promethazine). Neuroleptic activity of these compounds is lost if a fourth carbon atom is added to existing chain, or if one or two of the methyl or other substituents of the tertiary amino group of the side chain are removed as is the case with some of the metabolites of chlorpromazine.

Of the butyrophenones, the most intensively studied group includes substituted piperidine compounds such as haloperidol. Spiroperidol is the most potent compound of this group. Droperidol is a short-acting tetrahydropyridine derivative (Fig. 11.5.1-1) that is almost exclusively used in combination with a narcotic analgesic, fentanyl, in neuroleptic anesthesia, most often in a precompounded mixture (INNOVAR). A closely related family of interesting drugs, the diphenylbutylpiperidines (e.g., pimozide and fluspirilene) are currently under clinical investigation for antipsychotic potency.

Depot forms of fluphenazine (e.g., the enanthate and decanoate) are used as long-acting parenteral neuroleptic agents. These agents are esterified long-chain fatty acid derivatives that are slowly absorbed and metabolized.

Penfluridol, an investigational drug, is chemically unrelated to all other antipsychotic drugs but is similar to piperazine-type phenothiazines and the butyrophenones with respect to its pharmacological and adverse effects. It is a long-acting antipsychotic drug even when administered orally (60-100 mg) once a week in chronic schizophrenia and is comparable with depot fluphenazine preparations administered parenterally every 2 weeks (1).

Clozapine (LEPONEX) is a dibenzodiazepine derivative (Fig. 11.5.1-1) with some atypical neuroleptic properties. It does not produce extrapyramidal side effects (16), and elevates prolactin levels only when administered in very large doses. The drug has low cerebral dopamine antagonist action and high inherent anticholinergic activity. It is an investigational antipsychotic drug, and its use is limited because of its occasional bone marrow toxicity (8).

PHARMACOLOGICAL EFFECTS

The pharmacological effects of various antipsychotic agents are more or less similar, only differing in their intensity to some extent from agent to agent. To facilitate description of their effects, chlorpromazine will be taken as a prototype for the group, and later differences between the various agents with respect to certain pharmacological effects will be pointed out. Table 11.5.1-1 presents neuroleptics of various groups with their dose and side effects.

Central Nervous System. The brain is the main site of action of the neuroleptic drugs that produce a number of behavioral and neurophysiological effects.

Behavioral Effects. Delay and Deniker (5), who originally investigated the effects of chlorpromazine in psychiatric patients, described the drug's effects as a *neuroleptic syndrome*, characterized by psychomotor slowing, emotional quieting and affective indifference.

Initially, subjects may show drowsiness and apparent indifference or some slowness in response to external stimuli. However, subjects can be easily aroused and will respond to direct questions. There is a diminution of initiative and of anxiety without a change in consciousness or of intellectual facilities. Psychotic patients become less agitated; their aggressiveness and impulsiveness decrease and psychotic symptoms of hallucinations, delusions and disorganized thinking gradually disappear. Along with these antipsychotic effects, the neurological effects (e.g., parkinsonism, akathisia and others to be described later) may appear at an early stage.

An early recognized effect of neuroleptics was their ability to tame animals. For example, rhesus monkeys, which are usually intractable, become easy to handle once injected with a neuroleptic. At low doses, neuroleptics reduce exploratory behaviors and spontaneous locomotor activities. At higher doses, they produce *catalepsy*, an abnormal motor state in which an animal can be positioned in unusual postures; for example, rats will remain with their paws placed on rubber stoppers for minutes at a time.

Neuroleptics selectively disrupt active conditioned avoidance responding. For this test, animals are trained to respond to a light or a tone (conditioned stimuli) that precedes a punishing foot shock from an electrified grid floor (unconditioned stimulus). Once trained, the animal will avoid the unconditioned stimulus by seeking a safe region (climb a pole, move to an unshocked portion of the cage, and so on). Low doses of neuroleptics will interfere with the ability of the animal to avoid the shock (conditioned response) but not with the ability to escape the shock once it is applied (unconditioned response). On the other hand, central nervous system depressants such as alcohol or barbiturates disrupt both avoidance and escape responses to the same extent, probably because these depressants cause greater deficits in motor performance than do the neuroleptics.

Because neuroleptics are dopaminergic antagonists, it is not unexpected that they block the central effects of drugs that either stimulate dopamine receptors directly (e.g., apomorphine) or cause the release of dopamine (e.g., d-amphetamine). Thus, in rodents, neuroleptics block enhancement of locomotor activity caused by low doses of apomorphine and d-amphetamine as well as the stereotyped gnawing and sniffing caused by higher doses of these dopaminergic agonists.

Table 11.5.1-1
Neuroleptic Drugs: Dosage, Side Effects, and Dosage Forms

Nonproprietary Name	Trade Name	Antipsychotic: Dose Range[a] (mg)	Antipsychotic: Initial Dose (mg)	Side Effects[b]: Sedation	Side Effects[b]: Extrapyramidal Effects	Side Effects[b]: Hypotensive Effects	Dosage Forms[c]
PHENOTHIAZINES							
Aliphatic							
Chlorpromazine HCl[d]	THORAZINE	200-800	25-100 p.o. 25, 50 i.m.	+++	++	++ p.o. +++ i.m.	T, C, L, I
Triflupromazine HCl	VESPRIN	50-200	20-50	++	+++	++	T, C, L, I
Piperidine							
Thioridazine HCl	MELLARIL	200-800	25-100	+++	+	+++	T, L
Mesoridazine Besylate	SERENTIL	100-400	25-50	+++	+	+++	T, L, I
Piperacetazine	QUIDE	20-160	20-50	++	++	+++	T
Piperazine							
Acetophenazine Maleate	TINDAL	40-100	20-40	++	++	+	T
Butaperazine	REPOISE	20-80	10-20	++	++	+	T
Carphenazine	PROKETAZINE	75-400	25-75	+	+++	+	T
Fluphenazine HCl	PERMITIL PROLIXIN	2-10	2.5-5	+	+++	+	T, L, I
Fluphenazine Enanthate or Decanoate	PROLIXIN ENANTHATE or DECANOATE	25-100 q. 2 weeks	12.5 i.m.	+	+++	+	I
Perphenazine	TRILAFON	8-32	5-10	++	+++	+	T, L, I
Prochlorperazine	COMPAZINE	75-100	5-10	++	+++	+	T, C, L, I
Trifluoperazine HCl	STELAZINE	4-40	2-4	+	+++	+	T, L, I
THIOXANTHENES							
Chlorprothixene	TARACTAN	50-400	25-50 p.o.	+++	++	++	T, L, I
Thiothixene	NAVANE	6-30	2-4	++	++	++	C, L, I
BUTYROPHENONES							
Haloperidol	HALDOL	2-20	2-5 p.o. 5 i.m.	+	+++	+	T, L, I
DIHYDROINDOLONES							
Molindone HCl	MOBAN	75-225	25-50	+	++	+	T
DIBENZOXAZEPINES							
Loxapine succinate	LOXITANE	40-200	10-20	++	+++	++	C

[a] This is the dose range that benefits most patients. Much higher doses have been used safely and effectively for most drugs (with the exception of thioridazine) in selected cases unresponsive to doses in the usual range.
[b] Strong = +++; moderate = ++; weak = +.
[c] T = tablet, C = capsule, L = liquid (syrup, elixir, concentrate), I = injection (ampul, vial, syringe).
[d] hydrochloride.

Sedation. Neuroleptics have other actions in the central nervous system (e.g., sedation, hypothermia) that do not appear to result from the blockade of dopamine receptors.

Some neuroleptics (e.g., aliphatic or piperidine phenothiazines) have rather pronounced sedative effects, whereas others (e.g., piperazine phenothiazines and butyrophenones) cause little sedation. Thus, sedation is not essential for antipsychotic action. The mechanism of the sedative effect is unknown, but it may relate to the ability of these drugs to block histamine or α-adrenergic receptors. The sedation can be differentiated from the antipsychotic action in that the latter may take days or weeks to develop fully, whereas tolerance generally develops to the sedation. Furthermore, promethazine, a phenothiazine derivative devoid of antipsychotic and dopamine receptor-blocking properties, does cause sedation. Increasing the dose of neuroleptics does not cause a progressively more severe depression (loss of consciousness, stupor, and so on). Thus, unlike many other sedatives, neuroleptics have a very wide margin of safety. The sedation produced by the phenothiazines differs from that of barbiturates or general anesthetics in that there is minimum motor incoordination and patients can be easily aroused. The sedation produced by neuroleptics, which is characterized by drowsiness, dizziness, lethargy and apathy, is generally unpleasant. Accordingly, these drugs do not have an abuse potential; there are no reports of psychological dependence in humans, and animals do not self-administer neuroleptics. As might be expected, however, neuroleptics disrupt the self-administration of drugs that enhance dopamine transmission (d-amphetamine, cocaine).

Seizure Threshold. Unlike antianxiety agents, antipsychotic drugs do not possess anticonvulsant properties, and they may even exacerbate convulsive disorders. Some neuroleptics, such as aliphatic phenothiazines with low potency (especially chlorpromazine), can lower seizure threshold and induce epileptiform seizure discharge. These agents increase the incidence of seizures in untreated epileptic patients and in patients undergoing withdrawal from CNS depressants such as barbiturates and alcohol. More potent phenothiazines, such as piperazine derivatives, thioxanthenes and molindone, appear to have the least effect on seizure threshold.

Motor Activity. Chlorpromazine causes skeletal muscular relaxation in some types of spastic disorders possibly by blocking γ-motoneuron discharges (Chapter 9.2). In some schizophrenics, neuroleptics can induce *catatonia* similar to the cataleptic immobility observed in animals. Extrapyramidal disorders induced by neuroleptics are discussed later.

Body Temperature. Neuroleptics interfere with the normal regulation of body temperature probably by disrupting regulatory mechanisms in the hypothalamus.

Emesis. Apomorphine and certain ergot alkaloids are known to produce vomiting by stimulating dopaminergic receptors in the chemoreceptor trigger zone (CTZ) in the area postrema of the medulla. Neuroleptics can specifically prevent such drug-induced emesis and certain other types of vomiting (see later).

Autonomic Nervous System. Some neuroleptics possess potent α-adrenergic blocking properties (e.g., chlorpromazine) whereas others (e.g., haloperidol) are essentially without effect. Blockade of these receptors may play a role in the impairment of ejaculation, nasal stuffiness, and hypotension that can accompany the administration of aliphatic or piperidine phenothiazines. Orthostatic hypotension and mild tachycardia may also result, in part, from the depression of vasomotor centers in the medulla. Epinephrine should not be used to treat hypotensive states in patients pretreated with chlorpromazine and other α-adrenergic blockers because with the α-adrenergic receptors blocked epinephrine is only able to activate β-adrenergic receptors, thereby causing peripheral vasodilation and a further drop in blood pressure (epinephrine reversal).

Some neuroleptics (e.g., thioridazine) have rather pronounced muscarinic cholinergic-blocking properties; these compounds exhibit very few extrapyramidal symptoms (see Table 11.5.1-1). On the other hand, blockade of muscarinic receptors by some neuroleptics can result in dry mouth, blurred vision, decreased sweating and constipation.

Cardiovascular System. The assessment of the cardiovascular effects of neuroleptics is complex because of their direct effects on the heart and indirect effects through the autonomic reflexes. The overall effect is orthostatic hypotension, to which tolerance soon develops and blood pressure returns to normal. The hypotensive effect is due to the direct depressant action on the heart observed as a negative inotropic action. Chlorpromazine also has a direct vasodilating action due to α-adrenergic blockade centrally and peripherally.

Kidney. Neuroleptics have a slight diuretic effect, possibly due to direct inhibition of reabsorption of water and electrolytes in the nephron or inhibition of secretion of antidiuretic hormone. However, there is little change in glomerular filtration rate.

Liver. Sometimes obstructive jaundice is produced due to hypersensitivity reaction to the drugs. Neuroleptics do not produce any other effect on the liver and can be used with caution, in persons with impaired hepatic function.

Endocrines. The chronic administration of neuroleptics can produce marked changes in the endocrine system. Prolactin secretion is increased. The concentrations of gonadotropins, estrogens and progestins in urine are reduced. These agents depress the secretion of adrenocorticotropic hormone (ACTH) and growth hormone from the adenohypophysis, but no effect on growth and development has been noted. In addition, these drugs impair insulin release and glucose tolerance in some prediabetic patients.

MECHANISM OF ACTION AND BIOCHEMICAL EFFECTS

The behavioral effects of the neuroleptics are currently believed, but not unequivocally proven, to be related to the antipsychotic properties of neuroleptics, which in turn result from the blockade of dopaminergic receptors in limbic forebrain regions. Some of the other pharmacological actions of neuroleptics appear to result from the blockade of dopamine receptors in other regions. For example, extrapyramidal effects (see "Adverse Effects") result from blockade of dopamine receptors in the basal ganglia (caudate nucleus and putamen), antiemetic effects result from blockade of dopamine receptors in area postrema, and endocrinological effects result from blockade of dopamine receptors in the anterior pituitary (prolactin).

Some of the biochemical properties of neuroleptics can be demonstrated *in vitro* (4, 7). Cell membrane fragments from dopamine-rich regions of brain (e.g. striatum) will respond to the addition of dopamine or dopamine agonist by the activation of adenylate cyclase resulting in the formation of cyclic adenosine monophosphate (AMP). This dopamine-stimulated adenylate cyclase is blocked by the addition of neuroleptics to the incubation medium. In addition, these cell membrane fragments will bind radioactive dopamine or dopamine agonist and antagonist. Dopaminergic agonists and antagonists will displace the specific binding of these radioactive ligands. The relative concentrations of different neuroleptics required to displace radioactive dopamine agonists or antagonists from binding sites, or to block dopamine-stimulated adenylate cyclase are roughly correlated with the relative clinical doses of these same compounds (Fig. 11.5.1-2).

The biochemical properties of neuroleptics can also be characterized *in vivo*. The activities of most dopaminergic nerves in the brain appear to be regulated, in part, by a dopamine receptor-mediated feedback mechanism. For example, when dopaminergic agonists are administered, the activity of nigrostriatal dopaminergic nerves decreases, as evidenced by direct electrophysiological recordings or by indirect biochemical measurements. That is, dopamine agonists reduce the rate of dopamine turnover and the concentrations of dopamine metabolites such as dihydroxyphenylacetic acid (DOPAC) and homovanillic acid (HVA). On the other hand, dopaminergic antagonists cause just the opposite effects. Thus, concentrations of DOPAC and HVA are elevated in the CSF of patients treated with neuroleptics. This compensatory increase in the activity of dopaminergic neurons in response to the administration of dopamine receptor-blocking drugs can be used as a neurochemical index of neuroleptic activity.

Another sensitive indicator of dopamine receptor blockade is the plasma concentration of prolactin. Dopamine that is released from tuberoinfundibular nerves (see Fig. 7.4-1) is carried by the hypophyseal portal blood to the anterior pituitary where it inhibits the release of prolactin. Neuroleptics block dopamine receptors in the anterior pituitary and thereby remove the tonic inhibitory input to the prolactin-secreting cells which causes a marked increase in the circulating concentration of prolactin. By blocking dopaminergic receptors in the medio-

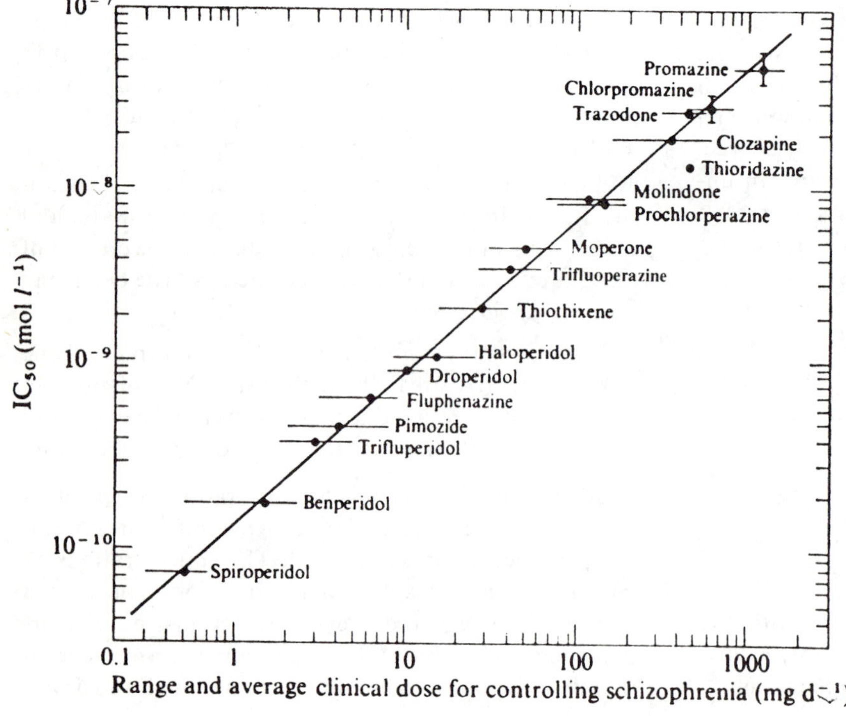

Fig. 11.5.1-2

Comparison of the clinical potencies of neuroleptic drugs, measured as average daily dose in treating schizophrenia with potencies of the same drugs in displacing ^{3}H-haloperidol from dopamine receptor sites in vitro in calf caudate nucleus membranes (IC50 = drug concentration required to displace 50% of specific ^{3}H-haloperidol binding). (From Ref. 15, by permission).

basal hypothalamus, neuroleptics also interfere with the normal control of growth hormone release from the anterior pituitary. Thus, patients treated with neuroleptics will generally have elevated serum concentrations of prolactin and reduced concentrations of growth hormone.

PHARMACOKINETICS

Most antipsychotics have variable and unpredictable absorption patterns when given orally and are frequently administered parenterally to increase the bioavailability of active drug. These agents are highly lipid-soluble, tightly bound to membranes and plasma proteins, and accumulate in organs with rich blood supply (i.e. brain, lung, and so on). Neuroleptics have a long half-life in the body and can be well tolerated in high oral doses. This usually permits medication to be given once or twice a day. Elimination follows a multiphasic pattern. Chlorpromazine is eliminated in a biphasic fashion with half-lives of 2 and 30 hours. Most neuroleptics are initially oxidized by hepatic microsomal and nonmicrosomal enzymes and are then conjugated with glucuronic acid. More than 100 metabolites of chlorpromazine have been postulated, and many of these have been identified in the urine of patients long after the administration of the drug has stopped. The metabolites are excreted via the kidney and to a limited quantity in the bile.

TOLERANCE AND PHYSICAL DEPENDENCE

Tolerance develops to the neuroleptic-induced sedative effects. Tolerance and cross-tolerance are also observed in behavioral and biochemical effects particularly related to blockade of dopaminergic receptors in the basal ganglia (2). These drugs are not addicting; however, a mild degree of physical dependence is manifested by muscular discomfort, and difficulty in sleeping may occur several days after abrupt discontinuation.

ADVERSE EFFECTS

Neuroleptics have relatively flat dose-response curves and thus a high therapeutic index. Many of the side effects of these compounds are merely extensions of their pharmacological actions, which have been discussed earlier. Particularly some of these effects (e.g., extrapyramidal reactions, endocrine dysfunction) may be closely related to the mechanism of action of these agents (i.e. their antidopaminergic effect). However, extrapyramidal reactions, as well as side effects due to other biological actions of the neuroleptics, do vary from agent to agent.

Sedation and Hypotension. Sedation and hypotension are mainly the result of the α-adrenoceptor blocking properties of the neuroleptics. Neuroleptics can produce sedation in psychotic and generally more frequently in nonpsychotic individuals. Aliphatic and piperidine phenothiazines and chlorprothixene are the most sedative of the neuroleptics (Table 11.5.1-1). The sedative effect of even these agents diminishes over a period of weeks but initially can be very severe.

Thioridazine is particularly hypotensive, whereas trifluoperazine produces little or no hypotension. The hypotension is frequently orthostatic in nature. Norepinephrine, or phenylephrine, which are α-adrenergic agonists, or dopamine, can be used to treat neuroleptic-induced hypotension in an emergency.

Inhibition of Ejaculation. Inhibition of ejaculation is also due to the antiadrenergic effects of the neuroleptics. This has been reported most frequently with mesoridazine and thioridazine.

Extrapyramidal Side Effects

Early-Onset Effects. The adverse effects of neuroleptics that cause the most concern are classified as *extrapyramidal effects;* these are disorders of muscle tone, movement, and posture (2, 11). These effects are believed to result from the ability of neuroleptics to disrupt dopamine transmission at the terminals of the nigrostriatal nerves. It has been proposed that the anticholinergic properties of the neuroleptics can partially overcome the results of dopamine receptor blockade, thus accounting for the low incidence of extrapyramidal symptoms with thioridazine and the high incidence due to haloperidol or fluphenazine. Most extrapyramidal effects, if they develop, will occur within several days to 2 months after the initiation of therapy. These acute effects can be divided into three types: parkinsonism, dyskinesias, and akathisia.

Some extrapyramidal reactions may develop within a few days after initiating treatment with neuroleptics, sometimes even after the first dose. These are usually acute dystonic reactions, including opisthotonos, facial grimacing, uncontrolled protrusion of the tongue, and oculogyric crises (eye rotating back in the orbit due to spasms of the extraocular muscles). Acute dyskinesias and dystonias occur in less than 5% of all patients. After 1-2 weeks of neuroleptic treatment, parkinsonism (akinesia, rigidity, resting tremor, increased salivation), and akathisia (restless legs) may develop.

Parkinsonian symptoms, which resemble closely those seen in idiopathic Parkinson's disease, occur in 10-15% of patients maintained on neuroleptics. Akathisia, a compelling need to be in motion, accompanied by discomfort, occurs in approximately 20% of all patients. The symptoms may disappear spontaneously, and they generally subside within 1 or 2 weeks after neuroleptic administration is stopped.

Treatment of the acute dystonic reactions generally requires administration of intravenous or intramuscular diphenhydramine (25-50 mg) or an anticholinergic drug. In general, anticholinergic drugs should not be given prophylactically when neuroleptic drugs are started, but only after extrapyramidal symptoms have developed. They should be stopped within 8-12 weeks to see if the patient still has extrapyramidal symptoms because tolerance develops to some of the extrapyramidal effects of neuroleptics in the striatum. It is possible that patients may develop toxic psychoses from excessive anticholinergic therapy, which could be confused with exacerbations of the psychoses. The risk of such psychoses is usually low but may be increased by concomitant administration of several drugs with anticholinergic effects (e.g., an anticholinergic agent, a tricyclic antidepressant, and thioridazine). Such psychoses can be successfully managed by reducing the dose of anticholinergic drugs or by administration of physostigmine.

Amantadine is a novel drug that can diminish parkinsonian symptoms due to neuroleptic administration. Doses of 100-300 mg/day orally may be used as an alternative to anticholinergic therapy; its mechanism of action is unknown. It is believed to cause dopamine release (Chapter 7.4).

Tardive Dyskinesia. Tardive dyskinesia is a symptom complex of involuntary repetitive choreiform movements of the tongue, mouth, facial, limb, and truncal muscles (e.g., lip sucking, chewing, tongue thrust or protruding, lateral jaw movements, sucking maneuvers) that often persists indefinitely after the neuroleptic is withdrawn. It can develop during or following the cessation of neuroleptic treatment; usually prolonged treatment precedes its appearance, but cases have developed after only a few months of treatment. The incidence is not well known, but a range of 1-50% has been proposed; it is higher in the elderly. Mild cases may be unnoticed by the patient, but severe cases may be socially and motorically disabling. This dyskinesia disappears during sleep and is aggravated by stress. One of the most widely accepted theories of its etiology is that tardive dyskinesia is due to development of supersensitivity in striatal dopamine receptors following prolonged blockage by neuroleptics (pharmacological denervation). However, it may be mentioned that whereas receptor supersensitivity is reversible, tardive dyskinesia is not. Moreover, because there is some evidence for dopamine receptor supersensitivity in schizophrenics, it is possible that it could occur in schizophrenics even without neuroleptic treatment. Tardive dyskinesia may develop in any patient population treated with neuroleptics. Orofacial movements similar to tardive dyskinesia have been reported following chronic antihistamine use and with toxic levels of phenytoin.

All neuroleptics currently approved for use in the United States have been implicated in the development of tardive dyskinesia, so there is no reason to choose a particular drug on this basis. Discontinuation of anticholinergic therapy when it is not indicated is another step that may prevent tardive dyskinesia, since some evidence suggests that the use of anticholinergic agents increase the risk of tardive dyskinesia. Intermittent therapy with neuroleptics, interrupted by so-called drug holidays that last for a few days, weeks, or months, would be a useful strategy to detect early tardive dyskinesia, but there is some evidence this may enhance the risk of its developing or its severity. Patients and their families should be apprised of the risk of tardive dyskinesia when long-term neuroleptic use is recommended.

Tardive dyskinesia frequently emerges for the first time as drug dosage is reduced. Thereafter, the symptoms may resolve entirely or persist and worsen. There is no way at the present time to predict the outcome at this phase.

The use of agents that enhance cholinergic activity has been proposed in the treatment of tardive dyskinesia because the striatal cholinergic neurons can inhibit dopaminergic neurons. Deanol and choline have been studied for this purpose. There is evidence that 15-20 g of choline per day can alleviate tardive dyskinesia in some patients, but it, too, has unwanted side effects, such as a fishy odor or enhanced peripheral cholinergic stimulation. Lecithin is currently being evaluated in tardive dyskinesia.

Cardiotoxic Effects. There is some evidence that chlorpromazine has an antiarrhythmic effect upon the heart, but because of a significant incidence of sudden death in young patients treated with neuroleptics, there is a suspicion that these agents may precipitate ventricular tachyarrhythmias. Thioridazine has been suspected as the causal agent more frequently than other neuroleptics. It produces a high incidence of T-wave changes in the ECG that resemble hypokalemia and can be reversed by potassium administration. The clinical significance of these changes is not clear. However, there is no firm evidence indicating the neuroleptics as the cause of sudden death.

Allergic Reactions. Although a high incidence of allergic-type obstructive jaundice had been reported with neuroleptics, especially chlorpromazine, the incidence of this adverse reaction appears to have decreased in recent years. It usually develops within 3-4 weeks of initiating neuroleptic treatment and is associated with skin reactions, jaundice, fever, and eosinophilia. Patients may be immediately switched to another class of neuroleptics, although the obstructive jaundice apparently may spontaneously remit, even without a switch in neuroleptics. Neuroleptics may be used in patients with diseased livers, with caution paid to the reduced ability of these individuals to metabolize the drug.

Endocrine Effects. Neuroleptic drugs can interfere with gonadotropin regulation and produce amenorrhea, but this is relatively infrequent. Prolactin elevations are marked in females receiving therapeutic doses of neuroleptics; males have lesser increases. Galactorrhea may occur in both males and females as a consequence of the prolactin elevations but usually, although not always, ceases upon discontinuation of neuroleptic medication. Gynecomastia in males and breast engorgement in females may occur with chronic neuroleptic treatment. These symptoms readily respond to discontinuation of the neuroleptic medication. Small doses of bromocriptine may be useful to counteract the effect of neuroleptics on prolactin secretion but may interfere with the antipsychotic effect of the neuroleptics.

Neuroleptic Malignant Syndrome. The use of neuroleptics, especially parenteral high potency neuroleptics, or discontinuation of dopamine agonists, e.g. L-DOPA or amantadine may rarely produce the *neuroleptic malignant syndrome,* characterized by fever (to 42° C), rigidity, altered consciousness (including delirium and coma) and autonomic instability (tachycardia, labile hypertension, diaphoresis and pallor). It usually begins within two weeks of administering neuroleptics and may last 1-4 weeks. It may be fatal (20% mortality), although if recognized, can be treated by cessation of neuroleptic administration, *bromocriptine, dantrolene* and body cooling. It is usually associated with increased serum creatine kinase activity due to muscular rigidity, primary or secondary changes in muscle cell physiology or intramuscular injections. It is not a hypersensitivity response. Neuroleptic administration has been cautiously restarted in recovered patients without incident. The pathophysiology appears to be a marked decrease in dopaminergic activity.

THERAPEUTIC USES

Therapy of Schizophrenia

Choice of Drugs

Oral and Short-Acting Intramuscular Drugs. As is apparent from Table 11.5-1, the various classes of neuroleptics differ in potency, side effects, and availability of dosage forms. The aliphatic and piperidine phenothiazines, as well as chlorprothixene, are the most sedating of the neuroleptics. For this reason, they have frequently been used when beginning treatment with agitated schizophrenic and manic patients. Less sedating drugs may be just as calming, without being as soporific. The injectable form may be preferred because it acts more rapidly than the oral form and because some patients refuse to take oral medication. However, these injections are painful (especially chlorpromazine), and the oral form should be used whenever possible. The liquid oral form acts more rapidly than capsules or tablets. As will be discussed subsequently, rapid tranquilization with haloperidol is widely used for the treatment of agitated, acutely psychotic patients because multiple injections may be given over a relatively brief period of time with less risk of hypotensive episodes than with chlorpromazine. It should be noted that chlorprothixene has less hypotensive effect than chlorpromazine, and that thioridazine is not available in an injectable form and has a high incidence of hypotensive reactions.

A general rule of thumb is that the more potent the neuroleptic, regardless of class, the fewer sedative, hypotensive, and anticholinergic side effects, and the higher the incidence of extrapyramidal side effects (Table 11.5.1-1).

At the current time, there is no scientific basis to predict which drug may be of the best long-term benefit to a given patient. Other than avoiding the drugs with serious hypotensive properties in patients who already have low blood pressure, are dehydrated, or are otherwise in poor physical health, one could use any of these drugs to begin treatment with a previously unmedicated patient. If a patient has had an allergic reaction to a particular drug, or has a history of good or poor response to a particular drug, these factors should influence the choice of an agent. The availability of parenteral as well as oral, and of liquid as well as capsule or tablet, forms might influence drug choice if patient compliance with an oral regimen is considered to be a factor.

There is no rationale for administering more than one neuroleptic to a patient because all compounds are thought to act by a common mechanism (i.e., by blocking dopamine receptors). Although the drugs do vary in anticholinergic, antiadrenergic, and antiserotonergic properties, and no doubt in other properties as well, it is not yet clear if any of these additional properties contributes to their antipsychotic effects. If a specific aspect of their pharmacology is useful in a particular patient, that should be empirically discovered through an appropriate trial after thoroughly examining the effect of a wide range of dosages. When second or third neuroleptics are added to the treatment regimen of a patient who has not responded well to a given neuroleptic and there is a subsequent good response, it is not clear what, if anything, the initial medications were providing to the overall result. When patients fail to respond to a particular neuroleptic and there is evidence that the drug has been ingested or that there are adequate blood levels or serum prolactin elevations, it is best to discontinue the initial drug and to initiate treatment with a drug of a different chemical class. If the initial drug was a phenothiazine, it might be appropriate to try a butyrophenone, thioxanthene, molindone, or loxapine.

Long-Acting Depot Neuroleptics. Depot forms of fluphenazine are widely used both in the treatment of acutely psychotic patients and for maintenance treatment where there is concern about compliance with oral medication or possible difficulties with absorption. Fluphenazine enanthate should provide adequate blood levels of fluphenazine for 10-14 days; fluphenazine decanoate should provide adequate blood levels for 2-3 weeks. Dosage varies from 12.5 mg every 4 weeks subcutaneously or intramuscularly to 100 mg s.c. or i.m. every week. The lowest dose necessary to prevent relapse should be used. Although no especially adverse consequences to such high doses have been reported, dosage should be kept as low as possible consistent with optimal clinical benefit. Approximately 5 mg of fluphenazine orally per day is equivalent to 25 mg fluphenazine enanthate or decanoate given every 10 or 14 days, respectively. Penfluridol is an orally administered long-acting neuroleptic that is not yet available in the United States. It should be noted that several recent controlled studies in the United States have failed to find significant advantage of depot over oral medication in the maintenance treatment of schizophrenia. Because depot medication is slowly absorbed, resulting in an increase in serum prolactin only after 6 hours, it should not be used as a substitute for i.m. injections of conventional neuroleptics for rapid control of symptoms.

Regulation of Dosage. It is frequently useful to begin the administration of neuroleptic treatment with a small test dose such as 100 mg p.o. or 25 mg i.m. of chlorpromazine or the equivalent dose of another neuroleptic. This will permit the observation of the development of an idiosyncratic reaction or orthostatic hypotension. If no such reactions occur within 1-2 hours, further drug administration can proceed with greater assurance that no serious adverse effects will ensue.

Clinically significant differences in patient requirements for neuroleptic drugs have been amply documented. This is due in large part to pharmacokinetic factors such as variations in drug absorption, metabolism, distribution, and protein binding. There are considerable individual variations in the pharmacokinetics and pharmacodynamics of the neuroleptics in psychotic patients. Children were reported to attain lower plasma levels of neuroleptics than adults at a given dose (13). Measurements of serum neuroleptic concentrations are useful for adjusting the dose of the drug in patients who are not showing therapeutic response, for assessing adverse reactions, and for monitoring patient compliance. Because of bioavailability factors, chronically ill adult patients and children often require high doses of neuroleptics (14). Variations in blood levels have been noted after the same doses have been given to different patients. Dosage requirements will vary with body weight and size. There is some evidence that females respond better to neuroleptics independently of differences in body weight and size, and thus may respond to lower doses. The stage of the illness and the severity of the symptoms are clearly factors in determining overall dosage. The use of these agents should be integrated with a comprehensive treatment plan that includes attention to psychosocial factors in the patients' daily life (12). Patients who are more acutely psychotic and who have very florid symptomatology often require higher doses of neuroleptics to achieve a remission than patients who have passed the acute stage of their illness and require some type of maintenance treatment. Table 11.5.1-1 gives an approximate guide to dosage, but the physician should be alert to the need to utilize more or less than the listed doses as circumstances indicate. Thioridazine, however, should not be given in doses greater than 800 mg/day because of the possibility of pigmentary retinopathy.

There have been several recent reports of the use of megadoses of neuroleptics (e.g., for tranquilization). The technique usually involves use of the high-potency neuroleptics, which lack potent effects on blood pressure. Haloperidol i.m. every 30-60 minutes may be sufficient to control severely agitated and belligerent psychotic patients, but the dose and timing must be individualized, based upon response to the previous dose. As much as 100 mg of haloperidol has been given over a 24-hour period. Improvement may occur in most but not all patients in most of the major areas of psychopathology, including thought disorder, delusions, and hallucinations, but it is rare for this improvement to be of major proportion. Side effects include dystonic reactions and cogwheel rigidity, which usually respond to anticholinergic agents. Sedation and hypotension are slight. This approach has been useful in manic as well as schizophrenic patients.

Frequency of Administration. Most neuroleptics have a long half-life in the body and can be well tolerated in high oral doses. This usually permits medication to be given on a twice- or even once-a-day schedule, which is very convenient for both patients and nursing staff and increases patient compliance. In the early stages of treatment, more frequent administration may be needed to control behavior and to avoid the development of hypotension from a large single dose. Prescribing neuroleptics in tablet or capsule form of higher strength is also cost effective. Administration of the dose prior to sleep will not only help a patient fall asleep but will minimize discomfort due to anticholinergic or antiadrenergic effects; extrapyramidal symptoms are actually reduced during sleep (as in idiopathic parkinsonism).

Duration of Neuroleptic Treatment. It usually requires 4-12 weeks for antipsychotic medication, together with milieu and other forms of social therapies, to bring about the remission of acutely psychotic symptoms. Even at this point, many patients will still have significant remnants of their delusional symptoms, thought disorder, and hallucinations, which they may or may not be willing to share with their physicians or other professional staff. The decision to decrease medication dose at this stage is difficult. There are no controlled studies to indicate the relative benefit of continuing higher or lower doses. It is current clinical practice to begin to reduce the dose slowly and steadily at this point and to observe the effect of the reduced dose on psychotic symptomatology. Should symptoms reemerge, dose should be raised. In some instances, it may be possible to give neuroleptic medication 4-5 days a week or to omit an entire week's or month's medication without any apparent adverse effect on symptomatology. These so-called drug holidays may be of use in reducing the risk of long-term side effects such as tardive dyskinesia, but there is no solid evidence to substantiate this. In fact, some evidence suggests that variation in dopamine receptor blockade (as occurs in short but frequent drug holidays) may increase the risk of tardive dyskinesia. Patients should receive the lowest dose needed to maintain them at their optimal level of functioning.

Relapse after withdrawal of antipsychotic drugs usually requires 1-6 months to develop. The reason for this long duration is not continued dopamine receptor blockade, since neuroendocrine studies have demonstrated that the responsiveness of dopamine receptors returns 2-4 days after discontinuing neuroleptic drugs.

Utilization of Other Psychotropic Medications. During the initial evaluation period before starting neuroleptic medication, it may be useful to utilize chloral hydrate or a benzodiazepine for sleep purposes, but this should not be necessary during the period when neuroleptic medication is utilized. If the patient is still experiencing serious anxiety or sleep disturbance 5-7 days after starting medication or raising the dose, this is an indication that a higher dose is warranted. Antianxiety drugs such as the benzodiazepines have little or no place at the current time in the treatment of the acute psychoses except for the acute treatment of phencyclidine psychoses or drug-induced psychoses for which the identity of the injected agent is unknown. However, massive doses of diazepam (up to 200 mg/day) have been reported to be useful as a supplement to neuroleptic treatment in some schizophrenic patients.

Lithium carbonate may be utilized with neuroleptics in the treatment of manic-depressive patients and schizoaffective patients.

Tricyclic antidepressants or other antidepressants, including the monoamine oxidase inhibitors, should not be routinely administered to schizophrenic patients. Tricyclic antidepressants can sometimes cause exacerbation of psychotic symptoms in schizophrenia. This is particularly true of agitated patients who may become more hostile, have increased auditory hallucinations, and develop more bizarre delusions and behavior within days after starting tricyclic antidepressant treatment. Patients who present with mixed depressive and schizophrenic symptomatology, but with no clear history of affective disorder in themselves or in their immediate family, frequently require only neuroleptic therapy and should not be given antidepressants initially. Similarly, schizophrenic patients who develop depressive symptoms after recovering from an acute psychosis often fail to respond to addition of tricyclic antidepressant medication. On the other hand, patients with bipolar or unipolar affective illnesses who present a mixture of depressive and schizophrenic symptomatology respond much better to neuroleptic and tricyclic antidepressant combination treatment than to either drug alone. The reasons for these discrepancies are unknown but suggest that the etiology of depressive symptomatology in schizophrenics is different than that in primary depressed patients. It is recommended, therefore, that depressive symptoms in a schizophrenic patient be treated with an adequate trial of neuroleptic alone before consideration of an antidepressant.

Pregnancy and Neuroleptic Drugs. There is mixed evidence about the safety of neuroleptic drug administration during pregnancy. In 166 patients who received chlorpromazine or haloperidol during a part of their pregnancies, the overall incidence of abortion, neonatal survival, and birth defects did not exceed that of the control groups. Neuroleptics have been used during pregnancy to prevent nausea and vomiting, and there is no increased association with fetal damage that has been reported as a result. There is some clinical evidence that suggests neuroleptic administration during the last trimester may be somewhat more dangerous than during the first two trimesters. Several cases in which neuroleptic-treated mothers gave birth to children who manifested various extrapyramidal symptoms have been reported. If neuroleptics are required to prevent a pregnant woman from doing harm to herself or others, or to maintain adequate physical care of herself during the period of gestation, it would appear that the weight of current evidence is in favor of neuroleptic use. The possible risks should be explained to the patient and family members so that informed consent for the relatively minimal known risks can be balanced by the patient and her family against the potential benefits.

Other Forms of Somatic Treatment. Electroconvulsive treatment (ECT) is sometimes useful in the treatment of schizophrenia, although its major role is in the treatment of severe depressions. ECT may be helpful in treating the extremely excited catatonic patient who does not respond to rapid tranquilization with haloperidol or chlorpromazine or who cannot tolerate such treatment because of the side effects. ECT, because it usually produces immediate effects, may be useful in treating patients who are intensely suicidal or self-destructive. The procedures for ECT administration in schizophrenics are identical to those for the treatment of depression. The frequency of ECT can vary. Multiple ECT on a single day may be needed to treat the most severely agitated or self-destructive patients, but multiple ECT to induce regression in preparation for reintegrative therapy is not widely accepted.

Dopamine receptors (autoreceptors) on terminals of dopaminergic neurons can inhibit the synthesis and release of dopamine. Stimulation of these autoreceptors by low doses of dopamine agonists may be of therapeutic value in the treatment of acute psychosis and tardive dyskinesia. Low doses of apomorphine (1.5-3 mg, s.c.) have been used for this purpose. The effects are short lasting and tolerance may develop. Bromocriptine has been used, with minimal success. More specific autoreceptor agonists are being developed.

Reserpine, which depletes the stores of dopamine as well as of norepinephrine and 5-hydroxytryptamine, was once widely used to treat schizophrenic psychosis. Now it is used only as a supplement to neuroleptic treatment in patients who do not respond to neuroleptic agents alone. Hypotension and depression may occur with reserpine use.

Propranolol, a β-adrenergic blockers, has been used to treat acute schizophrenia. Very high doses are required, necessitating constant cardiac monitoring. Because of the negative results shown in most of the studies with this drug, its use should be avoided.

Peptides such as *β-endorphin, des-try-gamma-endorphin, des-enkephalin-gamma-endorphin, cholecystokinin* and *vasopressin* have been used to treat schizophrenics, usually as a supplement to neuroleptic medication. The results have been very mixed, with non-United States investigators often reporting favorable results in small samples. The positive effects reported have been subtle in most cases but may persist after the medication is stopped. The possibility that the results of peptide therapy were non-specific placebo effects has not been excluded but further efforts in this area of research are indicated.

The so-called orthomolecular school of psychiatry is based upon numerous claims that megavitamin therapy (high doses of niacin, ascorbic acid and B_{12}) is useful in the treatment of most or all schizophrenics. Although it is possible that along the spectrum of biological diseases that comprise the schizophrenic syndrome, a rare disease may be benefited by megavitamin therapy, controlled studies have failed to demonstrate that such treatment is useful. There have been reports that glutens contained in wheat may be etiologically involved in schizophrenia. Anecdotal claims, not well substantiated, of other dietary allergies frequently appear in the literature.

The use of insulin coma and psychosurgery for the treatment of schizophrenia, once widespread in the United States and elsewhere, has now all but ceased.

Hemodialysis has also been extensively investigated and not found to be successful.

Other Uses

Antagonism of Effects of Other Drugs. Neuroleptics have some utility in treating the symptoms of milder forms of alcohol withdrawal, but the anxiolytics (chlordiazepoxide and diazepam) are now generally the preferred drugs for treating this condition. Neuroleptics have been used in treating the hallucinations induced by large doses of amphetaminelike drugs, but symptomatic treatment is preferred.

Nausea amd Vomiting. Neuroleptics block vomiting associated with various disease processes (uremia, gastroenteritis, radiation sickness) and with a variety of chemicals (e.g., apomorphine, narcotic analgesics, tetracyclines, estrogens, disulfiram, antineoplastic agents). This property of neuroleptics appears to result from their ability to depress the chemoreceptor trigger zone in the medulla. These drugs do not block nausea or vomiting caused by vestibular stimuli (motion sickness). In addition, possibly because of the depression of sites in the medulla, some neuroleptics are useful in the treatment of intractable hiccough. Chlorpromazine has been used to treat nausea and vomiting of pregnancy but should not be given for such purpose during pregnancy. Thioridazine is the only neuroleptic that does not have any antiemetic effect in humans.

Preanesthetic Medication. Phenothiazine and butyrophenone neuroleptics that are devoid of hypotensive properties have some utility as preanesthetic agents because of their sedative and antiemetic properties, and because they enhance the effects of other commonly used preanesthetic agents (e.g., barbiturates, narcotic analgesics). Butyrophenones in combination with a narcotic analgesic have been used to produce *neurolept analgesia,* a state of quiescence and indifference to environmental stimuli. During this state, simple manipulative and surgical procedures can be performed. More complicated surgical procedures can be performed if the effects of the neuroleptic-analgesic combinations are supplemented with nitrous oxide. A popular combination for this purpose consists of the butyrophenone droperidol and the analgesic fentanyl (INNOVAR).

Miscellaneous. Methotrimeprazine (LEVOPROME) is an aliphatic phenothiazine derivative that is administered parenterally to recumbent patients to relieve pain. Its usefulness as an analgesic resides in the fact that it is nonaddicting and causes neither respiratory depression nor vomiting. On the other hand, its usefulness is limited by its marked sedative and hypotensive actions. Haloperidol has proven useful in controlling the tics and vocal utterances of Gilles de la Tourettes syndrome.

DRUG INTERACTIONS

Antacids such as aluminum hydroxide and magnesium trisilicate may decrease the absorption of the neuroleptics from the gastrointestinal tract by physical adsorption of the neuroleptic to the antacid. *Anticholinergic drugs* may decrease the rate of absorption of neuroleptics by slowing down intestinal motility, leading to a more extensive metabolism of neuroleptics by the intestinal mucosa. *Barbiturates,* through their capacity to induce liver microsomal enzymes that metabolize neuroleptics, can also cause decreased blood levels of neuroleptics. There is also some evidence that cigarette smoking may have the same effect as barbiturates on microsomal enzymes.

Phenothiazines have been reported to reverse the antihypertensive effects of *guanethidine* by interfering with the transport of guanethidine into adrenergic nerve endings. Neuroleptics may enhance the action of *tricyclic antidepressants* by inhibiting the enzyme that metabolize these drugs. *Epinephrine* can produce a worsening of hypotension in neuroleptic-treated patients because the neuroleptics block the α-adrenergic properties of epinephrine, leaving unopposed the β-adrenergic stimulation of receptors in peripheral vasculature; the resulting vasodilation in skeletal muscle causes blood pooling. Neuroleptics combined with alcohol, narcotic analgesics, or general anesthetics may have more than additive sedative properties; combinations may have produced severe central nervous system depression, coma and sometimes death. Patients receiving neuroleptics should be cautioned to restrict their alcohol ingestion to no more than 1 or 2 oz of 80-proof alcohol.

REFERENCES

1. *AMA Drug Evaluations,* 5th ed. Chicago: American Medical Association, 1983, p. 213.
2. Baldessarini, R.J. and Tarsy, D. Relationship of the actions of neuroleptic drugs to the pathophysiology of tardive dyskinesia. *Int. Rev. Neurobiol.* 21:1, 1979.
3. Caldwell, A.E. History of psychopharmacology. In: *Principles of Psychopharmacology,* 2nd ed. (Clarke, W.G. and del Guidice, J., eds.): New York Academic Press, 1978, p. 9.
4. Creese, I., Burt, D.R. and Snyder, S.H. Biochemical actions of neuroleptic drugs: Focus on the dopamine receptor. In: *Handbook of Psychopharmacology,* Vol. 10 (Iversen, L.L., Iversen, S.D. and Snyder, S.H., eds.). New York: Plenum Press, 1978, p. 37.
5. Delay, J. and Deniker, P. Trente-huit cas de psychoses traitees par la cure prolongée et continue de 4560 RP. Le Congrès. Paris: Masson et Cie, 1952.
6. Fielding, S. and Lal, H. Behavioral actions of neuroleptics. In: *Handbook of Psychopharmacology,* Vol. 10 (Iversen, L.L., Iversen, S.D. and Snyder, S.H., eds.). New York: Plenum Press, 1978, p. 91.
7. Iversen, L.L. Catecholamine-sensitive adenylate cyclases in nervous tissue. *J. Neurolchem.* 50:237, 1977.
8. Jenner, P. and Marsden, C.D. Neuroleptics. In: *Clinical Psychopharmacology, Part 1* (Hippius, H. and Winokur, G., eds.). Princeton, N.J.: Excerpta Medica, 1983, p. 180.
9. Laborit, H., Huguenard, P. and Alluaume, R. Un nouveau stabilisateur vegetatif, le 4560RP. *Presse Med.* 60:206, 1952.
10. Lehmann, H.E. and Hanrahan, G.E. Chlorpromazine, a new inhibiting agent for psychomotor excitement and manic states. *Arch. neurol. Psychiatry* 71:227, 1954.

11. Marsden, C.D., Tarsy, D. and Baldessarini, R.J. Spontaneous and drug-induced movement disorders in psychotic patients. In: *Psychiatric Aspects of Neurologic Disease* (Benson, D.G. and Blumer, D., eds.). New York: Grune & Stratton, 1976, p. 219.

12. Meltzer, H.Y. Regression is unnecessary. In: *Psychotherapy of Schizophrenia* (Gunderson, J.G. and Mosher, L.R., eds.). New York: Jason Aronson, 1975, p. 123.

13. Meyers, B., Tune, L. and Coyle, J. Clinical response and serum neuroleptic levels in childhood schizophrenia. *Am. J. Psychiatry* 137:4, 1980.

14. Rivera-Calimlin, L. and Hershey, L. Neuroleptic concentrations and clinical response. *Ann. Rev. Pharmacol. Toxicol.* 24:361, 1984.

15. Seeman, P., Lee, T., Chau-Wong, M. and Wong, K. Antipsychotic drug doses and neuroleptic/dopamine receptors. *Nature* 261:717, 1976.

16. Simpson, G.M. and Varga, E. Clozapine a new antipsychotic agent. *Curr. Ther. Res.* 16:679, 1974.

CHAPTER
11.5.2

DRUGS FOR THERAPY OF AFFECTIVE DISORDERS

Elaine Sanders-Bush, Herbert Y. Meltzer
and
Fridolin Sulser

Affective disorders, including bipolar and unipolar endogenous depression and mania (18), are universal human illnesses known to occur in every society and culture. The *catecholamine* hypothesis proposes that affective disorders result from abnormalities in central noradrenergic systems [norepinephrine (NE) deficiency and/or abnormalities in noradrenergic receptor regulation], whereas the *indolealkylamine* hypothesis postulates that abnormalities in central serotonergic pathways [serotonin (5-HT) deficiency or excess] may occur in selective subgroups of patients with affective disorders (1). Drugs with proven clinical efficacy in the treatment of depression include:

1 Tricyclic antidepressants
2 Monoamine oxidase (MAO) inhibitors
3 Some miscellaneous new compounds

The antimanic drugs include mainly lithium salts.

ANTIDEPRESSANTS

TRICYCLIC ANTIDEPRESSANTS

History and Chemistry. Clinically effective tricyclic antidepressants are either tertiary or secondary amines, the latter of which can be formed *in vivo* by oxidative N-demethylation (Fig. 11.5.2-1). The antidepressant activity of the prototype of this group of drugs, imipramine, was fortuitously discovered in 1957 by Kühn (11) while he was investigating the drug as a potential antipsychotic agent. At that time, the antidepressant activity could not have been predicted from the pharmacological profile of the drug. Indeed, the initial data on the pharmacology of imipramine in normal animals suggested that this drug was a weak phenothiazine-like antipsychotic agent with sedative and antihistaminic properties.

Table 11.5.2-1 contains a number of miscellaneous drugs with established or potential antidepressant activity and pharmacological properties pertinent to the discussion of the mode of action of the tricyclic antidepressants.

Pharmacological and Biochemical Properties. In normal animals imipramine, the prototype of tricyclic antidepressants, exerts anticholinergic and antihistaminic properties similar to the phenothiazine-like antipsychotic drugs. These effects explain many of the side effects observed following the administration of tricyclic antidepressants but probably have little relevance to the clinical therapeutic activity. Recently, it has been observed that tricyclic antidepressants block histamine H_2-receptors in brain and responses mediated by histamine H_1-receptors in cultured mouse neuroblastoma cells. The relevance, if any, of these acute antihistamine effects of the drugs to their therapeutic efficacy is unknown. Like the phenothiazines, tricyclic antidepressants decrease spontaneous motor activity, potentiate the action of barbiturates and alcohol, slow the frequency of the EEG, and reduce the arousal reaction to sensory stimuli. With regard to these pharmacological properties, the difference between tricyclic antidepressants and phenothiazine-like antipsychotic drugs is quantitative rather than qualitative in nature.

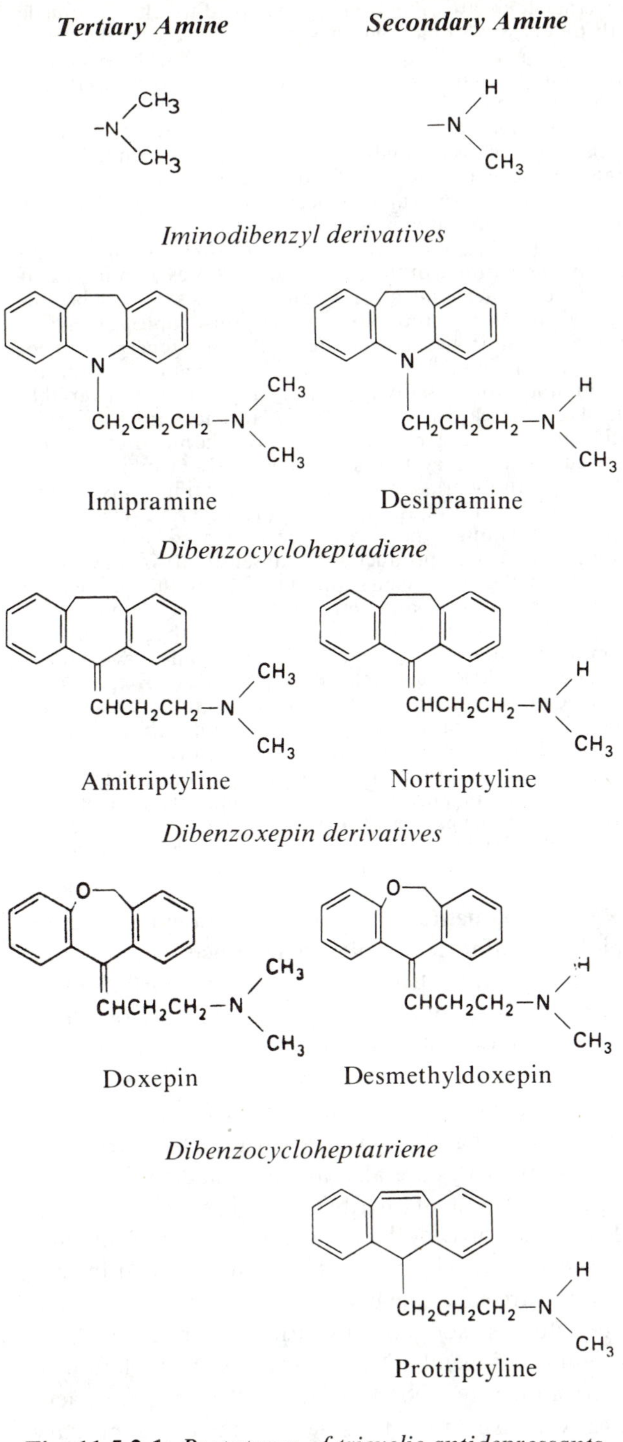

Tertiary Amine ***Secondary Amine***

$-N(CH_3)_2$ $-N(H)CH_3$

Iminodibenzyl derivatives

$CH_2CH_2CH_2-N(CH_3)_2$ — Imipramine

$CH_2CH_2CH_2-N(H)CH_3$ — Desipramine

Dibenzocycloheptadiene

$CHCH_2CH_2-N(CH_3)_2$ — Amitriptyline

$CHCH_2CH_2-N(H)CH_3$ — Nortriptyline

Dibenzoxepin derivatives

$CHCH_2CH_2-N(CH_3)_2$ — Doxepin

$CHCH_2CH_2-N(H)CH_3$ — Desmethyldoxepin

Dibenzocycloheptatriene

$CH_2CH_2CH_2-N(H)CH_3$ — Protriptyline

Fig. 11.5.2-1: *Prototypes of tricyclic antidepressants.*

Imipramine-like drugs enhance and prolong (over a wide dose range) noradrenergic responses elicited by pre- or postganglionic sympathetic stimulation. Generally, secondary amines are more potent in enhancing these responses than the corresponding tertiary amines which, in higher concentrations, exert chlorpromazine-like adrenoceptor-blocking properties.

Although it is difficult to show qualitative differences in the pharmacological profile of tricyclic antidepressants and the structurally related phenothiazine derivatives in normal animals, such differences become apparent in animals with abnormal CNS activity. Thus, tricyclic antidepressants antagonize or prevent various autonomic effects elicited by reserpine [e.g., decreased sympathetic activity (hypothermia, ptosis), increased parasympathetic activity (miosis, diarrhea, bradycardia), and decreased motor and/or exploratory activity]. The reserpine antagonism by tricyclic antidepressants is caused by their potentiation of norepinephrine at noradrenoceptor sites and by their anticholinergic activity.

Mode of Interaction with Adrenergic and Serotonergic Mechanisms

Inhibition of Neuronal Reuptake of Biogenic Amines. Though tricyclic antidepressants have been reported to inhibit monoamine oxidase (MAO) *in vitro* there is little or no convincing evidence that these drugs block MAO under *in vivo* conditions; the levels of brain norepinephrine, dopamine, and serotonin are not increased following their administration.

Tricyclic antidepressants inhibit the neuronal reuptake mechanism for biogenic amines (10). Generally, tertiary amine tricyclic antidepressants are more potent than the corresponding secondary amines in blocking the reup-

Table 11.5.2-1
Inhibition of Monoamine Uptake by Established and Potential Antidepressants[a]

Drug	Norepinephrine	Serotonin	Dopamine
Amitriptyline	+	++	0
Nortriptyline	+++	+	0
Imipramine	++	+++	0
Desipramine	++++	+	0
Protriptyline	+++	+	0
Chlorimipramine	++	++++	+
Desmethylchlorimipramine	+++	+	0
Doxepin	++	++	0
Iprindole	0	0	0
Mianserin	0	0	0
Fluoxetine	0	+++	0
Nisoxetine	++++	0	+
Zimelidine	+	+++	0
Nomifensine	+++	+	+++
Amoxapine	+++	++	0
Maprotiline	+++	+	0
Trazodone	0	+	0

[a] 0 = Inactive; + = weak inhibitor; ++ = moderate inhibitor; +++ = strong inhibitor; ++++ = potent inhibitor.

take of serotonin, and secondary amines are more potent inhibitors than their corresponding tertiary amines of the neuronal reuptake of norepinephrine (Table 11.5.2-1). Tricyclic antidepressants act as competitive inhibitors of the high-affinity uptake of norepinephrine. This increases the availability of norepinephrine at noradrenoceptor sites and can explain many of the pharmacological actions of the drugs, such as the potentiation of exogenous norepinephrine or of norepinephrine released by sympathetic nerve stimulation as well as the antagonism of decreased sympathetic activity caused by reserpine. The blockade of serotonin reuptake by tricyclic antidepressants results in an accumulation of this amine at postsynaptic serotonergic receptor sites. The different potencies of tertiary and secondary amines of tricyclic antidepressants as inhibitors of the neuronal uptake of norepinephrine and serotonin are reflected in the effect of these drugs on the firing rate of norepinephrine- or serotonin-containing cells. Tertiary amines (preferential serotonin-uptake inhibitors) decrease the firing rate of serotonergic raphe neurons, whereas secondary amines exert minimal or no effect in equivalent doses. In contrast, the spontaneous activity of norepinephrine-containing cells in the locus ceruleus is markedly depressed by secondary amines of tricyclic antidepressants, whereas their corresponding tertiary amine analogs are much weaker. With the exception of nomifensine, tricyclic antidepressants do not appreciably inhibit the uptake of dopamine into dopaminergic neurons.

Inhibition of Neuronal Reuptake and Therapeutic Activity. The question of whether the clinical therapeutic activity of tricyclic antidepressants is more closely related to inhibition of norepinephrine or serotonin reuptake cannot be unequivocally answered because these drugs affect transport mechanisms of both amines or are converted *in vivo* to metabolites that, in concert with the parent drug, will inhibit the uptake of both amines. If differences in the relative inhibition of the uptake of serotonin and norepinephrine are indeed of clinical therapeutic significance, controlled clinical trials with more selective uptake inhibitors such as maproptiline (selective norepinephrine-reuptake inhibitor) and fluoxetine (selective serotonin-uptake inhibitor) should provide more definite answers to the problem.

Adaptive Regulation at Pre- and Postsynaptic Sites. The inhibitory effects of tricyclic antidepressants on the uptake of norepinephrine and/or serotonin occur within minutes, whereas clinical therapeutic action requires treatment for several weeks. The reported adaptive changes occurring after chronic but not acute administration of tricyclic antidepressants may be clinically relevant. Thus, repeated administration of desipramine produces a significant decrease in the activity of tyrosine hydroxylase in brain areas with noradrenergic projections, whereas no significant changes in enzyme activity occur 24 hr following the administration of a single dose of the drug. Such adaptive changes in biosynthetic capacity are compatible with findings of a decreased rate of turnover of norepinephrine following chronic administration of tricyclic antidepressants.

Besides the discrepancy in the time-course between uptake inhibition and the clinical therapeutic action of tricyclic antidepressants, there are other findings that are difficult to reconcile with the classic amine hypothesis of affective disorders. For example, the tricyclic iprindole does not inhibit the uptake of either norepinephrine or serotonin and the therapeutic efficacy of the tetracyclic mianserin appears not to be related to inhibition of monoamine uptake. Thus, an acute increase in the availability of catechol and/or indolealkylamines is not directly related to the therapeutic activity of antidepressant drugs, nor is a blockade of neuronal uptake mechanisms for biogenic amines a prerequisite for antidepressant activity.

Recent results have provided evidence that tricyclic antidepressants, regardless of their acute effect at presynaptic sites, if administered on a clinically relevant time basis cause subsensitivity of the postsynaptic noradrenoceptor-coupled adenylate cyclase system in brain structures with noradrenergic projections (22, 23). This delayed action of tricyclic antidepressants on noradrenoceptor sensitivity is generally but not invariably linked to a decrease in the density of β-adrenoceptors. Tricyclic antidepressants share this delayed action on the noradrenoceptor-coupled adenylate cyclase system with MAO inhibitor-type "atypical" antidepressants such as maprotiline, nisoxetine, zimelidine, mianserin and iprindole (Table 11.5.2-1) and also with ECT. Though the role of the decreased density of β-adrenoceptors in the production of subsensitivity is not yet fully understood, the results lend support to the view that the delayed therapeutic action of antidepressants may be related to this delayed change in noradrenoceptor function, thus leading to a deamplification of the norepinephrine cyclic adenosine monophosphate (cAMP) mediated information flow. Extrapolated to the clinical situation, one is tempted to speculate that depression-prone patients may suffer from an inability to regulate properly or, more precisely, to down-regulate central noradrenergic receptor activity rather than from a simple deficiency in norepinephrine and/or serotonin. Treatment with antidepressant drugs and ECT would then depend on the successful induction of subsensitivity of the noradrenergic receptor system.

Pharmacokinetics The tricyclic antidepressants are rapidly and almost completely absorbed from the gastrointestinal tract. Because a significant portion of an oral dose is metabolized during the first pass through the liver, the bioavailable dose is less than 100%. The tricyclic antidepressants are extensively bound to plasma proteins, with the free fraction accounting for less than 10% of the total drug concentration in plasma. These very lipid-soluble drugs are also highly bound to tissue and have large volume of distribution values.

The action of tricyclic antidepressants is terminated almost exclusively by biotransformation to polar metabolites that are subsequently excreted in urine. Less than 5% of a dose is excreted in the urine as unchanged drug. The routes of metabolism involve N-demethylation of tertiary amines to secondary amines that are pharmacologically active, and, to a lesser extent, to primary amines; N-oxidation; dealkylation of the entire side chain; and ring hydroxylation of either the parent compound or the demethylated products with subsequent excretion in the urine as conjugates. The latter pathway of inactivation accounts for 50-75% of the dose in the urine. Marked species differences in the pattern and rate of metabolism of imipramine and desmethylimipramine are found. For example, after imipramine administration, desipramine accumulates in the tissues of humans and rats, but not in rabbits or mice. Studies on the metabolic fate of amitriptyline have shown that N-demethylation and hydroxylation are also the major metabolic reactions for this tricyclic antidepressant. However, whereas imipramine is hydroxylated in position 2 of the aromatic ring, amitriptyline is hydroxylated at the ethylene bridge, thus forming the alcoholic metabolite 10-hydroxyamitriptyline.

Metabolism in Humans. The half-lives of tricyclic antidepressants in humans listed in Table 11.5.2-2 show that the rate of metabolism of these drugs decreases with age, perhaps partially accounting for the greater incidence of side effects in elderly patients. Given the relatively long half-lives, several days of treatment are required to reach steady-state plasma levels. Single daily doses are adequate and even preferred because of greater patient compliance.

The steady-state plasma levels of these drugs show a 10- to 20-fold variation among patients taking the same dose, suggesting that dose alone is not a reliable indicator of the amount of drug at the active site. Further, for at least one tricyclic (nortriptyline), the relationship between plasma levels and clinical response is curvilinear; at either low or high plasma levels, only a small percentage of the patients respond relative to the percentage of patients who improve at plasma levels between 50 and 150 ng/ml. However, not every investigation has found evidence for a "therapeutic window" for nortriptyline, and certainly this may not be true for every tricyclic antidepressant. For example, imipramine is the only other tricyclic that has been extensively studied in this way; the available data suggest a linear relationship between plasma level and clinical outcome. However, most investigators agree that measurements of the plasma levels of tricyclic antidepressants are valuable, indeed perhaps necessary, for the proper management of the patient (6). This should be done at least once, preferably about 2-3 weeks after initiation of treatment, when steady-state plasma levels are obtained; the therapeutic response should be near maximum at a given dose.

Table 11.5.2-2
Plasma Half-Lives of Commonly Used Tricyclic Antidepressants

Drug	$t_{1/2}$ (Hours)
Imipramine	9-28
Desmethylimipramine	20-25
Amitriptyline	20-30
Nortriptyline	35-45
Chlorimipramine	15-20
Desmethylchlorimipramine	25-50
Protriptyline	72-120

Role of Metabolites. It is generally assumed that, other than the demethylation of tertiary amines to secondary amines, the metabolism of tricyclic antidepressants yields inactive products. However, recent evidence suggests that the ring-hydroxylated products are also pharmacologically active. Furthermore, the hydroxylated metabolites of imipramine, desipramine and nortriptyline attain levels in blood and tissues that are nearly equal to those of the parent compounds, so they may partially mediate both therapeutic and cardiotoxic effects of tricyclic antidepressants. Because there are marked differences between tertiary and secondary amines of tricyclic antidepressants with regard to modifying noradrenergic and/or serotonergic neuronal activity, any of the multitude of factors known to alter hepatic metabolism can influence the ratio of tertiary/secondary amine and thus the pharmacological profile of this type of drug.

'Interaction with Other Drugs. The blockade of catecholamine uptake by tricyclic antidepressants may enhance the actions of the catecholamines themselves and of directly acting sympathomimetic drugs, even to the point of causing a hypertensive crisis. Further, the initiation of antidepressant therapy in patients who are chronically taking the antihypertensive drugs guanethidine, bethanidine, or debrisoquin will interfere with or nullify the antihypertensive action, as the latter drugs are actively transported into sympathetic nerve terminals and tricyclic antidepressants block their access to the site of action. Careful monitoring of patients on anticoagulants is required, since tricyclic antidepressants have been reported to increase the half-life of oral anticoagulants. Phenobarbital has been reported to decrease the plasma levels of tricyclic antidepressants, whereas methylphenidate and phenothiazines may increase their plasma levels.

The early literature contains alarming reports of potentially fatal complications (hypertensive and hyper pyretic episodes, convulsions and death) in patients simultaneously treated with MAO inhibitors and tricyclic antidepressants. More recently, the combined use of these drugs has been reexamined with the conclusion that the hazards are possibly exaggerated.

Adverse Effects. Except for allergies and idiosyncratic reactions, side effects generally are an extension of each drug's pharmacological actions and occur more frequently at higher doses. Elderly patients are more sensitive to the adverse effects, particularly urinary retention and paralytic ileus. Some degree of tolerance to most of the side effects usually develops within 2 weeks, although symptoms related to the CNS, such as drowsiness and tremor, may persist.

The most frequent side effects are related to the anticholinergic activity of tricyclic antidepressants and include blurred vision (myopia and loss of accommodation), dryness of mouth, sweating, urinary retention, constipation and, rarely, paralytic ileus. Precipitation of acute glaucoma may occur, but this is rare and usually occurs in narrow-angle glaucoma.

The most common CNS effects are drowsiness and a fine tremor that occurs in about 10% of elderly patients. Epileptiform seizures may occur in patients without a prior history of seizure disorders, but these occur infrequently and only after high doses. In some individuals, a latent schizophrenia may become overt, and tricyclic antidepressants can occasionally precipitate hypomania or mania in patients with bipolar illness. The therapeutic maneuver is to stop the tricyclic drug as the patient is emerging from depression.

Cardiovascular effects include orthostatic hypotension, which may force discontinuation of therapy, tachycardia, and a number of ECG changes including flattened or inverted T-waves and prolonged PR and QRS intervals that may occur at therapeutic serum levels. With large overdoses, severe cardiotoxicity, including cardiac arrhythmias, bundle branch and complete heart blocks, may occur. In view of these known effects of tricyclic antidepressants on cardiac conduction, their use in persons with known cardiac disease should be carefully considered.

Neuroendocrine effects including galactorrhea, amenorrhea, loss of libido in men, and excessive weight gain occur relatively infrequently, although the latter is one of the main reasons for noncompliance. Allergic and idiosyncratic reactions are rare and include cholestatic jaundice that subsides upon discontinuation of the drug, skin rashes, bone marrow depression and agranulocytosis.

Acute overdose may lead to life-threatening cerebral excitation, respiratory depression and myocardial toxicity. As little as 10 times the daily dose may be fatal. Treatment is symptomatic, although gastric lavage may be helpful. The onset of the symptoms is rapid, so speed is of utmost importance. Early signs of anticholinergic poisoning may include mydriasis, hyperpyrexia, hyperreflexia, confusion, agitation and delirium. ECG changes with an anticholinergic origin range from sinus tachycardia to atrial arrhythmias that respond well to neostigmine methylsulfate; ventricular arrhythmias may be treated cautiously with lidocaine or phenytoin. A profound hypotension may develop but usually disappears if the cardiac arrhythmias are corrected. Convulsions, if they occur, are treated with i.v. diazepam. Patients should always be monitored for at least 72 hr because symptoms may reoccur.

Patients treated with 150 mg of imipramine or more for 2 months or longer frequently show symptoms of withdrawal within 2-4 days following abrupt discontinuation of treatment. These symptoms, consisting of nausea, vomiting, diarrhea, cramps, chills, insomnia and anxiety, can be avoided by gradual discontinuation of the drug.

Preparations. *Imipramine,* USP (TOFRANIL, PRESAMINE) oral or i.m. (150-300 mg/day). *Amitriptyline,* USP (ELAVIL, ENDEP) oral or i.m. (150-300 mg/day). *Doxepin,* USP (SINEQUAN) oral (75-200 mg/day). *Desipramine,* USP (NORPRAMINE, PERTOFRANE) oral (150-250 mg/day). *Nortriptyline,* USP (AVENTYL) oral (75-150 mg/day). *Protriptyline,* USP (VIVACTYL) oral (15-60 mg/day).

MONOAMINE OXIDASE INHIBITORS

Monoamine oxidase (MAO) catalyzes the oxidative deamination of a large number of monoamines, some of which (norepinephrine, epinephrine, dopamine, serotonin) are believed to function as neurotransmitter substances in the central and peripheral nervous systems. Other substrates for MAO may have physiological roles as modulators of nerve function or are pharmacologically active if ingested in food (phenylethylamine, tryptamine, tyramine). MAO is predominantly localized in the outer membrane of mitochondria and catalyzes the conversion of an aliphatic amine to an aldehyde, which is then converted rapidly to the corresponding carboxylic acid by aldehyde dehydrogenase (oxidation) or to the corresponding alcohol by alcohol dehydrogenase (reduction).

Based on substrate and inhibitor specificity, two forms of MAO have been defined. *Type A* MAO prefers norepinephrine and serotonin as substrates and is preferentially inhibited by clorgyline. *Type B* MAO prefers phenylethylamine and benzylamine and is preferentially inhibited by deprenyl. Tyramine, tryptamine and dopamine are substrates of both forms. Substrate and inhibitor selectivities for MAO A or MAO B are relative rather than absolute characteristics. Most tissues, including brain, contain various proportions of both type A and type B enzymes, whereas human platelet MAO is electrophoretically homogeneous and appears to consist only of the B form. It has not yet been resolved whether these two forms represent distinct enzymes, polymers, or different conformations of the same enzyme or the same enzyme in different membrane environments.

The mood-elevating (antidepressant) effects of the first potent MAO inhibitor, iproniazid, became apparent during its use as a chemotherapeutic agent for the treatment of tuberculosis. The clinical use of MAO inhibitors as antidepressants has, however, been limited because of severe side effects such as the precipitation of hypertensive crises resulting from interaction with dietary factors (e.g., tyramine in cheese). However, in recent years they have been used more frequently for treatment of atypical depression with predominant anxiety and phobic symptoms.

Classification and Metabolic Fate. For practical purposes, MAO inhibitors can be classified as hydrazine derivatives and a heterogenous group designated as nonhydrazines (Fig. 11.5.2-2). Details in chemistry and structure-activity relationships are discussed by Maxwell and White (14).

The MAO inhibitors are readily absorbed after oral administration. The onset of enzyme inhibition may be delayed for the hydrazine type, perhaps because these drugs are cleaved to active products. A major pathway of metabolism of hydrazine drugs, such as phenelzine, is acetylation. Marked differences in the rate of acetylation are found in phenelzine-treated patients, and some studies suggest differences in therapeutic and toxic effects in slow and fast acetylators. Isocarboxazid is metabolized by cleavage to benzylhydrazine and subsequent excretion in the urine as hippuric acid. Hippuric acid is a major urinary metabolite of tranylcypromine formed by oxidative cleavage of the side chain to benzoic acid and conjugation with glycine. These drugs are irreversible inhibitors of MAO, so the duration of their action is determined by enzyme regeneration, a process that takes several weeks.

Biochemical Effects. The administration of MAO inhibitors causes an increase in the concentration of various amines in animals and humans. Inhibition of MAO in rats, mice, rabbits and monkeys leads to an elevation of cerebral serotonin, nore-

Hydrazide derivatives

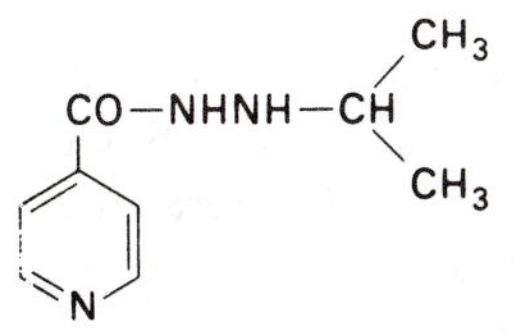

Iproniazid

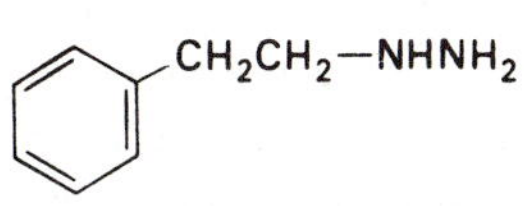

Phenelzine

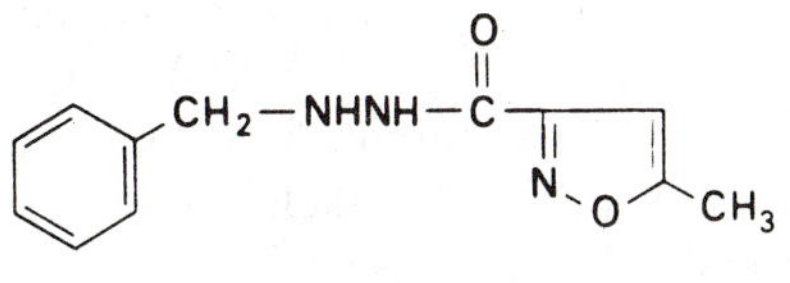

Isocarboxazid

Nonhydrazide derivatives

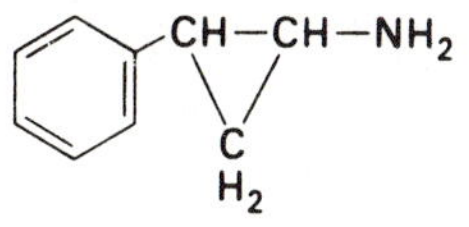

Tranylcypromine

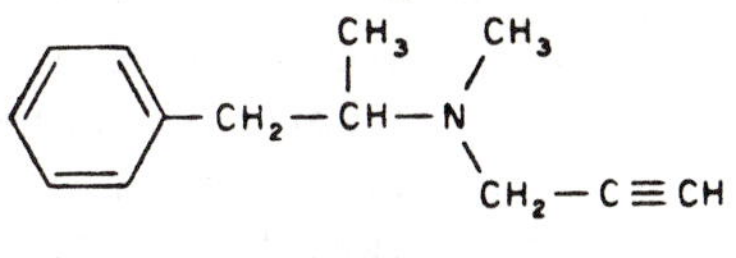

Deprenyl

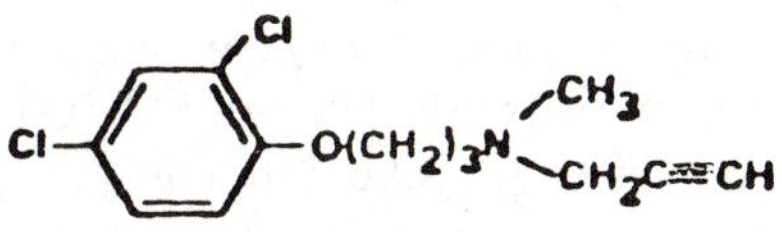

Clorgyline

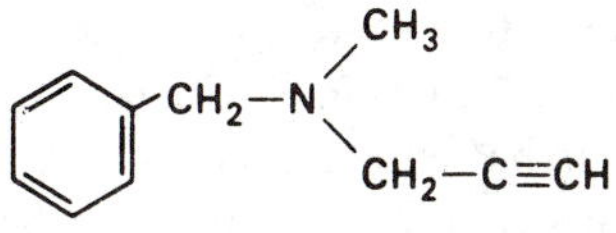

Pargyline

Fig. 11.5.2-2: *Chemical structures of MAO inhibitors.*

pinephrine and dopamine, whereas in cats and dogs only the level of serotonin is elevated. Because marked CNS stimulation occurs in rats, mice and rabbits, but not in cats and dogs, the hypothesis has been advanced that CNS stimulation and perhaps the antidepressant activity in humans are the consequence of an increased level of brain catecholamines or serotonin that, in turn, increases the availability of the physiologically active amines at central catecholaminergic or serotoninergic receptor sites. A number of monoamines (tryptamine, octopamine) whose levels in tissue are extremely low have been shown to accumulate following the administration of MAO inhibitors. In addition to increasing the concentration of monoamines, MAO inhibitors concomitantly decrease the formation and excretion of the deaminated metabolites of norepinephrine [dihydroxymandelic acid, vanillylmandelic acid (VMA), 3-methoxy-4-hydroxyphenylglycol (MHPG)], serotonin (5-hydroxyindoleacetic acid) and dopamine [homovanillic acid (HVA)]. MAO inhibitors are also known to inhibit the neuronal uptake of neurotransmitters, although this effect is not common to all. Although the acute administration of MAO inhibitors increases the availability of norepinephrine at receptor sites and thus enhances noradrenergic activity, the chronic administration of these drugs causes subsensitivity of noradrenoceptor systems in brain, linked to a reduction in the density of β-adrenoceptors.

MAO inhibitors, particularly the hydrazines, interfere with a variety of other enzymes, including diamine oxidase, cholinesterase, amino acid decarboxylase and hepatic drug-metabolizing enzymes.

Pharmacological Effects. The pharmacological actions of MAO inhibitors of practical importance are:

1. CNS stimulation
2. Lowering of blood pressure
3. Antianginal effects

In most species, MAO inhibitors increase locomotor activity and prevent the sedative and hypothermic effects of reserpine. A casual relationship between CNS stimulation and MAO inhibition is fairly well established and generally related to the increased availability of catecholamines or serotonin. Some MAO inhibitors (e.g., tranylcypromine and phenelzine) exert amphetaminelike sympathomimetic effects.

Many MAO inhibitors reduce arterial blood pressure. However, the fact that some but not all MAO inhibitors cause hypotension may indicate that enzyme inhibition is not responsible for this effect. A bretylium-like activity, accumulation of the false transmitter octopamine, and ganglionic blockade have been suggested as possible explanations. The antianginal effect is poorly understood but could be the consequence of decreased cardiac work resulting from lowered blood pressure.

Mechanism of Antidepressant Action. Although some investigators report that depression is associated with lower platelet and brain MAO activity, others have found no difference or significantly increased MAO levels. The mechanism(s) of action of the MAO inhibitors in human depression are not known, but the biochemical consequences of enzyme inhibition (increased availability of catecholamines and serotonin) at central adrenergic or serotoninergic receptor sites can accommodate both the catecholamine hypothesis (deficiency of catecholamines) and the indolealkylamine hypothesis (serotonin deficiency) of affective disorders.

It is of interest that MAO inhibitors, if administered on a clinically relevant time basis, share with various prototypes of tricyclic and other antidepressants, and with electroconvulsive treatment (ECT), the ability to cause subsensitivity of central noradrenoceptor systems linked to a down-regulation of β-adrenoceptors. The decreased noradrenoceptor function resulting from prolonged therapeutic administration of different prototypes of drugs that alleviate depression in humans suggests that their therapeutic action may be related to this common delayed postsynaptic change in noradrenoceptor function rather than to their acute and often opposite action (or lack of action) at presynaptic sites.

Interaction with Other Drugs. MAO inhibitors interfere with the metabolism of barbiturates, aminopyrine, acetanilide, cocaine and meperidine and thus prolong the effects of these drugs. They also potentiate the action of anticholinergic agents, sympathomimetic amines, and amphetamine-like drugs. A life-threatening hypertensive crisis may be initiated by the latter in combination with MAO inhibitors. Caution is urged in using MAO inhibitors in combination with tricyclic antidepressants, but early reports of adverse consequences have not been substantiated.

An important interaction between these drugs and diet is the "tyramine-cheese" reaction in which a hypertensive crisis is precipitated in patients treated with MAO inhibitors who ingest foods rich in tyramine or other pressor agents such as phenylethylamine and L-DOPA. Tyramine occurs in many foods (cheeses, wines, pickled products) as a byproduct of certain fermentation reactions; its pressor action is normally terminated by metabolism by liver MAO, and blockade of this inactivation leads to the hypertensive attack. The syndrome consists of sudden onset of a severe headache usually occipital in location, vomiting, hyperpyrexia, chest pain, muscle twitching, and restlessness. The attack usually disappears in a few hours, but it may cause fatal intracranial bleeding. Patients and family members should be warned and given lists of dietary items and drugs that may lead to this reaction. If a hypertensive crisis develops, the MAO inhibitor should be withdrawn immediately. Because the MAO inhibition caused by hydrazine-type inhibitors is irreversible, several weeks must elapse before tyramine-containing foods are safe. Severe cases of hypertension may require the administration of an α-adrenoceptor-blocking drug, such as phentolamine.

Adverse Effects. Numerous side effects and adverse reactions, some of which may be related to MAO inhibition, may occur in patients treated with MAO inhibitors. CNS side effects include insomnia, irritability, motor restlessness, tremor, agitation, and seizures, which can be viewed as an extension of the CNS-stimulating properties. MAO inhibitors have been reported occasionally to precipitate an acute exacerbation of psychotic symptoms in patients with a history of schizophrenia, to initiate hypomania, and to convert a retarded depression into an agitated or anxious depression. These effects may require withdrawal of MAO inhibitors and/or the addition of an antipsychotic drug. Autonomic side effects are variable and include orthostatic hypotension, dry mouth, constipation, delayed bladder and bowel function, impotence, and delayed ejaculation. Serious liver toxicity may occur, producing a clinical syndrome similar to viral hepatitis with jaundice, diffuse hepatocellular damage, elevated serum liver enzymes, and bile stasis. Hepatic toxicity is apparently not related to dose or duration of treatment or to MAO inhibition per se. Hepatotoxicity was more common with MAO inhibitors such as iproniazid and pheniprazine, which have been removed from the market, than with the currently available MAO inhibitors. MAO inhibitors should be discontinued at any indication of abnormal liver function. Other side effects such as blood dyscrasias, red-green color blindness, and severe skin reactions have occurred following the use of some of the hydrazine derivatives.

Toxic signs of acute overdose include agitation, hallucinations, hyperpyrexia, hyperreflexia, convulsions, and blood pressure changes with both hypertension and hypotension being reported. Gastric lavage and maintenance of cardiopulmonary function may be required. Conservative treatment aimed at maintaining body temperature, blood pressure, and proper fluid and electrolyte balance is frequently successful.

Therapeutic Uses. The slow onset of the therapeutic action of MAO inhibitors (2-3 weeks) and the high incidence of spontaneous improvement of depressive episodes make it difficult to compare the efficacy of various MAO inhibitors. MAO inhibitors are often used to treat depressed patients with phobic, anxious, and obsessive-compulsive manifestations. Considering the potential toxicity of this class of antidepressants and that tricyclic antidepressants produce the same or possibly higher rate of improvement, it is generally felt that MAO inhibitors should be reserved for refractory patients who fail to respond to tricyclic antidepressants.

Preparations. MAO inhibitors marketed for use in depression (with their oral effective dose range) include: *Tranylcypromine*, USP (PARNATE): oral, 20-40 mg/day. *Isocarboxazid*, USP (MARPLAN): oral, 10-60 mg/day. *Phenelzine*, USP (NARDIL): 50-100 mg/day. *Pargyline* (EUTONYL) is marketed as an antihypertensive drug, though its pharmacological profile is similar to other MAO inhibitors that are used for the treatment of depression.

MISCELLANEOUS ANTIDEPRESSANTS

In recent years several new antidepressants (2) have been introduced in the United States, which are discussed next.

AMOXAPINE

Amoxapine (ASENDIN) is chemically a dibenzoxazepine derivative (Fig. 11.5.2-3). In experimental animals, amoxapine reduces the uptake of NE and 5-HT by the presynaptic nerve endings. It also possesses blocking effects on histamine (H_2), muscarinic acetylcholine, α_1-adrenergic and dopamine (D_2) receptors in human brain (17). Antidepressant properties of amoxapine are attributed to the 8-hydroxy metabolite of the compound.

The drug is well absorbed after oral administration and reaches the peak blood levels in about 90 min. About 90% of the drug binds to serum protein, and it has a half-life in the range of 8-30 hours. Amoxapine itself is a metabolite of an antipsychotic compound loxapine. It is almost completely metabolized and its major metabolite is 8-hydroxyamoxapine. The metabolites of amoxapine are excreted in the urine as glucuronide conjugates.

Amoxapine is indicated in patients with psychotic depression. The recommended effective dose of the drug is 200-300 mg/day and the starting dose is 50 mg three times daily. Elderly patients require lower dosage of the drug.

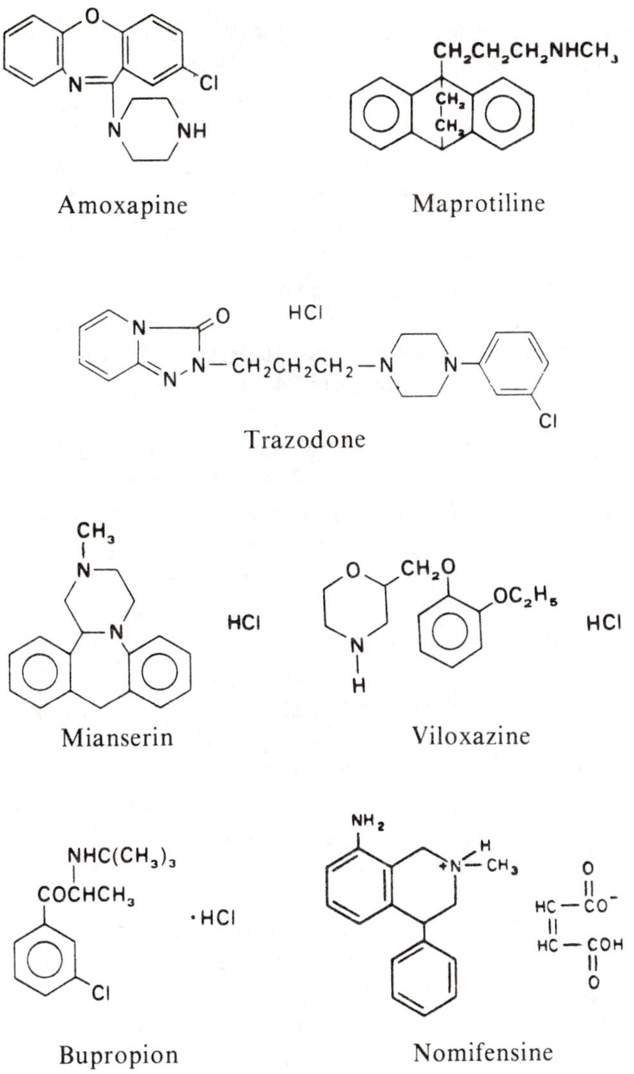

Amoxapine

Maprotiline

Trazodone

Mianserin

Viloxazine

Bupropion

Nomifensine

Fig. 11.5.2-3: *Miscellaneous antidepressants.*

The frequent adverse effects of amoxapine are drowsiness, dry mouth, constipation, and blurred vision. Because of its dopamine receptor-blocking effects, amoxapine increases serum prolactin levels, produces extrapyramidal side effects, and may induce tardive dyskinesia. It should therefore not be used routinely for treating nonpsychotic depressions.

Amoxapine is available as 50-, 100-, and 150-mg tablets.

MAPROTILINE

Maprotiline (LUDIOMIL) belongs to a new chemical series, dibenzo-bicyclooctadiens (Fig. 11.5.2-3). Maprotiline blocks neuronal uptake of both NE and 5-HT; the potency of blockade of NE uptake is higher than that of 5-HT. The drug also possesses varying degrees of blocking effect on histamine (H_2), α_1-adrenergic, and muscarinic cholinergic receptors of human brain (17).

It is rapidly absorbed from the gastrointestinal tract and has a variable half-life ranging from 27-58 hours (8). The drug has been claimed to have a rapid onset of action, but no real difference in clinical efficacy has been found between imipramine and this drug. Anticholinergic and sedative side effects and cardiotoxicity of maprotiline are said to be less than tricyclics. The usual daily dose of maprotiline ranges between 75 and 300 mg. Lower doses of the drug (50-75 mg/day) should be used in elderly patients over 60 years of age. Maprotiline is available as 25- and 50-mg tablets.

TRAZODONE

Trazodone (DESYREL) is a triazolopyridine derivative and chemically unrelated to tricyclic or other antidepressant drugs (Fig. 11.5.2-3). Trazodone has a moderate blocking effect on neuronal uptake of 5-HT. The drug has a peripheral α-adrenergic- and 5-HT-blocking activity (12).

Clinical efficacy of trazodone in depression has been reported to be comparable with other antidepressants. The drug has fewer side effects compared with conventional antidepressants. The drug is administered initially at a daily dose of 150 mg (in divided doses), and the maximum dose varies between 400 and 600 mg/day. Trazodone is available as 50- and 100-mg tablets.

MIANSERIN

Mianserin is a tetracyclic, originally developed as an antihistamine agent (Fig. 11.5.2-3). Its proposed mechanism of action is blockade of presynaptic α_2-receptors, resulting in block of autoinhibitory mechanism of NE synthesis. Its marked H_1-blocking action is probably responsible for the sedative action. Its antidepressant action is relatively weak. The drug has no anticholinergic side effects (16).

ZIMELIDINE

Zimelidine is a bicyclic agent with a selective inhibitory action on 5-HT uptake (Table 11.5.2-1). Because of its neurological toxicity, the drug has been taken off the market.

FLUVOXAMINE

Fluvoxamine is a unicyclic agent with a potent inhibitory action on 5-HT uptake and a minimal effect on NE uptake. In clinical trials, the drug has been reported to be effective at doses of 50-300 mg/day. The main side effects of the drug include nausea and a sense of fatigue without sedation (13).

VILOXAZINE

Viloxazine is a bicyclic tetrahydroxazine compound with a primary inhibitory action on 5-HT uptake (Fig. 11.5.2-3). It has no anticholinergic effects. It appears to be equally effective as tricyclic antidepressants. Like tricyclics, viloxazine also lowers the convulsive threshold. It has a short half-life (2-5 hours), and its cardiovascular side effects are less compared with tricyclic compounds (3).

BUPROPION

Bupropion is a chlorpropiophenone with a relatively weak inhibitory action on NE and 5-HT uptake, but with a potent inhibitory action on DA uptake (21) (Fig. 11.5.2-3). It has a rapid onset of action, and its antidepressant effects appear to be equal to those of tricyclics. Its main side effects are dryness of the mouth and insomnia, and it has been reported to exacerbate psychotic symptoms.

NOMIFENSINE

Nomifensine is a tetrahydroisoquinoline with primary inhibitory action on both NE and DA uptake, and a weak action on 5-HT uptake (Fig. 11.5.2-3). It is also reported to be a 5-HT receptor antagonist. It has been reported to elicit amphetamine-like actions in animal studies, which may account for its side effects such as insomnia, restlessness, tachycardia, and nausea in humans (19).

THERAPY OF DEPRESSION

Somatic treatment is one of the cornerstones of the treatment of depressive illness. However, even more so than with the treatment of schizophrenia, the judicious use of psychosocial treatments such as individual psychodynamic, behavioral, or cognitive therapy, group therapy, family therapy, and activity therapy may be necessary and sufficient for the optimal treatment of some depressed patients (9).

The treatment of most depressed patients does not require hospitalization. Some form of psychosocial treatment and administration of adequate doses of an antidepressant medication are usually sufficient to restore most depressed patients to their previous level of functioning. The monoamine oxidase (MAO) inhibitors are not the first antidepressant drugs to prescribe because they are generally less efficacious than the tricyclic antidepressants. MAO inhibitors are also potentially more dangerous because of their ability to potentiate the toxic effect of ingested biogenic amines such as tyramine. However, patients with atypical depressions (e.g., those characterized by marked phobic and anxious symptoms) may respond better to MAO inhibitors than to tricyclic antidepressants.

The most widely used drugs for the treatment of depression on an outpatient basis are the tricyclic antidepressant or related agents, iprindole and doxepin (7, 15). These drugs may be most efficacious in the treatment of patients with retarded depression rather than those who have marked agitation. Therapy is generally begun with small divided doses to determine the nature and extent of any untoward side effects. Sedation and anticholinergic side effects tend to be higher with amitriptyline and lower with desipramine. Some depressed patients with manic-depressive (bipolar) illness may escalate into a manic phase within several days or weeks of beginning treatment with tricyclic antidepressants.

Although there are proposals for biochemical predictors of good clinical response to imipramine [e.g., low levels of 3-methoxy-4-hydroxyphenylglycol (MHPG) in 24-hour urine collections] or to amitriptyline (high levels of MHPG), such suggestions require further verification before they can be recommended for routine use. Any one of the approved tricyclic antidepressants, or related drugs such as doxepin or iprindole, may be utilized. The usual starting dose is 50 mg/day. A dose of 150 mg should be reached by the end of the first week of treatment. The dose should be increased if there is little or no response within 2 weeks. The usual maximum therapeutic doses are in the range of 250-300 mg, although some patients may require doses as high as 450-600 mg/day. An exception is protriptyline, which is effective in doses of 10-60 mg/day.

Because the half-life of these drugs is approximately 24 hours, they may be given in a single dose several hours before bedtime to minimize the anticholinergic and sedative effects during daytime, take advantage of the sedative effects to induce sleep, and increase patient compliance.

Clinical improvement may be noted within a week but not infrequently requires 2-3 weeks of treatment. If a patient fails to respond to the usual maximum dose of an antidepressant, one of the new antidepressants such as trazodone may be utilized.

In treating depressed patients, one must be ever alert to the possibility of suicide. It is incumbent upon the physician to clarify the suicidal plans of depressed patients. Hospitalization is indicated when patients cannot provide believable assurance that they do not plan to commit suicide.

The somatic treatment of hospitalized depressed patients usually involves the use of tricyclic antidepressant medication or the equivalent, such as trazodone or amoxapine. Not infrequently, depressed patients are hospitalized only after they have failed to respond to an outpatient trial of antidepressant medication. Often the problem has been that the dose was insufficient to achieve adequate blood levels. Thus, a second trial of tricyclic antidepressant—possibly a secondary tricyclic if the first trial was with a tertiary tricyclic, or vice versa, and at higher dosages—may be successful.

Some patients with major depressive disorder fail to respond to any tricyclic antidepressant despite adequate blood levels. There is no single sequence of treatment that can be universally applied in such treatment-resistant patients. It should be recognized that if the depression is severe, manifesting vegetative symptoms and suicide risk, electroconvulsive therapy (ECT) may be indicated.

If the tricyclic-resistant patient has bipolar illness, the addition of lithium carbonate to the tricyclic antidepressant has recently been reported to produce very rapid improvement in some patients. If this fails, the combination of a tricyclic antidepressant with an MAO inhibitor or with a neuroleptic drug may be tried next. The combination of an MAO inhibitor and a tricyclic antidepressant is not approved by the Food and Drug Administration because there is some evidence that the combination may be toxic. However, there have been a number of reports that the combination is safe when used cautiously, and it may be effective in patients who fail to respond to either drug alone.

In a female with unipolar major depressive disorder who does not respond to tricyclic antidepressants, the addition of L-triiodothyronine (LT_3) sodium 25 μg/day has been reported to increase the efficacy of a tricyclic alone. Failure of trial(s) with tricyclic antidepressants, with or without LT_3, can be followed by a trial with an MAO inhibitor or combined MAO inhibitor and tricyclic antidepressant therapy. If the patient is psychotically depressed, as evidenced by the presence of delusions or hallucinations, the addition of an antipsychotic drug to the tricyclic antidepressant is often effective. Neuroleptic drugs by themselves have definite antidepressant properties.

Amoxapine, a recently introduced antidepressant that also has neurolepticlike properties. Because of this, it may contribute to the development of tardive dyskinesia. Amoxapine may be indicated in cases where the combination of a neuroleptic and a tricyclic antidepressant is indicated.

ECT has been shown to be more effective than chemotherapy alone in patients with severe depression (5). Although antidepressant medications are always used first in depressed outpatients, ECT is sometimes administered on an outpatient basis, particularly in patients who had a good response to ECT for a previous episode of depression, or in patients requiring maintenance treatment following a course of ECT as inpatients. ECT has an important role in the treatment of severely depressed, suicidal patients, particularly when antidepressant medications as well as one of the various forms of psychotherapy or other nonsomatic treatments have failed.

In depressed patients who have responded to an antidepressant, it is common clinical practice to continue lower doses of maintenance medication for an additional 3-5 months after the initial course of treatment. In patients with recurrent depressive episodes, it may be necessary to continue treatment for much longer periods of time. If a depressed patient has a history of prior manic episodes, treatment with lithium carbonate in addition to the antidepressant drug should be considered. After 4-6 months, lithium alone may be adequate for prophylactic purposes.

ANTIMANIC DRUGS

LITHIUM SALTS

Lithium salts were used in the late 1940s as popular substitutes for patients on sodium-free diets. In 1949, Cade (4) reported the successful treatment of manic patients with lithium carbonate, and then lithium's value in the treatment of affective illness was seriously considered. It is of interest that the disease-specific antimania effect of lithium was recognized in this first report on the use of this alkali ion in psychiatry.

Lithium belongs to the alkali metals, having the smallest cation radius (0.60 Å) of this group. It occurs in trace amounts in the body.

Pharmacological Effects and Mode of Action. In therapeutic amounts, lithium does not exhibit marked sedative or excitatory actions in laboratory animals. Lithium enters excitable cell membranes through the Na^+ channels or ionophores. It has been suggested that lithium entry through the Na^+ channel may inhibit calcium entry during the action potential and thereby inhibit the stimulus-coupled release of norepinephrine or other putative neurotransmitters. Once lithium is inside the cell, it is removed by the active cation pump at one-eighth to one-twenty-fifth of the rate of Na^+; consequently, lithium accumulates intracellularly. Most likely for this reason, a better correlation exists between the lithium level in red blood cells and that in brain than between plasma and brain levels.

The acute administration of lithium results in an increased turnover and deamination of norepinephrine, whereas chronic administration of lithium decreases the rate of norepinephrine turnover and enhances norepinephrine reuptake by synaptosomal fractions. Lithium has also been found to inhibit the release of norepinephrine from brain slice preparations. All these mechanisms would tend to decrease the availability of the physiologically active norepinephrine at noradrenoceptor sites. Finally, lithium has been found to inhibit the basal and norepinephrine-stimulated adenylate cyclase activity and to slightly decrease β-adrenergic-receptor binding.

Short-term administration of lithium increases the high-affinity uptake of tryptophan into synaptosomes of brain, an increase associated with a proportional increase in the conversion of tryptophan to serotonin. Chronic treatment with lithium, though not affecting the increased uptake of tryptophan, causes a reduction in the activity of tryptophan hydroxylase. In accordance with the data,clinical studies demonstrate an increased accumulation of 5-hydroxyindoleacetic acid in the CSF following administration of probenecid in patients acutely treated with lithium and a return to control values or below after prolonged administration of lithium.

Pharmacokinetics. Lithium is readily absorbed from the gastrointestinal tract following oral ingestion. Peak plasma levels occur 2-4 hours after a single oral dose of lithium carbonate. Lithium rapidly distributes to the liver and kidney and is more slowly absorbed by muscle, bone, and brain. The lithium concentration in the thyroid gland reaches two to five times that in serum. Elimination takes place predominantly through the kidneys; after glomerular filtration, lithium is reabsorbed with Na^+ and water in the proximal tubules. Dietary Na^+ restriction can lead to the accumulation of lithium and severe intoxication, whereas the addition of salt to the diet increases the excretion of lithium. Severe toxicity has been observed in patients using diuretics that cause Na^+ loss.

Therapeutic Uses. The therapeutic efficacy of lithium in the treatment of mania is well established, with an improvement rate of 60-100%. Lithium has a more specific effect against mania than neuroleptics, which cause a "drugged" state. Also, lithium is disease-specific, whereas the neuroleptics generally act on all cases of excitation regardless of etiology. The onset of therapeutic action is gradual over a period of 6-10 days, with normalization occurring in 1-3 weeks. In emergency cases, as in acute manic episode, chlorpromazine, and particularly haloperidol, may be preferred to initiate treatment, as these drugs cause a rapid, effective suppression of the manic overactivity and restlessness. Subsequently, maintenance treatment with lithium can be substituted.

Although lithium has demonstrated superior efficacy over placebo in the maintenance treatment of bipolar recurrent affective illness, decreasing the frequency, severity, and duration of episodes, the prophylactic use of lithium in recurrent unipolar depression is controversial. It is not as effective as the tricyclic antidepressants in treating depression in bipolar or unipolar depressed patients, but because tricyclic antidepressant drugs frequently induce manic episodes in patients with manic-depressive illness, it may be necessary to treat depressed bipolar patients simultaneously with lithium and antidepressant medication or to use lithium alone. The therapeutic value of lithium in the treatment of schizophrenia, schizoaffective disorders, anxieties, phobias, and obsessive-compulsive disorders is inconclusive. Lithium treatment must be sufficient to give plasma levels ranging from 0.6 to 1 mEq/l but should be kept below 2 mEq/l to prevent toxicity. There is some evidence that the prophylactic effects of lithium are just as great at blood levels close to 0.6 mEq/l as at higher levels. Because of concern about possible long-term toxic effects of lithium on renal function, it may be most prudent to reduce the dosage to the amount needed to produce the lower blood levels.

Adverse Effects. The side effects at therapeutic serum concentrations of lithium are generally mild and include nausea, muscular weakness, fine tremors of the hands, and fatigue. Lithium frequently produces polyuria and polydipsia, which are fully reversible on discontinuation of the medication. When serum levels of lithium rise to values above 2 mEq/l, more severe toxicity may develop including ataxia, slurred speech, drowsiness, confusion, impaired consciousness, and coma. A few patients have developed a state of hypothyroidism with diffuse nontoxic goiters following chronic treatment with lithium. Because the kidney is the only important route of lithium excretion, the treatment of severe lithium poisoning has to be aimed at increasing the lithium clearance (e.g., by saline infusion). In cases of very severe poisoning, the benefits of dialysis, either peritoneal dialysis or hemodialysis, may outweigh the risks.

Preparations. The most readily available salt is lithium carbonate; 1 millimole of lithium is equal to 6.9 mg of lithium and is contained in 37 mg of lithium carbonate. Commercially available preparations are in the form of 300-mg capsules (LITHANE, ESKALITH, LITHONATE). The dosage in adults with normal kidney function ranges between 25 and 50 millimoles/day that equals 300-500 mg lithium carbonate t.i.d., which will normally produce an effective serum lithium level ranging between 1 and 1.5 mEq/l.

REFERENCES

1. Akiskal, H. S., and McKinney, W. T. Overview of recent research in depression. *Arch. Gen Psychiatry* 32:285, 1975.
2. *AMA Drug Evaluation,* 5th ed. Chicago: American Medical Association, 1983, p. 241.
3. Ban, T. A., McEvoy, J. P., and Wilson, W. H. Viloxazine: A review of the literature. *Int. Pharmacopsychiatry* 15:118, 1980.
4. Cade, J. F. J. Lithium salts in the treatment of psychotic excitement. *Med. J. Aust.* 2:349, 1949.
5. Fink, M. *Convulsive Therapy: Theory and Practice.* New York: Raven Press, 1979, p. 1.
6. Glassman, A. H., and Perel, J. M. Tricyclic blood levels and clinical outcome: A review of the art. In: *Psychopharmacology: A Generation of Progress* (Lipton, M. A., Dimascio, A., and Killam, K. F., eds.). New York: Raven Press, 1978, p. 917.
7. Hollister, L. E. Tricyclic antidepressants. *N. Engl. J. Med.* 229:1168, 1978.
8. Hollister, L. E. Current antidepressant drugs: Their clinical use. *Drug* 22:129, 1981.
9. Klerman, G. L., DiMascio, A., Weissman, M., Prusoff, B. A., and Paykel, E. S. Treatment of depression by drugs and psychotherapy. *Am. J. Psychiatry* 131:186, 1971.
10. Koe, B. K. Molecular geometry of inhibitors of the uptake of catecholamines and serotonin in synaptosomal preparations of the rat brain. *J. Pharamacol. Exp. Ther.* 199:649, 1976.
11. Kuhn, R. Uber die Behandlung depressiver Zustande mit einem Iminodibenzylderivat (G-22355). *Schweiz. Med. Wochemschr.* 87:1135, 1957.
12. Lapierre, Y. D. New antidepressant drugs. *J. Clin. Psychiatry* 44(8, sec. 2):41, 1983.
13. Lapierre, Y. D., Oyewumi, L. K., and Coleman, B. The efficacy of fluvoxamine as an antidepressant. *Clin. Trials J.* 18:313, 1981.
14. Maxwell, R. A., and White, H. J. Tricyclic and monoamine oxidase inhibitor antidepressants: Structure-activity relationships. In: *Handbook of Psychopharmacology,* Vol. 4 (Iversen, L. L., Iversen, S. D., and Snyder, S. H., eds.). New York: Plenum Press, 1978, p. 83.
15. Morris, J. B., and Beck, A. T. The efficacy of antidepressant drugs. *Arch. Gen. Psychiatry* 30:667, 1974.
16. Pinder, R. M., Blum, A., Stulemeijer, S. M. et al. A double blind multicenter trials comparing the efficacy and side-effects of mianserin and chlorimipramine in depressed in and outpatients. *Int. Pharmacopsychiatry* 15:218, 1980.
17. Richelson, E. Pharmacology of antidepressants to use in the United States. *J. Clin. Psychiatry* 43:4, 1982.
18. Roth, M. The classification of affective disorders. *Pharmakopsychiatry Neuropsychopharmakol.* 11:27, 1978.
19. Sharma, S. D. A double-blind clinical evaluation of nomifensin, a new dopaminergic antidepressant. *Curr. Ther. Res.* 27:157, 1980.
20. Shaw, D. M. The practical management of affective disorders. *Br. J. Psychiatry* 130:432, 1977.
21. Soroko, F. E., Mehta, N. B., Maxwell, R. A. et al. Bupropion hydrochloride [(±) α-t-butylamino-3-chloropropriophenone HCl]: A novel antidepressant agent. *Common. Pharm. Pharmacol.* 29:767, 1977.
22. Sulser, F. New cellular mechanisms of antidepressant drugs. In: *New Frontiers of Psychotropic Drug Research* (Fielding, S., and Lal, H., eds.). New York: Futura Publishing, 1979, p. 29.
23. Sulser, F. Mode of action of antidepressant drugs. *J. Clin. Psychiatry* 44(sec. 2):14, 1983.

ADDITIONAL READING

Barbaccia, M.L., Ravizza, L., and Costa, E. Maprotiline: An antidepressant with an unusual pharmacological profile. *J. Pharm. Exp. Therap.* 236:307, 1986.

Frazer, A. et al. Pharmacologic mechanisms of action of antidepressants. *Psychiatr. Clin. North Am.* 7:575, 1984.

CHAPTER

11.5.3

DRUGS FOR THERAPY OF ANXIETY

Steven M. Paul, Paul J. Marangos and Phil Skolnick

Anxiety is a ubiquitous emotion experienced throughout life. Though it may be defined as an unpleasant feeling characterized by uneasiness and apprehension, anxiety is also a strong motivating force in many forms of behavior and, like fear, may have fundamental adaptive and perhaps evolutionary significance. Excessive or pathological anxiety is clearly undersirable and is a very frequent medical complaint either alone or in combination with other psychiatric disorders such as depression. Physiological and psychiatric perspectives of anxiety have been extensively reviewed by Lader (18) and Lehmann (20). Drugs used in the treatment of anxiety (anxiolytics or minor tranquilizers) comprise the largest class of prescribed drugs in the world (24). In 1977, for example, nearly 70 million prescriptions were written for diazepam (VALIUM) and chlordiazepoxide (LIBRIUM) in USA alone; this represents nearly 8000 tons consumed in a single year.

HISTORY

The earliest antianxiety agents in clinical use, the bromides, various alcohols (including ethanol), and other closely related analogs (such as chloral hydrate and paraldehyde), were largely supplanted by the barbiturates, which are still occasionally used for this purpose. These latter compounds are used primarily as sedative-hypnotics and have been largely replaced by safer and more efficacious drugs.

The era of modern antianxiety agents began with the introduction of the propanediols in the early 1950s. The development of the agents derived from efforts to find a nonaddicting anxiolytic lacking the potentially lethal respiratory depressant properties of the barbiturates. Meprobamate, a propanediol carbamate that became available in 1955, is regarded as the first relatively specific antianxiety agent. Although still used extensively, it has been largely overshadowed by the benzodiazepines, a group of compounds that represents the most important class of antianxiety agents in terms of both utilization and efficacy.

CLASSIFICATION

Chemical and pharmacological classes of drugs used in the treatment of anxiety are listed in Table 11.5.3-1 with their doses. Pharmacology of these drug classes will be described; relative attributes of the broad groups and individual classes will be discussed in the last section.

PROPANEDIOL CARBAMATES

MEPROBAMATE

Meprobamate was synthesized by Berger and coworkers as a potential muscle relaxant in an attempt to find a more potent and long-lasting derivative of mephenesin (4). It is a simple aliphatic compound (Fig. 11.5.3-1) that is rapidly absorbed after oral administration. Peak plasma levels are attained within 1-2 hr after ingestion, and complete elimination usually occurs within 24-36 hr (half-life of approximately 11 hr). Only 10% of the drug is excreted unchanged; most is oxidized to hydroxymeprobamate or eliminated as the glucuronide conjugate. Meprobamate is widely and rather uniformly distributed throughout the body as well as in various regions of the brain.

Pharmacological Effects. In general, the pharmacological effects of meprobamate are similar to other CNS depressants, such as the barbiturates (3). In common with other antianxiety agents, the drug has potent muscle-relaxant and anticonvulsant properties. Both of these effects are observed at subsedative doses, but their relationship to the antianxiety effects of the drug is unclear. Behaviorally, meprobamate does not affect classically

Table 11.5.3-1
Chemical and Pharmacological Classes and Dosage for Antianxiety Drugs

Class and Drug	Bedtime Dose [a] (mg)	Daytime Dose (mg) (1-2 times)	Maximum[b] Total (mg)
1. Sedative-hypnotic			
Barbiturates			
Phenobarbital	32-65	16	100
Propanediol carbamate			
Meprobamate	400-800	200-400	1600
Benzodiazepines			
Chlordiazepoxide	10-50	5-25	100
Diazepam	2-10	2-5	20
Oxazepam	15-30	10-15	60
Prazepam	20	10-20	60
Clorazepate	7.5-30	3.75-30	45
Halazepam	40	20-40	160
Lorazepam	1-4	1-2	10
Alprazolam	0.5	0.25-0.5	4
2. Sedative-autonomic			
Diphenylmethane antihistamines			
Hydroxyzine	25-50	10-25	100
Diphenhydramine	25-50	10-25	100
Phenothiazine antipsychotics			
Trifluoperazine	5-10	2-5	20

[a] Wherever possible, use sngle daily dose at night with doses during day taken only as required.
[b] All doses are a rough guide. Maximum doses may be less than required by some patients; they are unlikely to lead to any physical dependence.

Source: Modified from Ref. 15.

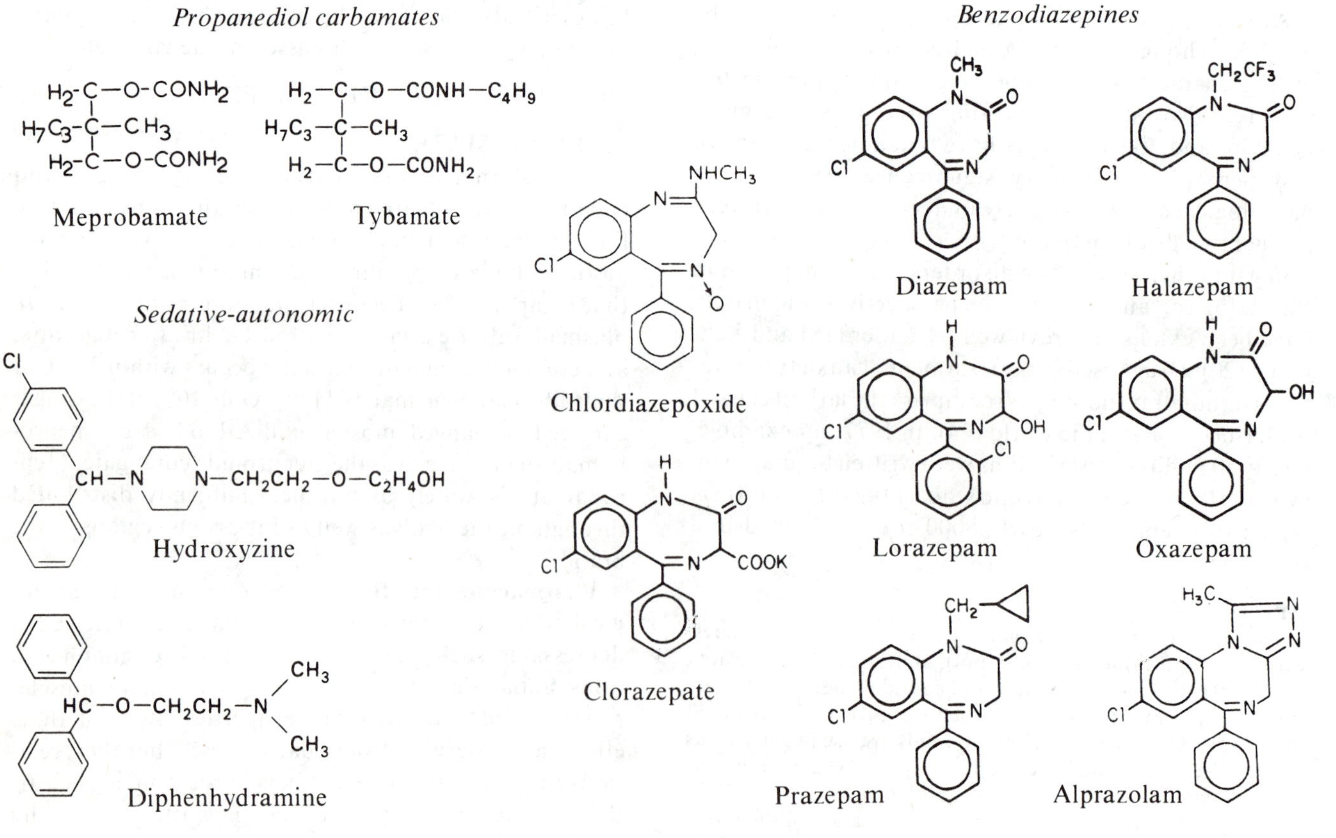

Propanediol carbamates

Meprobamate

Tybamate

Chlordiazepoxide

Benzodiazepines

Diazepam

Halazepam

Sedative-autonomic

Hydroxyzine

Lorazepam

Oxazepam

Clorazepate

Diphenhydramine

Prazepam

Alprazolam

Fig. 11.5.3-1: *Chemical structures of commonly used antianxiety drugs.*

conditioned responses but suppresses the autonomic (i.e., visceral) responses that accompany conditioned reflexes. Similar autonomic responses are seen in anxious patients or in normal subjects as a response to stressful situations.

Mechanism of Action. The exact mechanism of action of meprobamate is unknown. Its muscle-relaxant and anticonvulsant (and perhaps anxiolytic) properties may stem from a depressant effect on nerve conduction in interneurons (3). For example, meprobamate depresses various multineuronal reflexes such as the flexor or crossed extensor reflex but has little effect on monosynaptic reflexes such as the knee jerk. In relatively low doses, meprobamate will counteract the neuronal hyperexcitability produced by strychnine and tetanus toxin, effects believed to be mediated through central interneurons. The biochemical basis for these neurophysiological actions is unknown. Meprobamate has been shown not to exert significant effects on central biogenic amine release, turnover or metabolism. It has been noted that the structures of many of the propanediol carbamates (i.e., mephenesin and mephenoxalone) bear a striking resemblance to the β-adrenergic blockers (12); whether this is simply coincidence or relates to the mechanism of action of the propanediol carbamates remains to be determined.

Tolerance, Dependence and Abuse. It is generally accepted that *tolerance* develops to the clinical effects of meprobamate (2). As with the barbiturates, meprobamate will induce the hepatic microsomal drug-metabolizing enzymes, increasing its own metabolism and contributing to the development of tolerance. *Addiction* to meprobamate can occur after prolonged use at high doses. Serious withdrawal reactions (probably related to the drug's relatively short half-life) have been reported and should be carefully considered in patients being managed during chronic use of the drug. Physical signs of withdrawal, not unlike those seen during alcohol withdrawal, have been reported following discontinuation of doses in the therapeutic range (1200-2400 mg/day). Serious signs of withdrawal (e.g., seizures) are not uncommon after discontinuing larger doses (>3000 mg/day).

Adverse Effects. These reactions of meprobamate are, in general minor. Serious adverse reactions include allergic and dermatological reactions such as urticarial or maculopapular rashes; these idiosyncratic reactions are uncommon and are usually observed after only a few doses. Meprobamate is less dangerous with respect to acute toxicity than the barbiturates, but its therapeutic index (ratio between lethal and therapeutic dose) is much less than for the benzodiazepines. Because meprobamate induces the hepatic drug-metabolizing enzymes, it can alter the metabolism and pharmacological effects of many other drugs, a fact that should be considered when prescribing it with other agents.

Preparations. *Meprobamate* (MILTOWN, EQUANIL) comes in 200-, 400- and 600-mg tablets. It is also marketed as a suspension for oral use. The usual daily dose is 1200-1600 mg. Other propanediol carbamates include *tybamate* (TYBATRON), *carisoprodal* (SOMA, RELA) and *metbutamate* (CAPLA).

BENZODIAZEPINES

History. The benzodiazepines are a rather remarkable group of compounds used not only as anxiolytics, but also as hypnotics, anticonvulsants and muscle relaxants (24). Clinically active benzodiazepines were first synthesized by Sternbach and colleagues in the late 1950s (29). Chlordiazepoxide (LIBRIUM), the first 1,4-benzodiazepine introduced into clinical use (1960), was followed a few years later by a more potent derivative, diazepam (VALIUM), and more recently by the popular hypnotic flurazepam (DALMANE). As a result of the economic incentives resulting from the development of safe antianxiety agents, literally thousands of benzodiazepine derivatives have been synthesized and tested. At the present time there are approximately a dozen benzodiazepines (including the triazolobenzodiazepines and 1,5-benzodiazepines) in therapeutic use throughout the world. Eight of them are currently available in the United States as anxiolytics (Table 11.5.3-1). Although the various benzodiazepines differ significantly in their clinical potencies, there is no evidence that at behaviorally equivalent doses there are any major differences in efficacy. Furthermore, although several benzodiazepines such as flurazepam (DALMANE) and nitrazepam (MOGADON) are marketed specifically as hypnotics, recent reports suggest that these agents are no more effective as hypnotics than diazepam.

Chemistry. The benzodiazepines were derived from a group of compounds described in the early German literature as the 4,5-benzo-hept-1,2,6-oxidiazines (12, 29). The parent 1,4-benzodiazepine and some of the more common benzodiazepines are pictured in Fig. 11.5.3-1. Most clinically effective benzodiazepines contain a phenyl substituent at the 5 position. Electron-withdrawing substituents at position 7 are essential for anxiolytic activity, whereas substitutions at positions 6, 8 and 9 lead to a marked diminution or complete loss of activity. Substitution of a methyl group in position 1 of the B ring (i.e., the amide nitrogen) also enhances anxiolytic activity while further increasing the size of the alkyl group in this position results in a decrease in activity. Substitution(s) at the ortho position of the C ring by electron-withdrawing groups (e.g., halogens) enhances anxiolytic activity, while substitution at the meta- and para-positions decreases activity. The phenyl group (C ring) does not appear to be essential for anxiolytic activity, since bromozepam, which contains a pyridine substituent, is reported to be an effective antianxiety agent with little or no sedating effects. The addition of a triazolo moiety on the B ring (triazolobenzodiazepines) produces compounds that have been reported to be more potent than diazepam. The chemistry of benzodiazepines has been extensively studied; the reader is directed to other more comprehensive reviews for more detailed structure-activity relationship (12, 29).

Pharmacological Effects. In humans the benzodiazepines have a spectrum of pharmacological actions that include (a) anxiolytic, (b) anticonvulsant, (c) muscle-relaxant and (d) sedative-hypnotic effects. Although they have been demonstrated to be superior to placebo in reducing anxiety in numerous well-controlled clinical studies (14), not all studies have shown significant drug-placebo differences, a fact that is probably related to the highly variable and episodic nature of anxiety (14).

In animals the antianxiety effects of the benzodiazepines are readily demonstrable in a number of experimental paradigms. Perhaps the most impressive effect(s) of the benzodiazepines is their ability to "release" conditioned and unconditioned behaviors previously suppressed by punishment (22). These behavioral paradigms are called *conflict situations* because the behavioral response(s) of the animal are both rewarded and punished. In the conflict paradigm, untreated animals will normally be influenced by punishment and will suppress responses for the rewarding stimulus (e.g., food and water in hungry and thirsty rats). Benzodiazepines (as well as other anxiolytics) characteristically enhance the behavioral responses for the rewarding stimulus during conditions of punishment. The major clinical effects of the benzodiazepines in humans also involve a decrease in the behavioral and autonomic consequences of frustration, fear and punishment; thus, the conflict test may represent a useful animal model of anxiety (21). This assumption is further supported by the relatively specific anticonflict effect of the benzodiazepines where other psychotropic drugs (e.g., phenothiazines, analgesics, antidepressants) are without effect. Other animal tests, including antagonism to pentylenetetrazol and cat muscle-relaxant tests, are extremely good predictors of anxiolytic activity in humans and are generally used as initial screening tests for potential antianxiety agents (22).

Mechanism of Action. Benzodiazepines have been shown to affect many neurotransmitter systems within the brain and spinal cord, including cholinergic, noradrenergic, serotonergic, dopaminergic and glycinergic pathways. Despite well-documented effects on these systems, it is questionable whether these effects are directly related to the drugs' mechanism of action, or are simply epiphenomena.

Neurophysiological evidence suggests that the benzodiazepines selectively facilitate the transmission of the major inhibitory neurotransmitter γ-aminobutyric acid (GABA) at multiple levels in the brain and spinal cord (13). More recent biochemical studies (see later) also support an important role for GABA in potentiating benzodiazepine action at the neuronal or cellular level (7). It is likely that some of the pharmacological effects of the benzodiazepines (although it is not clear which effects) are mediated via actions on this neurotransmitter system. Although the facilitory action of benzodiazepines on GABAergic transmission may be of importance for the anticonvulsant properties of the benzodiazepines, behavioral studies have failed to demonstrate synergistic actions between GABA and the benzodiazepines (6). In contrast to the neurophysiological studies, which fail to support a role for serotonin in the mechanism(s) of action of the benzodiazepines, behavioral studies suggest a role for serotonin in mediating the anticonflict activity of the benzodiazepines in animals (28). Nonetheless, because complex behavioral states such as anxiety may involve multiple neurotransmitter systems, it may be too simplistic to postulate that only one neurotransmitter system is involved in all of the actions of these drugs.

The recent demonstration of high-affinity, saturable and stereospecific binding sites for benzodiazepines in the CNS has provided perhaps the most useful information concerning the biochemical mechanisms of action of these compounds (27, 31). The good correlations obtained between the antianxiety (clinical) potencies of a series of pharmacologically active benzodiazepines and their abilities to bind to these sites suggest that they are, in fact, pharmacological receptors. The presence and pharmacological importance of benzodiazepine receptors in the brain has now been confirmed by many investigators (30). It is generally accepted that binding to these receptors represents the first step in a cascade of events responsible for the pharmacological action(s) of the benzodiazepines.

The existence of these receptors and the absence of any known normally occurring compounds capable of interacting with them further suggest the presence, in the brain, of a heretofore unidentified benzodiazepine-like substance(s). Recently, a number of compounds capable of displacing radioactively labeled benzodiazepines from receptor sites have been isolated from brain tissue. These substances have been identified as the purines (inosine, hypoxanthine and nicotinamide). Both electrophysiological as well as behavioral evidence suggest a benzodiazepinelike action for these compounds. However, whether or not these effects occur under physiological conditions has not been determined. Furthermore, other more potent inhibitors of diazepam binding to benzodiazepine receptors have been isolated but are as yet unidentified (30).

Although initial studies on the benzodiazepine receptor failed to support a pharmacological interaction between the receptor and any of the known neurotransmitters, more recent evidence suggests a role for GABA (30) in the regulation of this receptor. Incubation of brain membranes with GABA (or GABA-like compounds) *in vitro* results in a marked increase in the affinity of radioactive benzodiazepines for the benzodiazepine receptor. This phenomenon has also been shown to occur *in vivo* by administering drugs that elevate brain GABA levels (30). It has been reported that benzodiazepine receptors enhance GABA-mediated chloride conductance allosterically across the neuronal membrane (26). These biochemical studies support previous neurophysiological and pharmacological ones, implicating GABA in the mechanism(s) of action of the benzodiazepines.

It has been suggested that two pharmacologically distinct receptors exist for benzodiazepines. These receptor sites are termed type I and type II. Type I receptors have been proposed to mediate anxiolytic actions of benzodiazepines. Type II receptors may mediate actions like ataxia and sedation (9).

The search for a naturally occurring ligand to the benzodiazepine receptor and the ultimate characterization of such a substance will have broad implications in neurobiology. In this regard, the use of the benzodiazepine receptor assay as a rapid screening test for new antianxiety agents has already resulted in the development of two new nonbenzodiazepine drugs that have been shown to have anxiolytic effects in animal screening tests (30). One of these agents, a triazolopyradizine, apparently lacks many of the undesirable side effects (e.g., sedation) observed with the benzodiazepines themselves.

Pharmacokinetics. Subtle structural modification of the benzodiazepines results in alterations in absorption, distribution and metabolism. Diazepam (the most widely used benzodiazepine) will be discussed as a prototype. It appears to be completely and rapidly absorbed, reaching peak plasma concentrations within 1 hr after oral administration. The benzodiazepines are extremely lipophilic compounds, which explains their accumulation in adipose tissue and rapid uptake into brain. In experimental animals, for example, brain levels of diazepam at 1 min after intravenous administration are higher than the corresponding blood levels (8). This fact probably accounts for the efficacy of benzodiazepines in the acute management of seizure disorders such as status epilepticus (5). The rate and completeness of absorption of benzodiazepines following intramuscular injection are variable (11).

Diazepam metabolism proceeds by N-demethylation and hydroxylation at the 3 position. Both the N-demethylated (nordiazepam) and hydroxylated (oxazepam) metabolites of diazepam are pharmacologically active and probably account for the long-acting effects of the parent drug. Oxidation reactions are impaired in old age, hepatic cirrhosis, and during concurrent therapy with drugs such as cimatidine, estrogens, disulfiram, or isoniazid (11). Excretion of the benzodiazepines and their hydroxylated and demethylated metabolites usually occurs in urine as the glucuronide conjugate. The elimination of diazepam from the body is biphasic, with a rapid elimination phase ($t_{1/2}$ of 2-3 hr), followed by a slower phase ($t_{1/2}$ 2-8 hr).

Tolerance, Dependence and Abuse. The question of whether tolerance develops to the behavioral effects of the benzodiazepines is somewhat controversial. Although most clinical investigators agree that tolerance develops to the major side effects (sedation), there is little evidence documenting the development of tolerance to the anxiolytic effects (21). These observations are supported by studies in experimental animals where tolerance has been shown to develop to the sedation and ataxia observed after acute or subacute administration of relatively high doses of the benzodiazepines, but not to their anticonflict or antipentylenetetrazol activity, pharmacological effects that are highly indicative of anxiolytic activity in humans (21, 22). Nevertheless, clinical studies on the development of tolerance are difficult to carry out because of the episodic and vascillating nature of anxiety. In addition, the benzodiazepines are most useful in the short-term treatment of "relatively transient forms of anxiety, fear and tension" (2); thus, chronic use is generally not indicated for most patients.

Serious questions have been raised concerning the incidence of psychological and/or physical dependence to the benzodiazepines (2, 23). There appears to be little doubt that psychological dependence can develop, especially after chronic use of relatively high doses. Furthermore, serious withdrawal reactions (e.g., seizures) have been reported after discontinuing similar doses. Physical dependence to the benzodiazepines, however, is not likely unless dosages between 10 and 20 times the recommended daily dose are used. Recent study, however, has shown that definite withdrawal symptoms can occur on discontinuation of long-term normal doses of benzodiazepines (19). The clinician should be aware that the onset of withdrawal symptoms after discontinuing such doses is considerably later than that seen with meprobamate or the short-acting barbiturates. In summary, the potential for abusing benzodiazepines is more significant than was previously thought, and thus careful monitoring of the frequency and quantity prescribed is essential.

Adverse Effects. Fatal overdoses following ingestion of even large amounts of benzodiazepines are quite rare. Oral doses as high as 2-3 g have been reported to produce little or no serious respiratory or cardiovascular problems. However, most deliberate overdoses usually involve more than one agent, and the combination of benzodiazepines and other CNS depressants (e.g., alcohol) can be lethal. Although effective treatment of benzodiazepine overdose can be achieved by supportive measures only, it has been reported that CNS depression can be reversed by physostigmine (1).

The most common side effects of the benzodiazepines include daytime sedation and drowsiness. Ataxia or motor incordination is not uncommon, especially in the elderly. Idiosyncratic reactions including hepatic damage, blood dyscrasias, and dermatological reactions are quite rare. Stimulation of appetite is a not an uncommon side effect seen with the benzodiazepines as well as other anxiolytics.

The benzodiazepines readily pass the placental barrier and although no major developmental anomalies are reported to be associated with benzodiazepine use in pregnancy, subtle behavioral effects are known to occur in experimental animals (16). Diazepam, as well as its major metabolites, has been identified in human breast milk at concentrations approximately 10% of those in plasma. In most cases, these concentrations are probably too low to affect the nursing infant.

Preparations. *Chlordiazepoxide*, USP (LIBRITABS) and *chlordiazepoxide hydrochloride*, USP (LIBRIUM) are supplied in capsules of 5-, 10- and 25-mg sizes. Ampules containing 100 mg of chlordiazepoxide are also available for parenteral administration. The usual single dose ranges from 5 to 25 mg, and starting daily dosages are approximately 20-30 mg. *Diazepam*, USP (VALIUM) is available in tablet form (2, 5, 10 mg) as well as in 2-ml ampules (5 mg/ml) for i.v. or i.m. injection. Daily divided doses of 2-40 mg are administered according to the severity of symptoms and the age of the patient. *Oxazepam*, USP (SERAX) is available in capsules of 10, 15, 30 mg. The usual daily dose ranges from 30 to 120 mg, again depending on the severity of symptms.

Lorazepam (ATIVAN), 0.5-, 1-, 2-mg tables. For i.m. and i.v. injection 2- and 4-mg/ml cartridge needle units or 10-ml vials. *Prazepam* (CENTRAX), 5-, 10- and 20-mg capsuls and 10-mg tablets. *Halazepam* (PAXIPAM), 20- and 40-mg tablets. *Clorazepate dipotassium* (TRANXENE), 3.75-, 7.5- and 15-mg capsules and tablets. *Alprazolam* (XANAX), 0.25-, 0.5- and 1-mg tablets.

MISCELLANEOUS ANXIOLYTICS

A number of miscellaneous drugs, including some of the antihistaminics and β-adrenergic blockers, are also used in the treatment of anxiety. These compounds are usually prescribed for other purposes, but their continued, and in some cases increasing, use in anxious patients warrants discussion.

DIPHENYLMETHANE ANTIHISTAMINICS

The two most common drugs in this class are hydroxyzine and diphenhydramine. These drugs have also been called *sedative-autonomics* because, in contrast to other anxiolytics, they have significant effects on the autonomic nervous system (14). They differ from the classic antianxiety agents in that they tend to increase muscle tone, lower seizure threshold, and are not associated with physical dependence. Cross-tolerance, as seen among the more common sedative-tranquilizers, is not observed with these drugs.

Hydroxyzine is commonly given to relieve the temporary anxiety associated with medical and dental procedures. Because it also has antiemetic properties, it has been considered especially useful as a preoperative medication. The exact mechanism(s) of action of these drugs as anxiolytics is unknown, although they have been shown to depress neuronal activity in certain limbic areas of the brain that are believed to be involved in emotional behavior.

The diphenylmethane antihistaminics appear to be relatively safe, as few serious side effects have been reported. They do potentiate the effects of meperidine and barbiturates, and their use in early pregnancy is contraindicated.

Preparations. *Hydroxyzine hydrochloride* or *hydroxyzine pamoate* (ATARAX, VISTARIL) are available in tablet form (10, 25, 50, 100 and 500 mg) and as a syrup (10 mg or 25mg/5 ml). Dosages, depending on individual requirements, vary from 75 to 100 mg/day. *Diphenhydramine* (BENADRYL) is available in capsules of 25 and 50 mg.

β-ADRENERGIC BLOCKERS AND NEWER AGENTS

Recently, there has been increased interest in the use of β-adrenergic blockers, structurally related to the propanediol carbamates (Fig. 11.5.3-1) for the treatment of anxiety. The β-blockers seem to be particularly useful in the somatic manifestations of anxiety, such as tachycardia, trembling, sweating, and so on (12). Although a number of studies indicate that β-blockers are quite useful, especially in acute episodes of anticipatory anxiety (e.g., stage fright), their mechanism(s) of action remain contrtoversial, since practolol, a β-adrenergic blocker that does not cross the blood-brain barrier, has also been reported to be an effective anxiolytic (12). Whether the antianxiety effects of the β-adrenergic blockers involve central or peripheral mechanism(s) will require further investigation.

A number of newer potential anxiolytics have been shown to have *antianxiety* effects in animals (12, 30) and are currently being studied in humans. Glaziovine, a naturally found alkaloid, was reported to have anxiolytic properties similar to diazepam, apparently without significant sedative properties (12).

In recent years buspirone, an azaspirodecanedione, has been reported to possess consistent and significant efficacy in the treatment of generalized anxiety in several double-blind trials (10). The drug has both dopamine agonist and antagonist properties and has an anxiolytic spectrum similar to diazepam (25) with less abuse liability. It appears to have fewer side effects than diazepam.

TREATMENT OF ANXIETY

Anxiety is a primary symptom associated with many kinds of emotional disorders as well as a frequent secondary symptom of many medical and surgical conditions. Severe anxiety, whether primary or secondary, can be extremely disabling.

Most investigators report that between 2 and 5% of the general population in Western culture may be considered to have "pathological anxiety" (i.e., anxiety that interferes significantly with everyday functioning or is resulting in pathophysiological changes). However, within the subpopulation of psychiatric outpatients, somewhere between 6 and 27% have been diagnosed as having moderate-to-severe anxiety (14). The most important decision to be made prior to drug treatment concerns the magnitude of anxiety reaction, including both its intensity and chronicity. Because of its highly variable nature, anxiety may manifest itself in several ways. Autonomic signs of anxiety are particularly useful indicators of its intensity. The physiological or autonomic components of anxiety can also result in pathophysiological changes, including gastrointestinal disorders (e.g., colitis, ulcer), cardiovascular disorders (e.g., hypertension, tachycardia, and so on), and fatigue. Before initiating treatment with anxiolytics, it is imperative to rule out other major psychiatric disorders, such as depression and schizophrenia. This is because these disorders, including any associated anxiety, will usually respond better to antidepressants and neuroleptics, respectively.

It is also imperative to differentiate among the various subtypes of anxiety disorders (17). This is because some forms, particularly the spontaneous panic attack usually seen in agoraphobic patients, respond best to treatment with tricyclic antidepressants and monoamine oxidase inhibitors (17). Moreover, the severe anxiety frequently seen in patients with obsessive-compulsive disorder may respond better to behavioral treatment (desensitization) rather than pharmacological intervention.

Table 11.5.3-2
Comparative Favorable and Unfavorable Attributes of Some Drugs Used for Therapy of Anxiety

	Phenobarbital	Meprobamate	Benzodiazepines	Diphenhydramine	Phenothiazines
Favorable attributes[a]					
Sedative/anxiety ratio	+	++	++	±	±
Muscle relaxation	±	++	+++	0	–
Duration of action	+++	++	+++	+	++
Unfavorable attributes					
Tolerance, habituation	±	+++	±	0	0
Physical dependence	+	+++	+	0	0
Disturbed sleep pattern	++	++	±	++	++
Potential suicidal use	++	++	0	++	0

[a]Degree of probability: –, opposite effect; 0, none; ±, minimal; +, slight; ++, moderate; +++, great.
Source: Modified from Ref. 15.

Medication is indicated once it is ascertained that a patient has pathological anxiety. Nevertheless, psychotherapy (to learn the causes of anxiety and how to cope with them) and behavioral therapy should be considered as long-term treatment; environmental alterations (to avoid anxiety-producing situations) may be helpful. Anxiolytics are used for relatively short-term treatment.

Several types of drugs have been used for treatment of anxiety. Anxiolytic drugs of sedative-hypnotic type are preferred by patients and clinicians. The choice of a specific drug for an individual patient is best made on the basis of the patient's acceptance of the drug either from past experience or from experience obtained in an empirical clinical trial (15).

Benzodiazepines appear to be most extensively used. Table 11.5.3-2 shows relative favorable and unfavorable attributes of several classes of anxiolytic agents that may account for the popularity of these drugs. Of the benzodiazepines, older agents because of their long use may have been more thoroughly investigated. Chlordiazepoxide and diazepam have been used extensively in children. In the elderly and in patients with hepatitis, oxazepam and lorazepam may be favored.

A certain degree of tolerance develops to the sedative effects of the minor tranquilizers, whereas little or no tolerance has been shown for the beneficial antianxiety effects of the drugs. This group of drugs has some abuse potential and produces physical dependence. On the other hand, the sedative-autonomic group of drugs often produces feelings of inner restlessness and mental fuzziness as well as uncomfortable anticholinergic peripheral side effects, such as dry mouth and blurred vision. These effects may make these agents unlikely for abuse. Considering all these aspects, the benzodiazepines appear to be most preferable for therapy of anxiety; for a small number of patients, sedative-autonomic agents may prove to be beneficial. However, benzodiazepines are completely ineffective in 25-30% of all anxious patients (17). Some suitable combination of both types (one type promoted as a daytime sedative and the other type serving as a hypnotic being used during the night) may be useful. β-adrenergic agonists have been experimentally used to block peripheral autonomic manifestations of anxiety, but they do not show better results than benzodiazepines and need further evaluation.

REFERENCES

1. Avant, G. R., Speeg, K. V., Jr., Freemon, F. R. et al. Physostigmine reversal of diazepam-induced hypnosis: a study in human volunteers. *Ann. Intern. Med.* 91:53, 1979.
2. Baldessarini, R. J. Chemotherapy. In: *Harvard Guide to Modern Psychiatry* (Nicholi, A. M., ed.). Cambridge, Mass.: Harvard University Press, 1978, p. 424.
3. Berger, F. M. Meprobamate and other glycol derivatives. In: *Psychotherapeutic Drugs:* Part II. Applications (Usdin, E., and Forrest, I., eds.). New York: Marcel Dekker, 1977, p. 1089.
4. Berger, F. M., and Bradley, W. The pharmacological properties of α-β-hydroxy-γ-(2-methylphenyloxy) propane (Myanesin). *Br. J. Pharmacol.* 1:265, 1946.
5. Browne, T. R., and Penry, J. K. Benzodiazepines in the treatment of epilepsy. *Epilepsia* 14:277, 1973.
6. Cook, L., and Sepinwall, J. Behavioral analysis of the effects and mechanisms of action of benzodiazepines. In: *Mechanism of Action of Benzodiazepines* (Costa, E., and Greengard, P., eds.). New York: Raven Press, 1975, p. 1.
7. Costa, E., Guidotti, A., and Mao, C. C., and Suria, A. New concepts on the mechanism of action of benzodiazepines. *Life Sci.* 17:167, 1975.
8. Garattini, S., Marcucci, F., and Mussini, E. The metabolism and pharmacokinetics of selected benzodiazepines. In: *Psychotherapeutic Drugs:* II. Applications (Usdin, E., and Forrest, I. S., eds.). New York: Marcel Dekker, 1977, p. 1039.
9. Gershon, S., and Eison, A. S. Anxiolytic profiles. *J. Clin. Psychiatry* 44(11, Sec. 2):45, 1983.
10. Goldberg, H. L., and Finnerty, R. Comparison of buspirone in two separate studies. *J. Clin. Psychiatry* 43:87, 1982.
11. Greenblatt, D. J., Shade, R. I., and Abernathy, D. R. Current status of benzodiazepines. *N. Engl. J. Med.* 309:354, 1983.

12. Gschwend, H. W. Chemical approaches to the development of anxiolytics. In: *Anxiolytics* (Fielding, S., and Lal, H., eds.). Mount Kisco, N.Y.: Future, 1979, p. 1.
13. Haefely, W., Kulcsor, A., Mohler, H., Pieri, L., Polc, P., and Schaffner, R. Possible involvement of GABA in the central actions of benozdiazepines. In: *Mechanisms of Action of Benzodiazepines* (Costa, E., and Greengard, P., eds.). New York: Raven Press, 1975, p. 131.
14. Hollister, L. E. Clinical Use of Psychotherapeutic Drugs. Springfield, Ill.: Charles C. Thomas, 1973.
15. Hollister, L. E. Psychiatric disorders. In: *Drug Treatment*, 2nd ed. (Avery, G. S., ed.). New York: ADIS Press, 1980, p. 1057.
16. Kellogg, C., Tervo, D., Ison, J., Parisi, T., and Miller, R. K. Prenatal exposure to diazepam alters behavioral development in rats. *Science* 207:205, 1980
17. Klein, D. F. Anxiety reconceptualized. In: *Anxiety: New Research and Changing Concepts* (Klein, D. F., and Rabkin, J., eds.). New York: Raven Press, 1981, p. 235.
18. Lader, M. Behavior and anxiety: Physiologic mechanisms. *J. Clin. Psychiatry* 44(12, Sec. 2):5, 1983.
19. Lader, M. Dependence on benzodiazepines. *J. Clin. Psychiatry* 44:121, 1983.
20. Lehmann, H. E. The clinicians view of anxiety and depression. *J. Clin. Psychiatry* 44(8, Sec. 2):3, 1983.
21. Lippa, A. S., Greenblatt, E. N., and Pelham, R. W. The use of animal models for delineating the mechanisms of action of anxilytic agents in animal models. In: *Psychiatry and Neurology* (Usdin, E., and Hanin, I., eds.). New York: Pergamon Press, 1977, p. 279.
22. Lippa, A. S., Nash, P. A., and Greenblatt, E. N. Pre-clinical neuro-psycho-pharmacological testing procedures for anxiolytic drugs. In: *Anxiolytics* (Fieldings, S., and Lal, H., èds.). Mount Kisco, N.Y.: Futura, 1979, p. 41.
23. National Academy of Science, *Sleeping Pills, Insomnia, and Medical Practice*. Washington, D.C.: Report of a study of the Institute of Medicine, 1979.
24. Randall, L. O., and Kappell, B. Pharmacological activity of some benzodiazepines and their metabolics. In: *The Benzodiazepines* (Garattini, S., and Mussini, E., and Randall, L. O., eds.). New York: Raven Press, 1973, p. 27.
25. Rickels, K., Weisman, K., Norstad, N. et al. Buspirone and diazepam in anxiety: A controlled study. *J. Clin. Psychiatry* 43(12, Sec. 2):81, 1982.
26. Skolnick, P., and Paul, S. M. Benzodiazepine receptors in the central nervous system. *Int. Rev. Neurobiol.* 23:103, 1982.
27. Squires, R. F., and Braestrup, C. Benzodiazepine receptors in rat brain. *Nature* 226:732, 1977.
28. Stein, L., Wise, C. D., and Berger, B. D. Antianxiety action of benzodiazepines: Decrease in activity of central serotonin neurons in the punishment system. In: *The Benzodiazepines* (Garatini, S., Mussini, E., and Randall, L.O., eds.). New York: Raven Press, 1973, p. 299.
29. Sternbach, L. H. Chemistry of 1, 4-benzodiazepines and some aspects of the structure-activity relationships. In: *The Benzodiazepines* (Garatini, S., Mussini, E., and Randall, L. O., eds.). New York: Raven Press, 1973, p. 1.
30. Tallman, J. F., Paul, S. M., Skolnick, P., and Gallager, D. W. Receptors for the age of anxiety: Pharmacology of the benzodiazepines. *Science* 207:274, 1980.
31. Williamson, M., Paul, S. M., and Skolnick, P. Labeling of benzodiazepine receptors *in vivo*. *Nature* 275:551, 1978.

ADDITIONAL READING

Brown, J. T., Mulrow, C. D., and Stondemire, G. A. The anxiety disorders. *Ann. Intern. Med.* 100:558, 1984.

Chan, A.W. Effects of combined alcohol and benzodiazepine: a review. *Drug Alcohol Depend.* 13:315, 1984.

CHAPTER
11.6

DRUGS AND SUBSTANCE ABUSE

Sachin N. Pradhan, Samar N. Dutta and Leo E. Hollister

Drug abuse has been defined as "persistent or sporadic drug use inconsistent with or unrelated to acceptable medical practice" (76). Striking inconsistencies exist in the way the terms *use* and *abuse* are employed in different cultures. Thus, although smoking and nicotine are known to cause serious detrimental effects on user's health, its excessive use is only recently being taken seriously by some people. In Western society, while chronic intoxication with alcohol is usually considered drug abuse, acute intoxication on some occasions is not. However, such use does not only involve drugs used in therapy, but also many other nontherapeutic substances including marijuana, LSD, and other hallucinogenic substances.

In many cultures certain substances are used as social or religious practice and as such are not considered as abused (e.g., peyote in Mexico). It is thus difficult to define drug or substance abuse. However, when a modest amount of a chemical or a plant material is self-administered for pleasurable effects, or when use of a drug may be experimental just to test its effect out of curiosity or under peer pressure, it can then be considered as substance abuse. In general , this phenomenon results from a variety of cultural, social, psychodynamic, and behavioral factors, and each component differs from one abuser to another.

TERMINOLOGY

The various terms used in connection with substance abuse (previously termed drug abuse) have been confusing and have undergone modifications through the years.

Drug addiction is defined as a state of periodic or chronic intoxication, detrimental to the individual and society, produced by the repeated consumption of a drug (natural or synthetic). Its characteristics include: (a) an overpowering desire or need (compulsion) to continue taking the drug and to obtain it by any means; (b) a tendency to increase the dose; (c) a psychic (psychological) and sometimes a physical dependence on the effects of the drug.

Drug dependence, a single term introduced in 1964 by the WHO Expert Committee on Addiction-Producing Drugs, is defined as a state, psychic and sometimes also physical, resulting from the interaction between a living organism and a drug, characterized by behavioral and other responses that always include a compulsion to take the drug on a continuous or periodic basis in order to experience its psychic effects, and sometimes to avoid the discomfort of its absence. A person may be dependent on more than one drug (137).

Drug habituation or psychic dependence currently refers to a state of "a compulsion that requires periodic or continuous administration of a drug to produce pleasure or avoid discomfort" (56). It need not be detrimental to the individual or to the society.

Physical dependence is an altered physiological state, produced by repeated administration of a drug, that demands the continued administration of the drug in order to prevent a characteristic and specific group of symptoms (with respect to the drug), termed as the withdrawal or abstinence syndrome.

FACTORS INVOLVED IN DRUG ABUSE

In spite of extensive investigations carried out to understand the factors responsible for abuse of a drug, it has not been possible to pinpoint any particular factor or factors. A wide variety of factors have been suggested to initiate, encourage, or permit self-administration, e.g., environmental cues, personality, genetic factors, and psychological factors. The relative extent to which primary reinforcement, tolerance, physical dependence, and other factors encourage substance abuse in specific subsets of individuals are discussed briefly.

Drug as a Reinforcer. A number of psychoactive drugs serve as reinforcers to initiate a self-administration habit, and when the drug is repeatedly used it can cause a compulsive drug abuse behavior. In humans reinforcement may be in the form of a feeling of pleasure, relief of pain or discomfort, or an altered perception. The reinforcing behavior has been extensively studied in several animal specimens, e.g., rats, monkeys, and baboons in the laboratory environment. The dose, route of administration, presence of other agent(s), pretreatment with other agents, and the nature and the amount of effort required to receive a specific dose are known to modify drug-induced reinforcement (104). A drug or a substance shows certain patterns, of self-administration in experimental animals, and in humans it may act as a reinforcer even in absence of physical dependence or any preexisting psychopathological conditions.

TOLERANCE

Chronic administration of ethanol, opiates, barbiturates, benzodiazepines, and amphetamines is associated with the development of tolerance and/or physical dependence. The development of tolerance to the undesirable side effects often reinforced continued use of the drug. Chronic tolerance may not develop to all the predictable pharmacological actions of a drug. For example, with opioids tolerance develops against analgesia, euphoria, sedation and other CNS depressant effects, but not to miosis, constipation and convulsions. Indirectly, tolerance may contribute to the pattern of abuse by raising the dose in order to experience the reinforcing effects. The mechanisms involved in the development of tolerance are only partially identified and are further discussed in Chapter 3.

PHYSICAL DEPENDENCE/WITHDRAWAL SYNDROME

Physical dependence is generally viewed as a physiologic state of adaptation concomitant with the development of chronic tolerance, and sudden withdrawal of medication results in a characteristic set of withdrawal symptoms (abstinence syndrome).

The adaptational processes that finally lead to withdrawal manifestations are supposed to begin with the first dose in the case of opioids and CNS depressants. Withdrawal symptoms occur presumably due to drug-induced alterations in the CNS (predominantly), and to some extent in the peripheral nervous system. In the case of opioids withdrawal symptoms are known to occur in spinal subjects and decorticated dogs.

THEORIES OF PHYSICAL DEPENDENCE

Several theories have been put forward to explain the phenomenon of physical dependence (particularly with respect to opioids), and these are as follows:

Homeostatic Counter Adaptive Theory. Himmelsbach (50) proposed that the autonomic (especially hypothalamic) centers which are primarily responsible for maintaining homeostasis produce adaptive adjustments in response to effects of morphine. With its repeated administration, a condition of autonomic hyperreactivity is produced and the ability of morphine to disturb homeostasis is reduced, thus tolerance is developed. On withdrawal of the drug such autonomic hyperactivity is manifested representing the abstinence syndrome.

Enzyme Expansion Theory (45). Dependence-producing drugs, initially through feedback inhibition mechanisms, block the activity of enzyme(s) that synthesize certain neurotransmitter(s) which mediate important cellular functions. Resultant decrease in the transmitter concentration results in increased synthesis of new enzyme bringing it to predrug level and thus accounting for tolerance. During withdrawal of the drug the existing excess enzyme activity results in increased neurotransmitter synthesis and rebound cellular activity.

Receptor Increased Theory (24). Chronic use of dependence-producing drugs that decrease neuronal activity and inhibit synthesis of neurotransmitters, indirectly cause an increase in the number of receptors; either more receptors are synthesized or more 'silent' receptors are converted to the active form. During withdrawal the normal neurotransmitter activity together with excess receptors produces rebound effects.

Disuse Supersensitivity (23, 58). Drugs that produce tolerance and physical dependence may cause disuse supersensitivity directly or indirectly by decreasing the flow of impulses along neuronal pathways, similar in effect to peripheral denervation supersensitivity in the autonomic nervous system. During abstinence the flow of impulses resumes to supersensitivity resulting in rebound hyperexcitability.

Redundancy Theory. Martin (79) extended the homeostatic theory of Himmelsbach by postulating that there are two or more alternative pathways for mediating a physiological function in the CNS. Narcotics interrupt one of the pathways, and as a consequence, a secondary or redundant pathway may be induced to assume most portion of the function of the primary pathway and undergoes hypertrophy. During abstinence the primary pathway resumes its normal activity, and together with the redundant pathway produces an exaggerated response (hyperactivity).

Dual Action Hypothesis. Seevers and Deneau (105) postulated that binding of morphine to certain receptors on the surface of axons results in central depression, while binding to intracellular receptors in the cell body of the same or other neurons results in central stimulation. Tolerance develops to depressant effects, but not to the excitatory effects. Withdrawal of the drug precipitates the abstinence syndrome manifesting an imbalance in receptor function which is in favor of excitation.

Stereospecific Receptors (57). Two classes of opiate receptors might exist: one stereospecific and blocked by the antagonist, the other weakly specific and not blocked by naloxone. The abstinence syndrome could be partly due to selective inhibition of stereospecific receptors.

Receptor Conformation Change. Snyder (114) proposed that depending on the presence of sodium ion, the opiate receptor undergoes a transition between "no-sodium" or agonist state and "sodium" or antagonist state (which is normally existing, hypersensitive to antagonists, but subsensitive to agonists). Tolerance and dependence to opiates are postulated to be associates with a change in the receptor to no-sodium form. However, such receptor alteration has not been detected.

DRUGS OF ABUSE

The drugs of abuse will be discussed in this chapter in the following groups: (a) Heroin and other opioids; (b) Barbiturates and other CNS depressants including alcohol and solvents; (c) Psychomotor stimulants including nicotine; (d) Marijuana; and (e) LSD and other hallucinogens.

HEROIN AND OTHER OPIOIDS

History. Opiumlike agents were reported to be used in drinking in Greek mythology. In the 18th century, opium smoking was very popular and widespread in China. Beginning in the middle of the 19th century following isolation of pure alkaloids, and with the introduction of the hypodermic needle and parenteral use of morphine, nonmedical use of opium derivatives was further increased. In the United States minor "epidemics" of opiate use were reported during the Civil War, and approximately 4% of Americans abused opiates during the immediate post-Civil War period. Prior to World War I, nonmedical use of opiates was about 1 in 400 adults. The incidence and pattern of use was alarming enough to call for passage of the Harrison Narcotic Act in 1914.

Incidence of Opiate Abuse. A significant surge in the number of heroin abusers was witnessed between 1967 and 1970 in almost every major city in the United States. An estimated 626,000 to 724,900 abusers were reported between 1972 and 1974 and 500,000 to 600,000 abusers in 1975. In one study conducted by the University of Michigan it was reported that about 10% of high school seniors (sample population of 15,500) used opiates (other than heroin) in 1979, and about 1.1% of the sample admitted to using heroin (61).

Life-time ("ever-used") prevalence of heroin among young adults (age 18-25) declined from 4.6% in 1972 to 1.2% in 1982. Such prevalence in older adults (age 26-34) in 1982 was 3.5%. Current use (i.e., use in the month prior to the survey) in 1982 was shown to drop to less than 0.5% in all age groups (90).

Tolerance, Abuse Liability and Physical Dependence

Tolerance. Except for miosis, constipation and convulsions, tolerance develops to the other pharmacological actions of narcotics following repeated administrations. Even a single administration has been shown to result in the development of some degree of tolerance to some of its pharmacological responses. Frequency and size of the dose of narcotic analgesics generally influence the rate of development of tolerance; larger doses and frequent use promote rapid development of tolerance and the reverse happens when a low dose of the drug is used infrequently. Interruption in the repeated administration of drug is usually accompanied by reduction in the degree of developed tolerance. This is illustrated by the fact that an adult may be overdosed if he has missed self-administration of drugs for a few days. Tolerance to analgesia, euphoria, narcosis and respiratory depression are not absolute in nature and are developed in a "staircase" phenomenon. However, tolerance once developed to emesis, antidiuretic effect, and hypotensive actions is considered absolute in nature, and these responses cannot be elicited even by very high doses.

Development of cross tolerance is demonstrated among various narcotic analgesic agents (e.g., morphine, methadone, meperidine and their congeners).

It is generally agreed upon that tolerance developed to some action of narcotics has some direct bearings on the induction of physical dependence.

Abstinence Syndrome. Abrupt cessation of self-administration of narcotic analgesics (e.g., morphine, heroin) results in manifestations of withdrawal symptoms in dependent/tolerant individuals, newborn infants of dependent mothers (144), and several species of experimental animals (118). The nature of a narcotic analgesic, its daily intake, interval between doses, the duration of abuse habit, and the abusers personality and health status may influence the character and severity of narcotic withdrawal symptoms. Opioid withdrawal occurs in two recognized phases: i) acute, or primary, phase which lasts for about 4 to 10 weeks, and ii) chronic, or secondary, phase lasting for about 26 to 30 weeks. The acute, or primary, phase is composed of purposive and nonpurposive behavior (139). The purposive, goal-oriented symptoms are greatly influenced by the environment and directed toward obtaining more drugs, whereas the nonpurposive symptoms are independent of environment and without any goal. Purposive behaviors in morphine and heroin withdrawals are characterized by complaints, pleas, demands, and other activities to secure more drugs, starting shortly before the next expected dose and peaked at 36 to 72 hours after the last dose. Thereafter, these symptoms subside gradually. Nonpurposive symptoms mostly represent stimulation of the central and autonomic nervous systems and begin about 8 to 12 hours after the last dose, with lacrimation, rhinorrhea, yawning and sweating. Restless sleep ("yen") occurs in 12 to 14 hours. Peak manifestations occur between the second and third day, comprising weakness, insomnia, chills, nausea, vomiting, abdominal cramps, craving for sweets, muscle aches, rise in blood pressure and heart rate, hyperpnea, hyperthermia, and piloerection with waves of gooseflesh. Ejaculation in males and orgasm in females may manifest. Marked weight loss, dehydration, and acidosis may result from vomiting, anorexia, diarrhea, and sweating. If no treatment is initiated, most of the gross manifestations subside in 7 to 10 days.

The chronic, or secondary, phase of narcotic withdrawal symptoms is characterized by hypotension, bradycardia, low body temperature, mydriasis, and decreased sensitivity of respiratory center to carbon dioxide. This phase being stressful, it is likely to cause increased urinary excretion of epinephrine, hyperresponsiveness to stress, poor self-image and overreactions to physical discomfort. Signs and symptoms of abstinence of morphine and some representative narcotic agents are summarized in Table 11.6-1.

Table 11.6-1
Abstinence Syndrome For a Few Representative Narcotics and Narcotic Antagonists

Drugs	Drug seeking behavior	Primary abstinence syndrome: Manifestations	Primary abstinence syndrome: Onset; peak; duration	Substitution in morphine-dependent (240 mg/day) subjects	Precipitation of abstinence syndrome by nalorphine
Morphine	+	Weakness; restlessness; inability to concentrate; yawning; rhinorrhea; tearing; perspiration; gooseflesh; tremor; loss of appetite; vomiting; abdominal cramps; increase in pulse, blood pressure, body temperature, respiratory rate, and pupil size; malaise; joint and muscle pain	6-18 hr; 24-48 hr; 5-6 weeks	Suppresses	+
Methadone	+	Weakness, anxiety, anorexia, insomnia, abdominal discomfort, headache, sweating, pain in muscles and bones, hot and cold flashes, nausea, vomiting; increase in temperature, blood pressure, pulse, respiratory rate, and pupil size	24-48 hr; 3rd day; 6-7 weeks	Suppresses	+
Meperidine	+	Milder than those of morphine, autonomic signs not marked, pupils may not be widely dilated; usually little nausea, vomiting, or diarrhea. However, at peak, muscle twitching, restlessness, nervousness may be worse than during morphine withdrawal	3-hr; 8-12 hr; 4-5 days	Suppresses	+[a]
Codeine	+	Similar to morphine, but less intense: postural hypotension and fainting marked		Suppresses	+
Propoxyphene	+	Mild abstinence syndrome of rhinorrhea, myalgia, nausea, diarrhea, sweating, and irritability (4)	6-12 weeks	Suppresses	
Nalorphine	0	Less than and different from morphine, but close to cyclazocine: yawning, lacrimation, rhinorrhea, sweating, scratching, "electric shocks", chill, fever, diarrhea, loss of appetite and weight	8 hr; 1-5 days or more; 3-6 weeks	Precipitates	0
Cyclazocine	0	Resembles nalorphine more closely than morphine; loss of appetite and weight; increase in pulse rate, pupil size, temperature	3-4th days; 7th day; 6 weeks	Precipitates	0
Pentazocine	+	Resembles partially to nalorphine, but also to morphine: sweating, tremor, chills, muscular cramps (mainly legs), fever, abdominal cramps, nausea, vomiting, itching, lacrimation		Precipitates	0[b]
Naloxone, Naltrexone	0	None or a very few		Precipitiates	

Modified from Pradhan and Dutta (98).
[a] If daily intake of meperidine is 1,600 mg or more.
[b] Naloxone, not nalorphine or levallorphan, can antagonize pentazocine-induced respiratory depression.

Central Site(s) for Narcotic Tolerance and Dependence. Repeated intraventricular administration of morphine has been shown to cause development of tolerance to analgesia (17). Centrally morphine-treated animals can manifest withdrawal symptoms induced by peripheral administration of morphine antagonists (e.g., naloxone). It is generally recognized that narcotic physical dependence is not related to any specific area(s) of the brain, but changes are likely to occur throughout the entire neuroaxis. There are some suggestions that certain specific signs of withdrawal can be altered by acute lesions. Lesions in the centromedian and parafascicularis nuclei decrease the incidence of writhing and "wet-dog" shakes (2). Several studies have indicated that the limbic system is involved in some actions of morphine (27, 141). Ventromedial and ventrolateral hypothalamus, medial thalamus, and medial areas of the diencephalon have also been implicated in the development of narcotic tolerance and withdrawal symptoms (98). It has been implied that narcotic tolerance and dependence occur within opiate sensitive neurons wherever they may exist (25).

Mechanism of Development of Tolerance and Physical Dependence. Mechanism of narcotic tolerance and dependence is not clearly understood. A number of theories, as discussed earlier, has been proposed to this end. Kosterlitz and Hughes also suggested that reduced enkephalin release might explain tolerance and dependence to opiates (67). While mechanisms of narcotic tolerance and dependence appear to be inseparable, they differ from that of the acute effects of these agents. From various theories as well as other evidences it appears that the narcotic withdrawal manifestations can be considered as rebound effects that are produced as adaptive or homeostatic responses to counter acute effects of these drugs. Neurochemically, these manifestations are results of alterations in the metabolism and actions of several neurotransmitters particularly dopamine, serotonin, acetylcholine and GABA among others. It appears that the adaptive alterations in neurotransmitter metabolism may involve protein and RNA synthesis, since several inhibitors of such macromolecular synthesis can inhibit narcotic-induced tolerance-dependence thus suggesting that gene expression may play a significant role in these narcotic-related processes (134).

Diagnosis of Dependence. Dependence on narcotic analgesics can be clearly demonstrated by withholding administration of any narcotic in an institutional setting. Characteristic abstinence syndrome will appear over a period of 24 to 48 hours. Narcotic withdrawal syndrome can be promptly elicited by administering a narcotic antagonist.

Under certain circumstances the precipitation test by using a narcotic antagonist can give false results; for example, if this test is given 12 to 16 hours after the last dose, signs of precipitated abstinence may not appear (135). Naloxone and levallorphan can also precipitate abstinence syndrome within minutes in opiate-dependent persons, but there are no medical indications for the precipitation test for diagnostic purpose.

Treatment. Treatment include pharmacological or psychosocial methods or a combination of both. For long-term management of opiate dependence, two pharmacologic methods are basically employed: opiate maintenance and opiate antagonists. *Methadone maintenance* method, introduced by Dole and Nyswander over a decade ago, is still considered as the principal mode of treatment for heroin addicts in the United States (32). The aim of methadone maintenance is to achieve stabilization on the drug, gradually increasing the dose until a high degree of cross-tolerance develops such that the euphoric feeling even from high doses of other opioids is not experienced (narcotic blockade). The rationale for this approach stems from the belief that chronic use of an opioid produces a metabolic alteration in the person, so that after withdrawal (months even years) there is a feeling of abnormality (opioid hunger) experienced. In this program the patient is placed on methadone at a daily oral dose that will not cause sedation, constipation, or other side effects, but high enough to eliminate the craving of street opiate. The dose usually varies from 25 to 120 mg daily. Generally, two dosage levels have evolved, one "low" maintenance dose (40-50 mg/day) and the other "high" maintenance dose (80-100 mg/day). The rate of attrition seems to minimize if "high" maintenance dose is employed early in the treatment. The drug is administered daily under the supervision of a dispenser, and urine is checked for other illicit use of drugs. One problem with methadone therapy is that a patient on maintenance may seek additional opiates to have more positive drug effects. This results in receiving a dose to which he is not tolerant and fatal overdose may occur. A longer-acting synthetic congener of methadone, levo-alpha-acetylmethadol (LAAM), has been tried in place of methadone. LAAM has an approximate 72 hours of duration of action as opposed to 24 hours for methadone; thus daily visits to the clinic for methadone can be avoided (48).

Clonidine, a presynaptic central alpha-adrenergic receptor agonist used therapeutically as an antihypertensive agent, alleviates the opiate withdrawal symptoms. Presumably the action of the drug decreases the release of norepinephrine and therefore blocks the disturbances of the autonomic nervous system associated with withdrawal. Its major advantage is that, unlike methadone, it has no narcotic action and is not addicting. Some studies suggest that clonidine detoxification allows 100% of the addicts to become opiate-free and clonidine-free within 14 days but that treatment with naltrexone and group therapy may be needed to maintain a drug-free state (44, 131). Additionally, both cyclazocine and naltrexone narcotic antagonists have been used to prevent recurrent addiction after detoxification, but naltrexone is still an investigational drug (81). A synthetic partial agonist-antagonist, buprenorphine, has been shown to relieve the desire for opiate and at the same time block heroin effects (84).

Narcotic antagonists. are being used experimentally for management of narcotic addiction. When an opioid antagonist is given chronically, the receptor sites for the agonist are blocked, thus negating the pharmacological effects, particularly the euphoric effect. For most addicts the euphoric experience is the reinforcement for continued use of the opioid. Therefore, administration of an opioid without an effect would soon lead to extinction and drug use is discontinued.

Naltrexone is the preferred narcotic antagonist for treating opiate-dependent persons. It is orally active, has a long duration of effect, and lacks agonist properties. A single dose of 50 to 100 mg is adequate to block the effects of intravenously administered 25 mg of heroin for about 24 to 48 hours. The usual practice is to start with small daily doses, ultimately reaching three times weekly doses with 100, 100, and 150 mg (the latter dose to continue blockade of opiates over a weekend). The greatest drawback to use of this agent is that few addicts will accept it as a permanent treatment.

A variety of psychosocial approaches have been tried to narcotic-dependent persons on the assumption that drug use is symptomatic of some emotional disturbances or inability to cope adequately with normal lifestyle. The common technique used is *peer pressure group*, emphasizing confrontation. Other techniques include individual or group psychotherapy, didactic approach of communal living, transcendental meditation, Zen, or hypnosis.

A large-scale evaluation project (Drug Abuse Reporting Programme, DARP) was carried out on the effectiveness of drug abuse treatment, involving almost 44,000 clients in 52 treatment centers throughout the United States and Puerto Rico between 1969 and 1973 (107). The data from this study indicate that methadone maintenance, therapeutic community, and outpatient drug-free programs led to favorable results.

Acute Overdose. Acute overdose with narcotic agents is a frequent cause of death among addicts. The clinical manifestations include respiratory depression, coma, marked miosis of the pupils, pulmonary edema, and in some cases convulsion. The latter is commonly seen with meperidine and d-propoxyphene. The specific antidote is naloxone to reverse the respiratory and CNS depression. Naloxone does not possess any agonistic effect. Because of the short half-life of the antagonist, the patient should be kept under observation for 24 hours for possible return of CNS depression and apnea. Therapy of narcotic overdose is discussed in more detail in Chapters 10.1 and 32.

Medical Complications. Varieties of substances used to dilute the narcotic substances have been held responsible for the morbidity and mortality associated with narcotic abuse. Many pathological conditions have been reported as complications in narcotic-dependent persons.

Acute reactions may occur due to pharmacologic overdose of narcotics or many adulterants including quinine. Clinical manifestations of acute reactions due to narcotic overdose include respiratory difficulty, cyanosis, mental confusion leading to coma, constricted or fixed dilated pupils.

Subcutaneous injections of heroin frequently result in skin abscesses and cellulitis. One of the most common and serious systemic septic complications of parenteral narcotic abuse is bacterial endocarditis with involvement of either or both sides of the heart. In right-sided lesions *Staphylococcus aureus* is frequently the causative organism. Other septic complications include meningitis, arthritis, osteomyelitis, and metastatic abscesses in kidney, brain, liver, and spleen. Viral hepatitis due to the use of contaminated needles is also common in a community of addicts. Central nervous system complications include hemiplegia, aphasia, and facial paresis resulting from abscess formation, embolism from left-side valvular disease or mycotic aneurysm (ruptured). Meningoencephalitis and transverse myelitis may also be seen. Pulmonary complications of parenteral drug abuse include pneumococcal or aspiration pneumonia, septic emboli, effusion, and empyema.

Male heroin addicts frequently complain of decreased libido, impotence, and delayed ejaculation. Menstruation irregularities, toxemia of pregnancy, and prematurity in infants of addicted mothers have been reported. Homicide, suicide, and accidents have been implicated in 20 to 40% of narcotic-related deaths.

CNS DEPRESSANTS

BARBITURATES AND OTHER DEPRESSANTS

Incidence. In 1903 barbital was the first barbiturate introduced for clinical use, and its abuse was reported in 1904 (38). An estimated 200,000-2,000,000 abusers of sedative-hypnotics were reported in 1977 (78). Cooper in 1977 reported that out of a total of 219,064 admissions to federally funded treatment centers for various kinds of substance abuse, 10,764 were for barbiturate abuse and 6,442 for abuse of other sedative-hypnotics or anxiolytics (76). Recent use (in the month prior to survey) of sedatives increased from 1% in youth (age 12-17) and 1.6% in young adults in 1974 to 1.3% and 2.6% in respective age groups in 1982. Life-time ("ever used") prevalence in these age groups also increased from 3% and 10% in 1972 to 5.8% and 18.7% respectively in 1982 (90).

Patterns of Abuse. There are several types of subjects who may become sedative-hypnotic abusers. First, patients seeking alleviation from insomnia start using the drug in progressively increasing doses, resulting in persistent self-medication at a higher dose. The second group includes long-term users of the drug in recommended doses; about 15-20% of these subjects continue the drug intake beyond the initial use for a fixed period (e.g., 3 months) (16). The third includes individuals who have never received a prescription for initial therapeutic use of sedative-hypnotic drugs, but they procure the drug from street sources and use them in a social way with or without acquaintances. Barbiturates, benzodiazepines or other sedatives are taken frequently by opioid users to enhance the effects of weak street heroin and by some alcoholics to relieve their withdrawal symptoms. Each of these patterns of abuse may lead to physical dependence. Dependence on large doses of sedative-hypnotics is somewhat more common in women of middle age (4).

Some nonsleep effects, such as rapidity of onset of action to induce euphoria and a state of "total oblivion," and absence of unpleasant side effects, have been suggested to promote psychic dependence on these drugs. These drugs have also been demonstrated in monkeys and dogs to possess a self-reinforcing drive for repeated self-administration (40).

Tolerance, Habituation, and Dependence. Both acute and delayed tolerance emerge from the use of sedative-hypnotics. However, not all the CNS functions develop tolerance to the same magnitude. The mechanism(s) of chronic tolerance for sedative-hypnotics are discussed elsewhere in the book in connection with general consideration of development of drug tolerance (Chapter 3) and sedative-hypnotics (Chapter 11.2-1).

Physical dependence to sedative-hypnotics may be demonstrated in persons who have developed tolerance to the drug, and can be readily recognized by the emergence of characteristics symptoms in abstinence state. The neurophysiological mechanism to withdrawal symptoms is largely unknown (64). Clinical characteristics of withdrawal syndrome of sedative-hypnotics are well documented including their occurrence in newborn infants of dependent mothers (12, 140). Intensity and duration of prior drug abuse, rate of metabolism of the drug involved, and several other factors may influence the occurrence and severity of withdrawal symptoms. Prolonged use of larger doses of sedative-hypnotic drugs generally leads to severe withdrawal, and drugs like diazepam and phenobarbital which are slowly metabolized in the body are less likely to cause severe symptoms of abstinence. In the case of pentobarbital dependence, the major clinical symptoms of withdrawal appear usually 36 hours after the last dose and are rarely seen before 12 hours. The onset of withdrawal symptoms in the case of diazepam is delayed and takes several days. The manifestations of sedative-hypnotic withdrawal syndrome are presented in Table 11.6-2. Usually abrupt cessation of barbiturates in a physically dependent person is associated with the occurrence of seizures on the third day of abstinence and then recovery over the next several weeks. Because of these seizures, withdrawal of sedative-hypnotics is more potentially dangerous than narcotic withdrawal. Physically dependent persons usually manifest impairment of psychomotor function, sleep disorder, and possibly impairment of metabolic functions. Gross withdrawal symptoms simulate symptoms of widespread central denervation hypersensitivity or unregulated overreactivity of each of the brain areas. Symptoms related to the motor system are easily recognized; tremor and hyperreflexia are the early features of withdrawal, and seizures (of grand mal types) constitute the most severe response. The withdrawal seizures have certain characteristics; they are not continuous, not preceded by an aura, and the postictal phase is generally mild in nature. The sensory functions are usually clear and any impairment suggests injury to the brain resulting from hyperthermia, shock, or from the drugs used to treat the patient.

Complications of Chronic Abuse. Chronic use of high doses of sedative-hypnotics is characterized by classic "barb freak," utter neglect of self-care and intermittent occurrence of seizures. A variety of other symptoms may be evident in persons who are short of frank intoxication, these include a) impairment of psychomotor function, b) altered sleep patterns, and c) abnormalities of folate and vitamin D metabolism. Both barbiturates and nonbarbiturates (e.g., benzodiazepines) can interfere with psychomotor skills (such as those needed for automobile driving) (74). There are some reports to suggest that very large chronic dosages of many hypnotics induce changes in sleep EEG, characterized by slow-wave sleep with nitrazepam (1) or flurazepam. A sort of "partial drug withdrawal" phenomenon that has been attributed to chronic use of sedative-hypnotic is manifested by increased restlessness found in later phase of sleep in some persons. A biphasic REM sleep (initial decrease followed by an increase late at night) has been reported in sedative-hypnotic users (1, 65). Some studies have even demonstrated that cases of insomnia can be cleared in sedative-hypnotic users by withdrawal of the drug (10).

Table 11.6-2
Barbiturate Abstinence Symptoms

		Abstinence Symptoms	
Dose (g/day)[a]	Duration (months)	Minor[b]	Major
0.4	3	High voltage paroxysmal EEG discharge[c]	Convulsions in 10 to 25%
0.6 - 0.8	1-2	EEG abnormality, anxiety, muscle twitchings, intention tremor of hand and fingers, progressive weakness, dizziness, visual hallucination, nausea, vomiting, insomnia, anorexia and weight loss, orthostatic hypotension	
0.9 - 2.2	1-5	Intensity and incidence of the minor symptoms increase	Convulsions in 75%; delirium[d] and hyperthermia (100.6°F) in 66%

[a] Pentobarbital or secobarbital. Antiepileptic treatment with 0.2 g/day of barbiturates for 12 months showed no tolerance or physical dependence.
[b] Appear between 8 and 36 hours after the last dose of barbiturates, reach peak on the 2nd day, and decline in course of 2 to 15 days.
[c] Appears on the 2nd day and declines between 4th and 8th days.
[d] Occurs between 4th and 7th days.
Source: Adopted from Fraser (41).

Folate deficiency (associated with anemia) possibly due to defective conversion of tetrahydrofolate to 5-methyl-tetrahydrofolate has been reported in patients treated with anticonvulsants (e.g., phenobarbital) (80). Rickets in children and osteomalacia in adults have been reported to occur following long-term use of barbiturates in epileptics. The mechanism of development of vitamin D deficiency is believed to be due to accelerated phenobarbital-induced hepatic metabolism of active forms of vitamin D (48).

Diagnosis of physical dependence. A fairly acute appraisal of sedative-hypnotic dependence can be made on the following bases: a) a thorough history taking from close associates, e.g., friends and relatives, b) physical examination and search for symptoms and signs of withdrawal, c) presence of complications (e.g., cutaneous signs) or other disease entities such as cirrhosis of liver or malnutrition seen in drug abusers, d) presence of tolerance and cross-tolerance, e) EEG changes, and f) blood and urine tests (116).

Management of sedative-hypnotic dependence. In order to avoid emergence of serious withdrawal syndrome, gradual withdrawal of the offending drug over a period of ten days to three weeks is needed to minimize the withdrawal symptoms (nonsubstitutive treatment). If the drug and the daily dosage is known, then the dose is generally reduced at a rate of 10% a day (81).

In patients who are taking a mixture of drugs or an unknown sedative-hypnotic agent, their tolerance to pentobarbital (having a wide cross-tolerance) is determined by a diagnostic test (138). In this test 200 mg of pentobarbital is administered orally (100 mg for elderly or debilitated patients). The patient is then evaluated over the next hour for signs of intoxication (positive Romberg's sign, ataxia, incoordination, nystagmus, slurred speech, and drowsiness). Appearance of signs of intoxication provides presumptive evidence that the subject is not tolerant to sedative-hypnotics and there is little chance of withdrawal syndrome if the drug is withheld. This test is further extended by giving pentobarbital (100 mg) every 6 hours for 24 hours following the initial dose of pentobarbital. The lack of appearance of withdrawal symptoms when the drug is withheld, or intoxication is interpreted as evidence for absence of tolerance.

A positive test with pentobarbital indicates tolerance to sedative-hypnotics and withdrawal treatment is recommended. The patient should always be hospitalized for withdrawal treatment. Pentobarbital is commonly given by mouth (or i.m. if needed) at a dose of 200-400 mg every six hours until signs of mild intoxication appear. The patient is maintained for about two days at the mild intoxication dose level, and then the dose is gradually reduced daily by no more than 10% of the previously established stabilization dose or no more than 100 mg per day. Appearance of mild or moderate signs of intoxication requires temporary suspension of reduction schedule and the patient is sedated with optimal pentobarbital doses to suppress such manifestations.

To prevent recurrence of abuse, general procedures recommended for alcohol dependence are adopted, these will be discussed later in this chapter. In order to discourage development of drug-seeking behavior, drugs with habituation or addiction potential should be avoided, phenothiazines or antihistaminic class of compounds may be used.

ALCOHOL

Alcoholism. Alcoholism has been defined as both a behavioral disorder and a chronic disease state, both of which occur as a consequence of persistent and excessive use of alcohol leading to physical disability and impaired emotional, occupational and/or interpersonal adjustments. It denotes a series of problems which may range from alcohol abuse (as defined by the drinker's society) to alcohol addiction, and may include excessive drinking in normal social situations; drinking in isolation; drinking to reduce anxiety, apprehension, or anger; drinking to facilitate the induction of sleep during conditions of insomnia; early morning drinking; and alterations in memory function (blackout) during heavy episodic alcohol intake (86). Alcohol addiction may include both tolerance and physical dependence. With development of tolerance a person consumes progressively increasing amounts of alcohol to achieve the same state of psychological reinforcement previously induced by smaller doses of alcohol. Physical dependence on alcohol is fairly confirmed when a reduction in amount or complete cessation of alcohol consumption leads to the manifestation of signs and symptoms of alcohol withdrawal.

Epidemiology. In the year 1974-1975 several reports indicated that an estimated 5.5 to 9 million alcoholics were in the United States. The number of drinkers in the United States is reported to be gradually increasing (more so among women), and according to some estimates women alcoholics constitute about one-fifth to one-third that of men (88). The prevalence of alcoholism is lower in elderly than in middle-aged persons. Life-time ("ever used") prevalence of alcohol use increased from 54% in youth (age 12-17), 81.6% in young adults (age 18-25) and 73.2% in older adults (age 26 and more) in 1974 to 73.3%, 95.3% and 91.5% in respective groups in 1979. Current use (use in the month prior to survey) also increased from 34%, 69.3% and 54.5% in 1974 to 37.2%, 75.9% and 61.3% respectively in 1979. Compared to 1979 reports, life-time prevalence (65.2%, 94.6%, and 88.2%) as well as current use (26.9%, 67.9% and 56.7%) in 1982 was less in respective age groups (90).

Etiological Factors. It is generally recognized that an interplay of a cluster of factors such as physiological, psychological, and socioeconomical results in the development of alcoholism. A genetic factor has been suggested by some studies (46, 103). This genetic predisposition along with some personality traits (poor coping capacity under stress) often drive such individuals to alcohol for relief and pleasure, the latter functioning as a reinforcer.

Tolerance to Alcohol. Chronic use of alcohol leads to the development of tolerance, as with other CNS depressants including barbiturates, psychotropic drugs, and opiates. Tolerance to alcohol can be subdivided into categories: pharmacologic, behavioral, and cross-tolerance to other CNS depressants. *Pharmacologic tolerance* probably represents metabolic adaptive phenomenon as a consequence of long-term ingestion. There are several reports to indicate that with prolonged drinking episodes there is enhanced metabolism of alcohol, although the mechanism for accelerated metabolism is not fully understood. Pharmacologic tolerance plays an important role in the adaptive tolerance of the CNS and possibly also contributes to behavioral tolerance minimally.

Behavioral tolerance to alcohol is said to occur when a person even with high blood concentration of alcohol (following drinking a relatively large volume of alcohol) can perform complex behavioral and psychomotor functions. A subject who has developed tolerance to alcohol has also been shown to manifest *cross-tolerance* to other drugs such as barbiturates, volatile anesthetics, and minor tranquilizers.

Patterns of Alcohol Abuse. In an attempt to specify a therapeutic regimen for a particular type of alcohol abuse, alcoholism has been categorized into alpha, beta, gamma, delta, and epsilon alcoholism (59) (Table 11.6-3). Sometimes alcoholism is divided into reactive (similar to alpha or epsilon), essential (gamma and delta), and symptomatic (alpha and epsilon) types (108).

Diagnosis and Management of Acute Intoxication. Acute intoxication is readily recognized by thick slurred speech, nystagmus, ataxic gait, and associated psychological changes such as sluggish thoughts, poor concentration and memory, faulty judgment, and narrowed range of attention. There may be emotional episodes, e.g., laughing or crying easily, irritability, hostility, paranoia, and even suicidal tendencies. Severe intoxication is accompanied by coma and markedly depressed respiration.

In treating acute alcohol intoxication one should give careful consideration to the fact that often in addition to alcohol other CNS depressants may be involved, and this makes the clinical event less predictable. In such cases, the recommended treatment is to admit the patient to the intensive care unit of a hospital, support respiration by intubation, and start hemodialysis to reverse poisoning. In the case of a conscious and disruptive subject, haloperidol, 2-3 mg (i.m.), may be used, and repeated after 30 minutes (if behavior demands it) with close monitoring of vital signs.

Withdrawal Syndrome. Withdrawal syndrome varies from the common hangover to delirium tremens (DT) depending on prior history of nutritional state and alcohol intake. This may start with sweating, tremulousness, (as early 6-8 hours after cessation of drinking), insomnia, headache, nausea, tachycardia, muscle twitching, cramps, vomiting, diarrhea, and agitation in more severe cases. Manifestations of minor withdrawal syndrome subside greatly by 40 to 50 hours after cessation of drinking. The DT is clinical syndrome that most commonly appears 2 to 3 days after the patient has stopped heavy drinking, but it may be seen up to 3 weeks after stopping intake of alcohol. Its principal symptoms include disorientation and hallucination. Seizures may occur at any time up to about 10 days after cessation of drinking and may progress into status epilepticus. The seizures always precede the onset of DT, but once the DT becomes stabilized, convulsions no longer occurs. Other clinical find-

Table 11.6-3
Patterns of Alcoholism

Category	Psychological dependence	Withdrawal phenomenon	Physical complications
Alpha	Present, correspond with problem drinking — reacting to psychological stress	Absent	None
Beta	Not significant, but heavy drinking pattern	Minimal to absent, moderate physical tolerance	Present, liver damage
Gamma[a]	Present, model "alcoholism," loss of control	Marked withdrawal symptoms; tissue tolerance, sudden loss of tolerance seen	May be severe
Delta[a]	Present, no loss of control, more advanced form of beta type, no serious or psychological difficulties	Present	May be present
Epsilon	"Craving" at times only (episodic), classic "dipsomania"	Mild or absent; no tissue tolerance	Usually absent

[a] Constitutes the addictive disease process.

ings common in DT include tachycardia, diaphoresis, hypertension, fever, hyperactivity, and insomnia.

All patients with DT must be hospitalized. The aim of treatment is to calm the patient down and provide a gradual withdrawal from the depressant effects of alcohol. This is achieved by drugs that have close cross-tolerance with alcohol and a long and slowly dissipated depressant effect. Chlordiazepoxide or diazepam is generally used to meet the therapeutic needs. DT is clearly related to withdrawal and not to underlying nutritional, neurologic, or psychiatric disorders. Most DT is self-limiting and is over within 72 hours. In some alcoholics both the minor and major symptoms of withdrawal are present concurrently, the minor symptoms being blended into the major syndrome; in others, the two syndromes are distinct.

Physical Complications of Alcohol Abuse. Numerous physical disorders have been reported in the literature and are listed in Table 11.6-4.

Table 11.6-4
Complications of Alcohol Abuse

A. *Gastrointestinal disorders*
1. Esophagitis
2. Esophageal carcinoma
3. Gastritis
4. Malabsorption
5. Chronic diarrhea
6. Pancreatitis
7. Fatty liver
8. Alcoholic hepatitis
9. Cirrhosis (may lead to cancer of liver)

B. *Cardiac disorders*
1. Alcoholic cardiomyopathy
2. Beriberi

C. *Skin disorders*
1. Rosacea
2. Telangiectasia
3. Rhinophyma
4. Cutaneous ulcers

D. *Neurologic and psychiatric disorders*
1. Peripheral neuropathy
2. Convulsive disorders
3. Alcoholic hallucinosis
4. Delirium tremens
5. Wernicke's syndrome
6. Korsakoff's psychosis
7. Marchiafava's syndrome

E. *Muscle disorder*—alcoholic myopathy

F. *Hematologic disorder*—
megaloblastic anemia

G. *Vitamin deficiency disease*
1. Beriberi
2. Pellagra
3. Scurvy

H. *Metabolic disorders*
1. Alcoholic hypoglycemia
2. Alcoholic hyperlipemia

Diagnosis and Management of Chronic Alcoholic State. There are a number of screening tests that attempt to differentiate alcoholic from nonalcoholic population (6, 10). One of these is the Michigan Alcoholism Screening Test (MAST) (6). This test contains a series of 25 questions to be answered yes or no. A short Michigan Alcoholism Screening Test (SMAST) with 3 questions was developed and has been found to be accurate. A diagnostic algorithm with multiple discriminant analysis of several biochemical and hematological parameters has been reported to correctly differentiate alcoholics from nonalcoholics (103). A diagnosis can be based on the results of these two tests.

For long-term management of chronic alcoholics the primary aim is to match the right subject to the right rehabilitation program. These programs include psychotherapy, group psychotherapy, marital and family therapy, behavioral therapy, Alcoholics Anonymous, community resources, long-term living centers, and occupational programs (4). Details of the rehabilitative measures are beyond the scope of this book.

Drugs such as disulfiram, metronidazole and calcium carbimide are used in alcoholism treatment to deter alcohol consumption (92). These drugs inhibit hepatic aldehyde-NAD-oxidoreductase, the enzyme that catalyses oxidation of acetaldehyde to acetic acid. High level of acetaldehyde in the blood is associated with the appearance of tachycardia, tachypnea, hypotension, palpitation, nausea, and often vomiting. These aversive reactions start almost immediately after alcohol consumption (even less than 30 ml), and reach a peak within 30 minutes. Alcohol-sensitizing drugs are given to alcoholics who clearly seek them.

SOLVENTS

One method of introducing chemicals into the body is by inhalation of volatile substances; the large area of the lungs renders easy access and promotes rapid experience of the psychological components of systemic action. This method for substance abuse has been exploited by mankind over recent years. A case of gasoline inhalation was first described in the United States in the 1950s. Abuse of larger numbers of volatile substances has been reported recently. Although no age group can boast immunity from solvent abuse, the participants tend to be mostly the younger children, which is unlike the pattern of other hard drug abuse. Inhalant abusers usually do not belong to a drug subculture. In one study it was reported that by 1967 about 50% of Denver males aged between 10 and 17 years had experience with glue sniffing on at least one occasion (21). The spread of solvent abuse in North America has been discussed in an article published in 1980 (132). In a recent study the inhalation of fumes from typewriter correction fluids has been reported to be gaining popularity in almost every regions of the country (43).

Chemistry. Commercial solvents contain a variety of chemical ingredients. In adhesive and plastic cements the common organic solvent is toluene. Benzene, cyclohexane, hexane tricresyl phosphate, and xylene are also used in various combinations. These solvents are also present in lacquer thinners and enamels. Cleaning fluids usually contain one of the following: perchloroethylene, trichlorethane, trichloroethylene, and carbon tetrachloride. A mixture of aliphatic hydrocarbons especially naphtha is present in lighter fluid. In nail polish remover the usual ingredients are acetone and aliphatic acetates. Freons, a number of chlorinated-fluorinated hydrocarbons, are used as aerosol propellants and as refrigerants. These solvents, being readily soluble in fat, affect the lipid components of cells, particularly of the central nervous system.

Patterns of Abuse. The usual method employed for gasoline sniffing is direct inhalation from the gasoline tanks of cars or motorcycles (11). Although exact information on the frequency and duration of sniffing practice is lacking in the literature, according to some reports (132), the practice ranges from once every few months to 3-4 times weekly. In glue sniffing the users frequently use plastic or paper bags as dispensers of adhesives. In some instances, an additional plastic bag is placed over the head or the entire body in order to prolong the exposure. Aerosols are either inhaled directly from the spray or through some improvised device to aid direct inhalation.

Clinical Manifestations. In Chapter 28.2 the pharmacology and toxicology of a number of industrial solvents (e.g., isopropanol, glycols, aliphatic hydrocarbons, gasoline and kerosene, benzene, toluene, carbon tetrachloride) are discussed. These solvents and additional agents mentioned here share a common pharmacological effect; almost all of them cause CNS depression resembling ethanol intoxication in many aspects.

Solvent inebriation generally leads to initial psychic stimulation followed by depression. The psychic state is characterized by delirium, mental confusion, psychomotor clumsiness, conditional disinhibition, and impairment of perceptual and cognitive skills (22). Dizziness, staggering gait, and drunkenness are often early manifestations of solvent abuse. Gasoline sniffers are often referred to psychiatric assessment for strange behavioral patterns or hallucinations that are usually visual, but sometimes auditory (71). Case reports indicate development of model psychosis very similar to a condition induced by hallucinogenic drugs (122).

Sensations of numbness and of being "blank" or "dead" or floating or spinning in air have been experienced by some abusers. Although gasoline sniffing is usually a solitary activity, emotional manifestations vary from uncontrollable laughter to tears and then ending in profound depression. In a group situation sniffers may be involved in fighting or homosexual activity (22). The euphoric feeling of solvent inhalation may last for a few minutes to one or two hours. Unlike alcohol, a solvent abuser may get high several times a day because of short duration of experience. All psychic effects of solvent inhalation are reversible and no residual effect after discontinuation has been reported (31).

Pharmacokinetics. Solvents are readily absorbed from the lung into systemic circulation. A small portion of these may be absorbed from the gastrointestinal tract. Being lipid soluble, solvents are distributed quickly in the brain. Major portions of volatile solvents are excreted through lungs, imparting characteristic odor in the breath which may last for hours. Some solvents such as benzene undergo hepatic biotransformation to the extent that about 50% and the metabolites are excreted free or as glucuronic acid or sulfuric acid conjugates.

Tolerance and Dependence. Chronic abuse of solvents results in development of tolerance which may happen any time from three months to three years. Psychological dependence generally occurs with agents such as gasoline, lighter fluid, and glue, and is mostly related to the psychic experience rather than to any particular agent. There are rare reports of withdrawal manifestations to sniffing habits, but generally solvents are not considered to cause clear physical dependence.

Adverse Effects. Toxic manifestations of solvents (see also Chapter 28.2) can be divided into acute and chronic, as listed for some solvents in Table 11.6-5. Aromatic hydrocarbons like benzene and toluene are known to cause toxic effects related to hemopoietic, gastrointestinal and hepatic systems (22). Toluene has been reported to cause chromosomal damage. Chronic inhalation of metallic paints creates additional toxicity problems because of heavy metal ingredients such as copper and zinc; lead is also contained in some old paints.

Hepatic dysfunction has been reported in a chloroform sniffer for about seven years (136). Subjects with homozygous sickle-cell disease were reported to develop erythrocytic aplastic crisis as a result of glue sniffing (94). In glue sniffers transient abnormalities of EEG have been noted by some investigators; one toluene sniffer developed encephalopathy with diffuse EEG slowing (132). Polyneuropathy associated with sensorimotor disturbance and muscular atrophy are also infrequently reported in sniffers of glue containing n-hexane.

Extreme high level exposure to gasoline may cause some toxic effects, mostly resulting from its content of lead, benzene, or other additives. These effects are mostly neurological, gastrointestinal, or hemopoietic in nature. Presence of lead in gasoline may show signs of plumbism, especially encephalopathy (33, 70).

Prevention and Management. Attempts were made to add unpleasant chemical(s) to discourage sniffing, but this led the abuser to seek for other solvents. The major drive to build a negative attitude toward solvent sniffing at an early age is probably the right way. Rehabilitation of an abuser is really a multifaceted problem and requires careful planning and supportive measures as needed for other types of drug abuse.

PSYCHOMOTOR STIMULANTS

In recent years there have been epidemics of amphetamine abuse in the United States, Japan, and Sweden. None of the CNS stimulants included under the current Drug Enforcement Administration (DEA) Schedule (Chapter 5) has been shown to be free of the abuse potential, as in case of amphetamine. Repeated self-administration of amphetamines or amphetaminelike drugs intravenously lead to outbreaks of paranoid psychoses and violent behaviors in the users.

History. The stimulant effects of chewing coca leaves were discovered by folk medicinemen in the Andes centuries ago. The active component, cocaine, was discovered in 1860. Freud recommended it as a pain-killer to one of his colleagues who, following its long-term use, developed psychotic state, violent behavior, and hallucinations (62). Currently, cocaine probably is the most popular recreational drug in the United States. Although cocaine and amphetamine are similar in their acute effects, the former is preferred, because it has more potent euphoric effect and has a snob appeal as a more expensive drug.

Prevalence of Stimulant Abuse. The exact extent to which drugs of this class are abused is not clearly known. Amphetamine seems to maintain its popularity on college campuses as a means of preventing sleep and at the same time maintaining cognitive functions before examinations. One survey conducted in 1974 indicated that about 26% of university graduates used amphetamine as a study aid (99).

Truck drivers constitute another segment of the general population who abuse amphetamine quite frequently. However, there is some controversy regarding the resultant effects on driving and road accidents. Some believe that there have been fewer accidents due to drug-induced avoidance of fatigue. Among athletes, abuse of amphetamine has also been found widespread; one report indicated that about 60% of professional

Table 11.6-5
Reported Toxicity of Solvents

Solvents	Acute Toxicity	Chronic Toxicity
Volatile solvents		
Benzene	Respiratory arrest and cardiac arrhythmias occur with all volatile solvents	Bone marrow depression, leukemia, aplastic anemia, liver damage
Toluene		Anemia, encephalopathy; liver, kidney, cerebellar and chromosomal damage
Xylene		Liver damage
Naphtha		Emotional lability
Carbon tetrachloride		Hepatorenal syndrome (33)
Trichloroethylene, trichlorethane perchloroethylene		Neuropathy; kidney and liver damage (43)
Chloroform		Hepatotoxicity
Glue sniffing		Aplastic anemia (94), encephalopathy, polyneuropathy
Gasoline		Signs of lead poisoning (33, 70)
Aerosols	Laryngospasm, airway freezing and suffocation due to occluded airway, cardiac arrhythmias, "sudden-sniffing-death"	

Some of the information are based on Cohen (22).

football players regularly used them in game situation (60). Often, recreational users of amphetamine or cocaine resort to polydrug abuse.

There are two types of habitual users of amphetamine. One is the occasional or recreational user, who claims to be calm, confident, or alert and decisive while on the drug. The other type of abuser originates from the prescription use of amphetamine for anorexia or fatigue. The intravenous administration of amphetamine is considered to be the most serious form of abuse and usually a very high dose of amphetamine (up to 2 g) may be self-administered per day. This form of abuse has declined in recent years.

In order to counteract the stimulant effect of amphetamine and cocaine often barbiturates are abused concurrently. Combination of amphetamine during daytime and barbiturates at night is often practiced. Additionally, there are some reports that indicate concurrent use of narcotics and cocaine (37).

Life-time ("ever used") prevalence of cocaine use has gradually increased from 2% in youth (age 12-17) and also in old adults (age 26 or more) in 1972 to 7% and 9% in respective age groups in 1982, but its prevalence is most concentrated in young adults (age 18-25) in whom the increase was from 9% in 1972 to 28% in 1982. In age group 26-34, 22% tried cocaine on at least one occasion compared to 4% of persons aged 35 or older. In 1982 current use (in the month prior to the survey) was also high 7% and 3% in age groups 18-25 and 26-34, in contrast to 2% in persons aged 12-17 and 5% in persons aged 35 or more. In this group dramatic increase in life-time prevalence occurred up to 1979 after which it leveled off showing only about 1% increase (from 27.5% to 28.3%). About 12% of the entire 18 to 25 age group said that they had used cocaine more than ten occasions. In this young adult group cocaine use was more likely among males than females and among whites than among other races. Use of marijuana was common along with cocaine in the same occasion in every age group (90).

Behavioral Pharmacology of Stimulant Dependence. Cocaine and amphetamine both facilitate self-stimulation in rats (142), and both drugs can be self-administered intravenously by rats to the point of seizures and death (93). Brain catecholamines (NE and DA) have been implicated in the actions of these drugs on CNS reward sites (37). Long-term administration of amphetamine in monkeys has been known to cause prolonged depletion of dopamine in the central nervous system (106). In humans, following withdrawal from chronic use of amphetamine a decrease in the norepinephrine metabolite in the brain has similarly been demonstrated (133).

Acute effects of amphetamine and cocaine have great similarities. Oral amphetamine cause mydriasis, hypertension, diaphoresis, anorexia, tachycardia, and, in large doses, confusion and arrhythmias. Euphoria, alertness, hyper-vigilance, and feelings of heightened physical and mental capabilities also occur in most subjects, along with some degree of anxiety and in some instances dysphoria. Stimulant use leads to sharp definition of body image, rather than eliciting colorful subjective effects characteristic of psychotomimetics. The effects from intravenous administration do not differ from those after oral route, but the onset of these effects is rapid. Both amphetamine and cocaine have been reported to stimulate sexual behavior in both men and women (37).

Behavioral Complications. Psychosis usually develops as a result of chronic use of amphetamine and is characterized by paranoid delusions, hallucinations and bizarre behavior. Hallucinations usually cease 2 to 3 days after cessation of drug administration, though delusions may linger for weeks or months (36). There is a report of eliciting paranoid symptoms in individuals who have abstained from amphetamine abuse for some time by reintroduction of the drug, even a single dose (68). Differentiation of stimulant psychosis from paranoid schizophrenia is a difficult problem. However, the presence of paranoid delusions and visual hallucinations may provide distinguishing evidence for the stimulant psychosis. Subjects often manifest hyperactivity, aggressiveness, hostility and anxiety. Primary delusion is usually experienced suddenly with a feeling of conviction, and it is different from the rudimentary delusional moods seen with acute toxic reactions (37). The initial signs and symptoms of stimulant psychosis may occur in subjects who do not develop psychosis (35).

Curiosity, pleasurable suspiciousness, overfascination with details, and cataloging and collecting are some of the pastimes manifested by the abusers. In heavy users anxiety, fear and suspicion are often noted. Some investigators feel that if amphetamines are given in enough doses over time, a psychotic state can be elicited in a subject (5). Variation in the mood from warm friendliness to sudden hostility and rage may result in violent acts (37). Violent activity is frequently linked to an unstable and/or psychotic behavior. Sudden increase in dosage, fatigue, and use of other drugs such as barbiturates are believed to be contributing factors toward violent behavior (36). Stimulant abuse also elicits delusions and hallucinations in individuals with a schizophrenic diathesis (37). Several studies suggest that stimulants increase the chance of developing full-fledged psychosis in individuals with latent schizophrenia (35).

Chronic administration of amphetamines to experimental animals has been demonstrated to induce stereotyped behavioral changes characterized by investigatory activities (37). The latter has a logical resemblance to repetitions, hoarding, and stereotyped behavior and thinking observed in human abusers (35).

Adverse Effects of Chronic Abuse of Stimulants. Intermittent use of amphetamines or cocaine by sniffing may cause irritation of the nasal mucous membrane. Chronic abusers are generally nutritionally debilitated and develop excoriations of the skin and open sores from scratching and pinching due to delusion of "cocaine bugs". Chronic intravenous administration of methamphetamine has been implicated in genesis of necrotizing angiitis and occlusion of cerebral vessels in young subjects. There are other septic complications that may result from the use of nonsterile drug preparations (125).

Tolerance and Withdrawal Syndrome. With amphetamine, tolerance develops to the anorectic, hyperthermic and lethal effects, and a reverse tolerance to its local anesthetic-convulsant actions is generally recognized (37). Acute tolerance or tachyphylaxis has been demonstrated for cardiovascular and subjective effects of cocaine (39). While development of tolerance to some effects of cocaine is demonstrated in human as well as in animal studies, increased intensity is reported in other effects (for example, kindling) indicating a sensitization to cocaine (63). There is no cross-tolerance between amphetamines and cocaine, but between amphetamine analogs some degree of cross-tolerance may be seen.

Withdrawal of stimulants does not produce major abstinence symptoms. Depression, anxiety, increased appetite, fatigue and extended sleep may be considered as evidence of physical dependence. The EEG shows characteristic increase in REM sleep pattern during the extended sleep phase. In some abusers withdrawal shows headache, diaphoresis, muscle cramp, and mental confusion. Although it has been controversial in case of cocaine, a true withdrawal syndrome following its chronic use is gradually becoming evident. Depression, social withdrawal, craving, tremor, muscular pain, disturbance in eating and sleep and EEG changes are some indicative withdrawal manifestations (63).

Management of Toxicity and Overdosage. Chronic stimulant users present a wide variety of clinical manifestations based on the drug abused, dosage, surroundings and individual patient variations. Psychotomimetic amphetamines, DOM or MDA, produce typical symptoms such as panic, anxiety, or depersonalized episodes.

A flexible therapeutic approach is generally recommended for treatment of acute intoxication. Sympathomimetic stimulation may be counteracted by haloperidol or other depressant drugs. Fatal toxicity usually terminates with hyperthermia. Submersion in cold water, ice packing, or small doses of chlorpromazine are usually employed to prevent hyperthermia. Less life-threatening intoxication with amphetamine managed by initial gastric lavage or emesis, and acidification of urine by ammonium chloride to promote renal excretion of the drug.

In treating subjects with a history of i.v. self-administration of amphetamines or cocaine, one should also give consideration to hepatitis, endocarditis, pneumonia, lung abscess and tetanus.

In recent years several cases with cocaine "body packer" syndrome have been reported (82). This syndrome refers to the ingestion of multiple packages containing drugs for the purpose of transporting contraband. Rupture of packets in the gastrointestinal tract was reported to cause acute cocaine poisoning often with fatal outcome.

For the treatment of stimulant psychosis, neuroleptic drugs are commonly recommended only if the psychosis is sustained following cessation of drug. For amphetamine psychosis treatment, hospitalization is warranted for proper medical supervision. Patients on withdrawal schedule should be forewarned that a depression may follow and last for few weeks to a few months. Tricyclic antidepressants (e.g., desipramine) may be indicated for a long-standing depression. Psychologic approaches to treatment would be similar to those recommended for narcotic addiction.

NICOTINE AND TOBACCO SMOKING

Nicotine, 1-methyl-2-(3-pyridyl) pyrrolidine [$CH_3NCH(C_5H_4N)CH_2CH_2CH_2$], is the alkaloid obtained from the plant *Nicotiana tabacum*. The pharmacology of nicotine is discussed in detail in Chapters 8.1 and 11.3.

Constituents of Smoke Cigarette smoke contains a wide variety of compounds which exist in two phases: particulate and gas. However, many of them remain in a distribution equilibrium, i.e., partially in gas phase and partially in particulate phase. Compounds in cigarette smoke that are judged to contribute to health hazards are carbon monoxide, nicotine and "tar". Tar is defined as the total particulate matter collected by a Cambridge filter (CM-113) after deducting moisture and nicotine, and includes compounds that are known as polycyclic aromatic hydrocarbons (PAH) (129). One of the tar compounds, β-naphthylamine, is known to be a human bladder carcinogen, and it has been reported to be present in tobacco smoke in a very low concentration (0.002 μg/cigarette) (51). It is generally recognized that various compounds in the cigarette smoke may interact to produce a pathological condition. That may be quite different from that produced by these agents when given separately. This is particularly important with respect to carcinogenic effect, where a combined effect is produced by a cancer-initiating agent, a cancer-promoting agent, and a cancer-accelerating agent. The makers of low yield cigarettes often claim that this brand delivers less tar and nicotine than high-yield brands. A recent study has demonstrated that the smokers of low-nicotine cigarettes do not consume less nicotine (9).

Prevalence. Various reports on health consequences of tobacco smoking including carcinogenesis and cardiovascular diseases have significantly reduced incidences of smoking in recent years. Current prevalence (use in the month prior to survey) of cigarette smoking dropped from 22% in youth (age 12-17) and 47% in young adults (age 18-25) in 1977 to 15% and 39.5% in respective age groups in 1982 (90).

Absorption from Smoking Tobacco. There are some quantitative differences in inhaling practices between cigarettes, cigars and pipes. About three times the quantity of nicotine is excreted in the urine with customary cigarette inhalation than with cigars and pipes (not inhaled). However, there is no difference in mean nicotine excretion if all are inhaled or not inhaled. Of various constituents of cigarette smoke such as acetaldehyde, isoprene, acetone, toluene, particulate matter, and carbon monoxide, 86-90% of all compounds except carbon monoxide is retained in human lungs. Carbon monoxide is retained to the extent of 54% (29).

Nicotine, after being absorbed from smoke rapidly, leaves the blood to concentrate in various body organs and tissues, particularly in the brain, adrenals, liver, and kidneys (124). In monkeys placental transfer of nicotine occurs rapidly and concentration in fetal circulation exceeds maternal circulation (117).

Metabolism of nicotine is carried out mainly in the liver. Nicotine and certain of its metabolites are excreted in the urine and saliva (123).

Chronic toxicity. The important health consequences of cigarette smoking are development of premature coronary heart disease, lung cancer, chronic obstructive respiratory disease, and in pregnant women, stillborn children, and babies with lower average birth weight. Passive exposure to parental cigarette smoking has been shown to be associated with reduced levels of pulmonary functions in young children (119).

Coronary heart disease. Heavy smoking is considered as a potent risk factor for coronary, cerebral, and peripheral vascular disease. Both nicotine and carbon monoxide have been suggested as causative factors, but a clear understanding of this issue still remains to be arrived at. Several prospective and retrospective studies have reported that once smoking is stopped about 90% of cardiovascular risk is reversed in about 18 months (73). In about 15% of smokers, carboxyhemoglobin level of 5% or more has been shown to exist, and such individuals show about 20-fold increase in the prevalence of atherosclerotic vascular disease. Recent studies have indicated that there are some components of the tobacco leaf that are responsible for this pathophysiology rather than previously suggested nicotine (73). It has been suggested that genetic factors play some role in the development of coronary symptoms in man (14). Cigarette smoking has been shown to interfere with the efficacy of anti-anginal drugs such as propranolol, atenolol and nifedipine (30).

Bronchopulmonary Diseases. Three common respiratory ailments, chronic bronchitis, pulmonary emphysema, and bronchial asthma, have been related to smoking, to which high morbidity and mortality due to these disease conditions have been attributed (126). Both in experimental animals and humans inhalation of cigarette smoke has been demonstrated to induce acute and chronic changes in ventilatory functions and pulmonary histology (55, 145). An acute effect of tobacco smoking is to increase pulmonary resistance (145). Dust clearance is also considerably slower in smokers than in the nonsmokers. In one study smokers were observed to retain five times more dusts than nonsmokers (19). Slowing down of pulmonary clearance mechanism by the ciliotoxic action of smoking has been suggested (19) to be responsible for the synergistic effect of tobacco smoke and certain environmental carcinogens (e.g., asbestos); asbestos workers who smoke cigarettes had a 90-fold greater risk of mortality from bronchogenic carcinoma compared to nonsmoking asbestos workers. In addition to inhibition of clearance mechanism, effects of on proteolytic enzymes and its interference with immune mechanism may contribute to chronic obstructive lung disease (115).

Malignancy. A number of epidemiological studies have demonstrated that smokers have greatly increased risks of dying from lung cancer compared with nonsmokers (49, 69). Like asbestos, other substances have been identified or suspected to be tumorigenic in cigarette smokers; they are divided into two groups: (a) cancer initiator, and (b) tumor promoter. For the role of the cancer initiators, polycyclic aromatic hydrocarbons, nitrosamines, and certain pesticides and fungicides have been implicated. Tumor promoters are polymers of unknown structures, volatile phenols and N-alkylheterocyclic compounds have been identified (143). Smoking has been implicated in the development of other types of cancer in humans and these include cancer of larynx, oral cancer, esophageal cancer, bladder and pancreas cancer (127). Currently available evidence does not establish an association between smoking and the incidence of breast cancer (102).

Smoking and Pregnancy. Both retrospective and prospective studies have demonstrated a relationship between fetal growth retardation and cigarette smoking. Animal studies have shown that chronic exposure of rabbits to carbon monoxide during gestation leads to a dose-related reduction in the birth weight of their puppies (6). Several investigators have also suggested a strong relationship between cigarette smoking and spontaneous abortion and higher stillborn rate (128).

Tolerance and Physical Dependence. Chronic smokers develop partial tolerance to nicotine, and it is more due to pharmacodynamic actions rather than alterations in metabolism. Abrupt withdrawal of smoking results in the appearance of symptom complex within 24 to 36 hours, characterized by headache, nausea, diarrhea or constipation, lack of concentration, anxiety, and irritability. These withdrawal symptoms vary from one smoker to another. There are some reports to indicate partial suppression of withdrawal symptoms by nicotine.

MARIJUANA

Marijuana and hashish are derived from *Cannabis sativa,* the hemp plant that grows in many parts of the world. Cannabis was used as an intoxicant in India around 1000 B.C. The use of cannabis spread from the Indian subcontinent to the Middle and Near East during the next several centuries and finally reached the United States via North Africa, Latin America, and the Caribbean in the nineteenth century.

Prevalence and Pattern of Use. Marijuana may be the most frequently abused substance; current estimates vary between 200 and 300 million users throughout the world with the changing styles of youth culture. A 1971 survey indicates that in the United States about 24 million persons have at least once used cannabis, with more than 50% of the people being in the age group between 16 and 26 years and its use gradually increasing in the older people. About 2% of adults and 4% of youths between 12 and 17 years of age used it more than once a day (121). Life-time ("ever-used") prevalence of marijuana use increased from 14% in youth (age 12-17), 39.3% in young adults (age 18-25) and 9.2% in older adults (age 26 and more) in 1971 to 30.9%, 68.2% and 19.6% respectively in 1979. Current use of marijuana (use in the month prior to the survey) also showed increase from 6%, 17.3% and 1.3% in 1971 to 16.7%, 35.4% and 6% in 1979; in respective age groups in 1982. In 1982, life-time prevalence (26.7%, 64.1% and 23%) as well as current use (11.5%, 27.4% and 6.6%) of marijuana showed slight decreases in the youth and young adults, but slight increases in older adults. The 1982 survey shows that marijuana is frequently used in combination with alcohol or other drugs (90).

Probably males and females, in all socioeconomic and occupational groups, equally abuse marijuana with little variation. For occasional users there may not be other drug abuse, but in persons with a compulsive drive for the substance abuse, it may be used along with other drugs. Marijuana is smoked in cigarette form ("joints") and in a variety of ways using pipes and other paraphernalia.

Characteristics of Marijuana Users. Initial experimentation with marijuana usually happens through curiosity, easy availability, and peer pressure. Due to the fact that marijuana elicits pleasurable psychological effects, a certain percentage of users get almost totally preoccupied with the substance at the expenses of other daily duties and responsibilities (111). Very heavy users of marijuana almost always remain intoxicated and seek the pharmacological effects of the substance rather than its social experience. According to some reports marijuana users are more likely to abuse other prescription drugs such as minor tranquilizers and barbiturates, and polydrug abuse in a marijuana abuser is a consistent feature. Certain personality characteristics contribute to concurrent abuse of either narcotics or psychedelic drugs.

Source and Chemistry. *Cannabis sativa* grows annually in the tropical and temperate zones of the world. The plant exists in both male and female forms and usually the resin-covered flowering tops of the female plant and their adjacent leaves are considered to have highest concentration of the psychoactive principles (cannabinoids). In the United States, the term *marijuana* refers to any part of the hemp plant or extract therefrom. A resinous cannabis extract considerably rich in cannabinoids is referred to as *hashish* (means dry grass in Arabic) and *charas* (in India). Hashish is about 5 to 10 times as potent as "typical" marijuana. The resinous mass from small leaves and bracts of influorescence of the flowering top is called *ganja* in India. The dried leaves and flowering shoots of the plant containing less psychoactive plant have been variously termed *bhang* (in India and the Middle East), *kif* (in North Africa), *dogga* (in South Africa), and *macohna* (in parts of South America).

More than 20 psychoactive compounds have been isolated from *C. sativa* and collectively they are referred to as cannabinoids. Mechoulam and coworkers isolated the major active constituent of marijuana, 1, Δ^1-3, 4-trans-tetrahydrocannabinol (Δ^1-THC), in pure form, elucidated its structure, and synthesized it. The same compound was also isolated by other chemists and named Δ^9-THC. The difference in numbering the atoms is due to the fact that the compound was regarded as a monoterpene derivative by Mechoulam and a dibenz-α-pyran by others. (Fig. 11.6-1)

Pharmacological Effects. Cannabinoids induce certain gross behavioral changes in animals, including catalepsy, ataxia, and hyperactivity. Spontaneous motor activity and exploratory behavior have been shown to be suppressed. They decrease aggressiveness in nonstressed animals, but enhance aggression on stressed condition (77). Cannabinoids have also been reported to suppress learned behavior. The overall effect of various marijuana derivatives on the CNS is initial stimulation followed by depression. Many of the cannabinoids (e.g., Δ^9-THC, cannabinol and cannabidiol) have been reported to possess anticonvulsant activity (77). Δ^9-THC has been

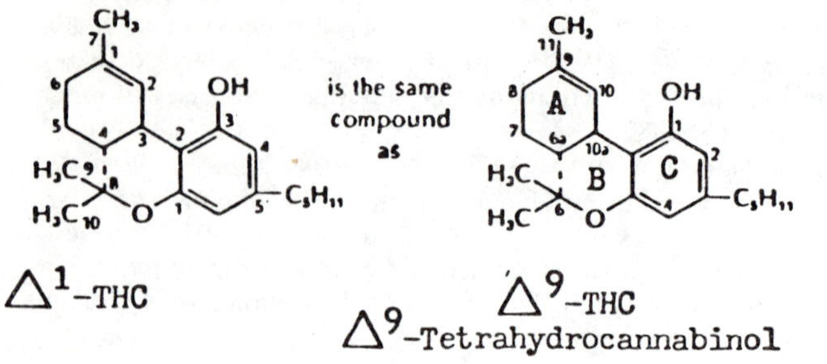

Δ^1-THC is the same compound as Δ^9-THC

Δ^9-Tetrahydrocannabinol

Fig. 11.6-1. *Chemical structures of Δ^9-tetrahydrocannabinol.*

shown to manifest analgesic and antipyretic effects in a number of animal species (75, 66). Both marijuana smoking and Δ^9-THC have been reported to cause a dose-related clinically significant fall in intraocular pressure in normal subjects. The exact mechanism of this effect is not clearly elucidated, though the ocular sympathetic system has been implicated (47).

There have been differences in the cardiovascular effects of marijuana between nonanesthetized animals and humans and anesthetized subjects (95). In humans the acute pharmacological actions of marijuana include conjunctival vascular congestion, tachycardia, fall in intraocular pressure, bronchodilatation, peripheral vasodilatation, and orthostatic hypotension. Sleep pattern may be altered. Acute behavioral effects of marijuana are variable and depend on the dose, route of administration, environmental and social setting, personality, and previous experience with the drug. Performance and cognitive functions are generally suppressed and driving ability is significantly impaired during marijuana intoxication.

Pharmacokinetics. The most common route of administration of marijuana is by smoking homemade cigarettes. A marijuana cigarette may weigh between 0.5 and 1 g and its THC contents may vary from less than 1% to 6% depending on the source. About 50% of THC in the smoke is absorbed through the respiratory system and the onset of action is very rapid (in less than a minute). Onset of action following oral ingestion is about 30 to 120 minutes, and the oral absorption is greatly influenced by the nature of vehicle used (95). Δ^9-THC binds strongly to plasma proteins. The half-life of Δ^9-THC has been shown to be about five days. Cannabinoids are extensively metabolized in the liver. The unchanged drug and its metabolites are mainly excreted in the bile and feces, and to a lesser extent in the urine (72).

Tolerance and Physical Dependence. A varying degree of tolerance develops to some of the psychologic and physiologic effects of the drug. Some evidence suggests that a mild form of physical dependence to cannabis occurs in man. Withdrawal symptoms may include hyperirritability and dysphoria (139). Anorexia, insomnia, sweating and hot flashes may also occur (63a).

Therapeutic Potentials. The most promising therapeutic potential for marijuana and tetrahydrocannabinol (THC) is in the treatment of nausea and vomiting induced by cytotoxic drugs in cancer chemotherapy (7, 28). Compared to prochlorperazine (COMPAZINE), a standard antiemetic drug, THC or its synthetic derivatives such as nabilone or levonantradol were found to be more effective in most of the studies. THC and its analogs, however, show substantial adverse effects, particularly drowsiness, dry mouth, dizziness, and hypotension; psychotic reactions also occur. These effects may be greater with increasing age of the patients.

THC has been claimed to reduce pain in cancer patients. Reduction of intraocular pressure in glaucoma is another possible therapeutic use of THC (Chapter 21.1). Potential effectiveness as bronchodilator, and anticonvulsant has also been reported. All these potential benefits are under investigations (7, 28).

Adverse Effects. Adverse reactions are generally behavioral and include depression, acute panic condition, and paranoid ideation. With very high doses acute toxic psychosis may result characterized by disorientation and auditory and visual hallucination. There is considerable disagreement regarding marijuana abuse and the development of a stable psychotic state (13) Rarely, "flashback" episodes as with psychedelic drugs may occur with marijuana. Frequent upper respiratory infections, low plasma testosterone levels, along with certain cellular changes in the sperm have been reported. But the clinical importance of the latter has not been understood clearly.

Diagnosis and Treatment. Although it is difficult to obtain a clear and definite history in most cases, a thoughtful history and a careful physical examination play important parts in providing clues for marijuana abuse. Among the laboratory methods used for detection of marijuana and its metabolites in the body fluids, gas chromatography and thin-layer chromatography are most frequently employed. However, specificity of these methods is very limited. In recent years radioimmunoassay and mass spectrofragmentography have been introduced for the purpose of marijuana detection.

The patient should be repeatedly reminded about the adverse effects of chronic marijuana abuse. Tranquilizers may sometimes be used to treat violent or aggressive state. Marijuana abuse rarely requires hospitalization except for severe and chronic disorder.

LSD AND OTHER HALLUCINOGENS

From time immemorial humans have searched for and succeeded in securing substances that would produce alterations in perception, thought, and mood without much affecting consciousness and orientation. These substances have been called hallucinogens, a term that is not completely satisfactory, since it overemphasizes the induced perceptual alterations compared with changes in mood and thought that are often much more prominent. They have also been given various other names, each of which has some limitations: psychotomimetic, although the drug-induced state does not truly mimic the naturally occurring psychosis; psychotogenic, although the concept of psychosis includes both endogenous and exogenous pychosis; deliriant, although the subjects taking these compounds are seldom delirious. They have also been inappropriately called psychedelic (mind-manifesting), mysticomimetic, and phantastica. The old term hallucinogen will be used here for such substances. They produce their effects depending on various conditions of *set* (psychological makeup of the subject) and *setting* (the physical, social, and emotional environment).

Source. Hallucinogens belong to diverse chemical groups. As such they are classified according to their chemical structure. Many of these hallucinogens are from plant origin; others are semisynthetic or synthetic. Of these lysergic acid diethylamide (LSD-25) is the most widely known hallucinogen. Phencyclidine is one of the most extensively used compounds in recent years. The chemical structures of some of these agents are given in Fig. 11.6-2.

LSD-25

History. In 1943 Albert Hofmann, a chemist in Sandoz laboratories at Basel, Switzerland, investigated the central stimulant properties of LSD because of its resemblance to nikethamide, which also contained the diethylamide structure. While working on this compound, he experienced some unusual effects described by him very vividly as follows:

> On a Friday afternoon, April 16th, 1943, while working in the laboratory, I was seized by a peculiar sensation of vertigo and restlessness. Objects, as well as the shape of my associates in the laboratory, appeared to undergo optical changes. I was unable to concentrate on my work. In a dreamlike state, I left for home, where an irresistible urge to lie down and sleep overcame me. Light was so intense as to be unpleasant. I drew the curtains and immediately fell into a peculiar state of "drunkenness," characterized by an exaggerated imagination. With my eyes closed, fantastic pictures of extraordinary plasticity and intensive color seemed to surge towards me. After two hours, this state gradually subsided and I was able to eat dinner with a good appetite.

Hofmann attributed these effects to a very small quantity of d-LSD that might have been ingested or inhaled. Stoll subsequently, through systematic study of this compound, confirmed Hofmann's original observation (100). LSD became available through illicit channels in the United States in 1960 and thereafter its abuse followed in increasing numbers.

Chemistry. Lysergic acid is an indole derivative and the chemical basis of the natural ergot alkaloids. It is the hydrolysis product of ergonovine (ergometrine) and its derivatives. There are four optically active isomers of LSD and among them d-LSD is the only potent hallucinogenic compound.

Pattern of Abuse. In the United States the abuse of LSD reached a peak in 1966-67 and thereafter gradually declined. LSD-type drugs have been considered as psychedelic (mind-manifesting) and have been used more by college students, the affluent, intellectuals, artists, and philosophy-minded persons. The common pattern of use of these drugs is an occasional trip every few weeks to months. Often other drugs such as marijuana or amphetamines are used in between.

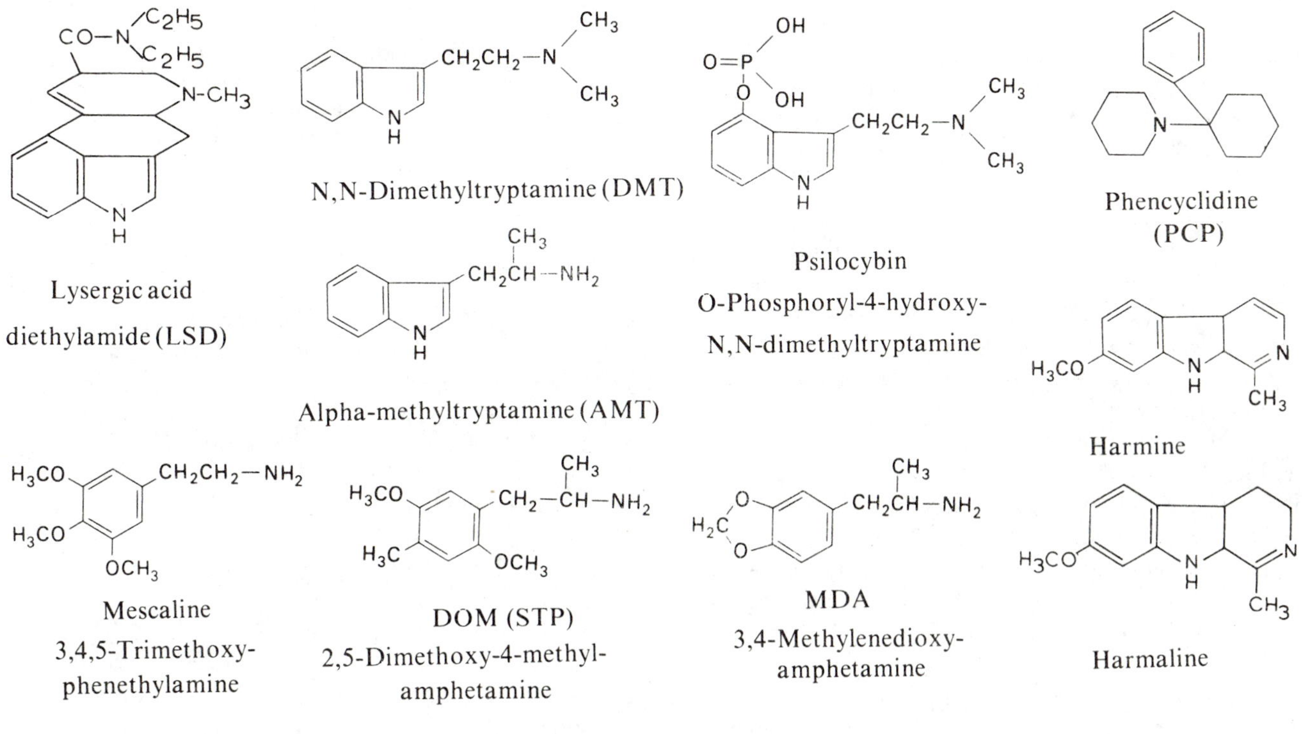

Lysergic acid diethylamide (LSD)

N,N-Dimethyltryptamine (DMT)

Alpha-methyltryptamine (AMT)

Psilocybin
O-Phosphoryl-4-hydroxy-N,N-dimethyltryptamine

Phencyclidine (PCP)

Harmine

Mescaline
3,4,5-Trimethoxyphenethylamine

DOM (STP)
2,5-Dimethoxy-4-methylamphetamine

MDA
3,4-Methylenedioxyamphetamine

Harmaline

Fig. 11.6-2. *Chemical structures of some hallucinogens.*

Prevalence of Hallucinogen Use. Life-time ("ever-used") prevalence of use of one or more hallucinogens (LSD, PCP, etc.) in the USA increased from 1974 to 1979 in all age groups: 6% to 7% in youth (age 12-17); 17% to 25% in young adults (age 18-25); 1% to 5% in older adults (age 26 or more). In 1982, the trend in their use showed a decrease; 5% of the youth, 21% of the young adults, 19% of older adults (age 26-34) and only 2% of the adults aged 25 or more used these drugs. Combined use of marijuana with hallucinogens was widely practiced. Current use (during the month prior to interview) of hallucinogens in 1982 was reduced to only 1.7% of the users among the young adults (age 18-25) (90).

Pharmacological Effects. LSD is the most potent hallucinogenic compound known, about 100 times more potent than psilocybin and 4,000times more potent than mescaline. At oral doses of 0.5 to 2 μg/kg, LSD effects are usually manifested. In susceptible individuals as low as a 20 to 25 μg dose can produce some CNS effects. The LSD effects in humans consist mainly of psychological effects and a few somatic effects. They usually follow a sequential pattern with somatic symptoms appearing first, perceptual and mood changes next, and psychic changes last.

The physiological effects usually appear in the initial phase within a few minutes of LSD intake, but some of them may continue to the end. These may include dizziness, weakness, tremor, nausea, hyperreflexia, occasional ataxia, paresthesias, some sympathomimetic effects (mydriasis, tachycardia, hypertension, hyperthermia, piloerection, dry mouth), and stimulated respiration. These are usually indicative of central effects of the drug. In this initial phase, an inner tension appears to occur, being relieved by laughing or crying; changes in pulse rate, blood pressure, or respiration may be caused by this induced anxiety state rather than by the primary drug effect. Several feelings appear to coexist at the same time and it becomes difficult to focus on them.

The perceptual and psychic changes induced by LSD not only depend on the dose, but also are greatly influenced by the set and setting. Perceptual symptoms begin to appear in about an hour or two after ingestion of the drug and become gradually prominent. Most markedly affected is the visual perception, although auditory, tactile, and other sensations may also be affected. Visual imagery becomes vivid and may appear to be beautiful or horrible. Color of objects become more intense and saturated. Visual illusions are common. Flat surfaces assume a depth and fixed objects undulate and flow. Body images become distorted, hands and feet may feel enormous, or the whole body may seem to be shrunken away. Perception of size, direction, or distance is altered. Sometimes a wavelike phenomena involving micropsia or macropsia may occur. Due to altered time perception, the visual changes may appear to continue forever. Afterimages are noticeably prolonged, sometimes producing overlapping of the ongoing and the preceding perception. Some subjects may elaborate such confluence into hallucinations. Auditory perception may be enhanced, but auditory hallucination is rare.

Synesthesia (merging of one sense modality with another) is common; sounds are seen, colors are heard or appear to have specific smells. During this stage there is often rapid mood changes. Commonly experienced are euphoric feelings, elation, bliss, and ecstasy. Mood may be labile, shifting from elation to apprehension, and depression to gaiety during the same session.

Psychic symptoms may be varied and diverse. The ego boundaries may dissolve partially or completely, to the extent that a realization of separation between self and the external world becomes subtle or sometimes nonexistent. Subjects may experience depersonalization and derealization. With many, there is a fear of fragmentation or disintegration of self, and there may be a need to lean on something or someone for structure and support. At the peak of experience, about 2 hours or more, there is difficulty in thought, expression, and concentration. The entire syndrome begins to clear in about 12 hours, although the half-life of the drug is about 3 hours.

Mechanism of Action. Recent works have shown that following administration of LSD, the concentration of 5-hydroxyindolacetic acid (5-HIAA), the principle metabolite of serotonin (5-HT) in the brain is decreased. The rate of 5-HT turnover in the brain is also reduced by LSD. In microelectrophoretic studies, application of 5-HT to 5-HT containing neurons in the dorsal raphe nuclei or in the forebrain to which the dorsal raphe neurons project inhibits neuronal activity in both sites. Extremely small i.v. doses (10-20 μg/kg) of LSD have been shown to inhibit firing of 5-HT neurons in the raphe nuclei in rats, presumably suggesting presynaptic agonistic action at the 5-HT receptors in these brain areas. This inhibition is reversible and exceedingly selective in respect to brain areas and drug itself. The resultant reduced impulse flow in 5-HT neurons has been suggested to cause depression of 5-HT turnover. Furthermore, LSD has been shown to block only the excitatory effects of 5-HT on the firing of randomly encountered cells in the reticular formation, cortex and other areas; the inhibitory effects of 5-HT in these areas are not affected by LSD or even may be potentiated by its high doses. Thus LSD appears to act also as a 5-HT antagonist in the central postsynaptic sites (3).

The mechanism of action of LSD is more complicated and needs further clarification. Its postsynaptic effects on 5-HT neurons have been shown to comprise a mixture of both agonistic and antagonistic actions. Moreover, other neurotransmitters such as catecholamines may also be involved in its action (42).

Pharmacokinetics. LSD is readily absorbed from the gastrointestinal tract and distributed widely in all tissues. The half-life in humans is about three hours. It is said to be completely metabolized in the liver to an inactive metabolite, 2-oxy-LSD, and only trace is excreted in the urine and stool.

Tolerance and Lethal Dose. Tolerance to LSD develops rapidly within three to four days of repeated use. Cross-tolerance has been demonstrated between LSD, mescaline, psilocybin, but none between LSD and amphetamines or LSD and scopolamine. Physical dependence on these drugs has not been observed. The lethal dose of LSD varies according to species of animals studied, and in humans LD_{50} is about 14 mg or 0.2 mg/kg.

Adverse Effects. Three groups of adverse reactions

have usually been observed in respect to LSD. (a) Acute panic reactions may occur initially and sometimes may continue during a "bad trip," subjects may feel helpless and afraid of losing control or of going crazy. It can be treated by reassurance in a supportive environment, and by antianxiety and sedative agents. (b) Flashback reactions or spontaneous recurrences of LSD effects in absence of the drug ("free trip") may occur. Treatment is the same as in acute panic reactions. (c) Prolonged psychotic complications including schizophrenic decompensations and prolonged hallucinosis may occur. Chlorpromazine has been found to be most effective for such psychosis.

Abuse of LSD has been claimed to enhance chromosomal breakage and results in potential risk of congenital birth defects in abusers' offspring. Substantial evidence seems to be lacking in this respect and controversy still exists. It has been suggested that spontaneous abortion rate is unusually high in pregnant women exposed to LSD. The immune system may be adversely affected, but this also requires confirmation.

PHENCYCLIDINE

History. Phencyclidine, also known as SERNYL, SERNYLAN, and PCP, was developed in the late 1950s as a "dissociative anesthetic" agent. Later on, it was found to produce postanesthetic excitement, visual disturbance, and delirium. It is now restricted to veterinary use only under the trade name of SERNYLAN.

The first "street" use of PCP was reported in 1967 when it rapidly gained reputation as a bad drug. For a while it was passed off as LSD, marijuana, or other varieties of hallucinogen. Since the mid-1970s it has found its place as a drug of abuse under its own label. It is known among the abusers by a number of street names such as angel dust, peace pill, crystal, PCP, and horse tranquilizer. It can be smoked or snorted.

Prevalence of Use. In a 1977 survey, 14% of 18 to 25 year-old youth in the U.S.A. were reported to have used PCP at least once. In 1979 the "ever-use" rate for youth (aged 12 to 17) was 3.9% and declined to 2.2% in 1982. For young adults (aged 18 to 25) the corresponding decline was from 14.5% in 1979 to 10.5% in 1982 (90). However, information from Drug Abuse Warning Network (DAWN) from National Institute on Drug Abuse (NIDA) shows that from January 1981 to July 1983, PCP and PCP combination cases showed an increasing trend from 1.95% to 3.65% among the drug-related emergency room patients.

Chemistry. Phencyclidine [1-(1-phencyclohexyl) piperidine HCl] is an arylcyclohexylamine. It is related to ketamine which is used as a dissociative anesthetic in humans. It is relatively easy to synthesize and has been prepared in many clandestine laboratories, possibly containing a wide variety of impurities.

Pharmacological Effects. In small doses the drug produces a state resembling alcoholic intoxication with ataxia and generalized numbness of extremities (96). In subanesthetic doses the psychological effects usually are experienced in three stages: (a) changes in body image accompanied by feeling of depersonalization, (b) perceptual distortions, visual or auditory, followed by (c) discomforting feeling of apathy or estrangement. Sensory disturbance produced by the drug has been described to resemble sensory deprivation (96). Amnesia for the episode may occur. Disorganization of thought and derealization are greater than with LSD. Increasing doses produce marked analgesia, anesthesia, stupor, or coma. Tachycardia, hypertension, hypersalivation, fever, muscle rigidity and convulsions may occur.

Mechanism of Action. Phencyclidine has been shown to inhibit uptake of norepinephrine, dopamine (DA) and serotonin (5-HT) *in vitro*. However, *in vivo*, only 5-HT uptake (in the brainstem) was found to be depressed by a single dose (10 mg/kg) of PCP; it did not affect DA uptake in the striatum at this dose (112). Like amphetamine, PCP produced a decrease in the number of [^{3}H]spiroperidol sites in the striatum after chronic treatment; this decrease could be due to chronic hyperactivity of dopaminergic neurotransmission leading to down regulation of D_2-dopamine (neuroleptic) receptors (101). PCP also inhibits tyrosine hydroxylase and decreases striatal DOPA level. It can release DA from striatal tissue slices, but its potency is quite less than amphetamine in this regard. For these and other reasons, PCP that does not appear to have a direct action on pre- or postsynaptic dopamine receptor, has been considered to be an indirect dopamine agonist, but its properties are closer to the non-amphetamine type than to amphetamine itself (85). In addition, PCP, following a single dose administration can cause some changes in the activity of choline acetyltransferase, acetylcholinesterase and glutamic acid dehydrogenase in the cerebellum and hippocampus indicating the involvement of also other neurotransmitters (54).

Pharmacokinetics. PCP is well absorbed from all routes of administration. It may be hydroxylated and metabolites are conjugated with glucuronic acid. There is considerable gastroenteric recirculation. Decreased plasma pH decreases drug concentration in cerebrospinal fluid. Thus in cases of overdose continuous gastric suction and acidification of urine are useful; they can reduce the half-life of the drug during overdose from about 3 days to about 1 day.

Tolerance and Dependence. Human users of PCP show tolerance, psychological dependence, but not physical dependence (97). Tolerance develops to the behavioral and toxic effects of PCP in animals as well as to subjective effects in human users. Psychological dependence is indicated by craving for a drug noted in users. This is supported by the ability of PCP to maintain self-administration behavior in dogs and monkeys and thus to serve as a positive reinforcer.

Although there is no clinical report of physical dependence in human users, such dependence has been induced in monkeys under experimental conditions (8). Withdrawal symptoms are manifested after abrupt discontinuation of PCP following long term intoxication; by 4 hours postdrug, animal showed decreased intoxication, started eating and became less ataxic. At 8-12 hr they showed marked hyperresponsiveness with a distinctive oculomotor hyperactivity that was different from nystagmus observed during intoxication. In addition to these, several of the following symptoms are observed during the peak hours (12-16 hr) of withdrawal: piloerection, tremor, diarrhea, continuous vocalization, priapism, bruxism and ear and facial twitches. Abdominal contraction, emesis and convulsions occurred in some animals. Symptoms which are gradually decreased over next 24 hr, could be immediately reversed by i.v. administration of 0.25 mg/kg of PCP.

Adverse Effects. Acute intoxication with phencyclidine has been reported to cause death. Manifestations of acute intoxication include excitation, nystagmus, hypertension, muscular rigidity and hyperreflexia. Cardiac arrhythmia, convulsions and coma may result from high doses. Chronic abuse of phencyclidine may lead to a syndrome of organic brain disorder characterized by disorientation, and visual and memory disorders (87). Infants with a history of in utero exposure to PCP have been reported to manifest sudden outbursts of agitation and rapid alterations in level of consciousness, similar to responses observed in adults following intoxication with the drug.

MISCELLANEOUS AGENTS

OLOLIUQUE

Ololiuque is the Aztec name given to seeds of certain species of wild American morning glory (family Convolvulacea or snake plant). Its history, chemistry and pharmacological effects have been reviewed by Cohen (20). The hallucinogenic effects are mainly due to the content of *d*-lysergic acid amide and *d*-isolysergic acid amide. In humans morning glory seeds produce facial flushing and increased light sensitivity at lower doses, and apathy, indifference, and sedation at higher doses (30 mg). Ergotism may be caused by ingestion of a large number of seeds.

TRYPTAMINE DERIVATIVES

Agents belonging to the class of tryptamine derivatives include α-methyl-tryptamine (AMT), N,N-dimethyltryptamine (DMT), and diethyltryptamine (DET) (Fig. 11.6-2). AMT is an analog of psilocybin, and the indole analog of amphetamine. It produces a prolonged effect considered to be pleasant but not as experienced with psilocybin. Early symptoms are anxiety and restlessness. DMT occurs with bufotenine in the seeds and leaves of the mimosacea plant (*Piptadenia peregrina Benth*).It is orally inactive, used by sniffing. Psychological effects include perceptual distortions, visual hallucinations, mydriasis, and hypertension. DET, an analog of DMT, is mainly a synthetic product. In humans given intramuscularly, it produces mild to moderate psychosis resembling mescaline, associated with sympathetic stimulation. Perceptual findings are prominent and mood is always euphoric. Aftereffects include lethargy, headache, depression and insomnia.

ALKYLHYDROXYTRYPTAMINE

Bufotenine. Bufotenine first isolated from the frog (*Bufo vulgaris*) skin, was also found to occur in seeds of mimosacea plants (*Piptadenia peregrina Benth*). Bufotenine at nontoxic doses produces visual disturbances, ataxia, blindness, and suppression of conditioned avoidance response in various animal species (96). In humans, bufotenine at doses ranging from 1 to 20 mg causes a feeling of tightness in the stomach, paresthesia of face, visual hallucinations, inability to concentrate, impairment of time and space perception, purple color of the face, nausea, nystagmus, mydriasis, and relaxation sequentially in increasing doses.

PSILOCYBIN AND PSILOCIN

Psilocybin and psilocin are alkaloids obtained from a mushroom belonging to the genus *Psilocybe* (Chapter 8.1). Psilocybin is the 4-O-phosphorylated and psilocin the 4-hydroxylated ester of DMT. Psilocin is the active metabolite of psilocybin. Hallucinogenic effects of psilocybin are similar to LSD in many respects, but the effects are short lasting (2 to 6 hours). However, LSD is about 150 to 200 times more potent than psilocybin which is about 1.5 times less potent than psilocin (96). Symptoms of psilocybin ingestion (60 to 209 μg/kg) include weakness, dizziness, nausea, anxiety, mydriasis, blurred vision, impaired coordination and hyperreflexia. There are also visual effects manifested by brighter colors, sharply defined objects, and colored patterns and shapes, often occurring with eyes closed. Tolerance develops to psilocybin and cross-tolerance among LSD, psilocin, and psilocybin has been demonstrated.

MISCELLANEOUS ALKALOIDS

A hallucinogenic drink used by South American Indians for ceremonial purposes has been found to contain alkaloids (harmine, harmaline and tetrahydroharmine) from the plant *Banisteria caapi*. In humans, it has been shown to cause visual hallucination. At higher oral doses it causes nausea, vomiting, tremors, buzzing noises, sinking sensation, a feeling of bodily vibrations, and numbness (96). Various other pharmacological actions have been reviewed by Hollister (53).

PHENYLETHYLAMINE

Mescaline. Mescaline is the primary active component of the peyote cactus. Peyote has been used by the Mexican Indians in their religious rites to experience visions for purposes of prophecy, divination, and a state of trance. Additionally, it has been used to relieve fatigue and hunger.

Mescaline is the principal alkaloid isolated from peyote cactus by Heffter in 1896 (96). There are about a dozen and a half alkaloids in peyote. Mescaline is a phenylethylamine derivative and structurally related to NE and epinephrine.

In normal subjects mescaline produces psychic effects very similar to LSD; the latter being 4,000 times more potent. Mescaline-induced hallucinations are visual and consist of brightly colored lights, geometric designs, animals and sometimes people. These are mostly illusions and pseudohallucinations. Anxiety, impairment of intellectual functions, and EEG disturbances may occur usually with higher doses. Like LSD it causes central sympathetic stimulation (characterized by mydriasis, hypertension and tachycardia), hyperreflexia, and static tremor. It is readily absorbed from the gastrointestinal tract and has a half-life of 6 hours. In humans about 60-90% of a single dose is excreted unchanged in the urine. Other pharmacological effects of mescaline have been reviewed by Hollister (53).

AMPHETAMINES

DOM (STP), DOE and MDA are chemically related to both amphetamines and mescaline. They are often referred to as "psychotomimetic amphetamines." The chemical structures are shown in Fig. 11.6-2.

DOM (STP) is 2,5 -dimethoxy -4-methylamphetamine. Like other hallucinogens, it produces an ambivalent feeling involving both euphoria and dysphoria, perceptual alterations including visual and auditory changes, uncontrolled laughter, and difficulty in controlling thoughts, expression, and emotion. At higher doses it produces hallucinations similar to LSD, mescaline, or psilocybin (96). DOM also causes manifestation of sympathetic hyperactivity. Tolerance develops to behavioral, electrophysiological, and biochemical actions of DOM.

Cross-tolerance between DOM, mescaline, and *d*-LSD has been shown to exist (130). Adverse effects of DOM include dry mouth, blurred vision and photophobia (atropine-like). Intoxication is managed by sedation (e.g., diazepam), chlorpromazine can counteract symptoms of smaller doses of DOM but has no effect on severe toxic symptoms.

MDA (3,4-methylenedioxyamphetamine) possesses minor sympathomimetic effects and causes a sense of well-being with heightened tactile sensation and increased urge to be with or talk to other people. Side effects of MDA are muscle ache, tightening of the jaw and grinding of teeth, delirium, and temporary amnesia.

ANTICHOLINERGIC ALKALOIDS

The leaves of *Datura stramonium* have been smoked for pleasure in various parts of Africa and India. Jimsonweed, as it is known in the United States, caused mass poisoning among British troops in Jamestown, Virginia, in 1676. There are several species of *Datura* and they contain the alkaloids atropine, hyoscyamine and scopolamine. Hallucinations produced by anticholinergic alkaloids are to some degree similar to LSD (and are associated with mydriasis, fever and tachycardia as in the case of LSD), but differ from the latter in that they cause simple and discrete as opposed to magnified and spectacular distortions.

PIPERIDYL BENZILATE ESTERS

Piperidyl benzilate esters are anticholinergic compounds synthesized in an attempt to substitute for the natural alkaloids. A series of piperidyl benzilate esters (JB-329, JB-318, JB-336) and piperidolate (96) have been found to possess potent central anticholinergic and psychotomimetic actions. Their clinical effects in humans resemble those of belladonna alkaloids. Hallucinations are primarily visual and not like LSD. Delirium rather than schizophrenialike condition is produced. In larger doses delirium persists for more than 24 hours. The peripheral anticholinergic effects are more pronounced than the sympathetic effects of LSD. The mode of action of these compounds is not clear. It has been suggested that psychotomimetic piperidyls may interfere with brain acetylcholine. Tolerance is produced as a result of repeated doses of DITRAN (JB-329).

OTHER AGENTS

Fly agaric, nutmeg, amantadine, and antihistamines are known to cause hallucinations. Their pharmacological actions have been reviewed by Pradhan (96).

ACUTE TOXICITY

Deaths directly related to LSD-like drugs have not been reported. Like LSD, acute toxicity from these drugs may include acute panic reactions and psychotic disorders. There is no systematic therapeutic regimen established for this class of drugs. Subjects with acute panic reaction should be left with someone in a calm and undisturbing state. Severely agitated subjects may need diazepam or chlorpromazine by one or more injections or orally to counteract the agitated state. Other therapeutic measures are directed toward supportive and symptomatic treatment.

MIXED SUBSTANCE ABUSE

It is a common practice among many substance abusers to use more than one drug or substance. Such "mixed substance abuse" which has also been called as "poly drug" or "multiple drug abuse" is prevalent among students, house wives, military personnel, doctors, alcoholics and narcotic addicts (34). About 5 to 25% of drug abuse subjects are mixed substance abusers (89).

Mixed drug abusers generally manifest worse psychiatric status and show significantly greater incidence of psychopathology than the opiate-only abusers. Of the two treatment modalities available for mixed abusers (i.v., drug-free therapeutic community, and methadone maintenance), mixed opiate-stimulant abusers have been reported to obtain greater benefits from the methadone maintenance program, and mixed opiate-depressant subjects showed more improvement when treated in drug free therapeutic program (83).

TOLERANCE AND DEPENDENCE LIABILITY

Information regarding development of tolerance and dependence with respect to a number of common drugs of abuse are summarized in Table 11.6-6.

Table 11.6-6
Parameters of Dependence and Tolerance of Some Common Intoxicants

Drug	Tolerance	Psychological Dependence	Physical Dependence
Alcohol	+	+++	+++
Barbiturates	++	+++	+++
Heroin	+++	++++	++++
D-Amphetamine	+/–	++	+
Cocaine	+/–	+++	+
Nicotine	+	++	+
Caffeine	+	++	0/+
Marihuana	+/–	++	0/+
LSD	+	+?	0
Nalorphine	+	0	+

+ (mild) to ++++ (severe); – reverse tolerance or sensitization.

REFERENCES

1. Adam, K., Adamson, L., Brezinova, V., et al. Nitrazepam: Lastingly effective but trouble on withdrawal. *Br. Med. J.,* 1:1558, 1976.
2. Adler, M. W., and Geller, E. B. Factors to be considered in using brain lesions to study the central sites of action of narcotics. In: *Factors Affecting the Action of Narcotics* (Adler, M. W., Manara, L., and Samanin, R., eds.). New York: Raven Press, 1978, p. 93.
3. Aghajanian, G. K., and Wang, R. Y. Physiology and pharmacology of central serotonergic neurons. In: *Psychopharmacology: A Generation of Progress* (Lipton, M. A., DiMascio, A., and Killam, K. F., eds.). New York: Raven Press, 1978, p. 171.
4. Allgulander, C. Dependence on sedative-hypnotic drugs: A comparative clinical and social study. *Acta Psychiat. Scand. Suppl.,* 270:1, 1978.

5. Angrist, B., and Gershon, S. The phenomenology of experimentally induced amphetamine psychosis: Preliminary observations. *Biol. Psychiat.*, 2:95, 1970.
6. Astrup, P. Pathologische wirkungen massiger kohlenmonoxid-konzen-trationen. *Staub-Reinhaltung der Luft*, 32:146, 1972.
7. Bateman, D. N., and Tawlins, M. D. 1982. Therapeutic potential of cannabinoids. *Br. Med. J.*, 284:1211, 1982.
8. Balster, R. L. and Wollverton, W. L. Tolerance and dependence to phencyclidine. In: *PCP (Phencyclidine): Historical and Current Perspectives* (Domino, E. F., ed.). Ann Arbor, MI: NPP Books, 1981, p. 293.
9. Benowitz, N. L., Hall, S. M., Herning, R. I., et al. Smokers of low-yield cigarettes do not consume less nicotine. *N. Engl. J. Med.*, 309:139, 1983.
10. Billiard, M., Besset, A., and Passount, P. Screening a population of insomniacs. *Sleep Res.*, 5:159, 1976.
11. Black, P. D. Mental illness due to the voluntary inhalation of petrol vapour. *Med. J. Austr.*, 2:70, 1967.
12. Bleyer, W. A., and Marshall, R. E. Barbiturate withdrawal syndrome in passively addicted infant. *J. Amer. Med. Assoc.*, 221:185, 1972.
13. Carney, P., and Lipsedge, M. Psychosis after cannabis abuse. *Br. Med. J.*, 288:1381, 1984.
14. Cederlof, R., Triberg, L., and Hrubec, Z. Cardiovascular and respiratory systems in relation to tobacco smoking: A study on American twins. *Arch. Environ. Health*, 18:934, 1969.
15. Chasnoff, I. J., Burns, W. J., Hatcher, R. P., and Burns, K. A. Phencyclidine: Effects on the fetus and neonate. *Dev. Pharmacol. Ther.*, 6:404, 1983.
16. Clift, A. D. Sleep disturbance in general practice. In: *Sleep Disturbance and Hypnotic Drug Dependence* (Clift, A. D., ed.). Amsterdam: Excerpta Medica, 1975, p. 155.
17. Clouet, D. H., and Iwatsubo, K. Mechanisms of tolerance to and dependence on narcotic analgesic drugs. *Ann. Rev. Pharmacol.*, 15:49, 1975.
18. Cochin, J., and Kornetsky, C. Factors in blood of morphine tolerant animals that attenuate or enhance effects of morphine in nontolerant animals. In: *The Addictive States* (Wikler, A., ed.). Baltimore: William and Wilkins, 1968, p. 268.
19. Cohen, D., Arai, S. F., and Brain, J. D. Smoking impairs long-term dust clearance from the lung. *Science*, 204:514, 1979.
20. Cohen, S. Psychotomimetic agents. *Ann. Rev. Pharmacol.*, 7:301, 1967.
21. Cohen, S. The volatile solvents. *Public Health Reviews*, 11:185, 1973.
22. Cohen, S. Abuse of inhalation. In: *Drug Abuse, Clinical and Basic Aspects* (Pradhan, S. N., and Dutta, S. N., eds.). St. Louis: C. V. Mosby, 1977, p. 290.
23. Collier, H. O. J. Supersensitivity and dependence. *Nature* (London) 220:228, 1968.
24. Collier, H. O. J. Drug Dependence: A pharmacological analysis. *Br. J. Addict.*, 67:277, 1972.
25. Collier, H. O. J. Dependence within the opiate-sensitive neuron. In: *National Institute on Drug Abuse Research Monograph* (Harris, L. S., ed.), Series 27. Washington, D.C.: DHEW, 1979, p. 219.
26. Cooper, J. R. *Sedative-hypnotic Drugs: Risks and Benefits.* National Institute on Drug Abuse, Rockville, MD., 1977, p. 69.
27. Costall, B., and Naylor, R. J. A role for the amygdala in the development of the cataleptic and stereotypic actions of the narcotic agonist and antagonist in the rat. *Psychopharmacologia*, 35:203, 1974.
28. Council on Scientific Affairs, AMA. Marijuana. Its health hazards and therapeutic potentials. *J. Amer. Med. Assoc.*, 246:1823, 1981.
29. Dalhamn, T. Retention of cigarette smoke components in human lungs. *Arch. Environ. Health*, 17:746, 1968.
30. Deanfield, J., Wright, C., Krikler, S., et al. Cigarette smoking and the treatment of angina with propranolol, atenolol, and nifedipine. *N. Engl. J. Med.*, 310:951, 1984.
31. Dodds, J., and Santostefano, S. A comparison of the cognitive functioning of glue sniffers and non-sniffers. *J. Pediatr.*, 64:565, 1964.
32. Dole, V. P., Nyswander, M. E., and Kreek, M. J. Narcotic blockade. *Arch. Intern. Med.*, 118:304, 1966.
33. Durden, W. D., and Chipman, D. W. Gasoline sniffing complicated by acute carbon tetrachloride poisoning. *Arch. Intern. Med.*, 119:371, 1967.
34. Dutta, S. N, and Kaufman, E. Multiple drug abuse. In: *Drug Abuse: Clinical and Basic Aspects* (Pradhan, S. N., and Dutta, S. N., eds.). St. Louis: Mosby, 1977, pp. 303.
35. Ellinwood, E. H., Jr. Amphetamine psychosis. In: Description of the individuals and process. *J. Nerv. Ment. Dis.*, 144:273, 1967.
36. Ellinwood, E. H., Jr. Assault and homicide associated with amphetamine abuse. *Amer. J. Psychiat.*, 127:1170, 1971.
37. Ellinwood, E. H., Jr. and Petrie, W. M. Dependence on amphetamine, cocaine, and other stimulants. In: *Drug Abuse, Clinical and Basic Aspects* (Pradhan, S. N., and Dutta, S. N., eds.). St. Louis: C. V. Mosby, 1977, p. 248.
38. Fernandez, G., and Clarke, M. A case of "veronal" poisoning. *Lancet*, 1:223, 1904.
39. Fischman, M. W. The behavioral pharmacology of cocaine in humans. In: *Cocaine: Pharmacology, Effects, and Treatment of Abuse* (Grabowski, J., ed.). Rockville, MD: National Institute on Drug Abuse, 1984, p. 72.
40. Fraser, H. F., and Jasinsky, D. R. The assessment of the abuse potentiality of sedative/hypnotics (depressants): Methods used in animals and man. In: *Drug Addiction I* (Martin, W. R., ed.). New York: Springer-Verlag, 1977, p. 589.
41. Fraser, H. F., Wikler, A., Essig, C. F., and Isbell, H. Degree of physical dependence induced by secobarbital or pentobarbital. *J. Amer. Med. Assoc.*, 166:126, 1958.
42. Freedman, D. X., and Halaris, A. E. Monoamines and the biochemical mode of action of LSD at synapses. In: *Psychopharmacology: A Generation of Progress* (Lipton, M. A., DiMascio, A., and Killam, K. F., eds.). New York: Raven Press, 1978, p. 347.
43. Greer, J. E. Adolescent abuse of typewriter correction fluid. *Southern Med. J.*, 77:297, 1984.
44. Gold, M. S. Pottash, A. L. C., Sweeney, D. R., and Kleber, H. D. Clonidine detoxification. A fourteen-day protocol for rapid opiate withdrawal. In: *Problems of Drug Dependence*, NIDA Research Monograph, 27:226, 1979.
45. Goldstein, A., and Goldstein, D. B. Enzyme expansion theory of drug tolerance and physical dependence. In: *Addictive States* (Wikler, A., ed.). Baltimore: Williams and Wilkins, 1968, p. 265.
46. Goodwin, D.W., and Guze, S.B. Heredity and alcoholism. In: *Biology of Alcoholism, Vol. 3., Clinical Pathology* (Kissin, B., and Begleiter, H., eds.). New York: Plenum Press, 1974.
47. Green, K., and Kim, K. Interaction of adrenergic blocking agents with prostaglandin E_2 and tetrahydrocannabinol in the eye. *Exp. Eye Res.*, 15:499, 1973.
48. Hahn, T. J., Hendin, B. A., Scharp, C. R., and Haddad, J. J., Jr. Effect of chronic anticonvulsant therapy on serum 25-hydroxycholecalciferol levels in adults. *N. Engl. J. Med.*, 287:900, 1972.
49. Hammond, E. C. Smoking relation to the death rates of 1 million men and women. In: *Epidemiological Approaches to the Study of Cancer and Other Chronic Diseases* (Haenszel, W., ed.). Bethesda, Maryland: U.S.P.H.S. National Cancer Institute, monograph 19, 1966, p. 127.
50. Himmelsbach, C. K. Morphine with reference to physical dependence. *Fed. Proc.*, 2:201, 1943.
51. Hoffman, D., Masuda, Y., and Wynder, E. L. Alpha-naphthylamine and beta-naphthylamine in cigarette smoke. *Nature*, 221:254, 1969.
52. Hollister, L. E. Structure activity relationships in man of cannabis constituent and homologues and metabolites of Δ^9-tetrahydro-

cannabinol (THC). *Pharmacology*, 11:3, 1974.

53. Hollister, L. E., Macnicol, M. E., and Gillespie, H. K. An hallucinogenic amphetamine analog (DOM) in man. *Psychopharmacologia*, 14:62, 1969.

54. Hsu, L. L., Smith, R. C., Rolstein, C., and Leelavathi, D. E. Effects of acute and chronic phencyclidine on neurotransmitter enzymes in rat brain. *Biochem. Pharmacol.*, 29:2524, 1980.

55. Ide, G., Suntzeff, V., and Cowdry, E. V. A comparison of the histopathology of tracheal and bronchial epithelium of smokers and nonsmokers. *Cancer*, 12:473. 1959.

56. Isbell, H., and Chrusciel, T. L. Dependence liability of "non-narcotic" drugs. *Bull. W.H.O.*, 43 (suppl.), 5, 1970.

57. Jacquet, Y. F., Klee, W. A., Rice, K. C., Iijima, I., and Minamikawa, J. Stereospecific and nonstereospecific effects of (+) and (−) morphine: Evidence for a new class of receptors. *Science*, 198:842, 1977.

58. Jaffe, J. H., and Sharpless, S. K. Pharmacological denervation supersensitivity in the central nervous system: A theory of physical dependence. In: *Addictive States* (Wikler, A., ed.). Baltimore: Williams and Wilkins, 1968, p. 226.

59. Jellinek, E. M. *The Disease Concept of Alcoholism*. New Haven: Hillhouse Press, 1960.

60. Johnson, L. A. Amphetamine abuse in professional football. *Dissert. Abstr. Internat.* Ann Arbor, Mich.: M-Films 73-11,437, 1973.

61. Johnston, L. D., Bachman, J. G., and O'Malley, P. Drugs and the nation's high school students. In: *Drug Abuse in the Modern World* (Nahas, G. G., and Frick, H. C., eds.). New York: Pergamon Press, 1979, p. 87.

62. Jones, E. *The Life and Work of Sigmund Freud* (Trilling, L., and Marcus, S., eds.). New York: Basic Books, 1961.

63. Jones, R. T. The pharmacology of cocaine. In: *Cocaine: Pharmacology, Effects, and Treatment of Abuse* (Grabowski, J., ed.). Rockville, MD: National Institute on Drug Abuse, 1984, p. 34.

63a. Jones, R. T., and Benowitz, N. The 30-day—Clinical studies of cannabis tolerance and dependence. In: *Pharmacology of Marihuana* (Braude, M. C., and Szara, S., eds.), Vol. 2. New York: Raven Press, 1976, p. 627.

64. Kalant, H, LeBlanc, A. E., and Gibbons, R. J. Tolerance to and dependence on some nonopiate psychotropic drugs. *Pharmacol. Rev.*, 23:135, 1971.

65. Kales, A., Kales, J. D., Scharf, M. B., and Tan, T. Hypnotics and altered sleep-dream patterns, II. All night EEG studies of chloral hydrate, flurazepam, and methaqualone. *Arch. Gen. Psychiat.*, 23:219, 1970.

66. Kaymakcalan, S., Turker, R. K., and Turker, M. N. Analgesic effect of delta-9-tetrahydrocannabinol and development of tolerance to this effect in the dog. *Psychopharmacologia*, 35:123, 1974.

67. Kosterlitz, H. W., and Hughes, H. Some thoughts on the significance of enkephalin, the endogenous ligand. *Life Sci.*, 17:91, 1975.

68. Kramer, J. C., Fischman, V., and Littlefield, D. C. Amphetamine abuse. Pattern and effects of high doses taken i.v. *J. Amer. Med. Assoc.*, 201:305, 1967.

69. Kreyberg, L. A. Aetiology of lung cancer. *Morphological and Epidemiological and Experimental Analysis*. Oslo: Universitetsforlaget, 1969, p. 99.

70. Law, W. R., and Nelson, E. R. Gasoline sniffing by an adult. Report of a case with unusual complications of lead encephalopathy. *J. Amer. Med. Assoc.*, 204:1002, 1968.

71. Lawton, J. J., and Malmquist, C. P. Gasoline addiction in children. *Psychiat. Quarterly*, 35:555, 1961.

72. Lemberger, I., and Rubin, A. The physiologic disposition of marihuana in man. *Life Sci.*, 17:1637, 1975.

73. Levy, R. I. Prevalence and epidemiology of cardiovascular disease. In: *Cecil Textbook of Medicine* (Beeson, P. B., McDermott, W., and Wyngaarden, J. B., eds.). Philadelphia: W. B. Saunders, 1979, p. 1059.

74. Linnoila, M. Effects of drugs and alcohol on psychomotor skills relative to driving. *Ann. Clin. Res.*, 6:7, 1976.

75. Liu, R. K. Hypothermic effects of marihuana, marihuana derivatives, and chlorpromazine in laboratory mice. *Res. Com. Chem. Pathol. Pharmacol.*, 9:215, 1974.

76. Malfroy, B., Swerts, J. P., Guyon, A., Rogues, B. P., and Schwartz, J. C. High-affinity enkephalin-degrading peptidase in brain is increased after morphine. *Nature* (London), 276:523, 1978.

77. Fifth annual report to the U.S. Congress. *Marihuana and Health*, Rockville, MD: National Institute on Drug Abuse, 1975.

78. Martin, W. R. General problems of drug abuse and drug dependence. In: *Drug Addiction I* (Martin, W. B., ed.). New York: Springer-Verlag, 1977, p. 3.

79. Martin, W. R. A homeostatic and redundance theory of tolerance to and dependence on narcotic analgesics. *Proc. Assoc. Res. Nerv. Ment. Dis.*, 46:206, 1968.

80. Mattson, R. H., Gallagher, B. B., Reynolds, E. H. and Glass, D. Folate therapy in epilepsy. *Arch. Neurol.*, 29:78, 1973.

81. Mayfield, D. G., and Johnston, R. G. M. Pharmacology treatment in drug abuse. *Rhode Island Med. J.*, 61:69, 1978.

82. McCarron, M. M., and Wood, J. D. The cocaine 'body packer' syndrome. *J. Amer. Med. Assoc.*, 25:1417, 1983.

83. McLellan, A. T., Woody, G. E., Evans B. D., and O'Brien, C. P. Treatment of mixed abusers in methadone maintenance: Role of psychiatric factors. *Ann. N.Y. Acad. Sci.*, 398:65, 1982.

84. Mello, N. K., and Mendelson, J. H. Buprenorphine suppresses heroin use by addicts. *Science*, 207:657, 1980.

85. Meltzer, H. Y., Sturgeon, R. D., Simonovic, M., and Fessler, R. G. Phencyclidine as an indirect dopamine agonist. In: *PCP (Phencyclidine): Historical and Current Perspectives* (Domino, E. F., ed.). Ann Arbor: NPP Books, P.O. Box 1491, 1981, p. 207.

86. Mendelson, J. H. Alcohol abuse and alcohol related illness. In: *Cecil Textbook of Medicine* (Beeson, P. B., McDermott, W., and Wyngaarden, J. B., eds.). Philadelphia: W. B. Saunders, 1979, p. 705.

87. Millman, R. B. Psychedelics. In: *Cecil Textbook of Medicine* (Beeson, P. B., McDermott, W., and Wyngaarden, J. B., eds.). Philadelphia: W. B. Saunders, 1979, p. 703.

88. Moore, R. A. Dependence on alcohol. In: *Drug Abuse: Clinical and Basic Aspects* (Pradhan, S. N., and Dutta, S. N., eds.). St. Louis: C. V. Mosby, 1977, p. 211.

89. National Institute on Drug Abuse. *Statistical Series.*, Q. Report 2 Washington, D.C.; U.S. Government Printing Office, (8 May), 1981.

90. Miller, J. D., and others. *National Survey on Drug Abuse: Main Findings 1982*, Rockville, MD: National Institute on Drug Abuse, 1983.

91. Paton, W. D. M. A pharmacological approach to drug dependence and drug tolerance. In: *Scientific Basis of Drug Dependence* (Steinberg, H., ed.). London: Churchill, 1969, p. 31.

92. Peachey, J. E., and Naranjo, C. A. The role of drugs in the treatment of alcoholism. *Drugs*, 27:171, 1984.

93. Pickens, R., and Thompson, T. Self-administration of cocaine and amphetamine by rats, reported to the NAS-NRC Committee on Problems of Drug Dependence, 1967.

94. Powars, D. Aplastic anemia secondary to glue sniffing. *N. Engl. J. Med.*, 273:700, 1965.

95. Pradhan, S. N. Marijuana. In: *Drug Abuse: Clinical and Basic Aspects* (Pradhan, S. N., and Dutta, S. N., eds.). St. Louis: C. V. Mosby, 1977, p. 148.

96. Pradhan, S. N., LSD and other hallucinogens. In: *Drug Abuse: Clinical and Basic Aspects* (Pradhan, S. N., and Dutta, S. N., eds.). St. Louis: C. V. Mosby, 1977, p. 174.

97. Pradhan, S. N. Phencyclidine (PCP): Some human studies. *Neurosci. Biobehav. Rev.*, 8:493, 1984.

98. Pradhan, S. N., and Dutta, S. N. Narcotic analgesics. In: *Drug*

Abuse: Clinical and Basic Aspects (Pradhan, S. N., and Dutta, S. N., eds.). St. Louis: C. V. Mosby, 1977, p. 49.

99. Rabins, P., Swanson, W. C., and Gallant, D. M. A comparison of two methods of determining drug use among university students. *J. Louisiana St. Med. Soc.*, 126:1, 1974.

100. Rinkel, M., Hyde, R. W., and Solomon, H. C. Experimental psychiatry. IV. Hallucinogens: Tools in experimental psychiatry. *Dis. Nerv. Syst.*, 16:229, 1955.

101. Robertson, H. A. Chronic phencyclidine, like amphetamine, produces a decrease in [^{3}H] spiroperidol binding in rat striatum. *Eur. J. Pharmacol.*, 78:363, 1982.

102. Rosenberg, L., Schwingl, P. J., Kaufman, D. W., et al. Breast cancer and cigarette smoking, *N. Engl. J. Med.*, 310:92, 1984.

103. Ryback, R. S., Eckardt, M. J., and Pautler, C. P. Biochemical and hematological correlates of alcoholism. *Res. Commun. Chem. Pathol. Pharmacol.*, 27:533, 1980.

104. Schuster, C. R., and Thompson, T. Self-administration of and behavioral dependence on drugs. *Ann. Rev. Pharmacol.*, 9:483, 1969.

105. Seevers, M. H., and Deneau, G. A. A critique of the "dual action" hypothesis of morphine physical dependence. *Arch. Int. Pharmacodyn.*, 140:514, 1962.

106. Sedien, L. S., Fischman, M. W., and Schuster, C. R. Changes in brain catecholamines induced by long-term methamphetamine administration in rhesus monkeys. In: *Cocaine and Other Stimulants* (Ellinwood, E. H., Jr., and Kilbey, M. D., eds.). New York: Plenum Press, 1977, p. 179.

107. Sells, S. B., and Simpson, D. D. The case for drug abuse treatment effectiveness, based on the DARP research program. *Br. J. Addiction*, 75:117, 1980.

108. Selzer, M. L. The Michigan alcoholism screening test: The quest for a need of diagnostic instrument. *Amer. J. Psychiat.*, 127:1653, 1971.

109. Sharma, S. K., Klee, W. A., and Nirenberg, M. Dual regulation of adenylate cyclase accounts for narcotic dependence and tolerance. *Proc. Nat. Acad. Sci. USA.*, 72:3092, 1975.

110. Sharma, S. K., Klee, W. A., and Nirenberg, M. Opiate-dependent modulation of adenylate cyclase. *Proc. Nat. Acad. Sci. USA*, 74:3365, 1977.

111. Smith, D. C., and Mehl, C. An analysis of marijuana toxicity. *Clin. Toxicol.*, 3:101, 1970.

112. Smith, R. C. Meltzer, H. Y., Arora, R. C., and Davis, J. M. Effects of phencyclidine on [^{3}H] catecholamine and [^{3}H] serotonin uptake in synaptosomal preparations from rat brain. *Biochem. Pharmacol.*, 26:1435, 1977.

113. Snyder, S. H. A model of opiate receptor function with implication for a theory of addiction. In: *Opiate Receptor Mechanism* (Snyder, S. H., and Matthysse, S., eds.). Cambridge, Mass.: MIT Press, 1975, p. 137.

114. Snyder, S. H. VIII. A model of opiate receptor function with implications for a theory of addiction. *Neurosci. Res. Prog. Bull.*, 13:137, 1975.

115. Department of Health, Education, and Welfare Publication No. (PHS) 79-50066, *Surgeon General Smoking and Health* (Office of Smoking and Health, eds.). Washington, D.C.: U.S. Government Printing Office, 1979.

116. Sutherland, E. W., III. Dependence on barbiturates and other CNS depressants. In: *Drug Abuse: Clinical and Basic Aspects.* (Pradhan, S. N., and Dutta, S. N., eds.). St. Louis: C. V. Mosby, 1977, p. 235.

117. Suzuki, K., Horiguchi, T., Comas-Urrutia, A. C., Muller-Heubach, E., Morishima, H. and Adamson, K. Placental transfer and distribution of nicotine in the pregnant rhesus monkey. *Amer. J. Obstet. Gynecol.*, 119:253, 1974.

118. Swain, H. H., Woods, J. H., Medzihradsky, F., Smith, C. B., and Fly, C. L. Annual Report: Evaluation of new compounds for opioid activity. In: *NIDA Research Monograph*, 27 (Harris, L. S., ed.). Washington, D.C.: DHEW, PHS, 1979, p. 356.

119. Tager, I., Weiss, S. T., Munoz, A., et al. Longitudinal study of the effects of maternal smoking on pulmonary function in children. *N. Engl. J. Med.*, 309:699, 1983.

120. Terry, J. G., and Braumoeller, F. L. Nalline: an aid in detecting narcotic users. *Calif. Med.*, 85:299, 1956.

121. Tinklenberg, J. R. Abuse of marijuana. In: *Drug Abuse: Clinical and Basic Aspects* (Pradhan, S. N., and Dutta, S. N., eds.). St. Louis: C. V. Mosby, 1977, p. 263.

122. Tolan, E. J., and Lingl, F. A. Model psychosis produced by inhalation of gasoline fumes. *Amer. J. Psychiat.* 120:737, 1964.

123. Tsujimoto, A., Kojima, S., Ikeda, M., and Dohi, T. Excretion of nicotine and its metabolites in dog and monkey saliva. *Toxicol. Appl. Pharmacol.* 22:365, 1972.

124. Tsujimoto, A., Nakashima, T., Tanino, S., Dohi, T., and Kurogochi, Y. Tissue distribution of (^{3}H) nicotine in dogs, and rhesus monkeys. *Toxicol. Appl. Pharmacol.*, 32:21, 1975.

125. Tuazon, C. U., and Sheagren, J. N. Septic complications. In: *Drug Abuse, Clinical and Basic Aspects* (Pradhan, S. N., and Dutta, S. N., eds.). St. Louis: C. V. Mosby, 1977, p. 332.

126. U.S. Public Health Service. *The Health Consequences of Smoking.* Washington, D.C.: U.S. Department of Health, Education, and Welfare, 1976, p. 163.

127. U.S. Public Health Service. *The Health Consequences of Smoking.* Washington, D.C.: U.S. Department of Health, Education, and Welfare, 1976, p. 263.

128. U.S. Public Health Service. *The Health Consequences of Smoking.* Washington, D.C.: U.S. Department of Health, Education, and Welfare, 1976, p. 411.

129. U.S. Public Health Service. *The Health Consequences of Smoking.* Washington, D.C.: U.S. Department of Health, Education, and Welfare, 1976, p. 625.

130. Wallach, M. B., Hine, B., and Gershon, S. Cross-tolerance of tachyphylaxis among various psychotomimetic agents in cats. *Eur. J. Pharmacol.*, 29:89, 1974.

131. Washton, A. M., Resnick, R. B., and Rawson, R. A. *Clonidine Hydrochloride: A Nonopiate Treatment for Opiate Withdrawal.* National Institute on Drug Abuse. Research Monogram, Series 27, 1979, p. 233.

132. Watson, M. J. Solvent abuse by children and young adults. *Br. J. Addiction*, 75:27, 1980.

133. Watson, R., Hartmann, E., and Schildkraut, J. J. Amphetamine withdrawal: Affective state, sleep patterns, and MHPG excretion. *Amer. J. Psychiat.*, 129:263, 1972.

134. Way, E. L., and Glasgow, C. Recent developments in morphine analgesia: Tolerance and dependence. In: *Psychopharmacology: A Generation of Progress* (Lipton, M. A., DiMascio, A., and Killam, K. F., eds.). New York: Raven Press, 1978, p. 1535.

135. Way, E. L., Mo, B. P. N., and Quock, C. P. Evaluation of the nalorphine pupil diagnostic test for narcotic usage in long-term heroin and opium addicts. *Clin. Pharmacol. Ther.*, 7:300, 1966.

136. Weinraub, M., Groce, P., and Karno, M. Chloroform. A new case of a bad old habit. *Calif. Med.*, 117:63, 1972.

137. *WHO Expert Committee on Addiction—Producing Drugs*, 13th report. Geneva: WHO Technical Report Series No. 273, 1964.

138. Wikler, A. Diagnosis and treatment of drug dependence of the barbiturate type. *Amer. J. Psychiat.*, 125:758, 1968.

139. Wikler, A. Drug dependence. In: *Clinical Neurology* (Baker, A. B., and Baker, L. H., eds.). Vol. 2, New York: Harper and Row, 1975, p. 1.

139a. Wikler, A. Aspects of tolerance to and dependence on cannabis. *N. Y. Acad. Sci.*, 282:126, 1976.

140. Wikler, A., and Essig, C. F. Withdrawal seizures following chronic intoxication with barbiturates and other sedative drugs. In: *Epilepsy and Modern Problems in Pharmacopsychiatry* (Niedermeyer, E., ed.). Vol. 4, Basel: Karger, 1970, p. 170.

141. Wikler, A., Norrell, H., and Miller, D. Limbic system and opioid addiction in the rat. *Exp. Neurol.*, 34:543, 1972.

142. Woods, J. H., and Downs, D. A. The psychopharmacology of

cocaine. In: *Drug Use in America: Problem in Perspective,* Second Report of the National Commission on Marihuana and Drug Abuse, Washington, D.C.: U.S. Government Printing Office, 1973.

143. Wynder, E. L., and Hoffmann, D. Experimental tobacco carcinogenesis. *Science,* 162:862, 1968.

144. Zelson, C., Rubio, E., and Wasserman, E. Neonatal narcotic addiction: Ten year observation. *Pediatrics,* 48:179, 1971.

145. Zwi, S., Goldman, H. I., and Levin, A. Cigarette smoking and pulmonary function in healthy young adults. *Amer. Rev. Resp. Dis.,* 89:73, 1964.

ADDITIONAL READING

Abel, E.L. Effects of prenatal exposure to cannabinoids. *Natl. Inst. Drug Abuse Res. Monogr. Ser.* 59:20, 1985.

Chan, A.W. Effects of combined alcohol and benzodiazepine: a review. *Drug Alcohol Depend.* 13:315, 1984.

Dans, A.T. Clinical experience with 781 cases of alcoholism evaluated and treated on an inpatient basis by various method. *Int. J. Addict.* 20:643, 1985.

Harclerode, J. Endocrine effects of marijuana in the male-preclinical studies. *Natl. Inst. Drug Abuse Res. Monogr. Ser.* 44:46, 1984.

Mason, A.P. et al. Cannabis: pharmacology and interpretation of effects. *J. Forensic Sci.* 30: 615, 1985.

Maykut, M.O. Health consequences of acute and chronic marihuana use. *Prog. Neuropsychopharmacol. Biol. Psychiatry* 9:209, 1985.

Straussman, R.J. Adverse reaction to psychedelic drugs. A review of the literature. *J. Nerv. Ment. Dis.* 172:577, 1984.

Ward, A., and Holmes, B. Nabilone. A preliminary review of its pharmacological properties and therapeutic use. *Drugs* 30:127, 1985.

Section III
DRUGS AFFECTING CHEMO-HUMORAL REGULATION OF FUNCTION

CHAPTER 12

HORMONES

Samar N. Dutta and Sachin N. Pradhan

Hormones are diverse chemical substances, synthesized through complex reactions by specialized cells and directly released into the circulation to act upon their target organs. Generally, hormones are secreted from the endocrine glands in their active form in which they act on the target tissue. In some instances the final active form of the hormone is produced in the peripheral tissues through biotransformation. In the circulation, most of the hormones are bound to plasma proteins, but in general it is the free hormone that is biologically active.

In most instances, multiple stimuli are responsible for the secretion of a given hormone. These stimuli include a major substrate such as plasma glucose for insulin release, plasma Ca^{2+} for parathyroid hormone secretion, and levels of trophic hormones [adrenocorticotropic hormone (ACTH), follicle-stimulating hormone (FSH), and thyroid-stimulating hormone (TSH)], whose synthesis and release are regulated by the central nervous system, via the hypothalamic-releasing hormones and factors. A number of nonspecific stimuli such as shock, stress, and various drugs in pharmacological doses also affect the production and release of hormones.

Functionally hormones belong to four principal classes (Table 12-1). Hormones can also be grouped into: (a) peptides, catecholamines, and releasing factors; (b) steroids including vitamin D metabolites; and, (c) thyroid hormones, in order to explain the molecular basis of their mechanism of action.

MECHANISM OF ACTION

The current concept of the mechanism of peptide and steroid hormone action is summarized in Fig. 12-1. It is now generally accepted that all five steroid hormone groups (adrenal glucocorticoids and mineralocorticoids, progesterone, estrogens, and androgens), as well as thyroid hormones and vitamin D, react with specific intracellular receptors, either cytoplasmic or nuclear. The hormone-receptor complex then induces a conformational change, prior to interacting with the chromatin in the nucleus. The chromatin-bound, hormone-receptor complex can increase (or possibly decrease) the transcription of specific messenger ribonucleic acids (mRNA).

The peptide hormones, releasing factors, and catecholamines bind to receptors located on the external surface of the plasma membrane. The specific receptors with high affinity for ligands undergo a conformational change after hormone binding and thereby activate membrane-related effector systems to elicit cellular response to hormonal stimulation. The major effector, adenylate cyclase, is activated by glucagon, glycopeptides [human chorionic

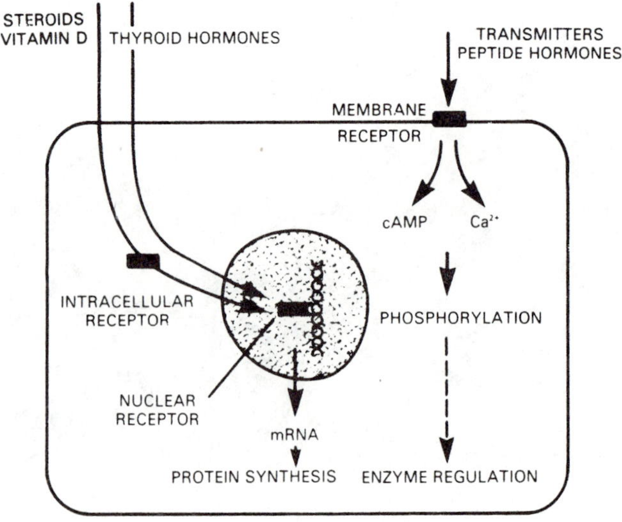

Fig. 12-1. *General mechanisms of target-cell activation by hormones acting on plasma-membrane receptors and those acting via cytoplasmic and nuclear receptors* (Taken from Ref. 2, by permission).

Table 12-1
Physiological Grouping of Hormones

Hormones Affecting Intermediary Metabolism and Growth	Hormones with Specific Functions and Trophic Hormones	Hormones Affecting Mineral and Water Metabolism	Hormones that Affect Cardiovascular or Renal Functions
Glucagon	TSH	Aldosterone	Glucocorticoids
Glucocorticoids (in excess)	HCG	ADH	Glucagon
Insulin	FSH	Parathyroid hormone	Angiotensin
Somatomedins and growth factors	LH	Calcitonin	Estrogens
	ACTH	Vitamin D	
Growth hormone	Angiotensin		
Prolactin	Hypothalamic-releasing hormones		
Androgens			
Progestins	MSH		
Estrogens	Oxytocin		

gonadotropin (HCG), FSH, TSH, and luteinizing hormone (LH)] releasing hormones [luteinizing hormone-releasing hormone (LHRH), thyrotropin-releasing hormone (TRH), parathyroid hormone (PTH), melanocyte stimulating hormone (MSH), and vasopressin (ADH)]. Activation of adenylate cyclase results in an accumulation of cyclic adenosine monophosphate (cAMP) and an increase in cytosolic calcium concentration. The mechanism by which the cytosolic calcium concentration is increased involves both influx of calcium from extracellular fluid and redistribution of intracellular calcium (2). Increased cytosolic cAMP activates protein kinases that phosphorylate various proteins at specific sites, and the altered proteins mediate the actions of the hormones. In reference to peptide hormones such as insulin, prolactin, growth hormone, and growth factors, cAMP does not appear to be involved in eliciting target cell response to these hormones. It has been suggested that a plasma membrane-derived peptide factor is possibly the mediator for changes in intracellular enzyme activities, which are induced by insulin in target cells (16).

In recent years isolation and characterization of receptors for insulin have been largely clarified (5). Cuatrecasas and colleagues (4) have postulated that a conformational change in the receptor after binding to hormone results in binding to and alteration of other membrane proteins such as adenylate cyclase.

Continuous or repeated exposure of target cells in many organs to the stimulatory hormone has been noted to elicit progressively decreasing response, which is generally termed as tachyphylaxis, refractoriness, or desensitization. This phenomenon is commonly encountered with hormones that are dependent on stimulation of adenylate cyclase for this cellular response. The desensitization process can be either heterologous (i.e., exposure to one hormone subsequently inhibits the response to other ligands mediated through adenylate cyclase) or homologous (i.e., the inhibition is hormone specific). The suggested mechanisms for heterologous desensitization include inhibition of adenylate cyclase by cAMP, a product of the activation process; increased phosphodiesterase activity and thereby increasing cAMP degradation; and/or deactivation of the nucleotide regulatory protein (2). Homologous desensitization is generally attributed to structural and/or functional changes at the receptor level.

ENDOCRINES AND AGING

Changes in the physiological functions of the endocrine glands during development and puberty are well known. In recent years, the physiological functions of these glands have been shown to be altered with aging, and several disease processes unique to the geriatric population are related to changes in hormonal status. The hormonal status commonly seen in elderly subjects is shown in Table 12-2. The incidence, manifestations, or response to therapy of some common endocrine and/metabolic disorders such as diabetes mellitus, thyroid dysfunction, impotence and male hypogonadism, polyglandular failure, and osteoporosis is markedly influenced by the aging process (12, 13). Because of higher incidence of neoplasms in the geriatric population, the incidence or ectopic hormone syndromes also rises. In recent years, arginine vasopressin, a neuropeptide, has been shown to improve memory in geriatric subjects and in patients with senile dementia (6).

CLINICAL USES

The naturally occurring hormones and their synthetic analogs are used mainly in replacement therapy for deficiency of a particular endocrine organ or system. They are also used as diagnostic aids to evaluate the functional status of one or more endocrine organs or in certain metabolic disorders associated with endocrine malfunction. Some peptide and steroid hormones are used in pharmacological doses to induce a hyperfunctional state, or to elicit an entirely new pharmacodynamic effect to treat some disease entities such as asthama, inflammatory conditions (e.g., rheumatoid arthritis), shock, neoplasms, and so forth.

Table 12-2
Hormonal Changes with Aging

Hormone	Status
Sex	
Male	
Testosterone	Normal or decreased
Gonadotropins	Increased, normal, or decreased
Estradiol	Increased
Female	
Estrogens	Decreased
Luteinizing hormone (LH)	Increased
Follicle-stimulating hormone (FSH)	Increased
Thyroid	
Thyroxine (T_4)	Normal or decreased[a]
Triiodothyronine (T_3)	Normal or decreased[a]
Thyroid-stimulating hormone (TSH, thyrotropin)	Normal or increased
Adrenal	
Cortisol	Normal[b]
Androgens	Decreased
Calcium-Metabolism-Related	
Parathormone (PTH)	
Intact hormone	Decreased
C-terminal fragment	Increased[c]
Calcitonin	Decreased
25-OHD$_3$ and 1,25-(OH)$_2$D$_3$[d]	Decreased
Posterior Pituitary	
Arginine vasopressin (AVP)	Increased[e]

[a]Decrease often associated with or due to concomitant illness (euthyroid sick syndrome).
[b]Cortisol secretion and disposal rates and tissue responsiveness are decreased.
[c]Sensitivity to action of parathormone is decreased.
[d]25-OHD$_3$, 25-hydroxy vitamin D$_3$; 1,25-(OH)$_2$D$_3$, 1,25-dihydroxy vitamin D$_3$.
[e]Sensitivity to AVP at renal tubule is decreased.
Source: Adopted from Ref. 12.

During the past decade, significant advances have been made in the clinical applications of gonadotropin-releasing hormone (GnRH). These investigations have led to increased successes in enhancing fertility in women with a deficiency of endogenous GnRH (17). The discovery that continuous activation of GnRH receptors by constant administration of the releasing hormone and its synthetic analogs results in inhibition of the pituitary-gonadal axis has led to their use for clinical control of fertility in both females and males (15), precocious puberty (9), endometriosis (11), breast cancer (8), and prostatic cancer (1).

In recent years considerable advances have been reported in the management of osteoporosis. Synthetic 1,25(OH)$_2$D$_3$ (calcitriol), the active form of vitamin D (7), synthetic human parathyroid hormone (1-34 fragment) (14), and synthetic salmon calcitonin (3) have been reported to be effective in the treatment of postmenopausal osteoporosis. Recently published findings have also suggested that calcitriol is involved in cell differentiation of hematolymphopoietic tissue; thereby, it may play a role in the chemotherapy of certain leukemias (10).

REFERENCES

1. Borgmann, V., Nagel, R., Al-Abadi, H, et al. Treatment of prostatic cancer with LH-RH analogues. *The Prostate* 4:553, 1983.
2. Catt, K. J., and Dufau, M. L. Introduction: The clinical significance of peptide hormone receptors. *Clin. Endocrinol. Metab.* 12:XI, 1983.
3. Chesnut, C. H., Baylink, D. J., Gruber, H. E. et al. Anabolic steroids and calcitonin, in the treatment of postmenopausal osteoporosis. In: *Clinical Disorders of Bone and Mineral Metabolism* (Frame, B., and Potts, J. T., eds.). Princeton, N.Y.: Excerpta Medica, 1983, p. 355.
4. Cuatrecasas, P., Hallenberg, M. D., Chang, K-J,. and Bennett, V. Hormone receptor complexes and their modulation of membrane function. *Recent Progr. Horm. Res.* 31:37, 1975.
5. Czech, M. P. Structural and functional homologies in the receptors for insulin and the insulin-like growth factors. *Cell* 31:7, 1982.
6. de Wied, D., and Van Ree, J. M. Neuropeptides, mental performance and aging. *Life Sci.* 31:709, 1983.
7. Gallagher, J. C., Jerpbak, C. M., Jee, W. S. S. et al. 1,25-Dihydroxyvitamin D$_3$: Short- and long-term effects on bone and calcium metabolism in patients with postmenopausal osteoporosis. *Proc. Natl. Acad. Sci. USA* 79:3325, 1982.
8. Klijm, J. G. M., and deJong, F. H. Treatment with a luteinizing-hormone-releasing-hormone analogue (buserelin) in premenopausal patients with metastatic breast cancer. *Lancet* 1:1213, 1982.
9. Luder, A. S., Holland, F. J., Costigan, D. C. et al. Intranasal and subcutaneous treatment of central precocious puberty in both sexes with a long-acting analog of luteinizing hormone-releasing hormone. *J. Clin. Endocrinol. Metab.* 58:966, 1984.
10. Manolagas, S. C., and Deftos, L. J. The vitamin D endocrine system and the hematolymphopoietic tissue. *Ann. Intern. Med.* 100:144, 1984.
11. Meldrum, D. R., Chang, R. J., Lu, J. et al. Medical oophorectomy using a long-acting GnRH agonist—a possible new approach to the treatment of endometriosis. *J. Clin. Endocrinol. Metab.* 54:108, 1982.
12. Morley, J. E. The aging endocrine system. *Postgrad. Med.* 73:107, 1983.
13. Nasr, H. Endocrine disorders in the elderly. *Med. Clin. North Am.* 67:481, 1983.
14. Reeve, J., Meunier, P. J., Parsons, J. A. et al. Anabolic effects of human parathyroid hormone fragment on trabecular bone in involutional osteoporosis: a multicenter trial. *Br. Med. J.* 2:1340, 1980.
15. Sandow, J. Clinical applications of LHRH and its analogues. *Clin. Endocrinol.* 18:571, 1983.
16. Seals, J. R., and Czech, M. P. Production by plasma membranes of a chemical mediator of insulan action. *Fed. Proc.* 41:2730, 1982.
17. Yen, S. S. C. Clinical applications of gonadotropin-releasing hormone and goanodotropin-releasing hormone analogs. *Fertil. Steril.* 39:275, 1983.

CHAPTER
12.1

PITUITARY HORMONES

Edward T. Knych and John A. Thomas

HISTORY

It was not until the very early 1900s that the surgical removal of the canine pituitary was shown to retard growth and development (1). Numerous studies in the early 1920s reported that injections of hypophysial extracts caused excessive growth in experimental animals. In 1933, Collip et al. employed anterior pituitary extracts to prevent atrophy of the adrenal cortex in hypophysectomized animals (3). During this same time, several investigators reported that anterior pituitary extracts could stimulate lactation and enhance the development of the mammary glands. The same pituitary extract that caused lactation in mammals could also stimulate the crop sac of the pigeon and was named *prolactin* by the avian physiologist Riddle (28). Through the years, many of the anterior pituitary hormones have been isolated, purified, and synthesized in the laboratory. Adrenocorticotropic hormone (ACTH) is commercially available and currently has a more widespread therapeutic usefulness than the other pituitary hormones.

The early investigations of Sir Henry Dale disclosed the presence of pressor substances in posterior pituitary extracts but did not immediately recognize the presence of antidiuretic activity (5). Other investigators reported that extracts of the posterior pituitary gland affected the rate of urine flow. Once the antidiuretic properties of posterior pituitary extracts were disclosed, they were successfully used to treat diabetes insipidus. By 1928, it was discovered that the posterior pituitary gland contained two hormonal substances, and in 1954 du Vigneaud confirmed this fact by synthesizing oxytocin and vasopressin (8).

ANATOMICAL CONSIDERATIONS

The pituitary gland is a very important regulatory organ lying in a bony-walled cavity of the skull called the *sella turcica*. The organ is situated at the base of the brain. The anatomic relationship between the hypothalamus and the pituitary allows for both neural and vascular communication. The anatomical region that joins the hypothalamus and the pituitary stalk is referred to as the *median eminence*. The pituitary gland is composed of the *adenohypophysis* (lobus glandularis, anterior lobe), *neurohypophysis* which consists of the lobus neurosus (posterior lobe) and the infundibulum (neural stalk). The pars intermedia is present in most mammals but is virtually absent in humans.

The adenohypophysis, which is embryologically derived from an invagination of Rathke's pouch, is supplied with blood by a portal system originating in the median eminence. This portal system provides the communication link between the hypothalamus and the adenohypophysis. Blood flow is primarily from the hypothalamus to the anterior lobe. Recent evidence suggests, however, that retrograde flow (i.e., flow from the anterior lobe to the hypothalamus) may also occur (11). If so, hypothalamic function could be regulated by adenohypophysial hormones.

The neurohypophysis, in contrast, originates from an invagination of the floor of the third ventricle of the embryonic brain. Its neural character is retained in the form of nerve tracts that originate in cell bodies of the paraventricular and supraoptic nuclei of the anterior hypothalamus and whose axons terminate in the posterior lobe. The neurohypophysial hormones, oxytocin and vasopressin (antidiuretic hormone, ADH), are synthesized in the magnocellular perikarya of the these two nuclei, transported in neurosecretory granules along the axons of the neurons and secreted at (a) the posterior pituitary into the systemic circulation, (b) the zona externa of the median eminence into the hypophysial portal circulation, and (c) the third ventricle into the cerebrospinal fluid (CSF). Each of the neurohypophysial hormones is synthesized, transported, and secreted in association with specific proteins, called neurophysins. The function of these acidic proteins, aside from binding the neurohypophysial hormone, is not yet known. Oxytocin and vasopressin are synthesized by different cell types having distinct regional localization within the supraoptic and paraventricular nuclei.

The various trophic hormones of the adenohypophysis are synthesized in specific cell types located within the anterior pituitary gland itself. The synthesis and/or release of the various trophic hormones is affected by specific substances (namely, hypothalamic-releasing hormones) that emanate from different regions of the hypothalamus (32).

HYPOTHALAMIC-RELEASING HORMONES

The nomenclature as well as the relationlship between the hypothalamic-releasing hormones and their respective adenohypophysial trophic hormones is depicted in Table 12.1-1. For every trophic hormone, at least one hypothalamic hormone has been shown to stimulate or inhibit its secretion (30). In some instances, a particular trophic hormone may be affected by both an inhibitory and a stimulatory substance.

Releasing hormones extracted and purified from the hypothalamus of several mammalian species, when injected into humans, seem to evoke the appropriate trophic hormone response. Because most of the hypothalamic releasing hormones are polypeptides (31), they have a short biological half-life and are usually ineffective following oral administration. Structural analogs of these polypeptides possessing releasing hormone-like activities have been synthesized in an effort to prolong their biological half-life and hence improve their pharmacological usefulness in selected pituitary disorders.

Corticotropin-releasing Factor (CRF). It has been more than 25 years since the demonstration that hypothalamic extracts contained corticotropin-releasing factor (CRF) capable of stimulating the release of adrenocorticotropin hormone (ACTH). Several substances, present in hypothalamic extracts, have been identified that stimulate the release of ACTH. These include vasopressin, norepinephrine, fragments of proteins such as hemoglobin, and modified amino acids (36). None, however, meets fully the characteristics expected of CRF. Recently, a 41-residue peptide, isolated from ovine hypothalamus, has been characterized and synthesized (34). Though it may be premature to refer to this peptide as CRF, it does have many of the properties expected of CRF and merits further study. The clinical usefulness of CRF may be restricted to assessing the pituitary reserve of ACTH and to counteracting pituitary suppression in patients who have been subjected to intensive adrenal cortical steroid therapy.

Thyrotropin-releasing Hormone (TRH). Thyrotropin-releasing hormone was the first hypothalamic-releasing factor to be isolated and synthesized. It has been studied extensively in both animals and humans (2, 24). The structure of this tripeptide is shown in Fig. 12.1-1. TRH stimulates the release of thyrotropin (TSH) from the anterior pituitary, resulting in an increase in serum triiodothyronine (T_3) and thyroxine (T_4). These circulating

Table 12.1-1
Relationship between Hypothalamic-Releasing Hormones and Trophic Hormones Emanating from the Adenohypophysis

Releasing Hormone	Trophic Hormone Affected
Corticotropin-releasing hormone (CRF)	ACTH (adrenocorticotropic hormone)
Thyrotropin-releasing hormone (TRH)	TSH (thyroid-stimulating hormone)
Gonadotropin-releasing hormone (GnRH)	FSH (follicle-stimulating hormone) and LH (luteinizing hormone)
Growth hormone-releasing factor (GRF)	GH (growth hormone)
Growth hormone inhibitory factor (GIF) (somatostatin)	GH (growth hormone)
Prolactin-releasing factor (PRF)	Prolactin
Melanocyte-stimulating hormone-releasing hormone (MRH)	MSH (melanocyte-stimulating hormone)
Melanocyte-stimulating hormone inhibitory hormone (MIH)	MSH (melanocyte-stimulating hormone)

GnRH

pyro-Glu-His-Trp-Ser-Tyr-Gly-Leu-Arg-Pro-Gly-NH_2

Somatostatin

NH_2-Ala-Gly-Cys-Lys-Asn-Phe-Phe
S-S
OH-Cys-Ser-Trp-Phe-Thr-Lys-Trp

Synthetic TRH

pyro-Glu-His-Pro-NH_2

Fig. 12.1-1. *Amino acid sequences of GnRH, somatostatin, and synthetic TRH.*

thyroid hormones, in turn, modulate TRH-induced TSH release in humans. The TSH response to TRH has been reported to be increased by theophylline and estrogens and decreased by corticosteroids (15). TRH also causes the release of variable amounts of prolactin, follicle-stimulating hormone (FSH), leuteinizing hormone (LH) and growth hormone (GH) (15). TRH is found not only in the hypothalamus but throughout the central nervous system, including the spinal cord, the gastrointestinal tract, testes, and placenta (21). It is not surprising, then, that pharmacological doses of TRH have been reported to have a wide variety of extrapituitary effects. TRH is active when given orally and parenterally, although it requires doses nearly 100 times greater when given orally than parenterally. It is inactivated in plasma within minutes by enzymatic cleavage of the amide group. Biochemical degradation of TRH is greatest in the hypothalamus, brain, and kidney. TRH can be used diagnostically to distinguish between hypothalamic and pituitary hypothyroidism, to evaluate pituitary function, and to assess prolactin reserve. Transient metallic taste, flushing of the face, and mild nausea are generally reported immediately after injection of TRH.

Gonadotropin-releasing Hormone (GnRH). Gonadotropin-releasing hormone is a decapeptide (Fig. 12.1-1) that promotes the rapid release of LH and to a lesser extent FSH (19). Because of this preferential action, GnRH is also known as luteinizing hormone-releasing hormone (LHRH). There is evidence that suggests the existence of a separate follicle-stimulating hormone-releasing factor (FSH-RH) (17). In humans, GnRH is active when given by several different routes of administration (22, 37). It is rapidly degraded in plasma and excreted in the urine with a half-life of about 4 min. Analogs of GnRH have been synthesized that are degraded more slowly and therefore have a longer duration of action. Some analogs are inhibitory and may prove to be useful as contraceptives. GnRH and its agonist analogs have been used to induce ovulation and spermatogenesis. Suitable regimens for the induction of ovulation use intermittent administration of GnRH in an attempt to mimic the normal pulsatile surges of GnRH. Prolonged administration of high doses of GnRH can lead to a reversible atrophy of the ovary or inhibition of spermatogenesis. Large doses of androgens and estrogens may suppress gonadotropin release after GnRH administra tion.

Growth Hormone-releasing Factor and Growth Hormone Release Inhibitory Factor (SOMATOSTATIN). The secretion of growth hormone is regulated by both an inhibitory substance and a stimulatory substance. Characterization of this stimulatory factor(s) is under investigation. The inhibitory factor, on the other hand, has been identified as a tetradecapeptide called somatostatin (Fig. 12.1-1) (4, 19). Bioassay, radioimmunoassay, and immunohistochemistry techniques reveal a widespread tissue distribution of somatostatin. The hypothalamus has the highest concentration. Infusion of somatostatin, in humans, leads to a prompt inhibition of the growth hor mone secretion that follows various stimuli. In addition, TRH-stimulated TSH release is also diminished. Somatostatin has been found in the GI tract, where it is capable of inhibiting the release of gastrointestinal hormones as well as gastric acid secretion and gastric emptying. Pancreatic somatostatin appears to be identical to hypothalamic somatostatin and is found in the D cells of the pancreas. It is capable of inhibiting the release of both glucagon and insulin in humans (also see Chapter 13.1-1). The clinical potential of somatostatin is limited by its short duration of action and multiple loci of action. Numerous analogs have been examined in an attempt to enhance duration and selectivity of action. Such analogs hold potential in the treatment of acromegaly, in pancreatic islet tumors, and in diabetes mellitus.

Prolactin-releasing Factor (PRF) and Prolactin Release Inhibitor Factor (PIF). Current evidence suggests that prolactin secretion is controlled by a hypothalamic-inhibitory substance (PIF, probably dopamine) and per haps by a hypothalamic-releasing factor (PRF). Prolactin secretion is inhibited by the administration of the dopamine precursor L-dopa and by the dopamine agonists bromocriptine and apomorphine. The suppression of prolactin secretion by bromocriptine has been used clinically in the treatment of hyperprolactinemia. Hyperprolactinemia is often associated with amenorrhea, galactorrhea, and male infertility. It should also be recognized that a wide variety of drugs stimulate prolactin secretion. These include hormones, antianxiety agents, analgesics, antidepressants, antihypertensives, anesthetics, and antihistamines.Though many of these agents are capable of decreasing the central nervous system levels of dopamine, it is also likely that other mechanisms are involved in the stimulation of prolactin levels.

HORMONE FEEDBACK SYSTEMS

A basic understanding of the hormonal relationship between the pituitary gland and various target organs (e.g., gonads, adrenal and thyroid glands) is necessary to therapeutically manipulate the endocrine system. Negative feedback systems are the principal controlling mechanisms. Usually the secretory response of the target organ is increased by its particular trophic hormone. In turn, the hormonal secretion of the target organ evoked by the trophic hormone acts back upon the hypothalamus and/or the adenohypophysis to suppress further secretion of the trophic hormone. This type of regulatory mechanism has been termed *long-loop negative feedback*. A *short-loop negative feedback* system is also possible in which the increased secretion of trophic hormone inhibits directly further release of its hypothalamic-releasing hormone. Thus, ACTH can stimulate the adrenal cortex to secrete cortisol (and other steriods), which in turn is blood-borne back to the pituitary gland to inhibit the further release of ACTH. Increased levels of ACTH also directly suppress further secretion of CRF from the hypothalamus. A similar feedback system exists between TSH and the secretion to thyroxine (T_4) or triiodothyronine (T_3). The feedback regulation of prolactin or growth hormone is less well defined. Gonadotropins (FSH and LH) can stimulate the ovaries and the testes to secrete estrogen and androgen, respectively. Generally, these sex hormones complete the negative feedback loop modulating the secretion of GnRH. However,the feedback system controlling the secretion of FSH and LH is more complex in the female because both positive and negative feedback effects of estrogens upon the hypothalamic-adenohypophysial axis may be involved, depending upon the phase of the menstrual cycle.

Pharmacological levels of natural or synthetic steroids, particularly if administered for extended periods of time, result in a suppression of trophic hormone secretion (7). Cortisol and synthetic glucocorticoids (i.e., antiinflammatory steroids) can suppress ACTH secretion. Similarly, pharmacological doses of progesterone, progesteronelike agents, estrogens, or testosterone can inhibit gonadotropin secretion. Oral contraceptives are very effective in causing an inhibition of LH secretion, thus blocking ovulation. Several drugs, without inherent hormonal activity, are also capable of disrupting hormonal feedback systems.

ADENOHYPOPHYSIAL HORMONES

ADRENOCORTICOTROPIC HORMONE (ACTH)

Chemistry. The chemical structure of ACTH reveals it to be a single-chain polypeptide consisting of 39 amino acids (Fig. 12.1-2). Peptides 1-20 are required for full biological activity. ACTH is generally extracted from animal pituitaries, although a synthetic preparation (cosyntropin) is available. Species variations appear limited to the region of the peptide chain from the 25th to the 32nd residue. ACTH is synthesized as part of a larger prohormone molecule of approximately 31,000 daltons molecular weight (10). This molecule serves as a precursor for not only ACTH but also α-MSH, β-MSH, CLIP (corticotropin-like intermediate-lobe peptide), 16-K fragment, β-LPH, γ-LPH, α-endorphin, β-endorphin, and γ-endorphin. The biological role of these peptides and the mechanisms controlling their release, in particular that of the opioid β-endorphin, are currently under active investigation. It is clear, however, that those stimuli that lead to a release of ACTH also cause the release of β-lipotropin and β-endorphin.

Natural ACTH

Ser-Tyr-Ser-Met-Glu-His-Phe-Arg-Try-Gly-
1 2 3 4 5 6 7 8 9 10

Lys-Pro-Val-Gly-Lys-Lys-Arg-Arg-Pro-Val-Lys-Val-Tyr-
11 12 13 14 15 16 17 18 19 20 21 22 23

Pro-Asp-Ala-Gly-Gln-Asp-Glu-
24 25 26 27 28 29 30

Ser-Ala-Glu-Ala-Phe-Pro-Leu-Glu-Phe-
31 32 33 34 35 36 37 38 39

Synthetic ACTH (Cosyntropin)

Ser-Tyr-Ser-Met-Glu-His-Phe-Arg-Try-Gly-
1 2 3 4 5 6 7 8 9 10

Lys-Pro-Val-Gly-Lys-Lys-Arg-Arg-Pro-Val-Lys-Val-Tyr-Pro-
11 12 13 14 15 16 17 18 19 20 21 22 23 24

Fig. 12.1-2. *Amino acid sequences of natural and synthetic ACTH*

Physiological Aspects. Normally, ACTH secretion is episodic, with several secretory pulses occurring throughout the day and night. A diurnal variation in ACTH release results in the highest corticosteroid levels at the beginning of the awake cycle and lowest at the onset of the sleep cycle. Thus, in humans with a normal day-night cycle, ACTH and cortisol levels are maximal early in the day with a gradual decline to a nadir in the evening. The oscillating level of ACTH, however, can be increased by several factors (hypoglycemia, metyrapone, vasopressin, alcohol) or stresses (exercise, pain, anesthesia). CRF modulates the synthesis and/or release of ACTH. An increase in ACTH secretion leads to a rapid stimulation of glucocorticoid secretion from the adrenal cortex. These steroids, in turn, feed back upon the hypothalamic-adenohypophysial axis, causing a suppression of ACTH secretion. Several synthetic steroids can interfere with this negative feedback system.

ACTH exerts a number of extraadrenal actions. Pharmacological doses of ACTH can stimulate lipolysis in adipose cells and enhance amino acid and glucose uptake in muscle.

Mechanism of Action. Specific receptors for ACTH are located on the surface of certain adrenal cortical cells. The binding of ACTH to its plasma membrane receptors, in the presence of calcium, leads to the activation of the adenylate cyclase (cyclic adenosine monophosphate, cAMP) system. The metabolic actions of ACTH on the adrenal are mimicked by cAMP. In particular, the stimulation of key enzymes leads to an increase in the conversion of cholesterol to corticosteroids. In addition, ACTH increases RNA and protein synthesis, resulting in an increase in adrenal weight and function.

Therapeutic Uses. Naturally occurring and synthetic ACTH are used more extensively for therapeutic and diagnostic purposes than any of the other anterior pituitary hormones (Table 12.1-2) (20). In part, the therapeu-

Table 12.1-2
Pharmacological Uses of Anterior Pituitary Hormones

Hormone	Suggested Indications
ACTH	Diagnosis of hypoadrenalism Antiinflammatory states (?) Epilepsy
GH	Pituitary dwarfism Renal failure Bone marrow hypoplasia Juvenile spontaneous hypoglycemia Burns Severe trauma
TSH	Diagnosis of thyroid disorders
HCG (LH-like activity)	Induce ovulation
HMG (FSH- and LH-like activity)	Induce ovulation
Prolactin	None

tic effectiveness of ACTH is achieved secondarily by stimulating the release of glucocortical steroids that possess antiinflammatory propertiers. Those inflammatory states requiring therapeutic attention, however, are best treated with synthetic antiinflammatory steroids and not with ACTH. Occasionally, ACTH has been used in selected cases of epilepsy where conventional anticonvulsant drugs have failed. Synthetic ACTH has been used as a rapid diagnostic test for hypoadrenalism. A single intramuscular injection of 0.25 mg of cosyntropin (equivalent to 25 IU of natural ACTH), followed by monitoring of plasma cortisol, is used to differentiate primary adrenocortical insufficiency from hypopituitarism. ACTH is ineffective orally and must be administered either i.m. or s.c. The plasma half-life of ACTH is approximately 30 min. SYNACTHEN-DEPOT is a longer-acting preparation of ACTH.

During the course of ACTH therapy, hypersensitivities, mild fever, and anaphylaxis have been reported. ACTH can produce sodium retention and hypokalemia, both of which are secondary responses to ACTH-induced increases in adrenocortical secretion.

GROWTH HORMONE (GH)

Chemistry. Human growth hormone is a polypeptide with a molecular weight of 22,000 daltons and consisting of 191 amino acid residues (18). Sufficient immunological differences exist between human and primate growth hormone to limit the therapeutic effectiveness of growth hormone obtained from animal sources. Although growth hormone has been synthesized, it is not yet available on a widespread commercial or therapeutic basis. Currently, recombinant DNA technology is being developed in an attempt to meet future demands for GH.

Physiological Aspects. Growth hormone plays an important role in the regulation of cellular metabolism (26). It enhances skeletal growth by stimulating the epiphysial plates, and it increases chondrogenesis. It also exerts a pronounced protein anabolic action and can stimulate hepatic glucose output leading to diabetogenic actions.

GH levels are regulated by a hypothalamic-releasing factor and an inhibitory factor, somatostatin. In addition, several physiological, pharmacological, and pathological factors can also affect GH secretion. Growth hormone secretion is inhibited by hyperglycemia and augmented by hypoglycemia. Pharmacological doses of insulin and vasopressin, as well as arginine and L-DOPA, can provoke the release of growth hormone. Insulin, arginine, and L-DOPA are used diagnostically to assess the pituitary reserve of GH.

Mechanism of Action. Whereas a growth hormone receptor has been described in cultured human lymphocytes, very little is known of its chemical nature, composition, or structure. The protein anabolic action of GH upon cells appears to be exerted at the ribosomal level, where the hormone affects either ribosomal translation or attachment. Growth hormone enhances the transport of amino acids. Growth hormone, unlike most other adenohypophysial hormones, does not seem to direct its stimulatory action at specific target cells.

Therapeutic Uses. A number of therapeutic uses have been suggested for human growth hormone (somatropin) (Table 12.1-2). Because of its limited supply, however, its use is limited to children with a proven deficiency of the hormone and accompanying short stature. Such hormone replacement therapy is usually initiated with a dose of 2 IU of human growth hormone (three times per week, i.m.). It is necessary to monitor height measurements and bone age closely for at least 6-12 months.

Growth hormone therapy has been of some value during specific phases of renal failure, in bone marrow hypoplasia, and in some cases of juvenile spontaneous hypoglycemia.

The therapeutic use of growth hormone can produce some side effects, including hyperglycemia and severe ketosis, which contraindicate its use in diabetics. Antibodies can develop even to human growth hormone, which can lead to a decrease in therapeutic effectiveness. Concomitant administration of GH and glucocorticoids results in the inhibition of the therapeutic effectiveness of GH.

THYROTROPIN (Thyroid-Stimulating Hormone, TSH)

Chemistry. TSH is a glycoprotein with a molecular weight of about 28,000 daltons secreted by cells of the anteromedial portion of the pituitary. It is composed of two subunits (27). The α-subunit consists of 96 amino acids and is nearly identical with that found in several other glycoproteins [i.e., FSH, LH, and human chorionic gonadotropin (HCG)]. TSH differs from these glycoproteins in the composition of its β-subunit that consists of 110 amino acids and in its carbohydrate content. Biological specificity appears to reside in the β-subunit. There are immunological differences among various mammalian species with respect to TSH. Besides TSH, several other endogenous substances have been reported to exert a thyroid-stimulatory effect, and these include human chorionic thyrotropin (HCT), long-acting thyroid stimulator (LATS), and human thyroid stimulator (HTS).

Physiological Aspects. TSH secretion is modulated in part by hypothalamic TRH and in part by the level of circulating thyroid hormones, thyroxine (T_4) and/or triiodothyroine (T_3). TSH stimulates both morphological and biochemical changes in the thyroid gland. Increased size and vascularity of the thyroid are seen following TSH administration. Within minutes of TSH administration, thyroid hormone secretion increases. TSH stimulates all phases of thyroid hormone synthesis, including iodide uptake, thyroglobulin synthesis, and thyroglobulin proteolysis. Daily production of TSH is about 165 μU.

Mechanism of Action. TSH interacts with specific, high-affinity receptors located on the membrane of thyroid cells. This interaction activates adenylate cyclase and subsequently elevates cAMP concentrations within the cell. Thus, cAMP acts as a second messenger and is capable of mimicking most of the actions of TSH on the thyroid.

Therapeutic Uses. Thyrotropin is isolated from bovine pituitary glands and possesses the same physiological effects as human TSH. It is used diagnostically to evaluate thyroid function. The *TSH stimulation test* generally involves the i.m. administration of 10 IU of TSH followed by a 24-hr radioiodine uptake. However, direct measurement of both basal and stimulated TSH levels by radioimmunoassay has decreased the use of the TSH stimulation test.

FOLLICLE-STIMULATING HORMONE (FSH)

Chemistry. FSH is a glycoprotein composed of two subunits and has a molecular weight of approximately 32,000 daltons. The α-subunit is nearly identical to that found in the other adenohypophysial glycoprotein hormones (33). The composition of the β-subunit and carbohydrate content differ from the other glycoprotein hormones. Human menopausal gonadotropin (HMG), which is isolated from the urine of postmenopausal women, also has FSH-like activity but only 1/25th the potency.

Physiological Aspects. To achieve optimal hormonal balance within either the male or female reproductive system, both FSH and luteinizing hormone (LH) are required. The timing and cyclic secretion of FSH and LH in the female are critical for the various hormonal events that occur during a normal ovulatory period and menstrual cycle. FSH secreted during the follicular phase of the menstrual cycle stimulates development of the ovarian follicles. FSH concentrations in plasma are highest during the follicular phase of the cycle and slowly decline before sharply increasing just prior to ovulation. Concentrations are lowest during the luteal phase of the cycle. In males, FSH is responsible for spermatogenesis and the integrity of the seminiferous tubules. It also appears to be required for optimal stimulation of testicular steroidogenesis induced by LH. FSH has a half-life in the blood of 3-4 hr.

Mechanism of Action. Specific receptors for FSH have been identified in both the ovaries and the testes. Some of the early biochemical events triggered by FSH involve the cAMP-adenylate cyclase system. The exact biochemical mechanism for the stimulation of development of the ovarian follicle is not fully understood.

Therapeutic Uses. Because human supplies of FSH are limited and FSH of animal origin exhibits immunological differences, human menopausal gonadotropin (HMG) has been used as a hormonal substitute. HMG, extracted from the urine of postmenopausal women, contains equal quantities of both FSH- and LH-like activity. The gonadotropins are used primarily to induce ovulation in anovulatory women (12). HMG, because of its FSH-like activity, is administered for 9-12 consecutive days to promote follicle development and prime the ovaries for the subsequent administration of human chorionic gonadotropin (HCG), which has biological activity similar to that of LH. The incidence of multiple births following such treatment is approximately 25%. An alternate method of attempting to induce ovulation in infertile women is the use of the nonsteroidal drug clomiphene (13). Ordinarily, clomiphene therapy (50 mg/day) is initiated on days 5 through 9 of the menstrual cycle. The mechanism of action of clomiphene appears to involve the release of endogenous FSH and LH, resulting in ovulation. Clomiphene can cause an excessive secretion of ovarian estrogens, produce abdominal and pelvic discomfort, and increase the incidence of multiple births.

Though oligospermia and azoospermia might respond to FSH therapy, male infertility due to reduced spermatogenesis is more often treated with testosterone or other androgens.

LUTEINIZING HORMONE (LH) AND HUMAN CHORIONIC GONADOTROPIN (HCG)

Chemistry. Like FSH, LH is a glycoprotein consisting of an α- and a β-subunit (33). Its molecular weight is approximately 30,000 daltons. The β-subunit appears to be responsible for hormonal activity. Human chorionic gonadotropin (HCG), a glycoprotein hormone of placental origin, has a slightly larger molecular weight than LH, but its pharmacological actions are similar. Therefore, HCG is a suitable hormonal substitute for LH.

Physiological Aspects. For LH to exert its optimal

stimulatory actions upon the female reproductive system, it is necessary first for FSH to prime the ovaries. In the male, this priming action of FSH is less conspicuous. Spermatogenesis depends upon FSH, whereas androgen production by the interstitial cells (Leydig cells) is stimulated by LH (also called interstitial cell-stimulating hormone, ICSH) in the male. LH and FSH levels are modulated by hypothalamic gonadotropin-releasing hormone (GnRH) and by the negative feedback regulation of the sex steroids. It is noteworthy that synthetic polypeptides exhibiting GnRH-like activity are receiving ongoing clinical assessment for their potential therapeutic usefulness in disorders of the endocrine system.

Mechanism of Action. In the corpora lutea and in the Leydig cells, LH (and HCG) promotes steroidogenesis by accelerating the conversion of cholesterol to pregnenolone. LH receptors are present on the membrane surface of cells in both the corpus luteum and the testes. Both LH and HCG stimulate the cAMP-adenylate cyclase system in the gonads.

Therapeutic Uses. Human chorionic gonadotropin is used as a substitute for human LH because of the limited supply of the latter hormone (12). HCG has LH-like activity, and therefore is often used in conjunction with HMG or clomiphene to induce ovulation. HCG can stimulate androgen production by viable Leydig cells, but male sex hormone deficiencies respond better to regimens employing testosterone. HCG has been used to aid testicular descent in cases where there is no anatomical obstruction (unobstructed cryptorchidism).

PROLACTIN

Chemistry. Prolactin is a single-chained polypeptide with a molecular weight of about 22,500. There are some chemical similarities as well as a physiological likeness between prolactin and GH. In fact, the first 40 amino acid residues of the prolactin sequence are the same as those present in GH (18). The plasma half-life of prolactin is also comparable with that of GH. Both hormones exhibit a plasma half-life of about 30 min.

Physiological Aspects. Prolactin causes the initiation and maintenance of lactation, but only after the mammary glands have been suitably primed with progesterone, estrogens, insulin, and adrenal cortical steroids. Prolactin influences the devlopment of the alveoli of the mammary glands. In nonhuman species, prolactin exerts a luteotropic action (e.g., rats), stimulates the growth of the crop sac (e.g., pigeons), and influences water balance (e.g., frogs) (28). Pharmacological amounts of prolactin possess growth hormone-like actions.

Secretion of prolactin is regulated by a hypothalamic prolactin-releasing factor (PRF). Dopamine inhibits prolactin secretion and may act physiologically as a hypothalamic-inhibitory factor (PIF). During certain physiological states, such as sleep, exercise, stress, pregnancy, and postpartum period, prolactin secretion is elevated. Normally, the most potent stimulus for prolactin secretion in the female is induced by suckling. Prolactin secretion is elevated in pituitary adenoma, in some patients with hypothyroidism, chronic renal impairment, hepatic failure, or anorexia nervosa. Drugs such as methyldopa and cimetidine are capable of stimulating prolactin secretion. Excessive prolactin secretion in males may cause decreased libido and galactorrhea, and in females amenorrhea, galactorrhea, and infertility. Bromocriptine, an ergot alkaloid possessing dopamine agonist activity, suppresses prolactin secretion.

Mechanism of Action. Because of the chemical similarity between GH and prolactin, it is not surprising that it produces some physiological actions similar to those produced by GH. Also, like GH, prolactin acts directly upon tissues and is not regulated by a feedback function of a target organ. Prolactin acts directly upon the mammary gland. Purified preparations of mammary cell membranes possess a high-affinity binding site for this hormone.

Preparations. *Corticotropin injection,* USP (ACTH, ACTHAR): available as sterile solution or lyophilized powder (ACTHAR); 25, 40, or 80 U i.m. or i.v. injection; 25 U infused over 8 hr.

Corticotropin injection, USP, repository form (ACTHAR GEL, CORTICOTROPIN GEL): 40 or 80 U/ml; 40 U i.m. or s.c.

Corticotropin zinc suspension, USP (CORTICOTROPIN ZINC): 40 U and 2 mg zinc/ml, i.m. injection.

Cosyntropin (CORTROSYN): synthetic peptide containing the sequence of human ACTH from residue 1-24; lyophilized powder with 0.25 mg peptide and 10 mg mannitol in 1 ml containers with diluent; administered i.m. or i.v.

Growth hormone (ASELLACRIN): powder (sterile, lyophilized) containing 10 IU hormone and 40 mg mannitol.

Thyrotropin-releasing hormone (RELEFACT TRH, THYPINONE): solution containing 0.5 mg/ml in 1-ml containers.

Thyrotropin (THYTROPAR): power (lyophilized) 10 IU with diluent; given i.m. for diagnostic purposes.

Human menopausal gonadotropin (menotropins, PERGONAL): each 2-ml ampul contains 75 IU each of follicle-stimulating hormone activity and luteinizing hormone activity; initially one ampul i.m. daily for 9-12 days.

Human chorionic gonadotropin (HCG, ANTUITRIN-S, A.P.L., FOLLUTEIN, PREGNYL): powder (lyophilized) with 5000, 10,000, 20,000, or 40,000 IU and 10-ml diluent; 1000-4000 IU given i.m. two to three times weekly.

FACTORS AND DRUGS AFFECTING ADENOHYPOPHYSIAL HORMONES

Aside from the naturally occurring hypothalamic-releasing hormones and their synthetic analogs, several endocrine pathologies can influence the levels of circulating adenohypophysial hormones. Giantism is characterized by elevated levels of GH and dwarfism may be manifested by low circulating levels of GH. ACTH levels may be elevated in Cushing's disease and decreased in Addison's disease. Panhypopituitarism can result in differential degrees of suppression of the various trophic hormones.

Besides a host of pathological endocrine disorders, a variety of pharmacological agents can alter circulating levels of the adenohypophysial hormones. For example, pharmacological doses of cortisol and synthetic glucocorticoids such as dexamethasone suppress the secretion of ACTH. Of course, the oral contraceptives and pharmacological doses of estrogens and androgens can suppress endogenous levels of FSH and LH. Clomiphene, on the other hand, can stimulate the release of pituitary gonadotropins (13).

Other pharmacological agents alter the levels of pituitary hormones yet have no inherent hormonal activity. Certain CNS drugs can alter the hypothalamic neural pathways that control the releasing hormones. For example, morphine can interfere with gonadotropin secretion and block ovulation. Phenothiazine tranquilizers alter dopaminergic activity and can produce elevated levels of prolactin leading to galactorrhea.

The circulating levels of GH can be altered by a wide variety of agents (Table 12.1-3). Some of these agents have inherent hormonal activity, whereas other drugs lack such activity.

Table 12.1-3
Agents Influencing Plasma Levels of Growth Hormone

Drugs Increasing Growth Hormone Levels	Drugs Decreasing Growth Hormone Levels
Estrogens	Glucocorticoids
Oral contraceptives	Chlorpromazine
Insulin	α-Adrenergic receptor blocking agents
Vasopressin	Bromocryptine
Arginine	Ethanol
Glucagon	
Norepinephrine	
Dopamine	
β-adrenergic receptor blocking agents	

NEUROHYPOPHYSIAL HORMONES

ANTIDIURETIC HORMONE (ADH) (VASOPRESSIN)

Chemistry. ADH is a nonapeptide with two half-cysteine residues forming a bridge between positions 1 and 6 (Table 12.1-4). The disulfide bridge is essential for biological activity. A basic amino acid in position 8 confers antidiuretic activity. Arginine is found in position 8 in all mammalian species except swine, which have lysine in this position. Digestion of vasopressin with aminopeptidase results in the loss of biological activity (8). Vasopressin has been synthesized (8, 29). The estimated plasma half-life is between 10 and 20 min with the liver and kidney being major sites of chemical inactivation.

Physiological Aspects. ADH is synthesized in localized cell populations within the supraoptic and paraventricular nuclei of the hypothalamus, transported to the neurohypophysis by exoplasmic flow, and released into the blood by a variety of stimuli, including stress and hyperosmolarity of the blood. The principal stimulus for ADH secretion is the osmotic pressure of the blood, which influences hypothalamic osmoreceptors. Hyperosmolarity leads to an increased secretion of ADH (to conserve water) and an accompanying sensation of thirst causing an increase in water intake). The increased intake and

Table 12.1-4
Structure Activity Relationship of Natural and Synthetic Antidiuretic Peptides

8-Arginine vasopressin (ADH)

Cys-Tyr-Phe-Glu-Asp-Cys-Pro-Arg-Gly(NH_2)
1 2 3 4 5 6 7 8 9

Peptides	AA Position/AA Substitution[a]	Activity[b] Antidiuretic	Pressor
c2Natural			
ADH (mammals)	As above	100	100
8-Lysine vasopressin (lypressin, swine)	8-Lys	80	60
Oxytocin	3-Ile, 8-Leu	1	1
Synthetic			
Desmopressin (DDAVP)	1-Deamino-Cys, 8-D-Arg	1200	0.39
DVDAP	1-Deamino-Cys, 4-Val, 8-D-Arg	1230	0

[a] AA = amino acids, positions with respect to ADH.
[b] Relative to ADH, assayed in the rat.

conservation of water lead to a reduction in the osmolarity of the blood and a blunting of the stimulus for ADH secretion.

The physiological site of action of ADH is the distal tubules and collecting ducts of the nephron. In the presence of ADH, the tubules are maximally permeable to water. Pharmacological amounts of this hormone can stimulate vascular smooth muscle contraction and enhance the secretion of ACTH. It has been reported that human neonates release vasopressin in stressful situations, and this could be used as an indicator for fetal stress (6).

Recent studies also indicate that ADH, along with oxytocin, may have actions in the central nervous system. These studies suggest a role for the neurohypophysial hormones in the modification of memory-related processes and in the induction of specific forms of behavior (35).

Mechanism of Action. Though the mechanism of action of vasopressin remains to be fully elucidated, this hormone appears to exert its antidiuretic action by regulating the permeability of the renal epithelium to water and urea. Through the actions of this hormone, water moves freely across the epithelium in response to the osmotic gradient that exists in the renal interstitium, resulting in a maximally concentrated urine. Currently available evidence suggests that ADH increases the size or number of pores through which water may traverse the membrane (16). Vasopressin increases the intracellular concentration of cAMP, but the exact role of the nucleotide in the action of vasopressin is not clearly understood.

Unitage and Preparations. Antidiuretic activity of vasopressin is assayed in terms of a pressor unit that is determined by measuring its pressor activity in rats and comparing the activity with that of a USP posterior pituitary standard.

Several pharmacological preparations of vasopressin are available (Table 12.1-5). Vasopressin tannate (PITRESSIN TANNATE) and the vasopressin analog desmopressin acetate (DDAVP) have longer duration of action than vasopressin. Vasopressin tannate is administered intramuscularly or subcutaneously, whereas desmopressin is administered intranasally. Aqueous vasopressin (PITRESSIN) is a water-soluble posterior pituitary extract containing variable amounts of arginine and lysine vasopressin. Synthetic lysine vasopressin (lypressin, DIAPID) is available for administration by nasal insufflation.

Therapeutic Uses. The principal therapeutic use for vasopressin is in the management of diabetes insipidus (9, 29). Diabetes insipidus is a disorder of renal water conservation due either to a deficiency in ADH (central diabetes insipidus) or to an inability of the kidney to

Table 12.1-5
Antidiuretic Hormone Preparations

Antidiuretic Hormone Preparations	Source	Usual Dose and Route of Administration	Duration	Indications	Side Effects
Vasopressin injection (Aq. sol. 20 pressor U/ml)	Synthetic	s.c./i.m./intranasal Adults: 5-10, U q.i.d. Children: 2.5-10 U q.i.d.	2-8 hr	Central diabetes insipidus	Angina, myocardial infarction, nausea, abdominal cramp, diarrhea, uterine cramp, allergic reactions, and inflammatory reactions at the injection sites
Vasopressin tannate injection (susp. in peanut oil, 5 pressor U/ml)	Synthetic	i.m. Adults: 2.5-10 U every 1-3 days Children: 1.25-2.5 U, as required	24-72 hr	Severe diabetes insipidus	Same as above and excessive water retention
Desmopressin acetate (DDAVP) solution 0.1 mg/ml	Synthetic	Intranasal Adults: 0.1 ml b.i.d. or t.i.d. Children: 0.05-0.3 ml/day, single or 2 divided doses	up to 20 hr	Severe diabetes insipidus, where other ADH preparations are ineffective	Transient headache, increase in blood pressure, nasal congestion, vulval pain
Lypressin (Solution, 50 pressor U/ml)	Synthetic	Intranasal: one spray (2 pressor units) each nostril, 3 to 4 times daily	3-4 hr	Mild to severe diabetes insipidus	Hypersensitivity; other side effects insignificant

respond to vasopressin (nephrogenic diabetes insipidus). This disorder is characterized by polyuria and polydipsia.

Vasopressin is used therapeutically in replacement therapy for central diabetes insipidus. Occasionally, its smooth muscle-stimulating properties are useful in patients with gastrointestinal distension and incomplete paralysis. Pharmacological amounts of vasopressin are also used as a diagnostic test for evaluating the pituitary reserve of ACTH. Analogs of vasopressin, which have reduced pressor action, have been used to stimulate the formation of various blood factors.

Large doses of vasopressin stimulate gastrointestinal smooth muscle and may produce nausea, diarrhea, and abdominal cramps. Uterine cramps are a common complaint following intensive therapy. The vasoconstrictor properties of large doses of vasopressin are such that the hormone is contraindicated for patients with histories of coronary artery disease. Water intoxication is possible in those patients who are unable to limit their water intake after therapy is initiated. Errors in dosage are possible when using vasopressin tannate because of separation of the drug from the oil vehicle. Local inflammatory reactions may occur if the same site of injection is repeatedly used. It is important, therefore, to rotate sites of administration. Nasal application of ADH preparations can cause irritation and congestion locally, rhinorrhea, nasal pruritus, and nasal ulceration.

Because nephrogenic diabetes insipidus is resistant to vasopressin therapy, several nonhormonal drugs, including chlorpropamide, clofibrate, and, somewhat paradoxically, the thiazide diuretics, may prove useful in reducing the polyuria.

OXYTOCIN AND OXYTOCIC AGENTS

Chemistry. Oxytocin, like ADH, is a nonapeptide (Table 12.1-4). It differs from vasopressin in two positions; position 8 contains leucine and position 3 isoleucine. The latter alteration appears to be important for oxytocic activity. The similarity in structure leads to an overlapping biological activity, especially when employing pharmacologic doses (8).

Physiological Aspects. Oxytocin stimulates the contraction of smooth muscles of the uterus and the myoepithelial cells surrounding the alveoli of the mammary glands. Oxytocin is much more potent than vasopressin in its milk-ejecting activity. The sensitivity of uterine smooth muscle to oxytocin fluctuates during the menstrual cycle and during pregnancy (29). When concentrations of estrogen are low, the utertus is quite insensitive to oxytocin. In pregnancy, the uterus is most sensitive to oxytocin during the last trimester.

Mechanism of Action. High-affinity receptor sites have been demonstrated in the mammary gland and the uterus. In the uterus, these receptor sites are located on the cell membrane of smooth muscle cells. Oxytocin can increase the release of prostaglandins in the uterus and increase the level of cAMP in the mammary gland. It is not known, however, if these represent primary actions of the hormone or are secondary to the induced response.

Adverse Effects. A major adverse effect of the obstetrical use of oxytocin is hyperstimulation of the uterus, which may progress to uterine tetany with marked impairment of uteroplacental blood flow, uterine rupture, cervical laceration, or trauma to the infant. Oxytocin may also lead to hypotension (25).

Presently available forms of oxytocin (PITOCIN, SYNTOCINON) are synthetic. They can be administered by slow intravenous infusion, intramuscularly, or in the form of a nasal spray.

Other oxytocic agents such as sparteine (TOCOSAMINE), prostaglandins (dinoprost tromethamine, PROSTIN F_2 ALPHA; Chapter 13.2), and ergot alkaloids (e.g., ergonovine; Chapter 19) have been used as uterine stimulants. Sparteine is not as effective and reliable as oxytocin even though it has a more rapid onset of action than oxytocin. The introduction of dinoprost tromethamine as an abortifacient in the second trimester of pregnancy represents the first clinical use of the prostaglandins.

Therapeutic Uses. The most important therapeutic use of oxytocin is in the induction of labor (9, 25). Oxytocin is effective in increasing both the force and frequency of uterine contraction. Following delivery, it can be utilized to increase uterine tone and decrease hemorrhage. Oxytocin may also be of value in relieving postpartum breast engorgement.

Unitage and Preparations. Oxytocic activity is assayed in terms of an oxytocin unit that is determined by measuring vasodepressor activity in anesthetized chickens and comparing the activity with that of a USP posterior pituitary standard.

FACTORS AND DRUGS AFFECTING NEUROHYPOPHYSIAL HORMONES

Several drugs and stimuli can influence the circulating levels of oxytocin and vasopressin (9) (Table 12.1-6). Many of the drug interactions involving vasopressin have been identified using indirect indices of vasopressin release such as the measurement of free water clearance. Ethanol is perhaps the most often studied drug with respect to inhibition of ADH secretion; in fact, ethanol inhibition of ADH secretion has formed a standard bioassay for vasopressin preparations.

Both pharmacological and physiological stimuli can increase the circulating levels of ADH and oxytocin. Suckling is a potent physiological stimuli leading to an increase in the secretion of oxytocin and subsequent contraction of the myoepithelial cells of the mammary glands. Nonspecific stress or ether-induced stress can increase ADH and reduce urinary output.

Table 12.1-6
Effects of Various Drugs and Stimuli upon the Blood Levels of Posterior Pituitary Hormones

ADH (Vasopressin)	
Increase Levels	*Decrease Levels*
Stress	Ethanol
Ether	Atropine
Morphine	α-Adrenoceptor agonist
Barbiturates	
Nicotine	
Suckling	
Vincristine	
Clofibrate	
Acetylcholine	

Oxytocin	
Increase Levels	*Decrease Levels*
Coitus	Ergocornine and other ergot alkaloids
Suckling	Ethanol
Prostaglandin E_1	
Prostaglandin $F_{2\alpha}$	

REFERENCES

1. Aschner, B. Über die Funktion der Hypophese. *Arch. Ges. Physiol.* 65:341, 1912.
2. Burger, H.G. and Patel, Y.C. Thyrotropin releasing hormone-TRH. *Clin. Endocrinol. Metabol.* 6:83, 1977.
3. Collip, J.B., Selye, H. and Thomson, D.L. Gonad-stimulating hormones in hypophysectomized animals. *Nature* 131:56, 1933.
4. Chakraverty, K. and Kar, K. Current status of hormone releasing and release inhibiting peptides of the hypothalamus. *Adv. Biosci.* 38:203, 1982.
5. Dale, H.H. The action of extracts of the pituitary body. *Biochem. J.* 4:427, 1909.
6. deVane, G.W. and Porter, J.C. An apparent stress-induced release of arginine vasopressin in human neonates. *J. Clin. Endocrinol. Metab.* 51:1412, 1980.
7. deWied, D. and deJong, W. Drug effects and hypothalamic-anterior pituitary function. *Ann. Rev. Pharmacol. Toxicol.* 14:389, 1974.
8. du Vigneaud, V. Hormones of the posterior pituitary gland: oxytocin and vasopressin. In: *The Harvey Lectures, 1954-1955.* New York: Academic Press, 1956.
9. Edwards, C.R.W. Vasopressin and oxytocin in health and disease. *Clin. Endocrinol. Metabol.* 6:233, 1977.
10. Eipper, B.A. and Mains, R.E. Structure and biosynthesis of pro-ACTH/endorphin and related peptides. *Endocrinol. Rev.* 1:1, 1980.
11. Flerko, B. The hypophysial portal circulation today. *Neuroendocrinology* 30:56, 1980.
12. Fracnhimont, P. Pituitary gonadotropins. *Clin. Endocrinol. Metabol.* 6:101, 1977.
13. Garcia, J., Jones, G.S. and Wentz, A.C. The use of clomiphene citrate. *Fertil. Steril.* 28:707, 1977.
14. Guillemin, R. and Gerich, J.E. Somatostatin: physiological and clinical significance. *Ann. Rev. Med.* 27:379, 1976.
15. Hall, R. and Gomez-Pam, A. The hypothalamic regulatory hormones and their clinical applications. *Adv. Clin. Chem.* 18:173, 1976.
16. Hays, R.M. Antidiuretic hormone and water transfer. *Kidney Int.* 9:223, 1976.
17. Hsueh, A.J.W. and Jones, P.B.C. Extrapituitary actions of gonadotropin-releasing hormone. *Endocrinol. Rev.* 2:437, 1981.
18. Li, C.H. The chemistry of human pituitary growth hormone: 1956-1966, In: *Growth Hormone,* Amsterdam, (A. Pecile and E. Mueller, eds.). Excerpta Medica Foundation, 1968, p. 3.
19. McCann, M. Physiology and pharmacology of LHRH and somatostatin. *Ann. Rev. Pharmacol. Toxicol.* 22:491, 1982.
20. Malone, D.N.S. and Strong, J.A. The present state of corticotropin therapy. *Practitioner* 208:329, 1972.
21. Morley, J.E. Neuroendocrine control of thyrotropin secretion. *Endocrinol. Rev.* 2:396, 1981.
22. Mortimer, C.H. Clinical applications of the gonadotropin releasing hormone. *Clin. Endocrinol. Metabol.* 6:167, 1977.
23. Ondo, J. and Pass, K. The effects of neurally active amino acids on prolactin secretion. *Endocrinology* 98:1248, 1976.
24. Okerland, M.D. and Greenspan, F.S. Clinical studies of thyrotropin and thyrotropin-releasing hormone. *Pharmacol. Therap.* (Part C) 2:79, 1977.
25. Pauerstein, C.J. Use and abuse of oxytocic agents. *Clin. Obstet. Gynecol.* 16:262, 1973.
26. Pecile, A. and Mueller, E.E. (eds.) *Growth Hormone and Related Peptides,* New York. Elsevier-North Holland Publ. Co., 1976.
27. Pierce, J.G. The subunits of pituitary thyrotropin — their relationship to other glycoprotein hormones. *Endocrinology* 89:1331, 1971.
28. Riddle, O. Prolactin in vertebrate function and organization. *J. Natl. Cancer Inst.* 31:1039, 1963.
29. Sawyer, W.H. and Manning, M. Synthetic analogs of oxytocin and the vasopressins. *Ann. Rev. Pharmacol. Toxicol.* 13:5, 1973.
30. Schally, A.V., Coy, D.H. and Meyers, C.A. Hypothalamic regulatory hormones. *Ann. Rev. Biochem.* 47:89, 1978.
31. Tager, H.S. and Steiner, D. Peptide hormones. *Ann. Rev. Biochem.* 43:509, 1974.
32. Terry, L.C. and Martin, J.B. Hypothalamic hormones: subcellular distribution and mechanisms of release. *Ann. Rev. Pharmacol. Toxicol.* 18:111, 1978.
33. Vaitukaitis, J.L., Ross, G.T., Braunstein, G.D. and Rayford, R.L. Gonadotropins and their subunits: basic and clinical studies. *Recent Prog. Horm. Res.* 32:289, 1976.
34. Vale, W., Spiess, J., Rivier, C. and Rivier, J. Characterization of a 41-residue ovine hypothalamic peptide that stimulates secretion of corticotropin and beta-endorphin. *Science* 213:1394, 1981.
35. Walter, R., Flexner, L.B., Ritzmann, R.F., et al. Central nervous system effects of posterior pituitary hormones, fragments and their derivatives on drug tolerance/dependence and behavior. In: *Polypeptide Hormones.* (Beers, R.F., Jr. and Bassett, E.G., eds.), New York: Raven Press, p. 321.
36. Yasuda, N., Greer, M.A. and Aizawa, T. Corticotropin releasing factor. *Endocrinol. Rev.* 3:123, 1982.
37. Yen, S.S.C. Gonadotropin-releasing hormone. *Ann. Rev. Med.* 26:403, 1975.

ADDITIONAL READING

Vickery, B. Comparison of the potential for therapeutic utilities with gonadotropin-releasing hormone agonists and antagonists. *Endocrine Rev.*, 7:115, 1986

Handelsman, D.J., and Swerdloff, R.S. Pharmacokinetics of gonadotropin-releasing hormone and its analogs. *Endocrine Rev.*, 7:95, 1986.

CHAPTER
12.2

CALCEMIC HORMONES

Alexander D. Kenny

CALCIUM HOMEOSTASIS

ENDOCRINE CONTROL OF CALCIUM HOMEOSTASIS

The plasma calcium concentration is held within narrow limits, close to 10.0 mg/dl, by homeostatic mechanisms which are mainly endocrine in nature. This control is effected on the plasma ionic calcium concentration which under normal circumstances represents about 50% of the total calcium concentration.

STATE OF CALCIUM IN PLASMA

The plasma total calcium exists in three main fractions:

1. Protein-bound Ca (mainly to albumin)	4.6mg/dl, 1.15 mM
2. Complexed Ca (with small anions):	0.6 mg/dl, 0.15 mM
3. Ionic Ca^{2+}:	4.8 mg/dl, 1.20 mM
Total:	10.0 mg/dl, 2.50 mM

Of these, complexed and ionic calcium fractions are ultrafilterable.

The protein-bound calcium does not pass through a semipermeable membrane and is referred to as the nondiffusible or nonfilterable calcium fraction. This fraction is primarily bound to albumin and is influenced by perturbations in plasma protein levels such as in hypoalbuminemia; for each 1 g/dl fall in plasma albumin the plasma total calcium concentration will decrease by an increment of 0.8-1.0 mg/dl. Those fractions that pass through the membrane (complexed and ionic) are known as the diffusible or ultrafilterable calcium fraction. The ultrafilterable calcium is not synonymous with the ionic calcium, but in the past, it has been equated with the ionic calcium for diagnostic purposes. The complexed calcium is associated with small anions such as bicarbonate, phosphate, and citrate. The complexed and protein-bound fractions are biologically inactive. On the other hand, the plasma ionic calcium is that fraction that is important for normal function of nerves, muscles, and secretory processes. It is this fraction that is held under tight homeostatic control. Plasma pH can influence the plasma ionic calcium level; a rise in pH causes a fall in plasma ionic calcium concentration, and a fall in pH increases the ionic fraction. Although changes in plasma pH modify slightly the affinity of albumin for calcium, their influence on the ionic calcium fraction is mediated largely through the effect on the interaction between calcium and the small anions, particularly orthophosphate (28). This phenomenon is undoubtedly related to the mild tetany sometimes experienced by individuals, often young women, who are hyperventilating.

The central nervous system appears to be more sensitive to changes in ionic calcium concentration than the peripheral nervous system. It is fortunate that the ionic calcium level in the cerebrospinal fluid (CSF) is protected from gross fluctuations in the plasma; it remains relatively constant in the face of major acute perturbations in plasma ionic calcium concentrations (20).

Diagnostically, the plasma ionic calcium concentration may prove useful. The original frog heart method of McLean and Hastings (26) for determining the ionic calcium fraction is impractical. Nevertheless, the technique led to the development of a means for calculating the ionic calcium level from a knowledge of the plasma concentrations of total calcium and protein (27). Indeed, this was the only approach before the advent of calcium selective electrode technology (33). This latter development, coupled with the availability of radioimmunoassay methods for determining parathyroid hormone (2, 35) permits greater precision in the differential diagnosis of disorders of calcium metabolism.

CALCIUM METABOLISM IN THE ADULT

Normal Adult. Calcium metabolism in the adult is summarized in Fig. 12.2-1. If a normal daily intake of 800 mg of calcium is assumed, then less than 50% is absorbed through the gastrointestinal tract. The remainder, together with an unabsorbed quantity of secreted calcium, passes into the feces. In addition, urinary calcium contributes to a daily loss which rarely amounts to more than 200 mg. The unabsorbed secreted calcium and the urinary calcium loss together have been termed the "endogenous loss" over which there is little control, endocrine or otherwise. Bone contains 99% of the total body calcium which is approximately 15-18% of the total body weight (1000-1200 g in the 70-kg male). About 500 mg of calcium enter and exit from bone per day.

Pregnancy. Additional calcium losses in pregnancy are minimal. The total calcium content of the neonate at birth is only 30-35 g, or less than 3% of the maternal stores of calcium. Most deposition of calcium in the fetus occurs during the last 4 months, and there is a tendency for the plasma total calcium to fall in later pregnancy and for the immunoreactive parathyroid hormone levels to rise progressively toward term (5, 35).

Lactation. Lactation represents a more severe strain on maternal calcium metabolism. Human milk has a calcium concentration (33 mg/dl, range 15-60 mg/dl) that is many times higher than that in plasma. The maternal calcium losses during lactation are difficult to estimate with precision due to variations in calcium concentration, daily milk output, and length of lactation period. From 40 to 80 g of calcium may be lost in the milk, so that in a normal pregnancy and lactation period a total of not more than 10% of the maternal stores of calcium are lost over a 15- to 18-month period. When compared with the egg-laying chicken, which loses 10% of its calcium stores daily, these losses in the human are relatively insignificant. Nevertheless plasma calcitriol concentrations are elevated in early pregnancy and continue elevated throughout pregnancy (21, 34) and lactation (21).

ENDOCRINE CONTROL OF CALCIUM METABOLISM

The endocrine control of calcium metabolism involves mainly three hormones and three target organs:

Calcemic Hormones	Major Target Organs
Parathyroid hormone (PTH)	Bone and kidney
Calcitriol [1,25-$(OH)_2D_3$]	Gut and bone
Calcitonin (CT)	Bone

It is now becoming clear that the kidney, through its hormone, calcitriol, may play a pivotal role in the endocrine control of calcium metabolism (Fig. 12.2-2). Which endocrine axis (PTH-bone; calcitriol-gut; PTH-kidney; calcitriol-bone; CT-bone) is important for acute (minute-to-minute) and chronic (day-to-day or week-to-week) regulation of calcium metabolism is not known with certainty. Classically the PTH-bone axis

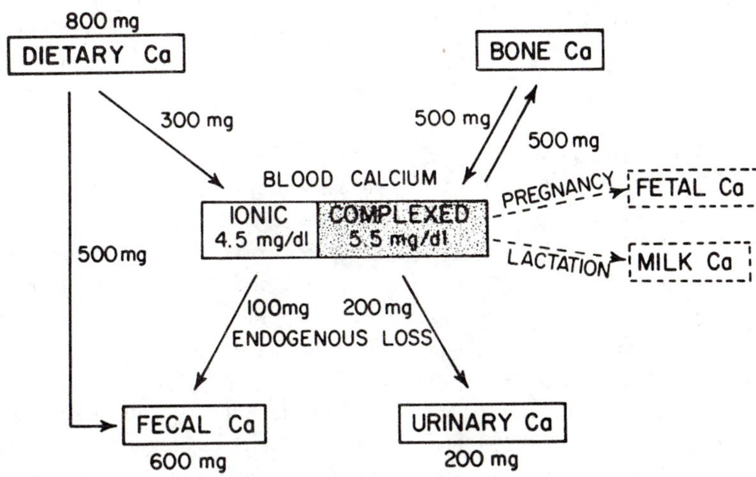

Fig 12.2-1. *Calcium metabolism in the human adult.*

Calcium metabolism varies widely between individuals; the above diagram represents a possible kinetic scheme for an individual consuming the Recommended Daily Dietary Allowance of 800 mg/Ca/day. All quantities indicated are on a per day basis. Normally less than 50% of the calcium intake is absorbed via the gastrointestinal tract; 300 mg or 37.5% of the intake is suggested. The remaining 500 mg passes unabsorbed into the feces and is joined by a net amount of approximately 100 mg which is secreted into the gastrointestinal tract and remains unabsorbed. The urinary loss of around 200 mg is that portion (1%) of the glomerular filtrate calcium which is not reabsorbed in its passage through the nephron. This loss, together with the net amount secreted by the gastrointestinal tract, is termed the endogenous loss. The body exercises little regulation over the endogenous loss of calcium. The turnover of bone calcium is represented as 500 mg/day^{-1}. Gut calcium transport and bone calcium turnover are under endocrine control. Pregnancy and lactation involve additional losses of calcium.

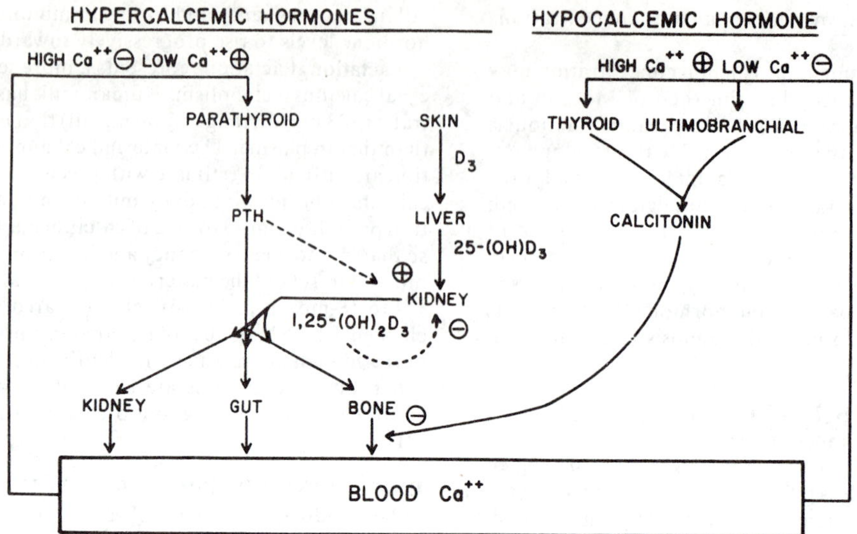

Fig. 12.2-2. *Endocrine control of calcium homeostasis.*

There are three major hormones and three major target organs involved in the endocrine control of calcium homeostasis. Two of the hormones, parathyroid hormone (PTH) and vitamin D_3 (D_3), are hypercalcemic agents. The third hormone, calcitonin, is hypocalcemic in action in mammals but has no such effect in submammalian vertebrate speies. Hypocalcemia stimulates the release of parathyroid hormone which acts on its target organs, bone, kidney, and gut, to mobilize calcium into extracellular fluid. As the plasma calcium rises in response to the hormone its further secretion is suppressed. Vitamin D_3 is synthesized in the skin and, together with dietary vitamin D_3 (animal sources) or vitamin D_2 (plant sources), enters the circulation. Vitamin D_3 is converted by the liver to 25-hydroxyvitamin D_3 [25-(OH)D_3] which is activated to its hormonal form, 1,25-dihydroxyvitamin D_3 [1,25-$(OH)_2D_3$], by the kidney which secretes the hormone for transport to its target organs, gut, bone, and kidney, where it, like parathyroid hormone, mobilizes calcium for the extracellular fluid compartment. Calcitonin acts mainly on bone to inhibit resorption. Secretion of this hypocalcemic hormone is stimulated by hypercalcemia and suppressed by hypocalcemia. Parathyroid hormone and 1,25-$(OH)_2D_3$ exert positive and negative feedback regulatory influences respectively on the production and secretion of 1,25-$(OH)_2D_3$.

has been considered of prime importance, but more recently the PTH-kidney axis has gained greater attention. We now know that PTH not only modulates renal handling of calcium and phosphate (19) but also exercises a regulatory influence on calcitriol production by the kidney (9, 17). In addition, calcitriol itself exerts a negative feedback influence on its own production. Calcitonin is considered to be of little physiological importance in humans, although this point of view is questioned by some.

CALCIUM REQUIREMENTS

The Food and Nutrition Board of the National Academy of Sciences and the National Research Council have published Recommended Dietary Allowances (RDAs) for calcium (Table 12.2-1). In general the RDAs for calcium have been determined by use of the calcium balance method, in which total dietary calcium intake is held at a constant and known level while total fecal and urinary calcium outputs are measured. That level of calcium intake resulting in a zero or slightly positive balance in a large pool of subjects is accepted as the RDA. The adult of either sex is recommended to ingest 800 mg of calcium per day. The latter figure has been questioned as being unnecessarily high. In 1962 the World Health Organization concluded (39) that in adult males "no frank signs of calcium deficiency have ever been described in any part of the world, even in populations with a habitually low calcium intake." There is reason to believe that the calcium balance method in the normal subject reveals only one piece of important information: the immediate dietary history of the subject with respect to calcium intake. In other words it reflects the average American or Western diet. In addition there is evidence to indicate that an individual can adapt in time to a low-calcium diet by increasing the efficiency of calcium absorption from the gut. An adult, when first placed on a low-calcium diet, goes into negative balance immediately, and after weeks or months of adaptation, finally exhibits a zero or even a positive balance (23). In fact, Peruvian males have been identified as living all their lives on calcium intakes of less than 300 mg/day with no evidence of calcium deficiency disease (11).

Calcium Requirements in Pregnancy. Although additional calcium losses in pregnancy are minimal, the RDA for the pregnant female is increased by 400 mg/day of calcium (Table 12.2-1). There is little objective evidence to back this recommendation. In fact the hypocalcemia of late pregnancy does not respond to extra dietary calcium or vitamin D, and there is no convincing evidence that a low-calcium intake during pregnancy is deleterious to the mother. Black African women undergoing multiple pregnancies (average 9: range 2-20 children) on very low calcium intakes showed no evidence of pathological bone loss (37, 38).

Calcium Requirements in Lactation. The RDA for the lactating female is increased by 500 mg/day of calcium (Table 12.2-1)

Table 12.2-1
Recommended Daily Dietary Allowances for Calcium

Subjects	Recommended Dietary Allowances for Calcium			
	NAS-NRC[a] (USA)		WHO[b] (UN)	
	Age (years)	Calcium (mg/day)	Age (years)	Calcium (mg/day)
Infants	0.0-0.5	360	0-1.0	500-600
	0.5-1.0	540		
Children	1-10	800	1-9	400-500
Males	11-18	1200	10-15	600-700
			16-19	500-600
	19+	800	19+	400-500
Females	11-18	1200	10-15	600-700
			16-19	500-600
	19+	800	19+	400-500
Pregnant	—	1200	—	1000-1200
Lactating	—	1200	—	1000-1200

[a]NAS-NRC: Food and Nutrition Board, National Academy of Sciences-National Research Council, USA.

[b]WHO: World Health Organization, United Nations.

and, as in pregnancy, there is little evidence to support this recommendation. Nevertheless, the recommended increase in intake is usually justified on the basis of margin of safety.

CALCIUM PREPARATIONS

Most of the calcium preparations described below are used either acutely or chronically to treat hypocalcemic conditions. Oral preparations include calcium carbonate, calcium chloride, calcium gluconate, and calcium lactate. Parenteral preparations include individual drugs (calcium chloride, calcium gluceptate, calcium gluconate) and various binary mixtures such as calcium gluconate-calcium ascorbate, calcium gluconate-calcium gluceptate, or calcium lactate-calcium glycerophosphate. In addition, calcium salts are marketed in combination with vitamin D. Dosages and routes of some of the preparations are presented in Table 12.2-2. Caution should be exercised in administering any of the parenteral calcium preparations in patients receiving cardiac glycosides because of the tendency of calcium to potentiate the action of these potentially toxic drugs.

Calcium Gluconate. Calcium gluconate, administered slowly by the intravenous route, is the drug of choice in the acute treatment of hypocalcemic crisis. It may be used chronically by the oral route. It is nonirritating by the oral and intravnous routes; the intramuscular route should be avoided. Calcium gluconate is available as a 10% solution for parenteral administration and as tablets ranging from 300 to 1000 mg for oral use.

Calcium Gluceptate. The calcium salt of glucoheptonic acid may be used intravenously for the acute relief of hypocalcemic crisis. It may also be injected intramuscularly in patients in which the intravenous route is not available. This agent is not used orally.

Calcium Lactate. Calcium lactate is administered only by the oral route and is indicated for the treatment of mild hypocalcemia and for maintenance therapy. It is available as 300- and 600-mg tablets.

Calcium Carbonate. Calcium carbonate may be given by the oral route only and is used for the control of mild hypocalcemic states and for maintenance therapy.

MANAGEMENT OF HYPOCALCEMIC AND HYPERCALCEMIC CRISIS

Hypocalcemic Crisis. Hypocalcemia may occur in many different situations with completely different etiologies. If severe enough and untreated, it can lead to death. Some of the conditions associated with hypocalcemia include: hypoparathyroidism, both idiopathic and iatrogenic (thyroid surgery); chronic renal failure; vitamin D deficiency of nutritional or malabsorption origin; chronic anticonvulsant therapy with phenytoin and phenobarbital; neonatal tetany; hemorrhagic pancreatitis; hypomagnesemia; and administration of calcium-complexing agents such as citrate that can occur during massive transfusions with citrated blood.

The treatment of hypocalcemic crisis, regardless of etiology, starts with the immediate intravenous injection of a parenteral calcium preparation such as 10% calcium gluconate solution (Table 12.2-2). This agent is given slowly until tetany is controlled and then may be followed by a slow infusion of a more dilute solution (0.3-0.8% solution of calcium gluconate diluted in isotonic sodium chloride or 5% dextrose) over 3-12 h. In those patients in which the calcium preparation cannot be administered intravenously for one reason or another, calcium gluceptate is available for the intramuscular route. Oral maintenance therapy may be instituted, once the crisis is over, with any of the oral preparations (calcium gluconate, calcium lactate, or calcium carbonate). Other therapy is initiated, if necessary, depending upon the etiology of the hypocalcemia. Plasma calcium levels should be monitored to avoid toxic hypercalcemic states. If hypomagnesemia is the etiological condition, then the tetany may not be controlled by calcium administration; in this case 2 ml of 50% magnesium sulfate should be administered intramuscularly.

Table 12.2-2
Calcium Preparations: Doses and Routes of Administration

Calcium Preparation	Ca Content (%)	Route	Available Form	Recommended Dose
Calcium gluconate, USP	9	i.v.	10% solution	Adults: 20-ml injection slowly of solution followed by slow infusion of 0.3-0.8% solution over 3-12 hr
		Oral	300- to 600-mg tablets	Adults: 15 g/day in divided doses Children: 500 mg/kg/day, in divided doses
Calcium gluceptate, USP	8	i.v. i.m.	18-mg/ml solution	Adults: 5-20 ml Adults: 2-5ml (gluteal region)
Calcium lactate, USP	13	Oral	300- to 600-mg tablets	Adults: 4.5-9 g/day in three divided doses with meal Children: 500 mg/kg/day in divided doses
Calcium carbonate, USP	40	Oral	Powder	Adults: 3-6 g/day in three divided doses with meals

Hypercalcemic Crisis. Chronic elevation of the plasma ionic calcium level can have serious pathophysiological effects that can be life-threatening. This is certainly the case if metastatic calcification of the kidney leads to irreversible impairment of renal function. Hypercalcemia is most commonly associated with neoplastic disease, but other etiologies include: hyperparathyroidism; sarcoidosis, hypervitaminosis D; thiazide diuretic therapy; milk-alkali syndrome; and hyperthyroidism.

Treatment depends on the etiology and therefore the control of the precipitating disorder. For example, primary hyperparathyroidism usually succumbs to surgical removal of a parathyroid adenoma. The immediate management of hypervitaminosis D includes the stopping of all vitamin D medication and the institution of other supportive measures described elsewhere in this chapter. Nevertheless, more immediate additional measures are often indicated in hypercalcemic crisis. These measures include: (1) rehydration of the patient and promotion of calcium diuresis; (2) administration of intravenous and oral inorganic phosphate; (3) treatment with mithramycin; and (4) administration of glucocorticoids in specific situations not requiring an acute lowering of the plasma calcium concentrate.

A routine for the treatment of hypercalcemic crisis, suggested by Newmark and Himathongkam (30), has the following salient features. The patient is immediately hydrated with physiological saline, and diuresis is further facilitated by administration of the loop diuretic, furosemide, every 4-6 hr as needed to maintain a urinary output of 100-200 mg/hr. Electrolytes should be monitored during this acute phase and replaced if necessary. Once the plasma calcium begins to fall, then an oral hypocalcemic agent such as inorganic phosphate is prescribed as required. On the other hand, if the acute treatment with hydration and furosemide fails to combat the hypercalcemia, then one of the following more drastic measures is indicated: (1) intravenous infusion of inorganic phosphate; (2) higher doses of oral phosphate; (3) rectal administration of inorganic phosphate; (4) intravenous injection of mithramycin and inorganic phosphate.

PARATHYROID HORMONE

Chemistry and Assay

Chemistry. Crude extracts of parathyroid hormone were first prepared in 1925, but the pure hormone was not isolated until 1960. The reason for this delay in purification of the hormone was mainly methodological; the late 1950s brought the development of the more convenient and sensitive rat bioassay method (15, 29).

Parathyroid hormone is a single-chain polypeptide containing 84 amino acids with a molecular weight of around 9500. Biological activity is associated with the N-terminal portion of the molecule. A biologically active synthetic N-terminal fragment ($PTH_{1\text{-}34}$) of both bovine and human parathyroid hormones is available commercially for experimental studies. The preparation of parathyroid hormone used clinically, Parathyroid Injection, USP is only about 0.5% pure and must be standardized by the USP dog bioassay method. The marketing of this preparation was discontinued in 1980 by the sole American manufacturer (Eli Lilly) due to insufficient clinical demand.

In the gland, parathyroid hormone is first synthesized in prohormone forms (pre-pro and proparathyroid hormones) that are considerably larger in molecular weight (8). Most of the additional amino acids are linked to the N-terminal portion of the molecule.

Once secreted, the 1-84 intact hormone is rapidly metabolized into a series of biologically active and inactive fragments with different plasma half-lives (35). These fragments embarrass interpretation of plasma parathyroid hormone levels as determined by radioimmunoassay. A biologically inactive fragment, with a molecular weight of around 7000 and associated with the C-terminal of the molecule, reacts immunologically with most of the parathyroid hormone antisera available. In addition, this fragment, due to its having the longest plasma half-life of the parathyroid hormone fragments, is usually the major circulating fragment. In spite of these serious theoretical complications in interpretation of radioimmunassay data, the latter do reflect the parathyroid status of the patient and are of practical use in diagnosis if interpreted cautiously by individuals familiar with the problem.

Assay. The official USP bioassay method must be used for the standardization of all preparations of parathyroid hormone used clinically; it also defines the USP unit. By definition, 100 USP units is that amount of parathyroid activity which will raise the serum calcium an average of 1.0 mg/dl 16-18 hr after subcutaneous administration to an adequate number of dogs of suitable size. Other assays used experimentally have been summarized by Kenny and Dacke (19). The radioimmunoassay for parathyroid hormone, in spite of its deficiencies discussed above, is by far the most sensitive assay method allowing the measurement of plasma hormone levels which are not amenable to simple detection by other methods (2).

Pharmacological Effects

Overview. Bone and kidney represent the major target organs of the hormone both physiologically and pharmacologically. Other minor sites include the gut and smooth muscle. The actions of parathyroid hormone on its target tissues are summarized in Table 12.2-3. Scrutiny of these responses reveals that some are in concert and some are in opposition with respect to the effects on plasma and urinary calcium and phosphate levels. Those in concert are therefore predictable. The overall effects of parathyroid hormone on mineral metabolism, after taking the responses at both bone and kidney into account, are presented in Table 12.2-4.

Effects on Bone. *Resorption.* Parathyroid hormone has effects on bone which can be viewed as biphasic. There is an immediate effect within minutes on existing bone cell activity, particularly the osteocyte population; this includes both embedded osteocytes and surface osteoprogenitor cells, which represent 95% of all bone cells. These cells are joined one with another and form a cellular membrane covering a major part of all bone surface. This increase in bone cell metabolic activity is called osteolysis and physiologically, at least, is associated with mineral homeostasis. Later, after 12-24 hr there is an increase in the number of remodeling cells (osteoclasts and osteoblasts) which normally represent only 5% of bone cells. At first the osteoclasts increase in number, followed later by an increase in the number of osteoblasts. The early phase does not require protein synthesis; the later phase does. The early phase of osteolysis is associated with an uptake of calcium by bone cells and an increase in cytosolic calcium and cyclic adenosine monophosphate (cAMP). The later phase is preceded by an increase in DNA, RNA, and protein synthesis prior to the increase in the number of multinucleated osteoclasts. The process by which bone cells dissolve bone mineral and collagen is not known with certainty. There is increasing evidence that the actions of parathyroid hormone on osteoclasts are mediated by the action of the hormone on osteoblasts as the direct target cells (36).

Formation. Parathyroid hormone eventually increases the pool size of the bone-forming cells, the osteoblasts, but this event occurs later than the increase in the number of osteoclasts.

Effects on Kidney. *Urinary Phosphate.* Parathyroid hormone has three major actions on the kidney involving phosphate, calcium, and vitamin D metabolism. Other minor effects are increased excretion of potassium, bicarbonate, and sodium, and decreased excretion of magnesium, ammonia, and hydrogen ions.

Parathyroid hormone causes a rapid increase in urinary cAMP and inorganic phosphate following intravenous injection. A rise in cAMP precedes that of phosphate; this supports the concept that the phosphaturic action is mediated through the cAMP second-messenger system. In isolated renal tubular cells, parathyroid hormone induces a rapid rise in cAMP and enhances calcium uptake. A parathyroid hormone-responsive adenylate cyclase is in the renal cortex, and the phosphaturic action is located in the proximal renal tubule where phosphate reabsorption is inhibited.

Table 12.2-3
Parathyroid Hormone: Specific Target Organ Responses

Target Organ	Mediator	Mechanism	Responses
Bone	cAMP[a]	Bone resorption ↑	Plasma Ca ↑ Plasma P ↑
Kidney	cAMP cAMP?	TRP[b] ↓ TRCa[c] ↑	Urinary P ↑ Urinary Ca ↓
Gut	$1,25\text{-}(OH)_2D_3$[d]	Gut Ca transport ↑ Gut P transport ↑	Plasma Ca ↑ Plasma P ↑
Vascular smooth muscle	cAMP	Relaxation ↑	Hypotension ↑ Renal plasma flow ↑

[a] cAMP: 3′,5′-cyclic adenosine monophosphate.
[b] TRP: tubular reabsorption of phosphate.
[c] TRCa: tubular reabsorption of calcium.
[d] $1,25\text{-}(OH)_2D_3$: 1,25-dihydroxyvitamin D_3.

Table 12.2-4
Parathyroid Hormone: Overall Effects

Response	Contributing Mechanism	Overall Effect
Predictable responses		
Plasma Ca ↑	Bone: resorption ↑	Hypercalcemia
↑	Kidney: TRCa[a] ↓	
Urinary P ↑	Kidney: TRP[b] ↓	Hyperphosphaturia
↑	Bone: resorption ↑[c]	
Unpredictable responses		
Urinary Ca ↑	Bone: resorption ↑[c]	Unpredictable
↓	Kidney: TRCa ↑	
Plasma P ↑	Bone: resorption ↑	Unpredictable
↓	Kidney: TRP ↓	

[a] TRCa: tubular reabsorption of calcium.
[b] TRP: tubular reabsorption of phosphate.
[c] Indirect effect; increased mobilization of the element from bone leads to an increase in the plasma concentration and hence an increase in the filtered load of the element.

Urinary Calcium. Parathyroid hormone enhances calcium reabsorption by the distal renal tubules and thereby causes a decrease in the urinary calcium excretion. This is a direct action of parathyroid hormone on the kidney. Whether the urinary calcium rises, falls, or remains unchanged in response to parathyroid hormone depends upon the relative contributions of this direct renal action and the other actions of parathyroid hormone on bone and gut which contribute to a hypercalcemic response with a long pharmacodynamic half-life and therefore to an increased filtered load. More often than not, the latter dominates in a pharmacological situation. This is illustrated in Fig. 12.2-3 taken from the work of Froeling and Bijvoet (14). As long as the infusion of parathyroid hormone is continued and the plasma calcium, and therefore the filtered load, continues to rise, there is no net loss of calcium in the urine. The direct action of parathyroid hormone causes calcium retention, but this is counteracted by the increased filtered load. However, once the infusion is stopped, the direct action, possessing a very short pharmacodynamic half-life, ceases immediately and the filtered load takes over, resulting in a dramatic increase in urinary calcium loss.

Vitamin D Metabolism. There is considerable evidence that parathyroid hormone regulates, physiologically and pharmacologically, the renal-vitamin D endocrine system by activating the 25-hydroxy-vitamin D_3-1-hydroxylase enzyme, leading to secretion of the hormone, 1,25-dihydroxyvitamin D_3. Further details of this action are discussed later in this chapter.

Gut. Parathyroid hormone increases absorption of calcium across the gut. This is neither an immediate nor a marked response, and there is reason to believe that this is not a direct action of parathyroid hormone on the gut. It is probably mediated by parathyroid hormone's stimulation of 1,25-dihydroxyvitamin D_3 secretion by the kidney.

Pharmacokinetics. Parathyroid hormone is ineffective orally and must be given parenterally (i.v. or i.m.). It has a short plasma half-life of around 30 min (1-84 intact molecule). Nevertheless, the hypercalcemic response to a single injection usually persists for several hours, indicating that the pharmacodynamic half-life is of much longer duration. At least three immunoreactive parathyroid hormone fractions have been identified in the plasma of hyperparathyroid patients; these fractions have molecular weights of around 9500 (PTH_{1-84}), 7000, and 4500, respectively. Of these, only the 9500- and 4500-fractions are considered to be biologically active (35). Some of the fragments have longer plasma half-lives of up to 4 hr.

Parathroid Hormone Receptor Classification. There is increasing evidence that parathyroid hormone may elicit its various actions through the mediation of more than one type of receptor. Simple oxidation of the two methionines at positions 8 and 18 in the PTH_{1-34} molecule leaves its hypercalcemic, hypocalciuric, and calcitriol-stimulating properties intact but partially or totally eliminates other important responses to the hormone. The oxidized agonist exhibits little or no activity with respect to renal adenylate cyclase, hyperphosphaturic, or smooth muscle relaxing (hypotensive) activities (18, 31).

Role of Parathyroid Hormone in Calcium Homeostasis. Although it is generally accepted that the endocrine

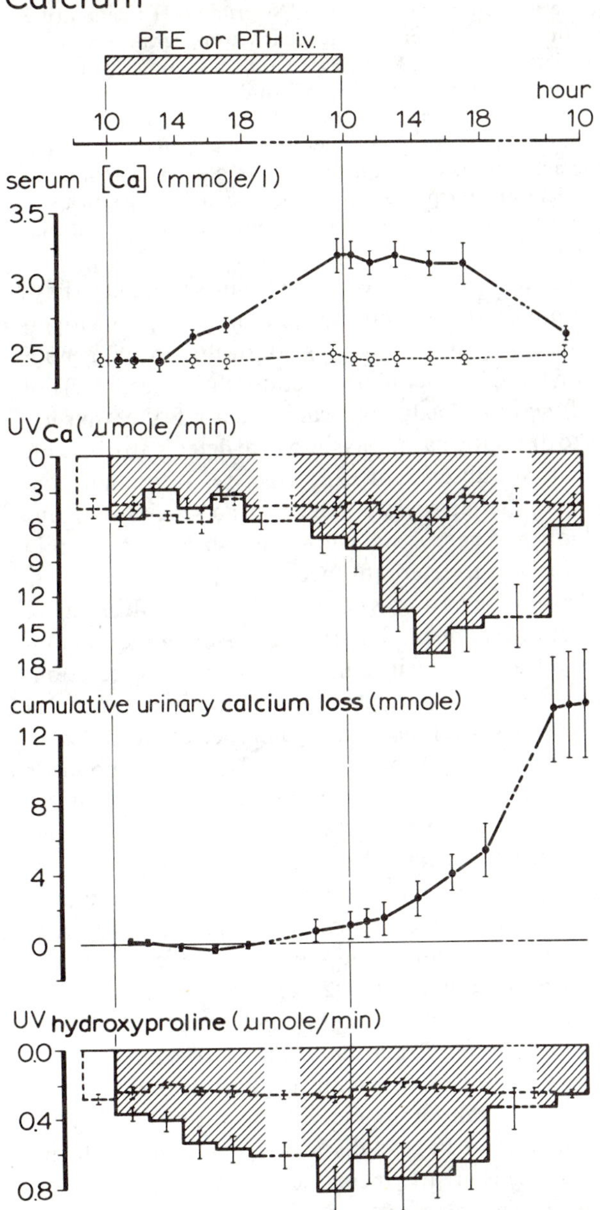

Fig. 12.2-3: *Effect of a 24-hr infusion of parathyroid hormone (PTE or PTH) in humans on serum calcium concentration, urinary calcium excretion rate, cumulative calcium loss (differences between control and experimental period), and hydroxyproline excretion.*

Dashed lines represent the data during the 24-hr preinfusion period; solid lines are the data during the infusion and postinfusion periods. The hormone was infused at the rate of 2 USP U/kg/hr. During the infusion period, there is essentially no calcium loss; the direct effect of parathyroid on enhancing tubular reabsorption of calcium is counterbalanced by the increased filtered load of calcium (increased serum calcium) resulting from the direct effect of the hormone on mobilization of calcium from bone. That bone is being mobilized is evidenced by the rise in urinary hydroxyproline during the infusion. Urinary calcium loss begins to occur only when the infusion is stopped; the increased filtered load is now unopposed by any direct action of the hormone on tubular reabsorption of calcium. (Reproduced from Ref. 14 by permission of the publisher).

control of calcium homeostasis involves three hormones (parathyroid hormone, calcitonin, and vitamin D) and three target organs (bone, gut, and kidney), it is not clear which of the possible hormone-target organ axes plays the major role in minute-to-minute, hour-to-hour, plasma calcium homeostasis. The parathyroid hormone-bone osteolysis and parathyroid hormone-kidney system are rapidly acting and therefore are probably of more importance in short-term homeostasis. The vitamin D-gut system, and the parathyroid hormone-bone osteoclastic actions, on the other hand, are slow to respond and may play a major role in long-term adaptation, particularly to calcium deprivation. Calcitonin is not considered to be of vital physiological importance in humans.

Therapeutic Uses. The therapeutic uses of parathyroid hormone are minimal; the vitamin D preparations are the agents of choice in the treatment of hypoparathyroidism. The official preparation, Parathyroid Injection, USP has been occasionally used diagnostically.

Adverse Reactions. Acute administration of parathyroid hormone causes hypercalcemia, muscular weakness, and cardiac dysfunction. Chronic administration induces in addition a condition resembling hyperparathyroidism; it is associated with excessive bone resorption (osteitis fibrosa) and metastatic calcification in the kidney (nephrocalcinosis and renal stones), stomach, bronchi, heart, and arteries.

Preparations. No official preparation of *Parathyroid Injection*, USP has been commercially available in the United States since 1980. Prior to that date the official preparation was a crude extract of the hormone prepared from bovine parathyroid glands and contained 100 USP U/ml. Synthetic bovine and human parathyroid hormone (1-34) fragments are available from several commercial sources but none is marketed for official clinical use.

Management of Parathyroid Dysfunction

Primary Hyperparathyroidism. Parathyroid adenoma is the most common (90%) form of primary hyperparathyroidism; the remaining cases are due to hyperplasia (8%) and to carcinoma (2%). The disease is characterized by hypercalcemia, normo- or hypophosphatemia, elevated urinary hydroxyproline and hypercalciuria, and elevated plasma parathyroid hormone levels. Renal metastatic calcification and stones are seen frequently; 5% of all cases (15% of recurrent cases) of renal stones have hyperparathyroidism. Bone disease (osteitis fibrosa) is seen in a significant number of patients. Primary hyperparathyroidism is seen with its greatest frequency in women between 40 and 50 years of age; its associated weakness, lassitude, anorexia, and mental symptoms can be confused with the menopause. Untreated acute hyperparathyroidism can lead rapidly to death. Surgical removal of the adenoma is the preferred and highly successful treatment.

Ectopic Hyperparathyroidism. Occasionally a nonparathyroid tumor, particularly lung and renal tumors, secretes a hypercalcemic agent, the nature of which is not always known with certainty. Prostaglandins and parathyroid hormone have been separately implicated. Removal or destruction of the tumor is the treatment of choice.

Secondary Hyperparathyroidism. Hyperplasia and hyperfunctioning of the parathyroid glands can result from either simple vitamin D deficiency secondary to gastrointestinal or renal disease. By far the most important is the secondary hyperparathyroidism associated with chronic renal failure. The enhanced secretion of parathyroid hormone, coupled with the disorder in vitamin D metabolism, leads to the development of a complicated bone disease referred to as renal osteodystrophy. Secondary hyperparathyroidism is treated according to the etiology.

Hypoparathyroidism. Hypoparathyroidism, whether it be idiopathic, iatrogenic (surgical), or pseudohypoparathyroidism (target cell subsensitivity) is characterized by hypocalcemia, hyperphosphatemia, decreased renal phosphate clearance, and neuromuscular symptoms, such as tetany and convulsions, which can eventually lead to asphyxia and death. Diagnosis can be assisted by eliciting latent tetany by tapping the facial nerves and producing a contraction of the facial muscles (Chvostek's sign), or application of a tourniquet leading to carpopedal spasm (Trousseau's sign). Treatment is to administer intravenous (in the case of an emergency) or dietary calcium, such as calcium gluconate, coupled with extremely large doses of vitamin D preparation such as ergocalciferol. The high doses of vitamin D would be extremely toxic in a normal subject. The plasma calcium level is monitored weekly to avoid toxic hypercalcemia resulting from hypervitaminosis D. Calcitriol, a commercial preparation of the hormone 1,25-dihydroxyvitamin D_3, may also be used to treat hypocalcemic states. The vitamin D analog, dihydrotachysterol, is occasionally used. Dihydrotachysterol and calcitriol have shorter half-lives than vitamin D; stopping the former medications allows a more rapid retreat from toxic hypercalcemia should it develop. Parathyroid hormone is never used as replacement therapy in hypoparathyroidism as it may lead to osteitis fibrosa.

CALCITONIN

The calcitonin-secreting cells (C cells) are located in the thyroid gland in humans and other mammals where they are also known as parafollicular cells. For this reason the hormone has been referred to also as thyrocalcitonin in the past. In submammalian species, such as birds, reptiles, amphibia, and fishes, the C cells are found mainly in the ultimobranchial gland; therefore the more general term, calcitonin, is preferred.

Chemistry. Calcitonin, in sharp contrast to the history of parathyroid hormone, was discovered, isolated, sequenced, and synthesized in a span of about 5 years (12). The calcitonins isolated from all species studied to date (human, salmon, bovine, ovine, porcine) are single-chain polypeptides with 32 amino acids with molecular weights around 3500 and a 1-7 intrachain disulphide bridge at the N-terminus. The similarities and differences between the calcitonins from the various species are depicted in Fig. 12.2-4. The structure of salmon calcitonin is much closer to that of human calcitonin. The complete structure of calcitonin is needed for biological activity; loss of the C-terminal amide group or either the C-terminal or N-terminal amino acid results in complete loss of biological activity. Salmon calcitonin, the preparation available for therapeutic use in the human, is many times more potent than mammalian calcitonins.

Pharmacological Effects. Calcitonin is thought to be of minor physiological importance in humans, except perhaps in emergency situations following an exogenous calcium load. Neither hypofunction (thyroidectomy) nor hyperfunction (medullary carcinoma of the thyroid) leads to dramatic pathophysiological defects attributable to calcitonin absence or excess per se. In humans and other mammalian species, calcitonin acts mainly on bone and kidney. There is no known action of calcitonin in submammalian vertebrate species.

Calcitonin secretion is controlled by a simple negative feedback mechanism. The rise of plasma ionic calcium causes release of calcitonin; a fall suppresses secretion. Other agents, including gastrin and glucagon, can act as secretagogues. In some mammalian species the ingestion of food can raise plasma calcitonin levels with no prior detectable rise in plasma calcium levels. Plasma gastrin levels, however, do rise in response to food ingestion and are assumed to mediate the release of calcitonin.

Bone. Calcitonin inhibits bone resorption, resulting in a rapid fall in plasma calcium and inorganic phosphate. The hypocalcemic and hypophosphatemic responses are rapid in onset and short (1-2 hr) in duration. The hormone can inhibit bone resorption independently of parathyroid hormone. Calcitonin is more effective in situations where bone has a high turnover rate, such as in young individuals or in individuals with pathological bone, such as in Paget's disease of bone, in which the turnover rate is greatly increased.

Kidney. The renal effects of calcitonin are species dependent. In humans there is a transient rise in urinary inorganic phosphate, calcium, magnesium, sodium, and chloride, a response which does not persist with repeated daily injections.

Pharmacokinetics. Calcitonin is ineffective by the oral route and must be administered parenterally (s.c. or i.m.). The plasma half-life depends on the type of calcitonin. Salmon calcitonin, the type used therapeutically, has a much longer half-life than human calcitonin, and this partially accounts for its greater potency and effectiveness.

Therapeutic Uses. Only one disease, Paget's disease of bone, has responded successfully to calcitonin therapy. Calcitonin is essentially nontoxic.

Paget's Disease of Bone. The major therapeutic use of calcitonin is in the treatment of Paget's disease of bone. This condition, which is characterized by a 10- to 20-fold

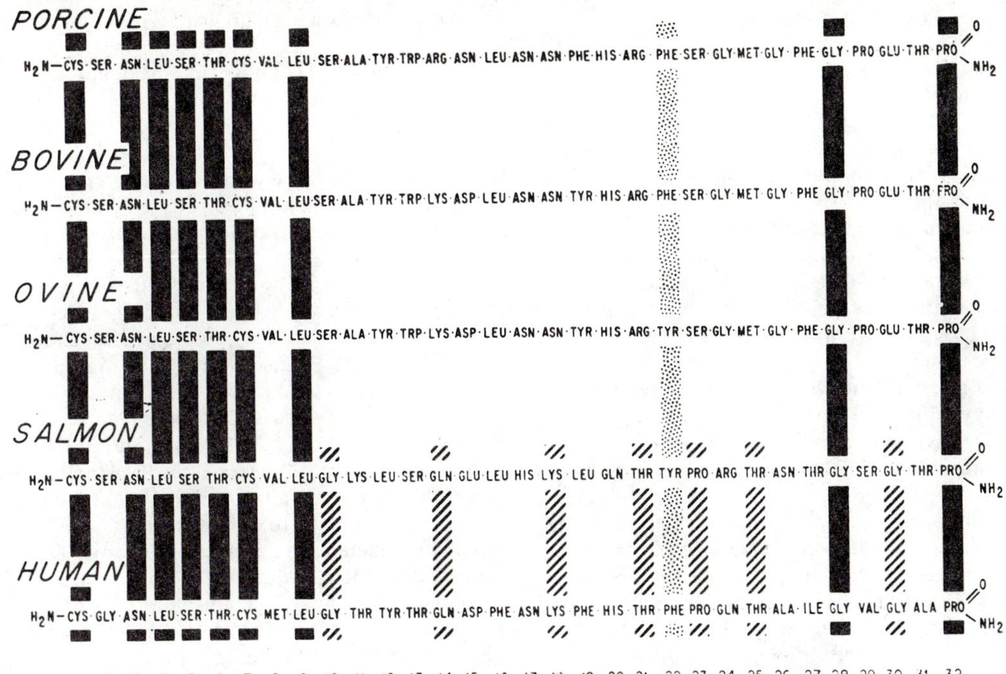

Fig. 12.2-4. *Comparison of amino acid sequences of porcine, bovine, ovine, salmon I, and human calcitonins.* Solid bars indicate sequence positions homologous among all five molecules; cross-hatched bars indicate salmon and human calcitonin similarities. [Reproduced from Potts, J.T., Jr., Niall, H.D., Keutmann, H.T., and Lequin, R.M. Chemistry of the calcitonins: Species variation plus structure-activity relations, and pharmacological implications. In: *Calcium, Parathyroid Hormone and the Calcitonins* (Talmage, R.V., and Munson, P.L., eds.). Amsterdam: Excerpta Medica, 1972, p. 121, by permission of the publishers].

increase in turnover rate in certain bones, is a logical therapeutic target for calcitonin. Clinical experience with salmon and human calcitonins is encouraging. In addition to an immediate subjective improvement, urinary calcium and hydroxyproline excretion fall rapidly and approach normal after several weeks of treatment (6). Plasma calcium and alkaline phosphatase levels fall more slowly. Bone pain is relieved and bone biopsies reveal a decrease in both resorption and formation rates; the latter results in a decrease in turnover rate. Effective treatment has been observed with doses of salmon calcitonin as low as 0.5 mg once a week.

Management of Calcitonin Dysfunction

Medullary Carcinoma of the Thyroid. The only known pathological condition associated with C-cell function is medullary carcinoma of the thyroid. Most patients are normocalcemic; chronic calcitonin hypersecretion in this condition leads to no overt calcium or bone pathology. Skeletal remodeling, both resorption and formation of bone, is markedly reduced, but there is no net increase in bone formation. Diagnosis is effected by determination of plasma calcitonin levels by radioimmunoassay; the levels can be 1000-fold above normal. Treatment consists in removal of the tumor by surgical or other means.

VITAMIN D

Very rapid developments in our understanding of vitamin D metabolism took place in the 3-year span 1968-1971. It was during this period that important contributions from the work of Kodicek, DeLuca, Norman, Haussler, and their associates led to our recognition of the renal-vitamin D endocrine system (9). The early reports indicated that vitamin D_3 was converted to a more polar metabolite that was identified as 25-hydroxyvitamin D_3 (3) and that the liver was the site of conversion (32). A second metabolite, subsequently known as 1,25-dihydroxyvitamin D_3, was detected in avian intestinal chromatin and was proposed as the active form of vitamin D_3 (10). This metabolite was subsequently shown to be formed exclusively in the kidney (7) and identified as 1,25-dihydroxyvitamin D_3 (13, 22). It is now accepted that vitamin D_3 and its liver metabolite, 25-hydroxyvitamin D_3, are physiologically inactive precursors or prohormones of 1,25-dihydroxyvitamin D_3, the active form of the vitamin. The latter is now designated as a hormone. Hence, vitamin D_3, or more specifically its active form, may be viewed as a hormone secreted by its endocrine gland, the kidney, and carried by the circulation to its target tissues, gut, bone, and kidney. It is largely within this endocrine framework that the pharmacology of vitamin D will be discussed.

Terminology. Vitamin D is a generic term, there being no specific compounds named vitamin D or vitamin D_1. The terminology of the vitamin Ds is relatively complex, compounded by a plethora of synonyms. There are two major series; those of animal origin (D_3 series) and those of plant origin (D_2 series). Within the animal series there are five major compounds: (a) the vitamin D_3 precursor or provitamin, 7-dehydrocholesterol; (b) vitamin D_3 itself; (c) the liver metabolite, 25-hydroxyvitamin D_3; (d) the active kidney metabolite, 1,25-dihydroxyvitamin D_3; and (e) the less active kidney metabolite, 24,25-dihydroxyvitamin D_3. Of these five compounds only one, 1,25-dihydroxyvitamin D_3, is considered to be the active hormonal form of vitamin D_3. The 24,25-dihydroxyvitamin D_3 metabolite is relatively inactive and the current concept is that 24-hydroxylation marks the beginning of the inactivation and excretion process. The terminology of vitamin D and related compounds is summarized in Table 12.2-5.

Chemistry. Vitamin D_3 and vitamin D_2 are secosteroids in which the steroid ring B has undergone fission. The structures of vitamin D_3, vitamin D_2, and related compounds are presented in Fig. 12.2-5. In the tachysterol series, represented by dihydrotachysterol$_3$, ring A is rotated 180° so that the hydroxyl group in position 3 occupies a location sterically equivalent to the 1-hydroxyl group of the active hormonal form, 1,25-dihydroxyvitamin D_3. This is important for understanding why these compounds are biologically active.

Renal-Vitamin D Endocrine System. The precursor, 7-dehydrocholesterol, is synthesized in the skin, and is converted to vitamin D_3 by a photochemical reaction catalyzed by ultraviolet light with a wavelength between 290 and 320 nm. Negro melanization and Oriental keratinization protect against excessive production of vitamin D_3 by excluding most ultraviolet light below 430 nm. Skin tan in Caucasians affords similar protection.

Vitamin D_3 is transported in the blood, bound to a specific protein, to the liver, where it undergoes conversion to 25-hydroxyvitamin D_3 on the hepatic smooth endoplasmic reticulum. The vitamin D_3-25-hydroxylase requires NADPH, molecular oxygen, and a cytoplasmic protein factor, but unlike the mixed function oxidases, does not require cytochrome P_{450}. Excess vitamin D_3 and 25-hydroxyvitamin D_3 are considered essentially inactive. However, if the level increases by 10-fold or more, 25-hydroxyvitamin D_3 begins to exhibit bone-mobilizing effects that can reach toxic proportions.

The liver metabolite, 25-hydroxyvitamin D_3, moves at physiologically inactive levels in the blood, bound to a specific protein, to the kidney where it undergoes conversion to either 1,25-dihydroxyvitamin D_3, 24,25-dihydroxyvitamin D_3, or possibly to a third metabolite, 25,26-dihydroxyvitamin D_3. There appears to be a reciprocal relationship between 1,25-dihydroxy-

Table 12.2-5
Vitamin D Terminology[a]

Form	Activity	Animal Series	Plant Series
Provitamin	Inactive[b]	7-Dehydrocholesterol (provitamin D_3)	Ergosterol (provitamin D_2)
Vitamin	Inactive[b]	Vitamin D_3 (cholecalciferol, USP; activated 7-dehydrocholesterol; calciol[e])	Vitamin D_2 (ergocalciferol, USP; CALCIFEROL; ercalciol[e])
Liver metabolite	Inactive[c]	25-Hydroxyvitamin D_3 [25-hydroxycholecalciferol; 25-(OH)D_3; calcifediol (CALDEROL); calcidiol[e]]	25-Hydroxyvitamin D_2 [25-hydroxyergocalciferol; 25-(OH)D_2]
Kidney metabolites	Very active	1,25-Dihydroxyvitamin D_3 [1,25-dihydroxycholecalciferol; 1,25-$(OH)_2D_3$; calcitriol[e] (ROCALTROL)]	1,25-Dihydroxyvitamin D_2 [1,25-dihydroxyergocalciferol; 1,25-$(OH)_2D_2$; ercalcitriol[e]]
	Less Active	24,25-Dihydroxyvitamin D_3; [24,25-dihydroxycholecalciferol; 24,25-$(OH)_2D_3$]	24,25-Dihydroxyvitamin D_2 [24,25-dihydroxyergocalciferol; 24,25-$(OH)_2D_2$]
Synthetic analogs			
	Inactive[d]	1α-Hydroxyvitamin D_3 [1α-(OH)D_3]	
	Inactive[d]	Dihydrotachysterol$_3$ (DHT$_3$; dihydroercalciol[e])	Dihydrotachysterol$_2$ (DHT$_2$; dihydrotachysterol, USP; HYTAKEROL)

[a] Synonyms or abbreviated forms are in parentheses.
[b] Physiologically inactive as such; must be converted eventually to the hormonal form for physiological or pharmacological activity.
[c] As with (b) but, in addition, 25-(OH)D_3 is active itself at pharmacological levels (50- to 100-fold normal).
[d] Pharmacologically inactive as such; requires 25-hydroxylation in the liver to render it active.
[e] Recommended trivial name by IUPAC-IUB Joint Commission on Biochemical Nomenclature (*Eur. J. Biochem.* 124: 223, 1982).

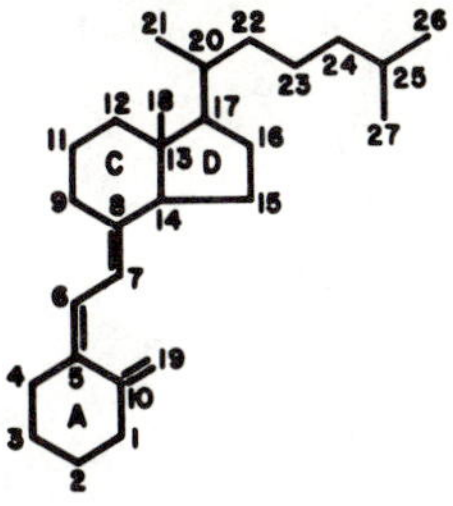

Secosteroid Numbering System

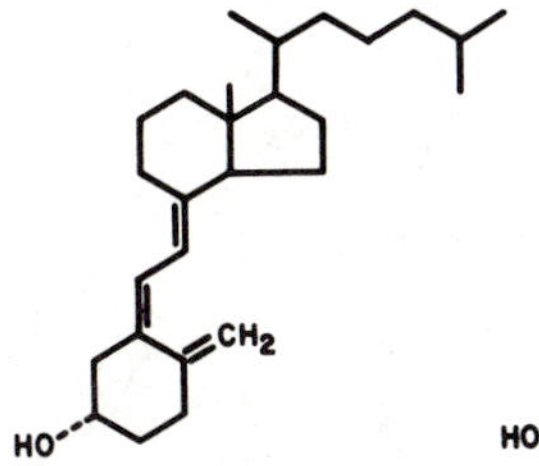

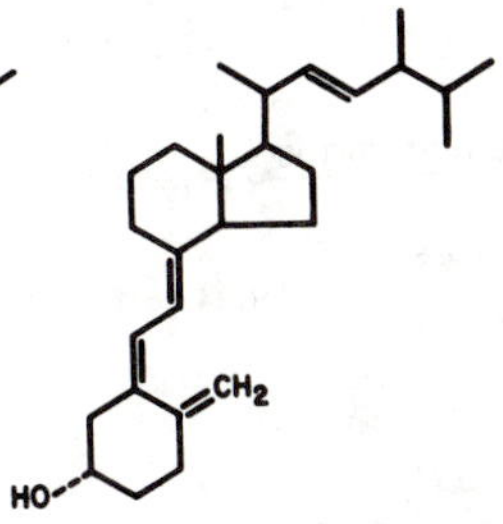

cholecalciferol vitamin D_3 Ergocalciferol vitamin D_2

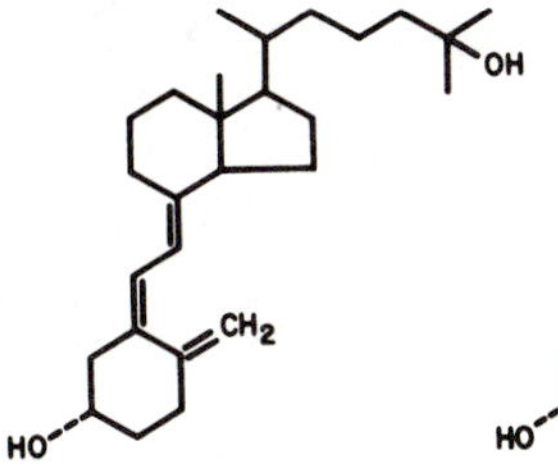

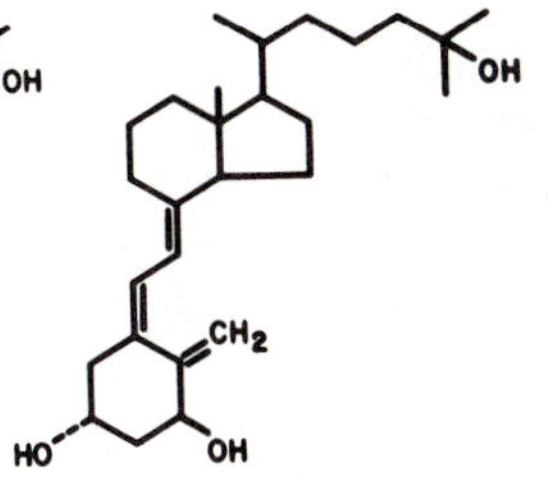

25-Hydroxyvitamin D_3 1,25-dihydroxyvitamin D_3

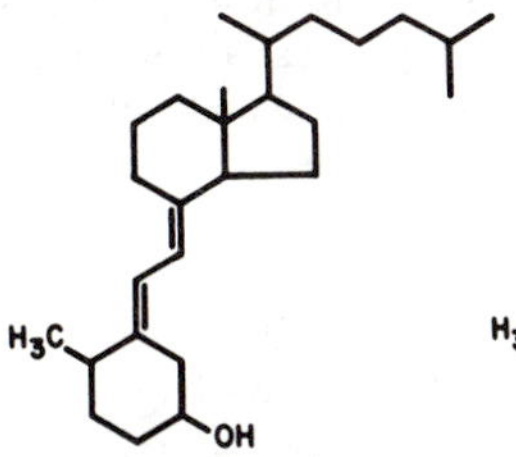

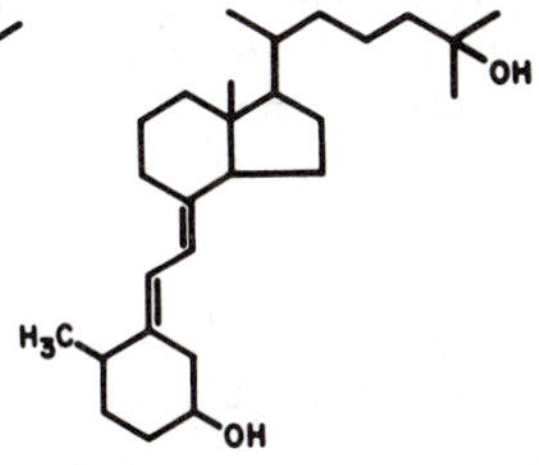

Dihydrotachysterol$_3$ 25-Hydroxydihydrotachysterol$_3$

Fig. 12.2-5. *Chemical structures of vitamin d and related compound.*

vitamin D_3 and 24,25-dihydroxyvitamin D_3. When the hormonal form is being actively synthesized and secreted, the production of the less active metabolite, 24,25-dihydroxyvitamin D_3, is essetially shut down. Conversely, when production of the hormone is suppressed then synthesis of the less active metabolite is increased (1, 16).

The two renal enzymes, 25-hydroxyvitamin D_3-1-hydroxylase and the 25-hydroxyvitamin D_3-24-hydroxylase, are located in the mitochondrion. The 1-hydroxylase, which has been studied more extensively, requires NADPH, molecular oxygen, and cytochrome P_{450}, and therefore resembles the hepatic mixed-function oxidases except for subcellular location. Secretion of 1,25-dihydroxyvitamin D_3 by the kidney probably occurs by passive diffusion. Once secreted, 1,25-dihydroxyvitamin D_3 is transported by the plasma, presumably bound to a protein, to its target tissues, gut, bone, and possibly kidney. In the context of the above scheme, it is understandable why the peak responses to injection of 1,25-dihydroxyvitamin D_3, 25-hydroxyvitamin D_3, and vitamin D_3 appear at increasingly larger intervals after administration. The components of the renal-vitamin D endocrine system are depicted in Fig. 12.2-6. The third renal metabolite, 25,26-dihydroxyvitamin D_3, which has been identified under certain circumstances in avian species, is inactive and, like 24,25-dihydroxyvitamin D_3, is considered to be a component of the process of elimination of vitamin D_3.

Control of the Renal-Vitamin D Endocrine System. When discussing the actions of either vitamin D_3 or vitamin D_2, it is assumed that the effects are mediated by the active metabolite of the vitamin unless specified otherwise. In this context, vitamin D has two major target tissues, gut and bone, with the kidney being of lesser importance. Physiologically, vitamin D maintains adequate extracellular fluid levels of calcium and phosphate so that normal mineralization and remodelding of bone can occur. It does this in two ways. First, it has a direct action on calcium and phosphate transport by the intestine. Second, its permissive action on bone allows parathyroid hormone to exert its normal homeostatic, that is osteolytic, effect on bone and maintain the proper ratio of plasma calcium and phosphate. In the face of hypocalcemia both parathyroid hormone and 1,25-dihydroxyvitamin D are secreted and mobilize calcium and phosphate from both bone and gut sources. In the presence of higher than normal parathyroid hormone levels the phosphate is rapidly excreted by the kidney as a result of the direct action of parathyroid hormone on inhibiting renal tubular reabsorption of phosphate. The net response is to restore only the deficiency in plasma calcium. On the other hand, in the face of hypophosphatemia only, 1,25-dihydroxyvitamin D is secreted. This hormone mobilizes both calcium and phosphate from the gut and permits the mobilization of these ions from bone. The rise in plasma calcium suppresses parathyroid hormone secretion and thereby causesd calcium excretion and phosphate retention by the kidney. The net result is that the excess calcium is excreted and phosphate is retained; the hypophosphatemia is restored to normal without disturbing the plasma calcium levels.

Pharmacological Effects

Gut. The action of vitamin D on the gut is to stimulate the intestinal transport of both calcium and phosphate. The active form, 1,25-dihydroxyvitamin D_3, is 10-100 times more potent than 25-hydroxyvitamin D_3 in stimulating transport of calcium. Parathyroid hormone is not required for the action of 1,25-dihydroxyvitamin D_3 on the gut. The mechanism by which 1,25-dihydroxyvitamin D_3 stimulates calcium absorption is not known with certainty. The hormone is thought to act by stimulating gene expression through its cytosolic receptor, resulting in the synthesis of specific proteins, which mediate and enhance transport of calcium from mucosal to serosal site. Calcium-binding protein is one of the specific proteins so synthesized. Glucocorticoids, such as cortisol, oppose vitamin D's action on the gut.

Bone. Vitamin D is required for the physiological actions of parathyroid hormone on bone. This permissive role of vitamin D allows parathyroid hormone to perform its normal homeostatic function through osteocytic osteolysis and its normal remodeling functions through osteoclastic and osteoblastic activity. The liver metabo-

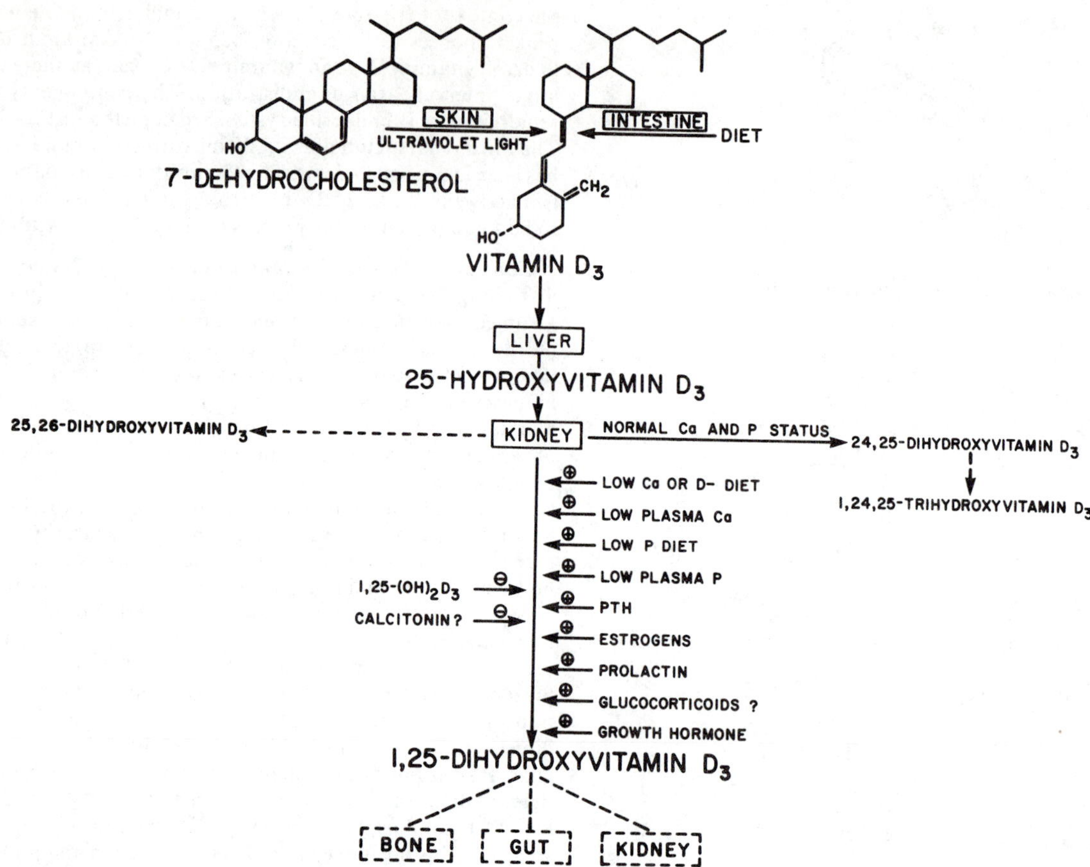

Fig. 12.2-6. *The renal-vitamin D_3 endocrine system.*
The renal metabolite, 1,25-dihydroxyvitamin D_3 [1,25-$(OH)_2D_3$], is the hormonal form of vitamin D_3, and the regulation of its production and secretion is the control point in vitamin D_3 metabolism. The following agents or conditions have been suggested as having physiological or pharmacological regulatory influences on this control point: parathyroid hormone (PTH); calcitonin (CT); estradiol; cortisol; prolactin; growth hormone; plasma calcium and phosphate; low calcium, phosphate, or vitamin D diets; and the hormone 1,25-$(OH)_2D_3$, itself. The proposed negative (-) and positive (+) influences are indicated by appropriate signs.

lite, 25-hydroxyvitamin D_3, is 50-100 times less potent, and therefore is of little physiological importance in this regard. Nevertheless, at pharmacological levels encountered in vitamin D_3 overdoses, this bone action of 25-hydroxyvitamin D_3 is of considerable therapeutic and toxicological significance. The renal hormone 1,25-dihydroxyvitamin D_3, can cause bone resorption in the absence of parathyroid hormone but only at pharmacological doses, that is 30- to 100-fold normal. This action, together with that of 25-hydroxyvitamin D_3, is the basis for vitamin D therapy in hypoparathyroidism. In the absence of vitamin D, parathyroid hormone can elicit certain initial biochemical responses in bone cells, such as an increase in cAMP levels and calcium uptake, but cannot effect the final morphological changes seen in bone cell pool sizes.

Kidney. Vitamin D increases calcium and phosphate reabsorption by the proximal renal tubule.

Pharmacokinetics. All three therapeutic forms of vitamin D, that is vitamin D_2, vitamin D_3, and 1,25-dihydroxyvitamin D_3, are adequately absorbed by the oral route and, in view of their slow onset of action, need not be given parenterally. Once absorbed, the drugs are handled pharmacokinetically as described above. Circulating levels of 1,25-dihydroxyvitamin D are a mixture of active derivatives of the vitamin D_2 and vitamin D_3 forms. The ratio depends upon the relative contributions of the former from dietary sources and of the vitamin D_3 from both endogenous (skin) and exogenous (dietary) sources. Whereas most assays measure the total of the two forms, some assays can discriminate. Under most circumstances discrimination is not necessary as both forms are considered equipotent biologically. Plasma 1,25-dihydroxyvitamin D levels, when determined by a nondiscriminating assay, should be expressed without the D_2 or D_3 subscript.

Vitamin D and Related Preparations

Ergocalciferol and Cholecalciferol. Ergocalciferol (vitamin D_2) and cholecalciferol (vitamin D_3) are by far the most common and least expensive of the vitamin D preparations. They are readily absorbed by the oral route and exhibit similar pharmacokinetic behavior in the liver and kidney. The half-life of cholecalciferol is measured in days (4.5 days) (24).

Calcitriol. Calcitriol (ROCALTROL), an oral preparation of 1,25-dihydroxyvitamin D_3, is now available for the treatment of hypocalcemic states, particularly those associated with chronic renal failure (25). It has a shorter half-life (measured in hours) than its prohormone, vitamin D_3, and for this reason is considered safer; overdosage hypercalcemia returns to normal more quickly. Initially, the plasma calcium level should be monitored twice weekly. Calcitriol does not depend upon functional kidney tissue for its activation; it is already in its active form.

Calcidiol. Calcidiol (calcifediol, CALDEROL) is an orally effective preparation of 25-hydroxyvitamin D_3 for the treatment of hypocalcemic states and certain metabolic bone diseases including chronic renal failure. At pharmacological levels, calcidiol directly increases gut calcium absorption and bone resorption but its metabolites, particularly 1,25-dihydroxyvitamin D_3, also account for a major part of the drug's action. Its half-life is measured in days (31 days), an elimination rate which is markedly decreased in vitamin D deficiency states (24).

1α-Hydroxyvitamin D_3. 1α-Hydroxyvitamin D_3 is a synthetic analog which acts in vivo on both gut and bone and is effective orally as replacement therapy in the treatment of renal osteodystrophy (4) by bypassing the metabolic block in the kidney. It is assumed that 1α-hydroxyvitamin D_3 is converted by the normally functioning liver to the active hormonal form, 1,25-dihydroxyvitamin D_3. Its pharmacodynamic effectiveness does not depend upon functional kidney tissue for its activation. Its clinical use is still in the experimental stage.

Dihydrotachysterol₂. Dihydrotachysterol$_2$ is a vitamin D analog sometimes called AT-10 (antitetanic preparation number 10). Dihydrotachysterol$_2$ is administered orally and is shorter-acting and therefore safer than vitamin D. It has been available for decades, but it is expensive and its pharmacodynamic actions are erratic and less predictable. Activation of dihydrotachysterol$_2$ requires only 25-hydroxylation by the liver; it does not depend upon functional kidney tissue for its activation.

Doses of Vitamin D Preparations. The types of preparations, doses, and therapeutic indications are summarized in Table 12.2-6.

Adverse Effects. Vitamin D intoxication, referred to as hypervitaminosis D, may be caused by extremely high doses (100,000 U/day or more) in normal adults. In infants, hypervitaminosis D may be induced with much lower doses (under 5000 U/day).

Management of Vitamin D Dysfunction

Vitamin D Deficiency: Rickets and Osteomalacia. Rickets and osteomalacia are vitamin D deficiency diseases found in children and adults, respectively, and exhibit a defect in the normal mineralization of bone and disturbances in calcium and phosphate metabolism. Hypovitaminosis D or vitamin D deficiency is characterized by hypocalcemia, hypophosphatemia, increased plasma alkaline phosphatase, hypersecretion of parathyroid hormone, phosphaturia, subsensitivitiy of bone to the osteolytic and remodeling actions of parathyroid hormone, and uncalcified osteoid in bone leading to bending and pseudofractures of the long bones. Many other factors, either singly or in conjunction, can lead to rickets or osteomalacia. These include malabsorption syndromes (impaired vitamin D absorption), inadequate sunlight, imbalance in calcium/phosphate ratio in the

Table 12.2-6
Vitamin D and Related Drugs: Therapeutic Indications and Doses[a]

Therapeutic Indications	Preparation	Recommended Dose (USP Units/day)
Prophylaxis	Ergocalciferol	400
Rickets: Deficiency	Ergocalciferol	1000-4000
Osteomalacia: Deficiency	Ergocalciferol	1000-4000
Malabsorption	Ergocalciferol	40,000-400,000
Vitamin D-resistant rickets (hypophosphatemic rickets)	Ergocalciferol[b]	40,000-160,000
Vitamin D-dependent rickets (1-hydroxylase rickets)	Ergocalciferol	3000-80,000
Anticonvulsant rickets (prophylaxis)	Ergocalciferol	4000-40,000
Renal osteodystrophy (chronic renal failure)	Ergocalciferol[c]	40,000-80,000
	Calcitriol[c]	0.25 μg/day
Distal renal tubular acidosis	Ergocalciferol	40,000-500,000
Hypoparathyroidism	Ergocalciferol[c]	25,000-100,000
	Calcitriol[c]	0.25 μg/day
	Dihydrotachysterol[c]	0.1-5 mg/day

[a]The plasma calcium should be monitored regularly to avoid hypervitaminosis D toxicity; use of calcitriol and dihydrotachysterol requires more frequent monitoring than for ergocalciferol because of their pharmacokinetic differences.
[b]Combined with oral phosphate therapy.
[c]Combined with other therapeutic measures including high-calcium diet, and phosphate-binding oral preparations, and in the case of chronic renal failure, hemodialysis.

diet, dietary factors which render calcium or phosphate unavailable for absorption, and drug interactions resulting in impaired vitamin D absorption or metabolism.

Treatment consists of administering moderate doses (1000 U/day) of vitamin D, usually in the form of ergocalciferol, together with adequate dietary calcium and phosphate. The plasma calcium and phosphate level should be monitored regularly for therapeutic control and to avoid overdosage. Initially the plasma calcium and phosphate may fall to the point of tetany due to immediate mineralization of the hungry osteoid. This is followed by a steady gradual rise in plasma calcium and phosphate levels and a return to normal in these parameters over a period of 6-12 weeks at which time the dose is reduced to prophylactic levels (400 U/day).

Iatrogenic Rickets and Osteomalacia. Long-term anticonvulsant therapy with either phenobarbital or phenytoin has led to a higher incidence of rickets and osteomalacia in epileptic patients. This has been attributed to induction of hepatic microsomal enzymes leading to an accelerated hepatic metabolism of vitamin D_3 to inactive metabolites and away from the normal pathway leading eventually to 1,25-dihydroxyvitamin D_3. Plasma 25-hydroxyvitamin D levels are lower, but paradoxically, 1,25-dihydroxyvitamin D levels tend to be normal or elevated (9). The precise etiology of the vitamin D deficiency syndrome is unclear.

Treatment consists of prophylactic administration of moderate (1000 U/day) to high (10,000 U/day) doses of vitamin D to all patients on long-term anticonvulsant therapy. All epileptic patients should be examined for hypoparathyroidism, as the combination of diseases constitues an extremely complicated therapeutic situation. Anticonvulsant therapy would only aggravate the hypocalcemic condition and associated convulsive tendencies linked to the hypoparathyroidism.

Renal Osteodystrophy. Chronic renal failure can lead to a relative deficiency in 1,25-dihydroxyvitamin D production by the kidney, which results in hypovitaminosis D, hypocalcemia, and secondary hyperparathyroidism. The associated bone disease is complex, exhibiting a spectrum of pathology ranging from osteitis fibrosa (secondary hyperparathyroidism) to rickets or osteomalacia (hypovitaminosis D). Treatment with vitamin D is not uniformly successful due to the presumed relative block in the renal conversion of 25-hydroxyvitamin D to 1,25-dihydroxyvitamin D. The disease responds to dihydrotachysterol$_2$, 1,25-dihydroxyvitamin D_3 (calcitriol), or to 1α-hydroxyvitamin D_3. Gut calcium absorption and urinary and plasma calcium levels rise and plasma alkaline phosphatase, phosphate, and immunoreactive parathyroid hormone levels fall. Other treatment consists in controlling plasma calcium and phosphate levels during an initial period of dialysis and in decreasing the parathyroid hormone levels which can be extremely high. Calcitriol (ROCALTROL) will probably become the drug of choice.

Vitamin D-Resistant Rickets (Hypophosphatemic Rickets). Vitamin D-resistant rickets is a familial disorder believed to be an X-linked recessive trait. The cause of the disease is unknown, but it is likely that the primary defect is a renal lesion characterized by impaired tubular reabsorption of phosphate. For this reason this disorder is sometimes called *phosphate diabetes*. Urinary phosphate is increased and plasma phosphate is decreased. Plasma parathyroid hormone, calcium, and 25-hydroxyvitamin D_3 levels are usually normal. Treatment consists of administering extremely high doses (100,000 U/day) of vitamin D, with or without neutral phosphate, aimed at restoring the plasma phosphate levels to normal or near normal.

Vitamin D-Dependent Rickets. Children with vitamin D-dependent rickets do not respond to the usual moderate doses used to treat vitamin D-deficiency rickets, but require 3-10 more times these doses to effect complete healing. The disease appears to be a genetic defect in the activity of the renal 1-hydroxylase enzyme, causing a relative block of the conversion of 25-hydroxyvitamin D_3 to 1,25-dihydroxyvitamin D_3.

Hypervitaminosis D. Vitamin D overdosage is a serious toxicity that may be caused by extremely high doses of the drug. However, much smaller doses can cause serious toxicity in infants. The condition is associated with hypercalcemia, hyperphosphatemia, anorexia, irritability, weight loss, fatigue, and irreversible metastatic calcification and nephrocalcinosis. It is treated by removing the sources of vitamin D, administering fluids to combat renal toxicity, placing the patient on a low-calcium diet, and administering glucocorticoids such as cortisol to lower the plasma calcium level.

REFERENCES

1. Baksi, S.N. and Kenny, A.D. Vitamin D_3 metabolism in immature Japanese quail: effects of ovarian hormones. *Endocrinology*, 101:1216, 1977.
2. Berson, S.A., Yalow, R.S., Aurbach, G.D. and Potts, J.T., Jr. Immunoassay of bovine and human parathyroid hormone. *Proc. Natl. Acad. Sci. USA*, 49:613, 1963.
3. Blunt, J.W., DeLuca, H.F., and Schnoes, H.K.: 25-Hydroxycholecalciferol. A biologically active metabolite of vitamin D_3. *Biochemistry*, 7:3317, 1968.
4. Chan, J.C.M., Oldham, S.B., Holick, M.F. and DeLuca, H.F. 1-α-Hydroxyvitamin D_3 in chronic renal failure. *J. Am. Med. Assoc.*, 234:47, 1975.
5. Cushard, W.G., Jr., Creditor, M.A., Canterbury, J.M. and Reiss, E. Physiological hyperparathyroidism in pregnancy. *J. Clin. Endocrinol. Metab.* , 34:767, 1972.
6. DeRose, J., Singer, F.R., Avramides, A., Flores, A., Dziadiw, R., Baker, R.K. and Wallach, S. Response of Paget's disease to porcine and salmon calcitonins. *Am. J. Med.*, 6:860, 1974.
7. Fraser, D.R. and Kodicek, E. Unique biosynthesis by kidney of a biologically active vitamin D metabolite. *Nature* (London), 228:764, 1970.

8. Habener, J.F. and Potts, J.T., Jr. Biosynthesis of parathyroid hormone. *N. Engl. J. Med.*, 299:580, 635, 1978.
9. Haussler, M.R. Vitamin D: metabolism, drug interactions and therapeutic applications in humans. In: *Nutrition and Drug inteactions*. Academic Press, New York, 1978, p. 717-705.
10. Haussler, M.R., Myrtle, J.F. and Norman, A.W. The association of a metabolite of vitamin D_3 with intestinal mucosa chromatin *in vivo. J. Biol. Chem.*, 243:4055, 1968.
11. Hegsted, D.M., Moscoso, I. and Collazos, C. A study of the minimum calcium requirements of adult men. *J. Nutr.* , 46:181, 1952.
12. Hirsch, P.F. and Munson, P.L. Thyrocalcitonin. *Physiol. Rev.*, 49:548, 1969.
13. Holick, M.F., Schnoes, H.K., DeLuca, H.F., Suda, T. and Cousins, R.J. Isolation and identification of 1,25-dihydroxycholecalciferol. A metabolite of vitamin D active in intestine. *Biochemistry*, 10:2799, 1971.
14. Froeling, P.G.A.M. and Bijvoet, O.L.M. Kidney-mediated effects of parathyroid hormone on extracellular homeostasis of calcium, phosphate and acid-base balance in man. *Neth. J. Med.*, 17:174, 1974.
15. Kenny, A.D. Parathyroid glands and calcium metabolism. *World Rev. Nutr. Dietet.*, 2:157, 1960.
16. Kenny, A.D. Vitamin D metabolism: physiological regulation in egg-laying Japanese quail. *Am. J. Physiol.*, 230:1609, 1976.
17. Kenny, A.D. Intestinal Calcium Absorption and Its Regulation. CRC Press, Boca Raton, Fla., 1981, pp. 1-176.
18. Kenny, A.D. and Pang, P.K.T. Response of the renal vitamin D endocrine system to oxidized parathyroid hormone (1-34). *Proc. Soc. Exp. Biol. Med.*, 171:191, 1982.
19. Kenny, A.D. and Dacke, C.G. Parathyroid hormone and calcium metabolism. *World Rev. Nutr. Dietet.*, 20:231, 1975.
20. Kirk, G.R., Breazile, J.E. and Kenny, A.D. Pathogenesis of hypocalcemic tetany in the thyroparathyroidectomized dog. *Am. J. Vet. Res.*, 35:407, 1974.
21. Kumar, R., Cohen, W.R., Silva, P. and Epstein, F.H. Elevated 1,25-dihydroxyvitamin D plasma levels in normal human pregnancy and lactation. *J. Clin. Invest.* 63:342, 1979.
22. Lawson, D.E.M., Fraser, D.R., Kodicek, E., Morris, H.R. and Williams, D.H. Identification of 1,25-dihydroxycholecalciferol, a new kidney hormone controlling calcium metabolism. *Nature* (London), 230:228, 1971.
23. Malm, O.J. Calcium requirement and adaptation in adult men. *Scand. J. Clin. Lab. Invest.* (Suppl. 36), 10:, 1958.
24. Mawer, F.B., Lumb, G.A., Schaeffer, K. and Stanbury, S.W. The metabolites of isotopically labelled vitamin D in man: The influence of the state of vitamin D nutrition. *Clin. Sci.*, 40:39, 1971.
25. Maxwell, D.R., Benjamin, D.M., Donahay, S.L., Allen, M.K., Hamburger, R.J. and Luft, F.C. Calcitriol in dialysis patients. *Clin. Pharmacol. Ther.*, 23:515, 1978.
26. McLean, F.C. and Hastings, A.B. A biological method for the estimation of calcium ion concentration. *J. Biol. Chem.* , 107:337, 1934.
27. McLean, F.C. and Hastings, A.B. Clinical estimation and significance of calcium-ion concentration in the blood. *Am. J. Med. Sci.*, 189:601, 1935.
28. Moore, E.W. Ionized calcium in normal serum, ultrafiltrates, and whole blood determined by ion-exchange electrodes. *J. Clin. Invest.*, 49:318, 1970.
29. Munson, P.L. Biological assay of parathyroid hormone. In: *The Parathyroids* (Greep, R.O. and Talmage, R.V., eds.). Charles C Thomas, Springfield, Ill., 1961, p. 94-113.
30. Newmark, S.R. and Himathongkam, J. Hypercalcemic and hypocalcemic crises. *JAMA*. 230:1438, 1974.
31. Pang, P.K.T., Yang, M.C.M., Keutmann, H.T. and Kenny, A.D. Structure activity relationship of parathyroid hormone: Separation of the hypotensive and hypercalcemic properties. *Endocrinology*, 112:284, 1983.
32. Ponchon, G., Kennan, A.L. and DeLuca, H.F. "Activation" of vitamin D_3 by the liver. *J. Clin. Invest.*, 48:2032, 1969.
33. Radde, I.C., Höffken, B., Parkinson, D.K., Sheepers, J. and Luckham, A. Practical aspects of a measurement technique for calcium ion activity in plasma. *Clin. Chem.*, 17:1002, 1971.
34. Reddy, G.S., Norman, A.W., Willis, D.M., Goltzman, D., Guyda, H., Solomon, S., Philips, D.R., Bishop, J.E. and Mayer, E. Regulation of vitamin D metabolism in normal human pregnancy. *J. Clin. Endocrinol. Metab.* , 56:363, 1983.
35. Reiss, E. and Canterbury, J.M. Emerging concepts of the nature of circulating parathyroid hormones: Implications for clinical research. *Rec. Prog. Hormone. Res.*, 30:391, 1974.
36. Rodan, G.A. and Martin, T.J. Role of osteoblasts in hormonal control of bone resorption: A hypothesis. *Calcif. Tiss. Int.*, 33:349, 1981.
37. Walker, A.R.P. Calcium balance in pregnancy. *Lancet*, 1:107, 1975.
38. Walker, A.R.P., Richardson, B. and Walker, F. The influence of numerous pregnancies and lactations on the bone dimensions in South African Bantu and Caucasian mothers. *Clin. Sci.*, 42:189, 1972.
39. World Health Organization Technical Report Series No.230: Calcium requirements, World Health Organization, Geneva, 1962.

ADDITIONAL READINGS

AMA Drug Evaluations. In: *Agents Affecting Calcium Metabolism*, 5th ed., American Medical Association, Chicago, 1983, p. 1195.

Aurbach, G.D. (ed.). Handbook of Physiology, Section 7, Endocrinology, Vol. VII, Parathyroid Gland. *Am. Physiol. Soc., Washington, D.C., 1976.*

Fraser, D.R. Regulation of the metabolism of vitamin D. Physiol. Rev. 60:551, 1980.

Kanis, J.A. Vitamin D metabolism and its clinical application. *J. Bone Joint Surg.*, 64-B:542, 1982.

CHAPTER
12.3

INSULIN, ORAL HYPOGLYCEMIC DRUGS AND GLUCAGON

Zulfiquar Merali

INSULIN

History. In the late 1800s, von Mering and Minkowski (75) demonstrated that pancreatectomy in dogs evoked a syndrome similar to diabetes mellitus in humans, implicating the lack of a pancreatic factor in the etiology of diabetes mellitus. Using 10 dogs, borrowed lab space, and no research funding, two Canadian researchers succeeded in extracting an active factor from the pancreas that, when injected into severly diabetic dogs, reduced the highly elevated blood glucose concentrations to almost normal levels. In 1922, Banting and Best demonstrated the therapeutic value of this pancreatic extract, insulin, in a young human diabetic patient with severe hyperglycemia (500 mg/dl) and polyurea (3-5 l urine/day), where an immediate improvement in the concentration and excretion of blood glucose was evident (4). Since then, although important insights into the nature of diabetes and its treatment with insulin have accrued, a universal method that produces continuous euglycemia for all patients has proven elusive. However, skillful use of insulin regimens is still vital to the treatment of all insulin-requiring patients.

Chemistry and Source. Insulin is a small protein with a molecular weight of about 6000. Human insulin consists of 51 amino acids arranged in two chains, A (acidic) and B (basic), cross-bridged by two disulfide bonds (Fig. 12.3-1). The sequence of amino acids and the arrangement of disulfide bridges were determined by Sanger and associates (68). Insulin is synthesized by the β cells of the islets of Langerhans. The source of therapeutically used insulin has been the pancreas of animals, most often that of cattle, pigs, or fish.

Specific activities of various mammalian insulins are similar, although species variations in amino acid sequence do exist and may be of clinical significance in the development of allergic reactions to commercial insulin preparations. The major sites of chemical difference between porcine, ovine, equine, and cetacean insulins are in positions 8, 9 and 10 of the A-chain. The porcine hormone is quite similar to that of humans as it differs only by the substitution of an alanine residue at the carboxy terminus of the B-chain (70).

Bovine insulin is intrinsically more antigenic to humans than porcine insulin because it differs from human insulin with respect to three amino acids, whereas porcine differs by only one. Some bovine insulins have been reported to contain substantial amounts of pancreatic glucagon, pancreatic polypeptide, vasoactive intestinal peptide (VIP), and somatostatin (23). In addition to these impurities, proinsulin and intermediates such as C-peptide may comprise as much as 5% of commercial insulin preparations. Chromatographic purification has led to production of two highly purified insulins: (a) single-peak insulin which is over 99% pure insulin plus desamids and arginine insulins, and (b) single-component or monocomponent insulin which is over 99% pure insulin (free of proinsulin and peptides with molecular weights over 10,000). The monocomponent insulins are less immunogenic in humans. There are some reports to indicate that the monocomponent insulins allow the insulin dosages to be lower and that they are helpful in avoiding insulin allergy and lipodystrophy or lipoatrophy (78). Although human insulin molecules can be synthesized chemically, the process is complex and expensive. Using porcine insulin as the starting material, however, human insulin can now be synthesized with relatively more ease (67). However, in an attempt to obtain a source of pure, less immunogenic, and readily available material not dependent upon the availability of cattle or pigs, research efforts have been directed toward microbial production of human insulin. Expression in *Escherichia coli* of chemically synthesized genes for human insulin has recently been achieved (13, 27), a technique that represents a good tool for production of future human insulin needs. Recent studies indicate that human insulin has reduced immunogenicity and that about half of the patients with severe allergy or resistance to commercial insulin preparations improve with human insulin. Thus, human insulin may have important immunological advantages over the animal insulins (23). However, more experience is required to determine the clinical significance of these findings in the usual insulin-taking patient (23).

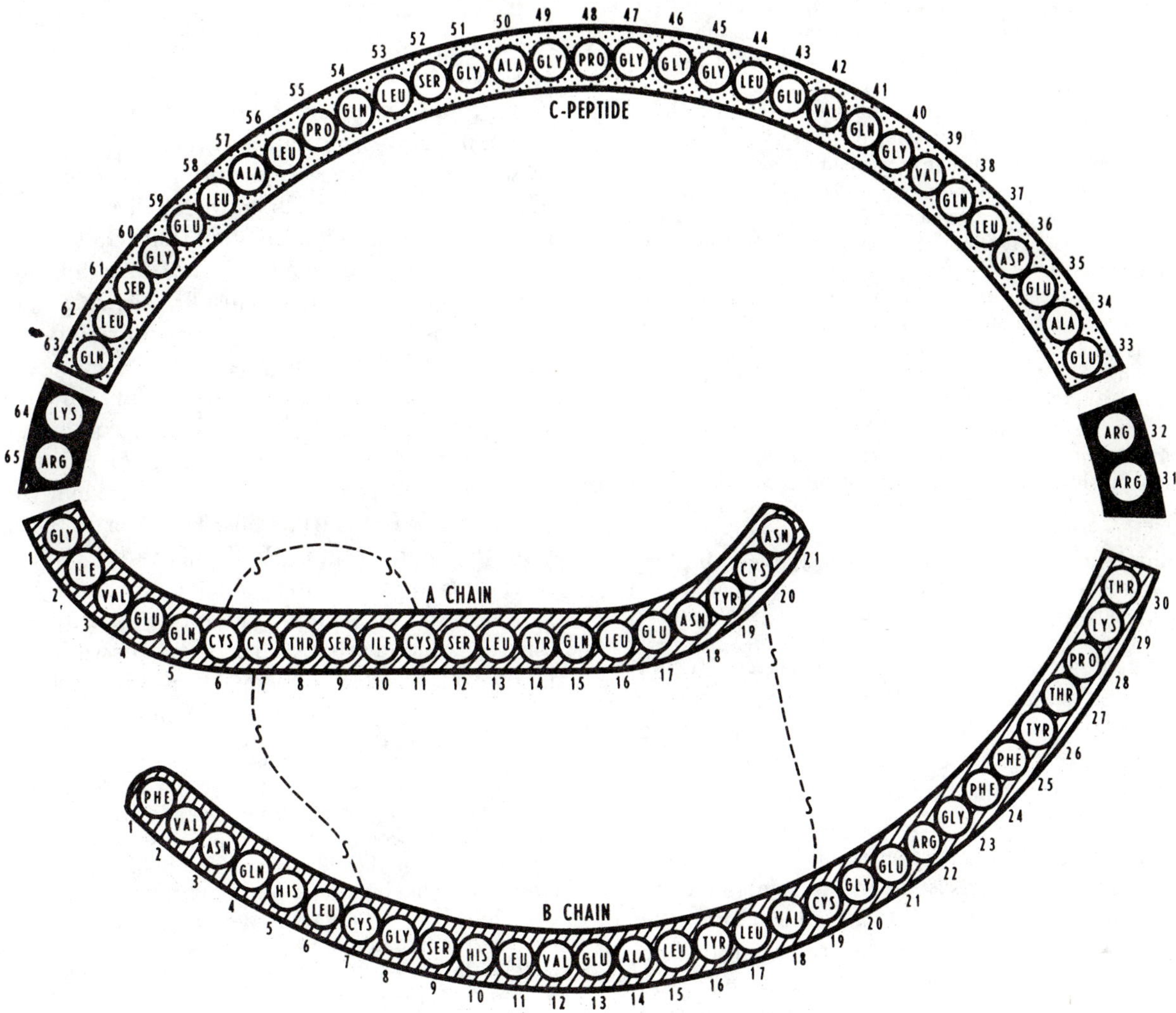

Fig. 12.3-1. *Structure of human proinsulin showing A-and B-chains of insulin molecule and C-peptide.*

Structural modifications that have been found to diminish biological activity of insulin include: (a) disruption of disulfide bonds by reduction or oxidation; (b) esterification of the carboxyl groups; (c) removal of C-terminal group of A- or B-chains; and (d) modification of the free amino groups or aliphatic hydroxyl groups. Insulin is vulnerable to proteolytic destruction by the digestive enzymes (such as trypsin or carboxypeptidase), thereby preventing its oral use.

Biosynthesis, Release and Metabolism. The pancreatic β cells synthesize a single-chain polypeptide precursor, proinsulin, which is biotransformed into insulin when four basic amino acids (arginine 31, arginine 32, lysine 64 and arginine 65) and the connector (C-peptide), made up of residues 31-65, are removed (Fig. 12.3-1). Proinsulin is synthesized in polyribosomal elements of the rough endoplasmic reticulum of the pancreatic β cells, whereas the conversion to insulin is achieved at the Golgi complex. The storage granules containing proinsulin and insulin bud off from the Golgi apparatus, and the enzymatic conversion of proinsulin to insulin plus C-peptide is completed. The granules may then be stored, destroyed, or released by exocytotic processes. During this process of secretion, the insulin-containing granules move to the cell membrane, which then ruptures, releasing the contents of the granules into the extracellular space (emiocytosis) (60).

The most important physiological stimulus for release of insulin is the concentration of glucose in the plasma. Glucose-induced insulin release has two components, an initial burst of release that peaks in minutes and rapidly declines, followed by a second, more sustained elevation of insulin levels dependent upon protein synthesis. The initial phase appears to be a more important determinant of the rate at which glucose is utilized in the body; selective impairment of this early phase of secretion has been noted in many prediabetic and diabetic patients (29).

Insulin secretion is stimulated by amino acids, fatty acids, and ketone bodies as well as by glucose. Other stimuli known to enhance the rate of insulin release are secretory products of the gastrointestinal tract such as secretin, gastrin, pancreozymin, glucagonlike factor, certain other hormones such as growth hormone and glucocorticoids, and some of the oral hypoglycemic agents.

In addition, autonomic mechanisms are also known to influence the secretion of insulin. The predominant effect of norepinephrine or epinephrine is to inhibit insulin secretion, a response mediated by α-adrenergic receptors. Selective stimulation of β-adrenergic receptors, on the other hand, stimulates the secretion of insulin. Administration of phentolamine, an α-receptor-blocking agent, results in marked elevation of circulating insulin levels, an effect attributed to concurrent inhibition of epinephrine effects via the α-receptors and stimulation of epinephrine effects via the β-receptors.

Exercise and pathological states associated with activation of the autonomic nervous system lead to suppression of insulin secretion through the α-receptor mechanism, whereas vagal nerve stimulation or cholinomimetic drugs enhance insulin release (49). The sympathetic and parasympathetic systems may thus control the basal rate of secretion of insulin as well as the reaction to stress.

The bulk of insulin in circulating blood appears as free hormone, although a small fraction may be bound to α- and β-globulins. The liver and kidney are of primary importance in degrading insulin. Minor quantities of insulin are bound in peripheral tissues such as muscle and fat. In the liver, the breakdown of insulin is accomplished by two systems: (a) action of glutathione-insulin transhydrogenase, which reduces and cleaves the disulfide bridges; and (b) proteolytic activity, which further cleaves the reduced and separated chains to smaller peptides and amino acids.

The uptake by tissues and rate of destruction may be diminised by antibodies and other proteins that may bind insulin under abnormal conditions, such as certain type(s) of diabetes mellitus.

Pharmocological and Physiological Effects. Insulin exerts several metabolic effects on a wide variety of tissues. It plays a key role in the intermediary metabolism, and its effects are most marked on three primary target tissues, namely the liver, adipose tissue, and skeletal muscle (Table 12.3-1). Metabolic events triggered by insulin in the major target tissues result from activation of cell-surface transport system for nutrients and ions along with intracellular enzymes that influence the latter through major metabolic pathways. Although the biochemical basis of insulin action has not been clearly established, it is now generally accepted that the cell-surface receptors initially react with the hormone followed by receptor clustering and passage of the insulin-receptor complex into the cell (internalization) (15). These receptors are composed of four subunits, contain two or more binding sites, and show features of negative cooperativity (17). Recent evidence has demonstrated that the transmembrane β-subunit of the insulin receptor is capable of expressing kinase activity. In addition to these receptors, distinct insulin binding sites have also been found on intracellular organelles, including the nucleus, endoplasmic reticulum, and Golgi apparatus. Although their functional role is currently unknown, there is some evidence that insulin may enter the target cells and interact within, raising the possibility that such intracellular binding sites may be involved in the long-term effects of insulin, such as those on protein, RNA, and DNA synthesis (28, 32). A synthesis of this information suggests that there are at least three distinct, but closely related, routes through which insulin receptors can elicit effects on target cells. They are: (a) the endocytosis of insulin receptor, (b) the activation of the insulin receptor tyrosine-specific protein kinase and (c) the activation of specific guanine nucleotide regulatory protein kinase(s). Such a proposal offers a means whereby insulin might exert a wide variety of actions within the cell (32).

Events at the level of plasma membrane triggered by insulin include the following:

Increased transport of sugars. Insulin accelerates the transport of hexoses across cell membranes and promotes the utilization of sugars. In muscle and adipose tissue, uptake is a rate-limiting step for the subsequent metabolism of glucose. The effects of insulin on hexose transport occur in minutes and are not inhibited by actinomycin, suggesting that synthesis of new proteins is not required. Although the molecular mechanism of hexose transport is not fully understood, it appears that a specific carrier molecule in the membrane is affected by insulin.

Increased transport of amino acids. Insulin enhances the active transport of amino acids, by processes as yet unknown.

Table 12.3-1
Summary of Insulin Effects on Target Organs

Tissue	Metabolism[a]		
	Carbohydrate	Protein	Lipid
Muscle	+ Glucose transport + Glycogen synthesis + Glycolysis	+ Amino acid uptake + Protein synthesis	
Liver	+ Glucokinase + Glycogen synthesis - Phosphorylase - Gluconeogenesis	- Proteolysis	+ Lipogenesis
Adipocytes	+ Glucose transport + Glycerol synthesis		+ Triglycerides + Fatty acid synthesis - Lipolysis

[a] +, increase; -, decrease.

Stimulation of amino acid transport by insulin results in increased inflow of amino acids into the cytosol, providing increased substrates for synthesis of proteins in liver and muscle cells.

Increased transport of ions across the plasma membrane. Insulin promotes increased efflux of sodium (Na+) and increased influx of potassium (K+) across the plasma membrane. This effect can be attributed to insulin stimulation of (Na+, K+) adenosine triphosphatase (ATPase). A similar effect on magnesium (Mg^{2+}) accumulation has also been demonstrated (77). Because K+ and Mg^{2+} are important in metabolism as, for example, in protein biosynthesis, it has been suggested that these cations may play roles as secondary messengers to mediate the actions of insulin.

Decreased level of cyclic adenosine monophosphate (cAMP) under some conditions. Insulin has been shown to lower cAMP levels in perfused liver and isolated rat liver cells, by unknown mechanism(s) (9, 47). This only partly explains the action of insulin on glycogen metabolism, as the hormone may also inhibit hepatic glycogenolysis by inhibiting the action of cAMP [or perhaps increased concentrations of cyclic guanosine monophosphate (cGMP) could explain many of the metabolic effects of insulin]. Inhibition of protein kinase could result in decreased phosphorylation of phosphorylase kinase, glycogen synthetase, and triglyceride lipase.

In addition to the events at the membrane level, insulin triggers rapid changes in a series of programmed enzymatic pathways in cellular metabolism. In principle, the influence on the metabolic programs is the same in different insulin-sensitive target cells. The final expression of the program, however, is somewhat different in different cell types, depending on their specialized functions. In general, insulin action results in overall anabolic effects with increased deposition of carbohydrates, lipids, and proteins. Some of the most characteristic effects of insulin on programmed cell metabolism are as follows.

Increased glycogen synthesis from glucose. Insulin increases the activity of glycogen synthetase and, consequently, enhances the conversion of glucose to glycogen (glycogenesis) in skeletal muscle, liver, and the adipocytes. Furthermore, insulin inhibits breakdown of glycogen (glycogenolysis) by inhibiting the activation of hepatic phosphorylation (48).

Decreased gluconeogenesis and hepatic glucose output. Insulin stimulates glycolysis and inhibits production of new glucose from proteins and amino acids (gluconeogenesis) by inducing formation of the enzymes controlling the former and suppressing those involved in gluconeogenesis (Fig. 12.3-2).

Increased synthesis of triglycerides from glucose. In adipose tissue, insulin increases formation of triglycerides by increasing fatty acid formation and increasing uptake of glucose, the immediate precursor of α-glycerophosphate, which is a requirement for triglyceride synthesis.

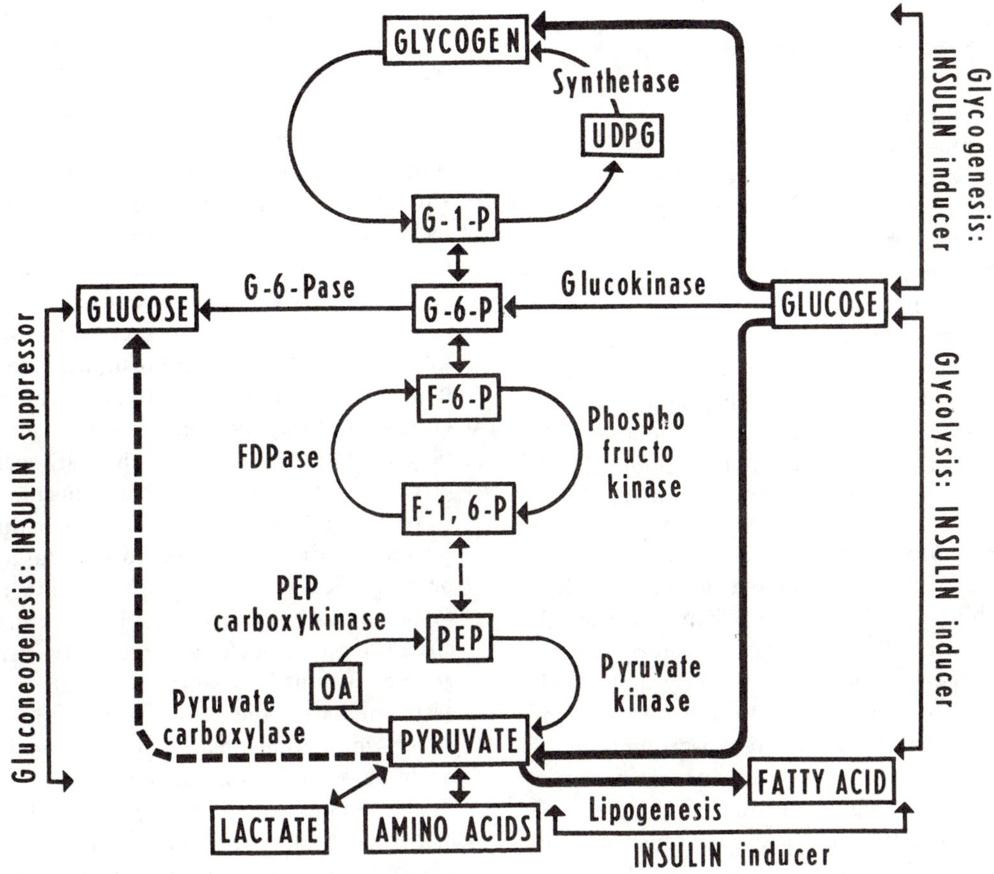

Fig. 12.3-2. *Influence of insulin on key enzymes controlling gluconeogenesis, glycolysis, and glycogenesis.*

Bold lines indicate induction; stippled lines indicate suppression of indicated processes. G-1-P = glucose-1-phosphate; G-6-P = glucose-6-phosphate; F-6-P = fructose-6-phosphate; F-1,6-P = fructose-1,6-diphosphate; PEP = phosphoenolpyruvate; OA = oxaloacetate; FDPase = fructose-1,6-diphosphatase; G-6-Pase = glucose-6-phosphatase; UDPG = uridine diphosphate glucose.

Inhibition of lipolysis. Insulin promotes fat synthesis in the liver and inhibits fat mobilization. In adipose tissue, the breakdown of triglyceride is decreased in the presence of insulin due to an inhibition of hormonally sensitive lipase activity, presumably via alterations in cAMP (37).

Increased synthesis of proteins from amino acids. In general, the effects on protein synthesis have been localized to translational events including polyribosome formation and peptide chain initiation. In muscle, insulin enhances the incorporation of amino acids into protein, independent of transport of amino acids.

Increased RNA synthesis. Insulin stimulation of precursor incorporation into RNA in rat diaphragm takes place even when the insulin effect on protein synthesis is blocked by puromycin. Conversely, insulin stimulation of incorporation of ^{14}C-labeled amino acids into proteins takes place even when RNA synthesis is blocked by actinomycin D.

Adverse Reactions

Hyperinsulinism. Overdosage of insulin can occur as a result of spontaneous or precipitated reduction in insulin requirement (e.g., omission of meals or increased exercise), or as a result of inadvertent administration of an excessive dose. The predominant symptoms, stemming from glucose deprivation, have a pattern and temporal sequence of signs and symptoms that are fairly, but by no means absolutely, constant. When the fall in blood glucose is rapid, the early symptoms, those produced by the compensatory secretion of epinephrine, include sweating, weakness, hunger, tachycardia, and "inner" trembling. When blood glucose falls more slowly, the symptoms are due to hypoglycemia in the brain and include headache, blurred vision, diplopia, mental confusion, incoherent speech, coma, and convulsions. If the fall in blood glucose is rapid, profound, and persistant, all such symptoms may be present.

Treatment of hypoglycemia consists of giving soluble carbohydrate or fruit juice orally; in comatose patients, intravenous administration of 50% glucose solution may restore consciousness. If glucose is not available, 0.5-1 mg of glucagon can be administered parenterally; it is effective only when hepatic glycogen is available.

Allergic Reactions. Local or systemic allergic reactions are often seen in patients receiving insulin. The local reactions (itching, swelling, and erythema) are usually mild and transient. Allergic urticaria, angioedema, and anaphylactic reactions occur infrequently and usually can be avoided by changing to insulin derived from another species. With the advent of newer, more highly purified preparations, allergic reactions are becoming less common. Thus, highly purified single-peak and single-component insulin may be used in sensitized individuals to minimize allergic reactions (22). Antihistamines are useful in the treatment of mild allergies. In more severe cases, however, treatment with corticosteroids, desensitization to insulin or, in certain maturity-onset cases, use of oral hypoglycemic agents may be required.

Therapeutic Uses

Diabetes Mellitus. Evidence that diabetes mellitus might be of pancreatic origin was initially furnished in the late 1800s by von Mering and Minkowski (75), who demonstrated that surgical removal of the pancreas in dogs evoked hyperglycemia, glycosuria, ketosis, and death. The next milestone was of course the discovery by Banting and Best of an active pancreatic extract capable of counteracting these effects which was of demonstrated therapeutic value in human diabetic patients (4). Although these observations did not prove that human diabetes is caused by the deficiency of a pancreatic secretion, their impact has dominated thinking about the etiology of diabetes. Indeed, at least until quite recently, there had been general agreement that human diabetes is entirely due to insulin deficiency.

The approach to the studies on the etiology of diabetes mellitus began to diversify in the 1930s, when Himsworth and coworkers provided evidence supporting the notion that insulin insensitivity, and not insulin deficiency, was present in many diabetic patients (31). This contention is further supported by the observation that, although in the case of insulin-dependent diabetes the islet tissue may show distinctive changes (characterized by pseudoatrophic islets and a marked reduction in the β-cell number) (25), such lesions are not universal. Indeed, no characteristic changes occur in the general appearance of islet organization between noninsulin-dependent diabetic patients and aging nondiabetic subjects. A reduced number of β cells can be found in these patients, but a similar reduction can also be found in many elderly subjects without clinical evidence of diabetes. There is some evidence to suggest that β cells in these patients may be less responsive to hyperglycemia.

Work by Houssay indicates that pituitary hormones interfere with the action of insulin and may contribute to hyperglycemia (33). Recently, it has been suggested that glucagon, the second islet cell (A or α) hormone, may also play an important role in the pathogenesis of hyperglycemia and hyperketonemia of insulin deficiency (63).

With respect to insulin resistance in diabetes, reduced insulin binding to its receptors on target cells has also been implicated. In fact, studies have demonstrated a remarkably close correlation between insulin binding to circulating monocytes and the *in vivo* sensitivity to exogenous insulin. Several cases of diabetes have also been associated with the presence of antiinsulin antibodies, which may bind insulin and prevent the necessary hormone-receptor interactions.

The recent search for the etiology of diabetes mellitus has focused on three interlocking mechanisms: viral, autoimmune, and genetic. Diabetes mellitus was found to be discordant in approximately 50% of identical twins when the propositus was initially diagnosed at less than 40 years of age. It was concordant, however, in up to 90% of cases diagnosed after 40 years of age, indicating that

(a) genetic influences may have a role in the development of diabetes mellitus and (b) environmental factors are involved in the expression of the disease (18).

Viral infections also have been considered likely causative or provocative agents in insulin-dependent diabetes for several years; the viruses implicated include mumps, Coxsackie B, cytomegalovirus, and those causing rubella, infectious mononucleosis, and varicella (64). Increased titers of antibodies to Coxsackie B virus have been noted in high frequency in diabetic patients. A variant of this virus has been isolated from the pancreas of a patient with acute-onset diabetes mellitus (79), and this virus has been found to be diabetogenic in some strains of mice (57). Epidemiological studies have shown both a seasonal incidence of insulin-dependent diabetes and a temporal relationship between certain viral infections and the subsequent development of diabetes, supporting the contention of viral involvement in the etiology of this disease (50).

Certain forms of diabetes may have an autoimmune explanation for islet-cell inflammation and damage. Several investigators have identified circulating islet-cell antibodies in patients with newly diagnosed insulin-dependent diabetes (14, 38). Studies involving family, twin, immunological, and human lymphocyte antigen (HLA) disease, and metabolic association clearly establish genetic heterogeneity between insulin-dependent and noninsulin-dependent types of diabetes. Furthermore, heterogeneity has been demonstrated with these two broad groups of patients (with respect to age of onset, islet antibodies, obesity, and chlorpropamide-alcohol flushing) (66).

Certain HLA types occur with increased frequency in patients with diabetes. The HLA locus on chromosome 6 is intimately involved in immunological integrity at both the cellular and humoral (antigen-antibody formation, or β-cell function) levels. Thus, a genetically mediated defect in immunological response appears to be a major cause of diabetes (12).

Classification of Diabetes Mellitus. During recent years, clinical, biochemical, pathological, genetic, and immunological findings have brought forth the realization that diabetes mellitus is a heterogenous syndrome with two dominant pathogenic lesions: (a) deficiency of insulin effect characterized by disordered β-cell function (and insulin deficiency) and/or a resistance to the effectiveness of insulin on peripheral tissue (characterized by normal or even elevated quantities of circulating insulin); and (b) the development of complications, including heart disease, blindness, cataracts, blood vessel damage, nerve disorders, and kidney damage. The precise relationship of these findings to each other is not known. The growth of knowledge of the etiology and pathogenesis have demanded a revision and unification of the classification of diabetes mellitus. A new classification scheme was proposed by a workgroup of the National Diabetes Data Group (NDDG) (56), and was subsequently adopted in a large part as recommendations of the World Health Organization (WHO) Expert Committee on Diabetes (77). This classification scheme, which is gaining international acceptance, was designed to keep the classes mutually exclusive. This scheme, summarized in Table 12.3-2, represents a consensus of the categories that, given present knowledge, were considered likely to be homogeneous, but it also recognizes that future developments may call for its modification (5, 69).

The characteristic signs of diabetes mellitus that are a consequence of relative or complete lack of insulin on intermediary metabolism include hyperglycemia, hyperlipemia, ketonemia, and azoturia.

Hyperglycemia. One characteristic common to all diabetic patients is an abnormally high blood glucose concentration. In the absence of insulin effects, there is (a) marked reduction of the rate of glucose transport across certain cell membranes, (b) reduction in enzyme systems catalyzing conversion of glucose to glycogen, and (c) abnormally high rate of glucose synthesis from amino acids and proteins. High blood sugar by itself may be the cause of diabetic complications; tight control of blood sugar may prevent, arrest, and possibly even reverse the progress of these complications. However, perfect blood glucose control (as in nondiabetic individuals) is not yet feasible; thus, the question remains whether the observed complications are due to the imperfect control, or whether they are correlated with, but not caused by, the excess sugar in the blood. Glucose can attach to proteins, and it has been suggested that at high concentrations such interactions may result in functional damage, particularly where proteins are slow to be replaced, such as the lining of blood vessels and the insulating material around nerve cells (6, 41). Complications of diabetes may also ensue from an overutilization of glucose in cells, such as those of nerve and lens, where glucose can enter even in the absence of insulin. During the presence of high glucose, minor metabolic pathways are employed by some cells, and one of these leads to accumulation of sorbitol (a sugar alcohol), which is metabolized slowly. Accumulation of sorbitol causes osmotic swelling of the lens, which is characteristic of cataracts. In diabetic rodents, cataracts can be prevented by drugs that inhibit aldose reductase, an enzyme that converts glucose to sorbitol (74). Sorbitol has also been shown to accumulate in cells lining of peripheral nerves of diabetic animals with subsequent swelling defects in conducting nerve impulses, effects that can be prevented with inhibitors of aldose reductase. High blood sugar may also be responsible for basement membrane changes through changes in protein configuration. The final answer to blood sugar control may come from the development of an artificial pancreas to inject insulin automatically in response to fluctuations in patients' blood sugar or from development of ways to transplant the islets of Langerhans (41). The development of the former is impeded by difficulties encountered in finding a biocompatible glucose sensor and the availability of an insulin that has long-term stability in implanted reservoirs. The main problem with the implanted β cells has been the lack of adequate source and immune rejection (23).

Hyperlipemia and Ketonemia. Increased plasma free fatty acids in diabetic subjects is largely due to increased mobilization from the peripheral fat depots, since in the absence of insulin, lipolysis facilitated by various hormones proceeds unchecked. The liver oxidizes these fatty acids to acetyl coenzyme A (CoA) and converts them to ketone bodies, some of which are organic acids. Although ketone bodies can be utilized as energy sources, when rate of production exceeds the rate of utilization, accumulation may cause metabolic acidosis (ketoacidosis).

Azoturia. The conversion of large amounts of protein to glucose is accompanied by increased production and excretion of urea and ammonia. The various metabolic changes are summarized in Fig. 12.3-3. These changes, in many instances, can be prevented or corrected by the administration of insulin. If the metabolic aberrations are not brought under therapeutic control, the loss of water and electrolytes and the accumulation of

Table 12.3-2
Classification of Diabetes Mellitus

Class	Clinical Characteristics
Insulin-dependent type (IDDM), type I	Dependent on injected insulin for the prevention of ketosis and preservation of life; onset usually < age 30; characterized by insulinopenia; islet cell antibodies frequently present
Noninsulin-dependent types (NIDDM), type II 1. Nonobese NIDDM 2. Obese NIDDM	Noninsulin-dependent and nonketosis prone (except under special circumstances such as stress); onset usually after age 40 and not secondary to other disease conditions; serum insulin levels may be normal, elevated, or depressed; about 60-90% of the subjects are obese and constitute the obese subtype which may improve by weight loss; hyperinsulinemia and insulin resistance characterize some patients this subtype
Other types[a]	
1. Pancreatic disease	Pancreatectomy, pancreatitis, carcinoma, etc.
2. Hormonal etiology	Cushing's syndrome, acromegaly, pheochromocytoma, primary aldosteronism, glucagonemia, somatostatinoma, etc.
3. Drug-induced condition	Diuretics, glucocorticoids, oral contraceptives, phenytoin (DILANTIN), phenothiazines, tricyclic antidepressants, etc.
4. Insulin receptor abnormalities	Abnormalities in numbers or affinity of insulin receptors or antibodies to receptors, with or without associated immune disorders
5. Certain genetic syndromes	Diabetes is found in increased frequency with a large number of genetic syndromes, such as hyperlipemias, myotonic dystrophy, lipoatrophy, leprechaunism, Friedreich's ataxia, Prader-Willi syndrome, etc.
Gestational diabetes	Onset or recognition during pregnancy; thus diabetics who become pregnant are not included in this class; condition probably due to complex hormonal and metabolic changes and/or insulin resistance

[a]For a more exhaustive list of diabetes caused by or associated with other categories of glucose intolerance, the reader is referred to Ref. 56.

hydrogen ion can lead to diabetic acidosis and coma, which can be fatal. Thus, the use of insulin as replacement therapy is indicated in treatment of insulin-dependent diabetes, and is also indicated in noninsulin-dependent diabetes that cannot be controlled by diet alone. In addition, insulin must often be substituted for an oral hypoglycemic agent (see later) in noninsulin-dependent diabetes complicated by acidosis, ketosis, and diabetic coma.

Insulin Resistance. In both obese subjects and noninsulin-dependent diabetes mellitus, insulin resistance is the characteristic feature. Impaired insulin action may result from prereceptor, receptor, or postreceptor defects.

In the prereceptor category, insulin resistance has been demonstrated due to secretion of an abnormal β cell product with diminished biological activity (26). Defective insulin production results in a hyperinsulinemic state. Within the β cells, an incomplete conversion of proinsulin to insulin has also been reported to cause increased proinsulin secretion (proinsulin has about 5% biological activity of insulin) (21).

Elevated levels of counterregulatory hormones (e.g., growth hormone, cortisol, glucagon, epinephrine, antiinsulin antibodies, or antiinsulin-receptor antibodies) have been associated with the insulin-resistant state (58). Available evidence indicates that due to target-tissue defects, the insulin-resistant state may exist. A decrease in the number of insulin receptors would result in reduced insulin action at a concentration that occupies fewer than the critical numbers of receptors needed to produce a maximal biological response (58). In obese subjects, decreased numbers of insulin receptors have been shown in different tissues (43). Recent studies seem to indicate that sulfonylureas may improve glucose tolerance by augmentation of both insulin secretion and insulin action (19, 20, 45).

Preparations and Therapeutic Regimen. Not long after the first patients were treated, the deficiencies of insulin treatment became evident. For instance pain, redness, itching, and induration at the injection site were common in patients who received the first extracts of animal pancreas (23), and it was with the advent of insulin purification technology of the 1970s that drastic reductions in frequency of the complications of insulin therapy became apparent. A second shortcoming of the early therapeutic insulin was that it was short-acting and required 4 to 6 injections daily, which was inconvenient, cumbersome, and fraught with the hazard of nocturnal hyperglycemia. In order to obviate multiple daily doses of insulin and to provide adequate insulin effects on glucose and nitrogen metabolism throughout the night, the insulin was modified by combination with a substance that would delay its absorption from the injection site. The first commercially available modified insulin, was an amorphous complex of protamine (harvested from fish testes), zinc, and insulin (PZI), from which insulin was released over a 24- to 36-hr period. In 1946 a crystalline complex of protamine, zinc, and insulin called neutral protamine hagedorn (NPH), which contained less protamine and zinc than PZI, became available, and had a duration of action of about 24 hr. Concern about protamine being foreign protein in insulin led to the

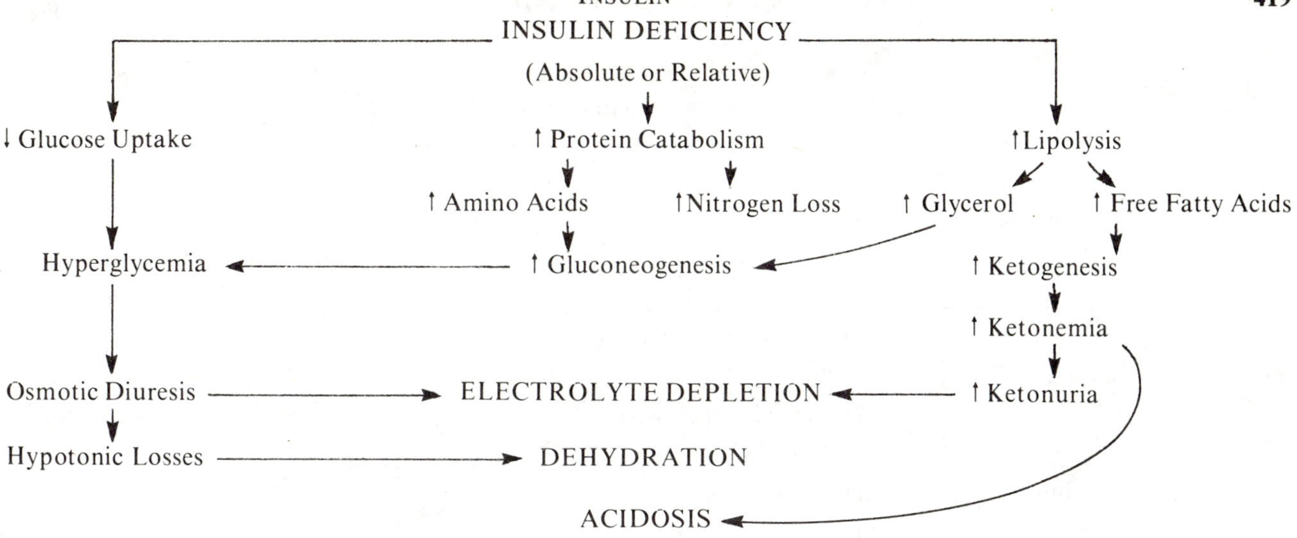

Fig. 12.3-3. *Interaction of effects resulting from insulin deficiency. (From Davidson, M.B. Diabetes mellitus and hypoglycemia. In: Endocrine Pathophysiology* (Hershman, J.M., ed.). Philadelphia: Lea & Febiger, 1977, p. 212.)

development of the lente insulins, which are suspensions of insulins with zinc concentrations about 10 times those of NPH.

Thus the types of insulin preparations available differ mainly in their rate of absorption and consequently in their onset, peak, and duration of action. The properties of rapidly absorbed insulin can be modified by various procedures, as listed here.

1. *Crystalline zinc insulin (regular insulin).* This preparation has a rapid onset (0.5-1 hr) and short duration of action (5-7 hr). It is the only preparation that can be used intravenously and, thus, can be used in the treatment of diabetic acidosis.

2. *Globin insulin.* This preparation is an acidic solution containing erythrocyte globin, zinc, and crystalline insulin. When injected, the solution neutralizes in tissue and the insulin-protein complex precipitates, resulting in a depot from which release of active insulin is slower and more sustained. Thus, this preparation has a slow onset and more prolonged duration of action (12-18 hr).

3. *Protamine zinc insulin (PZI).* In this preparation, crystalline insulin is combined with an excess of protamine (basic) in phosphate buffer to form a fine precipitate. The insulin is released from this complex in a steady prolonged manner (24-to 36-hr period).

4. *Isophane (neutral protamine hagedorn, NPH) insulin.* This too represents a crystalline complex of protamine, zinc, and insulins; however, it contains less protamine and zinc as compared with PZI format. Thus, its action is intermediate between that of PZI and regular insulin (24 hr in most patients).

5. *Insulin zinc suspensions.* Concern about protamine being a foreign protein in insulin led to the development of the lente insulins, which are suspensions of insulin devoid of protamine but with zinc concentrations about 10 times those of NPH. These preparations are made by substituting acetate for phosphate buffer, resulting in the formation of small amorphous particles or larger crystals. The amorphous preparation is called prompt insulin zinc suspension, USP (SEMILENTE), and has action between that of regular and NPH insulin. When the zinc is combined with the insulin to produce an all-microcrystalline material, the result is a form that is absorbed more slowly, having a duration of action slightly more prolonged than that of PZI, and it is called extended insulin zinc suspension, USP (ULTRALENTE). An intermediate preparation containing a 70:30 combination of ULTRALENTE and SEMILENTE results in LENTE, which has a time course comparable with that of NPH insulin. Regular insulin can be mixed with all types of insulin; SEMILENTE can also be mixed with LENTE or ULTRALENTE preparations. The various properties of available USP preparations of insulin are summarized in Table 12.3-3.

The insulins just described have endured as the principal tools of conventional insulin therapy. The most frequently employed regimen includes one dose of NPH or lente daily, either alone or in combination with regular insulin. For milder diabetics this program is frequently sufficient. For many noninsulin-dependent (type II) patients and most insulin-dependent (type I) patients of recent onset, two doses daily of NPH or lente alone or with combination with regular insulin are needed to achieve optimal glucose control over a 24-hr period without an increased risk of hypoglycemia.

Initiation of insulin treatment in all children and adolescents, pregnant women, and all adult diabetics with evidence of marked hyperglycemia, dehydration, ketonuria, or infection requires hospitalization. Generally, after establishing good control of plasma glucose with regular insulin, a split-dose regimen can be started. The total daily insulin dose is usually estimated by plasma glucose level and the degree of glycosuria. Two-thirds of the total estimated dose of insulin is given prior to breakfast and one-third before supper.

Patients with mild-to-moderate hyperglycemia but without ketosis, infection, or dehydration are selected for outpatient management, and insulin therapy is initiated as a split-dose regimen with two-thirds of total daily insulin in the morning and one-third in the evening. The total daily insulin requirement depends on several factors, including body weight and the degree of hyperglycemia. Further adjustment of dosage is made in the NPH and regular insulin based on plasma glucose (reflected by glycosuria) before supper and before breakfast, respectively.

Insulin requirement is increased in certain conditions, which include pregnancy, weight gain, infection, primary hyperparathyroidism, adrenal cortical hyperfunction, hyperthyroidism, acromegaly, and hypokalemia. During increased physical activity, renal or adrenal cortical insufficiency, and hypothyroid states, insulin requirement is decreased.

ORAL HYPOGLYCEMIC DRUGS

History. Oral hypoglycemic agents that would be effective in the management of patients with diabetes mellitus have been sought for over half a century. Several agents have been deve-

Table 12.3-3
Insulin Preparations (USP)

Action	USP Preparation	Hours after s.c. Injection		
		Approximate Time of Onset	Peak Action	Duration of Action
Rapid	Insulin injection (regular, crystalline zinc)	1	1-3	5-7
	Prompt insulin zinc suspension (SEMI-LENTE)	1	1-4	12-16
Intermediate	Isophane insulin suspension (NPH)	2	8-12	18-24
	Insulin zinc suspension (LENTE)	2	8-12	18-24
	Globin zinc insulin injection (globin)	2	6-10	12-18
Long	Protamine zinc insulin suspension	7	8-16	24-36
	Extended insulin zinc suspension (ULTRA-LENTE)	7	8-16	24-36

loped that are able to reduce the circulating levels of glucose and are in clinical use. However, many have proven toxic, and the use of some others is controversial as to whether they are effective and safe enough to warrant their widespread use.

The first serious attempt to synthesize an oral hypoglycemic agent occurred in 1926 when Frank and coworkers altered the guanidine molecule (21). This drug, SYNTHALIN, was used in Germany for several years to treat diabetes, but its use had to be discontinued because of toxicity. Subsequently phenformin, another biguanide, was found to have minimal toxicity and became widespread in use. Although biguanides are still in use in several parts of the world, the United States discontinued their general use as of October 1977 due to their toxic effects, particularly the high incidence of lactic acidosis (44).

During World War II, Janbon, a clinician from Montpelier, along with coworkers treated a number of patients suffering from typhoid fever with a new sulfonamide and noted that a number of them developed hypoglycemia (36). Thus carbutamide (an antibacterial) was the first effective oral hypoglycemic agent with less toxicity. Shortly thereafter, tolbutamide, which in contrast to carbutamide possessed no antibacterial activity and had less toxicity, was introduced. Tolbutamide and chemically related hypoglycemic agents, designated as sulfonylureas, are currently the only oral hypoglycemic agents available for general use in the United States.

SULFONYLUREAS

Chemistry. The more commonly used preparations of sulfonylurea compounds include tolbutamide, acetohexamide, tolazamide, chlorpropamide, and a more recently developed compound, glyburide. The first-generation sulfonylureas, which include tolbutamide, chlorpropamide, tolazamide, and acetohexamide, have an aliphatic side chain and a simply substituted aromatic ring at the other end. The introduction of a cyclohexyl group instead of the aliphatic side chain and addition of another ring structure to the aromatic ring led to the development of second-generation compounds with much higher intrinsic activity. More extensive cyclic substitutions at the benzene and/or urea groups of the sulfonylurea structure have led to the production of several more second-generation sulfonylureas (such as glyburide, glipizide, and glibornuride) that may soon enter the North American market. Molecular structures of the commonly used sulfonylurea drugs are shown in Fig. 12.3-4.

Pharmacological Effects. The acute hypoglycemic effect of sulfonylureas has largely been attributed to their ability to stimulate the islet tissue to secrete insulin. Sulfonylureas cause degranulation of β cells, a phenomenon associated with increased rate of insulin secretion. Clinical studies demonstrate that sulfonylureas have little effect in completely pancreatectomized and insulin-dependent diabetic subjects. They are effective, however, in noninsulin-dependent diabetic patients in whom the pancreas retains the capacity to secrete insulin. Although initial reports indicated that the sulfonylureas may cause the formation of new β cells in the pancreatic islets (β-cytotrophic effect), numerous other studies have failed to demonstrate such a β-cytotrophic effect (45). Furthermore, chronic sulfonylurea treatment has been found to decrease pancreatic insulin content and decreased *in vivo* and *in vitro* nutrient-stimulated insulin secretion. This effect of chronic treatment is believed to be due to the

First Generation Compounds

Second Generation Compounds

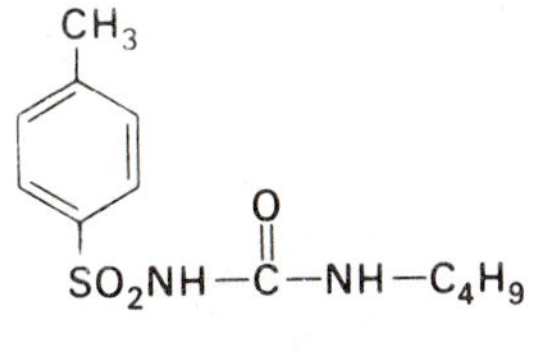

Tolbutamide

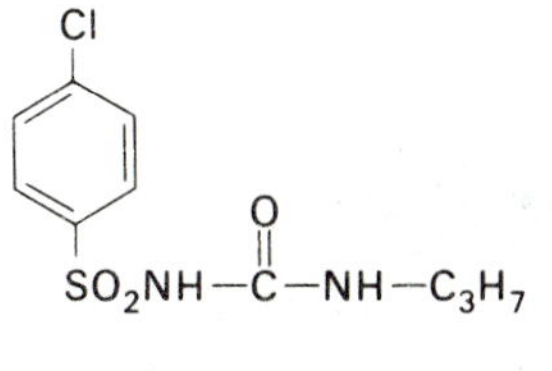

Chlorpropamide

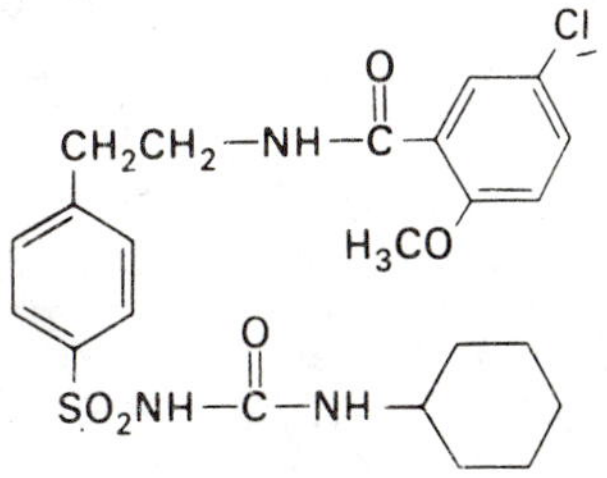

Glyburide

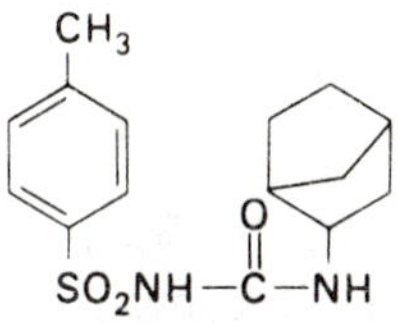

Glibornuride

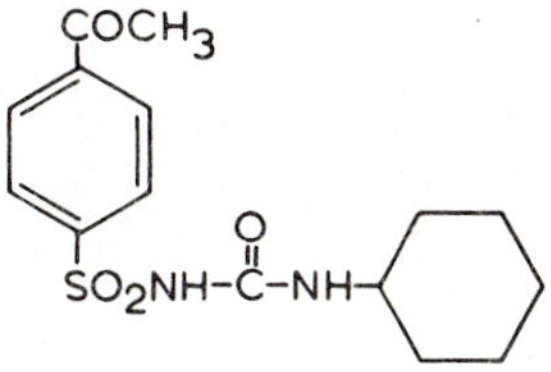

Acetohexamide

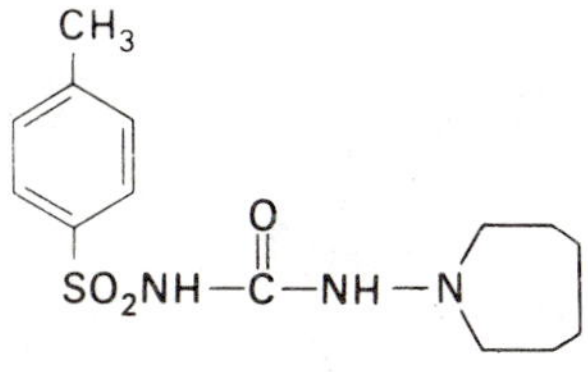

Tolazamide

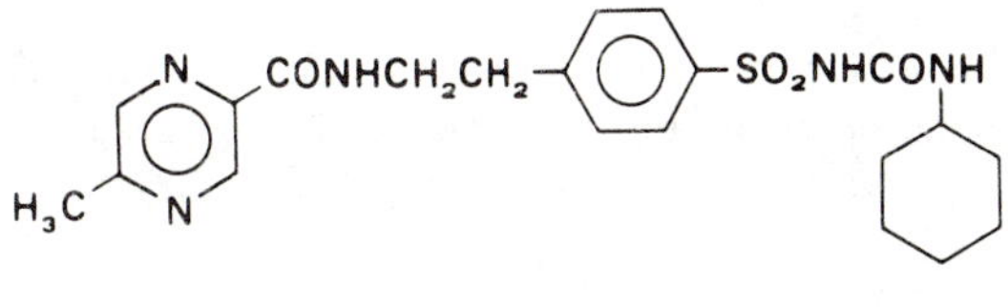

Glipizide

Fig. 12.3-4. *Chemical structures of sulfonylureas.*

reduced capacity of the islets for biosynthesis of proinsulin.

The sulfonylurea compounds also seem to affect blood sugar through extrapancreatic actions, such as a marked inhibitory effect on glucose release by the liver. More recent work on extrapancreatic actions of sulfonylureas has shown that these agents somehow enhance the sensitivity of peripheral target tissues to the effects of insulin and other hormones. Although the nature of these alterations remains to be elucidated, it is of interest that sulfonylureas have been found to increase the concentration of insulin receptor sites on the surface of blood cells and adipocytes (59). Such an effect could explain, at least in part, the potentiation of insulin action by sulfonylureas. Potentiation of insulin-mediated action persists for an unknown period. Significant amelioration of fasting hyperglycemia and glucose intolerance may persist until the absolute amount of insulin secretion becomes so low that its action, though potentiated, is insufficient for metabolic needs (45).

Pharmacokinetics. The sulfonylureas are well absorbed from the gastrointestinal tract and, after oral doses, are distributed throughout the extracellular fluid compartment, although partially bound to plasma proteins. The most important clinical difference among the sulfonylureas is their duration of action, which is determined in part by rate and route(s) of degradation of the individual drugs. Table 12.3-4 summarizes the pharmacokinetic characteristics of sulfonylurea compounds.

Adverse Effects. The incidence of untoward reactions estimated for this group of drugs is about 6%. The reported adverse effects include: severe hypoglycemia, which mimics acute CNS disorders, nausea, epigastric fullness, and heartburn (dose-related); jaundice; allergic skin reactions such as pruritus, erythema, urticaria, morbilliform or maculopapular eruptions; porphyria cutanea tarda and photosensitivity reactions; leukopenia, agranulocytosis, thrombocytopenia, hemolytic anemia, and aplastic anemia; hepatic prophyria and disulfiramlike reactions; and reduced radioactive iodine (RAI) uptake by the thyroid gland.

Drug Interaction. Administration of oral hypoglycemic agents concomitantly, or in close sequence with certain other drug(s), may interact to increase or diminish the intended hypoglycemic effect, or to cause an unintended reaction (Table 12.3-5).

Therapeutic Uses

Diabetes Mellitus. Recent doubts about the long-term safety of oral hypoglycemic agents have led to increased emphasis on the use of exercise and nutritional regulation in the management of the diabetic. Several studies have demonstrated that the degree of response seems to be related to successful weight reduction, particularly in the obese subtype of noninsulin-dependent diabetics. This may partly be related to the fact that obesity is associated with decreased insulin sensitivity (2, 76).

When dietary control and weight reduction are ineffective or not feasible, one must choose between insulin and

Table 12.3-4
Characteristics of Sulfonylurea Compounds

Compound	Daily Effective Dose Range (mg) (dose frequency)[a]		Half-life Approx. (hr)	Duration of action	Metabolizes	Excreted in 24-hr Urine	Residual Metabolite
Tolbutamide	500-3000	(D)	5	6-12	Rapidly	100%	None
Chlorpropamide	100-500	(S)	36	36-60	< 1%	80%	Unchanged
Acetohexamide	250-1500	(S or D)	6-7	12-24	Rapidly	60%	Minute amount[b]
Tolazamide	250-1500	(S or D)	7-8	10-15	Rapidly	85%	6 metabolites[c]
Glyburide	2.5-20	(S)	7-8	10-24	Rapidly	60%	None
Glipizide	2.5-15	(S)	2-4	12-24	Rapidly	68%	None

[a] S, single dose; D, divided dose.
[b] Metabolite, hydroxyhexamide, is 2.5 times more potent than original.
[c] Three of the metabolites are mildly hypoglycemic.

oral hypoglycemic agents. Some authorities consider insulin to be the safer and more effective approach. The sulfonylureas should only be used when a patient is unable or unwilling to take insulin. There is little evidence that oral hypoglycemic agents prevent cardiovascular complications from diabetes; on the contrary, available data, although still contrvoersial, suggest that the incidence of such complications may be increased in patients taking such drugs.

Oral hypoglycemics are contraindicated in ketosis-prone patients or in insulin-dependent diabetes mellitus, and they should never be used during ketoacidosis or in patients during pregnancy, surgery, stress, or infection, or in the presence of cardiac, renal, or hepatic disease (30).

Therapy is initiated using the minimum effective dose, increasing at weekly intervals until the desired degree of control is achieved. Patients who fail to respond to maximal doses within 1 month are considered to have primary failure, although some individuals may respond following weight reduction or a period of insulin therapy. Secondary failure refers to those patients who respond initially but later develop hyperglycemia.

Diagnostic Tests. In patients with pancreatic islet cell tumors, the blood glucose concentration drops rapidly after an intravenous injection of tolbutamide and remains low for about 3 hr. A similar effect is not observed in other hypoglycemic states, and tolbutamide administration can thus be used as a diagnostic test. Serum immunoreactive insulin determinations should also be performed. Extreme care is necessary in view of the possibility of fatal hypoglycemia.

Preparations. *Tolbutamide*, USP (ORINASE) tablets (250 and 500 mg); *tolbutamide sodium* (ORINASE DIAGNOSTIC) powder (1 g); *chlorpropamide*, USP (DIABINESE) tablets (100 and 250 mg); *acetohexamide*, USP (DYMELOR) tablets (250 and 500 mg); *tolazamide*, USP (TOLINASE) tablets (100, 250 and 500 mg); *glyburide* (DIABETA) tablets (1.25, 2.5 and 5 mg); *glipizide* (GLUCOTROL) tablets (5 and 10 mg).

Their effective dose range, dosage frequency, and duration of action are summarized in Table 12.3-4.

UNIVERSITY GROUP DIABETES PROGRAM CONTROVERSY

A cooperative clinical study in 2 university-based clinics (University Group Diabetes Program, or UGDP) was initiated in 1961 to determine if control of blood glucose prevents the development of vascular disorders in diabetic patients. For up to 8 years, the investigators followed obese adult diabetics randomly assigned to one of four treatment regimens: diet alone, diet plus two different insulin regimens, and diet plus tolbutamide. The results of these studies (summarized in Table 12.3-6) aroused much interest; the issue remains controversial (46).

BIGUANIDES

Chemistry. The discovery of the hypoglycemic effect of guanide compounds was fortuitous. It developed through the stage of monoguanidines and then diguanides, in which the two guanidine redicals were separated by a methylene bridge, and finally the biguanides were the two guanidine moieties that are directly linked. The general structure of biguanides is:

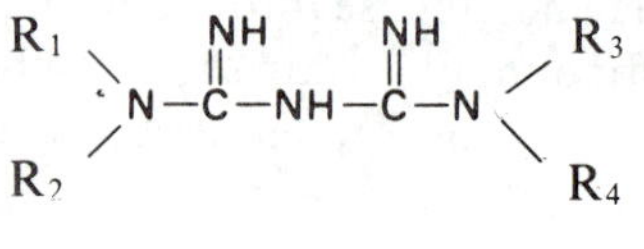

$$(R_1)(R_2)N-C(=NH)-NH-C(=NH)-N(R_3)(R_4)$$

Although phenformin was the only biguanide to be used widely in the United States, other biguanides such as methyl-phenformin (metformin) and butyl-phenformin (buformin) have been used in Canada and Europe. Because of the increasing number of reports of lactic acidosis associated with phenformin therapy, this drug was withdrawn from the Canadian market in early 1977, and from the general market in the United States by the Food and Drug Administration in 1978. It is now available through an investigational New Drug Application for carefully selected nonketotic diabetic patients.

Table 12.3-5
Drug Interactions with Oral Hypoglycemic Agents

Interacting Drug	Adverse Effect	Probable Mechanism
Alcohol	Minor disulfiramlike symptoms with sulfonylureas	Inhibition of intermediary metabolism of alcohol
	Increased hypoglycemic effect with ingestion of alcohol, particularly in fasting patients	Suppression of gluconeogenesis and glucagon release
	Lactic acidosis with phenformin	Synergism
	Decreased hypoglycemic effect with chronic alcohol abuse with tolbutamide	Increased metabolism
Anabolic steroids	Increased hypoglycemia	Not established
Anticoagulants, oral	Increased sulfonylurea hypoglycemia	Inhibition of microsomal enzymes
Chloramphenicol	Increased sulfonylurea hypoglycemia	Inhibition of microsomal enzymes
Clonidine	Decreased signs of hypoglycemia	Inhibition of catecholamine response to hypoglycemia
Contraceptive, oral	Possible hyperglycemia	Promotion of peripheral insulin resistance
Glucocorticoids	Possible hyperglycemia	Promotion of insulin resistance and increased gluconeogenesis
MAO inhibitors	Increased hypoglycemia	Not established
Phenylbutazone or oxyphenbutazone	Increased sulfonylurea hypoglycemia	Inhibition of microsomal enzymes
Propranolol	Prolonged hypoglycemia masks tachycardia and tremor	Decreased glycogenolysis β-receptor blockade
Rifampin	Possible decreased tolbutamide effects	Induction of microsomal enzymes
Salicylates	Increased hypoglycemia	Displacement from binding; additive effect
Sulfonamides	Increased sulfonylurea	Not established
Thiazides	Hyperglycemia	Supression of insulin release due to K^+ loss

Mechanism of Action. Biguanides do not reduce blood glucose levels significantly below normal, and they have no effect on plasma glucose in nondiabetic subjects (71); nor do they have any effect on the islet cells. The possible mechanism of hypoglycemia action of biguanides includes (a) decreased intestinal absorption of glucose (16), (b) inhibition of hepatic gluconeogenesis (11), and (c) increased peripheral glucose utilization (7).

Pharmacokinetics. Metformin is rapidly absorbed following oral administration, with its effects becoming apparent within 30 min. The blood concentration reaches a peak about 2 hr after absorption. Metformin is not metabolized, and most of the drug is excreted unchanged in the urine within 24 hr. Only small amounts are detected in the feces. Metformin is mainly concentrated in intestinal mucosa and salivary glands (10).

Table 12.3-6
The UGDP Study: Conclusion, Reactions, Counter-reactions

UGDP Conclusions and Supporting Data from Other Studies	Opposing Arguments
Tolbutamide caused an increase in the death rate due to myocardial infarctions in obese adult diabetic patients;similar results were obtained in studies from the Joslin Clinic and from England	The prevalence of myocardial disease may have been higher in the tolbutamide-treated group before the start of the UGDP treatment regimens; The death rate from myocardial infarction may have been exceptionally high at two UGDP centers; if the data from those centers are excluded, the UGDP report shows no increases in cardiac mortality due to tolbutamide
Tolbutamide may have caused an increase in the overall death rate in these patients; similar results were obtained in other studies	The increase in the overall death rate was statistically insignificant; without the data from two of the UGDP centers, there is no increase in overall death rate
Treatment with tolbutamide certainly did not improve survival, as compared with treatment with diet alone	Possible defects in the randomization of patients in the UGDP study may have weighed the tolbutamide-treated group in favor of an increased incidence of myocardial disease; furthermore, possible lack of close control of hyperglycemia with tolbutamide may have obviated any conclusions concerning the therapeutic efficacy of tolbutamide

Adverse Effects. Adverse reactions to biguanides include metallic taste in mouth, anorexia, nausea, diarrhea, weakness, weight loss, and muscle cramps. Phenformin-associated lactic acidosis is the most serious condition that appears to occur in diabetic patients (1, 3). Lactic acidosis usually occurs in diabetic patients with cardiac, liver, or kidney failure. Nevertheless, it also occurs in the absence of predisposing conditions.

Drug Interactions. Alcohol inhibits parahydroxylation of phenformin, thereby increasing the risk of hypoglycemia and aggravating lactic acidosis.

Therapeutic Uses. It is recommended that biguanide use be limited to the group of noninsulin-dependent nonketotic diabetes in whom the use of insulin poses special problems. These include patients who are symptomatic but cannot be controlled by diet and sulfonylurea alone; who cannot take sulfonylureas because of allergies and have none of the underlying risk factors that contraindicate the use of biguanides (such as impaired cardiovascular, hepatic, or renal function); whose symptoms are controlled by biguanides, but who cannot take insulin because of serious mental or physical disability; or whose occupation is such that the risk of hypoglycemia from insulin would threaten job performance or be a hazard to others.

Preparations. *Metformin* tablets (0.5 g); sustained-action tablets (0.85 g). *Buformin* tablets (0.05 g); sustained-action tablets (0.1 g).

GLUCAGON

In 1923, 2 years following the discovery of insulin, another pancreatic hormone was discovered by Murlin and coworkers (55). This hormone, glucagon, is looked on by many as a physiological antagonist of insulin. Immunocytochemical techniques employing relatively specific antisera to glucagon have identified α cells of the islets of Langerhans (and those of gastric fundus) as being the glucagon-containing cells. Exocytosis has been demonstrated to occur in pancreatic α cells as it does in β cells, and it is assumed that much, if not all, glucagon is secreted by this process. It is of interest, however, that "immunoreactive glucagon" can be demonstrated in totally depancreatized individuals; this extrapancreatic glucagon may originate from α cells of the gastric fundus or duodenum (39, 73).

Chemistry. Glucagon is a 29-amino acid polypeptide of identical primary structure in all mammalian species studied thus far, with the exception of the guinea pig. The biological activity of glucagon is believed to require the 3 C-terminal residues of this 29-amino acid peptide. This portion of glucagon appears to be necessary for its binding to the receptor site, whereas the N-terminal and perhaps the central portion of the glucagon molecule are involved both in binding to the receptor and in the activation of adenylate cyclase (34).

Pharmacological Effects. Interaction of glucagon with its receptor stimulates the production of cAMP through activation of adenylate cyclase. cAMP, in turn, binds to a regulatory subunit dimer of the cAMP-dependent protein kinase, thereby causing dissociation of two catalytic subunits of the enzyme. As a result, phosphorylase activity and glycogenesis are reduced.

Glucagon promotes gluconeogenesis, possibly through the enzyme pyruvate kinase, which if inhibited by glucagon would promote the formation of pyruvate and thus favor glucose synthesis (62) (Fig. 12.3-2). Glucagon appears to enhance net hepatic uptake of gluconeogenic precursors and increases the intrahepatic shunting of alanine into the gluconeogenic pathway. The gluconeogenic effect of glucagon, like the glycogenolytic effect, is inhibited by insulin (9). Glucagon also has a demonstrated role in ketogenesis. McGarry et al. (51) have proposed a bihormonal mechanism involving reduced insulin and increased levels of glucagon. Low insulin levels increase lipolysis and free fatty acid availability to the liver; in the presence of glucagon, free fatty acids are preferentially directed toward ketogenesis (51).

Glucagon also has a positive inotropic effect on the heart that differs from that of catecholamines, is not blocked by propranolol, and is not accompanied by ventricular irritability or increased peripheral resistance (61). Glucagon increases the release of several hormones including epinephrine (by the adrenal medulla), insulin (by the pancreatic β cells), as well as growth hormone and adrenocorticotropic hormone (ACTH) (by the anterior pituitary). The physiological significance of some of these observations is unclear (73)

Adverse Effects. Nausea and vomiting may occur with the administration of large doses. Hypersensitivity reaction to glucagon can occur, but is very rare.

Therapeutic Uses. Glucagon is used as an adjunct to glucose for treatment of acute hypoglycemic reactions. It is particularly useful when oral or intravenous administration of glucose is not possible. The response is rapid and can occur 5-20 min after its administration; if no response is seen within 25 min, a second dose may be administered. Glucagon and glucose may be administered concomitantly. Because glucagon has a positive inotropic effect on the heart under some circumstances, it has been found to be useful in the treatment of cardiogenic shock and congestive heart failure. Glucagon serves as a stimulus for the release of growth hormone and ACTH from the pituitary. It can also provoke insulin release from the pancreatic β cells for testing purposes. The ability of glucagon to stimulate calcitonin release may be of value in the recognition of medullary carcinoma of the thyroid. Glucagon can also be useful as a diagnostic agent in the detection of pheochromocytomas. An intravenous injection of 0.5-1 mg glucagon will usually provoke a paroxysm of hypertension in more than 90% of the patients with pheochromocytomas. The test appears to be as reliable as histamine and is devoid of the unpleasant flush and headache that usually accompanies the administration of histamine.

Preparation. *Glucagon* is available in lyophilized form (1- and 10-mg ampules) with accompanying solvent. The solution containing 0.5-1 mg of glucagon may be administered intramuscularly or intravenously, and may be repeated, if necessary.

REFERENCES

1. Alberti, K.G.M. and Nattrass, M. Lactic acidosis. *Lancet* 2:25, 1977.
2. Arky, R.A. Nutritional management of the diabetic. In: *Diabetes Mellitus* (Ellenberg, M. and Rifkin, H., eds.). New York: Medical Examination Publishing Co., 1983, p. 539.
3. Aro, A., Korhonen, T. and Halinen, M. Phenformin-induced lactic acidosis precipitated by tetracycline. *Lancet* 1:673, 1978.
4. Banting, F.G. and Best, C.H. The internal secretion of the pancreas. *J. Lab. Clin. Med.* 7:251, 1922.
5. Bennett, P.H. The diagnosis of diabetes: new international classification and diagnostic criteria. *Ann. Rev. Med.* 34:295, 1983.
6. Bunn H.F., Gabbay, K.H. and Gallop, R.M. The glycosylation of hemoglobin relevance to diabetes mellitus. *Science* 200:21, 1978.
7. Butterfield, W.J.H., Fey I.K. and Holling, E. Effects of insulin, tolbutamide, and phenethylbiguanide on peripheral glucose uptake in man. *Diabetes* 7:449, 1958.
8. Chance, R.E., Root, M.A. and Galloway, J.A. The immunogenicity of insulin preparations. *Acta Endocrinol* 83:185, 1976.
9. Claus, T.H. and Pilkis, S.J. Regulation by insulin of gluconeogenesis in isolated hepatocytes. *Biochem. Biophys. Acta* 421:246, 1976.
10. Cohen, A.M. and Shafrir, E. Comparison of free fatty acid and glucose response in diabetic patients treated with phenethylformamidinyliminourea HCl (DBI). *Israel Med. J.* 21:28, 1962.
11. Cook, D.E., Blair, J.B. and Lardy, H.A. Studies with phenethylbiguanide in isolated perfused rat liver. *J. Biol. Chem.* 248:5272, 1973.
12. Craighead, J.E. Current views on the etiology of insulin-dependent diabetes mellitus. *N. Engl. J. Med.* 299:1439, 1978.
13. Crea, R., Kraszewski, A., Hirose, T. and Itakura, K. Chemical synthesis of genes for human insulin. *Proc. Natl. Acad. Sci.* USA 75:5765, 1978.
14. Cudworth, A.G., Gamble, D.R. and While, G.B.B. Aetiology of juvenile-onset diabetes: A prospective study. *Lancet* 1:385, 1977.
15. Czech, M.P. Insulin action. *Am. J. Med.* 70:142, 1981.
16. Czyzyk, A., Tawecke, J., Sadowski, J., Ponikawska, I. and Szezepanik, Z. Effect of biguanides on intestinal absorption of glucose. *Diabetes* 17:492, 1968.
17. De Meyts, P., Roth, J., Neville, D.M., Gavin, J.R., III, and Lesniak, M.A. Insulin interactions with its receptors: experimental evidence for negative cooperativity. *Biochem. Biophys. Res. Commun.* 55:154, 1973.
18. Drash, A.L. The etiology of diabetes mellitus. *N. Engl. J. Med.* 21:1211, 1979.
19. Feinglas, M. and Lebovitz, H. Sulfonylurea treatment in insulin-independent diabetes mellitus. *Metabolism* 29:488, 1980.
20. Feinglas, M. and Lebovitz, H. Sulfonylureas increase the number of insulin receptors. *Nature* 276:184, 1978.
21. Frank, E., Nothmann, M. and Wagner, A. Die Synthalinbehandlung des Diabetes mellitus. *Dtsch. Med. Wochenscher.* 52:2067, 1926.
22. Galloway, J.A. and Bressler, R. Insulin treatment in diabetes. *Med. Clin. North Am.* 62:663, 1978.
23. Galloway, J.A. and deShazo, R.D. The clinical use of insulin and the complications of insulin therapy. In: *Diabetes Mellitus.* (Ellinberg, M. and Rifkin, H., eds.). New York: Medical Examination Publishing Co., 1983, p. 519.
24. Genuth, S. Classification and diagnosis of diabetes mellitus. *Med. Clin. North Am.* 66:1191, 1982.
25. Gepts, W. and Lecompte, P.M. The pancreatic islets in diabetes. *Am. J. Med.* 70:105, 1981.
26. Given, B.D., Mako, M.E., Tager, H. et al. Circulating insulin with reduced biological activity in a patient with diabetes. *N. Engl. J. Med.* 302:129, 1980.
27. Goeddel, D.V., Kleid, D.G., Bolivar, F., Jeuneker, H.L., Yansura, D.G., Crea, R., Hirose, T., Kraszewski, A., Itakura, K. and Riggs, D.A. Expression in *Escherichia coli* of chemically synthesized genes for human insulin. *Proc. Natl. Acad. Sci.* USA 76:106, 1979.
28. Goldfine, I.D. Insulin receptors and the site of action of insulin. *Life Sci.* 23:2639, 1978.
29. Grodsky, G.M. A threshold distribution hypothesis for packet storage of insulin and its mathematical modelling. *J. Clin. Invest.* 51:2047, 1972.
30. Hagg, S.A. Clinical use of oral hypoglycemic agents. *Am. J. Hosp. Pharm.* 33:943, 1976.
31. Himsworth, H.P. and Kerr, R.B. Insulin-sensitive and insulin-insensitive types of diabetes mellitus. *Clin. Sci.* 4:119, 1939.

32. Houslay, M.D. and Heyworth, C.M. Insulin: in search of a mechanism. *Trends Biochem. Sci.* 8:449, 1983.

33. Houssay, B.A. The hypophysis and metabolism. *N. Engl. J. Med.* 214:961, 1936.

34. Hruby, V.J., Wright, D.E., Lin, M.C. and Rodbell, M. Semisynthetic glucagon derivatives for structure-function studies. *Metabolism* (suppl.) 25:1323, 1976.

35. Humblin, T.J. Interaction between warfarin and phenformin. *Lancet* 2:1323, 1971.

36. Janbon, M., Chaptal, J., Vedel, A. and Schaap, J. Accidents hypoglycemiques graves par un sulfamidothiadiazol. *Montepell. Med.* 21:441, 1942.

37. Jeanrenaud, B. Adipose tissue dynamics and regulation, revisited. *Ergeb. Physiol.* 60:57, 1968.

38. Kaldany, A. Autoantibodies to islet cells in diabetes mellitus. *Diabetes* 28:102, 1979.

39. Kobayashi, S., Kujita, T. and Sasagawa, T. The endocrine cells of human duodenal mucosa. *Arch. Histol. Jap.* 31:477, 1970.

40. Koivisto, V.A. and DeFronzo, R.A. Exercise in the treatment of type II diabetes. *Acta. Endocrinol.* (suppl.) 262:107, 1984.

41. Kolata, G.B. Blood sugar and the complications of diabetes. Sugar itself may damage cells. *Science* 203:1098, 1979.

42. Kolata, G.B. Controversy over study of diabetes drugs continues for nearly a decade. *Science* 203:986, 1979.

43. Kolterman, O.G., Reaven, G.M. and Olefsky, J.M. Relationship between *in vivo* insulin resistance and decreased insulin receptors in obese man. *J. Clin. Endocrinol. Metab.* 48:487, 1979.

44. Krall, L.P. and Chabot, V.A. Oral hypoglycemic agent update: Symposium on diabetes mellitus. *Med. Clin. North Am.* 62:681, 1978.

45. Lebovitz, H.E. and Feinglos, M.N. The oral hypoglycemic agents. In: *Diabetes Mellitus.* (Ellenberg, M. and Rifkin, H., eds.). New York: Medical Examination Publishing Co., 1983, p. 591.

46. Leichter, S.B. Oral hypoglycemics: reexamining the controversy. *Drug Ther.* 8:87, 1978.

47. Liljenquist, J.E., Keller, V., Chiasson, J.L. and Cherrington, A.D. Insulin and glucagon actions and consequences of derangements in secretion. In: *Endocrinology* Vol. 2 (De Groot, L.G. et al., eds.). New York: Grune & Stratton, 1979, p. 981.

48. Mackrell, D.J. and Sokal, J.E. Antagonism between the effects of insulin and glucagon on the isolated liver. *Diabetes* 18:724, 1968.

49. Malaisse, W., Malaisse-Lagae, F., Wright, P.H. and Ashmore, J. Effects of adrenergic and cholinergic agents upon insulin secretion *in vitro. Endocrinology* 80:975, 1967.

50. Maugh, T.H. Virus isolated from juvenile diabetic. *Science* 204:1187, 1967.

51. McGarry, J.D., Mannaerts, G.P. and Foster, D.W. A possible role for malonyl-CoA in the regulation of hepatic fatty acid oxidation and ketogenesis. *J. Clin Invest.* 60:265, 1977.

52. Melander, A. and Wahlin-Bhol, E. Clinical pharmacology of oral antidiabetic agents. *Acta Endocrinol.* (suppl.) 262:119, 1984.

53. Merali, Z. and Singhal R.L. Protective effect of selenium on certain hepatotoxic and pancreotoxic manifestations of subacute cadmium administration. *J. Pharmacol. Exp. Ther.* 195:58, 1975.

54. Merali, Z and Singhal R.L. Diabetogenic effects of chronic oral cadmium administration to neonatal rats. *Br. J. Pharmacol.* 69:151, 1980.

55. Murlin, J.R., Clough, H.D., Gibbs, C.B.F. and Stakes, A.M. Aqueous extracts of pancreas. I. Influence on the carbohydrate metabolism of depancreatized animals. *J. Biol. Chem.* 56:253, 1923.

56. National Diabetes Data Group: Classification and diagnosis of diabetes mellitus and other categories of glucose intolerance. *Diabetes* 28:1039, 1979.

57. Nerup, J. HLA studies in diabetes mellitus: a review, *Adv. Metab. Disord.* 9:263, 1978.

58. Olefsky, J.M. and Kolterman, O.G. Mechanisms of insulin resistance in obesity and noninsulin-dependent (type II) diabetes. *Am. J. Med.* 70:151, 1981.

59. Olefsky, J.M. and Reaven, G.M. Effects of sulfonylurea therapy on insulin binding on mononuclear leukocytes of diabetic patients. *Am. J. Med.* 60:89, 1976.

60. Orci, L., Perrelet, A. and Gorden, P. Less understood aspects of the morphology of insulin secretion and binding. *Recent Progr. Horm. Res.* 34:95, 1978.

61. Parmley, W.W. The role of glucagon as a cardiovascular drug. *Drug Ther.* 2:16, 1972.

62. Pilkis, S.J., Claus, T.H., Rion, J.P. and Park, C.R. Possible role of pyruvate kinase in the hormonal control of dihydroxyacetone gluconeogenesis in isolated hepatocytes. *Metabolism* (suppl.) 25:1355, 1976.

63. Raskin, P. and Unger, R.H. Glucagon and diabetes. *Med. Clin. North Am.* 62:713, 1978.

64. Rayfield, E.J. and Seto, Y. Viruses and the pathogenesis of diabetes mellitus. *Diabetes* 27:1126, 1978.

65. Rotter, J.I. and Rimoin, D.L. Heterogeneity in diabetes mellitus. *Diabetes* 27:599, 1978.

66. Rotter, J.I. and Rimion, D.L. The genetics of the glucose intolerance disorders. *Am. J. Med.* 70:117, 1981.

67. Ruttenburg, M.A. Human insulin: Facile synthesis by modification of porcine insulin. *Science* 177:623, 1972.

68. Sanger, F. Chemistry of insulin. *Br. Med. Bull.* 16:183, 1960.

69. Smith, C.K. Current concepts in diabetes mellitus. *J. Fam. Pract.* 16:585, 1983.

70. Steiner, D.F., Kemmler, W., Clark, J.L., Oyer, P.E. and Rubenstein, A.H. The biosynthesis of insulin. In: *Endocrinology*, Vol. 1, *Section 7, Handbook of Physiology* (Steiner, D.F. and Freikel, N., eds.). Washington, D.C.:American Physiological Society, 1972, p. 175.

71. Taft, P. Rational use of oral hypoglycemic drugs. *Drugs* 17:134, 1979.

72. Unger, R.H. and Orci, L. Insulin, glucagon, and somatostatin secretion in the regulation of metabolism. *Ann. Rev. Physiol.* 40:307, 1978.

73. Unger, R.H., Dobbs, R.E. and Orci, L. Physiology and pathophysiology of glucagon. *Physiol. Rev.* 56:778, 1976.

74. Varma, S.D., Mizuno, A. and Kinoshita, J.H. Diabetic cataracts and flavonoids. *Science* 195:205, 1977.

75. von Mering, J. and Minkowski, O. Diabetes mellitus nach pankreas extirpation. *Centralbl. Klin. Med.* 10:393, 1889.

76. Vranic, M., Kemmer, F.W., Berchtold, P., Berger, M. Hormonal interaction in control of metabolism during exercise in physiology and diabetes. In: *Diabetes Mellitus* (Ellenberg, M. and Rifkin, H., eds.). New York: Medical Examination Publishing Co., 1983, p. 567.

77. World Health Organization Expert Committee on Diabetes Mellitus. Second report. *WHO Tech. Rep. Ser.* 646:1, 1980.

78. Wright, A.D., Walsh, C.H., Fitzgerald, M.D. and Malins, J.M. Very pure porcine insulin in clinical practice. *Br. Med. J.* 1:25, 1979.

79. Yoon, J.W., Austin, M., Onodera, T. and Notkins, A.L. Virus-induced diabetes mellitus. *N. Engl. J. Med.* 21:1173, 1979.

ADDITIONAL READING

Asmal, A.C., and Marble, A. Oral hypoglycemic agents. An update. *Drugs* 28:62, 1984.

Hale, P.J., Wright, J.V., and Nattrass, M. Differences in insulin sensitivity between normal men and women. *Metabolism* 34:1133, 1985.

Lebovitz, H.E. Clinical utility of oral hypoglycemic agents in the management of patients with noninsulin-dependent diabetes mellitus. *Am. J. Med.* 75:94, 1983.

Owens, D.R. effects of oral sulfonylureas on the spectrum of defects in noninsulin-dependent diabetes mellitus. *Am. J. Med.* 79:27, 1985.

CHAPTER
12.4

ADRENAL CORTICAL HORMONES

Gordon E. Johnson

The hormones of the adrenal cortex may be divided into three categories: the glucocorticoids, the mineralocorticoids, and the sex homones. The *glucocorticoids* exert major actions on carbohydrate, fat, and protein metabolism and act to modify cardiovascular function and the response to inflammatory stimuli. The *mineralocorticoids* are so named because of their effects on electrolyte and water balance. Many drugs have been synthesized to mimic in part or in whole the effects of the gluco- or mineralocorticoids. These drugs, together with the endogenous hormones, are called *corticosteroids*. They will be the subject of discussion in this chapter. Little will be said concerning the actions of the sex hormones, as they are discussed separately in Chapters 12.6 and 12.7.

SYNTHESIS AND RELEASE

The biosynthesis of the adrenal cortical hormones is described in Fig. 12.4-1. Although many steroids are synthesized in the adrenal cortex, the only steroids secreted in physiologically significant amounts are the glucocorticoids cortisol and corticosterone, the mineralocorticoid aldoosterone in its hemiacetal form, and the androgen dehydroepiandrosterone. The secretion of cortisol in humans is approximately sevenfold that of corticosterone. Corticosterone possesses about 30% of the glucocorticoid activity of cortisol but is many times more potent as a mineralocorticoid. Desoxycorticosterone is a mineralocorticoid with approximately the same quantities as aldosterone, its physiological effect on electrolyte metabolism is usually not significant. In disease conditions in which its secretion is markedly increased, the effects of desoxycorticosterone can be significant.

Regulation of Glucocorticoid Release

Hypothalamic and pituitary secretions control the release of cortisol from the adrenal cortex. The immediate stimulus to the release of cortisol is the secretion of adrenocorticotrophic hormone (ACTH) from the pituitary; the pituitary release of ACTH itself is controlled by corticotrophin-releasing factor (CRF) secreted by the hypothalamus and transported by the portal venous system of the hypothalamic-pituitary stalk to the anterior pituitary. Evidence of the importance of the hypothalamus to glucocorticoid secretion can be found in the fact that stress-induced activation of the pituitary-adrenal axis is reduced by hypothalamic lesions. Transposition of the anterior pituitary from its immediate proximity to the hypothalamus of the anterior chamber of the eye or the kidney reduces the concentration of CRF in the pituitary and significantly lowers adrenal weight and adrenal ascorbic acid concentration.

A rise in blood ACTH levels results in increased cortisol synthesis followed quickly by an increased release. Corticosteroids are not stored in the adrenal. The rate-limiting step in the synthesis of adrenocortical hormones is the conversion of cholesterol to pregnenolone. ACTH reacts with a specific hormone receptor of the adrenal cell plasma membrane, thereby stimulating adenylate cyclase activity. The resulting rise in cylic adenosine monophosphate (cAMP) increases the synthesis of pregnenolone and the adrenocortical hormones.

A major factor controlling the release of ACTH and cortisol is the circulating level of glucocorticoids. High levels of cortisol or synthetic glucocorticoids depress CRF and ACTH release. The ability of cortisol released from the adrenal to reduce the subsequent secretion of glucocorticoids maintains systemic levels in the normal physiological range. The feedback mechanism is counterproductive, however, in patients treated with large doses of glucocorticoids for periods in excess of 2 weeks. Hypothalamic-pituitary-adrenal function is depressed in these individuals, and several months free of exogenous corticoste-

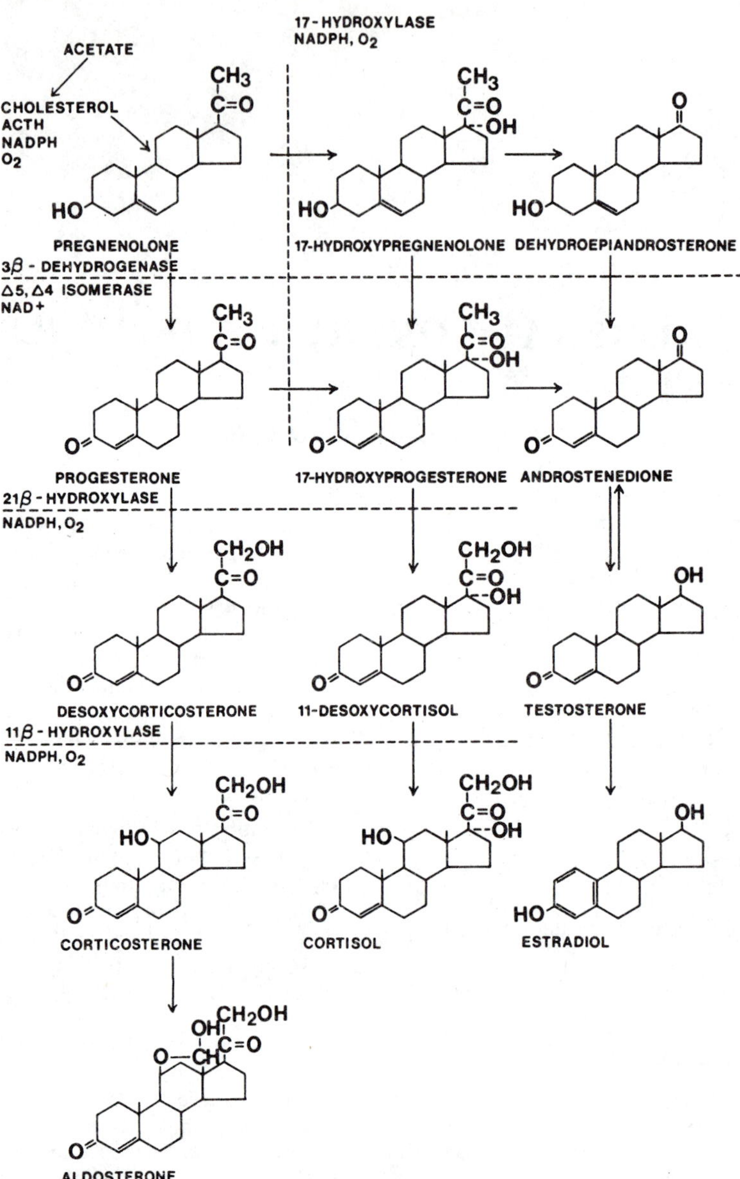

Fig.12.4-1. *Pathways for the synthesis of the adrenal steroids.*

roids may be required before the capacity of the adrenal cortex to secrete cortisol returns to normal.

Stress increases the release of glucocorticoids. Blood levels of ACTH increase rapidly, reaching a maximum about 2 minutes after encountering stress (40). Patients with Addison's disease or those treated for prolonged periods with high-dose glucocorticoid therapy, are unable to increase adrenocortical secretion during times of trauma, surgery, or infection, are less tolerant to stress, and may develop signs of adrenal insufficiency. In these circumstances, supplemental glucocorticoid treatment may be required.

A diurnal variation in the release of both ACTH and cortisol is apparent under normal physiological conditions. Responding to commensurate changes in circulating ACTH, high blood levels of cortisol are found in the early morning hours (10-25 μg cortisol/ 100 ml of blood at about 6:00 a.m.) and low levels in the late evening (5 μg cortisol/ 100 ml of blood by midnight) (50). Sleeping patterns play an important role in the diurnal variation. For example, individuals who work from 12 o'clock midnight to 8:00 a.m. and sleep throughout the day show peak levels of plasma cortisol just after arising (4:00 p.m.) and low levels just prior to retiring (9:00 a.m.).

Central neurotransmitters have also been implicated in the release of CRF, ACTH, and the subsequent synthesis and secretion of adrenocortical hormones. However, the involvement of such chemicals as acetylcholine, 5-hydroxytryptamine, noradrenaline, and dopamine in ACTH secretion is far from clear. It has been suggested that cholinergic and serotonergic mechanisms are involved in the circadian rhythm of ACTH, whereas stress responsiveness may have cholinergic and adrenergic or dopaminergic components.

Regulation of Mineralocorticoid Release

The secretion of aldosterone by the zona glomerulosa cells of the adrenal cortex is influenced by the renin-angiotensin system, plasma potassium levels, and the concentration of ACTH in plasma (17). Acting primarily on the distal convoluted tubules and collecting ducts of the kidney, aldosterone promotes sodium reabsorption in exchange for the secretion of potassium and hydrogen ions. In response to a decrease in renal artery pressure or plasma sodium or to sympathetic stimulation, the justaglomerular apparatus of the kidney secretes renin, which acts on a plasma substrate to produce first angiotensin I and subsequently angiotensin II. The latter is a potent vasoconstrictor and stimulus to aldosterone production. Following an increase in sodium and water reabsorption and potassium excretion, plasma aldosterone concentrations return to lower levels.

Hyperkalemia increases aldosterone secretion and hypokalemia reduces its release. The ability of potassium to stimulate aldosterone secretion is independent of the renin-angiotensin system.

During periods of stress, ACTH may stimulate the secretion of aldosterone. An example of this may be found in a study in which adrenal venous blood was collected from four conscious sheep immediately after acute jugular venous cannulation (11). Major fluctuations in cortisol and aldosterone secretion usually occurred concomitantly, whereas only small changes in plasma potassium and angiotensin were measured. Increased aldosterone is not sustained, however, by prolonged periods of elevated ACTH secretion. In patients with Cushing's syndrome, due to excess ACTH, aldosterone levels are usually normal or low. This may be due to decreased renin secretion in response to an initial sodium retention (19).

Aldosterone secretion exhibits a diurnal flucutation, being higher in the day and lower during the night. Posture is important in this regard, as the recumbent position is associated with lower serum aldosterone levels. Body position is not the only factor determining diurnal variation in aldosterone secretion, however. Subjects kept asleep for long periods of time also demonstrated slight variations in aldosterone production. Time of food consumption may also be important. Fruit eaten at night, instead of the usual times during the day, has been reported to eliminate the diurnal variation in plasma aldosterone levels, plasma renin activity, and urinary electrolytes.

EFFECTS OF GLUCOCORTICOIDS

Glucocorticoids produce a variety of effects. They influence not only the intermediary metabolism of carbohydrates, fats, and proteins but also salt and water balance. In supraphysiologic doses, glucocorticoids have marked anti-inflammatory and immunosuppressive effects. All tissues are not equally sensitive to the effects of glucocorticoids. Tissues with high concentrations of glucocorticoid receptors are more responsive than tissues with few receptors (Table 12.4-1)

Metabolic Effects. The metabolic actions of glucocorticoids are complex and involve both anabolic and catabolic effects. An overview of the metabolic effects of glucocorticoids is presented in Fig. 12.4-2. Glucose utilization is reduced and its synthesis increased. Evidence of the decreased utilization is seen in the reduced uptake of glucose into adipose tissue, skin, fibroblasts, and lymphoid tissue within 30 minutes of administration. The catabolic actions of glucocorticoids on fat and muscle increase the blood levels of free fatty acids, glycerol, and amino acids. Gluconeogenesis is increased. In addition to their catabolic actions on muscle, glucocorticoids reduce amino acid uptake into this tissue. The increased blood amino acid levels resulting from the antianabolic and catabolic effects of glucocorticoids stimulate the secretion of glucagon, which further accelerates hepatic glucose output (45). The increased levels of free fatty acids in the plasma provide an energy source, thereby conserving glucose as well as possibly inhibiting glucose uptake and utilization.

Table 12.4-1
Glucocorticoid-Responsive Tissue

A. *With specific glucocorticoid receptors*	
Brain	Fibroblasts
Heart	Intestine
Liver	Kidney
Lymphoid	Lung
Retina	Skeletal muscle
Smooth muscle	Stomach
Testes	
B. *With low concentrations of, or no detectable specific glucocorticoid receptor*	
Bladder	Uterus
Prostate	Seminal vesicle
Steroid-resistant fibroblasts	Steroid-resistant lymphoid cells

Source: From Ref. 2, with the permission of the authors and Dun-Donnelley Publishing Corp. Data obtained from various animal and red cell culture preparations.

Effects on Specific Tissues. *Liver.* In response to glucocorticoid stimulation, the liver hypertrophies and total protein content as well as RNA synthesis is increased. The two major metabolic actions of glucocorticoids in the liver are an increase in gluconeogenesis and glycogen deposition. Consistent with the metabolic complexity of the glucocorticoids, several factors are responsible for the increase in glycogen deposition (6, 16). Glucocorticoids stimulate glycogen synthesis from uridine-diphosphoglucose via glucose-l-phosphate. In addition, the hyperglycemia produced by glucocorticoids inactivates phosphorylase A, and stimulates the release of insulin, which in turn increases glycogen synthetase activity.

Adipose Tissue. Glucocorticoids also have lipolytic actions. They increase the release of glycerol and free fatty acids from adipose tissue, decrease glucose uptake, and lower free fatty acid production. These direct effects may be offset, in part, by insulin, which stimulates lipogenesis and inhibits lipolysis. The consequence of the antagonism between glucocorticoids and insulin is a redistribution of fat with steroid action predominating in areas of fat loss and insulin effects in regions of fat accumulation. A clinical manifestation of this is seen in the characteristic moon face and centripetal redistribution of fat observed following prolonged treatment with supraphysiological doses of glucocorticoids.

Muscle. As mentioned earlier, glucocorticoids are both antianabolic and catabolic on muscle. The decrease in

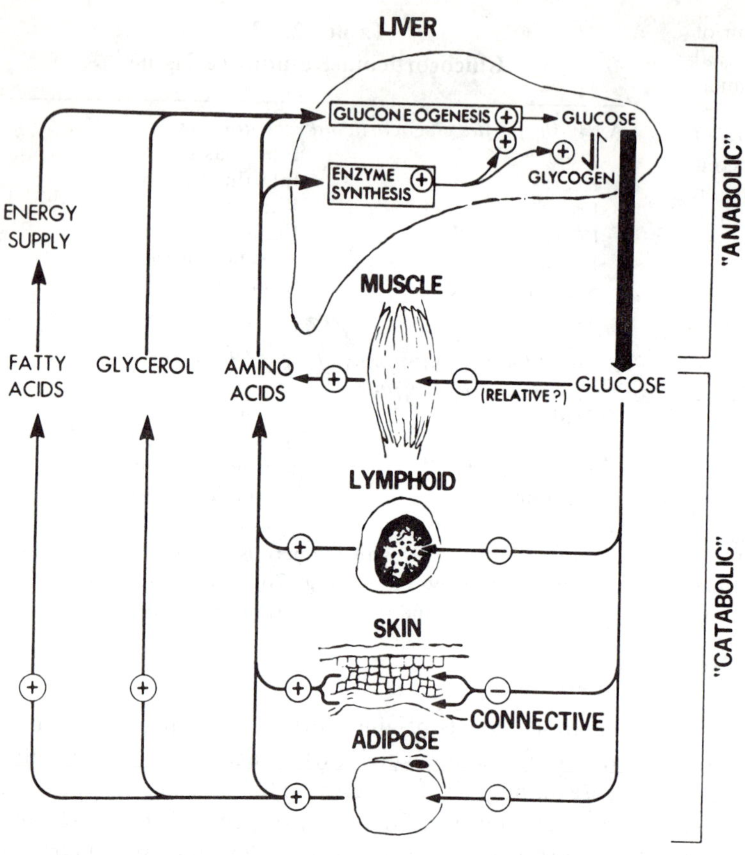

Fig. 12.4-2. *Glucocorticoid action on carbohydrate, lipid, and protein metabolism.* Arrows indicate the general flow of substrate in response to the catabolic and anabolic actions of glucocorticoids when unopposed by secondary secretions of other hormones. Not shown is increased gluconeogenesis by the kidney. The+ and - signs indicate stimulation and inhibition, respectively. (From. Ref. 2, with the permission of the authors and Dun-Donnelley Publishing Corp.).

glucose uptake and amino acid incorporation in muscle proteins, together with the increased rate of amino acid loss from muscle into blood (6), results in muscle wasting and myopathy when high doses of glucocorticoids are administered for prolonged periods.

Blood. Glucocorticoids increase neutrophils and thrombocytes in blood and decrease the numbers of circulating lymphocytes, eosinophils, and basophils. Both erythrocyte volume and hemoglobin mass are increased by glucocorticoids. Cushing's syndrome results in polycythemia with increased red cell precursors in marrow. Addison's disease, on the other hand, results in decreased red cell production. In this condition the resulting normochromic, normocytic anemia may be masked by hemoconcentration.

Skeleton and Bone. Glucocorticoids reduce the intestinal absorption of calcium, as a result of vitamin D antagonism, and increase the urinary clearance of the mineral. These effects, together with a steroid-induced reduction in the bone surface on which calcium might be deposited (2), lead to osteoporosis during long-term glucocorticoid therapy.

Cardiovascular System. The effects of glucocorticoids on the cardiovasculr system are complex and depend to a great extent on the state of adrenal function at the time of treatment. Glucocorticoids have a direct myocardial stimulant effect; their administration to normal individuals increases cardiac output and decreases total peripheral resistance (8). This action, together with the expansion of blood volume due to mineralocorticoid effects, increases glomerular filtration rate. In contrast, the acute administration of a glucocorticoid to patients with adrenal insufficiency decreases cardiac output and increases arterial pressure.

Further evidence for the complexity of glucocorticoid actions on the cardiovascular system may be seen in the fact that, although hypertension has been noted in 80-85% of patients suffering from Cushing's syndrome, the incidence of hypertension in patients treated with corticosteroids ranges from 4 to 25% (8). This may be simply a matter of a higher steroid level in the Cushingoid patient. The incidence of hypertension in patients treated with glucocorticoids appears to be related to the dose of steroid and the duration of therapy as well as to the presence of renal disease. The presence or absence of hypertension prior to steroid therapy does not appear to be a factor in the development of high blood pressure.

Central Nervous System. Glucocorticoids affect the central nervous system, although the mechanisms by which they influence brain function is not clear. The effects of the steroids include insomnia and increased fluctuations in mood, varying from depression to mania. Glucocorticoid receptors have been identified in several areas of the brain, with the highest concentrations being found in the hippocampus, amygdala, and cortex (42). Whether the effects of glucocorticoids on brain function result from their interaction with receptors or are secondary to metabolic changes is not known. Adrenal insufficiency is often accompanied by abnormalities in the electroencephalogram together with apathy, negativism, and inability to concentrate. Periods of drowsiness alternating with restlessness may also be observed (2).

Anti-inflammatory and Immunosuppressive Effects. Glucocorticoids owe much of their therapeutic usefulness to their marked anti-inflammatory effects. These actions are nonspecific and can be directed against inflammatory response to immunologically mediated disorders as well as to mechanical or chemical injury, or infection (44). Anti-inflammatory and immunosuppressive response to corticosteroids correlate with glucocorticoid potency. In developing new corticosteroids for the treatment of inflammatory disorders, efforts are made to design drugs with marked glucocorticoid and minimal mineralocorticoid effects.

Corticosteroids possess several pharmacological properties that contribute to their anti-inflammatory effects. The stabilization of lysosomal membranes within leukocytes and monocytes by glucocorticoids has been taken by many as an explanation of the anti-inflammatory effects of these drugs (4, 6, 9). However, the concentrations of corticosteroids required to produce this effect are beyond the normal therapeutic levels; therefore, alternate explanations must be sought.

Glucocorticoids modify both the vascular and cellular responses to inflammation. They decrease capillary permeability and increase the vasoconstrictor responsiveness to circulating catecholamines. By opposing the increases in capillary permeability produced by kinins and histamine, glucocorticoids reduce edema, caused by the leakage of protein and fluid into areas of injury, and decrease the initial inflammatory reaction.

A reduction in the migration of polymorphonuclear cells into areas of inflammation accompanies glucocorticoid treatment. The suppression of leukocyte accumulation at an affected site is important in reducing inflammation. This effect is a result of the decrease in capillary permeability and an alteration of the surface of granulocytes, which reduces their migration to sites of inflammation (14).

The administration of glucocorticoids results in a lymphocytopenia, involving primarily the T lymphocytes, and a decrease in the mass of lymphoid tissue (61). The lymphocytopenia produced by glucocorticoid treatment results from a redistribution of the recirculating lymphocytes from the circulation to other body compartments (13, 14, 61). As a result, the body is less able to respond to immunological challenge (Fig. 12.4-3).

Corticosteroid treatment results in an acute peripheral monocytopenia, probably due to a delayed release of bone marrow precursors and the disappearance of mature monocytes from the peripheral circulation (14). Glucocorticoids inhibit the response of macrophages to several chemotactic factors (Table 12.4-2), including a direct antagonism of the effects of the macrophage migration-inhibitory factor and the macrophage-aggregating factor (14). The clearance of both opsonized and nonopsonized material by the reticuloendothelial system is reduced by glucocorticoids (1). On the basis of *in vitro* evidence, it has also been suggested that glucocorticoids depress the bactericidal and fungicidal activity of macrophages (54).

Glucocorticoids interfere with the early stages of inflammation by reducing fibrin deposition, and the later manifestations of inflammation by minimizing capillary and fibroblast proliferation as well as the deposition of collagen and cicatrization. These drugs also assist in the maintenance of the integrity of the cell membrane and reduce the intracellular transfer of water that accompanies a local inflammatory response.

The use of glucocorticoids to treat inflammatory conditions is a double-edged sword. The suppression of inflammation may afford considerable relief or even prove lifesaving. By removing the signs of inflammation, however, conditions having an infectious origin may deteriorate without displaying appropriate symptoms to alert the physician. With a reduced immunological capability, patients on long-term high-dose corticosteroid treatment regimens are at a greater risk with respect to infections.

EFFECTS OF MINERALOCORTICOIDS

The actions of mineralocorticoids are mainly on the distal convoluted tubules and collecting ducts of the kidney to promote the reabsorption of sodium ions and the secretion of potassium and hydrogen. The increased secretion of aldosterone in hypercorticism produces a

Table 12.4-2
Soluble Mediators of Cell-Mediated Immunity Recognized to be Affected by Corticosteroids

Factors	Effects
Macrophage migration inhibitory factor	Localizes and (?) "activates" macrophages
Macrophage-aggregating factor	Same effect as macrophage migration-inhibitory factor (?)
Monocyte chemotactic factor	Attracts monocytes to inflammatory sites
Skin-reactive factor	Produces delayed hypersensitivity skin test in nonimmune subject
Lymphotoxin	Inhibits metabolism and growth of cellular targets

Source: From Ref. 14, with permission of the authors and the publisher.

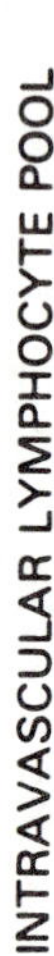

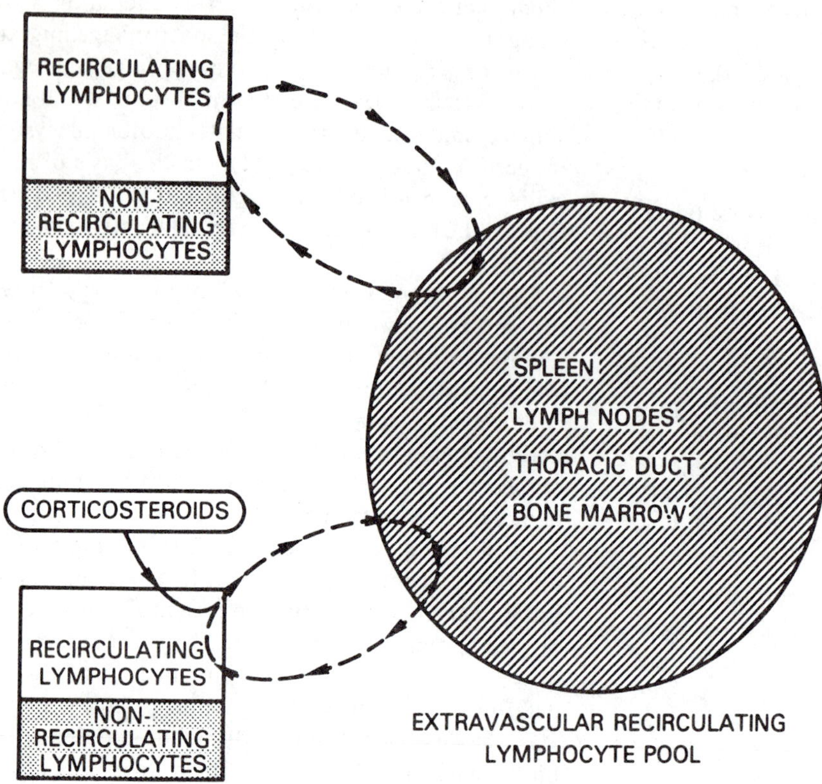

Fig. 12.4-3. *Schematic representation of the proposed mechanism of corticosteroid-induced lympho cytopenia.*

The equilibrium between the intravascular and extravascular portions of recirculating lymphocyte pool is affected by corticosteroid administration, so that the intravascular recirculating lymphocytes are depleted from the circulation and accumulate in the extravascular compartments of the recirculating lymphocyte pool. (From Ref. 14, with the permission of the authors and the publisher).

positive sodium balance and an expansion of the extracellular fluid volume. Sodium concentration in the plasma may remain normal or be slightly elevated. Hypokalemia and alkalosis are seen in about 20% of patients with Cushing's syndrome. In primary adrenal insufficiency, hyponatremia, hyperkalemia, and a contraction of the extracellular fluid volume occur. Water shifts from the extracellular into the intracellular compartment and cellular hydration takes place. In response to the reduced secretion of potassium and hydrogen ions, systemic acidosis may be seen. Under these conditions, appropriate therapeutic action, in the form of mineralocorticoids and/or sodium chloride, must be taken to prevent circulatory collapse, renal failure, and death.

Aldosterone-induced kaliuresis is dependent to a large extent on the presence of sodium; thus, it is not produced if the diet is totally lacking in sodium. In spite of the requirement for sodium in the distal convoluted tubule, evidence indicates that sodium reabsorption can change independently of potassium secretion. After several days of treatment, the kidney may "escape" from the sodium-retaining effects of a mineralocorticoid but not its kaliuretic action. Sodium escape is dependent on an expanded effective blood volume. Despite high aldosterone secretion, in subjects with low effective blood volumes, as in patients with congestive heart failure or cirrhosis with ascites and nephrosis, sodium escape does not occur.

The property of mineralocorticoids to retain sodium and lose potassium is also manifested in extrarenal tissues. Saliva and sweat show decreased sodium content and increased potassium levels following mineralocorticoid stimulation. Mineralocorticoids also cause decreased sodium and increased potassium content of stools.

SUBCELLULAR MECHANISM OF ACTION OF GLUCOCORTICOIDS AND MINERALOCORTICOIDS

Mineralocorticoids and glucocorticoids demonstrate the same general pattern of subcellular action (Fig. 12.4-4). After diffusing into cells, the drugs bind in a stereospecific manner to receptors in the cytoplasm with molecular weights between 50,000 and 150,000. Thereafter, the hormone (drug)-receptor complex enters the nucleus to produce its effects. The location of glucocorticoid receptors was described earlier (Table 12.4-1). Aldosterone receptors have been found in the renal nuclei. The aldosterone antagonist spironolactone blocks binding of aldosterone in the cytosol and nuclear fractions of rat kidney (12). In the absence of receptors, corticosteroids exert little activity.

The formation of the steroid-receptor complex stimulates new transcription of both mRNA and rRNA, a process essential to the physiological/pharmacological effects of the corticosteroids. Inhibitors of transcription (actinomycin D) or translation (cycloheximide) block chromatin template activity as well as precursor incorporation into RNA in steroid-exposed tissues (15). The formation of new protein by glucocorticoids has been demonstrated in liver, hepatoma cells, brain, retina, pancreas, mammary glands, lymphocytes, thymocytes, and fibroblasts. The physiological or pharmacological effects of the corticosteroids are mediated by the newly formed protein (15).

As might be expected from the preceding description of the subcellular mechanism of corticosteroid action, a latent period of at least 1 hour exists before the effect of the steroid can be

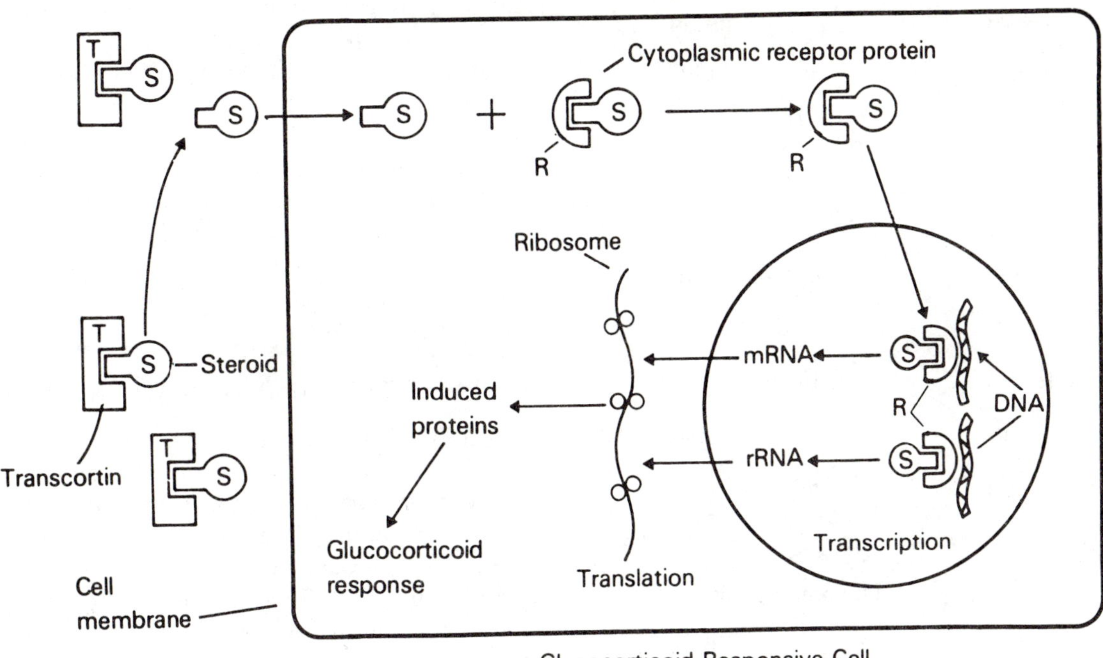

Fig. 12.4-4. *Schematic representation of the mechanism of action of glucocorticoids. (From Ref. 57, with the permission of the authors and ADIS Press).*

detected. Once the tissue has been stimulated, the effect will continue for some time after the steroid is removed. A more complete discussion of this topic can be found in the excellent reviews of Feldman et al. (15), Baxter and Forsham (2), and Fauci et al. (14).

SYNTHETIC CORTICOSTEROIDS

The introduction of cortisol as a drug provided a major therapeutic advance. However, since cortisol possesses significant mineralocorticoid actions, new steroids have been synthesized with the aim of accentuating glucocorticoid activity and reducing or abolishing mineralocorticoid properties.

Chemical groups essential to the anti-inflammatory or glucocorticoid activity of steroids are given in Fig. 12.4-5. Alteration in any of these groups results in loss of glucocorticoid activity. Cortisone is inactive itself and depends for its activity on *in vivo* metabolism to cortisol (Fig. 12.4-6). Herzog and coworkers (26) demonstrated that the introduction of a 1, 2-double bond into cortisone or cortisol increased glucocorticoid and anti-inflammatory potency approximately fourfold while reducing mineralocorticoid activity. The newly formed steroids were called prednisone and prednisolone, respectively. Prednisone must be metabolized to prednisolone to exert a pharmacological effect. Introduction of a halogen in the 9α-position increases glucocorticoid potency approximately eightfold (6), and mineralocorticoid potency several hundred times. The dramatic increase in mineralocorticoid activity mitigates against the use of the 9α-halogen derivatives as anti-inflammatory agents. 9α-Fluorocortisol (fludrocortisone) is used systemically as a mineralocorticoid. Subsequent studies revealed that 16α-hydroxy, 16α-methyl, or 16β-methyl groups eliminated the mineralocorticoid activity of 9α-fluorocortisol while leaving its glucocorticoid potency unchanged (10). The result of this research was the synthesis of triamcinolone, dexamethasone, and betamethasone, which possess 5-30 times the anti-inflammatory potency of cortisol and have minimal mineralocorticoid effects.

Two other structural modifications bear mention. The α-methyl and 6α-fluorine derivatives of prednisolone (methylprednisolone and paramethasone, respectively) have greater anti-iflammatory potency than the parent steroid.

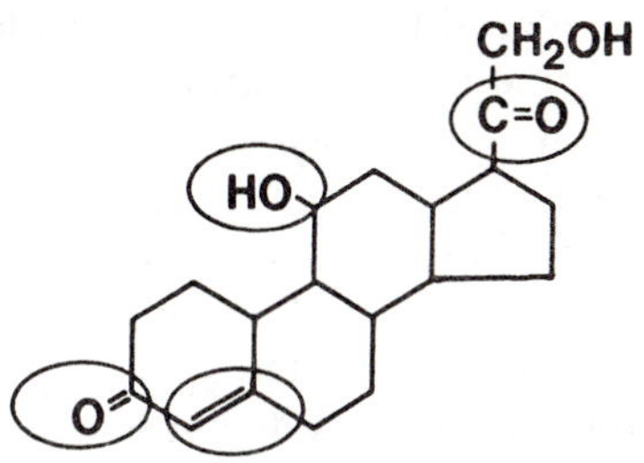

Fig. 12.4-5. *Steroid structure with groups essential to glucocorticoid activity circled.*

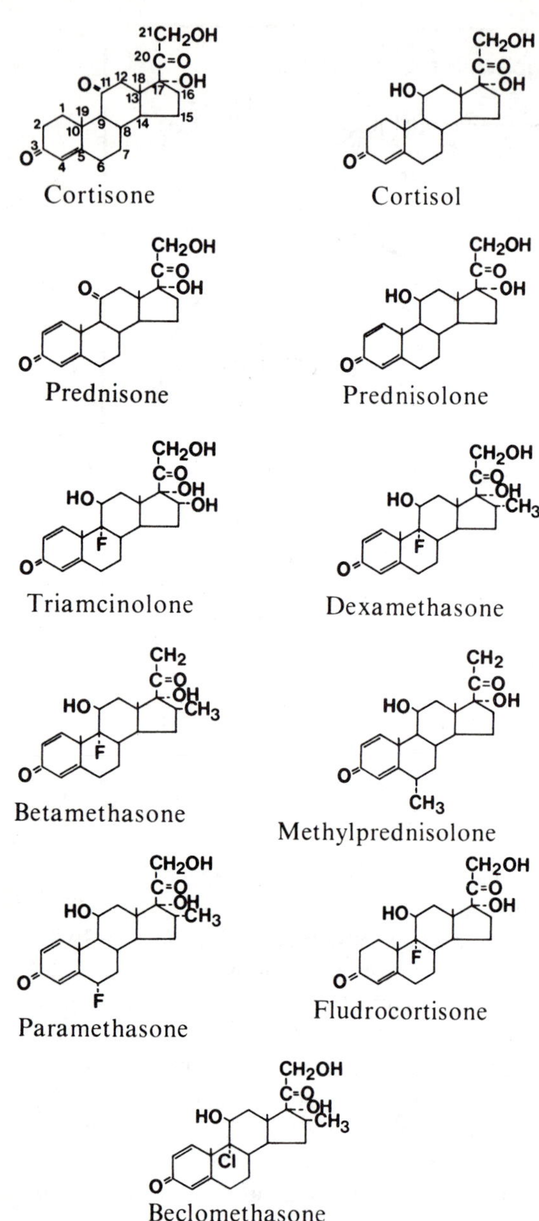

Fig. 12.4-6. *Structures of cortisone, cortisol, and their synthetic derivatives.*

The synthetic steroids differ from cortisol with respect to plasma protein binding and duration of action. Cortisol is extensively bound to plasma proteins with 80% attached to a high-affinity, low-capacity α_2-globulin called transcortin- or corticosteroid-binding globulin. An additional 10% of the cortisol in plasma is bound to albumin. The synthetic corticosteroids are less extensively bound to transcortin and albumin, and can diffuse more readily into tissue (57).

The corticosteroids are extensively metabolized, with reduction in ring A, reduction of the ketone at C-20, or cleavage of the side chain representing the major biotransformation; metabolites appear in the urine unconjugated or as glucuronides or sulfates. Although the plasma half-life of cortisol is 90 min (57), its biological half-life is from 8 to 12 hours. The synthetic corticosteroids are metabolized more slowly. Prednisone, prednisolone, methylprednisolone, and triamcinolone have biological half-lives between 18 and 36 hours and are classified as intermediate-acting steroids. Betamethasone and dexamethasone are considered long-acting steroids, with biological half-lives between 36 and 54 hours. The properties of several glucocorticoids are compared in Table 12.4-3.

THERAPEUTIC USE OF CORTICOSTEROIDS

REPLACEMENT THERAPY

Corticosteroids may be administered as replacement therapy in primary or secondary adrenal insufficiency. Primary adrenal insufficiency is characterized by inadequate cortisol production, in spite of the presence of large quantities of ACTH. The most frequent cause of Addison's disease is idiopathic atrophy of the adrenal glands, which results in a deficiency of both cortisol and aldosterone. Treatment for this condition involves the use of both a glucocortoid and a mineralocorticoid. An appropriate dosage regimen for the treatment of Addison's disease is 20 mg/day of cortisol and 0.1 mg/day of 9α-fluorocortisol.

Congenital adrenal hyperplasia (adrenogenital syndrome) results from enzyme deficiencies in the synthesis of cortisol. As a result of the low cortisol levels, ACTH secretion is increased, which elevates the synthesis and secretion of androgenically active steroids (Fig. 12.4-1). Evidence of the condition in the female is often seen at birth as masculinization of the external genitalia, whereas diagnosis of the adrenogenital syndrome in males may not be made until later in infancy or in childhood. Depending on the location of the enzymatic block, either salt loss or hypertension may accompany the adrenogenital syndrome. The most common form of the condition involves a deficiency in the C-21 hydroxylating enzyme, with a reduction in both glucocorticoids and mineralocorticoids. If the deficiency of aldosterone is sufficient, salt loss is seen and replacement must involve both gluco- and mineralocorticoids. Several dosage schedules have been suggested. In one, doses of 0.6 mg/kg day or cortisol are given in four equal doses, together with 0.05-0.1 mg/day of 9α-fluorocortisol acetate. Another protocol suggests a total daily dose of prednisone for an adult of 7.5-10 mg, with 50% of the dose given at bedtime and the remaining 50% divided equally between breakfast and supper. The rationale for the larger dose at bedtime is to suppress the nighttime increase in ACTH. In this regimen, 0.1 mg of 9α-fluorocortisol is also administered each morning. Regardless of the treatment protocol, doses of glucocorticoids should be adjusted to keep the 17-keto steroid excretion fully suppressed. If the block in steroid synthesis involves the C-11 hydroxylat-

Table 12.4-3
Adrenal Corticosteroid Preparations

Drug	Anti-inflammatory	Equivalent Potency[a] (mg)	Sodium-Retaining Potency	Daily Dose (mg) above which HPA Axis Suppression Possible[b]		Plasma Half-Life (min)	Biological Half-Life(hr)
				Males	Females		
Cortisol (hydrocortisone)	1	20	2+	20-30	15-25	90	8-12
Cortisone	0.8	25	2+	25-35	20-30	90	8-12
Prednisone	3.5	5	1+	7.5-10	7.5	200 or >	18-36
Prednisolone	4	5	1+	7.5-10	7.5	200 or >	18-36
Methylprednisolone	5	4	0	7.5-10	7.5	200 or >	18-36
Triamcinolone	5	4	0	7.5-10	7.5	200 or >	18-36
Paramethasone	10	2	0	2.5-5	2.5-5	300 or >	36-54
Betamethasone	25	0.6	0	1-1.5	1-1.5	300 or >	36-54
Dexamethasone	30	0.75	0	1-1.5	1-1.5	300 or >	36-54

[a] Potency is defined as a milligram for milligram equivalence with hydrocortisone.
[b] Intended as a guide only. The dose in an individual depends on total body surface area. The figures quoted are those that apply in general. HPA = hypothalamic-pituitary-adrenal.
Source: From Ref. 57, with the permission of the authors and ADIS Press.

ing step, greatly increased quantities of the mineralocorticoid 11-desoxycorticosterone are secreted. Under these conditions, hypertension can occur. Glucocorticoid therapy will reduce ACTH secretion and decrease the synthesis and release of 11-desoxycorticosterone and androgens.

Adrenal insufficiency secondary to pituitary insufficiency is characterized by low levels of both ACTH and cortisol. Aldosterone secretion is normal. Treatment involves replacement of the missing cortisol. Thirty-five to forty mg of cortisone or 20 to 25 mg of cortisol can be givn daily. The normal diurnal secretion of cortisol will be simulated if appropriately two-thrids of the daily dose is taken on arising in the morning and the remaining one-third around 4:00 p.m.

In patients requiring continuous steroid replacement therapy, acute adrenal insufficiency may occur if the dose of glucocorticoid is not increased during times of acute stress. Symptoms of acute adrenal insufficiency include anorexia, nausea, vomiting, dehydration, weakness, lethargy, tachycardia, and hypotension. Prompt treatment with cortisol (hemisuccinate or phosphate) i.v. is required. A bolus dose of 100 mg followed by a continuous infusion at a rate of 10-15 mg/hour is recommended (57). Glucocorticoids are essential to restore circulatory competence when shock has supervened.

SUPPRESSIVE THERAPY

Corticosteroids are used in numerous situations because of their anti-inflammatory or immunosuppressive effects. When used for the latter, corticosteroids are given either on a short-term high-dose, a long-term low-dose, or a long-term high-dose regimen.

Glucocorticoids may be used on a short-term high-dose basis for the treatment of medical emergencies, such as status asthmaticus and anaphylactic shock. Following a 48 to 72 hour course of intensive steroid treatment, the dosage either may be reduced rapidly or withdrawn abruptly, assuming the clinical condition has shown dramatic improvement. Used in this way, pituitary-adrenal suppression does not occur and other complications are relatively minor.

High-dose prednisone therapy, 2 mg/kg/day, for 1 month out of 4 months, for the treatment of leukemia in children is also followed by rapid recovery of the adrenal cortex (33).

Long-term low-dose corticosteroid therapy may be used with other forms of treatment in chronic conditions, such as rheumatoid arthritis. A dose of 2-10 mg of prednisone daily may be possible when the object of treatment is to relieve symptoms not associated with life-threatening conditions. The adverse effects of this dosage regimen are not as severe as if high-dose therapy is employed.

Conditions such as autoimmune hemolytic anemia and temporal arteritis require long-term high-dose glucocorticoid treatment. Glucocorticoids used in this manner are most likely to produce systemic toxicity. Patients requiring 75 mg of cortisol or equivalent doses of a synthetic steroid daily for more than 2 weeks will demonstrate pituitary-adrenal suppression. A gradual tapering of the dose will be required when steroid treatment is withdrawn because abrupt discontinuance of steroid therapy may produce acute adrenal insufficiency. When high-dose long-term glucocorticoid therapy is indicated, alternate-day treatment should be instituted when possible to reduce the incidence of adverse effects.

Alternate-Day Therapy. The concept of alternate-day steroid therapy was devised to minimize the consequences of chronic high-dose glucocorticoid treatment. Patients are started on daily corticosteroid therapy until relief is obtained. Thereafter, they can be converted gradually to an alternate-day regimen by doubling the daily glucocorticoid dose and administering it as a single dose on alternate mornings. Prednisone is an intermediate-acting corticosteroid with a biological half-life of 18 to 36 hours.

If administered on alternate mornings, its anti-inflammatory properties will be maintained for approximately 1.5 days. Hypothalamic-pituitary-adrenal responsiveness should return during the last 12 hours prior to the next dose.

The general principles involved in alternate-day therapy are as follows (57):

1. Use intermediate-acting steroids, such as prednisone or prednisolone. Long-acting steroids are not appropriate for alternate-day treatment.
2. Give the total daily dose as a single morning dose as soon as possible.
3. As soon as possible, move to an alternate-day treatment regimen by giving a 2-day dose every 48 hours and eliminating steroid therapy on the off day.

It may be necessary, if the disease suddenly worsens, to revert to daily steroid treatment. The complications of systemic lupus erythematosus, such as nephritis, thrombocytopenic purpura, and CNS involvement, may not respond to alternate-day therapy. Polymyositis, polymyalgia rheumatica and temporal arteritis, and severe rheumatoid arthritis generally do not respond well to alternate-day glucocorticoid treatment. Alternate-day corticosteroid therapy is controversial in renal transplant recipients (59).

Withdrawal of Glucocorticoid Therapy. If supraphysiological doses of glucocorticoids are used for longer than 2 weeks, suppression of the hypothalamic-pituitary-adrenal axis may persist for as long as 9-12 months. Following the cessation of steroid therapy, plasma levels of cortisol and ACTH remain low. Plasma levels of ACTH are the first to return toward normal over a period of several months. The return of plasma cortisol to normal levels may follow ACTH by an additional few months. Complete recovery from the effects of long-term glucocorticoid therapy can be assumed only when plasma cortisol levels rise into the normal range.

Withdrawal from glucocorticoid therapy should be gradual to avoid an acute adrenal crisis. The first step is to administer the total daily dose on a once-a-day basis. Thereafter, the dose can be decreased gradually to physiological levels. For example, cortisol can be administered as a single 20-mg dose every morning and then reduced by 2.5 mg/day once a week until the total daily dose is 10 mg. Because cortisol is a short-acting steroid, plasma cortisol levels determined at 8:00 a.m., immediately prior to the next dose, should reflect the endogenous release of the steroid. When endogenous cortisol levels rise above 10 mg/dl exogenous cortisol therapy can be discontinued.

Specific Indications for Systemic Glucocorticoid Therapy

Arthritis. Although the anti-inflammatory and immunosuppressive effects of glucocorticoids make them useful in the treatment of rheumatoid arthritis, they should never be used as the sole agent in the treatment of this condition. Physical therapy, salicylates, and other nonsteroidal anti-inflammatory agents should be tried first. If these measures fail to achieve satisfactory relief, glucocorticoid therapy can be instituted. The systemic toxicities of corticosteroids must always be borne in mind, and doses selected that, although offering relief, do not completely suppress arthritic symptoms. Prednisone is the most commonly used corticosteroid; the starting dose has been suggested as 5 mg daily, with increments of 2 mg every 4-7 days to a maximum of 10-12 mg daily. The infrequent intra-articular injection of corticosteroids can be used for the treatment of the acute inflammatory phases of osteoarthritis (17, 20).

Rheumatic Carditis. Patients who fail to respond to salicylates may be treated with corticosteroids. Glucocorticoids produce a more rapid onset of effects than salicylates and can be lifesaving in severely ill patients (with fever), or in patients suffering from arrhythmias, pericarditis, or acute congestive heart failure. Prednisone is most commonly employed, and the doses may range from 40 mg/day upward.

Collagen Vascular Diseases. Collagen vascular diseases include systemic lupus erythematosus, polymyositis, polymyalgia rheumatica, temporal arteritis, and mixed connective tissue disease syndrome. Glucocorticoids may be used to obtund the clinical consequences of these conditions. The general rule of "as low a dose as possible" holds true for many of these diseases, although conditions such as systemic lupus erythematosus and temporal arteritis may rapidly deteriorate to the point of causing irreversible tissue damage or threatening life. Under these situations, prednisone may be given in a dose of 1 mg/kg/day and increased at the rate of 20 mg/day if improvement is not noticed within 2 days. Two mg/kg/day of prednisone may be required in the treatment of systemic lupus erythematosus with central nervous system involvement. Progressive systemic sclerosis, although a disease of connective tissue and small blood vessels, is usually refractory to corticosteroids. The use of these agents may promote the development of malignant hypertension and progressive renal failure (60).

Renal Diseases. In patients with nephrotic syndrome resulting from systemic lupus erythematosus or primary renal disease, corticosteroid therapy may be beneficial. An exception is renal amyloidosis. The equivalent of 60 mg/day of prednisone may be used for 3 or 4 weeks. If evidence of a beneficial effect is seen (diuresis and decreased proteinuria), maintenance therapy involving prednisone administration on the first 3 days of each week is indicated.

Allergic Diseases. The anti-inflammatory effects of corticosteroids makes them of considerable value in the treatment of allergic diseases. However, because of their adverse effects, glucocorticoids are only indicated in situations not adequately controlled by less dangerous drugs, such as antihistamines. Because glucocortoids do not act immediately, life-threatening situations, such as anaphylaxis and angioneurotic edema of the glottis, should be treated with subcutaneous epinephrine.

Recently, two new formulations have been introduced for the symptomatic control of allergic rhinitis. These are sprays containing beclomethasone dipropionate or flunisolide. These preparations have potent topical anti-inflammatory properties. Furthermore, their safety is enhanced by the fact that the percentage of the administered dose that is swallowed is rapidly inactivated by the liver. As a result, few systemic side effects are observed.

Bronchial Asthma. Glucocorticoids can be of great value in the treatment of bronchial asthma. Because of concern for their adverse effects, glucocorticoids have been reserved for patients who have failed to respond adequately to previous therapy. In this situation, a glucocorticoid is usually added to existing drug regimens involving theophylline and a β_2 stimulant. Prednisone is often used in doses of 5 mg/day or higher. The daily ingestion of prednisone in these amounts is accompanied by pituitary-adrenal suppression and an increased susceptibility to infections, to mention but two of the possible consequences. The role of corticoids in chronic obstructive pulmonary disease is not clear. One study concluded that some patients with chronic obstructive pulmonary disease show significant improvement in response to systemic steroids; others fail to respond. Those patients who improved on steroids also responded later to β_2 stimulants (47).

The formulation of beclomethasone dipropionate in an aerosol product has assisted many patients who require steroid treatment. Beclomethasone dipropionate has excellent anti-inflammatory activity (Table 12.4-4); its therapeutic efficacy in the treatment of bronchial asthma has been documented (49). The clinical usefulness of the product is further enhanced by the fact that beclomethasone dipropionate is metabolized rapidly

Table 12.4-4
Topical Potency of Various Corticosteroids in Humans

Steroid	Skin-Blanching Activity (McKenzie's Method): (Relative Potency, Fluocinolone-16,17-Acetonide = 100)
Cortisol	0.1
Cortisol-21-acetate	1.0
Triamcinolone	0.01
Triamcinolone-16,17-acetonide	100.0
Fluocinolone-16,17-acetonide	100.0
Betamethasone	0.8
Dexamethasone	0.8
Dexamethasone-21-isonicotinate	8.0
Beclomethasone	0.8
Beclomethasone-17-propionate	360.0
Beclomethasone-17,21-dipropionate	500.0

Source: From Ref. 24, with the permission of the author and the publisher.

following absorption from the gastrointestinal tract. This is important in limiting its systemic effects, as approximately 80% of an inhaled dose of beclomethasone diproprionate is swallowed.

Beclomethasone dipropionate aerosol is of particular importance to children who have demonstrated a good response to prednisone but have suffered from a decreased growth rate. Children switched from oral prednisone to beclomethasone dipropionate aerosol have shown a marked increase in growth velocity. Many patients of all ages previously maintained on long-term systemic steroid therapy have been transferred to beclomethasone dipropionate aerosol with no deterioration in their clinical condition (48).

The use of the corticosteroid aerosol increases the susceptibility of the patient to *Candida albicans* infections in the mouth and throat. Beclomethasone dipropionate is contraindicated in active or quiescent untreated pulmonary tuberculosis or untreated fungal, bacterial, or viral infection. In this regard, it does not differ from the contraindications for the use of systemic steroids.

Short-term high-dose glucocorticoid treatment may be used to provide dramatic relief for patients in status asthmaticus. Cortisol sodium succinate can be given intravenously in doses of 100-500 mg. Plasma cortisol levels of 100-150 μg/100 ml are required for a therapeutic response. Prednisone, in a dose of 2 mg/kg/day orally, has also been shown to provide significant relief for patients suffering from an acute exacerbation of asthma (34). The treatment of respiratory difficulties with corticosteroids is not restricted to the amelioration of bronchial asthma. These drugs also increase the development of surfactant in the fetal lung (2) and are of value in the prevention of the respiratory distress syndrome in the newborn (32).

Cerebral Edema. The use of corticosteroids to treat cerebral edema is controversial. Many physicians feel that glucocorticoids produce a dramatic improvement in cerebral and spinal cord edema associated with surgical or other brain traumas. Dexamethasone is the drug of choice and is given i.m. in a loading dose of up to 8 mg as soon as possible after the insult. Others contend that there is little evidence to support the view that corticosteroid treatment improves cerebral edema, over and above that produced by mannitol or glycerol.

Malignant Hematological Disease. Glucocorticoids are used for the primary treatment of neoplastic disease in combination with various other cytotoxic drugs. They are also used as supportive therapy in complications such as hemolytic anemia, thrombocytopenia, and hypercalcemia. Their use in the treatment of cancer is discussed in Chapter 27.

Liver Disease. The use of glucocorticoids to treat liver disease is controversial. They have no place in the treatment of acute benign hepatitis (31). In the acute disease it has been suggested that glucocorticoids are of no value (23) and that they may interfere with the necessary immune response to infecting organisms.

Their value in massive hepatic necrosis or fulminant hepatitis has not been proven. In the opinion of some, subacute hepatic necrosis is improved with glucocorticoid therapy, although at least one study has indicated that their use may be detrimental in some patients (22). Glucocorticoids are of value in chronic active hepatitis. Prednisone, 40-60 mg, may be given daily for the treatment of chronic active hepatitis. This dose may be gradually tapered to 15-30 mg/day after 2-3 months as the condition improves. Under these circumstances, treatment may be continued for 12 months or longer after clinical and biochemical recovery to prevent a relapse.

Corticosteroids may be indicated for the treatment of severe alcoholic hepatitis, nonalcoholic cirrhosis without ascites in women, and severe progressive hepatic dysfunction associated with infectious mononucleosis (31). Glucocorticoids have been used together with prophylactic doses of antituberculosis agents in the treatment of sarcoidosis associated with hepatic granuloma. Although the symptoms of the disease appear to be controlled, little beneficial effect has been demonstrated on the hepatic lesions.

Shock. The effects of corticosteroids on the cardiovascular system have been discussed earlier. Although these drugs have often been used in the treatment of shock, the lack of well-designed controlled clinical trials has made it difficult to determine their efficacy, particularly in the case of cardiogenic shock and hemorrhagic shock (23). They do have a positive role when large doses (3 mg/kg of dexamethasone or 30 mg/kg of methylprednisolone have been suggested) are used in the treatment of septic shock. Treatment should begin as soon as shock is diagnosed and complemented by the appropriate use of antibiotics, fluid replacement, and repair of acid-base balance.

Intestinal Tract Diseases. If rest, diet, sedation, anticholinergic drugs, and chemotherapy prove ineffective in the treatment of chronic ulcerative colitis, corticosteroids may be indicated. Methylprednisolone acetate, 40 mg, or its equivalent in other glucocorticoids can be given nightly in a retention enema. Systemic corticosteroid therapy, 60-120 mg/day of prednisone or its equivalent, may be required in severely ill patients.

Celiac sprue is a chronic intestinal disorder caused by intolerance to gluten. Prednisolone, 30 mg/day, or one of its equivalents can be used together with a gluten-free diet if diet alone fails. Steroid therapy is usually continued for 3-4 weeks.

Topical Corticosteroids. Corticosteroids are incorporated into a variety of lotions, gels, creams, and ointments. They owe much of their popularity to their effectiveness as anti-inflammatory agents. In addition, glucocorticoids have an antimitotic action that enables them to reduce cell multiplication in psoriasis and decrese the formation of keratin cells. Although many dermatological disorders are treated topically with corticosteroids, their responsiveness to steroid therapy differs (Table 12.4-5).

The importance of halogenation to glucocorticoid potency has been discussed. The topical potency of a steroid is also influenced by the appropriate selection of the ester form. For example, betamethasone-17-valerate is 100 times more potent

Table 12.4-5
Response of Dermatological Disorders to Topical Corticoids

A. *Disorders generally responsive to topical corticoids*
- Seborrheic dermatitis
- Atopic dermatitis
- Lichen simplex chronicus (localized neurodermatitis)
- Pruritus ani (which is often a manifestation of psoriasis)
- Later phase of allergic contact dermatitis
- Xerosis (inflammatory phase)

B. *Disorders less responsive to topical corticoids*
- Discoid lupus erythematosus
- Necrobiosis lipoidica
- Lichen planus
- Hypertrophic lichen planus (mainly intralesional therapy)
- Alopecia areata (intralesional therapy)
- Hypertrophic scars (intralesional therapy only)
- Keloids (intralesional therapy only)
- Pemphigus
- Granuloma annulare
- Pretibial myxedema
- Psoriasis of palms, soles, elbows, knees
- Acne cysts (intralesional)

Source: From Tables 1 and 2 in Ref. 39, with the permission of the authors and W.B. Saunders Co.

in the vasoconstrictor skin assay, used to assess anti-inflammatory potency, than betamethasone itself. The increased potency results largely from the greater ability of the ester to cross the stratum corneum and reach the target tissues below. These results are not unique for betamethasone. Tests of cortisol, cortisol acetate, cortisol butyrate, and cortisol caproate demonstrated a progressive increase in anti-inflammatory activity as the partition coefficient increased (55). There is a limit, however, to the length to which the ester chain may be extended with the aim of increasing potency. Longer-chained esters of cortisol, such as cortisol pelargonate, cortisol laurate, and cortisol stearate, do not remain solubilized in the fluids of the stratum corneum following absorption of the vehicle and, as a result, have reduced topical activity. By combining halogenation of the steroid molecule with esterification, it is possible to increase significantly topical corticosteroid potency. It is possible to grade topical corticosteroids, on the basis of their anti-inflammatory potency, into one of four categories ranging from very potent to weak (Table 12.4-6).

The choice of vehicle is important in determining steroid absorption (38). Occlusion has long been recognized as an effective way of increasing topical corticosteroid activity. The increased hydration of the stratum corneum that accompanies occlusion facilitates the transport of the corticosteroid to the deeper skin tissues. Ointment bases are the most occlusive of the vehicles commonly used and tend to be most effective in promoting steroid penetration. Creams, although cosmetically more acceptable to the patient, are less occlusive and generally less effective in guaranteeing corticosteroid penetration. Lotions are least occlusive. These comments on vehicle suitability must also be weighed with the knowledge that creams, being oil in water vehicles, are more suitable for wet or weepy dermatoses. Ointments are often preferred for dry dermatoses. Fortunately, the wet or weepy skin problems usually offer less of a barrier to corticosteroid penetration, and therefore a cream is not only cosmetically acceptable but also able to provide adequate steroid penetration. Dry dermatoses offer greater impediment to corticosteroid penetration. In these conditions, an ointment is not only often more acceptable but also required for adequate drug efficacy. Lotions are often used in hairy areas of the body.

In choosing a topical corticosteroid preparation, attention should also be given to the regional differences that exist with respect to the ease with which drugs penetrate the skin. Areas of the body, such as the back, scalp, axilla, forehead, jaw angle, and scrotum, that present little impediment to drug absorption might best be treated with weaker steroids (39). The plantar surface of the foot and the ankle present greater barriers to absorption; stronger corticosteroids may be required at these sites.

Finally, the choice of corticosteroid preparation must take into account the fact that dermatological problems differ with respect to their sensitivity to steroid therapy (Table 12.4-5). Conditions that are very sensitive to steroid therapy may be treated adequately by weak glucocorticoids. Others more resistant to treatment may need a potent or very potent steroid.

Topical corticosteroid therapy can produce side effects (Table 12.4-7). Although theoretically such therapy can produce adrenal suppression, this is rarely encountered in adults. It represents a more serious threat in babies when a sizable percentage of the body surface is covered with glucocorticoids for prolonged periods (36). Dermal atrophy is a common adverse effect of steroids applied topically (37). Dermal collagen is damaged and striae will appear. This is more likely to occur in children and in adolescents (56). Thinning of the epidermis occurs with the more potent steroids. Rebound pustulation can also be seen when a strong corticosteroid is discontinued. Consistent with the effects of corticosteroids on the host defense mechanisms, the topical application of these drugs may encourage infections of the skin. Corticosteroid-antibiotic combination products are available to treat inflammation secondary to infection (27). Patients may rarely become sensitized to the steroid itself.

Table 12.4-6
Relative Clinical Potency of Commonly Used Topical Corticosteroid Preparations

Grade I: Very potent	Clobetasol propionate 0.05%
	Fluocinolone acetonide 0.2%
Grade II: Potent	Halcinonide 0.1%
	Betamethasone valerate 0.1%
	Fluocinolone acetonide 0.025%
	Fluocinonide 0.05%
	Beclomethasone dipropionate 0.025%
	Triamcinolone acetonide 0.1%
	Fluocortolone 0.5%
	Flumethasone pivalate 0.02%
Grade III: Moderately potent	Hydrocortisone butyrate 0.1%
	Clobetasone butyrate 0.05%
	Betamethasone valerate 0.05%
Grade IV: Weak	Hydrocortisone 1%
	Fluocortolone 0.2%

Source: From Ref. 56, with the permission of the author and ADIS Press.

Table 12.4-7
Summary of Local Adverse Effects of Topical Corticosteroids

1. Striae atrophicans
2. Dermal atrophy leading to telangiectasia
3. Dermal atrophy and fragility from prolonged occlusive techniques
4. Rebound pustulation on cessation of treatment
5. Perioral dermatitis
6. Increased incidence of all infections
7. Masking of infections such as tinea and scabies and herpes

Source: From Ref. 56, with the permission of the author and ADIS Press.

It is difficult for a student or physician, in these days of heavy advertising, to sift through information surrounding topical steroids and select the most appropriate product. A few simple rules may help:

1. Know the four basic classes into which steroids are grouped on the basis of potency and prescribe only one drug (or at the most two) from each class.
2. Understand the role of the vehicle and its effect on steroid efficacy.
3. Recognize the sensitivities of the various dermatological disorders to glucocorticoid treatment and select the weakest steroid possible that provides the benefit required.
4. Remember that topical corticosteroids may produce severe adverse effects. The more potent steroid preparations are more likely to produce toxicities.

Corticosteroids are used topically in the symptomatic control of ocular inflammatory disorders to control inflammation, reduce the amount of permanent scarring, and prevent visual loss. Corticosteroid therapy is, in general, indicated for all allergic ocular diseases, for most nonpyogenic inflammation, and for the reduction of scarring for certain types of severe injury (chemical or thermal corneal burns). Care must be taken to exclude infection as the cause of inflammation prior to applying a corticosteroid to the cornea. Inflammation secondary to infection must be treated with an antibacterial, possibly complemented with a steroid. Increased intraocular pressure, as a result of a decreased aqueous outflow, may occur after topical glucocorticoid therapy in the eye. Tlhe elevation is usually minimal, although in some individuals it is of a magnitude sufficient to induce glaucomatous changes with eventual loss of vision. The development of glaucoma after either ocular or systemic steroid administration may occur in as many as 40% of patients (18). Steroid treatment has also been implicated in the production of posterior, subcapsular cataracts.

INFLUENCE OF DRUGS OR DISEASES ON GLUCOCORTICOID EFFECTS

Disease states or concomitant drug therapy may alter corticosteroid action, usually because of a change in either corticosteroid distribution in the body or rate of clearance from the body. Interactions of corticosteroids with various drugs are summarized in Table 12.4-8.

The anticonvulsants phenytoin and phenobarbital can increase glucocorticoid metabolism (29) and reduce the therapeutic efficacy of the steroids. Not all corticosteroids are affected equally. The increase in the rate of metabolism of the steroid is proportional to the initial half-life. Thus, dexamethasone is affected more than prednisone and methylprednisolone, which in turn are more affected than cortisol (29). Phenytoin treatment doubled the mean midnight dose of prednisolone required to reduce 8:00 a.m. plasma cortisol levels below 5 μg/dl (40).

Concomitant treatment with phenytoin can lead to an erroneous diagnosis of Cushing's syndrome if a low-dose dexamethasone suppression test is used as a screening method (43). In these circumstances, cortisol is recommended as the steroid of choice for the screening test, as its effects are not altered significantly by phenytoin.

Cortisol is also the steroid of choice in the treatment of adrenal insufficiency in patients receiving antiepileptic drugs. In many patients it may not be necessary to modify the standard daily replacement dose of 30 mg of cortisol, whereas in others a dose of 40 mg daily may be required. When confronted with the necessity of using systemic glucocorticoid therapy to treat inflammatory diseases, it is recommended that the dose of steroid be doubled intially in an attempt to produce an effect comparable with that obtained in patients not receiving antiepileptic drugs (29, 53). Thereafter, further adjustments in dose can be made in accordance with the initial response.

Glucocorticoids have often been used with ephedrine in the treatment of bronchial asthma, although this practice is decreasing as more selective β-stimulants are developed. This is perhaps fortunate in view of the finding that ephedrine enhances dexamethasone metabolism in asthmatic patients (4). Ephedrine can also reduce the plasma concentration of cortisol.

Because rifampin increases the rate of metabolism of corticosteroids, it may be necessary to double the dose of glucocorticoids when rifampicin is used (29). A progressive deterioration of renal transplant function has been noted in tubercular patients receiving rifampicin. In addition, a reduced response to corticosteroids was recorded in patients treated for the nephrotic syndrome or tuberculosis pericarditis when rifampicin was given (29).

A decrease in plasma proteins accompanying liver disease results in a reduced binding of corticosteroids to albumin. The higher concentrations of prednisone and prednisolone in tissues increase the effects of the steroids (58); thus, dosages of these drugs should be reduced in accordance with serum albumin concentrations.

Steroid clearance is slowed in hypothyroidism and increased in hyperthyroidism (51). Usual doses of cortisol may produce Cushing's syndrome in the hypothyroid patient (51), whereas larger than normal doses of steroids may be required for replacement therapy or anti-inflammatory treatment in the hyperthyroid subject.

ADVERSE EFFECTS OF CORTICOSTEROIDS

Table 12.4-9 lists some of the more important complications of long-term high-dose suppressive corticosteroid therapy. In most cases, the adverse effects are a direct consequence of the major pharmacological properties of the corticosteroids and need not be explained in detail again.

The catabolic actions of glucocorticoids on muscle have been discussed. Following chronic steroid therapy, myopathy presents as a proximal muscle weakness; marked wasting of the musculature is seen, especially in the extremities.

An increased incidence of peptic ulceration is often

Table 12.4-8
Interaction of Corticosteroids with Various Drugs

Interacting Drugs	Effects of Interactions
Autonomic drugs	
Sympathomimetics	Increased intraocular pressure in patients under long-term treatment with corticosteroids
Anticholinergics	Increased intraocular pressure; hazardous in glaucoma patients
Anticholinesterases	Their effects in glaucoma antagonized by steroids
Antibiotics	
Amphotericin B	Deep fungal infection may emerge
Anesthetics	Increased hypotension during and after surgery
Antidepressants	Increased intraocular pressure and decreased metabolism of nortriptyline
Antihistaminics	
Chlorcyclizine	Increased metabolism of cortisteroids; increased intraocular pressure (after long-term treatment)
Diphenhydramine	Enzyme induction in the liver; decreased steroid activity
Barbiturates	Increased metabolism of corticosteroids Decreased corticosteroid activity; corticosteroid may potentiate sedation by barbiturates
Antiinflammatory drugs	
Indomethacin	Potentiation of corticosteroid action
Phenylbutazone	Displacement of corticosteroids from plasma protein-binding sites
Gold	Corticosteroids decrease therapeutic efficacy and increase toxicity of gold
Salicylates	Displacement of corticosteroid from the binding sites in plasma protein
Diuretics	
Chlorthalidone	Hypokalemia
Ethacrynic acid	Hypokalemia
Miscellaneous	
Digitalis	Hypokalemia, increased digitalis toxicity
Growth hormone (human)	Decreased anabolic effect
Insulin	Antagonism of blood sugar response
Vitamin A	Antogonism of antihealing effect of corticosteroid
Rifampin	Decrease of corticosteroid effect because of enzyme induction
Organophosphorous compounds	Corticosteroids may antagonize miotic effects

Source: Ref. 41.

cited as a consequence of glucocorticoid therapy, possibly as a result of a thinning of the protective gastric mucus and a potentiation of cholinergically mediated hydrochloric acid secretion. However, the ulcerogenic effect of glucocorticoids has not been demonstrated in well-controlled studies (7). One report suggests that 10-15% of patients taking steroids may develop nausea and vomiting (57).

The ability of glucocorticoids to affect central nervous system function has been described previously, with the symptoms varying from insomnia, nervousness, and slight mood changes to schizophrenia and suicide attempts. Reactions of this nature are generally more frequent and more severe in patients with known psychological difficulties.

It is not necessary at this time to reiterate the effects of corticosteroids on the cardiovascular system and the kidney. It is clear that the mineralocorticoid property of many steroids complicates their use in preexisting hypertension or cardiovascular disease. The use of drugs with minimal mineralocorticoid activity such as triamcinolone and dexamethasone, together with the restriction of dietary salt intake and/or the use of diuretic agents with supplementary potassium, may be preferable in patients with hypertension or cardiovascular problems.

Glucocorticoids have a marked effect on intermediary metabolism and, among other actions, stimulate the formation and diminish the utilization of glucose. Thus, latent diabetes mellitus may be unmasked by prolonged steroid therapy, and preexisting disease is often aggra-

Table 12.4-9
Complications of Cortiocosteroid Therapy

Musculoskeletal	*Metabolic*
Myopathy	Precipitation of clinical manifestations, including ketoacidosis, of genetic diabetes mellitus
Osteoporosis-vertebral compression fractures	Hyperosmolar nonketotic coma
Aseptic necrosis of bone	Hyperlipidemia
	Induction of centripetal obesity
Gastrointestinal	*Endocrine*
Peptic ulceration (often gastric)	Growth failure
Gastric hemorrhage	Secondary amenorrhea
Intestinal perforation	Suppression of hypothalamic-pituitary-adrenal system
Pancreatitis	
Central Nervous System	*Inhibition of fibroblasts*
Psychiatric disorders	Impaired wound healing
Pseudocerebral tumor	Subcutaneous tissue atrophy
Ophthalmological	*Suppression of the immune response*
Glaucoma	Superimposition of a variety of bacterial, fungal, viral, and parasitic infections in steroid-treated patients
Posterior subcapsular cataracts	
Cardiovascular and renal	
Hypertension	
Sodium and water retention (edema)	
Hypokalemic alkalosis	

Source: From Ref. 46, with the permission of the author and Annual Reviews, Inc.

vated. In one study, 17 children were shown to develop hyperglycemia and glycosuria following corticosteroid treatment (51). Steroid-induced diabetes is usually mild and can be managed by the appropriate use of diet and, if necessary, additional insulin therapy. Secondary to an alteration in adipose tissue metabolism, patients may accumulate fat in the supraclavicular area (buffalo hump) and acquire a moon face.

The property of glucocorticoids to induce osteoporosis by reducing the intestinal absorption of calcium and inhibiting the action of vitamin D as well as promoting the metabolism of bone matrix has been discussed. Prolonged glucocorticoid treatment of children results in reduced skeletal growth. Patients who are more likely to develop osteoporosis, such as postmenopausal women, elderly patients, immobilized patients, and diabetic patients, suffer a greater risk of compression fracture of the vertabral column. For these individuals, supplementary therapy with vitamin D and calcium is recommended.

The property of corticosteroids to attenuate significantly the host's defense mechanisms has been discussed in some detail. Attention should be given to the possibility of a preexisting infection before starting steroid treatment, not only for systemic administration of the drugs but also for their topical use. The application of a corticosteroid to the eye for conjunctivitis in the presence of an undiagnosed ocular infection may have disastrous consequences. It is important for a physician to determine if a topical inflammatory condition is secondary to an infection. When it is impossible to differentiate an inflammatory condition per se from inflammation secondary to infection, the physician would be well advised to combine steroid therapy with appropriate antibiotic treatment. Tuberculosis, if not recognized, may be reactivated by systemic corticosteroid therapy.

INHIBITORS OF SYNTHESIS

Metyrapone. Metyrapone is used as a diagnostic agent to determine ACTH reserve in patients with suspected disease of the anterior pituitary. This chemical inhibits the enzyme 11-β-hydroxylase, thereby reducing the conversion of 11-desoxycortisol to cortisol. Administration of metyrapone to a subject with normal pituitary function initially lowers plasma cortisol levels, thereby increasing ACTH secretion, resulting in the secretion of large amounts of 11-desoxycortisol, together with normal quantities of cortisol. Some of the metabolites of 11-desoxycortisol and cortisol are eliminated in the urine as 17-hydroxycorticosteroids (17-OHCS). The response to metyrapone in a normal individual is an increase in urinary 17-OHCS.

The failure of metyrapone to increase ACTH secretion, as reflected by an increase in urinary 17-OHCS, does not necessarily indicate a pituitary disorder. Before this diagnosis can be secured, it is necessary to measure the responsiveness of the adrenal to ACTH. ACTH administration should, therefore, precede the metyrapone test. It is also advisable to administer ACTH before metyrapone, as administration of the latter to a patient with primary adrenal insufficiency can precipitate an acute adrenal crisis.

After establishing the adrenal responsiveness to ACTH, two 24-hr urine samples are collected to determine the baseline excretion of 17-OHCS. Metyrapone is then given orally, 750 mg every 4 hr for six doses, and urine is collected for the 24 hr during which metyrapone is given and the 24 hr immediately following treatment. At least a twofold increase in urinary 17-OHCS above baseline values on either the day of metyrapone treatment or the next day is expected of normal subjects.

PREPARATIONS.

Mostly USP preparations are included. Abbreviation for the main drug is used for its preparations. Topical preparations include cream, ointment, lotion, suspension, and aerosol, but not enema and suppositories.

Glucocorticoids. *Cortisol*, USP (Hydrocortisone): tablet (5, 10, 20 mg), injection (25, 50 mg/ml), topical (0.125-2.5%); *C. Acetate*, USP: injection (25, 50 mg/ml), topical (1-2.5%); *C. Cypionate*, USP: oral (suspension 2 mg/ml); *C. Sodium Phosphate*, USP: injection (100 mg, 1 g powder). *Cortisone Acetate*, USP: tablet (5, 10, 25 mg), injection (25, 25 mg/ml, suspension), topical (1.5, 2.5% suspension). *Beclomethasone Dipropionate*, USP: inhaler (10 mg). *Betamethasone*, USP: oral, tablet (0.6 mg), syrup (0.6 mg/5 ml), injection (4 mg/ml), cream (0.2%); *B. Sodium Phosphate and Acetate*, USP: injection (6 mg/ml, suspension); *B. Dipropionate*, USP: topical (0.015-0.1%); *B. Valerate*, USP: topical (0.01-0.15%); *B. Benzoate*, USP: topical (0.25%). *Dexamethasone*, USP: oral, tablet (0.25-4 mg), elixir (0.5 mg/5 ml), topical (0.011-0.1%); *D. Sodium Phosphate*, USP: injection (4, 10, 25 mg/ml), topical (0.05-0.1%); *D. Acetate*, USP: injection (8 mg/ml). *Paramethasone Acetate*, USP: tablet (1, 2 mg). *Meprednisone*, USP: tablet (4 mg). *Methylprednisone*, USP: tablet (2-32 mg); *M. Acetate*, USP: injection (20, 40, 80 mg/ml, suspension), topical (0.25-1%); *M. Sodium Succinate*, USP: (40, 125, 500 mg, 1 g powder). *Prednisone*, USP: tablet (1-50 mg). *Prednisolone*, USP: tablet (1-5 mg), topical (0.5%); *P. Acetate*, USP: injection (25, 50, 200 mg/ml, suspension), topical (0.12-1%); *P. Sodium Phosphate*, USP: injection (20 mg/ml), topical (0.125-1%); *P. Sodium Succinate*, USP: injection (50-mg powder); *P. Tebunate*, USP: (20 mg/ml, suspension). *Triamcinolone*, USP: (1-16 mg); *T. Acetonide*, USP: injection (40 mg/ml, suspension), topical (0.025-0.5%); *T. Diacetate*, USP: oral, syrup (2, 4 mg/5 ml), injection (40 mg/ml, suspension); *T. Hexacetonide*, USP: injection (5, 20 mg/ml, suspension). Other topical preparations: *Desonide*: (0.05%); *Desoximetasone*, USP: (0.25%); *Flumethasone Pivalate*, USP: (0.025%); *Fluocinolone Acetonide*, USP: (0.01-0.2%); *Fluocinonide*, USP: (0.05%); *Fluorometholone*, USP: (0.025-0.1%); *Flurandrenolide*, USP: (0.025-0.05%); *Halcinonide* (0.025-0.1%); *Medrysone*, USP: (1%).

Mineralocorticoids. *Desoxycorticosterone Acetate*, USP: injection (5 mg/ml, oil; 125-mg pellets). *Desoxycorticosterone Pivalate*, USP: injection (25-mg/ml suspension). *Fludrocortisone Acetate*, USP: tablet (0.1 mg).

REFERENCES

1. Atkinson, J.P., Schreiver, A.D. and Frank, M.M. Effect of corticosteroids and splenectomy on the immune clearance and destruction of erythrocytes. *J. Clin. Invest.* 52:1509, 1973.
2. Baxter, J.D. and Forsham, P.H. Tissue effects of glucocorticoids; *Am. J. Med.* 53:573, 1972.
3. Breitenfield, R.V., Hebert, L.A., Lemann, J., Piering, W.F., Kaufmann, H.M., Sampson, D., Kalbfleish, J. and Beres, J.A. Stability of renal transplant function with alternate-day corticosteroid therapy. *JAMA* 244:151, 1980.
4. Brooks, S.M., Sholiton, L.J., Werk, E.E., Jr. and Altenau, P. The effects of ephedrine and theophylline on dexamethasone metabolism in bronchial asthma. *J. Clin. Pharmacol.* 17:308, 1977.
5. Burry, H.C. Use and abuse of corticosteroids in rheumatic diseases. *Drugs* 19:447, 1980.
6. Cahill, G.F. Action of adrenal corticosteroids on carbohydrate metabolism. In: *The Human Adrenal Cortex* (Christy, N.P., ed.). New York: Harper & Row, 1971, p. 205.
7. Conn, H.O. and Blitzer, B.L. Nonassociation of adrenocorticosteroid therapy and peptic ulcer. *N. Engl. J. Med.* 294:473, 1976.
8. David, D.S., Grieco, M.H. and Cushman, P.J. Adrenal glucocorticoids after 20 years: A review of their clinically relevant consequences. *J. Chron. Dis.* 22:637, 1970.
9. Dluhy, R.G., Lailer, D.P. and Thorn, G.W. Pharmacology and chemistry of the adrenal glucocorticoids. *Med. Clin. North Am.* 57:1155, 1973.
10. Elks, J. Steroids structure and steroid activity. *Br. J. Dermatol.* 94 (suppl. 12):3, 1976.
11. Espiner, E.A., Lun, S. and Hart, B.S. Role of ACTH, angiotensin, and potassium in stress-induced aldosterone secretion. *J. Steroid Biochem.* 9:109, 1978.
12. Fanestil, D.D. Mode of spironolactone action: Competitive inhibition of aldosterone binding to mineralocorticoid receptors. *Biochem. Pharmacol.* 17:2240, 1968.
13. Fauci, A.S. Mechanism of corticosteroid action on lymphocyte subpopulations. I. Redistribution of circulating T and B lymphocytes to the bone marrow. *Immunology* 28:669, 1975.
14. Fauci, A.S., Dale, D.C. and Balow, J.E. Glucocorticoid steroid therapy: Mechanism of action and clinical considerations. *Ann. Intern. Med.* 84:304, 1976.
15. Feldman, D., Funder, J.W. and Adelman, I.S. Subcellular mechanisms in the action of adrenal steroids. *Am. J. Med.* 53:545, 1972.
16. Fiegelson, P., Yu, F-L. and Hanoune, J. Effects of glucocorticoids on hepatic enzyme induction and purine nucleotide and RNA metabolism. In: *The Human Adrenal Cortex* (Christy, N.P., ed.). New York: Harper & Row, 1971, p. 251.
17. Friedman, D.M. and Moore, M.E. The efficacy of intraarticular steroids in osteoarthritis: A double-blind study. *J. Rheumatol.* 7:850, 1980.
18. Ganong, W.S., Biglieri, E.G. and Mulrow, P.J. Mechanisms regulating adrenocortical secretion of aldosterone and glucocorticoid. *Recent Prog. Horm. Res.* 22:381, 1966.
19. Ganong, W.F., Alpert, L.C. and Lee, T.C. ACTH and the regulation of adrenocortical secretion. *N. Engl. J. Med.* 290:1006, 1974.
20. Gifford, R.H. Corticosteroid therapy for rheumatoid arthritis. *Med. Clin. North Am.* 57:1179, 1973.
21. Giles, C.L. The ocular complications of steroid therapy. *Mich. Med.* 66:298, 1967.
22. Gregory, P.B., Knauer, M., Kempson, R.L. and Miller, R. Steroid therapy in severe viral hepatitis. *N. Engl. J. Med.* 294:681, 1976.
23. Gregory, P.B. The demise of corticosteroid therapy for acute viral hepatitis. *Gastroenterology* 80:404, 1981.
24. Harris, D.M. Some properties of beclomethasone dipropionate and related steroids in man. *Postgrad. Med. J.* 51 (suppl. 4):20, 1975.
25. Hendrickse, W., Lowe, J., McKiernan, J. and Pickup, M. Rifampicin-induced non-responsiveness to corticosteroid treatment in nephrotic syndrome. *Br. Med. J.* 1:306, 1979.
26. Herzog, H.L., Nobile, A., Tolksdarf, S., Charney, W., Hershberg, E.D., Perlman, G.L. and Pechet, M.M. New anti-arthritic steroids. *Science* 121:176, 1955.
27. Hodge, L. Corticosteroid/antibiotic combinations: When should they be used? *Drugs* 19:380, 1980.
28. Israel, H.L. and Goldstein, R.A. Hepatic granulomatosis and sarcoidosis. *Ann. Intern. Med.* 79:669, 1973.
29. Jubiz, W. and Meikle, A.W. Alterations of glucocorticoid actions by other drugs and disease states. *Drugs* 18:113, 1979.
30. Kotas, R.V. and Avery, H.E. Accelerated appearance of pulmonary surfactant in the fetal rabbit. *J. Appl. Physiol.* 30:358, 1971.
31. Lesesne, H.R. and Fallon, H.J. Treatment of liver disease with corticosteroids. *Med. Clin. North Am.* 57:1191, 1973.
32. Liggins, G.C. and Howie, R.N. A controlled trial of antepartum glucocorticoid treatment for prevention of the respiratory distress syndrome in premature infants. *Pediatrics* 50:515, 1972.
33. Lightner, E.S., Johnson, H. and Corrigan, J.J. Rapid adrenocortical recovery after short-term glucocorticoid therapy. *Am. J. Dis. Child.* 135:790, 1981.
34. Loren, M.L., Hyman, C., Leung, P., Rohr, C. and Brenner, A.M. Corticosteroids in the treatment of acute exacerbations of asthma. *Ann. Allergy* 45:67, 1980.

35. Luz, P.L., Weil, M.H. and Shubin, H. Current concepts on mechanism and treatment of cardiogenic shock. *Am. Heart J.* 92:103, 1976.
36. Maibach, H.I., Blank, H., Hooper, G., Marks, R. Stoughton, R.B. and Williamson, D.M. Topical corticoid therapy: A round table discussion. Part I. Adverse effects of topical corticoids: Systemic effects. *Cutis* 24:446, 1979.
37. Maibach, H.I., Blank, H., Hooper, G., Marks, R., Stoughton, R.B. and Williamson, D.M. Topical corticoid therapy: A round table discussion. Part II. Adverse effects of topical corticoids: Local effects. *Cutis* 24:633, 1979.
38. Maibach, H.I., Blank, H., Hooper, G. Marks, R., Stoughton, R.B. and Williamson, D.M. Topical corticoid therapy: A round table discussion. Part V: The base as a vehicle. *Cutis* 25:441, 1980.
39. Maibach, H.I. and Stoughton, R.B. Topical corticosteroids. *Med. Clin. North Am.* 57:1253, 1973.
40. Mangili, G., Motta, M. and Martini, L. Control of adrenocorticotrophic hormone secretion. In: *Neural Endocrinology* (Martini, L. and Ganong, W.S., eds.). New York, 1966, 297.
41. Martin, E.W. *Drug Interactions Index 1978/79.* Philadelphia: J.B. Lippincott, 1978, p. 116.
42. McEwen, B.S., Weiss, J.M. and Schwartz, L.S. Retention of corticosterone by cell nuclei from brain regions of adrenalectomized rats. *Brain Res.* 17:471, 1970.
43. Meikle, A.W., Stanchfield, J.B., West, C.D. and Tyler, F.H. Hydrocortisone suppression test for Cushing's syndrome: Therapy with anticonvulsants. *Arch. Intern. Med.* 134:1068, 1974.
44. Melby, J.C. Clinical pharmacology of adrenal steroids. In: *Steroid Therapy: A Clinical Update for the 1970's* (Thorn, G.W., ed.). New York: Medcom, 1971, 16.
45. Melby, J.C. Systemic corticosteroid therapy: Pharmacology and endocrinologic consideration. *Ann. Intern. Med.* 81:505, 1974.
46. Melby, J.C. Clinical pharmacology of systemic corticosteroids. *Ann. Rev: Pharmacol. Toxicol.* 17:511, 1977.
47. Mendella, L.A., Manfreda, J., Warren, C.P.W. and Anthonisen, N.R. Steroid response in stable chronic obstructive pulmonary disease. *Ann. Intern. Med.* 96:17, 1982.
48. Morrow Brown, H. and Storey, G. Treatment of allergy of the respiratory tract with beclomethasone dipropionate steroid aerosol. *Postgrad. Med. J.* 51 (suppl. 4):59, 1975.
49. Morrow Brown, H., Storey, G. and Jackson, F.A. Beclomethasone dipropionate aerosol in long-term treatment of perennial and seasonal asthma in children and adults: A report of five-and-half years experience in 600 asthmatic patients. *Br. J. Clin. Pharmacol.* 4:259S, 1977.
50. Ney, R.L. Modern concepts of adrenocortical function. In: *Steroid Therapy: A Clinical Update for the 1970's* (Thorn, G.W., ed.). New York: Medcom, 1971, 6.
51. Parfitt, A.M. Cushing's syndrome with normal replacement of doses of cortisone in pituitary hypothyroidism. *J. Clin. Endocrinol. Metab.* 24:560, 1964.
52. Perlman, K. and Ehrlich, R.M. Steroid diabetes in childhood. *Am. J. Dis. Child.* 136:64, 1982.
53. Petereit, L.B. and Meikle, A.W. Effectiveness of prednisolone during phenytoin therapy. *Clin. Pharmacol. Ther.* 22:912, 1977.
54. Rinehart, J.J., Balcerzak, S.P., Sagone, A.L. and LoBuglio, A.F. Effects of corticosteroids on monocyte function. *J. Clin. Invest.* 54:1337, 1974.
55. Schlagel, C.A. Penetration and action of glucocorticoids. In: *Advances in Biology of Skin, Vol. 12: Pharmacology and the Skin.* (Montagna, W., Van Scott, E.J. and Stoughton, R.B., eds.). New York: Appleton-Century-Crofts, 1972, p. 339.
56. Sneddon, I.B. Clinical use of topical steroids. *Drugs* 11:193, 1976.
57. Swartz, S.L. and Dluhy, R.G. Corticosteroids: Clinical pharmacology and therapeutic use. *Drugs* 16:238, 1978.
58. Uribe, M. and Go, V.L.W. Corticosteroid pharmacokinetics in liver disease. *Clin. Pharmacokin.* 4:233, 1979.
59. Wohlman, M, Allaben, R., Whitten, J., Edford, G., Baskin, S., McNichol, L. and Toledo-Perevra L.H. Alternate-day steroid therapy for renal transplant patients. *JAMA* 245:2493, 1981.
60. Yount, W.J., Utsinger, P.D., Puritz, E.M. and Ortbals, D.W. Corticosteroid therapy of the collagen mascular disorder. *Med. Clin. N. Am.* 57:1343, 1973.
61. Yu, D.T., Clements, P.J., Paulus, H.E., Peter, J.B., Levy, J. and Barnett, E.V. Human lymphocyte subpopulation: Effect of corticosteroids. *J. Clin. Invest.* 53:656, 1974.

CHAPTER
12.5

THYROID HORMONES AND ANTITHYROID DRUGS

Ram B. Rastogi and Radhey L. Singhal

THYROID HORMONES

The thyroid is the largest endocrine gland in humans weighing about 20 g in an adult. The thyroid hormones, namely, L-thyroxine (T_4) and L-triiodothyronine (T_3) (Fig. 12.5-1), are synthesized in the thyroid gland and subsequently released into the general circulation. In addition to T_3 and T_4, the gland secretes calcitonin (Chapter 12.2). T_3 and T_4 are vitally involved in the production and utilization of energy and play a major role in the process of growth and development of the organism; the former is the molecular form of thyroid hormone responsible for the initiation of most thyroid effects in humans. In the amphibian, metamorphosis will not occur in the absence of thyroid hormones. In the mammalian fetus, differentiation of the central nervous system requires the presence of thyroid hormones (5). In early neonatal life of lower mammals, this hormone is also required in the process of the myelination and organization of cellular architecture of the central nervous system (1). Excessive thyroid function in adults leads to a wide variety of clinical symptoms including weight loss, tachycardia, increased cardiac output, anxiety, mental agitation, and exaggerated response to environmental stimuli. On the other hand, deficient thyroid function results in weight gain, muscle weakness and fatigue, cold intolerance, apathy, and slowed mentation. The most dramatic effect found in either condition is that on oxygen consumption. Magnus-Levy (19) first reported the observation that respiratory exchange was depressed in Gull's disesae (hypothyroidism) and elevated in Graves' disease (hyperthyroidism).

SYNTHESIS AND RELEASE

The individual steps involved in the synthesis of thyroid hormones from iodine are as follows: (1) active transport of iodide (iodide trapping), (2) oxidation of iodine to free iodine and the iodination of tyrosyl groups of thyroglobulin, (3) coupling of iodotyrosine molecules within thyroglobulin matrix to form T_3 and T_4, (4) proteolysis of thyroglobulin and the release of free iodotyrosines and secretion of T_3 and T_4 into the blood, and (5) deiodination of iodotyrosines within the thyroid and reutilization of the liberated iodide. These processes are illustrated in Fig. 12.5-2. The main secretory product of thyroid gland is T_4 and the circulating pool of T_4 is larger than that of T_3.

Active Transport of Iodide. The active transport of iodide is the first step in the biosynthesis of thyroid hormone. The iodine ingested in the diet reaches the circulation in the form of iodide (I^-). The site of iodide transport in thyroid epithelial cells is most likely the basal membrane.

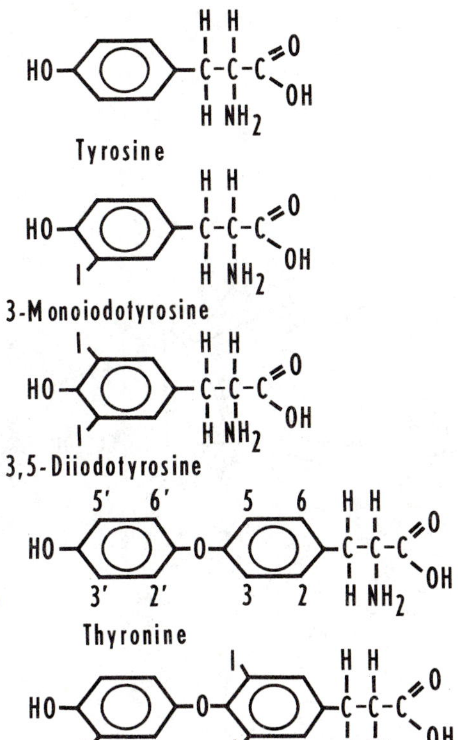

Tyrosine

3-Monoiodotyrosine

3,5-Diiodotyrosine

Thyronine

3′, 3,5-Triiodothyronine

3′, 3,5-Triiodothyroacetic acid (TRIAC)

3′, 5′, 3,5-Tetraiodothyronine (Thyroxine)

3′, 5′, 3,5-Tetraiodothyroacetic acid (TETRAC)

Fig. 12.5-1. *Structures of major thyroid iodoamino acids and their metabolites.*

Evidence suggests that thyroid I^- transport meets all the criteria for an active transport mechanism. The major points favoring this are: (1) I^- is concentrated against both a chemical and an electrical gradient, (2) I^- that is concentrated within the thyroid is not bound, (3) cellular integrity is essential, (4) I^- transport displays saturation kinetics, (5) the process is inhibited competitively by related ions, (6) oxidative metabolism and phosphorylation are required, and finally (7) the system possesses a high temperature coefficient. A number of anions such as perchlorate (ClO_4^-), thiocyanate (SCN^-), and pertechnetate (TcO_4^-) act as competitive inhibitors of iodide transport by the thyroid. Perchlorate is a very potent inhibitor of I^- transport and has been found effective in the treatment of hyperthyroidism.

Perchlorate and thiocyanate are clinically employed in the radioactive iodine (RAI) discharge test for the diagnosis of organification defects in the thyroid (33). Pertechnetate, which has a short half-life (6 hours), is widely used in the form of $^{99m}TcO_4$ for thyroid scanning and uptake studies to measure thyroid function. The iodide transport mechanism in the thyroid seems to require concurrent transport of potassium and is depressed by ouabain and other cardiac glycosides that inhibit the accumulation of potassium by tissue.

The iodide transport is regulated by thyroid stimulating hormone (TSH; thyrotropin). Hypophysectomy in rats is accompanied by decreased thyroid-to-serum iodide concentration ratio and this is increased by TSH. Furthermore, an autoregulatory system within the gland (i.e., the total organic iodine concentration within the gland) controls the iodide transport system of the thyroid.

Oxidation of Iodide and Iodination of Tyrosyl Groups of Thyroglobulin. Iodide (I^-), after entering into thyroid gland, is oxidized to iodine (I_2) by thyroid peroxidase. Of the known biological oxidizing agents, only H_2O_2 and O_2 are sufficiently potent to oxidize I^-. The generation of H_2O_2 in thyroid cells or any other tissue has not yet been elucidated. It is presumed to be formed in close proximity to its site of utilization. Tyrosyl groups of thyroglobulin readily react with the highly active iodine, forming monoiodotyrosine (MIT) and diiodotyrosine (DIT) (Fig. 12.5-2). Tyrosine is not iodinated while it is a free amino acid but is iodinated in linkage with thyroglobulin; the iodination *in vivo* probably occurs at the cell lumen interface. The congenital goiterous hypothyroidism has been reported to occur as a result of defective iodination in the thyroid. Thiourylene drugs such as propylthiouracil and methimazole are potent inhibitors of peroxidase activity involving iodide oxidation.

Coupling of Iodotyrosine Molecules Within Thyroglobulin to Form T_3 and T_4. Evidence indicates that thyroid peroxidase enzyme also plays an important role in the coupling reaction of two DIT molecules or one DIT and one MIT molecule, which aerobically condense to form T_4 and T_3, respectively, in the approximate ratio of 3:1. T_3 and T_4 are stored in the colloid of the follicular cavity as a moiety of the thyroglobulin molecule. Two MIT molecules do not condense because the nature of the biosynthetic reaction is such that DIT must remain in peptide linkage during the coupling reaction; consequently, DIT must be at least one of the two reaction partners. During iodine deficiency, a condition in which MIT is greatly increased relative to DIT in the thyroglobulin of the gland, the relative formation of T_3 is enhanced. It is presumed that in coupling-defect goiter the peroxidase enzyme involved in coupling is either inactive or absent. However, Inoque and Taurog (12) demonstrated that the coupling efficiency was depressed in extreme iodine deficiency and was restored to normal by a relatively small increase in iodine intake. Antithyroid drugs such as propylthiouracil and methimazole are potent inhibitors of thyroid peroxidase-catalyzed coupling reaction.

Proteolysis of Thyroglobulin and Release of Free Iodotyrosine. T_3 and T_4 are stored in the thyroid gland as a peptide-linkage amino acid in thyroglobulin, and because this protein molecule is too large to leave the thyroid, their secretion into the blood stream must be preceded by proteolysis of the thyroglobulin. The daily secretion of T_4 in normal humans is approximately 90 μg; that of T_3, about 25 μg. It is generally believed that TSH plays a crucial role in the secretion of thyroid hormones.

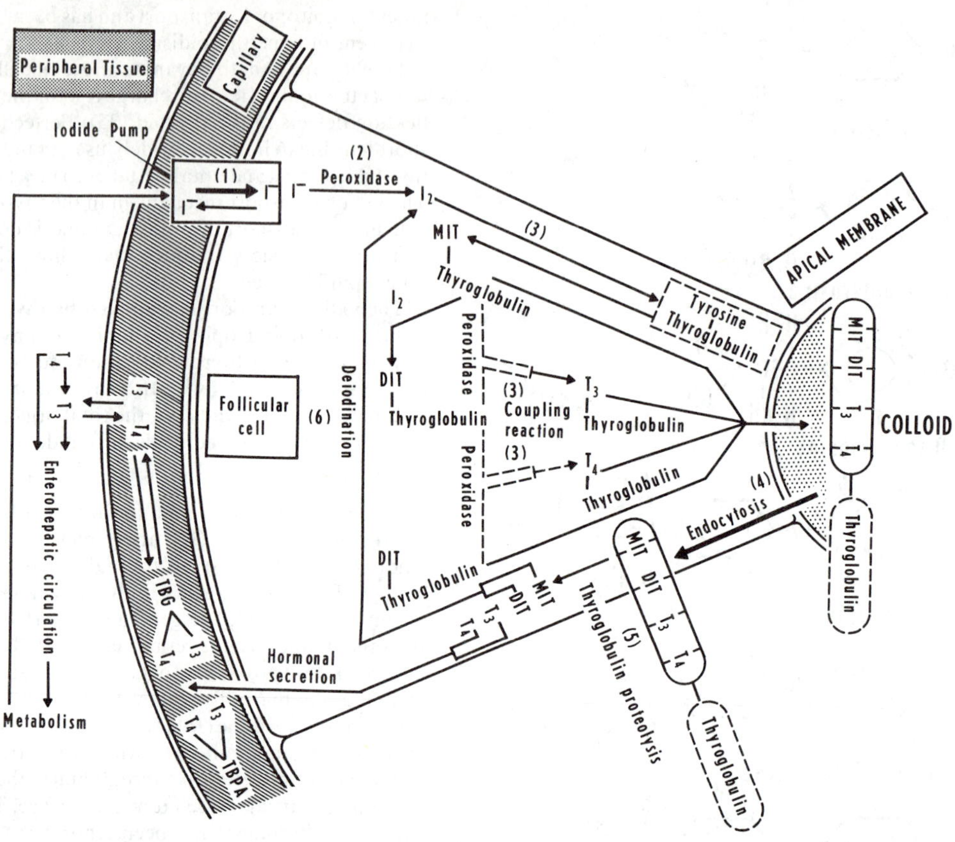

Fig. 12.5-2. *Steps in the biosynthesis and release of thyroid hormone.*
The number in parentheses represents the number of the metabolic step as follows: (1) iodide transport, ClO_4^-, SCN^-; (2) iodide oxidation, PTU, MMI; (3) iodination and coupling, PTU, MMI; (4) endocytosis, colchicine, Li, I^-; (5) thyroglobulin proteolysis, I^-; (6) deiodination, dinitrotyrosine. Abbreviations used: I^- = iodide; I_2 = iodine; T_3 = triiodothyronine; T_4 = thyroxine; MIT = monoiodotyrosine; DIT = diiodotyrosine; TBG = thyroxine-binding globulin; TBPA = thyroxine-binding prealbumin; ClO_4 = perchlorate; SCN^- = thiocyanate; PTU = propylthiouracil; MMI = methimazole; Li = lithium.

The release of thyroid hormone from the gland may be inhibited by a variety of agents. Foremost among these is iodide, which in high doses inhibits release of thyroid hormone in patients with hyperthyroidism. Lithium also inhibits thyroid hormone release, possibly through an action on the adenylate cyclase-cyclic adenosine monophosphate (cAMP) system (6). Secretion of thyroid hormone is also inhibited by colchicine and cytochalasin B.

Deiodination of Iodotyrosine in the Thyroid and Reutilization of the Liberated Iodide. The proteolysis of thyroglobulin results in release of free iodotyrosines as well as iodothyronines. Evidence shows, however, that iodotyrosines do not leave the thyroid gland, suggesting that iodotyrosines released from thyroglobulins are readily deiodinated within the gland by enzyme thyroid deiodinase. The purified enzyme is a flavoprotein, active toward DIT and MIT but not T_4. Studies in humans also suggest presence of enzymatic iodothyronine-deiodinating systems in the adenohypophysis that can convert T_4 to T_3 (14). Dinitrotyrosine is known to inhibit deiodination reaction. The iodide released from MIT and DIT by deiodination is partly reutilized for hormone synthesis and is partly lost from the gland as the so-called *iodide leak.*

THYROGLOBULIN

Thyroglobulin is a larger glycoprotein that serves as the substrate for iodination and hormonogenesis and is synthesized in the thyroid gland. The molecular weight of thyroglobulin is 660,000 (19S) and is made of 300 carbohydrate residues and 5500 amino acid residues, and it is stable between pH 5 and 11. Thyroglobulin serves two main purposes: the first function has to do with the process of hormone biosynthesis; the second is the storage within the gland of a considerable supply of hormone that is available for secretion at a steady rate or on demand and also the storage of iodine in a form that is available for reutilization in the thyroid cell for new hormone synthesis.

TRANSPORT, METABOLISM, AND EXCRETION: PATHOPHYSIOLOGICAL IMPLICATIONS

After their release into the circulation, T_3 and T_4 are almost instantaneously, but reversibly, bound to serum proteins. Under physiological conditions, most of the thyroid hormones are bound to an inter-α-globulin called thyroxine-binding globulin (TBG) and, to a lesser degree, to a thyroxine-binding prealbumin (TBPA). Albumin also serves as a carrier for thyroxine when other binding proteins are overburdened. Only about

1% of T_4 and T_3 circulates unbound. T_3 is predominantly bound to TBG and, to some extent, to albumin, but differs from T_4 by not being bound to any significant degree to TBPA (39). The binding proteins not only serve to prolong hormone availability at target organs, but also to dampen the effects of transient perturbations in T_4 secretion. This may partly explain why the circadian variation of serum TSH or thyroid iodine release does not produce detectable changes in circulating T_4 concentrations (2). In addition to retarding transport and buffering actions, binding proteins also serve a reservoir function for extrathyroid T_4 storage. At normal T_4 concentrations, 70% of TBG and more than 99% of TBPA and albumin-binding sites are unoccupied. This reservoir effect is demonstrated indirectly by a small rise in serum T_3 concentration that is observed after a single oral dose (2.5-3 mg) of levothyroxine (36). This aspect of T_4 binding may be of particular clinical importance where patient compliance is in question, both when replacement therapy is being considered and when thyroid hormone suppression tests are being performed on an outpatient basis.

Because T_4 is bound to serum carrier proteins, it assumes the diffusion properties similar to those of a moderately large serum protein such as albumin. As a result, the first step of T_4 transport from the organ of secretion to the target tissues is delayed for 4 or 5 days. On the contrary, the diffusion of T_3, which is not being bound to TBPA, requires only 22 hours, or approximately one-fourth of the time required for T_4. Moreover, the binding affinity of T_3 for the serum-binding proteins is 10-fold weaker as compared with T_4. These differences in kinetics may probably account for the fact that thyroxine elicits a slow onset but prolonged duration of action as compared with T_3. T_4 is catabolized by two pathways: The first involves deiodination of T_4 at the 5-position to form active T_3; in the second, deiodination at 5-position results in the production of inactive metabolite, reverse T_3 (rT_3). It is believed that 70-80% of the body's T_3 is formed from deiodination of T_4; the T_3 is four times as potent (calorigenically) as thyroxine. Certain drugs (estrogen) and physiological conditions such as pregnancy cause elevation in the concentration of TBG. This results in increased thyroxine binding and could lower the concentration of the free hormone. The feedback mechanisms compensate and increased thyroid secretion returns the free-hormone level to normal. Laboratory tests measuring total T_4 alone, therefore, would be subject to misinterpretation. Salicylates or dicumerol, which also bind to the serum protein, may result in higher free levels of T_4 and eventually a faster rate of metabolism. In nephrosis and hepatic cirrhosis, when there is reduced protein in plasma, the hormonal metabolism is accelerated.

In euthyroid individuals, the half-life of T_4 is about 6-7 days and that of T_3 is about 1.5 days. The half-life of T_4 is shortened (as little as 3 days) in patients with hyperthyroidism, whereas it may be somewhat prolonged (up to 10 days) in those with hypothyroidism. Thyroid hormones are mainly metabolized in liver, kidney, and muscle. In liver, T_4 is conjugated mainly as the glucuronide, whereas T_3 is conjugated mainly as a sulfate. After excretion via the bile duct, the conjugates are hydrolyzed in the intestine, possibly by bacterial enzymes, and most of the T_4 and T_3 reenter the blood via hepatic-portal circulation. Thus, there is an enterohepatic circulation of thyroid hormones. Approximately 20-30% of thyroxine is eliminated in the stool. Tetraiodothyroacetic acid (TETRAC) and triiodothyroacetic acid (TRIAC) are two important products of T_4 and T_3 metabolism, respectively, and are frequently measured in diagnostic tests. Like parent compounds, they are also conjugated and deiodinated before being finally excreted.

The quantity of T_4 metabolized daily appears to be related to the amount of T_4 that exists in the free state in serum. Chronic administration of drugs such as phenytoin (DILANTIN) and phenobarbital appear to induce degradative enzyme activity and thereby augment the disposal of T_4 (18).

PHYSIOLOGICAL AND BIOCHEMICAL ACTIONS

The thyroid gland exerts a powerful influence upon the body's activities. If the function of the gland is for any reason lost, serious disturbances in chemical and morphological structure arise and are manifested as physical and mental disorders. Thyroid hormones act on tissues through a variety of mechanisms that include transport of amino acids and electrolytes from the extracellular environment to the interior of the cell, synthesis or activation of specific enzyme proteins within the cell, and enhancement of intracellular events, including translation and transcription that lead to changes in cell size and cell number. Whether these actions are influenced by cyclic nucleotide is not clearly understood. Major sites of hormone action—the cell membrane, mitochondrion, ribosome, and nucleus—are similar in both the adult and neonate, but the effects are markedly different and tend to be tissue specific in both. More recently, Oppenheimer (22) suggested that triiodothyronine nuclear receptor complex is the basic unit of thyroid hormone action. This complex is believed to stimulate the formation of a diversity of messenger RNA sequences leading to the ultimate hormonal effects at the local cellular levels.

Growth and Development. It is believed that thyroid hormones play a vital role in the development of an organism. The absence of thyroxine or triiodothyronine, particularly at neonatal age, results in deficit in growth and causes mental retardation. However, thyroidectomy in the adult state does not produce such marked disturbances.

The restoration of growth in thyroidectomized animals is one of the most sensitive and specific responses to these hormones. In neonatally thyroidectomized rats, as little as 1-2 μg of T_3 injected daily, beginning from 5 to 10 days after birth, restores the growth to normal. A critical period of the first 10-15 days of neonatal life in rats or 3-6 months in children has been identified, during which optimal levels of thyroid hormones must be present for the normal growth and development of the body (30). Disturbances of growth are manifested chiefly in the skeleton. Growth of the whole body ceases prematurely in young animals and growth of long bones is particularly retarded. As a result, the thyroidectomized animal acquires the characteristic appearance of a dwarf.

Experimental thyroid ablation in early life results in decreased synthesis of protein, nucleic acid, and lipids, as well as in altered activity of a variety of enzymes in maturing nervous tissue (31). Examination of the brain of hypothyroid animals reveals deficient development, particularly of axonal and dendritic networks. It is assumed that axonal and dendritic deficiencies in thyroid hormone-deprived rats can account for as much as 80% of the reduction in the probability of neuronal interactions in sensorimotor cortex. This endocrine disorder also results in defective myelination. The contents of cerebroside, sulfatide, and cholesterol are lowered and the onset of sulfatide biosynthesis is delayed in young hypothyroid rats. Consistent with these observations is the finding in which excess thyroid hormone given to newborn rats resulted in an accelerated myelination and precocious development of brain, but caused a permanent deficit of DNA in both cerebrum and cerebellum.

Metabolism. The most constant and characteristic feature of thyroid insufficiency is the slowing of all metabolic processes and, in particular, a sharp decrease in the basal metabolic rate. This, in thyroidectomized animals, may be reduced by 30-45%. As a result of general slowing of all forms of energy metabolism, hypothermia is observed during hypothyroidism. By contrast, feeding thyroid extract or injecting thyroid hormones may cause profound increase in heat production in laboratory animals. Thermogenesis in patients with hyperthyroidism is increased by 200% or more. This calorigenic action is believed to be partly dependent upon protein synthesis.

There is much experimental evidence to show that thyroid hormones in moderate doses stimulate protein synthesis. A decreased incorporation of isotopic leucine into protein has been shown in the cerebral cortex of rats made hypothyroid at 1 day of age. By contrast, administration of L-thyroxine enhanced brain protein synthesis at the translation level in neonatal rats. Protein synthesis in the brain, however, remained unaffected in rats thyroidectomized in adulthood. Functional dissimilarities in the mitochondrial fractions have been presumed to be responsible for the varying effects in adult and developing rats, because the mitochondria of mature animals have been shown to be rather insensitive to the action of thyroxine (15).

Lipid and Carbohydrate Metabolism. Thyroid hormones accelerate the conversion of cholesterol into bile acids and enhance the elimination of cholesterol from the body. This may provide an explanation for decreased total and low-density lipoprotein (LDL) cholesterol of serum in hypothyroid patients. Hypothyroid patients exhibit a reduction in synthesis of cholesterol and in LDL catabolism. However, cholesterol reabsorption remains unchanged or even enhanced (21).

Thyroid hormones exert a profound effect on glucose homeostasis. A large percentage of hyperthyroid patients (40-70%) manifests an abnormal oral glucose tolerance. Hypothyroid patients often show decreased blood sugar levels in the postabsorptive state, with a slight increase after an oral glucose load; the intravenous glucose tolerance test reveals delayed disappearance of glucose. Thyroid hormone-induced changes in total body glucose metabolism involves: (1) increased intestinal absorption of carbohydrate, (2) increased glucose production by the liver and kidney, and (3) increased glucose utilization by muscle and adipose tissue (21).

Water and Electrolyte Metabolism. Disturbances of water and electrolyte metabolism are among the important clinical manifestations of thyroid disorders. In severe and prolonged thyrotoxicosis, the volume of urine excreted daily is much less than in the controls. Golber and Kandror (8) reported that severe thyrotoxicosis in rabbits induced by feeding thyroid extracts was accompanied by an increase in the water content of myocardium. The loss of extracellular fluid and sodium ions arising under the influence of small doses of thyroid hormone evidently leads to an extracellular dehydration of the body. Changes in thyroid function are also reflected in calcium and magnesium metabolism in the body. Thyroid hormones cause accumulation of intracellular calcium, possibly by altering membrane permeability to cations. In the brain, thyroid hormones also influence the Na^+-K^+ pump.

Cardiovascular System. The hyperfunctioning of the cardiovascular system is one of the striking features of hyperthyroidism and disturbance of the cardiac rhythm constitutes an invariable component of the clinical picture of hyperthyroidism. The heart rate and systolic pressure are elevated during hyperthyroidism. The cardiac hypertrophy seen during hyperthyroidism parallels increased oxygen consumption. By contrast, during hypothyroidism oxygen consumption falls with an accompanying lowering of stroke volume of the heart. More recently, it was demonstrated that thyroid hormone controls adenosine triphosphate (ATP) turnover in the heart (11). Thyroid hormones also influence electrophysiological parameters of the heart such as shortening of refractory period, a decreased duration of action potential. These changes along with a shortened atrioventricular conduction result in tachycardia and atrial fibrillation which are commonly seen in hyperthyroid patients.

An increased sensitivity of the sympathetic system of hyperthyroid dog has been reported (28). It has been suggested that enhanced adrenergic response of hyperthyroid heart is due to an increase in number of β-adrenoreceptors (38).

Central Nervous System. An abundance of information now exists emphasizing the importance of thyroid hormones in the structural and biochemical ontogeny of the central nervous system (30). The abnormalities observed in brains of cretins include hypoplasia of cerebral and cerebellar cortices, vascular dilation, deficiency of capillaries, and poor myelination. Neonatal thyroidectomy also produces marked interferences with the ontogenic increases of rate-limiting enzymes tyrosine hydroxylase, and tryptophan hydroxylase, and lowers the turnover of brain catecholamines and serotonin. Animals thyroidectomized at birth are listless, show lack of interest to environmental events, do not learn from experience and, like their human counterparts, can be considered mentally retarded. Behavioral studies in rats rendered hypothyroid from birth have shown not only an impairment in the capacity for adaptive behavior, but also concomitant alterations in the electroencephalogram (EEG). A human counterpart to manifest EEG changes and dendritic growth impairment reported in the neonatally hypothyroid rat may be the slow α rhythm and retardation in the ontogenic pattern of sleep EEGs reported in young hyperthyroid children. These findings raise the possibility that during hypothyroidism there may be defective neural connections between the brain stem and cerebral cortex (35).

By contrast, hyperthyroidism increases the turnover of catecholamines, serotonin, and acetylcholine in developing brain (30). Furthermore, thyroid hormone increases the sensitivity of catecholamine receptor sites in brain as well as in peripheral tissue (24, 27). These findings may partly explain the neurochemical mechanisms underlying anxiety, irritability, and exaggerated response to environmental stimuli generally seen during hyperthyroidism. Emotional disturbances as well as proneness to rapid fatigue have also been noted in patients with thyrotoxicosis. Employing hyperthyroid animals as a model of anxiety, it was reported that diazepam significantly reduced T_3-stimulated rise in excitability as well as serotonin and norepinephrine turnover in the brain.

REGULATION OF THYROID FUNCTION

The thyroid function is controlled by (1) suprathyroid and (2) autoregulatory mechanisms. Secretion of thyrotropin hormone, also called thyroid-stimulating hormone (TSH), which is the major modulator of thyroid function, is regulated at the level of pituitary thyrotropin by the antagonistic effects of thyroid hormones and thyrotropin-releasing hormone (TRH), a hypothalamic tripeptide neurohormone. Thyroid hormones inhibit whereas TRH stimulates the synthesis and secretion of TSH (Fig. 12.5-3). Thus, excess of thyroid hormone results in decreased secretion of TSH, whereas thyroid hormone insufficiency is associated with TSH hypersecretion. It remains a question whether T_4 itself is capable of inhibiting secretion of TSH or whether it acts only by giving rise to T_3. Animal studies have shown that somatostatin, a hypothalamic peptide that inhibits the release of growth hormone, decreases both basal and TRH-stimulated release of TSH.

The autoregulatory mechanism controlling thyroid function is independent of TSH secretion but is influenced by day-to-day variations in the availability of iodine. When moderate or large doses of iodide are administered chronically to human beings, adaptation occurs. Even though this adaptation is not complete and the quantity of iodine accumulated and organified is well in excess of normal, the rate of secretion of T_4 is not enhanced.

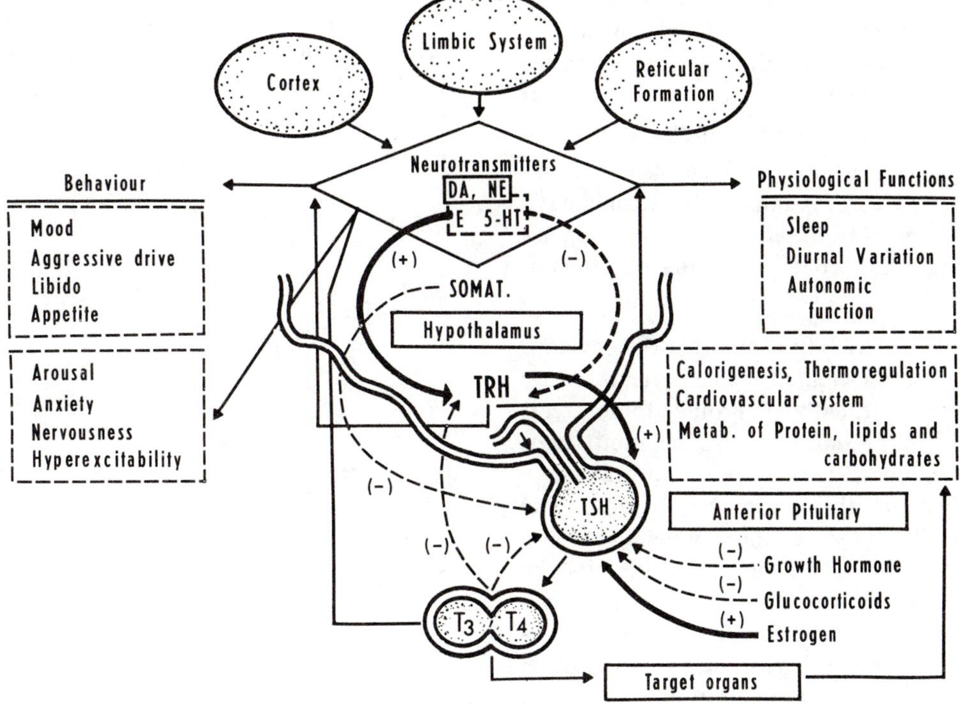

Fig. 12.5-3. *Inhibition of TSH secretion by thyroid hormones acting at the pituitary leve.*

TSH secretion is stimulated by the hypothalamic hormone TRH and inhibited by somatostatin (SOMAT), which is also synthesized in the hypothalamus. Secretion of both somatostatin and TRH is controlled by monoaminergic neurons in the brain. It is believed that epinephrine (E) = containing neurons stimulate, whereas serotonin (5-HT) = containing neurons inhibit the release of TRH from the hypothalamus. Whereas estrogens sensitize the pituitary to TRH effects, glucocorticoids and growth hormone reduce pituitary sensitivity to the action of TRH. Glucocorticoids also act on the hypothalamus to inhibit TRH release. Thyroid hormones thus released can influence the metabolism of certain neurotransmitters such as NE, DA, and 5-HT, which in turn can influence a number of behavioral activities and physiological functions. (Modified from Ref. 25).

ANTITHYROID AGENTS

Many organic compounds and inorganic ions have the ability to inhibit, directly or indirectly, the synthesis of thyroid hormones. Some of these exert their effects as part of a general toxic action (e.g., cyanide) or metabolic inhibitory action (e.g., antibiotics). Other drugs specifically influence certain steps of intrathyroidal or extrathyroidal metabolism of iodide or thyroid hormones. Several of the antithyroid agents are of great clinical value in the treatment of hyperthyroid state, whereas others are used primarily as research tools. Maintenance of an effective concentration of antithyroid drugs for sufficient time in hyperthyroid patients may lead to thyroid hypertrophy or goiter. This phenomenon gave rise to another common term for these compounds, namely, goiterogens.

CHEMICAL CLASSIFICATION

Complex Univalent Anions. A number of anions such as bromide (Br^-), thiocyanate (SCN^-) fluoborate (BF_4^-), perchlorate (ClO_4^-), and others whose ionic size is similar to that of iodide competitively inhibit the active transport of iodide both in the thyroid and extrathyroidal iodide-concentrating tissues. Among these, ClO_4^- and BF_4^- are most effective in interfering with the iodide transport. Patients who are treated with perchlorate must avoid ingestion of any iodine-containing compounds.

Other Anions and Cations

Calcium. Several studies have shown that excessive intake of calcium results in the development of endemic goiter. In experimental animals an increased thyroid ^{131}I-

uptake was found both *in vivo* and *in vitro,* which might be due to increased thyrotropic stimulation (17). However, the mechanism underlying the goiterogenic action of calcium is not clearly known.

Molybdate. Some signs of molybdenosis in rabbits resemble those of hypothyroidism. Widjajakusuma et al. (37) reported that molybdate significantly decreased the plasma T_4 concentration and T_4 secretion rate, whereas T_4 distribution space remained unchanged.

Cobalt. Several cases of thyroid hyperplasia among patients treated with cobaltous chloride for anemia have been reported (9). However, the effect seems species specific, since it failed to show a definite antithyroid effect in laboratory animals.

Lithium. Schou et al. (29) first reported the development of goiter in lithium-treated manic patients. More recently, it was demonstrated that chronic lithium treatment antagonized the T_3-induced rise in locomotor activity as well as catecholamine turnover in rat brain (26). The primary effect of lithium may be an iodide-like action to decrease thyroid secretion. However, some evidence suggests that this alkali metal also inhibits the synthesis of thyroid hormones. The doses of lithium carbonate (900-1500 mg/day) that are effective in hyperthyroidism appear also to interfere with peripheral hormone degradation. Thus, the clinical use of lithium salts as an antithyroid drug is still highly experimental.

Iodide. The Wolff-Chaikoff effect, in which large doses of iodide inhibit the binding of iodine to thyroid protein, was first demonstrated in 1948 (40). Thus, iodide resembles thionamide-type antithyroid agent in this respect. The Wolff-Chaikoff effect is transient in both humans and experimental animals and usually lasts only 1-2 days after iodide administration.

The ameliorating effect of large doses of iodide (as potassium iodide solution or Lugol's solution) in Graves' disease is due to an entirely different process involving inhibition of thyroid hormone secretion. This action is rapid and efficacious in severe thyrotoxicosis, and the effect is exerted directly on the thyroid gland. In a small proportion of individuals given large doses of iodide for a long period, as in the treatment of asthma or chronic bronchitis, goiter and hypothyroidism supervene. The thyroid gland shows hyperplasia and is depleted of stores of iodine. This could be corrected by giving thyroid hormone preparations. Asthmatic patients with thyroid antibodies and subjects with minor thyroid disturbances are more sensitive to iodine. Iodine also increases the blocking effect of other antithyroid drugs. Iodide, in conjunction with propranolol, is used in the treatment of thyrotoxic crisis.

Lugol's solution, which is widely used as an antithyroidal agent, consists of 5% iodine and 10% potassium iodide. Sodium iodide, USP and potassium iodide, USP are available in solid form, as is potassium iodide, USP for oral administration. The dosage of iodide can vary from 50 to 500 mg/day.

Organic Compounds. The organic compounds with antithyroid properties fall into three classes: (1) thioamides (e.g., thiourea); (2) aniline derivatives and aminoheterocyclic compounds (e.g., sulfonamides and sulfonylureas); and (3) substituted phenols (e.g., resorcinol). Of these, thioamides include all the currently used therapeutic agents (Fig. 12.5-4).

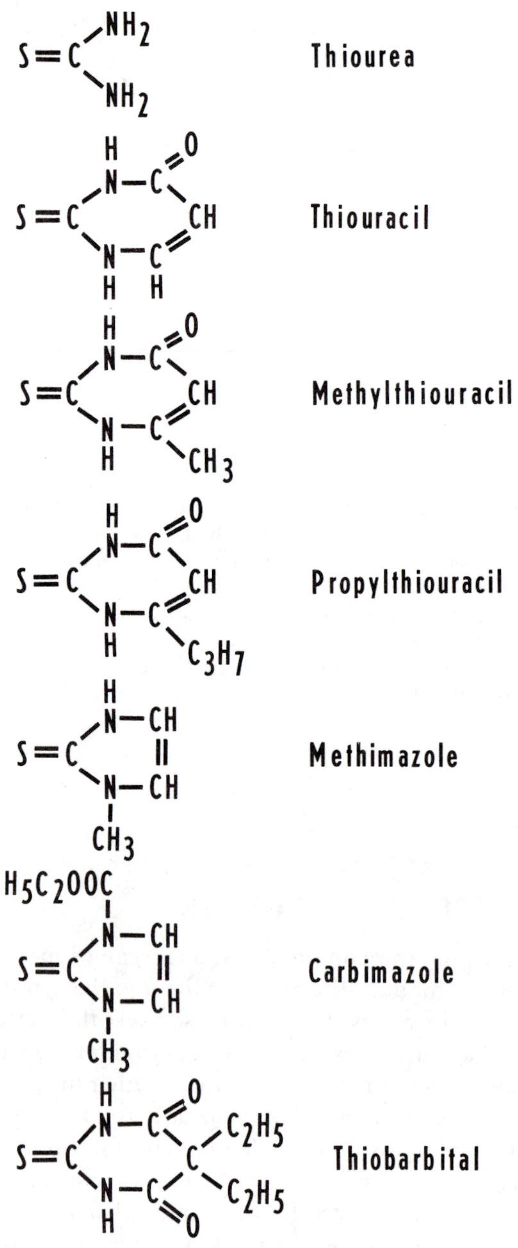

Thiourea

Thiouracil

Methylthiouracil

Propylthiouracil

Methimazole

Carbimazole

Thiobarbital

Fig. 12.5-4. *Structures of various thioureylenes used in the treatment of hyperthyroidism.*

Thioamides. Thiourea and its aliphatic derivatives as well as heterocyclic compounds containing a thiourylene group such as the thiouracils, propylthiouracil (PTU), methylthiouracil (MTU), methimazole, and carbimazole, are currently employed to treat hyperthyroidism. As shown in Fig. 12.5-4, it appears that the thiocarbamide group (S=C-N) is essential for antithyroid activity. The order of antithyroid potency in humans is as follows: methimazole > methylthiouracil > thiobarbital > thiourea = thiouracil > propylthiouracil. Thus, taking thiouracil as a standard, methimazole is about 100 times more potent. In rats, however, the order of relative activity is as follows: propylthiouracil > thiobarbital > methimazole > thiouracil = methylthiouracil > thiourea. In rats, taking thiouracil as a standard, propylthiouracil is 11 times more potent, followed by thiobarbital and methimazole, which are almost twice as potent as thiouracil in their antithyroid action.

MECHANISM OF ACTION

Thioamides inhibit the organification of iodide in the thyroid gland by interfering with oxidation of iodide to iodine by depressing peroxidase activity (34) and inhibiting the coupling of iodotyrosines (Fig. 12.5-5). Propylthiouracil or one of its metabolites binds to thyroglobulin in the thyroid gland, which in turn probably affects the structure of this thyroprotein, leading to inhibition of the coupling reaction (23). It has been proposed that coupling reaction is more sensitive to inhibition by antithyroid drugs than is the initial iodination of tyrosyl residues. Because all these compounds are strong reducing agents, they probably act by reducing active iodine back to iodide.

In addition to its primary effect of blocking oxidative iodination in the thyroid, propylthiouracil (PTU) decreases peripheral effectiveness of T_4 in the rat, and some evidence suggests that it also does so in hyperthyroid humans (7). This effect can be attributed to a significant inhibition in the rate of conversion of T_4 to T_3.

PHARMACOKINETICS

Propylthiouracil is about 75% absorbed orally, reaches peak blood levels in 1 hour, is distributed into a volume of greater than that of extracellular fluid but less than total body water, and is cleared with a half-life of about 1.5 to 2 hours (13). Biologically effective levels are achieved within 20-30 min. The overall bioavailability of the drug is estimated to be about 53-88% (3). It is believed that both liver and kidney play a major role in the metabolism of thioamide, particularly thiouracil, propylthiouracil, and methimazole. There is considerable individual variability with respect to absorption of methimazole and carbimazole from the gastrointestinal tract. Methimazole, unlike propylthiouracil, does not bind to plasma proteins. Serum half-life of methimazole is about 2 to 6 hours. Antithyroid drugs are concentrated in the thyroid tissue, and inhibition of iodide organification is depen-

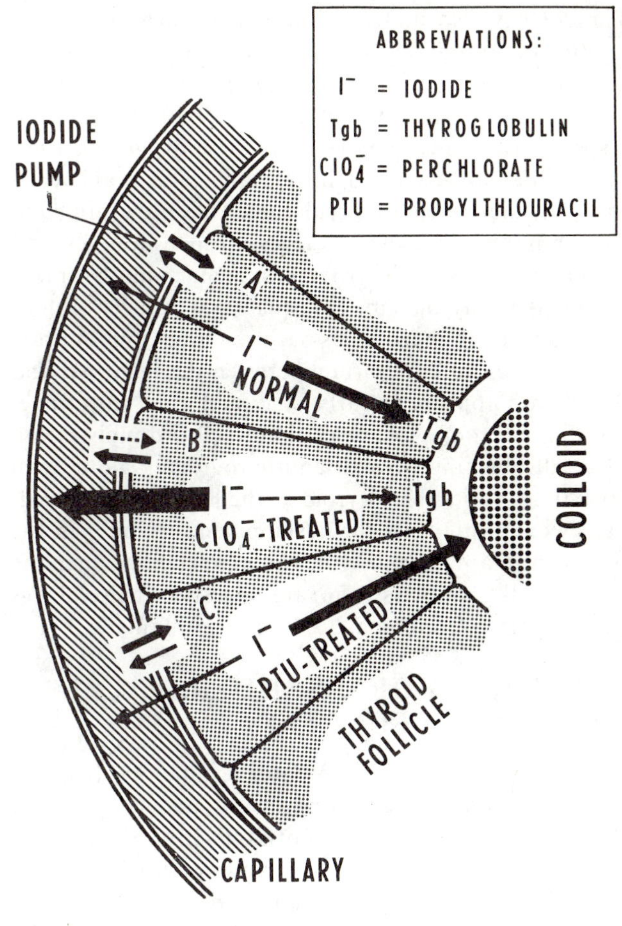

Fig. 12.5-5. *A diagram illustrating the effects of anion inhibitors (e.g., ClO_4^-) and organic iodination inhibitors (e.g., PTU) on the fate of iodide generated intrathyroidally from deiodination of iodotyrosines during the process of thyroid secretion.*

In all three cells of thyroid follicle, the iodide shown in the center is that which comes from intrathyroidal deiodination of iodoaminoacids, primarily monoiodotyrosine and diiodotyrosine. The direction and magnitude of the flux of the generated iodide is shown by the direction and size of arrows. The activity of the iodide pump is shown at the basal cell membrane, and the relative size of the arrows in ovals represents the magnitude of the flux in or out of the cell.

Cell A represents normal thyroid follicle of animals receiving no drug. In cell B the effect of ClO_4^- is illustrated. ClO_4^- inhibits the iodide pump at the basal cell membrane, allowing most of the intrathyroidally generated iodide to leave the thyroid effluent. Iodide moves more rapidly out of the follicle than it can be organically bound.

Cell C shows the effect of PTU, which inhibits the organic iodination, but produces no effect on iodide pump at the basal cell membrane. The pump prevents a massive exodus of iodide into the capillary. (Modified from Ref. 17).

dent on intrathyroid rather than blood levels of the drugs. These drugs also undergo intrathyroid metabolism by binding to thyroglobulin and stepwise oxidation (3). The main metabolites of propylthiouracil and methimazole are propylthiouracin-SO_2H and methylthiohydantoin, respectively. A major portion of these drugs and their metabolites are excreted in bile and later reabsorbed through entero-hepatic circulation. They are excreted in small amounts in urine and feces. Propylthiouracil and methimazole disappear from plasma much more rapidly during hyperthyroidism. Transplacental transfer of thiouracil and methimazole has been reported, and in pregnant females an equilibrium between the maternal and fetal blood appears as early as 30 min after an intravenous injection of ^{14}C-labeled thiouracil. Administration of a full blocking dose of antithyroid drug along with 60-120 mg desiccated thyroid to the hyperthyroid pregnant woman prevents the development of goiter in the newborn infant. Because the thioamides may enter the breast milk, mothers who are ingesting these drugs should refrain from breastfeeding their infants.

TREATMENT OF DISORDERS OF THYROID FUNCTION

Thyroid hormone disease states result either from an overproduction (hyperthyroidism) or underproduction (hypothyroidism) of thyroid hormone. In either case, the physical manifestation can be a goiter or swelling of the thyroid gland. In hypothyroidism, due to insufficient iodine intake, the negative feedback mechanism on the pituitary does not function; an increase in TSH secretion results, which causes the gland to hypertrophy. During hyperthyroidism, goiter may or may not be present. Hyperthyroidism with goiter indicates that either the negative feedback system that shuts off TSH release is not operative or that the long-acting thyroid-stimulating hormone (LATS) is being secreted. LATS, which is not controllable by feedback mechanisms of the thyroid and TSH, has been shown to exert identical stimulatory effects on thyroidal growth and iodine metabolism.

DRUGS FOR HYPOTHYROIDISM

Deficient circulating levels of T_4 and T_3 or impairment of their actions result in the clinical and biochemical features of hypothyroidism. There are several causes of hypothyroidism, which can be identified as primary (thyroidal), secondary (pituitary), or tertiary (hypothalamic). Primary hypothyroidism is characterized by low levels of thyroid hormones in serum, elevated basal TSH, and an exaggerated response to TRH. Secondary hypothyroidism is defined as a disorder of the pituitary gland resulting in low TSH levels, and this in turn results in lowering of T_3 and T_4. Tertiary hypothyroidism, in which the defect lies at the level of the hypothalamus, results in inadequate secretion of TRH as well as low TSH and thyroid hormone levels.

Cretinism and Pediatric Hypothyroidism. A permanent retardation in the development of skeleton or the central nervous system resulting from thyroid deficiency during fetal or early neonatal life has been termed cretinism. Cretinism is usually classified as endemic or sporadic. Endemic cretinism is geographically associated with endemic goiter and iodine deficiency. Sporadic cretinism is a condition of thyroid deficiency associated with retarded physical and mental development.

Cretinism may be associated with goiter, or without goiter when associated with a failure of development of the thyroid during fetal life, or with the presence of only a fragmentary thyroid at the base of the tongue. The following three methods are available for screening congenital hypothyroidism in a newborn child: (1) measurement of T_4 on filter paper spotted with blood at 2-3 days of age; (2) measurement of T_4 in umbilical cord blood; and (3) measurement of TSH in umbilical cord blood. An incidence of congenital hypothyroidism of 1 in 5000-6000 has been found with these screening methods (20). At birth, cretins may be recognized by a puffy and expressionless face and the presence of respiratory difficulty, cyanosis, persistent jaundice, umbilical hernia, poor feeding, hoarse crying, constipation, or large anterior or open posterior fontanels. Abnormalities of skeletal development such as absence of the distal femoral and proximal tibial epiphyses in a full-term fetus or neonate are regarded as a strong indication to determine the serum T_4 concentration as soon as possible.

It is known that treatment with T_4 (4.4-12.8 μg/kg/day) of congenital hypothyroidism prior to age 3 months yields a 78% chance of subsequent mental development into "normal range" (IQ greater than 85). The use of desiccated thyroid in children should be avoided. If treatment is postponed for 6 months, irreversible brain changes may occur. The child is dwarfed, the extremities are short, and he is mentally retarded, inactive, uncomplaining, and listless. The face is puffy and the enlarged tongue may protrude through the thickened lips of the half-opened mouth. The skin is dry and cool to the touch. The heart rate is slow, body temperature may be low, and the teeth erupt late.

Myxedema. Myxedema is a form of severe hypothyroidism in adults in which there is an accumulation of hydrophilic mucopolysaccarides in the ground substance of the dermis as well as other tissue, leading to thickening of the facial features and doughy induration of the skin. In adults, the manifestations of myxedema may develop gradually over a period of many years. Myxedema may result from the so-called primary atrophy of thyroid gland or lack of thyrotropin (TSH) secretion by the pituitary gland. In myxedema, the face is quite expressionless, puffy, and pallid. The skin is cold and dry, the scalp is scaly, and the hair coarse, brittle, and sparse. The fingernails are thickened and brittle, the subcutaneous tissue appears to be thickened, and there may be true edema. The voice is husky and low pitched, speech is slow, and the hearing is often faulty. The voluntary muscles are weak and flabby. The heart is often dilated and the cardiac output is diminished. The patient is prone to be drowsy and to sleep a great deal, and complains of cold in winter, but not of the heat in summer. Irrespective of the causes, hypothyroidism is treated by replacement with thyroid hormone. In addition to desiccated thyroid tissue preparations, synthetic T_4, synthetic T_3, and combinations of the two hormones are available. Most hypothyroid patients treated with L-thyroxine require between 0.1 and 0.2 mg/day. However, the dose should be individualized for each patient. The average daily dose of thyroid, USP required to treat myxedema is 120-180 mg.

Myxedema Coma. Myxedema coma can be readily recognized by the characteristic symptoms of severe hypothyroidism such as edematous face, large tongue, loss of eyebrows, alopecia, and slow reflexes. Mentation ranges from stupor to frank coma. Often, the patient has a history of gradual deterioration that becomes precipitous upon exposure to stress or cold, or with the onset of infection. The important feature of the disease is that hypotension is resistant to vasopressors unless thyroid hormone is given.

Myxedema coma has a mortality of up to 40%, even with modern modes of therapy. A loading dose of 0.4-0.5 mg of T_4 i.v. followed by a daily 0.1-mg T_4 i.v. dose is necessary until the patient can take oral medication. Improvement of vital signs can be seen within 6 to 12 hours, and return of consciousness occurs in 24 to 36 hours. Intravenous T_3 (25-50 μg daily) has been used with success; however, parenteral T_3 must be specially prepared from kits obtained only directly from the manufacturer.

Glucocorticoids are probably a valuable adjunct to thyroid hormone therapy for two reasons: (1) the possibility of hypopituitarism with adrenal insufficiency cannot be immediately excluded, and (2) it is possible that the return to normal metabolism could cause increased clearance of serum cortisol and consequent relative adrenal insufficiency, even in the absence of hypopituitarism. Hydrocortisone, 200-300 mg, is therefore given i.v. the first day and then tapered over the next few days.

Other Therapeutic Uses of Thyroid Hormones. Thyroid hormones have been used somewhat uncritically in the treatment of female infertility, menorrhagia, habitual abortion, and obesity. In the euthyroid woman, the ingestion of a replacement dose of desiccated thyroid (120-180 mg/kg/day) inhibits endogenous thyroid hormone production without altering the plasma-free T_3 levels. To achieve weight loss in a euthyroid obese patient, it is necessary to administer large amounts of thyroid hormone sufficient to produce hypermetabolism and iatrogenic thyrotoxicosis. Thyroid hormones have also been found useful to treat depressive illnesses when administered concurrently with tricyclic compounds (25).

Preparations. Preparations and dosages are listed in Table 12.5-1.

Side Effects and Drug Interactions. When used in proper dosages, thyroxine itself produces no side effects. Early symptoms of overdosage include palpitations, nervousness, diaphoresis, heat intolerance, headache, and insomnia. The overdosage may lead to hyperthyroidism, which is manifested by psychotic behavior, angina pectoris, cardiac decompensation, myalgia, severe diarrhea, and adrenal insufficiency.

Thyroid hormone potentiates the actions of oral anticoagulants, adrenergic agonists such as epinephrine, ephedrine, isoproterenol, and tricyclic antidepressants. Dosage adjustment of these agents may be necessary. Thyroid hormone increases catabolism of vitamin K-dependent clotting factors. Cholestyramine interferes with absorption of thyroid hormone from gastrointestinal tract. Thyroxine also decreases glucose tolerance in diabetic patients and may necessitate an increase in the dosage of oral hypoglycemic agents or insulin. Any patient taking steroids may be at risk for developing relative adrenal insufficiency when thyroid hormone is started; hence, steroid requirement should be closely monitored. Digitalized patients require increase in digoxin dose following concurrent treatment with thyroid hormone.

DRUGS FOR HYPERTHYROIDISM

Hyperthyroidism or thyrotoxicosis represents the clinical state produced by hypersecretion of the thyroid hormones, T_4 and T_3. There is also an increased production of T_3 from increased conversion of T_4 in the periphery. As a result, there is a sustained rise in plasma concentrations of both hormones. The most frequent types of this syndrome are: toxic diffuse goiter (also called exophthalamic goiter), Graves' disease, Parry's disease, or von Basedow's disease. Specific skin and eye changes are inherent manifestations of the disease. Toxic nodular goiter results from autonomous functioning of area(s), nodule(s), within the thyroid. In contrast to toxic diffuse goiter, toxic nodular goiter is a disease of the older age group. Furthermore, eye complications are rare in the toxic nodular goiter, and the disorder is often resistant to therapy.

Graves' disease in the newborn is manifested by irritability, flushing, supraventricular tachycardia, voracious appetite, poor weight gain or excessive weight loss, thyroid enlargement, and exophthalmos. Arrhythmias, cardiac failure, and death may occur if the thyrotoxicity is severe and the treatment is not adequate. The onset of symptoms and signs of Graves' disease may be delayed as long as 8-9 days in the newborn. The reason for this delay is not entirely clear. The treatment in the newborn includes sedation and digitalization. More specifically, iodide or thioamide drugs are administered to decrease thyroid hormone secretion. Propranolol HCl in an oral dose of 2 mg/kg/day, divided in two or three doses, can dramatically reduce cardiac and respiratory rates.

Thioamide Drugs. Thioamide derivatives such as propylthiouracil, methimazole and methylthiouracil are currently used as the principal therapy in Graves' disease in children and young adults. The preparations and dosages for initiation and maintenance of treatment are presented in Table 12.5-2.

Radioactive Iodine. ^{131}I can be employed for the treatment of Graves' disease, solitary toxic nodule, or toxic multinodular goiter in almost all patients past the childbearing age. The isotope is available as sodium radioiodide. It is generally taken orally, but intravenous preparations are available. Like stable iodine, ^{131}I is rapidly and efficiently trapped by the thyroid, incorporated into iodoamino acids, and deposited in colloid of follicles, from which it is slowly liberated. ^{131}I has a half-life of 8 days and emits both β and γ rays. The β rays have ionizing properties and thus destroy the cells, reducing both their functional and reproductive abilities. Patients who are severely hyperthyroid should be pretreated with a thioamide drug before radioactive ^{131}I is given; however, the antithyroid drug must be discontinued 3-4 days before treatment to avoid interference with the uptake of ^{131}I. Radioactive iodine is not used in pregnancy because of its passage across the placenta and potential damage to fetal thyroid. It is customarily used

Table 12.5-1
Thyroid Hormone Preparations and Dosages

Drugs	Trade Name	Replacement Dose/Day	Maintenance Dose/Day
Desiccated thyroid	THYRAR	Younger adults: 15-30 mg, p.o.; increase this amount by 15-30 mg at 2-week intervals Older adults: 7.5-30 mg, p.o.; dose is doubled at 6- to 8-week intervals until an optimal response is obtained	60-120 mg, p.o.
		Infants (1-4 months): 15-30 mg, p.o.; the amount is increased at intervals of about 2 weeks (4-12 months): 30-60 mg, p.o. (over 1 year of age): 60-180 mg	30-45 mg, p.o.
Thyroglobulin	PROLOID	Doses are the same as those given for desiccated thyroid	
Levothyroxine sodium	LEVOTHROID SYNTHROID	Young and middle-aged adults: 50-100 μg, p.o.; the amount is increased by 50-100 μg at 2- to 3-week intervals Older patients: 12.5-50 μg, p.o., for 6-8 weeks; this amount is then doubled every 6-8 weeks until the desired response is achieved Children: 3-5 μg/kg, p.o.; the dosage is increased at 2-week intervals	100-200 μg, p.o.
		Myxedema coma in adults and children: 200-500 μg, i.v.	100 μg, i.v., until patient can take oral medication
Liothyroine sodium (it has more rapid onset but shorter duration of action)	CYTOMEL	Young and middle-aged adults: 25 μg, p.o.; the amount is increased by 12.5-25 μg at 1-2 week intervals until the desired response is maintained Older adults: 2.5-5 μg, p.o., for 3-6 weeks; the amount is then doubled every 6 weeks Children: 5 μg, p.o.; this amount is increased no more than 5 μg at weekly intervals, until the desired response is maintained Myxedema coma: 10-25 μg every 8-12 hours	75-100 μg, p.o.
Liotrix (mixture of levothyroxine sodium and liothyroine sodium in a ratio of 4:1)	THYROLAR EUTHYROID	Young and middle-aged adults, and children: one tablet orally, containing 25 μg levothyroxine sodium and 6.25 μg of liothyroine sodium Older adults: one-fourth to one-half the amount given orally to younger adults; the dose is doubled at 6- to 8-week intervals until the desired response is maintained	

in patients unless surgery presents an unusual hazard, for example, in the presence of heart disease. A single dose (4-15 mCi) is often sufficient to treat hyperthyroidism, but repeated doses may sometimes be necessary, especially in patients with large nodular goiters. The most important complication following the use of radioiodine is hypothyroidism. In low doses (30 μCi), ^{131}I is also used for the diagnosis of thyroid dysfunction, because it measures uptake and localization of iodine with the use of external scanning devices.

Iodide. Iodides may be employed in the form of a strong iodine solution (Lugol's solution) or potassium iodide solution. Although small amounts of iodide are required for hormone synthesis, larger amounts block the synthesis. The action of iodide is primarily to inhibit the release of thyroid hormone, and secondarily to block the

Table 12.5-2
Thioamide Compounds

Compound	Initial Dose/Day	Maintenance Dose/Day	Incidence of Untoward Effects (%) Major[a]	Minor[b]
Carbimazole	30-50 mg, adults	5-20 mg, adults	0.7	2.0
Methimazole (TAPAZOLE)	15-60 mg, adults 0.4 mg/kg, children	10-30 mg, adults	0.3	5.0
Methylthiouracil	300-600 mg, adults	50-300 mg, adults	0.3	4.0
Propylthiouracil	300-600 mg, adults 150-300 mg, children 10 mg/kg in neonatal thyrotoxicosis	100-300 mg, adults	0.3	3.0

[a]Chiefly agranulocytosis.
[b]Chiefly skin rashes.

organic binding of iodine. However, when administered daily for a few weeks or months, the inhibition of thyroid hormone release is overcome, and the thyroid hormone stored in the gland starts to pour out, causing an acute hyperthyroid condition known as thyroid storm. To prepare hyperthyroid patients for thyroidectomy, either strong iodine solution, USP, 2-6 drops, or potassium iodide solution, USP, 5 drops, three times a day for 10 days prior ot surgery is used.

Ionic Inhibitors. As mentioned earlier, competitive inhibition of the iodide-trapping mechanism by the thyroid is achieved with a group of monovalent hydrated anions including thiocyanate (SCN^-), nitrite, and perchlorate (ClO_4^-). Potassium perchlorate in daily doses of 0.6-1 g may be used where toxic reactions to the thiocarbamide-type drugs have been encountered.

Miscellaneous Agents. Guanethidine, reserpine, and propranolol may be useful adjuncts to antithyroid agents in hyperthyroidism and thyrotoxic crisis. Of these, propranolol in doses of 20-40 mg/ day orally four times appears to be preferable because reserpine and guanethidine produce general sympathetic blockade whereas propranolol blocks only those β-adrenergic receptors that predominate in producing many of the symptoms of hyperthyroidism. However, propranolol probably has no effect on the underlying disease. Propranolol is indicated in the management of thyroid storm. It relieves tachycardia, palpitation, and hypertension and may help in preventing congestive heart failure, although it is contraindicated if myocardial failure is already present. Propranolol is also contraindicated in patients with asthma or history of hypersensitivity to this drug.

Preparations. The daily dose is ordinarily divided into three or four doses at intervals of 6 or 8 hours, because of the relatively short-lived effect of the drug. The 8 hour schedule is approximated by administration of a dose in the morning, in midafternoon, and at bedtime. However, Greer et al. (9) had reported several years ago that 300 mg propylthiouracil once a day was appropriate for effective therapy of most hyperthyroid patients. Methimazole, which has a relatively longer half-life, has also proved satisfactory in treating hyperthyroidism when given once daily in a dose of 30 mg. A possible explanation for this might be that in thyroid hormonogenesis the most sensitive point to the action of propylthiouracil is the coupling of iodotyrosines; a continuing action of the drug (that is actively concentrated by the thyroid gland) at this step over most of a 24 hour period would effectively reduce thyroid hormone formation but would not be reflected for the same length of time in changes in the uptake of radioiodine. The effect after a single daily dose is not entirely reliable, and it is better to initiate treatment with divided doses and switch, if desired, to a single daily dose for maintenance therapy. Therapy with antithyroid drugs requires medical supervision at intervals of 1-3 months. As a definitive therapy, with the object of inducing prolonged or permanent remission, the initial dose of an antithyroid drug (see Table 12.5-2) is continued until the patient is euthyroid or actually begins to be hypothyroid. Enlargement of the thyroid is often an early clue to overtreatment. Then the dose may be halved. However, too early and too great a reduction in dose is a common cause of failure to achieve satisfactory control of the disease. In pregnant women and in children, the use of antithyroid drugs alone is widely favored.

Selection of Antithyroid Drugs. Only a few of the large number of compounds known to possess antithyroid activity have been employed clinically. Some of these, including thiobarbital and thiouracil, were found unsuitable because of the high incidence of severe toxic reactions. Thiourea gives rise to an unpleasant odor and taste. The compounds most widely used today are PTU, methylthiouracil, methimazole and carbimazole. When compared with methimazole, PTU has a more rapid metabolism, limited lipid-solubility, lower potency, and limited placental transfer. However, we do not yet know whether any of these aspects really matter during clinical use of antithyroid drugs. Perhaps the only basis of selection is the incidence of sensitivity reactions to therapeutic doses rather than their relative potency.

Side Effects. The incidence of side effects from thioamide drugs is lower than from other antithyroid agents.

Except for the uniquely unpleasant odor and aftertaste imparted by thiourea, the side effects are qualitatively similar for all compounds. They may be classified as sensitivity reactions (which occur during the first 3 weeks of treatment) and the more serious complication of agranulocytosis (which occurs in 0.2-0.3% of patients treated with PTU or methimazole). Agranulocytosis most often appears after 4-8 weeks of treatment. Patients should immediately report the development of sore throat or fever, which usually heralds the onset of this reaction. The most common untoward reactions to thioamides consist of a mild, sometimes purpuric, papular rash that often subsides spontaneously without interrupting treatment but sometimes may call for changing to another drug, since cross-sensitivity is uncommon. Other rare reactions include fever, rhinitis, conjunctivitis, arthralgia, headache, thrombocytopenia, gastrointestinal manifestations, and Mikulicz's syndrome. Hepatocellular jaundice and periarteritis nodosa have also been occasionally reported. Another rare side effect is loss of scalp hair, which occurs within 2-3 months after starting the treatment. Spontaneous regrowth of hair occurs when the drug is stopped.

The side effects associated with the use of perchlorate include a high incidence of gastric irritation, nephrosis, and aplastic anemia. Thus, its only place in therapy has been in patients who cannot tolerate thioamides.

Remissions. The aim of treatment with antithyroid drugs is to achieve permanent remission of hyperthyroidism even after the treatment is discontinued. When treatment is continued for about a year, approximately one-half of the patients remain well for long periods, perhaps indefinitely thereafter. However, in 23% of the patients, hyperthyroidism returns promptly within 2 months. It is presumed that in these patients the disorder is still active and is merely controlled by the medication. Four years after the end of treatment, relapse is unusual. It is generally acknowledged that treatment with antithyroid drugs causes a loss of iodine from the thyroid, which results in a profound depletion of iodine from the body. The repletion of iodine stores is the possible underlying cause of the increased rate of relapse of hyperthyroidism. Patients are therefore advised to limit their intake of iodine during and a few months after the antithyroid therapy has been terminated. Patients treated with antithyroid drugs should be followed at yearly intervals to make sure that thyrotoxicosis has not relapsed. Studies have suggested that destructive therapy should be indicated if the thyrotoxicosis persists 2-4 years after the start of antithyroid treatment. However, if remission occurs after one course or two courses of antithyroid drugs, the destructive therapy is inappropriate.

OTHER THERAPEUTIC USES OF ANTITHYROID DRUGS

In addition to their wide application in the therapy of hyperthyroidism, antithyroid drugs are employed in the preparation for thyroidectomy. Most surgeons agree that thyrotoxicosis should be thoroughly controlled before subtotal thyroidectomy is undertaken. Propylthiouracil, in a dose of 0.1 g every 8 hour, is given for 1-3 months until the patient is euthyroid. At this time, potassium iodide or Lugol's solution may be added in a dose of three drops twice a day, and the two medication administered together for 1-3 weeks before the operation. The iodine decreases vascularity and friability of the thyroid gland so that the operative procedure is easier. Clinical evidence of the iodine effect is provided by an increase in firmness to palpitation and a decrease or disappearance of any residual bruit. Second, these compounds are also used as agents for controlling thyrotoxicosis in the pretreatment interval, or following treatment of patients receiving therapeutic doses of radioiodide. To lessen the incidence of later hypothyroidism, a trend has emerged toward employing an antithyroid drug for months or years while waiting for a gradual reduction in thyroid function caused by smaller doses of radioiodide. In severe hyperthyroidism, antithyroid drugs are given first, followed by radioiodide. The antithyroid drugs allow effective inhibition of thyroid hormone synthesis to begin immediately. They also prevent the delivery of large amounts of hormones into the blood from a radioiodide-damaged gland, as the radioiodide is given only after thyroidal hormone stores have been depleted. When this program is followed, the antithyroid drug is begun in a high dose, such as 600 mg PTU/day; after the patient is euthyroid or at least markedly improved, the drug is withdrawn for at least 3 days before administering the 4-10 mCi radioiodide (^{131}I) and may then be readministered starting 2-7 days later.

CHEMICAL FACTORS IN THE ENVIRONMENT AND THYROID

ANILINE DERIVATIVES AND AMINOHETEROCYCLIC COMPOUNDS

Potent antithyroid activity has been found in compounds with parasubstituted aminobenzene groups with or without aliphatic substitution on amino nitrogen. The antithyroid potency of these compounds is much less than that of thioamides, and none is currently used in the treatment of hyperthyroidism. These substances have a mechanism of action similar to that of thioamides, as they inhibit organic binding of iodine. However, there are apparently some major differences. Their action is markedly potentiated by small amounts of iodide, whereas thioamides are not. Para-aminobenzoic acid (PABA) has been successfully used in the treatment of thyrotoxicosis, and para-aminosalicylic acid, which is used extensively for the treatment of tuberculosis, has occasionally produced goiter in humans. The antithyroid activity of various sulfonylureas such as carbutamide and tolbutamide, which are used to treat diabetes, has been demonstrated in experimental animals and also in humans. However, they are considerably weaker than thioamides and are not employed in the treatment of thyrotoxicosis.

SUBSTITUTED PHENOLS

Aromatic compounds with metahydroxyl groups generally possess antithyroid activity (4). The most active of these compounds are resorcinol, phloroglucinol, and 2,4-dihydroxybenzoic acid.

IODINATED CONTRAST AGENTS

Sodium iopanoate and sodium opodate used orally for cholecystography induce marked decrease in serum T_3 and an increase serum T_4 and reverse T_3 (rT_3) levels in euthyroid subjects (16). The decrease in serum T_3 levels following administration of these contrast agents is due primarily to inhibition of peripheral 5-monodeiodination of T_4, and possibly, to a direct inhibitory effect on thyroid hormone (T_3) secretion.

NATURAL GOITEROGENS

One of the first reports of a possible role of natural goiterogen in the etiology of human goiter was the study of the relation between a high incidence of goiter and an extremely high consumption of cabbage. An increased incidence of goiter has also been reported in areas with high consumption of beet, kale,

Brassica seeds, soybeans, ground nuts, and walnuts. The antithyriod action of soy flour has been explained as resulting from an increase in fecal loss of thyroxine.

REFERENCES

1. Balazes, R., Booksbank, B. W. L., Davison, A., Eayrs, J. T., and Wilson, D. A. The effect of neonatal thyroidectomy on myelination in the rat brain. *Brain Res.* 15:219, 1969.
2. Balsam, A., Dobbs, C. R., and Leppo, L. E. Circadian variations in concentrations of plasma thyroxine and triiodothyronine in man. *J. Appl. Physiol.* 33:297, 1975.
3. Benker, G., and Reinwein, D. Pharmacokinetics of antithyroid drugs. *Klin.* Wochenschr. 60:531, 1980.
4. Berthezene, F., Fournier, M., Mernier, E., and Mornex, R. L'hypothyroidie induite par la resorcine. *Lyon Med.* 230:319, 1973.
5. Brasel, J. A., and Boyd, D. B. Influence of thyroid hormone on fetal brain growth and development. In: *Perinatal Thyroid Physiology and Disease,* (Fisher, D. A., and Burrow, G. N., eds.). New York: Raven Press, 1975, p. 59.
6. Emerson, C. H., Dyson, W. L. and Utiger, R. D. Serum thyrotropin and thyroxine concentration in patients receiving lithium carbonate. *J. Clin. Endocrinol. Metab.* 36:338, 1973.
7. Furth, E. D., Rives, K., and Becker, D. V. Non-thyroidal action of propylthiouracil in euthyroid, hypothyroid, and hyperthyroid man. *J. Clin. Endocrinol. Metab.* 26:239, 1966.
8. Golber, L. M., and Kandror, V. I. *Abstracts of Proceedings of the First All-Union Biochemical Congress.* No. 2. Izd. ANSSSR, 1964, p. 295.
9. Greer, M. A., Kendall, J. W., and Smith, M. *The Thyroid Gland,* Vol. 1. London: Butterworths, 1964, p. 357.
10. Harden, R. McG., and Alexander, W. D. The salivary iodide trap in man: Clinical applications. *Proc. R. Soc. Med.* 61:647, 1968.
11. Horwood, D. M., Rastogi, R. B., and Singhal, R. L. Effect of radiothyroidectomy and thyroid hormone replacement therapy on cardiac protein kinase activity and ATP hydrolysis. *Res. Comm. Chem. Pathol. Pharmacol.* 12:751, 1975.
12. Inoque, K., and Taurog, A. Acute and chronic effects of iodide on thyroid radioiodine metabolism in iodine-deficient rats. *Endocrinology* 83:279, 1968.
13. Kampmann, J., and Skovsted, L. The pharmacokinetics of propylthiouracil. *Acta Pharmacol. Toxicol. Metab.* 35:361, 1974.
14. Kaplan, M. M. The role of thyroid hormone deiodination in the regulation of hypothalamo-pituitary function. *Neuroendocrinology* 38:254, 1984.
15. Klee, C. B., and Sokoloff, L. Mitochondrial differences in mature and immature brain. Influence on rate of amino acid incorporation into protein and responses to thyroxine. *J. Neurochem.* 11:709, 1964.
16. Kleinman, R. E., Vagenakis, A. G., and Braverman, L. E. The effect of iopanoic acid on the regulation of thyrotropin secretion in euthyroid subjects. *J. Clin. Endocrinol. Metab.* 51:399, 1980.
17. Langer, P., and Greer, M. A. *Antithyroid Substances and Naturally Occurring Goiterogens.* S. Karger, New York, 1977, p. 3.
18. Larsen, P. R. Atkinson, A. J., Jr. Wellman, H. N., and Goldsmith, R. E. The effect of diphenylhydantoin on thyroxine metabolism in man. *J. Clin. Invest.* 49:1266, 1970.
19. Magnus-Levy, A. Ueber den respiratorischen gaswechsel unter dem einfluss der thyroidea sowie unter vers chiedeneu pathologische zustand. *Klin. Wochonschr.* 32:650, 1895.
20. Mitchel, M. L., Larsen, P. R., Levy, H. L., Bennett, A. J. E., and Madoff, M. A. Screening for congenital hypothyroidism. *JAMA* 239:2348, 1978.
21. Muller, M. J., and Seitz, H. J. Thyroid hormone action on intermediary metabolism. *Klin.* Wochenschr. 62:49, 1984.
22. Oppenheimer, J. H. Thyroid hormone action at the cellular level. *Science* 203:971, 1979.
23. Papapetrou, P. D., Mothon, S., and Alexander, W. D. Binding of the ^{35}S of ^{35}S-propylthiouracil by follicular thyroglobulin *in vivo* and *in vitro*. *Acta Endocrinol.* 79:248, 1975.
24. Prange, A. J., Jr., Meek, J. L., and Lipton, M. A. Catecholamines: Diminished rate of synthesis in rat brain and heart after thyroxine pretreatment. *Life Sci.* 9:901, 1970.
25. Rastogi, R. B. Thyrotropin releasing hormone influences on behavior: Possible involvement of brain monoaminergic systems. In: *Central Nervous System Effects of Hypothalamic and Other Peptides,* (Collu, R., Barbeau, A., Ducharme, J. R., and Rochefort, J. G., eds.). New York: Raven Press, 1978, p. 123.
26. Rastogi, R. B., and Singhal, R. L. Lithium: Modification of behavioral activity and brain biogenic amines in developing hyperthyroid rats. *J. Pharmacol. Exp. Ther.* 201:92, 1977.
27. Rastogi, R. B., Singhal, R. L., and Lapierre, Y. D. Effects of apomorphine on behavioral activity and brain catecholamine synthesis in normal and L-triiodothyronine-treated rats. *J. Neural Trans.* 50:139, 1981.
28. Rutherford, J. P., Watner, S. F., and Brunwald, E. Adrenergic control of myocardial contractility in conscious hypertrophied dogs. *Am. J. Physiol.* 237:590, 1980.
29. Schou, M., Amdisen, A., Jensen, S. E., and Olsen, T. Occurrence of goiter during lithium treatment. *Br. Med. J.* 3:710, 1968.
30. Singhal, R. L., and Rastogi, R. B. Neurotransmitter mechanisms during mental illness induced by alterations in thyroid function. *Pharmacol. Chemother.* 15:203, 1978.
31. Sokoloff, L. Roberts, P. A., Januska, M. M., and Kline, J. E., Mechanisms of stimulation of protein synthesis by thyroid hormones *in vivo*. *Proc. Natl. Acad. Sci. USA* 60:652, 1968.
32. Solomon, D. H. Treatment: Antithyroid drugs, surgery, radioiodine, selection of therapy. In: *The Thyroid* (Werner, S. C., and Ingbar, S. H., eds.). New York: Harper & Row, 1978, p. 814.
33. Stanbury, J. B., and Dumont, J. E. Familial goiter and related disorders. In: *The Metabolic Basis of Inherited Disease,* 6th ed. (Stanbury, J. B., Wyngaarden, J. B., Fredrickson, D. S., Goldstein, J. L., and Brown, M. S.,eds.). New York: McGraw-Hill, 1983, p. 231
34. Taurog, A. The mechanism of action of the thioureylene antithyroid drugs. *Endocrinology* 98:1031, 1976.
35. Topper, A. Mental achievement of congenitally hypothyroid children: Follow-up study of 20 cases. *Am. J. Dis. Child.* 81:233, 1951.
36. Wenzel, K. W., and Meinhold, H. Evidence of lower toxicity during thyroxine suppression after 3 mg L-thyroxine dose: Comparison to the classical L-triiodothyronine test for thyroid suppressibility. *J. Clin. Endocrinol. Metab.* 38:902, 1974.
37. Widjajakusuma, M. C. R., Basrur, P. K., and Robinson, G. A. Thyroid function in molybdenotic rabbits. *J. Endocrinol.* 57:419, 1973.
38. Williams, L. T., Lefkowitz, R. J., Watanabe, A. M. et al. Thyroid hormone regulation of beta-adrenergic receptor numbers. *J. Biol. Chem.* 252:2787, 1977.
39. Woeber, K., and Ingbar, S. H. Interactions of thyroid hormones with binding proteins. In: *Handbook of Physiology,* Vol. 3. Thyroids (Greer, M. A., and Solomon, D. H., eds.). Baltimore: Williams & Wilkins, 1974, p. 187.
40. Wolff, J., and Chaikoff, I. L. Plasma inorganic iodide as a homeostatic regulator of thyroid function. *J. Biol. Chem.* 174:555, 1948.

CHAPTER

12.6

MALE GONADAL HORMONES AND ANABOLIC STEROIDS

Edward T. Knych and John A. Thomas

ANDROGENS AND ANABOLIC STEROIDS

More than a century has elapsed since the German physiologist A. H. Berthold reported that castration-induced atrophy of the cockscomb could be prevented by implanting testes back into the abdominal cavity of the animal (2). Several decades later, extracts obtained from bull testes were observed to stimulate growth of the capon's comb. Subsequent purification and isolation of urinary steroids by several investigators eventually led to the crystallization of testosterone (4).

Testosterone is the principal hormonal product of the Leydig cells (interstitial cells) of the testes (5). Small amounts of testosterone are secreted by the adrenal gland. Two additional adrenocortical steroids, androstenedione and dehydroepiandrosterone, have weak androgenic activity. The seminiferous tubule has been known to have a weak capacity for testosterone synthesis.

Chemistry. Testosterone (or androstenolone), the principal endogenous androgen, is a C-19 steroid with a side chain at C-17 and two angular methyl groups (Table 12.6-1).

The testosterone molecule can be modified to increase its therapeutic usefulness. For example, alkylation of the 17α-position (e.g., methyltestosterone) decreases hepatic metabolism and produces a derivative that is orally active. Removal of the angular methyl group at C-19 results in a series of 19-nortestosterone derivatives that have a high protein anabolic activity and are active components in oral contraceptives (Table 12.6-2). The 19-norsteroids can be rendered orally active by the addition of alkyl groups at the C-17 position. Testosterone can also be esterified at the 17β-hydoxyl group (e.g., testosterone enanthate), which following its i.m. administration, leads to a more uniform pattern of absorption and an increase in the duration of action.

Physiological and Pharmacological Effects. Male sex hormones modulate sexual differentiation. Fetal androgens influence the development of the wolffian ducts and the urogenital sinus. Gonadal secretion of androgens is markedly increased at puberty and results in many physiological changes, leading eventually to sexual maturity (28). These changes include the development of facial and body hair, lowering of voice tone, and enhanced muscular and skeletal growth. At puberty, androgens are required for the initiation of spermatogenesis, development of external genitalia, and growth and maintenance of accessory sex organs. Sexual drive and libido are also increased by androgens. Other organs including the liver and kidney are affected by androgens.

Both endogenous androgens and certain derivatives can exert a generalized protein anabolic action. Testosterone causes the retention of nitrogen by increasing the rate of protein synthesis while decreasing protein catabolism. Synthetic anabolic steroids are weak androgens, and nitrogen retention may occur without significant virilization if intermittent therapy is employed. Androgens also cause the retention of sodium, potassium, and phosphorus and decrease the urinary excretion of calcium.

Under the influence of androgens there is a marked increase in skeletal growth resulting from stimulation of the epiphyseal plates of long bones (9). Epiphyseal centers appear and epiphyseal plates close earlier when stimulated by androgens. The mechanisms through which androgens stimulate growth and maturation of the skeleton are not clearly determined. It has been suggested that androgens stimulate release of growth hormone and thereby promote growth of the skeleton (18).

Administration of androgens to normal guinea pigs, rats, and fowl results in increases in hemoglobin, red blood cells, reticulocytes, and bone marrow erythroid activity. Increases in red cells, hemoglobin, and hematocrit have also been reported in castrated male subjects after the administration of androgens (10). In pharmaco-

Table 12.6-1
Some Androgenic Steroids Used in Therapy

Steroid	Preparations
Testosterone, USP	AS: 25, 50, 100 mg/ml, i.m. P: 75 mg, s.c.
Testosterone propionate, USP	T: 10 mg OS: 25, 50, 100 mg/ml, i.m.
Testosterone enanthate, USP	OS: 100, 200 mg/ml, i.m.
Testosterone cypionate, USP	OS: 50, 100, 200 mg/ml, i.m.
Methyltestosterone, USP	T: 5, 10, 25 mg C: 10 mg
Fluoxymesterone, USP	T: 2, 5, 10 mg
Danazol. USP	C: 200 mg

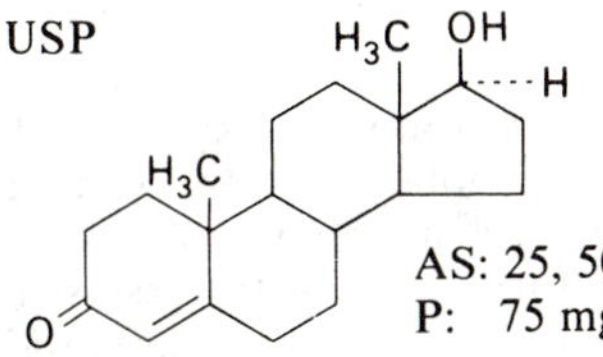

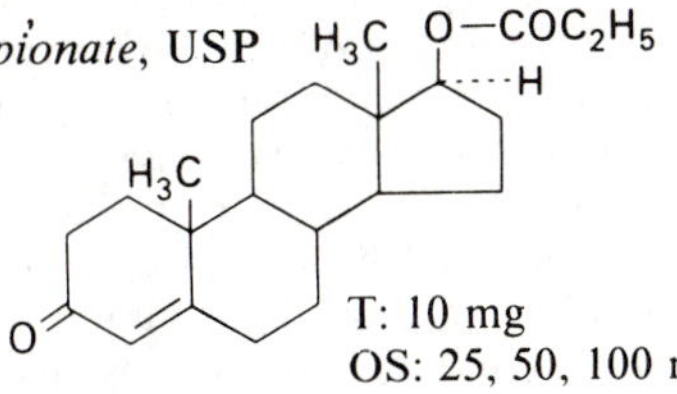

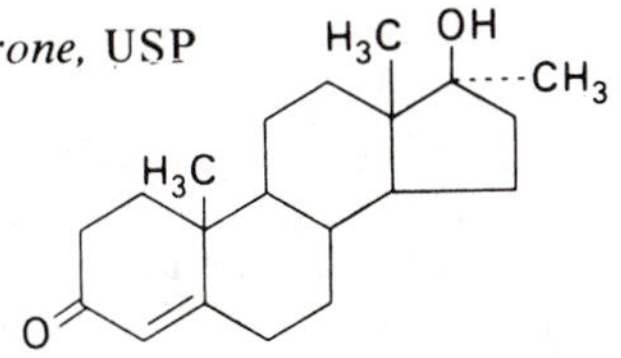

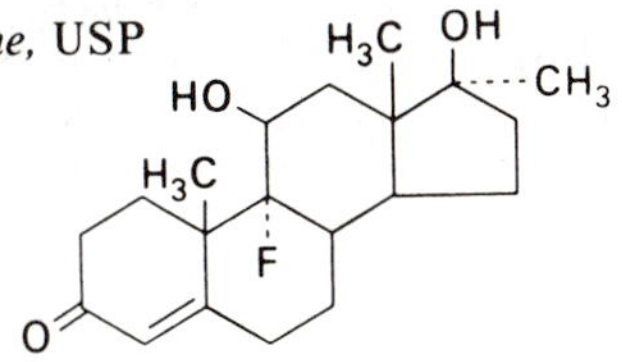

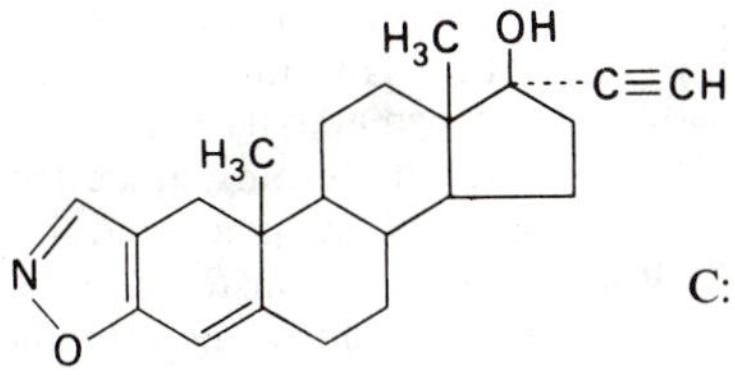

AS, Aqueous suspension; C, capsule; OS, oily solution; P, Pellets; T, Tablet.

logical doses, androgenic hormones may decrease levels of thyroxine-binding globulin (TBG), resulting in lowered total serum thyroxine (T_4) levels and increased resin uptake of T_3 and T_4. Androgens can stimulate salivary and sebaceous gland activity, although the specific biochemical events are poorly described.

The cellular actions produced by androgens or androgen-like steroids are best observed in the castrate animal treated with these hormonal agents. In fact, the response

Table 12.6-2
Some Anabolic Steroids Used in Therapy

Steroid	Preparations
Calusterone	T: 50 mg
Dromostanolone propionate, USP	OS: 50 mg/ml, i.m.
Ethylestrenol	E: 2 mg/5 ml T: 2 mg
Methandriol	AS, OS: 50 mg/ml, i.m.
Methandrostenolone, USP	T: 2.5, 5 mg
Nandrolone decanoate, USP	OS: 50, 100 mg/ml, i.m.
Nandrolone phenopropionate, USP	OS: 25, 50 mg/ml, i.m.

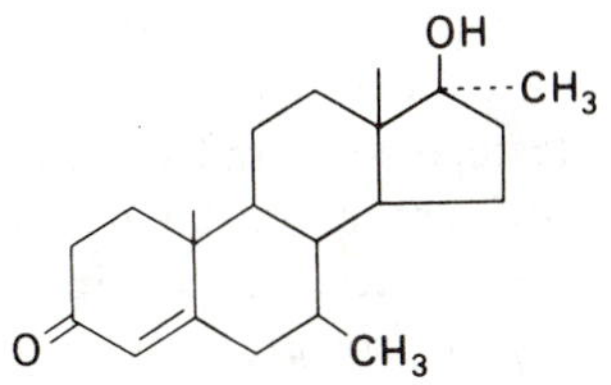

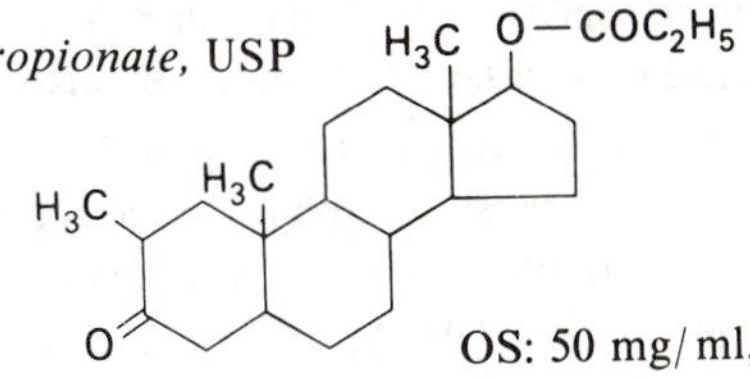

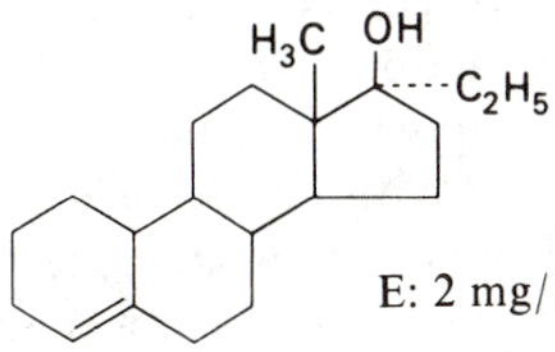

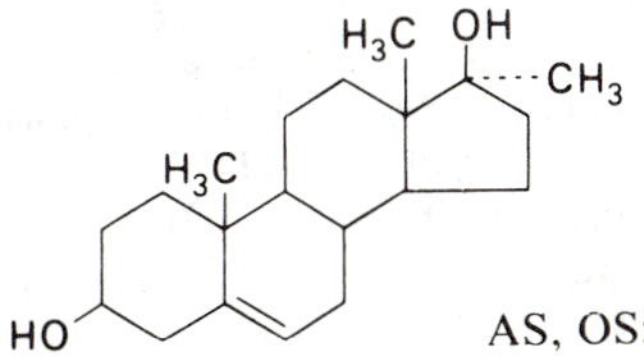

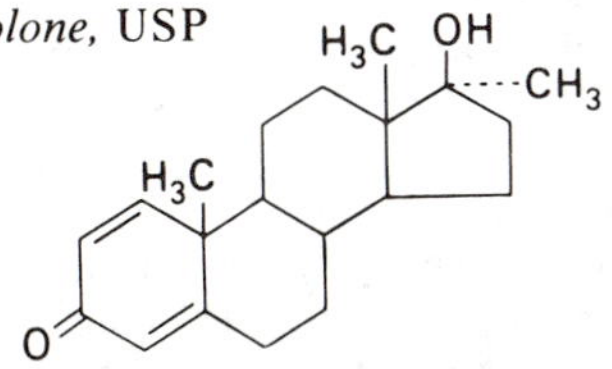

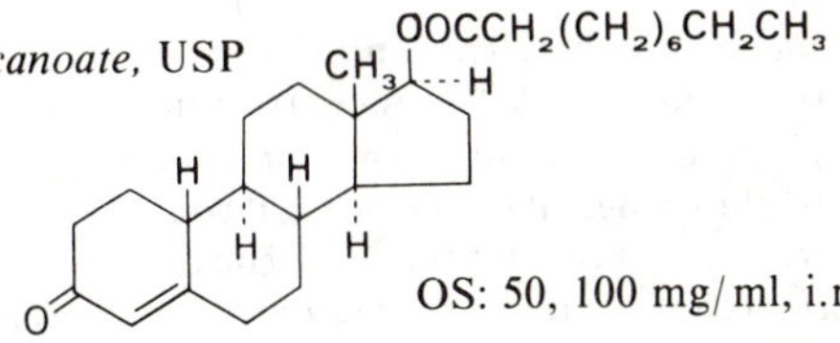

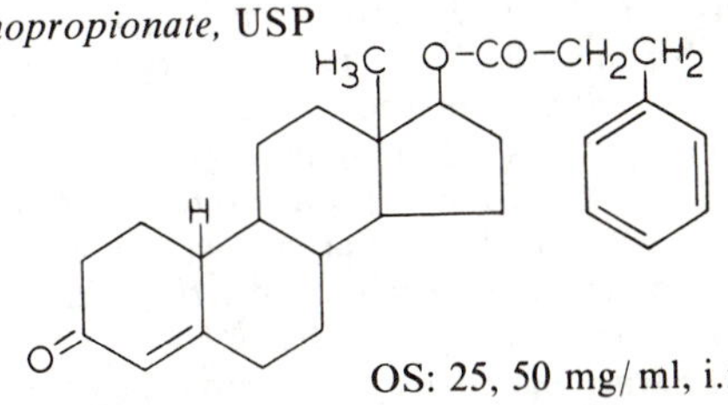

T, Tablet; Os, oily solution; E, emultion; AS, Aqueous suspension.

of sex accessory organs of the castrated animal provides the basis for androgen bioassays. Androgens cause a rapid increase in sex accessory organ RNA polymerase activity. The resulting RNA formed increases the synthesis of functional protein according to the genetic information coded in cellular DNA (12). The protein anabolic actions of testosterone and certain 19-norsteroids are particularly evident in skeletal muscles. DNA synthesis is also stimulated by testosterone in androgen-dependent organs such as the prostate and seminal vesicle. Lipid and carbohydrate metabolism is also increased by androgens in these organs. In particular, the androgen-induced increase in accessory sex gland fructose has been used as a chemical indicator of androgenic activity (17). Testosterone can increase intracellular concentrations of adenosine triphosphate (ATP) and cyclic adenosine monophosphate (cAMP). Androgens induce changes in cellular permeability that result in water imbibition and alterations in electrolyte content. Male sex hormones can exert a maintenance action upon spermatogenesis, but this action also requires the presence of follicle-stimulating hormone (FSH). Withdrawal of long-term administration of large doses of a long-acting testosterone preparation results in rebound spermatogenesis in subjects with oligospermia.

Biosynthesis. The biosynthesis of androgens occurs in the testes (Fig. 12.6-1) and in several other organs, including the ovary, adrenal, skin, and placenta (14). In the female, androgen synthesis is usually extragonadal. Androgens produced by the adrenal cortex consist primarily of androstenedione and dehydroepiandrosterone (DHEA), which are less potent than testosterone.

In the testes, steroidogenesis occurs primarily in the interstitial cells (Leydig cells) (6). Steroidogenesis is modulated by the pituitary gonadotropin luteinizing hormone (LH, ICSH). Acetate is the precursor for the androgens. It is converted to cholesterol, which is stored in lipid droplets in an esterified form. The cholesterol required for testosterone formation is transported into mitochondria, where pregnenolone is formed by the action of side-chain cleavage enzymes. The conversion of cholesterol to pregnenolone is the rate-limiting step in the formation of testosterone and is stimulated by LH. The action of LH is associated with activation of adenylate cyclase and increased intracellular cAMP concentrations. Pregnenolone, once formed, diffuses out of the mitochondria to the endoplasmic reticulum where it is converted, through a series of intermediate steroids, to testosterone. The conversion of pregnenolone to testosterone requires the action of five different enzymes: 17α-hydroxylase, 17,20-desmolase, 3β-hydroxysteroid dehydrogenase, 17β-hydroxysteroid dehydrogenase, and Δ 4, 5-3 ketosteroid isomerase. Daily production of testosterone by normal males ranges from 4 to 14 mg/24 hours. Aging may result in a decreased production of androgens.

The testes also secrete dihydrotestosterone (DHT), the A-ring reduced form of testosterone, which is about one and one-half to two times as potent as testosterone. About 50-100 μg of DHT is secreted daily by the testes.

Pharmacokinetics. Testosterone given orally is metabolized in the intestine and 44% is cleaved by the liver in the first pass. Oral doses as high as 400 mg/day are required to achieve clinically effective blood levels for full replacement therapy (8). Synthetic androgens with 17α-alkyl substitutions (e.g., methyltestosterone) are metabolized more slowly by the liver and are therefore more suitable than testosterone for oral administration.

Testosterone esters are less polar than testosterone. Esters of testosterone in oil (administered i.m.) are absorbed slowly; thus testosterone cypionate and enanthate can be given at intervals of several (2-4) weeks.

Nearly all of the circulating testosterone is bound to either sex hormone-binding globulin (SHBG) or to albumin. SHBG generally determines the distribution of testosterone between the free and bound forms, and the free testosterone concentration will determine its half-life, which varies widely, from 10 to 100 min.

Testosterone undergoes metabolic changes in both the liver and kidney (5). A number of hepatic enzymes can chemically modify the testosterone molecule, usually producing metabolites that are biologically active though less potent. In the liver, oxidation and conjugation render the testosterone molecule more water soluble and hence more readily excreted by the kidneys. Several drugs (e.g., barbiturates) and high doses of androgens can induce hepatic microsomal enzyme systems involved in androgen metabolism. The principle metabolites of testosterone are androsterone and etiocholanolone, which are measured in urine as 17-ketosteroids. However, a major fraction of 17-ketosteroids is derived from steroids secreted by the adrenal cortex. In androgen target organs such as the prostate, testosterone is metabolized by the enzyme 5α-reductase to DHT, which is the active form of the hormone (3). Testosterone may also be aromatized in several tissues (e.g., hypothalamus) to estradiol.

Androgen Receptors. Several organs contain specific high-affinity receptors for androgens (22). Androgen receptors are found in the cytoplasm of target organs such as the seminal vesicles and the prostate gland. The adenohypophysis and regions of the hypothalamus also contain androgen receptors.

Testosterone readily enters the cell by passive diffusion. Once inside most androgen-sensitive tissues, testosterone is converted to DHT by 5α-reductase. DHT appears to be the active form of the hormone in these tissues (3). In the hypothalamus, testosterone may also be aromatized to estrogen, which appears to play an important role in the negative feedback regulation of gonadotropin secretion. DHT readily forms a complex with the androgen receptor. This hormone-receptor complex is translocated to the nucleus, where it interacts with the proteins associated with chromatin. This interaction initiates the events characteristic of androgen activity (12).

Certain drugs, synthetic steroids, and estrogens can interfere with the uptake, metabolism, and binding of male sex hormones (27). Both steroid and nonsteroid estrogens can interfere with the assimilation of androgens into their target organs. Cyproterone acetate has antiandrogenic properties as a result of its ability to interfere with the formation of the androgen-receptor complex (19).

Adverse Effects and Contraindications. Excessive virilization is the most common adverse effect in the use of androgens, particularly in women and children. In females, facial hair, alopecia, and changes in voice pitch and body configuration are particularly distressing. Precocious puberty may develop in children of both sexes. Intensive androgen therapy in the prepubertal patient can result in premature closure of the epiphyseal plates and termination of long bone growth. Androgen therapy may also cause hypercalcemia. Priapism, acne, and gynecomastia may be troublesome in males.

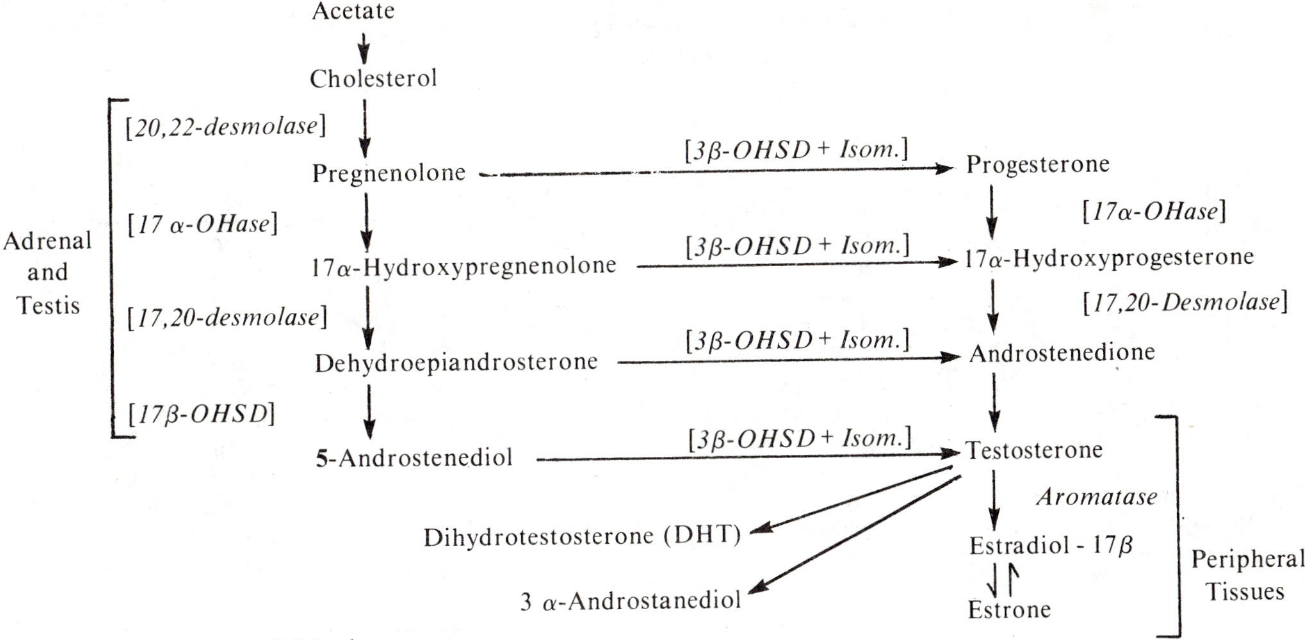

Fig. 12.6-1. *Biosynthesis of male sex hormones in the testes and conversion to other active hormones in peripheral tissues.*

Changes in hepatic function are seen with the use of those androgens containing a 17α-alkyl substitution. Such substitutions render the steroid orally effective. However, they also cause a decrease in liver function, usually reversible upon cessation of therapy, that may result in jaundice and/or biliary stasis. Primary hepatocellular carcinoma and peliosis hepatitis have been reported in patients treated with anabolic androgens for extended periods of time, although these reports are rare.

Androgens and anabolic steroids are contraindicated in males with carcinoma of the breast or with known or suspected carcinoma of the prostate. They are also contraindicated in pregnant women.

Therapeutic Uses. Hormonal replacement, in conditions associated with a deficiency or lack of endogenous testosterone, is the principle indication for the use of androgenic steroids and requires long-term therapy (13). These conditions include primary hypogonadism (testicular failure due to cryporchidism, bilateral torsion, orchitis, and vanishing testes syndrome), hypogonadotropic hypogonadism (gonadotropin or GnRH deficiency; pituitary-hypothalamic injury from trauma, tumors, or radiation), and delayed puberty (Table 12.6-3). In delayed puberty, replacement therapy should not be attempted prior to chronological age of twelve or a bone age of ten.

The ability of androgens to retard the aging process in males is somewhat dubious (29). The aging process in the male is not solely related to diminished blood levels of male sex hormones. Androgen levels in the male remain essentially unchanged until at least the seventh decade of life. Although there may be a reduction in androgen synthesis by the testes in advanced age, there is also a proportional decrease in the metabolic clearance rate of male sex hormones. There appears little justification for the use of androgens to slow the normal aging process.

Cooperative studies have established the ability of testosterone to induce objective regression of metastatic carcinoma of the breast in early postmenopausal women (16). Therapy with estrogens produces a similar response rate in these patients. However, since conventional chemotherapeutic agents produce higher remission rates, it is unclear whether androgens have a role in the treatment of breast carcinoma (23).

The protein anabolic agents have been used in a variety of conditions involving negative nitrogen balance. These agents are often used in these instances because they promote positive nitrogen balance but possess minimal virilizing activity. Androgens have been utilized in patients with debilitating diseases, after surgery, with severe trauma, and in instances involving corticoid-induced muscle wasting (25). The use of anabolic steroids to increase muscle mass and strength in normal healthy athletes lacks a therapeutic rationale and is highly questionable. Such "doping" of athletes may lead to suppression of gonadotropin release with subsequent inhibition of spermatogenesis and infertility. Anabolic steroids are probably effective as adjunctive therapy in the treatment

Table 12.6-3
Androgen Therapy

Drug	Route and Frequency of Administration	Replacement Therapy in Male Dose (mg)	Therapy in Breast Carcinoma Dose (mg)
Fluoxymesterone	p.o.,daily	5-20	10-40
Methyltestosterone	p.o., daily	10-50	50-200
	buccal, daily	5-25	25-100
Testosterone	s.c., pellets, q. 3-6 months	150-450	
Testosterone cypionate	i.m., q. 2-4 weeks	50-400	200-400
Testosterone enanthate	i.m., q. 2-4 weeks	50-400	200-400
Testosterone propionate	i.m., 2 to 3 times a week	25-50	50-100
	buccal, daily	5-20	200
Calusterone	p.o., daily		150-300
Dromostanolone	i.m., 3 times weekly		100
Testolactone	oral, daily		1000
	i.m., 3 times weekly		100

of postmenopausal osteoporosis when given with adequate dietary calcium and good general health-promoting measures.

Androgens exert an erythropoietic effect in certain types of refractory anemia (24). This effect is thought to result directly from stimulation of bone marrow cells and secondarily from increased synthesis of erythropoietin by the kidney. Large doses of androgens and anabolic steroids are used in the treatment of myelofibrosis, aplastic anemia, and anemias secondary to bone marrow depression following the use of myelotoxic drugs or radiation. Androgens have been used in the management of anemia due to renal failure in both anephric patients and those with intact kidneys (1). Danazol is frequently used in the treatment of endometriosis, fibrocystic disease of breast, and hereditary angioneurotic edema (15). In the latter condition stanozolol is also effective (26).

ANTIANDROGENS

An agent that can antagonize the action of testosterone is referred to as an antiandrogen (18) (Fig. 12.6-2). An antiandrogen does not necessarily have to exert its antagonistic action directly upon an androgen target organ. Rather, it may suppress pituitary gonadotropin release and thereby indirectly interfere with androgenic responses.

Estrogens and some progestational agents might be considered antiandrogenic when used in certain therapeutic circumstances. The chronic administration of estrogens to intact males leads to a castration-like effect upon androgen-sensitive tissues. The mechanism of estrogen action is probably related to its ability to suppress gonadotropin secretion, although estrogens can directly interfere with steroidogenesis and block several androgen-induced effects in accessory sex tissue.

Cyproterone acetate is a synthetic steroid that possesses some progestational activities (19). However, it is more widely known for its antiandrogenic action. This agent prevents the interaction of dihydrotestosterone with the androgenic receptor. Its clinical use in controlling androgen-dependent tumors (e.g., prostatic carcinoma) has not been too successful. Its use in the management of hirsutism and in severe acne has also been suggested. In addition to cyproterone acetate, the steroid BOMT (6α-bromol-17α-methyl-17β-hydroxy-14-oxa-5α-androstane-

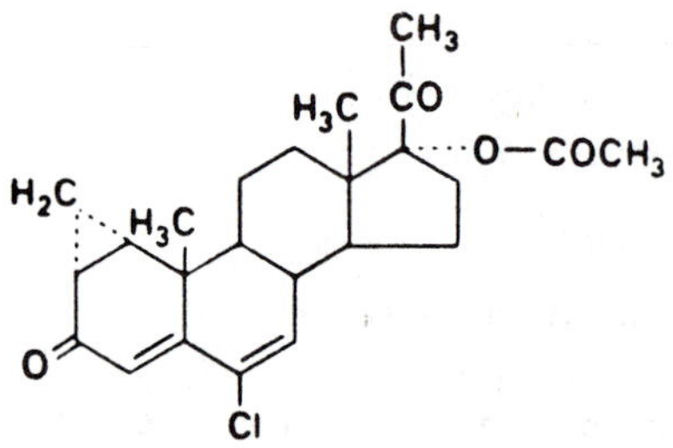

Cyproterone Acetate

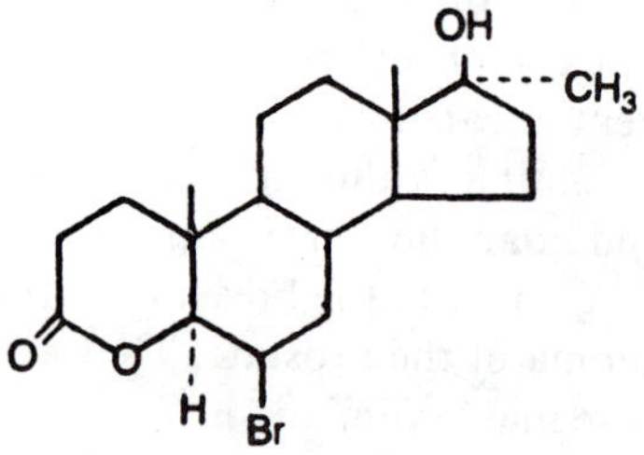

BOMT

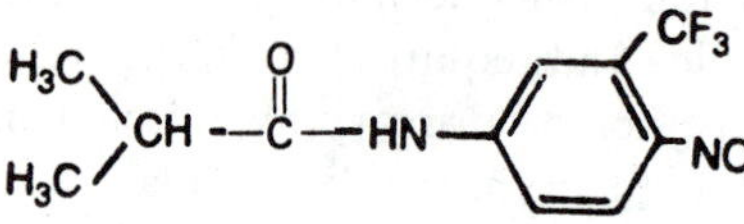

Flutamide

Fig. 12.6-2. *Some representative antiandrogens.*

3-one) and the nonsteroidal agent flutamide also interfere with the interaction of androgens and their receptors (20).

Antiandrogens and other agents are currently being studied for their ability to reversibly suppress spermatogenesis and thereby function as useful male contraceptives. A variety of agents can inhibit spermatogenesis (21, 29). These include the antiandrogens, alkylating agents, nitrofurans, dinitropyrroles, and chlorinated sugars. Unfortunately, their usefulness is limited by their irreversible action or toxicity. Nevertheless, interest has grown in the phenolic compound called gossypol, which the Chinese have isolated from various portions of the cotton plant. Although it is too early to evaluate the potential of gossypol as a male contraceptive, preliminary studies indicate its ability to reversibly inhibit spermatogenesis in humans. Interest is also being shown in the development of treatment regimens consisting of the administration of both a progestin and an androgen. The pharmacological basis for such a treatment regimen is the suppression of gonadotropin secretion by the progestin and the maintenance of secondary sexual characteristics by the androgen. All methods for male contraception remain investigational. However, it appears likely, that control of male fertility will be available in the foreseeable future.

REFERENCES

1. Anagnostou, H., and Fried, W. Anemia of renal disease. In: *Hematologic Problems of Renal Disease,* (Jepson, J. H., ed.). Menlo Park, Calif: Addison-Wesley, 1979, p. 1.
2. Berthold, A. H. Transplantation der holden. *Arch. Anat. Physiol.* 16:42, (1849).
3. Bruchovsky, N., and Wilson, J. D. The conversion of testosterone to 5α-androstan-17β-ol-3-one by rat prostate gland *in vivo* and *in vitro*. *J. Biol. Chem.* 243:2012, 1968.
4. Butenandt, A., and Tscherning, K. Über die chemische untersuchung der sexualhormons. *Z. Angen. Chem.* 44:905, 1931.
5. Eik-Nes, K. B. Production and secretion of testicular hormones. *Recent Prog. Horm. Res.* 27:517, 1971.
6. Hsueh, A. J. W. Current developments in the mechanism of action of reproductive hormones. *Clin. Obstet. Gynecol.* 21:53, 1978.
7. Huggins, C., Scott, W. W., and Hodges, C. V. Studies of prostatic Cancer. III. The effects of fever, of desoxycorticosterone and of estrogen on clinical patients with metastatic carcinoma of the prostate. *J. Urol.* 46:997, 1941.
8. Johnsen, S. G., Bennett, E. P., and Jensen, V. G. Therapeutic effectiveness of rat testosterone. *Lancet* 2:1473, 1974.
9. Kaplan, J. G., Moshang, R., Bernstein, R., Parks, J. S. and Bongiovanni, A. M. Constitutional delay of growth and development: effects of treatment with androgens. *J. Pediatr.* 82:38, 1973.
10. Kennedy, B. J. Stimulation of erythropoiesis by androgenic hormones. *Ann. Intern. Med.* 57:917, 1962.
11. Kennedy, B. J. Hormonal therapies in breast cancer. *Semin. Oncol.* 1:119, 1974.
12. Liao, S. Molecular actions of androgens. In: *Biochemical Actions of Hormones,* (Litwack, G., ed.). New York: Academic Press, 1977, p. 351.
13. Longson, D. Androgen therapy. *Practitioner* 208:338, 1972.
14. Lucas, W. M., Whitemore, W. F., and West, C. D. Identification of testosterone in human spermatic vein blood. *J. Clin. Endocrinol. Metab.* 17:465, !957.
15. Madanes, A. E., and Farber, M. Danazol. *Ann. Intern. Med.* 96:625, 1982.
16. McGuire, W. L. Physiological principles underlying endocrine therapy of breast cancer. In: *Breast Cancer, Vol. 1. Current Approaches to Therapy* (McGuire, W. L., ed.). New York: Plenum Press, 1977, p. 217.
17. Mann, T. *The Biochemistry of Semen and of the Male Reproductive Tract.* London: Metheum, 1964.
18. Martin, L. G., Clark, J. W., and Connor, T. B. Growth hormone secretion enhanced by androgens. *J. Clin. Endocrinol. Metab.* 28:425, 1968.
19. Martini, L., and Motta, M. *Androgens and Anti-Androgens.* New York: Raven Press, 1977.
20. Neumann, F., and Steinbeck, H. Antiandrogens. In: *Handbuch der Experimenter Pharmakologie,* Vol. 35, part 2, (Eichlar, O., et al., eds.). Berlin: Springer-Verlag, 1974, p. 235.
21. Nieschlag, E., Wickings, E. J., and Breuer, H. Chemical methods for male fertility control. *Contraception* 23:1, 1981.
22. O'Malley, B. W. Mechanism of action of steriod hormones. *N. Engl. J. Med.* 284:370, 1971.
23. Priestman, T., Baum, M., Jones, V., and Forbes, J. Comparative trial of endocrine vs cytotoxic treatment in advanced breast cancer. *Br. Med. J.* 1:1248, 1977.
24. Shahidi, N. T. Androgens and erythropoiesis. *N. Engl. J. Med.* 289:72, 1973.
25. Shahidi, N. T. Anabolic androgenic hormones. *Am. J. Med.* 62:546, 1977.
26. Sheffer, A. L. Fearon, D. T., and Austen, K. F. Clinical and biochemical effects of stanozolol therapy for hereditary angioedema. *J. Allergy Clin. Immunol.* 68:181, 1981.
27. Walsh, P. C., and Korenman, S. G. Mechanism of androgenic action: effect of specific intracellular inhibitors. *J. Urol.* 105:850, 1971.
28. Williams-Ashman, H. G., and Reddi, A. H. Actions of vertebrate sex hormones. *Ann. Rev. Physiol.* 33:31, 1971.
29. Wilson, J. D., and Griffin, J. E. The use and misuse of androgens. *Metabolism* 29:1278, 1980.
30. Wong, P. Y. D. Pharmacology of male contraception. *Trends in Pharmacol. Sci.* 1:254, 1980.

ADDITIONAL READING

Forbes, G.B. The effect of anabolic steroids on lean body meass: The dose response curve. *Metabolism* 34:571, 1985.

Haupt, H.A., and Rovere, G.D. Anabolic steroids: A review of the literature. *Am. J. Sports Med.* 12:469, 1984.

Hurley, B.F. et al. High-density-lipoprotein cholesterol in bodybuilders V power-lifters. *JAMA* 252:507, 1984.

Lamb, D.R. Anabolic steroids in athletics: How well do they work and how dangerous are they. *Am. J. Sports Med.* 12:31, 1984.

Snyder, P.J. Clinical uses of androgens. *Ann. Rev. Med.* 35:207, 1984.

Strauss, R.H., Liggett, M.T., and Lanese, R.R. Anabolic steroid use and perceived effects in ten weight-trained women athletes. *JAMA* 253:2871, 1985.

CHAPTER
12.7

FEMALE GONADAL HORMONES

Carol G. Smith and Michael T. Smith

THE NORMAL MENSTRUAL CYCLE

A schematic representation of hormone levels during the normal menstrual cycle is shown in Fig. 12.7-1. The menstrual cycle is divided into *menstrual, follicular, ovulatory,* and *luteal* phases, with the first day of menstruation designated as day 1 of the normal cycle. Ovulation occurs at approximately the middle of the cycle, whose length is shown as 28 days.

The initiation of the *follicular phase* of the normal menstrual cycle actually begins late in the previous cycle. Follicle-stimulating hormone (FSH) levels begin to increase late in the luteal phase. These increased levels of FSH are maintained throughout the menstrual phase and early follicular phase of the new cycle. During the follicular phase FSH and the slowly increasing luteinizing hormone (LH) levels stimulate follicular growth and development. Developing follicles begin to secrete estrogen as early as days 7-8 of the cycle; this estrogen secretion during the follicular phase of the cycle results in the proliferative growth of the endometrium. Concomitant with the rise of estrogens is a decrease in FSH (by negative feedback), whereas, in contrast, LH levels slowly increase, as the effects of estrogen on LH levels are thought to be mediated through both positive and negative feedback mechanisms. The rising estrogen levels late in the follicular phase cause a surge in the secretion of LH that persists for approximately 24 hr. There is also a concomitant but modest rise in FSH. The LH surge leads to the final steps in the maturation of the follicle and ovulation within 16-24 hr; LH also initiates the formation of the corpus luteum. Shortly after the onset of the LH surge, estrogen levels decline.

The *luteal phase* of the cycle is marked by an increase in plasma levels of progesterone and estrogen and the development of the secretory endometrium. The corpus luteum reaches full maturity at days 20-22; and, unless pregnancy intervenes, regression begins within several days. As the corpus luteum begins to regress, levels of progesterone and estrogen decrease. Coincident with the decreasing plasma concentrations of estrogen and progesterone, FSH and LH levels increase and a new cycle begins. The decrease in estrogen and progesterone levels also results in the initiation of menstruation.

CLASSIFICATION OF FEMALE SEX STEROIDS

ESTROGENS

Chemistry and Biosynthesis. The major source of endogenous estrogen in women is its synthesis and secretion (regulated by FSH) by ovarian follicles. In the normal menstrual cycle, the ovary synthesizes estrogen, primarily through cholesterol → pregnenolone → progesterone → 17-hydroxyprogesterone → androstenedione → estradiol. A reaction of major importance is the aromatization of the ring of androgenic precursors (androstenedione and testosterone) to form estrogens (Fig. 12.6-1). In certain pathological conditions, the aromatization reaction appears to be defective; the precursor androgenic steroids escape into circulation, producing virilizing effects (14). The aromatization of androgenic steroids of adrenal origin can occur in peripheral tissues, resulting in the production of estrogens of nonovarian origin; such peripheral production of estrone may be the major source of circulating estrogens in postmenopausal women (10). In pregnancy, the principal pathway of estrogen synthesis is placental conversion of androgens secreted by the fetal and maternal adrenals. The three main estrogens are *estradiol-17β* (the most potent of the ovarian estrogens), *estrone* (formed by the oxidation of estradiol and about one-half as potent as estradiol), and *estriol* (formed by the hydration of estrone). The latter conversions of estrogen take place mainly in the liver.

Chemical alterations in the natural estrogens have resulted in preparations that, in contrast to the endogenous hormones, are orally active (Fig. 12.7-2). Ethinyl estradiol is the C-17 ethinyl derivative of estradiol, and mestranol is the methyl ester of ethinyl estradiol. These modifications result in protection from inactivation by the liver, thereby enhancing the oral activity and increasing estrogenic potency. Conjugated estrogens are mix-

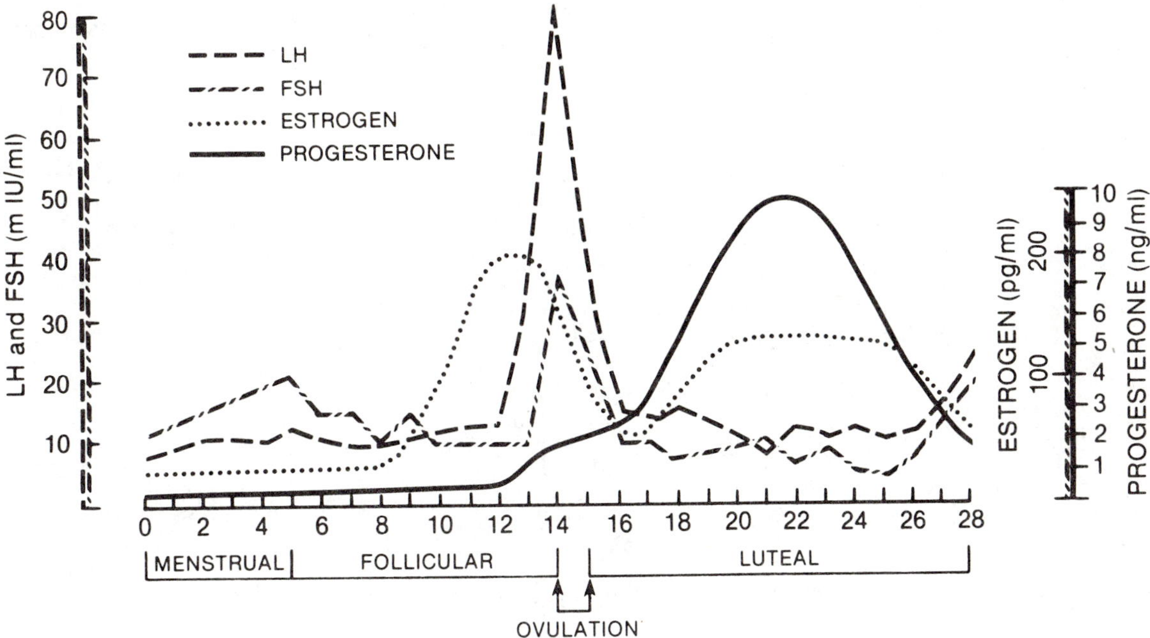

Fig. 12.7-1. *Schematic representation of the interactions of the gonadotropins and sex steroids during the normal menstrual cycle.*

Approximate hormone levels and days of the cycle demonstrate interrelationships of the gonadotropins and sex steroids during an ovulatory cycle.

tures of sodium salts of the sulfate esters of the estrogenic substances (principally estrone and equilin) excreted by pregnant mares. They contain 50-65% of sodium estrone sulfate, and 20-35% of sodium equilin sulfate, calculated on the basis of total estrogen content.

Approximately 80% of circulating estradiol is bound to sex hormone-binding globulin (SHBG); a carrier protein also transports testosterone. Natural and synthetic estrogens are metabolized in the liver to less pharmacologically active forms. These metabolites are excreted in the urine and bile as sulfates and glucuronides.

Other chemical compounds, including certain plant sterols, are also estrogens. Diethylstilbestrol (DES) is a potent, nonsteroidal estrogen with the following chemical structure:

$$\mathrm{HO{-}C_6H_4{-}C(C_2H_5){=}C(C_2H_5){-}C_6H_4{-}OH}$$

Diethylstilbestrol

It is orally active and metabolized slowly by the liver. DES has been extensively used as an estrogen and as an additive to cattle feed to accelerate weight gain. Recent studies have linked DES administration to the development of malignant tumors in reproductive tissues. A significant association between maternal ingestion of DES during pregnancy and the increased occurrence of vaginal adenosis and vaginal adenocarcinoma among female offspring (postpuberty) has been reported (7). Thus, DES and chemically related estrogens are now contraindicated during pregnancy. Other nonsteroidal estrogens with varying degrees of estrogenic potency include hexestrol, dienestrol, methallenestril, and chlortrianisene.

Estrogen Receptors. Interaction in target tissues between estrogens and the specific intracellular proteins called receptors is generally considered to follow the same scheme for all classes of steroid hormones. Steroids enter the cells of the target tissues by passive diffusion and then bind to specific receptors (cytosol proteins). The steroid hormone receptor complex then enters into the nucleus to bind with nuclear chromatin, which activates synthesis of messenger RNA (mRNA) molecules by a mechanism not clearly established. This hormone-receptor interaction is generally believed to be a necessary event in the mechanism of action of estrogens. Estrogen receptors bind both the natural and synthetic estrogens modulating physiological and pharmacological actions. There is some recent evidence to indicate that estrogen receptors may also be located on the surface of endometrial cell membranes (17) as well as within the nucleus (25).

The discovery of specific estrogen receptors has resulted in the development of steroid drugs that can bind to estrogen receptors and antagonize the actions of estrogens (antiestrogens). Clomiphene is an example of such a drug. It binds to estrogen receptors, for example in the hypothalamus, and blocks estrogen's inhibitory effect on gonadotropin secretion. By this mechanism, clomiphene increases LH and FSH levels and can be used as a potent fertility-inducing drug.

Physiological and Pharmacological Actions. Estrogens, during puberty in girls, cause the growth and development of the vagina, uterus, and fallopian tubes; stimulate the growth, fat deposition, and stromal development of the breasts; and also cause the growth of axillary and pubic hair and pigmentation of the skin of the genital region, nipples and areolae. Estrogen effects on growth include the puberal growth spurt and eventual closure of the epiphyses of the long bones.

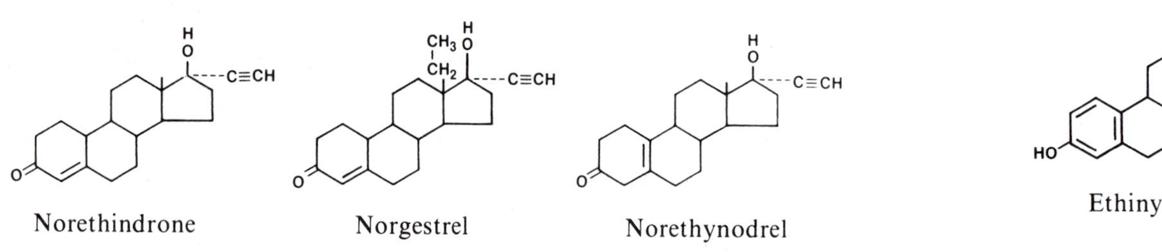

Fig. 12.7-2. *Chemical structures of the endogenous sex steroids, and some synthetic sex steroids used in oral contraceptive preparations.*

The synthetic estrogens are very similar to estradiol-17β, and the addition of substituent groups to the 3 and 17-β-positions potentiates their activity when taken orally. The synthetic progestins are formed in most cases by the removal of the 19 carbon atom of the testosterone molecule. These 19-nor derivatives have slight androgenic and anabolic activity. The progestational activity is further enhanced by the addition of substituent groups at the 3, 17, or 18-β-positions.

Estrogens, during the normal menstrual cycle, produce both inhibitory and stimulatory effects on pituitary gonadotropins. The inhibitory effects of pharmacological doses of synthetic estrogens on pituitary gonadotropin secretion provide an important therapeutic action (contraception). A synthetic estrogen, in combination with a progestin, can produce adequate inhibition of gonadotropins to inhibit ovulation. The estrogen in the oral contraceptive also serves as a replacement hormone for the deficiency in endogenous estrogen caused by oral contraceptives.

Estrogen Therapy in Menopause. Much controversy is associated with the use of estrogen in the treatment of the signs and symptoms of menopause (1). The term *menopause* refers to the cessation of menstrual cycles; the term *climacteric* refers to the premenopause (a period of irregular menses leading up to the cessation); and postmenopause (the cessation of menses for 1 year). The endocrine changes that occur during menopause are associated with declining ovarian function, decreases in ovarian estrogens and progesterone, and increases in the pituitary gonadotropic hormones. These endocrine changes are often associated with a series of complaints with no exact pathophysiological basis but are thought to involve steroid hormone deficiency, gonadotropin excess, autonomic nervous system imbalance, and psychogenic factors.

The signs and symptoms can be divided into *early manifestations*, including vasomotor symptoms, menstrual disorders, and psychic disturbances, and *late manifestations*, including atrophic changes of the lower genital tract (e.g., senile vaginitis), disorders of the lower urinary tract (e.g., urethritis, urethral atrophy, and cystitis), and senile osteoporosis.

Many of the signs and symptoms of menopause can be effectively relieved by hormonal replacement therapy (2, 9). In particular, the vasomotor symptoms, including hot flashes and sweating episodes, can be alleviated by estrogen therapy, although the mechanism is not well understood. The menstrual disorders (irregular uterine bleeding) associated with menopause are probably due to anovulatory cycles and the absence of progesterone. Low estrogen levels produce a hyperplastic pattern in the glands and stroma of the endometrium, which results in irregular uterine bleeding. Estrogen therapy, in fact, contributes to the hyperplasia of the endometrium (1). The addition of a progestational agent to the estrogen replacement therapy has been advocated as a better form of replacement therapy (22), as a cyclic estrogen-progestin therapeutic regimen provides for a more normal flow from a secretory endometrium (12).

Psychic disturbances such as irritability, anxiety, and depression can occasionally be relieved by estrogen replacement therapy. Sedatives, tranquilizers, and psychotherapy are also sometimes successful in relieving these disturbances.

Certain of the delayed manifestations of menopause can also be effectively treated with estrogen replacement therapy. The atrophic changes of the lower genital tract (due to estrogen deficiency) lead to the formation of a pale and thin vaginal mucosa that becomes more susceptible to inflammation and infection. Improvement of the vaginal mucosa is generally considered as one of the most sensitive indicators of adequate estrogen replacement. Tissues of the lower urinary tract are also responsive to estrogen stimulation; thus, urethritis and cystitis, when associated with estrogen deficiency, usually respond favorably to estrogen therapy.

The deficiency of steroid hormones may be associated with other metabolic disorders where estrogen therapy may be indicated. Thus, elevations in serum lipids and increased incidence of cardiovascular problems during the climacteric may be due to the lower levels of estrogen (21). In absence of anabolic effects of sex steroid, osteoporosis may result from the rapid loss of matrix or calcium from the bone (15) and may lead to fracture with minimum trauma. In adults, the most common types of osteoporosis are age-related (senile) and postmenopausal. The loss of ovarian function is the most important factor in the development of postmenopausal osteoporosis. Studies have shown that estrogen increases the secretion of calcitonin, which acts directly on bone to inhibit resorption (27). Loss of ovarian function with aging accelerates the decrease in calcitonin secretion and as a result the actions of the bone-resorbing hormones (e.g., parathyroid hormone) are unopposed. In severe postmenopausal osteoporosis, there is no treatment available that will restore bone mass to normal. However, further loss of bone mass can be retarded even when some years have elapsed after the onset of menopause. Although prevention of postmenopausal osteoporosis would be ideal, there is currently no clear method available for identifying women at risk of developing osteoporosis after natural menopause. The efficacy of estrogen has been demonstrated in preventing both loss of bone (11) and fractures (28) in postmenopausal osteoporosis. It is effective at doses as low as 0.625 mg/day (conjugated estrogen) or the equivalent. Adequate dietary calcium and exercise and nutrition may be important adjuncts. Riggs and coworkers have reported that calcium therapy alone could also reduce fracture rates by 50%, and that a combined therapy of calcium and estrogen could lower the rate to 25% of that in untreated women (20). Several other agents such as calcitriol (5), fluoride (19, 20), androgens (3), parathyroid hormone (18), and calcitonin (3) have been tried in the treatment of postmenopausal osteoporosis, but their effectiveness is equivocal.

The possible beneficial effects of cyclic estrogen administration or cyclic estrogen and progestin therapy have been discussed (2, 22). Continuous use of estrogens uniformaly produces endometrial hyperplasia, whereas cyclic administration does not; combined estrogen-progesterone therapy induces a withdrawal bleeding, with sloughing of the endometrium and perhaps a decreased risk of hyperplasia. At the present time, insufficient clinical evidence is available to make firm conclusions other than that the lowest dosage of estrogen that will relieve severe menopausal symptoms should be used, and that therapy should be interrupted periodically to allow sloughing of endometrium and to determine if the symptoms persist.

Other Uses of Estrogens. Replacement estrogen therapy is also useful in failure of ovarian development due to primary ovarian failure or hypopituitarism. Initial therapy consists of small doses (e.g., 0.02 mg ethinyl estradiol), which are increased slowly over a year or so, followed by the initiation of menstrual periods by cyclic treatment with larger doses of estrogens in combination with a progestin.

Functional uterine bleeding can occur during anovulatory cycles because of the continuous secretion of estrogen in the absence of progesterone. Estrogen therapy, or preferably estrogen and progestin combination therapy, can be useful in alleviating this syndrome. Dysmenorrhea can sometimes be relieved by inhibiting ovulation with estrogen administration, although combination therapy with a progrestin is preferred.

Estrogens have been used to suppress postpartum lactation and breast engorgement, presumably by a direct action on the mammary gland and an indirect action through inhibition of prolactin secretion. Doses of 0.1 and 0.2 mg of ethinyl estradiol for 5-7 days, or 5 mg of diethylstilbestrol for 5 days with additional tapered doses for several more days, seem adequate.

Estrogen therapy has been shown to be effective in the treatment of advanced breast cancer in postmenopausal (10 or more years) women whose tumor is estrogen-receptor positive. The usual dose of estrogen is at least 10 times the replacement dose. Therapy needs to be continued for at least 6-8 weeks before objective response becomes evident. Hormone-sensitive disseminated prostatic carcinoma is usually treated with estrogen. Estrogen therapy induces histological remission of tumor and regression of bone metastasis; the effect, however, is palliative. The mechanism of estrogen action probably involves an inhibition of the levels of androgens and an antagonism of the cellular actions of androgens.

Adverse Effects. In some women, estrogen replacement therapy may result in development of hypertension. Administration of pharmacological doses of estrogens in patients with breast or prostate cancer has been reported to be associated with increased incidence of thromboembolic phenomena. Patients with advanced breast cancer with metastases in the bone may develop hypercalcemia. Administration of DES during pregnancy is associated with vaginal adenosis and rarely adenocarcinoma in female offspring; in male offspring, infertility and developmental anomalies of the reproductive tract have been noted. There is some evidence to indicate that the risk of formation of cholesterol gallstone is increased in postmenopausal women receiving estrogens.

Potential Carcinogenic Effects. A number of recent studies has established an association between the incidence of endometrial cancer and the use of estrogen in menopausal and postmenopausal women (1). The risk of developing endometrial carcinoma has been reported as 4.5-13.9 times greater in postmenopausal women (6, 8, 13, 23, 26). Several studies have suggested that the problems associated with estrogen therapy in menopause may be related to the chemical form of the estrogen (i.e., estrone) and the continuous (not cyclic) manner in which the estrogen is administered.

Recent evidence indicates that the major endogenous estrogen in menopause is estrone, synthesized in adipose tissue from adrenal androstenedione. These studies have shown that estrone levels are increased in association with known predisposing factors for endometrial carcinoma (10, 24), suggesting that estrone might be the form of estrogen associated with the development of endometrial cancer.

Continuous use of estrogen causes a proliferation of the endometrium that, if prolonged, becomes hyperplastic, atypical, and finally neoplastic. Combined estrogen-progesterone therapy induces a withdrawal bleeding, with sloughing of the endometrium before atypical or neoplastic changes occur (12), and perhaps a decreased risk of hyperplasia. At the present time, insufficient clinical evidence is available to make firm conclusions other than that the lowest dosage of estrogen that will relieve severe menopausal symptoms should be used, and that therapy be interrupted periodically to allow sloughing of endometrium and to determine if the symptoms persist. The possible beneficial effects of cyclic estrogen administration or cyclic estrogen and progestin therapy have been discussed by Chabon (2).

Preparations. *Estradiol*, USP: (micronized) tablets (1 and 2 mg), pellets (25 mg, for s.c. implantation), and as various esters in aqueous suspension or oily solution for i.m. injection. *Estradiol Benzoate*: solution in sesame oil or aqueous (0.5 mg/ml, i.m. injections). *Estradiol Cypionate*: solution (aqueous; 5 mg/ml, i.m. injections). *Depo-Estradiol Cypionate*: solution in cottonseed oil (1 and 5 mg/ml, i.m. injections). *Estradiol Valerate*: solution (aqueous; 10, 20 and 40 mg/ml, i.m. injections), solution in sesame oil (10, 20 and 40 mg/ml, i.m. injections). *Estrone*, USP: aqueous suspension or solution in peanut oil (1, 2 and 5 mg/ml, i.m.); suppository (0.1 mg, intravaginal). *Estrone Piperazine Sulfate*: tablets (0.75, 1.5, 3 and 6 mg, p.o.). *Conjugated Estrogens*, USP (PREMARIN): contain 50-65% sodium estrone sulfate and 20-35% sodium equilin sulfate; tablets (0.3, 0.625, 1.25 and 2.5 mg, p.o.); lyophilized powder (25 mg, 5-ml diluent, i.v.); vaginal cream (0.625 mg/g). *Esterified Estrogens*, USP: tablets (0.3, 0.625, 1.25 and 2.5 mg, p.o.). *Ethinyl Estradiol*, USP: most active oral preparation known and about 20 times more potent than diethylstilbestrol; tablets (0.02 and 0.05 mg, p.o.). Its 3-methyl ester, *Mestranol*, USP, is as active and is extensively used in combination in oral contraceptives.

Nonsteroidal Estrogens. *Diethylstilbestrol*, USP (DES): preparations are most popular; capsules and tablets (0.1, 0.25, 0.5, 1 and 5 mg, p.o.); suppository (0.1 and 0.5 mg, vaginal). *Diethylstilbestrol Diphosphate*, USP (STILPHOSROL): 250-mg/5-ml ampul for injection; tablets (50 mg). *Chlortrianisene*: capsules (12, 25 and 75 mg p.o.). *Dienestrol*, USP: cream (0.01%, vaginal); suppository (0.7 mg, vaginal). *Hexestrol*: tablets (3 mg, p.o.).

The estrogenic response to equivalent doses of the estrogenic preparations is virtually the same. Choice of preparation is dependent upon cost and convenience. Oral therapy is usually preferred. Daily oral administration of ethinyl estradiol, diethylstilbestrol, and micronized estradiol is usually sufficient. Conjugated estrogens are less potent and may need to be given several times a day. Injection of long-acting estradiol esters may be useful in long-term, high-dose therapy for cancer. They are not suitable for treating menstrual disorders or in replacement therapy because the onset and cessation of action are slow.

PROGESTINS

Sources and Chemistry. The major source of endogenous progesterone is the corpus luteum during the luteal phase of the menstrual cycle and early in pregnancy, and the placenta during the remainder of pregnancy. A small amount of progesterone is produced by the adrenal cortex. During the luteal phase of menstruation, about 20-30 mg is secreted daily. The natural hormone, progesterone, is not effective after oral administration because of rapid metabolism by intestinal mucosa and by passage through the liver. Progesterone has a very short half-life (minutes) in the blood; though its metabolism is not fully understood, the major urinary products are water-soluble. Progestins, synthetic compounds having progestational effects, are obtained by the modifications of testosterone (e.g., norethindrone) and 17-α-hydroxyprogesterone (e.g., medroxyprogesterone acetate) and by altering the C-19 methyl group of progesterone to an α position. The structures of the synthetic progestins used in the oral contraceptives are shown in Fig. 12.7-2.

Physiological and Pharmacological Actions. Progesterone released during the luteal phase of the cycle leads to the development of a secretory endometrium. Abrupt decline in the release of progesterone from the corpus luteum at the end of the cycle is the main determinant of the onset of menstruation. In the target tissues, progesterone interacts with specific receptors in the same way as estrogen. Estrogen and progesterone act in concert to produce optimal endometrial development. Progesterone receptor numbers are increased by estrogen priming.

Although natural progesterone is poorly absorbed from the gastrointestinal tract, synthetic progestins are orally effective. The synthetic progestins commonly used in oral contraceptives all have similar progestational actions differing in potency (4). The degree of progestational potency and, to a lesser extent, the degrees of estrogenic and androgenic potency determine the contraceptive activity of the progestins and their ability to prevent breakthrough bleeding when given in combination with estrogen. For example, norgestrel is the *strongest* in progestional and androgenic potency, has no estrogenic activity and is in fact antiestrogenic. Norethindrone is an intermediate progestin with weak estrogenic and androgenic properties, and antiestrogenic activity (4, 7).

Therapeutic Uses. To test estrogenic stimulation of endometrium, progesterone is given i.m. 100 or 200 mg or medroxyprogesterone 10 mg, p.o., for 5 days. Withdrawal bleeding 3-5 days after indicates adequate estrogenic stimulations. Progesterone is administered along with estrogen to promote development or to maintain secondary sex characteristics. Progesterone is also used in dysfunctional uterine bleeding along with estrogens. Medroxyprogesterone is useful in the treatment of the obesity-hypoventilation syndrome.

Preparations. *Progesterone*: suspension (aqueous; 25 and 50 mg/ml); suspension in oil (25, 50 and 100 mg/ml, i.m. injections). *Dydrogesterone*, USP: tablets (5 and 10 mg, p.o.). *Hydroxyprogesterone Caproate:* (125 and 250 mg/ml, i.m. injections). *Medroxyprogesterone Acetate:* tablets (2.5 and 10 mg, p.o.). *Medroxyprogesterone Acetate:* aqueous suspension (100 and 400 mg/fl, i.m. injections). *Megestrol Acetate:* tablets (20 and 40 mg, p.o.).

REFERENCES

1. Antunes, C.M., Stolley, P.D., Rosenshein, N.B., et al. Endometrial cancer and estrogen use: Report of a large case-control study. *N. Engl. J. Med.* 300:9, 1979.
2. Chabon, I. The menopause and estrogen therapy. *J. Reprod. Med.* 11:233, 1973.
3. Chesnut, C.H. Treatment of postmenopausal osteoporosis: Some current concepts. *Scott. Med. J.* 26:72, 1981.
4. Dickey, R.P. and Stone, S. Progestational potency of oral contraceptives. *Obstet. Gynecol.* 47:106, 1976.
5. Gallagher, J.C. The use of calcitriol (1,25-dihydroxyvitamin D) in osteoporosis. In: *Clinical Disorders of Bone and Mineral Metabolism* (Frame, B. and Potts, Jr., J.T., eds.). New York: Excerpta Medica, 1983, p. 364.
6. Gordon, J., Reagan, J.W., Finkle, W.D. and Zick, H.K. Estrogen and endometrial carcinoma: An independent pathology review supporting original risk estimate. *N. Engl. J. Med.* 297:570, 1977.
7. Greenwald, P., Barlow, J.J., Nasca, P.C. and Burnett, W.S. Vaginal cancer after maternal treatment with synthetic estrogens. *N. Engl. J. Med.* 285:390, 1971.
8. Hanson, F.W. Oral contraceptives: A possible association with liver tumors and endometrial carcinoma. *Adv. Plan. Parent.* 12:86, 1977.
9. Hauser, G.A., Dahinden, U., Samartzis, S. and Wenner, R. Effects and side effects of estrogen therapy on the climacteric syndrome. In: *Ageing and Estrogens* (VanKeep, P.A. and Lauritzen, C., eds.). Basel: Karger, 1973.
10. Hemsell, D.L., Grodin, J.M., Brenner, P.F., Siiteri, P.K. and MacDonald, P.C. Plasma precursors of estrogen. II. Correlation of the extent of conversion of plasma androstenedione to estrone with age. *J. Clin. Endocrinol. Metab.* 38:476, 1974.
11. Lindsay, R., Hart, D.M. and Clark, D.M. The minimum effective dose of estrogen for prevention of postmenopausal bone loss. *Obstet. Gynecol.* 63:759, 1984.
12. Lucas, W.E. Causal relationships between endocrine metabolic variables in patients with endometrial adenocarcinoma. *Obstet. Gynecol. Survey* 29:507, 1974.
13. Mack, T.M., Pike, M.C., Henderson, B.E., et al. Estrogens and endometrial cancer in a retirement community. *N. Engl. J. Med.* 294:1262, 1976.
14. Mahesh, V.B. and Greenblatt, R.N. Steroid secretions of the normal and polycystic ovary. *Recent Progr. Horm. Res.* 20:341, 1964.
15. Meema, S. and Memma, H.E. Menopausal bone loss and estrogen replacement. *Israel J. Med. Sci.* 12:601, 1976.
16. Moghissi, K.S. and Marks, C. Effects of microdose norgestrel on endogenous gonadotropic and steroid hormones, cervical mucus properties, vaginal cytology, and endometrium. *Fertil. Steril.* 22:424, 1971.
17. Pietras, R.J. and Szego, C.M. Specific binding sites for estrogen at the outer surfaces of isolated endometrial cells. *Nature* 265:69, 1977.
18. Reeve, J., Meunier, P.J., Parsons, J.A. et al. Anabolic effect of human parathyroid hormone fragment on trabecular bone in involutional osteoporosis: A multicenter trial. *Br. Med. J.* 280:1340, 1980.
19. Riggs, B.L., Hodgson, S.F., Hoffman, D.L. et al. Treatment of primary osteoporosis with fluoride and calcium. Clinical tolerance and fracture occurrence. *JAMA* 243:446, 1980.
20. Riggs, B.L., Seeman, E., Hodgson, S.F. et al. Effect of the fluoride/calcium regimen on vertebral fracture occurrence in postmenopausal osteoporosis. *N. Engl. J. Med.* 306:446, 1982.
21. Rosenberg, L., Amstrong, B., Phil, D. and Jick, H. Myocardial infarction and estrogen therapy in post-menopausal women. *N. Engl. J. Med.* 294:1256, 1976.
22. Serious adverse effects of oral contraceptives and estrogens. *Med. Lett. Drugs Ther.* 18(5):21, Feb., 1976.
23. Shoemaker, E.S., Forney, J.P. and MacDonald, P.C. Estrogen treatment of postmenopausal women: Benefits and risks. *JAMA* 238:1524, 1977.
24. Siiteri, P.K., Ashby, R., Schwarz, B. and MacDonald P.C. Mechanism of estrogen action studies in the human. *J. Steroid Biochem.* 3:459, 1972.
25. Siiteri, P.K., Moriyama, I., Ashby, R. et al. Estrogen binding in the rat and human. *Adv. Exp. Med. Biol.* 36:97, 1973.
26. Smith, D.C., Prentice, R., Thompson, D.J. and Hermann, W.L. Association of exogenous estrogen and endometrial carcinoma. *N. Engl. J. Med.* 293:1164, 1975.
27. Stevenson, J.C., Abeyasekera, G., Hillyard, C.J. et al. Calcitonin and the calcium-regulating hormones in postmenopausal women: Effect of estrogens. *Lancet* 1:693, 1981.
28. Weiss, N.S., Ure, C.L., Ballard, J.H., Williams, A.R. and Daling, J.R. Decreased risk of fractures of the hip and lower forearm with postmenopausal use of estrogen. *N. Engl. J. Med.* 303:1195, 1980.

ADDITIONAL READING

Maggi, A., and Perez, J. Role of female gonadal hormones in the CNS: clinical and experimental aspects. *Life Sci.* 37:893, 1985.

CHAPTER
12.8

ORAL CONTRACEPTIVES

Carol G. Smith and Michael T. Smith

HISTORY

Demonstration of reversible inhibition of ovulation by use of progestational agents for a desired period of time and with great regularity was a fundamental contribution to the area of contraception and to the control of overpopulation in the world by Pincus (35). Initially, the derivatives of 19-nortestosterone were given orally in some arbitrary schedules from day 5 to day 25 of the menstrual cycle. Withdrawal bleeding occurred within a few days after completing the cycle, and the next pill cycle was then started. The effectiveness of such therapy was verified in an extensive field study in San Juan, Puerto Rico under the direction of Pincus and his associates by using ENOVID tablets (containing 10 mg of progestin norethynodrel and 0.15 mg of estrogen mestranol). The success of these studies has led to the development of a number of such hormone combinations and their worldwide use (36).

TYPES OF ORAL CONTRACEPTIVES

The combination oral contraceptives consist of a synthetic estrogen and a synthetic progestin (Table 12.8-1) taken for 20-21 days, usually beginning on day 5 of the cycle and covering what would have been the period of endogenous hormone function. The active pill cycle is followed by 7 days during which either no pills or inactive pills are taken, and then a new pill cycle is started. Patients taking oral contraceptives menstruate during the 7 days between pill cycles, usually beginning within 3 days after the last contraceptive dose.

Sequential oral contraceptive preparations available until several years ago consisted of estrogen given only during the first part of the pill cycle, followed by both estrogen and progestin for the remainder of the pill cycle. The assumption was that this sequential administration of steroids was closely similar to the normal menstrual cycle. Sequential contraceptives, however, were not as effective as the combination contraceptives and were shown to be associated with an increased incidence of endometrial pathology, including cancer (26, 30, 34), and they have been removed from the market.

Other preparations of oral contraceptives contain only a small dose of synthetic progestin (Table 12.8-1) taken daily without interruption. The contraceptive effect of these progestin-only pills is probably *not* inhibition of ovulation (17), but rather alteration in cervical mucus and endometrial secretions, thus inhibiting sperm penetration.

Postcoital contraceptives, which are often referred to as "morning-after" contraceptives, consist mostly of estrogen preparations alone. Various preparations that are employed include diethylstilbestrol (DES), ethinyl estradiol, estrone, conjugated estrogens, and a combination of ethinyl estradiol and norgestrel (1). The suggested mechanism for contraception is either interference with the passage of the ovum in the fallopian tube or alteration in the endometrial milieu to prevent nidation. Because estrogens are used for 5 days in larger doses, the risk of estrogenic side effects is also exaggerated. The common side effects of estrogens for use in postcoital contraception are nausea and vomiting. If DES is used for this purpose, its side effects, discussed in Chapter 12.7, should also be considered.

In recent years regimens other than oral contraceptives have been reported to have significant potential in fertility control. Synthetic agonistic peptide analogs of gonadotropin-releasing hormone (GnRH) have been shown to be potent luteolytic interceptives (45). The efficacy of agonistic analog of GnRH seems to be dependent

Table 12.8-1
Comparison of Some Oral Contraceptive Preparations

Trade Name	Steroid Components (mg)	Relative Activity[a]
Progestin-estrogen combination		
NORLESTRIN 2.5	Norethindrone acetate (2.5) Ethinyl estradiol (0.05)	P > E
OVRAL	Norgestrel (0.5) Ethinyl estradiol (0.05)	P > E
DEMULEN	Ethynodiol diacetate (0.05) Ethinyl estradiol (0.05)	P > E
NORINYL 1 + 50	Norethindrone (1.0) Mestranol (0.05)	P ≅ E
ORTHO-NOVUM, 10 mg	Norethindrone (10.0) Mestranol (0.06)	E > P
OVULEN	Ethynodiol diacetate (1.0) Mestranol (0.1)	E > P
ENOVID E	Norethynodrel (2.5) Mestranol (0.1)	E > P
Progestins only		
MICRONOR	Norethindrone (0.35)	P > E
OVRETTE	Norgestrel (0.075)	Only P effect

[a]The relative potency for each oral contraceptive is an estimate based on both the potency of each progestin (P) and estrogen (E) and the total amount of each component presents in the preparation. For a complete list of all available preparations, see Refs. 9 and 16.

on the timing of administration, variation in dose, and/or duration of treatment. The other novel approach in fertility control includes use of contraceptive vaccine that interferes with prefertilization reproductive processes (2).

MECHANISM OF ACTION

A number of steps in the reproductive process in women are amenable to interference, with the resulting effect of contraception. In the case of oral contraceptive steroids, at least three mechanisms may be involved in producing the desired response. The major pharmacological effect is inhibition of gonadotropin secretion that results in the absence of follicular development and ovulation. Measurements of circulating luteinizing hormone (LH) and follicle-stimulating hormone (FSH) show that the combination oral contraceptives suppress both the early follicular FSH and the midcycle surge of LH and FSH (40). A second contraceptive action, the effect of the progestational steroids on cervical mucus, is the production of thick cervical mucus hostile to sperm penetration. An additional contraceptive action is the effect of the progestins on the endometrium, causing less than optimum growth and development. If ovulation were to occur during contraceptive therapy, implantation would not be likely due to the altered endometrial state. Inhibition of gonadotropin secretion can be a pharmacological effect of either the estrogen or progesterone alone; in the combination oral contraceptives, however, the inhibition of ovulation is primarily due to the estrogen component, and the progestin component serves primarily to ensure a prompt withdrawal bleeding.

ADVERSE EFFECTS

When drugs such as oral contraceptives are administered to millions of healthy people, even a low incidence of adverse effects must be considered a cause for concern. Early animal and human studies demonstrated that oral contraceptives were safe and effective. After more than 20 years of use by patients, however, it has become apparent that a number of minor side effects and a few major side effects are associated with oral contraceptive use (11, 32, 41). The minor side effects, some of which can be alleviated by dosage adjustments and substitutions among the various oral contraceptive preparations, are the same as those symptoms that occur during natural periods of hormone excess or deficiency (9, 10). The symptoms of hormone excess, either progesterone or estrogen (Table 12.8-2) are similar to the symptoms and physiological changes associated with pregnancy. The symptoms of estrogen deficiency are similar to the symptoms associated with premenopause and menopause. The symptoms of progesterone deficiency are similar to those seen in anovulatory menstrual cycles. Individual patients differ in the amount of steroid required and tolerated. These differences in steroid responses may be due to normal levels of sex steroid secretion, individual rates of metabolism and excretion of steroids, or individual tissue sensitivities to steroids. Thus, the same oral contraceptive preparation may cause symptoms of hormone excess in one patient and symptoms of hormone deficiency in another.

If the minor side effects of oral contraceptives are interpreted as symptoms of hormone excess or deficiency, then it should be possible to switch patients to a preparation that more closely duplicates their natural requirements. Specifically, if an individual patient shows symptoms associated with estrogen deficiency, substitution of a preparation with greater relative estrogenic potency can be made. Substitution to a preparation with lower progestational potency may accomplish the same result because the symptoms of estrogen deficiency and progestin excess are closely related (10, 16). Certain side effects of oral contraceptives, especially those associated with *estrogen excess*, should be considered important and substitution should be made immediately, as most of the serious adverse effects caused by the oral contraceptives are associated with the estrogen component. Other minor side effects may disappear after several pill cycles.

The serious adverse effects of oral contraceptive therapy have received considerable attention because of their morbidity and mortality. The absolute incidence of the complications, though individually low, becomes overwhelmingly significant in view of the fact that an estimated 20 million women worldwide are treated with these drugs. These complications (or disease states) may also occur in women not taking oral contraceptives; in the medicated women, the disease states occur three to nine times more frequently and at a younger age. Life-threatening complications include thromboembolism, myocardial infarction, hypertension, and neoplastic changes (Table 12.8-3). Certain precautions and contraindications must be observed by patients and physicians alike. Nonfatal complications are less well understood. Some are simply lesser forms of the fatal complications, and others are complications having a reported

Table 12.8-2
Side Effects of Hormonal Excess or Deficiency Associated with Oral Contraceptive Therapy

Estrogen Excess	*Estrogen Deficiency*
Nausea, vomiting, dizziness visual changes	Spotting and bleeding (days 1-14)
Edema, bloating	Decreased menstrual flow, no withdrawal bleeding
Cyclic weight gain	Vasomotor symptoms (hot flashes)
Uterine enlargement	Atrophic vaginitis
Increased breast size, cystic breast changes	
Chloasma-hyperpigmentation	
Hypertension	
Vascular headache	
Dysmenorrhea, increased menstrual flow (also progestin deficiency)	
Progestin Excess	*Progestin Deficiency*
Increased appetite, noncyclic weight gain	Spotting and breakthrough bleeding (days 8-21)
Depression, fatigue	Dysmenorrhea, heavy flow, and clots (also estrogen excess)
Decreased libido	Delay in withdrawal bleeding
Breast tenderness, increased breast size (alveolar tissue)	Weight loss
Premenstrual syndrome (pelvic congestion)	
Aggravation of acne, oily skin and scalp	
Hirsutism	
Rash, pruritus	
Dilated leg veins	
Cholestatic jaundice	
Decreased days of menstrual flow	

Table 12.8-3
Association of Certain Complications of Oral Contraceptives with Hormone Components

Complication	Steroid
Benign liver tumors	Mestranol
Thrombosis/embolism	Estrogen
Myocardial infarction	Estrogen
Hypertension	Estrogen
Endometrial carcinoma	Estrogen (sequential contraceptives)
Fetal masculinization	19-Nortestosterone derivatives
Growth of uterine leiomyomata	Estrogen
Herpes gestationis	Progestin
Cholestasis	17-α-alkyl steroid

association with oral contraceptive therapy, but with no definite cause-effect relationship.

Cardiovascular System. ***Thromboembolic Events.*** A causal relationship between oral contraceptive therapy and thromboembolic disease has been established, including pulmonary embolism, stroke (cerebral thrombosis and cerebral embolism), and thrombophlebitis of the extremities. The risk is 3-11 times greater than in women not taking the pill (4, 11, 41, 42), and increases with the age of the patient. The development of thromboembolic events is not related to the duration of therapy, although there is evidence of a dose relationship. The incidence is statistically higher with preparations containing more than 50 μg of estrogen (3, 7, 33), resulting in a tendency to decrease the estrogen content of some preparations and a recommendation that physicians prescribe preparations with the lowest effective estrogen content possible.

The pathophysiological basis of thromboembolic events is through changes in (1) the vascular smooth muscle, (2) the clotting system, (3) fibrinolytic mechanisms and (4) vascular lumen diameter (18, 20, 21, 43, 46). The oral contraceptive agents cause a relaxation of venous smooth muscle that promotes stasis of the blood. In addition, estrogens increase fibrinogen, prothrombin, and five other clotting factors; the most prominent increase is in factor IX (14, 44). The platelets also tend to aggregate more readily in the presence of estrogen (28). Evidence also exists for a decrease in coagulation inhibitors normally present in the blood and specific vascular lesions consisting of intimal proliferation that actually decrease the functional lumenal diameter (21). The combination of venous stasis, increased coagulability and decreased anticoagulability, and decreased lumen diameter summate to increase thromboembolic tendencies. Similar complications have been noted in males treated with estrogenic compounds for prostatic cancer.

Myocardial Infarction. Myocardial infarction (MI) in young women of reproductive age is expectedly rare, with an increased incidence associated with oral contractptive use (31). This increased incidence is intimately related to cigarette smoking, the strongest risk factor for MI in women under 50 (24, 34). Oral contraceptives increase the risk of nonfatal myocardial infarction in healthy, nonpredisposed young women to three times that of nonusers (31); the risk increases to 4.5 times that of the nonusers for women who both smoke cigarettes and take oral contraceptives (34). The risk increases substantially for women in their 40s; estrogen medication other than in oral contracepitive preparations also has an increased risk of myocardial infarction in older women (39-45 years) (23).

Hypertension. An increased blood pressure has been observed, usually within the first few months of therapy, in some women on oral contraceptive steroids. The incidence and the actual rise in pressure are small. The blood pressure generally returns to normal following cessation of therapy, but in some women a hypertensive state remains. With preexisting hypertension, an additional incremental increase in blood pressure was noted (33). The incidence of hypertension increases with the duration of oral contraceptive use, so that 5% of users develop hypertension after 5 years of use (11, 25, 44).

Neoplasia. A definite oncogenetic association with oral contraceptive therapy exists for benign tumors of the liver, namely, hepatic adenomas. The tumors are usually in the right hepatic lobe and have been associated with mestranol administration. The incidence of the tumors is greatest in women with long-term oral contraceptive use. The danger of such tumors lies in their tendency to be a focus for fatal hemorrhage; the occurrence of the hemorrhage has often coincided with the patient's menstrual period (15, 27). An association with focal nodular hyperplasia, another benign liver tumor, has been suggested by some authors but rejected by others (22, 29).

Oral contraceptives frequently cause a polypoid hyperplasia of the endocervix; this lesion is benign but has been mistaken for carcinoma in the past. There is also unconfirmed evidence that oral contraceptive therapy causes dysplastic changes in the ectocervix (12, 13, 33).

Adenosis and adenocarcinoma of the vagina are distinctly rare entities, identified more frequently than usual in recent years. A clear association between these neoplasic states and diethylstilbestrol therapy in the patients' mothers has been shown (19, 32). DES had been used as therapy for threatened abortion but was banned from use in pregnancy by the FDA in 1971. Many young women, still under surveillance because they were exposed *in utero* to DES, are at increased risk for adenocarcinoma of the vagina. Males similarly exposed are at risk for cryptorchidism and hypoplastic testes, both of which are associated with an increased frequency of neoplasia (37).

Metabolism. The clinical significance of the metabolic effects of oral contraceptives is not obvious in all cases, but the drugs may, in some women, predispose to or accelerate the disease processes of diabetes mellitus and atherosclerosis (33).

The consensus of studies on carbohydrate metabolism (glucose tolerance tests and plasma insulin levels) in women taking oral contraceptives indicates a deterioration of carbohydrate metabolism (5). After 6 months of oral contraceptive use, women were noted to have significantly elevated oral glucose tolerance curves, although fasting blood sugar was usually normal. Plasma insulin levels were significantly elevated during the oral glucose tolerance test (39). Serum triglycerides and cholesterol, both substances that have been implicated in atherosclerosis, are also elevated by oral contraceptive therapy.

Thus, women who have signs of diabetes mellitus, prediabetes, or even a positive family history of diabetes should be carefully observed when given oral contraceptives, as the stress on carbohydrate metabolism caused by oral contraceptives could transform a prediabetic into a true diabetic state. Other forms of contraception should certainly be considered for such a woman, or for one who has a family history of premature heart attacks or stroke or a laboratory profile of any of the hyperlipidemic states. The added concentration of serum triglycerides in a preexistent hyperlipidemic state might certainly accelerate the disease process.

Nonfatal and Infrequent Complications. There are many nonfatal complications of oral contraceptive therapy (Table 12.8-4). Thrombosis of the retinal artery or retinal vein will lead to blindness, but such occlusion is not life-threatening. Similarly, vascular thrombosis in a different location may lead to ischemic colitis.

Another significant complication of oral contraceptive therapy is the effects on laboratory tests. Though most of these laboratory aberrations are due to actual metabolic changes induced by the steroids, some may be due to *in vitro* interference with the laboratory procedure. Some of the more important laboratory values that are elevated are serum triglycerides, serum thyroid-binding globulin, serum thyroxine, plasma cortisol, and serum iron. The urinary excretion of 17-hydroxycorticosteroids and 17-ketosteroids are usually decreased (32, 43).

Steroids that have an alkyl substitution at the 17-α-position, which includes both the estrogen and progestin components of the oral contraceptives, inhibit glucuronyl transferase. Thus, jaundice and elevated serum bilirubin may be observed in about 0.01% of women taking oral contraceptives (8). Women may also show elevated serum glutamate oxaloacetic transaminase (SGOT) and diminished bromsulphalein (BSP) excretion. Liver biopsies from such patients expectedly demonstrate bile stasis. Estrogen is considered to be the injuring agent in these effects on liver function.

Table 12.8-4
Non-fatal Complications or Infrequent Complications of Oral Contraceptive Therapy

Established Association with Oral Contraceptives
- Thromboembolism of minor vessels
  - Retinal artery occlusion
  - Mesenteric artery occlusion
- Ophthalmic disease
  - Corneal edema
  - Lid edema
  - Photophobia
  - Contact lens discomfort
- Gall bladder disease
  - Lithiasis
  - Cholecystitis
- Bacteriuria

Reported association with oral contraceptives
- Dermatitis
- Gingivitis
- Herpes gestationis
- Anemia
- Chloasma
- Psychiatric disturbance
- Congenital malformations
- Body contour change
- Weight gain
- Pancreatitis
- Chorea

DRUG INTERACTIONS

Oral contraceptives taken simultaneously with barbiturates, phenytoin, tetracyclines, ampicillin, or rifampin may result in breakthrough bleeding. These drugs probably increase estrogen metabolism by causing stimulation of hepatic mixed-function oxidases. Oral contraceptives decrease hypoprothrombinemic action of coumarin anticoagulants. Corticosteroid metabolism has been reported to be inhibited during oral contraceptive therapy. Oral contraceptives and tricyclic antidepressants given simultaneously require lowering of dose of the latter drugs.

REFERENCES

1. Adashi, E.Y. The morning after: novel hormonal approaches to postcoital interception. *Fertil. Steril.* 39:267, 1983.
2. Anderson, D.J. and Alexander, N.J. A new look at antifertility vaccines. *Fertil. Steril.* 40:557, 1983.
3. Andrews, W.C. Oral contraceptive and vascular thrombosis. *South. Med. J.* 70:519, 1977.
4. Bauer, R. Oral contraception and increased risk of cerebral ischemia or thrombosis: Collaborative group for the study of stroke in young women. *N. Engl. J. Med.* 288:871, 1973.
5. Beck, P. Contraceptive steroids modifications of carbohydrate and lipid metabolism. *Metabolism* 22:841, 1973.
6. Beral, V. Mortality among oral-contraceptive users: Royal College of General Practiotioners' oral contraceptive study. *Lancet* 2:727, 1977.
7. Carey, H.M. Principles of oral contraception. 2. Side effects of oral contraceptives. *Med. J. Aust.* 2:1242, 1970.
8. Corfman, P.A. Implications of contraception. A. Metabolic effects of oral contraceptives. *J. Med. Educ.* (suppl.2) 44:64, 1969.
9. Dickey, R.P. The pill: Physiology, pharmacology, and clinical use. In: *Seminar in family planning*, 2nd ed. (Isenman, A.W., Knox, E.G. and Tyrer, L., eds.). Chicago: American College of Obstetrics and Gynecology, 1974.
10. Dickey, R.P. *Managing Contraceptive Pill Patients.* Aspen, Colo: Creative Informatics, 1977.
11. Doll, R. and Vessey, M.P. Evaluation of rare adverse effects of systemic oral contraceptives. *Br. Med. Bull.* 26:33, 1970.
12. Drill, V.A. Oral contraceptives: Relation to mammary cancer, benign breast lesions, and cervical cancer. *Ann. Rev. Pharmacol.* 15:367, 1975.
13. Drill, V.A. Effect of estrogens and progestins on the cervix uteri. *J. Toxicol. Environ.* Health (suppl.1):193, 1976.
14. Dugdale, M. and Masi, A.T. Hormonal contraception and thromboembolic disease: Effects of the oral contraceptives on hemostatic mechanisms. *J. Chron. Dis.* 23:775, 1971.
15. Edmondson, H.A., Henderson, B. and Benton, B. Liver cell adenomas associated with use of oral contraceptives. *N. Engl. J. Med.* 294:470, 1976.
16. Freeman, W.S. When patients "can't" take the pill. *Am. Fam. Physician* 17:143, 1978.

17. Greenwald, P., Barlow, J.J., Nasca, P.C. and Burnett, W.S. Vaginal cancer after maternal treatment with synthetic estrogens. *N. Engl. J. Med.* 285:390, 1971.

18. Handin, R.I. Thromboembolic complications of pregnancy and oral contraceptives. *Prog. Cardiovasc. Dis.* 16:395, 1974.

19. Herbst, A.L., Poskanzer, D.C., Robboy, S.J., Friedlander, L. and Scully, R.E. Prenatal exposure to stilbestrol: A prospective comparison of exposed female offspring with unexposed controls. *N. Engl. J. Med.* 292:334, 1975.

20. Hougie, C. Thromboembolism and oral contraceptives. *Am. Heart J.* 85:538, 1973.

21. Irey, N.S. and Norris H.J. Intimal vascular lesions associated with female reproductive steroids. *Arch. Pathol.* 96:227, 1973.

22. Ishak, K.G. Hepatic neoplasms associated with contraceptive and anabolic steroids. In: *Recent Results in Cancer Research*, Vol. 66 (Lingeman, C.H., ed.). New York: Springer-Verlag, 1979.

23. Jick, H., Dinan, B. and Rothman, K.J. Oral contraceptives and nonfatal myocardial infarction. *JAMA* 239:1403, 1978.

24. Jick, H., Dinan, B., Herman, R. and Rothman, K.J. Myocardial infarction and other vascular diseases in young women: Role of estrogens and other factors. *JAMA* 240:2548, 1978.

25. Kaplan, N.M. Cardiovascular complications of oral contraceptives. *Ann. Rev. Med.* 29:31, 1978

26. Kaufman, R.H., Reeves, K.O. and Dougherty, C.M. Severe atypical endometrial changes and sequential contraceptive use. *JAMA* 236:923, 1976.

27. Klatskin, G. Hepatic tumors: Possible relationship to use of oral contraceptives. *Gastroenterology* 73:386, 1977.

28. Klopper, A. Developments in steroidal hormonal contraception. *Br. Med. Bull.* 26:39, 1970.

29. Knowles, D.M., II, Casarella, W.J., Johnson, P.M. and Wolff, M. The clinical, radiological, and pathologic characterization of benign hepatic neoplasms: Alleged association with oral contraceptives. *Medicine* 57:223, 1978.

30. Lyon, F.A. The development of adenocarcinoma of the endometrium in young women receiving long-term sequential oral contraception. *Am. J. Obstet. Gynecol.* 123:299, 1975.

31. Mann, J.I. Oral contraceptives and myocardial infarction in young women: A further report. *Br. Med. J.* 3:631, 1975.

32. Miale, J.B. and Kent, J.W. The effects of oral contraceptives on the results of laboratory tests. *Am. J. Obstet. Gynecol.* 120:264, 1974.

33. Mishell, D.R., Jr. Current status of oral contraceptive steroids. *Clin. Obstet. Gynecol.* 19:743, 1976.

34. Ory, H.W. Association between oral contraceptives and myocardial infarction: A review. *JAMA* 237:2619, 1977.

35. Pincus, G. Clinical effects of new progestational compounds. In: *Clinical Endocrinology I* (Astwood, E.B., ed.). New York: Grune & Stratton, 1960, p. 526.

36. Pincus, G. *The Control of Fertility*. New York: Academic Press, 1965.

37. Richmond, J.B. *Health Effects of the Pregnancy Use of Diethylstilbestrol*. Physician Advisory, HEW. Washington, D.C.: U.S. Government Printing Office, October 4, 1978.

38. Silverberg, S. and Makowski, E. Endometrial carcinoma in young women taking oral contraceptive agents. *Obstet. Gynecol.* 46:503, 1975.

39. Spellacy, W.N. Metabolic effects of oral contraceptives. *Clin. Obstet. Gynecol.* 17:53, 1974.

40. Swerdloff, R.S. and Odell, W.D. Serum luteinizing and follicle stimulating hormone levels during sequential and nonsequential contraceptive treatment of eugonadal women. *J. Clin. Endocrinol. Metab.* 29:157, 1969.

41. Vessey, M.P. Oral contraceptives and thromboembolic disease. *Am. Heart J.* 77:153, 1969.

42. Vessey, M.P. Thromboembolism, cancer, and oral contraceptives. *Clin. Obstet. Gynecol.* 17:1, 1974.

43. Weindling, H. and Henry, J.B. Laboratory test results altered by "The Pill." *JAMA* 229:1762, 1974.

44. Wood, J.E. The cardiovascular effects of oral contraceptives. *Mod. Con. Cardiovasc. Dis.* 41:37, 1972.

45. Yen, S.S.C. Clinical applications of gonadotropin-releasing hormone and analogs. *Fertil. Steril.* 39:257, 1983.

46. Zador, G. Estrogens and thromboembolic diseases: Present conception of a controversial issue. *Acta Obstet. Gynecol. Scand.* (suppl.) 54:13, 1976.

ADDITIONAL READING

Conn, P.M., Hsueh, A.J.W. and Crowley, W.F. Gonadotropin-releasing hormone: Molecular and cell biology, physiology, and clinical application. *Fed. Proc.* 43:2351, 1984.

Hogarth, P.J. Immunological Aspects of Mammalian Reproduction. New York: Praeger Scientific, 1982, p. 159.

CHAPTER
13

AUTOPHARMACOLOGY, ALLERGY AND IMMUNITY

Sachin N. Pradhan and Samar N. Dutta

In addition to a number of neurotransmitters (Sec. II) and hormones (Chapter 12) already discussed, the body possesses or can form many substances that can produce a wide variety of significant pharmacological effects. Although their physiological role may not be clear in most instances, these substances can be indirectly implicated in various functions in health and diseases because of their pharmacological actions. They have been called *autacoids* (Greek *autos* = self; *akos* = remedy). These substances that are of diverse chemical structures and pharmacological activities are the subject matters of this subsection. These include polypeptides, prostaglandins, histamine, serotonin, and other substances related to the immune mechanism.

In addition to polypeptide neurotransmitters (and/or neuromodulators) such as enkephalins and endorphins (Chapters 6 and 10.1) and hormones such as those of pituitary and parathyroid and also calcitonins and insulin (Chapters 12.1-12.3), there are some other polypeptides such as angiotensin (Chapter 13.1.2) and bradykinin (Chapter 13.1.3) whose functional roles are more or less established; however, there are many others that are diffusely distributed through brain, gut, and other parts of the body, and these peptides of the diffuse neuroendocrine system, as they are called, are of much potential importance (Chapter 13.1.1).

Roles of prostaglandins and other arachidonate metabolites are gradually being revealed (Chapter 13.2). Histamine and serotonin [5-hydroxytryptamine (5-HT); enteramine] have been discussed earlier as central neurotransmitters (Chapter 6), and also play some roles in peripheral functions. These amines and their antagonists are of much physiological, pathological, and therapeutic importance (Chapters 13.3 and 13.4).

In addition to the kinins and histamine, many other substances are involved in the complex immune responses that produce immunity and allergy. Pharmacology of immune system including drug allergy is discussed in Chapters 13.5-13.5.3.

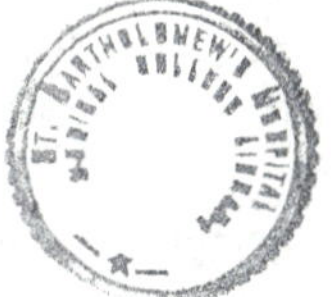

CHAPTER
13.1

POLYPEPTIDES

Sachin N. Pradhan and Samar N. Dutta

Polypeptides constitute a significant group of biologically active substances that are diffusely distributed in various functional systems. A number of hormones from the pituitary and other endocrine glands [e.g., adrenocorticotropic hormone (ACTH), oxytocin, vasopressin, calcitonin, insulin, glucagon] as well as hypothalamic-releasing hormones [thyrotropin-releasing hormone (TRH), luteinizing hormone-releasing hormone (LHRH), somatostatin], already described in earlier chapters, are polypeptides. Others, like enkephalin and substance P, which are localized in specific neuronal systems and fulfill at least some criteria for neurotransmitters, may be considered as the putative neurotransmitters of the peptidergic neuronal system (9, 12).

These and many other peptides along with several biogenic amines have been found to be localized in and secreted by cells of the CNS as well as gastrointestinal tract and other peripheral structures. The cytochemical and ultrastructural characteristics of these peptide-producing cells led Pearse to postulate that they contain biologically active peptides as well as biogenic amines (although there are exceptions) and are parts of the central and peripheral divisions of the amine precursor uptake and decarboxylation (APUD) cell system (5, 7). These cells have also been variously classified by different investigators (9). The central division contains cells of the pineal, the pituitary gland, and the two main cellular groups of the hypothalamus. The peripheral division is comprised mainly of the gastroenteropancreatic (GEP) endocrine cells and also the cells of lung, parathyroid, thyroid, adrenal medulla, sympathetic nervous system, and others. These scattered central and peripheral structures consisting of apparently unrelated cells that have similar histological properties and containing identical peptides and amines have been considered to constitute the diffuse neuroendocrine system (DNES) (6, 9).

In addition, there are other peptides, angiotensin which is known to occur in the kidney and certain areas of the CNS and which serves to control salt and water balance and act as a potent vasoconstrictor and hypertensive agent; centrally, it may mediate in the thirst drive, antidiuretic hormone secretion, and regulation of blood pressure (4). Furthermore, polypeptides of much pathophysiological interest include vasodilator kinins such as bradykinin and kallidin (10, 11, 13). These classes of polypeptides will be discussed in the following chapters.

CNS PEPTIDES

Various categories of CNS peptides are listed in Table 13.1-1. It is estimated that only 40% of the synapses in the CNS are served by the nonpeptide neurotransmitters. Investigations of the role of peptides both discovered and yet unknown may provide major insights in respect to the remaining synapses and the function of the CNS as a whole.

Immunocytochemical studies have shown that certain peptides are confined to the hypothalamus and preoptic area. These include: gonadotropin-releasing hormone; ACTH, β-lipotropin, and β-endorphin; vasopressin, oxytocin, and their respective neurophysins; and bradykinin. In contrast, thyrotropin-releasing hormone (TRH), somatostatin, neurotensin, substance P, cholecystokinin (CCK), vasoactive intestinal polypeptide (VIP), insulin, and enkephalins are distributed widely throughout the brain and spinal cord. Whereas the peptides of the former group because of their restricted distribution may function as neurohormones, those of the latter group may function as neurotransmitters or neuromodulators (Chapters 10.1 and 11).

POSSIBLE FUNCTIONAL ROLES

Recent investigations have indicated several possible functional roles of neuropeptides (1-3). Substance P, somatostatin, CCK, angiotensin II, and VIP are present in spinal ganglion neurons that have terminations in substantia gelatinosa. Presence of these peptides in areas containing afferent pain pathways may indicate their involvement in pain sensations. Particularly substance P has been shown to be a primary sensory neurotransmitter for pain (algesic). On the other hand, the ventrolateral periaqueductal gray (PAG) of the midbrain has been shown to possess opioid receptors, and its electrical stimulation produces analgesia that can be blocked by naloxone. Endogenous opioids (e.g., enkephalins and endorphins) may be active in this system. Analgesia can be produced by β-endorphin following its intraventricular administration in animals or intrathecal injection in humans.

Some peptides of the CNS such as substance P, VIP, neurotensin, bradykinin, oxytocin, and angiotensin that are known to be vasoactive are found in nerve terminals, some of which end on or near blood vessels suggesting their role in regulation of cerebral circulation.

Table 13.1-1
Various Categories of Peptides in CNS

Hypothalamic-releasing hormones	Brain-and-gut peptides
Thyrotropin-releasing hormone (TRH)[a]	Methionine enkephalin[a]
Gonadotropin-releasing hormone[a]	Leucine enkephalin[a]
Somatostatin[a]	Substance P[a]
Neurohypophyseal hormones	Neurotensin[a]
Vasopressin[a]	Somatostatin[a]
Oxytocin[a]	Bombesin
Neurophysin(s)[a]	Vasoactive intestinal polypeptide (VIP)
Pituitary peptides	Cholecystokinin (CCK-8)
Adrenocorticotropic hormone (ACTH)	Gastrin
β-Endorphin[a]	Secretin[b]
α-Melanocyte-stimulating hormone	Insulin
(α-MSH)	Glucagon[b]
Other pituitary peptides	Others
Prolactin	Angiotensin II
Growth hormone	Bradykinin
Luteinizing hormone	Carnosine[b]
Thyrotropin (TSH)	Sleep peptide(s)[b]

[a]Peptides first isolated and characterized in the CNS.
[b]Except these, other peptides listed here have been reported to be present in human cerebrospinal fluid (3, 8).
Source: Modified from Ref. 3

A number of peptides, particularly ACTH, melanocyte-stimulating hormone (MSH), vasopressin, and their analogs, have been shown to improve memory in experimental animals. Studies with ACTH 4-10 fragment, vasopressin, or its long-acting analog 1-desamino-8-D-arginine vasopressin appear to be encouraging in humans.

Several peptides have been shown in animal studies to be involved in regulation of feeding behavior and glucose metabolism. Food intake has been shown to be decreased by CCK, TRH, and insulin and increased by β-endorphin. Systemic administration of neurotensin and bombesin and intraventricular administration of CCK can produce hyperglycemia. Roles of such peptides in human obesity would be of interest.

Several brain peptides have been shown to be involved in thermoregulation. Intracisternal injection of TRH causes hyperthermia, whereas that of β-endorphin, neurotensin, and bombesin results in hypothermia. Somatostatin also causes hyperthermia.

Brain peptides may serve as a neural marker in pathogenesis of some diseases. Thus in Huntington's disease, in addition to decrease in the level of γ-aminobutyric acid (GABA) and activity of glutamic acid decarboxylase and choline acetyltransferase in the basal ganglia, there are also decreases in the levels of CCK and Met-enkephalin, and an increase in the levels of somatostatin and TRH. In Alzheimer's disease, in addition to decrease of acetylcholine content and choline acetyltransferase activity in the cortical regions, a selective decrease of somatostatin concentration in the hippocampus has been reported.

Although peptides may serve as neurotransmitters, they can also interact with other neurotransmitters and modulate their functions. Thus, vasopressin may modulate the neurotransmission in the central catecholaminergic system and produce its facilitatory effect on learning. β-Endorphin that has been implicated in states of increased food ingestion may interact with hypothalamic serotonin and dopamine in regulation of feeding behavior.

REFERENCES

1. Brown, M. and Tache, Y. Hypothalamic peptides: Central nervous system control of visceral functions. *Fed. Proc.* 40:2565, 1981.
2. Buck, S.H., Walsh, J.H., Yamamura, H.I. and Burks, T.F. Minireview. Neuropeptides in sensory neurons. *Life Sci.* 30:1857, 1982.
3. Krieger, D.T. and Martin, J.B. Brain peptides. *N. Engl. J. Med.* 304:876, 944, 1981.
4. Malvin, R.L. Physiological effects of angiotensin: Introduction. *Fed. Proc.* 38:2253, 1979.
5. Pearse, A.G.E. The cytochemistry and ultrastructure of polypeptide hormone-producing cells of the APUD series and the embryologic, physiologic, and pathologic implications of the concept. *J. Histochem. Cytochem.* 17:303, 1969.
6. Pearse, A.G.E. The diffuse neuroendocrine system and the APUD concept: Related "endocrine" peptides in brain, intestine, pituitary, placenta, and anuran cutaneous glands. *Med. Biol.* 55:115, 1977.
7. Pearse, A.G.E. and Takor Takor, T. Embryology of the diffuse neuroendocrine system and its relationship to the common peptides. *Fed. Proc.* 38:2288, 1979.
8. Post, R.M., Gold, P., Rubinow, D.R. et al. Minireview: Peptides in the cerebrospinal fluid of neuropsychiatric patients: an approach to central nervous system peptide function. *Life Sci.* 31:1, 1982.
9. Powell, D. and Skrabanek, P. Brain and gut. *Clin. Endocrinol. Metabol.* 8:299, 1979.

10. Rocha e Silva, M. Bradykinin and bradykininogen: Introductory remarks. In: *Chemistry and Biology of the Kallikrein-Kinin System in Health and Disease* (Pisano, J.J. and Austen, K.F., eds.). DHEW Publication No.76-791 (NIH); Washington, D.C.: U.S. Government Printing Office, 1977, p. 7.

11. Schachter, M. and Barton, S. Kallikreins (kininogenases) and kinins. In: *Endocrinology*, Vol. 3 (de Groot, L.J. et al., eds.). New York: Grune & Stratton, 1979, p. 1699.

12. Snyder, S.H. Brain peptides as neurotransmitters. *Science* 209:976, 1980.

13. Werle, E. A short history of the kallikrein-kinin system. In: *Chemistry and Biology of the Kallikrein-Kinin System in Health and Disease* (Pisano, J.J. and Austen, K.F., eds.). DHEW Publication No.76-791 (NIH). Washington, D.C.: U.S. Government Printing Office, 1977, p. 1.

CHAPTER 13.1.1

PEPTIDES OF THE DIFFUSE NEUROENDOCRINE SYSTEM

Sachin N. Pradhan and Samar N. Dutta

DIFFUSE NEUROENDOCRINE SYSTEM

The diffuse neuroendocrine system (DNES) (14) is made up of the central and peripheral divisions of the amine precursor uptake and decarboxylation (APUD) cell series, more than 40 in number. They were once presumed to be derived from a common neural ancestor, but now are thought to be "neuroendrocrine-programmed." The APUD cells produce more than 35 physiologically active peptides and a small number of active biogenic amines. A number of these peptides (17 or more) have been identified jointly in neurons and endocrine cells. These peptides with both neural and endocrine locations and site of production are called the *common peptides*. For the sake of brevity the principal sources of the common peptides can be referred to as brain and gut.

DNES is to be regarded as a third division of the nervous system whose products suppress, amplify, or modulate the activities of the neurons in the somatic and autonomic divisions (14). The cells of this system, widely dispersed in the neuraxis and GI tract, share the ability to secrete the same or similar peptide messengers. These regulatory molecules may (a) be discharged into the bloodstream to reach and act on the distant target cells (endocrine action), (b) diffuse locally through interstitial spaces to reach and act on the neighboring cells (paracrine action), and/or (c) cross a synapse to act on a postsynaptic cell (neurocrine or neurotransmitter action) (30).

POLYPEPTIDES OF THE BRAIN AND GUT

Several common peptides known to or suspected of mediating regulatory effects via endocrine, paracrine, or neurocrine action in the brain and gut to be discussed here are listed with their amino acid sequences in Table 13.1.1-1.

SUBSTANCE P (SP)

SP is a undecapeptide mainly present in the brain and gut with a role of a sensory transmitter of pain. SP was discovered by von Euler and Gaddum (28) in the extracts of gut and brain while studying the distribution of acetylcholine in the gut. It was purified, characterized, and synthesized in 1971 (27). It has been described in several recent reviews (16, 17, 24).

Distribution. SP occurs throughout the gut in the fine nerve fibers of the gut wall and in the scattered enterochromaffin cells of gut mucosa, which are rarely seen in adult human gut. It is present in pain-sensitive fibers in the tooth pulp and also in fine fibers beneath the epithelium of skin, tongue, and vagina. It occurs in 20% of the dorsal root ganglia cells with peripheral axons extending as free nerve endings in the skin and in relation to blood vessels, and the central portion of the axon terminates within the superficial layer in the dorsal horn of the spinal cord. In the spinal cord SP is concentrated in laminae I-III of the dorsal gray matter, areas known to receive most of the input from the central processes of primary afferent neurons. SP is also present in ventral gray of the cord (4). In the brain, amygdala, periaquiductal gray, raphe nuclei, and substantia nigra are rich in SP as well as serotonin and enkephalin. Such close association of these substances may be related to regulation of pain perception.

Physiological Role. SP plays a role as a sensory neurotransmitter of pain and in pain perception (9). By using as a tool the compound capsaicin (8-methyl-N-vanillyl-6-nonenamide), the principle active ingradient of hot peppers that causes release and nerve terminal depletion of SP from the spinal cord, it has been possible to substantiate the hypothesis that SP is an important neurochemical mediator for certain kinds of noxious peripheral stimuli (4). SP-immunoreactive neurons have been demonstrated in the afferent baro- and chemoreceptor pathways transmitting impulses from the peripheral receptors to the nucleus tractus solitarius. In addition, SP neuronal projections originating in the nuclei of ventral medulla have been shown to innervate the intermediolateral cell column of the spinal cord. These SP-containing neurons may have some role in central cardiovascular control (7). SP or a closely related peptide has been shown to be responsible for generation of the noncholinergic depolarization in autonomic ganglia. SP-containing fibers in the inferior mesenteric ganglia may be involved in a mechanism for peripheral reflex regulation of the gastrointestinal activity (10).

Pharmacological Effects. SP causes vasodilatation, cardiotonic effect (increased stroke volume and cardiac output), con-

Table 13.1.1-1
Amino Acid Sequences of Peptides with Dual Nervous and Endocrine Distribution[a]

Substance P (11)	Arg-Pro-Lys-Pro-Gln-Gln-Phe-Phe-Gly-Leu-Met-NH_2
Neurotensin (13)	pGlu-Leu-Tyr-Glu-Asn-Lys-Pro-Arg-Arg-Pro-Tyr-Ile-Leu-NH_2
Somatostatin (14)	Ala-Gly-Cys-Lys-Asn-Phe-Phe-Trp-Lys-Thr-Phe-Thr-Ser-Cys-NH_2
Bombesin (14)	pGlu-Glu-Arg-Leu-Gly-Asn-Gln-Trp-Ala-Val-Gly-His-Leu-Met-NH_2
Vasoactive intestinal peptide (VIP, 28)	His-Ser-Asp-Ala-Val-Phe-Thr-Asp-Asn-Tyr-Thr-Arg-Leu-Arg-Lys-Gln-Met-Ala-Val-Lys-Lys-Tyr-Leu-Asn-Ser-Ile-Leu-Ans-NH_2
Gastrin (17)	pGly-Gly-Pro-Trp-Leu-Glu-Glu-Glu-Glu-Glu-Ala-Tyr-Gly-Trp-Met-Asp-Phe-NH_2
Cholecystokinin (CCK, 34)	Lys-Ala-Pro-Ser-Gly-Arg-Val-Ser-Met-Ile-Lys-Asn-Leu-Gln-Ser-Leu-Asp-Pro-Ser-His-Arg-Ile-Ser-Asp-Arg-Asp-Asp-Tyr-Met-Gly-Trp-Met-Asp-Phe-NH_2

[a] In addition to these neuropeptides endorphins and enkephalins are listed in Fig. 10.1-1. Figures within parentheses indicate number of amino acids in the peptide.

traction of smooth muscles (e.g., in gut and lung), and stimulation of salivary secretion. SP has been shown to modulate synaptic transmission especially in cat α-motoneurons (12).

Pathology. In carcinoid syndrome, blood and tumor show high levels of substance P-like immunoreactivity. In animals dorsal root section or peripheral nerve lesions leads to a marked depletion of SP from the dorsal horn; similar loss of SP from superficial layers of dorsal horn from segments L4 to S2 was seen in two patients after leg amputation (8).

NEUROTENSIN

Neurotensin is a peptide containing 13 amino acids and has been described in some reviews (17, 24) and a monogram (13).

Distribution. It is distributed in various areas of the brain [hypothalamus, basal ganglia, cortex, thalamus, hippocampus, amygdala, stria terminalis, spinal cord (upper laminae I-IV of the dorsal horn)], anterior pituitary, endocrine cells of GI tract (from esophagus to colon), and also in adrenal medulla.

Physiological Role. Central administration of neurotensin has been shown in mice and rats to lower body temperature. It enhances the activity of sedatives and antagonizes the activity of stimulants. It lowers body temperature and reduces response to noxious stimuli (18). In the hypothalamus, it may participate in the release of pituitary hormones. Distribution of neurotensin bears a close resemblance to those of enkephalin in several areas of the brain. Both these peptides are closely distributed in the amygdala, although they are stored in distinct neurons. Their close distribution in dorsal gray and substantia gelatinosa of spinal cord implies a role in pain perception; such a role has been corroborated by potent analgesic effect of neurotensin (5). This analgesia is not blocked by naloxone and hence not related to opiate system.

In the GI tract, it may be a weak inhibitor of gastric acid secretion and gastric emptying and a mild stimulant of pancreatic bicarbonate secretion (1). It stimulates release of glucagon and inhibits release of pentagastrin-induced gastric acid. Since neurotensin binds with mast cells and some of its effects (e.g., hypotension, increased vascular permeability, smooth muscle contraction, prolactin release) are histamine-like and can be antagonized by H_1-histamine blockers, its actions may be mediated through histamine in some organs.

Thyrotropin-releasing hormone (TRH) antagonizes certain effects produced by neurotensin such as enhanced sleep after sedatives, hypothermia, antinociception, muscle relaxation, diminished avoidance behavior, diminished food consumption, catálepsy, and gastric cytoprotection (18), some of which are already mentioned previously.

SOMATOSTATIN

Somatostatin is a tetradecapeptide with an amino acid sequence 10-13 common to glucagon and secretin, and has been described in several reviews (15-17).

Distribution. It is distributed in the following areas: in the brain hypothalamus (especially median eminence), preoptic area, limbic system, periventricular area, brain stem, cerebral cortex, pineal gland, neurohypophysis; in the spinal cord in the dorsal horn at higher levels than in the ventral horn, and also in dorsal root ganglia along with SP, although in different cells (4); sympathetic ganglia and vagus nerve; in the GI tract in nerve terminals and endocrine cells of pancreas and stomach in close association with glucagon-secreting and insulin-secreting cells in the pancreas, and with gastrin-secreting cells in the stomach. The physicochemical and biological properties of the brain and the GI peptide are very similar.

Function. Somatostatin (and its analogs) act within the brain to influence parasympathetic and sympathetic outflow resulting in an increase in body temperature and gastric secretion and a decrease in adrenal epinephrine secretion and blood pressure (3).

Hypothalamic somatostatin inhibits release of growth hormone, thyrotropin, and several gastrointestinal hormones (e.g., gastrin, secretin, pancreatic polypeptide, insulin, glucagon, etc.). In neurohypophysis, it may modulate release of its hormones. In spinal cord and autonomic nervous system, it may be involved in the modulation of nociceptive and autonomic neurotransmission. Somatostatin applied directly inhibits neuronal firings in the cortex, hypothalamus, or spinal cord, but stimulates those in the hippocampus. It has been suggested that the depressant effects of somatostatin in the nervous system and on the endocrine cells may involve a common mechanism of interfering with calcium transport necessary for the stimulus-secretion coupling.

BOMBESIN

Bombesin is a tetradecapeptide isolated from the skin of the discoglossid frog, *Bombina bombina*. It is distributed in many tissues and has a wide spectrum of pharmacological action in mammals (see reviews in 16, 17, 29).

Distribution. Bombesin has been found to be present by both radioimmunoassay and immunohistochemistry in the brain, gut and lungs. It is present in high concentrations in the hypothalamus, thalamus, occipital cortex, medulla and pons, among many other brain areas, and in the antrum and fundus of the stomach, although it is also present in significant amounts in other parts of brain, throughout small and large intestines, and bronchial epithelium of neonatal lungs (5). It is present in 15-fold higher levels in the dorsal horn compared with the ventral horn of rat spinal cord (4).

Pharmacological Action. Intravenous infusion of bombesin produces a wide variety of actions in mammals including: a stimulation of pH-independent gastrin release and stimulation of gastric acid secretion (directly or gastrin-mediated); stimulation of pancreatic secretion (directly or mediated through cholinergic and other mechanisms); release of insulin, glucagon, and pancreatic polypeptide; stimulation of renin-angiotensin system and increase in systolic blood pressure; antidiuresis; gallbladder contraction, bronchoconstriction, and stimulation of intestinal motility. Its intracisternal administration in rats causes lowering of body temperature and hyperglycemia. Hyperglycemia appears to be mediated by central stimulation leading to release of adrenal catecholamines (16, 17, 29). Through its central action bombesin can also decrease gastric acid secretion, probably through increase of sympathetic outflow to gastric muscosa (3).

Bombesin may be involved in the central regulation of temperature, together with TRH and other peptides, and in the release of pituitary hormones (e.g., growth hormone or prolactin). Bombesin-induced hypothermia and growth-hormone release are antagonized by naloxone, thus indicating a link between bombesin and endorphins that is further strengthened by the analgesic properties of bombesin (2).

VASOACTIVE INTESTINAL POLYPEPTIDE (VIP)

VIP is a highly basic polypeptide containing 28 amino acids with close sequence similarity to the intestinal peptides, secretin and glucagon. Although it was originally extracted and partially purified from porcine lung, it was finally isolated as a powerful vasoactive substance from porcine duodenum, a richer source for the peptide (20). VIP has been the subject of several recent reviews (16, 17, 24) and a book (20).

Distribution. Large amounts of VIP are found in the brain, pituitary, gut, salivary gland, pancreas, and genitourinary tract. In the brain, highest level of VIP, like cholecystokinin (CCK), occurs in the cerebral cortex, although cortical VIP levels are only one-tenth those of CCK. It also occurs in high concentration in hippocampus amygdala and hypothalamus. VIP neurons appear to be contained in the cerebral cortex, hippocampus, suprachiasmatic nucleus, and periaqueductal gray. VIP nerve terminals are also localized in these same areas, but particularly dense terminals are found in the central amygdaloid nucleus and caudate nucleus. In the cerebral cortex, like CCK, VIP is stored in vesicles, released with neuronal depolarization, and is a potent, rapid, neuronal excitant in the CCK-rich hippocampus. VIP has also been demonstrated in dorsal root ganglion cell bodies and fibers as well as in the afferent vagal neurons with their cell bodies in the nodose ganglion. In the GI tract, its presence throughout its entire length (highest amounts being present in the colon and duodenum, 137 and 106 pmol/g, respectively) and in nerves of the stomach and esophagus may explain the relaxation of these parts after electric field stimulation.

Pharmacological Action. Besides vasodilatation, VIP causes relaxation of tracheobronchial and most gastrointestinal smooth muscles and stimulates secretion from pancreas and intestine. It inhibits gastric acid production and stimulates hepatic glycogenolysis and enhances lipolysis and insulin secretion. It causes neuronal excitation and releases prolactin, growth hormone, and renin (20). Intraventricular administration of VIP caused a significant depletion of catecholamine stores in periventricular nucleus of hypothalamus (6). VIP also causes marked stimulation of adenylate cyclase activity in many tissues, which probably underlies many of its biological effects (20).

Physiological Role. VIP can be released by depolarizing concentration of K^+, electrical stimulation of the vagus and chorda tympani, and field stimulation of isolated segments of the trachea and gut. VIP is a likely mediator of a nonadrenergic, noncholinergic inhibitory system at least in some organs. In some of its actions like vasodilatation and smooth muscle relaxation, VIP probably acts as a neurohumor, neurotransmitter, or neuromodulator rather than a classic hormone.

Pathology. VIP has been found to be responsible for the Verner-Morrison or watery diarrhea/hypokalemia/achlorhydria (WDHA) syndrome, which is always associated with an endocrine tumor, producing and secreting large quantities of VIP. The tumors are often found in the pancreas, but 25% of these are extrapancreatic. Morphologically, they are ganglioneuroblastomas. Intravenous infusion of VIP in normal nonfasting subjects has been reported to cause the symptoms of the pancreatic cholera syndrome (11).

Recently, Crohn's disease has been shown to be due to hypersecretion of VIP. In the bowel of patients suffering from the disease, the VIP-containing nerves are highly immunoreactive, and appear to be hyperplastic, thickened, and disorganized. Radioimmunoassay of colonic extracts shows 100% increase in their VIP contents (16).

CHOLECYSTOKININ AND GASTRIN

Cholecystokinin (CCK) is a substance originally isolated from duodenum that would contract gallbladder. It was found to be a polypeptide containing 33 amino acids. Gastrin, a heptadecapeptide, shares the same pentapeptide sequence with CCK at the COOH-terminal. They have been described in several reviews (17, 24).

Distribution. CCK occurs in the cerebral cortex, subcortical areas (hypothalamus, periaquiductal gray, amygdala, limbic system), spinal cord, and colon. Gastrin has been localized in the anterior and posterior lobes of pituitary; gastrin-like peptides have also been found in vagal, sciatic, and brachial nerves and nerve to the muscle wall of the proximal colon (17, 24). CCK and gastrin have also been shown in fibers of the vagus nerve and the cell bodies of the nodose ganglion and dosal root ganglion (4).

Physiological Role. CCK and gastrin have been considered to play a physiological role as neurotransmitters in central and peripheral nerves (19). CCK may act as a neurotransmitter involved in overall regulation of appetite (25). Very low doses of CCK-8 injected i.p. produce satiety, possibly working on some peripheral "satiety receptor" such as in the vagal nerves of the liver or stomach. CCK coexists with dopamine in the mesolimbic dopaminergic neurons, which are implicated in the action of antipsychotic agents, suggesting a role of CCK in schizophrenia.

Presence of gastrin in the pituitary may indicate its role in the release of pituitary hormones.

ENKEPHALINS AND ENDORPHINS

Two pentapeptides, methionine-enkephalin (Met-enkephalin) and leucine-enkephalin (Leu-enkephalin), which differ by only one amino acid at the carboxy terminal, as well as several larger polypeptides (isolated from brain and other tissues), interact with opiate receptors in the brain, gut and other tissues. The larger polypeptides that bind to the opioid receptors are generically known as endorphins (endogenous morphine); β-endorphin is one such polypeptide that contains 31 amino acids. The enkephalins and endorphins (Table 10.1.1) produce effects that are similar in many aspects to those of opioid drugs and hence are called opioid peptides, which are discussed in further detail in Chapter 10.1.

REFERENCES

1. Bloom, S.R. and Polak, J.M. Aspects of neurotensin physiology and pathology. *Ann. N.Y. Acad. Sci.* 400:105, 1982.
2. Brown, M., River, J., Kobayashi, R. and Vale, W. Neurotensin-like and bombesin-like peptides: CNS distribution and actions. In: *Gut Hormones* (Bloom, S.R. ed.). Edinburgh: Churchill Livingstone, 1978, p.550.
3. Brown, M. and Tache, Y. Hypothalamic peptides: central nervous system control of visceral functions. *Fed. Proc.* 40:2565, 1981.
4. Buck, S.H., Walsh, J.H., Yamamura, H.I. and Burks, T.F. Minireview: Neuropeptides in sensory neurons. *Life Sci.* 30:1857, 1982.
5. Clineschmidt, B.V., McGuffin, J.C. and Bunting, P.B. Neurotensin: antinocisponsive action in rodents. *Eur. J. Pharmacol.* 54:129, 1979.
6. Fuxe, K., Andersson, K., Hökfelt, T., Mutt, V., Ferland, L., Agnati, L.F., Canton, D., Said, S., Eneroth, P. and Gustafsson, J.A. Localization and possible function of peptidergic neurons and their interactions with central catecholamine neurons, and the central actions of gut hormones. *Fed. Proc.* 38:2333, 1979.
7. Helke, C.J. Neuroanatomical localization of substance P: implications for central cardiovascular control. *Peptides* 3:479, 1982.
8. Hunt, S.P., Rossor, M.N., Emson, P.C. and Clement-Jones, V. Substance P and enkephalins in spinal cord after limb amputation. *Lancet* 1:1023, 1982.
9. Jessell, T.M. The role of substance P in sensory transmission and pain perception. *Adv. Biochem. Psychopharmacol.* 28:189, 1981.
10. Jiang, Z., Dun, N.J. and Karczmar, A.G. Substance P: A putative sensory transmitter in mammalian autonomic ganglia. *Science* 217:739, 1982.
11. Kane, M.G., O'Dorisio, T.M. and Krejs, G.J. Production of secretory diarrhea by intravenous infusion of vasoactive intestinal polypeptide. *N. Engl. J. Med.* 309:1482, 1983.
12. Krivoy, W.A., Couch, J.R., Henry, J.L. and Stewart, J.M. Synaptic modulation by substance P. *Fed. Proc.* 38:2344, 1979.
13. Nemeroff, C.B. and Prange, Jr., A.R. (eds.). Neurotensin, a brain and gastrointestinal peptide. *Ann. N.Y. Acad. Sci.* 400:, 1982.
14. Pearse, A.G.E. and Takor, T.T. Embryology of the diffuse neuroendocrine system and its relationship to the common peptides. *Fed. Proc.* 38:2288, 1979.
15. Pimstone, B.L., Sheppard, M., Shapiro, B., Kronheim, S., Hudson, A., Hendricks, S. and Waligora, K. Localization in and release of somatostatin from brain and gut. *Fed. Proc.* 38:2330, 1979.
16. Polak, J.M. and Bloom, S.R. The neuroendocrine design of the gut. *Clin. Endocrinol. Metabol.* 8:313, 1979.
17. Powell, D. and Skrabanek, P. Brain and gut. *Clin. Endocrinol. Metabol.* 8:299, 1979.
18. Prange, Jr., A.R. and Nemeroff, C.B. The manifold actions of neurotensin: a first synthesis. *Ann. N.Y. Acad. Sci.* 400:368, 1982.
19. Rehfeld, J.F., Goltermann, N., Larsson, L.-I., Emson, P.M. and Lee, C.M. Gastrin and cholecystokinin in central and peripheral neurons. *Fed. Proc.* 38:2325, 1979.
20. Said, S.I. (ed.). Vasoactive Intestinal Peptide, New York: Raven Press, 1982.
21. Sharma, S.K., Klee, W.A. and Nirenberg, M. Dual regulation of adenylate cyclase accounts for narcotic dependence and tolerance. *Proc. Natl. Acad. Sci.* USA 72:3092, 1975.
22. Simon, E.J. and Hiller, J.M. The opiate receptors. *Ann. Rev. Pharmacol. Toxicol.* 18:371, 1978.
23. Snyder, S.H. The opiate receptor and morphine-like peptides in the brain. *Am. J. Psychiatry* 135:645, 1978.
24. Snyder, S.H. Brain peptides as neurotransmitters. *Science* 209:976, 1980.
25. Straus, E. and Yalow, R.S. Gastrointestinal peptides in the brain. *Fed. Proc.* 38:2320, 1979.
26. Terenius, L. Endogenous peptides and analgesia. *Ann. Rev. Pharmacol. Toxicol.* 18:189, 1978.
27. Tregear, G.W., Niall, H.D., Potts, J.T., Jr., Leeman, S.E. and Chang, M.M. Synthesis of substance P. *Nature (New Biol.)* 232:87, 1971.
28. von Euler, U.S. and Gaddum, J.H. An unidentified depressor substance in certain tissue extracts. *J. Physiol. (Lond.)* 72:74, 1931.
29. Walsh, J.H., Wong, H.C. and Dockray, G.J. Bombesin-like peptides in mammals. *Fed. Proc.* 38:2315, 1979.
30. Zimmermann, E.G. Peptides of the brain and gut. *Fed. Proc.* 38:2286, 1979.

ADDITIONAL READING

Hoebel, B.G. Integrative peptides. *Br. Res. Bull.* 14:525, 1985.

Jessell, T.M. Substance P in the nervous system. In: *Handbook of Psychopharmacology, Vol. 16 Neuropeptide* (Iversen, L.L., Iversen, S.D. and Snyder, S.H., eds.) New York: Plenum Press, 1983, p. 1.

Pernow, B. The putative role of neuropeptides in hyperreactivity and inflammation. *Eur. J. Anaesthesiol.* 2:155, 1985.

Miller, R.J. New perspectives on gut peptides. *J. Med. Chem.* 27:1239, 1984.

CHAPTER
13.1.2

ANGIOTENSIN

Sachin N. Pradhan and Samar N. Dutta

History. Nearly a century ago Tigerstedt and Bergman (11) showed that kidney contained a substance that when injected into another animal produced a hypertensive response; they named this pressor substance renin. Almost 40 years later, Goldblatt and his coworkers (6) produced persistent hypertension in dogs by constricting the renal arteries. Further studies of this experimental hypertension showed that renin itself was not the pressor substance, but acted as an enzyme responsible for formation of a pressor polypeptide, termed *angiotensin*, from a plasma substrate, *angiotensinogen* (1). Angiotensin has also been found to be distributed in the CNS. The renal and the brain renin-angiotensin systems have been of much interest because of their importance in hypertension and control of salt and water balance (7).

Chemistry. Angiotensinogen, a plasma α-globulin, is acted on by an enzyme renin present in the kidney, producing cleavage in the peptide link and yielding a (1-10) decapeptide, angiotensin I. The decapeptide is further cleaved by a converting enzyme, peptidyl dipeptidase (PDP), producing a highly potent (1-8) octapeptide, angiotensin II. Further hydrolysis of the latter by aminopeptidase produces a (2-8) heptapeptide, angiotensin III, also known as [des-Asp^1] angiotensin III, which is also pharmacologically potent. Further cleavage of angiotensin III by angiotensinase enzymes (e.g., carboxypeptidases, aminopeptidases, or endopeptidases) produces inactive peptide fragments. An alternate metabolic pathway may include initial conversion of angiotensin I by aminopeptidase to a (2-10) nonapeptide, [des-Asp^1] angiotensin I, with limited potency and then the cleavage of the latter by PDP to active angiotensin II. These biochemical processes in formation of angiotensin are illustrated in Fig. 13.1.2-1.

The structure of angiotensin has been modified, particularly with respect to residues in C terminal. In this regard, phenylalanine in position 8 is very important; its removal abolishes the agonist activity of the peptide. Replacement of this phenylalanine by alanine and further substitution of aspartic acid in position 1 by sarcosine, which makes the peptide resistant to degradation by some aminopeptidases and also increases its affinity for the receptor, produces a potent angiotensin II-blocking agent, [Sar^1, Val^5, Ala^8]-angiotensin (1-8) octapeptide, *saralasin*.

Physiological Role of Renal Angiotensin. The renin-angiotensin system is presently considered to modulate the homeostasis mechanisms involving regulation of hemodynamics and water and electrolyte balance (Fig. 13.1.2-2). Thus, decrease of plasma sodium concentration, renal perfusion pressure, or blood volume or pressure tends to stimulate secretion of renin from the kidney and vice versa. Renin is secreted by the granular juxtaglomerular cells (JG cells) in the walls of the afferent arterioles entering the glomeruli. JG cells secrete renin directly into the renal arteriolar bloodstream, thus behaving like endocrine cells, although renin is not a hormone but is an enzyme that stimulates formation of the hormone angiotensin. Secretion is influenced by three factors: (a) *Mechanical.* Any situation, systemic or local, lowering renal pefusion pressure and thus reducing tension in the wall of glomerular afferent arterioles stimulates renin secretion. (b) *Ionic.* Decreased concentration of sodium acts as a stimulus for renin secretion. The signal is mediated to the JG cells, through the macula densa cells of the corresponding juxtaglomerular apparatus. (c) *Neural.* Sympathetic sensorimotor innervation to the cells mediates influences of the CNS in response to emotional disturbances, painful stimuli, or reflex actions through volume receptors and baroreceptors.

Aldosterone Secretion. Aldosterone is secreted from the zona glomerulosa cells of the adrenal cortex directly in response to low concentration of sodium or high level of potassium or adrenocorticotropic hormone (ACTH); this effect can be demonstrated in absence of kidney. Such secretion in response to low sodium can also be promoted by angiotensin, which appears to exert some trophic effect on adrenal cortex. Both angiotensins II and III possess this trophic effect on glomerulosa cells, which show receptors for both polypeptides. Secretion of renin has been demon-

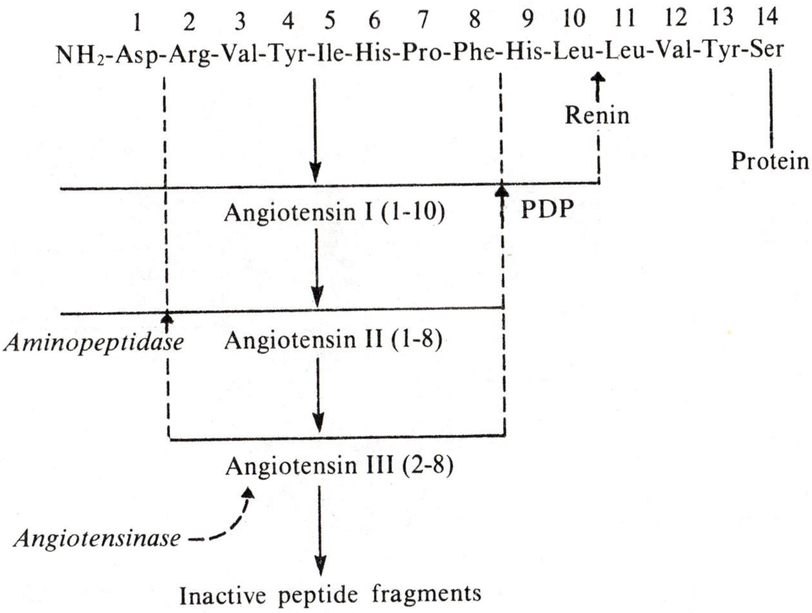

Fig. 13.1.2-1. *Metabolism of angiotensins.* Formation of angiotensins (Ang.) by the action of enzymes (renin, PDP or peptidyl depeptidase, aminopeptidase) at the cleavage sites (indicated by arrows with interrupted lines) in their respective substrates is illustrated. The classic pathway is shown by solid arrows. The alternate pathway (Ang. I ——— [des Asp I] ang. I ——— Ang. III, see text) is not presented. Amino acid sequences of angiotensins in this figure represent those of humans, horse, pig, and rat; the bovine form contains valine in position 5.

strated to be increased in patients on low-sodium diet and reduced by β-adrenergic blocking agents.

Angiotensin, formed locally within the kidney, and through its vasoconstrictor effect on glomerular arterioles, can influence the glomerular rate; it can also directly affect tubular reabsorption. Thus, urine formation can be influenced by angiotensin.

Renin secretion is stimulated through sympathetic reflex mechanism induced by lowering of blood pressure or volume (through volume receptors or baroreceptors) or other conditions (e.g., hemorrhage, exercise, hypoglycemia, emotional stress, and so on). The renin-angiotensin system, along with other factors, has been implicated in the causation of hypertensive states. It is known to play an important role in experimental renal hypertension produced by renal artery occlusion (Goldblatt hypertension) and in some hypertensive patients. However, plasma renin activity has been found to be elevated only in a few (about 16%) patients with essential hypertension and commonly in hypertensive patients with renal artery stenosis. However, recent development of angiotensin antagonists such as saralasin, which can lower blood pressure in hypertensive conditions, lends support to the proposed role of this system in hypertension.

Extrarenal Sources. ***Central Nervous System.*** Brain contains reninlike activity, angiotensin-converting enzyme, and other components of the renin-angiotensin system (see Fig. 13.1.2-2), which is independent of the classic renal system (9). Angiotensin receptor binding in the brain is also higher than in any other tissue in the body, although endogenous angiotensin level is found to be very low. Angiotensinlike immunoreactivity has been visualized by fluorescence histochemical techniques at many CNS sites including nerve terminals, suggesting a neurotransmitter or neuromodulator role of angiotensin II (5). Presence of angiotensin has been shown in some cells in paraventricular and perifornical areas in the hypothalamus, and with dense terminal patterns in the substantia gelatinosa of spinal cord, spinal nucleus of trigeminal nerve, central amygdala, locus ceruleus, and periventricular gray. The pattern of distribution resembles that of substance P, enkephalin, and neurotensin. Reduction of angiotensin staining in the dorsal spinal cord after dorsal root lesion indicates its presence in sensory neurons.

Microiontophoretic application of angiotensin II produced excitation in cells of brain sites (such as subfornical organ and organum vasculosum lamina terminalis) in rats; such excitation can be inhibited by saralasin, which also decreased the spontaneous firing rate of these cells, indicating that the spontaneous firing rate of these cells is being maintained by brain angiotensin.

Other Sources. Other tissues, besides the brain and kidney, showing reninlike (isorenin) activity include blood vessels, salivary gland, adrenal cortex, uterus, placenta, amniotic fluid, and some lung tumors. Although functional significance of such

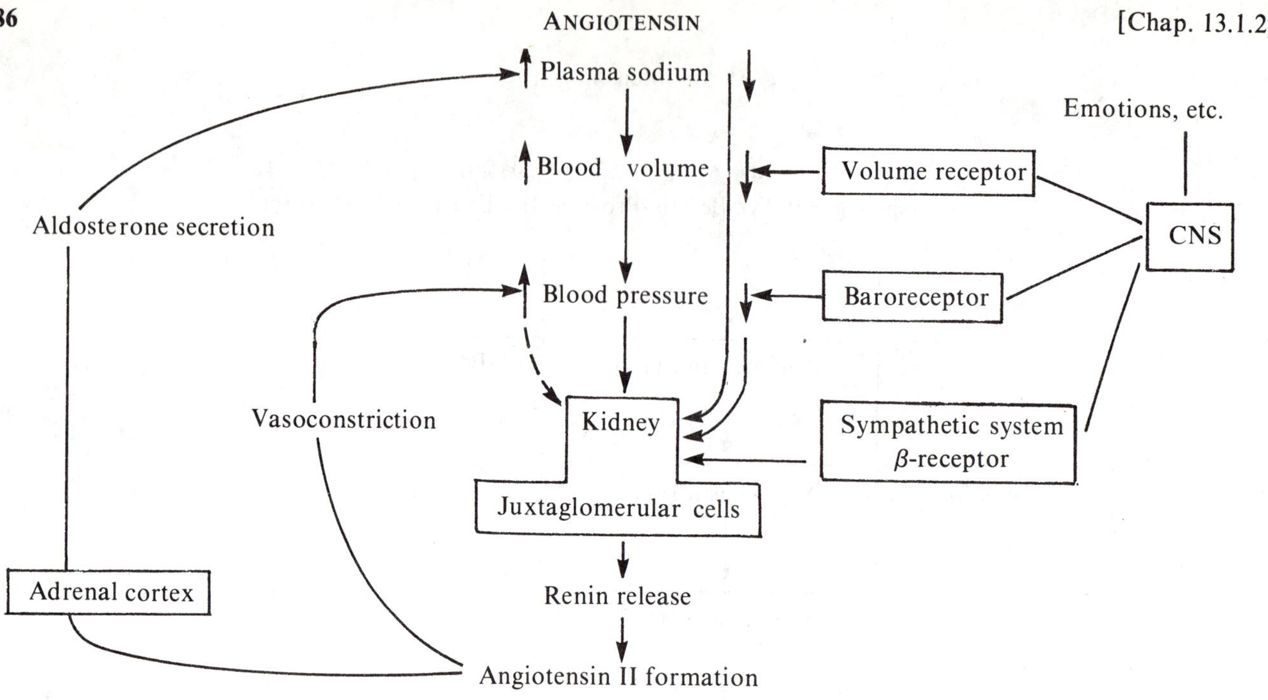

Fig.13.1.2-2. *A schematic showing homeostatic role of renin-angiotensin system in regulation of salt and water balance and blood pressure* (dashed arrow indicates feedback inhibition of kidney due to increased blood pressure).

renin is not known, such sources can account for reninlike activity in blood of nephrectomized animals and patients.

Pharmacological Effects.

Cardiovascular System. Angiotensin II is one of the most potent pressor agents known. On molar basis, its pressor effect is about 40 times more than norepinephrine. It has a rapid onset and brief duration of action. The pressor effect is mainly due to its vasoconstrictor effect on the skin, splanchnic area, and kidney, and to resultant increase in peripheral resistance. The constrictor effect, which is mainly exerted on the precapillary arterioles and to a lesser extent on the postcapillary venules, is due to direct action on the vascular smooth muscle, but also mediated indirectly through the sympathetic nervous system. On heart, angiotensin tends to increase the rate and force of contraction through central and adrenergic stimulation, as well as by direct stimulant action on the myocardium. However, due to reflex vagal activity, cardiac output usually falls.

Central Nervous System. When angiotensin is administered in the third ventricle (and in some cases intravenously in physiological range of concentrations), it causes increased thirst, increase in appetite for sodium, and release of antidiuretic hormone (ADH) (and possibly ACTH); all these effects tend to restore and conserve the blood volume, suggesting a hormonal role for maintenance of blood volume. Saralasin and SQ-20881 (a converting enzyme blocker) given in the ventricle reversed the central effects of angiotensin (2). Infusion of small doses of angiotensin into the vertebral arteries induces a pressor effect lasting up to a week. Since ablation of the area postrema in the medulla abolishes this effect, this area has been considered to produce the pressor effect by adrenergically mediated vasoconstriction and cardiac stimulation. Since area postrema is not protected by the blood-brain barrier, it may be affected by intravenous administration of drugs. It is interesting to note that an antagonist of angiotensin II ([Sar^1, Ile^8] angiotensin II) can lower blood pressure in rats made hypertensive by aortic coarctation, when administered intraventricularly, but not intravenously, indicating that its stimulatory effect on central sympathetic outflow is contributory to hypertension (10). Furthermore, such effect of centrally administered angiotensin can be verified in nephrectomized spontaneous hypertensive (SH) rats to show that peripheral renin-angiotensin is not involved in hypertension (9). Finally, in the spontaneously hypertensive rats an increased activity of the brain angiotensin has been demonstrated, which can be reduced by intraventricular administration of saralasin and converting enzyme inhibitors (4, 8).

Adrenergic System. Angiotensin stimulates central adrenergic outflow and facilitates sympathetic ganglionic and neuroeffector transmission, resulting in increased output of norepinephrine from the sympathetic nerve terminals. It also stimulates the release of catecholamines from adrenal medulla.

Clinical Use and Adverse Effects. Angiotensin amide (amide of angiotensin II) is the preparation (not available commercially in the United States) that has been used clinically as a pressor agent. It is given by slow intravenous infusion to restore blood pressure in several hypotensive conditions, but its value in the treatment of shock is highly controversial. Compared with norepinephrine, it is more potent, more sustained in its action, and less liable to be followed by hypotension. It does not produce arrhythmias or cause spasm of infused vein or tissue necrosis after extravasation at site of infusion. Sometimes it causes dizziness, headache, evidence of coronary insufficiency (depression of ST segment in ECG), profound bradycardia, and occasionally ventricular irregularities at high doses (due to high blood pressure and excessive vagal reflex).

In order to reduce the level of angiotensin II for treatment of hypertension, inhibitors of angiotensin-converting enzyme (ACE) have been developed. Two prototypes of such agents are: captopril, a sulfhydryl (SH)-containing compound, and MK-421 (enalapril), a recently developed non-SH-containing prodrug. It has been reported (3) that compared with captopril, ACE inhibition produced by MK-421 in tissues and plasma is stable on storage, antihypertensive activity of MK-421 occurs in absence of central ACE inhibition, and MK-421 has delayed onset of activity.

REFERENCES

1. Braun-Menendez, E. and Page, I.H. Suggested revision of nomenclature: Angiotensin. *Science* 127:242, 1958.
2. Brooks, V.L. and Malvin, R.L. An intracerebral, physiological role for angiotensin: Effects of central blockade. *Fed. Proc.* 38:2272, 1979.
3. Cohen, M.L. and Kurz, K. Captopril and MK-421: Stability on storage, distribution to the central nervous system, and onset of activity. *Fed. Proc.* 42:171, 1983.
4. Ganong, W.F. The brain renin-angiotensin system. *Ann. Rev. Physiol.* 46:17, 1984.
5. Ganten, D., Fuxe, K., Phillips, M.I., Mann, J.F.E. and Ganten, U. The brain isorenin-angiotensin system: Biochemistry, localization, and possible role in drinking and blood pressure regulation. In: *Frontiers in Neuroendocrinology*, Vol. 5 (Ganong, W.F. and Martini, L., eds.). New York: Raven Press, 1978, p. 61.
6. Goldblatt, H., Lynch, J., Hanzal, R.F. and Summerville, W.W. Studies on experimental hypertension. I. Production of persistent elevation of systole blood pressure by means of renal ischaemia. *J. Exp. Med.* 59:347, 1934.
7. Malvin, R.L. Physiological effects of angiotensin introduction. *Fed. Proc.* 38:2253, 1979.
8. Phillips, M.I. New evidence for brain angiotensin and for its role in hypertension. *Fed. Proc.* 42:2667, 1983.
9. Phillips, M.I., Weyhenmeyer, J., Felix, D., Ganten, D. and Hoffman, W.E. Evidence for an endogenous brain renin-angiotensin system. *Fed. Proc.* 38:2260, 1979.
10. Sweet, C.S., Columbo, J.M. and Gaul, S.L. Central antihypertensive effects of inhibitors of the renin-angiotensin system in rats. *Am. J. Physiol.* 231:1794, 1976.
11. Tigerstedt, R. and Bergman, P.G. Niere und kreislauf. *Scand. Arch. Physiol.* 8:223, 1898.

CHAPTER 13.1.3

KININS

Sachin N. Pradhan and Samar N. Dutta

Kinins are a group of potent endogenous vasodilator polypeptides. Two important kinins, bradykinin found in plasma, and kallidin found in plasma as well as in tissues, are prominent mediators of pharmacological responses and are of much physiological interest (5).

HISTORY

Werle and his associates in Germany showed the presence of a hypotensive substance in saliva, plasma, and other tissues (6); because of its high content in the pancreas, this substance was called kallikrein (*kallireas*, Greek, pancreas) and was shown to be an enzyme. The German group later showed the active substance produced by the action of this enzyme to be a decapeptide that they called kallidin. Rocha e Silva and his associates in Brazil independently showed that a substance produced by the action of snake venom or trypsin on plasma globulin could cause slow contraction of guinea pig ileum. This was found to be a nonapeptide that was termed bradykinin (*bradys*, slow) (4).

CHEMISTRY

The chemical structures of three kinins that have been identified in mammals are as follows:

Arg-Pro-Pro-Gly-Phe-Ser-Pro-Phe-Arg
1 2 3 4 5 6 7 8 9
Bradykinin

Lys-Arg-Pro-Pro-Gly-Phe-Ser-Pro-Phe-Arg
Lysylbradykinin (kallidin; Lys-bradykinin)

Met-Lys-Arg-Pro-Pro-Gly-Phe-Ser-Pro-Phe-Arg
Methionyllysylbradykinin (Met-Lys-bradykinin)

Each of these kinins contain bradykinin in their structure. Kallidin has an additional lysine molecule in the N-terminal position of the bradykinin molecule; hence, it is called lysylbradykinin.

Kinins are formed by the action of enzymes called kallikreins or kininogenases on the protein substrate, kininogens.

Kininogens or the kinin precursors are present in plasma, lymph, and interstitial fluid. Plasma kininogens are acidic glycoproteins consisting of a single polypeptide chain. They are grouped into two forms on the basis of their molecular weight; a low-molecular-weight form (LMW kininogen, 50,000 or less) and a high-molecular-weight form (HMW kininogen, ~ 100,000). HMW kininogens are thought to cross the capillary walls and get into tissues where they serve as the substrate for tissue kallikreins.

Kallikreins are enzymes present in plasma as well as in several tissues including pancreas, kidneys, intestine, salivary glands, and sweat glands. All kallikreins are serine proteases and are similar to other serine protease enzymes (e.g., trypsin, chymotrypsin, plasmin, and so on) in respect to their active sites and catalytic properties.

Plasma kallikrein originates from its precursor, prekallikrein, which is produced by liver and circulates in blood. Formation of plasma kallikrein can be facilitated by activated Hageman factor (HF, factor XII) (or a component of activated HF), trypsin, and possibly kallikrein itself. Plasma kallikrein preferably cleaves HMW kininogen circulating in the blood to yield the vasoactive polypeptide bradykinin. Some glandular kallikreins are present as prekallikreins and others exist in active forms. Their biochemical properties are generally different from plasma kallikreins. These tissue kallikreins act preferably on LMW kininogens to produce kallidin or Lys-bradykinin.

FORMATION

Bradykinin is a short-acting pathological hypotensive agent that is rapidly formed following any injury to the vascular system. As already mentioned, it is released into the bloodstream by plasma kallikrein which is activated by Hageman factor that is also involved in blood clotting. Thus, everytime the blood clotting system is activated, bradykinin formation occurs.

Kallidin (Lys-bradykinin) is produced by tissue kallikrein and is converted to some extent to bradykinin by aminopeptidase. It is the major urinary kinin and is probably formed by the action of renal kallikrein.

Methionyllysylbradykinin is formed from kininogen by the action of pepsin and pepsinlike enzymes. It has been isolated from acidified plasma. In acidified urine, acid-activated uropepsinogen catalyzes the release of methionyllysylbradykinin from urinary kininogen.

PHARMACOLOGICAL EFFECTS

Although kinin formation occurs as a localized phenomenon and half-life of the polypeptides in the circulation is very short (less than 15 sec), plasma kinin may exert a high degree of pharmacological activity. Pharmacological properties of kallidin and bradykinin appear to be mostly similar.

Cardiovascular System. Kinins are about 10 times more active than histamine on molar basis in causing vasodilatation due to their direct action on arteriolar smooth muscle and release of histamine from the mast cells. Administered intravenously in humans, they can cause flushing and congestion of conjunctiva. Dilatation occurs in blood vessels of muscle, kidney, and other viscera, and various glands, and also in coronary and cerebral blood vessels. These vasodilator effects may cause a sharp fall in systolic and diastolic blood pressure. In contrast to dilatation of the fine resistance vessels, kinins tends to produce contraction of large arteries, and large as well as small veins. The resultant hypotension and increased venous return cause a reflex tachycardia and increase in cardiac output.

The plasma kinins increase vascular permeability in the microcirculation, favoring efflux of fluid from blood to the surrounding tissue spaces. Their effect, like that of histamine or serotonin, is exerted on the postcapillary small venules rather than on true capillaries by causing contraction of endothelial cells and separation at their boundaries permitting free passage of fluid and plasma protein through the gaps, which is further facilitated by induced increase of venous pressure.

Extravascular Smooth Muscles. Kinins cause contraction in various isolated smooth muscles (e.g., rat uterus, guinea pig ileum and bronchus). On the other hand, rat duodenum is relaxed. In humans, kinin, especially after inhalation, causes respiratory distress in asthmatics.

Endocrine and Exocrine Glands. Active kinins or the related enzymes are present in intestine, pancreas, and salivary and sweat glands from which they may diffuse to the blood and act as local modulators of blood flow. Because of their action on smooth muscle, the released kinins may modulate the tone of salivary and pancreatic ducts and regulate gastrointestinal motility. Kinins also influence the transepithelial transport of water, electrolytes, glucose, and amino acids in the gastrointestinal tract. Kallikreins may also play a role in the physiological activation of various prohormones such as proinsulin.

Kidney. The essential synthetic and catabolic components of the glandular kallikrein-kinin system have been identified in the kidney and in the urine. However, the role of this system in renal function is not clear. Kallidin or bradykinin administered intravenously or intraarterially in humans, in anesthetized dogs, or isolated perfused kidney has been shown to cause renal arteriolar vasodilatation. But vasodilatation induced by pharmacological doses of kinin does not necessarily reflect the function of the renal kinin system *in situ*. Localization of the components of the kallikrein-kinin system along the nephron, and other tissues where transmembrane electrolyte movements are major functional activities, indicate a role of kinins in electrolyte transport and excretion in the kidney (2).

Sensory Nerves. The plasma kinins are potent algesic agents. They cause burning pain on application to the exposed base of a blister. Intraperitoneal or intraarterial injections of kinin in animals or humans also elicit pain response.

Role in Tissue Injury and Inflammation. Kinins have been found to be implicated in tissue injury and inflammation as endogenous substances evoking a coherent but nonspecific pattern of defense mechanism (1). Kinins act on resistance blood vessels causing vasodilatation and increasing local blood flow; and they also increase vascular permeability and promote exudation (i.e., passage of blood fluid, proteins, and eventually cells to the extravascular space). Thus, they may be considered as peptidic autacoids along with other plasma-derived inflammatory peptides such as anaphylatoxins and fibrin degradation products.

RECEPTORS

The kinins are thought to exert their biological actions mediated by their effects on specific receptors located in the membranes of the target tissues. The development of new analogs as well as the pharmacological intervention of bradykinin actions at different targets have permitted the characterization of at least two types of B- (for bradykinin) receptors: B_1 (e.g., in rabbit aorta) and B_2 (e.g., in cat ileum and rat uterus). These B-receptors should not be confused with β-adrenoceptors. Of these, the B_1-receptor is specific for kinin metabolites generated by kininase I. Actions mediated by the respective receptors are mentioned in Fig. 13.1.3-1 (1).

An homogeneous B_2-receptor population was demonstrated to be involved in the exudation-promoting effect of kinins in rabbit and rat dermis. Bradykinin showed highest affinity in most of the B_2-receptor systems, followed by Lys-bradykinin and then by Met-Lys-bradykinin, with the exception of the B_2-receptor mediating contraction of venous smooth muscle, which appears to be sensitive to Lys-bradykinin. On the other hand, on B_1-receptors Met-Lys-bradykinin and Lys-bradykinin are approximately 76 and 10 times more potent than bradykinin, respectively; the octapeptide, des-Arg^9-bradykinin (an active fragment from breakdown of bradykinin by action of Kininase I) is 10 times more potent, while the heptapeptide, des-Phe^8-des-Arg^9-bradykinin is inactive.

It has been possible to find out a specific competitive inhibitor for B_1-receptors; Leu^8-des-Arg^9-bradykinin is an example. So far such inhibitors for B_2-receptor have not been available.

METABOLISM

Kinins are metabolized rapidly by nonspecific endo- or exopeptidases, known as kininases. Their half-life is less than 15 sec. Two plasma kininases are well known. Kininase I is synthesized in the liver and is a carboxypeptidase (carboxypeptidase N) that acts at the C-terminal of the kinin by releasing lysine and arginine residues. By removing the C-terminal Arg, kininase I produces

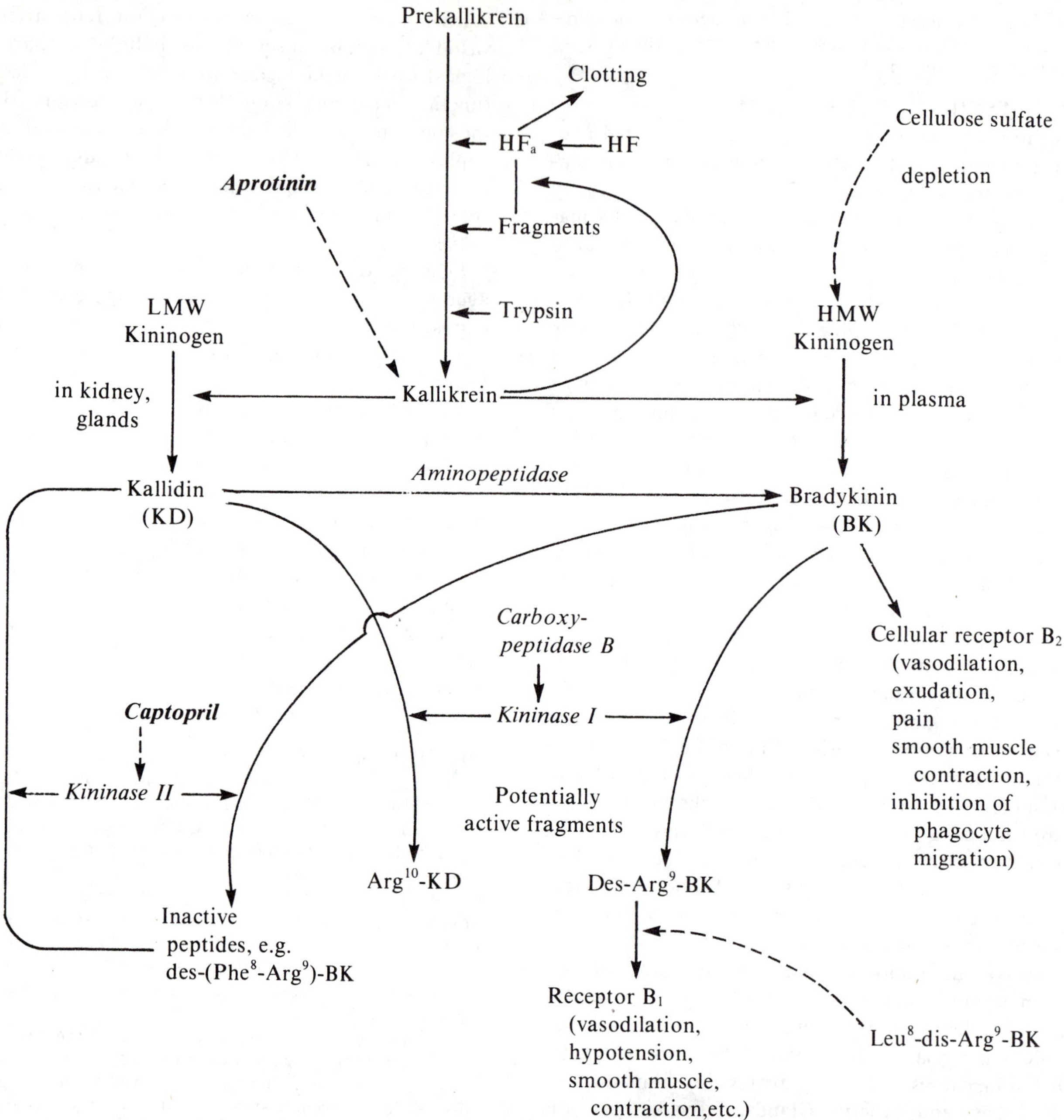

Fig. 13.1.3-1. *The kinins: their metabolism, actions, and pharmacological manupulations.*
(HF,Hageman factor; HF$_a$, activated HF; LMW and HMW,low molecular weight and high molecular weight kininogens. ——►,indicates stimulation and – – – ►,inhibition).

metabolites (e.g., des-Arg^9-bradykinin, des-kallidin), which are potent stimulants of B_1-receptors. Kininase II, which is present in plasma and vascular endothelial cells throughout the body, inactivates kinins. It is identical with angiotensin-converting enzyme (peptidyl dipeptidase) (discussed in Chapter 13.1.2) that cleaves the C-terminal phenylalanyl-arginine and activates the renin-angiotensin system by promoting conversion of angiotensin I to angiotensin II.

PHARMACOLOGICAL MANIPULATION

Various pharmacological approaches (1) have been made in animal experiments to modify (inhibit or potentiate) the activity of the kallikrein-kinin system. Intravenous injection of negatively charged cellulose sulfate causes depletion of the kinin precursor. Ellagic acid also depletes the plasmatic reservoir of kininogen. Such treatment has been shown to delay bacterial endoxtoxin-induced death in dogs and to some extent retard carragenin-induced development of edema in the rat paw, indicating thereby a role of kinins in endotoxin shock and local edema. Inhibitors of trypsinlike proteases, such as aprotinin (TRASYLOL, a polypeptide of bovine origin), have been shown to reduce carragenin-induced edema and endotoxin-induced shock, presumably by inhibiting the kallikreins to produce kinin; however, such action of aprotinin is not specific.

A competitive inhibitor for B_1-receptor has also been available. The actions of kinins that are mediated by the production of prostaglandins can be blocked by inhibitors of prostaglandin synthesis (e.g., aspirin, indomethacin).

Injection of purified pancreatic carboxypeptidase B is known to enhance the activity of kininase I. Such treatment has been shown to reduce hypotensive effect of exogenous bradykinin in animals and carragenin-induced edema in rat paw. Finally, the action of kinins can be enhanced by blocking the enzymes that cause their degradation. Agents like teprotide and captopril inhibit kininase II (angiotensin-converting enzyme) and prolong half-life of the kinins.

CLINICAL SIGNIFICANCE

High-molecular-weight (HMW) kininogen and prekallikrein are now known to be important for functioning of Hageman factor-dependent blood coagulation and fibrinolysis. There are individuals who are lacking in HMW kininogen (Fletcher trait) or prekallikrein (Fitzgerald, Flaujeac, and Williams traits), leading to minor bleeding disorders. Hyperbradykininemia may be related to episodic flushing syndromes and carcinoid. Other pathological conditions associated with excessive kinin formation include hereditary angioedema, septic and anaphylactic shock, and inflammatory reactions.

Attempts to reduce the inflammatory actions of kinins have been concentrated on the enzyme plasma kallikrein. Aprotinin, the inhibitor of kallikrein, has been under investigation in various clinics to reduce inflammatory conditions caused by kinin release in conditions such as acute pancreatitis and carcinoid syndrome.

Of major importance in the role of kinins in causing pain and increased tissue fluid accumulation is the fact that prostaglandins of the E and F series potentiate or amplify the pain-producing and permeability-increasing characteristics of kinins. These responses appear to be mediated through release of prostaglandins. In guinea pig lung, prostaglandins were shown to be released in response to bradykinin (3). Thus, agents such as aspirin, ibuprofen, and indomethacin are effective analgesics because they reduce the formation of prostaglandins and thus probably reduce the "amplifier" of the pain produced by kinins. These analgesics have no effect on kinin activity itself.

The current use of converting enzyme inhibitors such as captopril as antihypertensive drugs results in dramatically prolonged half-life of bradykinin leading to the still unproved suggestion that the antihypertensive action of captopril is, in fact, due to increased circulating levels of kinins.

LEUKOKININS

In addition to bradykinin, other kinin peptides are released during immunological or chronic inflammatory diseases. Leukokinins are examples of kinins that are formed by leukocyte enzymes acting on pathological proteins. These leukokinins are no doubt involved in pain and edema as seen in chronic diseases where white cells are in constant attendance.

The leukokinins also play an important role in neoplastic diseases where metastatic cells invade the peritoneal or pleural cavities. The ascitic fluid accumulation seen in these disease states is believed to be a function of the pharmacological actions of leukokinins formed by enzymes of the cancer cell.

REFERENCES

1. Marceau, F., Lussier, A., Regoli, D., and Giroud, J. P. Pharmacology of kinins: Their relevance to tissue injury and inflammation. *Gen. Pharmacol.* 14:209, 1983.
2. Margolius, H. S. The kallikrein-kinin system and the kidney. *Ann. Rev. Physiol.* 46:309, 1984.
3. Piper, P. J., and Vane, J. R. Release of additional factors in anaphylaxis and its antagonism by anti-inflammatory drugs *Nature* 223:29, 1969.
4. Rocha e Silva, M. Bradykinin and bradykininogen: Introductory remarks. In: *Chemistry and Biology of the Kallikrein-Kinin System in Health and Disease* (Pisano, J. J., and Austen, K. F., eds.). DHEW Publication No. 76-791 (NIH). Washington, D.C.: U.S. Government Printing Office, 1977, p. 7.
5. Schachter, M., and Barton, S. Kallikreins (kininogenases) and kinins. In: *Endocrinology,* Vol. 3 (de Groot, L. J. et al., eds.). New York: Grune & Stratton, 1979, p. 1699.
6. Werle, E. A short history of the kallikrein-kinin system. In: *Chemistry and Biology of the Kallikrein-Kinin System in Health and Disease* (Pisano, J. J., and Austen, K. F., eds.). DHEW Publication No. 76-791 (NIH). Washington, D.C.: U.S. Government Printing Office, 1977, p. 1.

CHAPTER
13.2

PROSTAGLANDINS AND OTHER ARACHIDONIC ACID METABOLITES

Adam K. Myers, Ulla-Maija Mäkilä and Peter Ramwell

HISTORY

Kurzrok and Lieb (11) discovered highly biologically active substances in human semen in 1930, which a few years later were named prostaglandins (PGs) by von Euler (1934) in the belief that these new substances in seminal plasma came from the prostate (4). The name has endured, although PGs in semen are known to originate in the seminal vesicles rather than the prostate. Nearly 30 years after their discovery, the first PGs, PGE_1 and $PGF_{1}\alpha$, were isolated and their chemical structures determined (1).

A major event in PG pharmacology occurred in 1971, when Vane (18) discovered that aspirinlike drugs inhibit the synthesis of PGs. This provided a mechanistic explanation for the therapeutic action of aspirin as well as an experimental tool for studying the functions of PGs in human subjects. The next important advance was the discovery of the cyclic endoperoxides, PGG_2 and PGH_2, which are the labile intermediates in PG synthesis (7). Thromboxane A_2 (TxA_2) was discovered 2 years later (8) and the structure and synthesis of prostacyclin (PGI_2) was determined a year after that (13). The most recent members of the family of arachidonic acid metabolites, the leukotrienes, were described by Samuelsson and coworkers (16) in 1979.

CHEMISTRY AND BIOSYNTHESIS

The most important precursor for the synthesis of PGs and related substances (eicosanoids) is arachidonic acid (eicosatetraenoic acid), which is abundantly present in cell membranes. Its release through activation of acyl hydrolases initiates PG synthesis, which is tissue specific. The scheme for the biosynthesis of the major arachidonic acid products is depicted in Fig. 13.2-1. The biologically important metabolites include the primary prostaglandins (PGE_2, $PGF_{2}\alpha$, and PGD_2) (Fig. 13.2-2), prostacyclin (PGI_2), thromboxane A_2 (TxA_2) (Fig. 13.2-3), and the leukotrienes (LTB_4, LTC_4, LTD_4 and LTE_4) (Fig. 13.2-4). In addition there are a number of hydroxylated arachidonate products that are termed hydroxy eicosatetraenoic acids (HETEs). 12-HETE (Fig. 13.2-1) is a major product of platelets, although its function is not known.

The subscripts in eicosanoid nomenclature refer to the number of double bonds. As opposed to the common bisenoic (PGs) and tetraenoic (LTs) products of arachidonic acid, analogous products with differing degrees of unsaturation can also be formed if the fatty acid substrate is dihomolinolenic acid or eicosapentaenoic acid. For example, PGE_1 and PGE_3 are products of these two substrates, respectively. However, such products are much less abundant and usually have reduced biological activity. In addition to these synthetic routes, pathways exist for the enzymatic or spontaneous degradation of arachidonic acid products. The metabolism of PGs is initiated by PG-15-dehydrogenase, and it occurs primarily in the lungs, kidney, and liver (17). Many of the eicosanoids are short-lived. This is especially true for PGI_2 and TxA_2, which are usually measured in terms of their inactive breakdown products, 6-keto-prostaglandin $F_{1}\alpha$ and thromboxane B_2, respectively. The degradation products of eicosanoids are typically more hydrophilic and less active.

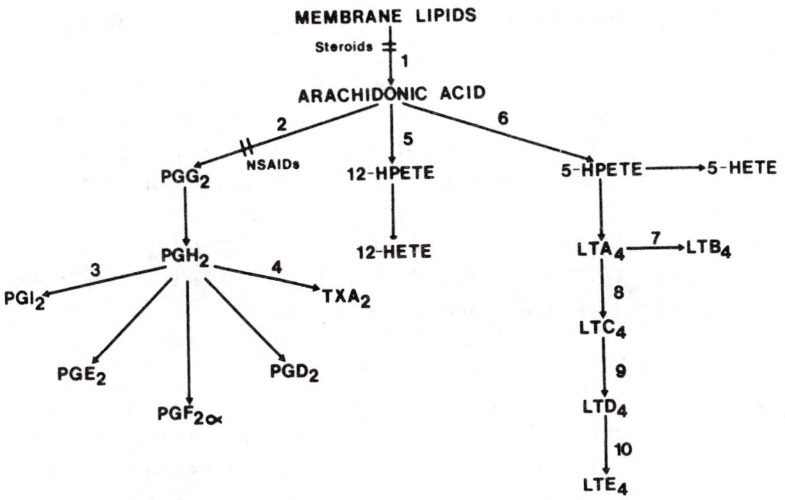

Fig. 13.2-1. *Pathways for the biosynthesis of the major active products of arachidonic acid.*

The enzymes in the arachidonic acid cascade include: (1) acyl hydrolases (phospholipases), (2) cyclooxygenase, (3) prostacyclin synthetase, (4) thromboxane synthetase, (5) 12-lipoxygenase, (6) 5-lipoxygenase, (7) hydrolase, (8) glutathione-S-transferase, (9) γ-glutamyl transpeptidase, and (10) dipeptidase. The nonsteroidal antiinflammatory drugs (NSAID) inhibit the cyclooxygenase enzyme. Glucocorticoids inhibit the acyl hydrolases.

REGULATION OF ARACHIDONIC ACID CASCADE

The complexity of the arachidonic acid cascade results in numerous points for biological regulation and pharmacological intervention. The first step in eicosanoid synthesis is the liberation of arachidonate from membrane lipids by acyl hydrolases, such as phospholipase A_2 or phospholipase C. This step is promoted by mechanical factors such as tissue injury, as well as humoral factors, including catecholamines, histamine, bradykinin, thrombin, and calcium ions, among others. Biological inhibition of arachidonate release is effected by the glucocorticoid hormones through nuclear transcription and the synthesis of specific antiphospholipase proteins (5). Pharmacological inhibition can be achieved by such agents as prednisolone, quinacrine, and chloroquine (14).

Free arachidonate is either reesterified to membrane lipids, or is acted on by lipoxygenase or cycloxygenase enzymes. Biological regulation of these steps is not well understood. However, it is clear that biological regulation of these and subsequent enzymes occurs, since the spectrum of arachidonate products can vary greatly

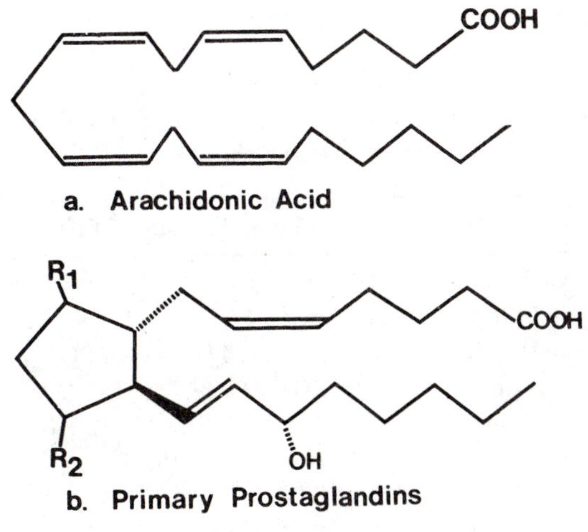

a. Arachidonic Acid

b. Primary Prostaglandins

Fig. 13.2-2. *The chemical structures of (a) arachidonic acid and (b) the primary prostaglandins (PGD_2, PGE_2, $PGE_{2\alpha}$), which differ only in the substituents designated R_1 and R_2 in the diagram above.*

R_1 = hydroxyl, R_2 = keto in PGD_2; R_1 = keto, R_2 = hydroxyl in PGE_2; R_1 and R_2 = hydroxyl in $PGF_{2\alpha}$. In each of these primary prostaglandins, the hydroxyl groups are oriented below the plane of the ring.

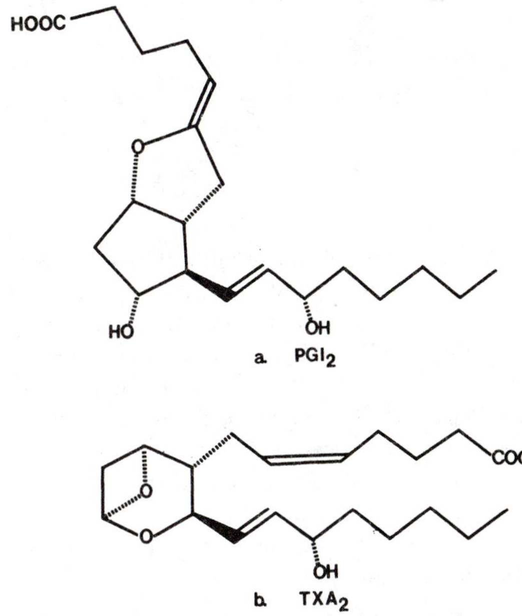

a. PGI_2

b. TXA_2

Fig. 13.2-3. *The chemical structures of (a) vasodilatory, antiaggregatory prostacyclin (PGI_2) and (b) vasoconstricting, proaggregatory thromboxane A_2 (TxA_2).*

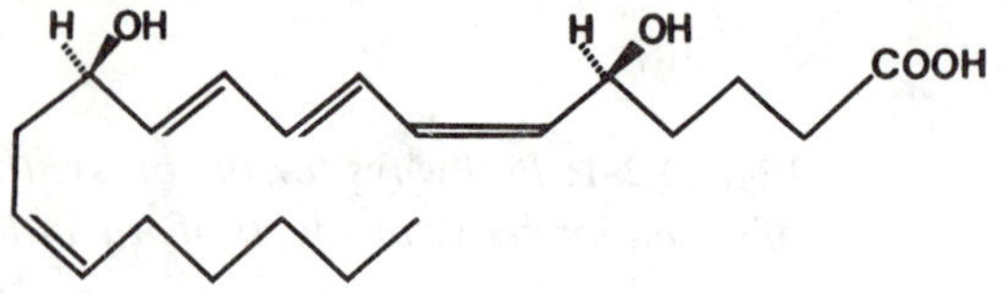

a. Leukotriene B_4 (LTB_4)

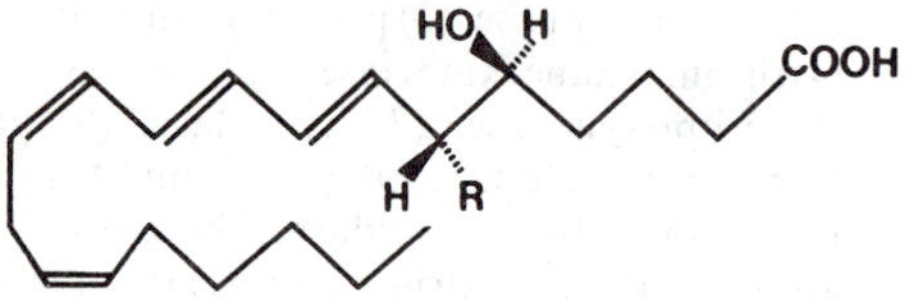

b. LTC_4 R = S-Cys-Glu-δ (Gly)

LTD_4 R = S-Cys-Gly

LTE_4 R = S-Cys

Fig. 13.2-4. *The chemical structures of the biologically important leukotrienes (LTs), including (a) the dihydroxy arachidonate products, LTB_4, and (b) the peptidoleukotrienes, LTC_4, LTD_4, and LTE_4.*

between cell types. Pharmacologically, the cyclooxygenase enzyme is inhibited by aspirin, indomethacin, and other nonsteroidal antiinflammatory agents (12). Drugs that specifically block lipoxygenase enzymes are currently in the developmental stage. Experimentally, both the cyclooxygenase and lipoxygenase enzymes can be blocked by eicosatetraynoic acid, which acts as a false substrate. Pharmacological manipulation of enzymes subsequent to the cyclooxygenase and lipoxygenase steps is also an area of current research interest because of the therapeutic implication.

BIOLOGICAL ACTIONS

Primary Prostaglandins

The primary PGs, PGE_2, $PGF_{2\alpha}$, and PGD_2, are formed from cyclic endoperoxides through enzymatic and nonenzymatic pathways in nearly all tissues and cells except lymphocytes. They have diverse physiological and pharmacological effects, and they are involved in both physiological and pathophysiological processes, often opposing each other in the same organ. Thus, it is impossible in the limited space available to discuss all of the actions of PGs. Since PGs act locally at the site of release, it is difficult to interpolate the data derived from peripheral blood measurements, *in vitro* studies, and animal studies to the actual *in vivo* situation. Some representative pharmacological actions of PGs and other arachidonate products are listed in Table 13.2-1.

Primary PGs are known to be involved widely as modulators in reproductive physiology (10). PGE_2 and $PGF_{2\alpha}$ are potent contractors of the uterus, and they are involved in the process of parturition. In addition they play a role in ovulation, luteolysis, and lactation as well as male fertility.

In the gastrointestinal tract, PGs promote motility and inhibit water and electrolyte absorption and acid secretion. They also have a cytoprotective role; this property of PGs is thought to account in part for the ulcerogenic action of nonsteroidal antiinflammatory drugs. The inhibition of absorption and promotion of motility account for the diarrhea observed as a side effect when PGs are administered as drugs.

Although it was formerly believed that primary PGs might be involved in regulation of the cardiovascular system, it is now recognized that they are not normally present in the circulation in concentrations sufficient for a regulatory role. Rather, the more potent and abundant eicosanoids PGI_2 and TxA_2 are more important physiologically (3). Pharmacologically, however, PGE_2 and PGD_2 are vasodilators, whereas $PGF_{2\alpha}$ is a vasoconstrictor. PGD_2 is also a potent inhibitor of platelet aggregation, but the physiological relevance of this effect is controversial.

Whereas primary PGs are probably not important in the regulation of vascular tone in the adult, PGE_2 along with PGI_2 seems to be involved in the maintenance of patency of the fetal ductus arteriosus (2). It is possible in newborns with certain types of congenital heart diseases to manipulate the ductus arteriosus pharmacologically by keeping it open with PGE_2 or its analogs. Accordingly, it is possible to close a persistent ductus arteriosus in preterm babies with indomethacin.

Table 13.2-1
Representative Pharmacological Actions of Arachidonate Metabolites

Pharmacological Action[a]	Primary Eicosanoid Effectors
Platelet aggregation	TxA_2
Platelet inhibition	PGI_2, PGD_2
Bronchoconstriction	LTC_4, LTD_4, TxA_2, $PGF_{2\alpha}$
Bronchodilation	PGE_2, PGI_2
Vasoconstriction[b]	TxA_2, $PGF_{2\alpha}$, LTC_4, LTD_4
Vasodilation[b]	PGI_2, PGE_2, PGD_2
Chemotaxis	LTB_4
Uterine contraction	PGE_2, $PGF_{2\alpha}$, TxA_2
Gastrointestinal contraction	PGE_2, $PGF_{2\alpha}$
Gastrointestinal cytoprotection	PGE_2, PGI_2, PGD_2

[a] Listed in the approximate order of potency. Effects can vary widely with species, method and duration of exposure, hormonal status, etc.
[b] Systemic actions; regional responses can be different.

Primary PGs have been implicated in a number of pathophysiological states, including pain, fever, and inflammation. Thus the analgesic, antipyretic, and anti-inflammatory properties of aspirinlike drugs have been attributed to the inhibition of PG synthesis. Similarly, glucocorticoids, which inhibit the release of arachidonic acid and, hence, the formation of all its products, share some of the therapeutic actions of the nonsteroidal drugs.

Prostacyclin

Prostacyclin (PGI_2; epoprostenol; Fig. 13.2-3) was first identified from vessel walls, where it is the major arachidonate product (13), but it can also be synthesized by other tissues. PGI_2 relaxes vascular smooth muscle and is the most potent inhibitor of platelet aggregation known. Thus, it may control blood flow and hemostasis together with its physiological antagonist TxA_2. Although PGI_2 was once speculated to be a circulating hormone, its actions are now thought to be local in nature, as is the case for other arachidonate metabolites. Unlike the primary PGs, however, PGI_2 is not significantly metabolized during pulmonary transit. It has a wide spectrum of other effects such as stimulation of the renin-angiotensin system, and it may be involved in cytoprotection along with the primary PGs. PGI_2 exerts its effects by increasing cyclic adenosine monophosphate (cAMP). Stable analogs of PGI_2 have been developed and are under extensive investigation for therapeutic applications for peripheral vascular disease (19).

Thromboxane A_2

Thromboxane A_2 (TxA_2) is formed from the cyclic endoperoxide, PGH_2, by the enzyme thromboxane synthetase, particularly by platelets, during the aggregation process (8), but also in other tissues. It differs significantly in structure from the primary PGs in that a six-membered oxane ring replaces the cyclopentane ring of PGs (Fig. 13.2-3). TxA_2 induces platelet adhesion and aggregation and is a potent vasoconstrictor and bronchoconstrictor. The actions of TxA_2 are hypothetically mediated by its inhibition of intracellular cAMP levels and promotion of calcium ion flux into cells. The overproduction of TxA_2 by platelets is speculated to contribute to the pathophysiology of various vascular and hemostatic disorders, and therefore inhibitors of TxA_2 synthetase (e.g., imidazole derivatives) might be therapeutically beneficial (6). The potential benefit of specific TxA_2-receptor antagonists in vascular diseases is also a subject of current investigation.

Lipoxygenase Products

The peptido-leukotrienes, LTC_4, LTD_4, and LTE_4, are the principal active components of the slow-reacting substance of anaphylaxis, and their major biological roles are apparently in immediate hypersensitivity and inflammatory reactions (15). These leukotrienes are potent bronchoconstrictors and also promote vascular permeability and, hence, edema in the presence of vasodilatory arachidonate metabolites. In addition, LTC_4, LTD_4, and LTE_4 are vasoconstrictors, although the pathophysiological relevance of this effect is yet to be clearly demonstrated.

LTB_4, a dihydroxy lipoxygenase product, is a potent inducer of neutrophil adhesion and chemotaxis. In combination with vasodilatory PGs and the vascular permeability-promoting peptido-leukotrienes, LTB_4 is thought to be an important mediator of inflammatory and immunological reactions. LTB_4 itself induces vascular permeability but is less potent than LTC_4 or LTD_4.

Because leukotrienes are involved in asthma and acute inflammation, there is great potential for selective leukotriene inhibitors and receptor antagonists. The therapeutic efficacy of the corticosteroids in immunological and inflammatory diseases probably stems, at least in part, from their inhibition of lipoxygenase product formation via their effect in inhibiting the release of arachidonic acid from membrane lipids.

DRUG PREPARATIONS FOR THERAPEUTIC USE

Currently, there are four PG preparations available for therapeutic use in the U.S. market, although many new analogs are being tested. Due to the nature of the applications, the adverse reactions, and recent introduction of these drugs, they should be used only by obstetricians, gynecologists, and neonatologists at facilities with specialized surgical and intensive care units.

Gynecological and Obstetric Applications

The ability of E- and F-series PGs and their analogs to terminate pregnancy at any stage by promoting uterine contractions has been adapted to routine clinical use in gynecology and obstetrics. They are used in termination of first- and second-trimester pregnancy, priming of cervix prior to abortion, and in induction of labor in pregnancies with intrauterine fetal death or hydatiform mole. Generally they can be administered intramuscularly, intravenously, intra- and extra-amniotically, and vaginally. Because primary PGs have many mutual effects, adverse reactions to various PGs used as drugs are also similar. Uterine pain, vomiting, diarrhea, fever, headache, and dyspnea are seen most often.

Systemic administration of PGs is not recommended to patients with pulmonary, cardiovascular, renal, or hepatic disease, diabetes, or epilepsy. Great care should also be taken when administered to patients with acute pelvic inflammatory disease or a previous cesarean section.

Carboprost Tromethamine. Carboprost (15-methyl $PGF_{2\alpha}$) is a methylated analog of $PGF_{2\alpha}$, and as such has the same spectrum of activity as $PGF_{2\alpha}$. The methyl group at C-15 results in prolonged biological activity. Carboprost is used to induce abortion in the second trimester, between the thirteenth and twentieth weeks of pregnancy. Repeated intramuscular injections totaling a mean dose of 2.6 mg are required to produce abortion, which occurs after an average of 16 hr.

Dinoprost Tromethamine. Dinoprost is the THAM [tris(hydroxymethyl)aminomethane] salt of $PGF_{2\alpha}$ and shares its pharmacological actions. Like carboprost, it is used to promote second-trimester abortion, usually after week 15. Dinoprost is administered intraamniotically at an initial dose of 40 mg and produces 86% complete abortions, requiring an average of 20 hr.

Dinoprostone. Dinoprostone is synthetic PGE_2 and has the pharmacological activity of the natural PG. Dinoprostone is available as a vaginal suppository and is used to induce therapeutic or elective abortions in the second trimester or in cases of intrauterine fetal death. The usual dose is 20 mg, repeated at 3- to 5-hr intervals, depending on the response of the uterus. Abortion can usually be achieved within 90 hr, with 25% being incomplete. When used to stimulate labor in cases of fetal death, the drug is nearly 100% effective.

Neonatal Applications

Alprostadil. Alprostadil (PGE_1) is structurally related to PGE_2, but has only one double bond; it is a minor natural product of the cyclooxygenase pathway, derived from dihomolinolenic acid. Its pharmacological actions resemble those of PGI_2 or PGE_2 in many systems. Thus, it is a vasodilator and inhibitor of platelet aggregation much like PGI_2 and contracts uterine and intestinal smooth muscle like PGE_2. Alprostadil is used in neonates with certain rare cases of congenital heart disease to temporarily maintain the patency of the ductus arteriosus before surgery. It has no absolute contraindications, but use in cases of respiratory distress syndrome is not recommended. Most common side effects include apnea, bradycardia, hypotension, and hyperpyrexia. Because of rapid pulmonary metabolism, the drug should be continuously infused intravenously at an initial dose of 0.05-0.10 μg/kg of body weight/min, and can be increased to 0.40 μg/kg. The duration of administration and dose should be minimized. Prolonged usage has been associated with ductal fragility and rupture.

REFERENCES

1. Bergström, S. and Sjövall, J. The isolation of prostaglandin F from sheep prostate glands. *Acta Chem. Scand.* 14:1693, 1960.
2. Coceani, F. and Olley, P.M. Prostaglandins and the circulation at birth. In: *Cardiovascular Pharmacology of the Prostaglandins* (Herman, A.G., Vanhoutte, P.M., Denolin, H. and Goossens, A., eds.). New York: Raven Press, 1982, p. 303.
3. Dusting, G.J., Moncada, S. and Vane, J.R. Prostaglandins, their intermediates and precursors: cardiovascular actions and regulatory roles in normal and abnormal circulatory systems. *Prog. Cardiovasc. Dis.* 21:405, 1979.
4. von Euler, U.S. Zur Kenntnis der pharmakologischen Wirkungen von Nativsekreten und Extrakten mannlicher accessorischer Geschlechtsdrüsen. *Arch. Exp. Pathol. Pharmakol.* 175:78, 1934.
5. Flower, R. and Blackwell, G.J. Anti-inflammatory steroids induce biosynthesis of a phospholipase A_2 inhibitor which prevents prostaglandin generation. *Nature* 278:456, 1979.
6. Granström, E., Diczfalusy, U., Hamberg, M., Hansson, G., Malmsten, C. and Samuelsson, B. Thromboxane A_2: Biosynthesis and effects on platelets. In: *Advances in Prostaglandin, Thromboxane, and Leukotriene Research*, Vol 10. (Oates, J.A., ed.). New York: Raven Press, 1982, p. 15.
7. Hamberg, M. and Samuelsson, B. Detection and isolation of an endoperoxide intermediate in prostaglandin biosynthesis. *Proc. Natl. Acad. Sci.* USA 70:899, 1973.
8. Hamberg, M., Svensson, J. and Samuelsson, B. Thromboxanes. A new group of biologically active compounds derived from prostaglandin endoperoxides. *Proc. Natl. Acad. Sci.* USA 72: 2994, 1975.
9. Johnson, R.A., Morton, D.R., Kinner, J.H., Gorman, R.R., McGuire, J.C., Sun, F.F., Whittaker, N., Bunting, S., Salmon, J., Moncada, S. and Vane, J.R. The chemical structure of prostaglandin X (prostacyclin). *Prostaglandins* 12:915, 1976.
10. Karim, S.M.M. and Hillier, K. Physiological roles and pharmacological actions of prostaglandins in relation to human reproduction. In: *Prostaglandins and Reproduction* (Karim, S.M.M., ed.). Lancaster: MTP Press, 1975, p. 23.
11. Kurzrok, R. and Lieb, C.C. Biochemical studies of human semen. II. The action of semen on the human uterus. *Proc. Soc. Exp. Biol. Med.* 28:268, 1930.
12. Metz, S.A. Anti-inflammatory agents as inhibitors of prostaglandin synthesis in man. *Med. Clin. North Am.* 65:713, 1981.
13. Moncada, S., Gryglewski, R., Bunting, S. and Vane, J.R. An enzyme isolated from arteries transforms prostaglandin endoperoxides to an unstable substance that inhibits platelet aggregation. *Nature* 263:663, 1976.
14. Ramwell, P.W., Leovey, E.M.K. and Sintetos, A.L. Regulation of the arachidonic acid cascade. *Biol. Reprod.* 16:70, 1977.
15. Samuelsson, B. Leukotrienes: Mediators of immediate hypersensitivity reactions and inflammation. *Science* 220:568, 1983.
16. Samuelsson, B., Borgeat, P., Hammarström, S. and Murphy, R.C. Introduction of a nomenclature: Leukotrienes. *Prostaglandins* 17:785, 1979.
17. Samuelsson, B., Granström, E., Green, K., Hamberg, M. and Hammarstrom, S. Prostaglandins. *Ann. Rev. Biochem.* 44:669, 1975.
18. Vane, J.R. Inhibition of prostaglandin synthesis as a mechanism of action for aspirin-like drugs. *Nature* (New. Biol.) 231:232, 1971.
19. Vane, J.R. Prostacyclin in physiology and pathophysiology. *Int. Rev. Exp. Pathol.* 23:161, 1982.

ADDITIONAL READING

Moncada, S. Prostacycline, from discovery to clinical application. *J. Pharmacol.* 16(Suppl. 1):1, 1985.

CHAPTER
13.3

SEROTONIN

Roger P. Maickel

Almost 50 years ago, extensive investigation began on a substance found in blood that had significant vasoconstrictor properties (4). This substance, first isolated from blood (9) and later found in thrombocytes (11), brain (1), and the enterochromaffin cells of the gastrointestinal mucosa (5), was originally called *serotonin* by some groups of investigators and *enteramine* by others. Subsequently, the compound was identified as an indole, 5-hydroxytryptamine (5-HT), and chemically synthesized in pure form (7). Its biosynthesis (Fig. 6-14) and catabolism (Fig. 6-16), distribution in the brain (Fig. 6-15), and role in some CNS functions and drug action(s), have been presented in Chapter 6.

As in the case of other biogenic amines (see Chapter 6), effects of serotonin are considered to be mediated through its action on serotonin receptors. A number of recent studies have suggested that two receptor types exist for serotonin in rodent brain (5-HT_1 and 5-HT_2); these receptors have differing roles in brain serotonergic function (8). The 5-HT_1 receptors have lower affinities for tryptamines (serotonin agonists), whereas the 5-HT_2 receptors have lower affinities for serotonin antagonists. Whether multiple serotonin receptors exist at peripheral sites has not yet been established.

The metabolic pathways of serotonin, including the side pathway of conversion of serotonin to melatonin that occurs in the mammalian pineal gland are summarized in Fig. 13.3-1. In addition to these major pathways, a number of minor metabolic pathways have been identified, leading to products such as various substituted tryptamines and tryptophols; for a complete discussion, the reader should consult the detailed review by Bosin (2).

PHARMACOLOGICAL EFFECTS

Serotonin per se has only limited investigational and no actual clinical therapeutic usage. Its actions in the body are in predominantly three loci: the brain, the circulatory system, and smooth muscle systems. A summary chart of the physiological activities of endogenous serotonin is presented in Table 13.3-1. It should be emphasized that most of these relationships have been developed as a result of research with experimental animals. With the exception of the limited uses of cyproheptadine and methysergide discussed later in this chapter, the status of serotonin in human medicine is literally that of an endogenous substance in search of a disease state.

PHARMACOKINETICS

Any serotonin that is administered orally or consumed in the diet is poorly absorbed from the stomach and subject to chemical degradation at acidic pH. What reaches the intestine, to be absorbed there, is subjected to active uptake by the enterochromaffin cells and/or degradation in the intestinal wall. Any minute amount reaching the bloodstream is destroyed by liver MAO or is taken up by the lungs or thrombocytes. Even after intravenous administration, the major part of the dose is rapidly oxidized to 5-hydroxyindoleacetic acid (5-HIAA) and excreted in the urine.

With the exception of the thrombocytes, which contain virtually no biosynthetic capacity for serotonin, all of the amine present in body sites is synthesized from l-tryptophan by the first two steps of the process shown in Fig. 13.3-1; the rate-limiting step is the action of tryptophan-5-hydroxylase. The thrombocytes possess a very active and highly efficient active uptake process, unlike that of nerve endings in serotonergic and catecholaminergic neurons. This process permits the thrombocytes to

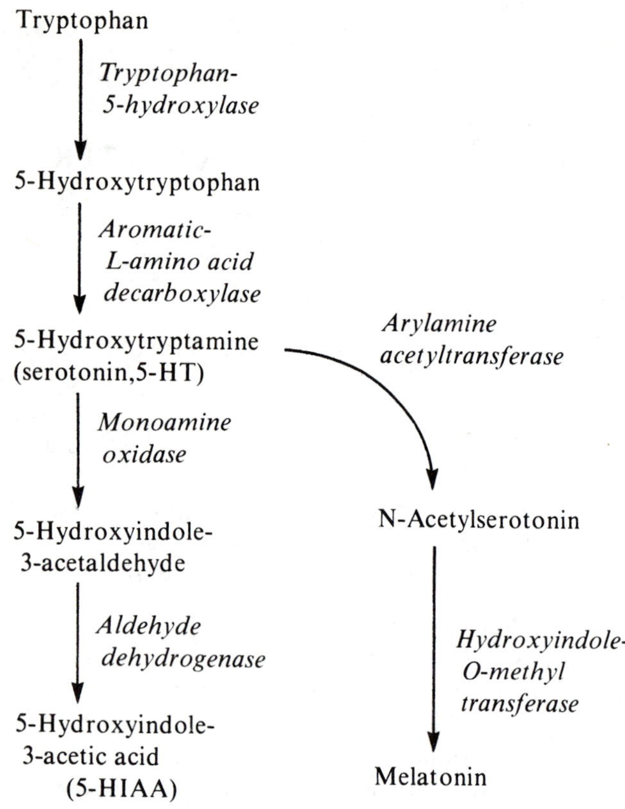

Fig. 13.3-1. *Serotonin metabolism.*

pick up serotonin as they pass through the intestinal circulation.

Serotonin stores in neuronal tissues are basically similar to those of catecholamines, releasable by reserpine and with reuptake processes that are impaired by the tricyclic antidepressants (6). A unique differential effect can be seen in the effect of guanethidine on serotonin levels in brain and intestine. When administered parenterally, guanethidine has no effect on intestinal levels of serotonin, although it depletes the heart of norepinephrine; when given into the lateral ventricles (to bypass the blood-brain barrier), guanethidine lowers both serotonin and norepinephrine in rat brain with equal facility (3).

CLINICAL ROLE

The most significant clinical role for serotonin is in the carcinoid syndrome. Massive tumors, generally of enterochromaffin cells and localized in the respiratory system or gastrointestinal tract, synthesize and release large quantities of serotonin. These amounts are so large that significant flushing, abdominal cramping, and diarrhea are seen; urinary levels of 5-hydroxyindoleacetic acid are often markedly elevated.

DRUGS INFLUENCING SEROTONERGIC FUNCTIONS

Table 13.3-2 contains a summary listing of the major classes of drugs that are known to influence serotonin in mammalian systems. The majority of these either are not in clinical use or have been discussed elsewhere in this text, and will not be further discussed. Two of the agents do, however, need further discussion, although they have been mentioned in other chapters.

Cyproheptadine. Cyproheptadine is an H_1-receptor blocker, discussed in more detail in Chapter 13.4, that also possesses significant serotonergic receptor blocking activity. This potency makes it useful in treatment of some conditions involving endogenous release of sero-

Table 13.3-1
Summary of Physiological Effects of Serotonin

Locus	Type of Action(s)	Relevance
Central nervous system	Neurotransmitter in serotonergic and tryptaminergic systems	Involved in control/modulation of sleep and other behavior and pituitary hormone secretion
Cardiovascular system	Positive inotropic and chronotropic actions on heart; strong constricting action on veins; promotes platelet aggregation	Acts as endogenous vasoconstrictor substance
Endocrine systems	Modulatory neurotransmitter	Implicated in control of release of *all* anterior pituitary hormones
Exocrine systems	Modulatory neurotransmitter	Reduces volume and acidity of gastric secretion in response to vagal stimulation; increases mucus flow
Intestinal system	Smooth muscle-stimulating substance present in enterochromaffin cells	Stimulates intestinal motility
Respiratory system	Stimulation of smooth muscle	Bronchoconstriction (in asthmatics)

Table 13.3-2
Drugs Influencing Serotonergic Functions

Site/Locus of Action	Drug	Mechanism(s) of Action	Effect(s) on Endogenous 5-HT Content	Clinical Use(s)
Synthesis	p-Chlorophenylalanine	Inhibition of tryptophan hydroxylase	↓	None
	p-Chloroamphetamine		↓	None
Storage	Reserpine	Inhibition of storage, release and depletion	↓	Antihypertensive Antipsychotic
	Tetrabenazine		↓	None
Receptor interaction	Cyproheptadine	Antagonistic	0	Antihistamine
	Methysergide	Antagonistic	0	Prophylactic use in migraine
	Lysergic acid diethylamide	Antagonistic (?)	0	None
	Quipazine	Agonistic	0	None
Reuptake mechanism(s)	Chlorimipramine	Nonspecific inhibition of amine reuptake	?	None
	Amitriptyline	Nonspecific inhibition of amine uptake	?	Antidepressant
	Imipramine	Nonspecific inhibition of amine uptake	?	Antidepressant
	Fluoxetine	Specific inhibition of 5-HT reuptake	?	None
	Fluvoxamine	Specific inhibition of 5-HT uptake	?	None
Metabolism	Isocarboxazid	MAO inhibition	↑	Antidepressant
	Phenelzine	MAO inhibition	↑	Antidepressant
	Tranylcypromine	MAO inhibition	↑	Antidepressant
	Fenfluramine	Not clearly defined	?	Anorexigenic Agent
Neurotoxin	5,6-Dihydroxytryptamine	Specific damage to 5-HT neurons	↓	None
	5,7-Dihydroxytryptamine		↓	None

tonin, such as the intestinal hypermotility associated with the carcinoid syndrome or the "dumping syndrome" seen in postgastrectomy patients.

Methysergide. Methysergide is also discussed with the other derivatives of the ergot alkaloids in Chapter 19. It is effective as a prophylactic agent for migraine and cluster headaches, but unlike other ergot derivatives such as ergotamine, this drug has no use in the treatment of such headaches (10). It is definitely indicated for those patients in whom vascular headaches are of sufficient frequency and severity to justify prophylactic therapy.

The exact mechanism of this action of methysergide is unknown. For example, although considered to be a serotonin antagonist, methysergide may actually enhance the vasoconstrictive action of serotonin in scalp arteries, just as it potentiates the vasoconstrictor action of catecholamines. Methysergide is known to interfere with vasomotor reflexes in the brain as well as inhibiting the serotonin-stimulated release of prostaglandins.

ADVERSE EFFECTS

Methysergide produces a variety of side effects that include the following:

1. Fibrotic changes occur in cardiac, pleuropulmonary, and retroperitoneal sites. Cardiac fibrosis can occur in the aortic or mitral valves or the root of the aorta, leading to murmurs and dyspnea; pleuropulmonary fibrosis can cause chest pain and pleural effusions. Retroperitoneal changes are most damaging, often leading to urinary tract obstruction; symptoms include dysuria and pain in either or both flank areas.

2. Vasoconstrictor effects common to many ergot derivatives produce peripheral vascular insufficiency resulting in coldness, numbness, pain in the extremities, and paresthesia.

3. CNS effects indicate modest stimulation, presumably because the molecule contains the lysergic acid polycyclic nucleus. These effects include nervousness, dizziness, insomnia, altered thinking, and even hallucinations.

4. Gastrointestinal effects include nausea, vomiting, diarrhea, and abdominal pain and occur early in therapy.

In general, patients on chronic therapy with methysergide should be seen on a frequent, regular basis and should be instructed to report all symptoms. A 3- to 4-week drug-free period, preceded by a gradual dosage reduction over 2-3 weeks, should be imposed on the patient in each 6-month therapy period.

Preparations. *Methysergide maleate* (SANSERT) is available in 2-mg tablets; the recommended daily dosage is 2 mg, b.i.d. or t.i.d., with meals.

REFERENCES

1. Amin, A. H., Crawford, B. B., and Gaddum, J. H. Distribution of substance P and 5-hydroxytryptamine in the central nervous system of the dog. *J. Physiol.* (London), 126:596, 1954.
2. Bosin, T. R. Serotonin metabolism. In: *Serotonin in Health and Disease, Vol. 1.* (Essman, W. B., ed.). New York: SP Medical and Scientific Books, 1968, p. 181.
3. Cox, R. H., Jr., and Maickel, R. P. Effect of guanethidine on rat brain serotonin and norepinephrine. *Life Sci.* 8:1319, 1969.
4. Erspamer, V. Pharmacology of enteramine. I. Action of acetone extract of rabbit stomach mucosa on blood pressure and on surviving isolated organs. *Naunyn Schmied. Arch. Exp. Pathol. Pharmakol.* 201:337, 1940.
5. Erspamer, V., and Asero, B. Identification of enteramine, the specific hormone of the enterochromaffin cell system, as 5-hydroxytryptamine. *Nature* 169:800, 1952.
6. Fuller, R. W. Pharmacology of central serotonin neurons. *Ann. Rev. Pharmacol.* 20:111, 1980.
7. Hamlin, K. E., and Fischer, E. E. The synthesis of 5-hydroxytryptamine. *J. Am. Chem. Soc.* 73:5007, 1951.
8. Peroutka, S. J., and Snyder, S. H. Multiple serotonin receptors and their physiological significance. *Fed. Proc.* 42:213, 1983.
9. Rapport, M. M., Green, A. A., and Page, I. H. Serum vasoconstrictor (serotonin). IV. Isolation and characterization. *J. Biol. Chem.* 176:1243, 1948.
10. Raskin, N. H. Pharmacology of migraine. *Ann. Rev. Pharmacol.* 21:463, 1981.
11. Twarog, B. M., and Page, I. H. Serotonin content of some mammalian tissues and urine. *Am. J. Physiol.* 175:157, 1954.

CHAPTER 13.4

HISTAMINE AND ANTIHISTAMINES

John H. McNeill

HISTAMINE

History. Histamine has been known to pharmacologists for three-quarters of a century. The compound was first used as a synthetic drug and its pharmacological properties were investigated by Sir Henry Dale (9). Later, histamine was found in tissue extracts, but it was first believed that its presence was due to putrefaction. It was not until 1927 that Dale and his colleagues were able to clearly demonstrate the presence of histamine in fresh tissue (9). Early interest in histamine was stimulated by the discovery of the many pharmacological effects of the amine and also by its wide distribution in a variety of tissues (hence its name, from the Greek *histos,* or tissue). Despite 75 years of research, the actual role of histamine in the body remains uncertain, and it has been characterized as "an amine looking for a function." There is evidence for a role of histamine in gastric secretion, inflammation, allergy, and anaphylaxis. There are also suggestions that histamine may function as a local "hormone" and as a neurotransmitter (28, 29).

Histamine Receptors. For many years, it was puzzling that certain of the effects of histamine (for example, contraction of smooth muscle) could be completely antagonized by antihistamines, whereas other effects (such as the decrease in blood pressure) could be only partially antagonized; still others (stimulation of gastric secretion) could not be antagonized at all. The recent introduction by Black and his colleagues of a new group of antihistaminic compounds has supported the existence of two types of histamine receptors, H_1 and H_2 (3). H_1 (not H_2) receptors are blocked by the classic antihistamines, whereas H_2 receptors are selectively blocked only by a very few recently synthesized compounds (e.g., cimetidine). Further support for the hypothesis has come from the development of selective H_1 and H_2-agonist drugs. Although none of these is of therapeutic importance at the present time, their development and use have furthered our knowledge of histamine receptors (39). Table 13.4-1 lists some organs or tissues and their functions involving these two types of histamine receptors.

Biosynthesis of Histamine. Histamine is 5-(2-aminoethyl)-imidazole, also known as β-imidazolyl ethylamine. Histamine is formed from L-histidine through decarboxylation by the enzyme histidine decarboxylase (Fig. 13.4-1). This enzyme exhibits a specific affinity for L-histidine and requires pyridoxal 5-phosphate as a cofactor. Aromatic amino acid decarboxylase (Dopa decarboxylase) has a low affinity for L-histidine. Pyridoxine deficiency and certain other chemical compounds that react with pyridoxal phosphate (e.g., hydrazine) inhibit histidine decarboxylase (2). Because histidine decarboxylase is an inducible enzyme, high enzyme activity results following release of histamine from various mammalian tissues (20).

Distribution and Release of Histamine. Histamine is widely distributed throughout the animal kingdom and there are marked species differences with regard to its distribution. In humans, the highest concentrations are found in lungs, skin, stomach, and nasal mucous membranes (28, 37). Histamine is believed to exist in two pools, one consisting of storage in mast cells found widely distributed in connective tissue and in circulating basophils, and a second, more recently recognized, pool of nonmast cell histamine, such as that of the gastric mucosa.

Mast cell and basophil histamine is highly concentrated within granules that also contain heparin and proteolytic

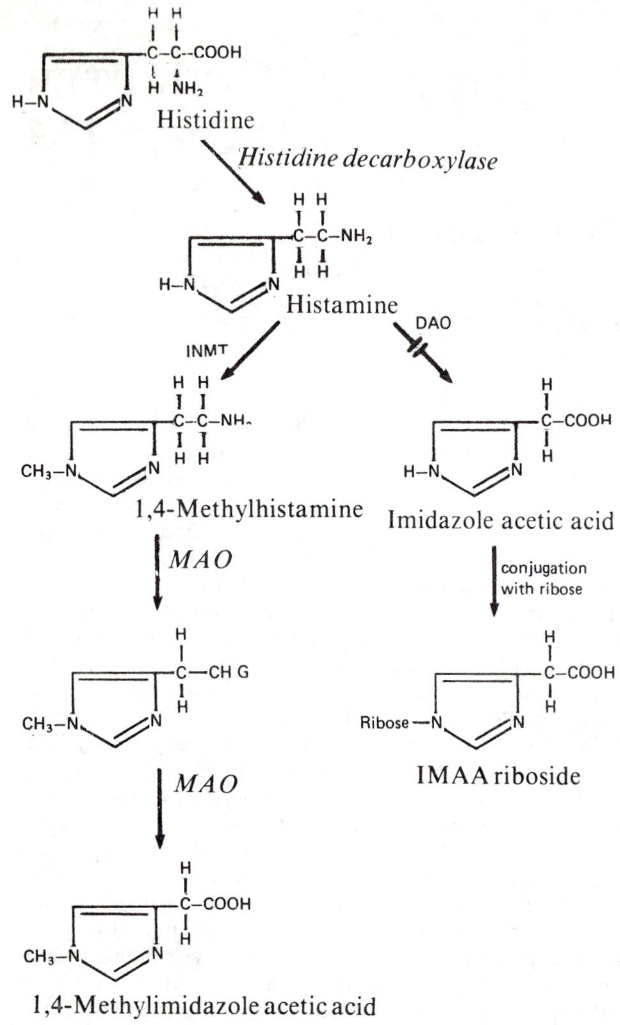

Histidine

Histidine decarboxylase

Histamine

INMT DAO

1,4-Methylhistamine Imidazole acetic acid

MAO conjugation with ribose

IMAA riboside

MAO

1,4-Methylimidazole acetic acid

Fig. 13.4-1. *Biosynthesis and major pathways for catabolism of histamine.*

enzymes (28). Release of histamine occurs in response to a variety of stimuli, including antigens and various basic drugs. Antigens appear to interact with IgE on the surface of the cell and drugs interact with specific receptors. Following such interactions, there is increased calcium influx into the cell with resulting exocytosis of the granules and the subsequent release of histamine. Therapeutic agents known to release histamine include the curare alkaloids, narcotic analgesics, and hydralazine (26). Drugs known to increase cyclic adenosine monophosphate (cAMP) (such as the catecholamines and theophylline) have recently been shown to decrease histamine release (22). The usual mechanism of action of these drugs in treating allergic responses and asthma is believed due to a physiological antagonism, although prevention of histamine release may also play a role. Sodium cromoglycate also decreases histamine release (18) by preventing degranulation of the mast cells.

Pharmacological Effects. In humans, injected histamine or the release of endogenous histamine has a marked effect on smooth muscle, particularly in the vasculature and bronchioles, on the cardiovascular system, and on gastric secretion. An increase in cerebrospinal fluid pressure may also result.

Smooth Muscle. Histamine causes a contraction of most smooth muscles, including those of the bronchioles and the gastrointestinal tract, by stimulating H_1 receptors. There are marked species variations in the response of smooth muscles to histamine. Bronchiolar constriction is of considerable clinical importance because it may occur following allergic reactions to drugs or other antigens resulting in the release of histamine. However, in normal individuals, the smooth muscle of the bronchus is least sensitive to histamine. Even though antihistamines can counteract the histamine response, more rapidly acting agents that will relax the smooth muscle, such as epinephrine, are the drugs of choice.

Cardiovascular System. In humans, injections of histamine cause a transient but marked decrease in blood pressure, tachycardia, flushing of the skin, and headache. Though histamine is known to constrict larger blood vessels, it will relax the vessels of microcirculation. This action is often referred to as capillary dilatation, but the vessels involved are primarily arterioles. The decrease in blood pressure and the flushing of the face and upper body can be attributed to vasodilatation. The effect is primarily on H_1 receptors, but H_2 receptors are also involved. Tachycardia results from both a reflex effect and from the stimulation of cardiac H_2 receptors. An increase in permeability of small venules, generally referred to as increased capillary permeability, also occurs and results in loss of plasma protein and fluid with formation of edema (28). Although cerebral vessels dilate in response to histamine, resulting in a pounding, throb-

Table 13.4-1
Histamine Receptors

Organ/Tissue	Receptor Type(s)
Smooth muscle of intestine and bronchi (contraction)	H_1
Smooth muscle of gallbladder (guinea pig), bovine stomach, trachea, and bronchus in different species (relaxation)	H_2
Rat uterus (relaxation)	H_2
Guinea pig right atrium, *in vitro* (chronotropic effect)	H_2
Decrease in blood pressure in cat	H_1, H_2
Mast cells, basophils, T lymphocytes, and neutrophils (immunoregulation)	H_2
Gastric secretion	H_2
Brain (putative neurotransmitter function)	H_1, H_2

bing headache, a role for endogenous histamine in headache has not been established (19).

Intradermal injections of histamine or local release of histamine in the skin results in the so-called triple response of Lewis. The triple response consists of a small red spot at the site of injection surrounded by a larger (approximately 1 cm) flushed area. The original red spot is rapidly replaced by edema fluid resulting in a wheal. The first two responses are due to dilatation of blood vessels, and the wheal is due to an increase in permeability of the vessels (21).

Large doses of histamine may release endogenous catecholamines from both nerve endings and the adrenal medulla. This is usually seen only in experimental animals.

Gastric Secretion. Histamine is a potent and effective stimulant of gastric secretion. Subcutaneous doses of histamine that produce few other effects can produce profound increases in gastric secretion by stimulating H_2 receptors in the parietal cells of the gastric mucosa. H_2 receptors are associated with adenylate cyclase, and the release of acid appears to be related to an increase in intracellular cAMP (32, 38). Histamine also stimulates salivary and lacrimal secretions.

Role of Cyclic Nucleotides in the Actions of Histamine. H_2-receptor stimulation is always associated with an increase in cAMP in all H_2-receptor-containing tissues where the response has been studied (13, 38). Thus, histamine stimulates adenylate cyclase obtained from the gastric mucosa of most species and from guinea pig heart. The positive inotropic effect of histamine in guinea pig heart is preceded by an increase in cAMP (38). Histamine also increases cAMP in the central nervous system, although a definite transmitter role for histamine has not been established. Both H_1 and H_2 receptors appear to be involved in the latter effect. Other tissues where stimulation of H_2 receptors results in an increase in cAMP include rat uterus, human leukocytes, canine fat cells, and rat renal cortex. H_1-receptor stimulation has been shown to increase cyclic guanosine monophosphate (cGMP) in human and guinea pig lung (13). An increase in cGMP does not always occur following H_1-receptor stimulation, however.

A number of drugs can elevate cAMP and cGMP in histamine-containing cells and can affect histamine release. As a general rule, drugs increasing cAMP, such as β-adrenoceptor agonists, histamine itself, and the methylxanthines, tend to decrease release. Drugs increasing cGMP, such as acetylcholine, increase release.

Pharmacokinetics. Orally administered histamine is essentially inactive even when administered in large doses because most of it is converted to N-acetylhistamine in the intestine. Any absorbed free histamine will be inactivated as it passes through the intestinal walls or by the liver.

The principal pathways for biotransformation of histamine in mammalian tissues involve ring methylation and oxidative deamination (Fig. 13.4-1). In the first reaction, histamine in the presence of imidazole N-methyltransferase (INMT) is methylated to form 1-methyl-4-[β-aminoethyl]-imidazole (methylhistamine) through transfer of a methyl group from S-adenosylmethionine. Methylhistamine is subsequently deaminated by monoamine oxidase to form 1-methylimidazole-4-acetic acid (methylimidazole acetic acid) (25). In the other pathway, deamination of histamine results by the enzyme diamine oxidase (DAO) to form imidazole acetic acid, which is conjugated and excreted as 1-ribosyl-imidazole-4-acetic acid (ribosyl imidazole acetic acid). Both INMT and DAO are widely distributed in most mammalian tissues and share the responsibility for termination of biological actions of histamine.

Histamine and its metabolites are excreted in the urine. In humans, approximately 55% of an injected dose of histamine can be accounted for as ring-methylated metabolites.

HISTAMINE-LIKE COMPOUNDS

Betazole, an isomer of histamine (a pyrazole derivative), is only one-fiftieth as potent as histamine but has more selectivity for H_2 receptors. Its chemical structure is:

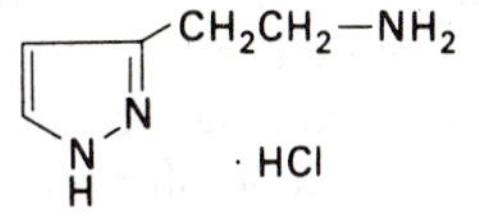

$CH_2CH_2{-}NH_2$
N
N
H
$\cdot$ HCl

Betazole

Although cardiovascular and bronchiolar effects are minimized, betazole induces maximum gastric secretion; caution is still recommended in using the drug in asthmatics. Side effects of betazole include flushing of the face and a sense of warmth, headache, urticaria, and weakness. More selective H_2 agonists are being developed for use in testing for gastric secretion, such as impromidine, a potent and selective H_2 agonist (11).

Pentagastrin, a synthetic pentapeptide derivative of the physiological gastric secretagogue gastrin may act by releasing endogenous histamine in the gastric mucosa or by stimulating gastrin receptors (32). Side effects (usually minor and transient) include dizziness, nausea, faintness, flushing, shortness of breath, and a desire to defecate.

A number of histamine analogs have been synthesized which have a high degree of specificity for either the H_1 or the H_2 receptor. Examples include pyridylethylamine (H_1) and impromidine (H_2). Such drugs are currently used as pharmacological tools for studying histamine receptors.

DRUGS PREVENTING THE ALLERGIC RELEASE OF HISTAMINE

Sodium cromoglycate (also known as cromolyn sodium) has proven valuable in the prophylaxis of bronchial asthma (2). Its effect is thought to depend on a temporary stabilization of the membrane of the mast cells without any influence on the reaction between antigen and cell-fixed antibodies (34). The release of histamine and slow-reacting substance in anaphylaxis (SRS-A) from lung mast cells is thus prevented. This drug has the following chemical structure and will be further discussed in Chapter 17.

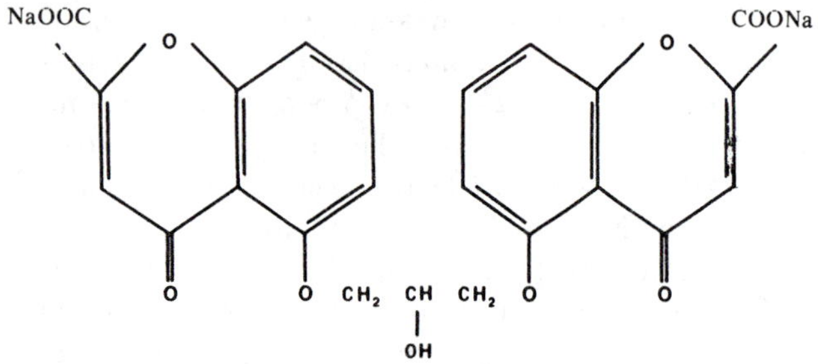

Sodium cromoglycate

ANTIHISTAMINES

Antihistamine drugs are of two types, H_1 blockers and H_2 blockers. Both groups act by competitively blocking histamine at the respective receptor sites. H_1 blockers do not resemble histamine in structure and have been available for nearly 40 years. H_2 blockers do resemble histamine chemically and have been made available only recently. An interesting analogy between histamine-blocking agents and adrenergic-blocking agents can be made in that α-adrenoceptor blocking drugs do not resemble the adrenergic drugs in structure, whereas β-adrenergic blocking agents do bear a resemblance.

In addition to blocking the actions of histamine, the H_1 antihistamines also possess anticholinergic and sedative properties. Antihistamines do not interfere with antibody formation, antigen-antibody interactions, release of histamine, or the actions of other mediators such as eosinophil chemotactic factor of anaphylaxis (ECF-A) and slow-reacting substances of anaphylaxis (SRS-A).

HISTAMINE H_1-RECEPTOR ANTAGONISTS

Chemistry. Most H_1 antihistamines are substituted ethylamines. Their general structure is depicted in Fig. 13.4-2.

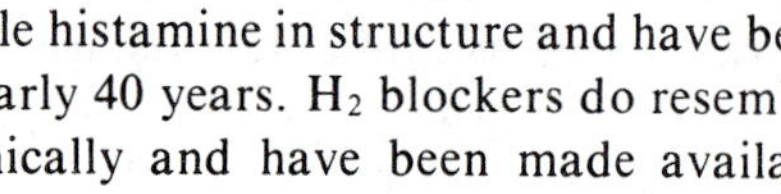

$$>X-CH_2-CH_2-N<{R \atop R}$$

Fig. 13.4-2. *General structure of H_1*-receptor antagonists.

The R groups are predominantly CH_3. The X substituent can be either N, O, or C. Depending on the X substitution, the drugs are commonly divided into several groups: alkylamines, ethanolamines, ethylenediamines, phenothiazines, piperazines, and a miscellaneous group. Table 13.4-2 lists selected drugs from each group with their duration of action, dose, and general comments. Representative structural formulas are shown in Fig. 13.4-3.

H_1-Receptor Blocking Effect. H_1 antihistamines will competitively block all the H_1 actions of histamine. They are particularly useful in treating the symptoms of allergy such as rhinitis, allergic dermatoses, urticaria, and angioedema, and some are useful antipruritics. They are of no value in the treatment of the common cold unless an allergic component is present. The anticholinergic effects of the antihistamines, which theoretically would be useful in drying up secretions in conditions such as the common cold, are in fact seldom prominent enough at therapeutic doses to be useful. Topical application of antihistamines has been used for both the antipruritic and antiallergic effects of the drugs. In such cases, the local anesthetic effect of the agents is an added useful factor. However, a higher incidence of drug sensitization reactions occurs with topical use.

Other Effects. In addition to blocking H_1 receptors, the antihistamines can produce a number of other effects. Prominent among these are effects on the central nervous system, anticholinergic effects, local anesthetic effects, and antiserotonin properties.

Most antihistamines produce some sedation, which is usually considered as a side effect. Diphenhydramine at a dose of 50 mg has been shown to be as good a hypnotic as 60 mg of secobarbital. Increasing the dose beyond 50 mg, however, does not increase the sedation (36). Promethazine also has prominent CNS depressant effects and is occasionally used as a sedative agent. One antihistamine, hydroxyzine, is used so often as an antianxiety agent that it is usually discussed with other antianxiety drugs. It should be noted that the amounts of antihistamine in many over-the-counter sleeping preparations are less than the therapeutic dose. The effectiveness of such preparations is thus highly questionable. At high dose of the antihistamine, stimulant effects occur, especially in children; hallucinations, excitement, ataxia, incoordination, athetosis, and convulsions occur accompanied by flushing, hyperpyrexia, and fixed dilated pupils. Depression, coma, and death can follow. The fatal dose in a child can be as little as 20-30% of adult doses. The effects described for high doses of antihistamines are mainly due to the anticholinergic effects of the drugs.

The anticholinergic effects of certain of the antihistamines probably account for their usefulness as antiparkinsonism agents, as well as for their useful effects in treating motion sickness (5, 6), vertigo, and Ménière's disease (8). Dimenhydrinate, diphenhydramine, cyclizine, meclizine, thiethylperazine, and promethazine have proven particularly useful in treating motion sickness and vertigo. As with all drugs, caution is advised in using these agents in pregnancy. Teratogenic effects have been noted in animals following administration of the piperazine compounds (29). Doxylamine is often used to treat the nausea and vomiting of pregnancy. Diphenhydramine is used in the treatment of parkinsonism.

The local anesthetic effect of the antihistamines makes

Table 13.4-2
H_1 Antihistamines

Generic Name	Representative Trade Name	Duration of Action	Single Dose (adult, mg)	Comments
Alkylamines				
Chlorpheniramine	CHLOR-TRIMETON	4-6	2-4	Effective in low doses;
Dexchlorpheniramine	POLARAMINE	4-6	2	less drowsiness as a side effect
Brompheniramine	DIMETANE	4-6	4-8	
Dimethindene	FORHISTAL	6-8	1-2	
Triprolidine	ACTIDIL	6-8	2.5	
Ethanolamines				
Carbinoxamine	CLISTIN	4	4	Significant anticholinergic effects;
Dimenhydrinate	DRAMAMINE	4-6	50	drowsiness often reported
Diphenhydramine	BENADRYL	4-6	50	
Diphenylpyraline	NOVAHISTINE[a]	4-6	2	
Ethylenediamines				
Antazoline	ANTISTINE	3-4	25-50	Some sedation; gastrointestinal side
Mepyramine				effects common
(pyrilamine)	NEO-ANTERGAN	4-6	25-50	
Tripelennamine	PYRIBENZAMINE	4-6	50	
Phenothiazines				
Methdilazine	TACARYL	12	8	Prominent sedation; useful anti-
Promethazine	PHENERGAN	4-6	25-50	nauseants
Thiethylperazine	TORECAN	—	10[b]	
Piperazines				
Cyclizine	MAREZINE	4-6	50	Sedation occurs; useful anti-
Meclizine	BONINE	12-24	25-50	nauseants; do not use in pregnancy
Others				
Azatadine	OPTIMINE	12	1	Are also antiserotonin
Cyproheptadine	PERIACTIN	6-8	4	

[a]Trade preparation contains ingredients in addition to the antihistamine.
[b]Antinauseant dose.

them useful as antipruritic agents. As mentioned previously, sensitization to the drugs occurs at a greater frequency following topical application.

Cyproheptadine is an antihistamine that also possesses marked antiserotonin properties.

Most antihistamines also possess cocainelike properties in that they can block the uptake of adrenergic amines (24). This property, however, does not seem to contribute to either their therapeutic or toxic effects.

Pharmacokinetics. H_1 antihistamines are well absorbed from the gastrointestinal tract. Effects are noted within 30 min after an oral dose; absorption is complete within 4 hours. The majority of H_1 antihistamines are lipid-soluble, distributed throughout the body, and readily enter the central nervous system. Localization occurs in the lung, a characteristic of many basic drugs. Metabolism is primarily via the liver oxidative drug enzymes, with excretion of unchanged drug and metabolites in the urine. In animal studies, some H_2 antihistamines have been found capable of inducing the drug-metabolizing enzymes of the liver (17, 28).

Adverse Effects. The most common side effects of antihistamines is sedation, characterized by drowsiness, lack of mental concentration, dizziness, ataxia, and lack of sound sleep. Marked sedation is produced by ethanolamines and a phenothiazine (promethazine). Alkylamines are least sedating and may stimulate the CNS. Anticholinergic effects of antihistamines may result in insomnia, tremors, nervousness, irritability, dryness of mouth, blurred vision, urinary retention, tachycardia, and constipation. Gastrointestinal complaints (e.g., anorexia, nausea, and vomiting) are common with ethylenediamines. There are rare reports of agranulocytosis, leukopenia, and thrombocytopenia associated with long-term use of antihistamines.

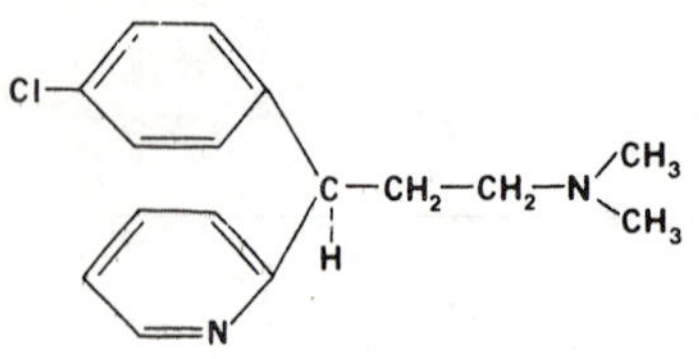

Chlorpheniramine

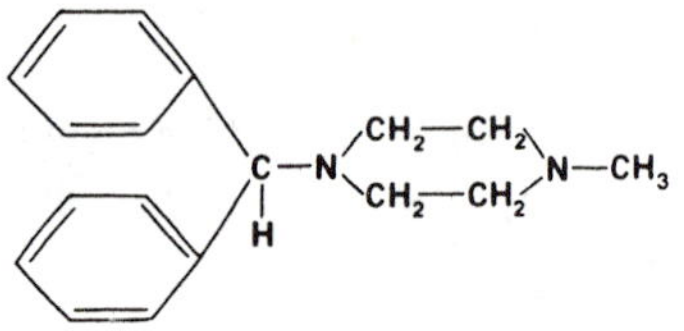

Cyclizine

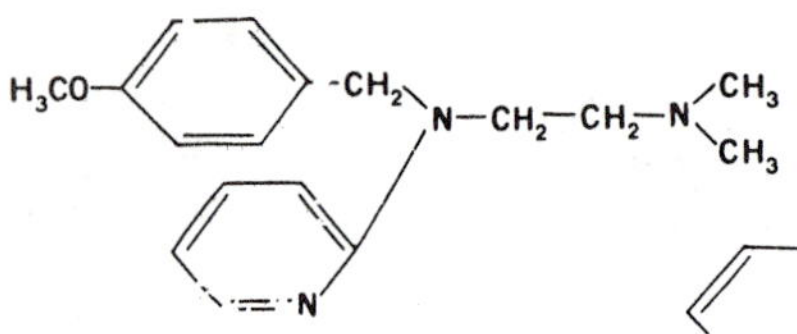

Mepyramine

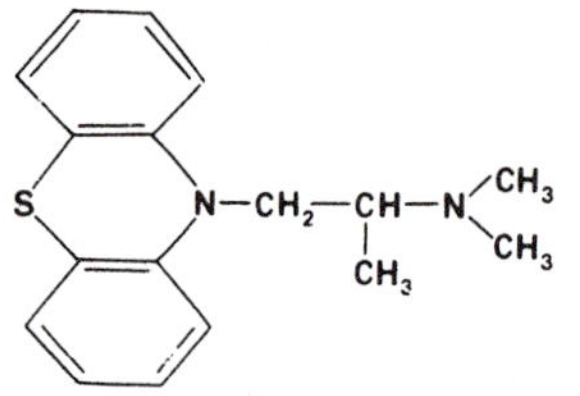

Promethazine

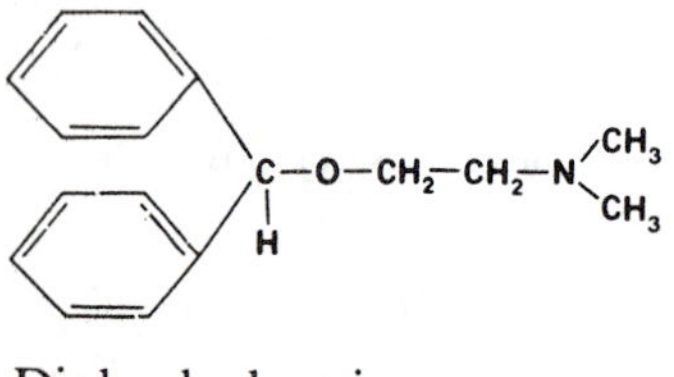

Diphenhydramine

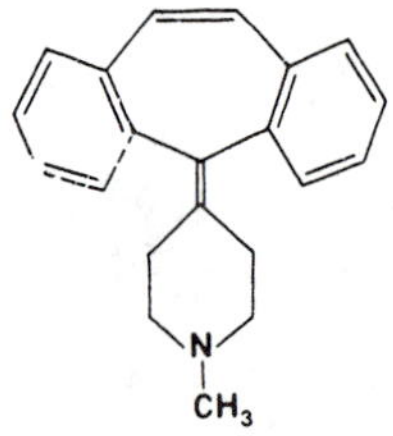

Cyproheptadine

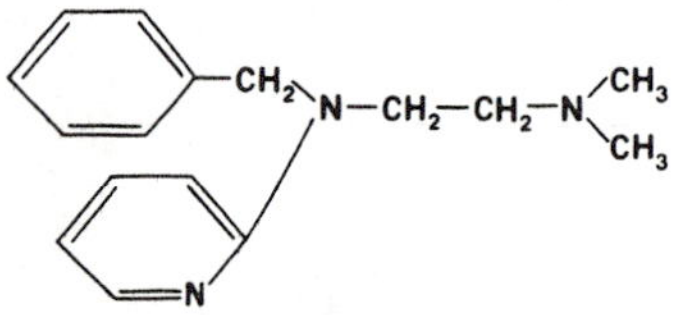

Tripelennamine

Fig. 13.4-3. *Structures of representatives of H_1*-receptor antagonists.

Acute overdosage may cause dryness of mouth and upper respiratory tract, pyrexia, mydriasis, hallucination, convulsions, respiratory failure, and death.

Drug Interactions. Antihistamines with a marked sedative effect potentiate the effects of barbiturates, nonbarbiturate sedatives, tranquilizers, narcotics, and anesthetics. The action of anticholinergics may be potentiated by antihistamines. Monoamine oxidase inhibitors clinically potentiate central depressant actions of antihistamines. The latter may also antagonize the actions of anticholinesterases. Hepatic microsomal enzyme induction by long-term use of some antihistamines may increase metabolism of glucocorticoids, phenytoin, and anticoagulants.

Therapeutic Uses. The major therapeutic uses of the antihistamines are in treating allergic rhinitis, urticaria, and other allergic phenomena including drug-induced allergic reactions. Additional uses include motion sickness and other conditions in which nausea is a problem. The drugs have been used as well in treating the withdrawal from depressant drugs including alcohol. This is a pharmacologically unsound use of the drugs, for they are not truly depressants. Antihistamines lower the threshold for convulsions and may actually make the withdrawal syndrome more severe by increasing the chance for seizures in severe depressant withdrawal (27).

Cyproheptadine has some usefulness in patients with gastric carcinoid tumor due to its antiserotonin properties. It may also have an effect on the hypothalamus to increase appetite and cause weight gain.

Preparations and Dosage. Preparations and dosage are listed in Table 13.4-3. Most preparations are for oral use, but some antihistamines are available as injectable preparations. Topical creams and ointments and nasal sprays are also available.

HISTAMINE H_2-RECEPTOR ANTAGONISTS

Specific antagonists have been designed to block the H_2 receptors that are involved in gastric acid and pepsin secretion. The H_2-receptor antagonists retain the imidazole ring of histamine but have bulky aliphatic side chains. The first such compound to be used clinically, burimamide, had to be given parenterally to suppress acid secretion. The second, metiamide, was active when given orally but was abandoned when it was noted to cause agranulocytosis, which resulted in its withdrawal from the market. H_2-receptor antagonists currently used in therapy include cimetidine and a recently approved newer drug, ranitidine.

CIMETIDINE

Cimetidine [N″-cyano-N-methyl-N′-[2[[(5-methyl-1H-imidazol-4-yl) methyl] thio]-ethyl]-guanidine] has a cyanoguanidine group in its side chain. Cimetidine suppresses acid secretion when given parenterally or orally, reduces symptoms of peptic ulcer disease, and accelerates healing rate of peptic ulcers. Its chemical structure is:

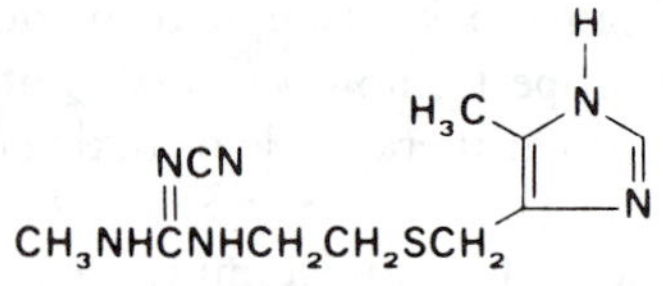

Cimetidine

Pharmacological Effects and Mechanism of Action. Cimetidine is an effective inhibitor of spontaneous gastric acid secretion, which is reduced by 80-90% for 6 to 8 hours following a 300-mg dose. It also reduces pepsin output and may have a specific gastric mucosal protective effect. Cimetidine also decreases secretion stimulated by histamine, betazole, gastrin and pentagastrin, cholinergic agents (bethanechol), insulin, caffeine, and test meals. Because cimetidine is a specific H_2-receptor blocking agent with no other blocking effects at therapeutic doses, it has been suggested that all of these agonists may produce gastric secretion by releasing histamine from the gastric mucosa, making histamine the final common mediator of gastric secretion (3, 7, 23). It has also been suggested that each agonist has its own receptor on the parietal cell. Because cimetidine can decrease gastric stimulation by histamine, gastrin, and acetylcholine, it is suggested that in addition to blocking histamine receptors, cimetidine decreases the affinity of gastrin and acetylcholine for their respective receptors (15). It has also been suggested that there is a positive interaction between histamine and either gastrin or acetylcholine. When histamine occupies the H_2 receptor, the action of gastrin or acetylcholine on their receptors is enhanced. If the binding of histamine to the H_2 receptor is blocked by cimetidine, the effect of gastrin or acetylcholine is greatly reduced (15, 31). The second messenger for histamine is believed to be cAMP (38). Second messengers for acetylcholine and gastrin are not known at this time (15, 31).

Pharmacokinetics. Following oral administration, cimetidine is absorbed from the proximal small intestine. Because the rate of gastric emptying affects the rate of cimetidine absorption, absorption of the drug is protracted when given with meals, and plasma levels of the drug and gastric acid suppression are sustained (34). After oral ingestion, peak cimetidine levels are reached in 60-90 min with 70-90% absorbed as compared with intravenous administration (14).

Cimetidine has an elimination half-life of approximately 1.5 to 2 hours. It is a polar molecule and primarily excreted via the kidneys in unchanged form as well as after conversion to sulfoxide and hydroxymethyl metabolites (12). Because the kidneys are the main site of cimetidine elimination, the dose in renal failure should be reduced from 300 mg four times a day to 300 mg twice daily; this reduced dose results in blood levels similar to those obtained in normal subjects (4). Patients undergoing hemodialysis clear cimetidine by this process and also require appropriate dose adjustment.

Adverse Effects. Side effects, relatively rare with cimetidine, include headache, dizziness, fatigue, skin rash, diarrhea, constipation, and muscular pain. These effects were also reported in patients receiving placebo. Reversible gynecomastia in males and galactorrhea in females have occurred in a very small number of patients. There have also been reports of agitation, mental confusion, and disorientation in elderly patients taking the drug at regular doses and in younger persons at higher than recommended doses. Improvement occurred when the drug was stopped (12). Increased serum transminases and creatinine levels occur in some patients. In a small number of cases, cimetidine produces dermatitis and/or allergic erythema. It has been suggested that in patients with hepatic and renal dysfunction, cimetidine crosses the blood-brain barrier and possibly alters mental status by blocking H_2 receptors in the brain (16).

As experience with cimetidine has increased, a number of drug interactions have been reported. Cimetidine does interfere with the metabolism of other drugs. This has clinical importance with drugs with a narrow therapeutic index, such as phenytoin, warfarin, and theophylline. Increases in steady-state blood levels and concomitant increases in toxicity and side effects of these agents have been reported when cimetidine has been administered. Careful monitoring of the patient with adjustment of dosage is necessary when such drugs are combined with cimetidine (33).

Therapeutic Uses. Cimetidine has been effective in treating duodenal ulcer, nonmalignant gastric ulcer, gastroesophageal reflux disease, and hypersecretion states such as Zollinger-Ellison syndrome. It also enhances the effectiveness of oral enzymes and decreases steatorrhea in patients with pancreatic insufficiency. The usefulness of the drug in all of these states is due to prevention of gastric secretion (12). Cimetidine has now been approved for prophylaxis in preventing duodenal ulcer in certain patients.

Cimetidine may also be of use in decreasing the flushing reaction seen in patients with gastric carcinoid tumor when given in combination with an H_1 blocker.

Preparations and Dosage. *Cimetidine* (TAGAMET) is available in 300-mg tablets and 300-mg single-dose vials (2 ml). The standard dose is one tablet three times daily with meals with 300-400 mg at bedtime. The intravenous dose is 200-300 mg every 6 hours. The dose may have to be increased in severe hypersecretory states such as Zollinger-Ellison syndrome, but it cannot exceed 2 g daily. The daily dose should be reduced in the elderly and in patients with renal failure by prolonging the interdose interval to 12 hours.

RANITIDINE

Ranitidine (ZANTAC) is a new H_2-receptor blocking antihistamine that inhibits gastric secretion with a potency four- to eight-fold that of cimetidine (3a, 23a). It has recently been approved for short-term oral use in the treatment of duodenal ulcer and for unrestricted use in hypersecretary states such as Zollinger-Ellison syndrome. Its chemical structure is distinct in having a furan ring as shown in its formula which follows, instead of the imidazole ring common to cimetidine and histamine.

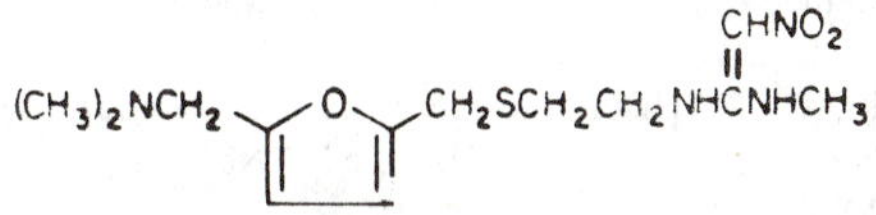

$$(CH_3)_2NCH_2\text{-[furan]-}CH_2SCH_2CH_2NH\overset{\overset{CHNO_2}{\|}}{C}NHCH_3$$

Ranitidine

Oral bioavailability of ranitidine is about 50%, and peak effect usually occurs within 1 hour. Plasma half-life after oral administration is 2.7 hours, somewhat longer than cimetidine. It has pharmacological effects similar to cimetidine, but because of its high potency it is given in a lower dose (150 mg twice daily equivalent to 1200 mg of cimetidine). Ranitidine is safer than cimetidine; minimal side effects have been reported in early clinical trials. There are reports of infrequent occurrence of gynecomastia or impotence during treatment with high doses of cimetidine; treatment of these patients with ranitidine leads to reversal of these effects in most cases. Ranitidine has lesser effect on cytochrome P-450-mediated drug metabolism, and as such it is expected to have fewer drug interactions. It is less lipophilic than cimetidine and as such is expected to cause less neurological problems occasionally seen with cimetidine; however, some central nervous system effects such as mental confusion and hallucination have been reported (see also Chapter 18.1).

REFERENCES

1. Bernstein, I. L., Siegel, S. C., Brandon, M. L., Brown, E. B., Evans, R. R., Feinberg, A. R., Friedlaender, S., Krumholz, R. A., Hadley, R. A., Handelman, N. I., Thurston, D., and Yamate, M. A. Controlled study of cromolyn sodium sponsored by the Drug Committee of the American Academy of Allergy. *J. Allergy Clin. Immun.* 50:235, 1972.
2. Bevan, M. A. Histamine. *N. Engl. J. Med.* 294:30, 1976.
3. Black, J. W., Duncan, W. A. M., Durant, G. J. Ganellin, C. R., and Parsons, M. E. Definition and antagonism of histamine H_2-receptors. *Nature* (London) 236:385, 1972.

3a. Brogden, R. N., Carmine, A. A., Heel, R. C. et al. Ranitidine: A review of its pharmacology and therapeutic use in peptic ulcer disease and other allied diseases. *Drugs* 24:267, 1982.

4. Canavan, J. S. F., and Briggs, J. D. Cimetidine clearance in renal failure. In: *Cimetidine: Proceedings of the Second International Symposium on Histamine H_2-Receptor Antagonists* (Burland, W. C., and Simkins, M. A., eds.). Amsterdam: Excerpta Medica, 1977, p. 75.
5. Chinn, H. I., and Oberst, F. Effectiveness of various drugs in prevention of air sickness. *Proc. Soc. Exp. Biol. Med.* 73:218, 1950.
6. Chinn, H. I., and Milch, L. J. Comparison of air sickness preventives. *J. Appl. Physiol.* 5:162, 1952.
7. Code, C. F. Histamine and gastric secretion: A later look. *Fed. Proc.* 24:1311, 1965.
8. Cohen, B., and deJong, J. M. B. V. Meclizine and placebo in treating vertigo of vestibular origin: Relative efficacy in a double blind study. *Arch. Neurol.* (Chicago) 27:129, 1972.
9. Dale, H. H. *Adventures in physiology*. London: Pergamon Press. 1953.
10. Dale, H. H., and Laidlow, P. P. The physiological action of β-iminozolethylamine. *J. Physiol.* 41:318, 1910.
11. Durant, G. J., Duncan, W. A. M., Ganellin, C. R., Parsons, M. E., Blackmore, R. C., and Rasmussen, A. C. Impromidine (SK & F 92676) is a very potent and specific agonist for histamine H_2 receptors. *Nature* (London) 276:403, 1978.
12. Finkelstein, W., nad Isselbacher, K. J. Cimetidine. *N. Engl. J. Med.* 299:992, 1978.
13. Ganellin, C. R. Histamine receptors. In: *Annual Report of Medicinal Chemistry* (Hess, H. J., ed.). New York: Academic Press, 1979, p. 91.
14. Griffiths, R., Lee, R. M., and Taylor, D. C. Kinetics of cimetidine in man and experimental animals. In: *Cimetidine: Proceedings of the Second International Symposium on Histamine H_2-Receptor Antagonists* (Burland, W. L., and Simkins, M. A., eds.). Amsterdam: Excerpa Medica, 1977, p. 38.
15. Grossman, M. I., and Konturek, S. J. Inhibition of acid secretion in dog by metiamide: A histamine antagonist acting on H_2 receptors. *Gastroenterology* 66:517, 1974.
16. Ivey, K. J. H_2 receptor antagonists. *Int. J. Dermatol.* 19:175.
17. Kuntzman, R. Drugs and enzyme induction. *Ann. Rev. Pharmacol.* 9:21, 1969.
18. Kusner, E. J., Dunnick, B., and Herzog, D. J. The inhibition by disodium cromoglycate *in vitro* of anaphylactically induced histamine release from rat peritoneal mast cells. *J. Pharmacol. Exp. Ther.* 184:41, 1973.
19. Lecomte, J. Liberation of endogenous histamine in man. *J. Allergy* 28:102, 1957.
20. Levine, R. J. Serotonin and the carcinoid syndrome: Histamine and mastocytosis. In: *Duncan's Diseases of Metabolism Endocrinology*, 7th ed. (Boncy, P. K., and Rosenberg, L. E., eds.). Philadelphia: Saunders, 1974, p. 1651.
21. Lewis, T. *The Blood Vessels of the Human Skin and Their Responses*. London: Shaw and Sons, 1927.
22. Lichtenstein, L. M., and Margolis, S. Histamine release *in vitro:* Inhibition by catecholamines and methylxanthines. *Science* 161:902, 1968.
23. MacIntosh, F. C. Histamine as a normal stimulant of gastric secretion. *Q. J. Exp. Physiol.* 28:87, 1938.

23a. McCarthy, D. M. Ranitidine or cimetidine. *Ann. Intern. Med.* 99:551, 1983.

24. McNeill, J. H., and Brody, T. M. The effect of various drug pretreatments on amine-induced phosphorylase activation and amine uptake. *J. Pharmacol. Exp. Ther.* 162:121, 1968.
25. Nilsson, K., Lindell, S. E., Schayer, R. W., and Westling, H. Metabolism of 14C-labelled histamine in pregnant and non-pregnant women. *Clin. Sci.* 18:313, 1959.
26. Paton, W. D. M. Histamine release by compounds of simple chemical structure. *Pharmacol. Rev.* 9:269, 1957.
27. Robertson, C. C. and Sellers, E. M. Alcohol intoxication and the alcohol withdrawal syndrome. *Postgrad. Med.* 64:133, 1978.
28. Rocha e Silva, M. (ed.). Histamine II and anti-histamines. In: *Handbuch der Experimentatellen Pharmakologie*. Vol. 18. Berlin: Springer-Verlag, 1978, p. 27.
29. Sadusk, J. F., and Palmisano, P. A. Teratogenic effect of meclizine, cyclizine, and chlorcyclizine. *JAMA* 194:987. 1965.
30. Seppala, T., Linnoila, M., and Mattila, M. J. Drugs, alcohol, and driving. *Drugs* 17:389, 1979.
31. Soll, A. H., and Grossman, M. I. Cellular mechanisms in acid secretion. *Ann. Rev. Med.* 29:495, 1978.
32. Soll, A. H., and Walsh, J. H. Regulation of gastric acid secretion. *Ann. Rev. Physiol.* 41:35, 1979.
33. Somogyi, A., and Gugher, R. Drug interactions with cimetidine. *Clin. Pharmacokinetics* 7:32, 1982.
34. Spence, R. W., Creak, D. R., and Celestin, L. R. Influence of a meal on the absorption of cimetidine: A new histamine H_2-receptor antagonist. *Digestion* 14:127, 1976.
35. Svedmyr, N., and Simonsson, B. G. Drugs in the treatment of asthma. *Pharmacol. Ther. B.* 3:397, 1978.
36. Teutsch, G., Mahler, D., Brown, C., Forrest, W., James, K., and Brown, B. Hypnotic efficacy of diphenhydramine, methapyrilene, and pentobarbital. *Clin. Pharmacol. Therap.* 17:195, 1975.
37. Van Arsdel, P. P., Jr., and Beall, G. N. The metabolism and functions of histamine. *Arch. Intern. Med.* 106:714, 1960.
38. Verma, S. C., and McNeill, J. H. Histamine H_2-receptors and the adenylate cyclase-cyclic AMP system. *Can. J. Pharm. Sci.* 13:1, 1978.
39. Yellin, T. O. (ed.). *Histamine Receptors*. New York: SP Medical and Scientific Books, 1979.

ADDITIONAL READING

Hirschowitz, B.I. An update on histamine receptors and the gastrointestinal tract. *Dig. Dis. Sci.* 30:998, 1985.

CHAPTER 13.5.1

THE IMMUNE SYSTEM

William L. West and Sachin N. Pradhan

For action in defense against toxic and infectious materials in the environment, the body mobilizes a specialized cell system called the immune system (immunity from the Latin *immunis* meaning "exempt from"). Although this system that is composed of a complex network of cells and depends for its function on the interaction of many cells and soluble factors provides resistance against many disease processes, functional derangement of this system leads to many allergic as well as autoimmune disorders. Immunological mechanisms have also been shown to be involved in many disease processes such as cancer (2) and several genetic disorders, and the possibility of immunotherapy for some such diseases has been suggested (1-3). A significant development has been the new approach to control and manipulate the immunological mechanisms by drugs causing immunostimulation or immunosuppression and their application in therapy (3).

COMPONENTS OF IMMUNE SYSTEM

Immunological capability is implemented by a variety of cell types, cellular receptors, and sequential enzymatic activators, as well as resultant cellular chemical products. Many of these cellular chemical products are biologically active, and their bioactivity and functions are covered in Chapter 13.5.2. The immune responses of the host defense system, although very complex, may be grossly classified as *nonspecific* and *specific*. The nonspecific, or primary immune responses to causative agents of disease, may be subdivided into two processes—namely, inflammation and phagocytosis. Participating in the primary response are cellular components such as polymorphonuclear leukocytes, including neutrophils and eosinophils, and marcophages. Many foreign substances (i.e., nonvirulant bacteria) are effectively cleared by phagocytosis alone, and the efficiency of clearance is greatly enhanced in the immunocompetent host (1, 2, 4). In the presence of virulent bacterial organisms, however, phagocytosis alone is inadequate, and hence specific immune responses including antibody and complement must act in concert in order to facilitate this action to eliminate such pathogens.

The specific, or secondary, immune responses are carried out by many subtypes of cells working together (1, 2). These subtypes are from two component cell types, both of which originate as stem cells in the bone marrow but, on passing into the body systems, take divergent pathways. One group of stem cells in birds migrates to the bursa of Fabricius, and in mammals its equivalent exerts this bursal function. These cells differentiate into bursa-dependent, intestine-dependent, or B lymphocytes possessing immunocompetent cell surfaces capable of responding to foreign antigens, as shown in Fig. 13.5.1-1.

On antigenic stimulation, B cells proliferate and differentiate into plasma cells that form specific antibodies releasing them into the serum, or into a subtype, small lymphocytes, responsible for immunological memory. Specific antibodies bind with an antigen in the plasma or in secretions from mucous membranes of the immune individual, neutralizing the bioactivity of an antigen. The specific antibody activity resides in plasma protein molecules called *immunoglobulin* (Ig), or *gamma globulins.* Five major classes of immunoglobulins are found in the adult and may be designated by IgG, IgM, IgA, IgD, and IgE, as shown in Table 13.5.1-1, which also lists some of their biological and molecular characteristics as well as their roles in certain responses. These antibodies are responsible for the humoral immunity (HI).

The other group of stem cells migrates to and is under the influence of the thymus gland. These cells differentiate into thymus dependent or T lymphocytes, which possess immunocompetent surfaces that differ from B lymphocytes (Fig. 13.5.1-1). After differentiation in the primary lymphoid organ, immunocompetent cells leave and a few return. On antigenic stimulation, T lymphocytes react in one of two ways. First, either the T cell or its products interact with B cells and help them to differentiate into plasma cells (Fig. 13.5.1-1). The mechanisms responsible for this cell-to-cell cooperation have not been completely elucidated. Overall, stimulated T cells release bioactive substances that may react with receptors on B cells, or proliferate to form sensitized lymphocyte populations (Fig. 13.5.1-1) that participate in cell-mediated immunity. The effector substances in cell-mediated immunity are lymphokines (including interferon) and monokines, factors that affect cellular proliferations, activations, and motility (6). Lymphokines are secreted primarily by stimulated T cells when they are acted upon by the specific sensitizing antigen. In humoral immunity, antibodies secreted by plasma cells interact with their specific antigens neutralizing them. In contrast, lymphokines secreted by sensitized T cells act nonspecifically on other lymphocytes, macrophages, and muscle cells, but not with the sensitizing

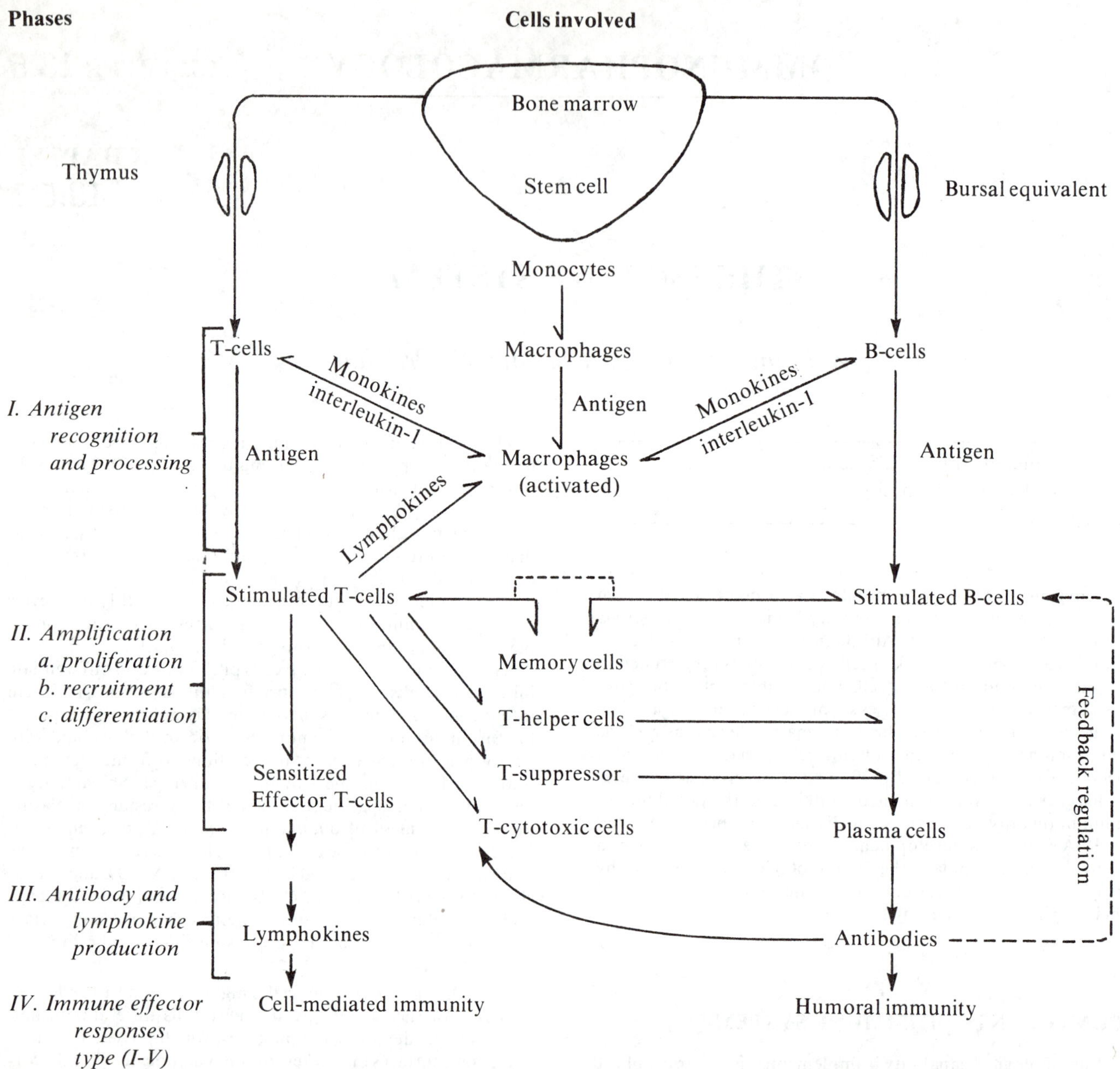

Fig. 13.5.1-1. *Specific defense response.*

antigen. The numerous T-cell subsets are differentiated by marker molecules in their cell surfaces (1, 2, 5, 6).

PHASES OF DEFENSE RESPONSE

The defense response can be divided into four phases: (1) antigen recognition and/or processing, (2) amplification, (3) antibody production and (4) immune responses. The initial phase or antigen recognition and processing, probably resides with macrophages, T cells, or B cells (Fig. 13.5.1-1). Cooperative interactions between these cellular components occur with subsequent amplification of the immune system that occurs by clonal proliferation of specific B-cell or T-cell populations. Recruitment and activation of other cell lines may occur as an orderly process [i.e., macrophages may be activated by sensitized T-cell subpopulations through elaboration of a macrophage-activating factor (MAF)]; and differentiation of the stimulated cells also follows proliferative responses [i.e., differentiation into plasma cells, T-*suppressor cells, T-effector cells,* or *T-helper cells* (Fig. 13.5.1-1)]. These components of the cellular immune system and their subtypes are critical to developing a specific immunological capability.

The immunological effector mechanisms or the actual pathways through which the immune response expresses itself have been grouped into five types: type I = immediate hypersensitivity; type II = cytotoxic reactions; type III = immune complex reactions; type IV = cellular immune responses; and, type V = antireceptor responses. These mechanisms are discussed in detail in Chapter 13.5.2.

Table 13.5.1-1
Some Characteristics of Immunoglobulins

Type of Immuno-globulin	Binds Comple-ment	Normal Serum Concentra-tion[a] (mg%)	Half-Life $t_{1/2}$ (days)	Molecular Weight ($n \times 10^3$)	Role	Placental Transport
IgG	Yes	1200 (80%)	23	150	Immunoprotection of fetus; enhances phagocytosis; neutralizes toxin	Yes
IgA	No	275 (7%)	6	170	Occurs also in saliva; protects external body surfaces	No
IgD	No	5	2.8	150	May serve as lymphocyte antigen receptor (?)	No
IgM	Yes	120 (7%)	5	890	Participates in agglutinating and cytolytic reactions	No
IgE	No	0.03	1.5	196	Associated with allergic disorders	No

[a]Numbers in parentheses represent percentage of total immunoglobulins.

REFERENCES

1. Hadden, J. W. The immunopharmacology of immunotherapy: An update. In: *Advances in Immunopharmacology* (Hadden, J., Chedid, L., Mulle, P., and Spreafico, F., eds.). New York: Pergamon Press, 1981, p. 327.
2. Haskell, C. M. Immunologic aspects of cancer chemotherapy. *Ann. Rev. Pharmacol. Toxicol.* 17:179, 1977.
3. Lewis, A. J., Carlson, R. P., and Chang, T. Therapeutic modulation of cellular mediated immunity. *Ann. Rep. Med. Chem.* 17:191, 1982.
4. Pesce, A. J., and Dosekum, K. Interrelation between the immune systems, complement, coagulation and inflammation. *Clin. Physiol. Biochem.* 1:92, 1983.
5. Rumjanek, V. M., Hanson, J. M., and Morely, J. Lymphokines and monokines. In: *Immunopharmacology* (Turk, J., Sirols, P., and Rola-Pleszczynski, R., eds.). New York: Elsevier, 1982, p. 267.
6. Spreafico, F., and Anaclero, A. Immunosuppressive agents. In: *Comprehensive Immunology and Immunopharmacology* (Hadden, J. W., Coffey, R. G., and Spreafico, F., eds.). New York: Plenum Press, 1977..

ADDITIONAL READING

Wechter, W.J. et al. Immunology in drug research. *Prog. Drug Res.* 28:233, 1984.

CHAPTER
13.5.2

PHARMACOLOGY OF IMMUNE RESPONSES

Michael A. Kaliner and Charles H. Kirkpatrick

INTRODUCTION

The immune system provides one of the essential mechanisms for defense against toxic and infectious materials in the environment. The discoveries of recent years have revealed that the system is highly specialized, extraordinarily sensitive, and very specific. Moreover, we now recognize that optimal function of this system depends on the interaction of a complex network of cells and soluble factors.

It is also known that the function of the immune system may be either beneficial or harmful. The responses to vaccines against poliomyelitis and smallpox, for example, have markedly reduced the impact of these diseases on humankind. At the opposite end of the spectrum are the patients with impaired immune responses who are exquisitely susceptible to infections with common bacteria, fungi, and viruses. In other patients, aberrant responses of the immune system create a unique hypersensitivity state that is illustrated by the common allergic disorders such as allergic rhinitis, asthma, or anaphylaxis and by the hypersensitivity pneumonitides that occur after occupational exposures. An extreme expression of the allergic state occurs in patients with a variety of autoimmune disorders such as hemolytic anemias, certain renal diseases, and many rheumatic diseases in which disturbances of the normal homeostatic process apparently allow a subject's immune system to damage its own tissue.

Complete texts are devoted to immunology, and extensive coverage of all facets of the immune response is clearly beyond the scope of a single chapter. Instead, we will restrict this chapter to aspects of the immune system that produce biological effects and to approaches to pharmacological manipulation of these effects. The reader is referred elsewhere for more extensive approaches to immunology (43, 48, 55).

IMMUNOLOGICAL EFFECTOR MECHANISMS

The actual pathways through which the immune response expresses itself have been conveniently classified by Gell and Coombs (21). As in any generalization, there are exceptions to this classification. However, their model provides an excellent method for analysis of the various components of the immune system. Immunological effector mechanisms may be divided into four distinct types (Fig. 13.5.2-1): type I = immediate hypersensitivity; type II = cytotoxic reactions; type III = immune complex reactions; and, type IV = cellular immune responses. An additional mechanism, in which antibody directed against a receptor site acts to either activate the receptor or prevent the usual agonist-receptor interaction, is operative in diseases such as myasthenia gravis (12) and some forms of diabetes, and constitutes an additional type V not included in the original classification. The reader is referred elsewhere for reviews of this reaction (14).

IMMEDIATE HYPERSENSITIVITY (TYPE-I REACTIONS)

COMPONENT PARTS

The allergic diseases are by far the commonest immunological diseases of humans, with more than 20% of the population having allergic rhinitis, allergic asthma, and/or urticaria. The basic immunological mechanism underlying the allergic reaction is the interaction of allergens with immunoglobulin E (IgE) molecules that are fixed to receptor sites on the surface of mast

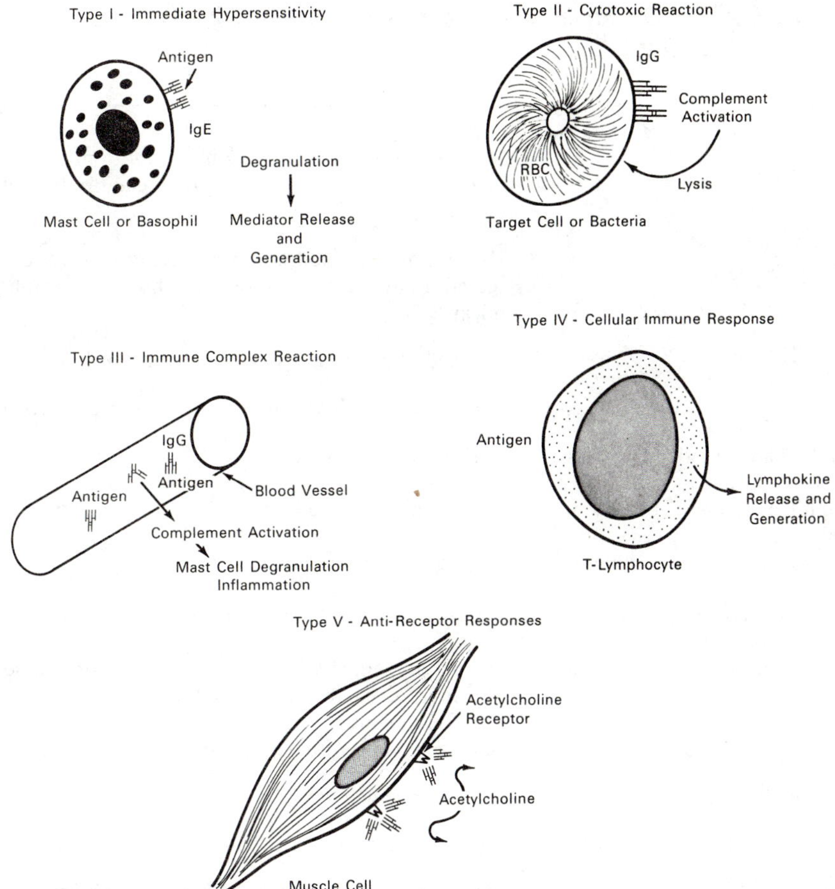

Fig. 13.5.2-1. *Classification of immunological effector mechanisms.*

Reactions of Types I-IV are based upon Gell and Coombs'original scheme (21) whereas Type V is a newly appreciated mechanism. Type I, which involves allergen interaction with mast cell- or basophil-fixed IgE antibodies, initiates the release and generation of the mediators of allergy (summarized in Table 13.5.2-1). Type II is the cytotoxic reaction induced by the fixation of IgG or IgM upon an antigenic component of a target cell with the consequent activation of complement and lysis of the cell. Type III, or immune complex disease, involves circulating complexes of allergen and IgG that fix and activate complement; this type of reaction leads to mast cell degranulation, increased vascular permeability, localization of the complexes in or near the vascular wall, and a subsequent inflammatory response. Type IV reactions, which are the delayed responses involving antigen stimulation of sensitized T lymphocytes, lead to the release and/or generation of the lymphokines. Type V reactions are antireceptor reactions that are induced by IgG antibodies directed at hormones of their receptors and interfere with the function of the hormone or its receptors.

cells or basophilic leukocytes. This interaction initiates a series of reactions (31) that lead to cytoplasmic granule secretion. The cytoplasmic granules of the mast cell and basophil are a virtual pharmacopoeia of mediators that, once released, produce multiple effects (Table 13.5.2-1). The diseases produced by these reactions are determined by the sites of the allergen-IgE interaction. Thus, ingested allergens may induce intestinal reactions (diarrhea, obstipation, cramps); inhaled allergens may induce upper airway (rhinitis or sinusitis) or lower airway reactions (asthma); and, systemically distributed allergens may induce anaphylaxis or, in milder forms, urticaria or angioedema.

Although immediate hypersensitivity reactions are most evident in allergic diseases, the mast cell and basophil may also contribute to immune complex (7, 38) and cellular immune responses (1). Further, immediate hypersensitivity is a mechanism of host defense in certain parasitic diseases (6). The theory that immediate hypersensitivity is the initial immune response to many invasive parasites is suggested by three factors: the increased serum levels of IgE in patients with parasitic infestations; the distribution of the mast cell in areas exposed to the external environment (skin, respiratory, and GI mucosae); and the ability of mast cell-derived mediators to recruit polymorphonuclear leukocytes and to regulate vascular permeability.

THE MEDIATORS OF IMMEDIATE HYPERSENSITIVITY

There are three distinct sources of the mediators of allergy (Table 13.5.2-1): (1) preformed mediators such as histamine, which are stored ready for release in the mast cell or basophil granules; (2) secondary or newly generated mediators, which are formed or activated after mast cell or basophil degranulation as a consequence of the actions of primary mediators upon

Table 13.5.2-1
The Mediators of Immediate Hypersensitivity

	Actions
I. *Preformed or Primary Mediators*	
Histamine	H-1 responses: vascular leakage, smooth muscle spasm, increases in cGMP, pruritus, prostaglandin formation, vasodilation
	H-2 responses: vasodilation, gastric acid secretion, mucus secretion, increases in cAMP, inhibition of lymphokine release
	H-1 and H-2 responses: hypotension, flush, headache
	Other: eosinophil chemotaxis, irritant-receptor stimulation
Eosinophil chemotactic factors of anaphylaxis	Eosinophil chemotaxis
Neutrophil chemotactic factors of anaphylaxis	Neutrophil chemotaxis
Superoxide-generating enzyme	Superoxide generation
II. *Newly generated or secondary mediators*	
Prostaglandins and thromboxanes	Bronchospasm ($PGF_{2\alpha}$, PGD_2, TxA_2); bronchodilation (PGE_1, PGI_2); increase cGMP ($PGF_{2\alpha}$), increase cAMP (PGE_1); mucus secretion ($PGF_{2\alpha}$, TxA_2, PGD_2); vascular leakage and dilation (PGE); potentiate pain perception (PGE)
Leukotriene B_4	Neutrophil chemotaxis
Leukotriene C_4, D_4, and E_4 (SRS-A)	Bronchospasm, vascular leakage, mucus secretion
Bradykinin	Vasodilation, vascular leakage, bronchospasm
Acetylglycerophosphorylcholine (PAF)	Vasopermeability, bronchospasm, platelet aggregation
Acetylcholine	Bronchospasm, mucus secretion
Prostaglandin-generating factor	Prostaglandin and HETE formation
III. *Constituents of the granule matrix*	
Heparin	Anticoagulant, modifier of complement activation
Superoxide dismutase	Facilitates superoxide conversion to reactive by-products
Peroxidase	Converts hydrogen peroxide to reactive by-products
Chymase	Chymotrypsin-like enzyme
Arylsulfatases	Sulfohydralases
β-Glucuronidase	Disrupts glucuronide bonds
Low- and high-molecular-weight inflammatory factors	Induce polymorphonuclear infiltrates followed by mononuclear infiltrates

target tissues (e.g., histamine stimulation of H_1 receptors includes prostaglandin formation) (50); and (3) the secretory granule matrix itself, once released into connective tissue, dissolves slowly and releases a number of firmly bound, potent molecules such as chymotrypsin, peroxidase, and heparin.

The biological responses induced by mast cell-derived mediators produce diseases including allergic rhinitis, asthma, urticaria, anaphylaxis, and food hypersensitivity and quite likely contribute to a variety of other phenomena. There is some redundancy in the biological effects of the mediators of allergy (Table 13.5.2-1) such that histamine, leukotrienes, several prostaglandins and thromboxane A_2, and bradykinin are all able to induce bronchospasm. Perhaps this redundancy explains why antagonism of the H_1-histamine receptor alone is insufficient therapy for asthma. On the other hand, the classic antihistamines are generally helpful in allergic rhinitis, suggesting that H_1 stimulation produces a significant portion of the symptoms in that disease. It is also evident from Table 13.5.2-1 that there are far too many mediators of allergy, each acting through independent mechanisms, to permit synthesis of specific antagonists for each mediator. Thus, only the most important mediators may be approached individually, and theoretically, it would be more efficacious to suppress mast cell degranulation itself. In Fig. 13.5.2-2 various possible approaches for intervention in allergic reactions are outlined.

MODULATION OF THE IMMUNOLOGICAL RELEASE OF THE MEDIATORS OF ALLERGY

Extensive examination of the biochemical events initiated by the IgE-allergen interaction within mast cells has revealed that the reaction begins with the activation of an external calcium-requiring serine esterase, leads to energy utilization (preferably over glucose-dependent pathways), and then to an intracellular calcium-requiring event followed by a step that is modulated by the intracellular levels of cyclic adenosine monophosphate (cAMP) and cyclic guanosine monophosphate (cGMP) (Fig. 13.5.2-3) (31, 32). It appears that this latter step regulates the polymerization-depolymerization of mast cell microtubules (33). Thus, the secretory reaction in mast cells may be prevented under conditions associated with an increase in cAMP, and conversely, the response is increased when cellular cAMP is reduced or cGMP is elevated (Fig. 13.5.2-4) (32).

Membrane-associated events triggered by aggregation of IgE receptors (34) include an evanescent rise in cAMP, transmethylation of phosphatidylethanolamine to phosphatidylcholine, activation of phospholipases with the cleavage of arachidonic acid from phosphatidylcholine, formation of prostaglandin D_2 (PGD_2), and generation of several fatty acid molecules capable of facilitating membrane fusion (28, 35). Pharmacologically, the mast cell responds to β_2 adrenergic agents, especially β_2 agents (see Chapter 8.1), phosphodiesterase inhibitors (see Chapter 17), PGE (see Chapter 13.2), cholera toxin, or cAMP itself, with reduction in the capacity of antigen to cause degranulation (32). α-Adrenergic stimulation, produced either by combining β-adrenergic blockade with epinephrine or norepinephrine or by employing phenylephrine alone, reduces mast cell cAMP and augments the release reaction. Agents such as muscarinic agonists (see Chapter 9.1) or $PGF_{2\alpha}$ (see Chapter 13.2) increase cGMP levels and augment the release reactions (32). It appears that the agents that are useful in the treatment of asthma act either by affecting the mast cell release reaction or by counteracting the action of mediators upon bronchial smooth muscle (see Chapter 17). An additional drug, disodium cromoglycate, acts solely on the mast cell, preventing antigen-induced degranulation, and has proven effective in preventing asthma in a portion of the population (46) (see Chapter 17). This agent may also be effective in allergic conjunctivitis, allergic rhinitis, food allergy, and in reducing the symptoms of systemic mastocytosis (46). These observations suggest that prevention of mast cell degranulation may be an effective mechanism for modulating allergic reactions.

Several novel, but as yet unsuccessful, approaches to allergic reactions have been studied and may become available. The allergic response requires the presence of IgE on the mast cell surface. Recent studies have identified as many as 500,000 IgE receptor sites on each mast cell (27). Structural identification of the receptor is underway, and it is known that it consists of four interacting glycoproteins. Further, it appears that cross-linking of the receptor, even in the absence of IgE, is sufficient to trigger the mast cell secretory reaction (29, 34). Thus, it may be possible

Approaches to Intervention in Allergic Reactions

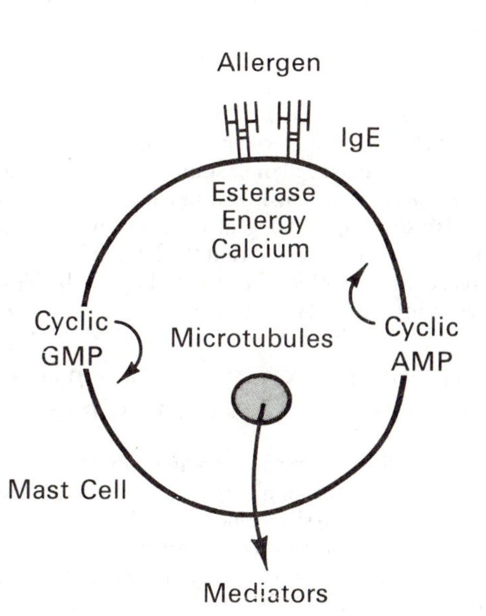

Prevent Allergen From Reaching Mast Cell
Avoid Allergen Contact
Reduce IgE Production
Prevent IgE Fixation to Mast Cell
Interfere with Intracellular Biochemical Events Necessary for Degranulation
- Raise Cyclic AMP
- Prevent Lowering of Cyclic AMP
- Prevent Raising Cyclic GMP

Prevent Synthesis of Mediators

Antagonize Specific Mediators
Enhance Degration of Mediators
Reverse or Prevent Biologic Effects of Mediator Action

Fig. 13.5.2-2. *Approaches to intervention in allergic reactions.*

The various approaches to modify each of the major steps in allergic reactions are outlined. Only a few of these approaches have been studied, thus many new and unique methods for modifying the immediate hypersensitivity response still require analysis.

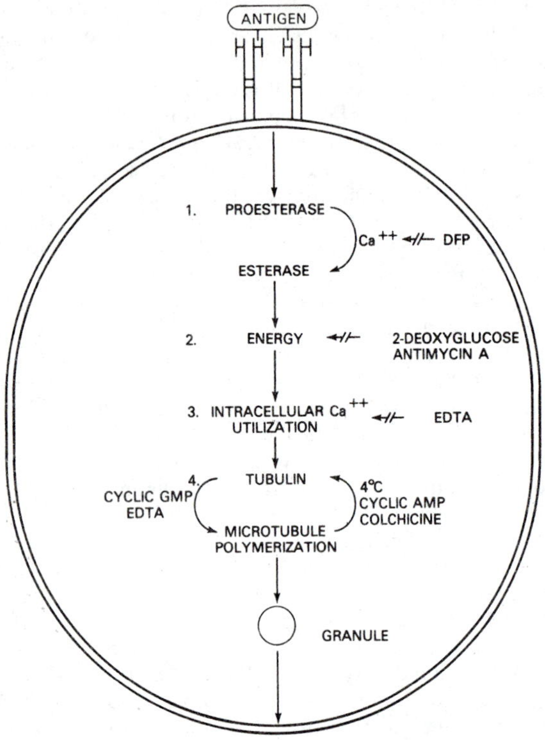

Fig. 13.5.2-3. *Sequential steps in mediator release.*

The immunological stimulation of mast cell degranulation proceeds along an orderly sequence of events that begins with antigen coupling to mast cell-bound IgE and progresses to the release of secretory granules. The fourth step in the sequence, microtubule polymerization, appears to be the stage at which cyclic nucleotides exert their modulating influence. (Adopted from Ref. 33).

to approach the allergic reaction by attacking the receptor site and preventing IgE-receptor linkage. One such attempt with a synthetic pentapeptide that interfered with IgE binding (25) was unsuccessful (3). However, the concept is exciting and potentially applicable once more information regarding the IgE-receptor interaction is available.

The immunological event that triggers the mast cell requires bridging of at least two IgE molecules with aggregation of their respective receptors (29). It is potentially plausible to develop univalent antigens that would fix to single IgE molecules and thereby prevent their aggregation. Such an approach has been tried with penicillin hypersensitivity with apparent success (57) and needs to be attempted with other allergens.

Another possible approach is to regulate IgE synthesis itself. As with other immunoglobulins, the synthesis of IgE by plasma cells requires T-lymphocyte helper factors and may be reduced by suppressor factors (30). Conditions that reduce specific IgE antibody synthesis have been identified in experimental animals (41) and suggest that this approach may be possible in humans (56).

IMMUNOTHERAPY OR HYPOSENSITIZATION

Long before the immunological components of the allergic response had been identified, the use of immunotherapy had been tried with apparent success in the treatment of allergic rhinitis (17, 45). Over the years, allergy immunotherapy achieved the status of an acceptable form of therapy for allergic conditions although little quantitation of either the allergy extracts or the results of injection of these materials was attempted. Recently, scientifically acceptable studies have been published demonstrating the therapeutic usefulness of hyposensitization (47, 53).

With the identification of IgE as the immunoglobulin responsible for the immunological specificity of allergic reactions, a test for quantitation of antigen-specific IgE was developed (58). This radioallergosorbent test (RAST) is useful in quantitating not only IgE, but also the antigen against which the IgE is directed. Thus, the RAST assay permits the development of standards for allergy extracts, not only in regard to antigenic content but also potency (24). The development of quantitation of allergy extracts by RAST is just beginning, but promises to overtake the older methods of allergenic standardization.

Hyposensitization or allergy immunotherapy has been the subject of numerous investigations (reviewed in 47 and 53). Adequate discussion of the experimental designs, patient selection, and experimental results requires more space than can be provided in this chapter. However, several general results are evident. Therapy of patients with allergic rhinitis due to pollens has been successful. Dust hyposensitization has generally been successful, but the use of mold and fungal extracts needs more analysis; bacterial desensitization is ineffective. The guidelines for successful immunotherapy are careful patient selection, the use of relatively concentrated extracts, and the continuation of therapy for several years. The immunological responses induced by immunotherapy include a reduction in allergen-specific IgE levels, an increase in circulating IgG-blocking antibodies directed against the allergens in the extract, and a reduction (desensitization) in mast cell and basophil responsiveness to allergen exposure. This last response may be manifested by a reduction in immediate-type skin test responses.

Perhaps the clearest demonstration of the effectiveness of desensitization comes from the recent series of experiments involving stinging-insect hyposensitization (26). These studies have clearly demonstrated that adverse reactions induced by bees, hornets, yellow jackets, and wasps are mediated by allergen-IgE-mast cell or basophil reactions and can be remarkably reduced by desensitization with specific venoms. The studies also showed that desensitization with whole body extracts is much less effective and that the effectiveness is reflected in an increase in IgG-blocking antibodies, a decrease in antigen-specific IgE, and mast cell or basophil desensitization.

CYTOTOXIC AND IMMUNE COMPLEX REACTIONS (TYPE-II AND TYPE-III REACTIONS)

This portion of immunopharmacology combines two distinct immunological mechanisms that lead to the activation of complement. In the first mechanism, which involves the cytotoxic reactions, antibody directed against an antigenic component of the cell membrane or basement membrane leads to complement activation with subsequent cellular lysis or inflammatory responses. The classic examples are hemolytic disease of the newborn, transfusion reactions, certain forms of glomerulonephritis, and autoallergic cytotoxicity. The second mechanism involves circulating immune complexes, usually complexed at a ratio of antigen/antibody of 3:2 (the resulting aggregate is small blood vessels or the renal glomeruli; they activate complement

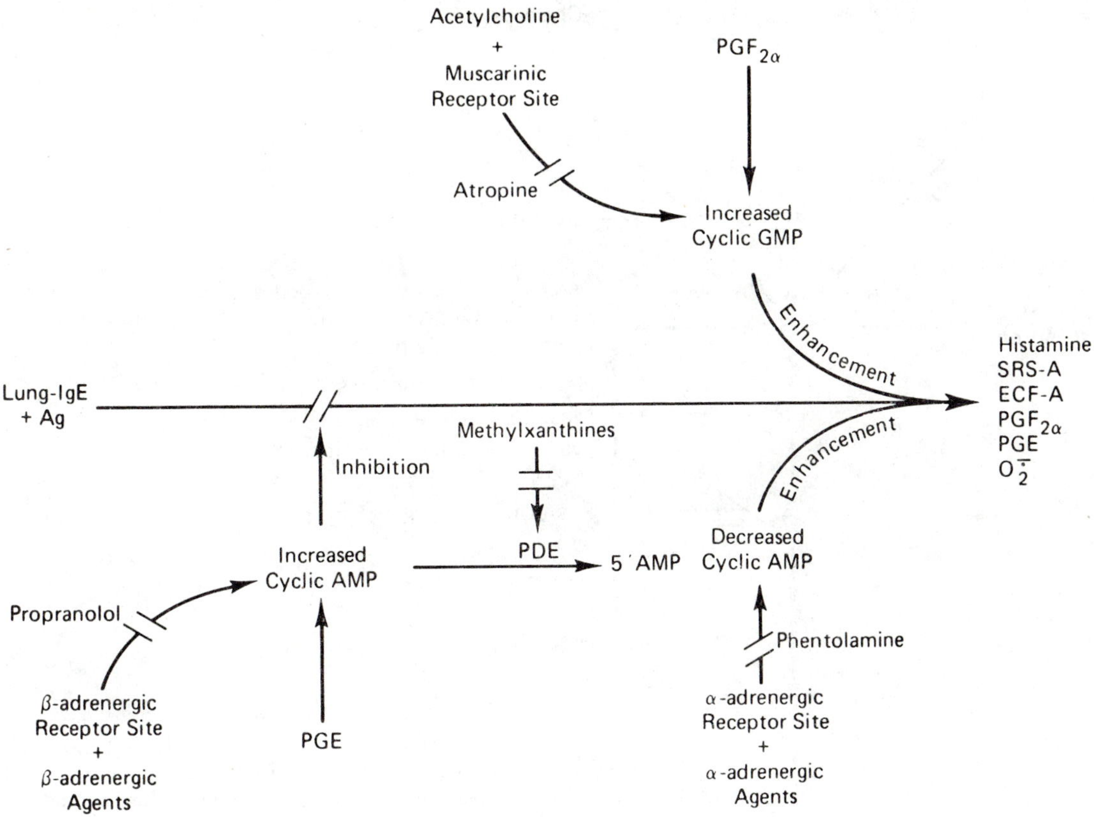

Fig. 13.5.2-4. *Pharmacological modulation of the immunological release of mediators.*
The secretion of the mediators of allergy from human lung mast cells sensitized with IgE and challenged with antigen may be modulated by the intracellular levels of cyclic nucleotides. An increase in cGMP or reduction in cAMP results in increased mediator release whereas in cAMP produce decreased release.

and an inflammatory reaction ensues (38, 39). Examples include serum sickness, certain forms of glomerulonephritis, and vasculitis. In both of these immunological mechanisms, the immunoglobulin provides the specificity of the reaction, and the target organ (either a cell, basement membrane, or circulating antigen) determines the type of reaction and disease manifestation produced. However, it is the activation of the complement system that produces the biological consequences.

COMPLEMENT ACTIVATION

The complement system consists of 14 separate proteins involved in the activation process and at least 3 inhibitors or regulatory proteins. The classic complement pathway (Fig. 13.5.2-5) is activated by antigen-antibody complexes, C-reactive proteins, and certain enzymes (11, 16). The activation involves the first component of complement, C_1, which consists of three distinct molecules, C_{1q}, C_{1r}, and C_{1s}. Once activated, C_1 interacts with and activates C_4, which leads to C_2 and C_3 activation. Once C_3 is in its active form, C_5, C_6, C_7, C_8, and C_9 are sequentially activated.

An alternative complement pathway (Fig. 13.5.2-5) also exists; this mechanism is activated by certain bacterial cell walls, trypsinlike enzymes, and aggregated immunoglobulins. The activation sequence is analogous to the classic pathway in that three factors, D, B, and C_{3b}, interact with each other in sequence and in turn activate C_3, which leads to the same terminal sequence of activation (C_5-C_9) as the classic pathway (11, 16). Thus, there are two mechanisms for initiating activation of the complement cascade. These pathways respond to distinct stimuli, thereby providing more flexibility to the complement system, and the two pathways converge to produce similar final results, frequently referred to as the membrane-attack complex.

There are three regulatory proteins that tend to suppress portions of the cascade: the C_1 esterase inhibitor (C_1 INH), the C_{3b} inactivator, and the anaphylatoxin inactivator. Finally, there is an antibody in certain patients with nephritis, termed C_3 nephritic factor, that stabilizes one of the intermediates in the alternative pathway leading to enhanced C_3 cleavage.

COMPLEMENT BYPRODUCTS

It is evident that the complement pathway is a potent mechanism for immunological expression. Classically, the end product of this system is cell lysis, usually illustrated by lysis of red blood cells (RBCs) but evident in bacteria and other cells. However, a number of noncytotoxic biological activities are generated during the activation sequence. It is these complement byproducts that may be approached pharmacologically (Fig. 13.5.2-5).

Cleavage of C_2 by C_4 leads to a small product known as C_2 kinin (11), which is capable of increasing vascular permeability. In the disease hereditary angioedema (HAE), an inhibitory pro-

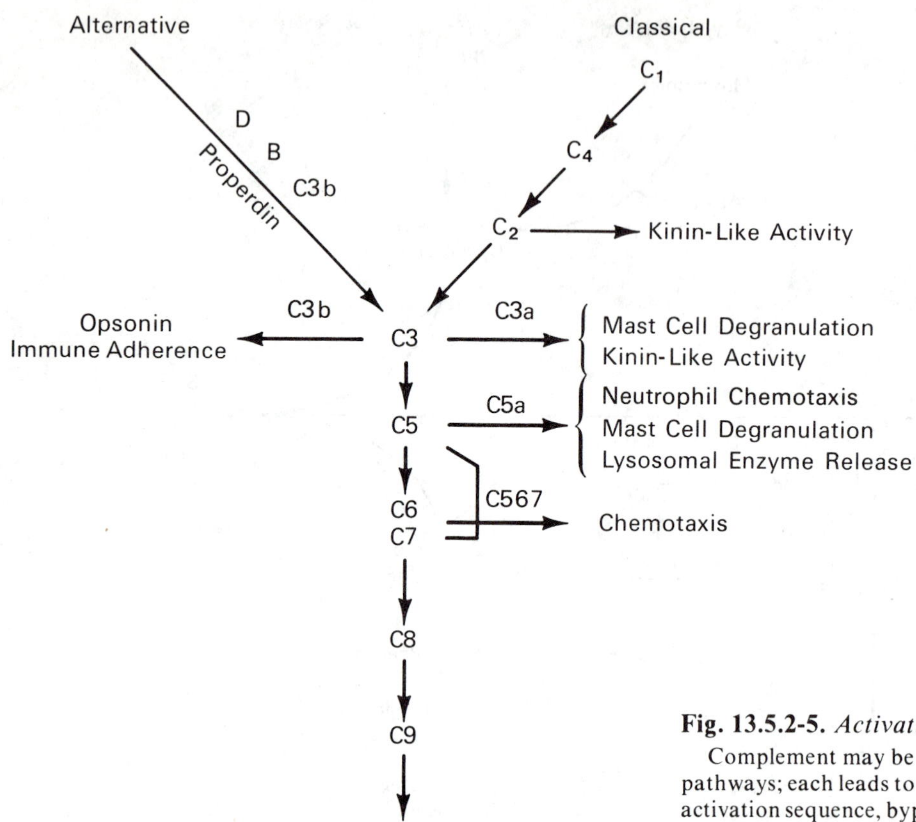

Fig. 13.5.2-5. *Activation of complement.*

Complement may be activated through alternative or classic pathways; each leads to C3 activation. During the course of the activation sequence, byproducts are formed that generate many of the complement-related biological events.

tein (C_1 INH) is functionally absent, and the early steps in the classic complement cascade are thereby unregulated. Activation of this pathway ensues due to minor trauma such as dental extractions, as well as from other ill-defined stimuli. The early complement components are activated, but the reaction does not proceed beyond C_3 as there is sufficient C_{3b} inactivator to regulate this step. The pathological consequences of C_1-C_4-C_2 activation may be partly due to the generation of the C_2 kinin, which causes marked edema of the face and throat as well as the GI tract. Attempts to control HAE have included infusions of fresh plasma to replace the C_1 INH (15), antifibrinolytic agents such as ϵ-aminocaproic acid, and androgens. Impeded androgens such as danazol are an especially effective therapy for this disease (15). HAE is inherited as an autosomal-dominant trait, and danazol apparently acts by stimulating normal (recessive) gene product formation, thereby producing sufficient C_1 inhibitor to prevent C_1 activation.

Two anaphylatoxins generated by the complement cascade are C_{3a} and C_{5a}. Both of these molecules are able to induce mast cell degranulation, leading to release of the mediators of anaphylaxis noted in Table 13.5.2-1. In addition, C_{5a} is a potent chemotactic agent attracting polymorphonuclear leukocytes and also stimulating lysosomal enzyme release from these cells. The C_{567} trimolecular complex may also be chemotactic. Thus, complement activation leads to a number of proinflammatory events in addition to cell lysis.

PHARMACOLOGICAL APPROACHES TO COMPLEMENT ACTIVATION

Other than modulating production of C_1 INH with danazol, little pharmacological manipulation of these activities has been attempted. There are some exciting suggestions that pharmacological antagonisms of histamine's effects upon the vascular bed with H_1 antagonists may modify and reduce the consequences of immune complex disorders (38), although these possibilities need greater exploration in the light of histamine H_2-induced vascular responses. The mast cell-anaphylatoxin interaction needs to be examined to determine whether this pathway is amenable to pharmacological manipulation. Identification of the molecular events involved in the actual lytic process of the terminal complement components is under active investigation and should provide possibilities for modification of this step, an avenue of investigation that will allow a new approach to the treatment of autoimmune hemolytic anemia, glomerulonephritis, and certain of the vasculitides and collagen vascular diseases.

CELL-MEDIATED IMMUNITY (TYPE-IV REACTIONS)

Each of the immunological reactions described in the preceding sections has a property in common—specific antibody molecules are essential for the pathogenesis of tissue injury. This section will consider the fourth class of reactions described by Gell and Coombs (21). These reactions are unique because there is no role for antibody molecules. Instead, the lesions are produced either directly by intimate contact between the target cells and cytotoxic lymphocytes, or indirectly by mediators known as lymphokines or monokines that are produced in small quantities at the sites of interactions between antigen and sensitized lymphocytes (Table 13.5.2-2).

The most familiar clinical expressions of cellular immunity

Table 13.5.2-2
Partial List of Lymphokines and Monokines

I. Factors that affect macrophage function
  1. γ-Interferon: probably responsible for previously identified activities such as: migration-inhibitory factor (MIF); macrophage-activating factor (MAF); macrophage-aggregation factor; and the factor that causes disappearance of macrophages from peritoneal cavity
  2. Macrophage chemotactic factor (MCF)
  3. Factors that alter surface tension
  4. Antigen-dependent MIF
II. Factors that affect neutrophil function
  1. Chemotactic factor
  2. Leukocyte-inhibitory factor (LIF)
III. Factors that affect lymphocyte function
  1. Interleukin-1 (lymphocyte-activating factor)
  2. Interleukin-2 (T-cell growth factor)
  3. Interleukin-3 (mast cell growth factor)
  4. B-cell growth factor
  5. Chemotactic factor
  6. E-rosette-augmenting factor (E-RAF)
  7. Transfer factor (TRF)
  8. Antigen-dependent helper factor
  9. Antigen-independent helper factor
  10. Antigen-dependent suppressor factor
  11. Antigen-independent suppressor factor
IV. Factors that affect eosinophil function
  1. Immune complex-dependent chemotactic factor
  2. Eosinophil-stimulation promoter (ESP)
V. Factors that affect basophil functions
  1. Chemotactic factor
VI. Factors that affect cells other than leukocytes
  1. Lymphotoxin (LT)
  2. Osteoclast-activating factor (OAF)
  3. Colony-stimulating factor (CSF)
  4. Collagen-producing factor
  5. Histamine-releasing factor
VII. Skin-reactive factor

are delayed cutaneous hypersensitivity reactions to substances such as tuberculin, contact allergic reactions such as those induced by the pentadecyl catechols of poison ivy, and rejection of foreign tissues and organs after transplantation. There is also evidence that the cellular immune system is important in resistance to infections with certain fungi, bacteria, and viruses; is involved in tissue injury in some autoimmune diseases; and participates in immune surveillance against neoplastic cells.

PATHOGENESIS OF CELLULAR IMMUNITY

For many years it was known that immune responses such as anaphylaxis, resistance to infections, or protection against certain toxins could be transferred to normal recipients with serum from immune donors. Repeated attempts to transfer other reactions such as tuberculin sensitivity or contact allergy with serum were unsuccessful. In 1942, Landsteiner and Chase (40) reported the experiments that demonstrated the phenomenon of cell-mediated immunity. They showed that contact sensitivity and tuberculin reactivity could be passively transferred to nonimmune guinea pigs with viable lymphoid cells from sensitive donors. A second important discovery concerning the mechanisms of cell-mediated immune reactions was the finding that only a minor fraction of the cells that comprised the infiltrates in delayed cutaneous hypersensitivity reactions are specifically antigen-sensitive (42, 44). The majority of cells apparently migrate into the infiltrate through nonspecific mechanisms.

It was known that migration of macrophages from tissue explants or cell suspensions containing antigen-sensitive lymphoid cells was inhibited when antigen was present (22, 52), and in the 1960s, it was demonstrated that this effect was mediated by an extracellular soluble factor (5, 9). Production of this factor occurred only when the lymphoid cells came from antigen-sensitive donors, and the phenomenon itself was antigen-specific. Thus, there was a mechanism through which a small number of cells from an antigen-sensitive donor could inhibit migration of a large number of macrophages. Other experiments showed that the factor was newly synthesized rather than stored for later release. This is in contrast to some of the mediators of the type I reactions (Table 13.5.2-1).

The factor that inhibited migration of macrophages was named macrophage migration-inhibitory factor (MIF). Other factors such as macrophage-aggregation factor and macrophage-activating factor (MAF) are probably identical. Indeed, current evidence indicates that all of these effects on macrophages are mediated by γ-interferon. Subsequently, many additional lymphokines and monokines have been described. Table 13.5.2-2 lists the factors that are either most intensively studied or are considered to have the most significant biological functions. In addition to the products of activated lymphocytes, products of nonlymphoid cells such as mononuclear phagocytes and fibroblasts (monokines and cytokines) (4, 23) provide important regulatory influences in cellular immunity.

PROPERTIES OF THE LYMPHOKINES

Few lymphokines have been isolated in pure form, and their chemical nature is only partly known. However, several lymphokines have been purified to a state of functional homogeneity. That is, the preparations were free from contamination by certain other lymphokines (19, 60). All of the lymphokines that have been characterized are proteins, and their activities are sensitive to proteolytic enzymes. Several lymphokines exist in multiple molecular forms with different molecular weights, and in some cases there is evidence that these molecules are actually different proteins and not merely dimers or polymers of a basic molecule. Noteworthy examples are guinea pig MIF, which exists as three or four species with molecular weights of 25,000-43,000 and 65,000 (19), and human lymphotoxin (LT), which occurs as four species designated as α, β, γ and δ.

A major step toward isolation and characterization of individual lymphokines has been the production of antilymphokine antisera. For example, Geczy and associates (20) have prepared an antiserum against guinea pig MIF that does not affect guinea pig LT or mitogenic factor (MF). Yoshida (60) prepared an anti-MIF serum that was devoid of activity against LT and MF, but was active against the chemotactic factor for macrophages. Conversely, the anti-LT antibody prepared by Gately and coworkers (18) had no activity against MIF or MF.

Certain lymphokines have unique physical or chemical properties. The chemotactic factor for macrophages that is produced by human lymphocytes is sensitive to heating at 56°C for 30 min; all other lymphokines resist this treatment. It has been reported that guinea pig MIF is sensitive to neuraminidase, but human MIF is not. Human LIF, a factor that inhibits the migration of polymorphonuclear leukocytes, has properties of a serine esterase and is sensitive to diisopropylfluorophosphate (54).

REGULATION OF LYMPHOKINE PRODUCTION

Lymphokines are products of activated lymphocytes. *In vivo* activation is antigen-mediated and dependent upon the presence of specific antigen-reactive lymphoid cells and antigen-presenting cells such as macrophages, dendritic cells, vascular endothelial cells, or Langerhans' cells of the epidermis. The interaction between antigen-presenting cells and antigen-responsive cells requires a genetic identity that is encoded by the I-region genes of the major histocompatibility complex. Expression of these I-region determinants is enhanced by exposure of macrophages to γ-interferon and reduced by prostaglandins such as PGE_1. In addition, many substances such as the plant lectins phytohemagglutinin and concanavalin A can nonspecifically activate T lymphocytes to produce lymphokines. Nonlymphoid cells such as fibroblasts also produce substances with lymphokinelike activities (4), as well as a number of other factors that affect cell growth.

Under proper conditions, both T lymphocytes and B lymphocytes can produce lymphokines (54). However, some instances of lymphokine production by B lymphocytes seem to require a small number of T cells, and these cells may produce critical helper factors. The observations in patients with immunodeficiency diseases strongly suggest that lymphokine production is primarily a T-cell-dependent phenomenon.

There is somewhat less information concerning pharmacological regulation of lymphokine production. Early experiments with agents such as actinomycin D and puromycin provided evidence that MIF (and presumably other lymphokines) production was dependent on new protein synthesis. Other experiments showed that lymphokine production occurs independently of cell division, and these results raised the possibility that the lymphocytes that respond to antigens by producing lymphokines reside in different cellular subsets from those that respond by cell division.

It is known that drugs that cause accumulation of cAMP usually have inhibitory effects on effector functions of lymphocytes. A similar effect has been found on MIF production. Histamine inhibits the production of MIF by lymphocytes, and this effect can be blocked by antagonists of H_2, but not H_1 receptors. It is not known whether this effect is expressed through changes in cellular cAMP. Glucocorticoids do not have direct effects on MIF production (2).

EFFECTS OF LYMPHOKINES ON TARGET CELLS

The interleukins are lymphokines that have important regulatory or differentiative roles in lymphocyte biology.

Interleukin-1 (IL-1). Macrophages regulate T-lymphocyte activities through antigen presentation, expression of I-region determinants, and through production of interleukin-1. IL-1 is a protease-sensitive molecule with a molecular weight of 12,000-16,000. Macrophages *in vitro* are induced to produce IL-1 by nonspecific stimuli such as lipopolysaccharide and immunomodulators such as muramyl dipeptide; there is little information about IL-1 production *in vivo*. The major biological activity of IL-1 may be induction of interleukin-2 production. When highly purified T lymphocytes are stimulated with antigen or mitogen, the cells undergo morphological changes, but DNA synthesis does not occur. Addition of IL-1 to the cells allows production of interleukin-2, and the cells then undergo mitosis.

Interleukin-2 (IL-2). IL-2, or T-cell growth factor, is a necessary second signal for proliferation of T lymphocytes in response to stimulation by antigens and mitogens. It is produced by T cells through specific interactions with receptors on the cell membrane. The effects of IL-2 on T cells of the helper and suppressor phenotype are well known, and there is some evidence that IL-2 may also regulate growth of B lymphocytes. Resting T cells do not express IL-2 receptors, but they appear shortly after the exposure of cells to lectins or antigens. Human IL-2 is protein with a molecular weight of 14,500.

Interleukin-3 (IL-3). IL-3, a lymphokine, is a potent inducer of 20 α-steroid dehydrogenase and is apparently related to maturation of corticosteroid resistance in T cells. There are suggestions that IL-3 is required for mast cell proliferation *in vitro*.

Lymphotoxins (LTs). Lymphotoxins may have two mechanisms of cell lysis. One is accompanied by a slow balloonlike swelling of the cells, and the other occurs in minutes and is expressed as a rapid shrinkage of the cells. The lytic effects of LTs are not accompanied by changes in synthesis of DNA, RNA, or protein, but there is a three- to four-fold increase in the rate of calcium influx. The effects of LTs may be inhibited by dimethylsulfoxide, cardiac glycosides, and local anesthetic agents.

Migration-Inhibitory Factors (MIF,). MIF has received a great deal of study, and it produces many morphological, physiological, and biochemical effects on macrophages (10, 49) (Table 13.5.2-3). One migration-inhibitory factor, LIF, contains serine esterase activity (52), but the natural substrate for this activity is unknown. MIF does not have a similar activity. There is now rather convincing evidence that the biological activities that were once attributed to MIF are due to γ-interferon.

REGULATION OF THE ACTIVITY OF LYMPHOKINES ON TARGET CELLS

Although the system that has received the most attention is the interaction between MIF and macrophages, it is probable that certain pharmacological manipulations will apply to other lymphokines. For example, addition of drugs that increase cAMP reduces the responsiveness of macrophages to MIF, and it is probable that similar drugs would reduce responses to mitogenic factors and lymphotoxin.

Effects that are more specific for MIF are summarized in Table 13.5.2-4. For example, addition of the sugar fucose to macrophages prevents inhibition of migration by MIF. Treatment of the macrophages, but not the MIF, with fucosidase produces a similar effect and suggests that fucose is an essential

Table 13.5.2-3
Effects of Lymphokines on Macrophages

I. Morphological
   - Increased spreading and stickiness
   - Increased ruffled membrane activity
   - Decreased electron-dense material
   - Increase in cytoplasmic granules

II. Biochemical
   - Increase in adenylate cyclase
   - Increase in cGMP
   - Increased uptake of Ca^{2+}
   - Increased transport of glucose, glucosamine, and leucine
   - Increase or decrease of lysosomal enzymes
   - Increased glucose-1-C oxidation
   - Increase in LDH and collagenase
   - Increased production of prostaglandin and plasminogen activator
   - Decrease in electrophoretic mobility

III. Physiological
   - Increased or decreased phagocytosis
   - Increased pinocytosis
   - Increased microbacterial activity
   - Increased cytotoxicity for tumor cells

Table 13.5.2-4
Pharmacological Modulation of Action of MIF

Class of Agent	Example
I. Agents that affect interaction between MIF and target cell	Fucose *Lotus* agglutinin Trypsin Neuraminidase Fucosidase
II. Agents that affect MIF metabolism	Protease inhibitors
III. Agents that affect cAMP	Theophylline
IV. Agents that influence polymerization of microtubules	Colchicine Vinca alkaloids
V. Other	Glucocorticoids

Source: Derived from Ref. 51.

component of the macrophage receptor for MIF. The observation that *Lotus* agglutinin binds to the macrophage receptor and produces MIF-like effects supports this concept. The macrophage receptors are also sensitive to proteases such as trypsin, and guinea pig MIF may be degraded by neuraminidase. Glucocorticoids do not affect MIF production by antigen-stimulated lymphoid cells (2), but they interfere with the effect of preformed MIF on macrophage migration. The mechanism of the effect is unknown.

IMMUNOMODULATORS

A number of substances modulate the intensity of immune responses by inducing maturation of potentially immunocompetent cells, expression of epitopes on the cell membranes, differentiation of responsiveness to specific antigens, or regulation of cell metabolism.

Thymic Hormones. Peptides from the epithelial cells of the thymus gland induce maturation of pre-T cells into cells that express the membrane-associated antigens of mature T cells and function as mature T cells. The structures of several of these hormones are known, and in the case of thymopentin, the biological activity resides in a pentapeptide. Little is known about the mechanisms of action of thymic peptides. There are reports of cases in which treatment with thymic peptides has provided improvement in immunological functions and clinical benefits to patients with immunological deficiency diseases.

Transfer Factor. Transfer factor is a low-molecular-weight (< 6000 daltons) substance that is extracted from the blood leukocytes of donors who have delayed hypersensitivity to the antigen under study (37). When it is injected into recipients who do not have delayed hypersensitivity, they become responsive. The effect appears to be antigen-specific. The mechanism of this effect is unknown. *In vivo* studies of lymphocytes from recipients of transfer factor show that these cells acquire the ability to respond to stimulation with the test antigen by producing lymphokines. This effect parallels the changes in responses to skin tests.

Transfer factor has been used successfully in the treatment of immune deficiency syndromes such as chronic mucocutaneous candidiasis, in the prophylaxis of varicella in children with leukemia, and in the treatment of recurrent herpes simplex infections. Transfer factor treatment prolongs the quality of life but not the survival of patients with the Wiskott-Aldrich syndrome.

Reserpine. In mice, expression of delayed hypersensitivity is dependent upon products of T cells and vasoactive amines from mast cells. Administration of reserpine to sensitive mice causes release of the amines into the cytosol where they are degraded by monoamine oxidase. Reserpine-treated mice are unable to express delayed hypersensitivity, but spleen cells from these mice will transfer sensitivity to nonimmune recipients. Thus, the effect of reserpine is on the expression of hypersensitivity and not the development of hypersensitivity.

Indomethacin. Studies in mice have shown that prostaglandins such as PGE_1 reduce expression of Ia antigens on macrophages. This impairs their function as antigen-presenting cells. Mycobacterial infections, leishmaniasis, and coccidioidomycosis are among the few human diseases in which the patients have deficient cell-mediated immunity. Administration of antiinflammatory drug indomethacin, which impairs production of prostaglandins, to the cells from these patients results in significant improvements in T-cell functions. Presumably, this improvement is due to improved antigen presentation although formal proof of this effect is not yet available. There is some recent evidence that indomethacin may also improve immune responses *in vivo,* but the possible application of this drug to long-term immunotherapy of these diseases is unknown.

Antihistamines. Histamine-binding lymphocytes have immunosuppressive activities. Their *in vivo* significance is unknown, but improvement in cell-mediated immune responses during cimetidine therapy has been reported in a few immunodeficient patients. This is presumably due to interference with suppressor T-cell function.

Levamisole. Levamisole, an imidazole drug, has been shown to improve chemotactic responses *in vitro* and *in vivo* and to enhance the expression of delayed hypersensitivity in patients with diseases that are associated with immunodeficiency. The mechanism is unknown, but may be related to accumulation of cGMP by levamisole-treated cells.

Isoprinosine. Isoprinosine is a complex of inosine and an organic salt that was originally developed as an antiviral agent. It has been reported to enhance the expression of surface antigens on T lymphocytes and to enhance T-cell responses to mitogens. In experimental animals, administration of isoprinosine enhances macrophage activity and responses by both T cells and B cells. Studies in immunodeficient subjects and in normal persons have shown that isoprinosine enhances a number of immunological and inflammatory activities including T-cell proliferation responses to mitogens and antigens, phagocytosis, and chemotaxis. It has been associated with enhanced antibody responses to viral vaccines. The mechanisms of these effects are unknown.

Interferon. Interferons were first described as antiviral substances. Subsequent studies have shown that interferons also have potent, antitumor activities, both in laboratory animals and in some human tumors. γ-Interferon enhances the expression of I-region gene products on macrophages and has potent macrophage-activating activity.

Other immunomodulators including immunosuppressants and immunoenhancers are discussed in Chapter 13.5.3.

CLINICAL CONSIDERATIONS

The majority of studies with lymphoid cells from healthy, normal subjects has shown a very close concordance between a person's reactivity to an antigen *in vivo* (shown by a positive delayed-type skin test) and the responses of his cells to that antigen *in vitro.* Normally, antigen-reactive cells respond to antigenic stimuli *in vivo* with lymphokine production, enhanced

DNA synthesis (lymphocyte transformation), and cellular cytotoxicity. The same responses may be induced by normal lymphocytes by the nonspecific T-cell mitogens phytohemagglutinin and concanavalin A.

These tests of lymphocyte function are useful in defining functional defects in patients with immunodeficiency diseases. As expected, patients with the lymphopenic forms of severe combined immunodeficiency are usually unable to express any lymphocyte-dependent responses to antigens or mitogens.

In the more common forms of cellular immune deficiency, delayed skin test responses are usually negative, and antigens do not activate patient's cells to DNA synthesis, cytotoxicity, or lymphokine production. However, there is a great deal of heterogeneity of lymphocyte function in these patients. In some patients, the lymphocyte transformation reactions are intact, but lymphokine production is impaired. Other patients fail to react to selected antigens, but have apparently normal responses to others. These observations suggest selective defects in specific cell maturation, antigen presentation, or defective integration of antigenic signals across the lymphocyte membranes.

Even though this situation seems confusing and very complex, certain conclusions may be warranted. If the information derived from patients with chronic mucocutaneous candidiasis (36) is applicable to other syndromes of defective cellular immunity, then failure of host cells to produce MIF in response to appropriate antigens reflects the fundamental deficiency of the disorder. Conversely, correction of cellular immune defects is usually accompanied by reconstitution of MIF-producing ability.

At the present time, we have essentially no information about the relative contributions of the individual lymphokines to the generation of positive delayed skin tests, to resistance to infectious diseases, or to immune surveillance. Acquisition of this information may be anticipated and will add an additional dimension to the treatment of cellular immunodeficiency syndromes.

REFERENCES

1. Askanese, P. W., and Kantor, K. S. Mechanisms of inflammation in delayed hypersensitivity. In: *Allergy—Principals and Practice* (Middleton, E., Reed, C. E., and Ellis, E. F., eds.). St. Louis: C. V. Mosby, 1978, p. 139.
2. Balow, J. E. and Rosenthal, A. S. Glucocorticoid suppression of macrophage migration inhibitory factor. *J. Exp. Med.* 137:1031, 1973.
3. Bennich, H, Ragnarsson, V., Johansson, S. G. O., Ishizaka, K., Ishizaka, T., Levy, D. A., and Lichtenstein, L. M. Failure of the putative IgE pentapeptide to compete with IgE for receptors on basophils and mast cells. *Int. Arch. Allergy Appl. Immunol.* 53:459, 1977.
4. Bigazzi, P. E. Cytokines: Lymphokine-like mediators provided by nonlymphoid cells. In: *Biology of the Lymphokines* (Cohen, S., Pick, E., and Oppenheim, J. J., eds.). New York: Academic Press, 1979, p. 243.
5. Bloom, B. R., and Bennett, B. Mechanism of a reaction *in vitro* associated with delayed-typed hypersensitivity. *Science* 153:80, 1966.
6. Capron, M., Rousseaux, J., Mazingue, C., Bazin, H., and Capron, A. Rat mast cell-eosinophil interaction in antibody dependent cytotoxicity Schistosoma mansoni schistosomula. *J. Immunol.* 121:2518, 1978.
7. Cochrane, C. G., and Koffler, D. Immune complex disease in experimental animals and man. *Adv. Immunol.* 16:185, 1973.
8. Cohen, S. Pick, E., and Oppenheim, J. J. (eds.). *Biology of the Lymphokines.* New York: Academic Press, 1979, p. 666.
9. David, J. R. Delayed hypersensitivity *in vitro:* Its mediation by cell-free substances formed by lymphoid cell-antigen interaction. *Proc. Natl. Acad. Sci. USA* 56:72, 1966.
10. David, J. R., and Remold, H. G. The activation of macrophages by lymphokines. In: *Biology of the Lymphokines* (Cohen, S., Pick, E., and Oppenheim, J. J., eds.). New York: Academic Press, 1979, p. 121.
11. Day, N. K., and Good, R. A. *Biologic amplification systems in immunology.* New York: Plenum Press, 1977, p. 325.
12. Drachman, D. B. Myasthenia gravis. *N. Engl. J. Med.* 298:136, 186, 1978.
13. Dumonde, D. C., Wolstencroft, R. A., Panayi, G. S., Mathew, M., Morley, J., and Howson, W. T. "Lymphokines": Non-antibody mediators of cellular immunity generated by lymphocyte activation. *Nature* 24:38, 1969.
14. Flier, J. S., Kahn, C. R., and Roth, J. Receptors, antireceptor antibodies and mechanisms of insulin resistance. *N. Engl. Med.* 300:413, 1979.
15. Frank, M. M., Gelfand, J. A., and Atkinson, J. P. Hereditary angioedema: The clinical syndrome and its management. *Ann. Intern. Med.* 84:580, 1976.
16. Frank, M. M. The complement system in host defense and inflammation. *Rev. Infect. Dis.* 1:483, 1979.
17. Freeman, J. Further observations on the treatment of hay fever by hypodermic innoculations of pollen vaccine. *Lancet* 2:814, 1911.
18. Gately, M. K., Gately, C. L., Henney, C. S., and Mayer, M. M. Studies on lymphokines: The production of antibody to guinea pig lymphotoxin and its use to distinguish lymphotoxin from migration inhibitory factor and mitogenic factor. *J. Immunol.* 115:817, 1975.
19. Gately, M. K., and Mayer, M. M. Purification and characterization of lymphokines: An approach to the molecular mechanisms of cell-mediated immunity. *Progr. Allergy* 25:106, 1978.
20. Geczy, C. L., Friedrich, W., and de Weck, A. L. Production and *in vivo* effect of antibodies against guinea pig lymphokines. *Cell. Immunol.* 19:65, 1975.
21. Gell, P. G. H., and Coombs, R. R. A. *Clinical Aspects of Immunology.* Philadelphia: F. A. Davis Co., 1964.
22. George, M., and Vaughn, J. H. *In vitro* cell migration as a model for delayed hypersensitivity. *Proc. Soc. Exp. Biol. Med.* 111:514, 1962.
23. Gery, I., and Davies, P. Immunoregulatory products of macrophages. In: *Biology of the Lymphokines* (Cohen, S., Pick, E., and Oppenheim, J. J., eds.). New York: Academic Press, 1979, p. 347.
24. Gleich, G. J., and Yunginger, J. W. The radioallergosorbent test: Its present place and likely future in the practice of allergy. *Adv. Asthma Allergy* 2:1, 1975.
25. Hamburger, R. N. Peptide inhibition of the Prausnitz-Kustner reaction. *Science* 189:389, 1975.
26. Hunt, K. J., Valentine, M. D., Sobotka, A. K., Benton, A. W., Amodio, F. J., and Lichtenstein, L. M. A controlled trial of immunotherapy in insect hypersensitivity. *N. Engl. J. Med.* 299:157, 1978.
27. Ishizaka, T., Adachi, T., Chang, T., and Ishizaka, K. Development of mast cells *in vitro.* II. Biologic function of cultured mast cells. *J. Immunol.* 118:211, 1977.
28. Ishizaka, T., Conrad, D. H., Schulman, E. S., Sterk, A. R., and Ishizaka, K. Biochemical analysis of initial triggering events of IgE-mediated histamine release from human lung mast cells. *J. Immunol.* 130:2357, 1983.
29. Ishizaka, T., Chang, T. H., Taggart, M., and Ishizaka, K. Histamine release from rat mast cells by antibodies against rat basophilic leukemia cell membrane. *J. Immunol.* 119:1589, 1977.
30. Ishizaka, K., and Ishizaka, T. Immunology of IgE-mediated hypersensitivity. In: *Allergy—Principles and Practice* (Middleton, E., Reed, C. E., and Ellis, E. F., eds.). St. Louis: C. V. Mosby, 1983, p. 43.

31. Kaliner, M. A., and Austen, K. F. The sequence of biochemical events in the release of chemical mediators from sensitized human lung tissue. *J. Exp. Med.* 138:1077, 1973.

32. Kaliner, M., and Austen, K. F. Immunologic release of chemical mediators from human tissue—pharmacologic controls and biochemical concomitants. *Ann. Rev. Pharmacol.* 15:179, 1975.

33. Kaliner, M. Human lung tissue and anaphylaxis. Evidence that cyclic nucleotides modulate the immunologic release of mediators through effects on microtubular assembly. *J. Clin. Invest.* 60:951, 1977.

34. Kanner, B. I., and Metzger, H. Crosslinking of the receptors for immunoglobulin E depolarizes the plasma membrane of rat basophilic leukemia cells. *Proc. Natl. Acad. Sci. USA* 80:5744, 1983.

35. Kennerly, D. A., Sullivan, T. J., and Parker, C. W. Activation of phospholipid metabolism during mediator release from stimulated rat mast cells. *J. Immunol.* 122:152, 1979.

36. Kirkpatrick, C. H., and Sohnle, P. G. Chronic mucocutaneous candidiasis. In: *Immunodermatology* (Safai, B., and Good, R. A., eds.). New York: Plenum Press, 1981, p. 495.

37. Kirkpatrick, C. H. Greenberg, L. E., and Petersen, E. A. Transfer factor. *Lymphokines* 8:1, 1983.

38. Kniker, W. T., Guerra, F. A., and Richards, S. E. M. Prevention of immune complex disease (serum sickness) by antagonists of vasoactive amines. *Pediatr. Res.* 5:381, 1971.

39. Kohler, P. F. Immune complexes and allergic disease. In: *Allergy—Principles and Practice* (Middleton, E., Reed, C. E., and Ellis, E. F., eds.). St. Louis: C. V. Mosby, 1983, p. 167.

40. Landsteiner, K., and Chase, M. W. Experiments on transfer of cutaneous sensitivity to simple compounds. *Proc. Soc. Exp. Biol. Med.* 49:688, 1942.

41. Lee, W. Y., and Sehon, A. H. Abrogation of reaginic antibodies with modified allergens. *Nature* 267:618, 1977.

42. McClusky, R. T., Benacerraf, B., and McClusky, J. W. Studies on the specificity of the cellular infiltrate in delayed hypersensitivity reactions. *J. Immunol.* 90:466, 1963.

43. Middleton, E., Reed, C. E., and Ellis, E. F. (eds.). *Allergy—Principles and Practice.* St. Louis: C. V. Mosby, 1983.

44. Najarian, J. S., and Feldman, J. D. Passive transfer of tuberculin sensitivity by tritiated thymidine-labeled lymphoid cells. *J. Exp. Med.* 114:779, 1961.

45. Noon, L. Prophylactic innoculation for hay fever. *Lancet* 1:1572, 1911.

46. Orr, T. S. C. Mode of action of disodium cromoglycate. *Acta Allergol.* 32 (suppl. 13):9, 1977.

47. Patterson, R. Lieberman, P., Irons, J. S., Pruzansky, J. J., Metzger, W. J., and Zeiss, C. R. Immunotherapy. In: *Allergy—Principles and Practice* (Middleton, E., Reed, C. E., and Ellis, E. F., eds.). St. Louis: C. V. Mosby, 1983, p. 1119.

48. Paul, W. E. *Fundamental Immunology.* New York: Raven Press, 1984.

49. Pick, E. Mechanism of action of migration inhibitory lymphokines. In: *Biology of the Lymphokines* (Cohen, S. Pick, E., and Oppenheim, J. J., eds.). New York: Academic Press, 1979, p. 59.

50. Platshon, L., and Kaliner, M. The effect of the immunologic release of histamine upon human lung cyclic nucleotide levels and prostaglandin generation. *J. Clin. Invest.* 62:1113, 1978.

51. Rich, A. R., and Lewis, M. R. The nature of allergy in tuberculosis as revealed by tissue culture studies. *Bull. Johns Hopkins Hosp.* 50:115, 1932.

52. Rocklin, R. Human leukocyte inhibitory factor (LIF): A lymphocyte mediator with esteratic properties. *Fed. Proc.* 37:2743, 1978.

53. Rocklin, R. E. Clinical and immunological aspects of allergen-specific immunotherapy in patients with seasonal allergic rhinitis and/or allergic asthma. *J. Allergy Clin. Immunol.* 72:323, 1983.

54. Rosenstreich, D. L., and Wahl, S. M. Cellular sources of lymphokines. In: *Biology and the Lymphokines* (Cohen, S., Pick, E., and Oppenheim, J. J., eds.). New York: Academic Press, 1979, p. 209.

55. Samter, M. *Immunological Diseases.* Boston: Little, Brown, 1978.

56. Sehon, A. H. Specific suppression of IgE antibodies. *J. Allergy Clin. Immunol.* 62:257, 1978.

57. de Weck, A. L., and Schreider, C. H. Specific inhibition of allergic reactions to penicillin in many by monovalent hapten. *Int. Arch. Allergy Appl. Immunol.* 42:782, 1972.

58. Wide, L., Bennich, H., and Johansson, S. G. O. Diagnosis of allergy by an *in vitro* test for allergen antibodies. *Lancet* 2:1105, 1967.

59. Yoshida, T., Bigazzi, P. E., and Cohen, S. The production of antiguinea pig lymphokine antibody. *J. Immunol.* 114:688, 1975.

60. Yoshida, T. Purification and characterization of lymphokines. In: *Biology and the Lymphokines* (Cohen, S., Pick, E., and Oppenheim, J. J., eds.). New York: Academic Press, 1979, p. 259.

CHAPTER
13.5.3

IMMUNOSUPPRESSANTS, IMMUNOENHANCERS, AND DRUG ALLERGY

William L. West and Sachin N. Pradhan

In Chapter 13.5.2 some discussions have been made in respect to immunomodulators including both immunosuppressants and immunoenhancers. This chapter provides further discussion on other agents belonging to both of these groups.

IMMUNOSUPPRESSANTS

Those immunosuppressants, or agents that suppress the immune system, available at present are primarily used as anticancer drugs, although they are also used in the therapy of other diseases (7, 12, 14). The clinically useful anticancer drugs that can also be used as immunosuppressants in other diseases are discussed in part in Chapter 27 in terms of their pharmacological effects, mechanisms of action, and other aspects; these are listed in Table 13.5.3-1.

ANTIMETABOLITES

PURINE ANALOGS

Azathioprine and mercaptopurine are the most extensively studied immunosuppressive agents. Following metabolic activation, these agents are known to depress antibody proliferative responses, to delay allograph rejection, and to prevent the development of delayed hypersensitivity reactions (7, 14). However, in cancer patients, established delayed hypersensitivity responses are not affected (4). These compounds are most active during phase II of the immune response as shown in Table 13.5.3-2, and, though often not the drug of choice, they are useful in the treatment of acute glomerulonephritis, systemic lupus erythematosus, and in the management of organ transplantation (7, 14).

Azathioprine and 6-mercaptopurine are absorbed from the gastrointestinal tract following oral administration. Azathioprine is metabolized to 6-mercaptopurine, and both are converted to active nucleosides and nucleotides that are cytotoxic to sensitive cells. An enzyme, xanthine oxidase, converts much of the active material to 6-thiouric acid, and hyperuricemia may result. Thus, xanthine oxidase plays a major role during therapy in the inactivation of these purine antimetabolites, and hence allopurinol may be used to control the resulting hyperuricemia and/or to reduce the dose. The dose of thioguanine, on the contrary, is not affected by allopurinol because lesser amounts of 6-thiouric acid are formed via this metabolic pathway in humans.

Azathioprine is reported to have a more desirable therapeutic index compared with other antimetabolites, and hence deserves more specific comments on uses and dosages (7, 14). Azathioprine is effective in the treatment of

Table 13.5.3-1
Classification of Drugs Used in Diseases with an Immunological Basis

Antimetabolites
Purine Analogs
Azathioprine (IMURAN)
Mercaptopurine (PURINETHOL)
Thioguanine (TABLOID)
Pyramidine analogs
Azaribine (TRIAZUR)
Cytarabine (CYTOSAR)
Folic acid analogs
Methotrexate (AMETHOPTERIN)
Alkylating agents
Cyclophosphamide
Cytimun
Antibiotics
Cyclosporin A
Corticosteroids and analogs
Hydrocortisone (cortisol)
Prednisolone
Methylprednisolone
Triamcinolone
Betamethasone
Dexamethasone
Paramethasone

Wegener's granulomatosis, temporal-cranial arteritis, polymyalgia rheumatica, and in patients with active rheumatoid arthritis. Azathioprine is widely used in the treatment of systemic lupus erythematosus with multiple organ involvement (i.e., lupus nephritis), although the results are not dramatic and at times are equivocal. In lupus, following azathioprine therapy, improvement in the ultrastructural and hematological manifestations occurs consistently.

The dose of azathioprine in active rheumatoid arthritis and in systemic lupus is 2-3 mg/kg. In the treatment of both chronic diseases, objective clinical criteria for improvement must be selected. Although a change may be evident after 1 week of therapy, the onset of the and adverse effects of thiopurines may be delayed.

The potential adverse effects of azathioprine include both mutagenesis and carcinogenesis, and hence there is a reluctance to use this agent in children for prolonged therapy. All thiopurines are partially metabolized in the liver, and in patients with compromised liver function the dose should be reduced. The thiopurines may produce idiosyncratic cholestatic hepatitis, which is reversible when the drug is withdrawn. Also, a few patients show an intolerance or hypersensitivity to the thiopurines that is manifested by urticarial skin rashes, gastrointestinal disturbances, and CNS manifestations. If either of these situations develop, other classes of immunosuppressive drugs may be in order.

A clinical remission is the primary objective of the therapy in rheumatoid arthritis and systemic lupus. Once this has been achieved, the dose should be reduced and some minimal dose established in order to maintain the remission for a prolonged period of time with fewer adverse effects. The abrupt withdrawal of medication after prolonged therapy should be avoided, as exacerbation of the disease may occur.

This approach to therapy is applicable in patients with chronic active hepatitis, ulcerative colitis or Crohn's disease, and regional enteritis, as well as autoimmune hemolytic anemia and chronic idiopathic thrombocytopenic purpura refractory to steroids. Whereas azathioprine may not be the drug of choice in the diseases mentioned, in combination with steroids it reduces the dose and adverse effects of the latter.

OTHER ANTIMETABOLITES

Other antimetabolites (e.g., 5-fluorouracil, cytarabin, and methotrexate) are also immunosuppressant in therapeutic doses and can be administered orally. Their use as immunosuppressants has been confined to patients with idiosyncratic responses to the purine antimetabolites. They affect phase II of the immune response, as does azathioprine (Table 13.5.3-2). In reference to selective effects on immunity (6, 7, 14), 5-fluorouracil in subtherapeutic doses in mice was shown to enhance tumor growth and suppress secondary antibody responses. Methotrexate was also shown to suppress humoral antibody response in humans; cytarbine has been extensively studied for its ability to selectively inhibit humoral immunity in tumor-bearing mice. Methotrexate and cytarabine do not appear to block the expression of established delayed hypersensitivity, or acquisition of new delayed hypersensitivity, but may alter the intensity of these reactions as is indicated by an effect on phase IV of the immune response (Table 13.5.3-2).

ALKYLATING AGENTS

CYCLOPHOSPHAMIDE

Cyclophosphamide, following its metabolic activation, has been studied extensively for effects on humoral and cell-mediated immunity (7, 11, 13). It was shown initially to be selectively toxic to B cells, and more recently, on certain suppressor T-cell populations. In addition, and depending on dose, effects on B cells may be reversible, whereas those on suppressor T-cell function are not. Several explanations have been suggested e.g., certain suppressor T-cell populations may not contain enzyme-mediated DNA repair mechanisms, and/or there are no reserve suppressor T cells. Though the exact mechanisms for these selectively desirable effects on immunity are not known, many active metabolites such as 4-hydroxycyclophosphamide, aldophosphamide, phosphoramide mus-

Table 13.5.3-2
Effect of Drugs on Phases of Immune Response

Phases of Immune Response (cells involved)	Effect of Drug[a]	
	Suppressant	Stimulant
I. *Antigen recognition and/or processing* (macrophages, activated B cells, T cells)	Cyclophosphamide Cytimun Corticosteroid	BCG *C. parvum* Levamisole
II. *Amplification* (lymphocytes in blastogenesis, macrophages, B cells, T cells)	Cyclophosphamide Cytimun Antimetabolites 5-FU 6-MP Cytarabine L-asparaginase Corticosteroids	Levamisole Concanavalin A
III. *Antibody Production*	Cyclophosphamide Cytimun Corticosteroids Cyclosporin A	Lipopolysaccharides Levamisole
IV. *Immune effector responses* (plasma cells, small lymphocytes, B cells, T cells)	Cyclophosphamide Cytimun Corticosteroids Methotrexate Cytarabine Cyclosporin A	Levamisole *C. parvum*

[a] 5-FU, 5-fluorouracil; 6-MP, 6-mercaptopurine; *C. parvum*, *Corynebacterium parvum*; BCG, bacillus Calmette-Guérin.

tard, acrolein, and possibly nornitrogen mustard are believed to be responsible for antineoplastic and immunosuppressive responses (13). Another interesting finding in reference to the mechanism is that suppressor T-cell functions are inhibited by doses of cyclophosphamide that have no measurable effects on B cells; hence inhibition of clonal proliferation may not be the only mechanism for its effects, assuming proliferative responses of both cell types should be equally sensitive. Thus, from this brief discussion cyclophosphamide appears to be one of the most suitable drugs for exploration of selective effects on the immune system (11, 13). Cyclophosphamide affects all phases of the immune response, as shown in Table 13.5.3-2.

Alkylating agents in general are known to be cytotoxic to lymphocytes by alkylating nucleic acids and forming cross-links between two macromolecules (polypeptide or polynucleotide chains) with relative stable bonds. In addition, they are known to inhibit protein and nucleic acid (DNA) biosynthesis, and selectively to alkylate purine bases, which not only results in depurination but also in errors during transcription and replication (Chapter 27).

Cyclophosphamide, or its active metabolites, though promising for selective effects throughout the immune system, must await further evaluation in this regard. However, as a general immunosuppressant, it has yielded clinically desirable results in several diseases of immunological origin. In those patients who may be refractory to steroid therapy or whose disease process exacerbates during withdrawal from steroid therapy, cyclophosphamide is known to be beneficial. In addition, improvements are obtained in (a) Wegener's granulomatosis, (b) selected patients with rheumatoid arthritis, and (c) nephrotic syndrome.

Cyclophosphamide is given orally in 2-mg/kg doses in the diseases just mentioned. A rigid monitoring program for clinical improvement and adverse effects should be established before the physician begins the regimen. A moderate leukopenia [2500-4000/cm^3 white blood cell (WBC) count] should be induced and maintained throughout the course of therapy. On the contrary, a fall in polymorphonuclear leukocytes to less than 1000/cm^3 predisposes the patient to infections as a complication, and a fall in platelet count below $10^5/cm^3$ is a signal to discontinue therapy.

After the selection of a dose, it should not be increased during the first 4 weeks of therapy; further, raising the dose more often than 3 weeks thereafter may provide an unnecessary risk for the patient. Blood counts should be monitored every 2 weeks throughout the therapeutic regimen.

As with other cytotoxic drugs, cyclophosphamide has an enormous potential for adverse effects on the gonads and blood-forming organs (reticuloendothelial system). Testicular atrophy and azoospermia have been reported in male patients. Severe hair loss (alopecia), occasional hemorrhagic cystitis (increase in fluid intake may reduce incidence), gastrointestinal intolerance, and mucositis have been reported in male and female patients. In addition, the physician must take into consideration the age of the patient and/or the patient's desire for procreation before selecting cyclophosphamide as the immunosuppressant. Also, cyclophosphamide is in part activated to alkylating molecular species in the liver smooth endoplasmic reticulum, and toxicity may be altered by other drugs or conditions that activate or inhibit these enzymes.

CYTIMUN

Cytimun is an analog of cyclophosphamide believed to have a better therapeutic index, and it is especially effective against B cells (3).

ANTIBIOTIC

CYCLOSPORINE

Cyclosporine (cyclosporine A) is a unique immunosuppressant indicated in the prevention of allograft rejection following organ transplantation (3). Initially proposed for use as an antifungal agent, cyclosporine A was found to possess more marked immunosuppressant effects than its antibiotic potential. It is an unusual cyclic peptide isolated from fungi *Cylindrocarpon lucidium* and *Trichoderma polysporum* and composed of 11 amino acids (2) with the following chemical structure.

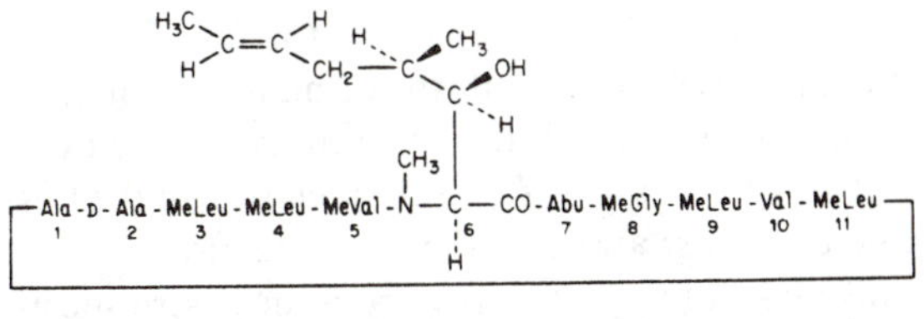

Ala - D - Ala - MeLeu - MeLeu - MeVal - N — C — CO - Abu - MeGly - MeLeu - Val - MeLeu
(1 2 3 4 5 6 7 8 9 10 11)

Cyclosporine

Cyclosporine specifically inhibits the generation of effector T lymphocytes without affecting the expression of suppressor lymphocytes and is not known to affect the functions of B cells. The drug is not cytotoxic; it must be administered before proliferation of T cells occurs due to exposure to a specific antigen.

In many studies, use of cyclosporine has resulted in slightly higher patient and graft survival than obtainable with conventional forms of immunosuppression (9). Experience with the drug has been obtained mostly with patients receiving renal transplants, but it has also been used in liver, pancreas, bone marrow, and heart recipients.

Adverse Effects. Cyclosporine has been reported to depress renal function that may be due to nephrotoxicity or a low-grade rejection reaction. Nephrotoxicity, which has been the most serious side effect, ranges from a mild elevation in serum creatinine levels to oliguric renal failure. This effect has been managed either by reduction of the dose of cyclosporine or by its substitution to other immunosuppressors (e.g., azathioprine and steroids) (9).

Gum hypertrophy is a common side effect. Other effects include hirsutism, tremor, neurasthenia, hepatotoxicity, benign breast tumors, and depressive psychosis.

Cyclosporin has been used at oral doses of 15-20 mg/kg along with other immunosuppressive agents (1).

STEROIDS

Glucocorticoids such as cortisol (hydrocortisone) and many of its synthetic analogs possess antiinflammatory, immunosuppressant, or immunomodulator properties, and are known to be of value in the treatment of inflammatory and allergic disorders as well as the management of patients after organ transplantation (8, 14, 15). Although the precise mechanisms through which these desirable effects are achieved during treatment are unknown, most investigators agree that these agents are immunoregulators and immunomodulators since their activity on the immune system may involve stimulating and suppressing effects on altered immune functions.

Corticosteroids in pharmacological dosages appear to affect all phases of the defense response, as shown in Table 13.5.3-2. Suppression of the inflammatory response after injury is characterized by (a) maintenance of integrity and permeability characteristics of the endothelium of the capillary beds, resulting in a decrease in leakage of edema-forming fluids and proteins as well as inhibition of exudation of inflammatory cells (neutrophils and mast cells); (b) stabilization of lysosomal membranes protecting the membrane from rupture following injury to the cells; and, (c) inhibition of chemotactic responses of neutrophils, resulting in the impedance of movement of neutrophils and monocytes toward the injury site (5). Most of the effects of glucocorticoids are mediated by actions on cytologic receptors that lead to alterations in proteins synthesis. The antiinflammatory mechanisms of these steroids may be in part due to the blocking of the release of arachidonic acid from phospholipids in the cell membrane and hence preventing the conversion of arachidonic acids to various metabolites [i.e., prostaglandins (PGE, PGF, PGD, PGI), thromboxane (TxA), hydroxy-eicosatetraenoic acid (HETE) derivatives, or leukotrienes], many of which are highly bioactive compounds. For example, the prostaglandins have an important regulatory role in lymphokine production, and lymphokines are involved in the regulation of immune and inflammatory responses (15). Suppression of all phases of the immune response is characterized by (a) an interference with phagocytosis and antigen processing (b) impeding cell migrations and/or (c) inhibition of cell-mediated immune reactions. The thymus-derived T lymphocytes are more susceptible to lower pharmacological doses of the steroids, and antibody production (B cells and plasma cells) is not significantly affected, except with large pharmacological doses where adverse effects limit their usefulness. Overall, glucocorticoid therapy is indicated in a variety of disorders in the immune system (see Chapter 12.4).

Structural analogs of cortisol, a major product of the adrenal cortex, include prednisolone, methylprednisolone, triamcinolone, betamethasone, dexamethasone, and paramethasone. The advantage of these compounds over cortisol at equipotent antiinflammatory dosages is that the adverse effect of sodium retention is reduced. All other potentially adverse effects associated with pharmacological dosages of steroids are still present.

IMMUNOENHANCERS

BACILLUS CALMETTE-GUÉRIN

Bacillus Calmette-Guérin (BCG) vaccine has been used in the treatment of melanoma and acute lymphocytic leukemia in humans and in a variety of experimental tumors (4, 5, 11). BCG is widely accepted as an immunological enhancer or a nonspecific adjuvant and has been shown to have antigens in common with human and animal tumor cells. Hence, it can stimulate specific and nonspecific immune responses in humans.

BCG is known to directly stimulate macrophage functions, resulting in increased macrophage cytotoxicity against neoplastic cells, increased phagocytic activity, increased lysosomal enzymes, activated phospholipase A, increased production of lymphocyte-activating factor (LAF) that enhances T-cell helper function and T-cell cytotoxicity, and increased chemotaxis. The main effect of BCG is on phase I of the defense response (Table 13.5.3-2).

The route and time of administration are crucial, and BCG contact with the tumor is important. For example, injection of BCG intralesionally in sites drained by lymph nodes increases the potential for favorable response.

BCG alone and in combination has shown exciting results in several diseases.

CORYNEBACTERIUM PARVUM

Corynebacterium parvum (*C. parvum*) has been used as an enhancer or adjuvant in cancer chemotherapy (4, 5, 11) and may be effective in patients with lung or breast cancer. *C. parvum*, unlike BCG, is effective either as killed bacteria or vaccine.

C. parvum was shown to increase antibody production against both T-cell-dependent and independent antigens and to increase the immunogenicity of small doses of antigens. *C. parvum* depresses allograft rejection and graft-versus-host reactions. This depression of the cellular immune response occurs concomitantly with stimulation of the humoral immune response. Overall stimulation of the reticuloendothelial system (RES) by *C. parvum* is characterized by hepatosplenomegaly, accelerated phagocytosis, macrophage proliferation or cloning efficiency, augmented antigen-processing efficiency, accumulation of lysosomal enzymes, activation of phospholipase A, and a nonspecific cytostatic effect on tumor cells. *C. parvum* has a profound effect on phase I of the immune response, as shown in Table 13.5.3-2.

C. parvum may be administered i.v., i.p., or intralesionally. Serious side effects have been recorded when given i.p. and include chills, fevers, and changes in blood pressure.

The available data on *C. parvum* from animals and humans suggest that it may be a useful agent in cancer, but the patient population studied to date in this country is small.

LIPOPOLYSACCHARIDES

Lipopolysaccharides (LPSs) are known to produce the characteristic biological activities of endotoxins from gram-negative bacteria (4, 5, 11). Although the immunoenhancement and antitumor effects reside in an active structural component, lipid A, which is common to a variety of bacteria, unacceptable toxicity of this purified lipid A has prevented its clinical trial. LPSs have their maximum effect on phase III of the immune response, as shown in Table 13.5.3-2.

LEVAMISOLE

Levamisole, a phenylimidazole derivative, is a potent anthelmintic agent (Chapter 16.4) that is known to stimulate the immune system in immunologically incompetent animals and humans (4, 5, 11, 12). Levamisole affects all phases of the immune response as shown in Table 13.5.3-2. Levamisole has no intrinsic antibacterial or antiviral properties, and hence these effects are mediated via immunoenhancement.

Levamisole is known to act on cyclic nucleotide metabolism increasing the breakdown of cyclic adenosine monophosphate (cAMP) and decreasing the breakdown of cyclic guanosine monophosphate (cGMP). It affects the proliferative responses of lymphocytes, antibody production to sheep red blood cells, lymphokine production, cytotoxicity, and phagocytosis by macrophages. Increased levels of cGMP are correlated with lymphocyte proliferation and augmentation of chemotactic responses after administering this drug to laboratory animals. Overall precursor T lymphocytes are facilitated in their differentiation into mature cells, and cell-mediated immunity is in some way restored.

Levamisole is a potent inhibitor of mammalian alkaline phosphatase and diamine oxidase. However, whether these effects are important in relation to the host defense system must await further investigation.

Levamisole is rapidly absorbed from the gastrointestinal tract in humans. An average dose for immunoenhancement in adults may be 150 mg/kg (orally). Peak plasma levels of 0.7 mg/l are obtained in 1-2 hr, and the plasma half-life is equal to 4 hr. Levamisole is metabolized in the liver. Parenteral administration (e.g., i.m.) of the drug will give higher (2x) peak plasma levels. Urinary excretion of levamisole (parent drug) is slow and is influenced by pH (low pH increasing elimination). Overall elimination of a single dose is complete within 48 hr (10).

Immunodeficiency diseases such as Job's syndrome or

hyperimmunologlobin E syndrome, lazy leucocyte syndrome, Wiskott-Aldrich syndrome, ataxia telangectasis, chronic granulomatous disease, and cyclic neutropenia all have been treated with some success. Infectious diseases such as recurrent herpes infections, recurrent furunculosis, acne conglobata, and chronic pyogenic skin infections have been improved by treatment with levamisole as indicated by an improvement of the lesions. Diseases associated with immunological mechanisms such as rheumatoid arthritis, Reiter's syndrome, systemic lupus erythematosus, aphthous stomatitis, and Crohn's disease have in some cases been improved following treatment.

DRUG ALERGY

The term *drug allergy (hypersensitivity)* is applied to adverse reactions that are immunologically mediated as opposed to reactions resulting from pharmacological idiosyncrasy, side effects, toxicity, or drug interactions (10). Allergy is not the most common cause of adverse drug reactions; however, some serious drug reactions may be due to allergy.

Drug allergy differs from drug toxicity in several ways: The lesion produced in a given population occurs in low incidence; the occurrence is very unpredictable; prior exposure (1-3 weeks) to an antigen (drug) may cause sensitization, and desensitization may also occur; the lesion is dose independent; and a high incidence of rash, fever, eosinophilia, and other blood dyscrasias is associated with therapy.

The differences between immune responses to drugs (drug allergies) and to foreign proteins are that in the case of drug allergy, (a) the incidence is low, (b) *in vitro* and *in vivo* tests or assays are often negative, and (c) the patterns of allergic responses are varied.

The etiology of drug allergy is not clear; the nature of the antigen and immunogenetic defects (atopy) in patients may be factors. For most drug allergies, the antigen has not been clearly and completely identified. However, most investigators agree that the drug or its metabolites serve as a hapten via covalent binding to an endogenous protein as a carrier, although polysaccharides or polynucleotides may probably serve in a similar way.

The immunogenicity of the carrier itself appears to be important because haptens combined with foreign proteins are better immunogens than haptens bound to a native protein (10). The carrier appears to interact with T lymphocytes initiating the response. Once T cells are activated, hapten-specific activation is produced in B lymphocytes and antihapten antibodies are formed.

As a rule, drugs do not have intrinsic protein reactivity; reactivity with protein usually takes place after formation of activated derivatives during metabolic processing of the drug. As an example, in the case of penicillin allergy, antibodies can be demonstrated in the serum of penicillin-treated patients, not to penicillin itself, but to its metabolic products capable of existing in covalent linkage to protein, especially the penicilloyl group (Chapter 24.2). Thus, a drug may be degraded to a reactive immunogen.

A requirement for metabolic processing of the drug can explain some otherwise puzzling aspects of drug allergy, such as its low incidence, variation in its frequency with different drugs, and its occurrence in specific organ systems (10). A drug may be metabolized by enzymatic degradation in some organ or tissue where the antigenically active metabolite (hapten) may accumulate or the hapten may combine with an intrinsic protein in a specific organ. These may result in organ- or tissue-specific allergic reactions. A drug may have many metabolites; only microgram amounts of highly reactive metabolites are sufficient for induction of immune reactions, and the proimmunogen derivatives are reactive to proteins, making them difficult to detect in the body fluids. All these factors make the precise identification of responsible antigens in drug allergy seldom possible.

CLINICAL MANIFESTATIONS

Various manifestations of drug allergy have been reviewed by Parker (10) and are briefly described here.

Anaphylaxis. Systemic anaphylaxis is an immunologically mediated, acute, life-threatening reaction in which the following manifestations may occur in combination or in isolated manner: hypotension, cardiac arrhythmias, bronchospasm, laryngeal edema, hyperperistalsis, urticaria, diffuse erythema, and pruritus. The reaction develops rapidly, reaching maximum within 5-30 min after i.v. or i.m. administration. In highly sensitive persons oral, cutaneous, or even respiratory exposure may produce the response.

Anaphylaxis is due to type I, or immediate hypersensitivity, reactions and is mediated in humans largely by IgE and some by a certain IgG subclass of antibodies. An important example of a drug producing such reaction is penicillin. Anaphylactoid reactions mimic anaphylaxis, being induced by mast cell (and basophil) degranulation, but in the absence of an IgE-mediated immunological reaction. A number of drugs are mast cell secretagogues capable of causing anaphylactoid reactions. Examples of these agents include organic mercurials, opiates (particularly heroin), organic iodides used in radiopaque contrast mediums, dextran, antibiotic bases including amphotericin B, and histamine H_1 antagonist.

Serum Sickness. Serum sickness is a systemic allergic reaction characterized by fever, lymphadenopathy, rash, arthritis, nephritis, edema, and neuritis. Its symptoms develop after a latent period of 6 days or more following initial exposure to a drug; the latent period reflects the time required to synthesize an adequate amount of antibody. The antibodies involved in the reaction probably include largely IgG and possibly IgM. In this reaction, antigen remains in circulation for a prolonged period; when antibody is formed after the latent period, any intravascular antigen still present reacts with the antibody. The reaction induces circulating immune complexes (type III reaction; see Chapter 13.5.2), producing the symptoms of serum sickness. Agents causing this reaction include penicillins, sulfonamides, thiouracils, cholecystographic dyes, phenytoin, aminosalicylic acid, and streptomycin.

Cytotoxic Reactions (Tissue or Organ Specific). Whereas anaphylaxis and serum sickness provide examples of systemic allergic drug reactions, immunological reaction to drugs may be directed toward a target organ (or tissue) such as formed elements of the blood, skin, kidney, lungs, heart, liver, muscle, and peripheral nerves.

The mechanism of these cytotoxic (or type II) reactions are threefold: (a) the drug may react chemically with the tissue, introducing a haptenic group on the cell surface and making the tissue susceptible to the antibody; (b) the antigen-antibody complex, after being formed in the fluid phase, may be localized on the cell surface; or, (c) replacement of organ-specific proteins by hapten may render them immunogenic and produce organ-directed autoimmunity. Thus, cytotoxicity may be produced immunologically on various formed elements of blood, producing (a) hemolytic anemia (drugs: penicillin, quinine, quinidine, dipyrone, aminosalicylic acid, mephenytoin, stibophen, cephalothin, and phenacetin); (b) thrombocytopenia [drugs: quinine, quinidine, meprobamate, chlorothiazide, thiouracils, chloramphenicol, sulfonamides, and allyl-isopropylacetylcarbamide (sedormid)]; or (c) granulocytopenia (drugs: aminopyrine, phenylbutazone, phenothiazines, thiouracils, sulfonamides, anticonvulsants, and tolbutamide).

Immunologically mediated cytotoxicity in blood may be differentiated from direct cytotoxicity. Examples of the latter include genetic variants in metabolism such as congenital glucose-6-phosphate dehydrogenase deficiency, in which acute hemolytic anemia is produced by antimalarials, analgesics, and a number of other drugs.

Skin Reactions. Drugs can produce every known type of skin reaction. They frequently accompany visceral drug reactions or may occur as an isolated manifestation. Such skin reactions described in the previous sections include involvement of a specific antibody. A different type of reaction in which no antibody involvement has been described includes cell-mediated immunity (type IV reactions). An example may include allergic contact dermatitis such as produced by poison ivy and many drugs.

Relationships of various manifestations of drug allergy to the type of immune responses and their diagonostic tests are briefly discussed in Chapter 31.

PREVENTION AND TREATMENT

Acute anaphylaxis can be treated by epinephrine or its congeners. Epinephrine is given s.c. (0.3-0.5 ml aqueous epinephrine in dilution of 1:1000) without any delay, since seconds may be vital in controlling the response. Epinephrine may be required every 20 min for several doses. Symptomatic treatment may be required for hypotension, cardiac arrhythmia, laryngeal edema, asthma, and other signs and symptoms.

Because the hypotension accompanying histamine release in anaphylaxis involves both H_1- and H_2-receptor sites (Chapter 13.4), both types of receptor antagonists should also be administered: diphenhydramine 50 mg i.v. and cimetidine 300 mg i.v. both given over several minutes are suggested. Corticosteroids are helpful, if allergic manifestations persist. Milder allergic reactions may be managed more conservatively by antihistamines or simply by withdrawing the drug.

Prophylactic antihistamines may be useful in prevention of serum sickness and milder allergic conditions. Desensitization has been successful in prevention or reductions of seriousness of allergic manifestations for several drugs including penicillin, p-aminosalicylic acid, isoniazid, phenytoin, penicillamine, tetracycline, and streptomycin (10).

REFERENCES

1. *AMA Drug Evaluation, 5th ed.* Chicago: American Medical Association, 1983, p. 1448.
2. Borel, J.F., Feurer, C., Magnée, C. and Stähelin, H. Effects of the new anti-lymphocytic peptide cyclosporin A in animals. *Immunology* 32:1017, 1977.
3. Calne, R.Y. Review/commentary immunosuppression for organ grafting. *Int. J. Immunopharmacol.* 1:163, 1979.
4. Crispen R.G. (ed.). *Neoplasma Immunity: Theory and Application.* Chicago: ITR, 1975.
5. Hadden, J.W., Delmonte, L. and Oettgen, H.F. Mechanism of immunopotentiation. In: *Comprehensive Immunology and Immunopharmacology* (Hadden, J.W., Coffey, R.G. and Spreafico, F., eds.). New York: Plenum Press, 1977.
6. Haskell, C.M. Immunologic aspects of cancer chemotherapy. *Ann. Rev. Pharmacol. Toxicol.* 17:179, 1977.
7. Kaplan, S.R. and Calabresi, P. Drug therapy: Immunosuppressive agents (part I and II). *N. Engl. J. Med.* 289:952, 1234, 1973.
8. Melby, J.C. Clinical pharmacology of systemic corticosteroids. *Ann. Rev. Pharmacol. Toxicol.* 17:511, 1977.
9. Merion, R.M., White, D.J.G., Thiru, S. et al. Cyclosporine: Five years' experience in cadaveric renal transplantation. *N. Engl. J. Med.* 310:148, 1984.
10. Parker, C.W. Drug allergy. *N. Engl. J. Med.* 292:Part I, 511; part II, 733; part III, 957, 1975.
11. Renoux, G. Trend in immunopotentiation. *Int. J. Immunopharmacol.* 2:1, 1980.
12. Schnieden, H. Levamisole - A general pharmacological perspective. *Int. J. Immunopharmacol.* 3:9, 1981.
13. Shand, F.L. Immunopharmacology of cyclophosphamide. *Int. J. Immunopharmacol.* 1:165, 1979.
14. Spreafico, F. and Anaclero, A. Immunosuppressive agents. In: *Comprehensive Immunology and Immunopharmacology* (Hadden, J.W., Coffey, R.G. and Spreafico, F., eds.). New York: Plenum Press, 1977.
15. Stenson, W.F. and Parker, C.W. Prostaglandins. In: *Immunopharmacology* (Turk, T., Sirols, P. and Rola-Pleszczynski, M., eds.). New York: Elsevier, 1982, p. 75.

ADDITIONAL READING

Drews, J. The pharmacology of the immune system; clinical and experimental perspectives. *Prog. Drug Res.* 28:83, 1984.

Goldman, M.H. et al. Cyclosporine in cardiac transplantation. *Surg. Clin. North Am.* 65:637, 1985.

CHAPTER
14

ESSENTIAL EXOGENOUS SUBSTANCES

VITAMINS: INTRODUCTION

Lalita Kaul and Yousef Tizabi

Vitamins are essential diverse organic substances that the body lacks or cannot synthesize in adequate amounts and therefore depends on exogenous sources for their supply. Vitamin deficiency may result from inadequate intake (poor diet, e.g., of alcoholics), malabsorption, or increased metabolic need. The significance of vitamins was probably realized as early as the middle of the sixteenth century. It was noted then that lemon juice could be used with remarkable success as an antiscorbutic agent in sailors who were kept on monotonous diets at sea for relatively long periods of time. However, the term *vitamine* was introduced with the discovery of thiamine during the first decade of the twentieth century. This term was derived on the false notion that all these essential substances contained amines; hence, vitamine, or vital amine. The final "e" was dropped later to preserve the nomenclature yet to repudiate the amine theory.

For simplicity, vitamins have been classified into two groups: (1) water-solubles (e.g., vitamins B complex and C which are little stored in the body); (2) fat-solubles (e.g., vitamins A, D, E, and K which are stored by the body). These groups are discussed in the following two chapters.

It has been the general belief that vitamins can only be beneficial to health if taken in large doses. This has been the cause of several toxic symptoms that have come to the attention of the medical profession as well as the public recently. It is therefore very important to consider the risk-benefit ratio in prescribing high-dose vitamin supplementation in cases where the actual deficiency or proof of efficacy is lacking.

CHAPTER
14.1

VITAMINS: FAT SOLUBLE

Lalita Kaul and Yousef Tizabi

The fat-soluble vitamins include vitamins A, D, E, and K. Vitamin D has been discussed separately in Chapter 12.2; the remaining vitamins will be discussed in this chapter.

VITAMIN A

History. In 1913 two groups (McCollum and Davis; Osborne and Mendel) independently reported that rats failed to grow and developed necrosis of the cornea when they were fed diets containing carbohydrate, protein, lard, and salts. When an ether extract of butter or egg yolk was added to the diet, growth resumed and the eye condition was corrected. Drummond later suggested that this fat-soluble factor be named vitamin A.

In 1919, Steenbock demonstrated an association between vitamin A and plants containing the yellowish color carotene pigment. A study conducted by Moore in 1930 showed that the carotenes were structurally related to vitamin A and were converted to the vitamin in the body. In 1933, Wald demonstrated a link between vitamin A and the visual process with the later discovery that rhodopsin, the pigment responsible for sight in dim light, contained vitamin A in combination with protein (40). His demonstration of the reactions involved in bleaching and regeneration of rhodopsin, won him the Nobel Prize for Medicine in 1967. Pure vitmain A was synthesized in 1947 by Isler and his colleagues. In 1950, Karrer and Inhoffen reported the synthesis of β-carotene, and 2 years later Farrar and associates prepared vitamin A_2.

Sources. The animal sources of vitamin A are liver, kidney, butter, whole milk, and eggs. One of the richest sources of vitamin A is fish liver oils, but these are primarily used as supplements. Margarine and skimmed milk are fortified with vitamin. A.

The major sources of carotene are yellow and green vegetables and fruits. Vitamin A content of fruits and vegetables is generally proportional to the intensity of color; thus, the deeper the green or yellow, the higher the vitamin A content.

Chemistry. Pure vitamin A is a pale yellow crystalline compound that exists in nature in several forms, as shown in Fig. 14.1-1. It occurs largely as retinol (vitamin A_1), a primary alcohol that is found in mammals and saltwater fish, mainly in the liver. Another structurally similar compound, 3-dihydroretinol (vitamin A_2), usually occurs mixed with retinol in tissues of freshwater fish. Vitamin A is soluble in fat and fat solvents but insoluble in water; it is relatively stable to heat and to acids, but is easily oxidized. Rapid destruction occurs on exposure to high temperatures in the presence of air, by ultraviolet irradiation, or in rancid fats. The β-ionone ring (as in retinol) or a more unsaturated ring (as in 3-dehydroretinol) is essential for vitamin A activity. *In vivo,* retinol is converted to retinaldehyde (retinal), which has been isolated from the retina of the eye. In this form, the vitamin functions in dark adaptation. Retinal may be further oxidized irreversibly to retinoic acid which does not have any significant role in the visual process (see Fig. 14.1-2).

In plants, vitamin A exists mainly as β-carotene, the structure of which is given in Fig. 14.1-1. Upon hydrolysis, each molecule of β-carotene should theoretically yield two molecules of vitamin A. The actual biological activity between the chemical structure and the biological activity is due partly to inefficiency of carotene absorption and partly to the oxidation of some of the retinal formed from carotene to retinoic acid.

Measurement. Vitamin A is measured in international units (IU). The equivalents are:

1 IU = 0.3 μg retinol = 0.6 μg β-carotene = 1.2 μg other carotenoids. Recently, the Food and Nutrition Board has recommended that retinol equivalents (RE) should be used in place of IU because this method of measurement takes into account the amount of absorption of the carotenes and the degree of conversion to vitamin A. These equivalents are:

1 RE = 1 μg retinol (3.33 IU) = 6 μg β-carotene (10 IU) = 12 μg other carotenoids (10 IU).

Functions. Vitamin A is necessary for growth, reproduction, maintenance of epithelial tissues, and normal vision.

One of the best defined roles of the vitamin is its requirement for normal vision (40). The human retina contains two photoreceptor systems: Rods which are sensitive to light of low intensity, and cones which receive

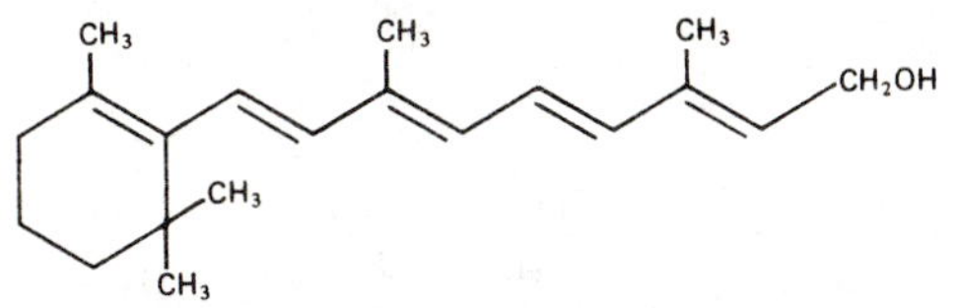

Vitamin A. [Retinol; 3,7-dimethyl-9-(2,6,6-trimethyl-1-cyclohexen-1-yl)-2,4,6,8-nonatetraen-1-ol.].

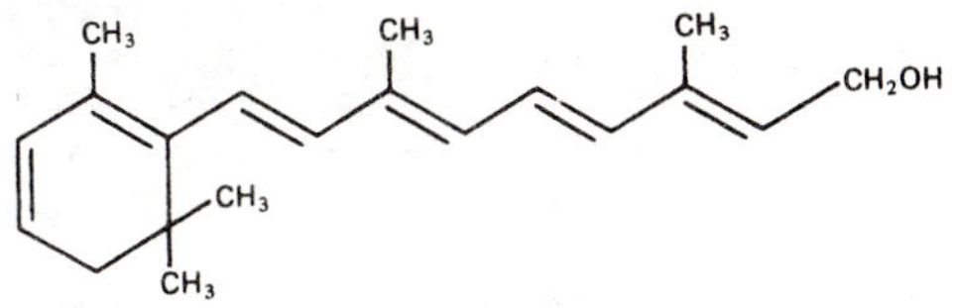

Vitamin A_2. (3,4-Didehydroretinol; retinol$_2$; dehydroretinol.)

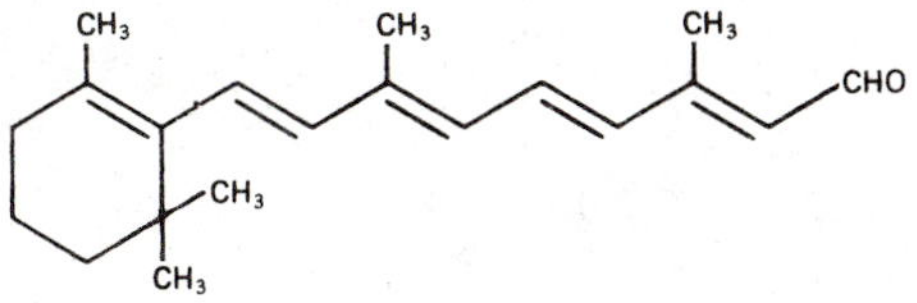

Vitamin A Aldehyde. (Retinal; retinaldehyde).

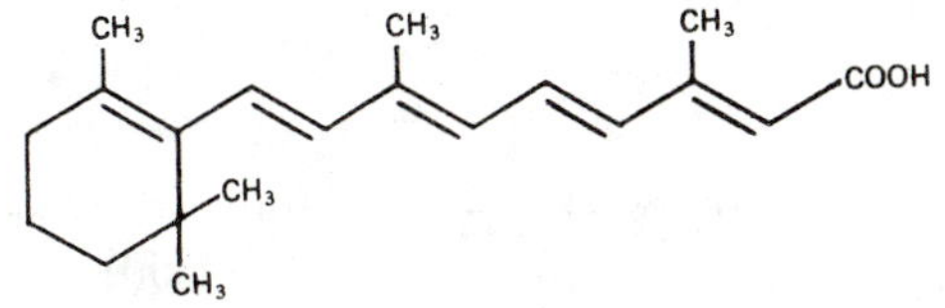

Retinoic acid

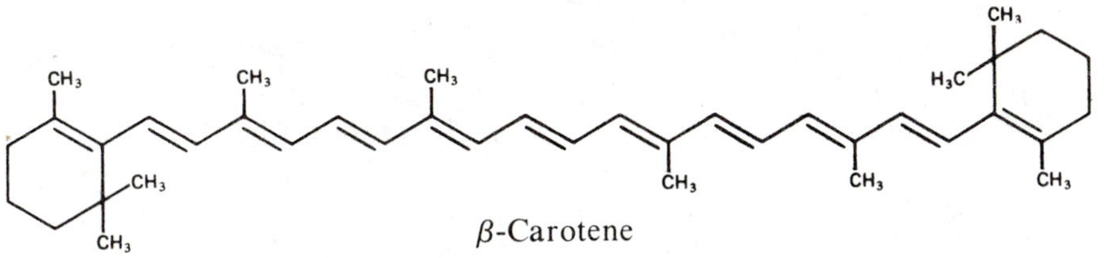

β-Carotene

Fig. 14.1-1. *Chemical structures of vitamin A and related compounds.*

light of high intensity and colors. Retinal is the prosthetic group of photosensitive pigments in both rods and cones. The major difference between the visual pigments in rods (rhodopsin) and cones (iodopsin) is due to the nature of the protein associated with retinal. Rhodopsin is bleached by light, causing the separation of protein and retinaldehyde in the all trans form. In the dark, the pigment is regenerated by the isomerization of retinaldehyde back to the *cis* form. In healthy persons, the rates of bleaching and regeneration are equal. Some retinaldehyde is lost in each cycle, and night blindness results when there is not sufficient vitamin A present for regeneration of the rhodopsin (Fig. 14.1-2 and 14.1-3).

Both retinol and retinal (retinaldehyde) will prevent night blindness, but as mentioned earlier, retinoic acid is not effective in this case. The role of vitamin A in the growth process is not very clear although its involvement in variation of metabolic reactions has been documented (41).

Studies on experimental animals have shown that vitamin A (with the exception of retinoic acid) is essential for spermatogenesis in the male and normal estrus cycle in the female. In humans, vitamin A has been shown essential for normal skeletal and tooth development, and seems to participate in the development of the enamel-forming cells of the teeth.

Vitamin A is necessary for the maintenance of the epithelial cells' integrity, thus its deficiency results in hard and dry epithelial tissues. This in turn may lower the body's resistance to infection (37). Vitamin A may also have a role in maintaining the immune competence of the individual (5, 20). It is possible that retinoids (synthetic as well as naturally occurring vitamin A compounds) may act through glycoprotein formation mechanism or by affecting the gene expression of the target cells (15).

Absorption, Transport, and Storage. Dietary vitamin A (*cis*-retinyl ester) is hydrolyzed in the intestinal tract to retinol and then passes across the mucosal wall of the cell. Within the cell, retinol combines with palmitic acid. Retinyl palmitate passes from the intestinal wall into the lymph system via the thoracic duct, then into the bloodstream, and finally into the liver.

β-Carotene is partly absorbed via the lymphatic system and is partly converted to vitamin A in the intestinal mucosa. The absorption of carotene and vitamin A from the intestinal wall is on the one hand adversely affected by the amount and the quantity of protein in the diet and on the other hand is facilitated by the dietary fat and bile secretion. The major pathways for biotransformation of vitamin A are summarized in Fig. 14.1-3.

About 95% of the body's vitamin A reserves are found in the liver; this normal supply will last for several months without any additional intake of the vitamin. In the bloodstream most of vitamin A circulates in a retinol-binding protein and retinol-prealbumin (transthyretin) complex, and some of it circulates in a lipoprotein complex (15). The plasma concentration of vitamin A is regulated by liver stores of the vitamin as well as the liver enzymes (23).

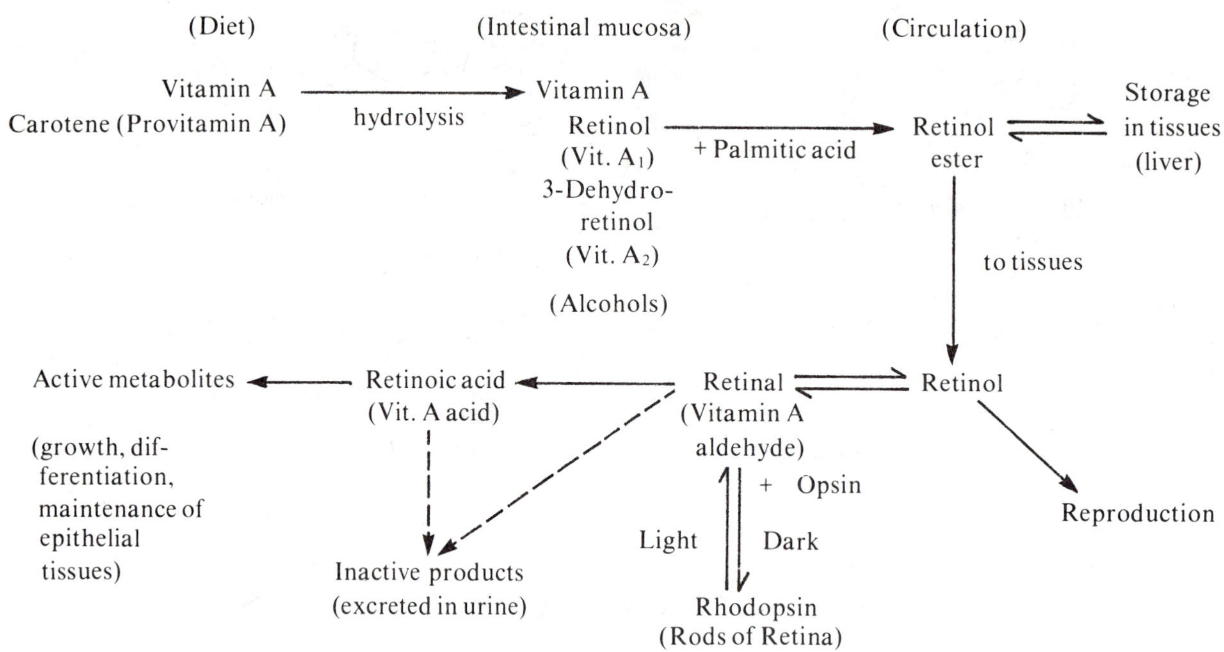

Fig. 14.1-2. *Major biotransformations of vitamin A in the body.*

Deficiency. Among the earliest signs of vitamin A deficiency are skin lesions, such as hyperkeratosis and infections. Skin becomes rough, dry, and scaly. Goose pimple-like follicles first appear on the upper forearms and thighs, and then spread along the shoulders, back, and abdomen. However, the most important manifestations of vitamin A deficiency are night blindness or nyctalopia and xerosis or drying of the conjuctiva (xerophthalmia). With continued deficiency, xerosis and distortion of the cornea occur. In untreated cases, the cornea undergoes degeneration, keratinization, and ulceration; such advanced changes are known as keratomalacia (26).

In addition to the skin and eye lesions, vitamin A deficiency may cause changes in the epithelial tissues throughout the body, with keratinization or hardening, the progressive degeneration of the cells, thus increasing susceptibility to severe infection of nasal passages, lungs, and genitourinary tract.

Adverse Effects. Overdose of vitamin A results in a serious condition known as hypervitaminosis A. The common symptoms of toxicity are anorexia, hyperirritability, fatigue, weight loss, headache, vomiting, abdominal pain, growth failure, xerosis, itching, hair loss, bone and joint pains, and drying and desquamation of the skin. Other manifestations include polydipsia, polyuria, enlargement of the liver, spleen, and lymph glands, hypercalcemia, hypoplastic anemia, leukopenia, decreased clotting time, and increased intracranial pressure. In the rat embryo, excess vitamin A is a known teratogen (22). Acute toxicity has been reported in Arctic explorers who consumed large quantities of polar bear liver. Several reports have shown acute hypervitaminosis A in infants due to single, massive doses of 1,300,000 IU or more of the vitamin (32).

Chronic hypervitaminosis A in adults has been reported in cases where more than 50,000 IU were ingested daily for months or years (6, 12). This condition occurs most frequently in patients who receive large doses of this vitamin as treatment for dermatological conditions and in food faddists who include large doses in their daily diet.

Massive doses of carotene are not converted to vitamin A rapidly enough to cause vitamin A toxicity, but can cause the skin to become yellow. It is thought that the vitamin A toxicity is mostly due to the retinal that circulates with lipoproteins and effects the cell membranes in a nonspecific manner (15).

Requirements. The recommended allowance for vitamin A for males over 11 years is 1000 RE or 3300 IU, for females over 11 years, 800 RE or 2640 IU. The requirement is greater in patients with diseases in which the absorption, storage, or mobilization of vitamin A is impaired or excretion of the vitamin has greatly increased.

Therapeutic Uses. Prophylactic doses of vitamin A are given during infancy, pregnancy, and lactation. It is recommended that infants should receive 400-700 RE of the vitamin daily. Pregnant and lactating mothers should receive additional 200 and 400 RE daily, respectively.

Vitamin A therapy may be used in conditions such as steatorrhea, cirrhosis of the liver, total gastrectomy, biliary obstruction, kwashiorkor, and infection of the respiratory tract (15). It has also been prescribed for the local

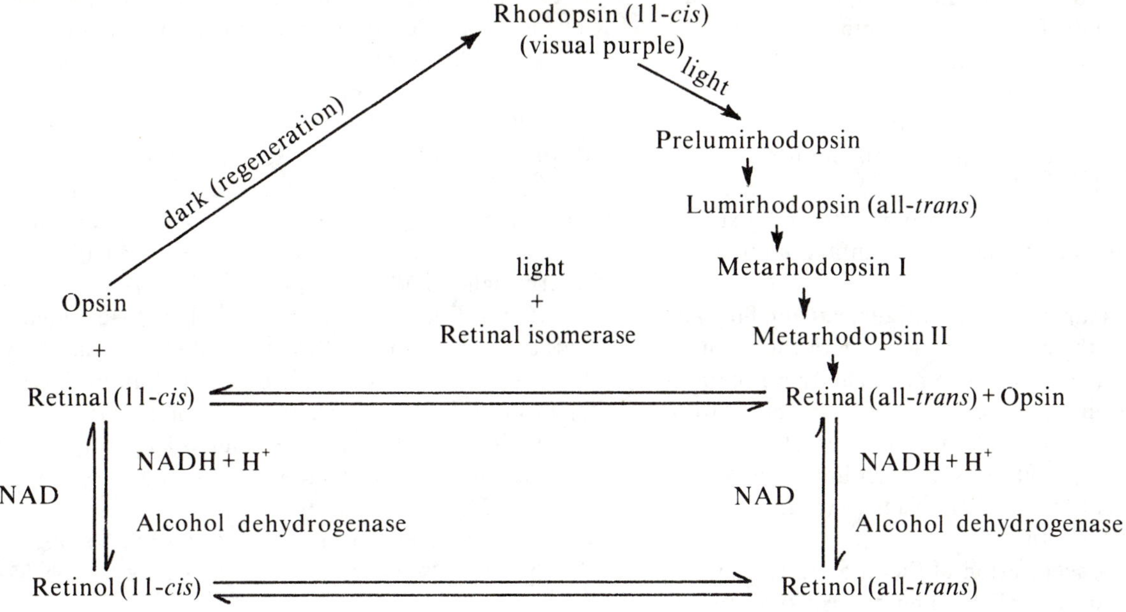

Fig. 14.1-3. *Role of vitamin A in visual cycle (32a).*

treatment of infections, burns, wounds, and acne vulgaris (15, 19).

Animal experiments have shown that retinol may be effective in the prevention of carcinomas; however, such use for the treatment of human carcinomas has been largely abandoned because of massive (toxic) dose requirement for any beneficial effect. The development of new synthetic retinoids may overcome this obstacle (15, 29, 42).

Preparations. Vitamin A capsules USP contain 1.5-15 mg of retinal or (5000-50,000 USP vitamin A units) per capsule. Tretinoin, USP (all *trans*-retinoic acid, RETIN A) for topical use in skin diseases as a 0.1% cream and a 0.05% lotion.

VITAMIN E

History. In 1922, Evans and Bishop discovered a fat-soluble substance, the absence of which from the rat diet caused irreparable damage of the germinal epithelium in males and termination of pregnancy in females (10). This substance necessary for reproduction was referred to as antisterility vitamin and was later called tocopherol (Greek: child bearings).

Sources. Vitamin E is found in a wide variety of foods. The principal sources are vegetable oils, whole grains, dark green vegetables, nuts, legumes, soybean, cottonseed, corn, sunflower, and wheat germ oils. Human milk also contains vitamin E which is at higher concentration than the cow's.

The amount of tocopherols present in oils is proportional to the amount of linoleic acid. There is considerable loss of vitamin E during food processing and storage, including freezing. The milling of grains removes about 80% of vitamin E; deep-fat frying also destroys some of the vitamin.

Chemistry. There are two families of vitamin E compounds. The first series (the tocopherols) derive from tocol which contains a 16-carbon saturated isoprenoid side chain. The second series (tocotrienols) contain three unsaturated side chains. Within each series, the compounds differ only in the number and position of methyl groups in the ring structure. Since α-tocopherol (5, 7, 8-trimethyl tocol) the structure of which is as follows, comprises about 90% of the tocopherols and shows the greatest biological activity in animal tissue, it is considered the most important tocopherol. The activity of tocopherols is affected by optical isomerism, thus the d-forms are more active than the l-forms. Vitamin E is stable to heat and acid but unstable to alkali, ultraviolet light, and oxygen.

Alpha-tocopherol

Measurement. Vitamin E is measured in international units or in milligrams of α-tocopherol. One IU of vitamin E is equivalent to 1 mg synthetic dl-2-tocopherol acetate. The activity of the natural form, d-α-tocopherol acetate, is 1.36 IU/mg.

Functions. The metabolic roles of vitamin E are not well understood, although the principal function appears to be that of an antioxidant that inhibits the oxidation of unsaturated fatty acids. Vitamin E helps to protect red blood cells against hemolysis by oxidizing agents. It also facilitates the absorption, storage, and utilization of vitamin A as well as counteracting some effects of hypervitaminosis A (2). Vitamin E is also required for the incorporation of pyrimidines into nucleic acid, especially in the formation of red blood cells in the bone marrow.

Because of the striking structural and biological similarity between vitamin E and some members of the coenzyme Q (quinone) groups, it has been suggested that vitamin E may be mimicking the action of this coenzyme (35). Coenzyme Q functions as an electron carrier in terminal electron transport and has an important role in oxidative phosphorylation. Vitamin E can be partially substituted for by selenium, chromanols, some sulfur-containing amino acids, and certain antioxidants found in food (3, 6, 39).

Absorption, Transport, and Storage. Fat and bile salts are essential for the efficient absorption of the vitamin, which is carried from the gastrointestinal tract in combination with the chylomicrons into the lymph circulation and to the liver. The adult plasma tocopherol level ranges from 0.5 to 1.2 mg/100 ml. Newborn infants have low tissue stores because of little transfer of vitamin E from the placenta to the fetus.

The highest concentration of the vitamin is found in the pituitary, adrenal gland, and testes, and storage occurs mostly in the muscle and adipose tissue.

Deficiency. In adults the incidence of vitamin E deficiency is rather rare because of the adequate nutritional supply and considerable storage of the vitamin. Clinical evidence of vitamin E deficiency has been noted mostly in premature infants (11, 16, 27) or in individuals, particularly children suffering from protein-calorie malnutrition, malabsorption syndromes, steatorrhea, celiac disease, lipoproteinemia, fibrocystic disease of the pancreas, and biliary atresia. The signs of vitamin E deficiency include: enhanced hydrogen peroxide hemolysis, creatinuria, and necrosis of striated muscle. Recently, reports of areflexia, gait disturbance, diminished proprioception, diminished vibrating sense, and ophthalmoplegia associated with vitamin E deficiency have appeared (4). Several studies have shown that infants consuming a formula with an inadequate dose of vitamin E become irritable and develop edema and anemia; treatment with vitamin E alleviates these symptoms (8).

Adverse Effects. No evidence of significant vitamin E toxicity in humans consuming up to 800 IU of the vitamin for more than 3 years has been detected. The most common complaints in such cases are those of gastrointestinal disturbances (e.g., diarrhea, nausea, and flatulence) which are transitory (4). Recently, reports of higher incidence of necrotizing enterocolitis in vitamin E-treated infants have appeared. It is therefore recommended that caution be exercised with regard to the use of high-dose vitamin E supplementation in premature infants (4, 36).

Requirements. The Food and Nutrition Board recommends 8 and 10 mg α-tocopherol for women and men, respectively.

The need for vitamin E is increased if the diet is high in polyunsaturaed fatty acids. At the present time, however, no recommendations have been made about the ratio of vitamin E to polyunsaturated fatty acids.

Therapeutic Uses. Vitamin E has been used at times in a wide range of conditions where adequate experimental evidence is lacking. Among these are: heart disease, muscular dystrophy, fibrositis, Dupuytren's contracture, scleroderma, lupus erythematosus, acne, menopausal disorders, senile vaginitis, sexual impotence, nephritis, diabetes, ulcer, wound healing, and others (4, 18, 25, 29, 34). At present, however, there is enough evidence to support prolonged vitamin E treatment in patients with intermittent claudication (4, 29).

Vitamin E has been shown to reduce the incidence of induced tumors in some animal studies (7). This has been the rationale for using large doses of vitamin E in treatment of various cancers. However, most of the human studies have yielded negative results. Therefore convincing evidence for such modes of therapy are presently lacking (29, 42).

Preparations. Vitamin E, USP (AQUASOL E, E-FEROL, etc.), capules and tablets (30-1000 IU); injectable forms (100 or 200 IU/ml).

VITAMIN K

History. Vitamin K was discovered in 1935 by Dam, who observed that chickens maintained on a low-fat diet developed spontaneous bleeding. This fat-soluble substance, a dietary antihemorrhagic factor, was named vitamin K (koagulation vitamin). The purified compound was isolated from alfalfa in 1939 (38).

Sources. Alfalfa is the richest source of vitamin K. Leafy green vegetables, such as kale and spinach, are excellent sources of the vitamin. Cabbage, cauliflower, egg yolk, soybean oil, and liver are also good sources of the vitamin. In plants, vitamin K is present mostly in the green or photosynthetic portions.

Chemistry. In nature, vitamin K exists as phylloquinone (vitamin K_1) and menaquinone (vitamin K_2). Menadione (vitamin K_3), is a synthetic analog which is almost as active as the naturally occurring vitamins K_1 and K_2. Vitamin K_1 or phylloquinone, also known as phytonadione, is 2-methyl-3-phytyl-1-4-naphthoquinone. It is found in green plants and is the only natural vitamin K available for therapeutic use. Vitamin K_2 represents a series of compounds (the menaquinones) that contain polyunsaturated side chain with 30-45 carbon atoms comprised of 6-9 isoprenoid units (2-methyl-3-difarnesyl-) and that are synthesized by microorganisms including bacteria of the intestinal tract. Coprophagic animals may benefit from fecal vitamin K_2, which is largely of bacterial origin, but it is doubtful that the vitamin produced by the bacteria is directly absorbed. In ruminants, bacterial vitamin K may be absorbed directly and represents an important nutritional source of the vitamin.

The structures of vitamin K_1, K_2, and K_3 are given as follows:

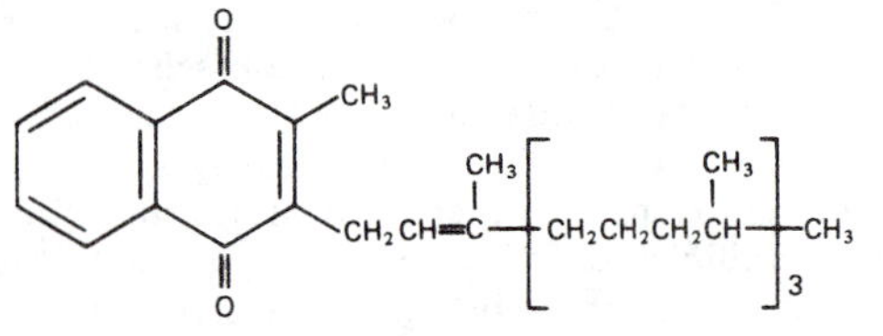

O, CH3, CH3, CH3, $CH_2CH{=}C{-}[CH_2CH_2CH_2CH]_3{-}CH_3$, O

Vitamin K_1 (2-Methyl-3-phytyl-1,4-naphthoquinone; 3-phytylmenadione; phytomenadione; phytonadione; phylloquinone).

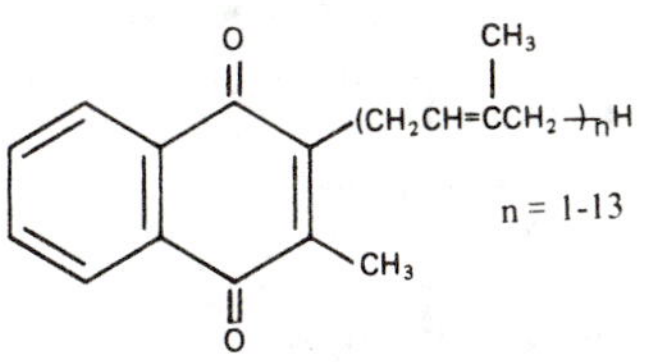

Vitamin K_2 (Menaquinone series)

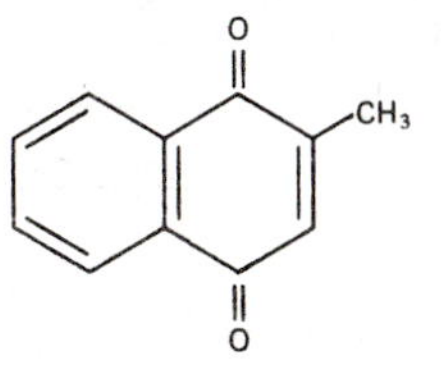

Vitamin K_3 (Menadione).

Vitamin K is stable to heat but easily destroyed by acid, alkali, light, and oxidizing agents.

Measurement. The biological activity is measured by the ability to prevent hemorrhage in young chicks. Menadione (vitamin K_3) is used as the standard for measuring vitamin K_1 and vitamin K_2 potency. Nonbiological methods of analysis include spectrophotometry, polarography, thin layer chromatography, and gas chromatography.

Functions. The primary function of vitamin K is the synthesis of prothrombin (factor II), proconvertin (factor VII), plasma thromboplastin component (PTC, Christmas factor, factor IX), and the Stuart-Prower factor (factor X), all of which are essential for the coagulation of blood (33, 38) (also see Chapter 15.6).

The precise biochemical role of vitamin K in the synthesis of blood coagulation factors remains unclear. Studies with actinomycin D have suggested that vitamin K is involved in the control of DNA-directed mRNA synthesis, and further experiments have shown that vitamin K acts at the ribosomal level or in the transformation of a precursor protein to a final product (24). The vitamin-dependent clotting factors are present in the liver as completed polypeptide chains. It has been suggested that vitamin K functions by attaching the carbohydrate moiety to the completed polypeptide chain of the glycoprotein, prothrombin (17). Vitamin K also seems to function in electron transport and oxidative phosphorylation (38).

Absorption, Transport, and Storage. The absorption of vitamin K occurs via the lymphatic system, and like other fat-soluble vitamins requires the presence of bile and pancreatic juice. Thus, obstruction of the bile duct will reduce the absorption of vitamin K. Also, the ingestion of mineral oil will cause greater excretion of the vitamin in the feces. As mentioned before, vitamin K can be synthesized by intestinal bacteria, and this is an additional source of the vitamin available to the host.

Deficiency. The first signs of vitamin K deficiency were observed in chicks: delayed blood clotting, hemorrhages under the skin, and internal bleeding. In humans, dietary deficiency of vitamin K is not likely, because it can be synthesized by intestinal bacteria and is provided in adequate amounts in the diet. The deficiency in adults is invariably caused by a failure in absorption, following long-term intravenous feeding, antibiotic use, obstruction of the biliary tract, and severe diarrhea. Low prothrombin levels can also be due to inability of the liver to synthesize this factor.

Vitamin K deficiency is frequently seen in newborn infants because of inadequacy of the vitamin present in mother's milk and lack of intestinal bacteria (1, 14). Infants whose mothers take anticoagulants are also likely to develop deficiency symptoms. Hemorrhagic disease of the newborn infant can be prevented by administering a single dose of vitamin K_1 immediately after birth. The practice of giving vitamin K to the mother prior to delivery is not recommended because excessive dosage leads to hemolytic anemia in the infant.

Dicumarol, an anticoagulant (Chapter 15.6) frequently used to treat coronary thrombosis, prevents the formation of prothrombin and carries the risk of hemorrhage. Vitamin K may be given to counteract the excessive intake of the anticoagulant.

Adverse Effects. Large doses of menadione have produced toxic symptoms in rats and jaundice in human infants. Also hemolytic anemia, hyperbilirubinemia, and kernicterus in premature and newborn infants have been observed following large doses of vitamin K_3. Phytonadione and the menaquinones have not exhibited signs of toxicity. However, phytonadione may cause flushing, cyanosis, shock, hypersensitivity, or anaphylactic reactions in i.v. administration.

Requirements. No dietary allowances have been established because of the variations in intestinal synthesis and the adequate presence of the vitamin in the diet.

The minimum requirement for patients with vitamin K deficiency due to antibiotic therapy is approximately 0.03-15 μg/kg of body weight daily.

Therapeutic Uses. Vitamin K is the most effective antidote to hemorrhage due to coumarin overdosage. It may also be used in the newborns as prophylactic or therapeutic treatment of hemorrhagic disorders associated with hypoprothrombinemia. Since vitamin K has been shown to inhibit the growth of tumor cells in culture (30) and to interfere with normal leukocyte function *in vitro* (13), future therapeutic uses in control of tumors might prove feasible.

Preparations. Phytonadione, USP (vitamin K_1, phylloquinone, AQUAMEPHYTON, KONAKION, MEPHYTON): tablets (5 mg); ampules (2 or 10 mg/ml) of phytonadione, dispersed in a solution of buffered polysorbate and propylene glycol (KONAKION, given i.m. only), or in polyethylated fatty acid derivatives and dextrose (AQUAMEPHYTON, given by any parenteral route).

Menadione, USP (vitamin K_3): tablets (5 mg); solution in oil (25 mg/ml, for i.m. injection). Menadione sodium bisulfite, USP (HYKINONE): tablets (5 mg); ampules (5-10 mg/ml). Menadiol sodium diphosphate, USP (KAPPADIONE, SYNKAVITE): tablets (5 mg); injection (5, 10, or 37.5 mg/ml).

DRUG INTERACTIONS

Interaction of various drugs with vitamins A, D, and K are summarized in Table 14.1-1.

Table 14.1-1
Interaction of Various Drugs with Fat-Soluble Vitamins Altering Their Requirements

Vitamins	Interacting Drug	Possible Mechanisms	Possible Symptoms
A, D, K	Mineral oil	Lipid solvent interferes with absorption	Rickets for vitamin D
A, D, K	Cholestyramine	Interferes with action of bile salts and reduces uptake of fat-soluble vitamins	
A	Neomycin	Causes damaged intestinal wall; inhibits pancreatic lipase; binds bile salts	
D	Glutethimide	Causes enzymes induction probably due to similarity of structure to phenobarbital	Osteomalacia
D	Irritant cathartics	Increase peristalsis; damages intestinal wall	Osteomalacia
D, K	Anticonvulsant	Induces certain enzymes, increasing breakdown of vitamins and (in case of vitamin D) its active metabolite	
K	Broad-spectrum antibiotics	Reduces formation of vitamin K in the distal part of small intestine	Scanty clinical evidence
K	Salicylates Cinchona alkaloids	Cause not known; act synergistically with coumarin vitamin K antagonists	

Source: Ref. 28.

REFERENCES

1. Aballi, A. J. Vitamin K and the newborn. *Lancet* 1:1358, 1978.
2. Bauernfeind, J. C., Newmork, H., and Brin, H. Vitamin A and E nutrition via intramuscular or oral route. *Am. J. Clin. Nutr.* 27:234, 1974.
3. Bieri, J. G. In: *Present Knowledge in Nutrition.* Washington, D.C.: The Nutrition Foundation, 1876, p. 98.
4. Bieri, J. G., Gorash, L., and Hubbard, V. S. Medical uses of vitamin E. *N. Engl. J. Med.* 308:1063, 1983.
5. Brown, K. H., Rajan, M. M., Chakraborty, J., and Aziz, K. M. A. Failure of a large dose of vitamin A to enhance the antibody response to tetanus toxoid in children. *Am. J. Clin. Nutr.* 33:212, 1980.
6. Committee on Drugs and on Nutrition. American Academy of Pediatrics. The use and abuse of vitamin A. *Nutr. Rev.* (Suppl. 1) 32:41, 1974.
7. Cook, M. G., and McNamara, P. Effect of dietary vitamin E on dimethylhydrazine-induced colonic tumors in mice. *Cancer Res.* 40:1329, 1980.
8. Dicks-Bushnell, M. V., and Davis, K. C. Vitamin E content of infant formulas and cereals. *Am. J. Clin. Nutr.* 20:262, 1967.
9. Drape, H. H., and Csallary, A. S. Metabolism and function of vitamin E. *Fed. Proc.* 28:1690, 1969.
10. Evans, H. M. The pioneer history of vitamin E. *Vit. Horm.* 20:379, 1963.
11. Farrell, P. M. Vitamin E deficiency in premature infants. *J. Pediatr.* 95:869, 1979.
12. Fisher, G., and Skillern, P. G. Hypercalcemia due to hypervitaminosis A. *JAMA* 227:1413, 1974.
13. Gallin, J. I., Seligmann, B. E., Cramer, E. B., Schiffmann, E., and Fletcher, M. P. Effects of vitamin K on human neutrophil function. *J. Immunol.* 128:1399, 1982.
14. Goldman, H. I., and Amadio, P. Vitamin K deficiency after the newborn period. *Pediatrics* 44:745, 1969.
15. Goodman, S. D. Vitamin A and retinoids—health and disease. *N. Engl. J. Med.* 310:1023, 1984.
16. Hassan, H., Hashim, S. A., Van Itallie, T. B., and Sebrell, W. H. Syndrome in premature infants associated with low plasma vitamin E levels and high polyunsaturated fatty acid diet. *Am. J. Clin. Nutr.* 19:147, 1966.
17. Johnson, H. V., Martinovic, J., and Johnson, B. C. Vitamin K and the biosynthesis of the glycoprotein in prothrombin. *Biochem. Biophys. Res. Commun.* 43:1040, 1971.
18. King, R. A. Vitamin E therapy in Dupuytren's contracture. *J. Bone Joint Surg.* 31B:443, 1949.
19. Klegman, A.M., Mills, O.H., Leyden, J.J., Gross, P.R., Allen, H.B., and Rudolph, R.I. Oral vitamin A in acne vulgaris. Preliminary report. *Int. J. Dermatol.* 20:278, 1981.
20. Krishnan, S., Bhuyan, U. N., Tawlar, G. P., and Ramaligaswami, V. Effects of vitamin A and protein-calorie malnutrition on immune responses. *Immunology* 27:383, 1974.
21. March, B. E., Wong, E. Seier, L. et al. Hypervitaminosis E in the chick. *J. Nutr.* 103:371, 1973.
22. Morris, G. M. Vitamin A and congenital malformations. *Int. Zeitschrift Vitamin Errahrungsforschung* 46:220, 1972.
23. Olson, J. A., Gunning, D., and Tilton, R. The distribution of vitamin A in human liver. *Am. J. Clin. Nutr.* 32:2500, 1979.
24. Olson, R. E. Studies of the *in vitro* biosynthesis of vitamin K-dependent clotting proteins. In: *The Fat-Soluble Vitamins* (DeLuca, H. F., and Suttie, J. W., eds.). Madison: University of Wisconsin Press, 1970, p. 463.
25. Olson, R. E. Vitamin E and its relation to heart disease. *Circulation* 48:179, 1973.
26. Oomen, H. A. P. C. Vitamin A deficiency, xerophthalmia, and blindness. *Nutr. Rev.* 32:161, 1974.
27. Oski, F. A., and Barnes, L. A. Vitamin E deficiency: A previously unrecognized cause of hemolytic anemia in premature infants. *J. Pediatr.* 70:211, 1967.
28. Ovesen, L. Drugs and vitamin deficiency. *Drugs* 18:278, 1979.

29. Ovesen, L. Vitamin therapy in the absence of obvious deficiency. What is the evidence? *Drugs* 27:148, 1984.

30. Prasad, K. N., Prasad, E. J., and Sakamoto, A. Vitamin K_3 (menadione) inhibits the growth of mammalian tumor cells. *Life Sci.* 29:1387, 1981.

31. Pike, R. L., and Brown, M. L. *Nutrition; An Integrated Approach,* 2nd ed. New York: Wiley, 1975, p. 147.

32. Review: Vitamin A intoxication in infancy. *Nutr. Rev.* 23:263, 1965.

33. Review: Vitamin K and prothrombin structure. *Nutr. Rev.* 32:279, 1974.

34. Roberts, H. J. Vitamin E and thrombophlebitis. *Lancet* 1:49, 1978.

35. Smith, J. L., Bhagavan, H. N. Hill, R. B., Gaetani, S. et al. Biological activities of compounds in the vitamin E, vitamin K and enzyme Q groups in chicks, rabbits and rats. *Arch. Biochem. Biophys.* 101:388, 1963.

36. Sobel, S., Gueriguian, J., Troendle, G., and Nevius, E. Vitamin E in retrolental fibroplasia. *N. Engl. J. Med.* 306:867, 1982.

37. Somer, A., Hussaini, G., Tarwotjo, I., and Susanto, D. Increased mortality in children with mild vitamin A deficiency. *Lancet* 2:585, 1983.

38. Suttie, J. W. Vitamin K and prothrombin synthesis. *Nutr. Rev.* 31:105, 1973.

39. Tappel, A. L. Lipid peroxidation damage to cell components. *Fed. Proc.* 32:1870, 1973.

40. Wald, G. The biochemistry of vision. *Ann. Rev. Biochem.* 22:497, 1953.

41. Wasserman, R. H., and Corradine, R. A. Metabolic role of vitamin A and D. *Ann. Rev. Biochem.* 40:501, 1971.

42. Willett, W. C., Polk, B. F., Underwood, B. A., Stampfer, M. J. et al. Relation of serum vitamins A and E and carotenoids to the risk of cancer. *N. Engl. J. Med.* 310:430, 1984.

CHAPTER
14.2

VITAMINS: WATER SOLUBLE

Lalita Kaul and Yousef Tizabi

VITAMIN B COMPLEX

The original vitamin B, distinguished from the antiscorbutic vitamin (vitamin C), was actually comprised of a group of different substances that were later identified and named appropriately. This section discusses the components of vitamin B complex with the exception of vitamin B_{12} (cyanocobalamin) and folic acid (pteroylglutamic acid) which are covered in Chapter 15.7.

THIAMINE (VITAMIN B_1)

History. In the late nineteenth century, Takaki demonstrated that the incidence of beriberi, a form of polyneuritis in the Japanese navy, could be markedly reduced by the addition of fish, meat, and whole grains to the customary naval ration of polished rice (40). In 1847, Eijkman demonstrated that beriberi could be cured by the addition of the rice polishings to the diet. In 1911, Funk isolated the active factor in a concentrated form and coined the term vitamine to refer to a class of essential food factors. In 1926, crystalline thiamine was isolated from rice polishings, and 10 years later its structure was determined (48).

Sources. Rich sources of thiamine include lean pork, liver, dry beans and peas, soybeans, whole grains, and enriched breads and cereals. Brewer's yeast and wheat germ are excellent sources of thiamine, but do not form an important part of most American diets. Egg yolk, milk, and green leafy vegetables are also fair sources of thiamine.

Chemistry. The thiamine molecule is composed of a pyrimidine and a thiazole (Fig.14.2-1).

Thiamine is available commercially as both hydrochloride and mononitrate. Thiamine hydrochloride is a crystalline white powder with a faint yeast-like odor and a salty, nutlike taste.

Thiamine is stable in dry heat and acid solution but decomposes rapidly in alkaline solution. The mononitrate salt is more heat stable than the hydrochloride.

Functions and Mechanism of Action. Thiamine functions as part of the coenzyme thiamine pyrophosphate (TPP), also known as cocarboxylase. TPP is required for the oxidative decarboxylation of α-keto acids, including pyruvate and α-ketoglutarate, and for transketolase functions in the pentose phosphate pathway. It also serves as a cofactor in the condensation of glyoxylate and α-ketoglutarate to form 2-hydroxy-3 ketoadipate (48) (Table 14.2-1).

Thiamine exerts specific effects in nerve tissue that are independent of its coenzyme function. It has been shown that stimulation of nerve fibers results in release of free thiamine and thiamine monophosphate (19). In cultured glial cells thiamine deficiency impairs synthesis of fatty acids and cholesterol. This defect could be the basis of degenerative changes seen in glial cells in early thiamine deficiency (28).

Absorption, Transport, and Storage. The absorption of thiamine takes place principally in the upper part of the duodenum. The total amount of thiamine in the human body is approximately 30 mg, with the liver, kidney, heart, brain, and muscles having higher concentrations than the blood. Excess thiamine is excreted in the urine. When thiamine intake is very low, little or none is excreted.

Deficiency. The early symptoms of thiamine deficiency include fatigue, irritability, depression, anorexia, and loss of weight and strength. The increasing deficiency affects the gastrointestinal, cardiovascular, and peripheral nervous systems. The patient may complain of indigestion, constipation, headaches, insomnia, and tachycardia after moderate exercise and cramping of the calf muscles with burning and numbness.

Severe thiamine deficiency leads to the condition called beriberi, the chief symptoms of which are polyneuritis. Beriberi may occur in dry or wet form. Dry beriberi

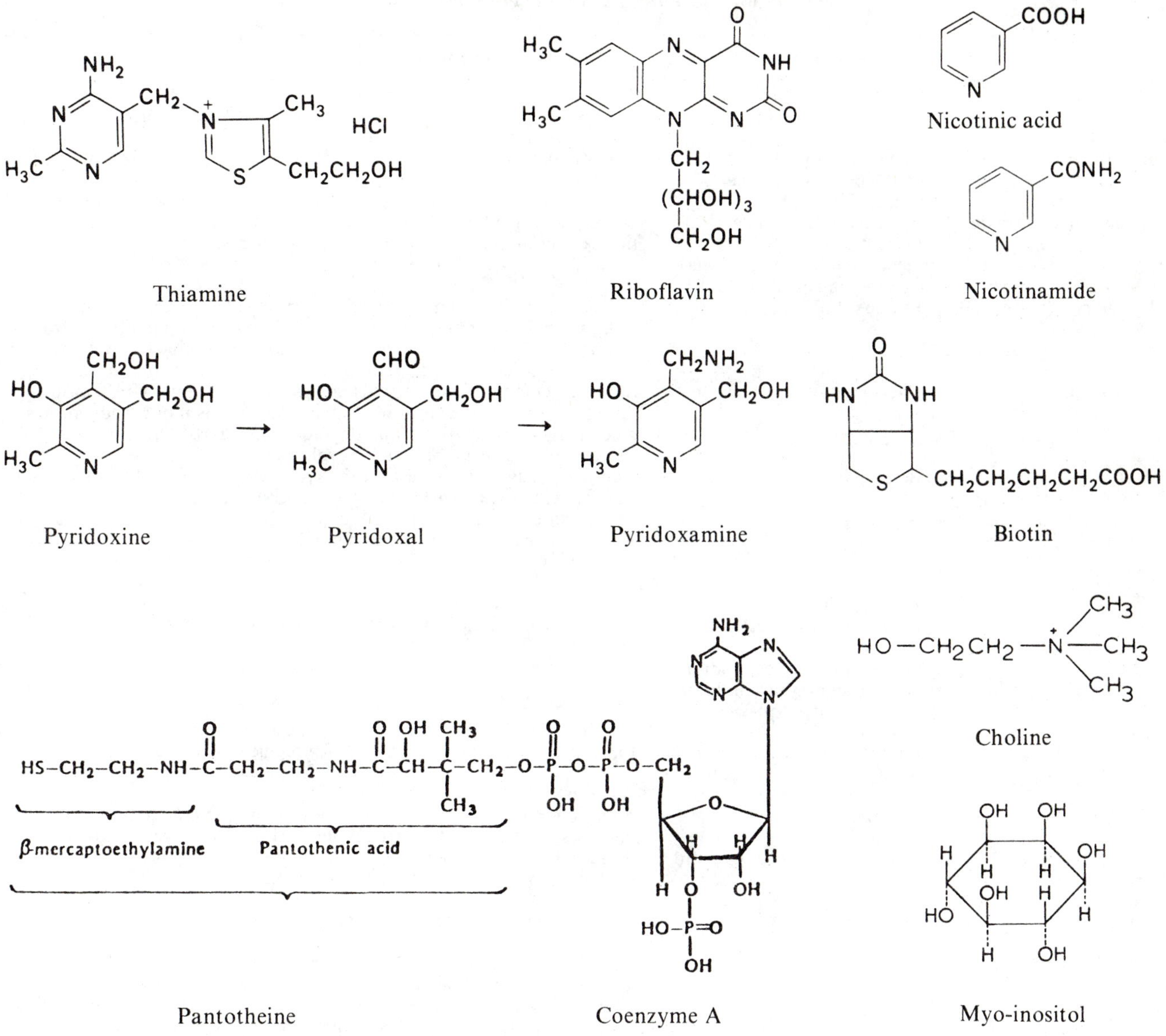

Thiamine

Riboflavin

Nicotinic acid

Nicotinamide

Pyridoxine → Pyridoxal → Pyridoxamine

Biotin

Pantotheine

Coenzyme A

Choline

Myo-inositol

Fig. 14.2-1: *Chemical structures of components of vitamin B complex and related compounds.*

is characterized by nervous lesions accompanied by emaciation. Wet beriberi, on the other hand, is characterized by severe edema that masks the emaciation, but may be associated with cardiac failure. The symptoms of infantile beriberi, as frequently seen in the Far East, are facial edema, irritability, vomiting, abdominal pain, loss of voice, and convulsions (47).

One of the serious complications of alcoholism associated with severe thiamine deficiency is Wernicke's encephalopathy. Certain signs of this syndrome, notably ophthalmoplegia, nystagmus and ataxia, respond well to prompt treatment with thiamine. However, Wernicke's syndrome is usually accompanied by Korsakoff's psychosis which is characterized by impairment in learning and memory; these changes are usually irreversible.

Determination of the activity of erythrocyte transketolase enzyme is useful in detecting marginal thiamine deficiency before clinical signs become apparent (5).

Requirements. The minimum requirement for thiamine is about 0.35 mg/1000 kcal, and the recommended allowance is 0.5 mg/1000 kcal. The daily allowance for men aged 23-50 years is 1.4 mg and for women of the same age is 1 mg.

Adverse Effects. Although there is a limited number of reports on adverse effects of thiamine in humans, starting at approximately 125-350 mg/kg dosage, the following

Table 14.2-1
Water-Soluble Vitamins and Their Mechanism of Action

Vitamin	Active Form	Mechanism of Action
Thiamine (vitamin B_1)	Thiamine pyrophosphate	Acts as coenzyme to (1) decarboxylase for α-keto acids (i.e., pyruvate and α-ketoglutarate), (2) transketolase for utilization of pentose in the hexose monophosphate shunt
Riboflavin (vitamin B_2)	Flavin mononucleotide (FMN); flavin adenine dinucleotide (FAD)	Acts as enzyme to a variety of respiratory enzymes; oxidizes reduced pyridine nucleotides (NAD)
Niacin (nicotinamide)	Nicotinamide adenine dinucleotide (NAD); nicotinamide adenine dinucleotide phosphate (NADP)	Serves as coenzyme for a wide variety of enzymes that catalyze oxidation-reduction reactions essential for tissue respiration
Pyridoxine (vitamin B_6)	Pyridoxal phosphate	Acts as coenzyme for amino acid decarboxylation, transamination, as well as other metabolic conversions involving tryptophan (to hydroxytryptamine, xanthurenic acid, and others), methionine (to cysteine), and other sulfur-containing amino acids and hydroxyamino acids
Pantothenic Acid	Coenzyme A	Serves as cofactor for enzyme-catalyzed reactions involving transfer of acetyl (two-carbon) groups in oxidative metabolism of carbohydrates, gluconeogenesis, synthesis and degradation of fatty acids, synthesis of sterols, steroid hormones, and porphyrins
Biotin	Biotin	Acts as coenzyme for several carboxylase enzymes (involving CO_2 fixation) (e.g., pyruvate carboxylase and acetyl coenzyme A carboxylase)
Choline	Choline	Acts as methyl donor (supplies methyl group to homocysteine to form methionine); affects mobilization of fat from the liver (lipotropic action)
	Acetylcholine	Serves as neurotransmitter
	Phospholipids (such as lecithin), plasmalogen (abundant in mitochondria) and sphingomyelin (in brain) and lipoprotein (plasma)	Serve as structural components of biological membranes and plasma lipoproteins
Inositol	Inositol	Lipotropic action on fatty liver and intestine
	Phosphatidylinositol in phospholipids (cell membrane) and lipoprotein (plasma)	Important structural component of biological membrane and tissues
Cyanocobalamin (vitamin B_{12})	Methylcobalamin	Acts as methyl donor for conversion of homocysteine to methionine; interacts with intracellular metabolic pathways that involve folate
	5-Deoxyadenosyl cobalamin	Required for the isomerization of L-methylmalonyl CoA to succinyl CoA needed for lipid and carbohydrate metabolism
Folic acid	Folinic acid	Acts as coenzyme for transmethylation: required for (1) synthesis of nucleoproteins, (2) maturation of red blood cells
Ascorbic acid (vitamin C)		Functions in a number of biochemical reactions, mostly involving oxidation e.g., facilitation of conversion of certain proline residues to hydroxyproline in collagen synthesis; oxidation of lysine to provide hydroxytrimethyllysine for carnitine synthesis; coenzyme for dopamine-β-hydroxylase Acts in synthesis of steroids by the adrenal cortex Acts in conversion of folic acid to folinic acid Facilitates microsomal drug metabolism Protects p-hydroxyphenylpyruvic acid oxidase from inhibition by its substrate tyrosine in tyrosine metabolism

symptoms may be manifested: edema, nervousness, tremor, sweating, tachycardia, vascular hypotension, herpes, allergic reactions and fatty liver (21).

Therapeutic Uses. Simple deficiency can be treated with moderate doses of thiamine. Some inborn errors of metabolism, however, respond to larger doses of thiamine. These include thiamine-responsive megaloblastic anemia, lactic acidosis, branched-chain ketoaciduria, and subacute necrotizing encephalomyelopathy. The Wernicke-Korsakoff's syndrome represents a very severe deficiency and daily doses of 100 mg should be administered intravenously (24).

Preparations. *Thiamine hydrochloride,* USP (viamine B_1 hydrochloride): white crystals or crystalline powder. Tablets, USP (5-500 mg); injection, USP (100 mg/5 ml); *thiamine mononitrate,* USP is used in some multivitamin preparations.

RIBOFLAVIN (VITAMIN B_2)

History. In 1932, Warburg and Christian isolated an enzyme from yeast that was necessary for cell respiration; the enzyme had two components: a protein and a yellow pigment. In 1933, Kuhn and his associates identified the heat-stable yellow pigment portion of the enzyme as flavin or vitamin B_2. The significance of flavin as an essential growth factor was demonstrated by György in 1954 (13). The vitamin was later termed riboflavin because of the presence of ribose in its structure.

Sources. Milk and milk products are excellent sources of riboflavin. Other sources include organ meats, eggs, lean meat, leafy green vegetables, and whole grain and enriched cereals.

Chemistry. Chemically, riboflavin is 6,7-dimethyl-9 (D-1-ribityl) isoalloxazine (Fig. 14.2-1). It is an orange-yellow crystalline substance, soluble in water or acid. The vitamin is destroyed in the presence of alkali or on exposure to ultraviolet light. Riboflavin is relatively stable to heat, especially in an acid solution.

Functions and Mechanism of Action. Riboflavin is a constituent of the coenzymes, flavin mononucleotide (FMN) and flavin adenine dinucleotide (FAD). These coenzymes, together with a number of oxidases, serve as carriers in electron transport. During this process, hydrogen is transferred from one compound to another until it reaches oxygen and forms water.

Riboflavin is also a part of L- and D-amino acid oxidases that oxidize amino acids and hydroxy acids to α-keto acids, and of xanthine oxidase that catalyzes the oxidation of a number of purines (32) (Table 14.2-1).

Absorption, Transport, and Storage. Riboflavin is phosphorylated and absorbed from the upper part of the small intestine. In the body tissues it is present as a coenzyme or as a flavoprotein. The major portion of the vitamin is stored in the liver, kidney, and heart.

Urinary excretion is proportional to the dietary intake of the vitamin, and increases markedly if intake exceeds 0.75 mg/1000 kcal.

Deficiency. The most characteristic signs of riboflavin deficiency are greasy dermatitis around the nose, cracking of the lips at the corners (cheilosis), glossitis, and increased vascularization of the cornea. The lips and tongue turn purplish red. The eyes become sensitive to light, and there is blurring of vision. Scrotal and vulvar lesions with scaly, pruritic dermatitis are also commonly seen (38). These conditions are followed by anemia and neuropathy. Deficiency may also appear in patients with severe gastrointestinal diseases that interfere with the absorption of the vitamin (32).

Requirements. The minimum requirement for riboflavin is 0.3 mg/1000 kcal. The recommended daily allowance for males 23-50 years is 1.6 mg and for females is 1.2 mg.

Adverse Effects. Riboflavin is essentially nontoxic in humans; however, isolated cases of paresthesia and itching may occur (21, 43).

Therapeutic Uses. To cure riboflavin deficiency disease, 5-10 mg of the vitamin is given orally every day. A parenteral route may be used if there is an absorption problem.

Drug Interactions. Thyroid and adrenal hormones regulate the enzymatic conversion of riboflavin into its active coenzyme derivatives. Interactions of phenothiazine, boric acid, and oral contraceptives (33) are summarized in Table 14.2-2.

NIACIN (NICOTINIC ACID)

History. In 1735, Casals described a disease, *mal de la rosa*, which later became known as pellagra (Italian for rough skin). In the early nineteenth century, pellagra was a leading cause of death in the United States, especially in the South.

In 1922, Goldberger concluded that black tongue in dogs was similar to pellagra in humans. In 1937, Elvehjem et al. discovered the effectiveness of nicotinic acid in curing black tongue in dogs (8). Following this discovery, Spies et al. reported dramatic clinical improvements in patients with pellagra by giving them nicotinic acid (39). The term niacin was suggested by Cowgill to avoid association with the nicotine to tobacco.

Sources. Tryptophan is a precursor of niacin (60 mg of tryptophan yields 1 mg of niacin). Some foods such as liver, lean meat, fish, and poultry are the chief sources of niacin and tryptophan. Milk is a poor source of preformed niacin but rich in trytophan. Plant sources of both niacin and tryptophan include beans, legumes, and nuts.

Chemistry. Niacin (pyridine-3-carboxylic acid) is easily converted to the physiologically active compound, nicotinamide (or niacinamide) (Fig. 14.2-1). The amide derivative is more soluble than niacin in both alcohol and water.

Functions and Mechanism of Action. Niacin serves as a component of the coenzymes nicotinamide adenine dinucleotide (NAD) and nicotinamide adenine dinucleotide phosphate (NADP). Like the flavin coenzymes, NAD and NADP function in the transfer of hydrogen and participate in biochemical reactions. For example, decarboxylation of pyruvic acid and the formation of acetyl coenzyme A require NAD, and dehydrogenation reactions in the Krebs cycle require both NAD and NADP. Some of the enzyme systems in which NAD participates are alcohol dehydrogenase, glyceraldehyde-3-phosphate dehydrogenase, lactic dehydrogenase, and glycerophosphate dehydrogenase. NAD and NADP are also involved in many other biochemical reactions.

Absorption, Transport, and Storage. Both niacin and niacinamide are well absorbed from the intestinal tract. There is a limited storage of the vitamin in the tissues, and the excess is excreted in the urine as N-methylnicotinamide and N-methyl pyridone. In the deficiency state, metabolites in the urine would be either decreased or absent.

Some nicotinamide is excreted into the gastrointestinal tract, where it is converted by intestinal bacteria to nicotinic acid; this may be absorbed and returned to the general circulation.

Deficiency. Clinical deficiency of niacin leads to the condition called pellagra characterized by the "three Ds": dermatitis, diarrhea, and dementia. Early signs include fatigue, headache, anorexia, and sore tongue, mouth, and throat. There is a characteristic symmetric dermatitis, especially on the exposed surfaces of the body, hands, forearms, elbows, feet, legs, knees, and neck. At first the skin becomes red, swollen, and tender. If the condition remains untreated, the skin becomes rough and ulcerated. Sunshine and exposure to heat aggravates the dermatitis.

The gastrointestinal symptoms include enteritis and diarrhea. The CNS effects are dizziness, depression, insomnia, delusions, hallucinations, and dementia. Motor and sensory disorders may also occur. As mentioned

Table 14.2-2
Interaction of Water-Soluble Vitamins with Various Selective Agents Increasing Their Requirements

Vitamin and Interacting Drug	Possible Mechanisms	Possible Symptoms
Thiamine (vitamin B_1)		
Estrogen-containing oral contraceptives	Reduced erythrocyte transketolase activity	
Manganese sulfate	Large concentration destroys vitamin B_1	
Riboflavin (vitamin B_2)		
Oral contraceptives	Reduced erythrocyte glutathione reductase activity	
Phenothiazines	Inhibited flavin coenzyme biosynthesis; increased vitamin excretion	
Boric acid	Formation of complex and increase of riboflavinuria	
Niacin		
Isoniazid	Reduced formation from tryptophan and inhibition of coenzyme function	Pellagra
Pyridoxine (vitamin B_6)		
Isoniazid	Hydrazone-vitamin complex formation; leading to increased urinary excretion; decreased production of pyridoxal phosphate (PP) and inhibition of PP-containing enzymes, and also direct toxic effect of complex on neural tissue.	Peripheral neuropathy
Penicillamine, hydralazine	?Complex formation and similar mechanism as that of isoniazid	Peripheral neuropathy
Levodopa	?Also enhanced decarboxylation of levodopa by vitamin	Burning feet syndrome; reduced effectiveness of levodopa in Parkinsonism
Oral contraceptives	Induction of tryptophan oxygenase; competition for binding sites on apoenzymes	Depression; also indicated by oral tryptophan load test
Folate		
Anticonvulsant	Decreased absorption (45); competitive inhibition of vitamin coenzymes; enzyme induction	Megaloblastic anemia
Methotrexate	Inhibits dihydrofolate reductase	Megaloblastic anemia (7, 45)
Pyrimethamine, triamterene, trimethoprim	Inhibit dihydrofolate reductase	Megaloblastic anemia, but not high risk
Oral contraceptives	Reduction of folate absorption by inhibiting peptidase activity; increase in synthesis of folate-binding macroglobin; enzyme induction accelerating folate metabolism	Megaloblastic anemia
Cholestyramine	Complex formation and decreased absorption	Reduction in serum folate level
Alcohol	Interference with absorption and transport of activated form; inhibition of the hemopoietic activity of folate (6, 29)	
Sulfasalazine (salicylazosulfapyridine)	Decreased absorption (due to associated diseased condition of intestines)	Low serum folate
Vitamin B_{12}		
Cholestyramine	Decreased absorption	
Neomycin	Damage to intestinal wall; inhibition of intrinsic factor function	
Potassium chloride (slow release)	Decreased absorption, probably due to decreased ileal pH	
Biguanides (metformin, phenformin), p-aminosalicylic acid, colchicine	Reduced absorption (41) possibly by inhibiting enzymes related to absorption	
Oral contraceptives	Possible altered tissue distribution	Low serum level
Vitamin C		
Oral contraceptives	Decreased absorption; increased plasma concentration of ceruloplasmin, which has ascorbate oxidase activity; increased concentration of reducing substances (glutathione); changes in tissue distribution	Lower plasma concentration
Salicylates	Reduced uptake in thrombocytes and leukocytes	Lowered plasma concentration
Tetracycline	Increased excretion	Reduced concentration in leukocytes

Source: Refs. 21 and 30.

earlier, tryptophan is a precursor for niacin. However, in carcinoid tumors the conversion of tryptophan to 5-hydroxytryptamine (serotonin) is favored over its conversion to nicotinic acid, and therefore symptoms of pellagra may be precipitated in carcinoid patients.

Requirements. The symptoms of pellagra can be prevented by daily intake of 4.4 mg of niacin per 1000 kcal. The recommended daily allowances are 18 mg for the adult male and 13 mg for the adult female.

Adverse Effects. Niacin has a limited adverse effect in humans with doses of 1-4 g/kg. The following effects may be observed: burning, itching, peripheral vasodilatation, hypotension, tachycardia, tachypnea, increased cerebral blood flow, decreased serum cholesterol, and fatty liver (21).

Therapeutic Uses. Niacin or niacinamide may be used prophylactically or therapeutically for treatment of pellagra. Niacinamide, however, is the preferred agent since it does not produce the flushing reactions or the tingling sensations caused by niacin. Large doses of niacin (3-6 g daily) reduce the plasma level of cholesterol, β-lipoproteins, and triglycerides (5, 27). However, prolonged usage of such a high dose may cause gastrointestinal irritation and liver damage (4). Niacin has also been used therapeutically to induce cerebrovascular dilatation in senile ataxia (5).

PYRIDOXINE (VITAMIN B_6)

History. In 1936, György coined the term vitamin B_6 for the factor which prevented acrodynia (skin lesions) in rats (14). The structure of the vitamin was elucidated in 1939 (15) and the Council on Pharmacy and Chemistry assigned the name pyridoxine to it.

Sources. Meat, poultry, and fish are the primary sources of vitamin B_6 and account for 45% of the total intake. Vegetables (particularly potatoes), dairy products, flour, and cereals are also rich in vitamin B_6. However, most of the pyridoxine content in whole grains is lost in the milling process.

Chemistry. Vitamin B_6 consists of a group of related pyridines: pyridoxine, pyridoxal, and pyridoxamine (Fig.14.2-1). These may appear in free form, or combined with phosphate, or with phosphate and protein.

Pyridoxine is soluble in water and less so in alcohol and acetone. It is stable to heat in acid solution, but is unstable to visible and ultraviolet light in neutral and alkaline solution.

Functions and Mechanism of Action. All three forms of vitamin B_6 are converted to pyridoxal phosphate by pyridoxal kinase. Pyridoxal phosphate acts as a cofactor for many enzymes involved in amino acid metabolism, including the conversion of tryptophan to 5-hydroxytryptamine and that of methionine to cysteine.

Pyridoxal phosphate is also required for the activity of glycogen phosphorylase, for the formation of antibodies, for the synthesis of δ-aminolevulinic acid, a precursor of heme, and possibly for the conversion of linoleic acid to arachidonic acid (9, 10).

Absorption, Transport, and Storage. All the three forms of the vitamin are readily absorbed from the gastrointestinal tract. In humans, pyridoxine and pyridoxamine may be converted to pyridoxal, which is then oxidized by hepatic aldehyde oxidase. The principal metabolite which is excreted in urine is 4-pyridoxic acid.

Deficiency. The tryptophan load test is frequently used to measure vitamin B_6 adequacy. Xanthurenic acid, an intermediary metabolite of tryptophan metabolism, is excreted in the urine when there is insufficient vitamin B_6. Reduced levels of serum and red blood cell transaminases and decreased excretion of pyridoxic acid are also indicative of the deficiency.

The deficiency symptoms of vitamin B_6 in adults include seborrheic dermatitis around the eyes, eyebrows, and the corners of the mouth. Deficiency of vitamin B_6 in infants causes nervous irritability, convulsive seizures, vomiting, weakness, ataxia, and abdominal pain (10, 26).

Requirements. The requirement for vitamin B_6 is proportional to the amount of protein metabolized. The recommended daily allowance of vitamin B_6 for women and men is 2 and 2.2 mg, respectively. This provides a margin of safety and allows a protein intake of 100 g. People who consume a low-protein diet require less vitamin B_6.

Drug Interactions. There are a number of compounds that interfere with the action of vitamin B_6. Thus, the use of isoniazid (INH) or cycloserine in the treatment of tuberculosis may cause peripheral neuritis that can be prevented by vitamin B_6 supplementation.

The requirement for vitamin B_6 is also increased during pregnancy or in women who use steroid contraceptives as well as in patients receiving penicillamine, hydralazine, corticosteroids (35).

Adverse Effects. Sensory neuropathy from daily ingestion of megadoses of vitamin B_6 (2 g or more) has recently been reported (36).

Therapeutic Uses. There is a very small group of vitamin B_6-dependent individuals who require 200-600 mg of pyridoxine hydrochloride daily to prevent convulsive seizures. Some cases of chronic anemia accompanied by hyperferremia and abnormal tryptophan metabolism also respond favorably to vitamin B_6 supplementation.

Preparations. *Pyridoxine hydrochloride,* USP, colorless or white crystals, or white crystalline powder. Tablets, USP, (5-100 mg); injection, USP (sterile solution of pyridoxine hydrochloride in water, 50 or 100 mg/ml).

BIOTIN

History. In 1936, Kögel and Tonnis isolated from egg yolk an active factor in crystalline form that they named biotin because it was needed for yeast growth and that also could protect against egg white toxicity. Biotin was synthesized in 1942 (23, 34).

Sources. Dietary sources include organ meats, egg yolk, legumes, and nuts.

Chemistry. Biotin is a monocarboxylic acid (Fig.14.2-1) resistant to heat, light, and weak acids. Three forms of biotin have been derived from natural sources. These are biocytin (ϵ-N-biotinyl-L-lysine) and the D and L sulfoxides of biotin. As a coenzyme, biotin is covalently linked to an ϵ-amino group of a lysine residue of the apoenzyme.

Functions and Mechanism of Action. As a coenzyme, biotin participates in carboxylation, decarboxylation, and deamination reactions. It is essential for the synthesis of fatty acids, fixation of CO_2 in the conversion of pyruvate to oxaloacetate, and the synthesis of purines. It is also required for the deaminases for threonine, serine, and aspartic acid (23) (Table 14.2-1).

Absorption, Transport, and Storage. Biotin is rapidly absorbed from the gastrointestinal tract, and because of minimal metabolism it appears in the urine in the intact form. Synthetic biocytin is hydrolyzed to biotin in the body. There is some storage of biotin in the kidneys, liver, brain, and adrenal glands. Intestinal bacteria also synthesize biotin.

Deficiency. Biotin deficiency does not occur frequently in humans but can be induced by ingestion of large quantities of raw egg whites as the main source of dietary protein. The egg whites contain avidin, a glycoprotein that binds biotin and prevents its absorption from the intestinal tract. Heating of the egg white inactivates avidin. Biotin deficiency symptoms include dermatitis, loss of hair, hyperesthesia, muscle pain, anorexia, slight anemia, hypercholesterolemia, and changes in the ECG (1).

Requirements. The requirements for biotin have not been established. The average American diet contains 150-300 μg of biotin, which is considered adequate by the Food and Nutrition Board (46).

Therapeutic Uses. Synthetic biocytin has been given in various conditions, but no beneficial results have been reported. The main therapeutic use of biotin has been in the treatment of infantile seborrhea and in the condition of genetic abnormality of biotin-dependent enzymes. In such cases 5-10 mg of biotin may be administered daily.

Preparations. Biotin is available commercially, although there is no USP preparation.

PANTOTHENIC ACID

History. Pantothenic acid, a substance essential for the growth of yeast, was identified in 1933 and was isolated in 1939 by R. J. Williams and associates. The name pantothenic (Greek word for from everywhere) signifies its wide distribution in nature. In 1950 Devries et al. showed pantothenic acid as the constituent of coenzyme A (49).

Sources. Most of the pantothenic acid in animals is found as a part of coenzyme A. Good food sources of the vitamin are whole grains, legumes, liver, yeast, egg yolk and meats. Significant amounts of the vitamin are lost from grains during milling and in dry processing of foods.

Chemistry. The pantothenic acid molecule consists of β-alanine and a hydroxyl- and methyl-substituted butyric acid, pantoic acid.

In the free form, pantothenic acid is an unstable, viscous yellowish oil that is soluble in water. Commercially it is available as a white crystalline calcium or sodium salt.

The structures of the vitamin and coenzyme A are presented in Fig. 14.2-1.

Functions and Mechanism of Action. As a part of coenzyme A, pantothenic acid is involved in transfer of acetyl groups and participates in the oxidation of pyruvate, α-ketoglutarate, and fatty acids. Coenzyme A is also important in the synthesis of cholesterol, other sterols, fatty acids, and porphyrin in the hemoglobin molecule (Table 14.2-1).

Absorption, Transport, and Storage. Pantothenic acid is readily absorbed from the gastrointestinal tract and is present in all tissues in concentrations from 2 to 45 μg/g.

Coenzyme A is synthesized in all cells. Liver, kidney, brain, adrenal, and heart tissues contain high concentrations of the vitamin.

Deficiency. Pantothenic acid deficiency is not frequently seen in humans but can be induced by feeding a semisynthetic diet, with or without pantothenic acid antagonists, such as ω-methyl-pantothenic acid. The symptoms include fatigue, malaise, headache, insomnia, nausea, abdominal and leg cramps, epigastric distress, and vomiting. The eosinopenic response to adrenocorticotropic hormone (ACTH) is impaired, and the sedimentation rate becomes elevated. There is also increased sensitivity to insulin.

It has been suggested that neuropathy observed in alcoholics is due to pantothenic acid deficiency (18).

Requirements. The daily requirement is not known. The Food and Nutrition Board suggests a daily intake of 5-10 mg of pantothenic acid.

Adverse Effects. Pantothenic acid is essentially nontoxic in humans except for increase in blood histamine and sensitivity of joints (21).

Therapeutic Uses. No therapeutic use has been recommended.

Preparations. *Calcium pantothenate,* USP tablets (10-250 mg); recemic calcium pantothenic, USP.

CHOLINE

History. Choline was first identified as a component of lecithin in 1862, and its lipotropic activity was demonstrated by Best and associates in 1932 (11). Besides its function in lipid metabolism, choline is also the precursor of acetylcholine. However, since choline has not been shown to act as a cofactor in any enzymatic reaction and because of lack of evidence of a choline deficiency syndrome in humans, there is some doubt whether choline may be regarded as a true vitamin.

Sources. Egg yolk is the richest source of choline. Legumes, organ meats, milk, muscle meats, and whole grain cereals are also good sources.

Chemistry. Choline, or trimethylethanolamine (Fig. 14.2-1), occurs in free form and as a component of lecithin and some of the plasmalogens and sphingomyelins. Choline can be synthesized in the body via methylation of phosphatidylethanolamine.

Functions and Mechanism of Action. Choline has an important role in the transport of fat as well as being a source of labile methyl groups. It is a part of lecithin, and is also the precursor of acetylcholine (Table 14.2-1).

Absorption, Transport, and Storage. Part of the choline administered orally to rats or humans is converted to trimethylamine and its oxide by intestinal bacteria before absorption. There is very little excretion in the urine.

Deficiency. Choline deficiency has not been demonstrated in humans. Its deficiency in rats causes fatty liver and renal degeneration, which can be prevented by other methyl donors (betaine and methionine) or by folic acid and vitamin B_{12} (11).

Requirements. Requirements for humans are not known. A typical American diet furnishes from 200 to 600 mg daily.

Therapeutic Uses. Choline in doses of 150-300 mg/kg has been used in the treatment of fatty liver and hepatic cirrhosis (11) as well as certain disorders of the nervous system such as tardive dyskinesia, Huntington's disease, Gilles de la Tourette's disease, Friedreich's ataxia, and presenile dementia (2, 12). However, it has not proven to be consistently effective in such disorders.

Preparations. Choline is not an official drug. It is, however, available as choline bitartrate, choline dihydrogen citrate, and choline chloride.

INOSITOL

History. In 1944, Walley recognized the importance of inositol in animal nutrition (25). In 1957, Eagle and associates demonstrated that inositol is an essential substance for the growth of all human as well as other animal cells in tissue culture. Again, for the same reasons as given for choline, there is some doubt whether inositol may be considered a true vitamin.

Sources. Inositol is found in fruits, vegetables, whole grains, meats, and milk.

Chemistry. Inositols are cyclic alcohols chemically related to the sugars (Fig. 14.2-1). There are seven optically inactive and one pair of optically active stereoisomeric forms of inositol. The optically inactive myoinositol is nutritionally active.

Functions and Mechanism of Action. Myoinositol is widely distributed in the human body and has been shown to exert a lipotropic action in patients with fatty infiltration of the liver (25) (Table 14.2-1).

Absorption, Transport, and Storage. Inositol is converted to glucose and vice versa. Inositol is only one-third as effective as glucose, however, in treating ketosis during starvation. The normal human plasma concentration is about 0.5 mg/100 ml of blood. There is very little excretion in the urine.

Deficiency. Deficiency symptoms have been observed in animals. In rats, the deficiency results in alopecia, retarded growth, and impaired lactation.

Requirements. There is no evidence that myoinositol is required in the diet of humans.

Therapeutic Uses. Inositol has been used in diseases associated with fat metabolism. However, solid evidence for its therapeutic efficacy is lacking.

ASCORBIC ACID (VITAMIN C)

History. The dietary prevention of scurvy was shown by Lind in 1750. In 1928, ascorbic acid was first isolated from orange, cabbage, and adrenal cortex by Szent Györgyi, who named the compound hexuronic acid. In 1932, the vitamin was isolated again by Waugh and King, who demonstrated its antiscorbutic activity in guinea pigs (44).

Sources. Citrus fruits are excellent sources of vitamin C. Other sources include cabbage, tomatoes, strawberries, cantaloupe, pineapple, potatoes, sweet potatoes, and dark green and deep yellow vegetables.

Chemistry. Ascorbic acid is a hexose derivative closely related to the monosaccharide sugars. Plants and most animal species synthesize it from glucose and other simple sugars.

Ascorbic acid is easily oxidized; the process is accelerated by heat, light, alkalies, oxidative enzymes, copper, and iron. Ascorbic acid is highly soluble in water and is stable in acid solutions below pH 4.

The structure of the vitamin is:

HO OH
O= O —CHOH
CH_2OH

Functions and Mechanism of Action. Vitamin C has a significant role in collagen synthesis and conversion of cholesterol to bile acids.

As an antioxidant, ascorbic acid protects vitamins A and E and polyunsaturated fatty acids from oxidation. It aids in the conversion of ferric to ferrous iron and in the release of iron from transferrin in the circulation, and in transfer of iron to the liver for its incorporation into the storage form, ferritin (17). Furthermore, it is required for the conversion of folic acid to folinic acid, and participates in the synthesis of catecholamines and steroid hormones by the adrenals (17) (Table 14.2-1).

Absorption, Transport, and Storage. Ascorbic acid is rapidly absorbed from the gastrointestinal tract. High concentrations are found in the adrenal gland and the retina of the eye. Spleen, intestine, bone marrow, pancreas, thymus, liver, pituitary, and kidney also contain some vitamin C. The plasma concentration is related to dietary intake and is about 12 mg/l in a diet containing 100 mg of ascorbic acid. Plasma concentrations of less than 1 mg/l indicate that the subject is at a high risk of developing scurvy (20).

Deficiency. Only humans, monkey, guinea pig, Indian fruit bat, and the red-vented bulbul bird (native of India) have thus far been shown to require ascorbic acid in the diet. Scurvy, the state of vitamin C deficiency, is more prominent in infants and young children. The symptoms are mostly related to defective formation of collagen and include: swollen, tender, and hemorrhagic gums and faulty bone calcification. Additionally, in infants there may be signs of tenderness and swelling in the thighs as well as anemia. Deficiency symptoms in adults also include bleeding of gums, cramps in the leg, anemia, and petechial hemorrhages (37, 42).

Requirements. The minimum daily requirement is 10 mg for adults. The recommended daily allowance is 60 mg for both males and females over 14 years. Requirements are increased during tuberculosis, rheumatic fever, and burns.

Adverse Effects. Megadoses of vitamin C may cause the formation of cystine or oxalate stones, particularly in gouty individuals, increased absorption of iron, and increased mobilization of some minerals. Inhibitory effect on mitosis, possible change to β-cells of pancreas, and decreased insulin production by dehydroascorbic acid have been reported. Also, high doses of vitamin C may lead to diarrhea, allergies, reproductive failure, vitamin C dependency, thrombosis, aciduria (oxalic, folic, uric) and vitamin B_{12} inactivation (16, 21).

Therapeutic Uses. Therapeutic doses of vitamin C are used in the treatment of scurvy. It has also been used in the treatment of idiopathic methemoglobinemia and in the treatment of high levels of tyrosine and phenylalanine in premature infants receiving a high-protein and low-ascorbic acid diet. Recently, evidence has been accumulated on efficacy of vitamin C therapy in the treatment of pressure sores (30).

The use of large doses of ascorbic acid in the prevention and treatment of colds and upper respiratory infection is controversial (22, 30, 42). There is still inadequate evidence of any effect of vitamin C in prophylaxis or therapy of cancer. However, since there is a low level of vitamin C in patients with malignant diseases, it is important to ensure adequate intake of the vitamin by such individuals (31).

Preparations. *Ascorbic Acid,* USP white or slightly yellow crystals or powder; tablets, USP (CEVALIN, etc., 25, 50, 100, 250, 500, 1000 mg); injection, USP (50, 100, 200, 250, 500 mg/ml).

MECHANISM OF ACTION

Mechanisms of action of various members of vitamin B complex and vitamin C are summarized in Table 14.2-1.

DRUG INTERACTIONS

Interactions of various drugs with different members of vitamin B complex and vitamin C are listed in Table 14.2-2.

REFERENCES

1. Balnave, D. Clinical symptoms of biotin deficiency in animals. *Am. J. Clin. Nutr.* 30:1408, 1977.
2. Barbeau, A. Emerging treatments: Replacement therapy with choline or lecithin neurological disease. *Can. J. Neurol. Sci.* 5:157, 1978.
3. Brin, M. Erythrocytes as a biopsy tissue for functional evaluation of thiamine adequacy. *JAMA* 187:762, 1964.
4. Christensen, N.A., Archor, R.W.P., Berge, K.G. and Mason, H.L. Hypercholesterolemia: Effects of treatment with nicotinic acid for three to seven years. *Dis. Chest.* 46:411, 1964.
5. Darby, W.J., McNutt, K.W. and Todhunter, E.N. Niacin. In: *Present Knowledge in Nutrition.* Washington, D.C.: Nutrition Foundation, 1976, p. 167.
6. Eichner, E.R. and Hillman, R.S. Effect of alcohol on serum folate level. *J. Clin. Invest.* 52:584, 1973.
7. Ellegaard, J., Esmann, V. and Henriksen, L. Deficient folate activity during treatment of psoriasis and methotrexate diagnosed by determination of serine synthesis in lymphocytes. *Br. J. Dermatol.* 87:248, 1972.
8. Elvehjem, C.A., Madden, R.J., Strong, S.M. and Wolley, D.W. The isolation and identification of the anti-black tongue factor. *J. Biol. Chem.* 123:137, 1938.
9. Gershoff, S.N. Effect of dietary levels of macronutrients on vitamin requirements. *Fed. Proc.* 23:1077, 1964.
10. Gershoff, S.N. Vitamin B_6. In: *Present Knowledge in Nutrition.* Washington, D.C.: Nutrition Foundation, 1976, p. 149.
11. Griffin, W.H. and Nye, J.F. Choline X: Effects of deficiency. In: *The Vitamins, Vol. 3* (Sebrell, W.H. and Harris, R.S., eds.). New York: Academic Press, 1971, p. 81.
12. Growdson, J.H. and Wortman, R.J. Dietary influences on the synthesis of neurotransmitters in the brain. *Nutr. Rev.* 37:129, 1979.
13. György, P. Early experiences with riboflavin: A retrospect. *Nutr. Rev.* 12:97, 1954.
14. György, P. Developments leading to the metabolic role of vitamin B_6. *Am. J. Clin. Nutr.* 24:1250, 1971.
15. Harris, S.A. and Folkers, K. Synthesis of vitamin B_6. *J. Am. Chem. Soc.* 61:1245, 1939.
16. Herbert, W. and Jacob, E. Destruction of vitamin B_{12} by ascorbic acid. *JAMA* 230:241, 1974.
17. Hodges, R.E. Ascorbic acid. In: *Present Knowledge in Nutrition.* Washington, D.C.: Nutrition Foundation, 1976, p. 119.
18. Hodges, R.E., Bean, W.B., Ohlson, M.A. and Bleilen, R. Human pantothenic acid deficiency produced by omega-methyl pantothenic acid. *J. Clin. Invest.* 38:1421, 1951.
19. Itokawa, Y. and Cooper, J.R. Ion movements and thiamine, II. The release of the vitamin from membrane fragments. *Biochem. Biophys. Acta.* 196:274, 1970.
20. Kallner, A., Harman, D. and Horning, D. Steady-state turnover and body pool of ascorbic acid in man. *Am. J. Clin. Nutr.* 32:530, 1979.
21. Krumdieck, C.L. Folic acid. In: *Present Knowledge in Nutrition.* Washington, D.C.: Nutrition Foundation, 1976, p. 175.
22. Kutsky, R.J. Handbook of vitamins, minerals and hormones. New York: Van Nostrand Reinhold Co., 1981.
23. McCormick, D.B. Biotin. In: *Present Knowledge in Nutrition.* Washington, D.C.: Nutrition Foundation, 1976, p. 217.
24. McLaren, D. Metabolic disorders. In: *Current Therapy* (Conn, H.F., ed.). Philadelphia: W.B. Saunders Co., 1978, p. 409.
25. Milhorat, A.T. Inositol. XI. Deficiency effects in human beings. In: *The Vitamins, Vol. 3* (Sebrell, W.H., Jr. and Harris, R.S., eds.). New York: Academic Press, 1971, p. 398.
26. Mueller, J.F. and Vilter, R.W. Pyridoxine deficiency in human beings induced with desoxyperidoxine. *J. Clin. Invest.* 29:193, 1950.
27. *Nutr. Rev.* (editorial). Treatment of hypercholesterolemia with nicotinic acid. 19:325, 1961.
28. *Nutr. Rev.* Role of thiamine in regulation of fatty acid and cholesterol biosynthesis in cultured brain cells. 37:24, 1979.
29. *Nutr. Rev.* Inhibition of the hemopoietic activity of folic acid by ethanol. 37:254, 1979.
30. Ovesen, L. Drugs and vitamin deficiency. *Drugs* 18:278, 1979.
31. Ovesen, L. Vitamin therapy in the absence of obvious deficiency. What is the evidence? *Drugs* 27:148, 1983.
32. Rivlin, R.S. (ed.). *Riboflavin.* New York: Plenum Press, 1975.
33. Rivlin, R.S. Hormones, drugs, and riboflavin. *Nutr. Rev.* 37:241, 1979.
34. Robinson, C.H. *Normal and Therapeutic Nutrition, 15th ed.* New York: Macmillan, 1977, p. 184.
35. Rose, D.P. The interactions between vitamin B_6 and hormones. *Vit. Horm.* 36:53, 1978.
36. Schaumburg, H., Kaplan, J., Winderband, A., Vick, N., Rasmus, S., Pleasure, D. and Brown, M.J. Sensory neuropathy from pyridoxine abuse (a new megavitamin syndrome). *N. Engl. J. Med.* 309:445, 1983.
37. Schorah, C.J. The level of vitamin C reserves required in man: Towards a solution to the controversy. *Proc. Nutr. Soc.* 40:147, 1981.
38. Sebrell, W.H. and Butler, R.E. Riboflavin deficiency in man. *Pub. Health Rep.* 54:2121, 1939.
39. Spies, T.D., Cooper, C. and Blankenhorn, A. The use of nicotinic acid in the treatment of pellagra. *JAMA* 110:622, 1938.
40. Takai, K. Health of the Japanese navy. *Lancet* 2:86, 1887.
41. Tomkin, G.H. Malabsorption of vitamin B_{12} in diabetic patients treated with phenformin: A comparison with metformin. *Br. Med. J.* 2:673, 1973.

42. Vilter, R.W. Nutritional aspects of ascorbic acid: Uses and abuses. *West J. Med.* 133:485, 1980.
43. Vitale, J.J. Vitamins. Kalamazoo, Mich.: Upjohn Co., 1976.
44. Waugh, W.A. and King, C-G. Isolation and identification of vitamin C. *J. Biol. Chem.* 97:325, 1932.
45. Waxman, S., Corcino, J.J. and Herbert, V. Drugs, toxins, and dietary amino acids affecting vitamin B_{12} or folic acid absorption and utilization. *Am. J. Med.* 48:599, 1970.
46. Whitehead, C.C. The assessment of biotin status in man and animals. *Proc. Nutr. Soc.* 40:165, 1981.
47. Williams, R.R. *Toward the Conquest of Beriberi.* Cambridge, Mass.: Harvard University Press, 1961.
48. Williams, R.R. and Cline, J.K. Synthesis of vitamin B_1. *J. Am. Chem. Soc.* 58:1504, 1936.
49. Wright, L.D. Pantothenic acid. In: *Present Knowledge in Nutrition.* Washington, D.C.: Nutrition Foundation, 1976, p. 226.

ADDITIONAL READING

Levine, M. New concepts in the biology and biochemistry of ascorbic acid. *New Eng. J.Med.* 314:892, 1986.

McCay, P.B. Vitamin E: interactions with free radicals and ascorbate. *Ann. Rev. Nutr.*, 5:323, 1985.

Petrie, W.M. and Ban, T.A. Vitamins in psychiatry. Do they have a rate? *Drugs* 30:58, 1985.

CHAPTER 14.3

MINERALS

Lalita Kaul and Yousef Tizabi

Minerals are chemical elements or compounds occurring naturally as a product of inorganic processes. The human body contains 50 or more chemical elements, 4 of which (oxygen, hydrogen, carbon, nitrogen) form and make up 96% of the body weight. The remaining 4% of the body weight is composed of the essential and nonessential minerals and mineral contaminants. In accordance with the recommendation of the National Academy of Sciences for their nutritional requirements (19), minerals may be classified into four groups:

1. Essential macronutrients (needed in amounts of 100 mg/day or more), (e.g., calcium, phosphorus, potassium, sulfur, sodium, chloride, magnesium)
2. Essential micronutrients (trace elements needed in amounts no more than a few milligrams a day (e.g., iron, manganese, copper, iodine, fluoride, cobalt, molybdenum, selenium, chromium, zinc)
3. Micronutrients that may be essential for the human (e.g., nickel, silicon, tin, vanadium, cadmium)
4. Trace contaminants (e.g., aluminum, arsenic, barium, boron, bromide, gold, silver, lead, mercury, strontium, and others)

Physiological functions and pharmacological and toxicological effects of some of these minerals are of importance. Some of these have been discussed in other chapters (calcium, Chapter 12.2; iron, Chapter 15.7; mercury, lead, arsenic, and others, Chapter 28.1). Physiological and pharmacological aspects of magnesium, zinc, manganese, copper, fluoride, phosphorus, iodine, silver will be discussed here.

It is appropriate to note that since toxic concentrations of some minerals are rather close to the therapeutic or required dosages, it is important to have medical supervision with mineral pill supplements.

MAGNESIUM (Mg)

The adult body contains about 20-35 g of magnesium. About 55-60% is present as phosphates and carbonates in the bones, and about 27% is found in muscle and 18% in nonmuscle soft tissues and body fluids. Extracellular fluid contains 2% of magnesium.

In addition to its function in the skeleton structures, magnesium acts as a catalyst in several metabolic reactions. It is involved in the phosphorylation of glucose in its anaerobic metabolism and in its oxidative decarboxylations in the citric acid cycle. Magnesium is a catalyst for enzymes involved in the oxidative phosphorylation of adenosine diphosphate (ADP) to adenosine triphosphate (ATP) and also for the enzymes that are involved in the transfer of phosphate from ATP to a phosphate acceptor. It is also involved in protein synthesis through its action on ribosomal aggregation. Magnesium plays an important role in neuromuscular transmission and activity (26).

Magnesium is absorbed by active transport and competes with calcium for carrier sites. Therefore a high intake of either one of them interferes with the absorption of the other. The other factors that influence its absorption are the amount of phosphate and lactose in the diet, intestinal transit time, rate of water absorption, and resultant luminal magnesium concentration.

Under normal conditions, 3-5% of the magnesium is excreted in the urine every day. There is also some excretion of magnesium via the gastrointestinal tract, in saliva, and in milk. In case of magnesium deficiency, its excretion through the kidneys and the intestinal mucosa is considerably reduced (5).

The recommended dietary allowance of magnesium is 350 mg for the adult man and 300 mg for women. Good dietary sources are nuts, vegetables, grains, chocolate, cocoa, etc. (14).

Magnesium deficiency is frequently observed in chronic alcoholism, cirrhosis of the liver, malabsorption syndromes such as sprue, kwashiorkor, severe vomiting, prolonged use of magnesium-free parenteral nutrition, diabetic acidosis, diuretic therapy, hyperaldosteronism, diarrhea, nasogastric suction, parathyroid hypofunction or hyperfunction, malignant osteolytic lesions, excess vitamin D, thyrotoxicosis, and in burn patients with daily saline bath. Deficiency symptoms include neuromuscular hyperirritability, twitching, tremors, tetany, nystagmus, and dysphagia (5, 6, 26). There are also behavioral (psychosis) and cardiac disturbances.

Hypermagnesemia can occur if there is an unusual increase in absorption or decrease in urinary excretion. This condition occurs if the serum level exceeds 96 mg/l. Symptoms of this condition include muscle weakness, hypotension, atrial fibrillation or drowsiness, a curarelike effect at the myoneural junction, and blockade of release of catecholamine from adrenal medulla. At a very high concentration there is respiratory failure and cardiac arrest. This condition can be corrected by giving calcium gluconate.

Therapeutic doses of magnesium are used in the treatment of seizures associated with acute nephritis and with eclampsia of pregnancy. Magnesium salts are used commonly as cathartics and antacids.

Preparations. *Magnesium Sulfate* Injection, USP. Magnesium citrate and sulfate are most frequently used in gastrointestinal symptoms (see previous discussion). Other preparations include carbonate, chloride, hydroxide, and oxide. For parenteral administration, USP $MgSO_4 \cdot 7H_2O$, 10, 12.5, 25 and 50% solutions are used. One gram of this salt contains 8.12 mEq of magnesium.

ZINC (Zn)

The adult body contains about 2 or 3 g of zinc. High concentrations are found in the choroid of the eye, prostate, liver, bone, and hair.

Zinc is an integral part of several metalloenzymes. Some of these are: carbonic anhydrase, lactic dehydrogenase, alkaline phosphatase, carboxypeptidase, and aminopeptidase. As a cofactor, zinc is essential in the synthesis of DNA and RNA, in the mobilization of vitamin A from the liver, and in the enhancement of the action of follicle-stimulating hormone and luteinizing hormone. Zinc is also essential for the maintenance of the immune systems. It has been suggested that zinc may in some way participate in the uptake of glucose by cells (8, 18) and be involved in the secretion of insulin. There is enough evidence to suggest an important role for zinc in the maintenance of special senses, taste, smell (see Chapter 21.3) and vision (24).

Zinc is primarily absorbed from the duodenum and jejunum. Excessive intake of calcium, vitamin D, and phytate interferes with its absorption. After absorption, zinc combines loosely with plasma albumin for transport. The normal serum concentration is about 100-140 μg/100 ml. The concentration of zinc in plasma is reduced in a low-zinc diet, in pregnancy, and in women on oral contraceptives.

Zinc is excreted primarily by pancreatic and intestinal secretions and finally via the feces. Under normal conditions, urinary excretions range from 450 to 500 μg daily. In burns and following starvation, a significant amount of zinc is excreted in the urine; also, marked losses may occur through sweat (25). The recommended dietary allowance for adults is 15 mg daily. High dietary sources include: sea food, meat/organs, nuts/seeds, dairy products, grains, etc. (14).

The primary features of zinc deficiency are growth failure and hypogonadism characterized by delayed sexual development, short stature, hepatosplenomegaly, spoon nails, and anemia. In some people, endocrine function tests are consistent with hypopituitarism. Other symptoms include hypogeusia, dysgeusia, and hyposmia. These conditions are severe in acute viral hepatitis, cirrhosis of the liver, hepatic coma, and kwashiorkor. Severe zinc deficiency in pregnant rats has been reported to cause high incidence of birth defects and abortion (10). Also, microophthalmia, anophthalmia, and optic nerve abnormalities have been detected in the offspring of the female rats maintained on a zinc-deficient diet (24).

Conditioned zinc deficiency appears to be a problem in patients with alcoholism, cirrhosis, chronic renal disease, hemolytic anemias (thalassemia, sickle cell disease), chronic inflammatory disease, and malabsorption syndrome. Zinc deficiency can also be caused by abnormal losses due to proteinuria and zinc depletion associated with the use of histidine, penicillamine, phenytoin, thiamazole, thiazides, or aminoaciduria and protein-losing enteropathy. It has been suggested recently that the measurement of leukocyte zinc may be a far more reliable assessment of the body's zinc store than the conventional measurement of its concentration in tissue or body fluids (23).

Suggested dietary intake for adults (23-50 years) is 10-15 mg/day. In addition, supplementation will be required for abnormal gastrointestinal losses (11). Excessive intake of zinc (225-450 mg or more) will induce vomiting, cramps, and diarrhea. Acute toxicity is characterized by dehydration, electrolyte disturbance, gastric pain, weakness, muscular incoordination, and renal failure.

Zinc Salts. Zinc salts are used as astringents, emetics, corrosives, styptics, antiperspirants, and mild antiseptics. Highly soluble ionizing salts such as zinc chloride are quite irritating. Their action may be due to the ability of the zinc ions to precipitate protein, although other mechanisms may be involved. Also, zinc as well as chromium can be made available in a stable sterile solution as a component of various total parenteral nutrition infusates (29).

Preparations. *Zinc Acetate*, USP (astringent, styptic); *Zinc Chloride*, USP (0.5-2% solution, astringent).

Zinc Oxide, USP (mild astringent and antiseptic, used as powders, ointment, paste for skin diseases); *Zinc Oxide Ointments*, USP (20% zinc oxide); *Zinc Oxide Paste*, USP (25% zinc oxide); *Zinc Oxide and Salicylic Acid Paste*, USP (zinc oxide paste with 2% salicylic acid); *Calamine*, USP pink powder containing zinc oxide (not less than 98%) with about 0.5% ferric oxide; *Calamine Lotion*, USP (8% calamine and 8% zinc oxide); *Phenolated Calamine Lotion*, USP (calamine lotion with 1% phenol).

Zinc Sulfate, USP; *Zinc Sulfate Ophthalmic Solution*, USP (0.25% solution for angular conjunctivitis); *Zinc Sulfate* (4% solution for skin diseases, and 0.25-4% as vaginal deodorant, also used as deodorant antiperspirant and for acceleration of wound healing). *White Lotion*, USP (contains 4% zinc sulfate with equal concentration of sulfurated potash).

MANGANESE (Mn)

The adult human body contains about 10-20 mg of manganese. The good sources are whole grain cereals, nuts, and legumes. Manganese concentration of fetal tissues at term is about equal to that of the adult. Fecal loss of manganese, however, is five times greater than intake of this mineral from breast milk during the first week of life.

Manganese is primarily stored in liver, skin, and skeletal muscle. It is also stored in kidney, pancreas, and pituitary.

Manganese is poorly absorbed from the small intestine. It is bound to protein and transported as transmanganin (lactoglobulin). There is a dynamic equilibrium between intracellular and extracellular manganese. Whole blood cell level is 1.5-3 mg/1150 ml. Absorbed manganese is excreted through the intestine via bile and much of this is again reabsorbed. There is very little excretion in the urine.

Studies on experimental animals have shown that manganese is essential for normal bone growth, normal lipid metabolism, reproduction, and regulation of nervous irritability. Manganese is also an activator for a number of enzymes, including pyruvate carboxylase. Manganese can substitute for magnesium in a number of enzymes required for oxidative phosphorylation (1, 30).

Manganese can affect the brain by either its deficiency or its excess. Manganese-deficient rats develop convulsions and the toxicity produces neurological disturbances similar to those of Parkinson's disease. In humans its deficiency may cause glucose intolerance and its excess ($>$ 1000 mg/kg) can cause varieties of symptoms including psychic and neurological disorders, nephritis, pneumonia, lung hemorrhage, liver cirrhosis, anemia, and impotence (14, 15).

Recommended daily intake for adults is 2.5-5 mg. Concentrations for parenteral use are unknown at this time (15).

COPPER (Cu)

The adult human body contains about 75-150 mg of copper. The highest concentrations of this mineral are found in the liver, kidney, gastrointestinal tract, brain, and heart.

Normal daily diet contains roughly 2-5 mg copper. About 32% of this copper in foods is absorbed from the upper gastrointestinal tract. Plasma copper level is about 100 ng/100 ml. Absorption of stable complex is greater than free copper ion. Elements like calcium, cadmium, mercury, and zinc compete with copper for absorption. After absorption, the main copper fraction is carried to the liver. Within the hepatic cells, copper is needed for the synthesis of ceruloplasmin and other copper-containing proteins. Both high and low molecular weight complexes are excreted via the bile. Metal ions (e.g., molybdenum), anions (e.g., sulfide), and hormones (e.g., corticosteroids) are known to influence copper metabolism (22). Ascorbic acid also interferes with its absorption. Approximately 95% of the copper in blood plasma is bound to protein complex, ceruloplasmin, and 5% is bound to albumin or amino acids. Increased intakes of molybdenum and zinc increase the requirement for copper. Most of the copper is excreted in the feces, primarily through the excretion of bile. Up to 98% of an orally administered dose of copper is recovered in the feces and about 1-2% in the urine.

Copper is essential for iron absorption and mobilization prior to hemoglobin synthesis, melanin pigment formation, electron transport, integrity of the myelin sheath, maturation of collagen, elastin formation, phospholipid synthesis, and bone development. Copper proteins are involved in electron transfer reactions, and enzymes such as monoamine oxidase, tyrosinase, and dopamine-β-hydroxylase. Copper is an essential component of the butyryl coenzyme A dehydrogenase required for fatty acid oxidation, tyrosinase required for melanin pigment formation, and uricase required in purine metabolism. It is also required in the cytochrome oxidation system for energy production (2).

Copper deficiency in humans is rare but has been observed in kwashiorkor, the nephrotic syndrome, sprue, and sometimes in patients with iron deficiency anemia and adults on long-term total parenteral nutrition following bowel surgery. The deficiency symptoms include hypochromic anemia, skeletal abnormality, connective tissue dysfunctions, bone fragility, cardiovascular disorders, nervous disorder, and lack of pigmentation (21, 27).

Copper metabolism is disrupted in two genetic diseases, Menkes' syndrome and Wilson's disease. Hypocupremia occurs in spite of adequate dietary copper intake. In Menkes' syndrome, there are low concentrations of copper in serum, liver, and brain and depressed levels of serum oxidase activity. There is defect in the transport of copper across membranes. Wilson's disease is characterized by low plasma copper associated with excessive accumulation of copper in liver, brain, kidney, and cornea. The excess copper in these tissues leads to hepatitis, lenticular degeneration, renal malfunction, and neurological disorders. Acute toxicity may cause tachycardia, hypotension, hemolytic anemia, oliguria, uremia, coma, cardiovascular collapse, and death. Chronic excess dosage may lead to nausea, vomiting, epigastric pain, yellow watery diarrhea, jaundice, dizziness, and general debility (14, 27).

No recommended dietary allowances have been set, but a daily allowance of 2-3 mg is considered to be satisfactory for adults. Recommended daily intake for infants is 0.5-0.7 mg and for children 1-2.5 mg.

Copper Salt. Cupric sulfate, $CuSO_4.5H_2O$, is available as blue crystalline granules or powder and is soluble in water, forming blue solution with a disagreeable metallic taste. It is given as an emetic in a 0.3-g dose dissolved in 100 ml of water. In excessive doses, it may cause colic and diarrhea. It is also given in the treatment of phosphorus poisoning in which it reacts with phorphorus to form an insoluble copper phosphate. Copper is used as a molluscicide to kill snails and thereby control transmission of schistosomiasis to humans.

FLUORIDE

Fluoride occurs in the body chiefly as a fluoroapatite in the bones and tooth enamel. It elevates resistance of tooth enamel to caries and may increase the strength of the bone.

The average daily U.S. diet contains approximately 0.25-0.30 mg of fluoride. Fluoride is passively transported from the gastrointestinal tract. There is also absorption through lungs and skin. Fluoride administration has been shown to stimulate new bone formation in both humans and animals. The predominant effect of fluoride on the skeleton is osteoblastic stimulation (12). The newly formed bone during fluoride therapy has been shown to be poorly mineralized and presents the histological picture of osteomalacia. Administration of fluoride to several species of animals (rats, dogs, and calves) has been reported to cause increased bone resorption, parathyroid hyperplasia, and increased parathyroid hormone secretion. Whether or not fluoride increases the strength of bone has not been clearly demonstrated. About 75% of ingested fluoride is absorbed in the first hour. It is also absorbed through the lungs following inhalation. The degree of absorption of fluoride correlates well with its solubility. Most of the ingested fluoride is excreted in the urine (50-60%) and this accounts for daily excretion of about 3 mg. Renal excretion and skeletal sequestration are the principal mechanisms that regulate circulating fluoride levels. There are small losses through sweat and feces.

Fluorides have been used for the treatment of involutional osteoporosis, but the therapeutic benefits have not been established. In otolaryngology, fluorides have been shown to slow down or arrest the process of otospongiosis (otosclerosis). Currently, dental caries prophylaxis is the only effective and safe indication for fluorides (3). The doses of fluoride ion generally employed in the treatment of otospongiosis and osteoporosis are about 10-100 times more than that for prophylaxis of caries (7).

Acute fluoride toxicity (2000 mg/day) results in weakness, gastrointestinal symptoms (nausea, diarrhea, vomiting, hypocalcemia, hypoglycemia, and convulsions). Death may be due to paralysis or cardiac failure (9). Excessive intake of fluoride (20-80 mg/day or more for 10-20 years) can cause osteosclerosis (elevated bone calcium and overgrowth) and bone fluorosis with symptoms resembling arthritis (9, 17). Other signs of fluoride toxicity (2.5-5 g) are retinopathy, optic neuritis, atopic dermatitis, and edema.

Dental fluorosis results, if the concentration of fluoride in drinking water is in excess of 1.5 ppm. The teeth become mottled. About 25-50% of the ingested fluoride is deposited in skeleton daily. Parenteral fluids therefore should not supply more fluoride than that usually supplied by normal consumption of food and water (20).

Adequate daily dietary intake of fluoride for children and adolescents is 0.5-1.5 mg, and for adults 1.5-4 mg.

Preparations. *Sodium Fluoride*, USP: Oral solution, USP, tablet, USP. Stannous Fluoride, USP. The fluoride salts used in dentifrices include Sodium Fluoride, Stannous Fluoride, and *Sodium Fluoride and Phosphoric Acid Topical Solution*, USP.

PHOSPHORUS (P)

Phosphorus is widely distributed in foods. Meat and milk groups are the principal sources.

Physiologically and biochemically, phosphorus is one of the

most essential elements of the body. About 85% of phosphorus is in inorganic combination with calcium as the insoluble apatite of bones and teeth, the rest is distributed in skeletal muscle, skin, nervous tissues, and other organs. Calcium to phosphorus ration in the bones is 2:1. Soft tissues contain higher amounts of phosphorus than calcium. Phosphorus in the soft tissue is mostly in the form of organic esters and in the bone almost all in the mineral phase as orthophosphate.

Phosphorus is a constituent of DNA and RNA and as a part of phospholipids it is an integral component of cell membranes. Phosphorylation is a key reaction in several metabolic processes involving carbohydrates, lipids, and proteins. As part of the ADP-ATP system, phosphorus is essential for the storage and controlled release of energy in the form of "high-energy phosphate compounds." Inorganic phosphates in the body act as buffers in the regulation of acid-base equilibrium in plasma and within cells, play a role in H-ion excretion in the urine, and modify the effects of vitamin D.

Of dietary phosphorus, 60-70% is absorbed as free phosphate. Dietary organic phosphate esters (e.g., phytic acid of cereals and seeds) are not readily available to humans because of relative deficiency of the enzyme phytase in the intestinal lumen. Aluminum may interfere with intestinal phosphate absorption. Organic phosphate esters may themselves interfere with intestinal calcium absorption. Dietary phosphorus absorption is mainly regulated by variations in intake and renal excretion. The inorganic phosphorus level of serum is between 2.5 and 4.5 mg%, and it is slightly higher in children. Administration of insulin, glucagon, or epinephrine results in reduction in serum phosphate by stimulating the cellular glucose utilization and by increasing intracellular phosphate ester formation. Systemic alkalosis also leads to lowering of serum phosphate presumably due to a shift of phosphate out of the extracellular fluid compartment. Marked catabolism of body tissue in starvation and destruction of neoplastic lymphoid cells (lymphoblasts) following initiation of therapy with cytotoxic drugs may lead to cellular release of phosphate (hyperphosphatemia and reciprocal hypocalcemia) (4).

With normal kidney function, the urinary phosphorus represents roughly two-thirds of the dietary phosphorus and is excreted in the form of inorganic phosphate. Urinary excretion of phosphate is increased by digoxin, estrogens, thyroid hormone, parathyroid hormone, and long-term corticosteroid therapy. Growth hormone and short-term corticosteroids, on the other hand, reduce renal excretion of phosphates by increasing tubular reabsorption.

The recommended daily allowances of phosphorus for adults in the United States is 800-1200 mg. The calcium to phosphate ratio of milk is important in infant formula feeding. Cow's milk with a ratio of 1.3:1 compared with breast milk (calcium to phosphate ratio 2:1) may cause idiopathic hypocalcemia and tetany in infants.

Phosphate depletion can result from vitamin D deficiency, disorders in metabolism of vitamin D due to genetic abnormalities, liver disease, abnormalities of renal tubular reabsorption of phosphate, as in Fanconi's syndrome, and pharmacological agents such as the anticonvulsants, diphenylhydantoin, phenobarbital, and nonabsorbable antacids.

Phosphorus deficiency results in poor bone mineralization, with development of rickets in the growing bone and osteomalacia in adult bone. Severe hypophosphatemia may also cause muscle weakness due to reduction of organic phosphates in muscle cells, anorexia, and skeletal pain (16).

Hyperphosphatemia can result from renal insufficiency with marked reduction of glomerular filtration rate. To control this condition, patients are given aluminum hydroxide or calcium carbonate. This reduces phosphate absorption. In patients with normal kidney function, ingestion of large amounts of aluminum hydroxide, calcium carbonate, lactate, or gluconate can lead to severe hypophosphatemia. Also, excessive intake of antacids can lead to severe muscle weakness as a result of hypophosphatemia (4, 16).

Chronic excess of P intake may lead to secondary hyperthyroidism, bone resorption, hypocalcemia, and calcification of heart and kidneys (14).

IODINE (I)

The principal dietary source of iodine is iodized salt and breads in which iodates or iodides are added. About one-third of the iodine in the body is found in the thyroid gland as thyroglobulin. The most important function of iodine is as a constituent of the thyroid hormones, thyroxine and triiodothyronine. These hormones are important in the regulation of the rate of oxidation within the cells (see Chapter 12.5). Iodine is also found in salivary, mammary, and gastric glands, and kidneys.

Iodine is ingested in foods as inorganic iodides and as organic compounds. Elemental iodine is split from organic compounds and is reduced to iodide in the gastrointestinal lumen. The degree of absorption depends upon the amount of circulating thyroid hormone. Soybean products interfere with reabsorption of thyroxine, causing depletion and goiter.

Iodine is transported as free iodide and as protein-bound iodine (PBI). PBI rises during pregnancy and with hypertrophy of the thyroid gland and falls when the gland is underactive.

The kidneys are the main route of iodide excretion. Small amounts of iodide may also be excreted from the body in sweat, feces, and milk. There is no renal threshold for iodide as indicated by continuous loss even under serious deficiency.

Iodine deficiency occurs in areas where the iodine content of the soil is very low. The deficiency causes an increase in the size and number of epithelial cells in the thyroid gland and the condition is called endemic goiter (13). Severe deficiency of iodide can cause cretinism which is characterized by a low basal metabolism, weakness, dry skin, enlarged tongue, and severe mental retardation. Recently, it has been suggested that low dietary iodine may be correlated with increased risk of breast carcinoma (28). Excess iodine intake acutely may result in gastrointestinal irritation, angioedema, hemorrhage, and hypersensitivity. Chronic overdose may lead to brassy taste, burning sensation of mouth and throat, pulmonary edema, skin lesions, and gastric irritation (14).

Preparations. *Strong Iodine Solution*, USP (Lugol's solution; 5% iodine in 10% potassium iodide). *Sodium Iodide*, USP and *Potassium Iodide*, USP are available in solid form. *Potassium Iodide Oral Solution*, USP: oral dose 50-500 mg/day. Iodine is used in antiseptic preparations (e.g., *Iodine Tincture*, USP, contains 2% iodine and 2.4% sodium iodide diluted in 50% ethanol); *Iodine Topical Solution*, USP (contains 2% iodine and 2.4% sodium iodide). Iodine is also contained in some compounds used as radiographic contrast media (Chapter 33).

SILVER SALTS

Silver salts are used as antiseptics, astringents, and caustics. This applies particularly to the soluble, highly ionizable salts. The mechanism of their action appears to be, in part, precipitation of protein in the bacterial and other cells. Silver ions also interfere with metabolic activities in the cell by combining with biologically important chemical groups (e.g., sulfhydryl, phosphate, amino, and others) and can alter the bacterial cell surface and plasma membrane thus contributing to their germicidal effect. Silver salts are particularly germicidal for gonococci. Even in very low concentration (0.05 ppm), silver can produce marked bactericidal action. This oligodynamic action, as it is termed, is also produced by many heavy metals.

Preparations. *Silver Nitrate*, USP: caustic, antiseptic, and astringent; used either in solid form or in solution (0.01-10%). The solid form, *Toughened Silver Nitrate*, USP (lunar caustic), is used as pencils for cauterization of wounds and removal of warts and granulation tissue. In 1:1000 solution it rapidly destroys most microorganisms on contact. *Silver Nitrate Ophthalmic Solution*, USP (1%) is routinely used for the prophylaxis of gonococcal *Ophthalmia Neonatorum* by conjunctival instillation in newborn infants. However, it may cause chemical conjunctivitis. Alternatively, penicillin has been used, but sensitization and development of resistance to the antibiotic may be problems. In burns, 5% solution is used along with antimicrobial agents to prevent infection and rapid eschar formation. Removal of chloride to form insoluble silver chloride may lead to hypochloremia and consequently hyponatremia. Absorbed nitrate can cause methemoglobinemia. Silver salts stain tissue black due to deposition of reduced silver (argyria).

Silver Sulfadiazine can be used in the treatment of burns in place of silver nitrate. Its low solubility prevents hypochloremia and hyponatremia, but it does readily penetrate the eschar and has marked antibacterial action against *Pseudomonas*. Also, it does not produce argyrial staining of wounds and clothings. Colloidal preparations of silver [e.g., *Mild Silver Protein* (19-23% silver)] are less injurious and have been used as antiseptics.

REFERENCES

1. Asling, C.W. and Hurley, L.S. The influence of trace elements on the skeleton. *Clin. Orthoped.* 27:213, 1963.
2. Cartwright, G.E. and Wintrobe, M.M. Copper metabolism in normal subjects. *Am. J. Clin. Nutr.* 14:224, 1964.
3. Daily fluoride supplements and dental caries. *Nutr. Rev.* 36:329, 1978.
4. Ettinger, D.S., Harker, W.G., Gerry, H.W. et al. Hyperphosphatemia, hypocalcemia, and transient renal failure. *JAMA* 239:2472, 1978.
5. Flink, E.B. Magnesium deficiency: Etiology and clinical spectrum. *Acta Med. Scand.* 647:125, 1978.
6. Hamed, I.A. and Linderman, R.D. Dysphagia and vertical nystagmus in magnesium deficiency. *Am. Int. Med.* 89:222, 1978.
7. Harrison, H.E. and Harrison, H.C. Heredity metabolic bone disease. *Clin. Orthoped.* 33:147, 1964.
8. Hendricks, D.G. and Mahoney, A.W. Glucose tolerance in zinc deficient rats. *J. Nutr.* 102:1079, 1972.
9. Hodge, H.C. and Smith, F.A. Fluoride. In: *Disorders of Mineral Metabolism, Trace Minerals, Vol. I*(Bronner, F. and Coburn, J.W., eds.). New York: Academic Press, 1981, p. 439.
10. Hurley, L.S. Tetratogenic aspects of manganese, zinc, and copper nutrition. *Physiol. Rev.* 61:249, 1981.
11. Jeejeebhoy, K.N. Zinc and chromium in parenteral nutrition. *Bull. N.Y. Acad. Med.* 60:118, 1984.
12. Jowsey, J., Riggs, L.B., Kelly, P.J. and Hoffman, D.L. Effect of combined therapy with sodium fluoride, vitamin D, and calcium in osteoporosis. *Am. J. Med.* 53:43, 1972.
13. Kelly, F.C. and Snedden, W.W. Prevalence and geographical distribution of endemic goiter. In: *Endemic Goitre.* Geneva: WHO Monograph Series No.44, 1960, p. 27.
14. Kutsky, R.J. *Handbook of Vitamins, Minerals and Hormones.* New York: Van Norstrand Reinhold Co., 1981.
15. Leach, R.M. Manganese in enteral and parenteral nutrition. *Bull. N.Y. Acad. Med.* 60:172, 1984.
16. Lotz, M., Aisman, E. and Barter, F.C. Evidence for a phosphorus-depletion syndrome in man. *N. Engl. J. Med.* 278:409, 1968.
17. Messer, H.H. and Singer, L. Fluoride. In: *Present Knowledge in Nutrition.* Washington, D.C.: Nutrition Foundation, 1976, p. 325.
18. Mills, C.F., Quarterman, J.B., Chesters, J.K., Williams, R.B. and Dalgamo, A.C. Metabolic role of Zinc. *Am. J. Clin. Nutr.* 22:1240, 1969.
19. National Academy of Sciences. *Recommended Dietary Allowances, 8th ed.* Washington, D.C., 1974.
20. Nielsen, F.H. Fluoride, vanadium, nickel, arsenic, and silicon in total parenteral nutrition. *Bull. N.Y. Acad. Med.* 60:177, 1984.
21. O'Dell, B.L. Biochemistry and physiology of copper in vertebrates. In: *Trace Elements in Human Health and Disease, Vol. I* (Prasad, A.S., ed.). New York: Academic Press, 1976, p. 391.
22. Osterberg, R. Physiology and pharmacology of copper. *Pharmacol. Ther.* 9:121, 1980.
23. Prasad, A.S. and Cossack, Z.T. Neutrological zinc: An indicator of zinc status in man. *Am. J. Clin. Nutr.* 35:835, 1982.
24. Russell, R.M., Cox, M.E. and Solomons, N. Zinc and the special senses. *Ann. Int. Med.* 99:227, 1983.
25. Sandstead, H.H., Prasad, A.S., Schulert, A.R. et al. Human zinc deficiency: Endocrine manifestations and response to treatment. *Am. J. Clin. Nutr.* 20:422, 1967.
26. Schroeder, H.A., Nason, A.P. and Tipton, I.H. Essential metals in man: Magnesium. *J. Chron. Dis.* 21:815, 1969.
27. Shike, M. Copper in parenteral nutrition. *Bull. N.Y. Acad. Med.* 60:132, 1984.
28. Stadl, R.C. Dietary iodine and risk of breast, endometrial cancer. *Lancet* 2:890, 1976.
29. Tsallas, G.I. Availability and physiochemical stability of zinc and chromium in total parenteral nutrition solution. *Bull. N.Y. Acad. Med.* 60:125, 1984.
30. Underwood, E.J. A Trace Elements in Human and Animal Nutrition. New York: Academic Press, 1971, p. 172.

ADDITIONAL READING

Abu-Hamdan, D.K. et al. Zinc tolerance test in uremia. *Ann. Intern. Med.* 104:50, 1986.

Editorial. Copper deficiency induced by megadoses of zinc. *Nutr. Rev.* 43:148, 1985.

Kanis, J.A. and Meunier, P.J. Should we use fluoride to treat osteoporosis?: A review. *Quatr. J. Med.* 210:145, 1984.

Mills, C.F. Dietary interactions involving the trace elements. *Ann. Rev. Nutr.* 5:173, 1985.

Rude, R.K. et al. Low serum concentrations of 1,25-Dihydroxyvitamin D in human magnesium deficiency. *J. Clin. Endocrinol. Metal.* 61:933, 1985.

Spencer, H.C. Intestinal transport of minerals in renal failure: zinc absorption. In: *Nephrology: Proceedings of the IXth International Congress of Nephrology* (Robson, R.R., ed.). New York: Springer-Verlag, 1984, p. 1420.

Subba Rao, G. Dietary intake and bioavailability of fluoride. *Ann. Rev. Nutr.* 4:115, 1984.

Valberg, L.S. et al. Does the oral zinc tolerance test measure zinc absorption? *Am. J. Clin. Nutr.* 41:37, 1985.

CIRCULATORY SYSTEM

CHAPTER 15

CHAPTER 15.1

DIGITALIS GLYCOSIDES

Claire M. Lathers and Jay Roberts

The therapeutic indication for digitalis includes the treatment of congestive heart failure and atrial arrhythmias such as atrial flutter, paroxysmal atrial tachycardia, and atrial fibrillation. Digitalis and related compounds are the major drugs employed to treat congestive heart failure, though many other agents such as catecholamines, glucagon, cyclic adenosine monophosphate (cAMP) and phosphodiesterase inhibitors, veratrum alkaloids, amrinone, imidazoles, indoles, steroids, taurine, prostaglandins, and the calcium ion have been screened as the search continues for new cardiotonic agents that may provide a suitable substitute for digitalis.

HISTORY

As early as 1500 B.C., the Egyptians mentioned squill in Eber's Papyrus, and for centuries the Chinese noted that the dried skin of the common toad could be used therapeutically. The early Romans wrote of using digitalis as a diuretic, heart tonic, emetic, and rat poison; around the time of the First Crusade (A.D. 1000), the Saxon *Herbarium* included "Foxes Glofe." Other lay terms such as foxglove, folk's glove and ladies' glove, purple foxglove, and fingerhuth were modified to *digitalis purpurea* in 1542 by the botanist Leonhard Fuchs. Until 1630, digitalis was recommended for use to "cut and consume flegme and humours, and to scour and clean the breast;" as a gargle to correct inflammation and fever and to cure bowel problems; and for treatment of epilepsy, scrofulus, and ulcers. In the late 1700s, when William Withering employed an herb (foxglove) that an old Welsh woman used to treat dropsy, a dramatic medical transformation, described as a diuresis and a decrease in heart rate, began within hours. During the 10-year period between 1775 and 1785, Withering experimented with this herb and summarized his findings in a book entitled *An Account of the Introduction of Foxglove into Modern Medicine* (65). In 1799, John Ferriar found that digitalis exerted a primary action on the heart and a secondary effect on the kidneys. An early view of the mechanism of digitalis action noted a glycoside-induced constriction of hepatic veins, said to result in pooling of the blood in the liver and the portal system, which then reduced the circulating blood volume and venous pressure to relieve the right side of the heart of the overdistension imposed by the venous congestion. The decrease in heart size occurring after administration of digitalis was also suggested to result from an increase of the diastolic tone of the myocardium. Cattell and Gold (8) in 1938 attributed the drug's primary mode of action in relieving congestive heart failure to a direct action to increase the force of contraction.

SOURCE

The term digitalis implicitly includes a large number of naturally occurring steroid glycosides, aglycones, and semisynthetic derivatives that have similar therapeutic and toxic cardiac effects; the expressions "cardiac glycoside", "digitalis glycoside", and "glycosides" are used interchangeably for digitalis. The materials are found in dried plant leaves, seeds, bulbs, and in the secretion of the glands in the skin of Bufo toads. The cardiac glycosides digoxin, deslanoside, and lanatoside C are obtained from the foxglove plant leaves of *digitalis lanata*, whereas the glycosides digitoxin, gitalin, and digitalis leaf are obtained from the leaves of *digitalis purpurea*. Of these, digoxin and digitoxin are the most widely used clinically. The seeds of *strophanthus gratus* are the source of the glycoside ouabain; the bulb of *urginea maritima* provides the glycoside proscillaridin

A (squill); and acetylstrophanthidin is a semisynthetic aglycone (Fig. 15.1-1). The compounds obtained from toads are not ordinarily used in medicine.

CHEMISTRY AND STRUCTURE-ACTIVITY RELATIONSHIP

The digitalis glycosides all contain a steroid nucleus, a 5-or 6-membered unsaturated lactone ring attached to the C-17 position of the steroid nucleus, and a sugar moiety that is attached to the C-3 position (Fig. 15.1-1). The cardiac glycosides form aglycones by hydrolytic release of the sugar moiety; the resulting aglycones, also called genins, are responsible for the cardiotonic activity. When compared with the glycoside containing the sugar moiety, the aglycones exhibit more transient and less potent cardiac actions but manifest similar toxic effects. The sugar moiety governs drug absorption, accumulation, passage through biological membranes, and potency. When the unsaturated lactone ring is saturated, cardiotonic activity is reduced by 10-fold or more, but the onset of the cardiotonic action is delayed. Cardiotonic activity is completely eliminated if the lactone ring is opened.

Hydroxyl groups are found at position 14 in the naturally occurring aglycones; additional hydroxyl groups may be found at position 3, where the sugar moieties are generally attached. The number of hydroxyl groups on the genin influence the pharmacological characteristics of the digitalis material; for example, the five hydroxyl groups on the genin of ouabain make this molecule the most polar. Digoxigenin has two hydroxyls and digitoxigenin has only one hydroxyl group. Semisynthetic digitalis has been prepared by substituting the hydroxyl group at position 3 with organic acids, sugars, and other chemicals. A review of Tamm (60) provides an in-depth discussion of the relationship between chemical structure and biological activity.

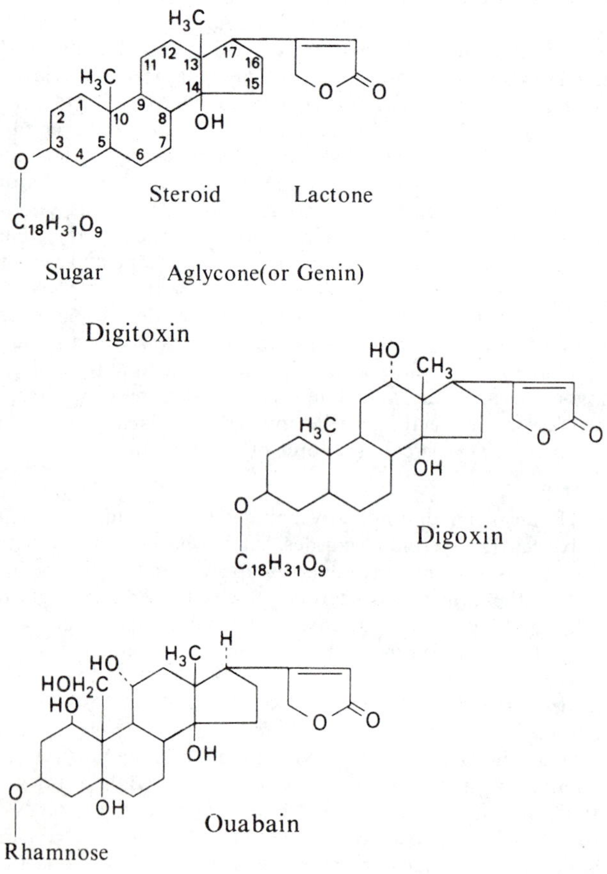

Steroid Lactone

$C_{18}H_{31}O_9$

Sugar Aglycone(or Genin)

Digitoxin

Digoxin

$C_{18}H_{31}O_9$

Ouabain

Rhamnose

Fig. 15.1-1. *Structural formula of some glycosides.*

PHARMACOLOGICAL EFFECTS

Heart. ***Contractility.*** Digitalis increases both the force and velocity of cardiac contractility in both normal and failing hearts (Table 15.1-1); the increased force of systolic contraction is termed the *positive inotropic action of digitalis* and accounts for the increase in cardiac output, the diuretic effect (indirect), and the decrease in cardiac size, preload, venous pressure, and blood volume observed after administration of digitalis to an individual suffering from congestive heart failure. Fig. 15.1-2 illustrates left ventricular function curves before and after acetylstrophanthidin; demonstrating increased contractility in the isolated heart preparation and that the increased force of contraction can be independent of extracardiac factors. An increased rate at which tension of force is developed, rather than a prolonged duration of the contractile process, characterizes the positive iniotropic effect.

Cardiac Output. Starling's *law of the heart* states that an increase in the initial myocardial fiber length or tension in the time period just preceding systole will increase the force of contraction of the ventricles; this relationship holds no matter what degree of sympathetic neural tone exists. Thus, an increase in the end-diastolic pressure or volume of the ventricles will cause an increase in the work capacity of the ventricular muscle (work = cardiac output X heart rate). In a failing heart (Fig. 15.1-3), the ability of the ventricular muscle to do work is decreased at all end-diastolic pressures or volumes, with a consequent decrease in stroke volume and an increased end-diastolic volume and pressure. Myocardial fiber tension increases, and the force of systolic contraction is enhanced; thus, the heart compensates for the decreased work capacity by progressive dilatation. This will continue until the heart can no longer compensate through this mechanism. Additional compensatory changes occur in the body as a result of increased sympathetic discharge. These changes, including an increased heart rate, venomotor tone, and peripheral arteriolar resistance, help to maintain arterial blood pressure and cardiac output. Compensatory increased renal arteriolar resistance forces a major amount of the renal blood flow to go to other organs, causing retention of water and electrolytes. These symptoms, which characterize congestive heart failure (Fig. 15.1-4), are altered as digitalis increases the force of systolic contraction (i.e., the increased cardiac work causes less blood to be retained in the ventricle at the end of systole: ventricular dilation is decreased; left ventricular end-diastolic pressure is decreased; venous pressure falls; the reflex sympathetic effects are decreased; and renal blood flow increases so that body water and electrolyte balances are again established through diuresis).

Table 15.1-1
Effect of Digitalis in the Normal and Failing Heart

Normal Heart	Failing Heart
1. ↑ In cardiac oxygen demands	1. ↓ Overall cardiac oxygen consumption and ↑ cardiac efficiency
2. ↑ Contractility	2. ↑Contractility
3. ↑ Total peripheral resistance due to direct vasoconstriction, arteriolar and venous smooth muscles and a centrally mediated ↑ in sympathetic tone	3. Peripheral resistance is already high because of the ↓ cardiac output and ↑ sympathetic tone
4. Step 3 opposes the increased cardiac contractility by ↑ peripheral impedance to ventricular ejection; net effect = no change in cardiac output	4. There is no peripheral impedance to increase in cardiac output to counter the effect of the ↑ total peripheral resistance
5. May ↓ venous pressure 6. May slow the sinus rate 7. Thus, under these circumstances, no ↑ in cardiac output can be demonstrated in spite of the positive inotropic effect	5. Thus, the ↑ contractility leads to ↑ cardiac output because the tone of peripheral vessels is lowered as a result of ↓ sympathetic tone

↑ = increase; ↓ = decrease.

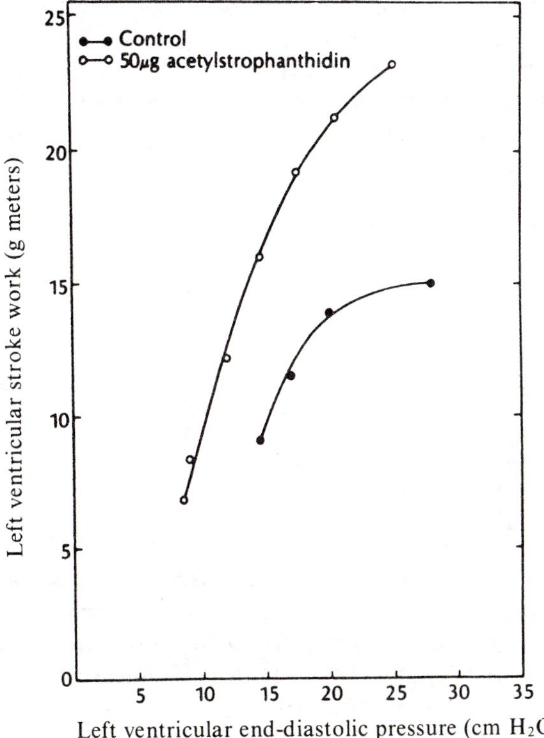

Fig. 15.1-2. *Left ventricular function curves before and after injection of 50 μg acetylstrophanthidin into the left coronary artery in the isolated supported heart preparation.*

Mean aortic pressure constant at 65 mm Hg; heart rate constant at 162 beats/min. Stroke work was changed by varying stroke volume. Acetylstrophanthidin shifted the ventricular function curve upward and to the left (i.e., increased myocardial contractility). (From Ref. 52 by permission).

Although digitalis increases cardiac contractility in both normal and failing hearts, its effect on cardiac output in normal individuals is not evident or may even result in a decrease, probably due to the reaction of digitalis to increase afterload. In patients with congestive heart failure, increased cardiac output (Table 15.1-1 and Figs. 15.1-3 and 15.1-4) is due to the fact that afterload decreases when congestive failure is relieved [i.e., due to a decreased sympathetic reflex (peripheral resistance)].

Oxygen Consumption. Following digitalization in the normal heart, the increased force of contraction produces an obligatory increase in oxygen consumption. In the failing heart, despite an obligatory increase in oxygen consumption, there is a net reduction in oxygen consumption following digitalization because the ventricular wall tension is reduced; the lower the wall tension, the lower the oxygen consumption. The end result is little or no change in oxygen consumption.

Conduction and Refractory Period. *Role of Autonomic Nervous System.* The effects of digitalis result from a direct action on the myocardium (23), as modified by its action on the autonomic nervous system and result in a reduction in sympathetic tone through an action on the baroreceptors (46, 64) and an antisympathetic effect at the cardiac receptor, particularly at the AV junctional area. An increased sympathetic activity has been reported as a result of an action on central autonomic centers (20), sympathetic ganglia (45), and the adrenergic nerve terminal (19). These effects have a variable action on the sympathetic nerves innervating the heart (35, 36) (i.e., increases or decreases). In addition to an action on the sympathetic division of the autonomic nervous system, digitalis also influences the parasympathetic nervous system by acting centrally, on the ganglia, and on the choli-

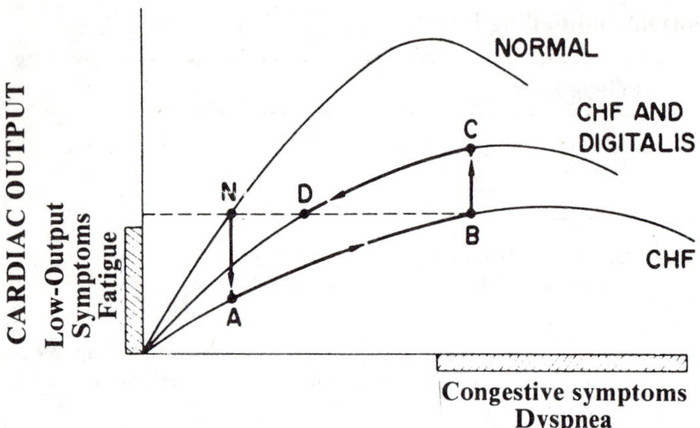

Fig. 15.1-3. *Operation of the Frank-Starling mechanism in the preload compensation for heart failure.*

The three curves represent ventricular function curves in normal, congestive heart failure (CHF), and heart failure after treatment with digitalis. Points N-D indicate in sequence: depression of contractility with decompensated heart failure (A), Frank-Starling compensation (B), increase in contractility with digitalis (C), and reduction in use of Frank-Starling preload compensation that digitalis allows (D). Points N, D, and B indicate the same cardiac output on the vertical axis, but each point is at a different end-diastolic pressure on the horizontal axis. The excessive end-diastolic pressures causing congestive symptoms and the lowered levels of cardiac performance resulting in low output symptoms are shown by the hatched areas. (Adopted from Ref. 41 by permission).

nergic nerve terminal. Furthermore, digitalis reflexly induces vagal slowing, mediated by the carotid sinus and aortic nerves.

Atrial Muscle. Digitalis actions on the atria may be modified by its vagal effects; release of acetylcholine and the sensitivity of the atrial muscle fibers to this neurotransmitter may be increased (43.) In the heart with intact vagal innervation, the atrial refractory period will be shortened and the atrial conduction velocity will be increased in the presence of digitalis. If the heart is denervated or if atropine has been given, digitalis may increase the refractory period and slow conduction in the atria.

Conducting Tissue and Ventricular Muscle. Low doses of digitalis slow AV conduction through an action on the vagal innervation of the heart; atropine will reverse this effect. In addition, increase in AV conduction velocity caused by sympathetic stimulation and catecholamines is reduced by digitalis. Recent evidence indicates that the action of digitalis to depress AV nodal conduction in denervated hearts depends largely on its effects on the autonomic nervous system (22, 63). A direct depressant effect becomes evident only after extremely high doses; this is not reversed by atropine, but is synergistic with the effect produced through vagal activation.

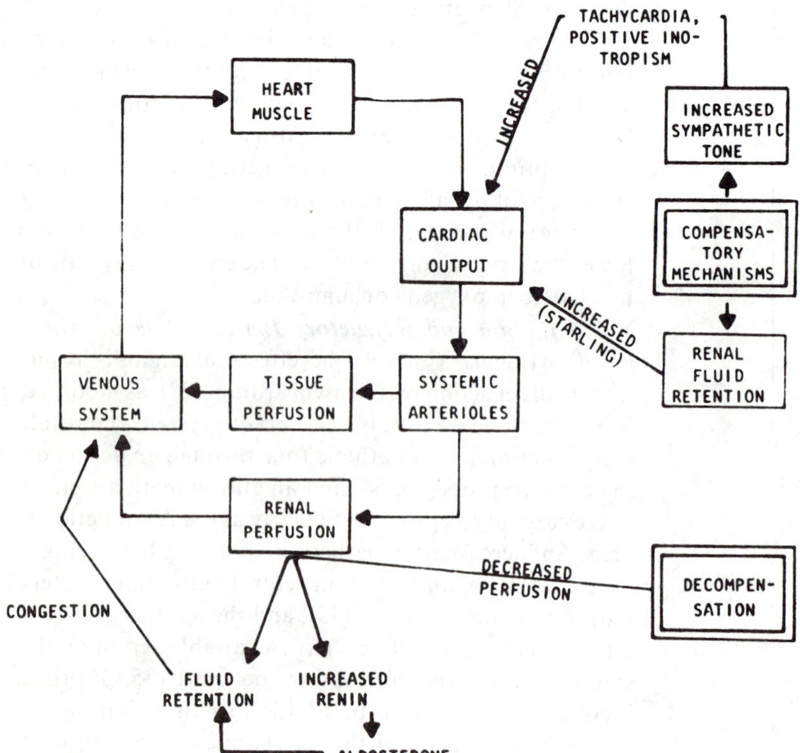

Fig. 15.1-4. *Schematic representation of the heart as a pump and the various mechanisms operating in cardiac failure.* (From Ref. 28 by permission).

Digitalis also increases the AV nodal refractory period. The action on the AV junction will decrease the number of impulses reaching the ventricles (22). The latter is important in patients exhibiting a rapid supraventricular rate due to atrial flutter or atrial fibrillation. In Purkinje fibers and ventricular muscle, digitalis shortens the duration of the action potential, decreases the refractory period, and may produce spontaneous pacemaker activity (Fig. 15.1-5). The effect on conduction is seen first in the Purkinje fibers, where it is more likely to occur if potassium is low or if the fibers are stretched.

Heart Rate. In animals, the sinus rate is slowed by digitalis due to an action on the vagus nerve and an antisympathetic effect and, in very large doses, through an extravagal action that probably involves a direct depressant effect on the node (62). In humans, however, cardiac slowing is a significant feature of digitalis action only when congestive neural heart failure is present. The increased sympathetic neural discharge, caused by the decreased cardiac output, may produce a sinus tachycardia; when digitalis is administered, cardiac output is increased, the sympathetic drive to the sinoatrial node is decreased, and the heart rate is slowed.

Cardiac Rhythm. Digitalis may induce every known type of cardiac arrhythmia by influencing impulse formation, conduction, or both. In general, arrhythmias developing from digitalis are classified as triggered (depending on the presence of an initiating impulse) or automatic (in a quiescent heart) (11). In respect to automatic rhythms, it should be noted that vagal stimulation may unmask digitalis enhancement of ventricular ectopic activity at a time when overt signs of digitalis toxicity have not appeared (47). In addition ouabain shortens the interval required for the ventricle to escape after arrest has been induced by vagal stimulation. If, on the other hand, the ventricle shows coupled extrasystoles or salvos of extrasystoles (i.e., presumably triggered impulses), vagal stimulation may lead to prolonged quiescence not only of the atrium but also of the ventricle, for without an initiating impulse there can be no triggered activity (11).

The basic electrophysiological mechanisms involved in digitalis-induced cardiac arrhythmias stem from three fundamental changes in cardiac electrical properties. First, increased automaticity may occur due to changes in increased rate of diastolic depolarization, particularly in specialized conducting systems such as Purkinje tissue.

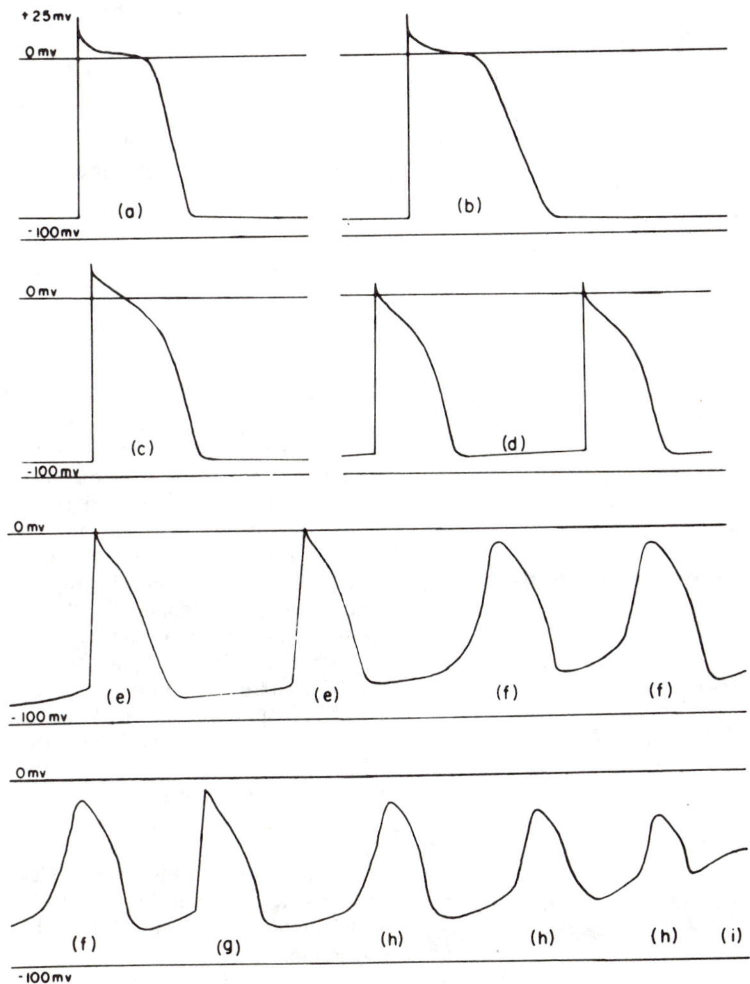

Fig. 15.1-5. *Sequence of changes in the transmembrane action potential of an isolated preparation of canine Purkinje fibers caused by ouabain.*

Driving stimuli are applied at a rate of 30/min (a) control; (b) increased action potential duration due to prolongation of phase 3; (c) onset of progressive decrease in action potential duration due to shortening of phase 2; (d, e) further shortening of the action potential accompanied by development of depolarization during phase 4, a decrease in the level of maximum diastolic potential, and an associated decrease in the rate of rise and amplitude of the action potential; (f) onset of spontaneous activity due to phase 4 depolarization and a further decrease in maximum diastolic potential; (g) a single-driven response, interrupting the spontaneous activity, demonstrates a higher rate of rise and greater amplitude than the spontaneous action potentials but further deterioration in comparison with earlier records; (h) recurrence of spontaneous action potentials of progressively lower amplitude, due to the progressive decrease in maximum diastolic potential, and leading to arrest and inexcitability in (i). (From Ref. 26 by permission).

Although ectopic beats have been observed in cardiac muscle exposed to ouabain, these developed in the absence of slow diastolic depolarization and are dependent on the preceding driven responses. A constant coupling to the preceding beat was also evident. This combination of characteristics indicates that the occurrences of ectopic beats in muscle are caused by reentry due to nonuniformity in conduction and/or refractoriness in a particular segment of cardiac muscle, or of the conducting system. For any given dose of digitalis, toxicity will appear sooner in the Purkinje fibers than ventricular muscle. Thus, the concept of *tissue dependence* (i.e., the tissue in which the alterations occur, namely, the atrium, specialized conducting system, and ventricles) should be considered an important variable in digitalis toxicity.

Several recent studies using microelectrode recordings of the Purkinje fibers suggest that a mechanism other than phase 4 depolarization is involved in the digitalis—induced automaticity, namely, *oscillatory afterpotentials* (Fig. 15.1-6). The effect of digitalis on automaticity depends on conditions such as potassium concentrations and heart rate. It has been reported that at slow rates, phase 4 depolarization and oscillatory afterpotentials coexist, whereas oscillatory afterpotentials dominate at faster rates. In any case, regardless of the underlying electrophysiological mechanisms, the arrhythmia induced not only results from direct actions of the drug on the heart but also involves action of the agent on both divisions of the autonomic nervous system (34, 36, 48, 49, 61).

The effect of toxic doses of digitalis to produce arrhythmia has been related to the ability to alter the activity of the sympathetic nerves innervating the heart; both enhancement and depression of nerve activity has been reported after the administration of digitalis (45, 62). The effects of ouabain on sympathetic nerve discharge have been demonstrated (33, 35, 36). Ouabain initially decreased spontaneous discharge of the sympathetic preganglionic filaments, but increased nerve activity was associated with the development of arrhythmia. Roberts and co-workers (50) suggested that digitalis influences autonomic neural activity in the heart in a dose-related manner to produce local changes in neural function; this *discordant* neural activity would alter conductivity, automaticity, and excitability in different areas of the myocardium. These effects would impede the normal "flow of the cardiac impulse" culminating in arrhythmia (23).

Electrocardiographic Changes. Electrocardiographic manifestations of digitalis effects (some of which are demonstrated in Fig. 15.1-7) include: prolonged PR interval (decreased AV conduction), shortened QT interval (shortening of repolarization time), AV dissociation (slowing of AV conduction), ventricular arrhythmias such as premature ventricular contractions, bigeminal rhythm, and ventricular fibrillation.

Peripheral Vascular Resistance. Digitalis exerts a moderate direct constrictor action on peripheral arterial and venous smooth muscle; thus, the digitalis-induced increase in contractility in the normal heart does not

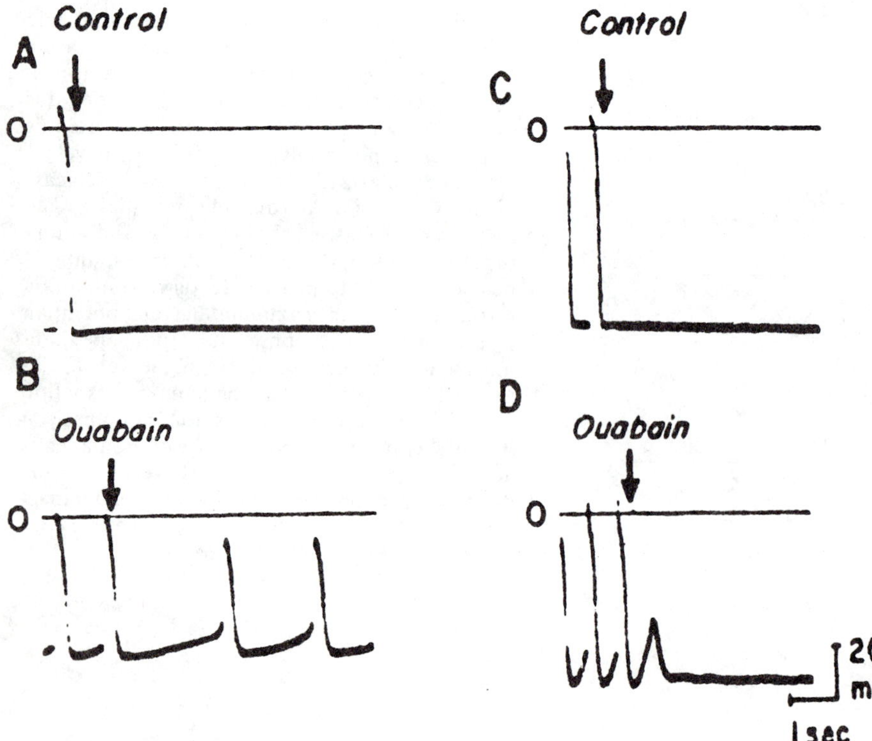

Fig. 15.1-6. *Digitalis-induced changes in phase 4 depolarization.* Panels A and C controls showing two different Purkinje fibers superfused with Tyrode's solution. The drive stimuli are discontinued at the arrows, followed in both panels by electrical quiescence. Panels B and D were recorded following 35 min of superfusion with ouabain, 2 x 10^{-7} M. Phase 4 depolarization is occurring in both fiberts. In B, discontinuation of the drive (arrow) is followed by the onset of a spontaneous rhythm at a cycle length longer than the basic drive. In D, discontinuation of the drive (arrow) is followed by a delayed after depolarization and subsequent electrical quiescence. Drive cycle length, 1000 msec; temperature, 37°C; Tyrode's $[K^+]_o$ = 2.5 mM in A and B, 4 mM in C and D. (From Ref. 51 by permission).

result in a rise in cardiac output. When given intravenously to a normal individual, ouabain produces: a rise in mean blood pressure; a decrease in forearm blood flow; an elevation of forearm vascular resistance; an increase in forearm venous tone: an increase in peripheral vascular resistance; and, a slight fall in cardiac output.

Cellular Mechanism. ***Therapeutic Effect.*** The possible subcellular mechanism(s) of action for the positive inotropic effect of digitalis has been reviewed by numerous authors (1, 7, 29, 40, 44, 48, 53, 55). Two effects that are manifested by digitalis, and that are thought to be related to its positive inotropic as well as its electrophysiological and toxic actions, include inhibition of cardiac Na^+, K^+-ATPase, and increased intracellular concentration of Ca^{2+}. Inhibition of the Na^+, K^+-ATPase activity results in inhibition of the Na^+ pump and causes an increase in the intracellular concentration of Na^+. The enhanced Na^+ may increase the magnitude of intracellular free Ca^{2+} available for excitation-contraction coupling (1). The latter is the mechanism by which the cardiac impulse gives rise to contraction and thus produces a positive inotropic effect (Fig. 15.1-8). A number of papers, however, disagree with this hypothesis (7, 44). Digitalis may increase the available intracellular Ca^{2+} by releasing intracellularly bound Ca^{2+} and by increasing the entry of Ca^{2+} into the cell from storage sites in the plasma membranes (Fig. 15.1-9). Indeed, digitalis and calcium may be synergistic to the point that the administration of Ca^{2+} may be dangerous in the digitalized patient.

The myocardial contractile apparatus consists of several proteins that include a regulatory complex composed of troponin and tropomyosin and involves Ca^{2+} for its action. The sequestration of Ca^{2+} into or in the sarcoplasmic reticulum from troponin occurs as the contractile apparatus relaxes. This, if Ca^{2+} is involved in the control of contraction and relaxation, then any of the systems involved in the modulation of internal Ca^{2+} may be sites for digitalis action. Na^+, K^+, and Ca^{2+} ions that flux between the outside and the inside of the cardiac cell actually move across the sarcolemma via the T system. The T system provides a means for ready access of digitalis to the sarcoplasmic reticulum especially involved in the intracellular transport of calcium in the vicinity of the contractile proteins found throughout the cardiac cell. The increased Ca^{2+} influx would provide a greater quantity of calcium to the contractile proteins, and this would enhance excitation-contraction coupling to result in a more forceful contraction (i.e., a positive inotropic action). A recent report indicates that cardiac nerves do contribute to digitalis-induced inotropic action and that

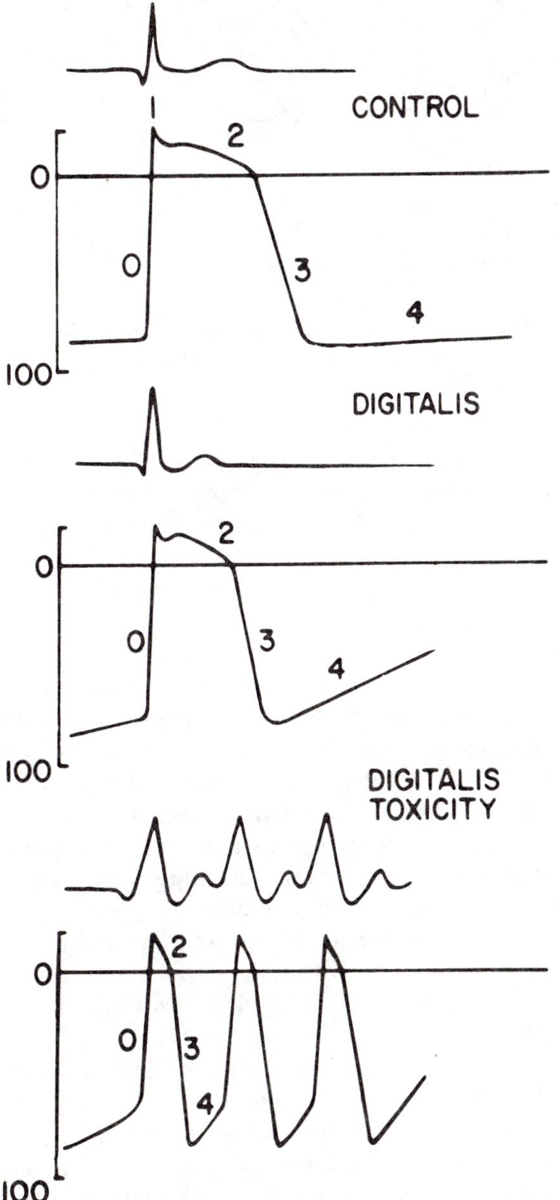

Fig. 15.1-7. *ECG and Purkinje fibers.* Note increase in phase 4 depolarization after digitalis administration. Lower strip: ventricular tachycardia occurs. (From Ref. 15 by permission).

Digitalis glycosides
↓
Na^+,K^+-ATPase inhibition
↓
Na^+-pump inhibition
↓
Enhanced $[Na^+]_i$ transient
↓
Enhanced $[Ca^{++}]_i$ transient
↓
Enhanced Ca^{++} binding to troponin-tropomyosin
↓
Enhanced activation of actomyosin system
↓
Enhanced contraction

Fig. 15.1-8. *Proposed mechanism for the inotropic action of digitalis.* (From Ref. 6 by permission).

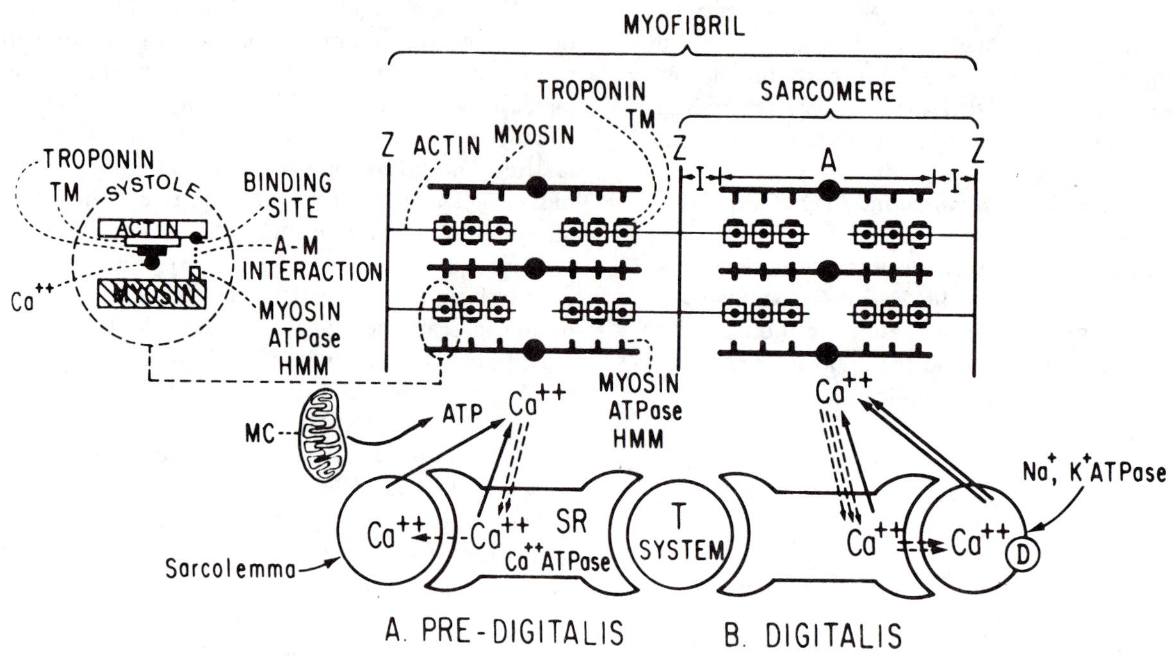

Fig. 15.1-9. *Schematic diagram of a cardiac cell, showing the proposed subcellular mechanism of the contractile, stimulating action of digitalis.*

D = digitalis site of action in the sarcolemma membrane (Na^+, K^+-ATPase receptor). SR = sarcoplasmic reticulum; MC = mitochondria; HMM = heavy mermyosin; A-M = actin-myosin; TM = tropomyosin. (From Ref. 40 by permission).

both adrenergic and cholinergic mechanisms are responsible for this modulation (10).

Adverse Effects. Digitalis, in doses that cause cardiac arrhythmias, has uniformly been reported to result in a loss of potassium from the cardiac cell, a loss attributed to the influence of digitalis on the Na^+, K^+-ATPase system, although in relation to time, recovery of the enzyme from inhibition is somewhat faster than the restoration of normal K^+ levels (1). Inhibition of Na^+, K^+-ATPase results in accumulation of sodium inside the cell and loss of K^+ from the cell, and the resting membrane potential decreases and repolarization time (primarily a K^+-dependent event) will also decrease. The lower the resting membrane potential, the slower the rate of rise of the action potential. Increased Na^+ inside the cell also contributes to the slower rate of rise. An action potential with a slow rate of rise would be conducted at a slower conduction velocity than those that have faster rates of rise. Slowed conduction could lead to reentrant arrhythmia. Within the specialized conducting systems, a decrease in conduction velocity will favor the independent discharge of multipacemakers as well as the development of circuitous paths of excitation that may predispose to reentry systems and eventually to fibrillation.

The onset of digitalis toxicity occurs earliest in hearts or preparations driven at faster rates. This earlier development of toxicity may be due to: (1) a greater uptake of digitalis by the tissue; (2) enhanced ionic exchange with faster rates in the presence of a poisoned Na^+, K^+ pump; or, (3) the enhancement of yet unidentified ionic currents (61). In this regard, it should be pointed out that because Ca^{2+} movements seem to contribute to the late stage of depolarization of the action potential and to the plateau phase during repolarization, the electrophysiological changes that accompany digitalis toxicity may be due, in part, to alteration in transmembrane exchange of calcium ions. The synergistic actions of calcium and digitalis in their capacity to produce cardiac abnormalities are well known. It is interesting that a number of agents that are capable of blocking current flow through the slow channels also diminish the toxic actions of digitalis. Among these agents are manganese and verapamil (17). Verapamil has been shown to terminate repetitive spontaneous activity primarily due to underlying digitalis-induced oscillating afterpotentials, whereas automaticity due to normal phase 4 depolarization was only slightly depressed under the same conditions (17).

In addition to its direct effects on ionic flux across the cardiac membranes, there is evidence that indicates that rhythm disturbances may also be initiated by an action of digitalis on the adrenergic nervous system. Ouabain has been shown to produce inhibition of the amine pump of the adrenergic nerve membrane, which appears to involve a Na^+, K^+-ATPase system. As a result of this inhibition of the amine pump by ouabain, the uptake of catecholamines into the neural binding sites is reduced. *In vivo*, this action is not readily demonstrable (16), unless procedures such as DC current shock are used.

Digitalis causes sensitization of the heart to arrhythmias following direct current shocks. Digitalis sensitization is thought to result from increased amounts of norepinephrine becoming available when the nerve terminals are depolarized by the DC current shock and the transmitter is not taken up in the nerve, as digitalis inhibits the amine pump. It would seem, therefore, that at the cellular level effects of digitalis not only on cardiac muscle but also on adrenergic neuronal structures must be taken into account. Indeed, recent studies indicate that for the protective effect of sympathectomy against ouabain-induced arrhythmias to develop the adrenergic nerve terminal must be present, although not functional as far as adrenergic neurotransmission is concerned (31, 32).

PHARMACOKINETICS

The basic differences in the pharmacokinetic properties of the digitalis materials (i.e., differences in water- or lipid-solubility, gastrointestinal absorption, metabolism, and excretion) are explained by the chemical differences discussed previously (Fig. 15.1 – 1). For example, digitoxin is highly lipid-soluble, completely absorbed from the GI tract, highly bound to plasma protein, and metabolized in the liver: it undergoes enterohepatic circulation, being excreted in bile and subsequently reabsorbed. Its long half-life (7 days) is increased by hepatic diseases or hepatectomy in animals. Digoxin and ouabain have different pharmacokinetic properties than digitoxin (Table 15.1-2). The disappearance of these compounds from the body is a first-order reaction (i.e., the total loss from the body will be proportional to the total amount present).

ASSAY OF DIGITALIS GLYCOSIDES

Powdered digitalis from leaf and other relatively impure preparations are assayed in pigeons, as stated in USP. Pure preparations (e.g., digitoxin, digoxin, and ouabain) are assayed spectrophotometrically and compared with their respective standards. Radioimmunoassay methods (2, 3) to determine serum concentrations of digoxin or digitoxin may indicate whether the patient has recently received digitalis and if the plasma level falls within toxic range which overlaps the therapeutic range (Fig. 15.1-10). Determination of plasma level has shown variations in bioavailability of different lots of digoxin and other preparations (due to differences in the tablet dissolution rates), resulting in unpredictable therapeutic response (37). The problem associated with digoxin bioavailability has recently been reviewed.

THERAPEUTIC USES

General. Digitalis is of most value in the treatment of heart failure characterized as *low output*, such as that seen in patients with a depressed cardiac output secondary to ischemic, valvular hypertension and congenital heart disease, cardiomyopathies,

Table 15.1-2
Pharmacokinetic Properties of Glycosides in Humans

Glycoside	Solubility	Polarity	Gastro-intestinal Absorption	Plasma Binding (%)	Plasma Half-Life[a]	Onset of Action (min)[b]	Peak Effect (hr)	Therapeutic Serum Concn. (ng/ml)	Route of Metabolism or Excretion
Digitoxin	Lipid	Low	Completely (90-100%)	90-97	5-7 days	25-120	4-12	10-25	Liver,[c] renal excretion of metabolites
Digoxin	Less lipid than digitoxin	Low	Not well[d,e] (60-85%)	25	1.5 days	15-30	1.5-5	0.5-2	Renal, some G.I., 25% excreted by nonrenal
Ouabain	Water	High	Unreliable; given i.v.	25	21 hr	5-10	0.5-2	0.4-0.64	Renal, some GI
Deslanoside	Slightly lipid	Low	Unreliable; given i.v.	22-25	33 hr	10-30	1-2		Renal
Digitalis leaf			Approx. 40%		4-6 days	120-240	8-10		Similar to digitoxin

[a] For normal subjects (prolonged by renal impairment with digoxin, ouabain, and deslanoside and probably by severe hepatic disease with digitoxin and digitalis leaf).
[b] For intravenous dose.
[c] Enterohepatic cycle exists; excreted in bile and reabsorbed.
[d] For tablet form of administration (may be less in malabsorption syndromes and in formulations with poor bioavailability).
[e] Highest concentrations found in heart, liver and kidney.
Source: Adopted from Ref. 55 by permission).

and cor pulmonale. *High output failure*, associated with anemia, arteriovenous fistulas, hyperthyroidism, beriberi, Paget's disease, and pulmonary emphysema, does not respond well to digitalis. Digitalis is also of limited value in the treatment of mitral stenosis with normal sinus rhythms, constrictive pericarditis, or pericardial tamponade and idiopathic hypertrophic subaortic stenosis. As indicated earlier, the symptoms associated with congestive heart failure are diminished or reversed by the action of digitalis that increases the force of contraction (Fig. 15.1-3).

In chronic ischemic heart disease with ventricular dysfunction, digitalis may be observed to exert an antianginal effect due to its action to lower ventricular wall tension and the associated reduction in oxygen consumption.

The use of digitalis in the treatment of myocardial infarction-induced failure is controversial (39) as digitalis may actually aggravate the arrhythmias associated with infarction, increase the size of infarction and subendocardial necrosis due to increased myocardial oxygen consumption, and cause coronary vasoconstriction. This favors the formation of left ventricular aneurysms due to the positive inotropic stimulation of the myocardium that has survived the infarction.

Digitalis is also of benefit when treating atrial flutter because it slows the ventricular rate. Slowing of the ventricular rate by digitalis is due to its effect on AV conduction, which results in fewer impulses being conducted to the ventricle. The depressant effect on AV conduction is primarily due to a vagomimetic and an antisympathetic action. It is important to note that digitalis usually will not convert the atrial arrhythmia to normal sinus rhythm; in fact, its vagomimetic action may convert atrial flutter to fibrillation. Digitalis may also be used to treat paroxysmal atrial tachycardia; this is due to its vagal effect. Digitalis, however, does not consistently prevent or terminate this arrhythmia.

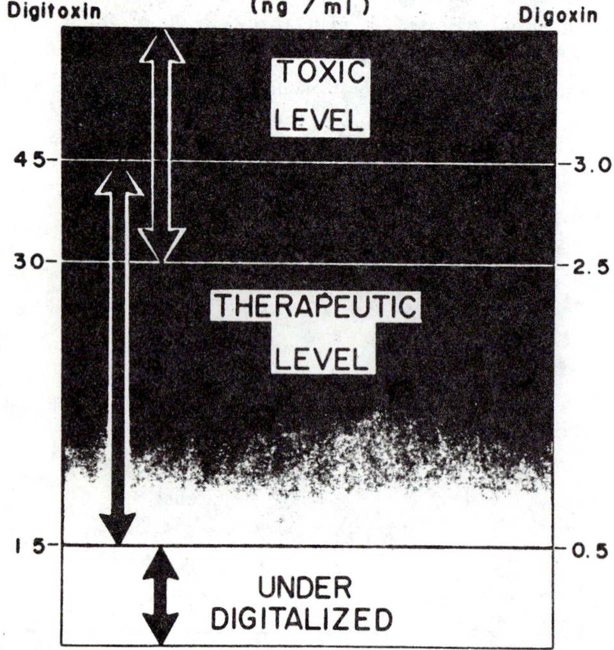

Fig. 15.1-10. *Serum digitalis levels.*

Note that the scale for digitoxin is shown on left vertical axis, digoxin on the right, in nanograms per milliliter. Because considerable degree of overlap is present, it is necessary to apply clinical judgment for appropriate evaluation. (From Ref. 13 by permission).

Therapy with digitalis is complicated by the small therapeutic index for the drug; this fact, coupled with the problem that in many individuals it is difficult to evaluate whether the dose regimen employed is optimal, accounts, in part, for the fact that digitalis intoxication occurs so frequently.

Pediatric. The pediatric and geriatric patient pose different problems for the physician prescribing digitalis. Pediatric patients in Europe or South America most probably will receive digoxin or digitoxin, whereas those in the United States are likely to receive digoxin (57) which is commercially available in oral or parenteral pediatric doses, is inexpensive, controls congestive heart failure and arrhythmias in the pediatric patient, and because of its rapid rate of excretion facilitates treatment of overdose cases. Absorption of digoxin from the gastrointestinal tract does not appear to be influenced by the feeding schedule; drug administration, however, should be done at times other than just before or after feeding, because regurgitation or vomiting will cause unpredictable losses of the drug. It has recently been suggested that pediatric preparations containing digoxin in alcohol solution may be completely absorbed from the gastrointestinal tract. Other investigators failed to find supporting evidence (12).

Although the consensus among American pediatric cardiologists is that infants and children are generally best managed with digoxin, intravenous lanatoside C is often used for rapid digitalization because the onset of action and the time to peak effect of intravenous lanatoside C are similar to those actions of digoxin. The advantage of digoxin over lanatoside C is that digoxin can be given intravenously for a rapid effect in an emergency and allows a smooth transition to either parenteral or oral maintenance digoxin at a later time. The transition of digoxin maintenance after initial treatment with lanatoside C is more difficult, however, because lanatoside C is employed only in a parenteral form and is excreted more rapidly than is digoxin. Due to the short half-life of lanatoside C, suboptimal serum levels may occur when the change to maintenance digoxin is effected. It has yet to be established if a loading rather than a maintenance dose of digoxin should be employed when following digitalization with lanatoside C.

It is known that children require more digitalis than do adults (i.e., about 50% more drug calculated on the basis of body weight must be given in order to obtain similar results) (42). The premature infant, however, requires a smaller digitalis dose due to decreased renal function (59). Table 15.1-3 indicates the recommended digitalizing doses for infants and children and includes a summary of serum digoxin concentrations reported by numerous authors. Detailed discussions of dose regimens for the pediatric patient may be found elsewhere (54, 59) (see also Chapter 30).

Geriatric. The use of digitalis in the elderly is complicated by reduced renal function, and thus the dose regimen should be reduced. Many patients are discharged from general hospitals to enter nursing homes where they may continue to receive digitalis and/or potassium supplements, but with proper adjustment of dose regimen.

DIGITALIZATION PROCEDURES

It has generally been considered that all digitalis materials have the same type of myocardial action and approximately the same therapeutic index. The rapid onset of action exhibited by ouabain permits its use in an emergency situation; deslanoside or digoxin have slightly longer times to the onset of action but may also be used. When initiating long-term treatment, a *loading* or *digitalizing dose* may be given to obtain the desired body glycoside level immediately. A lower *maintenance dose*, calculated to replace the daily loss of the glycoside, is then used to sustain the desired level (Table 15.1-4). Maintenance levels are

Table 15.1-3
Recommended Dosage of Digitalis Preparations in Pediatric Patients

		Loading Dose (mg/kg body weight)			
Preparation	Route of Administration	Prematures and Newborns	1 mo.-2 yrs. of Age	Over 2 yrs. of Age	Maintenance Dose
Digoxin	p.o.	0.03-0.05	0.06-0.08	0.04-0.06	1/10-1/5 of loading dose in newborns; 1/5-1/3 of loading dose in two divided doses in infants and children
	i.v.	0.03-0.05	0.04-0.06	0.02-0.06	Maintenance dose p.o., as above
Digitoxin	p.o. or i.v.	0.015-0.03	0.04-0.06	0.02-0.04	1/10 of loading dose in two divided doses daily

Source: From Ref. 54 by permission.

easier to sustain with a digitalis material that has a longer duration of action (i.e., digitoxin). With a drug exhibiting a long duration of action, however, toxic effects that develop may persist even after the digitalis is stopped; to avoid this possibility, a digitalis material with a shorter duration of action (i.e., digoxin) may be used. It should be noted that Table 15.1-4 includes only mean values; the physician must always consider individual patient variation when selecting a maintenance dosage schedule.

Individuals with severely impaired renal function (creatinine clearance less than 10 ml/min) may manifest digoxin toxicity when receiving one-fourth or less of the normal maintenance dose. When employing digoxin in such patients, it is generally recommended that the maintenance dose also be reduced by one-half or more. In patients with slightly impaired renal function (i.e., creatinine clearance values of 50-80 ml/min), one-half of the normal maintenance dose of digoxin or a full dose of digitoxin does not usually cause toxic symptoms. In patients with moderate or severely impaired renal function, the loading dose of digitoxin does not have to be adjusted because it is metabolized by the liver. The hypothyroid patient and the hypokalemic patient are generally also more sensitive to the effects of digitalis.

If a fixed daily maintenance dose but not a loading dose of digitalis is given, body drug levels will gradually accumulate until the amount removed from the body each day is equivalent to the maintenance dose (Fig. 15.1-11). This is because digitalis agents are removed from the body via a first-order reaction (i.e., the amount removed will be proportional to the total amount present in the body). Fig. 15.1-11 clearly shows that the curves for digitalis accumulation and removal are mirror images of each other; approximately 5 half-lives are required to reach kinetic equilibrium.

DIGITALIS TOXICITY

General. ***Cardiac.*** As summarized by Spector (58) the occurrence of digitalis toxicity is substantial. In the Boston Collaborative Drug Surveillance Program, 3828 hospitalized patients received digoxin, and approximately 9% of these patients developed cardiac toxicity. The toxicity was life-threatening in 2% of the patients, and several fatalities occurred; 3% exhibited gastrointestinal disturbances including anorexia, nausea, vomiting, and diarrhea. Studies done in Canada and Ireland also

Table 15.1-4
Adult Glycoside Loading and Maintenance Doses (mg)

Glycoside	Average Digitalizing Dose		Usual Daily Oral Maintenance Dose
	p.o. (mg)[b]	i.v. (mg)[c]	(mg)[a]
Digitoxin	0.7-1.20	1	0.1
Digoxin	1.25-1.50	0.75-1	0.25-0.5
Ouabain	—	0.3-0.5	—
Deslanoside	—	0.8	—
Digitalis leaf	0.80-1.20		0.10

[a] Average dose for adult patients without renal or hepatic impairments; will differ widely among individual patients and requires close medical supervision.
[b] Divided doses over 12-14 hrs at intervals of 6-8 hrs.
[c] Given in increments for initial subcomplete digitalization, to be supplemented by further small increments as necessary.
Source: From Ref. 55 by permission.

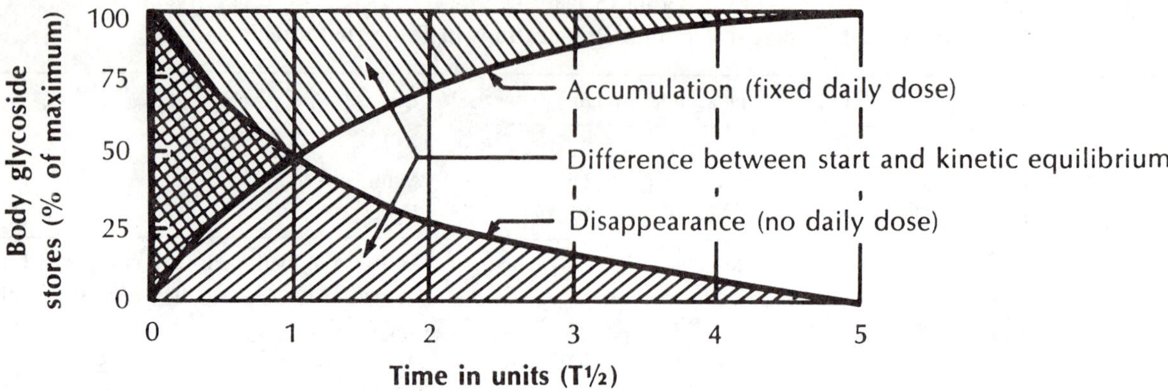

Fig. 15.1-11. *Accumulation of a digitalis glycoside on a fixed daily dose compared with its disappearance after dosage is stopped.* Time is expressed in units of half-times. (From Ref. 27 by permission).

indicate a similar incidence of toxicity associated with digitalis administered to hospitalized patients (58). In the study of Beller et al (2), digitalis toxicity was diagnosed in 31 (23%) of 135 outpatients receiving digitalis; another 8 individuals (6%) were classified as "possible toxic." Thus, the prevalence of digitalis toxicity in outpatients appears to be higher than that for inpatients.

Fig. 15-1-8 demonstrates the electrocardiographic changes associated with digitalis-induced toxicity. Extrasystoles that usually originate in the ventricle but may also arise from the atrium constitute the most common sign of digitalis cardiac toxicity in adults; the frequency of extrasystoles and ventricular tachycardia is less in children. Extrasystoles may also develop following a small dose of digitalis, however. In patients with atrial fibrillation, extrasystoles may occur coupled to each regular systole; this is called *pulsus bigeminus* or *digitalis coupling* and indicates digitalis toxicity. The digitalis bigeminy may occur alone or may precede, follow, or develop simultaneously with other signs of toxicity. Pulsus trigeminus may also develop. Patients in digitalis toxicity may manifest occasional dropped beats or partial or complete atrioventricular (AV) block.

Paroxysmal tachycardia, originating in either the atria or the ventricle, requires cessation of the digitalis. Paroxysmal atrial tachycardia with block is one danger signal. Nonparoxysmal tachycardias are more common than paroxysmal episodes. Atrial tachycardia generally arises from an ectopic focus in the atrium rather than from the sinoauricular (SA) node. If the patient manifests ventricular tachycardia, the digitalis must be stopped immediately to prevent the development of more ominous types of arrhythmia. *Bidirectional tachycardia* may be produced by digitalis in severly damaged hearts and is thought to originate supraventricularly with an alternating block in the major branches of the ventricular conduction system. Digitalis toxicity may produce atrial fibrillation, but this does not prevent the use of digitalis in the treatment of this arrhythmia. Ventricular fibrillation is the most common mode of death due to digitalis toxicity and may explain sudden deaths that occur in individuals receiving high doses of a digitalis agent. Additional arrhythmias that may be associated with digitalis toxicity include: AV nodal (junctional) tachycardia, intraventricular dissociation, parasystole, heart block, and atrial standstill.

Extracardiac. Digitalis toxicity is considered to be a prevalent adverse drug reaction due to the low therapeutic index of the drug and the development of hypokalemia during therapy of congestive failure. Hypokalemia, characterized by a decreased cardiac intracellular potassium concentration, is thought to be the most common cause of digitalis intoxication and may be due to excessive doses of digitalis, diuretic treatment, malnutrition, corticosteroid therapy, or hemodialysis. In addition to hypokalemia, hypomagnesemia, hypercalcemia, hypoxia, or increased acidity may precipitate digitalis toxicity. The development of digitalis toxicity may occur after the use of a large dose administered with diuretics for the treatment of severe arrhythmias or following the cumulative effect of maintenance doses taken for a long time. Table 15.1-5 summarizes the extracardiac symptoms of digitalis toxicity. Anorexia is usually the first sign of toxicity; nausea and vomiting generally develop several days later and may be accompanied by copious salivation. The episodes of nausea and vomiting may begin and end abruptly and then recur with greater severity. Digitalis stimulation of the chemoreceptor trigger zone elicits vomiting (5); it may develop without advance warning signs of anorexia or nausea. In addition, not all patients will exhibit vomiting. Gastrointestinal effects of digitalis toxicity may include diarrhea, abdominal discomfort, or pain: these disappear in several days following drug cessation.

Pediatric. Younger children accidentally poisoned by the ingestion of digitalis have been reported to display "rather innocuous electrocardiographic changes" at the same time that they succumb to seizures, coma, and respiratory arrest. Vagal stimulation, producing sinus arrhythmia, is generally seen in the young. Older children, like adults, complain of visual disturbances that include photophobia, hazy vision, color disturbances, and blind spots (Table 15.1-5).

If a child on digitalis begins to vomit, the possibility of digitalis toxicity must be considered. Disturbances of atrioventricular conduction and atrial ectopic activity have been reported for infants. Premature and newborn infants often show sinus slowing, with cardiac rates of less than 100 beats per minute, due to increased vagal activity. Other symptoms of digitalis toxicity in the infant include an exaggerated arrhythmia, supraventricular ectopic beats, and paroxysmal atrial tachycardia with variable ventricular response. Ventricular ectopic beats and tachyarrhythmias occur but are the exception (59). Reasons for differences between cardiac toxicities seen in the adult and the newborn are not certain.

Geriatric. Toxicity may develop in the geriatric patient given amounts of digoxin that would be well tolerated by younger individuals (9, 21). This difference may be due to: an age-induced increase in myocardial sensitivity to normal concentration; higher myocardial digitalis levels even though an usual dose was given; hypokalemia from diuretic therapy or laxative abuse; smaller body size; or, decreased renal excretion of digoxin due to age-induced

Table 15.1-5
Extracardiac Symptoms of Digitalis Toxicity

Symptoms	Characterization of Symptoms	Time of Appearance as Digitalis Toxicity Develops	Comments
Neurological			
Neuralgic pain	Usually involves lower third of face and stimulates trigeminal neuralgia; may involve extremities and lumbar area	May be the earliest sign	Most patients will complain of extreme fatigue and weakness
Generalized fatigue	Headache, fatigue, malaise, drowsiness, muscle weakness	Early symptoms	
Mental symptoms	Disorientation, confusion, aphasia; delirium, hallucinations; rarely convulsions		More commonly seen in elderly atherosclerotic individuals; may improve when fluid and electrolyte abnormalities are corrected and when digitalis and potent diuretics are discontinued
Vision	Blurred white borders or halos may appear on dark objects ("white vision"); may be alterations in colored vision: chromatopsia most common for yellow and green but red, brown, and blue vision can occur; transitory amblyopia, diplopia, and scotomata may occur		Most patients will complain of some type of vision disturbance
Papillomacular fibers of the optic nerve	Retrobulbar neuritis		
Miscellaneous			
Skin lesions	Urticarial or scarlatiniform	Rarely occur	Antihistamines have no effect
Eosinophilia			Atropine decreases, pilocarpine increases
Gynecomastia	Seen in men and women		Digitalis, because chemically similar to the sex hormones, is thought to exhibit estrogenic activity
Coagulation time	Therapeutic doses may decrease without influencing prothrombin time or clot retraction		Very rarely, digitalis may cause thrombocytopenia

decreases in the glomerular filtration rate causing an increased half-life for plasma levels of digitalis. After administration of a single dose, blood concentrations of digoxin and metabolites are almost twice as high in the geriatric patient when compared with younger individuals and, when related to body weight, were significantly higher in the elderly after 24 hours. The half-life of digoxin in the blood of elderly and younger patients was 73 and 51 hours, respectively (9). A recent review of clinical studies provides information on the relationships between age, dose, and plasma levels of digitalis in therapeutic and toxic populations.

Clinical Conditions Affecting Digitalis Toxicity. Patients with chronic pulmonary heart disease exhibit an increased frequency of toxicity to digitalis that is thought to be related to systemic arterial hypoxemia. In general, digitalis intoxication will occur at a lower plasma level of digitalis than that seen in patients with normal pulmonary function.

The effect of digoxin and digitoxin is increased in a patient who is hypothyroid (i.e., myxedema) because the decrease in plasma clearance produces a higher plasma level for comparable doses of digitalis based on body weight. The opposite situation exists in the hyperthyroid patient who manifests hypermetabolism and would therefore require a larger-than-normal dose of digitalis. Propranolol is generally thought to be effective in heart failure associated with thyrotoxicosis and in controlling the ventricular rate in atrial fibrillation or flutter; digoxin is unlikely to be beneficial.

Treatment of Digitalis Toxicity. When digitalis intoxication is diagnosed, digitalis and diuretic therapy should be discontinued. If the arrhythmias do not reverse or if they increase in severity, antiarrhythmic agents may be employed (38) (Table 15.1-6). Phenytoin or lidocaine are considered to be the treatment of choice for digitalis-induced tachyarrhythmias. Both of these drugs, in low doses, do not exert a depressant action on AV conduction. Therapeutic concentrations do not change or may improve conduction in the His-Purkinje system. Phenytoin has been shown to abolish ventricular tachycardias induced by acetylstrophanthidin and, at the same time, improve the AV conduction impairment induced by digitalis. Furthermore, it controls digitalis-induced arrhythmias without counteracting the inotropic action of digitalis (4). Procainamide or propranolol are alternative antiarrhythmic agents, although they may make heart block worse by causing a complete atrial-ventricular dissociation. If toxicity is produced by a short-acting digitalis preparation, tachyarrhythmias will be selflimited when the drug is stopped. An in-depth discussion of the clinical management of digitalis toxicity may be found elsewhere (18).

The use of potassium should be discouraged because it, like digitalis, depresses AV conduction.

A current innovative method employed to reverse human digitalis toxicity that was considered to be life-threatening and did not respond to conventional measures involved the administration of purified Fab fragments of bovine digoxin-specific antibodies (56).

Table 15.1-6
Dosage of Drugs to Counteract Digitalis Toxicity

Drug	Dosage/Form	Route	Dose
Lidocaine (XYLOCAINE)	Ampules 2% solution 20 mg/ml	i.v.	1 mg/kg (bolus injection) 1 mg/kg/min by continuous infusion
Phenytoin (DILANTIN)	Vials 50 mg/ml	i.v.	5 mg/kg (given over 5 minutes)
	Capsules 100 mg	p.o.	3-5 mg/kg/day in 3 divided doses
Propranolol (INDERAL)	Vials 1 mg/ml	i.v.	0.01 mg/kg (given over 10 minutes)
	Tablets 10, 40 mg	p.o.	0.02-0.05 mg/kg/day (in 3 or 4 divided doses)
Procainamide (PRONESTYL)	Vials 100 mg/ml	i.v.	100 mg in 5% glucose/water given slowly by drip; repeat effective dose every 5-10 minutes
		i.m.	7-10 mg/kg
	Capsules 250 mg	p.o.	15 mg/kg stat. 50-300 mg q. 6 hr for maintenance
Isoproterenol (ISUPREL)	Ampules 0.2 mg/ml	i.v.	1 mg in 250 ml 5% glucose/water 4 μg/ml by slow drip until desired effect
Quinidine sulfate	Tablets, 100, 200, 300 mg	p.o.	3-6 mg/kg every 2-3 hr x 5, can increase to 12 mg/kg every 2-3 hr x 5
Quinidine gluconate (QUINAGLUTE)	Tablet 0.33 g	p.o.	10-30 mg/kg/day
Potassium	Vials 44.6 mEq/50 ml	i.v.	1 g (13 mEq) in 250 ml 5% glucose/water 0.5 mEq/kg/hr (do not exceed 2 mEq/kg)
		p.o.	1-5 g/day; 1-2 mEq/kg/day

Source: From Ref. 59 by permission.

Table 15.1-7
Drugs that Interact with Digitalis Glycosides

Drug	Effect of Digitalis	Suggested Mechanism
I. *Cardiovascular agents*		
Diuretics	Increased toxicity	Hypokalemia; the magnesium deficiency that can follow diuretic therapy may also contribute
Heparin	Digitalis glycosides may antagonize the anticoagulant activity of heparin	
Phenytoin	May increase metabolism of digitoxin	Induction of hepatic microsomal enzymes
Quinidine	Enhances digoxin serum levels	Quinidine decreases renal glycoside clearance; although controversial, quinidine may also displace digoxin from tissue binding sites
Reserpine (parenteral)	Increased tendency for arrhythmias in the digitalized patient	Consequence of sudden catecholamine release
II. *Chemotherapeutic agents*		
Amphotericin B	Increased toxicity	Hypokalemia
III. *Gastrointestinal (GI) agents*		
Antacids (p.o.)	Decreased digoxin plasma level	Decreased absorption
Cathartics	Decreased effect of digitalis	Rapid passage of digitalis through the gut and decreased absorption
	May potentiate the effect of the absorbed digitalis	Hypokalemia
Cholestyramine	Decreased digitoxin plasma level and half-life	Binding of digitoxin in the intestine and interference with its enterohepatic circulation
Phenobarbital or phenylbutazone	Decreased plasma digitoxin level and half-life	Increased metabolism of digitoxin due to induction of hepatic microsomal enzymes
Kaolin-pectin	Decreased digoxin plasma level	Decreased absorption
Metoclopramide	GI absorption of slowly dissolving brands of digoxin may be decreased	Increased GI motility
Propantheline	GI absorption of slowly dissolving brands of digoxin may be increased	Decreased GI motility
IV. *Hormonal agents*		
Insulin	May increase toxicity	Hypokalemia
Thyroid	Underdigitalization if thyroid given to digitalized patient	Thyroid hormone increases metabolism leading to increased plasma clearance of digitalis
	May potentiate the toxic effects of digitalis	Sinus tachycardia may be caused by thyroid drugs
V. *Sympathomimetic agents*		
Ephedrine, epinephrine, and probably others	Increased risk of digitalis toxicity	Sympathomimetics may cause cardiac arrhythmias (i.e., ectopic pacemaker activity)
VI. *Miscellaneous*		
Calcium (parenteral)	Increased tendency for ectopic pacemaker activity; fatalities reported	Calcium may enhance positive inotropic effect of digitalis
Glucose infusions	Increased toxicity	May cause intracellular shift of K^+ with resultant decrease in serum K^+
Sulfasalazine	Possible decrease in digoxin plasma level	Decreased absorption
Succinylcholine	Potentiate digitalis effects on conduction that increases ventricular irritability	May be due to effect on cholinergic receptors that release catecholamines; depolarizing muscle relaxants may produce a sudden shift of K^+ from inside the digitalized myocardium muscle cell to outside to produce arrhythmias

Digoxin was bound to the Fab fragment and was then rapidly excreted.

POTENTIAL DRUG INTERACTIONS

Patients treated for heart failure (especially elderly patients) have often taken several other drugs in addition to digitalis. Many reports describe potential interactions with such drugs and the relationship to digitalis intoxication (14, 24, 25, 30). Table 15.1-7 summarizes those drug interactions that are currently thought to be the most important.

REFERENCES

1. Akera, T., and Brody, T.M. The role of Na^+, K^+-ATPase in the inotropic action of digitalis. *Pharmacol. Rev.* 29:187, 1978.
2. Beller, G.A., Smith, T.W., Abelmann, W.H. et al. Digitalis intoxication: A prospective clinical study with serum level correlations. *N. Engl. J. Med.* 284:989, 1971.
3. Besch, H.R., and Watanabe, A.M. Radioimmunoassay of digoxin and digitoxin. *Clin. Chem.* 21:1815, 1975.
4. Bigger, J.T., and Strauss, H.C. Digitalis toxicity: Drug interactions promoting toxicity and the management of toxicity. *Semin. Drug Treat.* 2:147, 1972.
5. Borison, H.L., and Wang, S.C. Physiology and pharmacology of vomiting. Pharmacol. Rev. 5:193, 1953.
6. Brody, T.M., and Akera, T. Relations among Na^+, K^+-ATPase activity, sodium pump activity, transmembrane sodium movement, and cardiac contractility. *Fed. Proc.* 36:2219, 1977.
7. Busse, F., Lullman, HJ., and Peters, T. Concentration dependence of the binding of ouabain to isolated guinea pig atria. *J. Cardiovasc. Pharmacol.* 1:687, 1979.
8 Cattell, M., and Gold, H. Influence of digitalis glycosides on force of contraction of mammalian cardiac muscle. *J. Pharmacol. Exp. Ther.* 62:1116, 1938.
9. Cervoni, P., and Chen, P.S. The digitalis glycosides. In: *Handbook on Pharmacology of Aging* (Goldberg, P.B., and Roberts, J., eds.). Fla.: CRC Press, 1983, p. 15.
10. Cook, L.S., Caldwell, R.W., Nash, C.B., et al. Adrenergic and cholinergic mechanisms in digitalis inotropy. *J. Pharmacol. Exp. Ther.* 223:761, 1982.
11. Cranefield, P.F. Action potentials, afterpotentials, and arrhythmias. *Circ. Res. Monog.* 62:56, 1978.
12. Doherty, J.E. Digitalis glycosides: Pharmacokinetics and their clinical implications. *Ann. Intern. Med.* 79:229, 1973.
13. Doherty, J.E., Dalrymple, G.V., Murphy, M.L. et al. Pharmacokinetics of digoxin. *Fed. Proc.* 36:2242, 1977.
14. Dohety, J.E., Straub, K.D., Murphy, M.L. et al. Digoxin-quinidine interaction: Changes in canine tissue concentration from steady state with quinidine. *Am. J. Cardiol.* 45:1196, 1980.
15. Dreifus, L.S., and Watanabe, Y. Clinical correlates of the electrophysiologic action of digitalis on the heart. *Semin. Drug Treat.* 2:197, 1972.
16. Eikenburg, D.C., and Stickney, J.L. Inhibition of sympathetic neuronal transport and ouabain-induced cardiac arrhythmias. *Res. Comm. Chem. Path. Pharmacol.* 18:587, 1977.
17. Ferrier, G.R. Digitalis arrhythmias: Role of oscillatory afterpotentials. *Prog. Cardiovasc. Dis.* 19:459, 1977.
18. Frankl, W.S., Roberts, J., and Lathers, C.M. Congestive heart failure. In: *Cardiovascular Therapeutics in Clinical Practice* (Frankl, W.S., Roberts, J., and Lathers, C.M., eds.). New York: Wiley, 1984, p. 115.
19. Gabriel, K.L., Kelliher, G.J., Roberts, J. and Oerton, R. Involvement of adrenergic nervous influence in ouabain-induced nonuniformity of ventricular repolarization. *J. Pharmacol. Exp. Ther.* 207:1, 1978.
20. Gillis, R.A., Raines, A., Sohn, Y.J. et al. Neuroexcitatory effects of digitalis and their role in the development of cardiac arrhythmias. *J. Pharmacol. Exp. Ther.* 183:154, 1972.
21. Goldberg, P.B., and Roberts, J. Pharmacology. In: *The Aging Heart* (Weisfeldt, M.L., ed.) New York: Raven Press, 1980.
22. Goodman, D.J., Rossen, R.M., Cannom, D.S. et al. Effect of digoxin on atrioventricular conduction: Studies in patients with and without cardiac autonomic innervation. *Circulation* 51:251, 1975.
23. Han, J., and Moe, G.K. Nonuniform recovery of excitability in ventricular muscle. *Circ. Res.* 14:44, 1964.
24. Hansten, P.D. *Drug Interactions,* 5th ed. Phildelphia: Lea and Febiger, 1985.
25. Hirsh, P.D., Weiner, H.J., and North, R.L. Further insights into digoxin-quinidine interaction: Lack of correlation between serum digoxin concentration and inotropic state of the heart. *Am. J. Cardiol.* 46:863, 1980.
26. Hoffman, B.F., and Singer, D.H. Effects of digitalis on electrical activity of cardiac fibers. *Progr. Cardiovasc. Dis.* 7:226, 1964.
27. Jelliffe, R.W. An improved method of digoxin therapy. *Ann. Intern. Med.* 69:703, 1968.
28. Joubert, P.H. Digitalis in clinical practice. *S.Afr. Med. J.* 50:146, 1976.
29. Katz, A.M. *Physiology of the Heart.* New York: Raven Press, 1977.
30. Kim, D.H., Akera, T., and Brody, T.M. Tissue binding sites involved in quinidine-cardiac glycoside interactions. *J. Pharmacol. Exp. Ther.* 218:357, 1981.
31. Lathers, C.M., Gerard-Ciminera, J.L., Baskin, S.I. et al. The action of reserpine, 6-hydroxydopamine, and bretylium on digitalis-induced cardiotoxicity. *Eur. J. Pharmacol.* 76:371, 1981.
32. Lathers, C.M., Gerard-Ciminera, J.L., Baskin, S.I. et al. Role of the adrenergic nerve terminal in digitalis-induced cardiac toxicity: A study of the effects of pharmacological and surgical denervation. *J. Cardiovasc. Pharmacol.* 4:91, 1982.
33. Lathers, C.M. Effect of timolol on autonomic neural discharge associated with ouabain-induced arrhythmia. *Eur. J. Pharmacol.* 64:95, 1980.
34. Lathers, C.M., and Roberts, J. Minireview: Digitalis cardiotoxicity revised. *Life Sci.* 27:1713, 1980.
35. Lathers, C.M., Kelliher, G.J., Roberts, J., et al. Nonuniform cardiac sympathetic nerve discharge: Mechanism for coronary occlusion and digitalis-induced arrhythmia. *Circulation* 57:1058, 1978.
36. Lathers, C.M., Roberts, J., and Kelliher, G.J. Correlation of ouabain-induced arrhythmia and nonuniformity in the histamine-evoked discharge of cardiac sympathetic nerves. *J. Pharmacol. Exp. Ther.* 203:467, 1977.
37. Lindenbaum, J. Bioavailability of digoxin tablets. *Pharmacol. Rev.* 25:229, 1973.
38. Lipski, J.I. Digitalis. In: *Drugs in Cardiology*, Vol. 1 Part 2, Donoso, E., ed. New York: Stratton Intercontinental, 1975, p. 42.
39. Lown, B.M., Klein, M.D., Baur, I., et al. Sensitivity to digitalis drugs in acute myocardial infarction. *Am. J. Cardiol.* 30:388, 1972.
40. Mason, D.T. Digitalis pharmacology and therapeutics: Recent advances. *Ann. Intern. Med.* 80:520, 1974.
41. Mason, D.T. Regulation of cardiac performance in clinical heart disease. In: *Congestive Heart Failure* (Mason, D.T., ed.) New York: York Medical Books, 1976, p. 111.
42. Mathes, S., Gold, H., Marsh, R., et al. Comparison of the tolerance of adults and children to digitoxin. *J. Am. Med. Assoc.* 150:191, 1952.
43. Mendez, C., Aceves, J., and Mendez, R. The antiadrenergic action of digitalis on refractory period of the AV transmission systems. *J. Pharmacol. Exp. Ther.*131:199, 1961.
44. Okita, G.T. Dissociation of Na^+, K^+-ATPase inhibition from digitalis inotropy. *Fed. Proc.* 36:2225, 1977.

45. Perry, W.L.M., and Reinert, H. The action of cardiac glycosides on autonomic ganglia. *Br. J. Pharmacol.* 9:324, 1954.
46. Quest, J.A., and Gillis, R.A. Carotid sinus reflex changes produced by digitalis. *J. Pharmacol. Exp. Ther.* 177:650, 1971.
47. Roberts, J., Ito, R., Reilly, J., and Cairoli, V.J. The influence of reserpine and βTM10 on digitalis-induced ventricular arrhythmia. *Circ. Res.* 13:149, 1963.
48. Roberts, J., and Kelliher, G.J. The mechanism of action of digitalis at the subcellular level. *Semin. Drug Treat.* 2:203, 1972.
49. Roberts, J., Kelliher, G.J., and Lathers, C.M. Role of adrenergic influences in digitalis-induced ventricular arrhythmia. *Life Sci.* 18:665, 1976.
50. Roberts, J., Levitt, B., and Standaert, F.G. Autonomic nervous system and control of cardiac rhythm. *Nature* (Lond.) 214:912, 1967.
51. Rosen, M.R., Wit, A.L., and Hoffman, B.F. Electrophysiology and pharmacology of cardiac arrhythmias. IV. Cardiac antiarrhythmics and toxic effects of digitalis. *Am. Heart J.* 89:391, 1975.
52. Sarnoff, S.J., Gilmore, J.P., Wallace, A.G., et al. Effect of acetylstrophanthidin therapy on cardiac dynamics, oxygen consumption, and efficiency in the isolated heart with and without hypoxia. *Am. J. Med.* 37:3, 1964.
53. Schwartz, A. Newer aspects of cardiac glycoside action. *Fed. Proc.* 36:2207, 1977.
54. Singh, S. Clinical pharmacology of digitalis glycosides: A developmental view point. *Pediatr. Ann.* 5:578, 1976.
55. Smith, T.W., and Haber, E. Digitalis. *N. Engl. J. Med.* 289:945, 1010, 1063, 1125; 1973.
56. Smith, T.W., Haber, E., Yeatman, L., et al. Reversal of advanced digoxin intoxication with Fab fragments of digoxin-specific antibodies. *N. Eng. J. Med.* 294:797, 1976.
57. Soyka, L.F. Clinical pharmacology of digoxin. *Pediatr. Clin. North Am.* 19:241, 1972.
58. Spector, R. Digitalis therapy in heart failure: A rational approach. *J. Clin. Pharmacol.* 19:692, 1979.
59. Steinfeld, L., and Dimich, I. Digitalis: A pediatric viewpoint. In: *Drugs in Cardiology*, Vol. 1 Part 2 (Donoso, E., ed.) New York: Stratton Intercontinental, 1975, p. 124.
60. Tamm, C. The stereochemistry of the glycosides in relation to biological activity. In: *New Aspects of Cardiac Glycosides* (Uvnas, B., and Wilbrandt, W., eds.). Proc. of the 1st International Pharmacological Meeting, Vol. 3. New York: Pergamon Press, 1967, p. 11.
61. Tanabe, T., and Saito, H. *Cardiac Glycosides and Adrenergic Activity.* Hokkaido University Medical Library Series Vol. 8. Hokkaido, Japan: Hokkaido University School of Medicine, 1975.
62. Ten Eick, R.E., and Hoffman, B.F. Chronotropic effect of cardiac glycosides in cats, dogs, and rabbits. *Circ. Res.* 25:365, 1969.
63. Wallace, A.G., Schaal, S.F., Sugimoto, T., et al. The electrophysiological effects of β-adrenergic blockade and cardiac denervation. *Bull. N.Y. Acad. Med.* 43:1119, 1967.
64. Weaver, L.C., Akera, T., and Brody, T.M. Digoxin toxicity: Primary sites of drug action on the sympathetic nervous system. *J. Pharmacol. Exp. Ther.* 197:1, 1976.
65. Withering, W. An account of the foxglove and some of its medicinal uses: With practical remarks on dropsy and other diseases. *Med. Class.* 2:305, 1937.

ADDITIONAL READING

Applefeld, M.M., and Roffman, D.S. Digitalis and other positive catecholamine-like inotropic agents in the management of congestive heart failure. *Am. J. Med.* 80(2B):40, 1986.

Baughman, K.L. Calcium channel blocking agents in congestive heart failure. *Am. J. Med.* 80(2B):46, 1986.

Colucci, W.S., Wright, R.F. and Braunwald, E. New positive inotropic agents in the treatment of congestive heart failure. *N. Eng. J. Med.*, 314:290, 1986.

Muller, J.E., Turi, Z.G., Stone, P.H. et al. Digoxin therapy and mortality after myocardial infarction. *N. Eng. J. Med.*, 314:265, 1986.

Tommaso, C.L. Nonglycoside, noncatecholamine inotropic in the treatment of congestive heart failure. *Am. J. Med.* 80(2B):36, 1986.

Valdes, R., Jr. Endogenous digoxin-like immunoreactive factors: impact on digoxin measurements and potential physiological implications. *Clin. Chem.* 31:45, 1985.

CHAPTER
15.2

ANTIARRHYTHMIC DRUGS

Peter E. Dresel

Classification of Antiarrhythmic Drugs
Mechanism of Cardiac Arrhythmias
  Automaticity
  Reentry
Drugs Used for Supraventricular Arrhythmias
  Edrophonium
  Adrenergic Agents
  Digitalis
  Verapamil
  Quinidine
Drugs Used in Treatment of Ventricular Arrhythmias
  Lidocaine
  Procainamide
  Disopyramide
  Bretylium
  β-Adrenoceptor Blockers
  Phenytoin
New Drugs
  Amiodarone
  Tocainide
  Mexiletine
  N-Acetylprocainamide
  Encainide
  Flecainide
  Meobentine

CLASSIFICATION OF ANTIARRHYTHMIC DRUGS

There have been many attempts to classify the antiarrhythmic drugs according to the specific changes in the cardiac action potentials that result from their administration. Each new development has called for their revision, but the latest version is included in Table 15.2-1, which adds to it an entirely different approach, based on the type of arrhythmia for which the drugs are used.

MECHANISM OF CARDIAC ARRHYTHMIAS

To understand the manner in which drugs affect cardiac arrhythmias, it is essential to understand the mechanisms that cause these disturbances. Knowledge of the shape and duration of cardiac action potentials and the major ionic currents determining them is assumed here. Two general mechanisms have been identified: automaticity and reentry.

Automaticity. Cells in the sinoatrial node and the specialized conduction systems depolarize spontaneously, which causes the generation of an action potential when a threshold potential is reached. The most rapid spontaneous depolarization in normal hearts occurs in cells within the sinoatrial (SA) or "sinus" node, and the slowest such rate in the most peripheral Purkinje (conducting tissue) cells (Fig. 15.2-1). Normal muscle cells do not

Table 15.2-1
Classification of Antiarrhythmic Drugs

A. *Classification by types of arrhythmias*
- I. Supraventricular
  - A. Sinus tachycardia or bradycardia
    - **Rarely requires drug treatment**
  - B. Paroxysmal atrial tachycardia
    - Cholinesterase inhibitors, α-adrenergic agents, β_1-adrenoceptor blockers, digitalis, verapamil
  - C. Atrial flutter or fibrillation
    - Digitalis, quinidine, amiodarone
- II. Ventricular
  - A. Occasional extrasystoles
    - Not to be treated
  - B. Frequent or multiple extrasystoles and ventricular tachycardia
    - Lidocaine, procainamide, disopyramide, quinidine, β_1-adrenoceptor blockers, new drugs
  - C. Ventricular fibrillation
    - Bretylium (?)

B. *Classification by mechanism of action*

Type	Mechanism	Example
Ia	↓ Rapid sodium current	Quinidine, disopyramide
Ib	As above, plus ↑ time-related recovery from inactivation	Lidocaine
II	Adrenergic blockade	Propranolol
III	↑ Duration of AP	Amiodarone
IV	↓ Calcium current	Verapamil

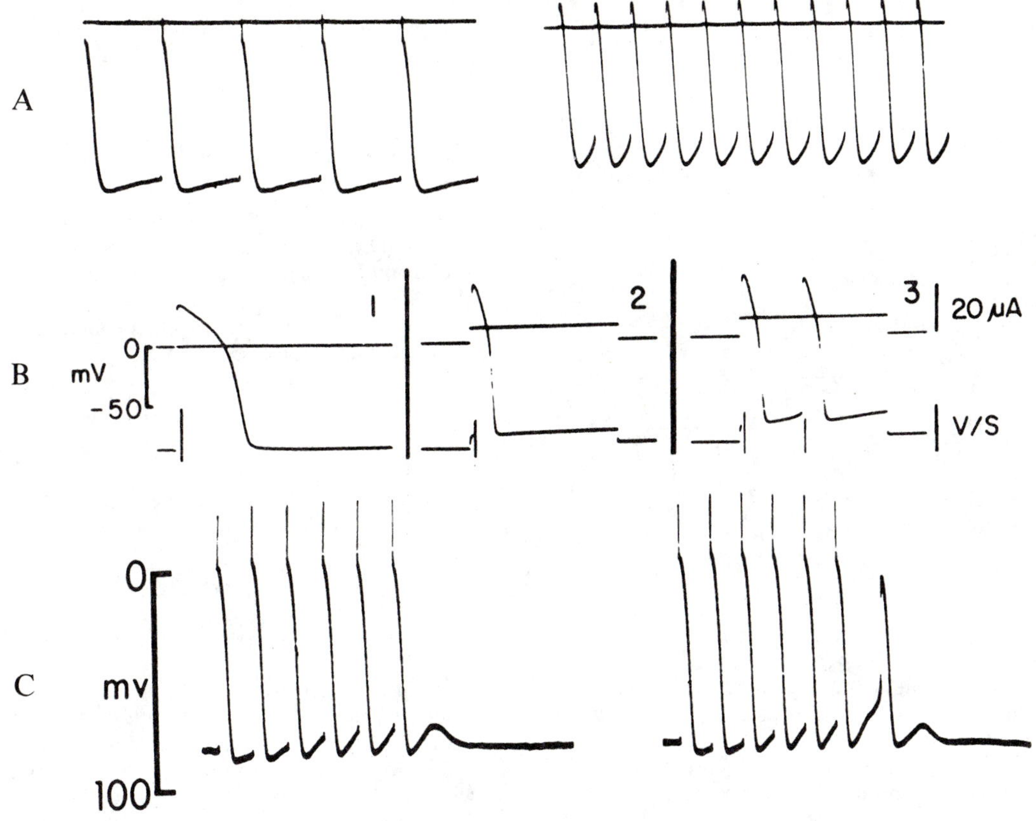

Fig. 15.2-1. (A) *Automaticity.* Left: slow diastolic depolarization (phase 4) in a Purkinje fiber is interrupted at varying intervals by depolarization conducted from a different pacemaker. This cell is called a latent pacemaker. Right: a true pacemaker in the sinus node. (Courtesy Dr. A.K. Reynolds). (B) *Automaticity caused by depolarization.* 1: normal action potential on a faster time scale than the other records. 2: slow diastolic depolarization induced by a depolarizing current (top trace). 3: repetitive activity induced by somewhat greater depolarization. This is a model for automaticity due to depolarization resulting from infarction. Drugs may increase membrane potential or decrease spontaneous depolarization. (From Ref. 6, with permission). (C) *Afterpotential in Purkinje cell treated with a toxic concentration of digitalis.* Left: cessation of a relatively slow rate of stimulation results in a nonpropagated afterpotential. Note that afterpotentials may be observed after each action potential. Right: cessation of a more rapid rate of stimulation results in an afterpotential of a size sufficient to cause a propagated unstimulated response. Drugs block the afterdepolarizations. (From Ref. 3, with permission).

depolarize spontaneously. Pathological processes such as myocardial infarction or drugs are able to increase automaticity, and the pacemaker may therefore change. The ionic current causing the spontaneous depolarization of these cells is primarily inactivation of a potassium outward current, but an inward calcium current has also been implicated in pacemaker activity. Automaticity of Purkinje cells is increased due to sympathetic drive or to partial depolarization caused by ischemia after a myocardial infarction. It is also increased by stretching tissue. The vagus has little effect on structures below the atrioventricular node. However, large increases in vagal tone can be effective in ventricular arrhythmias in a few cases.

Whereas the process of automaticity is entirely spontaneous, another type of unstimulated activity has been described in Purkinje and muscle cells partially depolarized by ischemia. A series of action potentials results in what appears to be spontaneous depolarization that is sufficient for one or more new action potentials to be generated (Fig. 15.2-1). A different mechanism applies when digitalis poisoning causes the appearance of afterpotentials that may reach threshold for an unstimulated beat to occur (Fig. 15.2-1). Although calcium entry through its channel is important to these afterdepolarizations, this may be secondary to an abnormal transient sodium current.

Recent work indicates that many complex arrhythmias may be explainable by the occurrence of a parasystolic focus. Unlike the classical description of this mechanism, such foci have now been shown to be modulated by the activity of nearby tissue. Even electrophysiological tests that were thought to distinguish between automatic and reentry mechanisms no longer appear to be reliable since the response of such a modulated focus is the same as may be expected from reentry. The effect of drugs on such foci has not been studied.

Reentry. The reentry mechanism is presently considered to be the most important one in the causation of both supra- and idioventricular arrhythmias. Reentry is totally different from the competition of pacemakers in arrhythmias due to changes in automaticity. It is based on changes in conduction velocity caused by pathological conditions (Fig. 15.2-2). The absolute requirement for reentry to occur is a site of (unidirectional) block and a section of tissue in which conduction has been

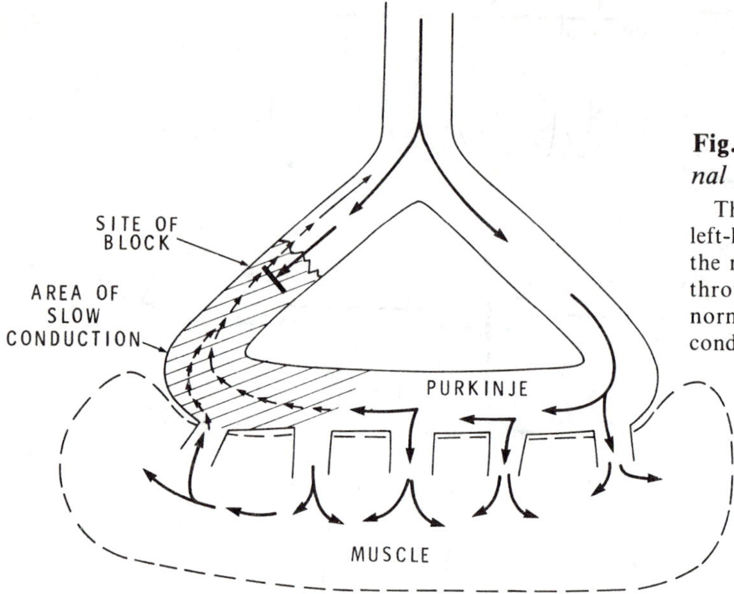

Fig. 15.2-2. *Schematic drawing of a reentry in the terminal Purkinje system.*

The normal impulse enters from the top, is blocked in the left-hand branch, but travels retrogradely through it to reexcite the normal tissue. Drugs may prevent retrograde conduction through the damaged branch or may prolong refractoriness in normal tissue sufficiently for the retrograde impulse not to be conducted after it exits.

slowed. Although it is simple to understand that a cell can be too severely damaged to conduct, it is more difficult to understand how slowed conduction can occur or how a block can be unidirectional. The explanation lies in the fact that conduction velocity in cardiac tissue is a continuous function of refractoriness; the action potentials, when they can be elicited, will be propagated with decreased velocity in partially refractory tissue. The *cause* of this is probably cellular excitability, but the most commonly used *correlate* of the rate of conduction through a series of cardiac cells is the maximum rate of rise of the upstroke of the action potential ($\dot{V}_{max}$) that is due to the rapid sodium current. This is a function of the membrane potential at which the action potential is elicited and of the time since the last action potential. Thus, a cell that has been partially depolarized by ischemia will have a less rapid $\dot{V}_{max}$, as will a cell in which a second stimulus arrives before repolarization is complete. In addition, $\dot{V}_{max}$ may be decreased for as long as 75 msec after complete repolarization. This is known as time-related recovery of the fast sodium current. Any influence that prolongs the refractory period by, for example increasing the duration of the action potential as does ischemia, or that partially depolarizes the cells, will cause a decrease in $\dot{V}_{max}$ and slowing of conduction.

The rapid inward sodium current determines $\dot{V}_{max}$ in normal cells and in abnormal cells that have membrane potentials as low as 50 mV. When cells are depolarized more severely and are exposed to high levels of norepinephrine, propagated action potentials are observed that have extremely slow conduction velocities and a very low $\dot{V}_{max}$. These are due to current carried by the calcium ion. Slow conduction through the atrioventricular (AV) node is also due in part to the role of calcium as a major carrier of the depolarizing inward current.

It is essential to the understanding of the mechanism of action of antiarrhythmic drugs to realize that cells are ordinarily excited by the rate of change of voltage of several adjacent cells. The threshold current that is required is a measure of the *excitability* of the cell. Many experiments have shown that injured cells have decreased excitability. $\dot{V}_{max}$ is thus important both to the ability to excite adjacent cells and to the rate of conduction. $\dot{V}_{max}$ can be sufficiently depressed to be unable to activate adjacent cells whose excitability may be impaired. Thus, it is possible for an impulse to be slowed to the point where it "dies out" along a length of damaged tissue. This is called *concealed* or *hidden* conduction.

Reentry can thus be pictured as a wave of excitation reaching cells that do not have sufficient excitability to be activated but that continue to recover while the impulse is slowly conducted in alternate pathways. When this alternate route has been traversed, the cells where block had occurred have recovered sufficiently to conduct the impulse toward the normal tissue. If sufficient time has elapsed for these normal cells again to be excitable, the impulse will spread throughout the ventricles.

Drugs can act either by causing sufficient further depression of conduction in the already damaged tissue to cause hidden conduction, or by increasing refractoriness in the more normal tissue to prevent emergence of the reentrant impulse.

Another mechanism for reentry is shown in Fig. 15.2-3. It shows an area of cardiac *muscle* tissue that has been damaged so that an impulse entering it travels in a complex pathway for a long enough period of time for reentry to occur. This requires a relatively large area of damaged muscle fibers such as that caused by a myocardial infarction. Drugs would have to depress muscle conduction (rather than Purkinje) to stop reentry due to this mechanism.

DRUGS USED FOR SUPRAVENTRICULAR ARRHYTHMIAS (1, 7)

The most common supraventricular arrhythmias are paroxysmal atrial tachycardia (PAT), atrial flutter, and atrial fibrillation. The first of these is caused by reentry within the AV node or the SA node. The purpose of therapy is to stop the reentry, that is, to slow conduction in the node(s) sufficiently to prevent emergence back into the atria. Atrial flutter and fibrillation differ only by their rates, the former being limited to rates below 300 beats/min. Atrial flutter may be considered a special case of reentry in which an organized wavefront travels through the specialized atrial conducting tissue in an approximately circular fashion, from which we derive the concept of the *circus movement* as the mechanism for this arrhythmia. Adjacent atrial muscle cells are excited at each passage of the circuit. If, however, reentry also occurs at these atrial cells, the impulses become totally disorganized, the total atrial rate increases severalfold (i.e., there is atrial fibrillation). Decreases in refractory period (e.g., vagal activity) convert flutter to fibrillation. The AV node blocks many of the impulses that reach it during flutter, but the ventricular rate is increased nevertheless. In the case of atrial fibrillation, the ventricular rate is irregular as well as rapid.

The purpose of therapy is to increase the degree of AV nodal block in order to slow the ventricular rate and preserve reasonably normal hemodynamics. One way to increase nodal refractoriness is to increase the vagal influence and/or to decrease sympathetic influence. Only a brief increase in vagal tone is required to break a paroxysm of atrial tachycardia. If such paroxysms occur too frequently, or if one is faced with atrial fibrillation or flutter, the vagal tone to the AV node must be increased chronically. The carotid sinus reflex and the Valsalva maneuver are the most effective methods of increasing briefly the vagal tone to the heart. Drugs are only used when these reflex maneuvers have failed, or when chronic changes of the vagosympathetic balance are required.

EDROPHONIUM

Edrophonium, a short-acting cholinesterase inhibitor, is used to potentiate the vagal activity due to the reflexes mentioned earlier when this activity is not sufficiently intense to cause conversion of PAT to normal sinus rhythm. This agent is discussed in Chapter 8.2.

A test dose of 1-5 mg is given i.v.; if this is ineffective, then 5-10 mg may be repeated. Administration of edrophonium should be followed by carotid sinus massage. This drug should not be given in hypotensive patients.

ADRENERGIC AGENTS

Phenylephrine and methoxamine are pure α-adrenoceptor stimulants which therefore increase blood pressure without affecting cardiac automaticity or conduction. These agents are sometimes effective in eliciting sufficiently strong reflex vagal activity when other methods have failed to stop PAT. They are discussed in Chapter 7.1.

These drugs are given i.v. over a period of 2-5 min, and the usual dose of phenylephrine is 0.5-1.0 mg and that of methoxamine is 5-10 mg. These drugs are contraindicated in hypertensive patients.

DIGITALIS

The effect of digitalis to increase the refractory period of, and to block conduction through, the AV node is considered a side effect when this drug is used as an inotropic agent. It is the major therapeutic effect in prophylaxis of PAT and in the management of atrial flutter or fibrillation. The mechanism of this effect is primarily to increase the net vagal influence. This increase is caused by (1) a central effect to increase the activity of the vagal nucleus, (2) sensitization of the carotid sinus to pressure, and (3) some sensitization of the cardiac tissue to the effects of acetylcholine released by the vagus nerve. A direct effect of digitalis on AV nodal conduction is difficult to demonstrate but is in the same direction as the effect of increased vagal activity.

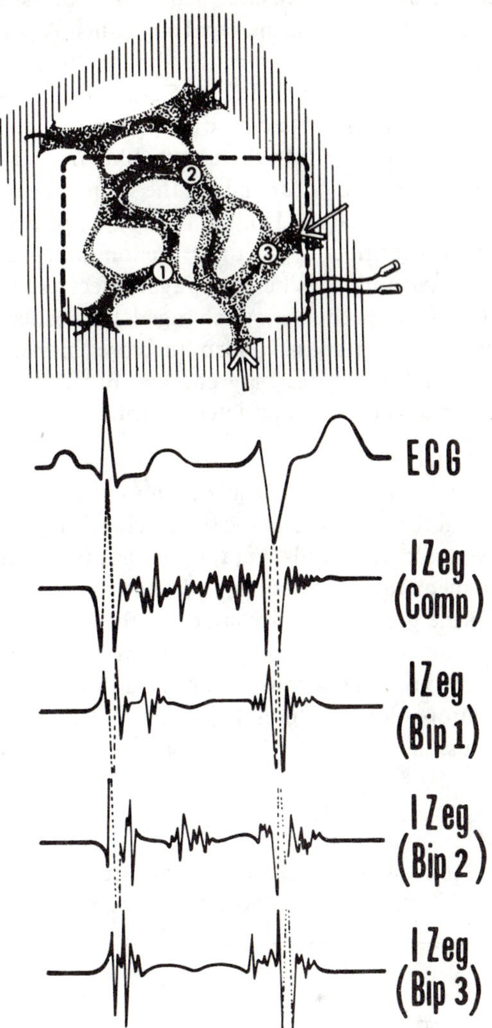

Fig. 15.2-3. *Reentry due to continuous activity in cardiac muscle.*

The diagram shows an infarcted area (IZ), the location within the dotted lines of a multicontact surface electrode (Comp), and three sets of bipolar surface electrodes (Bip 1,2,3). Activity is recorded by the bipolar electrodes at varying times after the normal QRS complex of the ECG. The composite electrodes shows this activity within the infarcted zone to be of sufficient duration to have caused the extrasystole in the ECG. Drugs cause decreased duration of continuous activity so that it ceases before reentry can occur. (From Ref. 2, with permission).

The effects of digitalis on electrical activity of the atria are more complex because the vagal mechanism operates in the opposite direction from the direct effect of the drug. This is summarized in Table 15.2-2. An increase in refractoriness results in a decrease in conduction velocity of a circus movement (atrial flutter). Slowing may be sufficient for block to occur and for the sinus pacemaker to reestablish dominance. Thus, in the 10% of patients in which the direct effect of the drug predominates, atrial flutter may terminate. When the vagal effect predominates, flutter is speeded or is changed to fibrillation; established fibrillation may also increase in net frequency. Ventricular rates may change, but AV nodal function remains their major determinant.

VERAPAMIL

The group of agents known as *calcium-channel blockers* differs in their specificity for the calcium channels of smooth versus cardiac cells. Verapamil was the first agent with this mechanism of action, and continues to be the drug with the greatest relative effect on the heart.

The importance of the calcium current in supporting conduction through partially depolarized Purkinje tissue and its major role in AV nodal conduction have already been discussed. One must also note the essential role of the calcium current in cardiac excitation-contraction coupling.

Table 15.2-2
Electrophysiological Effects of Drugs on Supraventricular Structures

	SA nodal automaticity	Atrium	AV-node
Digitalis			
Therapeutic doses			
Indirect (vagus)	↓	↓RP[a] ↑CV[b]	↑RP ↓CV
Direct	–	↑RP	Not Significant
Toxic doses	↓	↑RP	Block
Quinidine, disopyramide			
Indirect (anticholinergic)	↑	↓RP ↑CV	↓RP ↑CV
Direct	↓	↑RP ↓CV	↑RP ↓CV
Amiodarone	–	↑RP –CV	–RP –CV
Verapamil	↓	↑RP? ↓CV	↑RP ↓CV

[a] RP = Refractory period.
[b] CV = Conduction velocity.

Electrophysiological effects of verapamil and other antiarrhythmic drugs on supraventricular and ventricular structures are summarized in Tables 15.2-2 and 15.2-3.

Pharmacokinetics. Although it is completely absorbed from the GI tract after oral administration, only 10-20% of the administered dose appears in the blood because the liver sequesters the remainder (the first-pass effect). Intravenous administration results in an immediate, mild hypotensive response of short duration (10-20 min). Signs of interference with AV nodal conduction appear less rapidly but last up to 6 hr, indicating that the drug is slowly but preferentially bound to nodal tissue. The plasma half-life is 5 hr. Final excretion is largely by the kidney.

Adverse Effects. The major side effects are inherent in its mechanism of action. Patients with impaired sinus node or AV node function may develop bradycardia or sinus arrest, AV nodal block, and even asystole. Therapeutic concentrations of verapamil cause little change in cardiac contractile function because of reflex changes in sympathetic tone that oppose the drug effect in healthy hearts.

Contractile function may be severely compromised by the drug in the presence of heart failure or when sympathetic tone has been decreased by concurrent administration of β-adrenoceptor blockers. Severe bradycardias also occur with this drug interaction, even in healthy hearts. Although the drug is very effective in digitalis-induced ventricular arrhythmias, it must be used with great caution because complete AV nodal block may occur.

Therapeutic Uses. The major use for verapamil is in the management of supraventricular arrhythmias, especially PAT, in patients with otherwise normal hearts. Used intravenously, it will terminate this arrhythmia even when all other measures have failed, and it is very effective in prophylaxis when given orally. It will therefore probably emerge as the drug of choice in PAT. It has also been shown to be effective in some patients after myocardial infarction, but is not used except when other agents have failed.

The use of calcium-channel blockers in the management of angina is discussed in Chapter 15.4.

The drug is given by i.v. infusion (1 mg/min to a total dose of 10 mg). Oral doses of 40-120 mg three times daily are used in managing supraventricular arrhythmias.

QUINIDINE

Quinidine is the d-isomer of quinine, the antimalarial drug (Fig. 15.2-4). Although the first report of the use of these cinchona alkaloids in cardiac arrhythmias can be traced to the middle of the eighteenth century, the first systematic study indicating that quinidine is the more effective agent was done in 1918. Quinidine is thus the

Table 15.2-3
Effects of Drugs on Electrophysiology of His-Purkinje System and Ventricular Muscle

Drug	H-P Automaticity	Refractoriness		Conduction Velocity	
		Normal tissue	Damaged tissue	Normal tissue	Damaged tissue
Quinidine	Decrease	Increase	Increase	Slowed	Slowed
Procainamide	Decrease	Increase	Increase	Slowed	Slowed
Disopyramide	Decrease	Increase	More Increase	Slowed	More Slowed
Lidocaine	Decrease	Complex[a]	Increase	No change[b]	Slowed
Amiodarone	No change	Increase	?	No change	?
Verapamil	Decrease	No change	Increase	No change	Slowed

[a] Relatively refractory period but not effective refractory period is increased.
[b] Different effects depending on heart rate, presence of extrasystoles.

oldest and perhaps the best known antiarrhythmic drug. It is still the only presently available agent with proven effectiveness in converting, albeit temporarily, atrial flutter-fibrillation to normal sinus rhythm. Quinidine may be considered a general cardiac depressant, in that it decreases both the activation of and the recovery of all cardiac cells as well as the strength of contraction of cardiac muscle. Thus, quinidine increases the refractory period, the duration of the action potential, and the threshold to electrical stimulation, and decreases the $\dot{V}_{max}$, the speed of impulse propagation through all cardiac tissues, and the rate of impulse generation in automatic cells. Therapeutic blood levels cause electrocardiographic changes typical of slowing of ventricular conduction (widening of the QRS complex) and of changes in duration of action potentials (increases in QT interval corrected for heart rate by the formula $QT_c = QT/RR$ where RR = cycle length and QT is the period from the beginning of the QRS complex to the end of the T wave). The drug is effective acutely in the treatment of arrhythmias of ventricular origin but has been replaced by safer agents. It may be used orally for prophylaxis in patients at risk of multiple ventricular extrasystoles after myocardial infarction.

Pharmacokinetics. Quinidine is well absorbed from the GI tract and may be given intramuscularly but should not be given intravenously because sudden high blood levels may cause asystole. Oral absorption is influenced by the nature of the salt administered. Quinidine sulfate is more completely (80%) absorbed than the gluconate salt (70%), and the time to peak plasma levels is 1.5 hr for the former and 4 hr for the latter. The plasma half-life varies widely from 3-12 hr, in part because cardiac failure, present to some degree in many patients who require the drug, changes hepatic blood flow and secondarily hepatic metabolism. The drug is partially metabolized to a number of compounds, some of which retain pharmacological activity; 20-50% of the drug appears in the urine unchanged within 24 hr of administration, and 60-80% of the drug is bound to plasma protein. Tissue proteins have a high affinity to quinidine, and tissue/plasma ratios are very high.

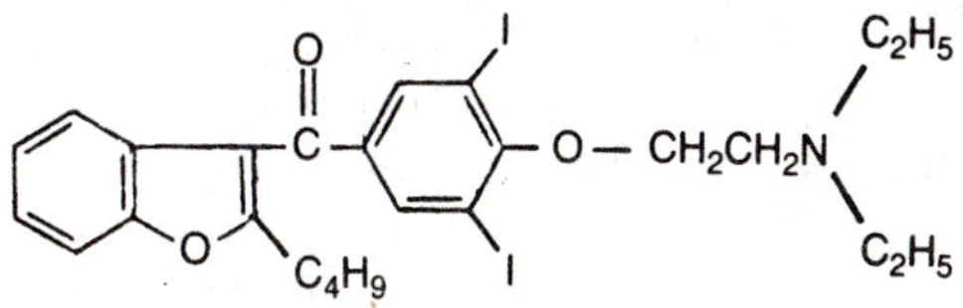

Amiodarone

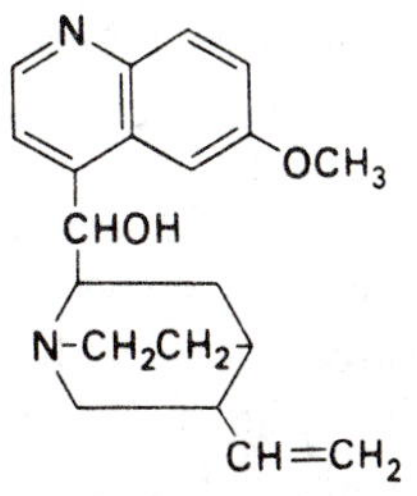

Quinidine

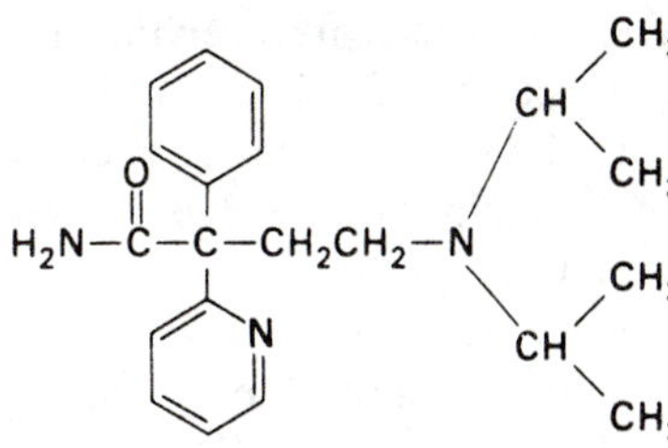

Disopyramide

Fig. 15.2-4. *Chemical structures of some antiarrhythmic agents.*

Adverse Effects. The most important side effects of quinidine are caused by its strong anticholinergic properties. Of these, the occurrence of tachycardias in patients with atrial arrhythmias and of urinary retention are probably the most important. The interactions of direct and anticholinergic effects of quinidine can be inferred from Table 15.2-2. There is no way to predict which will predominate in an individual. When quinidine is used to convert atrial fibrillation or flutter to normal sinus rhythm, the atrial rate tends to slow gradually. As the rate slows, AV-nodal block may be decreased (e.g., from 4:1 at an atrial rate of 400 beats/min to 2:1 at an atrial rate of 250 beats/min), and ventricular rate may therefore increase. This cause for ventricular speeding is additional to the anticholinergic effect of the drug which also decreases AV-nodal refractoriness and is the reason why patients are usually given digitalis before quinidine is used. The negative inotropic effect of quinidine may aggravate or induce cardiac failure unless digitalis has also been given. The effects on conduction can cause severe arrhythmias at high blood levels.

Quinidine, like quinine, causes a symptom complex known as *cinchonism*, the major signs of which are tinnitus, vertigo, photophobia, headache, nausea, diarrhea, and syncope. As with almost all drugs, a certain number of patients will be found to have hypersensitivity reactions as a result of administration of quite small doses.

Rare side effects of quinidine include blood dyscrasias, dermatological reactions, and unmasking or exaggeration of myasthenia gravis.

Some additional information on quinidine may be found in the sections on procainamide and disopyramide.

Drug Interactions. Administration of quinidine to digitalized patients causes sharp rises in digoxin blood levels that may reach toxic levels. Digitalis is displaced from cardiac and other tissue binding sites without displacement from the binding site on Na+-, K+-activated adenosine triphosphatase (ATPase). Digoxin half-life is increased primarily because of a decrease in the rate of renal excretion, in turn probably due to changes in renal secretion rather than filtration. Nonrenal clearance (metabolism and biliary excretion) may also be decreased. This important drug interaction also may occur when amiodarone or verapamil are given to patients receiving digitalis.

Quinidine may enhance the effects of antihypertensives, β-adrenoceptor blocking agents, and coumarin anticoagulants. A low serum potassium decreases quinidine efficacy. Antacids delay quinidine absorption from the GI tract. Phenobarbital and phenytoin reduce the plasma half-life of quinidine as a result of increased rate of hepatic metabolism.

Therapeutic Uses. Quinidine has been replaced by newer drugs for many indications. It is still being used, in part because of good oral absorption, in prophylaxis of atrial or ventricular arrhythmias, including tachyarrhythmias due to preexcitation (Wolff-Parkinson-White syndrome).

For adults, the oral dose of quinidine sulfate is 200-400 mg every 6 hr with a maximum daily dosage of 2.4 g; for children, 6 mg/kg, every 4-6 hr. Quinidine polygalacturonate and quinidine gluconate are administered at 8-12 hr intervals because of their different bioavailability. For severely ill patients, intramuscular administration of quinidine gluconate may be necessary, and the dose is 400 mg initially, to be repeated every 4-6 hr. The intravenous route is rarely if ever indicated, and employed only in hospitalized patients at a dose of 200-400 mg (given slowly at a rate of 10 mg/min) with continuous monitoring of electrocardiogram and blood pressure.

DRUGS USED IN TREATMENT OF VENTRICULAR ARRHYTHMIAS

LIDOCAINE

Lidocaine is the drug of first choice in the treatment of ventricular arrhythmias independent of etiology. Lidocaine had been used for over 20 years as a local anesthetic before it came into use as an antiarrhythmic agent.

Pharmacological Effects. Lidocaine has complex electrophysiological effects. It decreases Purkinje automaticity by decreasing the inactivation of the slow outward potassium current. It differs from other antiarrhythmic drugs in causing a shortening of the action potential (AP) of Purkinje fibers. This effect seems to be greatest in fibers with the longest action potentials so that the range of AP durations normally found in the heart is decreased. Lidocaine decreases the fast inward sodium current and is also the only major drug that slows the time-related recovery of the fast sodium current in normal Purkinje and muscle fibers. Thus, the decrease in refractory period to be expected from the shortening of the action potential tends to be counteracted by an increase in refractoriness due to the latter effect. The result is an increase of the ratio of refractory period/AP duration. This is one of the reasons for the effectiveness of the drug in aborting reentry arrhythmias. It slows the rate of rise of the action potential at any level of membrane potential. This is associated with slowing of conduction, especially in damaged fibers that have become partially depolarized. This depression of conductivity results in concealed conduction within the reentry pathway. Recent studies have indicated that lidocaine has a relatively selective effect on fibers that have been damaged but have survived myocardial infarction in experimental animals. It also appears to shorten the duration of tortuous conducted activity within muscle tissue sufficiently to prevent reentry from these areas. Lidocaine does not affect action potentials carried by the slow calcium current.

Lidocaine causes less depression of cardiac contractile force than do quinidine or procainamide. It is a vasodilator, but this effect is not of sufficient magnitude to cause significant hypotension when the drug is given intravenously. It is probable that lidocaine causes some increase in sympathetic nervous system tone, which would tend to counteract its direct vasodilator properties.

Pharmacokinetics. The most common route of administration is the intravenous one under constant ECG monitoring. A single intravenous bolus dose has a duration of action of approximately 20 min because it is redistributed throughout body water. The initial bolus is usually followed by a constant infusion of the drug. The plasma half-life of the drug after it has been equilibrated is approximately 2 hr due to the rapid metabolism of the drug. This short half-life allows "titration" of the patient to achieve the minimum effective blood level. Therapeutic blood levels are in the range of 1.5-5 μg/ml. Metabolism by dealkylation (Fig. 15.2-5) is done by the mixed-function oxidase system in the liver. Approximately 90% of the administered dose can be recovered from the urine as metabolites. The first metabolite, MEGX, is close to lidocaine in potency as an antiarrhythmic and is a CNS stimulant drug. Its plasma half-life is slightly longer. MEGX may therefore play some role in the therapeutic and toxic effects of lidocaine after prolonged infusions have led to high blood levels of the metabolite. The plasma half-life of lidocaine is grossly affected by the circulatory state of the patient. Overt congestive heart failure causes a significant increase in the half-life, most probably by decreasing hepatic blood flow. The variability in the rate at which the drug is metabolized emphasizes the importance of adjusting the rate of administration to the needs of the patient. Thus, abrupt fall in plasma levels may occur in patients previously well equilibrated with the drug when cardiac mechanical function improves and hepatic blood flow is increased. Intramuscular injections of lidocaine may also be effective in treating or preventing arrhythmias after myocardial infarction. It is more difficult to control blood levels with this route of administration, but certain advantages have been claimed when intensive care units are not available.

Adverse Effects. The most important toxic effects of lidocaine are referable to the central nervous system. Like all other local anesthetics, lidocaine is a CNS stimulant. It may appear to be paradoxical, but the therapeutic blood levels of the drug tend to cause sleepiness rather than overt CNS stimulation. Relatively small further increases in blood level cause anxiety and muscle twitching in the facial muscles and the extremities. If blood levels are allowed to increase further, frank convulsions will result. Again, a few patients will be found to have idiosyncratic and hypersensitivity reactions to the drug. Elderly patients may be more sensitive to the toxic effects, may display drowsiness, numbness, speech disturbances, and dizziness at plasma levels of 10 μg/ml or less.

Therapeutic Uses. Lidocaine is the drug of choice in ventricular arrhythmias; it is not effective in atrial arrhythmias. It has little effect on conduction through the AV node.

PROCAINAMIDE

The antiarrhythmic properties of the local anesthetic procaine were demonstrated in the early 1940s. Procainamide, in which an amide bond has been substituted for the ester bond of procaine, was found to be equally effective and to possess a longer half-life because of slower metabolism (Fig. 15.2-4).

Procainamide is very similar to quinidine. It differs from quinidine in that it is less likely to cause cardiac standstill on intravenous administration and in that it is only marginally effective against atrial arrhythmias. As with quinidine, possible differences between the effects of procainamide on damaged tissues versus normal tissues have not yet been studied.

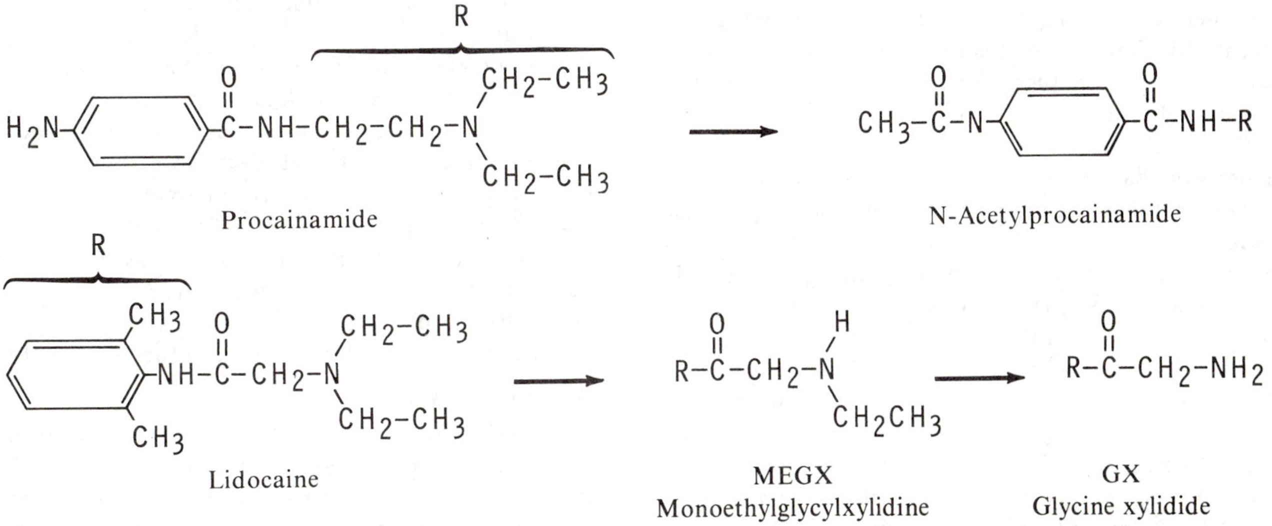

Procainamide → N-Acetylprocainamide

Lidocaine → MEGX (Monoethylglycylxylidine) → GX (Glycine xylidide)

Fig. 15.2-5. *Metabolism of procainamide and lidocaine.* The first metabolites of these drugs have antiarrhythmic activity.

Pharmacokinetics. Procainamide is known to be effective after oral administration, but absorption tends to be variable from day to day. The drug has a plasma half-life of 3-4 hr in patients with normal renal function. However, only approximately 60% of the drug is excreted unchanged, the remainder being metabolized primarily by the liver to a number of metabolic products. One of these, *N-acetylprocainamide* (Fig. 15.2-4) has considerable antiarrhythmic activity and a long biological half-life (6-8 hr). The genetic aspects of drug acetylation are discussed in Chapters 2 and 4. Accordingly the dose of procainamide may be reduced during chronic administration as the levels of N-acetylprocainamide rise. Only 15% of the unchanged drug is bound to plasma proteins. Protein binding to other tissues appears to be greater since a high tissue to plasma ratio is found. Therapeutic plasma concentrations are 4-10 μg/ml; toxic effects may be noted above 12 μg/ml.

Adverse Effects. The main side effect on intravenous administration of procainamide is hypotension. This is a serious disadvantage in patients whose coronary circulation is compromised. As with quinidine, high plasma concentrations are accompanied by disturbances in cardiac conduction as evidenced by a widening of the QRS complex and the induction of cardiac arrhythmias. Purkinje automaticity is also reduced. The drug has a dose-related negative inotropic effect of special importance in patients with heart failure. The degree of hypotension and of cardiac toxicity is a function of plasma level, and the drug must therefore be infused slowly. Intramuscular injections, though less likely to cause hypotension, are used relatively rarely because one loses control over the blood level. The drug can be used orally, but chronic oral administration has led to a number of unacceptable toxic reactions including the development of a symptom complex closely resembling systemic lupus erythematosus in as many as 25% of cases given high doses of the drug for long periods of time. This toxic sign occurs more frequently in that part of the population who are "slow acetylators." It is therefore probably caused by the unchanged drug rather than its active metabolite.

Rare toxic effects include blood dyscrasias, mental depression, hallucinations, and psychoses.

Therapeutic Uses. Procainamide must be considered a drug of second choice in the management of acute ventricular arrhythmias due to myocardial infarction. It is ineffective against atrial arrhythmias, and must be used cautiously because of its hypotensive effect.

Adult oral dose of procainamide is 250-500 mg every 3-4 hr. An initial loading dose of 750-1000 mg is sometimes necessary. For children, it is administered orally at a dose of 50 mg/kg in 4 to 6 divided doses. For intravenous administration in adults, about 100 mg of procainamide is infused slowly every 5 min, until the arrhythmia is corrected with a maximum loading dose of 1 g. For maintenance, the drug may be infused at a dose of 2-6 mg/min. Blood pressure and electrocardiogram should be continuously monitored. For intramuscular injection, it is given at a dose of 0.5-1 g every 6 hr. Patients with impaired renal function require reduced dosage.

DISOPYRAMIDE

Disopyramide is a relatively new drug with a quinidine-like spectrum of activity. It has been shown to be effective in some atrial arrhythmias.

Disopyramide shares the electrophysiological effects of quinidine in normal ventricular muscle and Purkinje fibers. It has recently been shown that disopyramide has additional effects on Purkinje fibers serving myocardial infarction. Not only are its effects on such fibers more profound than they are on normal ones, but the drug also has an effect on time-related recovery of the sodium channel that in normal tissue can only be observed after treatment with lidocaine.

Pharmacokinetics. The drug is well absorbed (80-100%) after oral administration and has also been used intravenously in place of procainamide for the management of arrhythmias after myocardial infarction. The drug is slightly more concentrated in the heart than in the plasma and appears to have greater concentration in ventricular than in atrial tissues. This may account for its greater effectiveness in ventricular arrhythmias. It is not highly bound to plasma proteins. Elimination is primarily by way of excretion, a total of 60-70% being eliminated unchanged in the urine. The remainder is metabolized by the liver. The half-life in normal subjects is approximately 4 hr whereas that in patients after acute infarction is 7-12 hr and that in patients with renal disease may exceed 14 hr. Therapeutic plasma levels range between 2.8 and 7.5 μg/ml.

Adverse Effects. The major side effects, like those of quinidine, are related to the atropinelike effect of the drug. Urinary retention is the most important of these. The present claim that these side effects are less serious than during the use of quinidine is subject to reevaluation as the drug comes into wider use. Recent data indicate that intravenous disopyramide in patients with heart failure may have a severe negative inotropic effect.

Therapeutic Uses. Disopyramide is used intravenously in the management of postinfarction arrhythmias as a drug of second choice, as is procainamide. Oral doses of 100-300 mg to a maximum of 1600 mg/day may be given in patients showing long-term arrhythmias. The drug has occasionally been used to suppress atrial flutter or fibrillation. Reduced dosage is recommended in patients with hepatic insufficiency, heart failure, or cardiomyopathies.

BRETYLIUM

Bretylium was developed, tested, and abandoned as an adrenergic neuron blocker similar to guanethidine. Like that compound, it causes an initial release of norepinephrine from sympathetic nerve endings. Thus, there may be an initial tachycardia, hypertension, and increases in severity of ventricular arrhythmias when the drug is used i.v. as an antiarrhythmic agent. This is quickly followed by bradycardia and hypotension due to the block of further release. It is useful only in ventricular arrhythmias and has been found to be effective when other agents have failed. This may be due to the fact that it has significantly more effect on normal than on depressed tissue and therefore prevents reentry by an "exit block," a mechanism of action different from the other agents.

Pharmacokinetics. The drug is not metabolized by the liver. Since renal excretion is the major determinant of plasma level and the patients given the drug often suffer from decreased renal function, the reported plasma half-life varies from 4 to 17 hr. Blood levels after intramuscular injection are maximal after 30-60 min. Plasma levels are not correlated with effectiveness because of preferential uptake by cardiac tissue that leads to a long duration of action.

Adverse Effects. Hypotension is the major side effect that may require cessation of therapy. Nausea and vomiting occur if the drug is injected rapidly i.v. A number of side effects, including parotid pain, skin rashes, and central nervous system dysfunctions, were associated with chronic use.

Therapeutic Uses. Bretylium has been stated to be the only agent able to reverse ventricular fibrillation when countershock has been ineffective. The drug is used only for refractory arrhythmias in intensive care facilities.

β-ADRENOCEPTOR BLOCKERS

Increased activity of the sympathetic nervous system is one of the factors causing arrhythmias after myocardial infarction. Nevertheless, the use of blocking agents has not been successful in the management of arrhythmias that occur within the first few days after infarction. Other drugs are more effective and potentially less toxic. Nevertheless, i.v. administration of a β-adrenoceptor blocker may be successful when other measures have failed.

The long-term sequelae of myocardial infarction, such as persistent arrhythmias and the occurrence of sudden death due to ventricular fibrillation, are a function of the size of the final infarcted zone and of the susceptibility of the healed or partially healed myocardium to changes in sympathetic tone. There is good evidence that β-adrenoceptor blockers decrease the incidence of sudden death, at least during the first year after infarction. Indications are that results are best when treatment is started very early, in some cases within hours of infarction. This indicates, as does some laboratory evidence, that these drugs may serve to limit the size of the infarct. Demonstration of a protective effect when they are started as late as 2 weeks after infarction shows the importance of protection from excessive sympathetic influence in the prevention of ventricular fibrillation.

β-adrenoceptor blockers are also effective in digitalis toxicity. The role of the sympathomimetic agents in digitalis toxicity is discussed in Chapter 15.1 (Table 15.1-7).

The drugs are sometimes used in the management of atrial arrhythmias, especially in prophylaxis in PAT. Here they act by decreasing the effects of the sympathetic nervous system on the refractory period of the AV node, thereby depressing conduction and abolishing reentry.

The details of the individual drugs are discussed in Chapter 7.2.

PHENYTOIN

This antiepileptic drug has proven effectiveness only in digitalis-induced ventricular arrhythmias. The i.v. use of phenytoin is complicated by the extreme alkalinity of its aqueous solutions. It has been demonstrated that reversal of digitalis cardiac toxicity occurs without reduction of the positive inotropic effect, but no clinical trials of this method of increasing the therapeutic ratio of digitalis have been reported.

Therapeutic Uses. Intravenous use of phenytoin for arrhythmias is indicated almost exclusively in severe digitalis intoxication. The dose is 50-100 mg given very slowly every 5 min until the arrhythmia disappears or toxicity occurs. The usual requirement is 700 mg. Constant monitoring of ECG and blood pressure are required. Oral doses equivalent to those in epilepsy control arrhythmias, but loading doses (1 g on day 1, 0.3-0.6 g on days 2 and 3) must be given in the rare case in which phenytoin is used chronically for this indication.

NEW DRUGS

A major effort is being made at present to develop a safe and effective, orally active drug that may be used for long-term therapy and prophylaxis against ventricular arrhythmias. Arrhythmias are the major cause of sudden death due to myocardial infarction, and the occurrence of sudden death is correlated with the frequency and severity of arrhythmias after recovery from a first infarction. Chronic oral therapy of such patients would probably be profitable. There does not appear to be enough information on any of these agents for one to predict which will survive. The names and brief pharmacological effects of some of these compounds are given here. Table 15.2-4 presents certain clinical pharmacological data for these and some other agents.

AMIODARONE

Amiodarone is still experimental despite intensive clinical investigation, especially in Europe. Its mechanism of action is different from all other known agents. It causes prolongation of the action potential in atrial and ventricular cells, thereby increasing greatly the refractory period. It has a negative inotropic effect and causes vasodilation, but it has a wide margin of safety even in the presence of severe congestive heart failure. It is effective against both atrial and ventricular arrhythmias on oral administration. Clinical trials indicate its great efficacy in the management of ventricular arrhythmias where other drugs have failed. It appears to be accumulated by various organs including the heart, so that plasma levels do not correspond to therapeutic effectiveness. Extremely long-lasting effects (30-45 days) have been observed after chronic treatment. Amiodarone is structurally similar to thyroxine and inhibits the conversion of this hormone to triiodothyronine. This indicates that thyroid-modulated functions may be decreased during chronic treatment. A major reason for the drug's present status is the finding of corneal microdeposits of the drug or one of its metabolites, (although these are reversible), of the development

Table 15.2-4
Clinical Pharmacology of Some Antiarrhythmic Drugs

Agent[a]	Therapeutic Plasma Level (mg/l)	Elimination Half-life	Maintenance Dose (mg)
Amiodarone	1.0-10.0[b]	25-55 days	200-800
Encainide	0.1-1.0[c]	6-8 hr	150-250
Flecainide	1.5-4.0	7-22 hr	150-350
Mexiletine	1.0-2.0	10-15 hr	600-1000
Tocainide	3.5-10.0	10-15 hr	400-1000
Verapamil	0.001-0.004	4-6 hr	320-480

[a] All except verapamil are well absorbed and have high bioavailability; verapamil bioavailability is 10-25% due to first-pass effect.
[b] Plasma level does not mirror therapeutic effect.
[c] Metabolites have high efficacy, make major contribution to effect.

of pulmonary fibrosis (whose relation to the drug has not been proven) and of neurological deficits.

TOCAINIDE

This congener of lidocaine shares many of its electrophysiological effects. The plasma half-life is 8-12 hr, long enough to allow twice or three times daily dosing, an important factor in compliance with chronic therapy. Initial i.v. studies indicated some incidence of cardiac failure, but oral studies show only some mild CNS toxicity (paraesthesia, sweats, tremor). The therapeutic ratio is not very high when minor toxicity is measured.

MEXILETINE

Mexiletine is another compound chemically similar to lidocaine. It is an effective drug after oral administration and has a plasma half-life that depends on the pH of the urine. When the patient's urine is acidic, a high proportion of the drug is excreted unchanged and the half-life is 3 hr. When the urine is alkaline, little unchanged drug is excreted. Metabolism by the liver is such that the half-life is changed to 8-9 hr. Cardiovascular and neurological toxic effects occur at doses close to the therapeutic, and include excessive bradycardia, hypotension, tremor, dizziness, blurred vision, nausea, ataxia, and confusion.

N-ACETYLPROCAINAMIDE

N-acetylprocainamide is the active metabolite of procainamide, as discussed earlier. It has been suggested that this drug is less likely to cause the systemic lupus erythematosus syndrome than the parent. It has a longer half-life (6-11 hr) and is more reliably absorbed orally than procainamide.

ENCAINIDE

Encainide is a very effective, orally absorbed antiarrhythmic drug with little negative inotropic effect. Its main cardiac side effect, widening of QRS complex, occurs even at therapeutic concentrations. Thus, it appears to have many of the characteristics of quinidine. It is metabolized to two major metabolites, both of which are 5-10 times more potent than the parent compound. They may also differ in their mechanism of action. It is probable that these metabolites make a major contribution to the effect of the drug after several days of treatment, but their pharmacokinetics have not been reported in detail. Their contribution to its toxic effects have also not been determined.

FLECAINIDE

Flecainide is effective in ventricular arrhythmias. It is well absorbed orally. It has a long half-life (18-20 hr). Early reports indicate a number of nonspecific side effects (e.g., blurred vision, dizziness, stomatitis) classified as minor but little cardiac toxicity.

MEOBENTINE

Meobentine is a new agent whose cardiac actions are like those of bretylium but which lacks that drug's effects on adrenergic nerve endings while sharing its long duration of action. This would greatly decrease the side effects of this type of antifibrillatory drug.

Preparations. *Quinidine Sulfate*, USP (CIN-QUIN, QUINORA): tablets 180, 200, and 300 mg; capsules 180 and 200 mg; (QUINIDEX) 300-mg extended-release tablets. *Quinidine Gluconate*, USP (QUINAGLUTE): 1-3 timed-release tablets of 324 and 330 mg; for i.v. injection, solution of 80 mg/ml (10 vials). *Quinidine Polygalacturonate* (CARDIOQUIN): tablets 275 mg (equivalent to 200 mg quinidine sulfate). *Procainamide Hydrochloride*, USP (PRONESTYL): capsules or tablets, 250, 375, and 500 mg; injection, 10-ml vials (100 mg/ml) and 2-ml vials (500 mg/ml). *Lidocaine Hydrochloride Injection*, USP (XYLOCAINE): solution, 20, 50, and 200 mg/ml. *Disopyramide Phosphate*, USP (NORPACE): capsules 100 and 150 mg (base). Preparations and dosage forms for *Bretylium Tosylate* (BRETYLOL), *Phenytoin Sodium* (DILANTIN), *Edrophonium Chloride* (TENSILON), *Methoxamine Hydrochloride* (VASOXYL), *Phenylephrine Hydrochloride* (NEOSYNEPHRINE), and *Propranolol Hydrochloride* (INDERAL) are listed in other chapters.

REFERENCES

1. Anderson, J.L., Harrison, D.C., Meffin, P.J. and Winkle, R.A. Antiarrhythmic drugs: Clinical pharmacology and therapeutic uses. *Drugs* 15:271, 1978
2. El-Sherif, N., Scherlag, B.J., Lazzara, R. and Hope, R.R. Reentrant ventricular arrhythmias in the late myocardial infarction period. *Circulation* 55:686, 1977.
3. Ferrier, G.R., Saunders, J.H. and Mendez, C. A cellular mechanism for the generation of ventricular arrhythmias by acetylstrophanthidin. *Circ. Res.* 32:600, 1973.
4. Hagemeijer, F. Verapamil in the management of supraventricular tachyarrhythmias occurring after a recent myocardial infarction. *Circulation* 57:751, 1978.

5. Heger, J.J. et al. Amiodarone: clinical efficacy and electrophysiology during long-term therapy for recurrent ventricular tachycardia or ventricular fibrillation. *N. Engl. J. Med.* 305:539, 1981.
6. Katzung, B. Effects of extracellular calcium and sodium on depolarization-induced automaticity in guinea pig papillary muscle. *Circ. Res.* 37:118, 1975.
7. Lucchesi, B.R. Key References—Antiarrhythmic drugs. *Circulation* 59:1076, 1979.

ADDITIONAL READING

Grant, A.O. et al. Antiarrhythmic drug action. Blockade of the inward sodium current. *Circ. Res.* 55:427, 1984.

Harrison, D.C. (ed.). Symposium on perspectives on the treatment of ventricular arrhythmias. *Am. J. Cardiol.* 52: 1c, 1983.

Muhiddin, K.A. et al. Is there an ideal antiarrhythmic drug? A review with particular reference to class I antiarrhythmic agents. *Postgrad. Med. J.* 61:665, 1985.

CHAPTER 15.3

DRUGS FOR THERAPY OF HYPERTENSION AND SHOCK

H. Lloyd Garvey

ANTIHYPERTENSIVE DRUGS

Untreated hypertension is a significant risk factor in a variety of cardiovascular diseases including atherosclerosis, angina pectoris, acute myocardial infarction, aortic aneurysm, strokes, renal failure, and heart failure. Follow-up studies have shown that the danger of potentially fatal cardiovascular disease increases proportionately to the elevation of diastolic pressure (30, 74, 75). In malignant hypertension that is characterized by very high blood pressure and neuroretinopathy, a progressive reduction in renal function is characteristic of the untreated course, with death resulting from uremia or cerebral hemorrhage.

In 90% of hypertensive patients, no clear etiology has been established. These are referred to as suffering from primary or essential hypertension. Hypertension of known causes such as tumor of the adrenal medulla (pheochromocytoma), tumor of the adrenal cortex (primary aldosteronism), and renal artery stenosis can be corrected surgically or treated with appropriate drugs. The following mechanisms are generally believed to be involved in the pathophysiology of primary hypertension: (a) high-sodium intake coupled with disturbances of sodium elimination, (b) hypersecretion of renin or overactivity of the renin-angiotensin system, (c) hyperactive central or peripheral autonomic nervous system, and (d) increased reactivity of peripheral arterial system to pressor agents. All accumulated data are consistent with the concept that cardiovascular damage is most likely to occur as a consequence of untreated hypertension and that partial reversal of these changes may be accomplished by control of the elevated pressure.

In most hypertensive patients, rational approach to therapy based on relating the mechanism of a drug's action to known pathophysiology is often not easily achieved, and thus the treatment of essential hypertension remains largely empirical. Because the homeostatic mechanisms for regulation of blood pressure remain intact in these patients, they will respond to physiological and pharmacological interventions. A large number of drugs that act upon various sites involved in blood pressure regulation are used for therapy of hypertension.

CLASSIFICATION

Drugs useful in the management of hypertension are usually classified according to their primary site or mode of action as shown in Table 15.3-1 and Fig. 15.3-1. The term *adrenoceptor* has been used in this table and in the text alternately in place of *adrenoreceptor* or *adrenergic*.

Table 15.3-1
Classification of Antihypertensive Drugs According to Their Primary Site and Mechanism of Action

A. Diuretics
- Thiazide-type
  - Chlorothiazide. benzthiazide, cyclothiazide
- Loop
  - Furosemide, ethacrynic acid
- Potassium-sparing
  - Spironolactone, triamterene, amiloride

B. Adrenergic-Depressant Drugs
- Centrally acting agents
  - Sedatives and hypnotics
    - Benzodiazepines, carbamates
  - Central α-adrenoceptor agonists
    - Clonidine, methyldopa, guanabenz, guanfacine
- Agents with both central and peripheral actions
  - Rauwolfia alkaloids
    - Reserpine, deserpidine
- Ganglionic-blocking agents
  - Trimethaphan, mecamylamine
- Adrenergic neuron-blocking agents
  - Guanethidine, guanadrel, bethanidine, debrisoquin
- Adrenoceptor-blocking agent
  - α-Adrenoceptor blocking agents
    - Prazosin, trimazosin, phenoxybenzamine, phentolamine
  - α- and β-adrenoceptor-blocking agents
    - Labetalol
  - β-Adrenoceptor-blocking agents
    - Propranolol
- Catecholamine synthesis blockers
  - Metyrosine
- Monoamine oxidase inhibitor
  - Pargyline

C. Direct-Acting Vasodilators
- Arterial vasodilators
  - Hydralazine, minoxidil, diazoxide
- Arterial and venous vasodilator
  - Sodium nitroprusside

D. Angiotensin antagonists
- Agent that blocks action of angiotensin II
  - Saralasin
- Agent that blocks formation of angiotensin II
  - Captopril, enalapril, teprotide

E. Calcium antagonists
- Nifedipine, diltiazem, verapamil

DIURETICS

Despite the fact that there is no definite evidence that sodium ingestion leads to hypertension, approximately one-third of patients with mild hypertension can be adequately controlled by the use of diuretics alone. Female hypertensive patients seem to tolerate diuretics better than male patients. These agents are usually recommended as the initial treatment for mild-to-moderate forms of essential hypertension. Regardless of their site and mechanism of action, all diuretics will lower blood pressure and potentiate other antihypertensive drugs. Consequently, they are frequently combined with more potent agents in the antihypertensive regimen.

Diuretics as a drug class are discussed in detail in Chapter 16.1, and their effects and doses are listed in Tables 16.1-2 and 16.1-3. In the following section the mechanisms of action and therapeutic uses of some of these agents in antihypertensive therapy will be briefly summarized.

Mechanism of Action. The mechanism of action of diuretics in promoting a reduction in blood pressure is not clear. A significant effect is sodium chloride depletion that leads to reduction in extracellular and plasma fluid volume with a consequent decrease in cardiac output. With chronic diuretic therapy hemodynamic adjustment occurs, cardiac output returns to normal, but the fall in diastolic pressure is maintained by a decrease in peripheral resistance.

Diuretics may also have a direct vasodilator action, but the mechanism of this vasodilation is not fully understood. It has been suggested that diuretics mobilize sodium from the arterial walls during a hypertensive state (104). However, this effect has not been demonstrated for the thiazide diuretics (96).

It is possible that diuretics may also promote arterial relaxation by a direct effect upon the smooth muscle of the arterial wall in a manner similar to diazoxide, a nondiuretic benzothiazide (see latter). Furthermore, the vascular responsiveness to angiotensin II is reduced during diuretic therapy (1). Diuretics also decrease the responsiveness of the cardiovascular system to catecholamines and to sympathetic nerve stimulation (32).

As a result of the drug-induced decrease in extracellular fluid volume, the secretion of renin is increased. The elevated renin level tends to oppose the action of the diuretic, but with continued use renin level will decrease to normal values. Although plasma volume will increase to near-normal values, a small volume deficit will persist (8, 95). It would therefore appear that the hypotensive action of diuretics is related to a combination of the reduction of extracellular and plasma volume as well as decreased ability of the cardiovascular system to compensate for the resultant hypovolemia.

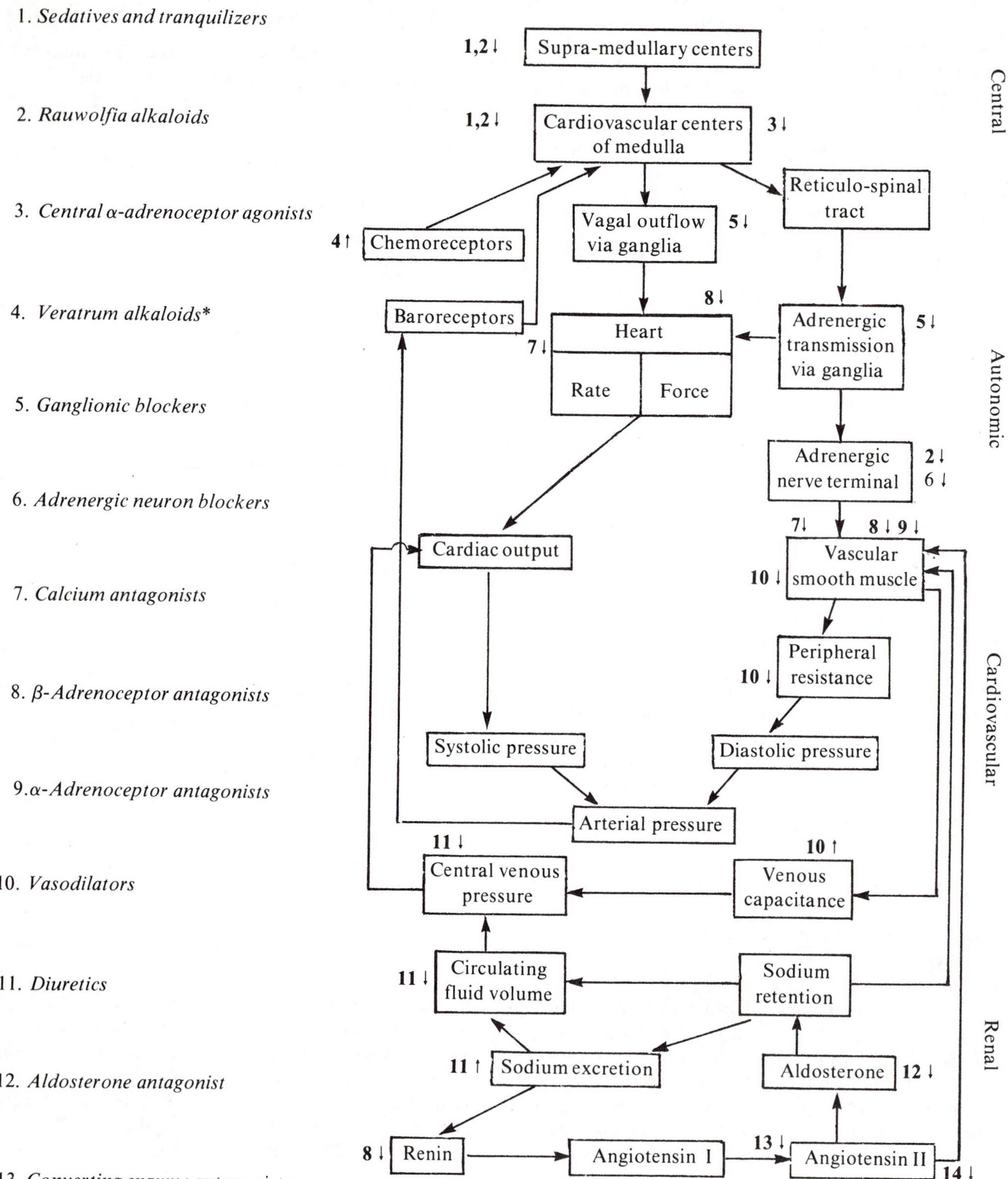

↑, Increase; ↓, decrease; *, not widely used.

Fig. 15.3-1. *Schematic representation of the main site of action of antihypertensive drugs.*

THIAZIDES

The thiazide diuretics were synthesized in 1957 and were the first orally active diuretics to be used for the control of hypertension. Structurally, they are similar to the sulfonamides and carbonic anhydrase inhibitors, and they cause saluresis by inhibiting sodium and chloride reabsorption in the distal nephron, and to a lesser extent, by inhibiting carbonic anhydrase. All thiazide diuretics produce similar pharmacological action. There is very little therapeutic advantage in choosing one agent over another. Differences are seen in their duration of action, and shorter-acting preparations must be administered at more frequent intervals to achieve maximum therapeutic benefit. They may be used orally as the sole drug for the management of mild hypertension or as adjunctive therapy in the management of more severe hypertension.

The most commonly encountered (5-10%) adverse effects of thiazide diuretics include tiredness, weakness, cramps, hyperuricemia, hypokalemia, hyperglycemia, and gastrointestinal distress (47, 87). Hypersensitivity reactions are seen in about 1-5% of patients whereas hypercalcemia, hyponatremia, and hypomagnesemia are rare. Thiazides should be cautiously used in the presence of severe renal or hepatic disease since azotemia and coma may result.

All benzothiazide diuretics are adequately absorbed orally and are distributed throughout the extracellular space. Diuresis is usually observed within an hour after administration. Chlorothiazide, the most widely used benzothiazide, is concentrated in the kidney and actively secreted in the proximal tubule (5, 9). Thiazides may also be eliminated through bile, especially when renal function is impaired.

LOOP HIGH-CEILING DIURETICS

The principal site of action of these rapid-acting and potent diuretics is on the ascending limb of the loop of Henle where they impair the ability of the kidney to reabsorb sodium and chloride (40, 92).

Furosemide is a monosulfamylanthranilic acid derivative, and ethacrynic acid is a phenoxyacetic acid derivative. Unlike the thiazides, due to their short duration of action, they must be administered at more frequent intervals to obtain equivalent antihypertensive action. Both drugs have very steep dose-response curves, hence diuretic efficacy increases with the dose throughout the therapeutic range even when glomerular filtration is severely impaired. In hypertensive patients with normal renal function the loop diuretic does not appear to be more effective than the thiazides but may produce even greater adverse effects. Consequently, they are usually reserved for patients with renal insufficiency who are refractory to the benzothiadiazides, for hypertensive crisis, and for patients with refractory congestive heart failure. In patients with severe renal insufficiency, furosemide is preferred to ethacrynic acid due to the higher incidence of gastrointestinal side effects associated with ethacrynic acid. Furosemide may also be used in conjunction with diazoxide in the management of hypertensive crisis in order to decrease the sodium-retaining property of diazoxide.

The major adverse effects of furosemide and ethacrynic acid are related to fluid and electrolyte depletion. They may induce a hypokalemic metabolic alkalosis that may be accompanied by hypotension and abnormal renal function. Electrolyte replacement and discontinuation of the drug usually alleviate these symptoms. Gastrointestinal disturbances such as nausea, vomiting, diarrhea, loss of appetite, and epigastric distress severely limit the oral use of ethacrynic acid. Hence, this drug is not usually given orally on a chronic basis. The incidence of these side effects is much less with furosemide. Furosemide possesses diabetogenic potential. During initial treatment most patients may complain of weakness, dizziness, fatigue, and muscle cramps. Both drugs elevate serum uric acid level through blockade of active renal uric acid secretion.

POTASSIUM-SPARING DIURETICS

The potassium-sparing diuretics (e.g., spironolactone, triamterene, and amiloride) possess weak antihypertensive action. Spironolactone, an aldosterone antagonist, binds to an aldosterone-binding protein in the cytoplasm of the distal tubular cells to inhibit the aldosterone-dependent sodium-potassium exchange. It is an effective antihypertensive agent, particularly when aldosterone production is elevated or when combined with other diuretic agents (e.g., thiazides) (17, 55). Spironolactone have been used in the following clinical conditions: (a) primary aldosteronism; (b) hypokalemia, especially as a result of chronic diuretic therapy; (c) hypertension and congestive heart failure (useful in combination with thiazides and is generally marketed as fixed combination of both drugs) (e.g., ALDACTAZIDE): and (d) cirrhosis and nephrotic syndrome. Due to its potassium-sparing property, spironolactone should be used with caution in patients with reduced renal function.

Both triamterene and amiloride are usually used in combination therapy with thiazide or loop diuretics because of their potassium-sparing action. Both drugs act on the distal convoluted tubule to cause a direct action upon the sodium-potassium exchange mechanism, instead of competitive antagonism with aldosterone.

Hyperkalemia is a common side effect of the potassium-sparing diuretics. Gynecomastia, breast tenderness, menstrual irregularities, and impotence—all related to the steroidal activity of spironolactone—may occur during chronic therapy with high doses. Triamterene and amiloride produce fewer side effects than spironolactone. However, deterioration of renal function and acidosis have been reported to occur when either drug is administered to azotemic patients. These drugs should not be given to patients with glomerular filtration rate less than 30 ml/min or to patients on potassium supplements.

Triamterene does not interfere with carbohydrate metabolism but can raise serum uric acid levels. Folic acid deficiency has also been reported during its use.

ADRENERGIC-DEPRESSANT DRUGS

CENTRALLY ACTING AGENTS

SEDATIVES AND HYPNOTICS

Sedatives and hypnotics (such as benzodiazepines, carbamates, and others) that depress the central nervous system reduce mental tension and produce calmness resulting in decrease of adrenergic outflow and lowering of blood pressure. These drugs are discussed in Chapters 11.2.1 and 11.5.3. They are more effective in combination with other drugs. As for an example, mebutamate (CAPLA), a hypnotic structurally related to meprobamate, is sometimes used with variable effectiveness in moderate as well as severe hypertension. Its effectiveness appears to be enhanced by concurrent hydrochlorothiazide therapy (16). Drowsiness, headache, xerostomia, and constipation appear to be the most frequently observed side effects, especially at higher dose levels.

CENTRAL α-ADRENOCEPTOR AGONISTS

Renewed interest in the central antihypertensive action of drugs was stimulated by the discovery that clonidine reduces central sympathetic outflow by stimulating medullary α-adrenoceptors. In animal experiments, clonidine has been shown to maintain antihypertensive action after midbrain section. Transection of the brain caudal to medulla abolishes its hypotensive effects (84). Since then a central action has been demonstrated for methyldopa (50). There is also some evidence for a central component in the antihypertensive action of β-adrenoceptor blockers such as propranolol (34, 35, 62).

CLONIDINE

Clonidine is an imidazole derivative closely related chemically to tolazoline and was synthesized during a search for nasal decongestant agents (Fig. 15.3-2).

Clonidine was initially studied as an α-adrenoceptor antagonist and indeed, in common with many structurally similar compounds, does possess α-adrenoceptor agonistic activity.

Mechanism of Action. Intravenous administration of clonidine produces an initial transient pressor response due to peripheral vasoconstriction (α-agonistic activity), followed by prolonged hypotension, negative chronotropic action, and sedation. Both cardiac output and peripheral resistance are also reduced, contributing to the hypotensive effect. It is the accepted hypothesis that clonidine stimulates presynaptic α_2-adrenoceptors at medullary centers thereby causing inhibition of central sympathetic outflow to the cardiovascular system (45). An α-adrenoceptor antagonist, such as tolazoline, readily reverses the hypotensive action of clonidine. Clonidine can also depress sympathetic transmission by a peripheral action, but this action contributes very little to the drug's antihypertensive effect.

Intravenous drug administration is also associated with a sharp decrease in plasma catecholamines that parallels the fall in blood pressure, and chronic therapy has been reported to reduce plasma renin activity possibly due to a centrally mediated decrease in sympathetic tone to renal blood vessels and to the juxtaglomerular apparatus (19). Naloxone can prevent the antihypertensive effect of clonidine in spontaneously hypertensive rats (23) indicating thereby an involvement of brain opioid peptides in the central regulation of blood pressures.

Pharmacokinetics. Studies performed mostly in normal volunteers indicate that the drug is well absorbed when given orally. Peak plasma levels occur within 2-4 hr. The hypotensive effect is usually maximal within 1 hr and lasts for 4-8 hr. In the brain tissue, clonidine is distributed in a manner similar to the catecholaminergic system, except for the cortex and hippocampal regions which show greater affinity. Peripherally, high concentrations occur in the liver, spleen, kidney and salivary, lacrimal, and parotid glands. Several metabolites have been identified in humans. About 45% of the unaltered drug is eliminated in the urine.

Adverse Effects. The most frequent side effect of clonidine is dryness of the mouth and eyes, sedation, and constipation. There is a low incidence of impotence as well as orthostatic hypotension. Sudden discontinuation of the drug in some patients may manifest signs and symptoms similar to those of pheochromocytoma (e.g., anxiety, nervousness, insomnia, tachycardia, rebound hypertension, and increased urinary catecholamines). Reinstatement of clonidine therapy or a combination of α- and β-adrenoceptor antagonists (not α-blocker alone) will effectively control these withdrawal effects. The mechanism of this phenomenon is unclear.

The antihypertensive effects of clonidine can be abolished by concurrent therapy with tricyclic antidepressants. Clonidine should not be employed in patients with depression. Alternative therapy should be instituted in patients who become depressed while taking the drug.

Therapeutic Uses. In addition to its efficacy in treating mild-to-severe hypertension, clonidine has also been advocated for the therapy of migraine headache as well as menopausal flushing.

Most hypertensive patients will respond to daily maintenance doses of less than 0.8 mg. The usual initial dose is 0.1 mg two to three times a day. The ability of clonidine to lower blood pressure without significant inhibition of homeostatic control mechanisms is highly desirable. However, the incidence of adverse effects and especially the propensity to induce withdrawal effects limits its use as a standard first-line drug.

Clonidine produces sodium and water retention with expansion of the plasma and extracellular fluid volume; these effects may counteract its antihypertensive effect. It

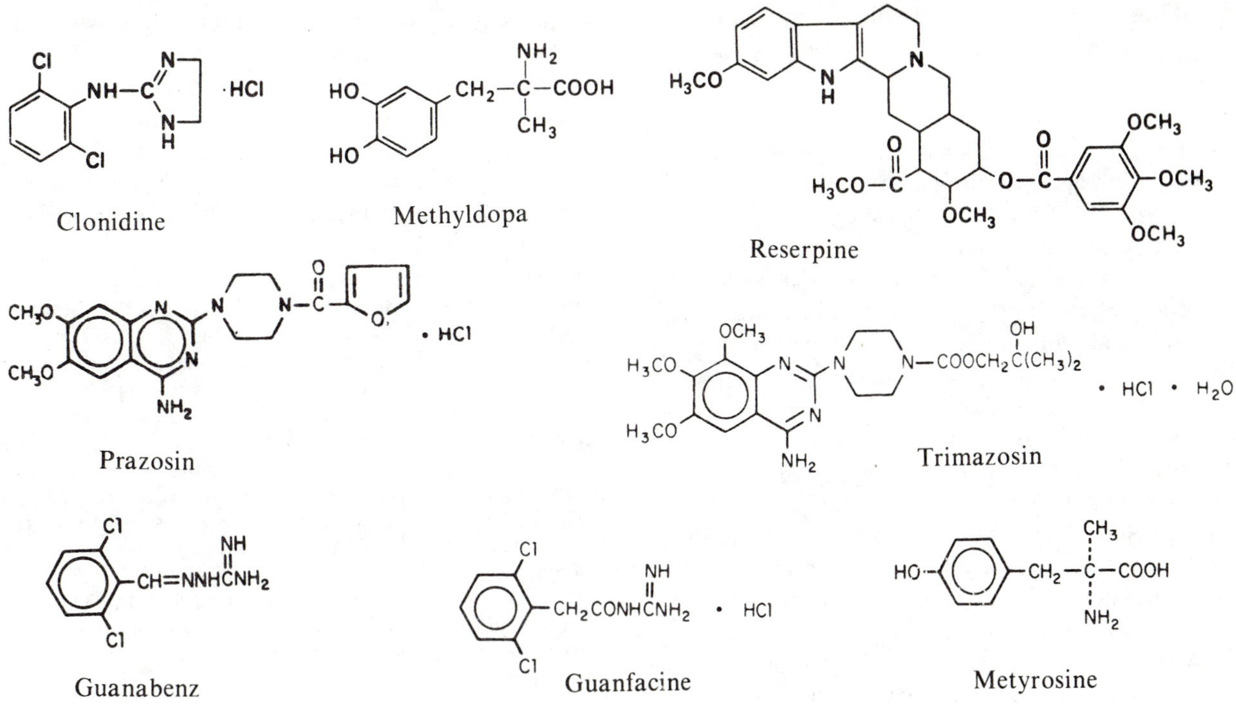

Clonidine

Methyldopa

Reserpine

Prazosin

Trimazosin

Guanabenz

Guanfacine

Metyrosine

Fig. 15.3-2: *Chemical structures of some adrenergic-depressant antihypertensive compounds.*

is therefore more effective when combined with a diuretic (105). Clonidine may be combined with a vasodilator in the treatment of resistant hypertension. In such instances reflex increases in both heart rate and cardiac output are reduced or abolished by clonidine. It is also a very useful agent for hypertension complicated by renal diseases.

Preparations. *Clonidine Hydrochloride*, USP (CATAPRES) is available in 0.1-0.2 mg tablets. The maximum daily dose is 1.8 mg. Because a single daily dose is usually inadequate to control blood pressure, the drug may be given in 3 divided doses of 0.15 mg. In order to minimize side effects, clonidine may be given in 2 unequal doses, the larger dose being given at bedtime and the smaller dose at noon (52).

Drug Interactions. The sedative effect of clonidine is synergistic with other centrally acting depressant drugs. Tricyclic antidepressant drugs such as imipramine and desipramine may nullify the effects of clonidine, hence their concurrent use should be avoided (10, 101).

METHYLDOPA

Methyldopa was developed as an inhibitor of dopa decarboxylase (91). Chemically, it is L-α-methyl-3,4-dihydroxyphenylalanine (Fig. 15.3-2).

The drug was first given to patients with malignant carcinoid tumors to decrease the production of serotonin (89). Its antihypertensive action was first noted in 1960 and subsequently confirmed in clinical trials (70).

Mechanism of Action. The antihypertensive action was originally attributed to dopa decarboxylase inhibition with a consequent reduction in norepinephrine stores. Later studies indicated that the CNS is the major site of the drug's antihypertensive action. Methyldopa is converted to α-methyldopamine and α-methylnorepinephrine, which stimulate central α-adrenoceptors in a manner similar to clonidine. Central sympathetic outflow is thus inhibited. Although it is apparent that the major effect of methyldopa is centrally mediated, a contribution of peripheral effects may play a minor role. It has been suggested that the observed reduction in renal vascular resistance may be related to the fact that α-methylnorepinephrine (a weaker vasoconstrictor than norepinephrine) accumulated in peripheral autonomic nerve endings. In addition, the drug lowers blood pressure in immunosympathectomized rats (25), which suggests a peripheral component of its effect.

Pharmacological Effects. Methyldopa administration reduces both supine and standing blood pressure. Exercise hypotension, postural hypotension, and diurnal blood pressure variations rarely occur. Although peripheral resistance is reduced, cardiac output, renal blood flow, and glomerular filtration rate are not significantly altered. Because of its minimal renal effects, methyldopa is especially valuable in treating hypertensive patients with renal insufficiency except for those with end-stage renal disease. In some patients heart rate is decreased while elevated plasma renin activity may decrease during therapy. Long-term therapy with α-methyldopa results in fluid retention, edema, and plasma volume expansion.

Pharmacokinetics. There is large interindividual variability in the absorption of orally administered methyldopa. Following an oral dose, peak plasma level occurs within 2 hr with a half-life of 3-4 hr. There is no demonstrable correlation between plasma levels of methyldopa and its antihypertensive action. This suggests an action mediated through a metabolite. The principal urinary excretory products are unaltered methyldopa, methyldopa mono-*o*-sulfate, and methyldopamine. Methyldopa and its metabolites may interefere with chemical tests for catecholamines. Thus, urinary excretion of metanephrines is doubled during methyldopa therapy. The plasma half-life is significantly increased in azotemic patients, hence the dose of α-methyldopa should be decreased in such patients.

Adverse Effects. The most frequently encountered side effects of methyldopa therapy include sedation, nasal congestion, and dry mouth. The incidence of sedation is initially high but usually decreases with continued therapy. However, a persistent lassitude and drowsiness may occur and be particularly disturbing to the patients who must remain mentally alert. Other effects relating to the central nervous system include extrapyramidal disturbances, vertigo, and psychic depression. Fluid and electrolyte retention with plasma volume expansion may occur, hence a diuretic is usually added to methyldopa therapy to control this side effect. Disturbances of sexual function including both impotence and failure to ejaculate have been reported. Postural hypotension may develop, but its incidence is very low when compared with more potent drugs such as guanethidine.

The drug may produce a variety of unique side effects unrelated to sympathetic depression, which may necessitate discontinuation of therapy. These include hemolytic anemia, fever and hepatitis. The drug is therefore not administered to patients with active hepatic disease. With chronic therapy the direct Coombs' test may be positive. However, this is rarely associated with hemolytic anemia. A rare drug-induced lactation associated with elevated prolactin level has been reported. Occasionally a flulike symptom that responds to salicylates may occur. As with clonidine, the abrupt withdrawal of methyldopa may result in hypertensive crisis. However, the incidence of this side effect is much less than that observed with clonidine.

Therapeutic Use. The clinical response to methyldopa is not always consistent. The majority of patients respond with a sustained decrease in blood pressure at a dose range of 0.5-2 g/day; a smaller population responds only to a higher dosage. A few patients who show an initial antihypertensive response later develop tolerance or resistance. Maximum reduction of blood pressure and heart rate occurs 4-6 hr after oral administration with a duration of up to 12-24 hr. Concurrent use of a thiazide diuretic will augment methyldopa's efficacy by reducing the tendency for sodium and water retention as well as the development of tolerance due to plasma volume expansion. The ethyl ester, methyldopate, is occasionally given intravenously in hypertensive emergencies. Methyldopa is indicated for moderate-to-severe hypertension and is particularly useful in hypertension complicated by renal disease. It is not recommended for patients with pheochromocytoma.

Preparations and Dosages. *Methyldopa*, USP (ALDOMET) is available in 125-, 250-, or 500-mg tablets for oral use. The average daily dose is 1 g, and little additional advantages can be gained by doses over 2 g. However, daily doses as high as 3 g have been employed. Although a single daily dose may be adequate, three divided doses of 375 mg are usually employed for effective blood pressure control. Somnolence is usually less troublesome if initial dose is low, and it is often more advantageous to reduce the dosage and add another drug rather than to exceed the maximum daily dose. Methyldopa may also be given by parenteral infusions in single doses of 0.5-1 g, adjusted to the need of the individual patient. The more soluble preparation *methyldopate hydrochloride,* USP (ALDOMET ESTER HYDROCHLORIDE) is also available for parenteral use in 5-ml vials (50 mg/ml).

GUANABENZ ACETATE

Guanabenz (WYTENSIN) is a guanidine derivative (Fig. 15.3-2) that lowers blood pressure by reducing adrenergic outflow from the brain by activation of central α_2-adrenoceptors. It appears to be as effective as methyldopa in patients with mild-to-moderate hypertension, but causes more frequent side effects. It is more useful and better tolerated (in reduced dosage) when given in combination with a diuretic. It is rapidly absorbed with a peak plasma concentrations at 4 hr after oral administration. The effect of a single dose lasts for 12-24 hr. About 80% of an oral dose is excreted in urine, largely as metabolites.

Most common adverse effects are sedation and dryness of mouth. Weakness and orthostatic hypotension may occur. Headache, palpitation, nasal congestion, and blurred vision are reported occasionally. Initial oral dose of 4 mg twice or 8 mg once daily is gradually increased. It is available in 4- or 8-mg tablets.

GUANFACINE

Guanfacine is a guanidine derivative (Fig. 15.3-2) that has a similar central action like clonidine. It enters and leaves the brain more slowly than clonidine. Its hypotensive effect is associated mainly with a fall in peripheral resistance; decrease in heart rate and cardiac output may also occur.

The drug is absorbed from the GI tract. Its plasma level is low due to its high tissue affinity and half-life is 14-17 hr. It is excreted mainly by kidney. It has been used alone or in combination with other agents as a step-2 drug for antihypertensive therapy. Its adverse effects resemble those of clonidine. Dryness of mouth and sedation are common. Tolerance develops frequently, and a withdrawal syndrome with rebound hypertension may occur (as in the case of clonidine) when the drug is withdrawn rapidly, particularly following therapy with high daily doses (4 mg or more).

Its initial oral dose is 0.5 mg twice daily to be increased gradually as needed. Daily maintenance dose is 1-3 mg. It is an investigational drug available in capsules of 0.5, 1, 2, and 3 mg.

AGENTS WITH BOTH CENTRAL AND PERIPHERAL ACTIONS

Rauwolfia Alkaloids

Several alkaloids are obtained from *Rauwolfia serpentina*, a climbing shrub indigenous to several Asiatic countries. Of these alkaloids reserpine and deserpidine are sometimes used in hypertension. The action of reserpine (Fig. 15.3-2) was first described by Moyer and Brest (68).

RESERPINE

Mechanism of Action. Reserpine depletes biogenic amines from postganglionic sympathetic nerve terminals, the adrenal medulla, and the central nervous system. The degree of residual adrenergic activity following reserpine appears to be related to the level of norepinephrine depletion (33). By inhibiting an adenosine triphosphate (ATP)-Mg^{2+}-dependent uptake mechanism, reserpine prevents storage of norepinephrine in storage granules of adrenergic nerve terminals. Norepinephrine will then be inactivated by cytoplasmic monoamine oxidase. The uptake of dopamine into storage vesicles is also prevented by reserpine. At large doses administered in experimental animals it will cause almost total catecholamine depletion. Following a single dose, complete recovery may be delayed for up to 14 days until new storage granules are synthesized (46). Reserpine does not inhibit norepinephrine reuptake from the synaptic cleft (88), nor does it interfere with the release process as guanethidine does. Despite the drug-induced depletion of brain serotonin and dopamine, central sympathetic outflow is not significantly altered (51).

Chronic reserpine therapy decreases arterial blood pressure, cardiac output, and peripheral vascular resistance. Whereas the vascular resistance remains reduced following its use, cardiac output gradually increases to predrug level (80, 83).

Pharmacokinetics. Reserpine is readily absorbed orally, and although it is widely distributed throughout most organs such as brain, liver, spleen, kidney, and adipose tissue, it is readily concentrated at adrenergic neuronal sites. There is no correlation between its plasma levels and antihypertensive effect. At the usual oral dose, adequate blood pressure control may require 2-3 weeks. Its metabolic fate is not known with certainty.

Adverse Effects. Excessive sedation and depression severe enough to cause suicide may occur even at the usual dose range of 0.25-0.5 mg/day (18, 28, 71). Reserpine is contraindicated in patients with a history of depression and, if symptoms of depression develop during its administration, should be discontinued. Other adverse effects include nightmares, aggravation of peptic ulcer due to increased gastric acidity, increased gastrointestinal motility, diarrhea, and impotence in males. Bradycardia and extrapyramidal symptoms suggestive of parkinsonism sometimes occur. Because reserpine depletes myocardial catecholamines, it has been implicated in the aggravation of congestive heart failure. There is some evidence to suggest that the long-term use of reserpine increases the risk of breast cancer by two to three times (3).

Therapeutic Use. In the treatment of ambulatory patients the usual initial dose is 0.25 mg/day. Maintenance dose should not exceed 0.25 mg/day to minimize side effects (29). Parenteral drug administration is very rarely employed. Maximal antihypertensive action usually occurs within 3 hr and will persist for approximately 24 hr. It is customary to administer a diuretic concurrently with reserpine to prevent false tolerance (22) and to minimize compensatory fluid retention. If during reserpine therapy sympathomimetic agents are required, they should be administered with care due to the drug-induced hypersensitivity (26). Agitated hypertensive patients may additionally benefit from its CNS-depressant properties.

Preparation and Dosage. *Rauwolfia Serpentina*, USP (whole root) and *reserpine*, USP are the most widely used official preparations. *Rauwolfia Serpentina* is available in 50- to 100-mg tablets for oral use; 200-300 mg of powdered roots is equivalent to 0.5 mg of reserpine. Reserpine (SERPASIL, SANDRIL) is available in tablets (0.1, 0.25, 0.5, or 1 mg) and in capsules (0.5 mg). A solution for injection (2.5 mg/ml in 2-ml ampules and 10-ml vials) and an elixir (0.2 mg/4 ml) are also available.

GANGLIONIC-BLOCKING AGENTS

Ganglionic-blocking drugs, although extremely potent, are rarely used as antihypertensive agents. A few of these agents, however, are reserved for severe or malignant forms of hypertension and for hypertensive emergencies. All ganglionic-blocking drugs block transmission in both parasympathetic and sympathetic ganglia. Thus they prevent onward impulse transmission to postganglionic autonomic nerves. The resultant decrease in sympathetic tone causes pooling of blood in venous capacitance vessels and a significant decrease in cardiac output (4). Total peripheral resistance may also be reduced. Pronounced orthostatic hypotension as well as symptoms due to associated parasympathetic blockade (blurred vision, constipation, impotence, urinary retention, paralytic ileus, and xerostomia) have severely limited the use of these agents in the therapy of hypertension. However, trimethaphan camsylate, a short-acting ganglionic-blocking drug is administered intravenously in hypertensive emergencies. Trimethaphan is also effective for the production of controlled hypotension during surgery and for the control of blood pressure in acute dissecting aortic aneurysm. It is administered by continuous intravenous infusion as a 0.1% (1 mg/ml) solution in 5% dextrose at a rate of 0.5-1 mg/min as determined by the patient's response. Because of rapid development of refractoriness to trimethaphan, patients should be treated with a potent orally acting antihypertensive agent as soon as possible. The use of trimethaphan is now being superseded by nitroprusside. A more complete description of the pharmacology of ganglionic-blocking drugs is presented in Chapter 8.4.

ADRENERGIC NEURON-BLOCKING AGENTS

These drugs interfere with the release of norepinephrine from the adrenergic nerve terminal. As a result, adrenergic influence on blood vessels and the heart rate are reduced.

GUANETHIDINE

The antihypertensive action of guanethidine (Fig. 7.3-1) was first reported by Maxwell et al. (63). McCubbin et al. (64) demonstrated guanethidine's effectiveness in both renal and neurogenic hypertensive dogs.

Mechanism of Action. Guanethidine impairs postganglionic sympathetic nerve function. It is transported into the neuronal storage granule by the same mechanism that transports norepinephrine. Its accumulation is associated with a reduction in adrenergic neuronal function. Reduction in neuronal function, however, occurs before demonstrable changes in tissue norepinephrine, suggesting the involvement of another mechanism in its action. It has been suggested that an inhibition of impulse transmission occurs at the level of the outer neuronal or vesicular membranes within the sympathetic nerve terminal (86). Thus, the process by which the action potential causes the release of stored norepinephrine is impaired. Intravenously administered guanethidine, especially in large doses, may produce an initial sympathomimetic effect due to displacement and release of norepinephrine. The effects of exogenously administered norepinephrine are also potentiated due to a combination of cocainelike effects (interference of norepinephrine uptake) as well as a denervation sensitivity of the neuroeffector junction (2). Because of guanethidine's poor CNS penetration, central catecholamines and serotonin are not affected. Adrenomedullary catecholamines are neither depleted nor released by guanethidine and plasma renin activity is not suppressed (24).

Following administration of guanethidine there is a progressive fall in systemic and pulmonary arterial pressure associated with a decrease in heart rate and cardiac output. The effect on systolic pressure in the erect posture or during exercise is marked (83). Glomerular filtration rate and renal plasma flow decrease initially, but during chronic treatment both return to pretreatment values. Often this drug leads to marked fluid retention. Its antihypertensive action is also associated with impairment of cardiovascular reflexes. Hence, postural and exercise hypotension are commonly encountered during therapy.

Pharmacokinetics. Patients vary in their responses due to variability in absorption (3-50%), biotransformation, and renal elimination of the drug. Following its absorption it is rapidly distributed to tissue storage sites including adrenergic neurons (65). Guanethidine has a half-life of about 5 days, and about 15% of the administered dose is eliminated each day. The drug is strongly basic, and renal tubular secretion plays a major role in its elimination. Hepatic microsomal metabolism of the drug occurs, especially after oral administration. Its metabolites are very polar, but with little antihypertensive activity. In patients with liver or kidney disease the dose of guanethidine should be reduced and the patient closely monitored to minimize drug overdosage.

Therapeutic Use. Guanethidine is employed as a potent orally active antihypertensive drug in the management of moderate-to-severe hypertension not responsive to other regimens. It is also employed in the management of hypertension due to renal amyloidosis. The usual dose range is 25-150 mg/day, but efficacy may be demonstrated at a dose as low as 5 mg/day. Concurrent diuretic or adrenergic receptor-blocking drugs will improve the drug's efficacy, lower its dosage, as well as minimize its side effects. In order to reduce the diurnal fluctuation of blood pressure that frequently occurs during therapy with large doses of guanethidine (61). It is often advisable to include methyldopa in the antihypertensive regimen.

Drug Interactions and Contraindications. Extreme bradycardia may occur if digitalis and guanethidine are used concurrently. Tricyclic antidepressants, methylphenidate, cocaine, and to a lesser extent phenothiazines block guanethidine's uptake and can reverse it's hypotensive action. Following concurrent use of guanethidine and an antidepressant drug, withdrawal of the latter drug may result in marked hypotension. Patients should be cautioned against using cold remedies containing indirectly acting sympathomimetic amines (e.g., ephedrine) while on guanethidine therapy, since these amines will not only prevent guanethidine uptake into the nerve terminals, but may also promote its release from intraneuronal sites. Potentiation of the effects of exogenously administered catecholamines with respect to blood pressure and predisposition to cardiac arrhythmia are frequent observations. Concurrent oral contraceptive therapy may reduce the hypotensive effect of guanethidine and make the satisfactory control of hypertension difficult. Concurrent use of alcohol, other vasodilators, or plasma volume-depleting drugs will accentuate the drug-induced postural hypotension.

Guanethidine is contraindicated in pheochromocytoma since severe hypertension may result. The drug is also contraindicated in the presence of congestive heart failure not associated with hypertension, since interference with the compensatory role of the sympathetic nervous system in this condition may occur. Drug therapy should be discontinued 2 weeks before general anesthesia and, if the patient is on monoamine oxidase (MAO) inhibitor therapy, the latter should be discontinued at least 1 week before starting guanethidine therapy.

Adverse Effects. Most of the adverse effects of guanethidine result from decreased sympathetic activity. These include orthostatic and exercise hypotension, lightheadedness, dizziness, ejaculatory failure, and fluid retention. Overt cardiac failure may be precipitated in patients with marginal reserve due to vascular volume expansion, edema, and reduction in cardiac sympathetic tone. Due in part to parasympathetic predominance, diarrhea is a common complaint. The incidence of diarrhea produced by this agent is greater than that observed with other adrenergic neuron-blocking agents, suggesting the involvement of other mechanisms. Guanethidine also produces neuromuscular blockade, which may account for the muscle fatigue and tremor observed in some patients.

Preparation and Dosage. *Guanethidine Sulfate*, USP (ISMELIN) is only available for oral use in 10- and 25-mg tablets. The daily dose varies widely, but its long duration of action makes a single daily dose convenient. The usual starting dose is 20 mg with increments at intervals of 5-7 days until the desired effects or unacceptable side effects occur. The usual daily dose is 25-50 mg, but doses exceeding 120 mg have been employed in hospitalized patients under careful supervision.

GUANADREL

Guanadrel (HYLOREL), a new adrenergic neuron-blocking drug, has a chemical structure (Fig. 7.3-1), mechanism of action, and hemodynamic effects similar to those of guanethidine, but has a more rapid onset and a shorter duration of action. It is recommended for step-2 therapy of moderate hypertension as an alternative to methyldopa. Information on its pharmacokinetics and adverse effects is given in Chapter 7.3.

BETHANIDINE AND DEBRISOQUIN

Two other adrenergic neuronal-blocking agents, bethanidine (ESTABAL) and debrisoquin (DECLINAX), are currently used on a limited basis as antihypertensive agents. They are structurally related to and similar in action to guanethidine (Fig. 7.3-1). Their mechanism of action and pharmacokinetics are described in Chapter 7.3. But their action is more rapid and shorter in duration (14, 35). It is thus possible to attain their maintenance dose more quickly, with less risk of developing prolonged hypotension, with these agents than with guanethidine.

These drugs are reliably absorbed when given orally and eliminated via kidney. Hence, reduction of dosage is necessary in the presence of renal failure. Some individuals have a genetic inability to metabolize debrisoquin, thus dosage requirement for this drug varies considerably among patients.

Like guanethidine, bethanidine and debrisoquin are effective in the management of hypertension. They show some minor differences from guanethidine in their effectiveness and side effects. Diarrhea is not observed with these drugs. Drug interactions and contraindications are similar to those described for guanethidine. There is less tendency with these drugs to produce hypertensive crisis in patients with pheochromocytoma. Neither drug is available for general use in the United States.

ADRENOCEPTOR-BLOCKING AGENTS

Adrenoceptor-blocking drugs have been investigated for their potential use as antihypertensive drugs. The limited efficacy of the classic α-adrenoceptor-blocking drugs as well as their side effects (postural hypotension and tachycardia) preclude their use in the chronic therapy of hypertension. Although the precise role of β-adrenoceptor mechanism in essential hypertension has not been defined, β-adrenoceptor-blocking drugs are widely used as antihypertensive drugs.

α-ADRENOCEPTOR-BLOCKING DRUGS

Two types of α-adrenoceptors have been defined: postsynaptic or vascular α_1-receptors and the presynaptic α_2-receptors. Currently, phenoxybenzamine, a noncompetitive long-acting agent, and phentolamine, a short-acting competitive blocking agent, are available for use in the therapy of hypertension. The pharmacological effects of both phenoxybenzamine and phentolamine on the circulation are almost identical to those of the direct-acting arterial vasodilators. They reduce peripheral vascular resistance and venous tone, and produce hypotension and reflex tachycardia. Both agents block postsynaptic α_1-adrenoceptors as well as presynaptic α_2-adrenoceptors, the effect of phenoxybenzamine being less significant on α_2-receptors. Phentolamine is a drug of choice for hypertensive crisis caused by excessive adrenergic activity, such as withdrawal from clonidine, MAO inhibitors, and excessive levels of sympathomimetic amines. Both agents are useful in preparing pheochromocytoma patients for surgery as well as to alleviate symptoms of hypertension in patients with inoperable tumors. The pharmacology of both agents has been previously discussed in Chapter 7.2.

PRAZOSIN

Prazosin is a quinazoline derivative (Fig. 15.3-2) and structurally related to both theophylline and papaverine, vasodilators that inhibit phosphodiesterase. It is an unusual vasodilator and is classified as both an arteriodilator and a venodilator. However, compared with phenoxybenzamine and phentolamine, it is less potent as a vasodilator.

Mechanism of Action. The mechanism of antihypertensive action of prazosin is poorly understood. Current hypothesis suggests a selective blocking action on postsynaptic α_1-adrenoceptors (106) with no affinity for the presynaptic α_2-adrenoceptors. Thus, the vasoconstriction produced by released norepinephrine is inhibited. On a molar basis, prazosin is about 10 times more potent than phentolamine. Its relative lack of activity at presynaptic α_2-adrenoceptors allows norepinephrine to exert a negative feedback control of its own release. Unlike hydralazine, diazoxide, or minoxidil, although prazosin reduces peripheral vascular resistance, a concurrent secondary reflex tachycardia or elevated plasma renin activity is not observed (43, 49, 58). Prazosin lowers blood pressure by decreasing peripheral vascular resistance. Cardiac output is usually unchanged, and renal blood flow and glomerular filtration rate are maintained (58). Plasma renin activity either is not affected or slightly increased.

Pharmacokinetics. Most of the drug is rapidly metabolized after oral absorption, and there is significant first-pass metabolism. Prazosin is metabolized by acetylation and glucuronide conjugation. About 90% of an administered dose is excreted in the feces. The half-life is about 3 hr, but when the drug is administered to patients with congestive heart failure or renal insufficiency higher blood levels are observed (11). Thus, the dosage should be reduced in these patients.

Adverse Effects. Adverse effects include orthostatic hypotension and syncope, which may occur with the first dose (first-dose effect). This phenomenon is believed to be due to inadequate venous return to the heart and is usually preceded by a rapid decrease in heart rate. The phenomenon can be minimized by giving the first dose in divided doses (i.e., 1 mg three times daily). Orthostatic hypotension occurs but is less prominent than with phenoxybenzamine or phentolamine and appears most frequently in patients with sodium deficiency. This may occur during intensive therapy with diuretics or in patients on low-sodium diet. Other adverse effects include drowsiness, dizziness, palpitation, headache, and easy fatigability. These side effects are usually well tolerated.

Therapeutic Use. Prazosin is effective in mild-to-severe hypertension. When the drug is used by itself, approximately 80% of patients with mild-to-moderate hypertension will have a significant fall in blood pressure.

Its efficacy may be increased by the addition of a diuretic and/or a β-adrenoceptor-blocking drug. Orthostatic hypotension may occur at the onset of treatment but disappears with continued therapy. Both prazosin and nitrates may cause syncope when used in combination. In addition, prazosin may precipitate angina in patients with ischemic heart disease. In such patients, prazosin should be combined with a β-adrenoceptor blocker or verapamil.

Preparations and Dosage. *Prazosin Hydrochloride* (MINIPRESS) is available in capsules (1, 2, or 5 mg). Antihypertensive dose ranges from 1.5 to 7.5 mg/day, given in two or five divided doses. Initial dose should not exceed 1 mg, and should be given at bedtime. The maintenance dose is generally 20 mg/day.

TRIMAZOSIN

Like prazosin, trimazosin is a quinazoline derivative (Fig. 15.3-2) and acts by dilating both arterioles and veins. However, its effect on α_1-adrenoceptor appears to be less marked than that of prazosin. Its antihypertensive action appears to be mainly due to a direct action on arterioles. Its effect on heart rate is variable. It may slightly reduce serum cholesterol levels and does not increase plasma renin activity.

Prazosin is rapidly absorbed with a peak plasma level at 1-2 hr after oral administration. It is 99% protein bound and metabolized in the liver. Its half-life is 2 hr and its major metabolite has a half-life of 4.8 hr.

Headache, dizziness, drowsiness, and weakness are common adverse effects. Trimazosin is an investigational drug that appears to have an efficacy like methyldopa and has been used alone or in combination with a diuretic to treat mild-to-moderate hypertension. Adult oral dose is 50-300 mg b.i.d. or t.i.d. It is available in capsules (25, 50, 100, and 150 mg).

α- & β-ADRENOCEPTOR-BLOCKING AGENTS

LABETALOL

Labetalol (Fig. 7.2-2) possesses both α- and β-adrenoceptor-blocking activity. The clinical trials have shown that labetalol is effective in lowering blood pressure in hypertension of mild-to-moderate severity (7, 57). It differs from propranolol in that it induces less slowing of heart rate, and its hypotensive action in the erect position is more pronounced than in the supine position.

Severe and resistant cases may respond to high doses, 1.2-4 mg/day. In hypertensive crisis, such as seen during clonidine withdrawal and in pheochromocytoma, labetalol is infused intravenously at a rate of 2 mg/min to a total of 1-2 mg/kg, followed by oral therapy (81). First-pass metabolism occur, and its metabolites are eliminated in the urine. The plasma half-life is 3-4 hr, and daily dosage should be lowered in patients with hepatic disease. Its bioavailability is increased by cimetidine. The drug is usually well tolerated. Labetalol may cause orthostatic hypotension, especially during initial therapy, when a diuretic is used concurrently, or when the patient is exposed to elevated temperature (e.g., during warm weather). Gastrointestinal disturbances, dizziness, nervousness, fatigue, and dryness of the mouth have also been reported. The drug should be cautiously used in patients with pheochromocytoma since a paradoxical increase in blood pressure may occur. Antinuclear antibodies have developed in some patients, but very few cases of a systemic lupuslike syndrome have been documented. Drug-induced tachycardia and fluid retention may be controlled by the use of a β-adrenoceptor-blocking drug and a diuretic, respectively.

β-ADRENOCEPTOR-BLOCKING AGENTS

The antihypertensive effect of pronethalol was first shown in 1964 by Prichard (77). In the same year Prichard and Gillam reported the antihypertensive action of propranolol (78). For several years β-adrenoceptor-blocking drugs were not generally accepted as therapeutic agents in the management of hypertension. At present, however, this class of drugs is very widely accepted.

PROPRANOLOL

Propranolol (Fig. 7.2-2) is the prototype of antihypertensive β-adrenoceptor-blocking drugs and is used for a variety of diseased states including angina pectoris, cardiac arrhythmias, and hypertension. The success of propranolol has prompted the introduction of several similar agents as potential antihypertensive agents (e.g., practolol, alprenolol, oxprenolol, timolol, acebutolol, sotalol, etc.) (Table 15.3-3). Their effectiveness and freedom from disturbing side effects common to most antihypertensive drugs have significantly aided their acceptance as first-line drugs in the management of hypertension.

Mechanism of Action. Propranolol antagonizes all β-adrenoceptor stimulation competitively. Some of the other agents (e.g., acebutolol, atenolol, metoprolol, and practolol) show selectivity for β_1-cardiac receptors and are therefore classified as cardioselective. In addition, some agents also exhibit partial agonistic activity—pindolol, acebutolol, alprenolol, oxprenolol, practolol, and timolol. Membrane-stabilizing activity is also exhibited by acebutolol, alprenolol, oxprenolol, pindolol, and propranolol. At the present time, however, it is considered doubtful that cardiodepression, partial agonistic activity, or membrane-stabilizing property resulting from inhibition of transfer of sodium across the membrane contribute to the antihypertensive action of these agents. In fact, the role of β-adrenoceptor blockade per se as the primary mechanism of the drug's antihypertensive action is quite controversial (34, 48). There are three current hypotheses that attempt to explain the antihypertensive action of propranolol and other β-adrenoceptor-blocking drugs.

1. A negative inotropic and chronotropic action on the heart to decrease cardiac output chronically (31, 100), with a rise in total peripheral resistance is the first hypothesis. Most β-adrenoceptor-blocking drugs decrease the rate of myocardial oxygen utilization. However, patients who fail to exhibit antihypertensive effect to propranolol still have decreased cardiac output (30). In addition, other β-adrenoceptor-blocking drugs reduce blood pressure without reducing cardiac output (60). Cardiac output may also be reduced in patients who do not show a fall in blood pressure. Hence, the reduction in cardiac output may not be totally responsible for the observed antihypertensive effects.

2. Chronic administration of β-adrenoceptor-blocking agents has been reported to inhibit plasma renin activity in both normotensive and hypertensive subjects (12, 59). β-Adrenoceptor-blocking drugs that do not significantly influence plasma renin activity will also lower elevated blood pressure. In addition, propranolol is an effective antihypertensive agent in patients with normal or low plasma renin activity, although higher doses may be needed. It is generally believed that in the majority of hypertensive patients lowering of plasma renin activity induced by β-adrenoceptor-blocking drugs contributes very little to their overall antihypertensive effects.

3. Propranolol readily crosses the blood-brain barrier and produces several effects attributed to inhibition of central sympathetic activity (76, 102). A central mechanism of antihypertensive action has been suggested by several studies (34, 35). It crosses the blood-brain barrier and produces CNS-related side effects. However, β-adrenoceptor-blocking drugs such as practolol, pindolol, and sotalol lower blood pressure without demonstrable CNS involvement. Side effects of β-adrenoceptor-blocking drugs such as nightmares and dreams and failure of these drugs to influence postural control of blood pressure are suggestive of a central mechanism of action.

In addition to the inhibition of peripheral adrenergic nerve function (65), an interaction with prostaglandins has also been suggested as a possible mechanism of the hypotensive action of β-adrenoceptor-blocking drugs (21).

Pharmacokinetics. Almost all of these drugs are adequately absorbed from the gastrointestinal tract with peak plasma levels achieved within 1-3 hr. The antihypertensive effects cannot be correlated with their plasma level; there is a significant lag between blood level and peak antihypertensive action. There is also no clear correlation between persistence of drug in the plasma and antihypertensive effect. With most agents, there appears to be a ceiling dose above which an increase in the dose does not produce greater antihypertensive action (102).

Propranolol and alprenolol are metabolized by hepatic degradation; about 50-80% of the oral dose of propranolol is subjected to hepatic first-pass metabolism. Thus, high doses are usually necessary to obtain a satisfactory response. Practolol and sotalol are excreted by renal mechanisms (50). Pindolol, acebutolol, atenolol, and timolol are excreted unchanged whereas metoprolol is biotransformed and its metabolites excreted by the kidneys. Detailed pharmacokinetics of β-adrenoceptor-blocking drugs have been discussed in Chapter 7.2.

Therapeutic Use. These agents reduce arterial blood pressure gradually over several days. Their action is additive with other antihypertensive drugs such as diuretics and vasodilators. The effective dose should be decided on the basis of the individual response. Satisfactory blood pressure control can be obtained in about 30% of hypertensive patients by the use of β-adrenoceptor-blocking drugs alone (67, 94). In combination with other agents, they can adequately control blood pressure of about 80% of all patients. This class of drugs is well tolerated by most patients; mild sedation is the only major side effect.

Adverse Effects and Contraindications. β-Adrenoceptor blocking drugs are contraindicated in patients with heart failure, bronchial asthma and obstructive airway diseases, intense bradycardia, or AV conduction disturbances. Overt congestive failure may be precipitated in patients with cardiac diseases due to the reduction in adrenergic support of the cardiovascular system. It should be used with caution in patients with diabetes mellitus. Central nervous system side effects such as hallucination, insomnia, depression, and nightmares can occur with drugs like propranolol and pindolol (102). The occurrence of an oculomucocutaneous syndrome has been associated with the use of practolol, which led to its withdrawal from general use.

CATECHOLAMINE SYNTHESIS BLOCKERS

METYROSINE

Metyrosine (α-methyl-p-tyrosine) (Fig. 15.3-2) blocks the rate-limiting step of catecholamine biosynthesis. It prevents conversion of tyrosine to dopa by inhibiting tyrosine hydroxylase. It is particularly useful for both preoperative treatment and long-term management of pheochromocytoma. Its administration will decrease catecholamine biosynthesis and reduce the severity of hypertension episodes. Metyrosine is not consistently effective in essential hypertension and, consequently, is rarely used for this disease. Sedation during initial therapy is a consistent adverse effect of metyrosine. Other adverse effects include anxiety, extrapyramidal reactions, breast swelling, galactorrhea, diarrhea, and sexual dysfunction.

The usual dose of metyrosine is 250 mg four times daily. The maximum daily dose is 4 g. Metyrosine does not eliminate danger of hypertensive crisis during manipulation of the tumor, hence, phentolamine should be available for use if needed. If the patient is not adequately controlled by metyrosine, phenoxybenzamine or prazosin may be added or substituted.

Metyrosine (DEMSER) is available in 250-mg capsules.

MONOAMINE OXIDASE INHIBITORS

Monoamine oxidase inhibitors that have been used as antidepressants frequently produce hypotension as a side effect. Pargyline has been used earlier for its antihypertensive action. However, these drugs are seldom used at present for antihypertensive therapy. They can produce serious adverse effects following ingestion of foods containing high levels of tyramine or cold remedies containing sympathomimetic amines.

DIRECTLY ACTING VASODILATORS

ARTERIAL VASODILATORS

In essential hypertension, the peripheral arterial system exhibits an increased reactivity to pressor agents such as epinephrine, norepinephrine, and possibly angiotensin. Such increased reactivity has been attributed to possible structural changes secondary to hypertension (27). However, increased vascular reactivity can precede hypertension and can also be subsequently reinforced by the development of hypertension. These drugs act directly upon vascular smooth muscle to cause relaxation and vasodilation. They act predominantly upon the arterial vascular bed to decrease total peripheral resistance and arterial blood pressure. The reduction in arterial pressure usually triggers a reflex increase in sympathetic activity, resulting in increases in heart rate and cardiac output. These baroreceptor-activated changes tend to oppose the reduction in arterial pressure. Whereas the venous bed is not usually dilated, reflex venoconstriction may occur, resulting in decreased venous return and cardiac output. A significant feature of most nonselective vasodilators is sodium retention. Drugs that dilate both arterial and venous vascular beds cause venous pooling and significant incidence of orthostatic hypotension as side effects. Orthostatic hypotension is not a prominent side effect of agents that act predominantly upon arterial smooth muscle.

HYDRALAZINE

Hydralazine is the only phthalazine derivative (Fig. 15.3-3) used clinically for the reduction of arterial pressure. Its pharmacological actions were first described in 1950 by Gross et al. (44), and its clinical efficacy was subsequently reported by Reubi (79).

Mechanism of Action. Hydralazine acts on smooth muscles in the arterial vascular bed to cause vasodilation. Its effect on the arteriolar vascular bed (precapillary) is greater than that on the venous bed (postcapillary). The drug is concentrated in the smooth muscle of the arterial wall, but the precise mechanism of its antihypertensive action is controversial. It may be related to the ability of the drug to chelate trace elements that may be required for smooth muscle contraction (68, 73). Vascular resis-

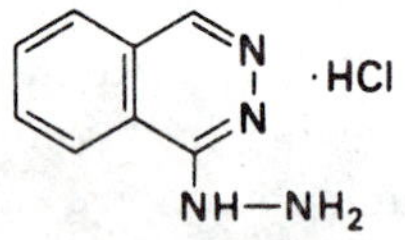

Hydralazine

Sar-Arg-Val-Tyr-Val-His-Pro-Ala

Saralasin

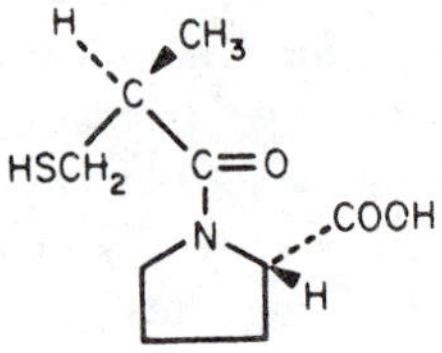

Captopril

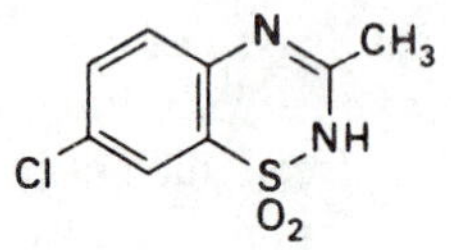

Diazoxide

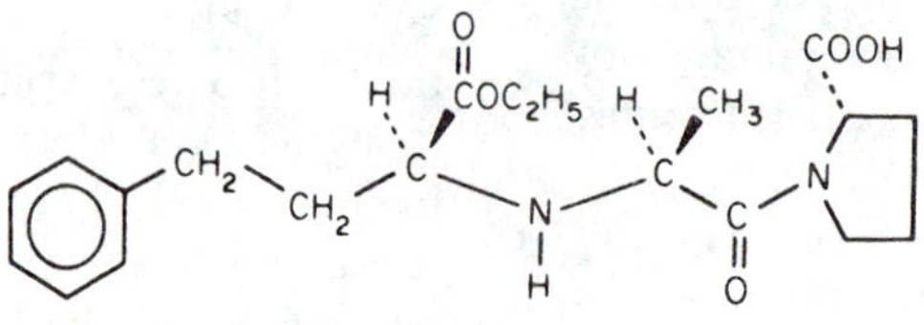

Enalapril

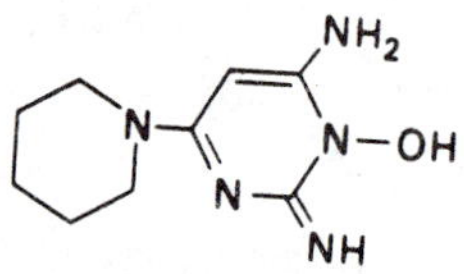

Minoxidil

5-oxoPro-Trp-Pro-Arg-Pro-Gln-Ile-Pro-Pro

Teprotide

Fig. 15.3-3: *Chemical structures of vasodilators, and angiotensin antagonists, used in antihypertensive therapy*

tance is reduced more markedly in the hepatic, portal, coronary, splanchnic, and renal vascular bed than in brain, skin, or skeletal muscle. Peripheral resistance is decreased and as a consequence pronounced stimulation occurs resulting in tachycardia and increases in stroke volume and cardiac output (82). The reflex activation of the sympathetic nervous system antagonizes the antihypertensive effects of hydralazine and is responsible for many of its adverse effects. The veins are not actively dilated and may reflexly constrict secondary to the reflex sympathetic activation, thus orthostatic hypotension is not a significant side effect of hydralazine. Sodium retention with expansion of the plasma and extracellular fluid volume may occur. In addition, plasma renin activity is increased (99). The combination of high cardiac output, elevated renin, and hypovolemia may limit the drug's effectiveness; hence, hydralazine is usually combined with a diuretic and β-adrenoceptor-blocking drug to increase its efficacy.

Pharmacokinetics. Hydralazine may be given orally or parenterally. Given orally, 65-90% of the drug is absorbed. Its antihypertensive effect develops within 15-60 min. The drug is metabolized in the liver by conjugation with glucuronic acid, ring hydroxylation, and N-acetylation. Genetically slow acetylators tend to have higher serum concentration than rapid acetylators. Because of extensive first-pass metabolism of the drug in the liver and intestinal mucosa, its bioavailability following oral administration is low; however, intake of hydralazine with meals usually increases its bioavailability. The half-life of the drug averages about 3 hr. About 15% of the drug is eliminated by the kidney unchanged.

Adverse Effects. Headache, palpitation, anorexia, nausea, dizziness, and sweating are the most common adverse effects. The hyperactive cardiovascular state may precipitate anginal attacks or myocardial infarction in patients with coronary heart disease. Other less frequent side effects include nasal congestion, flushing, lacrimation, edema, and muscle cramps. These side effects may be minimized by slowly increasing the dose. In addition, tolerance may develop with continued drug administration. Dyspnea on exertion is also reported by several patients. To minimize the cardiovascular side effects, hydralazine is usually given in combination with a β-adrenoceptor-blocking drug such as propranolol, or other drugs that reduce adrenergic function.

Prolonged drug administration at doses in excess of 200 mg/day may result in a lupuslike syndrome with joint pain, myalgia, and fever. The syndrome is usually reversible, but symptoms may persist for several months after cessation of therapy. The syndrome appears to be genetically related and occurs almost exclusively in Caucasians who are slow acetylators. Peripheral neuropathy related to pyridoxine deficiency has been described. Again, this effect is more apparent in slow acetylators as well as in patients with impaired renal function in whom the plasma half-life may be increased four- to five-fold.

Therapeutic Use. When hydralazine is used alone, the reflex sympathetic activation opposes its antihypertensive action, and accounts for most of the severe side effects. Hydralazine, therefore, forms part of a therapeutic regimen that includes a β-adrenoceptor-blocking drug and a thiazide diuretic. In this regimen the drug is effective in smaller doses starting with 10 mg (b.i.d. or t.i.d.) administered for long periods so that many of the side effects that normally limit its use are minimized.

Preparations and Dosage. *Hydralazine*, USP (APRESOLINE) is available as tablets (10, 25, 50, and 100 mg) for oral use and as ampules (20 mg in 1 ml) for parenteral (i.v. or i.m.) therapy. The usual oral dose is 100-200 mg/day, starting with an initial dose of 10-20 mg t.i.d. or q.i.d. with increments at 7- to 14-day intervals, until either the desired effect or unwanted side effects occur. Parenteral administration of the drug is usually started with 20-40 mg, and thereafter the later increment is adjusted according to the patient's response.

DIAZOXIDE

Diazoxide (HYPERSTAT) is a benzothiadiazine (Fig. 15.3-3) and a structural analog of the thiazide diuretics, but unlike the thiazide diuretics it causes sodium and fluid retention. Diazoxide is devoid of diuretic activity and is used predominantly for treatment of hypertensive emergencies.

Mechanism of Action. Intravenous administration of diazoxide to hypertensive patients results in prompt decreases in both systolic and diastolic pressures with associated reflex increases in heart rate and cardiac output. The drug directly relaxes arterial smooth muscle, possibly through antagonism of calcium action in smooth muscle with minimal effects upon venous bed. The function of the sympathetic nervous system is not impaired; hence, the reflex increase in activity may counteract its antihypertensive action (47). Diazoxide administration causes marked retention of sodium and water in both normotensive and hypertensive patients, and may expand plasma volume and produce edema, especially in patients predisposed to cardiac insufficiency. Like the thiazide diuretics, diazoxide inhibits tubular secretion of uric acid and decreases free water clearance. Plasma renin activity may also increase.

Pharmacokinetics. To produce maximum antihypertensive effects, the drug is usually administered by rapid intravenous infusion. It has been suggested that diazoxide is rapidly inactivated by protein binding and that slow infusions and oral administration are usually ineffective. When given by rapid intravenous injection, peak hypotensive effect occurs within 3-5 min and persists for up to 12 hr. However, it may not be necessary to give the drug as rapidly as was previously recommended, and the dose and rate of injection may be adjusted according to the blood pressure response (38).

The drug is eliminated by the kidney largely unchanged. In uremic patients the dosage should be reduced, otherwise a greater than normal fall in blood pressure may occur.

Adverse Effects. Marked hypotension and reflex sympathetic stimulation may occur; hence, patients receiving diazoxide should be closely monitored during the initial 15-20 min. Palpitation, diaphoresis, nausea, and vomiting are common side effects. Hyperglycemia due to inhibition of insulin release may occur. Hyperuricemia is another adverse metabolic effect of the drug. These effects are only of clinical significance if the drug is used for prolonged periods. Diazoxide is usually dissolved in an alkaline vehicle, and care should be taken to avoid extravasation at the injection site, which results in severe local pain.

Therapeutic Uses. Diazoxide is usually reserved for hypertensive emergencies. It is also occasionally used to treat hypoglycemia due to hyperinsulinemia. It is particularly effective when prompt reduction of blood pressure is desirable such as in hypertensive encephalopathy, malignant hypertension, and eclampsia. Because of extensive protein binding, the drug must be given rapidly to obtain high initial concentration of the free drug (85). When given at a dose of 5 mg/kg by rapid (within 30 sec) intravenous injection, maximum antihypertensive effect will occur within 5 min, and blood pressure will be reduced to normotensive levels in 75-85% of patients (66). Associated fluid retention may be controlled by the concurrent use of furosemide.

Caution should be exercised when diazoxide therapy is contemplated in patients with coronary or cerebral vascular insufficiency. In such patients a rapid reduction in blood pressure could precipitate ischemia (56). In patients with dissecting aortic aneurysm, diazoxide therapy is contraindicated due to its ability to increase cardiac output and left ventricular ejection velocity (shear force). Caution is also advised when used in diabetics because diazoxide may cause significant hyperglycemia.

Preparation and Dosage. *Diazoxide*, USP (HYPERSTAT IV) is available in ampules (300 mg in 20 ml) for i.v. use. Oral preparations for the management of hypoglycemia are available as capsules (50-100 mg) as well as a suspension (50 mg/ml).

MINOXIDIL

Minoxidil (Fig. 15.3-3) is an effective oral antihypertensive agent. It acts directly on arteriolar smooth muscle causing relaxation and reduction of peripheral vascular resistance, but has little or no effect on the veins. In this respect, its action appears to resemble that of hydralazine, but minoxidil-induced vasodilation is much greater. Its hypotensive effect is associated with reflex sympathetic activation, resulting in a marked increase in heart rate and cardiac output.

Plasma renin activity is also increased and pronounced retention of sodium and fluid occurs. Decrease in renal vascular resistance does not result in any significant reduction in glomerular filtration rate. The cardiac stimulation as well as elevated renin activity can be reduced by concurrent propranolol administration.

Pharmacokinetics. The drug is adequately (80-90%) absorbed from the gastrointestinal tract and is extensively metabolized in the liver. The metabolites (glucuronide conjugate) and the unaltered drug (about 10% of an administered dose) are eliminated in the urine (42). In circulation, minoxidil is not protein bound, and its rate of elimination is dependent on hepatic function and glomerular filtration. The drug does not appear to be reabsorbed or secreted within the renal tubule. Although its plasma half-life is 3-4 hr, the antihypertensive action of a single dose may persist for over 24 hr. The apparent discrepancy between plasma half-life and antihypertensive action may be related to the accumulation of the drug in the arterial wall.

Therapeutic Use. Minoxidil is a most potent vasodilator, and its combination with a β-adrenoceptor-blocking drug and a diuretic has proven to be most effective in patients with intractable malignant hypertension or with renal failure in whom bilateral nephrectomy would have been otherwise indicated (76). Renal failure does not influence either the plasma or therapeutic half-life. The usual dose range is 10-40 mg given once or twice daily.

Adverse Effects. Most of the adverse effects of minoxidil are similar to those of hydralazine and diazoxide, especially with respect to reflex sympathetic activation. In patients with some degree of renal failure fluid retention may be pronounced. The development of pericardial effusion is a potentially serious adverse effect associated with minoxidil therapy. Hirsutism of the face, chest, and brow may be quite disturbing in females. The hair growth becomes less pronounced with prolonged administration.

Preparations and Dosage. *Minoxidil* (LONITEN) is available as tablets (2.5 or 10 mg) for oral use. The initial daily dose is 5 mg with gradual increments to 10, 20, and 40 mg in single or divided doses. Maximal recommended daily dosage is 100 mg.

ARTERIAL AND VENOUS VASODILATORS

SODIUM NITROPRUSSIDE

The effectiveness of sodium nitroprusside [sodium nitroferricyanide $Na_2Fe(CN)_5NO.2H_2O$] as an antihypertensive drug was first described by Johnson (53) in 1929. The drug is an extremely powerful vasodilator and is currently used as the most consistently effective drug for the management of all hypertensive emergencies, regardless of their etiology (38).

Mechanism of Action. Nitroprusside differs from other vasodilators in that its direct vasodilator action is exerted on both the venous and arteriolar vascular beds with little effect upon the smooth muscle of the gastrointestinal tract or uterus. The venodilation results in increased venous capacitance and decreased cardiac preload. Venous pooling occurs when the patient is upright.

Renal blood flow and glomerular filtration rate are maintained, but the secretion of renin is increased.

Pharmacokinetics. The half-life of the drug is less than 30 min and the antihypertensive effect rapidly dissipates after cessation of intravenous infusion due to rapid inactivation of the drug. It is degraded by the liver to thiocyanate, which is excreted by the kidney. Thiocyanate toxicity may occur in hypertensive patients with impaired renal function. Due to its rapid onset and reliable antihypertensive action, the patient's blood pressure may be easily maintained at any desirable level by altering the rate of infusion.

Therapeutic Uses. Due to its venodilator effect resulting in reduction of preload, angina pectoris and heart failure usually improve during nitroprusside therapy. This is in marked contrast to drugs that do not affect preload (e.g., diazoxide, hydralazine, and minoxidil).

A disadvantage of nitroprusside therapy is that its infusion must be constantly monitored within the confines of the intensive care unit. When the drug is infused at a rate of 1-3 μg/kg/min in a solution of 5% dextrose, blood pressure decreases within seconds and can be maintained at the desired level by varying the rate of infusion. Upon discontinuation of infusion, the blood pressure returns to predrug levels within 2-3 min.

Nitroprusside is universally acceptable, and tolerance is very rare. Caution is advised in patients with dissecting aneurysm because the pulse pressure may widen and that may extend the dissection. Nitroprusside is the antihypertensive agent of choice for the management of hypertension associated with acute myocardial infarction and left ventricular failure due to its favorable effect upon cardiac performance (13, 64). It is also a better drug than other vasodilators such as a diazoxide and minoxidil for the management of hypertensive states where careful blood pressure regulation is necessary and hypotension might be detrimental (e.g., hypertension associated with acute coronary insufficiency, cerebrovascular insufficiency, and intracranial hemorrhage) (38).

Adverse Effects. Adverse effects are usually secondary to the excessive vasodilation and rapid hypotension. Symptoms include nausea, vomiting, sweating, restlessness, headache, palpitation, and substernal distress. Excessive accumulation of its metabolic product, thiocyanate, may produce twitching, disorientation, delirium, and psychosis. Prolonged therapy may result in causing symptoms of hypothyroidism because thiocyanate interferes with iodine transport by the thyroid gland.

Preparations and Doses. *Sodium Nitroprusside*, USP (NIPRIDE) is supplied in 5-ml vials containing 50 mg of the drug for reconstitution by first adding 2-3 ml of 5% dextrose solution to the vial; the content is then transferred to an infusion bottle containing the same diluent (500 ml). The bottle should be protected from light to prevent decomposition; preparations older than 4 hr should be discarded. The average adult dose is 3 μg/kg/min for patients who are not on concurrent antihypertensive medication. Maximum dose should not exceed 800 μg/min. Continuous monitoring of blood pressure is critical to successful drug use.

ANGIOTENSIN ANTAGONISTS

The renin-angiotensin system plays an important role in the maintenance of hypertension associated with elevation of plasma renin in humans. Agents that inhibit the production or action of angiotensin II have been studied as potential antihypertensive agents. These classes of compounds (e.g., renin inhibitors, angiotensin I-converting enzyme inhibitors, and angiotensin II antagonists) have shown promise as potentially useful agents (Chapter 13.1.2).

AGENT THAT BLOCKS ACTION OF ANGIOTENSIN II

SARALASIN

A synthetic analog such as saralasin [(Sar^1, Val^5, Ala^8) angiotensin II] (Fig. 15.3-3) competes with circulating angiotensin II for receptor sites within the vascular smooth muscle and the adrenal cortex (93). Its administration will block the pressor response to exogenous renin, angiotensin I, and angiotensin II in a dose-dependent fashion in experimental animals. In presence of a high level of angiotensin II, saralasin lowers blood pressure by displacing the potent vasoconstrictor from the vascular receptor site. In cases of low angiotensin II level, saralasin, which also acts as a partial agonist, can increase the blood pressure by binding to unoccupied receptor sites. Currently, saralasin is occasionally used in conjunction with other procedures as an aid to detect a renin-angiotensin factor in hypertension. Its usefulness is limited because of a high incidence of false-negative and false-positive results. Headache, nausea, malaise, light-headedness, and local discomfort at the site of injection are some of the adverse effects of saralasin. It can cause marked hypertension in pheochromocytoma patients.

AGENTS THAT BLOCK FORMATION OF ANGIOTENSIN II

CAPTOPRIL

Converting enzyme inhibitors such as captopril (SQ14225, CAPOTEN) (Fig. 15.3-3) inhibit the enzymatic conversion of inactive angiotensin I to angiotensin II, a potent vasoconstrictor (Chapter 13.1.2). Inhibition of angiotensin I-converting enzyme by captopril leads to a decrease in circulating angiotensin II and aldosterone, resulting in an increase in angiotensin I and renin levels. Its mechanism of action is believed to involve inhibition of the renin-angiotensin-aldosterone system, as well as a decrease in peripheral vascular resistance. It is effective in both essential and renovascular hypertension. Although blood pressure will decrease initially, optimal response may not be observed for several weeks. Its antihypertensive effect is enhanced by diuretics, especially thiazides.

During combination therapy captopril reduces diuretic-induced hyperaldosteronism and hypokalemia, but both drugs produce additive effects on plasma renin levels.

Captopril is absorbed (75%) given orally. Bioavailability is increased with chronic administration. About 25-30% of the drug is protein bound. It is excreted in the urine as unchanged drug (40-50%) or metabolites (35%) and in the feces (15%).

Side effects include skin rash, pruritus, loss of taste, nausea, vomiting, abdominal pain, proteinuria, and hyperkalemia.

Initial dose of captopril is 25 mg t.i.d., which may be increased. It is available in 25-, 50-, 100-mg tablets.

ENALAPRIL

Enalapril (MK-421) (Fig. 15.3-3) is a new angiotensin-converting enzyme inhibitor that, unlike captopril, does not have an SH group and also has different pharmacokinetic properties. Antihypertensive efficacy of enalapril appears to be similar to captopril; enalapril appears to be better tolerated and does not appear to have significant side effects like skin rash and loss of taste. It produces a better effect when combined with diuretics or methyldopa.

TEPROTIDE

Teprotide (Fig. 15.3-3) is another investigational converting enzyme inhibitor isolated from the venom of the snake, *Bothrops jararaca*. Its intravenous administration results in a decrease in blood pressure and orthostatic hypotension. Clinically, teprotide will effectively decrease blood pressure and plasma aldosterone levels in patients with renovascular hypertension or essential hypertension with elevated or normal plasma renin activity. Currently, these agents are important tools for investigating the participation of the renin-angiotensin system in the genesis of various forms of hypertension. They may also prove valuable in the management of patients with high levels of circulating angiotensin II (36).

CALCIUM ANTAGONISTS

In the plasma membranes of a variety of excitable cells such as cardiac cells and smooth muscle cells of the vasculature there are calcium-selective channels by which the calcium ion (Ca^{2+}) is carried to the cell interior, where calcium serves as an activator messenger and maintains a number of calcium-dependent processes including excitation-contraction coupling in both cardiac and vascular smooth muscle.

Calcium channel-blocking drugs, which are a group of compounds with diverse chemical structures, block the entry of Ca^{2+} through these channels and inhibit contractile function in the heart and vascular smooth muscle. These agents, therefore, appear to have applications in a number of cardiovascular disorders including arrhythmias (Chapter 15.2), angina (Chapter 15.4), and hypertension. Of the three agents now available for use in the United States (nifedipine, diltiazem, and verapamil), nifedipine has been used most frequently to treat hypertension.

NIFEDIPINE

Nifedipine, a dihydropyridine derivative (Fig. 15.4-1), causes coronary and peripheral arterial vasodilation, hypotension, and reflex tachycardia. It is an effective oral antihypertensive agent and, like other vasodilators, is most useful when given in combination with diuretics and adrenergic-depressant drugs, or methyldopa. Its pharmacological effects, pharmacokinetics, and adverse effects are described in Chapter 15.4.

THERAPY OF HYPERTENSION

For the purpose of therapy, hypertension is arbitrarily classified on the basis of level of diastolic blood pressure into mild (90-104 mmHg), moderate (104-114 mmHg), and severe (115 mmHg and above). Because arterial pressure rises continually throughout life, the usual definition of hypertension as being blood pressure greater than 140/90 is an oversimplification. Nonetheless, it has been demonstrated that the higher the blood pressure, the greater the mortality and morbidity resulting from stroke, heart attack, and renal failure. Morbidity can be significantly reduced by effective antihypertensive therapy. When hypertension is severe, it constitutes a medical emergency, and therapy must be immediate and rapid; mild-to-moderate hypertension can be approached in a less urgent manner, although therapy is mandatory.

In general the therapeutic goal is to achieve and maintain a resting diastolic pressure of less than 90 mmHg. This may not always be possible without producing severe adverse effects, in which case the most desirable diastolic pressure (usually 90-110 mmHg) should be aimed at.

The choice of a therapeutic regimen and the step by step manipulation of each patient's medication require skill and a thorough knowledge of the pharmacology of the individual antihypertensive agents. In the majority of patients it is not always possible to determine the etiological factors and mechanisms involved in the observed hypertensive state. Drug treatment is therefore largely empirical.

The following general principles govern antihypertensive therapy:

1. Blood pressure in the upright position should be kept as near normal as possible. In special situations (e.g., impaired renal function, impaired cerebral or coronary blood flow, and in some elderly patients) a higher blood pressure may have to be accepted.
2. A therapeutic regimen that reduces pressure in the supine as well as erect positions should be aimed at. Drugs that produce an appreciable incidence of postural hypotension are not readily accepted by patients.
3. Drug regimen should be changed only when there is a definite and valid reason for a change because most patients will readily tolerate a minor side effect rather than change to unfamiliar drugs.

4. Any change from the usual dosage should be gradual. Effective patient management is difficult, but once achieved, any rapid increment in dosage may precipitate adverse effects. Similarly, reduction in dosage may precipitate rebound effect as in the case of clonidine, or heart failure in some patients on diuretics.

5. Therapy should be continuous. Patients should be aware of the importance of and the need to take the medication faithfully.

6. The therapist should be aware of possible drug interaction, since the management of hypertension usually requires a double- or triple-drug regimen. Patients should be warned of possible side effects as well as potential interactions, not only between antihypertensive medications but with other drugs.

7. Patients on potent antihypertensive drug regimen should be adequately educated with respect to reduction in drug dosage if side effects develop, and to record their own blood pressure as a guide for adjustment in drug dosages.

A stepped-care program is currently the most widely accepted procedure for the management of the hypertensive patient and appears to provide adequate blood pressure control (Table 15.3-2). Table 15.3-3 provides summarized information on the major drugs currently used in the therapy of hypertension, their mechanism of action, side effects, and contraindications.

Management of Mild Hypertension. In a significant percentage of patients with mild hypertension, therapy with oral thiazide-type diuretics alone may reduce the elevated blood pressure to normotensive levels. Consequently, all patients with mild-to-moderate hypertension are usually started on a diuretic regimen (step 1). For practical purposes, a thiazide that is inexpensive and has a duration of action of at least 24 hr should be used (e.g., bendroflumethiazide 5 mg, or hydrochlorothiazide 50 mg/day). In patients taking digitalis glycosides or patients who develop symptomatic hypokalemia, a potassium-sparing diuretic or potassium supplements should be administered. Although the loop diuretics furosemide and ethacrynic acid are the most potent diuretics, they are less effective as antihypertensive agents and should be reserved for hypertension associated with renal failure or congestive heart failure. If the elevated pressure is not effectively controlled by a diuretic, a step-2 agent is usually added to the treatment regimen.

As step-2 agents, β-adrenoceptor-blocking drugs are well tolerated by most patients. The presence of asthma, congestive heart failure, and diabetes may contraindicate these drugs. If blood pressure is not reduced by one β-adrenoceptor blocker, it is unlikely to be reduced by another. The individual agent is usually chosen based on lack of side effects. In many instances β-adrenoceptor-blocking drugs may also be employed as step-1 agents in place of a diuretic.

Methyldopa, clonidine, and reserpine are adequate substitutes for β-adrenoceptor-blocking drugs. Methyldopa is of definite advantage in patients with obstructive airway disease, diabetes, and gout in whom a β-blocker or a thiazide is unsatisfactory. It is also the main antihypertensive drug for use during pregnancy. The usual starting dose is 250 mg b.i.d. with gradual increments at 2-day intervals to a maximum of 2 g/day.

Clonidine is just as effective as methyldopa. Careful patient compliance is mandatory in order to prevent rebound hypertension. Although its site of action is the same as that of methyldopa, both drugs have a characteristic spectrum of side effects. Clonidine is more likely to produce sedation, dry mouth, and fluid retention whereas methyldopa is more likely to produce orthostatic hypotension and impotence.

The combination of a diuretic with reserpine is also highly effective. However, although reserpine has the advantage of being long acting (requiring only one daily dose) and is the least expensive, it tends to cause a very high incidence of adverse effects (Table 15.3-3) and is therefore least tolerable by the majority of patients. There is also concern about the doubtful association between breast carcinoma and reserpine therapy. Its use in low doses in combination with a thiazide diuretic produces few adverse effects and appears to be a relatively inexpensive and effective regimen.

Moderate-to-Severe Hypertension. Although these patients often respond satisfactorily to the regimen outlined for mild hypertension, in several instances the combination of a diuretic and a sympathetic depressant (steps 1 and 2 of Table 15.3-2) agent may be insufficient. Vasodilators such as hydralazine or minoxidil that are usually reserved for the treatment of moderate-to-severe hypertensive patients may be cautiously added as a step-3 approach. The use of either agent is associated with reflex increases in sympathetic activity (e.g., increase in heart rate, cardiac output, and renin level). These responses that would otherwise obliterate the hypotensive action of the vasodilator are effectively controlled by adding a β-adrenoceptor blocker (e.g., propranolol and to a lesser degree by clonidine, methyldopa, and reserpine). The

Table 15.3-2
Stepped-Care Regimen

Step 1:	*Diuretics*
	a. Thiazide or related compound
	b. Furosemide or ethacrynic acid, if azotemia present
Step 2:	*Add a drug that interferes with sympathetic function*
	a. β-Adrenoceptor blocker: propranolol, metoprolol, etc.
	b. Methyldopa or clonidine
	c. Reserpine or other rauwolfia alkaloids
Step 3:	*Add a vasodilator*
	a. Hydralazine
	b. Prazosin[a]
	c. Other vasodilators[b]
Step 4:	*Add an adrenergic neuron blocker*
	a. Guanethidine,[c] bethanidine, debrisoquin

[a] First dose must be small, preferably at bedtime (see text).
[b] Minoxidil should be reserved for selected patients.
[c] Guanethidine is very potent but may be used in step 2 in small doses.

Table 15.3-3
Mechanisms of Action, Side Effects, and Contraindications for Antihypertensive Drugs

Drugs	Site of Action	Mode of Action	Major Adverse Effects	Contraindications
Diuretics				
Thiazide type	Distal nephron	Reduction of extracellular and plasma volume, mobilization of sodium, and decreased ability of cardiovascular system to compensate for hypovolemia	Hypokalemia, hyperuricemia, hyperglycemia, muscle weakness	Anuria, advanced renal failure, hyponatremia
Loop	Ascending loop of Henle		Fluid and electrolyte depletion, metabolic alkalosis, GI distress	Hyponatremia, severe GI disturbance
Potassium-sparing	Distal tubule		Hyperkalemia, gynecomastia, impotence, menstrual irregularities	Renal failure, hyperkalemia, hyponatremia
CNS drugs				
Clonidine	Medulla	α_2-Adrenoceptor stimulation to reduce sympathetic outflow, depression of peripheral sympathetic transmission	Rebound hypertension dry mouth, drowsiness, lethargy, impotence	None
Methyldopa	Medulla, periphery	α_2-Adrenoceptor stimulation, peripheral methylnorepinephrine formation	Sedation, lassitude, abnormal liver function, hypotension, anemia, positive Coombs' test	Hemolytic anemia, hepatic impairment
Ganglionic blockers	Sympathetic ganglia	Blockade of postganglionic sympathetic impulses	orthostatic hypotension, constipation, impotence, urinary retention	None
Adrenergic neuron-blocking drugs	Peripheral sympathetic nerve terminal	Prevention of neurotransmitter release, depletion of neurotransmitter	Hypotension, diarrhea, ejaculatory failure, dizziness	Tricyclic antidepressants, heart failure pheochromocytoma
Reserpine	Central and peripheral	Depletion of neurotransmitter	Depression, parasympathetic predominance, impotence, aggravation of peptic ulcer, parkinsonism	Depression, peptic ulcer, parkinsonism
α-Adrenoceptor blockers	Peripheral arterioles	Postsynaptic α-blockade	Orthostatic hypotension, syncope, drowsiness, dizziness, nausea	None
β-Adrenoceptor blockers	Peripheral, central	β_1 and β_2-Adrenoceptor blockade, antirenin effect, central action in medulla	Heart failure, bronchospasm, hallucination, nightmares	Bronchial asthma, bradycardia, heart block, heart failure, diabetes
Drugs acting on smooth muscle				
Hydralazine	Arterial vascular bed	Possible chelation of trace elements responsible for arterial tone	Aggravation of angina, palpitation, lupus-like syndrome, drug fever, bone marrow depression, anorexia, nausea, vomiting, edema, muscle cramps	Heart failure, atherosclerotic heart disease
Diazoxide	Arterial vascular bed	Possible antagonism of Ca^{2+} on arterial smooth muscle	Hypotention, reflex sympathetic stimulation, nausea, vomiting,	Dissecting aortic aneurysm, diabetes, care in coronary or cerebral insufficiency
Minoxidil	Arterial vascular bed	Possibly similar to hydralazine	Hirsutism, pericardial effusion, others as for hydralazine	As for hydralazine
Nitroprusside	Arterial and venous bed	Direct relaxation	Hypotension, nausea, vomiting, palpitation, hypothyroidism	Dissecting aortic aneurysm, hypothyroidism

vasodilator as a step-3 agent will therefore be very effective provided a sympathetic-depressant drug was included in the step-2 regimen. Prazosin when compared with minoxidil and hydralazine appears to produce less reflex increases in heart rate and plasma renin activity. It can be added whether or not a sympathetic-depressant drug is included in step 2. It appears to be more effective when used in conjunction with a diuretic and a sympathetic-depressant drug. This combination also permits the use of smaller doses of the individual agents and minimizes the side effects of each agent in the combination.

Blood pressure reduction in patients in this category should not be rapid, but be induced over a period of days. It is therefore customary to institute step-1 and step-2 approaches simultaneously. In patients with higher pretreatment pressures (125 mmHg), three levels of therapy (steps 1, 2, 3) may be initiated simultaneously.

Resistant Hypertension. A small group of patients will not respond to the conventional therapy outlined in steps 1-3. Careful reevaluation for compliance and underlying factors is mandatory before additional therapy is contemplated. If factors such as adequacy of the dosages of the antihypertensives used, plasma volume expansion, unfavorable drug interaction, and secondary forms of hypertension are ruled out, then the addition of an adrenergic neuron-blocking agent as a step-4 approach is justified. It must be remembered that guanethidine, bethanidine, and debrisoquin are potent agents with a very high incidence of adverse effects (e.g., diarrhea and orthostatic hypotension). These agents should therefore be reserved for the treatment of truly resistant severe hypertension that cannot be effectively controlled with any drug combination of steps 1-3. The combination of adrenergic neuron blocker with propranolol tends to increase the incidence of orthostatic hypotension. It is often advisable to reduce the dose of propranolol prior to guanethidine therapy. Minoxidil is sometimes advocated instead of guanethidine for these patients. It may be added in place of a vasodilator in step 3 or be simply added as a step-4 agent. Phenoxybenzamine is sometimes used in place of an adrenergic neuron blocker when a β-adrenoceptor blocker is used in step 2.

Hypertensive Emergencies. Certain features of hypertension may indicate the need for immediate and drastic therapy regardless of the etiology. Examination of the fundus of the eye is critical, because it will provide insight into events occurring in other vascular beds. One of the most significant pathognomonic signs of severe hypertension is necrotizing arteriolitis, usually manifested as hemorrhage and exudation in the retina (grade III changes). The presence of papilledema (grade IV) is required for the diagnosis of malignant hypertension. However, the prognosis of patients with retinal hemorrhage is just as poor because other organs such as the brain and kidney tend to show similar damage, and encephalopathy and renal failure are frequently present. The presence of grade III and/or IV retinopathy constitutes accelerated hypertension and requires immediate therapy even though the blood pressure may not be extremely high.

The major aim of therapy is to lower the blood pressure smoothly and quickly to near-normal levels in order to allow the arteriolitis to heal. Sodium nitroprusside and diazoxide are the agents of choice for hypertensive emergencies because of their prompt action and minimal effect upon CNS functions; nor does their administration preclude the use of other antihypertensive drugs with delayed actions. Although diazoxide is sometimes preferred when compared with sodium nitroprusside, there are several clinical contraindications to its use (see Table 15.3-4). If patients with malignant or accelerated hypertension also have coronary insufficiency or pulmonary edema, then sodium nitroprusside is a better choice, since by virtue of the drug-induced increased venous capacitance, both preload and subsequent cardiac oxygen demand will be decreased. In patients with hypertension associated with dissecting aortic aneurysm, trimethaphan, a ganglion-blocking agent, is a drug of choice with the most predictable effects (70). Diazoxide will increase heart rate and cardiac output due to reflex sympathetic stimulation that results in further damage to the aorta and as a consequence of that increases shear force.

Malignant hypertension not associated with severe complications may be treated as moderate-to-severe hypertension but as a real emergency. Oral therapy designed to reduce the blood pressure to 160/110 mmHg within 24 hr may be preferable to parenteral therapy. If parenteral therapy is employed, oral antihypertensive therapy should be initiated as soon as possible.

SPECIAL PATIENT GROUPS

Pediatric Hypertension. There is insufficient information to fully characterize hypertension in children, since essential hypertension may be the result of several separate entities in which genetic and environmental factors may interact to produce an elevation in blood pressure. Preliminary evidence suggests that abnormality of the renin-angiotensin system coupled with the handling of salt may play important roles in the genesis of hypertension in black children. In Caucasian children abnormal function of the autonomic nervous system appears to play a dominant role (6).

Until more conclusive evidence is available, clinicians are not sure of when to initiate treatment of hypertension in children. Children with borderline hypertension with coronary artery risk factors or a family history of early morbidity from hypertension or coronary artery diseases or evidence of early target organ damage are usually regarded as suitable candidates for antihypertensive drug therapy. Antihypertensive medication is definitely indicated in children and adolescents with diastolic pressures that would be considered abnormal even for adults. Management of these cases is the same as described for adults. Drug doses in children are usually based on age and weight. Maximum adult dose should not be exceeded.

Hypertension in the Elderly. Hypertension constitutes a significant cardiovascular risk factor in elderly patients. Most elderly patients are prone to the coexistence of two or more medical problems as well as the propensity to exhibit increased incidence of adverse effects to antihypertensive medications. Drug therapy in elderly patients may be influenced by inadequate metabolism or elimination, increased sensitivity, and/or impaired cardiovascular reflex mechanism resulting in an increased tendency to postural hypotension. Antihypertensive therapy in this age group requires special care and insight. Reduction of blood pressure should be gradual, and pressure should not be allowed to fall below the norm for the patient's age group. It is most important to avoid postural hypotension due to the resulting increased susceptibility to cerebral or coronary insufficiency, hence drugs that are prone to produce this side effect are not readily employed in this age group.

The choice of antihypertensive therapy should be tailored to the individual patient, taking into account coexistent diseases, other medication, and tolerance of the chosen antihypertensive drugs. In most cases oral diuretic of the thiazide type are used as the initial step; the high-ceiling loop diuretic exhibits a greater propensity to cause hypovolemia in this age group without effective blood pressure control. Hyperuricemia as a result of thiazide therapy should be carefully watched since many of these patients may be at the upper limit of normal uric acid levels or may already have had attacks of gout.

If in addition to weight loss and restricted salt regimen the diuretic regimen is not adequate, then a step-2 drug such as methyldopa or clonidine may be added. The use of these drugs is associated with little reduction in cardiac output. β-Adrenoceptor-blocking drugs may be employed as an alternative to clonidine or methyldopa. However, their effects in the elderly appear to be less predictable (19), possibly due to reduced β-adrenoceptor sensitivity. In addition, latent cardiac insufficiency may be further compromised by these drugs.

Vasodilators such as hydralazine may be cautiously added. The reflex tachycardia caused by hydralazine may not be as severe as in younger patients due to reduced β-adrenoceptor activity. Any significant increase in heart rate and fluid retention may be particularly bothersome in these patients. In addition the propensity of hydralazine to precipitate anginal episodes in patients with cardiac disease should be carefully evaluated.

Hypertension in Pregnancy. Hypertension that occurs during pregnancy should be treated. Similarly, patients who become pregnant while on antihypertensive therapy should have their medication continued. Drug therapy should be kept as simple as possible. A commonly employed regimen is a thiazide-type diuretic with reserpine or methyldopa if necessary. If this combination does not control the blood pressure, then hydralazine may be included. The sodium-retaining properties with subsequent volume expansion of antihypertensive drugs are of particular importance in pregnant hypertensive patients, especially in those who have a tendency for sodium retention when they are not pregnant. In these cases, sodium retention and volume expansion can be prevented by sodium restriction and the use of a loop diuretic such as furosemide.

DRUGS FOR THERAPY OF SHOCK

TYPES OF SHOCK

Circulatory shock is defined as a state of protracted underperfusion of vital tissues such as brain, myocardium, kidney, liver, and intestine. Persistent hypoperfusion will result in cellular dysfunction and organ damage. There are five types of circulatory shock.

Hypovolemic shock or hemorrhagic shock usually results from excessive loss of blood or plasma either externally, as in severance of a blood vessel, or internally, as occurs during severe gastrointestinal bleeding, fractures with hemorrhage into surrounding tissue, or major burns that attract large quantities of fluid to the burn site outside the circulation.

Neurogenic shock, otherwise called fainting, may result from strong stimuli (e.g., pain, fright, unpleasant sights) or severe cerebral trauma or hemorrhage that overwhelms the regulatory capacity of the nervous system. Vasodilation, bradycardia, and consequent hypotension would result in underperfusion of the brain and other vital organs; this would lead to fainting.

Allergic or anaphylactic shock is a severe and often fatal form of circulatory shock and is usually the direct result of exposure to foreign chemicals or proteins to which the patient is highly allergic. The resultant rapid decrease in blood pressure, and heart rate, and severe dyspnea are often fatal, if not treated.

Septic shock is produced by toxins elaborated by several bacterial (especially gram-negative bacilli) species, which when released, would cause pronounced vasodilation with pooling of blood and a rapid hypotension.

Cardiogenic shock results due to serious heart disease or myocardial infarction that would cause a rapid decrease in the ability of the heart to maintain normal cardiac output leading to a progressive decline in blood pressure.

The precise progression to the state of shock will depend upon the etiology of the disorder. In general, patients in shock usually exhibit mental obtundation, tachypnea, hypotension, tachycardia, pallor, cold and clammy skin, oliguria, and metabolic acidosis. Failure to reverse the underperfusion and subsequent ischemia will lead to deleterious changes. The onset of shock usually elicits compensatory mechanisms may accelerate and accentuate tissue injury, thereby contributing to the progression and perpetuation of the state of shock (90).

THERAPY OF SHOCK

The basic aim of drug therapy is to improve tissue perfusion by (a) expansion of blood volume, especially in cases where the blood volume is contracted, (b) augmentation of perfusion pressure and cardiac output (effective drug therapy will thus minimize the deleterious effects of underperfusion), and (c) reduction of arteriolar resistance in vital organs.

The following agents are usually employed in the management of shock and shocklike states:

1. Drugs that activate the sympathetic nervous system: epinephrine, norepinephrine, dopamine, dobutamine, isoproterenol, phenylephrine, and metaraminol
2. Vasodilators: sodium nitroprusside, nitrates, and phentolamine
3. Adrenocorticosteroids
4. Miscellaneous agents: glucagon, angiotensin, digitalis glycosides, and alkalinizing agents

SYMPATHOMIMETIC AMINES

The sympathomimetic amines are the class of drugs most widely used in the management of shock. Except in the presence of anaphylactic shock or severe hypotension, however, they should not be used as first-line drugs. Volume expanders should be administered when shock is caused by inadequate circulating blood volume. Patients who do not respond to volume replacement or are normovolemic, however, should be treated with sympathomimetic amines to improve and maintain perfusion of vital organs until the underlying cause is corrected or definitive therapy can be established. Effective therapy with sympathomimetic amines will result in improved perfusion of the heart, brain, kidney, and other vital organs. The sympathomimetic agents used for the management of shock include norepinephrine, epinephrine, dopamine, dobutamine, isoproterenol, and metaraminol.

Norepinephrine stimulates the myocardium to increase cardiac output by action on β_1-adrenoceptors (Chapter 7.1). Vasoconstriction of most vascular beds will occur by activation of α_1-adrenoceptors. The effect of norepinephrine on myocardial contractility is predominant at low doses sufficient to raise arterial pressure 100-110 mmHg. With larger doses, the peripheral vasoconstrictor action becomes more prominent, with a resultant decrease in blood flow to all areas except the heart and brain. Thus, norepinephrine has a limited role in the treatment of hypotension associated with cardiogenic shock.

Dopamine and dobutamine are useful agents in the management of cardiogenic shock (39). At lower doses (less than 10 μg/kg/min), dopamine increases cardiac output and causes vasodilation of the renal and mesenteric vascular beds. It is less potent than norepinephrine and metaraminol as a vasoconstrictor agent. Dobutamine is a synthetic sympathomimetic amine with prominent cardiac β_1-adrenoceptor-stimulant action. The drug produces minimal action upon β_2- and α_1-adrenoceptors (98). Its prominent inotropic action is not accompanied by a significant increase in heart rate or vasodilation as is observed with isoproterenol, nor does the drug cause endogenous release of norepinephrine as dopamine does. Dobutamine is usually infused at doses of 2.5-10 μg/kg/min, the duration of infusion being determined by the patient's response.

Epinephrine acts upon both α- and β-adrenoceptors (Chapter 7.1). In small doses, the vasodilator and cardiac inotropic actions predominate. Even in small doses, however, cutaneous and renal blood vessels are constricted. In large doses, a vasoconstrictor action predominates. Its α-adrenoceptor action in raising blood pressure and its β_2-adrenoceptor action on the bronchiolar smooth muscle make epinephrine a drug of choice for the management of anaphylactic shock.

Isoproterenol, a β-adrenoceptor agonist, is used primarily in low-output states such as shock resulting from myocardial pump failure. It may, however, produce intense tachycardia through a direct myocardial β-adrenoceptor-stimulant action as well as through the elicitation of baroceptor reflex mechanisms. The resultant disproportionate increase in myocardial oxygen requirement is a major disadvantage to its use in the presence of a compromised myocardium. Phenylephrine is the preferred agent for the management of neurogenic shock.

VASODILATORS

Because of the intense vasoconstriction associated with most shocklike states, the use of vasodilators has been advocated (15). Thus, vasodilators have been used in patients with pump failure, acute myocardial infarction, and severe left ventricular dysfunction. It is rational to assume that the use of vasodilators will improve cardiac performance by reducing peripheral vascular resistance. The resultant reduction in preload and afterload will in turn decrease cardiac work and oxygen demand. In addition, tissue blood flow will improve. Agents that produce both arterial and venodilation such as sodium nitroprusside, nitrates, and α-adrenoceptor-blocking drugs are more useful than agents with minimal actions on venous tone (e.g., hydralazine and diazoxide). Rapidly acting vasodilators, such as sodium nitroprusside may be preferred to α-adrenoceptor blockers because their use in part provides better moment-to-moment control. Phentolamine administration is a useful adjunctive measure with volume replacement in the management of hypovolemic shock. Its use will give a reliable indication of the adequacy of volume replacement and will permit administration of large volumes without overloading the myocardium.

ADRENAL CORTICOSTEROIDS

The use of adrenal corticosteroids (methylprednisolone or dexamethasone) is also advocated in bacteremic shock. The rationale for their use is based on the observations that these agents stabilize lysozomal membranes and reduce the elaboration of vasoactive substances. Their administration may also reduce the responses to endotoxins in septic shock (103).

OTHER AGENTS EMPLOYED

Glucagon has also been employed in the management of cardiogenic shock. Its positive inotropic action appears to be independent of activation of β-adrenoceptors. Although angiotensin can be used to restore blood pressure in a variety of hypotensive states, its value and place in the therapy of shock are highly controversial. The use of cardiac glycosides and alkalinizing agents in the management of shock is similarly controversial. In cardiogenic shock, digitalis glycosides may improve ventricular contractility. Although depressed cardiac contractility is frequently encountered in other forms of shock, the effectiveness of this class of agents in improving myocardial function has not been clearly established.

Metabolic acidosis may occur in shock due to underperfusion and the accumulation of metabolites. Improvement of tissue perfusion usually corrects the acidosis, and thus alkalinizing agents are not usually required. In selected cases, sodium bicarbonate may be cautiously administered.

REFERENCES

1. Abboud, F.M. Effects of sodium, angiotensin, and steroids on vascular reactivity in man. *Fed. Proc.* 33:143, 1974.
2. Abboud, F.M., Eckstein, J.W. and Wendling, M.G. Early potentiation of the vasoconstrictor action of norepinephrine by guanethidine. *Proc. Soc. Exp. Biol. Med.* 110:489, 1962.
3. Armstrong, B., Stevens, N. and Doll, R. Retrospective study of the association between use of rauwolfia derivatives and breast cancer in English women. *Lancet* 2:672, 1974.
4. Aviado, D.M. Hemodynamic effects of ganglion blocking drugs. *Circ. Res.* 8:304, 1960.
5. Baer, J.E., Leidy, H.L., Brooks, A.V. et al. The physiological disposition of chlorothiazide (Diuril) in the dog. *J. Pharmacol. Exp. Ther.* 125:295, 1959.
6. Berenson, G.S., Voors, A.W., Dalferes, E.R. et al. Creatinine clearance, electrolytes, and plasma renin activity related to the blood pressure of white and black children — The Bogalusa Heart Study. *J. Lab. Clin. Med.* 93:535, 1979.
7. Bolli, P., Waal-Manning, H.J., Wood, A.J. and Simpson, F.O. Experience with labetalol in hypertension. *Br. J. Clin. Pharmacol. (suppl. 3)* 3:765, 1976.
8. Bourgoignie, J.J., Catanzaro, F. J. and Perry, H.M., Jr. Renin-angiotensin-aldosterone system during chronic thiazide therapy of benign hypertension. *Circulation* 37:27, 1968.
9. Brettel, H.R., Aikawa, J.K. and Gordon, G.S. Studies with chlorothiazide tagged with radioactive carbon (C14) in human beings. *Arch. Intern. Med.* 106:57, 1960.
10. Briant, R.H., Reid, J.L. and Dollery, C.T. Interaction between clonidine and desipramine in man. *Br. Med. J.* 1:522, 1973.
11. Brogden, R.N., Heel, R.C., Speight, T.M. and Avery, G.S. Prazosin: A review of its pharmacological properties and therapeutic efficacy in hypertension. *Drugs* 14:163, 1977.
12. Buhler, F.R., Laragh, J.H., Vaughan, E.D. et al. Antihypertensive action of propranolol. *Am. J. Cardiol.* 32:511, 1973.
13. Chatterjee, K., Parmley, W.W., Ganz, W. et al. Hemodynamic and metabolic responses to vasodilator therapy in acute myocardial infarction. *Circulation* 48:1183, 1973.
14. Chrysant, S.G., Nishiyama, K., Adamopoulos, P.N. and Frohlich, E.D. Systemic hemodynamic effects of bethanidine in essential hypertension. *Circulation.* 52:137, 1975.
15. Cohn, J.N. and Franciosa, J.A. Vasodilator therapy of cardiac failure. *N. Engl. J. Med.* 297:254, 1977.
16. Corcoran, A.C. and Loyke, H.F. Mebutamate as antihypertensive agent in hospital outpatients. *JAMA* 181:1043, 1962.
17. Crane, M.G. and Harris, J.J. Effect of spironolactone in hypertensive patients. *Am. J. Med. Sci.* 260:311, 1970.
18. Deutsch, R.N. Depressive reactions of hypertensive patients: A comparison of those treated with rauwolfia and those receiving no specific antihypertensive treatment. *Circulation* 19:366, 1959.
19. Doyle, A.E., Anavekar, S.N., Louis, W.J. and Morgan, T.O. Antihypertensive drug treatment and plasma renin. In: *Systemic Effects of Antihypertensive Agents* (Samblhi, M.P., ed.). New York: Stratton Intercontinental, 1976, p. 185.
20. Dunn, F.G. Management of hypertension in the elderly. *Pract. Cardiol.* 7:112, 1981.
21. Durao, V., Pratta, M.M. and Goncalves, L.M.P. Modification of antihypertensive effect of beta-adrenoceptor-blocking agents by inhibition of endogenous prostaglandin synthesis. *Lancet* ii:1005, 1977.
22. Dustan, H.P., Tarazi, R.C. and Bravo, E.L. Dependence of arterial pressure on intravascular volume in treated hypertensive patients. *N. Engl. J. Med.* 286:861, 1972.
23. Farsang, C. and Kunos, G. Naloxone reverses the antihypertensive effect of clonidine. *Br. J. Pharmacol.* 67:161, 1979.
24. Ferguson, R.K., Rothenberg, R.J. and Nies, A.S. Patient acceptance of guanethidine as therapy for mild to moderate hypertension: A comparison with reserpine. *Circulation* 54:32, 1976.
25. Finch, L. and Haeusler, G. Further evidence for a central hypotensive action of alpha methyldopa in both the rat and cat. *Br. J. Pharmacol.* 47:217, 1973.
26. Fleming, W.W. and Trendelenburg, V. The development of supersensitivity to norepinephrine after pretreatment with reserpine. *J. Pharmacol. Exp. Ther.* 133:41, 1961.
27. Folkow, B. Haemodynamic consequences of adaptive structural changes of resistance vessels in hypertension. *Clin. Sci.* 41:1, 1971.
28. Fries, E.D. Mental depression in hypertensive patients treated for long periods with large doses of reserpine. *N. Engl. J. Med.* 251:1006, 1954.
29. Fries, E.D. Reserpine in hypertension: Present status. *Am. Family Physician* 11:120, 1975.
30. Fries, E.D. Treatment of hypertension: State of the art in 1979. *Clin. Sci.* 57:349S, 1979.
31. Frohlich, E.D., Tarazi, R.C., Dustan, H.P. and Page, I.H. The paradox of beta-adrenergic blockade in hypertension. *Circulation* 37:417, 1968.
32. Frohlich, E.D., Thurman, A.E., Pfeffer, M.A. et al. Altered vascular responsiveness: Initial hypotensive mechanism of thiazide diuretics. *Pro. Soc. Exp. Biol. Med.* 140:1190, 1972.
33. Gaffney, T.E., Chidsey, C.A. and Braunwald, E. Study of the relationship between the neurotransmitter store and adrenergic nerve block induced by reserpine and guanethidine. *Circ. Res.* 12:264, 1963.
34. Garvey, H.L. and Ram, N. Comparative antihypertensive effect and tissue distribution of beta adrenergic blocking drugs. *J. Pharmacol. Exp. Ther.* 192:220, 1975.
35. Garvey, H.L. and Ram, N. Centrally induced hypotensive effects of beta adrenergic blocking drugs. *Eur. J. Pharmacol.* 33:283, 1975.
36. Gavras, H., Brunner, H.R., Laragh, J.H. et al. An angiotensin converting-enzyme inhibitor to identify and treat vasoconstrictor and volume factors in hypertensive patients. *N. Engl. J. Med.* 291:817, 1974.
37. Gifford, R.W., Jr. Clinical application of new antihypertensive drugs. *Cleveland Clin. Q.* 42:255, 1975.
38. Gifford, R.W., Jr. Management and treatment of malignant hypertension and hypertensive emergencies, In: *Hypertension* (Genest, J., Koiw, E. and Kuchel, O., eds.). New York: McGraw-Hill, 1977, p. 1024.
39. Goldberg, L.I. Cardiovascular and renal actions of dopamine: Potential clinical applications. *Pharmacol. Rev.* 24:1, 1972.
40. Goldberg, M., McCurdy, D.K., Foltz, E.L. et al. Effects of ethacrynic acid (a new saluretic agent) on renal diluting and concentrating mechanisms: Evidence for site of action in the loop of Henle. *J. Clin. Invest.* 43:201, 1964.
41. Goldner, M.G., Zarowitz, H. and Akgun, S. Hyperglycemia and glycosuria due to thiazide derivatives administered in diabetes mellitus. *N. Engl. J. Med.* 262:403, 1960.
42. Gottleib, T.B., Katz, F.H. and Chidsey, C.A. Combined therapy with vasodilator drugs and beta-adrenergic blockade in hyper-

tension. A comparative study of minoxidil and hydralazine. *Circulation* 45:571, 1972.

43. Grahman, R.M., Muir, M.R. and Hayes, J.M. Differing effects of the vasodilator drugs, prazosin and diazoxide on plasma renin activity in the dog. *Clin. Exp. Pharmacol. Physiol.* 3:173, 1976.

44. Gross, F., Druey, J. and Meier, R. Eine neue Gruppe blutdrucksenkender Substanzen von besonderem Wizkungscharakter. *Experientia* 6:19, 1950.

45. Haeusler, G. Cardiovascular regulation by central adrenergic mechanisms and its alteration by hypotensive drugs. *Circ. Res. (suppl. 1)* 36:223, 1975.

46. Haggendal, J. and Dahlström, A. The recovery of the capacity for uptake-retention of (^{3}H) noradrenaline in rat adrenergic nerves after reserpine. *J. Pharm. Pharmacol.* 24:565, 1972.

47. Hambly, W.M., Jankowski, G.J., Pouget, J.M. et al. Intravenous use of diazoxide in the treatment of severe hypertension. *Circulation* 37:169.

48. Hansson, L. and Werko, L. Beta-adrenergic blockade in hypertension. *Am. Heart J.* 93:394, 1977.

49. Hayes, J.M., Grahman, R.M., O'Connell, B.P. et al. Experience with prazosin in the treatment of patients with severe hypertension. *Med. J. Aust.* 1:562, 1976.

50. Henning, M. Studies on the mode of action of alpha-methyldopa. *Acta Physiol. Scand. (suppl. 322)*, 75:1, 1969.

51. Iggo, A. and Vogt, M. Preganglionic sympathetic activity in normal and reserpine treated cats. *J. Physiol.* (London) 150:114, 1960.

52. Jain, A.K., Ryan, J.R., Vargas, R. and McMahon, F.R. Efficacy and acceptability of different dose schedule of clonidine. *Clin. Pharmacol. Ther.* 21:382, 1977.

53. Johnson, C.C. The actions and toxicity of sodium nitroprusside. *Proc. Soc. Exp. Biol. Med.* 26:102, 1929.

54. Johnson, G. and Regardh, C.G. Clinical pharmacokinetics of beta-adrenergic blocking drugs. *Clin. Pharmacokinet.* 1:233, 1976.

55. Johnston, L.C. and Greible, H.G. Treatment of arterial hypertensive disease with diuretics. V. Spironolactone, an aldosterone antagonist. *Arch. Intern. Med.* 119:225, 1967.

56. Kanada, S.A., Kanada, R.A., Hutchinson, R.A. and Wu, D. Angina-like syndrome with diazoxide therapy for hypertensive crisis. *Ann. Intern. Med.* 84:696, 1976.

57. Kane, J., Gregg, J. and Richards, D.A. A double-blind trial of labetalol. *Br. J. Clin. Pharmacol. (suppl. 3)* 3:737, 1976.

58. Koshy, M.C., Mickley, D., Bourgiognie, J. and Blaufox, M.D. Physiologic evaluation of a new antihypertensive agent: Prazosin HCl. *Circulation* 55:533, 1977.

59. Laragh, J.H. Vasoconstrictor volume analysis for understanding and treating hypertension. The use of renin and aldosterone profiles. *Am. J. Med.* 55:261, 1973.

60. Leishman, A.W., Thirkettle, J.L., Allen B.R. et al. Controlled trials of oxprenolol and practolol in hypertension *Br. Med. J.* 4:342, 1970.

61. Leonard, J.W., Gifford, R.W., Jr. and Humphrey, D.C. Treatment of hypertension with methyldopa alone or combined with diuretics and/or guanethidine. *Am. Heart J.* 69:610, 1965.

62. Lewis, P.J. and Hauesler, G. Reduction in sympathetic nervous activity as a mechanism for hypotensive effect of propranolol. *Nature* 256:440, 1975.

63. Maxwell, R.A., Plummer, A.J., Schneider, F. et al. Pharmacology of (2-octahydro-l-azocinyl)-ethyl-guanidine sulfate (SU 5864). *J. Pharmacol. Exp. Ther.* 128:22, 1960.

64. McCubbin, J.W., Kaneko, Y. and Page, I.H. The peripheral cardiovascular actions of guanethidine in dogs. *J. Pharmacol. Exp. Ther.* 131:346, 1961.

65. McMartin, C., Rondel, R.K., Vinter, J. et al. The fate of guanethidine in two hypertensive patients. *Clin. Pharmacol. Ther.* 11:423, 1970.

66. Miller, R.R., Vismara, L.A., Zelis, R. et al. Clinical use of sodium nitroprusside in chronic ischemic heart disease. Effects on peripheral vascular resistance and venous tone and on ventricular volume, pump, and mechanical performance. *Circulation* 51:328, 1975.

67. Morgan, T.O., Sabto, J., Anavekar, S.N. et al. A comparison of beta adrenergic blocking drugs in the treatment of hypertension. *Postgrad. Med. J.* 50:252, 1974.

68. Moyer, J.H. and Brest, A.N. Hydralazine in the treatment of hypertension. *Med. Clin. North Am.* 45:375, 1961.

69. Mylecharane, E.J. and Raper C. Further studies on the adrenergic neuron blocking action of some beta adrenoceptor antagonists and guanethidine. *J. Pharm. Pharmacol.* 25:213, 1973.

70. Oates, J.A., Gillespie, L., Udenfriend, S. and Sjoerdsma, A. Decarboxylase inhibition and blood pressure reduction by alpha-methyl-3, 4-dihydroxy-DL-phenylalanine, *Science* 131:1890, 1960.

71. Page, L.B. and Sidd, J.J. Medical management of primary hypertension. *N. Engl. J. Med.* 287:960, 1972.

72. Palmer, R.F. and Lasseter, K.C. Nitroprusside and aortic aneurism. *N. Engl. J. Med.* 294:1403, 1976.

73. Perry, H.M., Jr. A method of quantitating l-hydrazinophthalazine in body fluids. *J. Lab. Clin. Med.* 41:566, 1953.

74. Perry, H.M., Jr. Veterans Administration cooperation studies of hypertension. *Angiology* 29:804, 1978.

75. Perry, H.M., Jr. and Smith, W.M. Mild hypertension to treat or not to treat. *Ann. N.Y. Acad. Sci.* 304:472, 1978.

76. Pettinger, W.A. and Mitchell, H.C. Minoxidil—an alternative to nephrectomy for refractory hypertension. *N. Engl. J. Med.* 289:167, 1973.

77. Prichard, B.N. Hypotensive action of pronethalol. *Br. Med. J.* 1:1227, 1964.

78. Prichard, B.N. and Gillam, P.M. Treatment of hypertension with propranolol. *Br. Med. J.* 1:7, 1969.

79. Reubi, F.C. Renal hyperemia induced in man by new phthalazine derivative. *Proc. Soc. Exp. Biol. Med.* 73:102, 1950.

80. Reusch, C.S. The cardiorenal hemodynamic effects of antihypertensive therapy with reserpine. *Am. Heart J.* 64:643, 1962.

81. Rosei, E.A., Brown, J.J., Lever, A.F. and Robertson, A.S. Treatment of pheochromocytoma and clonidine withdrawal hypertension with labetalol. *Br. J. Clin. Pharmacol. (suppl. 3)* 3:809, 1976.

82. Rowe, G.C., Huston, J.H., Maxwell, G.M. et al. Hemodynamic effects of l-hydrazinophthalazine in patients with arterial hypertension. *J. Clin. Invest.* 34:115, 1955.

83. Sannerstedt, R. and Conway, J. Hemodynamic and vascular response to antihypertensive treatment with adrenergic blocking agents: A review. *Am. Heart J.* 79:122, 1970.

84. Schmitt, H. and Schmitt, H. Localization of the hypotensive effect of 2-(2,6-dichlorophenylamino) 2-imidazoline hydrochloride (ST 155, Catapresan). *Eur. J. Pharmacol.* 6:8, 1969.

85. Sellars, E.M. and Koch-Weser, J. Protein binding and vascular activity of diazoxide. *N. Engl. J. Med.* 281:1141, 1969.

86. Shand, D.G., Morgan, D.H. and Oates, J.A. The release of guanethidine and bethanidine by splenic nerve stimulation: A quantitative evaluation showing dissociation from adrenergic blockade. *J. Pharmacol. Exp. Ther.* 184:73, 1973.

87. Shapiro, A.P., Benedek, T.G. and Small, J.L. Effect of thiazides on carbohydrate metabolism in patients with hypertension. *N. Engl. J. Med.* 265:1028, 1961.

88. Shore, P.A. Transport and storage of biogenic amines. *Ann. Rev. Pharmacol.* 12:209, 1972.

89. Sjoerdsma, A., Oates, J.A., Zaltzman, P. Udenfriend, S. Serotonin synthesis in carcinoid patients: Its inhibition by alpha methyldopa with measurements of associated increases in urinary 5-hydroxytryptophan. *N. Engl. J. Med.* 263:585, 1960.

90. Sobel, B.E. Shock. In: *Heart Disease* (Braunwald, E., ed.). Philadelphia: W.B. Saunders, 1980.
91. Sourkes, T.L. Inhibition of dihydroxyphenylalanine decarboxylase by a derivative of phenylalanine. *Arch. Biochem.* 51:444, 1954.
92. Stason, W.B., Cannon, P.J., Heinemann, H.O. et al. Furosemide: A clinical evaluation of its diuretic action. *Circulation* 34:910, 1966.
93. Streeten, D.H., Dalakos, T.G., Anderson, G.H. and Freiberg, J.M. Use of angiotensin II analogs and converting enzyme inhibitors in management of hypertension. In: *Hypertension* (Genest, J., Koiw, E. and Kuchel, O., eds.). New York: McGraw-Hill, 1977, p. 1127.
94. Tarazi, R.C. and Dustan, H.P. Beta-adrenergic blockade in hypertension. Practical and theoretical implications of long-term hemodynamic variations. *Am. J. Cardiol.* 29:633, 1972.
95. Tarazi, R.C. and Dustan, H.P. Neurogenic participation in essential and renovascular hypertension assessed by acute ganglionic blockade: correlation with hemodynamic indices and intravascular volume. *Clin. Sci.* 44:197, 212, 1973.
96. Tobian, L., Janecke, J., Foker, J. et al. Effect of chlorothiazide on renal juxtaglomerular cells and tissue electrolytes. *Am. J. Physiol.* 202:905, 1962.
97. Turek, L.H. Clinical evaluation of mebutamate, an antihypertensive agent: Preliminary report. *Clin. Med.* 8:1335, 1961.
98. Tuttle, R.R. and Mills, J. Dobutamine: Development of new catecholamine to selectively increase cardiac contractility. *Circ. Res.* 36:185, 1975.
99. Ueda, H., Kaneko, Y., Takeda, T. et al. Observations on the mechanism of renin release by hydralazine in hypertensive patients. *Circ. Res. (suppl. 2)* 26:201, 1970.
100. Ulrych, M., Frohlich, E.D., Dustan, H.P. et al. Immediate hemodynamic effects of beta adrenergic blockade with propranolol in normotensive and hypertensive man. *Circulation.* 37:411, 1968.
101. Van Zweiten, P.A. The central action of antihypertensive drugs mediated via central alpha receptors. *J. Pharm. Pharmacol.* 25:89, 1973.
102. Waal-Manning, H.J. Hypertension, which beta-blocker? *Drugs* 12:412, 1976.
103. Weil, M.H. Current understanding of mechanisms and treatment of circulatory shock caused by bacterial infections. *Am. Clin. Res.* 9:181, 1977.
104. Winer, B.M. Antihypertensive mechanism of salt depletion induced by hydrochlorothiazide. *Circulation* 24:788, 1961.
105. Wollam, G.L., Gifford, R.W., Jr. and Tarazi, R.C. Antihypertensive drugs: Clinical pharmacology and therapeutic use. *Drugs* 14:420, 1977.
106. Wood, A.J., Phelan, E.L. and Simpson, F.O. Cardiovascular effects of prazosin in normotensive and genetically hypertensive rats. *Clin. Exp. Pharmacol. Physiol.* 2:297, 1975.
107. Zacharias, F.J., Cowen, K.J., Prestt, J. et al. Propranolol in hypertension: A study of long-term therapy, 1964-1970. *Am. Heart J.* 83:755, 1972.

ADDITIONAL READING

AMA Drug Evaluations, 5th Ed. Chicago: American Medical Association, 1983, pp. 685 and 699.

Ferguson, R.K. and Vlasses, P.H. Hypertensive emergencies and urgencies. *J.A.M.A.* 255:1607, 1986.

Finnerty, F.A. Jr. and Brogden, R.N. Guanadrel. A review of its pharmacodynamic and pharmacokinetic properties and therapeutic use in hypertension. *Drugs* 30:22, 1985.

Frohlich, E.D. Calcium channel blockers: A new dimension in antihypertensive therapy. *Am. J. Med.* 77(2B):1, 1984.

Gross, F. Present concepts and perspectives of antihypertensive therapy. *Clin. Exp. Hyperten.* (A) A4:1, 1982.

Handler, C.E. Cardiogenic shock. *Postgrad. Med.* 61:705, 1985.

Husseri, F.E. and Messerli, F.H. Adverse effect of antihypertensive drugs. *Drugs* 22:188, 1981.

Kaplan, H.R. Symposium on new antihypertensive drugs. *Fed. Proc.* 42:153, 1983.

Klein, W.W. Treatment of hypertension with calcium channel blockers: European data. *Am. J. Med.* 77:143, 1984.

Laragh, J.H. Converting enzyme inhibition for understanding and management of hypertensive disorders and congestive heart failure. *Am. J. Med.* 77(2A):1, 1984.

Pacy, P.J. et al. Nutrition and hypertension. *Ann. Nutr. Metab.* 29:129, 1985.

Prichard, B.N. and Owens, C.W. Mechanism of antihypertensive action of beta adrenergic blocking drugs. *Cardiology (suppl. 1)* 66:1, 1980.

Schier, O. and Marxer, A. Antihypertensive agents 1969-80. *Prog. Drug Res.* 25:9, 1981.

Stokes, G.S., Oates, H.F., and MacCarthy, E.P. Antihypertensive therapy: new pharmacological approaches. *Am. Heart J.* 100:741, 1980.

Symposium: Selection of initial antihypertensive therapy. New perspectives on coronary heart disease risk factors provide new insights. *Am. J. Med.* 80(2B):1, 1986.

Van Zwilten, P.A. et al. Pharmacological basis of the antihypertensive action of calcium entry blockers. *J. Cardiovascular Pharmacol. (suppl. 7)* 7:5105, 1985.

CHAPTER
15.4

ANTIANGINAL AGENTS

Atul R. Laddu and Prasad D.M.V. Turlapaty

Nitrates and Nitrites
β-Adrenoceptor Blocking Agents
Calcium Antagonists

Angina is manifested by sudden substernal pain often radiating to left shoulder and along the flexor surface of left arm. Anginal attack results from transient ischemia of a region of myocardium precipitated by an imbalance between myocardial oxygen demand and supply. In typical angina (angina pectoris) provoked by exercise or emotional stress and associated with other atherosclerotic lesions, oxygen requirements of the left ventricle exceed the capacity of the diseased coronary arteries to supply blood. Of the variables that determine the oxygen requirements of the left ventricle (heart rate, left ventricular systolic pressure, left ventricular volume, and myocardial contractility), heart rate and left ventricular systolic pressure play an important role in determining the myocardial oxygen consumption. In patients with angina pectoris, the double product (heart rate times systolic blood pressure), an index of the myocardial oxygen demand, is relatively constant whenever pain develops due to various stimuli such as exercise or emotional stress (23).

Use of pharmacological agents in the relief of angina is aimed to improve the balance between the supply and demand of oxygen in the myocardium. Agents which decrease either heart rate or systolic blood pressure (e.g., β-adrenoceptor blockers) reduce the oxygen requirements of the left ventricle and alleviate anginal pain. Other agents (e.g., nitrates and nitrites) that cause vasodilatation and consequently reduce preload and afterload of the heart, reduce the oxygen demand of the heart, although they also increase to some extent the oxygen supply of the ischemic myocardium.

In Prinzmetal's variant angina, the primary etiology is spasm of coronary arteries, but the precise mechanism for the vasoconstriction in individual patients is unknown. β-Adrenoceptor blocking agents and calcium antagonists have been found to be beneficial in patients with this type of angina, although the fundamental cellular mechanism is not yet clear.

NITRATES AND NITRITES

History. Amyl nitrite by inhalation was first used by Lauder Brunton in 1867 to treat patients with recurrent anginal pain, and its action was ascribed to an inhibition of the arterial tension. In 1879, William Murrell introduced sublingual nitroglycerin for relief of acute anginal attacks (15). Later, in 1933, Sir Thomas Lewis described the coronary dilatory effect of amyl nitrite and considered this as its mechanism in the relief of angina. In 1959, however, Gorlin and coworkers using xenon washout technique demonstrated that nitroglycerin did not alter coronary blood flow (9). In 1967, Robinson demonstrated that a certain value of the double product was associated with the precipitation of angina of effort, and indicated that agents with peripheral vascular effect could reduce angina by lowering the double product (23).

Chemistry. These compounds are salts or mixed esters of nitric acid or nitrous acid. They are listed in Table 15.4-1 with their chemical structure, preparations, dose, and duration of action and their chemical structures are presented in Fig. 15.4-1.

Pharmacological Effects

Cardiovascular System. The organic nitrates dilate both venous and arterial smooth muscle, although their action is predominantly on the venous system. Due to venodilation, blood pools in the veins, resulting in a decreased venous return to the heart and thereby decreased left and right ventricular end-diastolic pressures, left ventricular volume, and finally myocardial oxygen demand. Nitrates also decrease afterload (ventricular systolic wall tension) by decreasing peripheral arteriolar resistance, and thus effectively reduce myocardial oxygen consumption. Nitrates have a much weaker action on systemic vascular resistance. On the other hand, they reduce pulmonary vascular resistance consistently. Both experimental and clinical findings indicate that nitrates and nitrites do not have a predictably consistent effect on blood pressure in patients with hypertension. Nitrates often produce a reflex transient tachycardia. Adrenergic mechanisms involved in the control of cardiovascular functions are not affected by nitrates.

Nitrates may be used as effective antianginal agents. Because angina is usually precipitated by exercise or stress, either of which increases cardiac work and myocardial oxygen demand, nitrates function as antianginal agents possibly by increasing oxygen supply and decreas-

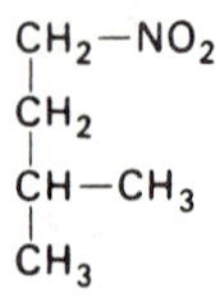

CH_2-NO_2
CH_2
$CH-CH_3$
CH_3

Amyl nitrite

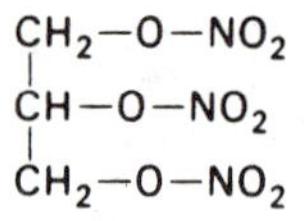

CH_2-O-NO_2
$CH-O-NO_2$
CH_2-O-NO_2

Nitroglycerin

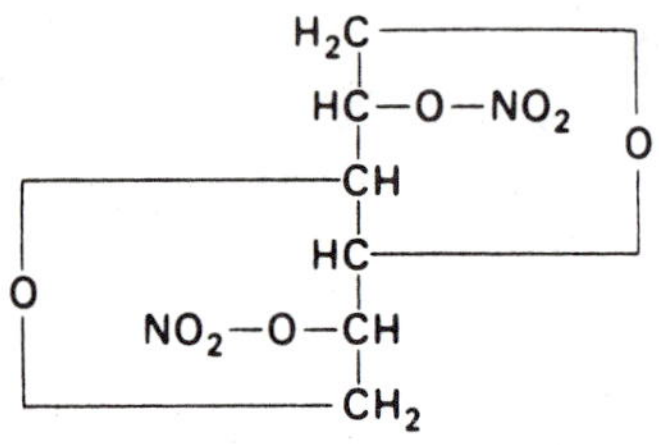

H_2C
$HC-O-NO_2$
CH
HC
NO_2-O-CH
CH_2
O
O

Isosorbide dinitrate

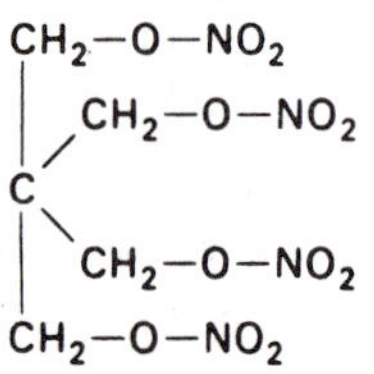

CH_2-O-NO_2
CH_2-O-NO_2
C
CH_2-O-NO_2
CH_2-O-NO_2

Pentaerythritol tetranitrate

CH_2-O-NO_2
$CH-O-NO_2$
$CH-O-NO_2$
CH_2-O-NO_2

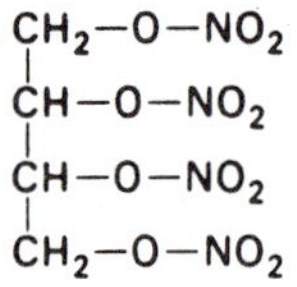

Erythrityl tetranitrate

Fig. 15.4-1: *Chemical structures of antianginal nitrates and nitrites*

ing oxygen demand. Nitrates increase oxygen supply by producing dilatation of large coronary arteries that would result in the redistribution of blood from normal to ischemic areas; they have minimal influence on the small intramyocardial coronary vessels that control autoregulation of the coronary vascular bed and that are responsible for coronary vascular resistance. Thus, nitrates play a little role in altering the process of autoregulation, as large coronary arteries do not take part in this process (28). Nitrates in animal models redistribute blood flow along collateral channels of large coronary arteries because these are effectively dilated by these agents; such effect in humans is not clearly defined. Nitrates decrease oxygen demand by reducing both preload and afterload on the heart, as myocardial oxygen demand increases proportionately with the increase of preload and afterload.

Other Regional Circulations. Nitrates produce relaxation of all vascular beds, although the magnitude of such an effect varies from one regional vascular bed to another. Bronchial smooth muscle is relaxed, irrespective of the preexisting tone. The biliary tract muscles, including those of the gallbladder, biliary ducts, and Oddi's sphincter are also effectively relaxed, as is the smooth muscle of the gastrointestinal tract. Nitrates reduce pulmonary arterial pressure as a result of pulmonary vasodilatation. In the cerebral vessels, nitrates produce vasodilatation and may elevate intracranial pressure. A decrease in systemic pressure results in a decrease in blood flow through the brain, which may account for nitrate headache. Retinal vessels are dilated following nitrate administration.

Mechanism of Action. The contractile mechanism of the smooth muscle is dependent on a Ca^{2+}-activated myosin adenosine triphosphatase (ATPase) similar to that present in the skeletal and the cardiac muscle. Calcium is necessary to activate the contractile mechanism; nitrates and nitrites appear to act by reducing calcium that is necessary for the activation of the contractile mechanism. It has been shown that sodium nitroprusside enhances the efflux of calcium from isolated blood vessels (29). Another mechanism of action of nitrates is due to increased cyclic guanosine monophosphate (cGMP) content in smooth muscle (16, 21). cGMP appears to stimulate a Ca^{2+}-binding process in smooth muscle, thereby reducing the concentration of free cytoplasmic calcium available to trigger muscle contraction.

Nitrites by their actions on the peripheral circulation reduce the demand for oxygen by the myocardium and thus relieve angina of effort. Nitrites have also been shown to cause release of prostaglandins and inhibit platelet function. They have minimal direct effect on cardiac muscle.

Nitrites have been used in treatment of effort angina, spontaneous angina, or variant angina and unstable angina (8).

Pharmacokinetics. Most of the nitrates used therapeutically are absorbed from the oral mucosa and less readily from the gastrointestinal tract. Following sublingual administration of nitroglycerin, clinical effects appear within a minute or two and last for about 1 hr (Table 15.4-1). Long-acting nitrate preparations (e.g., isosorbide dinitrate, pentaerythritol tetranitrate) when given orally in adequate dosage are absorbed from the intestine, and have a slower onset and longer duration of action. These are efficiently metabolized in the liver by the enzyme glutathione organic nitrate reductase to mononitro- and dinitro-metabolites, which are excreted by the kidney.

Following sublingual, intravenous, or transcutaneous administration of nitroglycerin, blood levels are achieved to an equal extent, although time to reach peak level varies between each route. Nitroglycerin ointment produces a reduction in left ventricular end-diastolic pressure both at rest and during exercise; the reduction persists for at least 1 hr after application, and it also increases exercise capacity for at least 3 hr. Effective levels of nitroglycerin are found in the blood for 8 hr after application of the ointment, indicating its continuous absorption. Patch formulations of nitroglycerin also maintain effective blood levels of nitroglycerin for about 24 hr.

Adverse Effects. Untoward effects of nitrates are secondary to their actions on the cardiovascular system. Headache, dizziness, flushing of the face, and postural

Table 15.4-1
Nitrates with Dose Regimen

Drug (trade name)	Preparation,[a] Route of Administration	Duration
Amyl nitrite, USP (Isoamyl nitrite)	P, 0.18, 0.3 ml, inhalation	10 sec - 10 min
Nitroglycerin, USP (Glyceryltrinitrate; NITROL; NITROSTAT, TRIDIL)	T(s), 0.3 mg	90 sec - 1 hr
	0.6 mg, 2% percutaneous (15 x 15 cm topical)	3-4 hr
	i.v. infusion (0.6-12 mg/hr)	8-12 hr during and 30 min postinfusion
Isosorbide dinitrate, USP (ISORDIL, SORBITRATE)	T(s), 2.5, 5 mg	Up to 1 hr
	T(s), 5, 10 mg	Up to 3 hr
	T(o), 5, 10, 20 mg	Up to 6 hr
	C, 40 mg	6-12 hr
	i.v., 1.25-5 mg/hr	Effective for short attacks of angina at rest
Pentaerythritol tetranitrate, USP (PENTRITOL, PERITRATE)	T(s), 10 mg	45 min
	T(o), 10, 20, 40 mg	Up to 6 hr
	C, 30, 45, 60, 80 mg	Up to 12 hr
Erythrityl tetranitrate, USP (CARDILATE)	T(s), 5, 10, 15 mg	10-45 min
	T(c), 30, 45, 60, 80 mg	Up to 12 hr

[a] P, pearl; T(s), tablet for sublingual use; T(c), chewable tablet; T(o), oral tablets; C, time-release capsules; O, ointment.

hypotension accompanied by syncope may develop in patients taking nitrate therapy. An occasional aggravation of anginal attacks may result due to reflex tachycardia following hypotension. Nitrite ions readily oxidize hemoglobin to methemoglobin, thus impairing the oxygen-carrying capacity of the blood. Halitosis may occur due to sublingual use of nitrates.

Contraindications. Nitrates are contraindicated in angina caused by hypertrophic obstructive cardiomyopathy, cor pulmonale, and arterial hypoxemia; nitrates may further decrease arterial oxygen tension by venous admixture. Amyl nitrite is contraindicated in the presence of glaucoma.

Tolerance and Withdrawal. Chronic use of nitrates produces tolerance to the antianginal efficacy. There is some evidence to indicate development of nitrate cross-tolerance. In munition workers, sudden withdrawal of nitrates may precipitate angina or death.

Therapeutic Uses. Nitrates are effective in the treatment of conditions such as variant angina (Prinzmetal type) and angina pectoris. They are also useful in the treatment of peripheral arterial disease such as Raynaud's disease, and occasionally in the management of biliary colic and ureteral spasm. Synergistic influence between nitrites and β-adrenoceptor blocking agents has been demonstrated in the treatment of angina. β-Adrenoceptor blockers inhibit reflex tachycardia induced by nitrites. Nitrites decrease the tendency of β-adrenoceptor blockers to cause ventricular enlargement and congestive heart failure by causing a decrease in venous return and thereby reducing left ventricular volume.

β-ADRENOCEPTOR BLOCKING AGENTS

β-Adrenoceptors are subclassified as β_1 receptors (present in cardiac muscle) and β_2 receptors (present in bronchial and vascular smooth muscle) (Chapter 7.2). Nonselective β-adrenoceptor blocking agents (i.e., having influence on both β_1 and β_2 receptors) that are marketed in the United States or are under clinical investigation include propranolol, nadolol, oxprenolol, pindolol, sotalol, and timolol. Cardioselective β_1-adrenoceptor blocking agents available for therapy or under clinical investigation include metoprolol, atenolol, and acebutolol (Table 15.4-2). Currently, only propranolol and nadolol are avialable in the United States for treatment of angina pectoris.

β-Adrenoceptor blockers produce a dose-dependent reduction in heart rate, systolic blood pressure, and double product during rest and exercise and thus reduce the cardiac work and oxygen demand. It has been shown that β-blockers with no intrinsic sympathomimetic activity (e.g., propranolol) cause an increase in left ventricular end-diastolic pressure by decreasing cardiac contractility, which in turn leads to an increase in ventricular volume and a subsequent increase in myocardial oxygen

Table 15.4-2
Plasma Half-Life and Doses of β-Adrenoceptor Blocking Agents for Angina Pectoris

β-Blocker (Trade Name)	Plasma half-life (hr)	Oral Dosage
Noncardioselective		
Propranolol (INDERAL)	1-6	120-480 mg/day
Nadolol (CORGARD)	12-17	80-240 mg/day
Oxprenolol (TRASICOR)	2	160 mg/day
Pindolol (VISKEN)	4	2.5-7.5 mg t.i.d.
Timolol (BLOCADREN)	4-5	15-45 mg/day
Sotalol	15-17	240-480 mg/day
Cardioselective		
Acebutolol (SECTRAL)	3-6	200-400 mg t.i.d.
Atenolol (TENORMIN)	6-9	50-100 mg/day
Metoprolol (LOPRESSOR)	3	150-300 mg/day

Source: Ref. 20.

consumption. This deleterious effect could probably be overcome by the concomitant reduction in heart rate and blood pressure. Experimental and clinical findings suggest, however, that β-adrenoceptor blockers with intrinsic sympathomimetic activity (e.g., acebutolol, pindolol, oxprenolol) may produce less incidence of an increase in left ventricular end-diastolic pressure. Both selective and nonselective β-blockers are effective in the treatment of angina pectoris. A limiting factor for the use of β-blockers in the treatment of angina is the appearance of bradycardia. The dose of these agents should be adjusted so that resting heart rate is 55-60 beats/min, and if in doubt, the attenuation of heart rate response to exercise should be used as an index of efficacy (3).

Adverse Effects. The major side effects of these drugs are an increase in airway resistance (specially in asthmatics), nausea, diarrhea, postural hypotension, claudication, sodium retention, potentiation of hypoglycemia, and precipitation of congestive heart failure in patients with borderline cardiac compensation. Cardioselective (β_1) adrenoceptor antagonists such as acebutolol, atenolol, and metoprolol may provide an additional advantage over propranolol for use in patients with chronic obstructive lung disease, asthma, or peripheral vascular disease. The β_1 specificity of the cardioselective drugs is only relative and is usually lost at higher dose levels.

β-Adrenoceptor antagonists are usually contraindicated in patients with diabetes mellitus requiring insulin, because they may augment the hypoglycemic action of insulin and mask the important signs of reflex tachycardia. Abrupt discontinuation of chronic therapy with β-blockers could result in exacerbation of angina, cardiac arrhythmias, resulting in ventricular tachycardia, myocardial infarction, and even sudden death. If therapy with these agents is to be discontinued, gradual withdrawal of the dosing regimen over a period of 1 or 2 weeks is recommended.

Combined therapy of nitrates and β-blocking agents in patients with angina could be beneficial. Nitrates increase myocardial oxygen supply; β-adrenoceptor blocking drugs decrease the oxygen demand. Furthermore, β-blockers by virtue of their influence on β_1 receptors would attenuate nitrate-mediated reflex tachycardia. The combination of β-blocking agents and nitrates allows the latter to be taken in high doses without producing reflex tachycardia or inotropic effects. The decrease in venous return resulting from the nitrates offsets the tendency of propranolol to cause increased left ventricular diastolic volume. The decrease in systolic vascular resistance due to nitrates lowers the blood pressure still further, the net result being a decrease in ventricular wall stress. The actions of the two types of drugs thus complement each other (see earlier).

CALCIUM ANTAGONISTS

These agents, also known as calcium-entry blockers or calcium-channel blockers, represent a new class of drugs having beneficial effects in the treatment of various cardiovascular disease states such as angina, arrhythmia, and hypertension. According to Fleckenstein et al., these drugs produce selective blockade of the slow channel of the cell membrane by interference with the transmembrane calcium influx (5). Calcium ions are known to play a pivotal role in the excitation-contraction coupling process of cardiac and vascular smooth muscle cells. Calcium antagonists, by inhibiting calcium influx, bring about important hemodynamic alterations that make them therapeutically valuable antianginal agents. Several agents (e.g., verapamil, nifedipine, diltiazem, perhexiline) that have been extensively studied have shown a variable degree of selectivity for cardiac muscle, atrioventricular conduction, peripheral blood vessels, and the coronary circulation. These agents represent a diversity of structures as illustrated in Fig. 15.4-2.

The calcium-channel blocking agents bring about changes in cardiovascular hemodynamics by (1) coronary arterial dilatation, (2) peripheral arterial dilatation, and (3) a negative inotropic and chronotropic effect. In addition, reflex mechanisms evoked due to peripheral dilatation may also be an important determinant of the net hemodynamic effect of these agents.

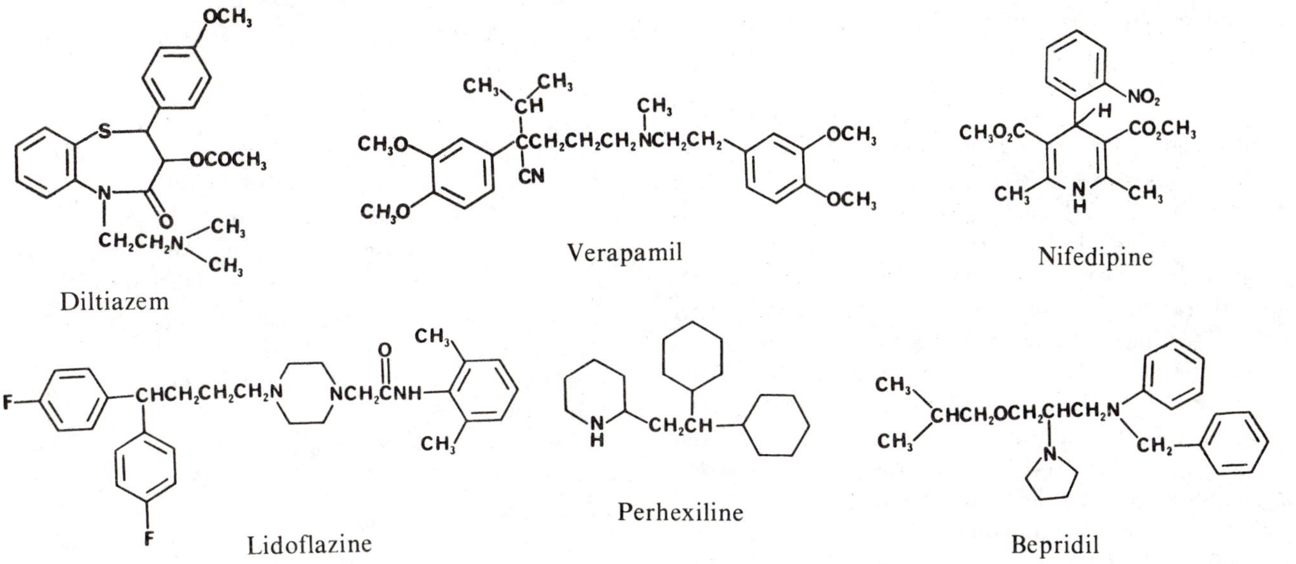

Diltiazem

Verapamil

Nifedipine

Lidoflazine

Perhexiline

Bepridil

Fig. 15.4-2: *Chemical structures of calcium antagonists.*

Effects on Coronary Circulation. All the calcium blocking agents reduce coronary vascular resistance, increase coronary blood flow by a direct dilatation of coronary arteries, and also increase flow through coronary collateral vessels. In equimolar doses, the order of potency for the vasodilator effect in the pig coronary arteries is: nifedipine > verapamil > diltiazem > perhexiline (6). The vasodilation induced by calcium-channel blocking agents is not influenced by β-adrenergic blockade, catecholamine depletion, or vagotomy (24).

Effects on the Peripheral Circulation. Calcium-channel blockers produce a significant reduction in total systemic vascular resistance, although their dilatory influence on the arterial side is more than on the venous side. The regional vascular beds dilated by these drugs are pulmonary, hepatic, hind limb, renal, and superior mesenteric in both animals and humans; in addition, nifedipine has been shown to dilate cerebral arteries in humans (17). Calcium-channel blockers have little effect on the responsiveness of cutaneous venous smooth muscle to sympathetic nerve stimulation, but they inhibit the adrenergic activation of splanchnic venous smooth muscle. Thus, by dilating both arterial and venous smooth muscle, these agents diminish afterload as well as preload to the heart.

Effects on Heart. All calcium-channel blockers exhibit direct negative inotropic effects on isolated cardiac muscle preparations (*in vitro*), the most potent in this regard being nifedipine and verapamil. In *in vivo* experiments, the net effect on myocardial contractility is a result of an interaction of direct and reflex-mediated phenomena. The direct negative inotropic effect is compensated for by the baroreceptor-mediated reflex positive inotropic and chronotropic responses triggered by the peripheral vasodilation.

Effects of calcium-channel blockers on heart rate and conduction are variable. In isolated tissues, verapamil produces negative chronotropic effect by depressing the SA node; *in vivo*, this effect is nullified by the reflex tachycardia due to vasodilation, the net effect being no change in the heart rate. In contrast, nifedipine has minimal depressant effect on the SA or the AV node. Of all the calcium-channel blockers, verapamil has the greatest affinity for the AV nodal tissue, through which it presumably exerts therapeutic effect in atrial fibrillation, flutter, and paroxysmal supraventricular tachycardia.

The calcium-channel blocking agents have differential influence on left ventricular end-diastolic pressure (LVEDP). If direct negative inotropic effects of these agents are not counterbalanced by reflex events, the LVEDP rises. In the case of verapamil, which induces less arterial hypotension than nifedipine, influence of reflex activity would be less than the negative inotropic effect, thus resulting in a rise of LVEDP. With nifedipine, because of its potent vasodilatory effects, reflex activity nullifies its negative inotropic influence, resulting in no change of LVEDP.

In summary, the hemodynamic effects of the calcium-channel blocking agents result from a complex interaction of direct and reflex effects on changes in heart rate, preload, afterload, cardiac contractility, and coronary blood flow. These agents, in addition to decreasing the double product and thereby oxygen demand, also increase the oxygen supply to the heart by direct coronary vasodilation.

Calcium antagonists have been clinically investigated in patients with classic angina pectoris, Prinzmetal-type variant angina, and unstable angina pectoris. Table 15.4-3 presents various calcium antagonists with their respective doses. Because coronary arterial contraction is dependent on calcium, these drugs might be the drugs of choice in patients with variant angina. In fact, many clinical trials have shown the effectiveness of nifedipine, verapamil, diltiazem, perhexiline, and lidoflazine in preventing pain due to variant angina (4, 26). In classic angina pectoris (angina due to effort), these agents may exert beneficial influence by decreasing peripheral vascular resistance (resulting in reduced afterload and preload on the heart), and by reducing myocardial contractility, thus improving the relationship between myocardial oxygen supply and demand (4, 26). In patients with unstable angina, coronary spasm also plays a role in the pathophysiological mechanism of pain and ischemia; these agents might prevent such spasm (26). Kimura and Kishida (14) demonstrated in a comparative study in patients with variant angina that calcium-channel blockers are more effective than β-adrenoceptor blockers. Calcium channel blockers are also more effective than nitrates in the treatment of variant angina associated with malignant ventricular arrhythmias and conduction disturbances. These drugs decrease the enhanced arterial smooth muscle tone (present during spasm) by inhibition of calcium influx.

In the presence of left ventricular failure, nifedipine, rather than verapamil, is beneficial since it does not affect AV conduction and does not depress myocardial contractility (11, 12).

The calcium antagonists have been found useful in preservation of ischemic tissue after acute myocardial infarction. These agents cause (1) reduction of myocardial oxygen requirements, (2) reduction of myocardial high-energy phosphate depletion, (3) coronary vasodilation, and (4) enhancement of collateral blood flow.

In a double-blind randomized study in patients with variant angina pectoris, Johnson et al. (11) demonstrated that verapamil compared with placebo (1) significantly decreased the frequency of anginal episodes, (2) decreased the consumption of nitroglycerin tablets, and (3) decreased the episodes of transient ST-segment elevation. These authors concluded that verapamil is a safe and effective agent in the treatment of variant angina pectoris and is also beneficial in patients with exertional angina and unstable angina.

In a double-blind randomized trial in patients with unstable angina, nifedipine added to either propranolol or long-acting nitrates significantly decreased the anginal episodes at rest when compared with placebo and conventional antianginal drugs (7). The beneficial effect of nifedipine was probably due to its influence on reducing coronary artery spasm rather than an effect on the afterload.

Table 15.4-3
Dosages of Calcium Antagonists in Angina Pectoris

Agent (trade name)	Indication	Dose
Verapamil (ISOPTIN, CALAN)	Angina pectoris (angina of effort)	80-120 mg, t.i.d.-q.i.d.
	Angina at rest, Prinzmetal's angina	80-120 mg, t.i.d.-q.i.d.
Nifedipine (PROCARDIA, ADALAT)	Angina pectoris	20-30 mg, t.i.d.-q.i.d.
	Angina at rest, Prinzmetal's angina	10 mg, t.i.d.
Diltiazem (CARDIZEM)	Angina pectoris	30-60 mg, t.i.d.-q.i.d.
Perhexiline (PEXID)	Angina pectoris	50-200 mg, t.i.d.

Source: Ref. 22.

In a trial involving patients with significant obstructive coronary artery disease, Daly et al. (1) demonstrated that nifedipine had a beneficial additive effect to β-blockers and that the two agents have an important place in the treatment of angina pectoris. Acute metabolic and hemodynamic responses were monitored at rest and during atrial pacing period of patients who were already on propranolol and receiving sublingual nifedipine. These indices revealed that nifedipine prolonged pacing time to angina, increased lactate extraction ratio, and produced coronary and peripheral vasodilation.

In a study (27) involving (a) patients with Prinzmetal's variant angina and documented coronary vasospasm, (b) patients with "mixed" angina, defined as those patients who exhibit evidence of both exertional angina as well as possible superimposed coronary vasospasm, and (c) patients with stable classic exertional angina whose symptoms are presumed to be due to fixed obstructive lesions alone, who were refractory to maximally tolerated doses of conventional antianginal therapy, nifedipine has been shown to be highly efficacious in decreasing the symptoms of angina pectoris. The mechanism of beneficial effect in patients with refractory angina may be due to an additional decrease in afterload and myocardial oxygen demand, as well as prevention of decrease in myocardial oxygen supply caused by coronary vasoconstriction (27).

Nifedipine in conventional doses in humans does not depress atrioventricular nodal conduction, whereas verapamil and diltiazem are known to cause depression. Nifedipine is thus less likely to cause electrophysiological side effects when combined with β-blockers. In patients with good left ventricular function, the incidence of adverse effects with combined therapy (β-blockers and calcium-channel blockers) is usually less than in patients with poor left ventricular function.

In a study (18) involving patients with recurrent angina occuring after acute myocardial infarction, diltiazem has been shown to suppress angina at rest as well as painless cyclic ST-segment elevation, indicating its effectiveness in the treatment of postinfarction angina caused by coronary artery spasm.

Bepridil is a newly synthesized calcium-channel blocker with antianginal effects. It slows SA node in a dose-dependent manner, prolongs atrial and atrioventricular refractory periods, increases coronary blood flow by decreasing coronary vascular resistance, and reduces left ventricular stroke work. *In vitro* studies suggest that it has an inhibitory effect on the fast Na^+ channels as well as slow Ca^{2+} channels. In clinical trials involving patients with chronic stable angina pectoris (2, 19), bepridil has been shown to be an effective and well-tolerated antianginal agent compared with placebo. Its mechanism of antianginal action appears to be due to increased coronary blood flow and reduction in afterload. The average effective total daily dose of oral bepridil is 300-400 mg.

In a double-blind, randomized, placebo-controlled, crossover trial, effects of bepridil on exercise tolerance in patients with chronic stable angina was investigated (10). When compared with placebo, bepridil administered 400 mg orally once a day prolonged total exercise time, time to onset of angina, time to ST-segment depression, and increased total workload achieved. Since the double product during placebo and bepridil therapy periods was similar, the mechanism of antianginal action could be primarily due to peripheral effect, thereby reducing myocardial oxygen demand. Bepridil has been shown to have systemic and coronary vasodilator properties (13).

Pharmacokinetics

Bepridil. Pharmacokinetic studies in normal human volunteers have revealed that the peak plasma concentration of bepridil after 400 mg once a day oral dosage is attained at approximately 2.4 hr after its administration, and steady-state plasma level is reached at approximately 6 days. The half-life for elimination of bepridil is approximately 42 hr and the route of elimination appears to be primarily renal.

Nifedipine (26). Nifedipine is absorbed greater than 90% after oral or sublingual administration. The onset of action is 3 min after sublingual and 20 min after oral dose. The plasma half-life is 4 hr; duration of action is 8-12 hr. About 90% of the circulating drug is protein bound; nifedipine is completely metabolized to inert metabolites, 80% of which are excreted via the kidneys. No adverse interactions with other drugs have been seen as yet, and it may be safely administered together with nitrates, β-blockers, digoxin, furosemide, anticoagulants, and antihypertensive and antidiabetic agents (26).

Verapamil (25). More than 90% of orally administered verapamil is absorbed, although the overall bioavailability of 10-20% suggests first-pass metabolism in the liver. In patients with hepatic cirrhosis, systemic availability of verapamil was reported to be greater than 50%. This was due to impaired ability to extract verapamil from plasma. Verapamil produces hypotension that is short lived, with an onset of action in less than 1-2 min and loss of activity by 10-20 min. The effect on the AV node lasts for up to 6 hr, suggesting preferential uptake and binding by the AV nodal tissue. Oral verapamil has an onset of action of 2 hr, and the effect lasts for 5 hr; the slow-release form of verapamil acts within 6 hr and lasts up to 14 hr. Both oral and intravenously administered verapamil are approximately 90% bound to plasma proteins and are extensively metabolized in the liver; the majority of the drug is excreted by the kidneys. Verapamil may have adverse interactions with β-adrenoceptor blocking agents or digoxin.

Diltiazem (26). Diltiazem is absorbed almost completely (greater than 90%) after oral administration (onset of action is within 30 min), with a plasma half-life of approximately 4 hr; about 80% is bound to plasma proteins. The majority of the drug is metabolized by the liver and the remainder is excreted by the kidneys. Some adverse reactions when diltiazem is combined with β-blockers have been reported.

Perhexiline (6, 26). Perhexiline is almost completely absorbed after oral administration with onset of action in 1 hr. Ninety percent of the circulating drug is bound to plasma proteins. It is extensively metabolized by the liver and excreted by the kidneys and the gastrointestinal tract.

Adverse Effects and Contraindications. The incidence of adverse effects with calcium antagonists reported so far is low: headache, dizziness, tinnitus, vomiting, flushing, ankle edema, and tiredness. Overdoses can cause significant decrease in ventricular performance. Because verapamil has potent effects on the SA and AV nodes, it is contraindicated in patients with sick sinus syndrome and in patients with severe defects of AV nodal conduction. With perhexiline, elevation of SGOT, SGPT, LDH, and alkaline phosphatase as a consequence of liver dysfunction and neuropathy has been reported.

REFERENCES

1. Daly, K., Bergman, G., Rothman, L., Atkinson, L., Jackson, G. and Jewitt, D.E. Beneficial effects of adding nifedipine to beta-adrenergic blocking therapy in angina pectoris. *Eur. Heart J.* 3:42, 1982.
2. DiBianco, R., Alpert, J., Katz, R.J., Spann, J., Chesler, E., Ferri, D.P., Larca, L.J., Costello, R.B., Gore, J.M., Eisenmann, M.J. and Cockrell, J.L. Bepridil for chronic stable angina pectoris:

Results of a prospective multicenter, placebo, controlled dose-ranging study in 77 patients. *Am. J. Cardiol.* 53:35, 1984.

3. DiBianco, R., Singh, S., Singh, J., Katz, R.J., Bortz, R., Gottdiener, J.S., Spodick, D.H., Laddu, A.R. and Fletcher, R.D. Effects of acebutolol on chronic stable angina pectoris. A placebo-controlled, double-blind, randomized crossover study. *Circulation* 62:1179, 1980.
4. Ellrodt, G., Chew, C.Y.C. and Singh, B.N. Therapeutic implications of slow-channel blockade in cardio-circulatory disorders. *Circulation* 62:669, 1980.
5. Fleckenstein, A. Specific pharmacology of calcium in myocardium, cardiac pacemakers, and vascular smooth muscle. *Ann. Rev. Pharmacol. Toxicol.* 17:149, 1977.
6. Fleckenstein-Grun, G., Fleckenstein, A., Byon, Y.K. and Kim, K.W. Mechanism of action of Ca++ antagonists in the treatment of coronary disease with special reference to perhexiline maleate. In: *Perhexiline Maleate: Proceedings of a Symposium.* Excerpta Medica, Amsterdam, 1976, p. 140.
7. Gerstenblith, G., Ouyang, P., Achuff, S.C., Bulkley, H.H., Becker, L.C., Mellits, E.D., Baughman, K.L., Weiss, J.L., Flaherty, J.T., Kallman, C.H., Llewellyn, M. and Weisfeldt, M.L. Nifedipine in Unstable Angina. A Double-Blind, Randomized Trial. *N. Engl. J. Med.* 306:885, 1982.
8. Giles, T.D. The current status of nitrites in management of angina pectoris. *Rational Drug Ther.* 15:1, 1981.
9. Gorlin, R., Brachfeld, N., MacLeod, C. and Bopp, P. Effect of nitroglycerin on the coronary circulation in patients with coronary artery disease or increased left ventricular work. *Circulation* 19:705, 1959.
10. Hill, J.A., O'Brien, J.T., Scott, E., Conti, C.R. and Pepine, C.J. Effects of bepridil on exercise tolerance in chronic stable angina: A double-blind, randomized, placebo-controlled, crossover trial. *Am. J. Cardiol.* 53:679, 1984.
11. Johnson, S.M., Mauritson, D.R., Willerson, J.T. and Hillis, L.D. A controlled trial of verapamil for Printzmetal's variant angina. *N. Engl. J. Med.* 304:862, 1981.
12. Karlsberg, R.P. Calcium channel blockers for cardiovascular disorders. *Arch. Intern. Med.* 142:452, 1982.
13. Kawada, M., Satoh, K. and Taira, N. Profile of coronary vasodilator and cardiac actions of bepridil revealed by use of isolated, blood-perfused heart preparations of the dog. *J. Cardiovasc. Pharmacol.* 5:506, 1983.
14. Kimura, E. and Kishida, H. Treatment of variant angina with drugs: A survey of 11 cardiology institutes in Japan. *Circulation* 63:844, 1981.
15. Krantz, J.C., Jr. Historical background. In: *Organic Nitrates* (Needleman, P., ed.). Handbuch der Experimentellen Pharmakologie, Vol. 40, Springer-Verlag, Berlin, 1975, p. 1.
16. Kukovetz, W.R., Holzman, S., Wurm, A. and Poch, G. Evidence for cyclic GMP-mediated relaxant effects of nitro-compounds in coronary smooth muscle. *Naunyn-Schmiedeberg's Arch. Pharmacol.* 310:129, 1979.
17. Lydtin, H., Lohmoller, G., Lohmoller, R., Schmintz, H. and Walter, I. Comparative hemodynamic studies with adalat and other antianginal drugs. In: *The Third International Adalat Symposium* (Jatene, A.D. and Lictlen, P.R., eds.). Excerpta Medica, Amsterdam, 1976, p. 98.
18. Nakamura, M. and Koiwaya, Y. Effect of diltiazem on recurrent spontaneous angina after acute myocardial infarction. *Circ. Res. (Suppl. I)* 52:158, 1983.
19. Narahara, K.A., Shapiro, W., Weliky, I. and Park, J. Evaluation of bepridil, a new antianginal agent: Clinical and hemodynamic alterations during the treatment of stable angina pectoris. *Am. J. Cardiol.* 53:29, 1984.
20. Opie, L.H. Drugs and the heart: I. Beta-blocking agents. *Lancet* 1:693, 1980.
21. Opie, L.H. Drugs and the heart: II. Nitrates. *Lancet* 1:750, 1980.
22. Opie, L.H. Drugs and the heart: III. Calcium antagonists. *Lancet* 1:806, 1980.
23. Robinson, B.F. Relation of heart rate and systolic blood pressure to the onset of pain in angina pectoris. *Circulation* 35:1073, 1967.
24. Ross, G. and Jorgensen, C.R. Cardiovascular action of iproveratril. *J. Pharmacol. Exp. Ther.* 158:504, 1967.
25. Singh, B.N., Ellrodt, G. and Peter, C.T. Verapamil: A review of its pharmacological and therapeutic use. *Drugs* 15:169, 1978.
26. Stone, P.H., Antman, E.M., Muller, J.E. and Braunwald, E. Calcium channel blocking agents in the treatment of cardiovascular disorders. Part II: Hemodynamic effects and clinical applications. *Ann. Intern. Med. 93:886, 1980.*
27. Stone, P.H., Muller, J.E., Turi, Z.G., Geltman, E., Jaffe, A.S. and Braunwald, E. Efficacy of nifedipine therapy in patients with refractory angina pectoris: Significance of the presence of coronary vasospasm. *Am. Heart J.* 106:644, 1983.
28. Winbury, M.M., Howe, B.B. and Hefner, M.A. Effect of nitrates and other coronary dilators on large and small coronary vessels: A hypothesis for the mechanism of action of nitrates. *J. Pharmacol. Exp. Ther.* 168:70, 1969.
29. Zsoter, T.T., Henein, N.F. and Wolchinsky, C. The effect of sodium nitroprusside on the uptake and efflux of ^{45}Ca from rabbit and rat vessels. *Eur. J. Pharmacol* 45:7, 1977.

CHAPTER
15.5

MANAGEMENT OF HYPERLIPOPROTEINEMIA

Donald B. Hunninghake, David J. Gordon, Israel Tamir and Basil M. Rifkind

LIPIDS AND LIPOPROTEINS

Lipids. Lipids are nonpolar compounds with metabolic and structural roles in living cells. *Fatty acids*, both unesterified and in the form of mono-, di-, and triesters of glycerol, are the major form of energy storage in humans and comprise approximately 40% of the average American's dietary caloric intake. Phospholipids, consisting of phosphatidic acid and its derivatives, are the structural basis of the lipid bilayer, which is ubiquitous in the membranes of all cells and cellular organelles. *Cholesterol* is the parent compound of the steroid hormones and, with its fatty acid esters, is an important structural component of plasma membrane.

Lipids are derived from both exogenous and endogenous sources in humans. Dietary triglycerides are hydrolyzed to monoglycerides and free fatty acids by pancreatic lipase in the intestinal lumen. Following absorption into the mucosal cells, reesterification occurs, and the newly formed triglycerides are carried by the lymph and then by the blood to tissues throughout the body, where they are metabolized or stored. In addition, synthesis of fatty acids from acetyl coenzyme A is carried out in the liver and other tissues.

The average American ingests about 450 mg/day of cholesterol; an additional 500-1000 mg/day is synthesized *de novo* in the liver and other tissues. Unlike the other lipids, which are completely catabolized to carbon dioxide and water, the end products of cholesterol catabolism are the bile acids, which are excreted into the gut, where they undergo cyclic absorption and excretion (the enterohepatic circulation), and only a small fraction is eliminated in the feces. Some cholesterol is also excreted unchanged by the liver into the enterohepatic circulation. The remaining excretion of cholesterol occurs via the shedding of epithelial cells from the gut and skin.

Lipoproteins. The aqueous insolubility of lipids requires biological mechanisms for transporting them from their sites of absorption and synthesis to the tissues where they are utilized. In humans, this is accomplished by the packaging of lipids with specific proteins (apoproteins A, B, C, D, and E) in macromolecular complexes called lipoproteins (Table 15.5-1, Fig. 15.5-1). In normal postprandial plasma, four major classes of lipoprotein can be identified by either ultracentrifugation or electrophoresis (Fig. 15.5-2). These are *high-density or α-lipoprotein* (HDL), *low-density or β-lipoprotein* (LDL), *very-low-density or pre-β lipoprotein* (VLDL), and *chylomicrons*. A fifth class, *intermediate-density lipoprotein* (IDL), has a short plasma half-life. It is present in normal plasma in only small quantities and is not routinely measured.

Table 15.5-1
The Lipoprotein Classes and Their Composition

Ultracentrifugal Classification	Density (g/cm^3)	Electrophoretic Mobility	Composition (%)			
			Cholesterol	Triglycerides	Phospholipids	Apoproteins
HDL	1.063-1.21	α	20	<2	30	50 (Apo A, C, D, E)
LDL	1.019-1.063	β	40-45	5-10	20-25	25 (Apo B)
IDL	1.006-1.019	β	30-35	35-40	15-20	15 (Apo B, C, E)
VLDL	0.95-1.006	pre-β	10-15	60-70	10-15	10 (Apo C, B, E)
Chylomicrons	<0.95	0	2-5	85-95	3-10	1-2 (Apo C, B, A)

Chylomicrons are the triglyceride-rich lipoproteins that transport dietary fat from the gut. Their triglyceride is hydrolyzed in the plasma by extrahepatic lipoprotein lipase. The metabolic fate of their lipoprotein remnants is incompletely understood; however, much of their apoprotein A passes to the HDL fraction. Chylomicrons are normally not present in the plasma of subjects who have fasted for 12 hours or more.

VLDL is synthesized primarily in the liver as a vehicle for endogenous lipids. Its content of triglyceride is five times its content of cholesterol, and it contains apoproteins B, C, and E. As its triglyceride content is progressively depleted by the action of extrahepatic lipoprotein lipase, it loses its apoproteins C and

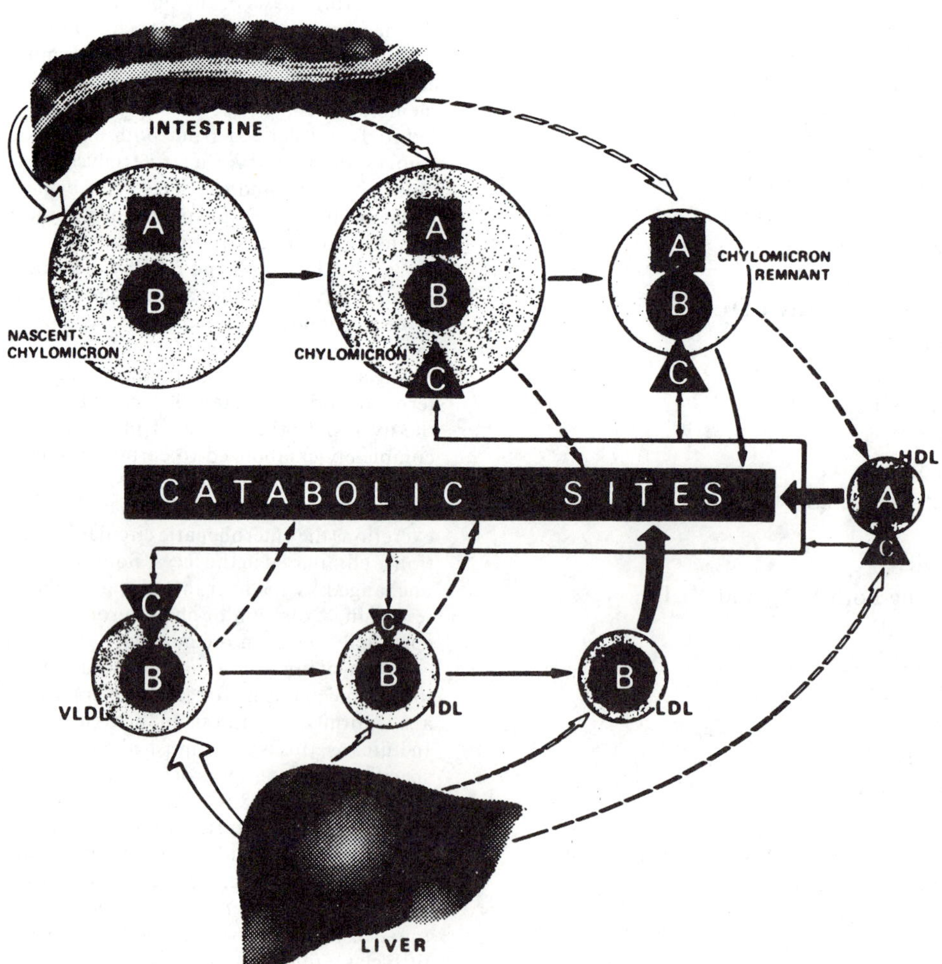

Fig. 15.5-1. *Schematic diagram of metabolism of lipoproteins and their major apoproteins (A, B, and C).* Dashed lines represent pathways that are not well defined experimentally. (From Ref. 46).

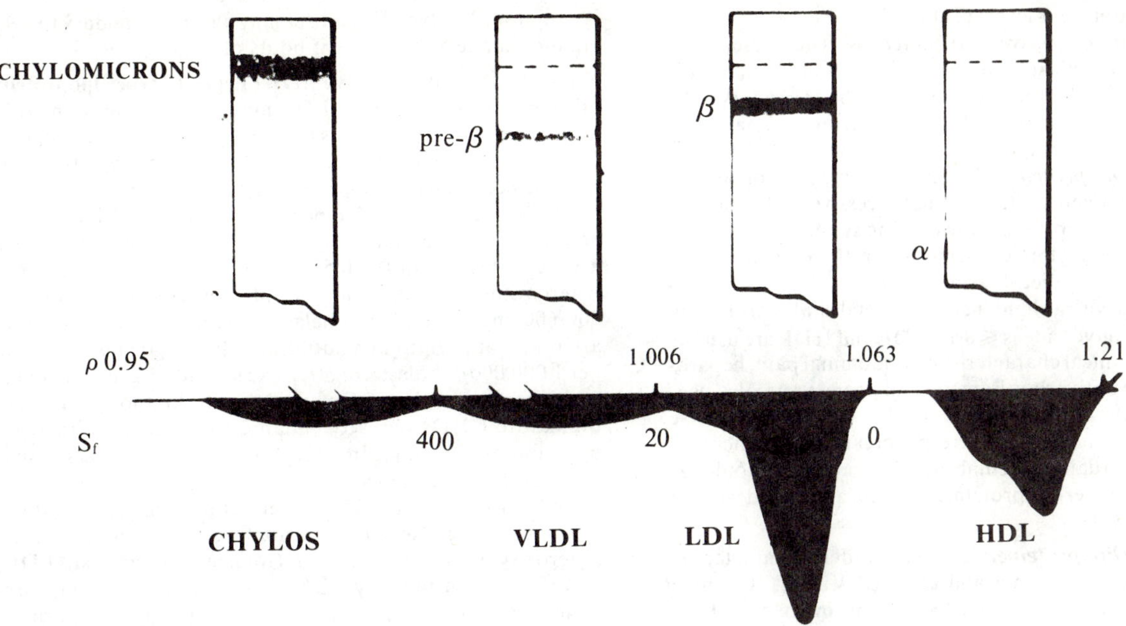

Fig. 15.5-2. *The lipoproteins.* Four classes of lipoprotein are distinguishable by ultracentrifugation of normal, postprandial plasma or serum. The electrophoretic mobility of each of these lipoprotein classes is displayed in the top half of the figure.

E to the HDL fraction and finally becomes LDL, a complex consisting primarily of cholesterol, phospholipid, and apoprotein B. IDL is the intermediate stage in this process. LDL is metabolized in the liver and in peripheral tissues and may accumulate in fatty deposits in fibrous tissues such as skin and tendons (xanthomata) and arterial walls (atherosclerotic plaques). Excessive levels of circulating LDL are known to be associated with a high incidence of coronary heart disease (CHD) and are a causal factor in the development of atherosclerosis (31, 34, 35).

HDL is a heterogeneous, relatively lipid-poor group of lipoprotein particles. At least three density subclasses of HDL exist ($HDL_{1, 2,}$ and $_3$), and further subdivisions are being made. The metabolic roles of HDL are poorly understood, but an inverse relationship has been demonstrated between HDL and CHD in prospective epidemiological studies (18). It is not known whether some component of HDL plays a direct protective role (e.g., by preventing deposition of cholesterol in arterial walls or by facilitating its removal) or whether an individual's HDL level is simply an indicator of the adequacy of his lipoprotein turnover. Preliminary evidence suggests that the beneficial effect may be associated with the HDL_2 subfraction. Although there is an inverse relationship between HDL levels and CHD incidence in prospective studies, conclusive evidence that increasing the plasma HDL levels is associated with a decreased incidence of CHD is lacking. Recent studies suggest that increasing the HDL or the ratio of HDL to either total or LDL cholesterol may be beneficial (5, 32); however, additional confirmation is required. Because of this uncertainty and because of the heterogeneity of HDL, therapeutic agents are not used for the sole purpose of increasing circulating HDL levels. (No suitable agent of this sort presently exists.) On the other hand, one would hesitate to employ a lipid-lowering drug that significantly lowers HDL cholesterol levels.

DISORDERS OF LIPID AND LIPOPROTEIN METABOLISM

General Comments. In clinical practice, the terms *hyperlipidemia* and *hyperlipoproteinemia* generally refer to lipid and lipoprotein levels above the ninty-fifth percentile for the population. An important question in a patient with elevated plasma lipids is, how are these lipids distributed in the lipoproteins? In 1967, Fredrickson et al. (16) introduced a system for classification of the hyperlipoproteinemias that was adopted by the World Health Organization (2) with minor modifications (Table 15.5-2). Judicious application of this system can greatly clarify diagnosis and rationalize the therapeutic approach. Although definitive classification requires the use of sophisticated techniques, inspection of plasma or serum that has been left undisturbed in the refrigerator overnight can provide useful diagnostic clues. Chylomicrons, when present, float to the top to form a "creamy" layer. High levels of VLDL impart overall turbidity to the sample. However, high levels of LDL are not detectable by inspection in this manner.

Hyperlipoproteinemia refers to lipoprotein patterns that are common to various underlying disorders and not disease entities attributable to well-characterized genetic and/or biochemical defects. A clear distinction has to be made between *primary* and *secondary* hyperlipoproteinemia (Table 15.5-2). Treatment of secondary hyperlipoproteinemia is aimed at the underlying disease, and it is the nature of this disease that determines the prognosis. In these cases, specific measures to lower circulating lipid levels are generally unnecessary. On the other hand, in primary hyperlipoproteinemia the prognosis of the patient depends on the sequelae of the disorder of lipid/lipoprotein metabolism, such as acceleration of atherosclerosis (types II, III, and IV) or pancreatitis (types I and V), and the aim of treatment is to prevent these sequelae by normalizing circulating lipid and lipoprotein levels (Table 15.5-3).

Disorders with Excessive Chylomicrons. The presence of chylomicrons in the plasma of fasting ($>$ 12 hours) subjects is always abnormal. Chylomicronemia may be secondary to a variety of underlying diseases (Table 15.5-2) and is a hallmark of two patterns of hyperlipoproteinemia (types I and V).

Type I Hyperlipoproteinemia. This rare lipoprotein pattern is usually due to a genetic (autosomal recessive) deficiency of the extrahepatic lipoprotein lipase enzyme system. It is characterized by massive chylomicronemia when the patient is on a normal fat-containing diet. Plasma triglyceride levels are enormously increased with a slight increase in total cholesterol (ratio of cholesterol/triglyceride is $\leqslant 0.1$). LDL and HDL are usually decreased. The clinical characteristics, abdominal pain, hepatosplenomegaly, eruptive xanthomata, and lipemia retinalis, usually appear by the second decade of life. The clinical course features recurrent bouts of severe pancreatitis, to which the patient may eventually succumb if not treated. It should be noted that type I hyperlipoproteinemia is *not* associated with an excess risk of CHD.

Type V Hyperlipoproteinemia. This disorder is characterized by fasting chylomicronemia and elevated VLDL. It is most frequently found as a secondary hyperlipoproteinemia (Table 15.5-2); but in some cases no underlying disorder can be found, and the abnormality is considered primary. The mode of inheritance is probably autosomal dominant, but the underlying metabolic defect is unknown. The type V disorder may be associated with an increased risk for CHD.

The clinical manifestations are similar to type I except that they usually present in adulthood. A high proportion of type V patients (25%) are obese with abnormal glucose tolerance, and a family history of hyperuricemia and carbohydrate intolerance is common. The type V disorder may also be secondary to heavy ethanol intake and recurrent bouts of pancreatitis.

Disorders with Excessive LDL (Type II Hyperlipoproteinemia). Elevation of plasma LDL may occur without any other abnormality in lipoproteins (type IIa) or may be accompanied by an increase in plasma VLDL (type IIb). The type II patterns may be secondary to a variety of causes (Table 15.5-2). The genetic form, or familial hypercholesterolemia (FHC), is characterized by an autosomal dominant mode of inheritance, with a gene frequency of 0.1-0.5% of the population (17). Among heterozygotes, plasma cholesterol is usually in the range of 300-600 mg/dl, and xanthelasma, xanthomata and corneal arcus may appear in early adulthood. In the rare homozygote (1 per 1,000,000), cholesterol often exceeds 800 mg/dl, and tendon and tuberous xanthomata may appear in childhood. The risk of premature CHD is greatly enhanced in patients with type II hyperlipoproteinemia. In FHC homozygotes, CHD is usually manifest before adolescence.

Cellular uptake of LDL is essential not only for its efficient catabolism, but also for regulation of several key steps in cholesterol synthesis. Brown and Goldstein found that LDL is bound to cell surfaces by LDL receptors that are along the cell membrane in coated pits that eventually pinch off to form sacs called coated vesicles. LDL bound in a coated vesicle is eventually deliver to lysosomes that then liberate the cholesterol from the LDL for cell use (6, 17). Thus, a defective receptor mechanism may led to accumulation of excessive levels of circulating LDL by slowing its catabolism and by interfering with the normal controls of cholesterol synthesis. FHC homozygotes lack functional receptors, whereas heterozygotes have one normal and one mutant receptor gene and can bind circulating LDL at

Table 15.5-2
Hyperlipoproteinemia: Definitions and Secondary Causes

	Lipid Criteria[a]			
Type	Cholesterol	Triglycerides	Lipoprotein Criteria	Secondary Causes of Hyperlipoproteinemia
I	0 or ↑	↑↑↑	Chylomicrons ↑↑↑	Systemic lupus erythematosus, dysgammaglobulinemias, diabetic ketoacidosis (all rarely)
IIa	↑ to ↑↑↑	0	LDL ↑ to ↑↑↑	Hypothyroidism, nephrotic syndrome, hepatic disease, dysgammaglobulinemias, acute porphyria, excess of dietary cholesterol and saturated fat
IIb	↑ to ↑↑↑	↑	LDL ↑ to ↑↑↑, VLDL ↑	
III	↑ to ↑↑	↑ to ↑↑	Presence of IDL (floating β)	Hypothyroidism, diabetes mellitus, obesity
IV	0 to ↑	↑ to ↑↑	VLDL ↑ to ↑↑↑	Excessive alcohol intake, diabetes mellitus, hypothyroidism, nephrotic syndrome, uremia, exogenous estrogens and progestins, pregnancy, exogenous corticosteroids, pancreatitis, storage diseases, dysproteinemias, systemic lupus erythematosus, recent myocardial infarction
V	↑ to ↑↑	↑↑↑	Chylomicrons ↑↑ VLDL ↑↑↑	Excessive alcohol intake, diabetes mellitus, hypothyroidism (rarely), nephrotic syndrome (rarely), exogenous estrogens and progestins (in primary type IV), pregnancy (in primary type IV), pancreatitis, glycogen storage disease, dysproteinemias, systemic lupus erythematosus

[a] 0 = normal levels; ↑ = slight elevation; ↑↑ = moderate elevation; ↑↑↑ = extreme elevation.

Table 15.5-3
Characteristics and Treatment of Hyperlipoproteinemia

Type	Clinical Features	Diet[a]	Preferred Drugs
I.	Abdominal pain, pancreatitis, hepatosplenomegaly, eruptive xanthomata, lipemia retinalis	Fat restriction; no alcohol	None
II.	Premature cardiovascular disease, tendinous and cutaneous xanthomata, xanthelasma; in type IIb disorder, obesity and glucose intolerance are common	Cholesterol and saturated fat restriction; caloric restriction, if appropriate	Cholestyramine; colestipol; nicotinic acid; (probucol and gemfibrozil are also used)
III.	Planar, tuberoeruptive, and other xanthomata, premature cardiovascular disease, obesity, hyperuricemia, glucose intolerance	Caloric and alcohol restriction	Clofibrate; gemfibrozil; nicotinic acid
IV.	Obesity, hyperuricemia, glucose intolerance, premature cardiovascular disease, eruptive xanthomata (rare)	Calorie restriction; alcohol restriction	Nicotinic acid; gemfibrozil; clofibrate
V.	Abdominal pain, pancreatitis, hepatosplenomegaly, premature cardiovascular disease, eruptive xanthomata, lipemia retinalis, obesity, hyperuricemia, glucose intolerance, peripheral neuropathy	Fat restriction; calorie restriction; no alcohol	Nicotinic acid; gemfibrozil; clofibrate

[a] Note that the current recommendation of the American Heart Association is a single diet for the treatment of all hyperlipoproteinemias (42). The features of this diet that are probably most important for the individual lipoprotein disorder are highlighted.

approximately half the normal rate. It should be noted that although there are defective LDL receptors in FHC, it has not been shown that this is the only biochemical defect in this disorder. LDL-receptor assays are not currently available for routine laboratory use.

Disorders with Abnormal IDL (Type III Hyperlipoproteinemia). Type III hyperlipoproteinemia is an uncommon disorder characterized by the presence in plasma of an abnormal LDL (often termed *floating β-lipoprotein*) with the electrophoretic mobility of LDL and the flotation characteristics of VLDL. Plasma levels of cholesterol and triglycerides are elevated due to the accumulation of remnant particles derived from the partial catabolism of VLDL and chylomicrons. Apoprotein E interacts with receptors that promote the uptake of remnant particles, and patients with the type III defect lack one component of the arginine-rich apoprotein E. The genetics of this disorder indicate a recessive mode of inheritance, but there are multiple alleles (7).

Clinically, type III hyperlipoproteinemia rarely presents before adulthood. Like many other lipoprotein disorders, it is frequently associated with obesity, glucose intolerance, and hyperuricemia, and often manifests itself by xanthomata, corneal arcus, and premature cardiovascular disease. However, the homozygous type III disorder has several clinical features that distinguish it from other lipoprotein disorders. Most striking are the peculiar yellow discoloration of the palmar creases (xanthoma striata palmaris) and tuberoeruptive xanthomas, which are virtually pathognomonic of type III hyperlipoproteinemia. Another distinctive feature is the tendency for the peripheral vasculature to be most affected by premature atherosclerosis.

Disorders with Excessive VLDL (Type IV Hyperlipoproteinemia). The type IV pattern is characterized by elevation in the concentration of endogenously synthesized triglyceride, which is transported in VLDL. It is a common and easily diagnosed disorder. The diagnosis is based on the presence of normal or near-normal plasma cholesterol levels and raised plasma triglyceride levels in the absence of chylomicrons or IDL.

Type IV hyperlipoproteinemia may be a secondary manifestation of many disorders and is most prevalent in women taking oral contraceptives. The primary form, inherited along autosomal dominant lines, shows late penetrance and is encountered only infrequently in childhood. Affected patients are usually obese and often show glucose intolerance. Although premature CHD frequently accompanies this disorder, it should be noted that prospective studies have generally failed to establish VLDL or triglyceride levels as *independent* coronary risk factors.

TREATMENT OF HYPERLIPOPROTEINEMIA

General Considerations. In the great majority of cases, hyperlipoproteinemia represents neither a discrete disease nor a group of diseases, but rather one end of a continuous distribution associated with a gradually increasing risk of cardiovascular disease. Therefore, the treatment of hyperlipoproteinemia is often not an effort to reverse a known established pathological process; it is an attempt to prevent not yet manifest CHD in a patient identified to be at high risk for that disease.

The results of the recently reported Lipid Research Clinics Coronary Primary Prevention Trial, coupled with previous information from a variety of cholesterol-lowering studies, provide clear evidence of the benefit of cholesterol (LDL) lowering in terms of preventing or delaying CHD morbidity and mortality (34, 35). This study, which was conducted in middle-aged, hypercholesterolemic males with no clinical evidence of CHD, demonstrated that a 1% reduction in cholesterol was associated with a 2% reduction in CHD risk. Evidence is also accumulating that cholesterol (LDL) lowering is of benefit for secondary prevention (5, 32).

The American Heart Association has issued preliminary guidelines for the management of hyperlipidemia (42). A Cholesterol Consensus Conference held at the National Institutes of Health in December, 1984 defined moderate risk cholesterol levels as the 75th percentile and high risk as the 90th percentile. Dietary therapy is always the first mode of treatment for all lipoprotein disorders and must be continued even if drug therapy is initiated. Cholesterol (LDL) lowering drugs are used as either primary or secondary preventive measures in terms of preventing or delaying the vascular complications of atherosclerosis. Reduction or prevention of recurring attacks of abdominal pain and pancreatitis may occur in patients with marked hypertriglyceridemia when these levels are reduced. Reduction in size or disappearance of xanthomas may provide cosmetic, psychological, or functional benefit. For example, drug therapy may yield prompt symptomatic improvement (resolution of xanthomata) in type III hyperlipoproteinemia.

The dose and specific drug used to treat the lipid disorder must take into account many diverse factors, including the lipoprotein pattern, cost, and availability of long-term safety data. In a particular patient, efficacy and side effects of the available drugs, the presence or absence of other metabolic disorders (e.g., diabetes, gout), and the motivation of the patient to embark on what is likely to be a lifelong therapeutic regimen must also be assessed. Because of the complexity of these factors and the incompleteness of our knowledge, lipid-lowering drugs are frequently prescribed inappropriately, a practice which we hope our readers will take care to avoid.

LIPID-LOWERING DRUGS

The lipid-lowering drugs may be conveniently divided into those whose primary effect is on LDL (mostly cholesterol), those primarily affecting VLDL (mostly triglyceride), and those affecting both of these lipoproteins (25). Although some of these drugs also affect HDL levels, no drug has been introduced specifically for this purpose and, for reasons described earlier, the clinical implications of these effects are not known.

DRUGS AFFECTING PRIMARILY LDL

CHOLESTYRAMINE

Cholestyramine was initially introduced in the early 1960s as a palliative treatment for patients with severe itching due to cholestatic jaundice. The incidental finding of marked reduction of serum cholesterol levels in these patients led to the application of this drug to the treatment of hypercholesterolemia. The efficacy, reliability, and specificity of this drug in reducing circulating levels of LDL-cholesterol have made cholesterol lowering its most important clinical application. Cholestyramine was used in the Lipid Research Clinics Study which documented that cholesterol (LDL) lowering reduced the risk for CHD.

Mechanism of Action. Cholestyramine is a high-molecular-weight polymeric resin containing quaternary ammonium groups that is not absorbed from the gut. The liver converts cholesterol to bile acids. Cholestyramine binds and prevents the absorption of bile acids and other anions from the gut (Fig. 15.5-3), by interrupting the enterohepatic circulation of bile acids and increases fecal excretion of bile acids by as much as 30-fold. Despite a compensatory increase in the rate of hepatic cholesterol synthesis, there is a net decrease in hepatic cholesterol that stimulates the production of LDL receptors by liver cells. This results in an increased rate of uptake and catabolism of LDL, with a decrease in circulating LDL levels.

Cholestyramine's major effect is to decrease the LDL fraction and increase the rate of cholesterol and LDL catabolism, and is primarily used for the treatment of type IIa hyperlipoproteinemia. Its action effectively complements the restriction of dietary cholesterol and saturated fat intake and the suppression of endogenous cholesterol synthesis produced by drugs such as nicotinic acid (see below). The combination of diet, cholestyramine, and nicotinic acid has been used frequently in FHC to obtain better results than could be with any of these regimens alone.

Cholestyramine also tends to raise HDL levels slightly. This effect is variable, but may be of some clinical importance (5, 32). Cholestyramine is not a useful drug in types III, IV, and V hyperlipoproteinemia because it frequently exacerbates hypertriglyceridemia. There is usually only a minor and variable increase in plasma triglycerides in the type IIa disorder; greater increases in triglycerides are more often seen in the type IIb disorder.

Administration and Dosage. Cholestyramine (QUESTRAN) is a hygroscopic, insoluble powder. It is usually provided in packets containing 4 g of the drug and 5 g of inert filler and weak orange flavoring for palatability. It is also available in bulk cans (QUESTRAN represents a distinct advantage in palatability over the earlier preparation, CUEMID, which had a strong fishy odor). Each packet is suspended in 2-4 oz of liquid (usually water or unsweetened juice) prior to ingestion. The adult dosage may be pushed as high as 32 g/day, but 24 g/day is a more typical tolerance limit. The average fall in total plasma cholesterol at this dosage is 20-25%, or a 25-30% in LDL-cholesterol. In children with FHC, the typical daily dose is 250-800 mg/kg.

Optimal cholesterol lowering is achieved by administration in at least two divided doses before meals. There is no demonstrable difference between a b.i.d. and q.i.d. regimen. Most patients elect a twice-daily schedule, but

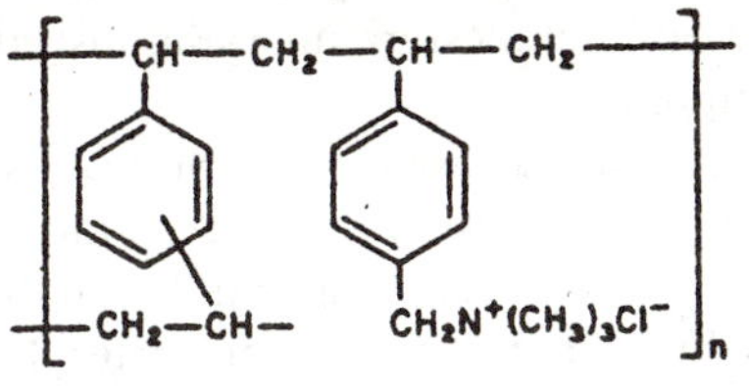

Cholestyramine resin

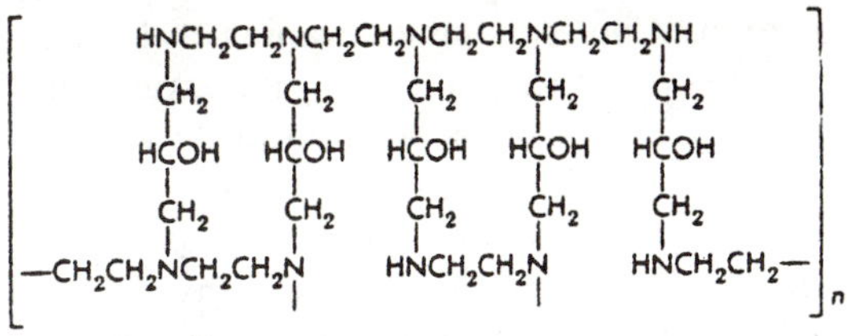

Colestipol

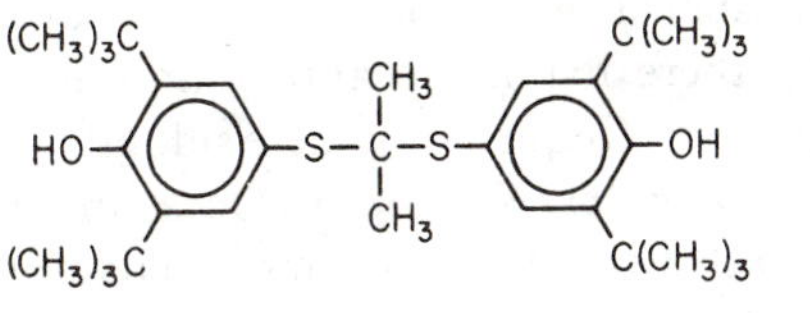

Probucol

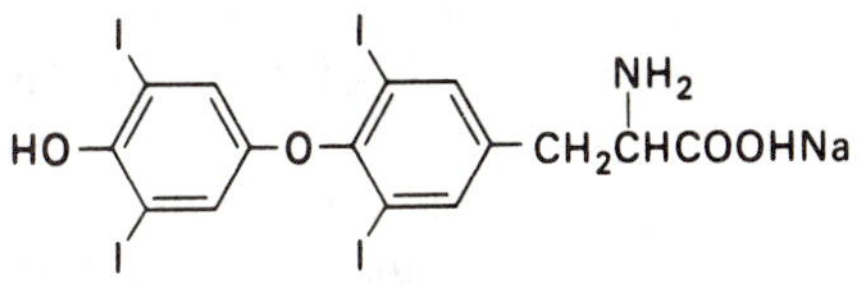

Dextrothyroxine sodium

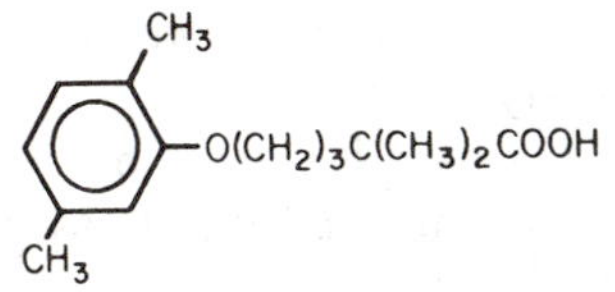

Gemfibrozil

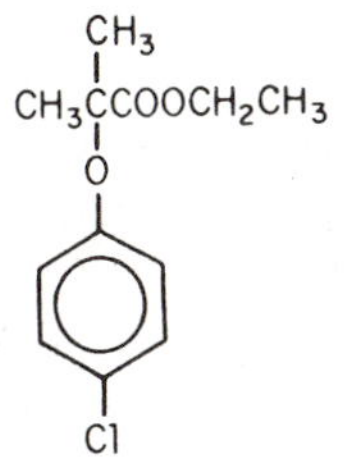

Clofibrate

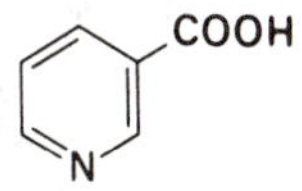

Niacin (nicotinic acid)

Fig. 15.5-3. *Chemical structures of hypolipidemic drugs.*

some patients prefer more frequent administration to decrease the volume ingested per dose.

Adverse Effects. Due to its nonabsorption from the gut, cholestyramine is relatively free of serious effects. Its known side effects relate mainly to the gastrointestinal system. Although these side effects are usually minor from the medical standpoint, they may interfere with drug adherence and must therefore be taken seriously.

Nonspecific Gastrointestinal Symptoms. The most common gastrointestinal side effect is constipation. Cholestyramine-induced constipation is usually alleviated by increased fluid intake, increased dietary fiber, and judicious use of stool softeners. If the patient has significant constipation, the patient should first be permitted to develop tolerance to a low dose of resin, and then the dosage of resin can be slowly increased.

Upper gastrointestinal symptoms, suh as nausea, gas, belching, or bloating and heartburn are not uncommon. Often these complaints are referable to the resin's bulkiness and marginal palatability. In such cases, modifying the flavoring or volume of the fluid vehicle, ingesting more slowly, and taking care to avoid excessive aeration in mixing the medication may alleviate these symptoms.

Malabsorption. Cholestyramine has occasionally been reported to interfere with the absorption of dietary fats, lipid-soluble vitamins (especially A, D, K), iron, calcium, and folate (23, 25). These effects are rarely (if ever) seen in the adult with uncomplicated type II hyperlipoproteinemia, but may occur in individuals with severe liver or small bowel disease. Children may also be more susceptible to these effects. Children and patients with malabsorption must be monitored, and administration of appropriate vitamins and mineral supplements may be required.

Adverse Effects in Pediatric Patients. As the drug of choice in FHC, cholestyramine is often administered to children and adolescents, in whom there may be special problems in addition to the potential for vitamin and mineral deficiency. Cholestyramine contains a large chloride load and may induce hyperchloremic acidosis. Large and sustained elevations in serum alkaline phosphatase and decreased serum folate levels have also been reported in children receiving this drug.

Gallstones. The effect of cholestyramine on biliary composition and stone formation is controversial. Animal studies have yielded conflicting results, and no lithogenic effect has been demonstrated in humans.

Miscellaneous. Cholestyramine administration is associated with mild increases in alkaline phosphatase, SGOT, and chloride and decreases in uric acid and serum carotenoids. The physiological mechanisms involved are not completely understood, and their clinical significance is not apparent. To date, no difference has been observed in the malignancy rates of cholestyramine and placebo-treated Lipid Research Clinic participants to date.

Drug Interactions. Cholestyramine, an anion exchange resin, can interfere with the absorption of a variety of anionic drugs (23). Drugs whose absorption has been shown to be altered by cholestyramine administration include cardiac glycosides, coumarin derivatives, β-adrenergic blockers, thiazide diuretics, and thyroxine; these drugs are also frequently used by potential candidates for cholestyramine therapy. Separating the time of administration of the resin and the concomitant drugs may minimize this interaction. However, a significant decrease in the absorption of drugs such as digitoxin, thyroxine, and the thiazides may still occur. The available information on drug interactions associated with cholestyramine usage should be reviewed and one must be prepared to make appropriate adjustments in the dosage of these drugs.

Contraindications. Cholestyramine is useful only in patients with type II hyperlipoproteinemia (mainly type IIa): it is ineffective and perhaps deleterious in other lipid disorders. It is poorly tolerated in patients with active gastrointestinal inflammation or with symptomatic anal disease (fissures, inflamed or bleeding hemorrhoids). In children and in patients with malabsorption due to gastrointestinal disease or surgery, nutritional status should be carefully monitored and supplemented as needed. Serum chloride should be monitored in pediatric patients and in patients with renal disease.

In summary, cholestyramine is presently a drug of choice in type II hyperlipoproteinemia. Its chief drawback is the reluctance of patients to take it because of its bulkiness, marginal palatability, and gastrointestinal side effects. Also, it is quite expensive. The drug will not be effective in an unmotivated or unreliable patient or in the hands of an impatient physician. Efforts to achieve good adherence should be made because cholestyramine has been shown to reduce the risk of myocardial infarction in hypercholesterolemic but otherwise healthy middle-aged men in the Lipid Research Clinics' Coronary Primary Prevention Trial (34, 35).

COLESTIPOL

Colestipol (COLESTID) is a more recently introduced bile acid sequestrant with essentially the same mechanism of action and side effects as cholestyramine (Fig. 15.5-3). This discussion will focus primarily on any known differences from cholestyramine.

Mechanisms of Action. Colestipol is also a high-molecular-weight anion exchange resin that interrupts the enterohepatic circulation of bile acids and increases cholesterol and LDL catabolism. Presumably, there is also an increase in the number of hepatic LDL receptors and increased hepatic LDL uptake and catabolism as reported with cholestyramine. The currently available preparation is not absorbed from the gut, and its main indication is type II hyperlipoproteinemia. It would appear that one can directly extrapolate the reduction in CHD risk produced by cholestyramine administration to the use of colestipol .

Dosage and Administration. Colestipol (COLESTID) is an insoluble, unflavored powder that is generally administered in either water or juice. It is available in individual packets (5 g) or bulk container. The cholesterol (LDL) lowering effect of 5 g of colestipol is equivalent to that produced by 4 g of cholestyramine (9 g with filler).

Adverse Effects. Colestipol has not been evaluated in a large, long-term trial such as was conducted with cholestyramine (34, 35), but there do not appear to be any major differences in the nature or frequency of these side effects.

Nonspecific Gastrointestinal Symptoms. Occasionally a patient may find one of the two resins more palatable than the other. No definite decrease in the incidence of upper gastrointestinal complaints has been reported with colestipol. However, colestipol does have antacid properties, and the total volume of resin that is administered is less than with cholestyramine

Malabsorption. No specific reports of malabsorption have occurred, but the same precautions as indicated for cholestyramine should be followed.

Drug Interaction. This is an area that requires further evaluation, and there may be some differences between colestipol and cholestyramine (23). Colestipol is a less highly charged molecule (mostly tertiary amines) than is cholestyramine and also has some antacid effect. The available data are not definitive, but suggest that colestipol interferes less than cholestyramine with the absorption of other drugs such as the thiazides. There may also be less need to separate the time of administration of other drugs when colestipol is substituted for cholestyramine.

Other. All of the comments regarding contraindications, precaution in children, and effects on laboratory tests that were made for cholestyramine appear to be applicable to colestipol.

DEXTROTHYROXINE

Dextrothyroxine (CHOLOXIN) is the sodium salt of the dextrorotatory optical isomer of naturally occurring thyroxine (Fig. 15.5-3). Its introduction as a lipid-lowering agent stemmed from the clinical observation that plasma cholesterol levels are inversely related to circulating levels of thyroid hormone. The dextrorotatory isomer shared the lipid-lowering activity of the natural hormone, with less tendency to produce a hypermetabolic state.

Mechanism of Action. Unlike the drugs previously discussed, dextrothyroxine is well absorbed from the gut, and its action is systemic. The best available evidence is that the drug, like the natural hormone, lowers plasma cholesterol primarily by enhancing LDL catabolism in the liver. Both isomers of thyroxine also enhance hepatic cholesterol synthesis, but not sufficiently to offset the increased catabolism. A 10-15% reduction in plasma cholesterol and LDL may be expected (3). There is usually no change or a modest reduction in plasma triglyceride levels.

Administration and Dosage. CHOLOXIN has been contaminated by varying amounts of the levorotatory isomer in the past but currently is stated to contain less than 0.5%. Dextrothyroxine has a plasma half-life approximating 24-36 hours which is significantly shorter than the levorotatory isomer. It is available in 1-, 2-, 4-, and 6-mg tablets. The initial dose is 1-2 mg/day and is increased slowly (no greater than a 1 mg/day increment each month) until an optimal dosage is reached. The single daily dose is a convenient schedule. Although the optimal adult dosage is 4-8 mg/day, this dosage may be excessive. Recent studies indicate that complete suppression of the hypophyseal-pituitary axis is usually achieved with daily dosages of 3-4 mg in adults. The drug is not recommended in children.

Adverse Effect. The clinical usefulness of dextrothyroxine is limited by its potentially adverse effects, as demonstrated by the experience of the Coronary Drug Project (10). In this study, the group receiving this drug showed an excess incidence (relative to the placebo group) of nonfatal myocardial infarction, a finding which necessitated terminating treatment of these patients. The drug was also associated with an excess incidence of cardiac arrhythmias, particularly in patients taking cardiac glycosides. These adverse effects were most marked in those patients with the most severe underlying myocardial disease at the onset of treatment. These results indicate that dextrothyroxine should not be administered to patients with myocardial disease.

About 1% of patients recieving the drug in the Coronary Drug Project developed a hypermetabolic syndrome (weight loss, sweating, shortness of breath, chest pain). Other side effects of uncertain clinical significance were sustained elevations in SGOT (serum glutamic oxaloacetic transaminase), serum bilirubin, and alkaline phosphatase, and impairment of glucose tolerance. Dextrothyroxine may also potentiate the action of the coumarin anticoagulants.

Contraindications. Dextrothyroxine is not an innocuous drug. It should be considered for use only in adult patients who are euthyroid and who are free of any indication of organic heart disease. Any history of myocardial infarction, angina pectoris, significant cardiac arrhythmias, rheumatic heart disease or congestive heart failure should be considered absolute contraindications to its use. Other contraindications include significant hypertension, advanced liver or kidney disease, pregnancy or lactation, hyperthyroidism, and history of iodism.

PROBUCOL

Probucol (LORELCO) was approved as a cholesterol-lowering drug by the FDA in 1978 (Fig. 15.5-3). Because it is relatively convenient to take and is generally well tolerated, it has become one of the more popular lipid-lowering drugs.

Mechanism of Action. Probucol is poorly absorbed from the gastrointestinal tract, but its action is systemic. The specific mechanism of action for the cholesterol-lowering effect is unknown, but may involve inhibition of endogenous cholesterol synthesis. There is no plasma accumulation of the immediate precursors of cholesterol (desmosterol and 7-dehydrocholesterol), suggesting that it must inhibit at an early step in cholesterol biosynthesis. It is highly lipid soluble and may accumulate in the various lipoproteins. Recent evidence suggests that probucol may accumulate in LDL. The biological activity of LDL is altered, and an increased rate of LDL removal occurs. Decreases of 10-20% in plasma cholesterol and LDL have been reported (1, 14), but more modest and inconsistent effects have also been observed. Probucol has no consistent effect on triglyceride levels.

However, probucol consistently lowers HDL levels (24). It appears that the reduction in HDL levels is due to decreased synthesis rather than an increased catabolic rate. Probucol may be used in combination with the bile acid sequestrants to obtain additional cholesterol lowering (14). Their action appear to be complementary.

Administration and Dosage. Probucol is available commercially as a 250-mg tablet. The usual adult dosage is 500 mg twice a day. However, the plasma half-life is on the order of weeks, and probucol may be present in the body for months after the drug is discontinued. The plasma lipid and lipoprotein values may also not return to pretreatment levels for 3-4 months after the drug is discontinued. This drug has not yet been established as safe or effective in children.

Adverse Effects. Clinical experience with this drug to date indicates no serious side effects. About 10% of patients experience diarrhea, and other gastrointestinal symptoms (i.e., flatulence, abdominal pain, nausea, vomiting) are not rare. However, these symptoms are usually mild and transient, and the vast majority of patients can tolerate the drug in the long run. Rare, idiosyncratic reactions featuring dizziness, palpitations, syncope, nausea, vomiting, and chest pain have been reported. An increased propensity to fatal ventricular arrhythmias has been observed with this drug in dogs and in monkeys, but not in its clinical use in humans. A final judgment of the safety of probucol for long-term use must await the accumulation of more clinical data. However, the long biological half-life of this drug, its HDL-lowering effect, and reports of cardiotoxicity in animals warrant some skepticism about whether long-term use of this drug is truly beneficial effect and/or long-term safety data are available for other drugs.

Contraindications. Known hypersensitivity to probucol is a contraindication.

β-SITOSTEROL

Sitosterols are plant sterols that are poorly absorbed from the gastrointestinal tract and were used as cholesterol-lowering agents. β-Sitosterol (CYTELLIN) was the most important sitosterol isomer. It was one of the earlier commercially available cholesterol-lowering drugs, but it was recently withdrawn from the market. It produced only a modest reduction in serum cholesterol, was expensive, and was used infrequently.

DRUGS AFFECTING PRIMARILY VLDL

The role of triglycerides in atherogenesis is controversial, but most studies indicate that triglycerides are not an independent risk factor for CHD. The extreme, often morbid, triglyceride elevations seen in type I or type V hyperlipoproteinemia are associated primarily with the chylomicron fraction and are best managed by dietary fat restriction. Hence, the clinical usefulness of drugs whose primary effect is to lower VLDL-triglyceride levels is limited.

CLOFIBRATE

Clofibrate is the ethyl ester of p-cholorphenoxyisobutyric acid (CPIB) (Fig. 15.5-3). It was the most effective of a series of substituted branched-chain fatty acids evaluated in the 1950s for their ability to lower serum cholesterol levels in rats. In 1962 it was reported to lower serum cholesterol and triglyceride levels, predominantly the latter, in men with CHD. Clofibrate was easy to administer and relatively inexpensive and was extensively and often uncritically prescribed. However, the evidence accumulated from two large multicenter clinical trials, the Coronary Drug Project (12) and the WHO-sponsored Clofibrate Study (8), indicated that there was significant toxicity associated with the long-term administration of clofibrate. Its use is currently limited to type III hyperlipoproteinemia, and it may be considered for use in individuals with marked hypertriglyceridemia.

Mechanism of Action. Although clofibrate has been available for many years, its pharmacological action is still poorly understood. Many mechanisms of action have been postulated, and it is possible that multiple mechanisms are involved. The proposed mechanisms have previously been extensively reviewed (25) and are only briefly and partially summarized here. They included displacement of lipid-active hormones such as thyroxine and androsterone from albumin; inhibition of lipolysis with a decrease in circulating free fatty acids; increased lipoprotein lipase activity; inhibition of VLDL synthesis and/or secretion from the liver; inhibition of hepatic cholesterol synthesis, increased conversion of VLDL to LDL, and increased cholesterol excretion.

In the Coronary Drug Project the clofibrate-treated group showed an average 6.5% reduction in serum cholesterol, as compared with 22% reduction in serum triglyceride levels (12). In the WHO study, where hypercholesterolemia was a criterion for inclusion, mean serum cholesterol reductions of 8-9% were reported (8). In patients with type III hyperlipoproteinemia and in some patients with the type II and type IV disorders, a more impressive drug response may be attained. Some patients with type IIb disorder may get a significant increase in both the total and LDL-cholesterol. Modest increases in HDL of 10-15% are noted following clofibrate administration.

Administration and Dosage. Clofibrate (ATROMID-S) is available in 500-mg capsules. The recommended adult dosage is 2 g/day, taken in two divided doses. The plasma half-life is approximately 12 hours in the adult. Clofibrate is primarily eliminated by renal excretion. The safety and efficacy of clofibrate in children and in pregnant women have not been established.

Adverse Effects. Clofibrate is very well tolerated by most patients. In the Coronary Drug Project, adherence to the drug and incidence of nonspecific symptoms in the clofibrate-treated group appeared to differ little from those in the group receiving a placebo (12). However, there were several trends in the clofibrate-treated group that were of potential concern. These included an increased incidence of pulmonary embolism, cardiac arrhythmias, angina pectoris, and nonfatal cardiovascular events. There was also an increased evidence of hepatic and splenic enlargement, abnormal liver function tests, and cholelithiasis. The latter is consistent with the known effects on biliary composition (i.e., reduction in bile acid concentration and increase in levels of biliary cholesterol). In addition, there was no significant benefit in the study either for total mortality, fatal or nonfatal myocardial infarction.

The results of the WHO study, a primary prevention trial, were also very disturbing. The clofibrate-treated group did show a 25% reduction in the incidence of nonfatal myocardial infarction relative to a comparable placebo-treated group. However, this trend was not present for fatal myocardial infarction or angina. Moreover, the clofibrate-treated group showed a significantly *higher* overall mortality rate than the placebo group. This difference was primarily attributed to elevated incidences of hepatobiliary disease (especially gallstones) and cancer. The final report on this study (9) indicates that, during the mean treatment period of 5.3 years, there was an excess mortality of 47% in the clofibrate-treated group. After an additional follow-up period of 7.9 years (13.2 years of total observation), there was an increased death rate of 11% in the clofibrate-treated group. The unexplained excess mortality occurred primarily during the period of active treatment with clofibrate.

Various nonspecific gastrointestinal complaints and skin rashes are not infrequent with clofibrate. Normally most circulating clofibrate is bound to albumin. In patients who are albumin depleted (e.g., nephrotic syndrome), high levels of free clofibrate may lead to polymyositis or lupus-like sydrome. A similar picture may be seen if the dose of clofibrate is not decreased in patients with reduced glomerular filtration. Another potential hazard of clofibrate is its potentiation of the coumarin anticoagulants, presumably by displacing them from albumin and increasing the amount of free anticoagulant. Severe ventricular arrhythmia is a very rare but serious side effect. Clofibrate has also been reported to be carcinogenic in rodents, but the implications of this finding for humans are controversial.

Contraindications. Clofibrate should not be given to pregnant or lactating women. It should be avoided in patients with significant hepatic or renal disease, particularly those with biliary cirrhosis, where the drug may further exacerbate the disease. Liver function tests should be monitored routinely in patients receiving this drug. Minimally, the dose of clofibrate must be reduced in patients with chronic renal disease.

In summary, *long-term administration of clofibrate is associated with significant toxicity, and the indications for its use are limited.* The only lipoprotein disorder where clofibrate (in combination with diet) appears to offer a consistent and marked benefit is type III hyperlipoproteinemia, where normalization of lipids and resolution of symptoms are often attainable. Clofibrate may be considered in certain patients with hypertriglyceridemia. Safer and more effective therapy is generally available for type IIa hyperlipoproteinemia.

GEMFIBROZIL

Gemfibrozil has recently been marketed in the United States. The chemical structure is depicted in Fig. 15.5-3. Its pharmacological properties, efficacy in terms of altering plasma lipids and lipoproteins, and indications for use and known drug interactions are very similar to those described for clofibrate. Only a few additional comments will be made.

Mechanism of Action. Like clofibrate, its mechanism of action has not been clearly defined. Gemfibrozil's primary effect is a reduction in plasma triglycerides and VLDL, and reductions of 40% or greater are commonly observed (15). Most studies indicate only a modest reduction in total and LDL-cholesterol ($<10\%$), but occasional studies indicate a greater effect (37). Gemfibrozil administration is also associated with a significant increase in HDL (20% or greater) that is somewhat greater than that reported with clofibrate. Again, increasing the HDL levels has not yet been demonstrated to definitely decrease the risk of CHD. The overall effect of all the plasma lipid and lipoprotein changes produced by gemfibrozil on CHD risk is currently being evaluated in a large-scale, long-term clinical trial (37, 38).

Administration and Dosage. Gemfibrozil (LOPID) is available in 300-mg capsules. The usual adult daily dose is 1.2 g/day, which is administered in a twice-daily schedule.

Adverse Effects. Gemfibrozil has few side effects and is well tolerated by most patients; abdominal discomfort, gastrointestinal complaints, and skin rashes are the most commonly encountered. A 5-year follow-up study revealed only a 6.3% dropout rate due to adverse experiences with the drug (37). The observed effects on bile composition make it theoretically less lithogenic than clofibrate, but its actual effect on the incidence of gallstones has yet to be established in practice. Long-term safety data or adverse experience information on a large number of patients, as are available for clofibrate, are currently unavailable. This information is being obtained in a long-term prospective clinical trial (37, 38).

Contraindications. Contraindications are probably similar to those for clofibrate and include severe renal or hepatic dysfunction (including primary biliary disease), preexisting gallbladder disease, and hypersensitivity to gemfibrozil.

DRUGS AFFECTING BOTH LDL AND VLDL

NICOTINIC ACID

Nicotinic acid (Fig. 15.5-3), also known as the B-vitamin niacin, can produce a marked reduction in plasma cholesterol, when administered at pharmacological doses. Side effects often pose a problem for adherence, but its ability to bring about substantial reductions in VLDL and triglyceride levels, total and LDL-cholesterol levels, and increases in HDL have made it a useful and inexpensive drug for patients who tolerate it.

Mechanism of Action. After many years of clinical experience with this drug, its complex effects on lipid metabolism are still only partially understood. It is well established that nicotinic acid inhibits the release of free fatty acids from adipose tissue. Increased lipolysis or delivery of free fatty acids to the liver stimulates hepatic synthesis of VLDL, and hence decreased lipolysis may be expected to result in decreased circulating VLDL and triglyceride levels. The decreases in triglyceride levels have also been reported to be due to increased lipoprotein lipase activity.

A fall in circulating levels of LDL and total cholesterol also occurs over a period of several days. A number of pharmacological mechanisms may contribute to this effect. VLDL is the precursor of most circulating LDL; therefore, the depletion of VLDL should reduce the rate of LDL synthesis. Nicotinic acid also inhibits cholesterol synthesis. Although nicotinic acid has been reported to stimulate oxidation of cholesterol, it does not appear to stimulate LDL catabolism in patients with type II hyperlipoproteinemia. Studies of LDL turnover in normal subjects and hypercholesterolemic subjects indicate that nicotinic acid decreases the rate of LDL synthesis (33). A reduction in the synthesis of VLDL would also result in decreased synthesis of LDL. Inhibition of lipoprotein synthesis appears to be an important mechanism.

In the Coronary Drug Project, the mean reductions in serum cholesterol and triglyceride were 10 and 26%, respectively, in the group receiving 3 g of nicotinic acid daily (12). Greater cholesterol lowering (20-30%) has been achieved when large doses of nicotinic acid are used to treat hypercholesterolemic patients in the usual clinic environment. Nicotinic acid also increases circulating HDL levels, and the magnitude of increase is generally greater than that observed with clofibrate and gemfibrozil. Again, the therapeutic benefit of pharmacologically induced increases in HDL has not been definitely proven.

Administration and Dosage. Nicotinic acid is commercially available in many forms under numerous brand names. Most preparations are available as 500-mg tablets, but smaller dosage forms are also available. A variety of nicotinic acid analogs have been evaluated, but none are superior to nicotinic acid. Some of these sustained-release preparations may be associated with more toxicity. Nicotinic acid is also available as a nonprescription drug. Nicotinic acid is generally well absorbed from the gut and has a very short plasma half-life. The use of 100-mg tablets has occasionally been recommended to enhance its absorption, but this does not appear to be necessary.

The usual and approved total daily dose of nicotinic acid is 3 g. However, daily doses of nicotinic acid as high as 6 g/day have been used to treat severely affected FHC heterozygotes and type V patients. (By contrast, the recommended daily requirement of niacin as a vitamin is 18 mg for adult males.) Nicotinic acid is usually administered three or four times daily because of its short plasma half-life. Some very preliminary evidence indicates that a twice-daily schedule may be effective in some patients. The drug is usually initiated at a low dosage and gradually increased (based upon the rapidity of development of tolerance to the side effects) until the therapeutic dose is achieved. The recommended pediatric dose for FHC homozygotes is 60-80 mg/kg/day.

Adverse Effects. The side effects of nicotinic acid are a major drawback to adherence. Continuous flushing in the first 2 hours after taking the drug is a nearly universal side effect when the drug is first administered, but the patient usually become tolerant to the flushing within several weeks. The flushing appears to be mediated by prostaglandins, and if it continues to be a major problem it can be alleviated by administration of an inhibitor of prostaglandin synthesis such as aspirin. Gastrointestinal symptoms include aggravation of peptic ulcer symptoms, diarrhea, nausea, and abdominal pain. Liver function abnormalities, hyperuricemia, and various degrees of glucose intolerance are potentially serious side effects. The latter two side effects frequently complicate or preclude its use in patients with types IV and V hyperlipoproteinemia, who are often hyperuricemic or hyperglycemic even without treatment. Persistence of liver function abnormalities necessitates either a reduction in dose or discontinuing the drug. Acanthosis nigricans was reported in 3.6% of Coronary Drug Project patients receiving this drug (12); however, the lesion was reversible and did not appear to be associated with subsequent malignancy. Nicotinic acid may also potentiate the hypotensive effects of the ganglionic blocking drugs.

Contraindications. Contraindications for use are in active peptic ulcer disease, liver disease, diabetes mellitus, hyperuricemia, and history of gouty arthritis.

In summary, adherence to nicotinic acid may be difficult to achieve, especially in the first few weeks. If tolerated, it is one of the more potent and versatile lipid-lowering agents. Because its inhibition of LDL synthesis complements the pharmacological effect of the bile acid sequestrants on LDL catabolism, the combination of cholestyramine or colestipol, nicotinic acid, and diet is frequently effective in the treatment of severe cases of FHC. Nicotinic acid is also a drug of choice in types IIb, IV, and V hyperlipoproteinemia for patients who can tolerate its side effects and have not obtained an adequate response from dietary measures.

INVESTIGATIONAL DRUGS

COMPACTIN AND MEVINOLIN

Compactin and mevinolin, which are fungal metabolites, represent a new class of hypolipidemic agents and appear to be very effective in terms of reducing total and LDL-cholesterol in many of the clinical trials that have been reported to date (27, 36). Both of these drugs interfere with the action of HMG CoA reductase, the rate-limiting enzyme in cholesterol biosynthesis. These drugs decrease cholesterol synthesis, and the associated decrease in hepatic cholesterol increases the production of hepatic LDL receptors. The increased number of LDL receptors results in an increase in the uptake and subsequent catabolism of LDL by the liver. These compounds produce a dramatic increase in the rate of LDL catabolism and a significant reduction in both total and LDL cholesterol. Preliminary studies indicate that if these drugs are combined with the bile acid-sequestering agents, there is an even greater increase in the number of LDL receptors and the rate of LDL catabolism.

Reductions ranging from 20 to 50% in plasma total and LDL-cholesterol have been obtained when varying doses of these drugs have been administered. Illingworth reported reductions in total and LDL cholesterol of 33 and 38%, respectively, when mevinolin was administered in a dosage of 40 mg b.i.d. (27). This type of response has been observed in FHC heterozygotes who are frequently resistant or only moderately responsive to currently marketed drugs, used or in combination. Mevinolin and compactin are available only for investigational use, and current studies are aimed at evaluating the appropriate dosages and dosage schedules. Future studies will have to determine whether there is any significant toxicity associated with long-term therapy. If absence of significant toxicity is demonstrated in long-term studies, this class of drugs will truly provide a major advance in the treatment of type II hyperlipoproteinemia.

NEOMYCIN

Neomycin, an aminoglycoside antibiotic, has been known to be an effective cholesterol-lowering agent for nearly 20 years (45). When administered in total daily doses of 1.5-2 g/day, reductions in serum cholesterol of 15-25% have been noted (40, 45). Earlier studies suggested that all density fractions of cholesterol were lowered, including HDL. A more recent study indicates that the reduction in total cholesterol is primarily related to a decrease in LDL-C and that there was no significant effect on HDL-C (22). The mechanism of action for the cholesterol-lowering effect is not known. However, since only 3-6% of an oral dose of neomycin is absorbed and since parenteral neomycin does not lower circulating cholesterol level, the drug appears to act primarily within the gastrointestinal tract.

Parenterally administered neomycin is associated with a variety of side effects, the more serious being ototoxicity and nephrotoxicity. The latter have not been observed in the reported studies of orally administered neomycin as a hypocholesterolemic agent (22, 40, 45). Malabsorption occurs when more than 2 g/day of neomycin are administered orally.

Neomycin is an inexpensive drug. The studies to date are very encouraging. Unfortunately, the drug cannot be recommended for routine use until larger controlled trials are conducted. It has not been approved for use as a hypocholesterolemic agent by the FDA.

SUCROSE POLYESTER

Sucrose polyester is an indigestible, negligibly absorbable triglyceride analog that consists of a mixture of hexa-, hepta-, and octaesters of sucrose with long-chain fatty acids. When given as a dietary fat substitute or supplement, this substance has shown considerable promise as an agent for lowering total and LDL-cholesterol (39). It does not appear to significantly affect triglyceride or HDL levels. Its use at this time is strictly investigational.

Sucrose polyester is unique among lipid-lowering drugs in that it is used as a dietary constituent. Depending on the saturation of its fatty acids, it may be provided as a solid substitute for butter or lard or as an oil to be used in salad dressings. Although only very small quantities of sucrose polyester are absorbed, they cannot be metabolized, and their chronic accumulation over years of therapy is of potential concern. Long-term safety data are not available for a significant number of patients to evaluate the preceding or many other factors such as the absorption of fat-soluble vitamins.

CLOFIBRATE ANALOGS

A number of phenoxyisobutyrate derivatives have either been marketed or extensively evaluated outside of the United States and also evaluated in clinical trials within the United States. The majority of the reports have focused on three compounds. Each has been reported to have some advantage over clofibrate in the treatment of hyperlipoproteinemia.

Bezafibrate. When compared with clofibrate, bezafibrate appears to produce greater reductions in plasma cholesterol and triglycerides (26, 41). The reports indicates a 15-25% decrease for cholesterol and a 20-50% reduction in triglycerides. In addition, it tends to raise HDL by 10-15 %. Bezafibrate is also active at plasma levels less than 4% of the therapeutic levels of clofibrate. Long-term toxicity data are not available.

Ciprofibrate. Ciprofibrate may be the most effective of the clofibrate analogs in reducing total and LDL-cholesterol. It is administered in a single daily dose and has been reported to be effective even in FHC (28). Reductions of over 30% in total and LDL-cholesterol and similar decreases in triglycerides have been reported. HDL has also been increased by about 10% with this drug. Clinical trials and long-term animal toxicity studies are currently in progress.

Fenofibrate. Significant reductions in plasma lipids in type II patients have also been reported with fenofibrate (13, 44). Reductions in cholesterol and triglycerides ranging from 20-30% and 25-60%, respectively, were noted. In type IV patients, long-term trials demonstrated triglyceride reductions in excess of 50%, an increase in HDL, and either a decrease or increase in LDL (13). The side effects reported to date have been minimal and usually do not require withdrawal of medication. Long-term safety data in large number of patients are not yet available.

ETOFIBRATE

Etofibrate is an ethylene glycol diester of clofibric and nicotinic acids that has been found to have pharmacological properties similar to combinations of clofibrate and niacin. Laboratory studies show that this drug's triglyceride-lowering activity is similar to that of clofibrate, but its ability to lower cholesterol in type II patients is greater (30). At therapeutic doses etofibrate reduces cholesterol by 15-20% and triglyceride levels by 25%. In type IV patients, etofibrate reduces triglyceride levels by $>$ 40%, but does not significantly affect cholesterol levels.

Etofibrate appears to have metabolic properties that are similar to a combination of clofibrate and nicotinic acid, and its biotransformation results in conjugates of both nicotinic acid and clofibric acid.

OTHER AGENTS AFFECTING LIPIDS AND LIPOPROTEINS

EICOSAPENTAENOIC ACID

Eicosapentaenoic acid (EPA), an ω-3 fatty acid, produces a significant decrease in plasma triglyceride and VLDL levels. The majority of the studies have used daily doses of 6-16 g of MAXEPA, but doses up to 30 g/day have been used in the treatment of type V hyperlipoproteinemia. MAXEPA is derived from fish oil with a high concentration of ω-3 fatty acids (approximately 28% of the total dose is ω-3 fatty acids). A recent study has established that EPA most likely acts by inhibiting hepatic VLDL synthesis (20).

EPA decreases platelet aggregability. Caution must be exercised when it is administered to patients who are taking other drugs that affect platelet function. EPA is derived from fish oil and is not being pursued as a drug but as a nutrition supplement.

HORMONAL AGENTS: ESTROGENS, PROGESTINS, AND ANABOLIC STEROIDS

The incidence of CHD in premenopausal women is lower than that observed for men of the same age. Differences in estrogen levels between the two sexes have been considered as a possible explanation. However, the use of estrogens in males in the Coronary Drug Project (11) was associated with an increase in total mortality. An increased incidence of nonfatal myocardial infarction, pulmonary embolism, and thrombophlebitis was also observed. Much of the emphasis has now switched to the potential effect of the use of various hormones on plasma lipid and lipoprotein levels and their potential for altering the incidence of CHD in women.

The effects of estrogen administration on plasma lipid and lipoprotein levels in women are generally dose dependent and related to menstrual status. Lower doses of estrogen are usually administered to premenopausal women, frequently in the form of oral contraceptives. Estrogen administration, in this situation, is associated with increases in total and LDL-cholesterol and triglycerides and no change in HDL levels. All of the preceding effects may be modified by the type and amount of the progestin that is administered (47).

The amount of estrogen that is administered to postmenopausal women is generally higher. A dose-dependent increase in HDL levels is observed with estrogen administration in postmenopausal women. LDL levels are also lower following estrogen administration although the total cholesterol levels may not be significantly different. There is currently a trend toward the use of estrogen-progestin combinations in postmenopausal women for endometrial protection. The effects of the amount and specific type of progestin being administered will have to be evaluated for its effect on plasma lipid and lipoprotein levels. There are currently no long-term, large-scale prospective studies available to assess the effect of estrogen or a combination of estrogen-progestin on CHD incidence in postmenopausal women.

Anabolic steroids are currently used in the treatment of osteoporosis in some postmenopausal women. There is currently some concern about their potential for increasing the incidence of CHD. The use of anabolic steroids is associated with increases in LDL levels, but the greatest concern is related to the marked reductions in HDL levels, which can range up to 50% (19, 48).

In the past, agents with hormonal effects were occasionally reported to be benefit in the treatment of type V hyperlipoproteinemia that was refractory to the use of diet and other drugs. Progestational agents, such as norethindrone acetate (NORLUTATE) and medroxyprogesterone acetate (PROVERA), were reported to be of benefit in women. Anabolic steroids, such as oxandrolone (ANAVAR), were reported to be of benefit in the treatment of adult males.

ANTIHYPERTENSIVE AGENTS

A wide variety of drugs, which are used for other indications, have been shown to alter plasma lipids and lipoproteins in recent years. Major attention has focused on the antihypertensive agents.

Although antihypertensive agents have been shown to effectively reduce total mortality, the incidence of cerebrovascular accidents, and prevent or arrest hypertensive renal damage, most studies do not indicate a decrease in either the morbidity or mortality for CHD. One hypothesis presented is that many antihypertensive drugs unfavorably affect plasma lipid and lipoprotein levels, thus comprising the advantage of controlled hypertension.

A number of studies have documented a rather consistent increase in cholesterol, LDL, and triglycerides with variable changes in HDL with diuretic therapy. Fourteen of 16 studies reviewed by Weidmann et al. (49), demonstrated increases in cholesterol ranging from 1 to 13% and increases in triglycerides from 2 to 33% (2 studies showed declines in triglycerides by 7 to 16%). All 10 investigations reviewing LDL and HDL changes found consistent increases in LDL from 3 to 21%. HDL responses varied from -7 to +13%. Furosemide also increased cholesterol and triglyceride and reduced HDL.

The β-adrenergic blocking agents produce increases in triglycerides and decreases in HDL (29). Preliminary, but inconclusive, evidence suggests that β-blockers with intrinsic sympathomimetic activity such as pindolol produce less of a change in plasma lipids than do the other agents, whether cardioselective or nonselective blockers. Vasodilators such as prazosin are reported to have no negative effect on lipids and lipoproteins. Further studies are required before the significance of these lipid changes on CHD incidence can be evaluated.

APPLICATION TO CLINICAL PRACTICE

The treatment of the *type I* disorder, in which lipoprotein lipase is deficient or absent, relies entirely on dietary measure—elimination of alcohol and severe restriction of long-chain fatty acids. Medium-chain triglyceride can be substituted for the usual fats. None of the known lipid-lowering drugs is of benefit.

Type II (especially type IIa) hyperlipoproteinemia is the disorder in which pharmacologic agents potentially have the most to offer, for it is associated with the greatest excess cardiovascular risk and is the disorder for which there are effective, nontoxic drugs. Also, there is definitive evidence of benefit that lowering of total and LDL-cholesterol is associated with a reduced risk for the development and progression of CHD (5, 32, 34, 35).

Diet is the initial form of therapy. The diet primarily emphasizes dietary restriction of cholesterol and saturated fat plus caloric restriction, if indicated. If the response to diet is not adequate, drug therapy may be necessary. Diet must be continued even if drugs are used. The biliary sequestrants (cholestyramine and colestipol) and nicotinic acid have been demonstrated to be safe in long-term studies involving many patients. These three drugs also produce the greatest decrease in LDL levels. Additionally, the administration of biliary sequestrants has been shown to decrease the risk for CHD. There is some suggestive evidence that nicotinic acid administration may also be associated with a reduced risk for CHD. Side effects and/or cost may limit the use of these drugs. The other drugs described in the text may then be considered.

Treatment of *type III* hyperlipoproteinemia also offers clear therapeutic benefits. Such treatment has reportedly resulted in marked improvement of peripheral vascular flow with corresponding symptomatic relief, although litte is known about whether treatment reduces the patient's risk of CHD. Moreover, the resolution of xanthomata in response to treatment is often dramatic. Diet, particularly weight reduction (in the obese) and alcohol restriction, is the first line of treatment. Clofibrate is generally stated to be the drug of choice for patients in whom dietary measures are insufficient. This is based upon the fact that there is a much longer and more extensive experience with the use of clofibrate. Long-term administration of clofibrate is associated with significant toxicity, however. Preliminary studies with both gemfibrozil and nicotinic acid indicate that both drugs effectively lower plasma cholesterol and triglyceride levels in type III patients.

It is difficult to justify treating *type IV* hyperlipoproteinemia aggressively with drugs. Dietary measures such as caloric restriction and alcohol restriction are frequently effective in correcting abnormal triglyceride levels. Triglyceride lowering has not been demonstrated to reduce the risk for CHD. Triglyceride lowering may occasionally be of benefit in individuals with marked increases in plasma triglycerides to reduce the risk of pancreatitis or for control of eruptive xanthomas. Clofibrate, gemfibrozil, and nicotinic acid may all produce significant reductions in circulating triglyceride levels, but chronic use may also be associated with adverse effects. Drugs should be used sparingly in the treatment of type IV hyperlipoproteinemia.

Type V hyperlipoproteinemia is also treated primarily by dietary restriction of fat and total calories and complete abstention from alcohol. Usually, drugs are not-needed. However, since affected patients are, like type I-patients, at risk of extreme, morbid hypertriglyceridemia if not successfully treated, aggressive treatment is called-for when diet fails. Nicotonic acid is the drug of choice in such cases, but its exacerbation of preexisting disorders of glucose and uric acid metabolism preclude its use in a substantial number of type V patients. Clofibrate is generally better tolerated by these patients but is often ineffective. One would predict that the effects of gemfibrozil would be similar to those for clofibrate. Investigational approaches such as eicosapentaenoic acid are currently being evaluated. The patient should be referred to a specialist in lipid disorders if standard therapy is unsuccessful.

Diet is the initial therapy for all lipoprotein abnormalities. The benefits and risks associated with the use of hypolipidemic agents should be considered in each patient. Drug therapy should be continued only if there is clear evidence of a beneficial effect in terms of changes in plasma lipids and lipoproteins. Many of the currently available drugs have significant disadvantages that include cost, difficulty of administration, adverse effects, and lack of efficacy. Hopefully drugs will be available in the future that minimize this problem. In the interim we hope that the material in this chapter will serve as a factual basis for the appropriate use of the current drugs.

REFERENCES

1. Atmeh, R.F., Stewart, J.M., Boag, D.E., Packard, C.J., Lirimer, A.R. and Shepherd, J. The hypolipidemic action of probucol: A study of its effects on high and low density lipoproteins. *J. Lipid Res.* 24:588, 1983.
2. Beaumont, J.L., Carlson, L.A., Cooper, G.R., Fejfar, G.R., Fredrickson, D.S., and Strasser, T. Classifications of hyperlipidemias and hyperlipoproteinemias. *Bull. WHO* 43:891, 1971.
3. Bechtol, L.D., and Warner, W.L. Dextrothyroxine for lowering serum cholesterol. *Angiology* 20:565, 1969.
4. Berge, K.G., Achor, R.W., Christensen, N.A. et al. Hypercholesterolemia and nicotinic acid. *Am. J. Med.* 31:24, 1961.
5. Brensike, J.F., Levy, R.I., Kelsey, S.F. et al. Effects of therapy with cholestyramine on progression of coronary arteriosclerosis: Results of the NHLBI Type II Coronary Intervention Study. *Circulation* 69:313, 1984.
6. Brown, M.S. and Goldstein, J.L. How LDL receptors influence cholesterol and atherosclerosis. *Sci. Am.* 251:58, 1984.
7. Brown, M.S., Goldstein, J.L. and Fredrickson, D.S. Familial type 3 hyperlipoproteinemia (dysbetalipoproteinemia). In: *The*

Metabolic Basis of Inherited Disease, 5th ed. (Stanbury, J.B., Wyngaarden, J.B., Fredrickson, D.S. and Goldstein, J.L., eds.) New York: McGraw-Hill, p. 655, 1982.

8. Committee of Principal Investigators. A cooperative trial in the primary prevention of ischemic heart disease using clofibrate. *Br. Heart J.* 40:1069, 1978.
9. Committee of Principal Investigators. WHO cooperative trial on primary prevention of ischemic heart disease with clofibrate to lower serum cholesterol: Final mortality follow-up. *Lancet* 2:600, 1984.
10. Coronary Drug Project Research Group. The Coronary Drug Project—Findings leading to further modification of its protocol with respect to dextrothyroxine. *JAMA* 220:996, 1971.
11. Coronory Drug Project Research Group. The Coronory Drug Project—Findings leading to discontinuation of the 2.5 mg/day estrogen group. *JAMA* 226:652, 1973.
12. Coronary Drug Project Research Group. Clofibrate and niacin in coronary heart disease. *JAMA* 231:360, 1975.
13. De Gennes, J.L., Cairou, F., Truffert, J. and Lavoie, M.A. Long-term (over 5 years) treatment of primary hyperlipidemias by fenofibrate alone or with cholestyramine. In: *Treatment of Hyperlipoproteinemia* (Carlson, L.A. and Olsson, A.G., eds.) New York: Raven Press, p. 175, 1984.
14. Dujoune, C.A., Krehbiel, P., Decoursey, S. et al. Probucol with colestipol in the treatment of hypercholesterolemia. *Ann. Intern. Med.* 100:477, 1984.
15. Fenderson, R.W., Deutsch, S., Menachemi, E., Chin, B. and Samuel, P. Effect of gemfibrozil on serum lipids in man. *Angiology* 33:581, 1982.
16. Fredrickson, D.S., Levy, R.I. and Lees, R.S. Fat transport and lipoproteins—an integrated approach to mechanisms and disorders. *N. Engl. J. Med.* 274:32, 94, 148, 215, 273, 1967.
17. Goldstein, J.L. and Brown, M.S. Familial hypercholesterolemia. In: *The Metabolic Basis of Inherited Disease*, 5th ed. (Stanbury, J.B., Wyngaarden, J.B., Frederickson, D.S. and Goldstein, J.L., eds.) New York: McGraw-Hill, p. 672, 1982.
18. Gordon, T., Castelli, W.P., Hjortland, M.C., Kannel, W.B. and Dawber, T.R. High Density lipoprotein as a protective factor against coronary heart disease: The Framingham Study. *Am. J. Med.* 62:707, 1977.
19. Haffner, S.M., Kushwaha, R.S., Foster, D.M., Applebaum-Bowden, D. and Hazzard, W.R. Studies on the metabolic mechanism of reduced high density lipoproteins during anabolic steroid thereapy. *Metabolism* 32:413, 1983.
20. Harris, W.S., Connor, W.E., Inkeles, S.B. and Illingworth, D.R. Dietary omega-3 fatty acids prevent carbohydrate-induced hypertriglyceridemia. *Metabolism* 33:1016, 1984.
21. Heel, R.C., Brogden, R.M., Pakes, G.F., Speight, T.M. and Avery, G.S. Colestipol: A review of its pharmacological properties and therapeutic efficacy in patients with hypercholesterolemia. *Drugs* 19:161, 1980.
22. Hoeg, J.M., Schaefer, E.J., Romano, C.A. et al. Neomycin and plasma lipoproteins in type II hyperlipoproteinemia. *Clin. Pharmacol. Ther.* 36:555, 1984.
23. Hunninghake, D.B. Drug interactions involving hypolipidemic drugs. In: *Cardiovascular and Respiratory Disease Therapy* (Petrie, J.C. ed.) New York: Elsevier/North Holland, 79, 1980.
24. Hunninghake, D.B., Bell, C. and Olson, L. Effect of probucol on plasma lipids and lipoproteins in type IIb hyperlipoproteinemia. *Atherosclerosis* 37:469, 1980.
25. Hunninghake, D.B. and Probstfield, J.L. Drug Treatment of hyperlipoproteinemia. In: *Hyperlipidemia—Diagnosis and Therapy*. New York: Grune and Stratton. p. 327, 1977.
26. Hutt, V, Wechsler, J.G., Klor, H.U. and Ditschuenit, H. Changes in the concentration and composition of lipids and lipoproteins in primary hyperlipoproteinemia during treatment with bezafibrate. *Arzneimittelforsch* 33:1185, 1983.
27. Illingworth, D.R. Mevinolin plus colestipol in therapy for severe heterozygous familial hypercholesterolemia. *Ann. Intern. Med.* 101:598, 1984.
28. Illingworth, D.R., Olsen, G.D., Cook, S.F., Sexton, G.J., Wendel, H.A. and Connor, W.E. Ciprofibrate in the therapy of type II hypercholesterolemia: A double blind trial. *Atherosclerosis* 44:211, 1982.
29. Johnson, D.B. The emerging problem of plasma lipid changes during antihypertensive therapy. *J. Cardiovas. Pharmacol.* 4(suppl. 2):5213, 1982.
30. Kaffarnik, H., Schneider, J. Schubotz, R., Zofel, P., Hausmann, L. and Goebel, K.M. Long-term treatment of hyperlipoproteinemia with etofibrate: clinical observations. *Artery* 8:537, 1980.
31. Kannel, W.B., Castelli, W.P., Gordon, T. and McNamara, P.M. Serum cholesterol, lipoproteins, and the risk of coronary heart disease: The Framingham Study. *Ann. Intern. Med.* 74:1, 1971.
32. Levy, R.J., Brensike, J.F., Epstein, S.E. et al. The influences of changes in lipid values induced by cholestyramine and diet on progression of coronary artery disease: results of the NHLBI Type II Coronary Intervention Study. *Circulation.* 69:325, 1984.
33. Levy, R.J. and Langer, T. Hypolipidemic drugs and lipoprotein metabolism. *Adv. Exp. Med. Biol.* 26:155, 1972.
34. Lipid Research Clinics Program: The Lipid Research Clinics Coronary Primary Prevention Trial Results. I. Reduction in incidence of coronary heart disease. *JAMA* 251:351, 1984.
35. Lipid Research Clinics Program: The Lipid Research Clinics Coronary Primary Prevention Trial Results. II. The relationship of reduction in incidence of coronary heart disease to cholesterol lowering. *JAMA* 251:365, 1984.
36. Mabuchi, H., Sakai, T., Sakai, Y. et al. Reduction of serum cholesterol in heterozygous patients with familial hypercholesterolemia. Additive effects of compactin and cholestyramine. *N. Engl. J. Med.* 308:609, 1983.
37. Manninen, V., Malkonen, M., Eisalo, A., Virtamo, J., Tuomilehto, J. and Kuusisto, P. Gemfibrozil in the treatment of dyslipidaemia: A 5-year follow-up study. *Acta Med. Scand.* 668(suppl.): 82, 1982.
38. Manninen, V., Manttari, M., Nikkila, E.A. and Gorringe, J.A.L. Helsinki Heart Study—advisory council report. *Res. Clin. Forums* 4(2):9, 1982.
39. Mellies, M.J., Jandacek, R.J., Taulbee, J.D. et al. A double-blind, placebo controlled study of sucrose polyester in hypercholesterolemic outpatients. *Am. J. Clin. Nutr.* 37:339, 1983.
40. Miettinen, T. Effects of neomycin alone and in combination with cholestyramine on serum cholesterol and fecal steroids in hypercholesterolemic subjects. *J. Clin. Invest.* 64:1485, 1979.
41. Mordasini, R., Riesen, W., Oster, P., Keller, M., Middelhoff, G. and Lang, P.D. Reduced LDL- and increased HDL-apoproteins in patients with hypercholesterolemia under treatment with bezafibrate. *Atherosclerosis* 40:153, 1981.
42. Nutrition Committee and Council on Arteriosclerosis: AHA Special Report. Recommendations for treatment of hyperlipidemia in adults. *Circulation* 69:1067A, 1984.
43. Parsons, W.B. Studies of nicotinic acid use in hypercholesterolemia. *Arch. Intern. Med.* 107:653, 1961.
44. Rossner, S. and Oro, L. Fenofibrate therapy of hyperlipoproteinaemia: A dose response study and a comparison with clofibrate. *Atherosclerosis* 38:273, 1981.
45. Samuel, P., Holtzman, C.M. and Goldstein, B.D. Long-term reduction of serum cholesterol levels of patients with atherosclerosis by small doses of neomycin. *Circulation* 35:938, 1967.
46. Schaefer, E.J., Eisenberg, S. and Levy, R.I. Lipoprotein apoprotein metabolism. *J. Lipid. Res.* 19:667, 1978.
47. Wahl, P.W., Walden, C.E., Knopp, R.H., Hoover, J.J., Wallace, R.B. and Rifkind, B.M. Relationship of estrogen/progestin potency to lipid and lipoprotein cholesterol concentrations in

oral contraceptive and menopausal estrogen users. The Lipid Research Clinics Program and Prevalence Study. *N. Engl. J. Med.* 308:862, 1983.

48. Webb, O.L., Laskarzewski, P.M. and Glueck, C.J. Severe depression of high density lipoprotein cholesterol levels in weight lifters and body builders by self-administered exogenous testosterone and anabolic-androgenic steroids. *Metabolism* 33:971, 1984.

49. Weidmann, P., Gerber, A. and Mordasini, R. Effects of antihypertensive therapy on serum lipoproteins. *Hypertension* 5(suppl. III):120, 1983.

CHAPTER
15.6

ANTICOAGULANTS

William L. West

An intimate knowledge of the hemostatic process is necessary in order to permit a rational approach to pharmacological intervention of hemorrhagic or thrombotic disorders. Hemostasis initiated by vascular injury not only involves the vasoconstriction of smooth muscle cells in small arteries, arterioles, and venules, but initiates many enzymatic interactions among the constituents of blood and the release of factors from the injured surrounding tissues. These in turn promote the formation of a mechanical plug composed of platelets, which is stabilized by the activation of the coagulation mechanism. Overall, the clotting or coagulation of blood is a vital modulatory mechanism in defense of vascular integrity. Occasionally, deficiencies in the constituents of blood exist that are associated with specific hemorrhagic or coagulation disorders. The pathophysiology of coagulation disorders and the clotting of blood are briefly reviewed in the following sections.

PATHOPHYSIOLOGY OF COAGULATION DISORDERS

Patients with bleeding disorders usually present with a deficiency in platelet number (thrombocytopenia) or function (thrombocytopathy, e.g., defect in glycoprotein, Glanzmann's thrombasthenia), and genetically altered or missing clotting factors (e.g., the hemophilias and von Willebrand's disease). In hemophilia A and von Willebrand's disease there is a deficiency in factor VIII, but von Willebrand's disease is further characterized by a deficiency in a humoral factor necessary for normal platelet function. Thrombocytopenia may be drug- or disease-induced, whereas the hemophilias are inherited diseases. Patients with an increased activation of the clotting mechanism by tissue and bacterial products often present with a tendency toward uncontrolled intravascular clotting and thrombus formation (e.g., disseminated intravascular coagulation, DIC).

A *thrombus* is an occlusive mass (plug or clot) attached to the wall of a vessel (artery or vein) or a chamber in the heart formed as a result of the coagulation of blood. Thromboembolism implies a secondary event in that the obstruction in the vessels occurs with a thrombus that arose from a site distant to the obstruction. Among the common causes of chronic pathological changes leading to thromboemboli are those related to atherosclerotic changes in the arterial wall; in contrast, venous stasis is a major factor contributing to venous thrombosis (9, 15, 18, 22). Thrombi, whether in arteries or veins, start as a result of a few platelets adhering to the lining surface of blood vessels with a sequential building up of platelets, eventually forming an aggregate. Platelets and fibrin are the essential constituents of a thrombus. Whereas the atherosclerotic changes in arteries seem to provide the nidus that activates the coagulation factors and the formation of arterial thrombi, such a nidus during venous stasis is unclear. The white (arterial) thrombus is composed primarily of platelets and fibrin; the nidus for its formation occurs in areas of rapid blood flow. The red (venous) thrombus is composed of fibrin, platelets, and erythrocytes; the nidus for its formation occurs in areas of low blood flow. Most experts now agree that platelet adhesion to subendothelial collagen may be the initial nidus in arteries and veins.

CLOT FORMATION

The clotting of blood is a series of complex events frequently referred to as the coagulation cascade that ultimately leads to hemostasis. *Hemostasis*, the arrest of bleeding, may be achieved physiologically by vasoconstriction, adhesion and aggregation of platelets, coagulation of blood, or some combination of these processes. *Coagulation* may be defined as the process of clot formation. Overall, the clotting of blood may be described as follows: acute vascular injury as well as certain chronic pathological changes in vessel walls cause the aggregation of platelets and release of clotting factors (a series of linked serine protease enzymatic reactions); these reactions culminate in the release of thromboplastin that converts prothrombin to *thrombin*, that in turn changes fibrinogen to fibrin. The reaction cascade is summarized in Fig. 15.6-1 and in the section on clotting factors that follows. It may be mentioned that factors VIII (antihemophilic factor), V (accelerator globulin), and III (tissue factor thromboplastin) are cofactors, whereas most of the activated factors are enzymes.

HEMOSTASIS AND PLATELETS

The primary hemostatic events begin with vasoconstriction after vascular tissue injury followed by *platelet adhesion* to the exposed subendothelial collagen fiber, and *platelet aggregation* culminates in a plug formation at the site of injury. The role of the clotting mechanism is to stabilize this primary hemostasis. Platelet adhesion and aggregation are stimulated by the release of adenosine diphosphate (ADP), thrombin, and epinephrine. Each of these soluble agents binds to specific receptors in the platelet membrane. Additional ADP release from platelet stores attracts more platelets to the aggregated mass that eventually forms into a platelet plug. Important morphological changes occur in these platelets, characterized by loss of individual cell membranes, discharge of platelet α and dense granules, and the formation of a thick gel-like mass. α-Granules contain platelet growth factor, platelet factor iv, β-thromboglobulin, fibronectin, von Willebrand's protein, and fibrinogen. Dense granules contain calcium, ADP, and serotonin. In addition, this mass of platelets provides a selective lipid surface referred to as platelet factor iii (PL-iii) which, along with other factors, facilitates coagulation reactions. The platelet plug formed as a result of the action of ADP is unstable; after initiation of the platelet adhesion and aggregation, the production of thrombin also occurs. Thrombin stimulates more ADP release from platelets and activates prostaglandin synthetase, a

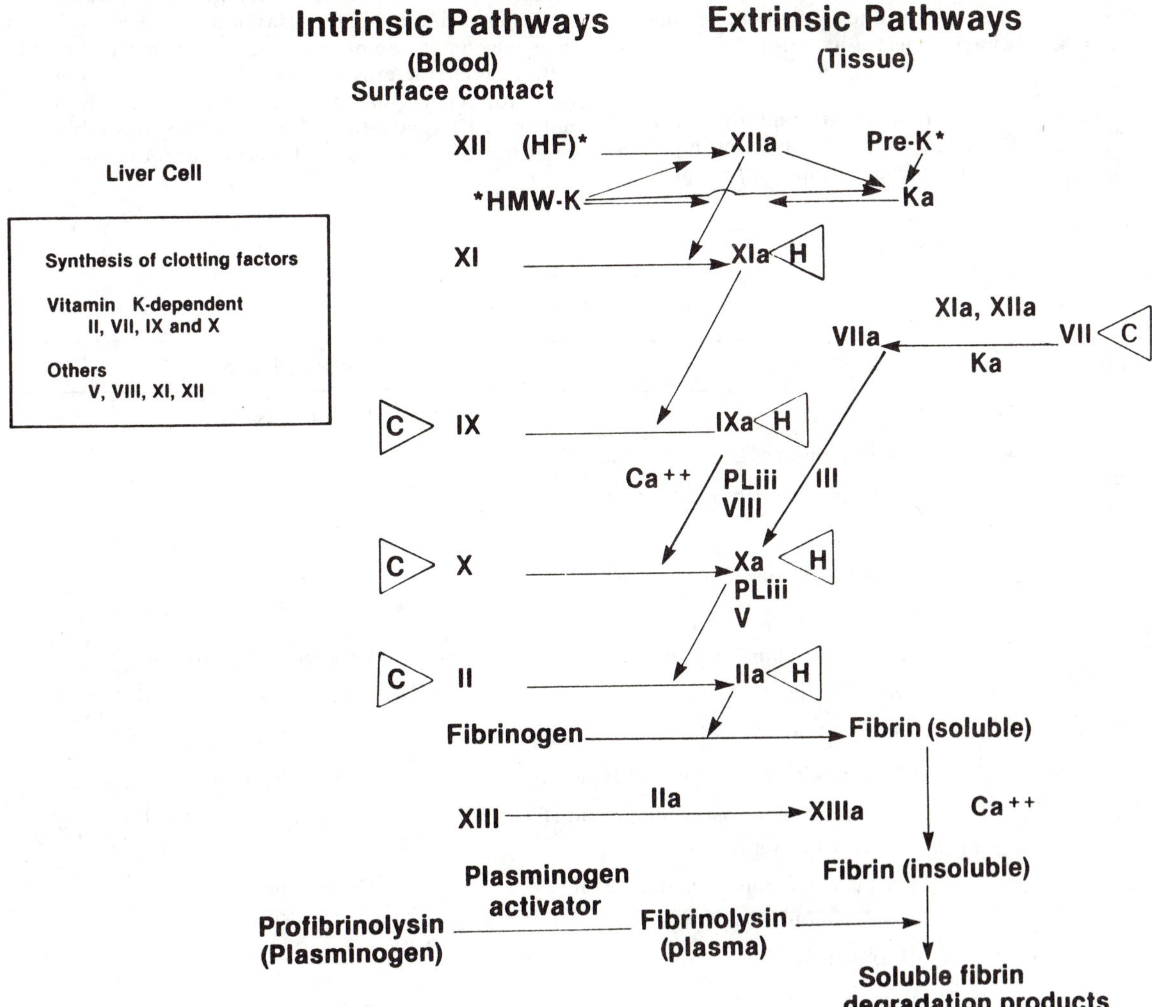

Fig. 15.6-1. *The coagulation cascade and sites of action of anticoagulants.*

Conversion of a factor (indicated by a Roman number) to its activated form by a series of linked serine proteases is indicated by the letter "a" after the factor number. Synthesis of vitamin K-dependent and independent clotting fators in liver cell is shown at the left of the diagram. Multiple sites of anticoagulant action of heparin and oral anticoagulants (coumarins) are indicated by H and C, respectively.

cyclooxygenase responsible for the formation of thromboxane A_2 (TXA_2) from arachidonic acid in the platelets that is a potent stimulus for the aggregation of platelets, and prostacyclin (PGI_2) from arachidonic acid in the blood vessel wall, which inhibits aggregation. These substances, TXA_2 and PGI_2, through their effects on platelet levels of cyclic adenosine monophosphate (cAMP), control the degree of aggregation and thrombus formation (14, 19). Increased levels of cAMP inhibit aggregation.

The platelet reactions triggered by ADP, epinephrine, and arachidonic acid metabolites are prevented by nonsteroidal antiinflammatory drugs, (e.g., aspirin) (see Chapter 10.2). These agents are classed as "weak" stimulators, whereas thrombin and collagen are "strong" stimulators of aggregation. Strong stimulators are known to overcome the effect of nonsteroidal antiinflammatory drugs to inhibit cyclooxygenase and still produce platelet reactions. As more and more thrombin becomes available, fibrinogen in the platelets is converted to fibrin. Thrombin also activates factor XIII (a transamidase) to XIIIa (active form) which cross-links adjacent fibrin monomers covalently to form insoluble fibrin (see Fig. 15.6-1). The overall role of thrombin is to increase the size and strength of the plug of platelets that are firmly interconnected by fibrin (7).

CLOTTING FACTORS

The conversion of the factor II to IIa (thrombin) can be achieved by intrinsic and extrinsic systems for the clotting of blood. Exposure of the subendothelial collagen after injury initiates the *intrinsic system* to cause clotting of blood via activation of Hageman factor XII to XIIa (Fig. 15.6-1 and Table 15.6-1). Hageman factor binds to the exposed surfaces of the subendothelial elements and is activated by proteolytic enzymes such as *kallikrein* (Ka) in the presence of high molecular weight kininogen (HMW-K) to factor XIIa (16). Activated factor (Hageman factor XIIa) performs two functions: (1) activates more Ka from prekallikrein (Fletcher factor) in the presence of HMW-K, and (2) activates factor XI to XIa in the presence of HMW-K. Activated factor XIa in the presence of ionized calcium (Ca^{2+}) becomes a protease that facilitates the conversion of factor IX to IXa. Factor IXa in the presence of Ca^{2+}, phospholipid (PL), and factor VIII stimulates the conversion of factor X to Xa. Factor Xa in the presence of Ca^{2+}, PL, and factor V stimulates the conversion of prothrombin (factor II) to thrombin (factor IIa). The conversion of factor II to IIa an *extrinsic system* is shown in Fig. 15.6-1. The release of tissue factors (TF) such as tissue thromboplastin (III) into the blood following injury activates factor VII to VIIa which then stimulates the conversion of factor X to Xa. Factors X and Xa play a pivotal role whether activation is induced by intrinsic or extrinsic systems, and thrombin (IIa) in the presence of Ca^{2+} stimulates the conversion of fibrinogen to fibrin. The fibrin formed initially is characterized as a soluble fibrin that in the presence of factor XIIIa and Ca^{2+} is converted to an insoluble fibrin polymer. This activation of factor XIII by thrombin (IIa) indicates that it has multiple actions in the clotting of blood.

Table 15.6-1
The Clotting Factors

Factor Number	Name	Cause of Deficiency
I	Fibrinogen	Liver disease
I′	Fibrin monomer (soluble and loose)	
I″	Fibrin polymer (insoluble and tight)	
II[a]	Prothrombin	Liver disease, vitamin K deficiency
III	Thromboplastin (tissue), tissue factor (TF)	
IV	Calcium, Ca^{2+}	
V	Accelerator globulin, labile factor	Parahemophilia (rare)
VII	Proconvertin	Liver disease, vitamin K deficiency
VIII	Antihemophilic factor A or hemophilia A factor	Genetic, hemophilia A
IX[a]	Christmas factor, hemophilia B factor	Genetic, hemophilia B
X[a]	Plasma thromboplastin component (PTC), Stuart-Prower factor	Liver disease, vitamin K deficiency
XI[a]	Plasma thromboplastin antecedent (PTA), antihemophilic factor C	Genetic, hemophilia C
XII[a]	Hageman factor	
XIII	Fibrin-stabilizing factor	Defective healing (rare)
	High molecular weight kininogen, Fitzgerald factor (HMW-K)	
	Kallikrein (K)	
	Platelet phospholipid (PL), platelet factor iii, PF iii	

[a] Endogenous inhibitors of coagulation (e.g., antithrombin III) have been identified as proteins with antithrombin action. Antithrombin III is a principal site of action of heparin.

INHIBITION OF CLOTTING

The inhibition of clotting may be achieved through the binding or neutralization of thrombin (IIa); such neutralization may be achieved *in vivo* through antithrombin III (heparin cofactor), an α_2-globulin, which is synthesized in the liver and widely distributed throughout the tissues of the body. Antithrombin III also binds or neutralizes other proteases in the coagulation cascade, namely, factors XIIa, XIa, Xa, and IXa, and is an important natural inhibitor of clotting. There are other natural inhibitors of proteases, such as the first component of complement (Cl inactivator), α_2-macroglobulin, α_1-antitrypsin, and α_2-antiplasmin (Hageman factor binds to Cl, plasmin binds to α_2-plasmin inhibitor and α_2-macroglobulin, and thrombin binds to antithrombin III). These factors that prevent fibrin formation may play a role in the localization of the fibrin clot by neutralizing coagulation factors that escape from the site of injury into the bloodstream. Further, the absorption of thrombin into fibrin may play a role in the termination of clot formation in that thrombin is not only associated with activation of enzymes and cofactors but also in some cases with their inactivation. As coagulation proceeds, certain of the reaction products released become inhibitory (e.g., high concentrations of thrombin can produce a prothrombin fragment that inhibits the activation of prothrombin by factor Xa, and fibrin degradation products have been shown to inhibit fibrin polymerization).

The deposition of fibrin is also associated with a fibrinolytic enzyme that causes lysis of both fibrin clots and fibrin. The proenzyme found in the plasma is called profibrinolysin or plasminogen. The activated enzyme is called fibrinolysin or plasmin. The profibrinolysin (plasminogen) seems to be associated with fibrinogen and is incorporated into the clot. Plasmin is formed by the proteolysis of plasminogen in the presence of fibrin by the natural tissue plasminogen activator. Fibrin's rate of dissolution by plasmin is determined by the α-chain cross-linking (e.g., fibrin that is not cross-linked is readily degraded, whereas completely cross-linked fibrin is resistant to degradation) (1, 7, 13). Thus, lysis of clot may be accomplished immediately after initiation, but becomes more refractory as the thrombus ages (increased cross-linking). Since plasmin free in the plasma is rapidly neutralized by an α_2-plasmin inhibitor, and fibrin binds the plasminogen activator and accelerates the activation plasminogen, the action of plasmin is localized at the thrombus site.

Agents used to modify the clotting mechanism may act by (1) enhancement of the natural inhibition of clotting (e.g., heparin), (2) intravascular enhancement of conversion of fibrinogen to fibrin [e.g., Malayan pit viper venum (Ancrod)], (3) suppression of synthesis of vitamin K-dependent clotting factors (e.g., warfarin), and (4) enhancement of fibrinolysis (e.g., streptokinase, plasmin, and urokinase).

EVALUATION OF CLOTTING

Tests for evaluation of clotting with some of their criteria are listed in Table 15.6-2.

The *prothrombin time* (PT of Quick) is a sensitive measure of changes in the extrinsic system, but not the intrinsic system in the common clotting pathway. The PT is prolonged by deficiencies in factors, V, VII, X, and II, by low levels of fibrinogen, or high levels of heparin. The normal PT ranges from 11.5 to 12.5 sec and is used to evaluate oral anticoagulant therapy. Therapeutic prothrombin times are expressed as an increase over the patient's control value (i.e., 1.5-2.5 times prolongation of patient's control PT is considered desirable). This test is unaffected by variations in factors XII, XI, IX, and VIII, or in platelets.

The *partial thromboplastin time* (PTT) is a sensitive measure of the intrinsic system, but not the extrinsic system in the common clotting pathway. It can detect deficiencies in all plasma factors except VII and XIII. The test is usually performed on platelet-poor plasma and hence tells nothing about the role of platelets in the clotting process. The normal PTT is 60-85 sec; prolongation of PTT is used to evaluate the effectiveness of oral anticoagulant therapy. PTT is prolonged by deficiencies of HMW-kininogen or kallikrein.

The *activated partial thromboplastin time* (APTT) is a sensitive measure of the intrinsic system, but not the extrinsic system in the common clotting pathway. It can detect deficiencies in all the plasma factors except VII and XIII. The test, also usually performed on platelet-poor plasma, tells nothing about the role of platelets in the clotting process. The normal APTT ranges from 24-36 sec, and unlike PTT, is widely used to evaluate heparin therapy.

The *activated coagulation time* (ACT) is a measurement of all of the factors except VII, and since it is a whole blood test, the role of platelets is also evaluated. The normal ACT ranges from 80 to 130 sec and is used to evaluate the effectiveness of heparin therapy.

The *whole blood clotting time* (WBCT, or Lee-White clotting time) is an insensitive measure of prothrombin deficiencies and moderately sensitive in measuring thromboplastin generation. WBCT is normal in the presence of a deficiency in factor VIII. Many variables that are difficult to control limit the usefulness of this test. Under ideal conditions, the WBCT ranges from 9 to 14 min, and is used to evaluate heparin levels.

HEPARIN

A PARENTERAL ANTICOAGULANT

Heparin is a mixture of mucopolysaccharide polymers containing D-glucosamine, D-glucuronic acid, and L-iduronic acid, in addition to sulfuric acid. The molecules are highly negatively charged, and molecular weights range from 5000 to 50,000 (average 15,000) daltons (17). In an effort to correlate the structure of heparin with its anticoagulant effects, only a small fraction (25-35%) of the molecular species in heparin binds to AT-III (α_2-globulin, heparin cofactor) with high affinity; this small fraction accounts for 85-95% of the total activity (17). In contrast, active forms of heparin had a molecular weight of 6000-8000 daltons. Analysis of the highly active small fraction revealed 1.1 additional residues of glucuronic acid per molecule, and 1.5 fewer residues of N-sulfated glucosamine per molecule (17). One of many possible active species is shown in Fig. 15.6-2.

Anticoagulant Action. Thrombin and antithrombin III combine in a molecular ratio of 1:1. The addition of heparin does not alter the combining ratio, but acceler-

Table 15.6-2
Test of Clotting Function

Test	Predictive Value	Normal Range	Factor(s) Evaluated	Drug Efficacy
Prothrombin time (PT)	+	11.5-12.5 sec	II, V, VII, X	Coumarins, indandiones
Partial thromboplastin time (PTT)	+	60-85 sec	All except VII, XIII	Coumarins, indandiones
Activated partial thromboplastin time (APTT)[a]	++++	24-36 sec	All except VII, XIII	Heparin
Activated coagulation time (ACT)	+	80-130 sec	All except VII	Heparin
Lee-White whole blood clotting time (WBCT)	++	9-14 min	All except VII	Heparin
Whole blood partial thromboplastin time (WBPTT)[b]	+++	84-140 sec	All except VII	Heparin

[a] Accurate, but requires approximately 2 hours to complete; heparin $t_{1/2}$ = 1.5 hours.
[b] Offers best combination for economy and accuracy.
Source: Modified from Ref. 11.

ates the rate of inhibition 1000-2000 times. Purified antithrombin III inhibits thrombin gradually in the absence of heparin, but the action is rapid in the presence of heparin. The thrombin-antithrombin complex formed is remarkably stable. The binding site for this complex involves serine residues at the active site on thrombin. The reactive site on AT-III contains an arginine residue. If heparin is present, it binds to lysine residues in the AT-III molecule accelerating the reaction between AT-III and thrombin. Thus, heparin may have an allosteric binding site on AT-III that alters the shape around the arginine reactive site in such a way that it becomes more accessible to thrombin (17). In addition, the affinity of heparin for the lysine site changes once the AT-III thrombin complex is formed, thus releasing heparin to combine with a second molecule of AT-III (17). These studies suggest that heparin may act as a catalyst.

Heparin has other pharmacological actions in addition to prolongation of the clotting time of blood, including: lipemia clearing, if heparin is injected postprandially; blockade of local or generalized Shwartzman and Arthus phenomena; inactivation of serotonin and some snake venoms; and interference with radioactive iodine uptake in red blood cells. More recently, heparin or a heparin fragment administered in combination with cortisone in some tumor-bearing animals was shown to inhibit angiogenesis, decrease tumor size, and to prevent metastases (6). The clinical efficacy of this combination needs to be established.

Pharmacokinetics. Heparin is poorly absorbed (less than 15%) from the gastrointestinal tract after oral administration; therefore, it must be given parenterally. Subcutaneous administration gives a relatively slow rate

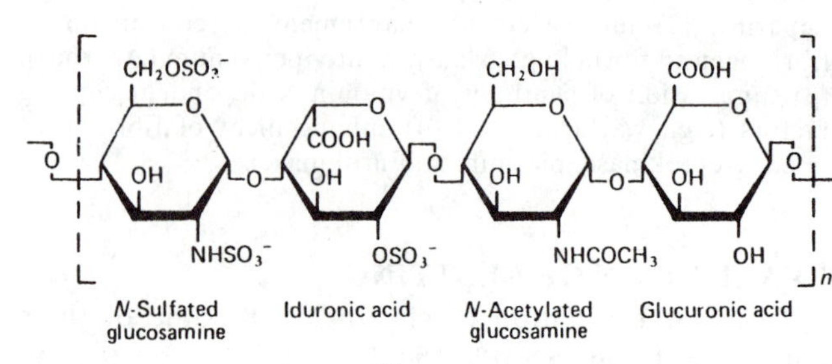

Fig. 15.6-2. *The chemical structure of heparin.*
The sequential arrangements of hexosamine and uronic acid residues represent only one of many possible existing within the polysaccharide chain of heparin.

of absorption of heparin. The intramuscular route of heparin administration is not recommended because of possible hematoma formation from local trauma caused by this acidic mucopolysaccharide. The site of action of heparin is reached rapidly by the intravenous route whether by intermittent bolus injections or sustained infusion techniques (5, 17).

Heparin does not appear in the milk of lactating mothers or cross the placental barrier. It is metabolized in liver by an enzyme, heparinase. Spontaneous or nonenzymatic breakdown of heparin also occurs, releasing sulfate groups into the total body water. These breakdown products, and the metabolite, uroheparin, are excreted in the urine. Unchanged (less than 10%) heparin appears in the urine only after large doses (5).

Heparin is largely bound (95%) to plasma proteins (lipoproteins, α-globulins, and fibrinogen). The plasma half-life of heparin is 1.5 hr. Its volume of distribution (0.05-0.2 l/kg) is limited to the intravascular space. The plasma clearance of heparin varies greatly in normal and diseased states and is dose dependent. Hence, the plasma half-life is dose-dependent, (i.e., it increases with dose). The uptake of heparin by the reticuloendothelial system may be important in plasma clearance. Some pharmacokinetic properties of heparin are given in Table 15.6-3. Following the administration of 100, 200, and 400 units per kilogram, the half-life of each dose was 56, 96, and 120 min, respectively. Effective therapy with heparin is designed to achieve an increase over the patient's pretreatment value by 1.5-2.5 times.

The kinetic behavior of heparin under three conditions of intermittent administration is shown in Fig. 15.6-3 (5). The administration of heparin in a fixed dose at 4-6 hr will not provide minimal anticoagulation for more than 50% of the time interval between doses. However, when the same dose is given every 1.5 hr, continuous anticoagulation is present. Unfortunately, using this dosing schedule, heparin has a tendency to accumulate. But, when a single loading dose is followed by smaller maintenance doses, continuous anticoagulation is present, and the clotting time returns more rapidly to the baseline value when the heparin is discontinued. Probably the most reliable method for assuring adequate amounts and constancy of effect from dosing is by intravenous infusion.

The duration of heparin therapy should not exceed 2 weeks (ideally 7-10 days). As soon as the patient prophylactically receiving heparin becomes ambulatory, oral anticoagulants should be started, usually 4-5 days before heparin therapy is ended (9).

Clinical Uses. The most frequent use of heparin is to provide an acute anticoagulant action prior to (prophylactically) and during the time oral anticoagulant therapy is becoming effective (usually 3 or 4 days) (9, 15, 18, 22). Therapeutic uses of heparin can be grouped as follows: (1) *venous thrombi* and *thromboembolism*; (2) *myocardial infarction* [the preferred route of administration in (1) and (2) is via constant infusion pump (20,000-40,000 U/day)]; and (3) *surgery*. Heparin in low doses has been shown to reduce the incidence of mortality (5%) from pulmonary embolization by inhibiting deep vein thrombosis (1, 9, 18, 22). The latter effect is related to the fact that low doses of heparin can neutralize activated factor X (Xa), especially when heparin levels are smaller than those required to inhibit the conversion of fibrinogen to fibrin by thrombin. Preoperative low-dose heparin prophylaxis is known also to reduce the incidence of deep vein thrombosis by over 50%. Patients with acute thrombosis, on the other hand, may require more heparin because of the binding of heparin to fibrinogen instead of antithrombin III.

Adverse Effects. The most important toxic or adverse manifestation from heparin therapy is uncontrolled bleeding, especially bleeding from undiagnosed lesions. Laboratory evaluation of heparin's effectiveness is required if the patient is to receive the maximum benefit from such therapy, except in the case of low-dose therapy. With continuous i.v. infusion as the route of administration, the anticoagulant effect should be regularly measured and used in adjusting dosages (1, 9, 18, 22).

True allergy or hypersensitivity to heparin is rare. Osteoporosis as an often-documented side effect occurs only after prolonged high-dose therapy; since there are no indications for prolonged therapy, this adverse effect is also rare. Heparin is contraindicated in hemophiliacs, severe malignant hypertension, and visceral malignancies.

Table 15.6-3
Comparative Pharmacokinetic Parameters of Anticoagulants

Generic Name	Route of Administration	Maintenance Dose (mg)	Half-life (hours)	Peak Effect (days)	V_d (l/kg)	Placental Transfer	Appearance in Breast Milk
Heparin	i.v. (bolus)	50	1-2	Immediate	0.05-0.2	No	No
Dicumarol	p.o.	25-100	60-100	2-3	0.14	Yes	No
Warfarin sodium	p.o.	2.5-10	35-45	0.5-1	0.10	Yes	No
Phenindione	p.o.	50-100	5-10	1-2	0.125	Yes	Yes

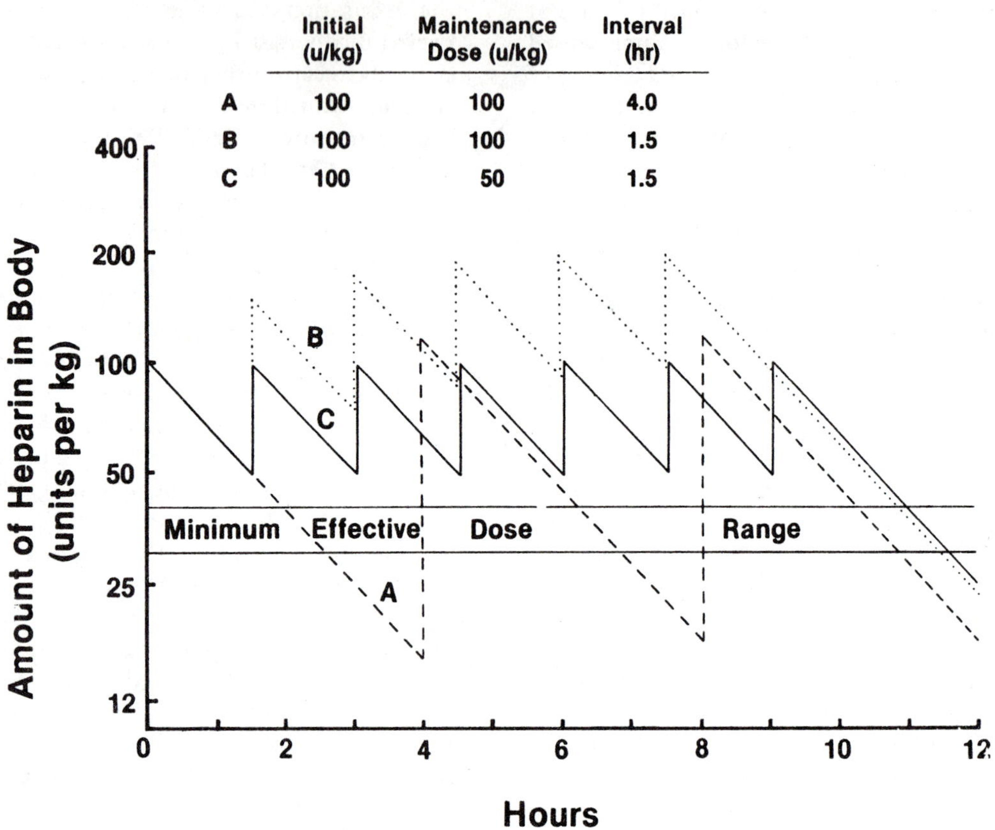

Fig. 15.6-3. *Kinetic behavior of heparin under three conditions of intermittent intravenous administration.* (From Estes,J.W.: ,*Adv.Exp.Med.Biol.* 52,181,1975. by permission).

Treatment of Heparin Overdose. Protamine, a highly positively charged peptide, neutralizes the negative charges of heparin that are responsible for the pharmacological actions. This basic protein rapidly forms a stable salt with acidic heparin in almost equal amounts [1 mg of protamine sulfate for each 1 mg of heparin (120 U)]. In a clinical situation, an amount of protamine equivalent to half of the previous dose of heparin is given at intervals of 10-15 min. Protamine is truly antidotal to heparin, but in most clinical situations heparin's activity disappears from plasma at a rate fast enough to obviate its need. If needed, a 1% solution of protamine sulfate is available for intravenous infusion. An excess of protamine sulfate also has anticoagulant action.

COUMARINS AND INDANEDIONES

ORAL ANTICOAGULANTS

Oral anticoagulants were introduced into clinical medicine almost a half century ago and were quickly reported useful in a variety of disorders, all characterized by a predisposition to the formation of thrombi. Basic science investigations of a hemorrhagic disease in cattle (discovered in 1922) revealed that the cattle consumed improperly cured sweet clover, and the active causative principle was identified to be a 4-hydroxycoumarin derivative called dicumarol. Since the discovery of the 4-hydroxycoumarin, a large number of compounds have been synthesized that inhibit the clotting of blood or plasma. All of these compounds have in common that their anticoagulant properties are related to their abilities to inhibit the biosynthesis of vitamin K (a fat-soluble vitamin) (8, 20, 21).

Vitamin K is responsible for the biosynthesis of factor II (prothrombin), factor VII, factor IX, and factor X, as is shown in Fig. 15.6-1. Oral anticoagulants are synthetic compounds of two chemical types; namely, coumarins and indanediones. Both types act by inhibiting the normal synthesis of these four factors, resulting in the accumulation of biologically inactive derivatives of these clotting factors (8, 20, 21). The decrease in the biologically active forms of VII, IX, X, and II therefore results in a decrease in the rate of clot formation. In the late 1960s, rapid progress was made in elucidating the mechanism of action of vitamin K through studying plasma obtained from patients who had been treated with oral anticoagulants. These studies, and others in laboratory animals, showed the presence of a prothrombin (II) precursor in livers of coumarin-treated individuals and suggested that the vitamin K-dependent step of prothrombin synthesis involved not protein synthesis but some other type of biochemical reaction (8, 20, 21).

The chemical characterization of normal prothrombin revealed that it contained 10 residues of an uncommon amino acid, γ-carboxyglutamic acid. These residues also form the calcium binding site on prothrombin (8, 20). In the presence of oral anticoagulants, γ-carboxyglutamic amino acid residues are not formed, but rather glutamic acid residues are inserted forming an "inactive" or "precursor" prothrombin. Subsequently, it was shown that subcellular preparations from rat liver catalyze the carboxylation of inactive prothrombin in the presence of vitamin K, resulting in clotting factors from their respective precursors. During this carboxylation vitamin K is oxidized to its epoxide (21). More specifically, oral anticoagulants inhibit the reduction of the biologically inactive vitamin K epoxide back to an active vitamin K, an action that causes the accumulation of vitamin K epoxide and depletion of vitamin K (see Fig. 15.6-4).

The structures of dicumarol, warfarin sodium, and phenidione are shown in Fig. 15.6-5. Phenindione is an indanedione. Dicumarol has two coumarin rings. The structural resemblance between dicumarols (or indanediones) and vitamin K (Chapter 14.1) is striking. However, since the regeneration of vitamin K from its epoxide is not a well-understood enzymatic step, and the nature of the reductant that serves as a cofactor remains unknown, the exact mechanism of action of these oral anticoagulants remains to be elucidated. The antagonism between oral anticoagulants and vitamin K is of the noncompetitive type. Oral anticoagulants are indirect-acting drugs. All show a long delay in their onset of action, directly related to plasma clearance of the four clotting factors, VII, IX, X, and II, and on the extent to which their formation is inhibited (21).

Pharmacokinetics. All oral anticoagulants are readily absorbed by passive diffusion from the upper gastrointestinal tract, except dicumarol, which is erratically absorbed with 15-30% recovered in the stool as unchanged drug. All coumarins and indanediones are highly bound to plasma proteins (90-99%) and are slowly metabolized. The volumes of distribution of both dicumarols and indanediones are low, 0.14 l/kg for dicumarol and 0.125 l/kg for phenindione. The rate of metabolism in the liver varies greately as does the effect of dose on elimination half-life (2, 4).

Dicumarol has a dose-dependent elimination half-life that increases with dose, but warfarin and phenindione do not exhibit this phenomenon. The pathways of metabolism differ, although most coumarins and indane-

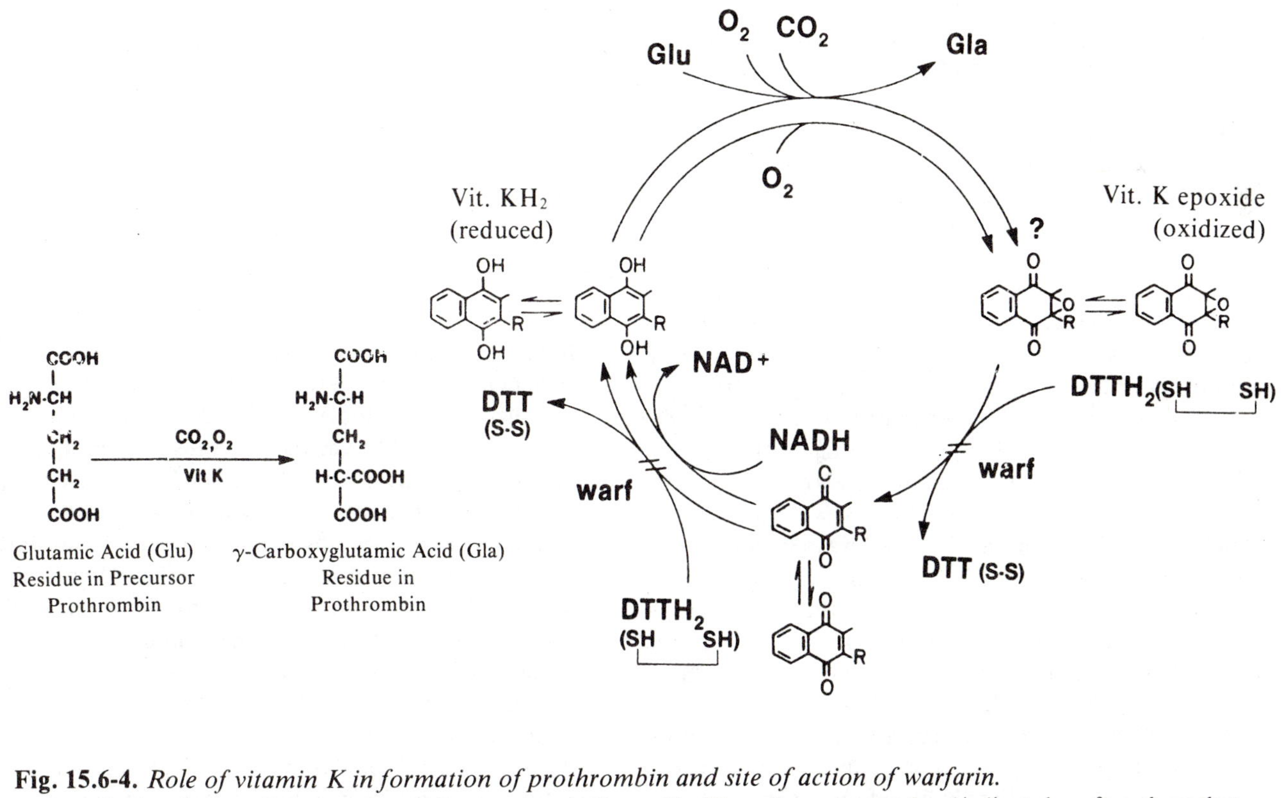

Fig. 15.6-4. *Role of vitamin K in formation of prothrombin and site of action of warfarin.*

Overall, vitamin K_1 or K_2 is stepwise oxidized to vitamin K epoxide. The pathways crossed and indicated warf are those that are sensitive to the action of the coumarin anticoagulants. The (?) in the figure indicates that the product of the involvement of vitamin K hydroquinone in the carboxylation reaction is not known. The figure indicates that the epoxide is reduced by a warfarin-sensitive pathway that used dithiothreitol (DTT) as a reducing agent, and that the quinone form of the vitamin can be reduced to the hydroquinone by either a warfarin-sensitive DTT-driven pathway or by a pyridine nucleotide-linked dehydrogenase. (From Suttie, J.W., *Fed. Proc.* 39: 2731,1980 , by permission).

diones are extensively metabolized in the liver. In some resistant individuals, the rate of elimination may vary 10-20 times. Liver metabolites and parent drugs are excreted by the kidney.

The elimination half-life of dicumarol is 60-100 hr, of warfarin sodium is 35-55 hr, and of phenindione is 5-10 hr. The longer elimination half-life of dicumarol and warfarin means that steady-state concentrations will be reached slowly, and with dicumarol, will vary with the size of the dose.

Even though the half-life of warfarin is less than dicumarol, the peak absorption time of both is 60-120 min. The V_d of both warfarin and dicumarol is similar and consistent with binding mainly to albumin. The V_d for albumin (0.1 l/kg) is similar, or 2.6 times the plasma volume. The mean half-life of warfarin is dose-independent, whereas dicumarol is dependent on plasma concentration. Since both are bound to plasma protein by greater than 90% and only the free drug is active or metabolized, it is important to know that no correlation exists between the dose of warfarin and the prothrombin time.

Warfarin is usually administered as a mixture of two isomers, called R and S. One isomer is about five times more potent as an anticoagulant than the other. The S-isomer is metabolized in the liver to 7-hydroxywarfarin and reduced to an alcohol. The R-isomer is metabolized by the reduction to an alcohol (RS alcohol). Both are metabolized to 6-hydroxywarfarin in small amounts. The hydroxylated metabolites are inactive. The half-life of the R-isomer is 45 hr, whereas the half-life of the S-isomer is 33 hr and the V_d is the same for both isomers. These facts are important, especially since the S-isomer is involved in many more stereospecific drug interactions (2, 3). The onset of action of oral anticoagulants is slow. Since phenindione, warfarin, and dicumarol act on the synthesis of vitamin K-dependent clotting factors, their onset of therapeutic efficacy depends not only on their own kinetics but also plasma clearance of the circulating clotting factors. The four vitamin K-dependent clotting factors have half-lives as follows: VII (6 hr), IX (24 hr), X (40 hr), and II (60 hr). Thus, factor VII from the extrinsic pathway disappears first because it has the shortest half-life, but factors IX and X from intrinsic pathways may be more important in thromboembolic diseases. Prothrombin time may be prolonged shortly after the beginning of therapy because of the rapid fall in factor VII, but the adequate anticoagulant effect will not occur for 3-5 days.

Anisindione is an indanedione derivative chemically related to phenindione. Its mechanism of action and uses are similar to other oral anticoagulants, and phytonadione (vitamin K), fresh whole blood, or plasma counteracts the anticoagulant effects. After an initial dose of 300 mg, the peak effect occurs between 48 and 72 hr and a maintenance dose of 25-150 mg daily should be given in order to keep the prothrombin time values between 2-2.5 times normal. After discontinuing the drug, the coagulation factors return to normal in 24-72 hr.

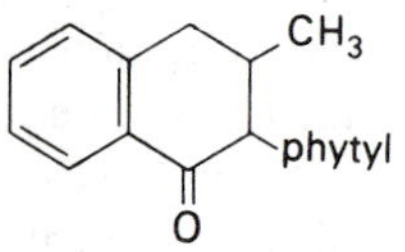

Vitamin K_1 (phytonadione)

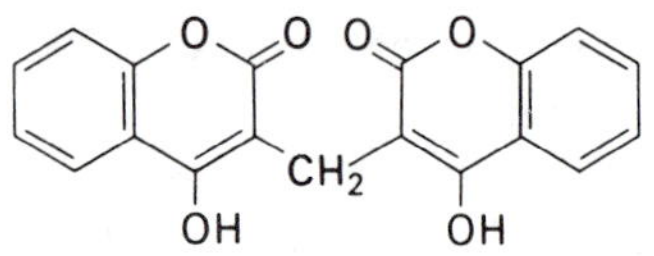

Dicumarol

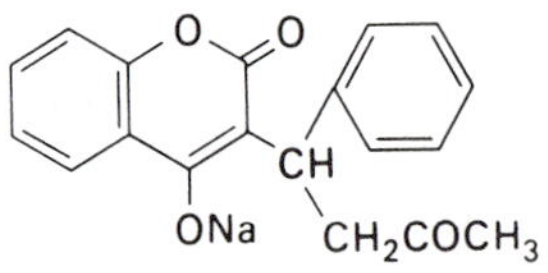

Warfarin sodium

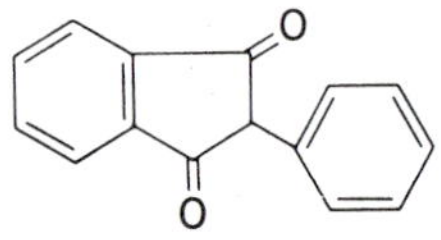

Phenindione

Fig. 15.6-5. *Structural formulas of coumarin anticoagulants and vitamin K.*

The characteristic severe adverse effects of phenindione, such as agranulocytosis, jaundice, and nephropathy, are not present with anisindione thus far, but if fever or rash occurs the drug should be discontinued. Dermatitis is the only consistent mild adverse effect reported.

Like phenindione, anisindione causes a discoloration (red-orange) of the urine when the pH is alkaline. Acidification of urine will cause the color to disappear, a property that distinguished this from hematuria.

Since the indanediones are potentially toxic as a chemical class, many suggest the use only in patients who cannot tolerate coumarins.

Some pharmacokinetic properties of oral anticoagulants are given along with those of heparin in Table 15.6-3.

Clinical Uses. Oral anticoagulants are used in the treatment of a variety of chronic vascular disorders such as pulmonary embolism and thrombophlebitis. The specific aim of the therapy is to prevent an extension of a clot that has already formed, since oral anticoagulants do not cause a previously formed clot to dissolve. Oral anticoagulants are used prophylactically in clinical situations that may lead to thromboembolic complication such as enforced bed rest in elderly patients, cardiac valve prosthesis, rheumatic mitral valve disease with atrial fibrillation, coronary thrombosis with atherosclerotic disease, severe chronic heart failure and venous stenosis, and several rare conditions (i.e., paroxysmal nocturnal hemoglobinuria and homocystinuria).

Through the use of a loading dose, a more rapid prolongation of the prothrombin time can be achieved, but this method does not necessarily offer more rapid protection against thrombi formation. Large loading doses increase the risk from hemorrhage in the patient, especially in patients with abnormal liver function or a genetic susceptibility. Most patients should be initiated on prophylaxis with oral anticoagulant therapy through the use of low maintenance doses. Such patients should be candidates for outpatient therapy and present no evidence of acute thrombotic episodes (2-4, 18). Warfarin has an intermediate half-life of 35 days. Using 5-10 mg/day of warfarin, therapeutic prothrombin times (1.5-2.5 times prolongation) should be obtained in 5-10 days. If an immediate anticoagulant effect is desired for any reason, heparin should be the drug of choice, not a loading dose of oral anticoagulant.

A maintenance dose of warfarin at a fixed dose level may not give the desired therapeutic result; rather, maintenance doses should be determined on an individual basis. The measurement of prothrombin time during oral anticoagulant therapy involves the determination of the time needed for the formation of a clot in citrated plasma after the addition of calcium, lipid extract, and tissue factor (emulsified rabbit brain). The normal plasma clotting time is 12 sec. Prothrombin times must be monitored regularly in order to identify patients who may be at risk for either excess bleeding or insufficient anticoagulant effect to prevent thrombi from forming. Patient compliance is crucial to success of therapy.

Management of an Overdose. Hemorrhage associated with excessive anticoagulation is a major adverse effect from oral anticoagulants. Vitamin K, either orally or parenterally, antagonizes these oral anticoagulants by converting the precursor proteins to fully formed clotting factors. Fortunately, reversal of excessive anticoagulation is rapid (6-8 hr) with the use of vitamin K_1 (phytonadione) when given in adequate doses. If an immediate effect is desired, prothrombin should be given in the form of fresh blood or fresh frozen plasma; both alternatives risk hepatitis.

Adverse Effects. Hemorrhage is by far the most frequent toxic effect, with bleeding from previously undiagnosed lesions or into a critical area the greatest hazard. Gastrointestinal disturbances such as mild diarrhea and soft stools as well as anorexia occur infrequently.

Oral anticoagulants are contraindicated in bleeding disorders, ulcers, local, regional, or lumbar anesthesia, possible cerebral hemorrhage, or bacterial endocarditis as well as in the presence of hepatic or renal disease. The primary bleeding sites are the kidneys, epidermis, and mucosa. Anticoagulants are usually discontinued before major surgical procedures, but minor surgical procedures can be done without great risk to the patient. Other complications are the rare and unusual purple toe syndrome, and a somewhat severe hemorrhagic vasculitis often involving the breast.

The oral anticoagulants warfarin and dicumarol cross the placental barrier reaching the developing fetus (10). Therapeutic doses in the mother will inhibit prothrombin formation in the fetal liver. The administration of oral anticoagulants during late pregnancy has been shown to cause fetal and placental hemorrhage. Warfarin given continuously to the mother during the first 8 weeks of gestation may result in congenital malformation.

DRUG INTERACTIONS

Unpredictable changes in the schedule of dosing are the most frequent cause of variation in a patient's prothrombin time. However, there are many drugs that alter both the plasma protein binding and metabolism of oral anticoagulants. There are several ways in which drugs interact with oral anticoagulants, as shown in Table 15.6-4. Some of the potentially important mechanisms are listed as follows:

1. Competing for binding sites on plasma proteins
2. Inhibiting degradative enzymes in the liver
3. Stimulating degradative enzymes in the liver
4. Decreasing synthesis of vitamin K
5. Increasing catabolism of clotting factors
6. Increasing formation of clotting factors
7. Stimulating bile flow

Phenylbutazone, indomethacin, and sulfisoxazole compete for binding sites on albumin and increase the effective free anticoagulant concentration. Barbiturates as a group/class stimulate drug-metabolizing enzymes in the liver and increase the rate of degradation. Chloramphenicol, phenytoin, and tolbutamide inhibit the degradation of oral anticoagulants in the liver and cause a rise in tissue and plasma levels. Antibiotics decrease bacterial flora, an important source of vitamin K (an antagonist to oral anticoagulants). Aspirin (acetylsalicylic acid) inhibits platelet function and may potentiate effects from oral anticoagulants.

FIBRINOLYSIS: PROMOTION AND INHIBITION

Agents used to reduce the size of thrombi such as urokinase, an endogenous activator, and streptokinase, an exotoxin from hemolytic streptococci, are used for therapeutic fibrinolysis (1, 13, 15). Streptokinase and urokinase are of equal efficacy in inducing thrombolytic activity but their molecular mechanisms differ. Streptokinase by combining with plasminogen in equal molar

Table 15.6-4
Some Important Drug Interactions with Oral Anticoagulants

Drugs that enhance actions	
1. Compete for binding on plasma proteins	2. Inhibit degradation of anticoagulant in liver
Sulfonamides Chloral hydrate Indomethacin Phenylbutazone	Chloramphenicol Phenytoin Tolbutamide Disulfiram Metronidazole Phenyramidol
3. Increase catabolism of clotting factors	4. Additive pharmacodynamic effect
Thyroid hormones Clofibrate	Salicylates
5. Unknown	
Cimetidine Anabolic steroids (methandrostenolone, norethandrolone, ethylestrenol)	
Drugs that depress action	
1. Stimulates degradation of anticoagulants in liver	2. Increase formation of clotting factors
Alcohol Barbiturates Glutethimide Griseofulvin	Estrogens Oral contraceptives Pregnancy
3. Stimulate bile flow	4. Unknown
Rifampin	Diuretics

Source: From Ref. 12.

amounts activates the conversion of plasminogen to plasmin, whereas urokinase causes the cleavage of plasminogen which releases an active fragment and also facilitates plasmin formation.

Streptokinase is given in intravenous infusion, 250,000-600,000 U over 20-30 min, then 100,000 U/hr for 3-5 days.

Urokinase is given by intravascular infusion, 2000-5000 IU over 11-15 min, then 2000-4000 IU/hr for 12-24 hr.

Urokinase is not antigenic. Streptokinase is known to cause allergic reactions, fever, and skin rashes.

Streptokinase and urokinase were shown to be of value in the treatment of pulmonary emboli and venous thrombosis.

Agents used to inhibit fibrinolysis are occasionally needed as an aid in management of hemophilia, a treatment in control of bleeding caused by fibrinolytic therapy, an aid to arrest bleeding associated with cranial aneurysms, and a means of limiting fibrinolytic activity associated with surgery of the prostate. The antifibrinolytic agents used are ϵ-aminocaproic acid and tranexamic acid (an alicyclic analog of aminocaproic acid). These agents are synthetic competitive inhibitors of plasminogen. They are rapidly absorbed from the intestine and cleared by the kidney. The loading dose for tranexamic acid is 15 mg/kg and aminocaproic acid is about 60 mg/kg. The maintenance dose for tranexamic acid is 30 mg/kg every 6 hr and for aminocaproic acid 85 mg every 6 hr. If the loading is given intravenously, it should be infused over a 30-min period in order to avoid a hypotensive response.

The adverse effects include hypotension, abdominal discomfort, nasal stuffiness, and thrombosis from inhibition of plasminogen activator. The tranexamic acid is believed to be more potent with fewer adverse effects.

Preparations. *Heparin.* The USP unit of heparin is the quantity that prevents clotting of 1 ml of citrated sheep plasma for 1 hr following addition of 0.2 ml of 1:100 $CaCl_2$ solution. *Heparin Sodium*, USP must contain at least 120 USP U/mg. *Heparin Sodium Injection*, USP, 250-40,000 USP U/ml in sterile water. *Calcium heparin injection* (CALCIPARINE) reported to cause lower incidence of local hematoma; widely used in Europe.

Oral Anticoagulants

Warfarin Sodium, USP (COUMADIN), 2-, 2.5-, 5-, 7.5-, 10-, and 25-mg tablets. *Warfarin Sodium for Injection*, USP available in vials of 50 mg containing sodium chloride and thiomersal and with ampules of sterile water. *Warfarin Potassium*, USP, 5-and 10-mg tablets. *Dicumarol*, USP (bishydroxycoumarin), 25-, 50-, 100-mg tablets and 25- and 50-mg capsules. *Urokinase* (ABBOKINASE), available in vials of 250,000 IU (50,000 IU/ml after reconstitution). *Streptokinase* (STREPTASE), available in vials of 250,000 and 750,000 IU. *Aminocaproic acid* (AMICAR), 500-mg tablets; syrup 250 mg/ml, vials 250 mg/ml. *Phenindione* (HEDULIN), 50-mg tablets. *Phenprocuomon* (LIQUAMAR), 3-mg tablets. *Anisindione* (MIRADON), 50-mg tablets.

REFERENCES

1. Albrechtson, U., Anderson, J., Einarsson, E. et al. Streptokinase treatment of deep vein venous thrombosis and post-thrombotic syndrome: Follow-up evaluation of venous function. *Arch. Surg.* 116:33, 1981.
2. Coon, W. and Willis, P. Some aspects of the pharmacology of oral anticoagulants. *Clin. Pharmacol. Ther.* 11:312, 1970.
3. Deykin, D. Warfarin therapy I. *N. Engl. J. Med.* 283:691, 1970.
4. Deykin, D. Warfarin therapy II. *N. Engl. J. Med.* 283:801, 1970.
5. Estes, J.W. Application of the kinetic of heparin to the formulation of dosage schedules. In: *Heparin* (Bradshaw, R.A. and Wessler, S., eds.). New York: Plenum, 1975, p. 181.
6. Folkman, J. Langer, R., Linhardt, R.J., Haudenschild, C. and Taylor, S. Angiogenesis inhibition and tumor regression caused by heparin or a heparin fragment in the presence of cortisone. *Science* 221:719, 1983.

7. Francis, D.W., Marder, V.J. and Barlow, G.H. Plasma degradation of cross-linked fibrin. Characterization of new macromolecular soluble complexes and a model of their structure. *J. Clin. Invest.* 66:1033, 1980.
8. Gallop, P.M., Lian, J.B. and Hauschka, P.V. Carboxylated calcium binding proteins and vitamin K. *N. Engl. J. Med.* 302:1460, 1980.
9. Gallus, A.S., Hirsh, J., O'Brien, S.E., McBride, J.A., Tuttle, R.I. and Gent, M. Prevention of venous thrombosis with small doses of heparin. *JAMA* 235:1980, 1976.
10. Hirch, J., Cade, J.F. and Gallus, A.S. Fetal effects of coumarin administered during pregnancy. *Blood* 36:623, 1970.
11. Kayser, S.R. Thrombosis. In: *Applied Therapeutics: The Clinical Use of Drugs*, 3rd ed. (Katcher, B.S., Young, L.Y. and Koda-Kimble, M.A., eds.). San Francisco: Applied Therapeutics, Inc., 1983, p. 333.
12. Koch-Weser, J. and Seller, E.M. Drug interactions with coumarin anticoagulants. *N. Engl. J. Med.* 285:487, 1971.
13. Matsuo, O., Rijken, D.C. and Collen, D. Thrombolysis by human tissue plasminogen activator and urokinase in rabbits with experimental pulmonary embolus. *Nature* 291:590, 1981.
14. Moncada, S. and Vane, J.R. Arachidonic acid metabolites and the interaction between platelets and blood vessel walls. *N. Engl. J. Med.* 300:1142, 1979.
15. Nemerson, Y. and Nassel, H.L. The biology of thrombosis. *Ann. Rev. Med.* 33:479, 1982.
16. Ratnoff, O.D. and Saito, H. Interactions among Hageman factor, plasma prekallikrein, high molecular weight kininogen and plasma thromboplastin antecedent. *Proc. Natl. Acad. Sci.* USA 76:958, 1979.
17. Rosenberg, R.D. and Lam, L.H. Correlation between the structure and function of heparin. *Proc. Natl. Acad. Sci.* USA 76:1218, 1979.
18. Sharma, G.V.R.K., Cella, G., Parisi, A.F. and Sasahara, A.A. Thrombolytic therapy. *N.Engl. J. Med.* 306:1268, 1982.
19. Smith, J.B. The prostanoids in hemostasis and thrombosis: A review *Am. J. Pathol.* 99:743, 1980.
20. Stenflo, J., Fernlund, P., Egan, W. and Roepstorff, P. Vitamin K dependent modification of glutamic acid residues in prothrombin. *Proc. Natl. Acad. Sci.* USA 71:2730, 1974.
21. Suttie, J.W. Mechanism of action of vitamin K: Synthesis of gamma-carboxyglutamic acid. *Crit. Rev. Biochem.* 8:191, 1980.
22. Wilson, J.E., Bynum, L.J. and Parkey, R.W. Heparin therapy in venous thromboembolism. *Am. J. Med.* 70:808, 1981.

CHAPTER
15.7

ANTIANEMIC AGENTS

Rudolph E. Jackson

TYPES OF ANEMIA

Anemia is generally characterized by a reduction in the number of circulating red blood cells and/or a depression of the total hemoglobin content per unit of blood volume. Classification of the anemias is based most commonly upon the underlying pathogenesis. Processes resulting in anemia may include a deficient production of red cells, excessive destruction of red cells, excessive blood loss, or a combination of deficient production and excessive destruction.

The nutritional anemias arise from deficiency of substances essential for erythropoiesis, such as iron, vitamin B_{12}, folic acid, protein, copper, cobalt, and others, and constitute the largest group of anemias affecting the populations of the world today (59, 60). The most widespread nutritional deficiency recognized in the United States today is iron deficiency. Evidence suggests that iron deficiency anemia occurs at a high frequency in infancy (3) and continues to be seen in adolescence and especially in women during the childbearing years. Inadequate intake, absorption, or utilization of essential substances may result in nutritional anemias.

Anemias can also be classified morphologically based on mean corpuscular size and hemoglobin concentration as follows:

1. Microcytic hypochromic
   a. Iron deficiency anemia
   b. Miscellaneous (thalassemia major, pyridoxine-responsive anemia, sideroblastic-refractory anemia)
2. Microcytic normochromic (as in subacute and chronic inflammatory condition)
3. Normocytic (as in sudden blood loss, hemolytic anemias, and other conditions)
4. Macrocytic
   a. Megaloblastic (deficiency of vitamin B_{12} or folic acid)
   b. Miscellaneous (chronic liver disease, hypothyroidism, etc.)

Such morphological classification helps in differential diagnosis of anemias and provides a preliminary guide to therapy particularly for the nutritional anemias. The hypochromic anemias are usually caused by iron-deficiency, and megaloblastic macrocytic anemias respond to vitamin B_{12} or folic acid therapy. For the rest of the anemias, therapy is difficult. This chapter will deal with agents effective in (1.) iron-deficiency and other hypochromic anemias, and (2) megaloblastic anemias caused by deficiency of vitamin B_{12} or folic acid.

AGENTS EFFECTIVE IN IRON-DEFICIENCY AND OTHER HYPOCHROMIC ANEMIC STATES

IRON

History. Iron, first mentioned in Greek mythology, was used therapeutically for many purposes including impotence, weakness and pallor. Iron itself was derived from water or wine in which a sword had rusted. The specific use of iron salts is credited to Sydenham who, in the later 1600s, recommended iron for treatment of chlorosis or "the green-sickness" often seen in girls between the ages of 14 and 17. The most prominent manifestation, a greenish pallor, was due to iron deficiency. In 1832, Pierre Blaud described the response of chlorosis to a mixture of ferrous sulfate plus potassium carbonate.

Another form of anemia, described in the early twentieth century, was *chronic hypochromic anemia*, which differed from chlorosis in developing later in life, around the fourth and fifth decades. Clinical features included epithelial changes involving the tongue and nails and achlorhydria. The anemia was most common among women with poor nutrition, multiple pregnancies, and excessive menstrual bleeding. Although it responded to iron, considerable disagreement arose on this point and for a period of time around 1920 iron therapy became discredited. After iron-deficiency anemia became more clearly distinguished from anemias due to other causes, the use of iron became more specific. The only important use of iron in modern medicine today is in the treatment of iron-deficiency anemia.

Iron Location in Body Compartments. The average adult body contains 3-4 g of iron (50 mg/kg of body weight) distributed in several major compartments including: (1) hemoglobin (70%); (2) body storage forms (ferritin, hemosiderin, and transferin, 25%); (3) myoglobin (4%); (4) cytochrome, catalase, and other iron-containing respiratory enzymes and plasma (1%). Body iron exists in two primary states: the inorganic, or loosely bound form, and the organic, or more tightly bound form. Iron-containing compounds may be grouped into those related to metabolic or respiratory-type functions and those related to storage and transport. Females in the childbearing period and later life tend to have body iron levels approximately one-half or less than those present in males.

Source of Iron. Iron is found in a variety of foodstuffs, with moderately high to high levels in meat, eggs, leafy vegetables, dried beans, cereals, and certain seafoods (especially oysters). Cow's milk and milk products, rice, fruits, and nongreen vegetables are especially low in iron.

The normal diet in the United States supplies approximately 18 mg/day of iron in males and 15 mg/day in females. Approximately 10% of this amount is absorbed; it is adequate to meet the body's daily requirement.

To decrease the high incidence of iron deficiency in infants and young children, proprietary milk preparations, cereals, and flour have been fortified with iron. Recommendations by the Committee on Nutrition of the American Academy of Pediatrics suggest that all infants in the first 6 months of life receive breast milk or an iron-fortified formula (12).

Iron Metabolism. ***Absorption.*** Iron is absorbed primarily in the duodenum and progressively less so as it moved down the bowel (13). Dietary iron is usually in the form of organic ferrous or ferric complexes that are subsequently reduced to inorganic ferrous forms in the stomach in the presence of the gastric acid pH. The alkaline pH of the small intestine favors the formation of ferrous hydroxide, which is the form in which dietary iron is absorbed. Absorption will vary according to the content of other foods, time relationship between the iron intake and intake of other foods, presence of various drugs in the gastrointestinal tract, or abnormalities of the gastrointestinal tract (Table 15.7-1).

The actual mechanism(s) controlling iron absorption from the gastrointestinal tract are not clearly understood. Ferrous hydroxide enters the mucosal cells of the small intestine where it is subsequently converted to ferric hydroxide, which combines with an intracellular protein, apoferritin, to form the compound ferritin. In the form of ferritin, the ferric iron is again reduced to the ferrous state, which has the capability of moving out of the cell into the portal circulation. Based on the action of apoferritin in combining with ferric hydroxide and converting it to ferritin, the *mucosal block theory* was advanced (5). This theory suggested that the degree of saturation of apoferritin or the amount of ferritin present served as a means of regulating the amount of iron absorbed from the gastrointestinal tract. A saturated apoferritin or ferritin state made the mucosal cell unable to absorb further iron. Unsaturation of apoferritin or decreased amount of mucosal cell ferritin resulted in increased uptake of iron into the mucosal cell.

Table 15.7-1
Gastrointestinal Factors Affecting Iron Absorption

Enhancers	Inhibitors
1. Vitamin C	1. Dairy products (milk, cheese, eggs)
2. Fats (PUF and SF)	2. High-fiber foods (brans, whole wheat)
3. Meats (relatively)	3. Tea
	4. Coffee
	5. Antacids (especially Mg trisilicate)
	6. Tetracyclines Oxytetracycline Methacycline Doxycycline

Although attractive, evidence now indicates that other factors including (1) the state of body stores of iron, (2) the degree of hemopoietic activity, and (3) how much iron is ingested regulate the rate and degree of the absorption of iron from the gastrointestinal tract (5, 8, 32).

Iron-deficiency states, alcohol, anoxia, ascorbic acid, amino acids, and fructose enhance the absorption of iron (32), whereas malabsorption diseases, amylophagia (starch eating), geophagia, phytates, phosphates, tetracyclines, and oral alkalis all interfere with iron absorption. The mechanism of action of several of the latter includes the formation of insoluble complexes or an alteration in pH resulting in the formation of insoluble iron hydroxides.

Transport. After entering the blood, iron in the ferrous state combines with transferrin, a β-globulin plasma protein. After conversion again to the ferric state and attachment to transferrin, it becomes part of the available plasma pool. This fraction, measured as serum iron, normally ranges from 50-150 μg%. Transferrin moves ferric iron from the plasma to the membranes of normoblasts in the bone marrow. From the membrane, iron enters the cell cytoplasm. Serum iron-binding capacity, a measure of the capacity of plasma to combine with iron, normally ranges from 250 to 350 μg%. Transferrin bands are easily recognized on starch-gel electrophoresis, with type C occurring most commonly (50).

The plasma pool is in a constant dynamic state, with approximately 30 mg of iron entering and leaving the plasma pool each day. Iron from dietary sources and from the breakdown of red cells enters the pools, whereas that going into storage sites or hemoglobin synthesis leaves the pool at a constant rate (37).

Distribution and Storage. The total content of iron in adult males is approximately 50 mg/kg of body weight, where as adult females have a slightly lower total body iron content, approximately 35 mg/kg of body weight. This difference occurs primarily because of a lower total average storage depot iron content of approximately 300 mg in females.

Iron is stored in liver, spleen, bone marrow, and other tissues. Stored iron represents approximately one-half of the total body iron and is found in two forms: ferritin, composed of ferric hydroxide molecules bound to the protein apoferritin; and hemosiderin, an ill-defined, chemically heterogeneous group of large iron-salt-protein aggregates. Iron in the ferritin form appears to be more easily mobilized than hemosiderin. Stored iron is available for use in the formation of hemoglobin in the marrow or extramedullary hematopoietic tissues.

The extreme conservation of iron results from the fact that iron is principally located intracellularly, where it is chelated in the porphyrin ring of hemoglobin, myoglobin, and various intracellular enzymes or bound in iron-protein complexes as ferritin and hemosiderin.

Excretion. Iron is excreted from the body in very small amounts, 0.5-1 mg/day (Table 15.7-2), mainly through exfoliation of iron-containing epithelial cells of the skin and gastrointestinal tract and also through loss of hair and nails, and fecal and urinary routes.

Table 15.7-2
Average Body Iron Losses

Route	Amount (mg/day)
Fecal	0.2-0.5
Urinary	0.1
Sweating (heavy)	0.5
Menstrual	3-4 (total = 20)

Females lose an average of 40 ml of blood during each menstrual cycle; thus approximately 20-40 mg of iron is lost during each cycle in addition to other normal losses. This accounts in part for the lower body iron content in females during the childbearing age and the greater prevalence of iron-deficiency anemia in this group. Further negative iron balance may occur during pregnancy and lactation, when there is a need for expansion of the total maternal red cell mass during the third trimester of pregnancy, the passage of iron across the placenta to the developing fetus, and the presence of iron in breast milk in the form of lactoferrin.

Iron Requirements. Approximately 10% of dietary iron is absorbed. As the normal dietary intake per day varies from 12 and 20 mg in males and between 8 and 15 mg in females, 0.8-2 mg of iron is absorbed. If there are no unusual requirements, the normal diet provides all the iron that is needed. During pregnancy, iron requirements are increased and the usual diet is inadequate; therefore, supplementation is required. Prematurity, the period of rapid growth during infancy, and a diet inadequate in iron during any stage of life all result in increased iron requirements.

Cow's milk is a poor source of iron, containing approximately 0.07 mg/100 ml. Cow's milk also contains heat-labile proteins that may damage the villi of the small intestine, causing additional blood loss (58). For these and other reasons, cow's milk is not recommended as the sole dietary intake for infants during the first 6 months of life and, according to some, throughout the first year of life. Breast milk supplemented with oral iron or iron-fortified proprietary forms of formula are better suited during early infancy.

Normal dietary iron requirements, taking into consideration 10% bioavailability, are presented in Table 15.7-3. A variety of dietary factors and abnormalities of the gastrointestinal tract may play a role in iron absorption. Gluten-sensitive enteropathy and other celiac diseases may impair iron absorption (31).

Iron Deficiency States. Iron deficiency may occur as a result of a variety of factors, including inadequate dietary intake, absorption abnormalities, blood loss, rapid growth, combinations of these factors, and other less commonly occurring conditions.

When a significant negative iron-balance state is present over a substantial period of time, a sequence of iron-deficiency changes occur in which iron stores are initially mobilized followed by a progressive depletion of functional body iron. Hillman and Finch have described these stages as: (1) iron depletion, (2) iron-deficient erythropoiesis, and (3) iron-deficiency anemia (9).

In the iron-depletion stage, the hemosiderin content of the reticuloendothelial cells in the marrow is decreased or absent. Mucosal absorption of iron tends to increase; plasma transferrin level increases; and plasma ferritin levels. As negative iron balance progresses, the iron-deficient erythropoiesis stage occurs. In addition to exhaustion of iron stores, there is a fall of plasma iron to a level below 30 $\mu g\%$, and the transferrin saturation drops to less than 15% accompanied by an increase in red cell protoporphyrin. Hemoglobin synthesis may be decreased, *although* there may not be recognizable anemia in this stage. In the iron-deficiency anemia stage, in addition to the previous abnormalities, there is a demonstrable anemia with characteristics red cell morphological changes including the presence of hypochromic, microcytic red cells, anisocytosis, and poikilocytosis (12).

In addition to the anemia and red cell changes in iron-deficiency anemia, a number of nonhematological manifestations have been described by various investigators. It has been suggested by some that growth is affected due to diet largely of milk (low in iron) resulting in a chubby infant. A large number of iron-deficient anemic infants were reported to be underweight (11, 14, 47). Iron compounds have been suggested to play a role in the mitotic process (20)

Koilonychia, angular stomatitis, and glossitis have been noted commonly in adults with iron-deficiency anemia (11). Also associated with iron deficiency are numerous biochemical abnormalities including decrease in heme proteins (myoglobin, cytochromes, catalase), decrease in activity of iron-containing enzymes (succinate dehydrogenase, monoamine oxidase. α-glycerophosphate oxidase), decrease in activity of enzymes in which iron serves as cofactor, and disturbed nucleic acid synthesis (41).

A possible relationship also exists between iron deficiency and alterations in behavior. Anemic iron-deficient 3- to 5-year-olds displayed decreased attentiveness, narrow attention spans, and perceptual restrictions (31). Moreover, iron-deficient infants and children increased their scores on the Bayley Scales of Infant Development within 5-7 days of therapy (41, 45). Iron deficiency was shown to have adverse effects on attention and memory control processes of older children (45).

Table 15.7-3
Daily Dietary Iron Requirements

Age (yr.)	Iron (mg)
0-0.5	10
0.5-3	15
4-10	10
11-18	18
Females: 19-50	18
51+	10
Males: 19+	10

Preparations

Oral Preparations. *Ferrous Sulfate,* USP: capsules, 150 mg (30 mg elemental iron); tablets, 192, 325 mg (39 and 65 mg elemental iron, respectively); *Ferrous Fumarate,* USP: tablets, 195 and 325 mg (64 and 107 mg elemental iron, respectively); *Ferrous Gluconate,* USP: tablets, 300 mg (38 mg elemental iron); *Ferrocholinate,* drops, 25 and 50 mg/ml; tablets, 40 mg; *Iron-Polysaccharide Complex,* capsules, 150 mg: elixir, 100 mg/5 ml; tablets, 50 mg.

The drug of choice for iron deficiency is oral ferrous sulfate. Any form of ferrous iron (gluconate, ascorbate, lactate, succinate, fumarate, glycine sulfate, etc.) is effective for oral administration, although only ferrous succinate is significantly better absorbed from ferrous sulfate without an increase in side effects (12). This increase in absorption over ferrous sulfate, which is much less expensive, does not constitute a critical therapeutic factor.

The amount of soluble elemental iron per dose rather than the form in which it is administered is most important in the occurrence of gastrointestinal symptoms: the largest amount that can be given without producing side effects is desirable. Ferric iron and heavily chelated iron are poorly and inefficiently absorbed. Vitamin supplementation or the use of other heavy metals is not necessary.

The adult dosage of ferrous sulfate is 300 mg for the hydrated salt and 200 mg for the dry salt, three times a day, to replenish body iron store within 6 months. Administration of iron at intervals throughout the day allows for more complete absorption. Dosages taken between meals also allow for greater absorption of iron, as most foods interfere with iron absorption. The hematological response to orally administered iron preparations generally becomes evident after 2 weeks of treatment. The pediatric dosage for iron is 4-6 mg/kg/day in three divided doses. This provides 1.5-2 mg/kg of elemental iron and is available in concentrated solutions that may be packaged in dropper or suspension forms.

Parenteral Preparations. *Iron dextran injection,* USP (IMFERON), is a parenteral preparation having a high-molecular-weight (5,000-7,000 daltons) complex of ferric hydroxide and dextran containing 50 mg/ml of iron. Iron dextran is available in 10-ml vials containing 0.5% phenol for i.m. injection and in 2-and 5-ml ampuls for i.m. and i.v. injection. It is safe, has few drawbacks, and is not commonly used. Dosage depends upon the starting hemoglobin level and the amount necessary to replenish stores. Dosages may be calculated as follows:

$$\frac{(\text{Norm. Hb} - \text{Init. Hb}) \times \text{bv (ml)} \times 3.4 \times 1.5}{100}$$

where Norm. Hb = Normal hemoglobin; Init. Hb = initial hemoglobin); and bv = blood volume.

Blood volume is approximately 80 ml/kg; the factor 3.4 converts grams of hemoglobin to milligrams of iron: and the factor 1.5 provides extra iron to replace depleted iron stores.

Other intramuscular preparations include: iron sorbitex injection, green ferric ammonium citrate, ferrous gluconate, iron adenylate, and iron polyisomaltose. Experience with these agents is limited. *Iron-poly* (sorbitol-gluconic acid) *complex* (FERASTRAL) (17, 52, 55) appears to be safe and effective intramuscular iron forms should be given deep i.m. in divided doses at daily intervals according to the weight and age of the patient. No preservative should be present in the agent when it is given i.v. The injection should be given very slowly, with close attention to any evidence of toxic or side effects.

Adverse Effects and Acute Overdose. ***Acute Iron Toxicity.*** Acute iron toxicity is not very common in adults, but serious problems occur in young children with the ingestion of doses in excess of 1 g. The mortality rate from acute iron poisoning in young children approaches 50% with ingestion of ferrous sulfate in excess of 2 g. Most commonly, these tablets are obtained from the mother's medication bottle and are ingested because they look like candy.

Signs and symptoms may have their onset within the first hour or later and consist most often of gastrointestinal irritation, bleeding, and necrosis. Other signs and symptoms include nausea, vomiting, lethargy, diarrhea with greenish then tarry or bloody stools, cardiovascular collapse and shock.

Treatment should start immediately after ingestion, if possible. Milk and eggs should be given to form iron-protein complexes with iron. The stomach should be lavaged (in the initial stages; this procedure is dangerous if gastric necrosis has already occurred). A chelating agent, such as deferoxamine, may be utilized for iron-chelating purposes.

Adverse Effects. Side effects of iron therapy may include diarrhea, constipation, nausea, and epigastric pain. Most of these symptoms occur as a result of the elemental iron content of the agent administered and may be decreased by reducing the dose by one-third to one-half. Administering the iron with meals may also reduce these side effects but may also reduce the amount of iron absorbed. Staining of teeth in young children and black discoloration of stools may occur, masking gastrointestinal bleeding.

Therapeutic Uses. The drug of choice for iron deficiency is oral ferrous sulfate which is effective and inexpensive. Given in an amount of 4-6 mg/kg per day in divided doses in infants and children, and 300 mg three times a day in adults, it is well tolerated and most effective. A response can be noted within the first 24 hours of therapy, with replacement of intracellular enzymes resulting in a number of subjective improvements including decrease in irritability and increase in appetite. This is later followed by improvement of blood parameters. Recent procedures for measuring serum ferritin level, transferrin saturation, and red cell protoporphyrin levels allow a more accurate determination than previously of the presence of iron store reduction or depletion. Iron therapy should continue until all peripheral blood parameters are returned to normal, and for at least an additional 4-6 weeks for repletion of iron stores. Every effort should be made to correct any underlying problem (blood loss, gastrointestinal absorption abnormality, etc.) that result in a return to a state of negative iron balance.

Failure to respond to oral iron may occur as a result of patient noncompliance, inadequate dosage, ineffective preparation, persistent loss of iron (e.g., continued G.I. bleeding), abnormal absorption or utilization of the iron, administration of iron along with an agent that will result in a nonabsorbable iron complex, or an incorrect diagnosis.

DEFICIENCY OF OTHER MINERALS AND VITAMINS

COPPER

Copper is essential in human metabolism, however, because it is present in so many forms and in such abundance, a copper deficiency is rare in humans. Anemia may occur as part of the picture of dysproteinemia in infancy. Low copper levels are also found in this syndrome; however, the anemia will respond to iron without the addition of copper (61).

COBALT

Cobalt deficiency has not been reported in humans, however, administration of cobalt may result in a rise in hematocrit, hemoglobin, and red cell indices in some patients with refractory anemia. The exact mechanism of this action is not known. Cobalt will stimulate erythropoietin production; however, erythropoietin levels are already elevated in these instances.

Toxic effects included cutaneous flushing, tinnitus, nausea and vomiting, nerve deafness, anorexia, weakness, and congestive heart failure. Cyanosis, coma, and death have occurred from cobalt chloride overdose.

PYRIDOXINE

Pyridoxine-responsive anemia (23) also called *sideroachrestic anemia*, is characterized by the presence of iron molecules in erythrocyte precursors frequently ringing the nucleus, a hypochromic microcytic anemia, elevated serum iron level with saturation of iron-binding protein, hemosiderosis, and an increased absorption of iron.

Although the picture of nutritional pyridoxine deficiency is lacking, therapy with either oral or intramuscular pyridoxine up to 200 mg daily results in a marked rise in hemoglobin and hematocrit. It is believed that pyridoxine may serve in the capacity of a coenzyme stimulating the incorporation of iron into the porphyrin ring to make heme (30).

ASCORBIC ACID

Severe ascorbic acid deficiency is often associated with hypochromic anemia, which may be microcytic in conditions of chronic blood loss, or macrocytic when associated with folic acid deficiency.

AGENTS EFFECTIVE IN MEGALOBLASTIC ANEMIAS

Megaloblastic anemias occur as a result of an asynchrony between the development of the red cell nucleus and the cytoplasm. This asynchrony results from a defect that causes a slowing in the synthesis of nuclear deoxyribonucleoprotein coupled with a relatively normal development of cytoplasmic RNA, and is characterized by the presence of megaloblasts in the bone marrow and macrocytes in the peripheral blood. The megaloblast is larger than the normoblast at a similar stage of red cell maturation. Morphological changes may also be present in leukocytes and megakaryocytes; polymorphonuclear leukocytes have hypersegmented nuclei, and platelets may be giant sized.

Normal cellular maturation is dependent upon two major classes of hemopoietic factors, the vitamin B_{12} coenzymes and the folates. Macrocytic anemia and megaloblastic dyspoiesis occur when one or the other is deficient. Other deficiencies that may also be characterized to a degree in a megaloblastic anemia include ascorbic acid, tocopherol, and thiamine.

Vitamin B_{12} and folate deficiency may rise from a variety of causes including inadequate intake, abnormal absorption, increased losses, increased requirements, and a variety of antagonistic agents to these factors. The abnormality present in B_{12} or folate deficiency affects all rapidly dividing cells, including those of the mucosa of the mouth, stomach, intestine, and vagina. Vitamin B_{12} deficiency may also result in neurological deficits.

History. In 1855, Addison initially discussed an idiopathic anemia that progressed to death; this anemia is frequently termed *addisonian anemia* (10). Biermer, in 1872, first used the term *pernicious anemia* in describing some 15 cases of progressive anemia. Neurological symptoms were first described by Gardner in 1877 and spinal cord involvement by Lichtheim in 1877 (10). Erlich first described the megaloblast in 1980 (10). Naegeli described hypersegmentation of the neutrophils in the peripheral smear in 1923 (10).

Minot, Murphy and Whipple were awarded the Nobel Prize in 1934 when Minot and Murphy (38) used raw liver by mouth to effect a dramatic response in pernicious anemia, following Whipple's earlier report of the addition of liver to the diet of anemic dogs and the beneficial effect on erythrocyte proliferation (56).

Castle (10) in 1929 showed that ground beef preincubated in normal gastric juice induced remission in 8 of 10 patients with pernicious anemia, whereas beef alone was ineffective. Thus, the concept of *intrinsic factor* in normal gastric juice and *extrinsic factor* in meats was introduced. It is now known that intrinsic factor from the stomach is required for the absorption of vitamin B_{12} from the diet.

Folic acid was isolated from a leafy vegetable by Mitchell et al. (39) in 1941 and found later to be effective in human patients with macrocytic anemia.

A recent concept suggests that pernicious anemia is a genetically determined autoimmune disorder that results from antibodies developed against the parietal cells of the stomach and the intrinsic factor.

VITAMIN B_{12} (Cyanocobalamin)

History. In 1948, crystalline vitamin B_{12} was isolated by Rickes et al. in the United States and Smith and Parker in England. In 1964, Dorothy Hodgkin won the Nobel Prize for her elucidation of the chemical structure of the vitamin by x-ray crystallography (6).

Chemistry. Vitamin B_{12} is a vitamin with the highest molecular weight (over 1300 daltons). It contains a central cobalt atom linked to four reduced pyrrole rings of a surrounding planar group or corrin nucleus—a porphyrinlike ring structure. It also contains a 5,6-dimethylbenzimidazolyl nucleotide linked at right angle to the corrin nucleus with a link to the cobalt atom. The cobalt atom is also connected to a variable R group that represents -CN and -OH in cases of cyanocobalamin (vitamin B_{12}) and hydroxycobalamin, respectively. The structure of the vitamin is shown in the next page.

Cyanocobalamin is the commercial form of the vitamin. The cyanide group attached to the central cobalt atom is present due to contamination from reagents used in isolation.

The vitamin is slightly soluble in water, ethyl alcohol, and phenols and is stable to heat. It is inactivated by light and by strong acid or alkaline solutions.

Sources and Requirements. Vitamin B_{12} differs from most other vitamins in that it is not synthesized by plants or animals. Only certain microorganisms can synthesize the vitamin. Vitamin B_{12} is synthesized by various bacteria present in the soil, sewage, and in the intestinal lumen. Bacteria such as *Propionibacterium shermanii, Streptomyces griseus*, and *Streptomyces*

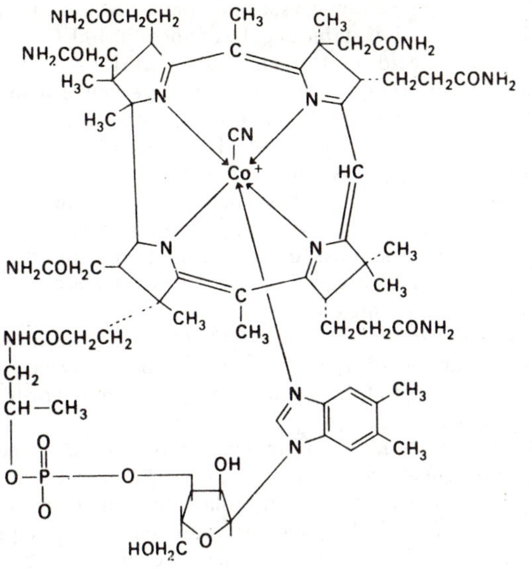

Cyanocobalamin

aureofaciens produce large amounts of the vitamin, whereas other organisms (*Lactobacillus lactis* and *leichmannii,* and *Euglena gracilis*) are unable to synthesize any and subsequently must obtain the vitamin from exogenous sources for optimal growth (37). These latter organisms are commonly used in vitamin B_{12} assay systems.

In humans, vitamin B_{12} is synthesized in the large bowel by bacteria. This material is not absorbed but is excreted in feces. In animals, vitamin B_{12} is absorbed from the intestine and is stored in liver and other tissues. Source of cyanocobalamin include animal liver, kidney, and seafoods that take in large quantities of vitamin B_{12}-synthesizing microorganisms in the sea. Moderate-to-smaller amounts are found in nonfat dry milk, the yolk of eggs, and in some cheeses (35). The daily minimum requirement of vitamin B_{12} is relatively small, between 3 and 7 μg/day (51). In the normal individual, even this amount supplies many times over the necessary amount when there are no problems with absorption. The daily requirement in infants is probably less than 0.5 μg (4).

Functions and Mechanism of Action. Vitamin B_{12} has been shown to be essential for a number of biochemical reactions in nature, most of which involve the intramolecular rearrangement of hydrogen or carbon (12). Vitamin B_{12} is essential for the functioning of all cells, especially those of the bone marrow, the nervous system, and the gastrointestinal tract. Vitamin B_{12} coenzymes are essential for the synthesis of methionine and choline (6) (Table 14.2-1). Reactions known to occur in humans include the biosynthesis of methionine and the isomerization of methylmalonate to succinate. The main importance of vitamin B_{12}-dependent methionine synthesis is probably in the regeneration of tetrahydrofolate from methyltetrahydrofolate. This then explains its relationship to folate metabolism (7, 25). The latter reaction plays an important role in gluconeogenesis utilizing cholesterol, fatty acids, as well as a number of amino acids via the Krebs cycle.

Absorption, Transport, and Excretion. Absorption of ingested vitamin B_{12} occurs chiefly in the ileum. Vitamin B_{12} taken in orally is bound to protein that has to be split before absorption takes place. Absorption may occur as a result of two mechanisms. An active process requires intrinsic factor and an intact ileal receptor site. It is the more important of the two mechanisms. Free vitamin B_{12} split from its peptide bond binds with intrinsic factor secreted by the parietal cells of the stomach. The complex of intrinsic factor (IF) and vitamin B_{12} (IF-B_{12}) goes through the small bowel to the distal ileum, where it is absorbed by specific receptor sites in a relatively neutral pH. Approximately 1 to 3% of the total amount ingested is absorbed passively by diffusion and occurs independent of IF. Absorption by this mechanism occurs along the entire small bowel.

IF is a glycoprotein of molecular weight 44,000-48,000 (1) secreted by parietal cells of the body and fundus of the stomach and has an avid attachment to vitamin B_{12}. One molecule of IF binds one molecule of vitamin B_{12}. The absorption of the IF-B_{12} complex in the small intestine requires a neutral pH and the presence of calcium which enhances receptor site attachment. Evidence suggests that only the vitamin B_{12} actually enters the cell. IF does not pass through the mucosal cells into the portal system (44); however, it is not clear whether it is digested off at the brush border or enters the mitochondria of the microvilli. In pernicious anemia, IF deficiency decreases absorption of vitamin B_{12}, resulting in its deficiency. In tropical sprue, celiac disease, regional enteritis, and other malabsorption syndromes, or after gastric resection, the absorption of vitamin B_{12} is subnormal.

Upon leaving the mucosal cells, vitamin B_{12} is transferred to the portal blood, where it primarily attaches to transcobalamin II and also probably in smaller fractions to transcobalamins I and III. Transcobalamin II is primarily a transport protein delivering vitamin B_{12} to the liver, bone marrow, and other tissues. It thus plays an important role in hematopoiesis, delivering vitamin B_{12} to developing cells undergoing active cellular protein synthesis. Transcobalamin I is considered as primarily a storage protein for vitamin B_{12} (46). The liver probably serves as the largest storage site of vitamin B_{12}. Total normal body stores measure approximately 2 to 5 mg.

The mean normal plasma concentration of vitamin B_{12} is 450 pg/ml with a nomal range of 200-900 pg/ml. The major routes of excretion of vitamin B_{12} are through the biliary tree and subsequently the gastrointestinal tract, and through renal excretion. Approximately 3 to 6 μg of vitamin B_{12} is secreted into the gastrointestinal tract daily, primarily in the bile. The greater amount of this is reabsorbed in the ileum by the IF mechanism. Unabsorbed vitamin B_{12} passes into the feces together with that synthesized by bacteria in the colon. The total amount from these two sources measures approximately 3 to 6 μg in feces daily. A much smaller amount is lost via the urinary tract.

Symptoms of Deficiency. Vitamin B_{12} deficiency may result from several processes, including inadequate intake, defective absorption, defective transport, or disorders of metabolism.

Clinical manifestations may have an insidious onset, with pallor, apathy, easy fatigability, and anorexia as early symptoms. Paresthesias are common and occur primarily because of a peripheral neuropathy associated in some cases with degeneration of the posterior and lateral tracts of the spinal cord. The biochemical basis for the neuropathy remains unclear but may be related to disturbed fatty acid metabolism secondary to a block in propionate metabolism (18).

In severe megaloblastic anemia secondary to vitamin B_{12} deficiency, total red cell number may be significantly decreased along with a decrease in leukocytes and platelets. The mean corpuscular volume of red cells in markedly increased and a proportion of the neutrophils show hypersegmented nuclei (i.e., more than five lobes). In the bone marrow there is an increased proportion of early cells with red cells in all stages of development and megaloblastic in appearance. The cytoplasm is comparatively more mature than the nucleus. Red cell life span is shortened with concurrent ineffective erythropoiesis.

In addition to neurological and hematological abnormalities, vitamin B_{12} deficiency may also be accompanied by atrophic glossitis, constipation, and elevation of serum bilirubin.

Adverse Effects. No serious adverse reaction has been reported with either cyanocobalamin or hydroxocobalamin. Allergic reactions to impurities in the preparations may occur rarely. Injection causes little or no pain, and no adverse local effects.

Drug Interactions. Neomycin, kanamycin, bacitracin, paromomycin, and phenformin produce vitamin B_{12} malabsorption (53). Vitamin B_{12} metabolism is increased in women taking oral contraceptives (48). Patients taking megadoses of vitamin C (1 g with each meal) have been reported to develop B_{12} deficiency (26, 27). The reactions of these and other drugs with vitamin B_{12} are given in Table 14.2-2.

Therapeutic Uses and Doses. Most patients with vitamin B_{12} deficiency have pernicious anemia, and these patients require treatment throughout life. In all cases of megaloblastic anemia, the correct underlying etiology should first be determined and specific therapy instituted.

The treatment of choice for vitamin B_{12} deficiency is the i.m. or deep s.c. injection of solutions of crystalline cyanocobalamin or hydroxocobalamin. For treatment of uncomplicated pernicious anemia, the dose is 30-50 μg daily for 1 week to 20 days, followed by 100 μg weekly until remission is complete; thereafter, 100 μg every 4 weeks will maintain remission.

For patients with demonstrable neurological damage, 1000 μg may be given once weekly for several months, then once or twice monthly for another year; neurological damage that is not reversed within 12-18 months must be considered irreversible.

The oral route of therapy should only be used for the treatment of dietary vitamin B_{12} deficiency.

Preparations. Cyanocobalamin, USP (RUBRAMIN, etc.): solution, 100 μg/ml and 1000 μg/ml for i.m. or deep s.c. injection.

Hydroxocobalamin, USP (ALPHAREDISOL, etc.): solution 1000 μg/ml i.m. or deep s.c. injection. In this compound, the CN group of cyanocobalamin is substituted by OH group.

FOLIC ACID (Pteroylglutamic Acid)

History. In the early 1930s, Willis in India observed megaloblastic anemia in pregnant women whose diets consisted mainly of white rice and bread. A similar condition was produced in monkeys. The unidentified factor was given many names, including Willis factor, vitamin M, factor U, and citrovorum factor. The name folic acid was given in 1941 by Mitchell et al. because of its presence in green leaves. The active material isolated was the same yellow substance isolated from butterfly wings by Hopkins in 1889 and purified and called xanthopterin in 1925 by Wieland; the growth factor was found in 1940 by Snell and Peterson. In 1946, the structure and synthesis of the vitamin were determined by Angier et al. and Pfiffer et al. (34).

Chemistry. Folic acid is the parent compound of a large group of naturally occurring, structurally related compounds, collectively called folates. Folic acid itself has a molecular weight of 441.4. Folic acid consists of a pteridine nucleus, p-aminobenzoic acid, and glutamic acid (Fig. 15.7-1). Pure folic acid is a bright yellow crystalline compound that is slightly soluble in water. It is stable at pH 5 or above at 100°C. It is easily oxidized in an acid solution and is light sensitive.

Sources and Requirements. Folates are widely distributed in nature. Foods having the highest concentrations of folate include yeast, liver, kidney, nuts, fresh green and yellow leafy vegetables, citrus fruits, and berries. Liver may contain up to 300 μg/100 g of folate. Milk is a very poor source of folate, and heating processes cause lowering or complete loss of folate content in milk and most foods. The total folate in a "normal" diet in America, as determined by the *L. casei* assay, is in the range of 1.0 to 1.2 mg daily.

Folic acid is readily absorbed from the gastrointestinal tract. For its metabolically active form, it must be converted from its conjugated state to folinic acid (citrovorum factor) or to tetrahydrofolic acid.

The minimal human requirement for folate is estimated to be 50 μg/day. The average store of folate in an adult is estimated to be approximately 7.5 mg. The folate content in the average daily diet is 200 to 300 μg. Dietary sources are thus adequate to maintain a positive folic acid balance. The folate requirement is increased in infants and pregnant women (infancy, 75-100 μg/day; pregnancy 300-400 μg/day), and patients with hemolytic anemia with rapid red cell turnover. Folic acid requirements may be increased severalfold in patients with malignant diseases (28), hyperthyroidism (36), paroxysmal nocturnal hemoglobinuria (42), and leukemia (49).

Functions and Mechanism of Action. Folic acid is converted by partial hydrogenation and addition of a formyl group to folinic acid (5-formyltetrahydrofolic acid, citrovorum factor) that is the carrier for single-carbon groups: methyl, hydroxymethyl, formyl, and formaldehyde (Fig. 15.7-1). One-carbon donors include formylglutamate, serine, glycine, methionine, and others. The single-carbon units transferred by folinic acid are important in the biosynthesis of methionine from homocysteine; methylation of nicotinamide of N_1-methylnicotinamide; methylation of pyrimidine intermediates to thymine; and, introduction of carbons 2 and 8 in the purine ring structure. Vitamin B_{12} is also involved in some of these reactions (34) (Table 14.2-1).

Absorption, Transport, and Excretion. Folate absorption occurs mainly through the duodenum and jejunum. Absorption is active in the case of small amounts of folic acid and by passive diffusion for large quantities. Folates are absorbed in the 5-methyltetrahydrofolate state, which is the main transport and storage form of folate in humans (43). Conversion to this state occurs through several biochemical reactions, namely, deconjugation, reduction, and methylations (22).

Specific physiological plasma binders of folate have not been clearly elucidated to date. When large amounts of folate are added to plasma, a large portion is found to be loosely bound to albumin (33). Measurements of normal plasma levels of folate by *L. casei* assay range from 3 to 20 ng/ml. Approximately one-third of the total body folate is found in the liver.

Folate is incorporated into red blood cells during erythropoiesis. The folate is largely in the polyglutamate form. Red cell folate remains fairly constant and is a useful tool for indicating approximate body folate levels. The average folate levels falls to approximately 1.5 μg/g in 130 days on a folate-deficient diet. Megaloblastic changes also occur (24). Initially there is a low serum folic acid level appearing around 3 weeks, followed by the appearance of hypersegmented neutrophils at 7 weeks, high urinary formiminoglutamic acid (FIGLU) excretion after histidine loading at 13 weeks; megaloblastic bone marrow changes

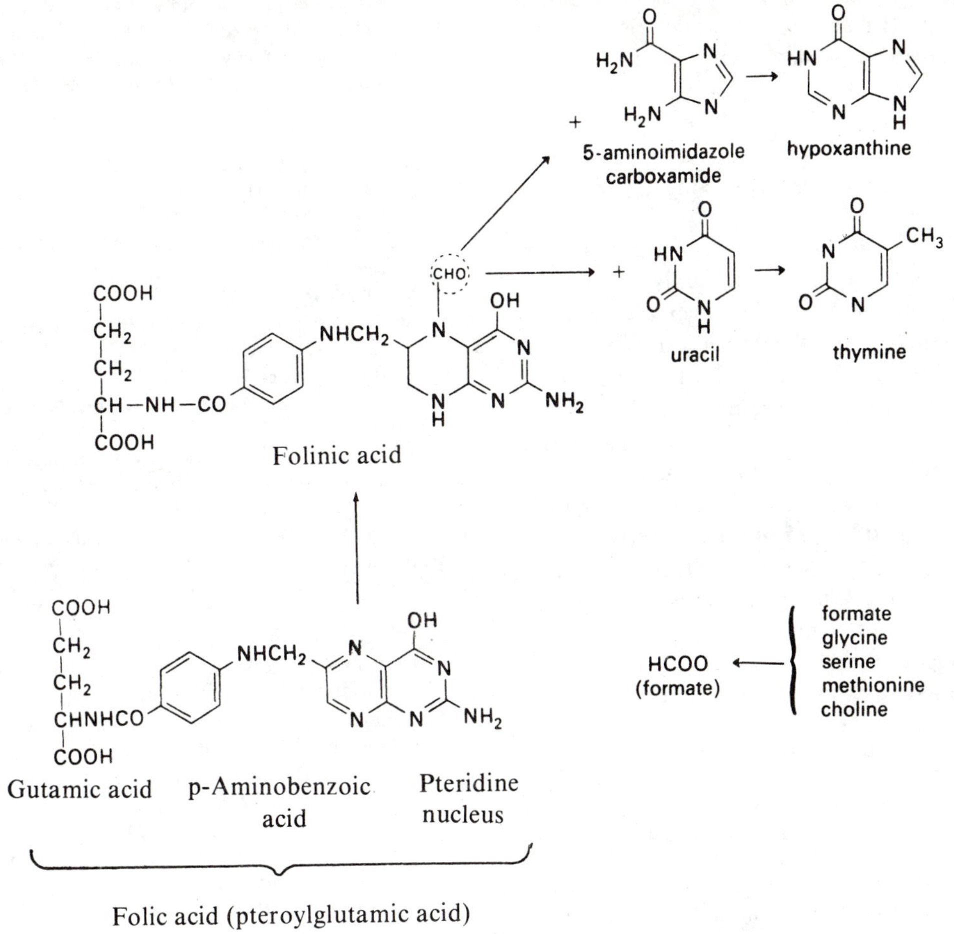

5-aminoimidazole carboxamide

hypoxanthine

uracil

thymine

Folinic acid

HCOO (formate) ← formate, glycine, serine, methionine, choline

Gutamic acid p-Aminobenzoic acid Pteridine nucleus

Folic acid (pteroylglutamic acid)

Fig. 15.7-1: *Folic acid and its metabolism.*

at 19 weeks; and anemia at 19.5 weeks (49). Clinical response following institution of folic acid therapy results in a reticulocytosis in 2 to 4 days and a return of hemoglobin levels to normal in 2 to 6 weeks. Megaloblastic changes of the marrow diminish within 24 to 48 hours.

Approximately 5 μg of folate is excreted daily in the urine. A smaller quantity appears in feces, bile, sweat, and saliva. There appears to be renal tubular reabsorption of folic acid by a carrier-mediated mechanism. The parent molecule is converted to pteridine and para-aminobenzoylglutamic acid by oxidative process.

Symptoms of Deficiency. Folic acid deficiency can result from inadequate dietary intake or from malabsorption. Deficiency of folic acid affects DNA synthesis; this results in a set of characteristic changes in the nuclear morphology of the cell, referred to as megaloblastic. This term usually applies to nucleated red blood cells that are increased in the blood, with a concurrent decrease in leukocytes and platelets.

Megaloblastic hematopoiesis in folate deficiency is indistinguishable from that in vitamin B_{12} deficiency. Glossitis, diarrhea, anorexia, and weight loss are prominent features. Unlike vitamin B_{12}-deficiency neurological signs indicative of myelin damage do not appear. For this reason the specific underlying deficiency should be uncovered, as folate therapy does not arrest the progression of neurological damage in cyanocobalamin deficiency and may initially mask such damage. Cell-mediated immunity is depressed in folate deficiency (19).

Adverse Reactions. Except for one questionable report of an allergic reaction, folic acid is essentially free of adverse effects in humans.

Drug Interaction. Some drugs such as methotrexate and trimethoprim inhibit dihydrofolate reductase in folic acid metabolism and cause megaloblastic anemia and pancytopenia (16, 57). Oral contraceptives cause folate-responsive megaloblastic anemia in some women. Phenytoin has been shown to interfere with the absorption of free folic acid (54).

Alcohol interferes with the normal absorption of folic acid and with the transport of N^5-methyltetrahydro-folic acid from storage areas (15). It has been suggested that alcohol blocks the hemopoietic activity of folic acid (40). Interaction of these and other drugs with folic acid is summarized in Table 1.2-2.

Therapeutic Uses and Doses. The only therapeutic use for folates is that of treatment of folate deficiency. An optimal response may occur with as little as 100 to 200 μg of folic acid daily in most patients; however, it is common to treat patients with 1 to 4 mg daily. In most patients,

0.5 to 1 mg of folic acid daily for 7 to 14 days induces a maximal hematological response. This may be given in the oral form. Malabsorption states will usually respond to this dose, as sufficient folate can be absorbed to replenish stores. Therapy should be maintained until a new population of cells appears, or in the case of chronic disease states maintenance doses of 1 to 5 mg/day may be required.

Although every effort should be made to avoid "shotgun" thereapy, occasionally in the critically ill patient with megaloblastic anemia and other severe symptoms immediate vitamin therapy is indicated before etiological diagnosis is available. In such cases, both cyanocobalamin, 100 μg, and folic acid, 15 mg, are given i.m. followed by 100 μg i.m. of cyanocobalamin and 5 mg p.o. of folic acid daily for a week. Every effort, otherwise, should be made to obtain a specific diagnosis with the utilization of specific treatment. Folic acid alleviates the megaloblastic anemias of infancy and pregnancy, nutritional macrocytic anemia, and most cases of tropical sprue or celiac disease. Folate may be indicated in those cases of megaloblastic anemia where there is a rapid turnover of red cells such as in hemolytic anemias.

Preparations. Folic acid, USP (FOLVITE): tablet containing 0.1 to 1 mg, p.o.; folic acid injection USP (folate sodium): 5 mg/ml in 10 ml vials, i.m., i.v., deep s.c., leucovorin calcium injection, USP (folinic acid, citrovorum factor), 1-ml ampule containing 3-mg, vial containing 50-mg powder to dissolve in 5 ml of sterile water to make 10 mg/ml solution for i.m. injection.

The sodium salt of folic acid (folate sodium) may be given by i.m., i.v., or deep s.c. injections. Parenteral administration provides no advantage over the oral route but may be used in selective states (i.e., the critically ill patient). Usual dosage for adults and children is up to 1 mg daily. When clinical symptoms have subsided and blood studies are normal, a maintenance dose of 0.1 to 0.25/mg/day should be given.

MEGALOBLASTIC ANEMIA NOT CAUSED BY VITAMIN B_{12} OR FOLATE DEFICIENCY

Megaloblastic anemia may be seen associated with several conditions not related to vitamin B_{12} or folate deficiency. These conditions include congenital disorders, such as hereditary orotic aciduria, thiamine-responsive megaloblastic anemia, pyridoxine-responsive megaloblastic anemia, çongenital familial magaloblastic anemia, congenital dyserythropoietic anemia, and the Lesch-Nyhan syndrome; acquired disorders, such as blood dyscrasias (sideroblastic anemia, hemochromatosis, leukemia, etc.), and drug-related megaloblastic anemia (purine antagonists, pyrimidine antagonists, inhibitors or ribonucleotide reductase, etc.).

REFERENCES

1. Allen, R.H. and Mehlman, C.S. Isolation of gastric vitamin B_{12}-binding protein using affinity chromatography. I Purification and properties of human intrinsic factor. *J. Biol. Chem.* 248: 3660, 1973.
2. *AMA drug evaluations*, 5th ed. Chicago: Am. Med. Assoc., 1983.
3. Andelman, M.B. and Sered, B.R. Utilization of dietary iron by term infants: A study of 1048 infants from a low socioeconomic population. *Amer. J. Dis. Child.* 111:45, 1966.
4. Baker, S.J. Human vitamin B_{12} deficiency. *World Rev. Nutr. Diet* 8:62, 1967.
5. Balcerzak, S.P. and Coreenberger, N.J. Iron content of isolated intestinal epithelial cells in relation to iron absorption. *Nature* 220:270, 1968.
6. Barker, H.A. and Coates, M.E. Vitamin B_{12} In: *The Vitamins*, 2nd ed. (Sebrell, W.H., Jr. and Harris, R.S. eds). New York: Academic Press, 1967.
7. Beck, W.S. The metabolic functions of vitamin B_{12}. *N. Engl. J. Med.* 266:708, 1962.
8. Brittin, G.M. and Raval, D. Duodenal ferritin synthesis during iron absorption in the iron deficient rat. *J. Lab Clin. Med.* 75:811, 1970.
9. Callender, S.T. Iron deficiency due to malabsorption of food iron. In: *Iron Metabolism and Its Disorders* (Kief, H., ed.). Amsterdam: Excerpta Medica, 1975.
10. Castle, W.B. Development of knowledge concerning the gastric intrinsic factor and its relation to pernicious anemia. *N. Engl. J. Med.* 249:603, 1953.
11. Chisholm, M. Tissue changes associated with iron deficiency. *Clin. Hematol.* 2: 303, 1973.
12. Committee on Nutrition: Iron fortified formulas. *Pediatrics* 47:786, 1971.
13. Conrad, M.E., Weintraub, L.R. and Crosby, W.H. The role of the intestine in iron kinetics. *J. Clin. Invest.*, 43:963, 1964.
14. Dallman, P.R. Tissue effects of iron deficiency. In: *Iron in Biochemistry and Medicine* (Jacobs, A. and Wormwood, M., eds.) Academic Press, New York, 1974.
15. Eichner, E.R. and Hillman, R.S. Effect of alcohol on serum folate level. *J. Clin. Invest.*, 52:584, 1973.
16. Ellegaard, J., Esmann, V., and Henriksen, L. Deficient folate activity during treatment of psoriasis and methotrexate diagnosed by determination of serine synthesis in lymphocytes. *Brit. J. Dermatol.* 87:248, 1972.
17. Evers, J.E.M. Iron-poly (Sorbitol-gluconic acid) complex and iron dextran in the treatment of severe iron deficiency anaemia. *Scand. J. Haematol.* Suppl. 32:377, 1977.
18. Frenkel, E.P. Abnormal fatty acid metabolism in peripheral nerves of patients with pernicious anemia. *J. Clin. Invest.* 52:1237, 1973.
19. Gross, R.L., Reid, J.V.O., Newberne, P.M. et al. Depressed cell-mediated immunity in megaloblastic anemia due to folic acid deficiency. *Amer. J. Clin. Nutr.* 225, 1975.
20. Guest, G.M. and Brown, E.W. Erythrocyte and hemoglobin of the blood. III. Factors in variability, statistical study. *Amer. J. Dis. Child.* 93:486, 1957.
21. Hallberg, L. and Sovell, L. Succinic acid as absorption parameter in iron tablets: Absorption and side effect studies. *Acta Med. Scand.* 459 (suppl.) 23, 1966.
22. Hardistry, R.M. and Weatherall, D.J. *Blood and Its Disorders.* Blackwell Scientific Publication, Ltd. Oxford, 1974.
23. Harris, J.W., Whittington, R.M., Weisman, R., Jr. and Horrigan, D.L. Pyridoxine responsive anemia in the human adult *Proc. Soc. Exp. Biol. Med.* 91:427, 1956.
24. Herbert, V. Experimental nutritional folate deficiency in man. *Trans. Assoc. Amer. Phys.* 75:307, 1962.
25. Herbet, V. and Zalusky, R. Interrelations of vitamin B_{12} and folic acid metabolisms: Folic acid clearance studies. *J. Clin. Invest.* 41:1263, 1962.
26. Herbert, W. and Jacob, E. Destruction of vitamin B_{12} by ascorbic acid. *J. Amer. Med. Assoc.*, 230:241, 1974.
27. Hines, J.D. Ascorbic acid and vitamin B_{12} deficiency. *J. Amer. Med. Assoc.*, 234:24, 1975.
28. Hoffbrand, A.V. Vitamin B_{12} and folate metabolism: The meg-

aloblastic anaemias and related disorders. In: *blood and Its Disorders.* (Hardisty, R.M. and Weatherall, D.J., eds.) Blackwell Scientific Publication, Ltd., Oxford, 1974.

29. Hoffbrand, A.V. et al. Incidence and pathogenesis of megaloblastic erythropoiesis in multiple myeloma. *J. Clin. Pathol.* 20:699, 1967.

30. Horrigan, D.L. Pyridoxine-responsive anemia: Influence of tryptophan on pyridoxine responsiveness. *Blood* 42:187, 1973.

31. Howell, D. Significance of iron deficiencies: Consequences of mild deficiency in children. (Extent and meaning of iron deficiency in the United States). In: *Summary proceedings of workshop of the Food and Nutrition Board*, National Academy of Sciences, 1971.

32. Jacobs, A. Digestive factors in iron absorption. In: *Progress in gastroenterology* (Glass, G.B.J., ed.) Vol. 2, Grune and Stratton, New York, 1970.

33. Johns, D.G., Sperti, S. and Burger, A.S.P: The metabolism of tritiated folic acid in man. *J. Clin. Invest.* 40:1684, 1961.

34. Krumdieck, C.L. Folic acid. In: *Present Knowledge in Nutrition.* Washington D.C.: Nutrition Foundation, 1976, p. 175.

35. Lichtenstein, H. et al. *Vitamin B_{12}* Microbiological Assay Methods and Distribution in Selected Foods. Home Economics Research Report, No. 13, USDA. Washington, D.C., 1961.

36. Lindenbaum, J., and Klipstein, F.A. Folic acid clearances and basal serum folate levels in patients with thyroid disease. *J. Clin. Pathol.* 17:666, 1964.

37. Miale, John B. *Laboratory medicine: Hematology.* 4th ed., C.V. Mosby Co., St. Louis, 1972.

38. Minot, G.R. and Murphy, W.P. Treatment of pernicious anemia by special diet. *J. Amer. Med. Assoc.* 87:470, 1926.

39. Mitchell, H.K., Snell, E.E. and Williams, R.J. The concentration of "folic acid." *J. Amer. Chem. Soc.* 63:2284, 1941.

40. *Nutrition Review.*: Inhibition of the hemopoietic activity of folic acid by ethanol. 37:254, 1979.

41. Oski, F.A. The nonhematologic manifestations of iron deficiency. *Amer. J. Dis. Child.* 133:315, 1979.

42. Pavlic, G.J. and Bouroncle, B.A. Megaloblastic crisis in paroxysmal nocturnal hemoglobinuria. *N. Engl. J. Med.* 273:789, 1965.

43. Perry, J. and Chanarin, I. Intestinal absorption of reduced folate compounds in man. *Br. J. Haematol.* 18:329, 1970.

44. Peters, T.J. and Hoffbrand, A.V. Absorption of vitamin B_{12} by the guinea pig. The role of the ileal mitochondrion. In: The cobalamins (a Glaxo Symposium) (Arnstein, H.R.V. and Wrighton, R.J., eds.). Churchill-Livingstone, Edinburg, 1971.

45. Pollitt, E. and leibel, R.L. Iron deficiency and behavior. *J. Pediat.* 88:372, 1976.

46. Retief, F.P., Gottlieb, C.W. and Herbert, V. Delivery of $CO^{57}B_{12}$ to erythrocytes from alpha and beta globulin of normal, B_{12}-deficient, and chronic myeloid leukemia serum. *Blood*, 29:837, 1967.

47. Robbins, F. and Pedersen, T. The role of iron in DNA and RNA synthesis. *Proc. Natl. Acad. Sci. U.S.A.* 66:1244. 1970.

48. Roe, D.A. Minireview. Effects of drugs on nutrition. *Life Sci.*, 115:1219, 1974.

49. Rose D.P. Folic acid deficiency in leukemia and lymphomas. *J. Clin. Pathol.* 29:29, 1966.

50. Smithies, O. and Hiller, O. The genetic control of transferrins in humans. *Biochem. J.* 72:121, 1959.

51. Sullivan, L.W. and Herbert, V. Studies on the minimum daily requirement for vitamin B_{12}: Hematopoietic responses to 0.1 microgm. of cyanocobalamin or coenzyme B_{12}, and comparison of their relative potency. *N. Engl. J. Med.* 272:340, 1965.

52. Svedberg, B. A clinical investigation of an iron-poly (sorbitol-gluconic acid) complex, Ferastral, for the treatment of iron deficiency anemia. *Scand. J. Haematol.* Suppl. 32:260, 1977.

CHAPTER
16

ROLE OF THE KIDNEY IN SALT AND WATER METABOLISM

Jerry B. Hook and William O. Berndt

The urinary system is made up of the kidneys, ureters, urinary bladder, urethra, and associated structures. In normal, healthy individuals the kidney is a highly dynamic organ. Although the two kidneys comprise less than 1% of total body weight, they receive 25% of the cardiac output. There are several consequences of this large perfusion. For example, to a large extent the susceptibility of renal mechanisms to nephrotoxicants is attributable to extensive exposure to these chemicals in the blood. In addition, the large perfusion leads to the formation of large quantities of glomerular filtrate most of which is reabsorbed (4). The examples in Table 16-1 were calculated for an adult man and demonstrate the magnitude of the normal physiological processes. The reabsorbed water and electrolytes are returned to the renal circulation permitting maintenance of normal fluid and electrolyte balance.

The major expenditure of renal energy is for reabsorption of normal plasma constituents (primarily sodium chloride). Indeed, it is estimated that more than 50% of the renal oxygen consumption is related to sodium chloride reabsorption. Because the amount of sodium chloride available for reabsorption is determined by the renal blood flow, this function can be viewed to regulate renal oxygen consumption (4). Because reabsorption of the glomerular filtrate is quantitatively the most important renal function, it is not surprising that in the main, disorders of the kidney are expressed as abnormalities in salt and water homeostasis. These disorders are often more complicated however, since some metabolic functions of the kidney may become deranged as well. Such functions as synthesis of erythropoietin and 1,25-dihydroxyvitamin D_3 may be reduced in certain renal disorders, as may be synthesis and/or release of renin and prostaglandins. Consideration of these disorders, however, is beyond the scope of these chapters.

NEPHRON FUNCTIONS

The primary role of the kidney is to maintain the volume and composition of the body fluids. To provide an appreciation as to how homeostasis is maintained (even when marked alterations of solute and water intake are experienced), an examination of the primary functions of the nephron will be undertaken.

For the sake of simplicity, renal pharmacologists and physiologists view the kidney in terms of its simplest functioning unit, the nephron. In reality, the nephron is not a single functional unit, but rather many functional units in series. Total renal function represents the sum of the integrated function of the many nephron segments and their associated vascular segments working in concert.

The three basic functions of the nephron are filtration, secretion, and reabsorption.

Table 16-1
Sodium, Chloride, Bicarbonate, and Water Balance in an Adult Man

	Filtered	Excreted	Reabsorbed Amount	Filtered load (%)
Sodium, mEq/day	25,200	152	25,048	99.4
Chloride, mEq/day	18,900	152	18,748	99.2
Bicarbonate, mEq/day	4,500	2	4,498	99.96
Water, l/day	180	1.5	178.5	99.2

Filtration. The glomerular capillary bed is similar to other capillary beds in the body with the exception that the hydrostatic pressure is probably higher and the efferent vessels of the glomerular capillary bed are arterioles rather than venules. Due to the high hydrostatic pressure within the glomerulus, fluid within the capillary is filtered into the tubule lumen.

This fluid contains all constituents of the plasma dissolved in the plasma water with the exception of large molecular weight proteins, lipids, and substances bound to plasma proteins. This glomerular selectivity based on molecular size occurs because the glomerular filtrate passes through capillary fenestrae, basement membrane, and slit membranes that offer little resistance to substances with molecular weights below 5000. Above that molecular weight various factors become important, such as molecular shape and charge. For example, negatively charged macromolecules do not penetrate as readily as neutral molecules of the same molecular size.

In humans, approximately 100-125 ml of plasma water is filtered per minute. The rate of glomerular filtration can be estimated by measuring the renal clearance of a material such as inulin. This substance is freely filtered at the glomerulus and is neither reabsorbed nor secreted by the tubule. Renal clearance of a substance, X, can be determined as the urinary excretion per unit time divided by the plasma concentration of that substance.

$$C_x = \frac{U_x V}{P_x}$$

Where:
C_x = clearance of substance X in ml/min
U_x = urinary concentration of substance in mg/ml
V = urine volume per unit time, ml/min
P_x = concentration of substance in plasma, mg/ml

Clearance, therefore, represents the number of milliliters of plasma from which the excreted material was extracted per unit time; for inulin, this clearance describes the glomerular filtration rate.

Secretion. Secretion is said to have occurred when the amount of a substance in the urine is greater than can be accounted for by filtration alone. This can occur because, in addition to entering the tubule by filtration, certain materials may also enter the tubular fluid by passage across the cells of the nephron. For example, it is widely recognized that there are active transport systems in the proximal tubule capable of translocating organic acids and organic bases from the plasma into the tubular urine. It is by this means that relatively large amounts of a variety of drugs (some of which may be bound to plasma proteins) may enter the tubular urine. However, because secretion has occurred one should not conclude that active transport was involved. For example, entry into the tubular fluid by passive means appears to account, at least in part, for the secretion of potassium. Ammonia may diffuse into the tubular urine where it is free to unite with hydrogen ion, forming ammonium ion which, because of its charge, will remain in the tubular urine. It should be clear that if a substance is actively secreted and not reabsorbed, its renal clearance will exceed the glomerular filtration rate (inulin clearance).

Reabsorption. The primary work of the kidney is to return to the vascular system the large variety of necessary plasma constituents that are filtered at the glomerulus. As indicated in Table 16-1, approximately 99% of the filtered salt and water are reabsorbed. Further, essentially all of the filtered bicarbonate, glucose, amino acids, etc., similarly are reabsorbed. Most of these reabsorptive mechanisms are energy-requiring processes; some materials, however, may be passively reabsorbed as well. For instance, along most of the nephron, active reabsorption of sodium induces an electrochemical gradient that favors the passive reabsorption of chloride. The reabsorption of water is similarly a passive event (2). As described in earlier chapters of this text, many drugs can be filtered at the glomerulus and then be passively reabsorbed as they are concentrated in tubular fluid subsequent to reabsorption of salt and water. For those substances where the reabsorptive process is the dominant one, renal clearance will be less than glomerular filtration rate.

To assess quantitatively the work done by the kidney, it is common to determine not only the clearance of a substance but also the filtered load. The product of the glomerular filtration rate (inulin clearance) and the concentration of freely filterable material in the plasma is referred to as the filtered load. If, for instance, we were concerned with the amount of sodium reabsorbed during any period of time, we would multiply the glomerular filtration rate (100 ml/min) times the sodium concentration of plasma (0.140 mEq/ml) to produce a filtered load of 14 mEq/min of sodium. Based on the excretion of sodium, the work done by the kidney, that is, the sodium reabsorbed per unit time, could be calculated.

RENAL HANDLING OF ELECTROLYTES

The primary cation in the plasma, sodium, is reabsorbed along the length of the nephron (1). Active transport of the electrolyte appears to occur from the intracellular compartment to the extracellular space (Fig. 16-1). This net transcellular movement of sodium, if unaccompanied by the movement of other ions, would soon generate a significant electrical potential across the cells and eventually sodium reabsorption would be retarded. Two types of ion fluxes, however, occur in conjunction with sodium reabsorption: (1) in several portions of the nephron, chloride is reabsorbed with sodium; and (2) sodium may be reabsorbed in exchange for movement of hydrogen or potassium into the urine. With both of these mechanisms, the electrical gradient established by net reabsorption of sodium will be minimized

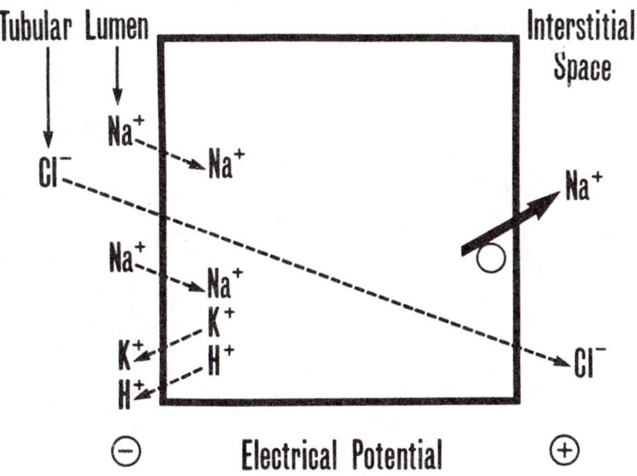

Fig. 16-1. *Simplified representation of electrolyte reabsorption across renal tubular cells.*

Active transport of sodium out of the cell establishes an electrical gradient with the outside of the cell slightly positive. Sodium in lumen diffuses down chemical gradient into the cell, rendering lumen slightly electronegative. The electrical gradient favors passive movement of chloride from urine to interstitial space. Excess of sodium over chloride in filtrate can be reabsorbed in exchange for potassium and hydrogen.

and salt will continue to be reabsorbed. Probably a similar mechanism is produced by active chloride transport in the ascending limb, except that a positive rather than negative electrical potential is generated by the primary ion transport process. The details of this reabsorptive process are poorly understood, however. In particular the precise relationship between sodium and chloride movement in the ascending limb is under intensive investigation.

Each portion of the nephron has specific functions (Fig. 16-2; Table 16-2) that may alter both the volume and composition of the tubular fluid as indicated in the segmental analysis given later. The final urine represents the algebraic sum of the specific reabsorptive and secretory functions which alter the composition of the glomerular filtrate. In addition, alterations in tubular function in one segment may alter functions in another (2, 3). To understand these interactions requires knowledge of function in each tubular segment.

Table 16-2
Filtrate Reabsorbed by Nephron Segment (%)

Nephron Segment	%
Proximal tubule	60-70
Loop of Henle	15-20
Distal tubule[a]	5-10
Collecting duct[a]	5-10

[a]Influenced by presence or absence of antidiuretic hormone.

SEGMENTAL ANALYSIS OF ELECTROLYTE AND WATER HANDLING BY THE NEPHRON

Proximal Tubule. The composition of fluid entering the proximal tubule is identical to that of the plasma with respect to substances of low molecular weights. Large proteins and lipids are absent. Thus, the concentrations of sodium (140 mEq/l), chloride (100 mEq/l), bicarbonate (27 mEq/l), potassium (4 mEq/l), etc., are approximately the same as in plasma water (4). The proximal tubule appears to act as a bulk absorptive surface, reabsorbing large quantities of all these materials such that at the end of the proximal tubule more than 60% of the filtrate has been reabsorbed, as have virtually all glucose and amino acids. Significant quantities of potassium and calcium also are reabsorbed in the proximal nephron.

Most filtered bicarbonate is reclaimed in the proximal tubule. This process requires participation of the enzyme carbonic anhydrase (Fig. 16-3). Carbonic acid is generated enzymatically in the cells of the nephron and rapidly dissociates to hydrogen and bicarbonate ions. Bicarbonate can diffuse into the extracellular space with sodium, and hydrogen moves into the tubular urine; the spontaneously formed carbonic acid is degraded to water and carbon dioxide. The carbon dioxide back diffuses, and in this manner, most filtered bicarbonate may be reclaimed. Additional bicarbonate may be generated by this process to resupply bicarbonate utilized as body buffer (4).

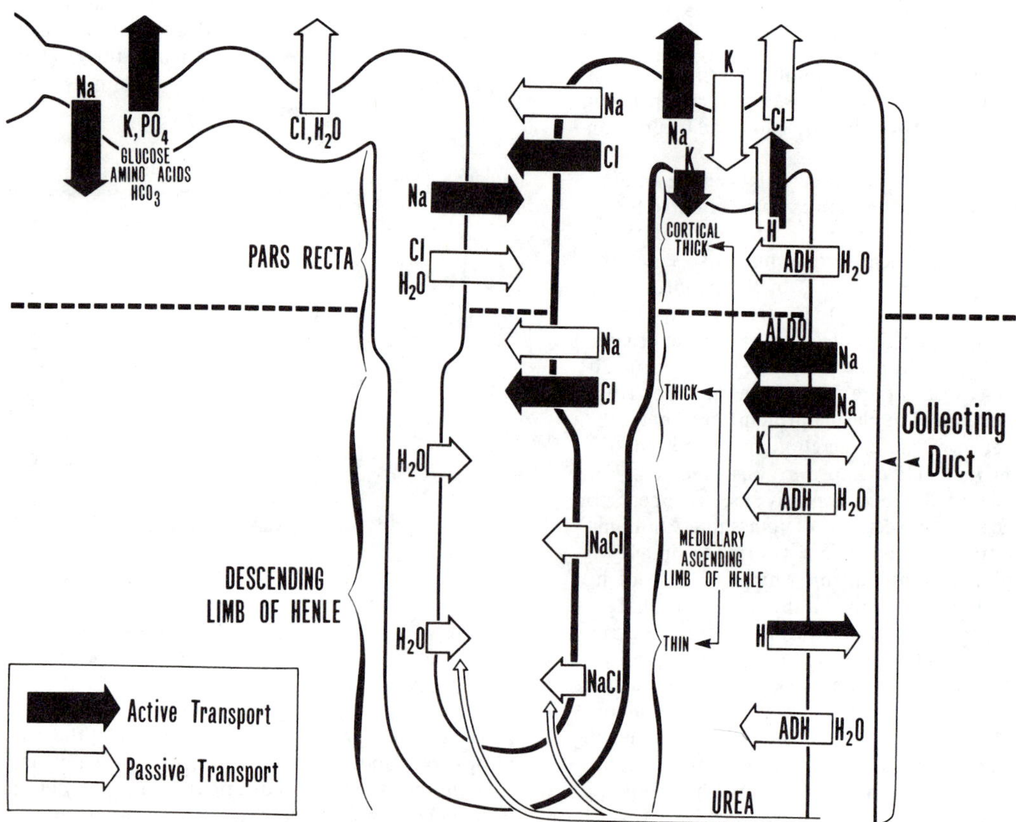

Fig. 16-2. *Schematic representation of segmental differences in electrolyte and water handling by the nephron (Modified from Ref. 2.).*

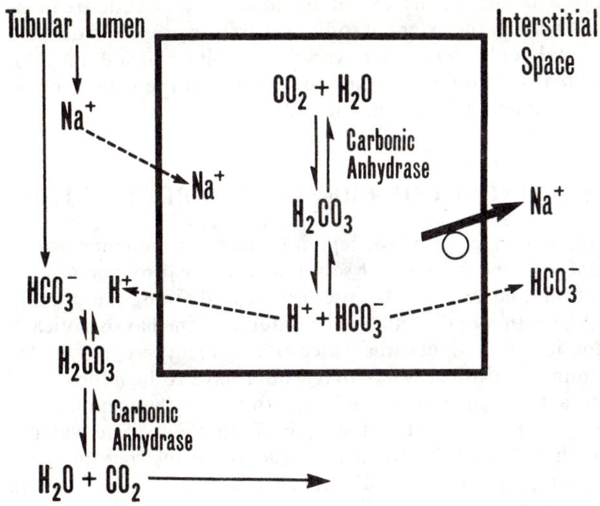

Fig. 16-3. *The renal handling of bicarbonate.*
Bicarbonate generated in cells is reabsorbed with sodium; hydrogen secreted into urine to form carbonic acid with filtered bicarbonate. Carbonic acid is catalytically degraded to H_2O and CO_2. CO_2 remains in urine or diffuses into cells. Generation of bicarbonate may proceed after filtrate is reabsorbed if the secreted hydrogen is buffered with phosphate or ammonia. Some evidence also exists for limited transcellular reabsorption of filtered bicarbonate.

Hydrogen ion secreted into the lumen may remain free in the urine. Most hydrogen ion in the proximal urine is buffered with phosphate

$$Na_2HPO_4 + H^+ \rightleftarrows NaH_2PO_4 + Na^+$$

or reacts with NH_3 to form NH_4^+. These buffering mechanisms allow for the elimination of significant quantities of H^+ without markedly altering pH of tubular fluid.

The major reabsorptive effort is directed at the movement of sodium, chloride, and water (1). Salt reabsorption appears to be related primarily to the active transport of sodium across the basolateral membranes of the proximal tubule cells. This active process provides the driving force for chloride movement as well as water transport. The pathway for chloride movement is, at least in part, through the cell, probably in association with sodium. It is thought that a sodium chloride-coupled transport process, or symport, exists driven by the sodium gradient. Water transport is a secondary process dependent on electrolyte movement and facilitated by the cellular architecture. Standing osmotic gradients develop in the deep intercellular channels which promote water flow into these channels. The increased hydrostatic pressure causes bulk fluid flow toward the open end of the channels. The high colloid osmotic pressure in the peritubular capillaries that results from the filtration of protein-free fluid promotes fluid absorption into the capillaries.

The proximal tubule cells are representative of a "leaky" epithelium not unlike that of the gallbladder. Only a small transepithelial potential difference is generated, and virtually no osmotic gradient is maintained across the cells. This latter point is important in that these considerations are essential to establish the proximal tubular fluid reabsorptive process as an isosmotic one. Thus, as electrolytes are reabsorbed from the tubular fluid, sufficient water is moved to maintain physiological osmotic relationships. At the end of the proximal tubule, the osmolality of the tubular urine is the same as that of the glomerular filtrate (i.e., approximately 300 mOsm/l).

Descending Limb of the Loop of Henle. Little active transtubular movement of electrolytes occurs in this segment of the nephron. Basically, it appears that as fluid moves down the descending limb of the loop of Henle, water is abstracted into the medullary interstitium (possible some urea moves into the urine). Therefore, the fluid increases in osmolality, reaching a maximum at the hairpin bend at the loop.

Thin Ascending Limb of the Loop of Henle. Recent physiological evidence indicates that due to differential membrane permeability, sodium chloride diffuses out of the ascending limb into the medullary interstitium as urea moves in. Permeability to urea is less than permeability to sodium chloride and the limb is impermeable to water. Thus, as the fluid moves up the ascending limb, osmolality decreases. It is noteworthy how dramatically the water permeability of the nephron has changed. The early nephron segments were leaky, whereas midway through the nephron the water permeability is extremely low.

Thick Ascending Limb of the Loop of Henle. The thick ascending limb of the loop of Henle has two segments, one in the outer medulla and one in the cortex. Both are relatively impermeable to water. The fluid is rendered dilute by the active extrusion of sodium chloride. This portion of the nephron is unique in that the electrochemical data suggest active chloride transport with sodium movement passive. Furthermore, the primacy of chloride is demonstrated by substitution of nitrate for chloride, which interferes with electrolyte transport. However, these observations do not explain the ability of ouabain to block NaCl movement, since ouabain is thought to act specifically on sodium transport. Probably a sodium chloride symport is involved in the transport process, but the nature of this transport is unknown.

Thus, as fluid reaches the end of the thick ascending limb, it is relatively dilute (osmolality approximately 100-150 mOsm/l) and sodium chloride concentrations approximately one-half of those in the interstitium. It is important to note that approximately this same situation pertains regardless of the state of hydration of the subject.

Distal Convoluted Tubule. By the time the original filtrate reaches the distal convoluted tubule, the volume has been reduced by 70-80% and the composition has been markedly changed. The distal convoluted tubule and the collecting duct that follows act as the final regulators of the composition of the tubular fluid, and it is these two areas of the nephron that are the most sensitive to hormonal regulation.

The distal segment of the nephron is complex: at least four cell types exist as well as many transport functions. The multiple transport processes and variable permeability characteristics may lead to a tubular fluid of markedly different composition than that in the proximal tubule.

Water permeability is relatively low in the distal convoluted tubules, so with continued salt reabsorption the urine is diluted further; indeed, tubular fluid osmolality may be as low as 75 mOsm/l at the end of the distal segment. In the presence of antidiuretic hormone, as much as 5-10% of the glomerular filtrate will be absorbed in this nephron segment. The concentration of chloride is relatively low in the fluid entering the distal tubule; the primary anions in the tubular fluid are those which are relatively impermeant (e.g., phosphate and sulfate). Thus, as sodium is reabsorbed actively and because of a relatively low passive permeability to sodium, an electrochemical gradient is established, favoring the delivery of hydrogen and/or potassium into the tubular fluid (see subsequent discussion).

The Collecting Duct. Electrolyte reabsorption continues throughout the collecting duct where the predominant active transport system is that for reabsorption of sodium. In this area of the nephron, sodium reabsorption is sensitive to the mineralocorticoid action of aldosterone. Sodium reabsorption here, as in the distal segment, generates an electrochemical gradient that favors the secretion of hydrogen and/or potassium. Whether potassium or hydrogen secretion predominates will depend upon existing physiological conditions. In an individual who is relatively acidotic, the predominant cation excreted will be hydrogen ion. In contrast, in alkalosis, the predominant cation to be excreted will be potassium. Although there is no doubt that potassium secretion can be passive, quantitative studies suggest that an active component also may exist. Which mechanism will be most important quantitatively will depend on physiological conditions and species.

The cells of the collecting duct are responsive to antidiuretic hormone (ADH). In the absence of ADH, dilute fluid entering the collecting duct will be rendered more dilute by salt reabsorption and a dilute urine will be excreted. On the other hand, in the presence of ADH, cells of the collecting duct become permeable to water, which will diffuse into the medullary interstitium and the urine will become concentrated.

Thus, the more proximal portions of the nephron (through the ascending limb of the loop of Henle) appear to act as bulk absorptive surfaces, reabsorbing large amounts of salt and water. Regardless of hormonal balance (assuming sufficient glomerular filtration), a dilute solution will be delivered into the distal tubule and collecting duct, a portion of the solute that was removed from the urine having been deposited in the medullary areas of the nephron. In the absence of ADH, as in patients with neurogenic diabetes insipidus, large volumes of very dilute urine will be excreted solely because the medullary collecting duct is impermeable to water. Conversely, an individual who is extremely dehydrated and producing a very concentrated urine is doing so because the collecting duct is highly permeable to water. Even here, the urine entering the collecting duct is as dilute as in the patient with diabetes insipidus.

This summary of physiology of the nephron should reinforce the concept that both volume and composition of urine, measured at the end of the nephron, reflect the sum of many different tubular events. The primary sites for the reabsorption of some electrolytes are given in Table 16-3. The complexity of the reabsorptive and secretory events suggests that changes in tubular function in one portion of the nephron may influence function in another. For instance, inhibition of sodium and chloride reabsorption in the proximal tubule or in the ascending limb of the loop of Henle will result in the delivery of increased amounts of sodium to the more distal portions of the nephron. A significant amount of this increased sodium delivered to the distal portions of the nephron may be reabsorbed; if this happens, increased excretion of potassium and/or hydrogen ion might be expected. Hence, the extent of potassium excretion can be influenced by the extent of sodium excretion or sodium delivery to distal nephron sites. Conversely, inhibition of sodium chloride reabsorption in the more distal area of the nephron may alter proximal tubular function (2).

THE CONCEPT OF FREE WATER PRODUCTION

Development of the concept of free water production helped clarify the mechanisms of salt and water reabsorption in the nephron and was of immense benefit in defining the primary sites of action of diuretics. Free water is defined as osmotically unobligated or solute-free water and, in reality, represents the amount of distilled water that would have to be added to or subtracted from a sample of urine to render that sample isosmotic with plasma. For the sake of simplicity, free water is usually calculated as the net production or loss per unit time and is represented as the difference between the urine flow and osmolar clearance.

$$\underset{(\text{ml/min})}{C_{H_2O}} = \underset{(\text{ml/min})}{V} - \underset{(\text{ml/min})}{C_{osm}}$$

where

$$C_{osm} = \frac{U_{osm}}{P_{osm}}$$

the renal clearance of osmotically active materials.

If urine were isosmotic with plasma (i.e., $U_{Osm}/P_{Osm} = 1$), the C_{H_2O} would be zero. During formation of a dilute urine positive free water would be generated (i.e., $V > C_{Osm}$ with a concentrated urine C_{Osm} would exceed urine volume and free water would be negative). By convention this is designated

$$T^c_{H_2O}$$

and defined as $T^c_{H_2O} = C_{osm} - V$.

The consequences of variations in free water formation or urine volume and urinary osmolar concentration are depicted in Table 16-4.

The mechanisms that underlie urinary concentration and dilution are important to the pharmacologist since alterations in free water excretion can be used to localize tubular sites of diuretic action. Although some studies have certified a tubular site of diuretic action on the basis of diuretic effects in a state of

Table 16-3
Tubular Electrolyte and Water Transfer Characteristics

	H_20 Permeability	NaCl Reabsorption	K^+ Reabsorption	K^+ Secretion	$NaHCO_3$ Reabsorption
Proximal tubule	High	Yes	Yes	No	Yes
Ascending loop of Henle	Low	Yes	Yes	No	No
Distal tubule	Variable[a]	Yes	Yes[b]	Yes[b]	Yes[c]
Collecting duct	Variable[a]	Yes			No

[a] Dependent on presence or absence of antidiuretic hormone.
[b] Exact locations poorly defined.
[c] Minimal, if at all.

maximal water diuresis, the certainty of localization is increased greatly if the effects of the diuretics are examined both under conditions of maximum water diuresis and maximum antidiuresis. The reasons for utilizing both experimental conditions are exemplied below in the discussion of diuretic actions on free water formation.

Free water is formed in the ascending limb of the loop of Henle, where electrolytes are reabsorbed but water reabsorption is minimal. Similarly, it is in the medullary portion of the thick ascending limb where active reabsorption of sodium chloride generates the high medullary tonicity responsible for urinary concentration (i.e, formation of $T^{c}_{H_2O}$). Indeed, it is this reabsorptive process that is thought to be the event which initiates the countercurrent multiplication process. The countercurrent multiplication is sustained though the action of the vasa recta acting as countercurrent exchangers. Urea also has an important, although still controversial, role in the countercurrent process.

In the cortical segment of the loop and in the distal convolution, tubular urine is rendered hypotonic. In the absence of ADH (i.e., maximal water diuresis), this tubular fluid passes on into the collecting ducts and is excreted without much modification. A diuretic that acted in the proximal tubule would lead to the delivery of larger than normal quantities of isosmotic fluid to the loop of Henle where much of the excess electrolyte would be reabsorbed. In the absence of ADH, this excess fluid would be excreted as an increased quantity of free water. A primary action of a diuretic in the cortical portion of the loop or in the distal convolution would decrease free water formation. That is, more salt would be retained in the tubular urine and, if there were no antidiuretic hormone, urine volume would not change. If urine volume did not change and salt excretion increased, that is C_{Osm} increased, free water would be decreased. Agents that act in the medullary portion of the ascending limb would similarly decrease free water clearance. That is, any agent that blocks salt reabsorption in regions of the nephron where water permeability is low would decrease positive free water formation.

In the absence of ADH, the major alteration in nephron behavior from that in its presence is the passive reabsorption of large quantities of water in the collecting ducts and perhaps distal tubules. Hence, there is the production of a hypertonic urine. A diuretic that acted in the proximal tubule would lead to the delivery to distal sites of a larger than normal volume of isosmotic fluid. As in the absence of ADH, most of the excess electrolyte would be reabsorbed in the ascending limb and distal tubule. Because collecting duct water permeability is high, the increased electrolyte reabsorption will lead to enhanced water reabsorption (i.e., an increased negative free water formation).

Table 16-4
Consequences of Alterations in Positive and Negative Free Water Formation

	Filtered H_2O Reabsorption (%)	24-hr Urine Vol. (liters)	Urine osmolality, μOsm/l
U_{osm}/P_{osm}[a] = 1	98.7	2.4	290
Maximal antidiuresis	99.7	0.5	1400
Maximal H_2O diuresis	88	23.3	30

[a] Urine osmolality/Plasma osmolality.

A diuretic that acts on sodium chloride reabsorption in the thick ascending limb of Henle's loop will decrease negative free water formation because this reabsorptive process initiates the urinary concentration mechanism.

In summary, to predict a tubular site of action of a new diuretic, experiments are required both in the absence and presence of ADH.

1. A diuretic with a proximal site of action will increase both positive and negative free water formation.
2. A diuretic that inhibits sodium chloride reabsorption in the thick ascending limb of Henle's loop will decrease both positive and negative free water formation.
3. A diuretic that blocks sodium chloride reabsorption in the cortical segments of the distal tubule (cortical diluting segment) will decrease positive free water formation, but have no effect on negative free water formation.

PATHOPHYSIOLOGY OF SALT AND WATER BALANCE

A primary disorder of concern to the physician is with salt and water homeostasis (2). Because the normal kidney handles such a large quantity of salt and water, an uncompensated change in function of only a few percent can have profound consequences. Salt and water homeostasis may become out of balance due to a primary renal disorder (failure of excretory mechanisms) or secondary to prerenal changes (low cardiac output, blood pressure, excessive intake of salt, etc.). In its simplest terms, either etiology will be associated with decreased renal blood flow (and decreased filtration) or increased salt reabsorption (such as due to mineralocorticoid excess). Regardless of the cause (assuming intake to be relatively constant), the patient will be in positive sodium balance (i.e., salt retention). The clinical challenge is to rid the patient of the retained salt as quickly and safely as possible. Whereas prerenal changes do occur and may be important, the scope of this and the next chapter deals primarily with problems of excretion.

Impairment of excretory processes may arise from a primary renal disorder or, secondarily, as in heart failure or shock, when delivery of water and electrolytes to the kidney is compromised. In either situation, the patient suffers from excessive retention of sodium chloride and water (i.e., edema formation). Because water moves in response to osmotic loads, therapy requires elimination of salt; water will then follow the excreted salt.

Therapy calls first for dealing with the etiology of the condition, such as digitalization in patients with congestive heart failure, or withdrawing salt-retaining therapeutic agents. In mild cases of fluid retention such treatment may be adequate. In more profound cases of fluid retention, however, when more extensive or more rapid elimination of fluid is required, the use of a diuretic may be indicated.

REFERENCES

1. Burg, M.B. The renal handling of sodium chloride. In: *The Kidney* (Brenner, B.M. and Rector, F.C., Jr., eds.) 2nd ed. Vol. 1. New York: W.B. Saunders, 1981, p. 272.
2. Jacobson, H.R. and Kokko, J.P. Diuretics: Sites and mechanisms of action. *Ann. Rev. Pharmacol. Toxicol.* 16:201, 1976.
3. Materson, B.J. Insights into intrarenal sites and mechanisms of action of diuretic agents. *Am. Heart J.* 106:188, 1983.
4. Sullivan, L.P. and Grantham, J.J. *Physiology of the Kidney.* Philadelphia: Lea and Febiger, 1982.

CHAPTER
16.1

DIURETICS

William O. Berndt and Jerry B. Hook

Diuretics are a widely used class of drugs that increase the rate of urine flow. A more important consideration, however, is the mobilization of solute, principally sodium, that underlies the fluid loss. All the important diuretics promote a saluresis or natriuresis in addition to diuresis (i.e., they are natriuretic as well as diuretic).

Diuretics may be used to enhance the removal of waste material from the body and to increase renal blood flow and glomerular filtration rate in certain cases of functional hypovolemia (e.g., shock, drug overdose, etc.). Most diuretics are employed acutely to remove excess salt and water from the body as in edema and ascites. Diuretics may also be employed chronically to prevent reaccumulation of fluid in chronic disease (e.g., congestive heart failure) and are widely employed in the treatment of hypertension. Indeed, despite changing concepts related to the cause of high blood pressure, treatment of this disease remains a major use for diuretics (2). The ability of diuretics to reduce blood pressure has been attributed to decreased plasma volume possibly complemented by subtle changes in blood vessel reactivity (see Chapter 15.3 for details).

Urine flow may be enhanced by increasing renal blood flow and glomerular filtration rate or by decreasing reabsorption of the filtrate. An increase in renal blood flow may be sufficient to produce clinically useful diuresis, as in hypotension, or in the diuretic effect of digitalis in patients with congestive heart failure. In most cases, however, the diuresis induced by increasing renal blood flow is not of sufficient magnitude or rapidity to achieve a significant or sustained loss of salt and water, the desired clinical result. Therefore, in the main, clinically useful diuresis is produced by decreasing tubular reabsorption of sodium and chloride (7).

Ideally, as with any drug, one wants to achieve the maximal therapeutic benefit at minimum risk. Unfortunately, given the nature of the diuretic response, it is not clear that a nontoxic diuretic can be developed. Achievement of the desired pharmacological effect (i.e., loss of sodium, chloride, and water) almost necessarily dictates a disruption in overall fluid and electrolyte balance. Whereas the retained fluid of edema or ascites was accumulated slowly and was a balanced solution of all the electrolytes normally found in plasma, most useful diuretics induced excretion of a fluid that contained primarily sodium chloride (1, 5, 7, 8). Thus, by their very nature diuretics tend to induce an abnormality in plasma composition. It is also useful to remember that the diuresis produced is, in essence, extracted initially from the plasma compartment. Therefore, care must be exercised so that diuresis is not so rapid that the effective volume of the plasma compartment is reduced faster than fluid can diffuse from interstitial space into this compartment.

For purposes of this presentation, the diuretic agents will be classified, somewhat arbitrarily, into two groups, major and minor diuretics. The major agents are those used extensively clinically and of considerable significance pharmacologically. The minor substances are those that have assumed a lesser status for one or more reasons.

MAJOR DIURETICS

OSMOTIC DIURETICS

The osmotic diuretics represent a special class of diuretic agents. These are relatively inert, usually nonreabsorbable materials that exert an osmotic effect due to their presence in the tubular urine. Increased filtration of an osmotically active, nonreabsorbable substance causes retention of water in the renal tubule. Hence, with less water reabsorbed the urine volume is increased. Despite the presence of significant quantities of a nonreabsorbable solute, the osmolar relationships within the tubular fluid remain the same as in the absence of the solute. Therefore, if isosmotic fluid reabsorption persists in the presence of significant concentrations of a nonreabsorbable solute, the tubular fluid concentration of some other solute must decrease. Indeed, direct measurements of tubular fluid sodium concentration have demonstrated a fall in its concentration. Because the proximal tubule reabsorbs sodium poorly against large concentration gradients, the reabsorption of this ion and chloride is limited. Reabsorption of salt in the loop of Henle is diminished similarly. Medullary blood flow also is increased during the diuresis. Increased delivery of sodium and water distally and washout of the medullary concentration gradients combine to decrease sodium and water absorption at distal sites (7, 8). Although there must be some effects of osmotic diuretics on electrolyte movement in the loop of Henle and distal segment, clearly the primary action is on the proximal tubule (Fig. 16.1-1). Finally, it should be noted that these diuretics can cause significant increases in potassium excretion since large quantities of sodium are delivered to the distal sites where potassium secretion occurs.

A well-recognized pathophysiological example of an osmotic diuresis is that produced by the enhanced glucose in the urine of patients with diabetes mellitus. The excess glucose in the urine cannot be reabsorbed after exceeding tubular reabsorptive capacity. Therefore, the glucose remains in the urine retaining water which leads to the well-known polyuria of diabetes mellitus.

Urea and a nonmetabolized sugar, mannitol, are examples of effective osmotic diuretics. Osmotically active diuretics such as mannitol are administered intravenously as hypertonic solutions. In contrast to all other diuretics, the first physiological response to mannitol or urea is an increase in plasma volume. In response to administration of the hypertonic solution, fluid is drawn from the extravascular space into the vascular compartment. This produced an increase in the vascular volume, increase in renal blood flow, and increase in glomerular filtration rate. The osmotically active material is filtered at the glomerulus, retains water in the tubular lumen, and is excreted. The primary use of these agents is to increase urine flow in cases of temporary hypovolemia such as in shock, or to increase urine flow following administration of poisons (i.e., in contrast to most other diuretics, mannitol increases the fraction of filtered fluid that exists in the proximal tubule). Osmotic diuretics also are used to reduce intracranial pressure temporarily in patients with brain edema and to reduce intraocular pressure and vitreous volume prior to ocular surgery (1).

Use of osmotic diuretics requires careful monitoring of renal function, for if the kidneys are unable to excrete the high osmotic load, the increased plasma volume may be detrimental to cardiac function. This may be particularly hazardous in patients with cardiac insufficiency.

BENZOTHIADIAZIDES

History and Chemistry. Because the therapeutic efficacy of acetazolamide as a diuretic was extremely limited (see later discussion), there persisted a search for a better diuretic that acted through inhibition of carbonic anhydrase. Partly through an accident of chemistry, the first of the thiazide series was synthesized. This compound, chlorothiazide, was an orally active agent with some effect on bicarbonate excretion. However, the primary anion excreted in response to chlorothiazide was chloride. There now exist many thiazide diuretics that have properties very similar to those of chlorothiazide except

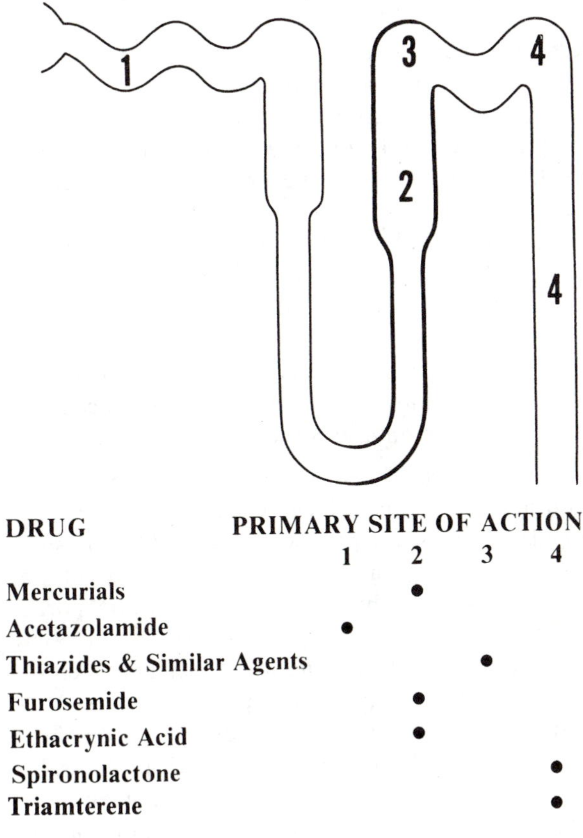

DRUG	PRIMARY SITE OF ACTION 1	2	3	4
Mercurials		•		
Acetazolamide	•			
Thiazides & Similar Agents			•	
Furosemide		•		
Ethacrynic Acid		•		
Spironolactone				•
Triamterene				•

Fig. 16.1-1. *Primary sites of action of the major diuretics.* (1) Proximal convoluted tubule; (2) thick ascending limb; (3) distal convoluted tubule (diluting segment); and (4) collecting duct.

for the action on bicarbonate excretion. Otherwise, the differences relate to the pharmacological characteristics of the compounds (5, 7, 8). The chemical structures of two of the many thiazides are given in Fig. 16.1-2.

Effects on Renal Function. These compounds act directly on the kidney. The primary action of these agents is to block the reabsorption of sodium chloride in the cortical-diluting segment of the nephron, either in the cortical segment of the thick ascending limb or in the distal convoluted tubule (Fig. 16.1-1). An action on the cortical-diluting segment is consistent with the reduction in positive free water formation, but no effect on negative free water formation (5). Earlier studies suggested both proximal and distal sites of action, but these involved stop-flow experiments that lacked specificity with respect to tubular sites of diuretic action.

The thiazides produce a marked and prompt increase in the excretion of sodium, chloride, and water. This action is noted regardless of the acid-base balance of the subject, although the urinary composition may vary somewhat depending on the acid-base status. For example, chlorothiazide will increase bicarbonate excretion at the expense of chloride in an alkalotic subject. In an acidotic subject, the urine is virtually free of bicarbonate after chlorothiazide. In either situation, however, a prompt and significant diuresis occurs (see Table 16.1-1). Furthermore, tolerance to the diuretic action does not develop, so they can be used for relatively long periods of time. Hence, these compounds are not only effective by oral administration, but will produce a reliable and predictable diuresis as well, regardless of the subject's acid-base balance (5, 7).

Little can be said about the mechanism(s) by which these compounds produce their effects on tubular transport. Although studies have been done on various aspects of intermediary metabolism, effects on transport enzymes, etc., except for the effects on carbonic anhydrase virtually nothing is known about the cellular or subcellular mechanism of action of this group of compounds.

Pharmacokinetics. The thiazides are well absorbed after oral administration, which accounts for much of their popularity. Most will produce a measurable diuresis within 1 hour after oral administration. All are organic anions and are secreted by the organic anion transport system in the proximal tubule. The secretion of these anions can be reduced by probenecid. The extent of secretion varies from compound to compound, as does the final urinary excretion, which depends in part on the extent of passive reabsorption. Agents with prolonged durations of action (e.g., bendroflumethiazide and polythiazide) show both high degrees of protein binding and lipid solubility. This latter characteristic leads to extensive passive reabsorption from the tubular fluid. Biliary excretion of chlorothiazide can occur in a nephrectomized animal. This drug also readily passes through the placental barrier.

Adverse Effects. In the main, the toxicity of the thiazides is an extension of their pharmacological effects. All thiazide diuretics will cause potassium loss: increased delivery of fluid and sodium to the more distal portions of the nephron brings about enhanced reabsorption of some of that sodium and increased secretion of potassium. Potassium loss can lead to muscle weakness, cardiac irritability, and other signs of disturbance of membrane potential. Similarly, loss of potassium may increase the toxicity of digitalis compounds. Urinary losses of potassium can be replaced by increasing dietary intake of foods high in potassium or with oral potassium supplements.

Thiazide therapy may be associated with hyperuricemia, which may trigger acute attacks of gout. The mechanism of this effect is not definitely established. Both uric acid and the thiazide diuretics are secreted into the urine, and competitive antagonism of urate secretion could lead to its increased plasma concentration. However, this may not be the only explanation since reabsorption of uric acid in the proximal tubule also appears to be enhanced during diuretic therapy. Hyperuricemia may be treated with probenecid, which enhances urate excretion by inhibiting the tubular reabsorption of urate, or with allopurinol, which blocks the enzyme xanthine oxidase and reduces uric acid synthesis (1).

Thiazides have been reported to cause hyperglycemia, hyperlipidemia, blood dyscrasias, hypersensitivity reactions, and pancreatitis (1). Lithium clearance is reduced by thiazides. Therefore, concomitant administration of these agents requires close monitoring of the concentration of lithium in serum. Caution also is in order when thiazides are administered with the neuromuscular blocking agents, tubocurarine or gallamine, because these diuretics may augment blockade of the neuromuscular junction. Prolonged administration of hydrochlorothiazide may produce hyperzincuria and zinc deficiency (Chapter 21.3).

In summary, the thiazides should be viewed as relatively nontoxic agents. Their extensive clinical use supports this statement. Of the adverse effects observed the following are most noteworthy:

(a) Potassium loss
(b) Hyperuricemia
(c) Hyperglycemia
(d) Hypersensitivity reactions

Therapeutic Uses. These agents are used commonly in the treatment of high blood pressure. A compound like chlorothiazide is relatively short-acting (6-12 hours) and may be used in the initial treatment of an edematous patients with congestive heart failure, nephrotic syndrome, or hepatic cirrhosis with ascites, conditions under which sensitivity of the distal tubule to increased sodium delivery may be enhanced. A longer-acting compound such as polythiazide (24-48 hours) or the nonthiazide, chlorthalidone (24-72 hours), may be employed in chronic therapy of hypertension. A newer nonthiazide, inda-

Thiazides

Chlorothiazide

Hydrochlorothiazide

Thiazide-like Diuretics

Chlorthalidone

Metolazone

Indapamide

Loop Diuretics

Furosemide

Bumetanide

Ethacrynic acid

Potassium-sparing Diuretics

Antialdosterone Compounds

Nonsteroidal Compounds

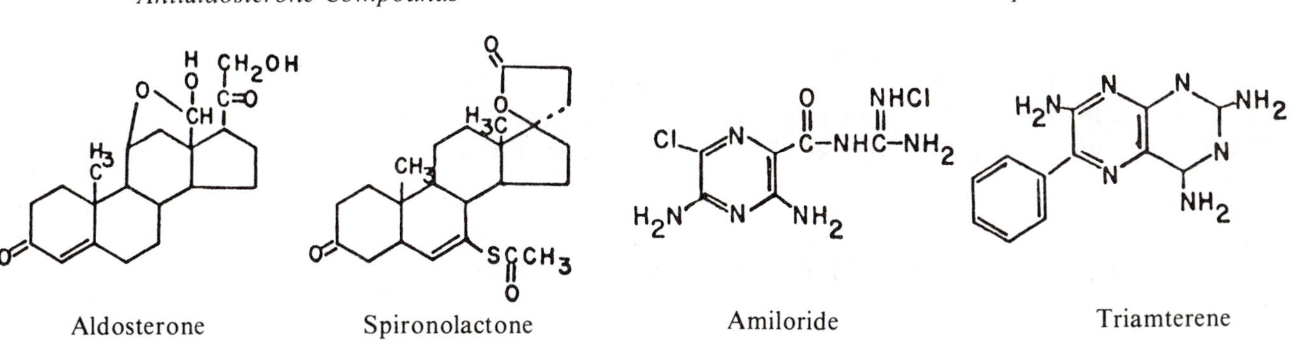

Aldosterone

Spironolactone

Amiloride

Triamterene

Fig. 16.1-2. *Chemical structures of various classes of diuretics.*

pamide (see later discussion), also may be used in treating high blood pressure. When administered chronically, thiazides seem to reduce vascular reactivity to sympathetic stimulation. Therefore, compensation by the sympathetic nervous system for any reduction in plasma volume does not occur (1).

An interesting therapeutic use of thiazide diuretics is in the treatment of diabetes insipidus. This is a condition in which production of antidiuretic hormone (ADH) is deficient (neurogenic) or the distal portions of the nephron do not respond to ADH (nephrogenic). Patients with neurogenic or nephrogenic diabetes insipidus excrete large volumes of dilute urine because essentially all of the fluid presented to the distal nephron is excreted. In such a patient, a compound like a thiazide further increases in urinary volume (i.e., decreased C_{H_2O}). Therapy in such a patient with a thiazide agent could lead to a significant reduction in plasma sodium concentration. The normal renal adaptation to a decrease in plasma sodium is enhanced reabsorption by the proximal tubule. Enhanced reabsorption of sodium in the proximal tubule will bring about enhanced reabsorption of water and therefore a decrease in urinary volume.

Thiazides also are useful in the chronic treatment of hypercalciuria to reduce stone formation (8). The reduction in calcium excretion appears to be due to increased proximal reabsorption of calcium. This effect of thiazides is a departure from the action of other diuretics where calcium excretion more or less parallels that of sodium.

As indicated previously, in addition to the thiazides, there are several diuretics that do not contain the benzothiadiazine nucleus yet are pharmacologically similar to the thiazides. Both chlorthalidone and metolazone produce effects nearly identical to the thiazides. A newer compound, indapamide, may prove particularly useful in the treatment of high blood pressure. It reduces vascular reactivity, possibly through a reduction in transmembrane calcium flux (10). Indapamide is excreted primarily by biliary mechanisms so that virtually no accumulation of indapamide or its metabolites occurs in dogs with both kidneys removed. Indapamide, as well as chlorthalidone and metolazone (Fig. 16.1-2), is well absorbed from the gastrointestinal tract. The diuretic action of these compounds is through inhibition of sodium-reabsorption in the distal cortical diluting segment.

HIGH-CEILING OR LOOP DIURETICS

History and Chemistry. In 1966 two new diuretics, furosemide and ethacrynic acid (Fig. 16.1-2), were approved for human use. These compounds, although markedly different in structure, appear to have very similar pharmacological actions on the kidney. Furosemide was developed to be another thiazide-like compound; its free sulfamyl group gave it a very minor action on carbonic anhydrase. Many studies had suggested that the organomercurials act by inhibition of renal sulfhydryl groups, and ethacrynic acid was designed to have a similar action (i.e., it was planned as a metal-free, sulfhydryl inhibitor). This diuretic was designed as an anion since it was reasoned that this characteristic might permit its more rapid delivery to a tubular site of action. Bumetanide (Fig. 16.1-2) was developed to have an action not unlike that of furosemide.

All of these compounds have similar pharmacological effects. They are termed *high ceiling* because each can mobilize large quantities of edema fluid, much larger quantities than with other diuretics presently in common use (Table 16.1-1). The description *loop diuretic* refers to the action of these substances on the thick ascending limb of the loop of Henle (see later discussion; Fig. 16.1-1).

Mechanism and Site of Action. In maximally effective doses, these agents are capable of inhibiting the reabsorption of as much as 30% of the filtered load of sodium and chloride, whereas thiazides inhibit about 10%. The ability of these agents to produce a rapid disruption of the renal concentrating mechanism as well as prevent the formation of dilute urine led to the conclusion that these agents

Table 16.1-1
Typical Urinary Electrolyte Excretion Patterns[a]

Diuretic	V (ml/min)	pH	mEq/min			
			Na^+	K^+	Cl^-	HCO_3^-
Control	1	6	50	15	60	1
Mannitol	8	6.5	720	120	880	32
Mercurial	7	6	1050	56	1120	7
Acetazolamide	3	8	210	180	50	350
Chlorothiazide	5	7.5	750	125	750	100
Ethacrynic acid	12	6	1800	120	1980	12
Triamterene	3	7.2	450	15	360	45
Aminophylline	3	6	450	45	510	3

[a] Data are representative of the responses seen in humans or dogs under conditions of normal acid-base balance. The excretion rates are those that would be expected at peak diuresis after a maximally effective dose.

act primarily in the thick ascending limb of the loop of Henle. This was subsequently confirmed by Burg and colleagues, who demonstrated that both of these agents selectively inhibit the active reabsorption of chloride in this segment of the nephron (5) and that this segment of the nephron is much more sensitive to these agents than is any other segment. All three compounds are organic anions and are actively secreted into the tubular urine. Indeed, the overall diuretics response appears to relate to the amount of drug with access to the site of action (3). Interestingly, it appears that a metabolite of ethacrynic acid, the cysteine adduct, is the active chemical moiety. Ethacrynic acid-cysteine is between 100 and 1000 times more effective as an inhibitor of chloride transport than is the parent compound (5).

These agents produce diuresis regardless of the state of acid-base balance. Interestingly, the compounds continue to produce saluresis (i.e., enhanced excretion of sodium and chloride at all plasma pHs). Unlike the organomercurials or acetazolamide, tolerance to the diuretic activity of the high-ceiling compounds is not related to alterations in acid-base. All loop diuretics markedly increase calcium excretion, which has led to their use in treating hypercalcemia. They also promote a significant loss of potassium, probably in response to the delivery of large quantities of sodium to distal sites. Loop diuretics appear to increase renal blood flow in certain circumstances. This effect is probably related to intrarenal prostaglandin release. It is uncertain whether or not the alterations in blood flow modify or regulate the diuretic response.

Two suggestions have been made concerning possible mechanisms of action, but neither suggestion is supported totally by the experimental data. Inhibition of sodium-potassium-activated adenosine triphosphatase (ATPase) may have a role in the diuretic action, but the action must be a very complicated one; there are several ATPase inhibitors which are not diuretic and it is unclear how these can be differentiated from the loop diuretics. Ethacrynic acid has certain actions on intermediary metabolism, and these effects were suggested early as possible mechanisms. However, not every diuretic has these actions, and the question of specificity is again unanswered.

Pharmacokinetics. All compounds in this group are absorbed well enough after oral administration to produce a diuretic response. Rapid excretion in the urine is accounted for both by glomerular filtration and tubular secretion. Ethacrynic acid is metabolized to a large extent (perhaps 60-70%), whereas furosemide and bumetanide are metabolized only minimally. As indicated previously, an ethacrynic acid metabolite may be the active form of the drug.

Resistance to these diuretics does occur, at least in part, because of modification of pharmacokinetic characteristics of the diuretics. Reduced glomerular filtration, for example, will decrease the amount of drug reaching sites of action. Also, the accumulation of organic acids will reduce tubular secretion. How these pharmacokinetic factors interact with pathophysiology-induced alterations in response to diuretics to produce resistance is unclear, but pharmacodynamic factors do appear to be important (3).

Adverse Effects. The primary adverse effects of these agents are an extension of the pharmacological action. Potassium loss occurs and may be of considerable magnitude. Similarly, excessive chloride and fluid loss can lead to hypochloremic metabolic alkalosis. The combination of rapid loss of volume, sodium, and chloride accompanied by little bicarbonate in the urine led to the concept of *contraction alkalosis*, a clinical term used to describe the patient whose plasma volume has been reduced rapidly by the extraction of essentially an isosmotic solution of sodium chloride. If plasma volume is contracted without a commensurate increase in bicarbonate excretion, bicarbonate concentration would be increased in the reduced plasma volume, thereby producing the alkalosis.

Like the thiazides, loop diuretics may induce hyperuricemia. Ototoxicity has been reported with these agents, but most commonly with ethacrynic acid. The severity of hearing loss depends on dose and may relate to a disruption of electrolyte balance in the endolymph. Finally, gastrointestinal bleeding has been reported most often with chronic use of these agents.

Therapeutic Uses. These agents have been used for the treatment of edema of cardiac or hepatic origin. Also, the management of acute pulmonary edema has been possible. No doubt in part this therapy relates to the diuretic effectiveness of the loop compounds, but there may be other important actions as well. It has been demonstrated that in patients with congestive heart failure, improved function in the cardiopulmonary circuit was achieved prior to the onset of diuresis. It has been suggested that this is due to the ability of furosemide, for example, to release vasoactive compounds, possibly prostaglandins, from the kidney which can influence cardiopulmonary function (3).

These substances have been used in clinical situations where acute renal failure has occurred or is anticipated. Uniform success with this therapeutic approach has not been achieved, although the use of loop diuretics or mannitol has proven useful in some experimental and clinical situations.

Furosemide has been used in attempts to remove noxious substances from the body. The rationale has been that the noxious material when dissolved in a larger volume would be less readily reabsorbed and therefore be excreted more rapidly. In fact, however, damage from noxious materials usually occurs in the proximal tubule. Even though the diuretics have a profound effect on urinary volume, that increased urine volume represents changes in function of more distal segments of the nephron. Actually, proximal reabsorption of salt and water may even be enhanced during diuresis, leading to greater, not lesser, concentration of toxic material in proximal areas of the nephron.

A new, high-ceiling diuretic, indacrinone, is of interest. The (-) enantiomer is a more potent natriuretic than the (+) enantiomer, while both enantiomers possess uricosuric activity. Alterations in the ratio of the (+) to (-) enantiomers has allowed optimization of both the natriuretic and uricosuric effects (11).

POTASSIUM-SPARING DIURETICS

Two groups of potassium-sparing compounds are available. These have fundamentally different mechanisms of actions, but both groups should be viewed as major agents, primarily of their utility in situations where loss of potassium should be prevented.

STEROIDAL AGENTS

Spironolactone (Fig. 16.1-2) is a complex steroid molecule that is a competitive inhibitor of the mineralocorticoid, aldosterone. The physiological effect of aldosterone is to enhance sodium reabsorption in the collecting duct and possibly in the distal convoluted tubule and to facilitate potassium excretion. Sodium reabsorption produces an electrical gradient favoring secretion of potassium and hydrogen in these areas of the nephron. Thus, the effect of spironolactone is to reduce sodium reabsorption and to decrease the excretion of potassium (5, 7, 8). Because aldosterone acts at sites other than the kidney, spironolactone would be expected to act on those sites as well (e.g., salivary glands).

When used alone, spironolactone is only mildly effective as a diuretic and is rarely used in this manner. Normally, it is used in combination with diuretics that promote potassium loss, such as the thiazides or loop diuretics. Spironolactone is particularly useful when administered in combination with other diuretics in the treatment of conditions involving secondary hyperaldosteronism, such as chronic congestive heart failure, the nephrotic syndrome, or cirrhosis with refractory fluid retention.

Careful monitoring of the concentration of potassium in serum is necessary during therapy with spironolactone. Hyperkalemia is likely to occur in patients with impaired renal function or excessive potassium intake.

Gynecomastia, impotence, and decreased libido have been reported in males treated with spironolactone. Menstrual disturbances may occur in women. Gastrointestinal disturbances and rashes also have occurred following administration of spironolactone (1).

NONSTEROIDAL COMPOUNDS

Like spironolactone, triamterene and amiloride (Fig. 16.1-2) exhibit sodium reabsorption in the more distal areas of the nephron (Fig. 16.1-1), with subsequent inhibition of potassium secretion. The actions of triamterene and amiloride, however, do not depend upon the presence of aldosterone and therefore must have fundamentally different mechanisms of action. Studies with model systems such as the toad bladder suggest that the effect of these agents is to prevent the entry of sodium from the luminal side of the cells (5, 9), but precise mechanisms are not understood.

In contrast to spironolactone, which requires 4 to 5 days for its full effect, triamterene or amiloride acts within hours of administration. Although more effective as a natriuretic than spironolactone, the nonsteroidal compounds are only mildly effective when used alone (Table 16.1-1). Their primary use is in combination with the more effective diuretics that facilitate potassium loss (5, 7).

The use of these nonsteroidal compounds in combination with other diuretics represents a rational use of fixed-dose combination therapy. However, caution must be exercised in the use of this combination since alterations in plasma potassium may occur.

MINOR DIURETICS

ORGANOMERCURIALS

The diuretic effect of heavy metals has been recognized by physicians for centuries. Because of the systemic and renal toxicity of the heavy metals, their use in medicine is now extremely limited. Beginning in the 1920s, however, a series of organomercurial compounds were widely used as diuretics. Until the mid-1960s, these agents (e.g., mersalyl and mercaptomerin) were the most effective and widely used diuretics available.

In usual therapeutic doses, the organomercurial compounds increase the excretion of sodium, chloride, and water and modify the excretion of potassium. Usually, if the potassium excretory rate is high when the drug is given, it falls; if the excretory rate is low, the organomercurial can cause it to rise. Although the increased potassium excretion probably relates to the increased delivery of sodium to distal sites, the decreased potassium excretion is generally taken to represent a direct action of the organomercurials on the distal tubule or collecting duct. The major diuretic response may be attributable to an action on the thick ascending limb of the loop of Henle, but data on this point are equivocal. Many believe the primary site of action to be the proximal tubule.

Probably the organomercurials produce their diuretic effect by releasing minute quantities of inorganic mercuric ion. It is thought that the free mercuric ion binds to sulfhydryl-containing receptors and through this interaction inhibits certain specific renal reabsorptive processes. This mercuric ion hypothesis has gone far toward explaining the development of refractoriness to the organomercurial compounds.

It is well established that repeated use of these diuretic substances can result in a systemic alkalosis, and once this condition develops, the organomercurials are ineffective. It is thought that the alkalosis that results in the production of an alkaline urine prevents or reduces the rupture of the carbon-mercury bond in the organomercurial compound, hence preventing or reducing the release of free mercuric ion. The diuretic responsiveness can be reestablished by the administration of acidifying salts such as ammonium chloride. Certain discrepancies have arisen with respect to the mercuric ion hypothesis, but this is still viewed as a useful working model.

Parenteral administration of the organomercurials was virtually essential for reliable results. In the hospitalized patient and under carefully controlled conditions, these compounds could produce a large and reliable diuresis. The organomercurials showed significant toxicity; they could not be administered intravenously because of cardiac toxicity. Prolonged use of mercurials in patients with impaired renal function could lead to renal failure or hemorrhagic colitis. Mercurial compounds also caused gastrointestinal disturbances, vertigo, fever, pruritus, and rash.

CARBONIC ANHYDRASE INHIBITORS

In the 1930s, it was recognized that the enzyme carbonic anhydrase catalyzed the hydration of carbon dioxide. Various sulfonamide antibacterials were found to inhibit this enzyme, producing an alkaline urine and eventually a metabolic acidosis. Through the use of various carbonic anhydrase inhibitors, the role of carbonic anhydrase in urinary acidification was established.

Table 16.1-2
Summary of Effects of Diuretics on Renal Function

Diuretics and their Groups	Efficacy[a]	Primary Site of Action[b]	Changes in Electrolyte Excretion[a]				Change in Na Reabsorption (%)	Comments
			Na	K	Cl	HCO_3		
MAJOR								
Osmotics								
Mannitol	+++	Prox. tub.	↑	↑	↑	—	20	Must be given i.v.
High-ceiling or loop								
Furosemide	+++	Th. ascend.	↑	↑	↑	↑/—	20-30	Produce isosmotic urine,
Ethacrynic acid	+++	Th. ascend.	↑	↑	↑	—	20-30	may produce alkalosis but still cause chloride loss
Thiazides	++	Dilut. seg.	↑	↑	↑	↑[c]	10	Differ in potency and duration of action.
Thiazidelike								
Chlorthalidone	++	Dilut. seg.						
Metolazone	++	Dilut. seg.						
Potassium-sparing								
Steroidal								
Spironolactone	+	Coll. duct.	↑	↓	↑	—	2	Requires aldosterone
Nonsteroidal								
Triamterene, amiloride	+	Coll. duct	↑	↓	↑	—	2-5	Aldosterone not required
MINOR[d]								
Mercurials	+++	Th. ascend., prox. tub., or both	↑	↑↓	↑	—	20	Given i.m. or s.c., may produce alkalosis and tolerance develops
Carbonic anhydrase inhibitors								
Acetazolamide	+	Prox. tub.	↑	↑	—	↑	5	May cause acidosis
Xanthines	+	Prox. tub.	↑	↑	↑	—	2-3	Tolerance develops quickly
Acidifying agents								
Ammonium chloride	+	Prox. tub.	↑	↓	↑	↓	2-3	Tolerance develops quickly

[a] High, +++; moderate, ++; least, +; ↑, increase; ↓, decrease; —, no change.
[b] Prox. tub., proximal tubule; th. ascend., thick ascending limb; dilut. seg., diluting segment; coll. duct, collecting duct.
[c] Seen with chlorothiazide only.
[d] Have no use as diuretics in medicine.

Several compounds (e.g., acetazolamide, ethoxyzoleamide) were developed as diuretics.

All of the pharmacological effects of this class of compounds are attributable to inhibition of carbonic anhydrase. This enzyme is present in considerable excess, and therefore nearly 99% of the renal activity must be blocked before any effects on renal function are noted.

These substances cause an increase in the excretion of sodium, bicarbonate, and water. Potassium output also is increased. In usual therapeutic doses chloride excretion is not increased. All of these actions result from blockade of the enzyme and the consequent failure of hydrogen ion production. Prolonged enzyme inhibition will result in a metabolic acidosis. Once the acidosis develops, the carbonic anhydrase inhibitors are totally inactive as diuretics. Even under ideal conditions, however, these agents have extremely low efficacy (see Table 16.1-1).

XANTHINES

The xanthines, caffeine, theophylline, and theobromine, are all mild diuretic agents. The most effective of these is theophylline. These agents seem to produce their diuresis by increasing renal blood flow, an effect complemented by a slight reduction of sodium reabsorption in the nephron. Tolerance develops to the diuretic effect of these compounds quite rapidly, and their use is restricted almost entirely to over-the-counter diuretic preparations.

ACIDIFYING DIURETICS

Agents such as ammonium chloride and calcium chloride will produce a mild natriuresis during the development of metabolic acidosis produced by the increased chloride load. They are rarely used as diuretics alone; historically they were used in combination with mercurial diuretics. Their current use is almost exclusively in over-the-counter diuretic preparations.

THERAPEUTIC CONSIDERATION

The information contained in Tables 16.1-1 and 16.1-2 and Fig. 16.1-1 relate to tubular sites of action, diuretic efficacy, urinary electrolyte patterns, etc. The information in Table 16.1-3 gives a representative list of proprietary names, dosage forms, etc. These data should allow the reader to put all the diuretics in perspective and to make appropriate generalizations about the consequences of the use of one or another of the agents. For example, some compounds are more likely to disrupt acid-base balance whereas others might have direct effects on potassium balance. These diversities might suggest the use of one agent over another for a particular clinical problem.

It is clear from Fig. 16.1-1 and Table 16.1-2 that the activity of virtually every nephron segment may be altered by one or another of the diuretics. This broad spectrum of activity is probably a reflection of there being a large variety of compounds with quite different efficacies. The most efficacious agents, however, have their primary effects in the more distal segments (e.g., the sensitivity of the thick ascending limb to the high-ceiling compounds).

Despite the variability in performance, there is little doubt that a greater potential for toxicity exists with the highly efficacious agents. A variety of toxic responses may be noted, but probably the more important ones (because of frequency of occurrence) relate to disruptions of fluid and electrolyte balance. Some of these problems are listed in the following discussion.

Sodium Depletion. Sodium depletion often results from very vigorous diuretic therapy (e.g., the persistent use of the more efficacious agents or the combined used of diuretics and salt restriction). This may occur without any appreciable alteration in the plasma sodium concentration, by the BUN, hematocrit, and potassium concentration may rise. This phenomenon is often associated with postural hypotension, weakness, etc.

Hypokalemia. Hypokalemia as a potential problem has been alluded to several times previously. Most likely this will occur in response to prolonged use of those agents which promote potassium loss (i.e., virtually every agent used chronically). This complication is even more serious if it occurs in a patient who receives digitalis. This difficulty is easily avoided or corrected by the use of potassium-sparing diuretics either alone (if adequate loss of edema fluid is produced) or in combination with more efficacious natriuretic agents. A direct approach to the resolution of this potential difficulty is the administration of potassium chloride or the consumption of a diet high in potassium.

Hyperkalemia. Although seen less frequently, elevation of plasma potassium is noted and can be very serious. This is usually seen as a complication in one of the following situations:

1. Prompt, excessive diuresis promoting a large loss of sodium, chloride, and associated water such as noted in acute sodium depletion
2. Dilutional hyponatremia
3. Therapeutic regimen designed to reduce potassium excretion (e.g., the use of potassium-sparing diuretics without adequate control).

Correcting this phenomenon often involves the restoration of the total fluid and electrolyte imbalance.

Chronic Dilutional Hyponatremia. Chronic dilutional hyponatremia is a very complicated syndrome, the underlying causes for which are not entirely clear. Hyponatremia probably results from rather greater loss of sodium and chloride than water, as is often seen with thiazides. In fact this complication is seen more often with thiazides than with other agents, but may also be a reflection of the underlying disease state and possibly may involve excessive secretion of antidiuretic hormone.

Finally, although not addressed directly in the tables and figures, it should be appreciated that many of the differences in diuretic response may relate to differences in pharmacological characteristics of the drugs. Some are better absorbed from the GI tract; some are more or less

Table 16.1-3
Representative Diuretic Preparations

Generic Name	Trade Name	Optimally Effective Dose (mg/day)	Dosage Form[a]
Amiloride	MIDAMOR	5-10	T, 5
Bendroflumethiazide	NATURETIN	2.5-15	T, 2.5, 5, 10
Benzthiazide	AQUATAG	25-200	T, 25, 50
Chlorothiazide[b]	DIURIL	500-2000	T, 250, 500
Chlorthalidone	HYGROTON	25-100	T, 25, 50, 100
Cyclothiazide	ANHYDRON	1-2	T, 2
Ethacrynic acid[b]	EDECRIN	50-200	T, 25, 50
Furosemide[b]	LASIX	40-200	T, 20, 40
Hydrochlorothiazide	HYDRODIURIL, ORETIC, ESIDRIX	25-100	T, 25, 50
Hydroflumethiazide	SALURON, DIUCARDIN	25-200	T, 50
Mannitol[c]	OSMITROL	50-200 g, i.v.	S, 5-25
Methyclothiazide	ENDURON, AQUATENSEN	2.5-10	T, 2.5-5
Metolazone	ZAROXOLYN, DIULO	5-20	T, 2.5, 5, 10
Polythiazide	RENESE	0.5-8	T, 1, 2, 4
Spironolactone	ALDACTONE	50-100	T, 25
Triamterene	DYRENIUM	200-300	T, 100
Trichlormethiazide	METHAHYDRIN, NAQUA	2-8	T, 2, 4

[a] T = tablet (mg); S = solution (%).
[b] Also available for injection.
[c] Only administered by i.v. infusion.

well absorbed from the renal tubule; some are more or less bound to plasma proteins. Whatever the details of these characteristics, it should be noted that the popular use of diuretics, especially in the treatment of high blood pressure, results in large part from these. Of course, the generally reduced toxicity of the newer compounds also has contributed to their general use. Certainly before the advent of the thiazides in the 1960s, diuretic use was neither safe nor convenient.

REFERENCES

1. *AMA Drug Evaluations,* 5th ed. Chicago: American Medical Association, 1983.
2. Baer, J.E. Diuretics, In: *Pharmacology of Antihypertensive Drugs* (Scriabine, A., ed.). New York: Raven Press, 1980, p. 1.
3. Bourland, W.A., Day, D.K. and Williamson, H.E. The role of the kidney in the early nondiuretic action of furosemide to reduce elevated left atrial pressure in the hypovolemic dog. *J. Pharmacol. Exp. Ther.* 202:221, 1977.
4. Brater, D.C. Pharmacodynamic considerations in the use of diuretics. *Ann. Rev. Pharmacol. Toxicol. 23:45, 1983.*
5. Burg, M.B. Mechanisms of action of diuretic drugs. In: *The Kidney* (Brenner, B.M. and Rector, F.C., Jr., eds.) Philadelphia: Saunders, 1976, p. 737.
6. Gerber, J.G. and Nies, A.S. Furosemide-induced vasodilation: Important of the state of hydration and filtration. *Kid. Intern.* 18:454, 1980.
7. Grantham, J.J. and Chonko, A.M. The physiological basis and clinical use of diuretics. In: *Sodium and Water Homeostasis: Contemporary Issues in Nephrology*, Vol. 1 New York: Churchill-Livingstone, p. 178.
8. Jacobson, H.R. and Kokko, J.P. Diuretics: Sites and mechanisms of action. *Ann. Rev. Pharmacol.* 16:201, 1976.
9. Laragh, J.H. Amiloride, a potassium conserving agent new to the U.S.A: Mechanisms and clinical reference. *Curr. Ther. Res.* 32:173, 1980.
10. Pruss, T. and Wolf, P.S. Preclinical studies of indapamide, a new 2-methylindoline antihypertensive diuretic. *Am. Heart J.* 106: 208, 1983.
11. Tobert, J.A., Cirillo, V.J., Hitzenberger, G., James, I., Pryor, J., Cook, T., Buntinx, A., Holmes, I.B. and Lutterback, P.M. Enhancement of uricosuric properties of indacrinone by manipulation of the enantiomer ratio. *Clin. Pharmacol. Ther.* 29:344, 1981.

CHAPTER
17

RESPIRATORY SYSTEM: ANTITUSSIVE, DECONGESTANTS AND ANTIASTHMATIC AGENTS

Thomas Bright and Frank Goodman

ANTITUSSIVE AGENTS

Cough has various meanings to the clinician. One extreme is the chronic cough in the bronchorrhea associated with chronic bronchitis, where cough serves as an important protective reflex. It is usually ignored by patients and is rarely bothersome to them. This cough should not be treated with antitussives. In the other extreme—in severe pulmonary hemorrhage or cough syncope—cough is not only *not* useful, but also may have fatal consequences. Such a cough obviously calls for aggressive antitussive therapy. Between these extremes lie many clinical conditions in which the patient may benefit by suppression of a bothersome cough.

The exact nature of all peripheral and central neural pathways in the physiology of cough remains unclear. It is clear, however, that chemical or mechanical irritation in either the upper or lower airway may initiate a coughing episode. Therapy of an individual cough depends upon the nature of the irritant, and upon the severity of the consequences of the cough in the individual. In practice, therapy is aimed at reducing afferent input and/or increasing the threshold of the central cough center.

Coughs due to upper airway irritation are best treated by removal of offending irritants. In instances in which nasal discharge is the offending agent, antihistamines or other antiallergic drugs may be useful. Soothing agents or demulcents may be used when cough stems from irritated pharyngeal mucosa. Agents such as guaifenesin or folk remedies based on liberal amounts of alcohol probably act by virtue of their local pharyngeal effects. Although topical anesthetics are occasionally employed, their anesthetic effects on the tongue and oral mucosa are usually undesirable. Coughs due to neoplasms or other intrapulmonary disease usually require potent central antitussives. Codeine, the standard by which other antitussives are evaluated, is usually employed in doses of 10 to 20 mg, in the form of a cough mixture.

AGENTS THAT REDUCE AFFERENT INPUT

SOOTHING AGENTS, DEMULCENTS

Coughs due to upper airway irritation are best treated by bland agents that dilute or modify the viscosity of pharyngeal secretions (*demulcents*). The popularity of liquid cough mixtures may be due in part to the demulcent effects of ingredients such as alcohol, propylene glycol, or expectorants such as guaifenesin. Where removal of irritants is not possible, soothing agents may help. Water, hard candy, or cough drops act in this manner. Such remedies usually suffice only for minor irritation or short duration, but they do have the virtue of being devoid of side effects.

Acetylcysteine. Acetylcysteine (N-acetyl-L-cysteine), a sulfur-containing amino acid, is a mucolytic drug that also reduces the viscosity in the respiratory tract and thereby promotes easier elimination. Its mucolytic action is said to be related to the SH group in the molecule, which presumably opens up the disulfide linkages in the pulmonary mucus secretion and thereby lowers the viscosity. Its mucolytic action is maximum between pH 7 and 9. The drug is indicated as an adjuvant therapy for patients with acute or chronic bronchopulmonary disease associated with excessive mucous secretions. Stomatitis, nausea, and rhinorrhea have been reported as side effects of acetylcysteine. Acetylcysteine is available as a 10 or 20% sterile solution.

TOPICAL ANESTHETICS

Weak topical anesthetics, such as benzocaine or phenol, are also employed for minor throat irritation. More potent topical anesthetics including cocaine, lidocaine, tetracaine, and dyclonine are used to suppress cough during instrumentation of the airway, such as bronchoscopy. Because of lower relative toxicity, lidocaine 0.5 to 4% as solution or jelly and dyclonine 0.5 to 1% as solution are most often employed for this purpose.

One agent with marked local anesthetic properties, benzonatate, is also orally active. It inhibits the intrapulmonary nervous component of the cough reflex in animals and presumably in humans as well. Benzonatate is employed sparingly in clinical medicine in favor of more reliable centrally active agents.

AGENTS THAT INCREASE CENTRAL COUGH THRESHOLD

OPIATES

The most potent central antitussives are opiates. In addition, these drugs display a wide variety of CNS and peripheral effects. The various opiates differ in relative potency for each effect, duration of action, and oral bioavailability. Morphine is the prototype analgesic molecule, and heroin (diacetylmorphine) is the prototype euphoriant. Codeine and its derivatives are, as a class, orally active, relatively weak analgesics with less addiction potential than morphine. Differences between derivatives are slight and are chiefly a matter of potency.

All opiates possess some respiratory depressant activity (i.e., decrease the sensitivity of brain chemoreceptors to carbon dioxide). This is rarely critical in patients with airway obstruction severe enough to produce chronic carbon dioxide retention. Such patients may be adversely affected even with the weak respiratory depressant effects of antitussive doses of codeine. It should be noted that such patients usually do not require or benefit from cough suppression, as an effective cough is essential to remove excessive airway secretions.

Adverse reactions to codeine include nausea, constipation, dizziness, palpitation, and drowsiness, and the side effects for hydrocodone, in addition to those for codeine, are dryness of throat and tightness of chest.

NONOPIATES

Other centrally active antitussives with clinical utility include dextromethorphan and noscapine. Dextromethorphan, the d-isomer of levorphanol (a codeine analog) is a centrally acting antitussive and equipotent to codeine, but rarely produces drowsiness or gastrointestinal disturbances like codeine. Noscapine is an opium alkaloid of benzylisoquinoline group, with no CNS action except antitussive effect. In dogs it produces histamine release and bronchoconstriction. Benzonatate, a polyglycol derivative chemically related to procaine, produces its antitussive effect by inhibiting afferent nervous input in the lung as well as by a central action. The antihistamine diphenhydramine may also have weak central antitussive activity (18). The chief virtue of these drugs is that they lack the respiratory depressant, euphoriant, and addictive potential of opiates. Their chief drawbacks lie in being less potent and less predictable in antitussive effect than the opiates. In the case of dextromethorphan, at least one source of unpredictability may be individual variations in metabolism (2). These compounds are more suitable than opiates for over-the-counter (OTC) self-medications; dextromethorphan is the most appropriate nonopiate for pediatric use.

MIXTURES

In clinical practice antitussives are usually employed in cough mixtures along with decongestants, antihistamines, and/or expectorants. There is no scientific rationale for shotgun use of most of these mixtures. Pragmatically, however, antitussive doses of codeine in combination with other ingredients are less subject to abuse (hence regulation) than a single-entity drug. As mentioned earlier, liquid cough mixture may have added benefit from local soothing or demulcent effects in the pharynx.

Properties of some antitussive agents with their doses are summarized in Table 17-1.

DECONGESTANT AGENTS

The nasal passages are lined with erectile tissue. Not only does the rich capillary bed of this tissue serve to warm inspired air, but by tumescence and detumescence it can alter the dimensions of nasal passages, thus modulating air flow through the nose. This process, carried out under neurohumoral control of the arterioles and venules that determine the blood volume of the nasal capillary bed, is mediated mainly through α-adrenergic mechanisms. When, through the inflammatory or allergic response, the erectile tissue becomes swollen, producing nasal obstruction, constriction of afferent arterioles can shrink the nasal capillary bed. The final common pathway for all current decongestant drugs is an α-adrenergic constriction of nasal precapillary vessels. Because excessive nasal secretions may also produce nasal obstructions, drugs that diminish these secretions are occasionally employed. The glands of the nasal and paranasal area are stimulated by a cholinergic mechanism; most antisecretory drugs are anticholinergic agents. The primary action of antihistamines in the relief of nasal obstruction

Table 17-1
Properties of Antitussives

Drug	Mechanism of Action	Oral Dose	Comment
Opioid			
Codeine	Central	Adult, 10-30 mg, q. 4-8 hr Children, 1 mg/kg in 4 divided doses	Available in over-the-counter mixtures in some states
Hydrocodone	Central	Adult, 5-10 mg, q. 4-8 hr	Schedule III narcotic more potent than codeine but may have more abuse potential
Nonopioid			
Benzonatate	Inhibits afferent nervous input; also central action	Adult, 100-200 mg, q. 8 hr	Prescription only
Dextromethorphan	Central	Adult, 15-30 mg, q. 4-8 hr Children, 1 mg/kg in four divided doses	May be less dependable than codeine; safe for OTC use; few effects
Noscapine	Central	15-30 mg, q. 4-8 hr	Few controlled studies; available OTC
Diphenhydramine	Central	25-50 mg, q. 4-6 hr	Weak antitussive

in nonallergic individuals may be through anticholinergic drying side effects.

DECONGESTANTS

TOPICAL DECONGESTANTS

Vasconstricting agents of various sorts have been applied to the mucous membranes of the nose for almost a century. The earliest of these used in Western medicine, cocaine, is still used to a limited extent to shrink the nasal vascular bed and provide anesthesia for examination of the nasal passages. Cocaine is a potent decongestant that has effects lasting up to several hours, although its effects on the central nervous system, its potential toxic problems, and its status as a controlled substance make it inconvenient to use. Furthermore, aside from painful examinations, its local anesthetic properties are undesirable. For this reason, the medicinal use of cocaine is limited to a great extent and other primarily sympathomimetic agents are usually employed. Topical decongestants are sympathomimetic drugs that produce α-adrenergic stimulation at low concentrations when applied to mucous membranes.

Ephinephrine. Epinephrine is occasionally used for its vasoconstricting properties, but its duration of action in the nasal mucosa is limited to a few minutes. Although it is used for hemostatic effects in packs or on saturated cotton applicators during surgery, it has little utility as a decongestant.

Other sympathomimetic drugs have proven more useful as topical decongestants because of their lack of other significant local effects, lack of systemic effects, and longer duration of action than epinephrine. The principal drugs are ephedrine (usually as a 1% aqueous solution), phenylephrine (solutions of 0.125-1%), and oxymetazoline (solution of 0.05%).

Ephedrine. Ephedrine applied topically has demonstrable decongestant effects, but tachyphylaxis appears rapidly, limiting its repeated topical use.

Phenylephrine. Phenylephrine, differing from epinephrine only in that it has no hydroxyl group on the ring structure, is perhaps the most commonly used short-acting topical decongestant. Pharmacologically, it is practically devoid of β-adrenergic effects but is a potent α-adrenergic agonist; its effects are primarily through direct stimulation of the receptor. When used topically, phenylephrine has minimal systemic action. It lacks the CNS depressant effects of other topical agents, which makes it suitable for infant use. Its chief drawbacks are limited duration of action (2-4 hours) and a tendency toward rebound congestion that is shared to an extent by all topical decongestants. Phenylephrine is also employed as a systemic decongestant (see later discussion).

Oxymetazoline. Oxymetazoline is one of the newer decongestant agents. When employed as an 0.05% solution, it has a longer duration of action than phenylephrine (up to 8 hours) and, like phenylephrine, has not shown CNS depressant activity in overdosage. With prolonged use, it may produce rebound congestion but is less of a problem in this regard than topical agents with a shorter duration of action.

Other less commonly employed topical agents, naphazoline (0.05% solution), tetrahydrozoline (0.05-0.1% solution), and xylometazoline (0.05-0.1% solution), share the common drawbacks of topical agents and have the additional problem of causing CNS depression in children with overdose.

Adrenergic agents should be given cautiously to patients with hyperthyroidism, hypertension, diabetes mellitus, and heart disease, or to those on tricyclic antidepressant drugs. Patients highly sensitive to adrenergic agents should not be given these drugs as they may manifest insomnia, dizziness, weakness, tremor, or cardiac arrhythmias after small doses.

SYSTEMIC DECONGESTANTS

Orally active α-adrenergic agonists in Western medicine date back to the mid-1920s. For the past 40 years, orally active decongestants have grown steadily in use because in most instances they possess a somewhat longer duration of action than the topical agents. In addition, they lack rebound congestion typical of topical agents. Tachyphylaxis is reported much less frequently with oral agents, which make them more suitable for repeated or prolonged use. The oral agents differ chiefly in their incidence of side effects, and, to a lesser extent, duration of action. All α-adrenergic drugs tend to aggravate hypertension and cause urinary retention by stimulation of the urinary sphincter. It should be noted, however, that pseudoephedrine is the only commonly used decongestant marketed as a single-ingredient remedy.

Phenylephrine. Phenylephrine exerts α-adrenergic effects on the nasal mucosa when taken orally. Large doses (probably 20 mg or more) are required in adults to exert a beneficial effect on the nose. Interestingly, its local vasoconstrictor effect may affect its absorption from the gut. The duration of phenylephrine effects on the nose are on the order of 2 to 4 hours. It is not marketed in oral form as a single drug but is found in combination with antihistamines (such as chlorpheniramine), and sometimes with additional decongestants (such as phenylpropanolamine). Adverse reactions to oral phenylephrine are rare except for aggravation of hypertension. Severe hypertension in patients taking MAO inhibitors has been reported. Unlike other oral agents, side effects of CNS stimulation are rare, which may have some advantage for a pediatric age group. It may also be advantageous to use in pregnant women because it is devoid of teratogenic effects (13).

Phenylpropanolamine. Phenylpropanolamine differs chemically from amphetamine by addition of a hydroxyl group in the β-methyl position. It has far fewer CNS-stimulating effects than amphetamine, little if any β-adrenergic activity, and has been employed as a nasal decongestant for over 30 years. As with many "old" drugs, little human research beyond anecdotal work has been performed. The effective decongestant dose in adults is 25 to 50 mg, though as with phenylephrine it is often combined with an antihistamine or other ingredient in cold or allergy preparations, making its nasal effects as a single ingredient difficult to ascertain. Its duration of action is estimated as 4 to 8 hours, although its presence as one ingredient of combination products clouds the issue. Like amphetamine, phenylpropanolamine has some anorectic properties, though it is much less potent in this regard than amphetamine. This effect is likely not important in adult decongestant therapy but may be undesirable, especially with prolonged use, in pediatric therapy. As with other α-adrenergic agonists, phenylpropanolamine may aggravate underlying hypertension.

Phenylpropanolamine has also been reported as causing hallucinations or toxic psychosis. Though this effect is rare, it seems more common with phenylpropanolamine than with other orally active decongestants (22). The possible potentiation of the CNS effects of phenylpropanolamine by anticholinergic drugs is also a cause of concern because most antihistamines and many other OTC preparations have anticholinergic properties (10).

Ephedrine. Ephedrine is one of several isomers of plant origin that was used for many centuries in clinical medicine: the l-isomer was introduced into Western medicine in 1924. It possesses both α- and β-adrenoceptor agonist activity and has been used extensively alone and in combination for asthma (see later discussion). It possesses some CNS stimulatory activity, and because of its β-agonist activity has cardiovascular and metabolic actions similar to epinephrine. Ephedrine has nasal decongestant activity in adults at oral doses of 25 mg, although it is rarely used for this purpose; it is more commonly used as a bronchodilator. It, too, has been reported to aggravate hypertension and may aggravate ventricular arrhythmias.

Pseudoephedrine. Pseudoephedrine (d-isoephedrine) differs from other ephedrine isomers in that it has primarily α-agonist effects. As such, it is a poor bronchodilator but is superior to ephedrine as an oral nasal decongestant. It is one of the more widely used modern decongestants and has been studied more extensively than any of the other systemic agents. Its effective oral dose in adults is 30 to 60 mg, with the latter being a more realistic dose. Pseudoephedrine is employed as a single-entity medication as well as in combination products. It has been reported to be effective in relieving eustachian tube obstruction and is employed clinically in this regard, although the role of decongestant therapy in such problems remains controversial.

Pseudoephedrine has some CNS-stimulating properties, but only at doses of 180 mg or greater, far in excess of the usual clinical dose. Pseudoephedrine lacks the anorectic effects of phenylpropanolamine but does have some measurable cardiovascular effects. In normal subjects, a mild increase in resting pulse rate has been observed at doses of 60 to 120 mg. No appreciable effect on blood pressure has been observed in normal subjects at doses of up to 180 mg, although pseudoephedrine has been reported to aggravate hypertension in some patients (11).

TOPICAL ANTIALLERGIC AGENTS

Congestion of the nasal mucosa can often be produced by immunoglobulin E (IgE)-mediated allergic reactions. These can be suppressed by glucocorticosteroids. Although systemic steroids can be employed, topical steroids are usually preferable in order to avoid the systemic steroid effects. Topical steroids are available in pressurized canister and pump nasal applicators.

Beclomethasone dipropionate 42 μg (one canister actuation) in each nostril two to four times per day; dexamethasone phosphate 0.2 mg (two canister actuations) two to three times a day; or, flunisolide one to two sprays of 0.25% solution two to three times a day are all effective in the treatment of nasal allergies.

As in the lung, the release of mediators of IgE-type reactions can be inhibited in order to blunt allergic nasal congestion. Topical disodium cromoglycate, although not a decongestant agent per se can be used to prevent allergic nasal congestion (8).

DRYING AGENTS

As mentioned in the preceding section, the α-adrenergic decongestants are often combined with other ingredients, the most common of which are antihistamines. Although this is a rational combination for allergic upper airway symptoms, the role of antihistamines in the common cold has been a matter of dispute for several years. The evidence now suggests that at least some antihistamines (e.g., chlorpheniramine) do have a drying effect in the common cold when watery secretions are present. In nonallergic individuals, this is almost certainly due to anticholinergic effects on the nose. For practical purposes, it is usually much less expensive and more efficacious to employ these medications on a trial basis than to try to sort out the relative contributions of allergens or viruses to a given cold.

Some specifically anticholinergic compounds (isopropamide, methscopolamine) are also added to decongestant mixtures. They are invariably found together with antihistamines in such mixtures, with presumably additive anticholinergic effects. The therapeutic wisdom of these additives has been questioned. Certainly they may increase atropinelike side effects, the most notable of which is dry mouth, thereby providing added efficacy when profuse watery nasal discharge is present.

The anticholinergic effects of drying agents are, of course, not confined to the nose; side effects of dry mouth and blurred vision are not uncommon. More serious side effects of urinary retention and excessive drying of lower respiratory tract secretions are seen (though not commonly) in "normal" individuals. Aggravation of asthma in some patients is often attributed to secretion retention, though the evidence for this is anecdotal.

The sedative properties of antihistamines vary not only among chemical groups but also among patients. This may offset (or be offset by) the CNS-stimulating properties of certain decongestants. Here again, trial and error is the usual method of assessing suitability of a particular mixture for any given individual.

ANTIASTHMATIC AGENTS

Bronchial asthma affects approximately 9 million people of both sexes and all age groups in the United States. It varies greatly from individual to individual in severity and duration of attacks. The classic form of the disease is characterized by reversible dyspnea and wheezing, which are usually short-lived and attributable to narrowing of the airways. The narrowing or obstruction consists of three main factors: (1) contraction of the smooth muscles in the bronchioles, (2) edema of the bronchiolar mucosa, and (3) increased mucus production.

Two pathophysiological mechanisms produce this obstruction: bronchial smooth muscle hyperreactivity and release of potent bioactive mediators [histamine, slow-reacting substance of anaphylaxis (SRS-A), eosinophil chemotactic factor, etc.] from mast cells in the lung in an immunoglobulin E (IgE)-related reaction. Abnormally severe constriction of bronchial smooth muscle, with its attendant reduction in airway caliber, can be demonstrated in asthmatics by challenge with histamine, cholinergic drugs, or allergens. Clinical inducers of bronchoconstriction may include exercise, aspirin, viral infections, occupational exposures (e.g., chemicals, animal danders), and emotional states. It can be reversed clinically and in the laboratory by bronchodilators. The cellular mechanism, debated for many years, revolves around the relative importance of the β-adrenergic receptor and the relative contribution of other systems in modulating smooth muscle cell calcium (17).

The release of mediators from mast cells produces a variety of physiological effects. Bronchoconstriction may be produced in the hyperactive smooth muscle, as previously described, and edema may be produced in the small, nonmuscle-containing airways through activation of the prostaglandin-thromboxane system. The leukotrienes C and D are important in mucus production. Eosinophils, which themselves contain granules of potent bioactive substances, are the hallmark of the abnormal mucus of asthma. They are drawn to the lung via the chemotactic mediator and degranulate (release mediators) in an antigen-antibody reaction of the IgE type. Clinically, this is blocked by stabilization of the mast cell or inhibition or suppression of the antigen-antibody reaction.

Because many factors may be involved in inducing an asthmatic episode, a rational approach for the treatment of asthma is theoretically possible at several points (9). The pharmacological approach to treating bronchial asthma, however, will be successful only when known precipitating factors have been removed from the patient's environment. Numerous drugs, along with other measures, have been effective in the management of asthma, with a goal of either preventing the onset or reversing bronchospasm (Fig. 17-1).

Bronchodilators, for the most part limited to the methylxanthines and the β-adrenergic agonists, are the major drugs used in the treatment of asthma. Although such usage is widely accepted as initial therapy, the limitations must be recognized. For example, airway

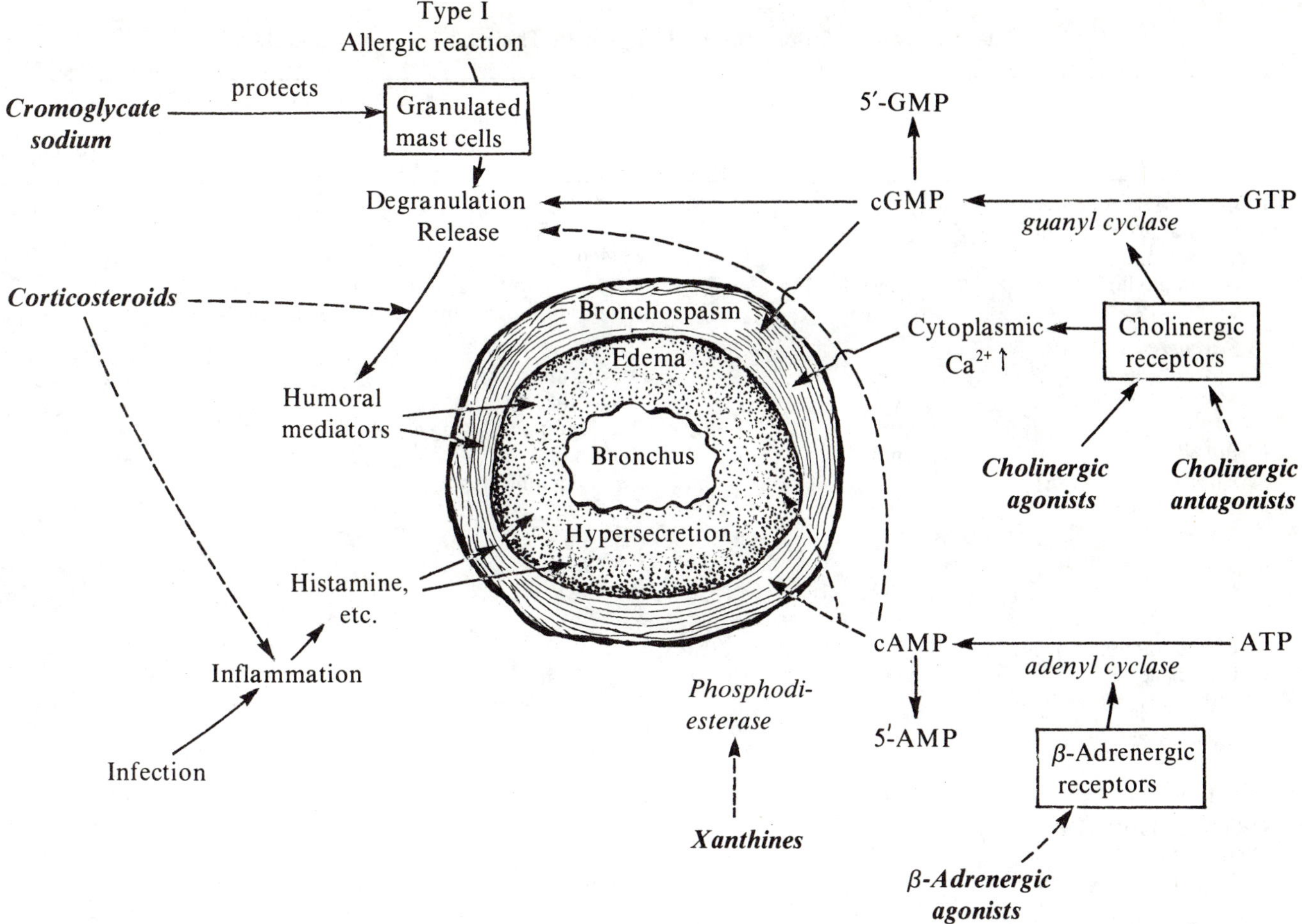

Fig. 17-1. *A schematic for site and mechamism of action of antiasthmatics.* Solid arrow (→) indicates stimulation or increase; interrupted arrow (--→) indicates inhibition or decrease. Humoral mediators released during allergic reactions include histamine, serotonin, SRS-A, ECF-A, PAF, kinins, and others.

obstruction is not always due solely to a bronchospasm: under these conditions, the obstruction will not respond to bronchodilators alone. Consequently, other therapeutic measures (e.g., corticosteroids and hydration) would be necessary for the total relief of the airway obstruction. Recognition is also increasing that, although some routine or standard approaches are useful in initiation of therapy, individualized regimes, frequently involving multiple drugs and routes of administration, are required for optimal control.

Antiasthmatic drugs are classified together with their dose and schedules in Table 17-2.

BRONCHODILATORS

The bronchodilator drugs vary in their therapeutic usefulness. The two major bronchodilator groups are sympathomimetics (adrenergic agonists) and methylxanthines. The mechanism of action of both groups of drugs appears related to increasing the level of cyclic adenosine monophosphate (cAMP), thereby modulating the calcium ions that control bronchial smooth muscle contraction. When combined, these agents should act synergistically (by virtue of their differing sites of actions), thus facilitating a greater relaxation. Although this is an appealing idea that is employed clinically, it has not been convincingly demonstrated in the laboratory.

XANTHINES

Theophylline and its ethylenediamine compound, aminophylline, have been effective in the treatment of asthma for many years. The presumed action of theophylline in asthma is its ability to relax bronchial smooth muscle by competitively inhibiting the enzyme phosphodiesterase, which breaks down intracellular, cAMP. The subsequent increase in the level of cAMP not only results in smooth muscle relaxation but also inhibits the release of SRS-A and histamine, known mediators of bronchoconstriction during IgE-mediated reactions (15). Theophylline also increases the force of skeletal muscle contraction (24). This may be useful in the treatment of respiratory muscle fatigue.

Table 17-2
Classification of Antiasthmatic Drugs with Their Doses and Schedule

Drug	Route[a]	Adult Dose	Approx. Duration of Action (hr)
BRONCHODILATORS			
Phosphodiesterase inhibitors			
Theophylline	p.o.	65-500 mg	6-12
Aminophylline	i.v. (slow)	5.6 mg/kg (= 5 mg/kg theophylline), initial loading dose followed by 0.25-0.9 mg/kg/hr	
β-Adrenergic agonists			
Epinephrine (α, β_1, β_2)	s.c.	0.2-0.5 ml	1-2
Metaproterenol (β_2)	p.o.	10-20 mg	4-8
	in.	2 to 3 puffs, (0.65 mg each)	3-4
Ephedrine (α, β_1,β_2)	p.o.	25-50 mg	4-6
Isoproterenol (β_1,β_2)	in.	up to 0.5 ml (5 mg/ml)	2-4
Terbutaline (β_2)	p.o.	2.5-5 mg	4-8
	s.c.	0.25 mg	4-6
	in.	0.4 mg	4-6
Albuterol (β_2)	p.o.	2-8 mg	4-6
	in.	0.18 mg	4-6
Fixed-combination drugs			
Ephedrine and theophylline	p.o.	6, 12, 25 mg 32.5, 65, 130 mg	
Anticholinergic			
Ipratropium[b]	in.	80 μg	4-6
Atropine	in.	200-400 μg	4-6
CORTICOSTEROIDS			
Systemic			
Prednisone or prednisolone	p.o.	Up to 1 mg/kg/day maximum; tape to smallest effective dose, 5-10 mg/day or 10-15 mg q. 2 days	
Methylprednisolone	p.o.	4/5 dose of prednisolone	
Hydrocortisone	i.v.	2-4 mg/kg loading dose, 3 mg/kg q. 6 hr	
Topical			
Beclomethasone	in.	Two puffs	6-8
Triamcinolone acetonide	in.	Maximum 20 puffs/day	
INHIBITORS OF MEDIATOR RELEASE			
Cromolyn sodium	in.	20 mg	6

[a] in. = oral inhalation; i.v. = intravenous; p.o. = per oral; s.c. = subcutaneous. Drugs are available in different forms (tablet, capsule, solution) in combination of different doses of these and other drugs.

[b] Investigational drug.

Although recognized as an effective bronchodilator for acute asthma, the use of theophylline was initially limited because of safety. The ability to assay serum theophylline levels and the demonstration of the relationship between the plasma concentration of theophylline and toxicity have permitted determination of the best dosage levels and more effective use. The optimum serum theophylline level appears to be in the range of 10 to 20 μg/ml; maintenance of this concentration by occasional measurements of the plasma concentration is recommended. This is especially important because pharmacokinetic studies indicate that many factors such as age, weight, smoking status, dietary habits, and various diseases influence theophylline metabolism. The average half-life for theophylline in serum is about 4 hours in children (with a range of 2-10 hours); in adults, the half-life is longer. Short half-lives are associated with rapid clearance of the drug and require more frequent dosing. The development of sustained-release theophylline preparations allows more constant plasma levels and avoids the large variations in serum peak and trough levels. Total daily doses usually range from 8 to 24 mg/kg/24 hours. The toxic level of theophylline also varies from one patient to another, although toxicity usually develops once the serum concentration exceeds 20 μg/ml, with nausea, vomiting, and diarrhea as the early signs. The more serious signs of theophylline toxicity such as convulsions and cardiac arrhythmias usually occur at levels of 30 to 50 μg/ml or higher. These serious side effects are usually preceded by the gastrointestinal signs, although seizures or even death, without warning symptoms, have been reported, especially in elderly patients.

Theophylline is employed as such or as the ethylenediamine salt, aminophylline; its enhanced solubility makes it suitable for intravenous use. Other salts, such as theoplylline-choline, are also used. Various claims for these salts are made, usually with regard to less gastrointestinal side effects, although the main difference between preparations is price. Each must be titrated to suit the individual patient.

Intravenous aminophylline is useful for emergency use where rapid blood levels are desirable and oral dosing may be difficult. Total daily theophylline dosage is similar to oral requirements; too-rapid infusion (greater than 50 mg/min) carries increased risk of major toxic reaction (20).

β-ADRENOCEPTOR AGONISTS

β-Adrenoceptor agonists act on the receptors of the smooth muscle and activate adenyl cyclase, which, in turn, converts adenosine triphosphate (ATP) to cAMP. The original sympathomimetic bronchodilators exhibited a variety of pharmacological effects because they acted on many different receptors. Epinephrine and ephedrine hve both α- and β-agonist activity. β-Receptors are also present in the heart; their stimulation increases heart rate and force of contraction. Stimulation of β-receptors relaxes smooth muscle of the bronchi and blood vessels. Long-term therapy with adrenergic agents has been made possible by the development of agents that are more specific for the β-receptors and have longer durations of action.

Isoproterenol has relatively pure β-receptor agonist activity. Unfortunately, isoproterenol stimulates both β-cardiac receptors and β-smooth muscle receptors. The attendant cardiac effects, including tachycardia, are major drawbacks; like epinephrine, isoproterenol has a relatively short duration of action and is best suited to acute therapy.

Isoetharine is relatively β-specific and has a duration of action of 4 to 6 hours, but is effective only by the inhalation route. Metaproterenol is orally active, has a duration of action of 4 to 8 hours, and is relatively β-specific when given orally.

Terbutaline is effective both by inhalation, parenterally, and orally in the treatment of exercise-induced bronchospasm and in the management of acute bronchospasm in stable asthmatic patients. Its bronchodilating effects last for about 5 to 6 hours. Long-term use of terbutaline has not been shown to cause clinically significant tolerance to its bronchodilating activity, although some tolerance to its tremorogenic activity may occur.

Albuterol (salbutamol) has been studied extensively by oral and inhalation routes, and it has been reported to be effective in the treatment of exercise-induced bronchospasm. Animal studies have shown no drug tolerance to albuterol.

Both terbutaline and albuterol are selective β-agonists. For rapid relief of an acute attack, epinephrine and terbutaline (both subcutaneously) are the drugs of choice. In case of mild attacks, inhalation of isoetharine or isoproterenol may be sufficient, although the more β-selective aerosols are rapidly gaining favor. Metaproterenol, terbutaline, or albuterol may be given orally for prolonged bronchodilator effects.

All β-agonists cause skeletal muscle tremors, a side effect that has limited the use of these agents, because it has been inseparable from the bronchodilator effects. In addition, ventricular arrhythmias have been reported following virtually all adrenergic agents, so they must be used with caution in patients who are prone to arrhythmia (1). Although it has not been demonstrated for all the β-agonists, there is a growing amount of evidence that, following continuous usage of these bronchodilators, tolerance and/or desensitization of some β-adrenoceptors can be demonstrated (21).

OTHER AGENTS

The use of anticholinergic therapy for asthma is based on the fact that some degree of airway tone is modulated by cholinergic innervation. The precise role of anticholinergics in the treatment of asthma has not been clearly established, however. Some studies have suggested a cholinergic-mediated reflex bronchospasm as an etiological factor in obstructive pulmonary disease (14).

Ipratropium bromide (not available in the United States) is a derivative of N-isopropyl noratropine. It probably reduces cholinergic bronchial spasm and thereby causes bronchodilation. It has little effect against 5-HT- or histamine-induced bronchial spasm. Pharmacological properties and therapeutic effects of ipratropium in asthma have recently been reviewed. The drug is less effective than β-adrenoreceptor agonist bronchodilators such as albuterol in asthma. It is generally well tolerated in usual inhaled doses, but dryness of mouth, bad taste, and tracheal irritation have been reported in some patients. One of the older anticholinergic drugs, atropine, has been found to have some chemical utility in the reversal of bronchospasm. Its nonpulmonary side effects can be lessened by delivery of the drug by the aerosol route.

The presence of prostaglandins in the lung and bronchial tissue suggest that prostaglandin E_2 might be a potential bronchodilator, but it is rapidly destroyed and irritating when inhaled. Prostacyclin, a naturally occurring inhibitor of platelet aggregation, has been shown to have marked bronchodilating action (3).

GLUCOCORTICOIDS

The glucocorticoids such as prednisolone and beclomethasone are the most reliable therapy for the treatment of asthma. Their action in asthma is not clear, but it is known that they reduce inflammation and potentiate the action of β-adrenergic agonists.

Because of the wide range of side effects, there is a reluctance among clinicians to prescribe chronic systemic steroids. They are utilized primarily in short-term therapy of patients with acute severe exacerbations who do not respond adequately to other available therapy. Initial doses of 20 to 60 mg/day of prednisone (or its equivalent) are given with tapering accomplished over 1-4 weeks. Long-term therapy is reserved for chronic asthma uncontrolled by other measures.

The complications of long-term systemic steroid therapy are uncommon when therapy is less than 1 month in duration. Certain acute effects do occur, including euphoria and increased appetite. Toxic psychosis has been reported as a rare acute side effect of large doses (40 mg prednisone equivalent).

Attempts have been made to minimize steroid side effects, including (1) alternate-day therapy, (2) use of short-acting steroids, and (3) use of steroids in inhaled form. Many patients who require systemic steroids do tolerate alternate-day therapy. The primary advantage of such therapy has been a reduction in the amount of pituitary-adrenal suppression, and in children, less effect on growth and development. Doses for alternate-day steroids, as initial therapy, average 50 mg/day of prednisone (or equivalent). Tapering to the minimal effective dose is accomplished over several weeks to allow recovery of normal pituitary-adrenal function. Prednisone and methylprednisolone are favored because of their short duration of action. Recently, methylprednisolone has been found to distribute more preferentially to the lung than prednisone and may therefore be the preferred drug for pulmonary applications (5).

The final approach to steroid therapy that minimizes systemic side effects is the use of inhaled (topical) therapy. Research in the use of inhaled steroids resulted in the introduction of beclomethasone dipropionate and triamcinolone acetonide for inhalation. This aerosol is used prophylactically and has been effective in reducing or eliminating the need for oral steroid in many patients (6, 12). Beclomethasone, in doses of 84 μg or triamcinolone, 200 μg every 6 hours, is solely prophylactic and has no place in the treatment of acute exacerbations. The chief side effect of beclomethasone is a predisposition to oral yeast infection. This can usually be prevented by having patients rinse their mouths with water following inhaled steroid. Patients receiving oral steroid must also be withdrawn slowly to avoid adrenal insufficiency.

Intravenous (short-term) glucocorticoids may be used to alleviate status asthmaticus or where oral dosing is not feasible. Doses of 125 mg of methylprednisolone every 6 hours have been shown to be more effective than lower doses in severe asthma. This intensive therapy should be discontinued within a few days to forestall serious toxic effects.

MEDIATOR RELEASE INHIBITORS

The use of disodium cromoglycate (DSCG) represents a different approach to the treatment of asthma. It has no bronchodilator effects, is not steroidlike, and is not a specific receptor blocker of mediators involved in IgE allergic reactions. DSCG is believed to exert its main action by stabilizing mast cells against degranulation, thereby inhibiting the release of mediators. DSCG is therefore designated a mediator release inhibitor. The drug is unable to prevent or reverse the effects once these agents are released and is not very effective for the treatment of asthma associated with chronic infection. The best responses to DSCG usually occur in younger patients with extrinsic or exercise-induced asthma. The presence of eosinophilia in blood or sputum and/or high circulating levels of IgE are also felt to be good predictors of success with DSCG (4).

Therapeutic response to DSCG may occur within a few days; however, some individuals may not benefit from DSCG until up to 6 weeks of therapy. After discontinuation of DSCG therapy, a residual effect may last for about 4 weeks. As mentioned previously, it is also used in perennial allergic rhinitis.

DSCG is poorly absorbed by the lung and by the gastrointestinal tract. Only about 8% of a dose is absorbed into the blood. Following inhalation, the plasma half-life of DSCG is about 60 to 90 minutes. Because it is poorly absorbed through the lung, initially four capsules or ampules (20-mg each) should be inhaled daily. Thereafter, the number of capsules should be reduced to a minimum that is adequate for the control of symptoms.

DSCG has been reported to cause severe anaphylaxis (rarely), urticaria, maculopapular skin rash, myositis, diarrhea, coughing, dizziness, nausea, vomiting, and wheezing. In a few patients, eosinophilic pneumonia has been reported to be associated with DSCG therapy.

Selection of antiasthmatic agents under different types of asthmatic states is summarized in Table 17-3, and their doses and schedules are given in both Tables 17-2 and 17-3.

DRUG INTERACTIONS

Interaction of several antiasthmatic agents with other drugs is summarized in Table 17-4.

Preparations. *Epinephrine HCl*: solution (1:1000 for s.c. injection), *Epinephrine Bitartrate*: suspension (7 mg/ml, oral inhalation). *Ephedrine Sulfate:* capsules (25 and 50 mg, p.o.); syrup 11 and 20 mg/5 ml, p.o.).

Isoproterenol HCl: solution (1:200, oral inhalation; 1:5000, i.v. infusion); tablets (10 and 15 mg); isoproterenol sulfate: suspension (2 mg/ml, oral inhalation).

Isoetharine HCl: solution (0.25 and 1.0% inhalation and 0.61% nebulizer inhalation).

Table 17-3
Selection of Antiasthmatic Drugs[a]

Asthmatic States	Drug and Schedule
Prophylactic in cold and exercise-induced asthma	Metaproterenol, in.; albuterol, in.; cromolyn sodium, in.
Chronic asthma, persistent wheezing, failure of β-adrenergic inhalations	Metaproterenol, p.o.; terbutaline, p.o.; albuterol, p.o.; theophylline, p.o.
Chronic asthma following failure of theophylline and β-adrenergics	Beclomethasone, in.; triamcinolone, in.; or alternate-day systemic corticosteroids, prednisone, prednisolone, methylprednisolone, p.o.
Acute severe attack	Epinephrine, s.c., 0.3-0.5 ml (1:1000) q. 20 min, 2 to 3 doses; terbutaline, s.c., 0.25-0.5 ml, q. 4-6 hr; methylprednisolone, i.v., 125 mg q. 6 hr; hydrocortisone, i.v., 0.25-1 g, initially, 100-300 mg q. 4-6 hr

[a]Dosage for the drugs not mentioned here are the same as in Table 17-2; abbreviations are the same as those for Table 17-2.

Metaproterenol Sulfate: tablets (10 and 20 mg); syrup (10 mg/5 ml); micronized powder (225 mg oral inhalation). *Terbutaline sulfate*: solution (1 mg/ml, s.c. injection); tablets (2.5 and 5 mg).

Albuterol: tablets (2 and 4 mg); micronized powder (90 mg per actuation for inhalation).

Theophylline: tablets (100, 125, 175, 178, 200, 225, 250, 300, and 500 mg, p.o.); tablets, time-release (100, 200, and 300 mg, p.o.); capsules, time-release, (50, 60, 75, 100, 125, 130, 200, 250, 260, and 300 mg, p.o.); aqueous suspension (250 and 500 mg/37 ml, rectally); suppository (120 and 500 mg, rectally). *Aminophylline*, USP: solution (25 mg/in 10 and 20 ml, i.v. infusion); solution (300 mg/5 ml, rectally); suppository (125, 250, 350, 450, and 500 mg, rectally). *Oxtriphylline*: tablets (100, 200 mg, p.o.); elixir (100 mg/5 ml, p.o.). *Dyphylline*: solution (250 mg/ml i.m. injection); tablets (200 mg, p.o.); elixir (100 mg/15 ml, p.o.); solution (100 mg/15 ml, p.o.).

Atropine Sulfate: ampules (0.4 mg/ml).

Cromolyn Sodium: capsules or ampules (20 mg, oral inhalation).

Beclomethasone Dipropionate: suspension (equivalent of 42-μg beclomethasone dipropionate per actuation, inhalation).

Triamcinolone Acetonide: suspension (100 μg per actuation for inhalation).

REFERENCES

1. Banner, A.S., Sunderrajan, E.V., Agarwal, M.K.A. and Whitney, W. Arrhythmogenic effects of orally administered bronchodilators. *Arch. Intern. Med.* 139:434, 1979.
2. Barnhart, J.W. The urinary excretion of dextromethorphan and three metabolites in dogs and humans. *Toxicol. Appl. Pharmacol.* 55:43, 1980.
3. Bell, S.C. and Capetola, R.J. Pulmonary and antiallergy drugs. In: *Annual report of medicinal chemistry* Vol. 13 (Clarke, F.H., ed). New York: Academic Press, 1978, p. 51.
4. Bernstein, I.L. Cromolyn sodium in the treatment of asthma: changing concepts. *J. Allergy Clin. Immunol.* 68(4):247, 1981.
5. Braude, A.C. and Rebuck, A.S. Prednisone and methylprednisolone disposition in the lung. *Lancet* 8356:995, 1983.
6. Brogden, R.N., Pinder, R.M., Sawyers, P.R. Beclomethasone dipropionate inhaler: A review of its pharmacology, therapeutic value, and adverse effect in asthma. *Drugs* 10:166, 1975.
7. Brooks, S.M., Werk, E.F., Ackerman, S.J., Sullivan, I. and Thrasher, K. Adverse effects of phenobarbital on corticosteroid metabolism in patients with bronchial asthma. *N. Engl. J. Med.* 286(21):1125, 1972.
8. Chandra, R.K., Heresi, G. and Woodford, G. Double-blind controlled trial of 4% intranasal sodium cromoglycate solution in patients with seasonal rhinitis. *Ann. Allergy* 49:131, 1982.
9. Cockroft, D.W. Mechanism of perennial allergic asthma. *Lancet* 8344:253, 1983.
10. Davis, W.M. and Pinkerton, J.T. Synergism by atropine of central stimulant properties of phenylpropanolamine. *Toxicol. Appl. Pharmacol.* 22:138, 1972.
11. Drew, C.D.M., Knight, G.T., Hughes, D.T.D. and Bush, M. Comparison of the effects of D (+) pseudoephedrine on the cardiovascular and respiratory systems in man. *Br. J. Clin. Pharmacol.* 6:221, 1978.
12. Falliers, L.J., and Petraco, A.J. Control of asthma with triamcinolone acetonide aerosol inhalations at 12 hour intervals. *J. Asthma* 19(4):241, 1982.

Table 17-4
Interaction of Antiasthmatics with Other Drugs

Antiasthmatic Drugs	Interacting With	Effects
Ephedrine	MAO inhibitors (e.g., isocarboxazid, phenelzine, tranylcypromine)	Hypertension
	Guanethidine	Antagonism of antihypertensive effects
β-Adrenergic agonists	Propranolol	Reduced efficacy of bronchodilators
	Diuretics	Decreased serum potassium (16)
Corticosteroids	Barbiturates	Increased metabolism of steroids (7)
Theophylline	Cimetidine, macrolide antibiotics	Increased blood level of theophylline (23)

13. Greenberger, P. and Patterson, R. Safety of therapy for allergic symptoms during pregnancy. *Ann. Intern. Med.* 89:234, 1978.
14. Gross, N.J. and Skorodin, M.S. Anticholinergic, antimuscarinic bronchodilators. *Am. Rev. Resp. Dis.* 129(5):856, 1984.
15. Hendeles, L. and Weinberger, M. Theophylline, a "state of the art" review. *Pharmacotherapy* 113(1), part 1:2, 1983.
16. King, M., White, J.R. and Barki, N.K. The effect of subcutaneously administered terbutaline on serum potassium in asymptomatic adult asthmatics. *Am. Rev. Resp. Dis.* 129:329, 1984.
17. Leff, A. Pathogenesis of asthma. *Chest* 81(2):224, 1982.
18. Lillienfield, L.S., Rose, J.C. and Princiotto, J.V. Antitussive activity of diphenhydramine in chronic cough. *Clin. Pharmacol. Ther.* 19:421, 1976.
19. Maran, Z., Shelhamer, J.H., Bach, M.K., Morton, D.R. and Kaliner, M. Slow-reacting substances, leukotrienes C and D, increase the release of mucus from human airways *in vivo*. *Am. Rev. Resp. Dis.* 126:449, 1982.
20. Mitenko, P. and Ogilvie, R.I. Rapidly achieved plasma concentration plateaus with observations on theophylline kinetics. *Clin. Pharmacol. Ther.* 13:329, 1972.
21. Morris, H.G. Densensitization of β-adrenergic receptors. *J. Allergy Clin. Immunol.* 65:83, 1980.
22. Norvenius, G., Eiderlov, E. and Lonnerholm, G. Mental disturbances with phenylpropanolamines: The Swedish experience. *Lancet* 2:1367, 1979.
23. Powell, J.R., Rogers, J.F., Wargin, W.A. Cross, R.E. and Eshelman, F.N. Inhibition of theophylline clearance by cimetidine but not ranitidine. *Arch. Int. Med.* 144:484, 1984.
24. Viires, N., Aubier, M., Murciano, D., Fleury, B., Talamo, C. and Pariente, R. Effects of aminophylline on diaphragmatic fatigue during acute respiratory failure. *Am. Rev. Resp. Dis.* 129(3):396, 1984.

ADDITIONAL READING

Eddy, N.D., Freibel, H., Hahn, K. and Halloch, H. The antitussive action of codeine-mechanism, methodology, and evaluation: Potential alternatives for cough relief. In: *Codeine and Alternatives for Pain and Cough Relief.* Geneva: World Health Organization, 1970, p. 127, 157.

Hendeles, L., Iafrate R.P. and Weinberger, M. A clinical and pharmacokinetic basis for the selection and use of slow release theophylline products. *Clin. Pharmacokinet.* 9:95, 1984.

Michaelides, D.N. Immediate hypersensitivity: The immunochemistry and therapeutics of reversible airway obstruction (a review). *Immunol. Allergy Practice* 2:133, 1980.

Myers, M. and Walsh, J.R. Pulmonary, anti-inflammatory and anticoagulant medications. *Prog. Drug Res.* 28:648, 1984.

Pavia, D. Effects of pharmacologic agents on the clearance of airway secretions. *Semin. Resp. Med.* 5(4):345, 1984.

Wilson, A.F. Drug treatment of asthma. *Prog. Drug Res.* 28:111, 1984.

Wilson, A.F. and McPhillips, J.J. Pharmacological control of asthma. *Ann. Rev. Pharmacol. Toxicol.* 18:541, 1978.

Ziment, I. Medications for coughs and colds. In: *Respiratory Pharmacology and Therapeutics.* Philadelphia: W.B. Saunders, 1978, p. 282.

CHAPTER
17.1

RESPIRATORY GASES

Samar N. Dutta and Sachin N. Pradhan

OXYGEN

Oxygen (O_2) was first introduced in 1727 by Stephen Hale, and almost five decades later Priestley indicated its beneficial effects in some disease states. In the 1780s Lavoisier reported pulmonary absorption of oxygen and its final metabolism into carbon dioxide and water in the body. In acutely ill patients, administration of oxygen to correct arterial hypoxemia is generally accepted as being of important clinical value. In recent years either continuous or intermittent chronic oxygen administration in patients with hypoxemia has also been reported to be widely used (1).

Effect of Oxygen Inhalation. Inhalation of 100% oxygen results in depletion of tissue nitrogen and interferes with the transport of CO_2, particularly at about 3 atmospheric pressure. In alveoli, when ventilated with oxygen, mainly the inert nitrogen is washed out, and the alveoli tend to collapse as oxygen is absorbed. Respiratory drive by aortic and carotid chemoreceptors is also inhibited by 100% O_2 inhalation, causing slight decrease in tidal volume and respiratory rate. Cardiovascular manifestations of oxygen inhalation include rise in systemic blood pressure, increase in peripheral resistance, mild bradycardia, and fall in cardiac output. Hyperoxia leads to constriction of cerebral and coronary vessels. Administration of oxygen in the presence of hypoxia causes dilatation of pulmonary blood vessels, but at high pO_2 there is vasoconstriction. Inhalation of 100% oxygen by normal subjects causes no appreciable effect on the hematopoietic system, but in patients with sickle cell anemia red cell formation may be inhibited.

Oxygen Therapy. The goal of oxygen therapy is to treat hypoxia, a state where tissues are inadequately oxygenated. Cellular metabolism, however, is maintained until tissue pO_2 is markedly reduced. Oxygen tension of mixed venous blood ($p\bar{v}O_2$) is an accurate determinant of tissue oxygenation and a $p\bar{v}O_2$ value below 30 mmHg generally shows tissue hypoxia. The relationship between oxygen saturation and arterial pO_2 bears an S-shaped curve with 90% saturation at pO_2 in excess of 60 mmHg. Clinically there is little advantage in raising pO_2 more than 60 mmHg. Oxygen therapy is primarily corrective in anoxic hypoxia that results from impaired respiratory exchange for oxygen. In both stagnant (due to circulatory failure) or histotoxic (as in cyanide poisoning) hypoxia the arterial pO_2 may be normal. In *diffusion hypoxia*, which occurs following long-term nitrous oxide anesthesia, arterial pO_2 may fall as much as 10%. This condition can be prevented by administration of 100% oxygen for a few minutes after termination of nitrous oxide anesthesia.

Clinical manifestations of hypoxia are relative to the degree of hypoxia (Table 17.1-1) and to the rate at which it develops. Inhalation of 100% oxygen is also used in the treatment of bowel, headache following pneumoencephalography, and to reduce the size of pulmonary air embolism. In these conditions, O_2 inhalation facilitates absorption of gas in closed body spaces. The fractional inspired concentrations of oxygen (FiO_2) required for therapy in various settings of acute hypoxemia are outlined in Table 17.1-2.

Response to Oxygen Therapy in Hypoxia. Clinical manifestations of hypoxia should be corrected by successful oxygen therapy. Hypoxic patients with low ventilation/perfusion ratio ($\dot{V}_A\dot{Q}_b$) are easily corrected by oxygen therapy. Serial arterial (paO_2) and venous ($p\bar{v}O_2$) measurements during oxygen therapy provide most reliable information regarding effectiveness of O_2 therapy. Furthermore, in order to obtain information regarding the efficiency of the oxygen transfer apparatus or about the adequacy of tissue oxygenation, one should also determine the difference between alveolar and arterial oxygen tension $p(A\text{-}a)O_2$, and "shunt" fraction. There are a number of other pulmonary measures [such as $paCO_2$, a product of respiratory rate and tidal volume, expiratory volume (VE), ratio of dead space to tidal volume (VD/VT)] and cardiac parameters (such as cardiac output and pulmonary capillary wedge pressure) that help in the evaluation and treatment of patients with acute hypoxia.

Adverse Effects. Several hypoxic patients who have lost the response of respiratory drive to CO_2 because of barbiturates, narcotic poisoning, or brain injury may develop apnea with the administration of oxygen. Similarly, marked hypoventilation may follow inhalation of supplemental oxygen in some patients with chronic obstructive pulmonary disease with CO_2 retention

Table 17.1-1
Relationship of Arterial pO_2 and Signs and Symptoms of Hypoxia

Arterial pO_2 (mmHg)	Nature of Development	Signs and Symptoms
<30	Acute	Circulatory failure, cardiac arrest, unconsciousness
30	Acute	Unconsciousness
>30 - <50	Acute	Emotional instability, loss of judgment, muscle incoordination, and visual disturbances
>30 - <50	Slow	Easy fatigability, weakness

(10). Long-term exposure of lungs to normobaric hyperoxia results in light-microscopic and ultrastructural pathological tissue changes (2, 3). Oxygen toxicity, however, shows great individual variation in susceptibility and resistance to the development of tissue damage, and related to the partial pressure of oxygen rather than to its percent concentration. Inhalation of 100% oxygen at about 2 atmosphere (atm) pressure leads to tracheobronchial irritation, and decreases in lung compliance, vital capacity, diffusing capacity, and pulmonary capillary blood volume (2). The initial symptoms of oxygen toxicity are sharp pleuritic substernal pain and dry cough occurring approximately 6 hours after exposure to 100% oxygen (9). At the molecular level, the mechanism of O_2 toxicity is generally attributed to free O_2 radical reactions with cellular components (3). Free radicals are unstable metabolites of oxygen that include superoxide ($O_2^{\cdot -}$), hydrogen peroxide (H_2O_2), and others. A vascular proliferative disease of developing retina (retrolental fibroplasia, RLF) has been reported to occur in some premature infants exposed to inhalation of high concentrations of oxygen. However, the etiology of this condition has been questioned by some investigators, and the subject has been thoroughly reviewed by James and Lanman (7). Other adverse reactions to normobaric oxygen are summarized in Table 17.1-3.

Hyperbaric Oxygen. The term hyperbaric oxygen refers to inhalation of 100% oxygen at greater than normal atmospheric pressure. Hyperbaric oxygen therapy overcomes the barrier to increased oxygen transport and causes an increase in physically dissolved oxygen in the blood. The pO_2 in blood is raised to about 2000 mmHg at 3 atmospheres absolute (ATA). Hyperbaric oxygen is bactericidal to anaerobes and facilitates removal of bubbles of gas from tissues.

Hyperbaric oxygen therapy has been used in acute carbon monoxide poisoning, acute cyanide poisoning, clostridial myone-

Table 17.1-2
Initial O_2 Therapy in Various Settings of Acute Hypoxemia[a]

Initial ABG	Interpretation	Initial FiO_2
pH $\uparrow$, pO_2 $\downarrow$, pCO_2 $\downarrow$ with baseline normal ABG	Hyperventilation secondary to hypoxemia (mild asthma, heart failure, pulmonary embolism)	Intermediate concentration ~ 40%. Exact FiO_2 is not important
pH normal or $\downarrow$, pO_2 $\downarrow$, pCO_2 normal or $\uparrow$ with baseline normal ABG	Early respiratory failure (tiring asthmatic, worsening congestive heart failure)	High FiO_2 of 50 - 100%
pH $\uparrow$, pO_2 $\downarrow$, pCO_2 normal or $\uparrow$, but <baseline pCO_2 with baseline $\uparrow$ pCO_2	Hyperventilation superimposed on COPD	28% by Venturi mask and $\uparrow$ to 31%, 35%, 40%, etc.; to achieve optimal ABG
pH $\downarrow$, pO_2 $\downarrow$, pCO_2 $\uparrow$ with baseline $\uparrow$ pCO_2	Early respiratory failure superimposed on COPD	24-28% by Venturi mask; if baseline pCO_2 $\uparrow\uparrow$ must start with 24% and $\uparrow$ incrementally to optimal ABG
pH $\downarrow\downarrow$, pO_2 $\downarrow\downarrow$, pCO_2 $\uparrow$ or $\uparrow\uparrow$ with baseline $\uparrow$ pCO_2	Impending respiratory failure	24% by Venturi mask and $\uparrow$ incrementally; if decision is made to intubate, give $\uparrow$ FiO_2 (100%) initially by IPPV; then aim at maintaining patient's normal baseline ABG; patient may be weaned to spontaneous ventilation via T piece

ABG = arterial blood gases; FiO_2 = fractional inspired concentration of oxygen; COPD = chronic obstructive pulmonary disease; IPPV = intermittent positive pressure ventilation;

pH $\downarrow$: 7.2-7.4	pCO_2 $\uparrow$: 40-50 mmHg	pO_2 $\downarrow$: 60-100 mmHg	low FiO_2 24-35%
$\downarrow\downarrow$: < 7.2	$\uparrow\uparrow$: >55 mmHg	$\downarrow\downarrow$: < 60 mmHg	intermediate : 35-50%
			high : 50-100%

Interpretation of ABG must be made with knowledge of age of patient and clinical setting. Baseline ABG can be inferred by determining whether disturbance represents acute or acute on chronic acidosis by standard techniques.

[a] *Source:* From Ref. 10

Table 17.1-3
Manifestations of Oxygen Toxicity (100% at 1 atm. pressure)[a]

Duration of Exposure	Clinical Manifestation
6 hour	Tracheobronchitis
18 hour	Slight abnormalities in pulmonary function testing. ↓ VC earliest. Later ↓ most lung volumes and capacities, ↓ compliance, ↑ RR, ↓ $paCO_2$, ↓ paO_2. No significant change in FEV_1. FEV_1/VC ↑.
24-28 hours	ARDS
Days to weeks	Hemolytic anemia ↓ Erythropoiesis Retinopathy of the newborn (retrolental fibroplasia) Pulmonary fibrosis (end stage of protracted ARDS) Diffuse organ damage including cardiac, renal, and hepatotoxicity

ARDS, acute respiratory distress syndrome; RR, respiratory rate; FEV_1, forced expiratory volume in 1 sec.;
↓, increase; ↑, decrease.
[a] *Source:* Ref.10

crosis, decompression sickness, air embolism (following pulmonary barotrauma or vascular cannulation), refractory osteomyelitis, and in the treatment of questionably vascularized skin grafts.

Humans can tolerate hyperbaric oxygen only for brief periods (less than 30 minutes at a time). CNS is primarily affected by hyperbaric oxygen, and the toxic manifestations are nausea, vertigo, tinnitus, paresthesia, anxiety, and involuntary movements. Both the duration of exposure and the ATA influence the severity of toxicity, and most individuals can tolerate up to 3 ATA for less than 30 minutes of exposure. Exposure of hyperbaric oxygen such as 3 atmospheres for about 35-95 minutes has been reported to induce grand mal seizure activity in humans (5). The mechanism for CNS toxicity of hyperbaric oxygen has not been clearly elucidated.

Drugs and Factors Affecting O_2 Toxicity. There are a number of drugs and chemicals that have been shown to increase the normobaric oxygen toxicity in mammals: paraquat (herbicide), disulfiram, dexamethasone, l-thyroxine, and diethyldithiocarbamate (7). The two antioxidant vitamins, α-tocopherol and ascorbate have been shown to provide some protection against normobaric oxygen toxicity. Both are reported to act by preventing oxidation of essential cellular components, or preventing formation of reactive metabolites such as hydroxyl and superoxide radicals and possibly lipid peroxides (7). The enzyme superoxide dismutase has been suggested to confer some protection against hyperoxic damage (4).

CARBON DIOXIDE

Carbon dioxide is the final product in catalysis of carbon-containing organic substances in the body. In the resting state about 200 mg of CO_2/min is excreted through the lungs. Due to the concentration gradient between arterial blood CO_2 and tissue CO_2, intracellular CO_2 diffuses out of the cell and enters the plasma and red blood cells. In venous blood, CO_2 is carried in four different forms: (1) dissolved CO_2, (2) carbonic acid, (3) bicarbonate ion, and (4) carbamino combinations. The pCO_2 in venous blood is about 46 mmHg, and CO_2 tension in blood serves as an important regulator of respiration.

Effect on Respiration. Carbon dioxide is a potent stimulator of respiration and increases the depth and rate of respiration even at 2% concentration. In normal subjects inhalation of CO_2 in increasing concentration causes graded increase in ventilation. Respiratory stimulation by CO_2 occurs within seconds, and peak response is usually achieved in 5 minutes. Mechanisms of respiratory stimulation by CO_2 involve two sites: (1) the brainstem respiratory integration areas which are acted on by impulses from (2) the medullary respiratory center that in turn is stimulated directly by CO_2 and also through the aortic and carotid chemoreceptor reflex. Hypercapnia has been shown to reduce the capacity of the unfatigued diaphragm to generate force during voluntary contractions, and to produce characteristic electromyographic changes of diaphragmatic fatigue, when breathing is performed against slight resistance (8).

Cardiovascular Effects. Circulatory effects of CO_2 result from its direct action on the heart and vascular smooth muscle and through involvement of the central and autonomic nervous systems. In humans the overall cardiovascular effects of CO_2 include increased cardiac output, tachycardia, and slight elevation in systolic pressure. On arterial smooth muscle the direct vasodilating action is opposed by sympathetic vasoconstrictive action. Both coronary and cerebral blood vessels are dilated in response to increased blood pCO_2 concentrations.

A slight increase in pCO_2 in blood may cause decreased excitability of the cerebral cortex and seizure activity, but sensory pain threshold is increased associated with headache, sweating, paresthesia, and a sense of discomfort. If pCO_2 in blood is higher than 25%, there is increased cerebral cortical activity that may lead to convulsions. Acute severe carbon dioxide poisoning is characterized by respiratory depression, lethargy, narcosis, and coma.

REFERENCES

1. Anthonisen, N.R. Long-term oxygen therapy. *Ann. Intern. Med.* 99:519, 1983.
2. Clark, J.M. The toxicity of oxygen. *Am. Rev. Resp. Dis.*, 110:40, 1974.
3. Deneke, S.M. and Fanburg, B.L. Normobaric oxygen toxicity of the lung. *N. Engl. J. Med.*, 303:76, 1980.
4. Deneke, S.M. and Fanburg, B.L. Oxygen toxicity of the lung: An update. *Br. J. Anaesth.*, 54: 737, 1982.

5. Frank, L. and Massaro, D. Oxygen toxicity. *Am. J. Med.* 69:117, 1980.
6. Gould, V.E., Tosco, R., Wheelis, R.F. et al. Oxygen Pneumonitis in man: Ultrastructural observations on the development of alveolar lesions. *Lab. Invest.*, 26:499, 1972.
7. James, L.S. and Lanman, JT. (eds.) History of oxygen therapy and retrolental fibroplasia. *Pediatrics* (Suppl.), 57:591, 1976.
8. Juan, G., Calverley, P., Talamo, C. et al. Effect of carbon dioxide on diaphragmatic function in human beings. *N. Engl. J. Med.* 310:874, 1984.
9. Sackner, M.A., Landa, J., Hirsch, J. et al. Pulmonary effects of oxygen breathing. *Ann. Intern. Med.* 82:40, 1975.
10. Tinits, P. Oxygen therapy and oxygen toxicity. *Ann. Emerg. Med.*, 12:321, 1983.

ADDITIONAL READING

Knighton, D.R., Halliday, B. and Hunt, T.K. Oxygen as an antibiotic. The effect of inspired oxygen on infection. *Arch. Surg.* 119:199, 1984.

Rashkin, M.C., Bosken, C. and Baughman, R.P. Oxygen delivery in critically ill patients. Relationship to blood lactate and survival. *Chest* 87:580, 1985.

Sugimoto, H., Ohashi, N., Sawada, Y. et al. Effects of positive end-expiratory pressure on tissue gas tensions and oxygen transport. *Crit. Care Med.* 12:661, 1984.

CHAPTER
18

THE ALIMENTARY SYSTEM

Drugs that are used in the treatment of disorders of the gastrointestinal tract may be classified according to their therapeutic indications. Drugs have produced beneficial effects in the management of peptic ulcer, constipation, vomiting, diarrhea, and other conditions. Accordingly, discussions in this section will be directed to drugs in the management of peptic ulcers (antacids, anticholinergics, and histamine H_2-receptor antagonists), laxatives and cathartics, antiemetics, and antidiarrheal agents.

CHAPTER
18.1

DRUGS USED IN THE MANAGEMENT OF PEPTIC ULCER

Constantine Arvanitakis and Aryeh Hurwitz

ANTACIDS

Antacids are compounds that neutralize hydrochloric acid secreted by parietal cells in the stomach. Until the advent of cimetidine and ranitidine, these drugs were the mainstay of treatment of acid peptic disease. Aluminum and magnesium hydroxide preparations are currently preferred for the treatment of peptic ulcer (7, 17). Antacids containing calcium carbonate are in disfavor because of acid rebound and stimulation of release of endogenous gastrin. Systemic antacids such as sodium bicarbonate may cause metabolic alkalosis and fluid retention, which limits their use for long-term therapy.

Pharmacological Effects. Antacids neutralize gastric acid and, when given in sufficient doses, raise pH to 4-4.5. This pH shift, from normal gastric pH of 1-2, reflects more than a 100-fold reduction in hydrogen ion concentration. Aluminum hydroxide gel, when given alone, delays gastric emptying, as shown in the experimental animal (10) and humans (11). The solubility of this antacid decreases markedly as pH is raised toward neutral. Aluminum hydroxide causes constipation. It binds and prevents the absorption of phosphate in the gastrointestinal tract, and is therefore used in the treatment of hyperphosphatemia in patients with chronic renal failure.

Magnesium hydroxide (milk of magnesia) rapidly neutralizes gastric hydrochloric acid with a neutralizing capacity of 30 mEq hydrogen ion per gram of drug. If taken in excess, it can raise gastric pH to over 9. Although it is a very potent antacid, its cathartic effect limits magnesium hydroxide use as an antacid to combinations with other antacids, especially aluminum hydroxide. The mixed antacid raises gastric pH to a maximum level of 6.5 -7.5. Combination antacids vary in composition, taste, cost, sodium content, and neutralizing capacity, all of which may be important factors in selecting a product for clinical use.

Pharmacokinetics. Nonsystemic antacids that contain magnesium and aluminum exert their pharmacological action in the stomach, pass into the small intestine, and are mainly excreted in the stool. These cations are poorly absorbed from the small intestine, and the fraction that is absorbed is excreted in the urine. By contrast, 37% of the cation in calcium carbonate is absorbed and excreted in the urine or deposited in bone.

Adverse Reactions. Aluminum hydroxide preparations cause occasional bloating, nausea, vomiting, constipation, and rarely, intestinal obstruction. Aluminum toxicity has been noted in patients with chronic renal failure. Some preparations contain significant amounts of sodium and may worsen hypertension and fluid retention in patients with cardiac, renal, or hepatic disease. Calcium carbonate, in addition to the rebound effect of additional acid output, may cause milk-alkali syndrome (hypercalcemia, calcinosis, renal failure, and azotemia). Hypophosphatemia and constipation have also been noted. Magnesium hydroxide may cause hypermagnesemia in patients with impaired renal function. Magnesium retention is manifested by neurological symptoms including somnolence and muscle weakness. Diarrhea is a common side effect of magnesium products.

Drug Interactions. Antacids affect the absorption and elimination of a variety of drugs including antibiotics, anticoagulants, psychotropic and antiinflammatory agents, glucocorticoids, iron, and vitamins. A list of some of these interactions that may alter the clinical efficacy of concomitantly ingested drugs in shown in Table 18.1-1. Antacid-drug interactions are mediated by altered gastric emptying, chelation, binding, adsorption, impaired dissolution or precipitation in the gastrointestinal tract, and modified renal elimination due to elevated urinary pH. It is therefore advisable to administer most drugs several hours before antacid ingestion whenever possible.

Therapeutic Uses. Antacids are used to relieve symptoms and accelerate healing of acid peptic diseases. The indications for antacid use include peptic esophagitis, gastric and duodenal ulcer, dyspepsia, gastritis, and upper gastrointestinal bleeding due to acid peptic disease; it also is used prophylactically in patients prone to develop stress ulcers or hemorrhagic gastritis. The specificity of antacid effect on ulcer pain and healing remains controversial. Two studies have shown accelerated healing of duodenal ulcer in patients given large doses of nonsystemic antacids for protracted period (9, 20). Despite the advent of H_2-receptor antagonists (cimetidine and ranitidine), antacids remain the most time-tested and safe drugs for effective treatment of acid peptic diseases.

Preparations. Antacid gels (liquid suspensions) are more effective than tablets. Many commonly used preparations contain 400 mg of magnesium and aluminum hydroxide in a 10 ml dose. This volume of such a product will neutralize 20-25 mEq hydrogen ion. For protracted neutralization in most subjects, 30 ml doses given at 1 and 3 hours after meals and at bedtime will suffice. Because antacids are taken for long periods in these large doses, factors other than neutralizing capacity must also be considered. These include taste, cost, and sodium content.

ANTISPASMODICS

The anispasmodic agents are anticholinergic drugs that inhibit the effects of acetylcholine released from postganglionic parasympathetic nerve endings (8). They block muscarinic actions of acetylcholine including smooth muscle contraction and exocrine gland secretion. Atropine is the prototype of this class of drugs that inhibits gastrointestinal motility.

Chemistry. The naturally occurring antispasmodic alkaloids are tertiary amines that are absorbed readily from the gastrointestinal tract, cross the blood brain barrier, and stimulate the medulla and cerebral cortex. The synthetic antimuscarinic drugs are cationic quaternary amines that are absorbed poorly from the intestine and do not readily cross into the brain.

Pharmacological Effects. In the gastrointestinal tract, the anticholinergics inhibit smooth muscle contraction and delay gastric emptying (12). When given in large doses, they inhibit gastric acid and pepsin secretion (21). Small intestinal and colonic motility is depressed accounting for their antispasmodic properties. Even when given at maximal doses (which invariably produce undesirable side effects), the anticholinergic drugs only suppress gastric acid output by 35-40%. In contrast, cimetidine inhibits acid by well over 60%, causes few side effects, but is less effective in reducing pepsin secretion.

Pharmacokinetics. Atropine is a tertiary amine that is well absorbed following oral administration with peak levels reached in 1 hour. Volume of distribution is 2-4 l / kg, and 50% is protein bound. Atropine is metabolized in the liver by N-demethylation and glucuronidation with 30-50% excreted in the urine. Its elimination half-life is 13-38 hours. Quaternary ammonium anticholinergic agents such as propantheline are slowly and poorly absorbed, with only 10% of an oral dose of this drug

Table 18.1-1
Antacid Drug Interactions Reported in Humans

Drug	Antacid	Change in Drug Level or Effect	Proposed Mechanism
Antimicrobials			
Isoniazid	$Al(OH)_3$	Depressed	Delayed gastric emptying
Sulfonamides	$NaHCO_3$, $Mg(OH)_2$	Enhanced	Increased dissolution
Tetracycline	$NaHCO_3$, $Mg(OH)_2$, $Al(OH)_3$, $CaCO_3$	Depressed	Poor dissolution, chelation
Cardiovascular			
Dicumarol	$Mg(OH)_2$	Enhanced	Faster Absorption of chelate
Digoxin	$Al(OH)_3$, $Mg(OH)_2$, $Mg(SiO_4)_3$	Depressed	?
Quinidine	Mg-Al-OH[a]	Enhanced	Decreased excretion in urine
Propranolol	$Al(OH)_3$	Depressed	?
CNS Agents			
Amphetamine	$NaHCO_3$	Enhanced	Decreased excretion in urine
Chlordiaze-poxide	Mg-Al-OH	Depressed	?
Chlorpromazine	Mg-Al-OH	Depressed	Adsorption of drug
Levodopa	Mg-Al-OH	Enhanced	Faster gastric emptying
Phenytoin	Unspecified	Depressed	?
Pseudoephedrine	$Al(OH)_3$	Enhanced	?
Nonsteroid Antiinflammatory			
Aspirin	Mg-Al-OH	Depressed	Increased excretion in urine
Naproxen	$NaHCO_3$	Enhanced	?
Vitamins/Minerals			
Calcium	$CaCO_3$	Enhanced	More calcium from antacid
Iron	$NaHCO_3$, $CaCO_3$	Depressed	Precipitation, poor dissolution
Phosphorus	$Al(OH)_3$	Depressed	Precipitation of calcium phosphate
Vitamin A	$Al(OH)_3$	Depressed	?

[a] Combination antacid containing aluminum and magnesium hydroxides.
Source: Summarized from Ref. 10.

reaching the blood, producing a maximal effect in 3-4 hours. In 24 hours, the fraction that is absorbed is excreted as parent drug or metabolites in the urine.

Adverse Reactions. The numerous undesirable side effects of the antispasmodic drugs are dose-dependent manifestations of their pharmacological actions, including dry mouth and skin, flushing, tachycardia, pupillary dilatation with blurred vision, cerebral excitement and delirium, and difficulty in micturition. The quaternary ammonium compounds may also cause postural hypotension and impotence because of their ganglionic blocking effects.

Drug Interactions. Antimuscarinic drugs delay gastric emptying and slow intestinal motility, thereby interfering with the absorption of rapidly absorbed drugs such as acetaminophen while enhancing the gastrointestinal uptake of slowly absorbed drugs like digoxin. Other drugs with anticholinergic properties, including antihistamines and tricyclic antidepressants, may have additive pharmacological effects with the antispasmodics, manifested as additive toxicity.

Therapeutic Uses. The anticholinergic drugs have been widely used in the treatment of peptic ulcer disease and irritable bowel and functional disorders, including diarrhea. The use in peptic ulcer disease should be limited to patients with persistent nocturnal pain who do not respond to antacids and H_2 antagonists given alone (13). Pirenzepine is an antimuscarinic agent with greater affinity for gastric receptors (5). It has been reported to accelerate ulcer healing while causing fewer antimuscarinic side effects. In treating irritable bowel syndrome, these drugs appear to be of greater benefit when abdominal pain is the predominant problem (14). The main contraindications to anticholinergic drug use are narrow-angle glaucoma, pyloric outlet obstruction, reflux esophagitis (because relaxation of the lower esophageal sphincter worsens acid regurgitation), and prostatic hypertrophy.

Preparations. Table 18.1-2 provides a list of some of the commonly used anticholinergic drugs, including trade names and dosages. Frequently, a maximal dose must be given to be effective. When given with cimetidine, the acid-suppressing effect of these drugs is additive at submaximal dosage. Anticholinergics may be used in combination with antacids.

HISTAMINE H_2-RECEPTOR ANTAGONISTS

Histamine H_2-receptors (1) which are involved in gastric acid and pepsin secretion, can be blocked by drugs like cimetidine or ranitidine which are the only currently available H_2-blocking agents used in the management of peptic ulcer. These drugs are discussed in detail in Chapter 13.4.

CIMETIDINE

Cimetidine is effective in the treatment of patients with duodenal ulcer, benign gastric ulcer, and hypersecretion states, as in Zollinger-Ellison syndrome. The drug is effective in reducing pain and promoting healing of peptic ulcer. It suppresses gastric acid secretion by blocking the interaction of histamine with the H_2 receptors of the parietal cells (6).

Cimetidine inhibits diurnal and nocturnal gastric acid secretion in basal state and after stimulation induced by various substances. Both gastric acid volume and hydrogen ion concentration are reduced by cimetidine. The drug also inhibits intrinsic factor secretion and reduces the amount of pepsin by lowering gastric fluid output. A single 300-mg dose of cimetidine inhibits meal-stimulated gastric acid secretion by 70% over a 3-hour period. The inhibitory effect exceeds that of anticholinergic drugs, which only reduce acid secretion by 25-30% when given at maximally tolerated doses. Cimetidine has no antimuscarinic effects and thus does not delay gastric emptying. Cimetidine may be given with antacids because neither drug reduces the effectiveness of the other.

Its minor side effects include headache, dizziness, fatigue, diarrhea, skin rash, and muscular pain. Gynecomastia and reduced sperm count may be caused by the weak antiandrogenic effects of cimetidine. The most serious problem is a rebound phenomenon of ulcer recurrence on cessation of therapy. Another problem is suppression of symptoms of malignant ulcer, causing a delay in making the proper diagnosis and instituting appropriate treatment.

RANITIDINE

A new histamine H_2-receptor antagonist, ranitidine (ZANTAC) is four- to eight-fold potent compared with cimetidine in reducing gastric acid secretion (2, 4, 16) (see Chapter 13.4). It has been approved for oral use in treatment of duodenal ulcer. In efficiency, ranitidine is comparable with cimetidine in healing ulcers and relieving pain. Because of its high potency, it is given in a lower dose (150 mg twice daily). It appears to have a lower incidence of toxicity and drug interactions.

SUBSTITUTED BENZIMIDAZOLES

OMEPRAZOLE

Omeprazole is a substituted benzimidazole which inhibits gastric acid secretion. It inhibits hydrogen-potassium-adenosine triphosphatase (ATPase), an enzyme located in the gastric parietal cell and involved in

Table 18.1-2
Anticholinergic Drugs in the Treatment of Peptic Ulcer

Generic Name	Trade Name	Dosage Unit	Usual Daily Dose
Tertiary Ammonium Compounds			
Atropine sulfate		0.4 mg	0.4-3 mg
Tincture of belladonna		0.03% solution (10 drops)	16-60 drops
Belladonna extract		15 mg	15-60 mg
Scopolamine (hyoscine)		0.4, 0.6 mg	0.4 -3 mg
Oxyphencyclimine	DARICON	5 mg	10-20 mg
Dicyclomine HCL	BENTYL	10 mg	30-60 mg
Belladonna + phenobarbital	DONNATAL	15 mg	45-90 mg
Quaternary Ammonium Compounds			
Glycopyrrolate	ROBINUL	1, 2 mg	2-8 mg
Poldine methosulfate	NACTON	4 mg	24-32 mg
Propantheline bromide	PRO-BANTHINE	7.5, 15 mg	15-60 mg
Hyoscine n-butyl bromide	BUSCOPAN	20 mg	80-120 mg
Mepenzolate bromide	CANTIL	25 mg	150-300 mg

Source: Adapted from Ref. 8.

acid formation. Omeprazole has been used to heal peptic ulcers in patients with Zollinger-Ellison syndrome who were refractory to other drugs (15).

AGENTS THAT ENHANCE MUCOSAL PROTECTION

CARBENOXOLONE

Carbenoxolone prolongs the life span of gastric epithelial cells and stimulates mucus secretion. It does not exert any effect on acid secretion, but it inhibits the action of pepsin. Carbenoxolone and the timed-release preparaation DUOGASTRONE accelerate the healing rate of gastric and duodenal ulcer and approximately 70-75% of ulcers are healed after treatment of 4 to 12 weeks.

Due to its aldosteronelike properties, carbenoxolone may induce sodium and water retention and hypokalemia.

COLLOIDAL BISMUTH PREPARATION

These preparations chelate the proteins of the ulcer base and form a protective coating against the activity of acid, pepsin, and bile. They enhance the healing rate of both gastric and duodenal ulcer and may be as effective as cimetidine.

SUCRALFATE

Sucralfate is a complex of sucrose octasulfate with aluminum hydroxide $[Al_2(OH)_5]^+$. Chemically, it is β-D-fructofuranosyl-β-D-glucopyranoside octakis (hydrogen sulfate) aluminum hydroxide complex with the following formula:

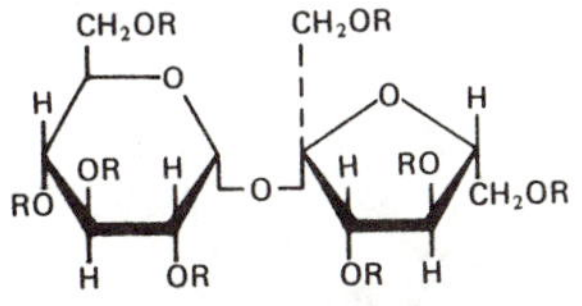

$R = SO_3[Al_2(OH)_5] \cdot 16H_2O$

Sucralfate

In the acidic environment of the stomach, some $[Al_2(OH)_5]^+$ ions dissociate from the parent compound. Subsequent polymerization of sucrose octasulfate molecules results in formation of a viscous and thick substance that is the active form of the drug.

Pharmacology. Sucralfate has been reported to act primarily by forming a protective cover over the ulcer crater and thereby shields the necrotic ulcer tissue from pepsin and probably gastric acid (19). The drug has a minimal acid-neutralizing property and reduces peptic activity in the lumen and at the ulcer site, but it does not reduce gastric acid secretion. At the necrotic ulcer sites, the drug is believed to attach to albumin, fibrinogen, damaged mucosal cells, and dead leukocytes. Other physicochemical properties may be involved in the process of adhesion of the active moiety of the drug to the ulcer base (22). The drug also adsorbs bile acids *in vitro*, but the exact role of this action *in vivo* has not been established. Less than 5% of the drug is absorbed from the gastrointestinal tract.

Side Effects. Less than 5% of patients treated with sucralfate were reported to manifest side effects. The most common side effect is constipation. Other infrequent side effects of the drug include diarrhea, nausea, dryness of mouth, skin rash, dizziness, vertigo, and sleepiness. Aluminum toxicity may be a potential problem in patients with renal insufficiency.

Drug Interactions. Sucralfate has been reported to reduce bioavailability of phenytoin by about 38% and interferes with the intestinal absorption of tetracycline when the two drugs are administered concurrently (22).

Therapeutic Uses. Several studies have demonstrated that sucralfate is superior to placebo and comparable with either cimetidine or antacid regimen in healing active duodenal ulcer (22). The drug is generally recommended at a dose of 1 g four times a day (30-60 minutes before meals) for 4-8 weeks. There is some evidence that sucralfate may be effective in the prevention of recurrent duodenal ulcer (18). The efficacy of the drug in the treatment of gastric ulcer has not been clearly determined. Furthermore, its efficacy has not been adequately tested in gastritis, bleeding ulcers, postoperative recurrent ulcers, and reflex esophagitis.

Preparations. Sucralfate (CARAFATE) is available as 1 g tablets.

PROSTAGLANDINS (PGs)

Prostaglandins of the group E_1 and E_2 inhibit gastric secretion in response to various stimuli such as histamine, pentagastrin, and food. In addition, prostaglandins exert a cytoprotective effect on gastric mucosa. The inhibition of gastric acid by PGs is related to a direct effect on the parietal cell that reduces the secretory response. This inhibitory effect is mediated by a systemic and local mechanism. Orally administered prostaglandins such as 16,16-dimethyl prostaglandin E_2 (16,16 DMPGE$_2$) have been shown to promote gastric ulcer healing. This group of agents demonstrates significant therapeutic potential for the treatment of peptic ulcer disease in the future.

REFERENCES

1. Black, J.W., Duncan, W.A.M., Durant, G.J. et al. Definition and antagonism of histamine H_2-receptors. *Nature* 236:385, 1972.
2. Brogden, R.N., Carmine, A.A., Heel, R.C. et al. Ranitidine: A review of its pharmacology and therapeutic use in peptic ulcer disease and other allied diseases. *Drugs* 24:267, 1982.

3. Brogden, R.N., Heel, R.C, Speight, T.M. and Avery G.S. Sucralfate: A review of its pharmacodynamic properties and therapeutic use in peptic ulcer disease. *Drugs* 27: 194, 1984.
4. Editorial. Cimetidine and ranitidine. *Lancet* 1:601, 1982.
5. Feldman, M. Inhibition of gastric acid secretion by selective and nonselective anticholinergics. *Gastroenterology* 86:361, 1984.
6. Finkelstein, W. and Isselbacher, K.J. Cimetidine. *N. Engl. J. Med.* 299:992, 1978.
7. Greenberger, N.J., Arvanitakis, C. and Hurwitz, A. Antacids and gastric antisecretory drugs. In: *Drug Treatment of Gastrointestinal Disorders* (Greenberger, N.J. et al. eds.) by Azarnoff, D. Edinburgh: Churchill-Livingston, 1978, p.1.
8. Greenblatt, D.J. and Shader, R.I. Anticholinergics. *N. Engl. J. Med.* 288:1215, 1973.
9. Hollander, D. and Harlan, J. Antacids vs. placebo in peptic ulcer therapy: Controlled double-blind investigation. *JAMA* 226:1181, 1973.
10. Hurwitz, A. Antacid therapy and drug kinetics. *Clin. Pharmacokinet.* 2:269, 1977.
11. Hurwitz, A., Robinson, R.G., Vats, T.S. et al. Effects of antacids on gastric emptying. *Gastroenterology* 71:268, 1976.
12. Hurwitz, A., Robinson, R.G. and Herrin, W.F. Prolongation of gastric emptying by oral propantheline. *Clin. Pharmacol. Ther.* 22:206, 1977.
13. Ivey, K.J. Anticholinergics: Do they work in peptic ulcer? *Gastroenterology* 68:154, 1975.
14. Ivey, K.J. Are anticholinergics of use in the irritable colon syndrome? *Gastroenterology* 68:1300, 1975.
15. Lamers, C.B.H.W., Lind, T., Moberg, S. et al. Omeprazole in Zollinger-Ellison syndrome: Effects of a single dose and of long-term treatment in patients resistant to histamine H_2-receptor antagonists. *N. Engl. J. Med.* 310: 758, 1984.
16. McCarthy, D.M. Ranitidine or cimetidine. *Ann. Intern. Med.* 99:551, 1983.
17. Morrissey, J.F. and Barreras, R.F. Antacid therapy. *N. Engl. J.* 1290:550, 1974.
18. Mosha, M.G., Spitaels, J.M and Khan, F. Short- and Long-term studies of duodenal ulcer with sucralfate. *J. Clin. Gastroenterol.* 3 (Suppl. 2):159, 1981.
19. Nagashima, R. Development and characteristics of sucralfate. *J. Clin. Gastroenterol.* 3 (Suppl. 2):103, 1981.
20. Peterson, W.L., Sturdevant, R.A.L., Frankel, H.D. et al. Healing of duodenal ulcer with an antacid regimen. *N. Engl. J. Med.* 297:341, 1977.
21. Piper, D.W. Antacid and anticholinergic drug therapy. In: *Peptic Ulceration Clinical Gastroenterology* (Sircus, W., guest ed.) Vol. 2, Philadelphia: Saunders, 1973, p. 2.
22. Richardson, C.T. Sucralfate. *Ann. Intern. Med.* 97:269, 1982.

ADDITIONAL READING

Carmine, A.A. and Brogden, R.N. Pirenzepine. A review of its pharmacodynamic and pharmacokinetic properties and therapeutic efficacy in peptic ulcer disease and other allied diseases. *Drugs* 30:85, 1985.

CHAPTER
18.2

LAXATIVES AND CATHARTICS

Mark McPhee, Aryeh Hurwitz and Constantine Arvanitakis

Laxatives, cathartics, purgatives, and stool softeners are administered to decrease stool consistency and to increase the frequency of defecation. Although traditionally these agents have been classified according to presumed mechanisms of action, little is really known about how and precisely where in the gut this laxative action takes place. Recent studies have served to confirm the fact that chemically diverse laxatives share, as a common pharmacological property, the ability to produce an increase in fecal water excretion. A working classification of the laxatives, based upon traditional categories of irritant-stimulants, osmotic cathartics, bulk-forming agents, and lubricants, will serve as a framework for this presentation. More satisfactory classification will become available only when mechanisms of action for these agents are more fully understood. A net increase in fecal water excretion may result from any combination of the following mechanisms.

Active Electrolyte Secretion. The major mechanism for active electrolyte secretion by the bowel is thought to be through stimulation of adenylate cyclase, resulting in increased intracellular concentrations of cyclic adenosine monophosphate (cAMP). Other potential intracellular mediators of active electrolyte secretion include stimulation of the guanylate cyclase-cyclic guanosine monophosphate (cGMP) system, or production of a rise in intracellular calcium concentration.

Decreased Absorption of Water and Electrolytes. Inhibition of sodium-potassium adenosine triphosphatase (Na-K-ATPase) activity with decreased capacity of the active intestinal sodium pump has been shown to result in net intestinal secretion of water and electrolytes.

Increased Intraluminal Osmolarity. An increase in intraluminal gut osmolarity may result in passive water secretion into the lumen along a concentration gradient. Increased osmotic load in the distal bowel may result from a variety of factors including malabsorption of nutrients, increased ingestion of poorly absorbed hyperosmotic substances, bacterial alteration of gut contents, or release of presumptive humoral agents.

Increased Motor Activity. Changes in gut motility may affect intestinal transport by decreasing contact time for mucosal absorption or by indirect alteration of tissue hydrostatic pressure or blood flow. Increasing coordinated and intestinal motor activity may lead to decreased transit time for gut contents. This decreases absorption, resulting in a net increase in fecal water excretion.

Increased Tissue Hydrostatic Pressure. Absorptive permeability may be altered by hydrostatic pressure within the bowel wall. A net secretion of water can result from the presence of increased tissue hydrostatic pressure as a driving force for increased water loss.

Mucosal Damage. Direct histological effects in intestinal mucosal damage can decrease the functional surface area available for active electrolyte and water absorption. Toxic enterocyte injury may also potentiate active gut electrolyte secretion, increased intraluminal osmolarity, and changes in hydrostatic pressure or motor activity.

CONTACT OR IRRITANT-STIMULANT CATHARTICS

ANTHRAQUINONES (Cascara, Senna, Aloe, Rhubarb, Danthron)

Chemistry. Anthraquinones are derived from boiling or aging of plant sources. These agents generally consist of 1,8-dihydroxyanthraquinones linked to glycoside residues. The drugs are stable in the acid milieu of the stomach and in the small bowel. Hydrolysis is accomplished by colonic flora, yielding biologically active aglycones or anthrones, plus glucose. Danthron (1,8-dihydroxyanthraquinone) is administered as a free anthraquinone rather than as a glycoside conjugate.

Pharmacological Effects. As a class, the anthraquinones inhibit Na-K-ATPase activity, resulting in decreased gut absorption of sodium and water. Colonic peristaltic activity is stimulated via a local effect on Auerbach's plexus. Small intestinal motility may also be accelerated and glucose absorption may be decreased. Other possible mechanisms have not been systematically studied. Oral administration of an anthraquinone laxative usually results in passage of a soft or semifluid stool 6 to 8 hours after ingestion. Considerable variability of effects exists among the various preparations.

Pharmacokinetics. Anthraquinone laxatives are most effective when given orally. The free anthraquinones are largely excreted in the feces, although some intestinal absorption does occur, and excretion in urine and breast milk may be demonstrated.

Adverse Effects. As with most laxatives, major toxic effects of the anthraquinones may result from excessive pharmacological action: diarrhea with loss of water and electrolytes in the stool, malabsorption of nutrients, and colicky abdominal pain. The use of aloe has largely been abandoned because of its propensity to produce severe abdominal cramping and (in excessive doses) nephritis. Chronic abuse of anthraquinones may lead to colonic motility disturbances (i.e., cathartic colon) and to a characteristic dark pigmentation of the colorectal mucosa (melanosis coli) that may be detected on sigmoidoscopic examination. The chemical nature of the pigmentation is in dispute, but it most probably consists of lipofuscin contained in mucosal macrophages. Melanosis may disappear within a period of 4 to 12 months following discontinuation of anthraquinone laxatives, but, when present, it is considered diagnostic of purgative abuse.

Drug Interactions. The effects of excess purgation, such as hypokalemia and extracellular volume depletion, may potentiate the toxicity of digitalis glycosides. Anthraquinones may decrease absorption of fat-soluble vitamins and synthesis of vitamin K, thus potentiating the effect of coumarin anticoagulants.

Preparations. A wide variety of proprietary and nonproprietary formulations are available for the anthraquinones. Aromatic cascara fluidextract is given as a 5-ml customary dose in adults; cascara extract (a powder) has a 300-mg recommended dose. Danthron is available in 75-mg tablets, with a usual adult dose of 75-150 mg. Senna may be given as a powder, fluidextract, or syrup, and is present in many proprietary preparations.

DIPHENYLMETHANES (Phenolphthalein, Bisacodyl, Oxyphenisatin)

Chemistry. The diphenylmethanes were developed as clinical cathartics on the basis of structural similarity to the parent compound, phenolphthalein. This product, a basic ingredient in many widely used proprietary laxatives and nostrums, is a diphenolic substitution of methane. Bisacodyl or 4,4'-(2-pyridylmethylene) diphenol acetate has the advantage of availability for rectal as well as oral administration. Oxyphenisatin acetate use has virtually been abandoned because of its propensity to cause jaundice and chronic hepatitis, especially when given with dioctyl sodium sulfosuccinate.

Pharmacological Effects. The diphenylmethanes decrease absorption of water and electrolytes by inhibiting Na-K-ATPase. Intestinal glucose absorption is also inhibited. Phenolphthalein may induce active electrolyte secretion, and bisacodyl has been shown to produce histological damage in the ileum and colon. As a class, the diphenylmethanes stimulate colonic motility. Oral administration usually results in one or two soft, formed stools 6 to 12 hours following ingestion. Rectally administered bisacodyl usually acts within 15 to 60 minutes.

Pharmacokinetics. Phenolphthalein is excreted largely unchanged in the feces, although 10-15% of an ingested dose is absorbed, conjugated, and excreted in the urine. A small fraction of the drug may be excreted in the urine in unconjugated form, and some of the absorbed dose is excreted into bile. The resulting enterohepatic circulation of phenolphthalein may prolong its cathartic effect. At alkaline pH, phenolphthalein-containing feces and urine may show a characteristic red discoloration that disappears upon acidification. This property may be used as a simple bedside diagnostic test to determine the presence of surreptitious phenolphthalein ingestion.

Approximately 5% of an administered dose of bisacodyl is absorbed, and some is excreted in the urine in glucuronide form. Biliary excretion and enterohepatic circulation do occur with a portion of the dose after deacetylation, intestinal absorption, and glucuronide conjugation. The remainder of an orally administered dose is excreted unchanged in the stool.

Adverse Effects. Major toxic effects of diphenylmethanes are similar to those of the anthraquinones (i.e., excess laxation producing fluid and electrolyte loss, malabsorption of nutrients, and chronic colonic motility disturbances). Phenolphthalein administration may cause allergic skin reactions such as dermatitis, fixed-drug eruption, Stevens-Johnson syndrome, or a systemic lupus erythematosus-like lesion with possible hematological side effects. Affected individuals should avoid further exposure to phenolphthalein.

Bisacodyl is administered in enteric-coated tablets that should not be chewed, as the drug is irritating to oropharyngeal and gastric mucosa. When given in suppository form, bisacodyl may cause a proctitis evident on proctosigmoidoscopy. Histological changes on rectal biopsy may include sloughing of epithelial cells and abnormal crypt architecture. A burning sensation in the rectum may be noted by the patient.

Preparations. Phenolphthalein is usually administered in oral tablet or capsule form containing between 60 and 100 mg of drug for adults. It is also available in a wide variety of proprietary preparations including gum and candy formulations. Bisacodyl is available as 5-mg enteric-coated tablets and as 10-mg rectal suppositories. The usual adult dose is 10 to 15 mg orally or 10 mg rectally.

HYDROXY FATTY ACIDS (Castor Oil)

Chemistry. The major example of this laxative class, castor oil, is obtained from the seeds of the plant *Ricinus communis* and is composed primarily (90%) of ricinoleic acid (12-hydroxy-9 octadecanoic acid) triglyceride.

Pharmacological Effects. Ricinoleic acid stimulates active electrolyte secretion by the small bowel, decreases glucose absorption, and alters intestinal permeability. Its effect on the intestinal adenylate cyclase-cAMP system is unclear. Small bowel motility is stimulated, and histological damage to the intestinal surface epithelial cells occurs. Caster oil acts rapidly following oral administration, producing copious, watery, semifluid stools 2 to 6 hours following ingestion.

Pharmacokinetics. The triglycerides in castor oil are hydrolyzed in the intestinal lumen by lipases to form glycerol plus free ricinoleic acid. At low doses (less than 4 g), nearly all of the free ricinoleic acid is absorbed in the small intestine and metabolized as a fatty acid. When the dose of castor oil is increased to the effective cathartic range, however, most of the drug is excreted unchanged or as ricinoleic acid in the feces.

Adverse Effects. Castor oil, by acting primarily on small intestinal function, may cause relatively severe abdominal cramping. Excessive purgation with electrolyte abnormalities, extracellular volume depletion, and dehydration is common—especially in children or elderly patients. Because of its rapid onset of action, the drug should probably not be administered at bedtime.

Preparations. Castor oil is usually administered orally as a flavored emulsion. The customary dose in adults may vary from 15 to 60 ml.

SURFACTANTS (Dioctyl Sodium and Calcium Sulfosuccinate)

Chemistry. Traditionally classified as stool softeners, the surfactants are surface-active emollient laxatives based upon salts of the anionic detergent dioctyl sulfosuccinate (DSS, docusate).

Pharmacological Effects. DSS stimulates active intestinal electrolyte secretion and increases mucosal cAMP content. Mild-to-moderate histological changes are produced. Alterations of intestinal motility or permeability by DSS are inconclusive in terms of clinical effect. Oral administration of the surfactants produces modest softening of solid stool following a delay of 12 to 72 hours.

Pharmacokinetics. DSS is primarily excreted unchanged in the feces. A fraction of an oral dose is absorbed, with significant concentrations found in the bile.

Adverse Effects. DSS is well tolerated in recommended doses. Massive oral doses have produced anorexia, vomiting, and diarrhea in animals, and DSS has been shown to be toxic to liver cells in tissue culture.

Drug Interactions. Surfactants may enhance absorption of mineral oil, so combined administration of these agents is contraindicated, DSS has been shown to potentiate the hepatotoxic effects of oxyphenisatin.

Preparations. The sodium salt of DSS is available in a variety of formulations including tablets, capsules, solutions, and syrups. The usual oral adult dose is 50 to 400 mg daily. Dioctyl calcium sulfosuccinate is available as 50- or 240-mg capsules, with a recommended adult dosage of 240 mg/day.

OTHER IRRITANT-STIMULANT CATHARTICS

Bile Salts. Bile salts, although not usually considered among the clinically useful laxatives, may have a major cathartic effect when administered orally in significant doses. Dihydroxy bile salts and unconjugated bile acids have been shown to stimulate adenylate cyclase and to induce active intestinal electrolyte secretion, presumably by increasing mucosal cAMP content. Bile salts may also alter intestinal permeability, increase motility, and produce histological epithelial damage.

Cathartic Resins. Cathartic resins such as jalap, colocynth, and podophyllum act primarily on the small intestine to stimulate motility and to decrease intestinal water and electrolyte absorption. These agents are quite irritating and may produce severe abdominal cramping and profuse, watery diarrhea, hypokalemia, dehydration, and prostration. Clinical use of cathartic plant resins should be avoided.

Calomel. Calomel (mercurous chloride) once enjoyed widespread use as a contact cathartic. Mercuric ions inhibit intestinal absorption of water and electrolytes; however, appreciable absorption of mercury may occur, and accumulation of tissue mercury can cause severe toxicity. Calomel has no valid use in modern therapeutics.

OSMOTIC CATHARTICS

SALINE CATHARTICS (Salts of Magnesium, Sulfate, or Phosphate)

Chemistry. The saline cathartics are inorganic compounds containing the cation magnesium or the anions sulfate or phosphate in combination with appropriate counterions. Magnesium salts used as laxatives include sulfate (Epsom salt), hydroxide (milk of magnesia), oxide, carbonate, and citrate. Other saline cathartics in common use are sodium phosphate, sodium sulfate (Glauber's salt), potassium sodium tartrate (Rochelle salt), potassium phosphate, and a combination of sodium phosphate plus sodium biphosphate (Fleet's phosphosoda).

Pharmacological Effects. Saline cathartics increase motility in both the small and large intestine. Altered intestinal permeability does occur. The production of increased intraluminal osmolarity is assumed as a primary mechanism for the laxative effect of the saline cathartics, but this has not been conclusively demonstrated. In fact, the amount of water eliminated in the stool following saline catharsis exceeds the amount required to render the ingested salt isotonic. Furthermore, the rapid onset of action of these agents (0.5-3 hours following ingestion) occurs well before the salt could be expected to reach the colon in appreciable concentrations. Recently, it has been postulated that magnesium salts may act through stimulation of endogenous cholecystokinin release, causing contraction of the gallbladder, increased pancreatic secretion, and altered intestinal water and electrolyte transport. This mechanism is in doubt, however, since other stimuli known to produce endogenous release of cholecystokinin do not cause diarrhea.

Pharmacokinetics. Saline cathartics are poorly absorbed in the intestine and are excreted for the most part unchanged in the feces. Approximately 5 to 20% of an administered dose of magnesium is absorbed through the gastrointestinal mucosa and eliminated in the urine. Phosphate and sulfate anions, as well as their corresponding cations, may also be absorbed to some degree. In the presence of normally functioning kidneys, the absorbed portion of the saline cathartic acts as a saline diuretic, promoting urinary excretion of water plus absorbed ions.

Adverse Effects. In addition to the possible side effects of excessive laxation, intestinal absorption of saline cathartic ions may lead to severe fluid and electrolyte imbalance. Magnesium-containing cathartics should not be given to patients with impaired renal function in whom toxicity with somnolence and coma may result. Sodium-containing cathartics should be used with caution in patients with underlying congestive heart failure, renal insufficiency, or hepatic failure.

Drug Interactions. Magnesium salts should not be used in combination with neomycin therapy because of the possibility of synergistic toxic neural effects.

Preparations. A wide variety of proprietary and nonproprietary saline cathartic preparations is available. For the magnesium salts, usual adult doses are 15 g sulfate, 30 ml hydroxide suspension, 4 g oxide, 8 g carbonate, and 200 ml citrate solution.

NONABSORBABLE SUGARS (Lactulose, Sorbitol, Mannitol)

Chemistry. Cathartics in this class are derivatives of disaccharides or monosaccharides that cannot be hydrolyzed or absorbed in the gut by carbohydrate transport pathways. The prototype compound is the synthetic disaccharide lactulose (1,4-β-galactoside-fructose). Reduction of monosaccharides to their corresponding alcohols yields a group of hexitols (sorbitol from glucose, mannitol from mannose) that resist absorption in the small intestine.

Pharmacological Effects. The nonabsorbable sugars are believed to be cathartic in the small intestine by osmotic effect. In addition, the products of bacterial degradation of lactulose lower colonic pH and increase intraluminal osmolarity even further, enhancing net secretion of water and electrolytes in the stool. Administration of an oral dose of nonabsorbable sugar usually results in passage of a soft, semiformed stool in 4 to 8 hours.

Pharmacokinetics. Nonabsorbable sugars pass through the small intestine intact, but are available for fermentative digestion by colonic bacteria. Fermentation of lactulose in the colon yields acetic and lactic acids plus hydrogen gas.

Adverse Effects. Nonabsorbable sugars are usually well tolerated in recommended doses, but side effects of excess laxative action may occur. Byproducts of colonic fermentation may produce bloating and increased intestinal gas. The presence of nonabsorbable hexitols in "dietetic" candy and other similar preparations may produce an undesired laxative effect. Systemic absorptions of sorbitol has been associated with the development of cataracts.

Preparations. The customary adult dosage for catharsis is 20-30 g of the sugar in suspension three times daily. Dosage is adjusted as necessary to maintain a frequency of two to three soft stools daily.

BULK-FORMING CATHARTICS

DIETARY FIBER (Bran, Psyllium, Carboxymethylcellulose, Agar, Tragacanth, Isphagula)

Chemistry. The bulk-forming cathartics, like the nonabsorbable sugars, compose a group of semisynthetic or naturally occuring plant polymers that do not undergo appreciable intestinal hydrolysis or absorption. Most of these agents consist of one or more subcomponents of substances nutritionally classed as dietary fiber: cellulose, hemicellulose, pectin, lignin, gum, or mucilage. Semisynthetic cellulose derivatives such as methylcellulose or sodium carboxymethylcellulose are glucose polymers. Cereal bran, the inner husk of the wheat kernel, consists primarily of hemicelluloses (polymers of xylose or uronic acids plus hexose and pentose sugars) and smaller quantities of cellulose and lignin (a polymer of substituted phenylpropanes). Psyllium, agar, tragacanth, and isphagula fall into the gum/mucilage class, consisting of polymers or uronic acids and hexose and pentose sugars.

Pharmacological Effects. Bulk-forming laxatives are thought to produce their cathartic effect by adsorption of water, yielding an increase in stool bulk and weight, softening of the stool, and changes in both colonic motility and intraluminal pressure. Subcomponents available for partial digestion by colonic flora have effects similar to those described for the nonabsorbable sugars (i.e., osmotic catharsis, flatus production, and lowering of stool pH). As a class, the bulk-forming laxatives increase net fecal water excretion and decrease intestinal transit time. Administration of recommended doses of one of the bulk-forming cathartics usually produces one or more soft, formed stools 8 to 24 hours following ingestion.

Pharmacokinetics. Bulk-forming dietary fiber components pass through the small bowel virtually unchanged. Some fiber subcomponents are available for fermentative digestion by colonic flora. Byproducts of bacterial action on dietary fiber may include organic acids such as lactic and acetic acids as well as colonic gas.

Adverse Effects. Bulk-forming cathartics are usually well tolerated. Abdominal cramping and intestinal gas production may be prominent with bran, and may persist for 2 to 8 weeks following initiation of therapy. Dietary fiber treatment should be avoided in patients with acute abdominal pain, active diverticulitis, dysphagia, or intestinal obstructive symptoms because of the possibility of mechanical obstruction of the GI tract. Generous amounts of oral fluid should accompany the administration of these agents. Bulk-forming cathartics may worsen symptoms in patients with inflammatory bowel disease or enteric fistulas. Decreased glucose absorption has been reported both in normal controls and in patients with diabetes mellitus on high-fiber diets. Dietary fiber treatment has also been shown to lower serum levels of zinc, calcium, iron, phosphate, magnesium, bile acids, triglycerides, and folic acid. These effects are of unknown clinical relevance.

Drug Interactions. High-fiber therapy with bran may increase the propensity for hypoglycemic reactions in diabetic patients treated with insulin.

Preparations. Bran is available in unprocessed form and as processed cereal. The customary adult dose for high-fiber bran therapy begins with a half cup of a commercially processed cereal or 15 g of unprocessed bran twice daily, increasing gradually over several days to 1.5 cups of cereal or 1 cup (6 oz) of unprocessed bran twice daily. Psyllium hydrophilic colloid should be administered as 1 tsp (7 g) to 3 tsp (21 g) in water or juice three times daily.

LUBRICANTS

MINERAL OIL

Chemistry. Mineral oil (liquid petrolatum) is a mixture of liquid hydrocarbons extracted and purified from petroleum.

Pharmacological Effects. Mineral oil retards intestinal absorption of water and electrolytes and softens the stool, possibly by reducing surface tension within the gut lumen. Administration of recommended doses of the drug usually results in passage of a soft, formed stool 6 to 8 hours after ingestion.

Pharmacokinetics. After oral administration, the majority of a dose of mineral oil is excreted unchanged in the feces. A small fraction of the dose is absorbed by intestinal mucosa and may be recovered either within intestinal epithelium or in mesenteric lymph nodes, liver, and spleen.

Adverse Effects. Liquid petrolatum is a lipid solvent, and this agent may interfere with intestinal absorption of the fat-soluble vitamins A, D, E, and K. Hypoprothrombinemia may result. Gastric emptying is retarded, and this effect has been associated with nausea and vomiting. Aspiration of mineral oil into the lungs may produce a severe lipoid pneumonia, especially in elderly or debilitated patients. Mineral oil may leak through the anal sphincter, resulting in anal incontinence, pruritus, and delayed healing of postoperative wounds or enteric fistulas. Absorbed mineral oil may elicit a foreign-body reaction in lymph nodes, liver, or spleen. This effect is of uncertain clinical significance.

Drug Interactions. Mineral oil should not be administered in conjunction with surfactant laxatives such as dioctyl sulfosuccinate, since intestinal absorption of the oil may be facilitated. Coumarin anticoagulant effects may be potentiated by mineral oil use. Absorption of a wide variety of drugs may be decreased or retarded by coadministration of mineral oil.

Preparations. Numerous proprietary and nonproprietary preparations of mineral oil are available. The customary adult dose is 15-45 ml taken orally at bedtime on an empty stomach.

THERAPEUTIC USE OF LAXATIVES

Laxatives and cathartics are widely used and abused. Because many of these agents are available without prescription, they are often mistakenly regarded as innocuous. Chronic use of the irritant-stimulant cathartics or the osmotic laxatives may result in serious fluid and electrolyte imbalances as well as long-term colonic motility dysfunction. The latter effect of habitual laxative use has been termed *cathartic colon* and is associated with a clinical syndrome of laxative-dependent chronic constipation. Therefore, as a general rule, chronic or frequent use of the contact cathartics, the saline laxatives, and mineral oil is contraindicated.

Bulk-forming agents as dietary fiber and osmotically active nonabsorbable sugars such as lactulose have not been associated with cathartic colon or with severe inhibition of nutrient absorption. In appropriate patients, bulk-forming laxatives may be effective during long-term use for control of symptoms of constipation, irritable bowel syndrome, or symptomatic diverticulosis of the colon. In fact, they may protect against the formation of colonic diverticula. Bulk laxatives are also useful in achieving stool softening in patients who should not strain during defecation (i.e., during pregnancy, postpartum, or postoperative states, and also in patients with hernia, hemorrhoids, cardiovascular disease, or painful rectoanal conditions). Lactulose administration is indicated in patients with acute or chronic portal-systemic encephalopathy.

Contact and saline cathartics should usually be reserved for situations requiring rapid, thorough evacuation of the intestinal tract (i.e., in preparation for surgery, radiological, or endoscopic procedures). These agents may also be used in patients with portal-systemic encephalopathy, for elimination of intestinal parasites following antihelminthic therapy, and in the management of some patients with drug or food poisoning. Occasionally, surfactant laxatives may be needed for more prolonged use in patients requiring stool softening. Long-term administration of mineral oil should be avoided in this situation. *It should be considered axiomatic that laxative administration is contraindicated in patients with undiagnosed acute abdominal pain or intestinal obstructive symptoms.*

GENERAL REFERENCES

Binder, H.J. Pharmacology of laxatives. *Ann. Rev. Pharmacol. Toxicol.* 17:355, 1977.

Binder, H.J. and Donowitz, M. A new look at laxative action. *Gastroenterology.* 69:1001, 1977.

Donowitz, M. Current concepts of laxative action: Mechanisms by which laxatives increase stool water. *J. Clin. Gastroenterol* . 1:77, 1979.

Fingl, E. and Freston, J.W. Antidiarrheal agents and laxatives. *J. Clin. Gastroenterol.* 8:161, 1979.

Greenberger, N.J., Arvanitakis, C. and Hurwitz, A. Laxatives. In: *Drug Treatment of Gastrointestinal Disorders* (Azarnoff, D. ed.). New York: Churchill-Livingstone, 1979, p. 42.

Klien, H. Constipation and fecal impaction. *Med. Clin. North Am.* 66:1135, 1982.

McPhee, M.S. Dietary fiber and intestinal disorders. In: *Harrison's Principles of Internal Medicine, Update II* (Isselbacher et al, eds.). New York: McGraw-Hill, 1982, p. 25.

CHAPTER
18.3

EMETIC AND ANTIEMETIC AGENTS

Herbert L. Borison and Lawrence E. McCarthy

MECHANISM OF VOMITING

Respiratory Mechanics of Retching and Expulsion. The forces that lift the upper gastrointestinal contents through the mouth in vomiting (or *emesis*) are generated by the somatic muscles of the thorax and abdomen (7). During the retching phase, repeated growing negative pressure pulses in the thorax coincide with positive pressure pulses in the abdomen to move the gastric contents by surges into the esophagus. This is followed in the expulsion phase by a sudden upward movement of the diaphragm that causes the intrathoracic pressure to turn positive even while the intercostal muscles remain in the inspiratory position. The result is delivery of vomitus through the open mouth with a force that may exceed the arterial blood pressure.

Neural Control of the Vomiting Act. Vomiting is controlled by a reflex coordinating center—the *vomiting center*—situated strategically in the reticular formation of the medulla oblongata where it is surrounded by neural centers for salivation, swallowing, retching, and other participating functions. Input and output connections of the vomiting center are illustrated schematically in Fig. 18.3-1. A novel departure from traditional thinking was made when it was shown that certain chemical agents (e.g., apomorphine) that were supposed to excite the vomiting center act instead upon the nearby chemoreceptor trigger zone (CTZ) (2). Thus, the vomiting center is not itself chemosensitive but it responds to excitatory neural inputs from specialized chemoreceptors wherever they are located, as for example in the nodose ganglion of the vagus nerve (activated by veratrum alkaloids). The CTZ is embodied in the area postrema of the fourth ventricle that is perfused simultaneously by blood and the cerebrospinal fluid.

Vomiting can still occur after all connections are severed between the forebrain and hindbrain. The perception of nausea and the transmission of certain emetic stimuli to the vomiting center are mediated by the limbic system ("visceral brain") in the cerebrum. Prominent among primary afferent pathways to the hindbrain are those concerned with visceral sensory activation, taste reception, and spatial orientation; in the case of motion sickness, the neural transmission route involves a synaptic link in the cerebellum.

On the output side of the reflex mechanism, vomiting can be executed only through the coordination of somatic and visceral effectors controlled by the vomiting center.

Neurotransmitters in the Vomiting Reflex Circuit. The best-known antiemetics fall into three main classes of receptor-blocking drugs—acting against cholinergic (muscarinic), histaminergic, and dopaminergic agents, respectively (Table 18.3-1). It has been suggested that a combination of antiemetic drugs directed at simultaneous blockade of the three receptor types would be the most effective form of therapy until a suitable multireceptor-blocking drug became available (8). This idea is supported by the observation that neurochemical radioreceptor-binding assays demonstrate high concentrations of one or more of the given receptor types in the vicinity of the chemoreceptor trigger zone, nucleus of the tractus solitarius, and vestibular nuclei (involved in motion sickness). Curiously, none of the corresponding putative transmitter substances has been identified in the primary afferent nerves that initiate emesis. Moreover, the elicitation of vomiting by drugs that activate the implicated receptor types is accomplished at specialized end-organs (e.g., the CTZ), not at synaptic relay points in the cranial nerve nuclei. Thus, a basic distinction must be made between actions of substances at afferent chemosensory elements and at interneuronal receptive elements in any meaningful neurochemical hypothesis for effective antiemetic therapy.

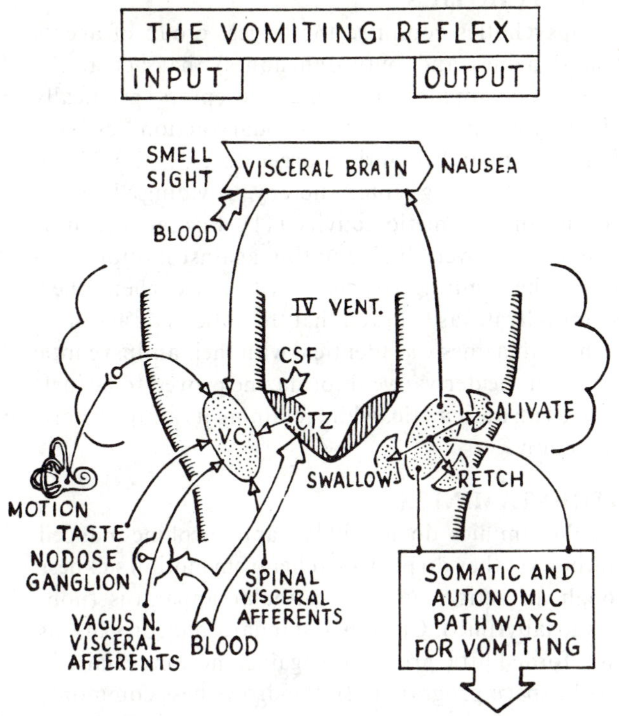

Fig. 18.3-1. *Input and output connections of the vomiting center utilized in the vomiting reflex.*

VC = vomiting center; CTZ = chemoreceptor trigger zone in the area postrema of the fourth ventricle. Chemical stimuli in blood can induce vomiting through the CTZ, nodose ganglion, and visceral brain. The CTZ can also be activated by substances in the cerebrospinal fluid.

Another hypothetical approach to the mechanism of emetic-antiemetic interactions is derived from a suggested role of enkephalin-modulated processes in the mediation of cancer chemotherapy-induced vomiting (5). In this case it is postulated that enkephalins (*endogenous opioids*) activate the CTZ and also inhibit the vomiting center, with the outcome dependent on the balance of the two influences. This balance is said to depend in turn on the relative activities of the enzymes involved in the turnover of the enkephalins at their respective sites of action. The functional relationship of the so-called endogenous opioids to the classic neurotransmitters as mediators of impulse transmission in the central nervous system remains to be elucidated.

EMETIC DRUGS AND OTHER CAUSES OF VOMITING

The use of drugs to evoke emesis has become obsolete except in certain cases of poisoning (4). If the victim is alert, syrup of ipecac may be given orally or apomorphine may be injected subcutaneously. Apomorphine does not depress the vomiting center; its emetic action on the CTZ is not antagonized by naloxone.

Major causes of vomiting are listed in Table 18.3-2. Although drugs are now rarely administered with the intent to produce vomiting, emesis occurs as a widespread unwanted pharmacotherapeutic side effect, especially of agents employed in cancer chemotherapy. Other drug classes with high-emetic potential include digitalis glycosides, ergot alkaloids, veratrum alkaloids, dopamin-

Table 18.3-1
Classification of Antiemetics

Class	Example[a]	Mechanism	Use[b]
Antipsychotic	Chlorpromazine (phenothiazine) Haloperidol (butyrophenone)	Dopamine-receptor blockade in CTZ of medulla and tranquilization	All types of nonphysiological vomiting
Antihistaminic	Dimenhydrinate	Depression of vestibular apparatus	Motion sickness mainly
Anticholinergic	Scopolamine	Unknown	Motion sickness mainly
Narcotic	Morphine	Depression of reticular formation	Not evaluated clinically
Cannabinoid	Δ^9-Tetrahydrocannabinol	Unknown	Vomiting in cancer therapy
Unclassified	Trimethobenzamide Metoclopramide	Dopamine-receptor blockade in CTZ of medulla	All types of nonphysiological vomiting
	Diphenidol	Depression of vestibular apparatus	Labyrinthitis mainly

[a] Example is the prototype but not necessarily best agent in class.
[b] Use may be limited by adverse reactions (see drug descriptions).

ergic-receptor agonists, antibiotics, narcotics, and general anesthetics. The expectation of gastrointestinal upset accompanying drug administration is so common that iatrogenic vomiting is often dismissed as a necessary evil.

It is estimated that 50% of normal women experience morning sickness during the early months of pregnancy. Treatment of this discomfort was responsible for the modern European calamity of birth defects produced by the nonspecific sedative drug, thalidomide (10). Motion sickness is a unique physiological type of emesis that can be severely disabling in ordinary daily pursuits. Remaining causes of vomiting, pathophysiological and toxic, encompass a wide variety of internal disorders and external noxious agents that can utilize single or multiple inputs to the vomiting center.

Table 18.3-2
Major Causes of Vomiting

Type	Examples
Iatrogenic	Treatment of cancer, heart failure, hypertension, parkinsonism, alcoholism, infectious diseases, and metabolic disorders
Physiological	Pregnancy, head motion and weightlessness
Pathophysiological	Uremia, cancer, endocrinopathies, migraine, allergies and inflammations
Toxic	Food poisons, industrial poisons, high-energy radiations, infections

ANTIEMETIC DRUGS

The extreme diversity of emetic-activating processes stands in sharp contrast to the stereotyped motor form of emesis, and helps to explain why none of the available antiemetic agents has been found effective in all situations (Table 18.3-2). The rational approach to antiemetic therapy is selection of an appropriate suppressant to fit the cause. Among drug inducers of vomiting, apomorphine (a dopaminergic-receptor agonist) is most susceptible to antiemetic blockade, whereas digitalis (a Na^+, K^+-ATPase inhibitor) has thus far proved to be invulnerable, even though both of these emetic agents act on the CTZ. Morphine activates still another receptor type in the CTZ, separately blocked by naloxone (3); the opiates also act as emetic suppressants downstream to the CTZ. This dual action accounts for the unpredictable nature of opiate-induced emesis. Naloxone can precipitate vomiting by preferentially antagonizing the antiemetic activity of a previously administered opiate.

ANTIPSYCHOTICS

Antipsychotics comprise the largest group of agents (phenothiazines and butyrophenones) that act at the CTZ to block dopaminergic emetic receptors specifically excited by apomorphine. A secondary action, less specific in nature and requiring larger doses, is thought to depress the vomiting center, thereby providing a broader spectrum of antiemetic activity (11). In practice, these agents have proved disappointing against motion sickness and the vomiting associated with cancer chemotherapy. Initially it was believed that the antiemetic action of the phenothiazines was identical with their antipsychotic action; but the derivative thioridazine proved to be ineffective as an antiemetic, while retaining its antipsychotic class action.

ANTIHISTAMINICS

Antihistaminics do not block apomorphine-induced vomiting, yet they do provide relief from motion sickness through an action on the vestibular apparatus (nonacoustic labyrinth). Curiously standard remedies in this class afforded little protection against motion malaise in the U.S. space program (12); the drowsiness commonly produced by such agents also detracted from their use by astronauts. Promethazine, the phenothiazine derivative with significant antihistaminic activity, was more effective for treating space flight discomfort, especially when combined with d-amphetamine.

ANTICHOLINERGICS

Belladonna alkaloids have long been used to alleviate travel sickness. When combined with d-amphetamine, scopolamine was found to provide best protection among all agents tested against motion discomfort in the space flight laboratory. Atropine was as effective as scopolamine, but the synthetic anticholinergics had little antiemetic potency.

NARCOTICS

The opiates have never become part of the antiemetic armamentarium despite the many indications of their potential usefulness coming from ancient folklore, clinical experience, and the scientific laboratory (6). This situation may be explained in part by the unwarranted identification of narcotic actions with those of apomorphine.

CANNABINOIDS

The pressing need for relief from vomiting in cancer chemotherapy has opened the door for the antiemetic use of marijuana and its derivatives. The cannabinoids can modify antineoplastic-induced vomiting, but at the price of mind distortion (9).

OTHER AGENTS

A number of other drugs that are less well classified are also able to block apomorphine-induced vomiting or to depress vestibular function. Metoclopramide in particular is a newer addition to the antiemetic armamentarium with the additional property of enhancing orthograde movement of the gastrointestinal contents (1). The injectable form of this drug has been approved for use in treating nausea and vomiting induced by cancer chemotherapy with cisplatin, but the drug is not effective in motion sickness (1).

In conclusion, the problem of giving relief from vomiting is as complex as the nature of vomiting itself, which ranges from the trivial to the life-threatening. Unfortunately, no reliable means are yet available to suppress vomiting in most serious circumstances.

REFERENCES

1. Albibi, R. and McCallum, R.W. Metoclopramide: Pharmacology and clinical application. *Ann. Intern. Med.* 98:86, 1983.
2. Borison, H.L. and Wang, S.C. Physiology and pharmacology of vomiting. *Pharmacol. Rev.* 5:193, 1953.
3. Costello, D.J. and Borison, H.L. Naloxone antagonizes self-blockade of emesis in the cat. *J. Pharmacol. Exp. Ther.* 203:222, 1977.
4. Gosselin, R.E., Hodge, H.C., Smith, R.P. and Gleason, M.N. *Clinical Toxicology of Commercial Products*, 5th ed. Williams and Wilkins, Co., Baltimore, 1984.
5. Harris, A.L. Cytotoxic-therapy-induced vomiting is mediated via enkephalin pathways. *Lancet.* 1:714, 1982.
6. Krueger, H., Eddy, N.B. and Sumwalt, M. *The Pharmacology of the Opium Alkaloids.* Public Health Reports (Suppl.) 165, U.S. Government Printing Office, Washington, D.C., 1941.
7. McCarthy, L.E. and Borison, H.L. Respiratory mechanics of vomiting in decerebrate cats. *Am. J. Physiol.* 226:738, 1974.
8. Peroutka, S.J. and Snyder, S.H. Antiemetics: Neurotransmitter receptor binding predicts therapeutic actions. Lancet. 1:658, 1982.
9. Sallan, S.E., Zinberg, N.E. and Frei, E. Antiemetic effect of delta-9-tetrahydrocannabinol in patients receiving cancer chemotherapy. *N. Engl. J. Med.* 293:795, 1975.
10. Taussig, H.B. A study of the German outbreak of phocomelia: The thalidomide syndrome. *JAMA.* 180:1106, 1962.
11. Wang, S.C. Emetic and antiemetic drugs. In: *Physiological Pharmacology* Vol. 2 The Nervous System—Part B (Root, W.S. and Hofmann, F.G., eds). Academic Press, New York, 1965, p. 255.
12. Wood, C.D. and Graybiel, A. Theory of antimotion sickness drug mechanisms. *Aerospace Med.* 43:249, 1972.

ADDITIONAL READINGS

AMA Drug Evaluations, 5th ed. American Medical Association, Chicago, 1983.

CHAPTER
18.4

ANTIDIARRHEAL AGENTS

Harbans Lal

Diarrhea may be defined as increased frequency, fluidity, or volume (weight) of fecal material; it may include the presence of abnormal constituents, such as blood, mucus, or pus, in the bowels. In diarrhea, mean daily fecal weight may increase from the normal 100-150 g to 150-300 g, and the water content of the fecal material may increase from a normal 60 to as much as 90%. Acute diarrhea is characterized by sudden onset of frequent, liquidy stools accompanied by weakness, gas, urgency, pain, and sometimes fever and vomiting. It is almost always caused by an acute intestinal infection. The common microorganisms that are responsible for causing acute secretory diarrheas are *Vibrio cholerae* and enterotoxigenic *Escherichia coli* (ETEC). The latter organisms have been reported as the most common cause of acute secretory diarrheas in small children in developing countries, and in travelers visiting certain parts of the world. Chronic diarrhea is the persistent passage of unformed stools and is generally caused by hormonal and nonhormonal factors.

ETIOLOGY AND PATHOPHYSIOLOGY OF DIARRHEA

Pathophysiologically, diarrhea is an abnormality of fluid secretion and/or absorption, often combined with abnormal bowel motility. Four major mechanisms can produce excess fecal fluid in lumen of the gastrointestinal tract: (a) secretion of solute and water; (b) exudation, (c) osmotic retention of water, and (d) disruption of adequate contact between chyme and the absorptive surface (6).

Secretory diarrhea (5) may result when the mucosa of the small or large intestine secrete abnormally (rather than absorb fluid) due to extra- or intraluminal stimuli. Increased intestinal secretion is the major cause underlying many forms of diarrhea. The secretory diarrheas may be produced by two broad groups of agents, with cholera toxin and the bile acids as prototypes (3). The cholera enterotoxin group has relatively selective effects on the intestinal tract, acting only on the small intestine primarily by activating adenylate cyclase. Other processes are largely unaffected, and mucosal permeability is not increased. This group includes *E. coli* and some other enterotoxins, theophylline and other inhibitors of phosphodiesterase, certain prostaglandins, vasoactive intestinal peptide (VIP) and other gastrointestinal hormones, and acetylcholine. In the Zollinger-Ellison syndrome, hypersecretion of gastric fluid is the major cause of diarrhea. Hypergastrinemia may also directly stimulate bowel secretion.

The bile acid group, which includes ricinoleic acid (the active metabolite of castor oil) and other fatty acids, and other anionic surfactants, has relatively nonselective effects on the intestinal tract and may represent nonspecific effect on cell membrane. They act on the small and large intestines in about the same concentrations and inhibit multiple transport processes. Absorption of sodium, glucose, other nutrients, and water are reduced; mucosal permeability to macromolecules is increased; adenylate cyclase activity is increased; and Na^+,K^+-adenosine triphosphatase (ATPase) activity may be inhibited.

Exudative diarrhea occurs due to the outpouring into the bowel of serum proteins, blood, mucus, or pus from sites of inflammatory, ulcerative, or infiltrative diseases. Such exudation is a factor in intestinal neoplasms, inflammatory bowel disease, bacterial and parasitic invasions (with *Salmonella*, amebae), and antibiotic-induced colitis (superinfection).

Osmotic diarrhea results from an excess of water-soluble molecules retained in the bowel lumen. Certain laxatives and some antacids increase water content in the bowel by providing slowly or incompletely absorbed polyvalent ions of magnesium sulfate and phosphate. Carbohydrate malabsorption also produces diarrhea by osmotic retention of fluid.

A number of metabolic diseases, such as hyperthyroidism, diabetes mellitus, adrenal insufficiency, and hypoparathyroidism, cause diarrhea for reasons that are as yet unclear.

Disruption of adequate contact between chyme and absorptive mucosal surface may cause diarrhea. For a required amount of absorption to take place, intestinal contents must be stirred properly and exposed to an adequate absorbing surface for a sufficient period of time. This is normally accomplished by a delicate balance between circular muscle activity, peristaltic movements, and propulsive reflexes. The well-regulated activity of intestinal wall musculature provides motility and mixing as well as propulsion of chyme. An increase in the transit speed (e.g., intestinal resection or bypass) causes inadequate mixing as well as inadequate contact with absorptive surface. It also alters the homeostatic millieu necessary for proper absorption and secretion. Prolonged transit leads to stasis (*fluid loop syndrome*), causing bacterial growth, malabsorption, and diarrhea. Intestinal motility can be altered abnormally not only by a large number of pathogenic factors but also by changes in hormonal activity, autonomic nerve function, emotional, and psychic factors. Abnormal colon motility provides a practical mechanism underlying diarrhea in many functional bowel diseases where the etiology of diarrhea otherwise remains unknown.

Many *pharmacological agents* are known to cause diarrhea as a side effect. Drug actions likely to result in diarrhea include: alterations in intestinal secretions (laxatives, fatty acids, autonomic drugs, prostaglandins); osmotic disturbances (laxatives, antacids, electrolytes, nutritional factors); disorders of motility (autonomic drugs, laxatives, psychoactive agents, irritants); alterations in bacterial flora (antibiotics, antimetabolites); and mucosal injury (salicylates, colchicine, antibiotics, radiation, antimetabolites, environmental toxicants).

Because of variable etiologies, diarrhea is often treated as a symptom of an undiagnosed and transient GI disorder. When appropriate diagnosis of the underlying disease is not possible in the time available, antidiarrheals are used for symptomatic relief. Following this, additional therapy may be indicated to treat the cause and the effect of the disease.

ANTIDIARRHEAL AGENTS

There is a number of specific antidiarrheal drugs available, as well as more than 100 over-the-counter (OTC) products used for symptomatic relief. The FDA warns that OTC products should not be used for more than 2 days in the presence of high fever, or in infants and children under 3 years of age, unless specifically desired by a physician. The FDA's tentative final monograph on OTC antidiarrheal drug products (1986) has recognized only activated attapulgite and polycarbophil as safe and effective, and not misbranded. The agency has proposed that the available data are insufficient to categorize opiate ingredients (in combination), charcoal, kaolin, pectin, belladonna alkaloids, alumina powder, bismuth salts, calcium carbonate, and sodium carboxymethylcellulose as safe and effective.

Following are the most frequently employed antidiarrheal agents.

OPIATES

The use of opium for relief of diarrhea preceded by many centuries its use as an analgesic. The constipating effect of opiates, regarded as an untoward action when the drugs are used for the relief of pain, is the basis of therapeutic desirability in patients with diarrhea.

Pharmacological Effects. Opiates, known to produce a very wide variety of pharmacological effects (see Chapter 10.1), have actions on the gastrointestinal tract (GIT) that are believed to result from their occupation of opiate receptors.

Stereospecific pre- and postsynaptic neuronal binding sites for opiates exist in the gastrointestinal wall, along with high concentrations of endogenous opioid peptides. Opiate-type antidiarrheals show high-affinity binding with their neuronal receptor sites located pre- and postsynaptically as well as on the glia cells. Glia cell binding may serve as a storage mechanism for subsequent release in the vicinity of the synaptic cleft. The affinity constant of an opiate-type antidiarrheal drug for the binding sites in the ileum directly correlates with its potency to inhibit electrically induced twitch tension of ileum preparations. The occupation of the opiate receptor also results in a decrease in evoked acetylcholine (ACh) release.

Specific actions of antidiarrheal opiates on the GIT include the following:

1. Stomach. Opiates reduce the secretion of hydrochloric acid as well as decrease motility associated with increasing the tone of the central portion of the stomach. There is also an increase in the tone of the first part of the duodenum, which often delays the passage of the gastric contents through the duodenum for as much as 12 hours.

2. Small intestine. After opiate administration, there is an increase in resting tone of the small intestine and induction of periodic spasms. The amplitude of the nonpropulsive type of rhythmic contractions is usually enhanced, but the more important propulsive contractions are markedly decreased. The tone of the ileocecal valve is enhanced. Water is more completely absorbed from the chyme because of the delayed passage of the bowel contents. Both biliary and pancreatic secretions are diminished, resulting in the delay of the food digestion.

3. Large intestine. Propulsive peristaltic waves in the colon are considerably diminished or abolished after opiates. The tone may increase to the point of spasm. The resulting delay in the passage of the contents causes desiccation of the feces, further retarding its advance through the colon. The amplitude of the nonpropulsive type of rhythmic contractions of the colon is usually enhanced. The tone of the anal sphincter is increased. There is also reduced attention to sensory stimuli for the defecation reflex.

All these factors acting in the stomach and small and large intestines contribute to antidiarrheal action of opiates.

Therapeutic Uses. The opiates are effective against diarrhea and are safe in doses of 15-20 mg of opium, or 1-2 mg of morphine. Codeine can also be used successfully in appropriate doses. Most opiate-containing OTC antidiarrheal drugs contain paregoric or its equivalent. In the usual dose, 1 tsp of paregoric contains 20 mg of powdered opium (2 mg of morphine).

In the usual antidiarrheal doses (given orally), addiction liability is low because morphine is not well absorbed; thus, the low dose is not large enough to produce analgesia or euphoria. Chronic use (as in ulcerative colitis, where the initial dose usually has to be increased to overcome tolerance) leads to the risk of physical dependence. Paregoric *per se* is a schedule III, prescription-only item; when combined with antidiarrheals that contain not more than 100 mg of opium (5 tsp of paregoric/100 ml of mixture), it is a schedule V item available for OTC purchase. Opium derivatives are potent CNS-acting drugs that may produce sedation, particularly when taken with other CNS depressants.

DIPHENOXYLATE AND DIFENOXIN

Diphenoxylate (9) (Fig. 18.4-1), a meperidine congener, was synthesized in 1956 as a specific antidiarrheal drug. At antidiarrheal doses, diphenoxylate produces no CNS effect characteristic of an opiate action. However, at doses several times higher than needed for antidiarrheal action, diphenoxylate elicits morphinelike central actions including euphoria, suppression of morphine abstinence, and a morphinelike physical dependence after chronic administration. In spite of this abuse potential, it is not abused, due in part to the fact that it is virtually insoluble in water, which obviates its abuse by the parenteral route. It is also available only in combination with atropine; the side effects and toxicity of the latter discourage use of excessive doses of the combination.

Difenoxin (9) (Fig. 18.4-1) is a metabolite of diphenoxylate that is rapidly hydrolyzed to its acid form in the body. Its actions are similar to those of diphenoxylate except that difenoxin is several times more potent than diphenoxylate. Difenoxin is also marketed in combination with atropine.

The mechanisms of the antidiarrheal action of diphenoxylate and difenoxin are similar to those of morphine, their action may be a consequence of the increased circular muscular activity of the intestine. Such increased activity favors segmentation or mixing of the bowel content and inhibits propulsion. Prostaglandins have been shown to cause diarrhea, presumably by enhancing transit of bowel contents and stimulation of intestinal secretion; diphenoxylate and difenoxin antagonize both of those actions.

Diphenoxylate provides rapid relief of symptoms in acute diarrhea and is effective in the management of chronic diarrhea. It is at least as effective as opiates but virtually without side effects or significant tolerance development when used in recommended doses. The preparations and doses are listed at the end of this chapter.

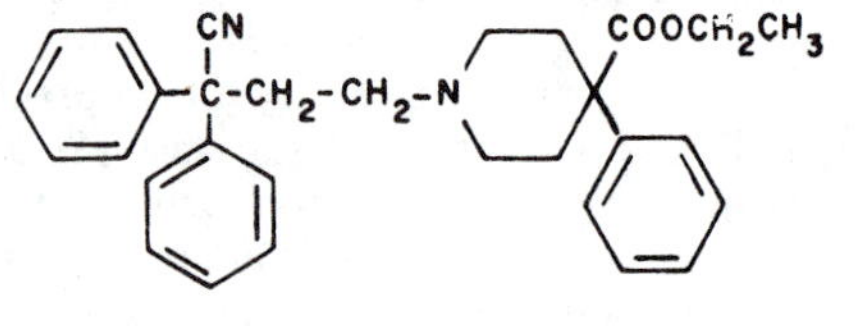

DIPHENOXYLATE

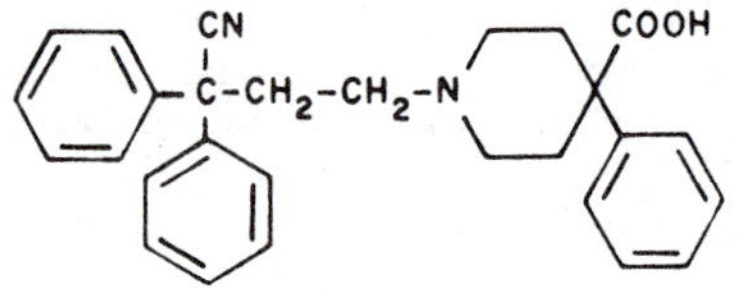

DIFENOXIN

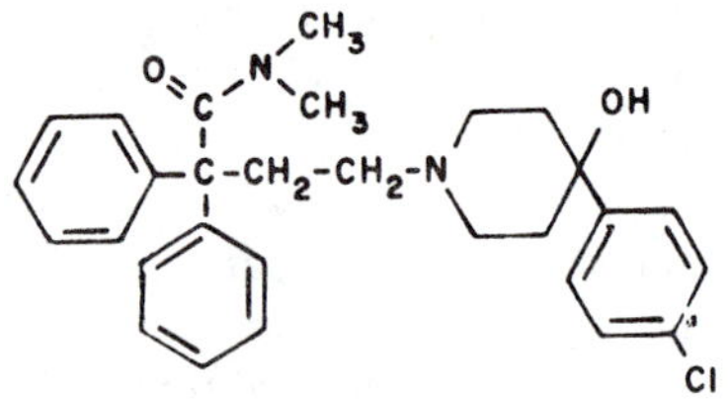

LOPERAMIDE

Fig. 18.4-1: *Chemical structures of some synthetic antidiarrheal drugs.*

LOPERAMIDE

Loperamide (Fig. 18.4-1) (7, 9), a piperidine derivative, is the most recently introduced antidiarrheal drug; not only surpasses older drugs in efficacy but is essentially free of opiatelike CNS effects even in maximally tolerated doses.

Mechanism of Action. Studies on the *in vitro* guinea pig ileum (the preparation chosen for the study of antidiarrheal drugs) show that loperamide is a potent inhibitor of peristaltic reflex activity, 47 times more active than morphine and 10 times more active than diphenoxylate. It is observed that when the intestinal lumen is distended, the longitudinal muscles contract; relaxation of the circular muscles results in shortening of the intestine (preparatory phase, mediated through cholinergic action). This phase is followed by a rapid phase (mediated through noncholinergic neurotransmission, possibly involving prostaglandin action) in which the circular muscles contract with relaxation of the longitudinal musculature, which propels the contents reflexly. Loperamide action consists of an inhibition of the initial slow cholinergic phase, followed by a depression of the propulsive phase; the total amount of bowel contents expelled is greatly reduced.

Loperamide directly antagonizes deoxycholic acid-induced secretion of sodium and water in the rat cecum, prostaglandin (PG) PGE_1-induced secretion, as well as cholera toxin-induced secretion in the rat jejunum. The variety of stimuli for hypersecretion that are antagonized by loperamide suggests, that the drug interferes with the mechanisms of fluid loss (which is important in controlling diarrhea) in addition to the inhibition of intestinal propulsions.

Therapeutic Uses. Loperamide is effective in both acute and chronic diarrhea caused by a large variety of etiological factors. The drug improves the consistency and reduces the frequency of stools; it normalizes reabsorption of water and electrolytes; and it inhibits intestinal secretions. It is useful in diarrhea associated with radiotherapy, prostaglandin action, trichuriasis in children, gastrointestinal surgery, and various cases of intractable diarrhea.

ABSORBENT: POLYCARBOPHIL

Polycarbophil is an absorbent that has a marked capacity to bind free fecal water. In diarrhea, it absorbs about 60 times its weight of water to produce formed stool. Paradoxically, the same action of polycarbophil is also useful in constipation as it prevents desiccation of fecal material and allows passage of soft stool. Polycarbophil is nontoxic and nonabsorbed, does not affect digestive enzymes and nutritional status, and is metabolically inactive.

ADSORBENTS

The adsorbents are the agents most frequently incorporated in OTC preparations for diarrhea. They are usually dispensed in liquid-suspension form to improve palatability because they are used in large doses. Adsorbents are useful only in mild diarrhea.

Adsorption is not a specific action; the materials possessing this property also adsorb nutrients, and digestive enzymes as well as toxins, bacteria, and other noxious materials. They may also adsorb drugs. The adsorbents, when used with ion exchange resins, combine their individual activities in relieving gastric distress and diarrhea. These agents are relatively inert and nontoxic.

KAOLIN

Kaolin is a native, hydrated aluminum silicate, powdered and freed from gritty particles by elution. It is used for the treatment of diarrhea and dysentery. Kaolin has been used in the treatment of chronic ulcerative colitis to adsorb bacteria and toxins in the colon, but it is doubtful whether appreciable activity is retained by the time the kaolin reaches the large bowel. Kaolin decreases the absorption of tetracyclines, anticholinergics, and other drugs.

Attapulgite. Attapulgite is a hydrous magnesium aluminum silicate, activated by thermal treatment and used in a finely powdered form.

Pectin. Pectin is a purified carbohydrate product obtained from acid extraction of the rind of citrus fruit or from apple pomace. Chemically, it consists chiefly of polygalacturonic acid, some of the hydroxyl groups of which are methylated. It is soluble in 20 parts of water to make a colloidal solution that is viscous, opalescent, and acidic in reaction. Pectin is widely employed in the symptomatic relief of diarrhea, often in combination with kaolin. The mechanism of action of pectin in diarrhea is unknown. In the bowel, pectin may act as an adsorbent and protective agent. It is decomposed in the colon by bacterial action to form acids and other as yet unidentified products that apparently provide an unfavorable environment for the bacterial flora that cause diarrhea.

MANAGEMENT OF ACUTE SECRETORY DIARRHEAS

Acute secretory diarrheas constitute a major source of morbidity and mortality throughout the world. Chronic secretory diarrheas are infrequent and will not be discussed here.

The following principles are generally adopted for the management of both cholera and travelers' diarrheas:

1. Treatment of fluid loss
2. Treatment of shock and acidosis, if present
3. Maintenance of nutritional status of the patient
4. Drug therapy

Depending on the severity of the diarrhea, one determines the relative importance of each of these principles.

Cholera. In patients with severe fluid loss due to cholera, repletion of fluid loss is achieved by intravenous therapy. After initial rehydration by i.v. therapy, these patients can be placed on oral fluids. Most patients with mild or moderate dehydration respond to rehydration by oral glucose-electrolyte solution (5). Adequate nutrition during acute diarrhea by either total parenteral nutrition or by oral route generally improves patients' condition.

Adjunctive antibacterial drug therapy for acute secretory diarrhea due to cholera includes tetracycline (at a dose of 50 mg/kg/day in children, 500 mg repeated every 6 hours for adults), or co-trimoxazole (8 mg/kg/day, trimethoprim and 40 mg/kg/day sulfamethoxazole in children, and 160 mg trimethoprim and 800 mg sulfamethoxazole every 12 hours for adults).

Travelers' Diarrhea. Travelers' diarrhea is mainly due to infection with ETEC and strains of *Shigella* (1). A relatively small percentage of patients suffer from infection due to intestinal parasites such as *Giardia lamblia* and *Entamoeba histolytica.* However, in many cases no microbial cause can be detected. The usual clinical features of travelers' diarrhea include sudden onset of mild-to-moderate watery bowel movement, abdominal cramps, tenesmus, fever, and sometimes vomiting.

Various antimicrobial agents [e.g., phthalylsulfathiazole, neomycin sulfate, doxycycline (200 mg on the first day of travel followed by 100 mg/day throughout the travel), co-trimoxazole, mecillinam (amdinocillin)] have been reported to have varying degree of success in the prevention of travelers' diarrhea.

Drugs that are commonly used in the treatment of travelers' diarrhea include absorbents such as bismuth

Table 18.4-1
Interaction of Antidiarrheal Agents with Other Drugs

Antidiarrheal Agents	Other Drugs	Effects
Opioids or congeners	CNS depressants	Additive CNS depression
Anticholinergics (antimuscarinics)	Tricyclic antidepressants, histamine H_1 antagonists, phenothiazines, procainamide, quinidine	Additive anticholinergic side effects
	Levodopa	Delayed gastric emptying caused by anticholinergic drugs may increase intragastric inactivation of levodopa
	MAO inhibitors	Increased anticholinergic effects reported with atropine
Kaolin-pectin	Digoxin, lincomycin, tetracyclines, anticholinergics, etc.	Adsorption in the intestine and reduced absorption
Attapulgite	Phenothiazines	Adsorption in the intestine and reduced absorption
Cholestyramine	Digitoxin and digoxin, warfarin, vitamin K, thyroxine and triiodothyronine, thiazide diuretics, iron, phenylbutazone	Binding in intestine and possible decreased absorption to varying degrees

Source: Ref. 3.

salicylate suspension (30-60 ml every 30 minutes); antisecretory antimotility agents such as diphenoxylate (usually in combination with atropine) and loperamide; and specific antimicrobials, co-trimoxazole, trimethoprim alone, and bicozamycin (2).

Opiates and their analogs have some potential risks, because they have been reported to be partly responsible for antibiotic-related diarrhea and pseudomembranous colitis (8). Use of loperamide in large doses in children has been reported to cause central nervous system side effects (4).

DRUG INTERACTIONS

Drug interactions are shown in Table 18.4-1.

Preparations. Some preparations involving commonly used antidiarrheal agents are listed with the trade names and active ingredients.

Morphine, INFANTILE PINK (opium camphorated, bismuth subsalicylate, pectin, calcium carrageenate, zinc phenolsulfonate); PABIZOL (paregoric, bismuth subsalicylate, aluminum magnesium phenyl salicylate, zinc phenolsulfonate); PARELIXIR (tincture of opium, pectin); PAREPECTOLIN (paregoric, kaolin, pectin); DONNAGEL-PG (powdered opium, kaolin, pectin); AMOGEL (powdered opium, bismuth subgallate, kaolin, pectin); CORRECTIVE MIXTURE WITH PAREGORIC (paregoric, bismuth subsalicylate, pepsin, phenyl salicylate, zinc phenolsulfonate); DIABISMUL (opium, kaolin, pectin); KIAQUEL (paregoric, pectin).

Diphenoxylate, LOMOTIL. Each tablet or 5 ml liquid contains 2.5 mg of diphenoxylate hydrochloride and 0.025 mg of atropine sulfate.

Difenoxin (difenoxin with atropine); not yet available in the United States.

Loperamide, IMODIUM (loperamide hydrochloride, 2 mg/tablet).

REFERENCES

1. DuPont, H.L., Olarte, J., Evans, D.G. et al. Comparative susceptibility of Latin Americans and United States students to enteric pathogens. *N. Engl. J. Med.* 295:1520, 1976.
2. Ericsson, C.D., DuPont, H.L., Sullivan, P. et al. Bicozamycin, a poorly absorbable antibiotic effectively treats travellers' diarrhea. *Ann. Intern. Med.* 98:20, 1983.
3. Fingl, E. and Freston, J.W. Antidiarrheal agents and laxatives. *Clin. Gastroenterol.* 8:161, 1979.
4. Friedli, G. and Haenggle, C.A. Loperamide overdose managed by naloxone. *Lancet* 1:1413, 1980.
5. Hughes, S. Acute secretory diarrheas. *Drugs* 26:80, 1983.
6. Matseshe, J.W. and Phillips, S.F. Chronic diarrhea. *Med. Clin. North Am.* 62:141, 1978.
7. Niemegeers, C.J.E., Colpaert, F.C. and Awouters, F.H.L. Pharmacology and antidiarrheal effects of loperamide. *Drug Dev.* 1:1, 1981.
8. Novak, E., Lee, J.G., Seckman, C.E. et al. Unfavourable effect of atropine-diphenoxylate (LOMOTIL) therapy in lincomycin-caused diarrhea. *JAMA* 236:1415, 1976.
9. Van Bever, W. and Lal, H. (eds.) *Synthetic Antidiarrheal Drugs.* New York: Marcel Dekkers, 1975.

CHAPTER
19

DRUGS AFFECTING UTERINE MOTILITY

Gautam Chaudhuri and Ira Silverman

Drugs affecting uterine contractility are especially useful to the obstetrician. Those that increase uterine contractions (oxytocics) are used to augment and induce labor; their use has decreased the rate of cesarean sections. Those, on the other hand, that inhibit uterine contractions (tocolytics) have been used to inhibit premature labor; their value lies in the fact that prematurity is the largest cause of perinatal morbidity and mortality.

In evaluating these groups of drugs, their effects on both the mother and the fetus must be considered.

ANATOMY AND PHYSIOLOGY

The muscular layer of the uterus (myometrium) is very thick and composed of an inner circular layer and an outer layer of longitudinal and oblique fibers. The myometrium, which undergoes marked hypertrophy during pregnancy, is heavily vascularized. The blood vessels run between the interstices of the muscle fibers; these act as a tourniquet when they contract, thereby controlling bleeding from the uterus.

The uterus is innervated by both the sympathetic and the parasympathetic nervous systems, the former by way of the postganglionic fibers from the inferior mesenteric and hypogastric ganglia, and the latter by way of the pelvic nerve. Both α-(excitatory) and β- (inhibitory) adrenergic receptors are present in the myometrium of mammals.

Uterine contractions are involuntary and, for the most part, are independent of extrauterine control. Paraplegics have normal, although painless, labor contractions, as do women after bilateral lumbar sympathectomy (38). The intensity and duration of each contraction are generally greatest in the fundal zone, followed by those in the midzone, and finally, least of all, the lower zone; this fundal dominance allows the expulsion of the fetus. If the intensity and duration of contractions were to be the same in all three zones, the pressure gradient would be absent and labor would not progress.

Drugs affecting uterine contractility can be conveniently classified into two groups: (1) those used for increasing uterine contractility (i.e., oxytocin, prostaglandins, ergot alkaloids, sparteine sulfate, and hypertonic solutions; and (2) those used for inhibiting uterine contractility (i.e., ethyl alcohol, β-adrenergic stimulants, prostaglandin synthetase inhibitors, magnesium sulfate, progesterone, and general anesthetics).

DRUGS INCREASING UTERINE CONTRACTILITY

The stimulus for uterine contraction, which must act on the myometrium, probably involves an increased intracellular concentration of free calcium to affect the contraction of the smooth muscle of the uterus similar to that involved in striated muscles. Accumulated evidence suggests that calcium exists in one or more bound forms in smooth muscle; one of the sequestering sites in the sarcoplasmic reticulum, which surrounds the myofibril and constitutes a storage system from which calcium is released to the myofibril. In the presence of free intracellular calcium, contraction occurs, whereas relaxation is associated with an adenosine triphosphate (ATP) energy-dependent mechanism that returns calcium to the sarcoplasmic reticulum (29).

Carsten (6) demonstrated that oxytocin, as well as prostaglandins E_2 and $F_{2\alpha}$, inhibits the ATP-dependent binding of calcium to the sarcoplasmic reticulum, an action that would give rise to an increased intracellular concentration of free calcium and lead to uterine contractions. There is a marked difference in the capability of oxytocin to inhibit calcium storage in uterine preparations of pregnant women when compared with its effect on nonpregnant women. By contrast, this difference is very modest, with both prostaglandins E_2 and $F_{2\alpha}$ (6) offering a possible explanation for the susceptibility of the myometrium to the effects of certain prostaglandins at all stages of gestation whereas there is a relative refractoriness to oxytocin-induced contractions of the human uterus until late in gestation.

OXYTOCIN

Chemistry. The structure of oxytocin, an octapeptide, was elucidated and synthesized in 1953 (10). DuVigneaud was awarded the Nobel Prize in Chemistry for synthesizing this first polypeptide hormone. It is a nonapeptide with two cysteine residues at position 1 and 6 connected with an -S-S- bridge (Fig. 12.1-4). Structurally similar compounds with varying amino acid sequences have been synthesized and found to have varying pharmacological properties. The oxytocic property is lost if the glutaminyl or asparginyl components are replaced by other amino acids. By contrast, replacement of isoleucine in the pentapeptide ring increases oxytocic activity (27). Synthetic oxytocin (SYNTOCINON), which has replaced extracts from the posterior pituitary for clinical use because it does not contain any vasopressin or foreign protein, is freely water-soluble and stable in acid solution.

Pharmacological Effects. ***Uterus.*** The contractile and electrical activity of the uterine smooth muscle is increased by oxytocin. This action, direct on the myometrium, is modified by the local estrogen-progestogen balance; estrogen increases oxytocin sensitivity, whereas progestogen dominance may block the myometrial response to oxytocin. When estrogen levels are low, the effects of oxytocin are markedly reduced. The immature uterus is quite resistant (8). Oxytocin can initiate or enhance rhythmic contractions at any time during pregnancy although the degree of responsiveness parallels the spontaneous motility, which is very low in the first and second trimester of pregnancy and increases sharply in the third trimester. There is an eightfold increase in responsiveness between the twentieth and thirtieth week (3). At an appropriate dosage, oxytocin increases the frequency and amplitude of contraction without raising uterine tonus: this property makes oxytocin suitable for the induction or augmentation of labor. Because higher dosages can produce uterine hypertonus, with grave consequences to the fetus as well as to the mother, the amount of oxytocin infused should be very closely monitored.

Cardiovascular System. The amount of oxytocin administered for most obstetrical purposes is insufficient to produce marked alteration of blood pressure. However, when a large dose is administered as a rapid intravenous bolus, there is a fall in both systolic and diastolic pressure, due to a direct vasodilator action (21).

Antidiuretic Effect. An important adverse effect of oxytocin is antidiuresis, caused primarily by the reabsorption of free water. Synthetic oxytocin as well as that derived from mammalian posterior pituitary glands possesses antidiuretic activity in both pregnant and nonpregnant women (1). Urinary flow can be markedly reduced when oxytocin is infused at a rate of 40-50 ml/min. With doses of this magnitude, it is possible to produce water intoxication if the oxytocin is administered in a large volume of electrolyte-free aqueous dextrose solution (11).

The antidiuretic effect of intravenously administered oxytocin disappears within a few minutes after the infusion is stopped. If high doses of oxytocin are to be administered, it is preferable to increase the concentration of the hormone infused rather than increasing the rate of flow of a more dilute solution.

Mammary Gland. Oxytocin contracts the myoepithelial cells of the mammary gland and, as a result, leads to milk ejection. This effect is seen only in pregnant women: as pregnancy advances, the sensitivity of the gland to this hormone increases (33).

Pharmacokinetics. Oxytocin is rapidly absorbed from mucosal surfaces, especially those of the buccal and nasal cavities. It is rapidly degraded by trypsin in the gut if administered orally. Its half-life in the nonpregnant woman is estimated to be about 10-15 minutes; in late pregnancy, it is said to be 1-3 minutes (29). The markedly short half-life in pregnancy is thought to be due to the presence in the circulation of a glycoprotein aminopeptidase referred to as both *oxytocinase* and *vasopressinase* and capable of inactivating both hormones. Plasma enzyme activity increases gradually until term and then declines after delivery. The placenta and pregnant uterine tissue show high oxytocinase activity and are thought to be the source of the circulating enzyme (22).

Diagnostic Use. Oxytocin is used for the stress test or oxytocin challenge test (OCT), where the fetal response to stress (i.e., three uterine contractions of 40-60 seconds duration over a 10-minute period after infusion of oxytocin) is observed. The fetal response is assessed by monitoring the fetal heart rate. An OCT is interpreted as positive when persistent and consistent late decelerations (fetal bradycardia occurring at the height of uterine contractions) are noted in association with most (more than half) of the adequate contractions. If no decelerations are noted, the test is termed negative and suggests that the fetus is not in jeopardy.

Therapeutic Uses: Oxytocin is used (1) for induction of labor when a definite obstetrical indication exists, (2) for augmentation of labor when the patient is definitely in labor, but the uterine contractions become weak, (3) to make the pregnant uterus firm at the time of evacuation of uterine contents, and (4) for control of postpartum and postabortal bleeding.

Preparations. *Oxytocin injection*, USP, contains 10 USP U/ml and may be administered either i.v. or i.m.; *oxytocin nasal spray*, 40 U/ml; *oxytocin citrate*, buccal tablets (PITOCIN CITRATE), 200 USP U.

Both the nasal spray and the buccal tablets are rarely used in obstetrics.

PROSTAGLANDINS

Prostaglandins, their source, chemistry, and pharmacological actions on various systems are dealt with in Chapter 13.2. The first report on the clinical application of prostaglandins appeared about 10 years ago regarding their use in the induction of labor. Since then, numerous excellent reviews and texts (14) have appeared that have discussed in great detail their applications to obstetrics and gynecology.

Pharmacological Effects. ***Uterus.*** Strips of myometrium from pregnant women uteri are contracted *in vitro* by both PGE_2 and $PGF_{2\alpha}$. In contrast, strips from nonpregnant human uteri are contracted by $PGF_{2\alpha}$ and show varied action to PGE_2.

Intravenous infusion of either PGE_2 or $PGF_{2\alpha}$ evokes sustained laborlike contractions with the tone falling between each contraction. In contrast to oxytocin, this action of prostaglandins is observed in the nonpregnant state as well as in all stages of pregnancy, although the sensitivity of the uterus to prostaglandins increases as pregnancy advances, quite similar to that seen with oxytocin. PGE_1 and PGE_2 are about 10 times more potent than $PGF_{2\alpha}$ in their oxytocic action during the last two trimesters of pregnancy (19). The pharmacological response of the uterus to these prostaglandins in late pregnancy very closely resembles that seen with oxytocin, although the prostaglandins show a narrower dose-response for production of physiological contractions and the occurrence of uterine hypertonus. Therefore, their administration needs very close monitoring.

The effects of the natural prostaglandins E_1, E_2, and $F_{2\alpha}$ on the isolated pregnant human cervix *in vitro* are variable and may be dose related. In a study on the stretch modules of the human cervix, $PGF_{2\alpha}$ effectively reduced cervical stiffness (7). In failed cases of prostaglandin-induced midtrimester abortions, the cervix is usually softened and at times dilated. PGE_2 and $PGF_{2\alpha}$ also lower the cervical resistance to mechanical dilation (18).

The mechanism by which prostaglandins contract the uterus is not exactly known. Csapo (9) hypothesized that prostaglandins are able to stimulate the myometrium tetanically, but progesterone withdrawal is necessary for the development of cyclic (high-frequency, high-amplitude) uterine activity.

Serum progesterone concentration is reduced prior to the onset of labor (39). There is a greater reduction in serum progesterone and elevation of estrogen in $PGF_{2\alpha}$-induced labor compared with oxytocin (23).

Smooth muscles. Prostaglandin E_2 and $F_{2\alpha}$ contract smooth muscles and can cause bronchoconstriction, vomiting, and diarrhea.

Adverse Effects. Nausea, vomiting, diarrhea, dizziness, rise or fall in diastolic pressure, tachycardia, flushing, tachypnea, and pyrexia have been reported. The vomiting can be controlled with the use of an antiemetic (e.g., chlorpromazine); the diarrhea is best treated with-diphenoxylate hydrochloride and atropine sulfate (LOMOTIL). Bronchoconstriction responds rapidly to the administration of a β-adrenergic stimulant such as salbutamol. The temperature returns to normal after discontinuation of prostaglandin administration.

An important side-effect is the rupture of the posterior wall of the uterus at the cervico-isthmic junction, and this can be prevented with gentle instrumental dilatation or by insertion of laminaria tents into the cervical canal (18). β-mimetic drugs inhibit prostaglandin-induced uterine activity, and these agents could prove useful in the prevention of impending uterine rupture (18).

Preparations. *Dinoprost tromethamine* (PROSTIN $F_{2\alpha}$): 40-mg vial (40 mg injected intraamniotically); *dinoprostone* E_2 (PROSTIN E_2): vaginal suppository (20 mg).

ERGOT ALKALOIDS

Ergot is the dried sclerotium of the fungus, *Claviceps purpurea* that grows on certain grains, particularly rye in moist warm seasons. The fungus is found in the grain fields of North America and Europe.

History. Epidemics of painful gangrene of the extremities due to vascular effects have been caused by consumption of bread made from infected rye. The disease was called St. Anthony's fire because sufferers experience relief by visiting the saint's shrine in Padua, Italy. The cure may have been affected because they left the area where the contaminated grain was being used.

Chemistry. Ergot contains a number of pharmacologically active alkaloids, as well as several bioactive amines such as histamine, tyramine, choline, and acetylcholine. All ergot alkaloids are derivatives of a tetracyclic compound, 6-methylergoline and, on hydrolysis, yield lysergic acid. The naturally occurring ergot alkaloids contain in the β-configuration and a substitution at position 8 and a double bond in ring D (Table 19-1). On the basis of their hydrolysis products, they have been designated as amine alkaloids and amino acid alkaloids (ergopeptines). Some of the pharmacologically active alkaloids of the two groups are shown in Table 19-2.

The naturally occurring alkaloids have been modified by addition of two H atoms in the double bond in the D-ring of lysergic acid. These have been termed dihydroergotamine, dihydroergotoxin, etc. Bromocriptine is another ergopeptine produced by bromo substitution at C_2 of α-ergokryptine. Methysergide is produced by methylation of the indole nitrogen (N_1) of methylergonovine.

Ergoline is basic to all ergot alkaloids and bears structural resemblance to the biogenic amines (norepinephrine, epinephrine, dopamine, and serotonin). It is, therefore, not surprising that ergot derivatives can act as agonists or antagonists, or both, at these amine receptors; these activities are discussed elsewhere in this text.

Pharmacological Effects. ***Uterus.*** All the natural ergot alkaloids contract the uterus. Ergonovine is superior with respect to the rapidity of the onset of uterine contractions when administered either intravenously or orally, and is also less toxic when compared with the other ergot alkaloids.

Ergot alkaloids increase the motor activity of the uterus and markedly stimulate myometrial contractions (which may last for hours). A characteristic feature is the marked increase in tonus where the muscles have tetanic contractions, leading to a blanching of the myometrium. Ergot alkaloids stimulate the gravid uterus at all stages of gestation, sensitivity increasing at term. They also stimulate the immature uterus; in this respect they resemble prostaglandins but differ from oxytocin.

Table 19-1
Natural Ergot Alkaloids and Their Congeners

A. Amine Alkaloids 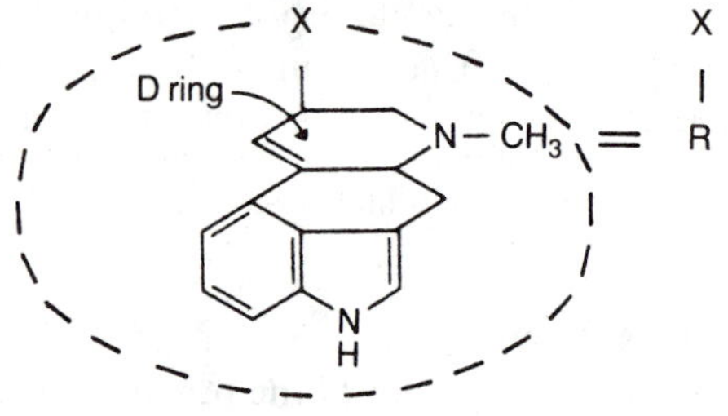	B. Amino Acid Alkaloids 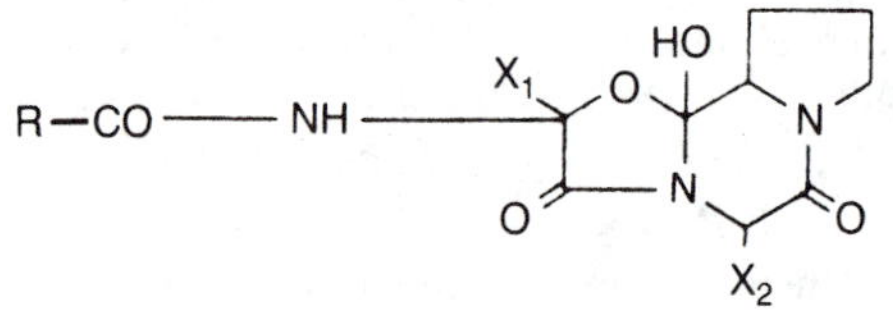

A. Amine Alkaloids	X	Predominant Effect
d-Lysergic acid	—COOH	
d-Lysergic acid diethylamide (LSD)	$—CON<(CH_2CH_3)(CH_2CH_3)$	Hallucinogen
Ergonovine (ergometrine)	$—CONHCH<(CH_2OH)(CH_3)$	Oxytocic
Methylergonovine	$—CONHCH<(CH_2OH)(CH_2CH_3)$	Oxytocic
Methysergide	Same as in methylergonovine + methyl substitution at N-1	5-HT antagonist

B. Amino Acid Alkaloids	$X_1(2')$	$X_2(5')$	Predominant Effect
Ergotamine	$—CH_3$	$—CH_2C_6H_5$	α-Adrenergic agonist
Ergotoxine group			α-Adrenergic agonist
Ergocornine	$—CH(CH_3)_2$	$—CH(CH_3)_2$	
Ergocristine	$—CH(CH_3)_2$	$—CH_2C_6H_5$	
α-Ergokryptine	$—CH(CH_3)_2$	$—CH_2CH(CH_3)_2$	
β-Ergokryptine	$—CH(CH_3)_2$	$—CH(CH_3)CH_2CH_3$	
Bormocriptine	Both same as in α-ergokryptine + substitution of a bromine atom at C-2		DA agonist

The dosage range between that increasing uterine motor activity and that producing hypertonus is much less compared with either oxytocin or prostaglandins; this precludes the use of ergot alkaloids for induction or augmentation of labor as well as for midtrimester abortion.

The increase in uterine tone produced by ergonovine is accompanied by only minor side effects and can be used to control postpartum and postabortal bleeding.

Cardiovascular System. Ergotamine produces vasoconstriction of both arteries and veins. It increases peripheral vascular resistance and decreases blood flow in various organs; it causes only slight hypertension. With dihydroergotamine, vasoconstriction, although less, is comparatively more on the capacitance than on resistance vessels, because of which this compound has been considered to be useful in the treatment of postural hypotension. Dihydrogenated derivatives of ergotoxine alka-

Table 19-2
Comparative Pharmacology of the Ergot Alkaloids and Their Derivatives

	Oxytocic Effect	Vasoconstriction	α-Adrenergic Receptor Activity
Ergonovine, methylergonovine	Highly active, onset rapid, orally effective	Slightly active	Weak partial agonist in blood vessels (less than ergotamine); little or no antagonistic action
Ergotamine	Highly active, onset slow even after i.v. injection, orally ineffective	Highly active	Partial agonist and antagonist
Dihydrogenated alkaloids	Active on pregnant human uterus (no activity observed in animals)	Much less active than parent compounds	Partial agonists in veins; antagonists in blood vessels

loids, on the other hand, are comparatively less active and produce hypotension through their CNS effects. Amine alkaloids such as ergonovine are much less active than the amino acid group and have only slight vasoconstrictor action; ergonovine caused slight blood flow in extremities in therapeutic doses. Methylergonovine, a synthetic derivative, has less hypertensive effect than ergonovine, with no difference in uterine actions; thus, methylergonovine is especially useful in cases of preexisting hypertension.

Adverse Effects. The parenteral administration of ergot alkaloids to postpartum women can sometimes initiate transient but severe hypertension, especially if conduction anesthesia is used during labor. These agents are avoided in preeclamptics or women with preexisting hypertension. Nausea is an occasional side effect.

Ergot Poisoning. Poisoning with ergot alkaloids can be acute or chronic. Acute poisoning, although rare, usually occurs following ingestion of a large amount of ergot in an attempt for abortion. Effects include vomiting, diarrhea, excessive thirst, cold and cyanotic skin, weak and rapid pulse, tingling, confusion, and coma. Death has been recorded with oral or intravenous doses of ergotamine.

Chronic poisoning has occurred in the past following ingestion of bread prepared from ergot-contaminated rye. It may also be produced by overdosage of ergot alkaloids taken over a prolonged period for migraine or in attempts for producing abortion. It may also occur in unusually susceptible persons, such as those with occlusive peripheral vascular disease and liver disease. Manifestations include gradually increasing circulatory changes leading to gangrene in feet and legs, and less frequently in hands. Drug-induced vasoconstriction and intimal lesion contribute to these changes. Other effects include nausea, vomiting, diarrhea, headache, dizziness, confusion, drowsiness, depression, rarely convulsions, hemiplegia, and miosis; these effects represent the depressant and stimulant effects on different CNS areas. Usual measures include withdrawal of the drug concerned and symptomatic treatment, particularly with use of a suitable vasodilator agent (e.g., sodium nitroprusside, an α-adrenergic blocker, etc.)

Therapeutic Uses. ***Labor and Puerperium.*** Ergonovine and methylergonovine are used for treatment of postpartum hemorrhage and postpartum uterine atony.

Migraine. Migraine is characterized usually by periodic painful headache and is considered to be due to increased blood flow in both intracerebral and extracranial blood vessels, resulting in increased pulsations of cranial arteries, particularly meningeal branches of external carotid. Pain is due to the arterial pulsations. The headache may be preceded by a subjective aura or some objective neurological symptoms corresponding to a period of unexplained vasoconstriction, decreasing the blood flow in some cerebral regions.

Ergotamine is effective in relief of migrainous headache in the majority of cases, due to its vasoconstrictor property. For this purpose it may be administered parenterally; relief is often dramatic, occurring in 15 minutes, Oral administration causes slower relief, requiring an average of 5 hours. This drug is not suitable for preventive purposes; given before, it may rather precipitate an attack by enhancing initial vasoconstriction.

Dihydroergotamine given intramuscularly is also effective in migraine but in fewer patients. Ergonovine is effective in half the number of cases relieved by ergotamine. It may be more useful given orally; however, it is not approved for therapy in migraine in the United States. Methysergide and propranolol are effective for prophylaxis of migraine. Caffeine enhances the effect of ergot alkaloids in migraine; this may be due to the twofold action of caffeine that (1) increases the oral and rectal absorption of ergotamine and (2) enhances vasoconstriction of cerebral blood vessels by causing release of catecholamines and antagonizing adenosine-induced vasodilation.

As Dopamine Agonist. Bromocriptine acts as a dopamine agonist and is used in the treatment of parkinsonism (Chapters 7.4 and 9.4) and for suppression of prolactin secretion (Chapters 11.5.1 and 12.1).

Other Uses. Dihydroergotoxine (HYDERGINE) has been used in senile dementia showing slight behavioral or psychological improvement in some patients. Its mechanism of action is not clearly understood.

Preparations. *Ergonovine maleate,* USP (ERGOTRATE): tablets (0.2 mg of the alkaloid salt); ampuls (0.2 mg, 1 ml). These preparations should be kept at temperatures of 0 to 12°C and away from light. *Methylergonovine maleate,* USP (METHERGINE): tablets (0.2 mg); ampuls (0.2 mg, 1 ml).

Ergotamine tartrate, USP (GYNERGEN, ERGOSTAT, etc.): tablets (1 mg, oral, or 2 mg, sublingual); aqueous solution (0.5 mg/ml) for injection. Solution is also available for inhalation (0.36 mg of salt per dose). *Ergotamine tartrate and caffeine,* USP: tablets (1 and 100 mg, respectively); suppositories (2 and 100 mg, respectively). *Methysergide maleate,* USP (SANSERT): tablets (2 mg).

Dihydroergotamine mesylate, USP: ampul (1 mg/ml) for injection. *Dihydrogenated ergot alkaloids* (HYDERGINE, CIRCANOL, DEAPRIL-ST): tablets (0.5 or 1 mg). Each 1-mg tablet contains 0.333 mg each of dihydroergocornine, dihydroergocristine, and dihydroergokryptine (dihydro-α-ergokryptine and dihydro-β-ergokryptine in the proportion of 2:1) as mesylates.

Bromocriptine mesylate (PARLODEL): tablets (2.5 mg).

THERAPEUTIC USES OF OXYTOCIC AGENTS

For *induction of labor* at term, the drug of choice is oxytocin. Given by intravenous infusion, it induces labor in the majority of cases. Combined with amniotomy, it is successful in 80 to 90% of cases. Prostaglandins ($PGF_{2\alpha}$ and PGE_2) are also equally effective in inducing labor, although they are not yet approved for use in the United States. Oxytocin has the potential advantage of stimulating uterine contraction and hence of being used at any stage of pregnancy. $PGF_{2\alpha}$ may occasionally produce uterine hypertonus.

For augmentation of labor, oxytocin has been used advantageously in some patients who are definitely in labor but whose uterine contractions have become weak.

After *delivery of fetus,* early administration of oxytocic agents can reduce the incidence of the postpartum hemorrhage. Ergonovine (or methylergonovine) is a preferred drug for this purpose because of its sustained duration and fairly rapid onset of action. These alkaloids have also been helpful for treatment of delayed involution and uterine atony, thereby reducing the possibility of bleeding and infection. Oxytocin has also been used in the past for these purposes, but its action is shortlasting.

For *therapeutic abortion,* during the *first trimester,* no drug is satisfactory; dilatation and suction curettage are commonly used. During the *second trimester,* intraamniotic injection of hypertonic (20%) saline, of prostaglandins (dinoprost, $PGF_{2\alpha}$, by intraamniotic injection), or of dinoprostone PGE_2 in vaginal suppository form has been used satisfactorily, although dilatation and evacuation have been found to be safer and more effective.

Table 19-3 summarizes the therapeutic characteristics of the three agents oxytocin, prostaglandin, and ergonovine.

DRUGS USED FOR INHIBITING UTERINE MOTILITY (TOCOLYTIC AGENTS)

The main indication for use of tocolytic drugs is to prevent premature labor; because little is known about the factors initiating labor, treatment is generally directed at inhibiting uterine contractions. Premature labor (defined as labor occurring before 37 weeks of gestation) may be spontaneous, or due to a complication of preg-

Table 19-3
Comparison of Oxytocic Agents

	Oxytocin	Prostaglandin	Ergonovine
Chemical nature	Physiological substance, octapeptide	Physiological substance, fatty acid derivative	Natural ergot alkaloid
Nature of uterine contraction	Contraction followed by relaxation	Contraction followed by relaxation	Tonic contractions
Sensitivity of uterus	Sensitivity increases with duration of pregnancy; most sensitive at term; immature uterus resistant	Contracts uterus in all stages of pregnancy and also nonpregnant and immature uterus	Sensitivity increases at term; nonpregnant and immature uterus stimulated
Route of administration	Given i.v., may be absorbed from buccal mucosa, and cannot be used orally	Can be given p.o., intravaginally, i.v., or intraamniotically	Can be given p.o., i.m., or i.v.
Onset of action	i.v. immediate i.m. in 2.5 minutes		i.v. immediate i.m. in 5 minutes
Duration of action	Very short		Prolonged, particularly after high dose
Uses	Induction of labor, postpartum uterine atony	Induction of labor and abortion	Prevention of postpartum uterine atony and hemorrhage

nancy; it accounts for a significant percentage of low-birth-weight babies. Early differentiation between true and false labor is often difficult before the uterus has contracted sufficiently to produce demonstrable effacement and dilatation of the cervix. For diagnosis of labor, uterine contractions must occur at least once every 10 minutes and last for at least 30 seconds. Progressive dilatation of the cervix is, of course, indicative of labor. Prevention is difficult becuse of the problems of identification of patients at risk; the alternative approach is effective treatment, but opinion is divided over the best method. Conservative treatment (bed rest and sedation) will be followed by cessation of contractions in 40-70% of cases, any more active treatment need to prove itself substantially better.

The gestational age through which labor should be stopped is reported in the literature as from 20 to 35 weeks, with estimated fetal weights ranging from 500 to 2000 g. Before using any drug to stop premature labor, one must be certain that the fetus is alive, that there is no medical or obstetrical contraindication to the arrest of labor, and that the cervix is less than 4 cm dilated.

Once the membranes have ruptured, treatment is rarely effective. Although some consider the practice to be contraindicated because of the risk of infection, others consider it worthwhile to try to delay labor for 24 to 48 hours to give the fetal lungs a chance to mature, especially if steroids have been given to stimulate the production of surfactant. Once a diagnosis of premature labor is made, it is important to start treatment immediately, for unnecessary delay might make the treatment ineffective. Although many agents are currently in use for the therapy of premature labor, none has achieved uniform success.

ETHYL ALCOHOL

In 1951, Van Dyke and Ames (40) demonstrated that ethanol inhibits the release of vasopressin from the posterior pituitary (37). Later, Fuchs (13) demonstrated the inhibitory influence of ethanol on the release of oxytocin. subsequently, in 1965, the inhibitory influence of ethanol on uterine contractions with prevention of premature labor was demonstrated (15).

Pharmacological Effects. ***Uterus.*** Ethanol probably inhibits uterine contraction by both a direct action on the myometrium as well as an indirect action of inhibiting oxytocin release.

In women in labor, oxytocin is released in a series of pulses that increase in frequency as labor progresses. The frequency of pulse release is reduced during i.v. infusion of alcohol at levels that produce no obvious direct effects on uterine activity. Ethanol inhibits uterine activity in spontaneous labor and uterine activity induced by PGE_2 and $PGF_{2\alpha}$ but not that induced by oxytocin (20). This might imply that spontaneous uterine contractility is mediated through prostaglandin release.

Adverse Effects. In the mother, symptoms of intoxication such as vomiting and restlessness, personality change, aspiration pneumonia, lactic acidosis, diuresis, incontinence of urine, and occasionally hypoglycemia and postalcohol headache syndrome are observed. Abnormal bone marrow morphology, fetal metabolic acidosis, and tendency to muscular hypotonia in neonates whose mothers received ethanol administration for control of premature labor have been reported.

Preparations. For the control of premature labor, a loading dose of 15 ml/kg of 10% ethanol in 5% dextrose is administered i.v. over 2 hours. A maintenance dose of 1.5 ml/kg/h is then continued for 10 hours or longer; if necessary. If labor recurs after the initial course of therapy, one or two additional courses may be utilized. If the onset of labor occurs within 10 hours of the previous infusion, it is necessary to reduce the loading dose.

β-ADRENERGIC STIMULANTS

Rucker (32) in 1925, noted that small doses of epinephrine inhibited uterine activity. The transient uterine response, as well as the marked cardiovascular side effects, prevented use of epinephrine for treatment of premature labor. Efforts to synthesize epinephrinelike agents with sustained uterine relaxation and fewer cardiovascular side effects resulted in a family of β-adrenergic agonists: isoxuprine, terbutaline, ritodrine, salbutamol, and fenoterol. Ritodrine will be discussed as the prototype β-adrenergic agonist and contrasted with related drugs where appropriate.

Pharmacological Effects. The ideal β-adrenergic tocolytic agent would activate uterine β_2-adrenoceptors and not influence β_1-cardiac receptors. Unfortunately, vascular smooth muscle also contains β_2-adrenoceptors, and pharmacological uterine tocolysis is accompanied by some hypotension and reflex tachycardia. The clinical usefulness of any specific β-adrenergic agonist is related to its effectiveness in promoting uterine relaxation but is limited by side effects caused by simultaneous β_1-adrenoceptor stimulation.

Uterus. Ritodrine hydrochloride has predominantly β_2-adrenergic activity and very weak β_1-adrenergic activity. It is a potent inhibitor of myometrial contractility in both the pregnant and nonpregnant uterus. Blood pressure responds with an increase in systolic and a decrease in diastolic pressure, resulting in a widened pulse pressure. Maternal cardiac output may be reflexly increased. Fetal heart rate increases slightly, probably secondary to transplacental passage of drug. By contrast, the use of isoxuprine, another β_2-adrenergic agonist, has been associated with hypotension that is thought to be due to α-adrenergic blocking effects. In one study, 20% of patients had severe hypotension, requiring cessation of isoxuprine therapy (35).

Pharmacokinetics. Absorption and excretion of ritodrine are similar in animals and humans, 30% of an oral dose is absorbed. In animals, 50 to 80% of a dose is excreted in the urine, and 90% of urine excretion is complete in 24 hours. The drug is lipid-soluble and crosses the placenta, with fetal levels approximately 20% that of the maternal serum.

Adverse Effects. The most common side-effects in the mother are cardiovascular and metabolic. Increases in maternal heart rate and reduction in blood pressure occur, but blunting of the maternal heart rate response may be seen with continued treatment. More severe tachycardia and hypotension occur with isoxuprine as compared with newer agents (4). Maternal response at a given concentration of ritodrine shows wide variability both between patients and within the same patient (5). Stimulation of β_2-adrenoceptor in liver and muscle results in glycogenolysis, causing mild hyperglycemia as well as elevations of lactate and free fatty acids. Insulin and glucagon secretion may also be increased.

Hypokalemia, as well as tremor, palpitations, and restlessness, is not uncommon. Earlier-generation β_2-adrenergic agonists, such as isoxuprine and terbutaline, are generally associated with more severe side effects than newer, more specific agents such as ritodrine, salbutamol, and fenoterol (12).

Transplacental passage of drug may cause fetal heart acceleration but is rarely of clinical significance. There has been no significant differences in umbilical pH, Apgar scores, head circumference, and neurological condition in ritodrine-treated neonates (16).

Drug Interactions. There are known cases of maternal pulmonary edema in patients treated simultaneously with ritodrine and corticosteroids (5). The mechanism of possible synergism remains unknown. Pulmonary edema has also been reported with other β-adrenergic agents, such as terbutaline or isoxuprine. Pulmonary edema occurs mainly in patients with unrecognized fluid overload or electrolyte imbalance (34). The hypokalemia caused by these agents may potentiate the toxicity of cardiac glycosides. The hyperglycemia caused may antagonize the effects of hypoglycemic agents.

Dose. Once the diagnosis of premature labor is established, ritodrine is given at an initial dose of 50-100 μg/min by i.v. infusion. The dose is increased by 50 μg/min every 10 min to a maximum dose of 35 μg/min until uterine contractions stop or unacceptable side effects occur. Dose is individualized to patient response, and the i.v. infusion is continued for 12-14 hours. Oral ritodrine is then given 10-20 mg every 4 hours.

Efficacy. There is no uniform agreement about the efficacy of β-adrenergic therapy for premature labor. In a series of double-blind prospective studies (2, 25), ritodrine was shown to be superior to placebo or ethanol infusion, and the ritodrine-treated group showed a significant decrease in perinatal mortality. These reports of greater efficacy and fewer side effects seem to establish ritodrine as the tocolytic agent of choice for treatment of preterm labor.

MAGNESIUM SULFATE

Parenterally administered magnesium sulfate is commonly used in the management of toxemic patients.

Pharmacological Effects. *Uterus.* A single study reported the effectiveness of magnesium sulfate in stopping premature labor (37). The effect seems to be directly related to the degree of dilatation of cervix at the time treatment is started. If treatment is started before the cervix is dilated more than 1 cm, it is very likely that premature labor will stop.

Side Effects. In the presence of high serum levels, CNS depressant action and curarelike action at the neuromuscular junction may be seen in the mother. Hypotonia may be seen in the newborn infant if delivery takes place while the drug is administered or very soon after its discontinuation.

The exact mechanism by which magnesium sulfate acts is not known. It is thought, however, that an elevated level of magnesium brings about a decrease in acetylcholine release and stabilizes muscle cytoplasm and its membrane.

Dose. A 2% solution of magnesium sulfate in 5% of dextrose in water is administered i.v. followed by administration of 1% magnesium sulfate solution infused at the rate of 100 ml/hr (1 g/hr).

PROGESTOGENS

In pregnant women, plasma progesterone levels gradually increase to a plateau at around 32 weeks of gestation. It has been postulated that parturition in women is preceded by a withdrawal of progesterone. Although a drop in progesterone may precede labor in some animal species, there is conflicting evidence for this in humans. Csapo (9) has reported low values of plasma progesterone in patients in premature labor. Progestational agents have been efficacious in the prevention of spontaneous abortion, although in gravid patients undergoing operations unrelated to delivery, no significant difference in abortion rate was noted between patients who received medroxyprogesterone acetate before and after surgery when compared with those who did not.

Recently, Johnson et al (17) have demonstrated in a well-controlled study the beneficial effect of 17-hydroxyprogesterone caproate over placebo in preventing premature labor when administered prophylactically in selected high-risk patients prone to develop premature labor. Although no complication attributable to the progestational agent was observed, the study population was too small for assessment of immediate or long-term safety.

Some studies indicate that administration of progestational compounds during the early stages of pregnancy may induce major congenital anomalies, further studies are therefore needed to clarify the risk/benefit ratio.

Chemistry. 17-Hydroxyprogesterone caproate (17-OHP-C) is the caproate ester of 17-hydroxyprogesterone, a naturally occurring progesterone compound.

Pharmacological Effects. *Uterus.* The exact mechanism by which a progestational agent may inhibit uterine contraction is not known. Recently, Turnball and associates (39) presented evidence that interrelation of progesterone and estradiol plasma concentrations might have a bearing on the initiation of spontaneous labor, since a reduction in maternal plasma progesterone level occurs 3-5 weeks before the onset of labor, whereas estradiol levels continue to rise during this time. Raja et al (31) observed that patients in premature labor have abnormally high plasma estradiol levels and normal plasma progesterone levels. Their findings would suggest that in human pregnancy, a dominant estrogen effect due either to a reduction in plasma progesterone or to a disproportionate rise in plasma estradiol concentration may bring about the onset of labor. It is, therefore, possible that progestogen supplementation under such circumstances might forestall premature labor.

Pharmacokinetics. 17-OHP-C is not absorbed orally and therefore must be given parenterally. Its metabolic fate remains to be determined, although some investigators reported an increase in the kidney excretion or pregnanediol after its administration to pregnant women.

Adverse Effects. The mother may experience a temporary discomfort at the site of injection. No definite effect on the fetus is known at this time.

Preparations. *17-Hydroxyprogesterone caproate injection* USP (DELALUTIN) is available in an oily solution of 125 mg/ml (in sesame oil) or 250 mg/ml (in castor oil) for i.m. injection. It has been injected at 250-mg dose once a week for prevention of premature labor.

PROSTAGLANDIN SYNTHETASE INHIBITORS

Prostaglandins E_2 and F_2, synthesized by the endometrium, are known to be powerful oxytocin agents. They are thought to play a role in parturition and have also been implicated in the spasmodic pain associated with dysmenorrhea (pain associated with menstruation). On this basis, drugs that inhibit prostaglandin synthesis have been evaluated for their efficacy in treatment of both premature labor and dysmenorrhea.

Pharmacological Effects. ***Uterus.*** *In vitro* studies have demonstrated that prostaglandin synthetase inhibitors inhibit spontaneous uterine contractions as well as prostaglandin production. In pregnant rats and in subhuman primates, these agents prolong both the time of onset of labor and the process of expulsion of the fetus. In women who had ingested high doses of acetylsalicylic acid for at least 6 months of pregnancy, the length of gestation, frequency of postmaturity, and mean duration of spontaneous labor were found to be greater than those in a group of women who did not consume aspirin (24).

In 40% of 50 women of 25-36 weeks gestation who were in preterm labor and who were given indomethacin suppositories and oral tablets, uterine contractions were abolished by the drug, irrespective of whether the membranes were intact or ruptured (42). Although the effectiveness of prostaglandin inhibitors in preterm labor is not completely established, it is interesting to note that indomethacin successfully inhibited uterine contractions for more than 7 days in 11 of 13 patients (85%) with ruptured membranes in preterm labor. In 9 of these 11 patients, pregnancy was continued until term. The reported premature closure of ductus arteriosus in some neonates has severely restricted the use of such therapy in this condition.

The presence of high amounts of prostaglandin F_2 in the menstrual blood of women suffering from dysmenorrhea has been demonstrated (28), and prostaglandin synthetase inhibitors have been used with success in the treatment of this condition, with the clinical efficacy correlated with diminished uterine contractions (41).

The prostaglandin synthetase inhibitors have not been approved by the FDA for use in premature labor. Zuckerman and associates (42) administered 100 mg of indomethacin rectally and followed this with 25 mg orally every 6 hours until contractions ceased. Repetitive doses of indomethacin were given and the total dosage used in their study ranged from 200 to 1100 mg.

Adverse Effects and Contraindications. Side effects that could be observed in the mother are discussed in Chapter 13.2. Fetal/neonatal side effects include premature closure of ductus arteriosus, transient primary pulmonary hypertension, and neonatal hemorrhage from abnormality of platelet function. Therapy is contraindicated in patients with active gastrointestinal lesions, the drugs should be used cautiously in patients with epilepsy and psychiatric disorders.

GENERAL ANESTHETICS

The uterine relaxant action of many general anesthetic agents limits their usefulness in obstetrics. Uterine relaxation can actually lead to uterine atony and increased postpartum bleeding, and is, therefore, avoided. However, in certain situations (breech decompositon and replacement of acutely inverted uterus) it may be useful.

MORPHINE AND MEPERIDINE

It is now accepted that morphine or meperidine, if used as analgesia in labor, may lead to a prolongation of the latent phase of labor. Once labor is established, it is unlikely to affect uterine contractility. Because these agents cross the placenta and can cause respiratory depression in the newborn, they are best avoided a few hours prior to expected delivery.

Table 19-4 summarizes characteristics of several tocolytic agents including their mechanism of action, side effects, and contraindications.

Table 19-4
Tocolytic Agents

Drug	Mechanism of Action	Route of Adminis-tration	Side Effects: Maternal	Side Effects: Fetal	Contraindications
Ethanol	Inhibition of endogenous oxytocin release; depression of myometrium; antagonism to prostaglandins	i.v.	Inebriation, respiratory depression, nausea, vomiting, aspiration pneumonia, hypoglycemia	Intoxication, CNS depression, muscular hypotonia	Liver disease, diabetes
β-Adrenergic stimulants (ritodrine)	Stimulation of β_2-adrenergic receptors in the myometrium, causing relaxation	i.v./ p.o. (?)	Tachycardia, hypotension, hypokalemia, nervousness	Mild tachycardia	Diabetes, cardiac patients on digitalis
Magnesium sulfate	Decrease in acetylcholine release, stabilizing muscle cytoplasm and its membrane	i.v.	Warmth, flushing, nausea, headache, respiratory depression	CNS depression, hypotonia	Cardiac disease, impaired renal function
Progesterone	Inhibition of myometrial contraction (?)	i.m.	Temporary discomfort at site of injection	Teratogenic effect (?)	
Prostaglandin synthetase inhibitors	Inhibition of prostaglandin synthesis, leading to decrease in uterine contraction	p.o.	GI bleeding, thrombocytopenia, allergic rashes, nausea, vomiting	Premature closing of ductus arteriosus (?), pulmonary hypertension (?), impaired platelet function leading to increased bleeding time (?)	GI tension, allergy, impaired platelet function

REFERENCES

1. Abdul-Karim, R. and Assali, N.S. Renal functions in human pregnancy.V. Effects of oxytocin on renal hemodynamics and water and electrolyte excretion. *J. Lab. Clin. Med.* 57:522, 1961.
2. Barden, T.P., Peter, J.B. and Merkatz, I.R. Ritodrine hydrochloride: A betamimetic agent for use in preterm labor. *Obstet. Gynecol.* 56:1, 1980.
3. Caldeyro-Barcia, R. and Posiero, J.J. Oxytocin and contractility of the human uterus. *Ann. N. Y. Acad. Sci.* 75:813, 1959.
4. Caritis, S.N., Edelston, D.I. and Mueller-Heubach, E. Pharmacologic inhibition of preterm labor. *Am. J. Obstet. Gynecol.* 133:557, 1979.
5. Caritis, S.N., Sheilin, L., Toig, G. and Wong, L.K. Pharmacodynamics of ritodrine in pregnant women during preterm labor. *Am. J. Obstet. Gynecol.* 147:752, 1983.
6. Carsten, M.E. Regulation of myometrial composition, growth, and activity. In: *Biology of Gestation Vol. 1. The Maternal Organism* (Assali, N.S., ed.). New York: Academic Press, 1968.
7. Conrad, J.T. and Euland, K. Reduction of the stretch modules of human cervical tissue by prostaglandin E_2. *Am. J. Obstet. Gynecol.* 126:218, 1976.
8. Csapo, A. Function and regulation of the myometrium. *Ann. N. Y. Acad. Sci.* 75:790, 1959.
9. Csapo, A.I. The prospect of prostaglandins in postconceptual therapy. *Prostaglandins* 3:245, 1973.
10. du Vigneaud, V., Ressler, C., Swan, J.M., Roberts, C.W., Katsoyannis, P.G. and Gordon, S. Synthesis of an octapeptide amine with the hormonal activity of oxytocics: Enzymatic cleavage of glycinamide from vasopressin and a proposed structure for this pressor antidiuretic hormone of the posterior pituitary. *J. Am. Chem. Soc.* 75:4879, 1953.
11. Feeney, J.G. Water intoxication and oxytocin. *Br. Med. J.* 285:243, 1982.
12. Freysz, H. et al. A long-term evaluation of infants who received a betamimetic drug while *in utero. J. Perinant. Med.*5:94, 1977.
13. Fuchs, A-R. Oxytocin and the onset of labor in rabbits. *J. Endocrinol.* 30:217, 1964.
14. Fuchs, A-R. Prostaglandins. In: *Endocrinology of Pregnancy*, 2nd ed. (Fuchs, F. and Clopper, A., eds.) Hagerstown: Harper and Row 1977, p. 294.
15. Fuchs, F., Fuchs, A-R, Poblete V.F., Jr. and Risk, A. Effect of alcohol on threatened premature labor. *Am. J. Obstet. Gynecol.* 99:627, 1967.
16. Huisjes, H.J. and Touwen, B.C.L. Neonatal outcome and treatment with ritodrine—A controlled study, *Am. J. Obstet. Gynecol.* 147:250, 1983.
17. Johnson, J.W.C., Austin, K.L., Jones, G.S., Davis, G.H. and King, T.M. Efficacy of seventeen alphahydroxy progesterone caproate in the prevention of premature labor. *N. Engl. J. Med.* 293:675, 1975.
18. Karim, S.M.M. and Amy, J.J. Interruption of pregnancy with prostaglandins. In: *Prostaglandins and Reproduction* (Karim S.M.M., ed.) Baltimore: University Park Press, 1975, p. 77.

19. Karim, S.M.M. and Hillier, K. Physiological roles and pharmacological actions of prostaglandins in relation to human reproduction. In: *Prostaglandins and Reproduction* (Karim, S.M.M., ed.). Baltimore: University Park Press, 1975, p. 23.

20. Karim, S.M.M. and Sharma, S.D. The effect of alcohol on prostaglandins E_2 and $F_{2\alpha}$-induced uterine activity in pregnant women. *J. Obstet. Gynecol. Br. Commonw.* 78:251, 1971.

21. Kitchin, A.H., Lloyd, S.M. and Pickford, M. Some actions of oxytocin on the cardiovascular system in man. *Clin. Sci.* 18:399, 1959.

22. Lauson, H.D. Fate of the neurohypophysial hormones. In: *International Encyclopedia of Pharmacology and Therapeutics*, Vol. 1, Section 41. *Pharmacology of the Endocrine System and Related Drugs.* (Heller, H. and Pickering, B.T., eds.) Oxford: Pergamon Press, 1970, p. 377.

23. Lamaire, W.J. Spellacy, W.N., Shevach, A.B. and Gall, S.A. Changes in plasma estriol and progesterone during labor induced with prostaglandin $F_{2\alpha}$ or oxytocin. *Prostaglandins.* 2:93, 1972.

24. Lewis, R.B. and Schulman, J.D. Influence of acetylsalicylic acid, an ihhibitor of prostaglandin synthetase, on the duration of human gestation and labor. *Lancet.* 2:1159, 1973.

25. Merkatz, I.R., Peter, J.B. and Barden, T.P. Ritodrine hydrochloride: A betamimetic agent for use in preterm labor. *Obstet. Gynecol.* 56:7, 1980.

26. Miller, F.C., Nochimson, D.J., Paul, R.H. and Hon, E.H. Effects of ritodrine hydrochloride on uterine activity and the cardiovascular system in toxemic patients. *Obset. Gynecol.* 47:50, 1976.

27. Passmore, R., and Robson, J. Drugs and the reproductive system. In: *A Companion to Medical Studies.* London: Blackwell Scientific Publications, 1968.

28. Pickles, B.R., Hall, W.J., Best, F.A. and Smith, C.N. Prostaglandins in endometrium and menstrual fluid from normal and dysmenorrhoeic subjects. *J. Obstet. Gynecol. Br. Commonw.* 72:185, 1965.

29. Pritchard, J.A. and Macdonald, P.C. Physiology of labor. In: *William's Obstetrics.* New York: Appleton-Century-Crofts, 1980, p. 369.

30. Pritchard, J.A. and Macdonald, P.C. Conduct of normal labor and delivery. In: *William's Obstetrics.* New York: Appleton-Century-Crofts, 1980, p. 405.

31. Raja, R.L.T., Anderson, A.B.M. and Turnbull, A.C. Endocrine changes in premature labour. *Br. Med. J.* 4:67, 1974.

32. Rucker, M.P. The action of adrenalin on the pregnant human uterus. *South Med. J.* 18:412, 1925.

33. Sala, N.L. The milk-ejecting effect induced by oxytocin and vasopressin during human pregnancy. *Am. J. Obstet. Gynecol.* 89:626, 1964.

34. Souney, P.F., Kaul, A.F. and Osathanondh, R. Pharmacotherapy of preterm labor. *Clin. Pharmacol.* 2:29, 1983.

35. Stander, R.W., Barden T.P., Thompson, J.F., Pugh, W.R. and Werts, C.E. Fetal cardiac effects of maternal isoxuprine infusion. *Am. J. Obstet. Gynecol.* 89:729, 1964.

36. Steer, M.L., Atlas, D. and Levitzki, A. Inter-relations between β-adrenergic receptors, adenylate cyclase and calcium. *N. Engl. J. Med.* 292:409, 1975.

37. Steer, C.M. and Petrie, R.H. A comparison of magnesium sulfate and alcohol for the prevention of premature labor. *Am. J. Obstet. Gynecol.* 129:1, 1977.

38. Theobald, G.W. Nervous control of uterine activity. *Clin. Obstet. Gynecol.* 11:15, 1968.

39. Turnbull, A.C., Flint, A.P.F., Jeremy, J.Y., Patten, P.T., Keirse, M.J.N.C. and Anderson, A.B.M. Significant fall in progesterone and rise in estradiol levels in human peripheral plasma before onset of labor. *Lancet.* 1:101, 1074.

40. Van Dyke, H.B. and Ames, R.G. Alcohol diuresis. *Acta Endocrinol.* 7:110, 1951.

41. Wiqvist, N. Prostaglandins and their synthetase inhibitors in primary dysmenorrhoea. In: *Practical Applications of Prostaglandins* (Karim, S.M.M., ed.). Baltimore: University Park Press, 1979, p. 217.

42. Zuckerman, H. and Harpaz-Kerpel, S. Prostaglandins and their inhibitors in premature labor. In: *Practical Applications of Prostaglandins* (Karim, S.M.M., ed.) Baltimore: University Park Press, 1979, p. 411.

CHAPTER
20

SKIN PHARMACOLOGY

Seven A. Kvorning, Jens Schou and Rebat M. Halder

The *skin* constitutes the barrier between the organism and the exterior that prevents foreign compounds from penetrating into the systemic circulation. Therefore, medications applied to the skin in dermatological preparations exert their effects mainly in the area where they are administered. For a drug to produce a systemic effect, the barrier must be penetrated by injection to instill the drug solution into the highly vascularized subcutaneous or muscular tissue where rapid absorption takes place.

ANATOMY AND PHYSIOLOGY

The human skin consists of three distinct layers, the epidermis, dermis, and subcutis.

Epidermis. The barrier function of the skin is mainly, due to the outermost keratinized layer of the stratified, squamous epithelium of the epidermis, the stratum corneum, consisting of 10-15 layers of keratinized cells. The stratum corneum protects the organism against water loss and also against entry of noxious compounds from the surrounding atmosphere as well as from liquids and solids getting in contact with the skin surface. The cells (keratinocytes) of the stratum corneum represent the final stage of epidermal cell proliferation in which the cells move toward the surface and finally end up being desquamated from the stratum corneum. The sequence of going from the actively dividing cell to reaching the surface as a keratinocyte takes about 1 month.

Dermis. While the epidermis is ectodermal epithelial tissue, the dermis (corium) is connective tissue derived from mesoderm. Dermis is much thicker than epidermis, but the relative cellular content is low whereas the amount of connective tissue fibers and ground substance is high. The fibroblasts produce the interstitial matrix of collagen fibers and hyaluronic acid that binds water in the connective tissue ground substance. There is a high degree of vascularization in this part of the skin, which also contains sensory nerve endings. The cutaneous appendages, such as the pilosebaceous follicles and sweat glands, are situated here as well. The secretory parts of the sweat glands are here and to some extent in the subcutaneous tissue (see later). Their excretory ducts penetrate the epidermis to reach the surface.

Subcutis. The subcutaneous tissue like dermis is of mesodermal origin and is characterized by a high-fat content in lipocytes forming a thermal insulation layer. It may be considered a specialized part of the dermis. The cellular density is low; besides lipocytes, fibroblasts are the dominant cells.

The function of the subcutaneous tissue, aside from thermal insulation, is to protect the viscera and bones against physical trauma (i.e., to function as a shock absorber).

PATHOLOGY AND THERAPY

The pathological disorders of epidermis and dermis are similar to the disease reactions shown by epithelial and connective tissues in any other part of the body. Like other epithelial tissues, epidermis may show hyperproliferation or hypoproliferation and delayed maturation. The characteristic reaction of connective tissue to infectious, mechanical, chemical, thermal, or other physical stimuli is inflammation. In this respect dermis and subcutis react as typical connective tissue. Further, allergic phenomena are often indicated both clinically and histopathologically. The most frequent pathological reaction of the skin is dermatitis, which may manifest itself in many different forms as seborrheic, eczematous, atopic, neuro- or contact dermatitis, to mention some examples. It is characteristic of the different forms of dermatitis for the pathological changes to involve the the epidermis, and the appendages.

Furthermore, many pathological reactions observed in the skin are only the apparent superficial signs of systemic diseases. Scaling of the skin may lead the dermatologist to diagnose hypothyroidism; hirsutism and acne may be initial signs of hormonal imbalance, and graying of the hair can be the first noticed sign of pernicious anemia. In other cases, the dermatologist has to institute systemic therapy against diseases where skin symptoms are dominant (e.g., when glucocorticoids are administered for very severe conditions or therapeutic doses of vitamins are administered for vitamin deficiencies with skin symptoms).

PREPARATIONS AND THERAPEUTIC EFFECT

Topical therapy used for skin disorders involves the use of the active ingredient(s) in a vehicle that is expected to be inactive. The therapeutic response, however, is very dependent not only on the active ingredient, but also on the qualities of the vehicle of the preparation. This is partly due to the importance of the vehicle for the uptake of the active ingredient from the preparation into the skin, and partly due to the healing influence of chemically inactive vehicles on skin disorders.

In general, topical therapy enables us to apply drugs in high concentration directly on the diseased skin. Systemic side effects depend on the absorption of the active ingredient; therefore, penetration into the skin to elicit the therapeutic response includes also the potential for production of systemic side effects (e.g., with topical adrenocorticosteroids).

Percutaneous Absorption. The mechanism of absorption from topical preparations is of relevance both for the potential of therapeutic responses and for the occurrence of side reactions. The passage of drug molecules through the stratum corneum depends on the hydration of this barrier layer. Hydration is maintained by continuous lipid layers and by most water-containing vehicles. The hydrated stratum corneum is much more permeable than it is in the unhydrated state. The distribution of a drug between a topical preparation and the stratum corneum follows the partition coefficient (skin/preparation) for the compound at steady rate conditions. This partition coefficient may be determined experimentally. The further passage through the skin follows Fick's law of diffusion. Accordingly, the following equation can be used to describe skin absorption, including the major factors involved in the kinetics:

$$\frac{dQ}{dt} = \frac{D(PC)C_v}{h}$$

where dQ/dt = steady rate of penetration; D = effective diffusion constant of the drug in the skin barrier; PC = effective partition coefficient (skin/vehicle); C_v = drug concentration in vehicle; and h = effective thickness of skin barrier.

The equation leaves out the blood flow in the area. This seems reasonable as it is generally agreed that the passage through the stratum corneum is the rate-limiting step in the process of skin absorption.

Whereas small molecules seem to be absorbed through the cells of stratum corneum, it is often assumed that the large molecules of corticosteroid hormones penetrate the appendages (sebaceous glands) as well as the cells of stratum corneum. But in general it can be said that skin is a slow route of absorption, although very special compounds such as liquid choline esterase inhibitors with high lipid-solubility may penetrate to toxic and even lethal amounts.

Intradermal and Subcutaneous Administration. The protective barrier of the skin is penetrated by injections. The drug solution is distributed just below the epidermis (intradermal injections) or infiltrates the loose and well-vascularized dermal and subcutaneous tissue (subcutaneous injections).

Intradermal injections lead to the formation of a wheal. Only amounts of 0.1 ml or less should be injected as close to the surface as possible, by use of a short and very thin needle. Intradermal injection of histamine solutions elicits the triple response of Lewis: localized redness at the site of injection due to direct vasodilation, surrounded by a bright red flush or flare due to indirect vasodilation resulting from axon reflexes, and subsequent replacement of localized redness by edema causing wheal formation (see Chapter 13.4). This reaction is also seen when histamine-releasing drugs such as morphine are injected intracutaneously. Intracutaneous injections are only used for diagnostic purposes, especially to diagnose antigen-antibody reactions in allergies.

Subcutaneous injections, on the other hand, give larger volumes of drug solutions (0.5-2 ml) into the tissue for absorption. The injections are given with a long slender needle into a fold of the skin raised between thumb and index finger. The solvent should be water; the solution should be isotonic; and pH should not differ too much from physiological conditions, especially not in buffered solution. Local anesthetics and epinephrine solutions can be rather acid (pH down to 3 by hydrochloric acid) without causing any harm to the tissue, as the solution is rapidly neutralized after injection. Alkaline solutions, however, should never be injected into the skin. Severe necrosis has resulted from injection of barbiturate solutions and also after accidental perivenous injections.

After subcutaneous injection, absorption is rapid, and the rate is inversely related to molecular size of the injected drug. However, the same amount of drug will be absorbed at a higher rate when given in a small volume with higher concentration than when a larger volume of a more dilute solution is injected. This seems to be due to the longer mean diffusion distance for the drug molecules to reach the capillaries in the latter case.

Transdermal Drug Administration. Transdermal drug administration is a therapeutic method to deliver drugs for systemic use through intact skin. Since the skin is the most extensive and accessible organ system of the body, and is separated by less than a millimeter of tissue from the underlying vascular system, it is ideal for drug administration.

The transdermal route of drug delivery eliminates variations in gastrointestinal absorption associated with oral administration. It also provides more efficient drug utilization and administers the drug at a controlled rate, thus eliminating pulse entry into the circulation. Transdermal delivery also gives the advantage of rapid termination of absorption of medication if needed.

The main barrier to transdermal absorption is the stratum corneum which because of its high-lipid content makes it impermeable to organic substances. Thus, by following Fick's law of diffusion, a proper balance in the partition coefficient is needed to give optimum flux for an administered drug. The absorption of a transdermally administrated drug is also dependent on the physical form of the drug. Low-molecular-weight drugs and nonionized drugs are more easily absorbed. Currently, scopolamine and nitroglycerine are available as transdermally administered drugs. Contraceptives, antihypertensive and anticancer drugs, and analgesics are currently being evaluated for transdermal administration.

Topical Therapy. Most skin therapy is used for symptomatic relief with the exception of antimicrobial therapy, which is instituted on a clear-cut indication. The major targets for symptomatic therapy are pruritus or itching, to be treated by antipruritic drugs or agents with local anesthetic effect: inflammatory reactions, against which the corticosteroid preparations have their main use; and finally, the uncontrolled proliferative conditions, including tumors, psoriasis, and condylomata, where cytotoxic and other growth-reducing therapies are used. Symptomatic skin therapy uses an advanced combination of vehicles and active ingredients.

There is no sharp distinction between drug preparations for skin diseases and cosmetic products marketed to promote the appearance of the body surface. Therefore, cosmetics are included for consideration in this chapter. The safety of cosmetics is regulated by the FDA and other regulatory authorities in different countries, the major purpose of regulation being to protect the population against hazardous effects of cosmetics.

AGENTS FOR TOPICAL USE

VEHICLES

Topical medications usually contain one or more active ingredients incorporated in a base that represents a drug form or vehicle. Although the vehicles consist of pharmacologically inert substances, many of them can influence the quality of the skin surface owing to their physical properties and can be therapeutically beneficial. On the other hand, the active ingredients interfere with chemical processes that control growth and function of living cells in epidermis and dermis. The principal constituents of vehicles include liquids (water, alcohol, organic solvents), powders, oils, and ointment bases. Besides the active ingredients, preservatives and cosmetics may be added to the vehicle.

Most vehicles have three major functions: (1) to form a reservoir storing the active ingredient; (2) to allow release and transport of suitable amounts of one or more therapeutic chemicals; and (3) to provide reasonable volume, consistency, and so on, for safe and practical application.

In addition to serving as carriers for active ingredients, many of the vehicles are used for their physical action alone, some giving relief from uncomfortable surface sensations, such as an ointment that makes a rough surface smooth. Correspondingly, a powder can reduce friction in skin folds, and an opaque liniment will shield an irritated skin from sun or irradiating heat.

The choice of local treatment demands a selection of vehicles as well as active chemicals. The factors influencing the selection of a vehicle include: hydrating, drying, or lubricating property of the vehicle; its ability to hold, release, or assist in the absorption (through stratum corneum) of the active ingredient; stability of the active agent in the vehicle; and the interactions, (physical and chemical) of the vehicle, stratum corneum, and active agents. Table 20-1 contains basic recommendations of the vehicle.

Depending upon the vehicle, dermatological formulations can be grouped as powders, wet dressings, liquid preparations (lotions, paints, shake lotions, tinctures), and lubricating preparations (gels, creams, ointments, paste).

Table 20-1
Basic Recommendations of Vehicles to Suit Various Skin Conditions

	Pastes	Ointments	Creams	Gels	Aqueous Solutions	Alcoholic Solutions	Shake Lotions	Powders
Dry scaling skin	(•)	•	•		•			
Moist skin[a]	(•)		•	•			•	
Oozing skin[a]			•		•		•	
Wounds		•		•	•			•
Scalp		•		•		•		
Skin folds	•		•				•	•

[a] Moist skin contains a small amount of water and low molecular solutes (e.g., in the axilla or during perspiration). In oozing skin, serous (protein-containing) exudate penetrates through micropores of stratum corneum (e.g., in acute eczema).

POWDERS

Powders consist of fine particles derived from plant products (polysaccharides, cellulose, silk protein), inorganic materials (boric acid, chalk, kaolin, talc, bentonite, titanium dioxide), or synthetic organicals (zinc or magnesium stearate). The function of a powder is physical (e.g., absorbing moisture and protecting the skin by avoiding friction). It can produce a local cooling effect by increasing evaporation. Some powders (e.g., of dextran) are hydrophilic and can exert high capillary activity. Applied on wounds, they serve as a chromatographic substance and remove different chemical products and reduce the microbial colonization. Powders are usually inert, but many of them change their qualities, if they become wet, not only mechanically but by making direct chemical contact. Mineral powders can induce granuloma formation if introduced under the epidermis, as in surgical wounds.

WET DRESSINGS

Wet dressings are used to treat acute inflammation with exudation, oozing, and crusting. For use, soft dressings are soaked in aqueous solution containing various ingredients [e.g., aluminium acetate (1:10-1:40 concentration), potassium permanganate (0.025-0.5%; astringent; stains skin), silver nitrate (0.1-0.5%); antimicrobial; stains skin and clothing)]. Other agents include copper or zinc sulfate, aluminum sulfate, and calcium acetate.

LIQUID PREPARATIONS

Lotions and paints are liquid medications. Their viscosity will usually be a little higher than for alcohol and water. They are suited for direct application of active drugs on the skin, particularly where an evanescent base is convenient. Lotions with glycerol and propylene glycol are used for dry and scaling skin, as they retain water in the epidermis. Shake lotions are suspensions of powder in a liquid, usually water with alcohol and glycerin that require shaking before application. Recently, commercial emulsions usually of thin uniform consistency have also been included in this category. Lotions are used to treat subacute inflammations after the severe exudation has stopped. The evaporation of this liquid provides intensive cooling; later, they have protective powder effect and can carry several active, dissolved, or dispensed ingredients. They are well tolerated, except when the skin feels dry, and allergic reactions are rare.

Zinc oxide, talc (mainly hydrous magnesium sulfate), glycerin, and water make a basic white shake lotion. A small amount of ferric oxide added to zinc oxide provides a pink color to the mixture—calamine which is used in shake lotion. Alcohol (added to a concentration of about 15%) and menthol (0.25-2%) enhance drying and cooling effects. Alcoholic or hydroalcoholic solutions of medicinal substances generally containing 10-20% (W/V) of the drug are known as tinctures. Phenol (0.5-1.5%) and camphor (1-3%), both of which affect cutaneous nerve transmission, and also menthol (0.25-2%), salicylic acid (1-2%), and coal tar solution (3-10%) impart antipruritic actions.

LUBRICATING PREPARATIONS

Lubricating preparations can vary from a low-viscosity oil to a stiff paste, depending on ingredients and pharmaceutical preparations. They are often named after their similarity to nonmedical products (cream, gel, and so on). The ingredients include some natural fats. Gels, oils, pastes, and waxes usually have a homogenous phase in which active ingredients will be dissolved or evenly distributed as particles, but creams, milks, and most ointments have two or more phases emulgated in each other. Theoretically, one of these phases will be water and the other an oil. Emulsions are described as oil in water (o/w; usually "cream") or water in oil (w/o; usually "ointment").

Fats include mineral fats (liquid, soft, and hard paraffin), animal fats (lard), wool wax (lanolin), beeswax, spermacet, and vegetable oil. Animal fats emulsify easily with detergents or soap. Wool waxes are hydrophilic and good emulgators and have a high "emollient" effect, but allergy is frequent, because their hydrophilic quality makes them particularly suited for treatment of weeping skin, which accelerates sensitization.

Gels are transparent or opaque, semisolid or solid (jellylike) colloidal dispersions. Examples are aqueous, acetone, alcohol, or propylene glycol gels of organic polymers such as agar, gelatin, cellulose, pectin, and others. On contact with skin, gel liquifies and dries to a greaseless nonocclusive film. *Jellies* are the subclass of gels containing a large amount of water and sometimes other ingredients, and are particularly applied to mucous membrane. They serve as lubricants for surgical gloves, finger cots, catheters, and for sexual intercourse. Gels can produce irritation (burning, stinging) or a drying sensation in some patients.

Creams and ointments are semisolid preparations that have protective and emollient properties and serve as vehicles for many drugs. They are particularly used for chronic inflammatory skin conditions with dry, thickened, scaling, pruritic, and lichenified lesions. These preparations hold or absorb water to promote skin rehydration; some of them repel water. Examples of different types of ointments include: *Hydrophilic Ointment,* USP, *Cold Cream,* USP, *Hydrophilic Petrolatum,* USP, *Anhydrous Lanolin,* USP, *Petrolatum,* NF, *White Petrolatum,* USP, *White Ointment,* USP, and *Hydrophilic Ointment,* USP.

Paste consists of a finely divided powder (listed earlier) incorporated into an ointment base (usually petrolatum). Such a mixture protects the skin against external irritants and sunlight. Titanium dioxide has particularly good sunscreen properties. *Zinc Oxide Paste,* USP is a commonly prescribed protective paste. Pastes protect the skin from friction caused by clothing and bandages.

ACTIVE INGREDIENTS

CAUSTICS

Caustics are destructive chemicals that cause denaturation of protein, dead or living. They are used against benign tumors and inflammatory granulation tissue. Silver nitrate (sticks or solution), trichloracetic acid, and bichloracetic acid (Kahlenberg solution) are used in concentrated solutions (30-50%). Caustic zinc choride paste is used for treatment of invading epitheliomas. Ferric subsulfate (Monsel's solution) and aluminium chloride can produce hemostasis during superficial surgical procedures by coagulating skin proteins.

KERATOLYTICS

SALICYLIC ACID

Salicylic acid is widely used in dermatological therapy as a keratolytic agent. Low concentrations of 1-5% are useful in acne vulgaris, seborrheic dermatitis, and psoriasis. Higher concentrations of 6-16% are useful for the treatment of calluses and warts, and 40% salicylic acid as a plaster is effective for corns and resistant warts.

The mechanism of action of salicylic acid in producing its keratolytic action is not well known. It is thought that salicylic acid may solubilize epidermal cell proteins that keep the stratum corneum intact. This results in desquamation of keratotic debris that helps in disorders with increased keratin production.

Salicylic acid is absorbed percutaneously with peak plasma levels occurring 6-12 hr after application (26). It is excreted slowly in the urine. To avoid salicylism, it should not be used over large areas or for prolonged periods of time.

Salicylic acid has been used to treat superficial fungal infections (Whitfield's ointment), but the antifungal effects are due to its keratolytic rather than fungistatic effects.

Patients who are allergic to salicylates may develop urticarial, allergic, or erythema multiforme-type reactions with topical application. Caution must be used in patients with peripheral vascular disease or diabetes as inflammation, ulceration, and necrosis may occur in these patients with excessive use or with high concentration.

PROPYLENE GLYCOL

Propylene glycol is used as a vehicle for topical organic compounds. However, in concentrations of 40-70% it works as a keratolytic agent by increasing the solubility of proteins in water and denaturing protein. Propylene glycol will alter keratin to hydrate and soften the skin (7). It is useful with or without salicylic acid to treat ichthyoses, keratodermas of palms and soles, keratosis pilaris, pityriasis rubra pilaris, and psoriasis. Propylene glycol in a 50% mixture with water is useful in treating tinea versicolor to remove scales.

Propylene glycol is minimally absorbed through the skin. Its main metabolite is pyruvic acid. Propylene glycol may cause an irritant contact dermatitis in some patients, especially those with eczema.

UREA

Urea is used as a cream or lotion form for dry and ichthyotic conditions of the skin. It hydrates the stratum corneum by disrupting the normal hydrogen bonding of keratin proteins.

Urea is absorbed through the skin and is excreted in the urine. Since urea is a natural byproduct of metabolism, systemic toxicity is unusual. Urea can be used to increase penetration of topical medications. Urea is available in cream and lotion form in 10% and 20% concentrations. Side effects include burning and stinging, particularly with the higher concentrations.

CYTOSTATIC AGENTS

Medications in this category are used mainly in the papulosquamous disorders, particularly in psoriasis. Photochemotherapy (PUVA) is discussed under the section "Systemic Drugs."

ANTHRALIN

Anthralin is used in psoriasis because it reduces epidermal cell mitosis and turnover by directly reducing DNA synthesis (11). Anthralin was developed as a substitute for chrysarobin. It is probably the most effective nonsteroidal topical agent for treating psoriasis. But, because of side effects and its high frequency of irritation, it must be used under supervised conditions.

Anthralin is absorbed percutaneously and should not be used in patients with renal function abnormalities since it may cause renal toxicity. Anthralin should be applied only to patches of psoriasis that are not acutely inflamed. Care should be taken not to apply anthralin on hair, face, intertriginous areas, or surrounding normal skin. If excessive irritation occurs, then therapy should be stopped.

Anthralin can stain clothing permanently and skin temporarily. Anthralin is available as an ointment in 0.1, 0.25, 0.5 and 1% concentrations. It is applied without occlusion at bedtime and washed off in the morning, followed by application of a corticosteroid cream to control irritation.

TARS

Tars are used to treat papulosquamous eruptions such as psoriasis, eczema, seborrheic dermatitis, and atopic dermatitis. Tars have a similar mode of action as anthralin, that is, suppressing DNA synthesis in the epidermis. Coal tar (liquor carbonis detergens; also known as LCD) is the most common form used.

Tars are available generally as liquor carbonis detergens (LCD) in a 20% solution that can be diluted or compounded for a bath or shampoo (12). Tars are also available as lotions, creams, gels, or ointments varying from a 1-7.5% concentration, as well as shampoos for the scalp.

Coal tars are not homogenous and may contain several thousand different compounds. Because of this complexity it is difficult to characterize coal tars. Folliculitis is a common adverse reaction from coal tars. Coal tars may have an unpleasant odor. They also stain clothing and skin. Allergic reactions may occur but are less common with coal tars than juniper tar, pine tar, or birch tar. Coal tars can also be photosensitizing; however, this may be used advantageously to treat psoriasis by using ultraviolet B light after removal of the tar from the skin (modified Goeckerman regimen). Crude coal tar preparations contain aromatic hydrocarbons and may be carcinogenic if used over a prolonged period of time.

CYTOTOXIC AGENTS

CANTHARIDIN

Cantharidin is a vesicant extracted from dried blister beetles (*Cantharis vesicatoria*) also known as Spanish fly. Cantharidin acts on mitochondrial enzymes and decreases adenosine triphosphate (ATP) levels. This results in epidermal cell membrane changes with acantholysis and blister formation.

This resultant intraepidermal vesiculation is helpful in treating warts (especially periungual and plantar types), and molluscum contagiosum (6). In treating periungual and plantar warts, cantharidin is applied to the wart surface and allowed to dry. A nonporous occlusive plastic tape is applied and left on for 24 hr. The blister that forms will rupture, crust, and fall off in 7-10 days, at which time the area can be debrided and any remaining wart can be retreated. It may require several such treatments to provide a cure. For molluscum contagiosum, a single application without occlusion is often effective. This method is especially good for children since it is painless.

Treatment with cantharidin does not result in residual scarring since its effect is entirely intraepidermal. However, a complication may be a ring of warts developing at the periphery of a cantharidin-treated lesion. This is a result of intraepidermal inoculation.

It is not known how much cantharidin is absorbed after topical application. It is excreted by the kidney. Systemic toxic effects do not occur with topical use. However, ingestion can result in abdominal pain, nausea, vomiting, and shock, as well as irritation of the urinary tract. Cantharidin is available in a 0.7% concentration in a liquid vehicle.

PODOPHYLLIN

Podophyllin resin is an extract of *Podophyllum peltatum* or May apple. Podophyllin acts as a cytotoxic agent by binding to the microtubule protein of the mitotic spindle and arresting epidermal mitosis in metaphase.

The main indication for podophyllin is in the treatment of condyloma acuminatum. A 25% concentration compounded with benzoin tincture is applied weekly and washed off in 4-6 hr. Care must be taken to apply it only to wart tissue to prevent erosion of normal tissue. It is suggested that white petrolatum be applied to surrounding normal tissue to provide protection from podophyllin.

Podophyllin should be applied sparingly on large lesions because it can be absorbed. Toxic symptoms include nausea, vomiting, psychotoxic confusional states, peripheral neuropathy, adynamic ileus, coma, and even death (3). Usage of podophyllin in pregnancy is contraindicated because it is teratogenic.

FLUOROURACIL

The systemic pharmacology of fluorouracil has been described in Chapter 27. It is used topically for multiple actinic keratoses and basal cell carcinomas.

Topical application of fluorouracil does not produce systemic toxic effects since only about 6% of a topically applied dose is absorbed percutaneously. Fluorouracil inhibits thymidylate synthetase and acts selectively against atypical epidermal cells by inhibiting DNA and RNA synthesis.

Fluorouracil is available in 1 and 5% creams and 1 and 2% solutions. Concentrations of 1 and 2% are effective for lesions on the face. Lesions on the hands and forearms may require a 5% concentration. Fluorouracil is applied twice daily for 2-4 weeks until a maximal inflammatory reaction occurs. Lesions initially become erythematous and then become eroded and ulcerated at which time treatment is stopped. Reepithelialization occurs and may take 1-2 months after therapy is stopped. A medium-potency nonfluorinated topical corticosteroid may be applied during therapy to reduce an excessive inflammatory response. Fluorouracil should be applied to an entire affected area, because lesions that may not be clinically apparent will respond as well.

Side effects from topical fluorouracil include pruritus, burning, tenderness, and postinflammatory hyperpigmentation. Exposure to sunlight should be avoided during treatment and for 1-2 months following cessation of therapy. Allergic contact dermatitis may occur, and it is suggested that a normal area of skin be tested with the fluorouracil preparation that is to be used.

PROTEOLYTICS

Proteolytics that hydrolyze necrotic protein in ulcerations and thrombi can be either nonspecific, like chlorinated alkali (Dakin's solution) and chloramine (0.25-0.5%), or they can be specific enzymes for protein (trypsin), fibrin (streptokinase), or deoxyribonucleic acids (streptodornase). In local therapy, these are applied as powders or as wet dressings.

ANTIPERSPIRANTS

Antiperspirants close the sweat ducts by denaturation of keratin in and around the opening of the gland. Aluminum hydroxychloride [$Al_2(OH)_5Cl.2H_2O$], the least acidic and least corrosive of the aluminum salts, has so far been most successful (23). A 20% alcoholic solution causes an obstructive gel to form in the sweat duct.

DRUGS USED IN PIGMENTARY DISORDERS

Hyperpigmentary conditions of the skin can be treated with hydroquinone preparations. Included in these conditions are postinflammatory states, melasma, freckles, and lentigines. Hypopigmentary conditions of the skin, including vitiligo and postinflammatory states, can be treated with psoralen compounds.

HYDROQUINONE

Hydroquinone is a bleaching agent that may be applied topically for hyperpigmentation (5). Its mechanism of action is to inhibit tyrosinase activity in melanocytes. This decreases melanin synthesis and transfer of melanocytes to keratinocytes. Hydroquinone is also directly toxic to melanocytes. Nonprescription hydroquinone-containing preparations are available in strengths up to 2%. Prescription preparations contain 4-5% hydroquinone. It is advisable to use a sunscreen while undergoing treatment with hydroquinone to decrease the effect of sunlight on the hyperpigmented area. Some hydroquinone preparations contain a sunscreen already mixed with it.

Side effects from hydroquinone occur in up to 15% of patients. This is usually an allergic contact dermatitis with erythema, burning, or peeling. Hydroquinone should not be used in children less than 12 years of age.

MONOBENZONE

Monobenzone is the monobenzyl ether of hydroquinone. Its mechanism of action is the same as that of hydroquinone; however, extensive destruction of melanocytes also occurs. Depigmentation can occur at sites distant from the area of application. For this reason, the only indication for the use of monobenzone is for extensive vitiligo in which there is little normally pigmented skin left (15). Monobenzone can be used to remove remaining pigmentation in this case. Side effects are similar to hydroquinone; however, the incidence is higher. Monobenzone is available as a 20% ointment. It is advisable to dilute this to 10% concentration with a vehicle such as aquaphor for the initial application. Gradually the concentration can be increased to 20% full strength if no adverse reactions occur.

Psoralens, which are used systemically and to some extent locally for treatment of pigmentary disorders, are discussed later in this chapter.

ANTIINFLAMMATORY CORTICOSTEROIDS

The advent of topical steroids in the 1950s brought a new era in dermatological therapy. Topical steroids are effective in various diseases of the skin due mainly to their antiinflammatory effects. They act by various mechanisms including local vasoconstriction, decreasing membrane permeability, and by decreasing mitotic activity of epidermal cells, which is especially important in proliferative diseases of the epidemis such as psoriasis (13). Other effects include stabilization of lysosomes. This may be important in inhibiting release of substances such as prostaglandins, histamine, and kinins which are responsible for itching and pain in the skin. The general pharmacology of corticosteroids is discussed in Chapter 12.4.

Hydrocortisone, the naturally occurring corticosteroid from the adrenal gland, was the first topical preparation used. Presently, many topical steroids are fluorinated compounds that are more potent but are also responsible for increased side effects. Table 20-2 shows selected topical corticosteroids based on their potency.

The choice of topical corticosteroid is dependent on the type of dermatological condition treated, the anatomical location, the age of the patient, and the acuteness or chronicity of the problem. The vehicle employed is also important. Topical steroids are available as creams, ointments, or gels.

The various forms of eczema including atopic dermatitis, irritant and allergic contact dermatitis, nummular eczema, and stasis dermatitis respond to low- to medium-potency topical steroids, as does seborrheic dermatitis. Stronger topical steroids are required for psoriasis, skin lesions of systemic and discoid lupus erythematosus, lichen planus, and sarcoidosis. Chronic dermatoses should be controlled with low-potency steroids; acute problems can be treated for short periods with high-potency steroids.

The anatomical location is important in terms of the potency of topical steroid used. There is much greater absorption through thin-skinned areas, such as the face, axilla, perianal, and genital areas (20). Conditions of the skin in which there is increased permeability such as in exfoliative dermatosis also require less potent topical steroid therapy. Children and elderly patients both have increased cutaneous absorption of topical steroids as well.

Topical corticosteroids in ointment form are more penetrating than gels or creams and are effective in treating thick, scaling, or keratotic lesions such as psoriasis. Creams and gels are more drying in nature and are helpful in conditions such as acute eczemas in which there is oozing and weeping of the lesion. For the scalp, an ointment or gel form is more cosmetically acceptable than a cream.

Systemic toxicity from topically applied corticosteroids is rare. It is usually seen with high-potency fluorinated topical steroids used over an extensive body area for prolonged periods. These systemic effects are discussed in Chapter 12.4. The total weekly dose required for a high-potency steroid to cause systemic effects is 30 g or greater in adults or 10 g or greater in children. However, children should really not be given high-potency steroids. Occlusion with plastic wrap or dressings will increase percutaneous absorption of steroids.

Table 20-2
Topical Steroids Ranked by Potency

Most Potent	1	Betamethasone diproprionate oinment 0.05%
	2	Fluocinonide cream, ointment, gel 0.05% Halcinonide cream 0.1%
	3	Triamcinolone acetonide cream 0.5% Betamethasone lotion, ointment 0.1%
	4	Fluocinolone acetonide ointment 0.025% Triamcinolone acetonide ointment 0.1%
	5	Betamethasone 17-valerate cream 0.1% Fluocinolone acetonide cream 0.025% Triamcinolone acetonide cream 0.1%
	6	Desonide cream 0.05% Flumethasone pivalate cream 0.03%
Least Potent	7	Topicals with hydrocortisone, dexamethasone, prednisolone

Adverse side effects with local steroid therapy are not rare. These include skin atrophy, telangiectasia, stria, hypopigmentation, acneiform eruption, perioral dermatitis, and hypertrichosis. The use of topical corticosteroids near the eye may cause an increase in intraocular pressure. For these reasons, the selection of a topical corticosteroid should be carefully made. Fluorinated steroids should not be used on the face.

Intralesional and sublesional corticosteroids should also be mentioned. These are steroid suspensions of 5-10 mg/ml concentration. They are injected with a small needle intralesionally and are useful when a potent steroid is necessary for such lesions as keloids, hypertrophic scars, hypertrophic lichen planus, alopecia areata, and cysts of acne.

ANTIMICROBIALS

NONSPECIFIC AGENTS

For initial treatment of skin infections, in most cases *nonspecific antimicrobials* that will not cause bacterial resistance and rarely contact allergy can be used. Many organic chemicals are antibacterial agents.

Salicylic acid, resorcinol, hydroxyquinoline, phenols, and precipitated sulfur have antiseptic properties (2-5% in ointments, pastes, and shake lotions). Synthetic dyes (e.g., magenta, malachite green, euflavine, gentian violet) can be painted on in 1-10% alcoholic or aqueous solution. Iodochlorohydroxyquinoline and congeners are active toward most bacteria and fungi (1-5% alone or in composite ointments).

ANTIBACTERIAL AGENTS

The majority of topical medications with specific local action are antibiotics (10). Bacitracin, gramicidin, neomycin, and polymyxin B are not absorbed from the intestinal tract and are useful topically. Gram-positive organisms are susceptible to neomycin, bacitracin, and gramicidin. Gram-negative organisms are susceptible to polymyxin B and neomycin. Neomycin has the broadest spectrum of activity. Bacitracin is available as an ointment in 500 U/g. Neomycin is available as 0.5% cream or ointment. There are several ointment mixtures of these antibiotics available. They are bacitracin and neomycin; bacitracin and polymyxin B; bacitracin, polymyxin B, and neomycin; neomycin, gramicidin, and polymyxin B.

Erythromycin and gentamicin are available as ointments in a 0.1% concentration. They have a more limited spectrum of activity. Gentamicin is effective especially for *Pseudomonas* skin infections.

Topical solutions and creams of tetracycline, and clindamycin are available in special formulations. These are used mainly in acne vulgaris and are discussed in that section.

Neomycin is responsible for a high incidence of allergic contact dermatitis, particularly in patients with stasis dermatitis of the legs. Bacterial resistance to topical antibiotics is not a problem routinely encountered in outpatient use.

ANTIVIRAL AGENTS

Acyclovir. The pharmacology and systemic use of acyclovir has been described in Chapter 25.1. Topically, acyclovir is available as a 5% ointment. The indications for usage are the primary episode of herpes genitalis and in limited non-life-threatening mucocutaneous herpes simplex infection in immunocompromised hosts (4). Acyclovir ointment is applied every 3 hr for 7 days. It is not beneficial if it is used in other than the primary episode of herpes genitalis. The goal of treatment of the primary episode of herpes genitalis is to prevent recurrent infection so that therapy should be instituted as soon as possible in primary herpes genitalis to prevent this from occurring. The indiscriminant usage of topical acyclovir has been reported to cause resistant strains of herpes simplex to develop.

ANTIFUNGAL AGENTS

The pharmacology and mechanisms of action of the drugs mentioned are discussed in Chapter 25.2. This section will focus on therapeutics of the drugs topically used in dermatological disorders, particularly imidazoles (e.g., clotrimazole), polyene antibiotics (e.g., amphotericin B, nystatin), haloprogin, and tolnaftate. Griseofulvin and ketoconazole, which are mainly used systemically, will be discussed later under systemic drugs.

Clotrimazole. Clotrimazole is used topically for pathogenic dermatophytes. These include *Epidermophyton, Microsporum,* and *Trichophyton* species. It is also useful for *Pityrosporon orbiculare* which is not a true fungus but is the agent responsible for tinea versicolor. It is also effective against *Candida albicans* on the skin and mucous membranes. Clotrimazole is available as a cream in a 1% concentration as well as a troche for oral use and suppository for vaginal use. Adverse topical reactions include pruritus, urticaria, erythema, and burning. Topical preparations should be used carefully around the eye. Clotrimazole is applied 2 to 3 times daily for 3-4 weeks.

Amphotericin B. Amphotericin B is primarily used intravenously for systemic mycosis. It is available, however, as a 3% ointment, cream, or lotion, and is effective for cutaneous and mucocutaneous candidiasis. Topical amphotericin B is not absorbed and has no systemic effects.

Nystatin. Nystatin is a polyene antibiotic that has antifungal properties by binding to sterols in the cell membrane of the fungus. This causes membrane permeability changes allowing leakage of cellular components. It is effective topically against *Candida* species and is available in cream, ointment, or powder form in a concentration of 100,000 units/g. Nystatin is applied 2 to 3 times daily.

Haloprogin. Haloprogin is useful as a 1% cream in the topical treatment of superficial dermatophytoses. The cure rate is better than with tolnaftate. It is available as 1% cream used twice or three times a day for 3-4 weeks.

Tolnaftate. Tolnaftate is an over-the-counter (OTC) preparation useful for superficial dermatophyte infections. Reactions are uncommon. Tolnaftate is available as a 1% cream.

SCABICIDES AND PEDICULOCIDES

LINDANE

Lindane (γ-benzene hexachloride) is an effective pediculocide and scabicide (22). There is no benzene ring present although the name γ-benzene hexachloride (GBH) suggests that. About 10% of topically applied lindane is absorbed percutaneously and excreted in the urine in a 5-day period. Lindane that is absorbed is concentrated in the brain and fatty tissues. The half-life is approximately 20-24 hr.

Lindane is available as a 1% cream, lotion, or shampoo. In pediculosis capitis or pubis the shampoo form is best suited and is lathered and left on the areas for 8-12 hr and washed off. If the parasites are present 1 week after treatment, then retreatment is needed. In scabies, the lotion or cream is applied to the entire body from neck to toes and is left on for 12 hr and washed off. Retreatment is indicated only if active mites are found at least 1 week after treatment.

Allergic contact dermatitis has not been reported with lindane, however, an irritant contact dermatitis may occur around the eyes or mucous membranes, or if it is applied excessively or too frequently. Lindane should not be used on acutely inflamed skin. Lindane, because it reaches high concentrations in the brain and fatty tissues, is potentially neurotoxic causing seizure abnormalities, particularly in children (19). It can also be hematotoxic and mutagenic. Because of the neurotoxicity of lindane, it is not suggested for usage in young children. Controversy exists about this; some say that if lindane is used according to instructions it would not be toxic. Others suggest use of lindane in half strength for half the amount of time as in adults. Lindane, however, should certainly not be used in pregnant or lactating females.

CROTAMITON

Crotamiton is a scabicide as well as an antipruritic agent. It is available as a 10% cream or lotion and is applied on the entire body from neck to toes. A second application is used 24 hr later, and a bath is taken 48 hr after the last application. Allergic and irritant contact dermatitis may occur. It should not be used on acutely inflamed skin or mucous membranes or around the eyes. Crotamiton is safe in all age groups and is an effective alternative to lindane (9).

SULFUR

Precipitated sulfur in a 6-10% concentration in white petrolatum is an effective scabicide. It is applied nightly for 3 nights. Sulfur has an unpleasant odor, but it is a safe alternative in children and pregnant females. Irritation is rare.

BENZOYL BENZOATE

Benzoyl benzoate may be used as a scabicide. It is available as a 50% emulsion and is usually diluted to a 25% emulsion that is applied on the entire body from neck to toes daily for 2-3 days. Benzoyl benzoate is not toxic systematically but may cause irritation around the eyes. Irritation on the skin may occur on the genitalia or scalp.

PYRETHRINS

Pyrethrins are available as an OTC preparation for the treatment of pediculosis. They are derived from chrysanthemum plants and are available in liquid and powder forms in 0.165 to 0.3% concentrations. These preparations are applied for 10 min and then washed off. They should not be used more than twice in a 24-hr period. Irritation is uncommon except when used around the eyes or mucous membranes.

DRUGS USED IN ACNE VULGARIS

Acne vulgaris is a disorder affecting pilosebaceous follicles of mainly the face, back, and chest. There is an increase in sebum production with a resultant breakdown by the skin bacteria *Propionibacterium acnes* into free fatty acids. Those free fatty acids are irritant and comedogenic causing production of comedones, pustules, and papules. Severe cases result in deep cystic and pustular lesions known as acne conglobata. There is also a disorder of keratinization in acne vulgaris with a resultant increase in follicular keratosis. Therapy of acne vulgaris is dependent upon the severity of disease. The main drugs used for acne are benzoyl peroxide, tretinoin, antibiotics (both systemic and topical), and isotretinoin.

BENZOYL PEROXIDE

Benzoyl peroxide is used in mild-to-moderate acne vulgaris for its keratolytic effect and also for its bacteriostatic effect against *Propionibacterium acnes*. Benzoyl peroxide is absorbed after topical application with benzoic acid being the main metabolite (16). There has been no reported systemic toxicity in humans from absorption.

Local irritation with dryness and erythema is not uncommon but is usually not severe enough to discontinue treatment. However, up to 3% of patients treated with benzoyl peroxide may develop an allergic contact dermatitis. This may be severe and requires discontinuation of therapy.

Benzoyl peroxide is available in concentration of 2.5, 5 and 10% as a cream, lotion, or gel. The gel contains alcohol and is more drying. The usual application of benzoyl peroxide is at night. Care should be taken to avoid contact with the eyes and mucous membranes.

RETINOIC ACID

Retinoic acid (tretinoin or transretinoic acid) is the acid form of vitamin A. It is a keratolytic and is effective in acne vulgaris by decreasing the cohesiveness of epidermal cells causing sloughing of the stratum corneum and increasing epidermal cell turnover. This in turn is thought to decrease follicular plugging (comedones).

Applied topically, retinoic acid remains mainly in the epidermis. Small quantities that are absorbed are metabolized by the liver and excreted in bile and urine. During the first 6 weeks of therapy, there may be an aggravation of acne with patients noting an increase in the number of comedones. However, this improves with continued therapy, and there is usually marked improvement in 12-16 weeks.

Retinoic acid can be very irritating to the skin. It should be used only on dry skin, and areas around the eyes and mucous membranes should not be treated. The initial treatment should be with the minimal concentration that is enough to cause mild erythema and peeling. Retinoic acid is available as cream, gel, or lotion in concentrations from 0.01 to 0.05%. The lotion form is particularly irritating. Side effects of retinoic acid include excessive dryness and an increased risk of sunburn. Retinoic acid is very useful in acne vulgaris where comedones predominate.

TOPICAL ANTIBIOTICS

Topical antibiotics are indicated for inflammatory acne vulgaris, which is characterized by pustules and papules (25). Clindamycin, erythromycin, and tetracycline are available as solutions having concentrations ranging from 1 to 2%. Tetracycline is also available as a cream form.

Topical absorption is generally low. There are reports of pseudomembranous colitis with topical clindamycin use, but the incidence is low. Patients having regional enteritis or ulcerative colitis, however, should not be treated with topical clindamycin (14). It seems that extemporaneous preparations using clindamycin hydrochloride are implicated more frequently than commercial preparations that use clindamycin phosphate.

Side effects from topical antibiotics are mainly due to the vehicle forms used. Those containing more alcohol and propylene glycol may cause erythema, dryness, burning, and pruritus.

Bacterial resistance may occur with topical antibiotics as well as a gram-negative folliculitis from bacterial overgrowth. Minocycline is usually given orally for these complications.

SYSTEMIC ANTIBIOTICS

Systemic antibiotics are discussed in detail elsewhere. Tetracycline is the main antibiotic used for acne vulgaris. It is effective for moderate-to-severe inflammatory acne vulgaris. Erythromycin is also effective and can be used if tetracycline is contraindicated. Dosage of both can be up to 250 mg four times a day with a response occurring within 6-12 weeks. Maintenance therapy usually consists of 250 mg twice a day.

RETINOIDS

Isotretinoin. Isotretinoin is 13-cis-retinoic acid and related to retinoic acid and retinol (vitamin A). Isotretinoin inhibits sebaceous gland function and keratinization. It is 99.9% bound in human plasma, almost exclusively to albumin.

Isotretinoin is indicated only in the treatment of severe recalcitrant cystic acne unresponsive to conventional treatment modalities (18). This is because of several severe side effects and potential for teratogenicity. The exact mechanism of action of isotretinoin is unknown, but reduction of sebaceous gland size and inhibition of sebaceous gland differentiation occur, leading to decreased cyst formation.

Twenty-five percent of patients on isotretinoin develop reversible elevation of plasma triglycerides. If this is clinically important is not known, but triglyceride levels should be obtained regularly. Elevations of liver enzymes, particularly SGOT and alkaline phosphatase, occur in 10-15% of patients. This is reversible with cessation of therapy; however, isotretinoin should be discontinued when these are elevated. Cheilitis occurs in 90% of patients and conjunctivitis in 40%. Dry skin, epistaxis, xerostomia, and dry nose occur in various degrees and combinations in up to 80% of patients. Musculoskeletal pain may also occur.

Since isotretinoin is related to vitamin A, patients should not take supplementary vitamin A which may lead to symptoms of acute hypervitaminosis A, including pseudotumor cerebri. Most importantly, there have been reports of teratogenicity in human fetuses in women taking isotretinoin while pregnant. It is essential to place women on contraceptive therapy while taking isotretinoin. Pregnancy must be avoided for at least 1 month after cessation of therapy. Isotretinoin dosage is given on a weight basis of 1-2 mg/kg/day. One course of treatment of 15-20 weeks' duration is usually sufficient to clear severe cystic acne permanently.

ANTIDANDRUFF SHAMPOOS

Dandruff and seborrheic dermatitis of the scalp (seborrhea capitis) are related in that both have an increased rate of proliferation of epidermal cells. However, they differ in that the scale in dandruff is dry whereas in seborrhea capitis it is greasy. Also, in seborrhea capitis there is erythema underlying the scale. However, both are treated with the same shampoos.

SELENIUM SULFIDE

Selenium sulfide is an effective shampoo in treating dandruff and seborrhea capitis. It has antimitotic activity and substantivity, that is, residual adherence to the scalp after the shampoo is rinsed out. Selenium sulfide is left on the scalp for 5-10 min and washed out. It is applied 1 to 3 times per week.

Toxicity has not been reported with selenium sulfide with prescribed usage. Allergic contact dermatitis has not been seen; however, irritation occurs on conjunctival mucosa and acutely inflamed skin. Selenium sulfide has been noted to discolor the hair with a brownish tint. It is available as a lotion in 1% concentration (OTC) and 2.5% (by prescription). Selenium sulfide is also effective for tinea capitis caused by *T. tonsurans* as it is sporocidal for this organism (1).

ZINC PYRITHIONE

Zinc pyrithione shampoos are effective in dandruff and seborrhea capitis probably because of their cytostatic activity. Toxicity has not been reported. They are available as an OTC product in 1 and 2% concentrations.

PROTECTIVE AGENTS AGAINST SKIN IRRITANTS

Protective skin preparations are intended to reduce hazards from environmental factors. Such preparations used against specific risk factors are described as follows.

Solutions of Acid, Alkali, and Detergent. The most frequent exposure will be in industrial or domestic work through either a brief immersion or prolonged exposure to toxic detergent, acid, or alkaline solution. Protection is obtained by covering the skin with a thin film of water-repellent grease. Petrolatum with well-controlled softening and melting points will be the basic ingredient of most preparations, often with addition of chemically inactive powder. Silicon fluid (e.g., methyl phenyl polysiloxanes), constituting up to 30% of the finished product, will improve the water repellency and facilitate application.

Organic Solvents, Oils, and Greases. Efficient protection against greases and organic solvents requires a continuous film that is insoluble in the substance it is being used to protect against. The principal ingredients that are usually dissolved or gelatinated in water consist of natural products like alginates, gum acacia, and casein, or synthetic cellulose derivatives.

Irritant Small Particles. Injuries caused by small particles (such as glass dust or fiberglass) that pierce the skin are prevented by a filler of kaolin, talc, or zinc oxide dusted on the skin with a moderately greasy surface of protective cream. The filler can also be incorporated in an ointment.

Contact Allergens. Protection against contact allergens can be very difficult because most of the allergens concerned are haptens of very small molecular size and therefore are easy penetrators. Either an impenetrable film as mentioned for highly irritant materials or the presence of a substance that can bind or neutralize such an allergen may be useful for protection; for example, sodium and calcium edetate serve as chelating agents for nickel, and washing with ascorbic acid solution reduces allergenic chromium to the trivalent ion which is nonallergic.

ULTRAVIOLET RADIATION

Sunscreens. Sunscreens are substances that protect the skin against ultraviolet light from the sun (8). The most commonly used sunscreens absorb ultraviolet light; less commonly used substances reflect light and are termed sunshades. Sunscreens are useful in patients with fair skin who burn easily, in individuals using topical or systemic photosensitizing drugs, or in patients with photosensitive diseases such as lupus erythematosus or porphyria.

Sunscreens absorb ultraviolet B (UVB) light whose wavelength is 280-320 nm. UVB is responsible for most of the erythema and tanning associated with sun exposure. Ultraviolet A (UVA) light which has a wavelength of 320-400 nm requires much more energy to produce a sunburn or tan, so that most sunscreens provide maximum protection against UVB.

The substances used as sunscreens are usually of two classes, para-aminobenzoic acid (PABA) and its esters, and the benzophenones. PABA protects mainly from light with wavelengths of 280-320 nm, whereas the benzophenones have a wider spectrum of protection (250-360 nm), although the benzophenones provide less protection in the UVB range.

Currently, sunscreens are classified by their protection factor (PF) or sun protection factor (SPF) which measures a sunscreen's ability to absorb ultraviolet light. The minimal erythema doses (MED) are measured with and without sunscreen, and their ratio determines the PF. The PF ranges from 4 to 15, with sunscreens with a PF of 15 having the maximum protection.

A sunscreen's effectiveness depends on the chemical used, its concentration, and the vehicle. Substantivity or the ability of the sunscreen and vehicle to resist removal during swimming or sweating is important. Esters of PABA are more substantiative than PABA alone.

Allergic contact dermatitis can occur with most sunscreens. Other side effects include tingling or burning with PABA preparations. PABA should not be used in persons allergic to benzocaine, procaine, paraphenyldiamine, and sulfonamides. Persons allergic to thiazides and sulfa drugs should not use PABA ester-containing sunscreens.

Sunshades or physical sunscreens are opaque and reflect light completely. These include titanium oxide, zinc oxide, and red veterinary petrolatum. These, however, are not cosmetically appealing.

Insect Repellents. The skin can be protected from stinging and biting insects with repellents that prevent insects from settling on the skin due to their odor. Repellents also can be used for impregnation of clothing, and this will usually give a much longer duration of effect (2-7 days instead of 4-6 hr). The substances used have a sharp, resinous smell and are moderately irritating to the skin of the face, axillae, and genitals. Important repellents (mainly against mosquitoes) in most temperate climates are dimethylphthalate, diethyltoluamide, and ethyl hexanediol. No repellents are available against bees, wasps, and spiders.

SYSTEMIC DRUGS

ANTIMICROBIALS

Systemic *antibacterial* treatment should be conducted after bacterial diagnosis where possible. Ordinary standard doses of oral or intramuscular chemotherapy will be sufficient unless local factors (defective vascularization, heavy edema, or infiltration) reduce the concentration at the site of infection. In such cases, higher doses than the standard are necessary.

Chemotherapy for skin diseases often starts before microbiological etiology has been verified. The initial choice of drug is supported by the experience that distinct clinical manifestations are seen by very few bacterial species.

Penicillin is the first choice in erysipelas and circumscribed cellulitis, which are usually due to streptococci. In impetigo with streptococci, staphylococci, or a mixture of both, penicillin is often effective. In erysipeloid, the situation is similar. Penicillin is empirically used in erythema migrans and acrodermatitis, both diseases of unproven infectious etiology. Penicillin may be contraindicated, primarily due to a history of allergy and also in the presence of massive mycotic infection, as some fungal allergens cross-react with antibodies to penicillin. In these cases, tetracycline and erythromycin can usually be substituted.

Tetracyclines are used against infection of contaminated lesions, where mixed infection cannot be avoided. In acne vulgaris, rosacea, and perioral dermatitis, tetracycline is used in a low dosage (250-500 mg/day) for weeks or months, after 2-4 days of 1000 mg/day. Although an accumulation of tetracycline in the sebaceous glands is demonstrated, the mechanism of action is not clear. Tetracyclines are contraindicated in children and in pregnant women, and they are photosensitizing for some patients (particularly demeclocycline). Further, they have multiple occasional side effects (nail color changes, onycholysis, and fixed eruptions) (see Chapter 24.4).

Sulfonamides and sulfones are rarely used for skin infections in temperate zones. Sulfones serve as antileprotic in the tropics. In dermatitis herpetiformis, disseminated vasculitis, and subacute lupus erythematosus, all immunologically mediated diseases, dapsone can be beneficial. This can be explained not by its antimicrobial activity, but by its effect on the immune system, most likely on complement activity.

The systemic antifungal agents used in therapy of dermatological disorders include griseofulvin and ketoconazole. Griseofulvin is the drug of choice for tinea capitis for which topical antifungals do not provide a cure. Griseofulvin taken orally is not indicated for usual superficial dermatophyte infection and has no action against *Candida* species. Griseofulvin is given in a dosage of 5 mg/lb of body weight in children and 1 g/day in adults.

Duration of therapy should be 6-8 weeks, and the hair should be cultured again to make sure that there is a complete cure. Griseofulvin is also indicated for tinea barbae and for resistant tinea infections of the skin, especially hands and feet involving *Epidermophyton, Microsporum,* and *Trichophyton* species. Nail infections with fungus (onychomycosis) respond only to systemic griseofulvin. However, onychomycosis requires from 6 to 16 months of continuous treatment, and adverse effects that have been mentioned in Chapter 25.2 should be kept in mind. In onychomycosis the micronized form of griseofulvin may be used with a dosage of 1 g/day.

Ketoconazole has been useful for chronic mucocutaneous candidiasis that is severe, debilitating, and unresponsive to usual modalities. Short-term use (7 days) has cleared chronic tinea versicolor. However, side effects must be kept in mind, which are mentioned in Chapter 25.2. It is not approved for dermatophyte infections.

HORMONES

Systemic corticosteroids and corticotropic hormones are used for several dermatological symptoms and diseases. The main indications fall into three groups:

1. Severe acute, life-threatening reactions such as anaphylaxis, generalized acute contact eczema, thrombopenic purpura, allergic vasculitis, erythema multiforme exudativum, Stevens-Johnson syndrome, toxic epidermal necrolysis, and intensive and widespread allergic reactions (e.g. to insect bites and stings). Steroids are then administered in moderate or high initial doses that are gradually tapered.
2. For some generalized subacute or chronic immunological reactions (exfoliative dermatitis, disseminated and systemic lupus erythematosus, periarteritis nodosa, dermatomyositis, pemphigus vulgaris, and bullous pemphigoid) where treatment is continuous with a dose graduated after the severity of the symptoms.
3. For several other dermatoses of incompletely understood etiology (e.g., psoriasis, lichen planus, atopic dermatitis, nummular eczema, and alopecia areata), but as these diseases often have a chronic course, the risk of multiple and severe side effects from hormone treatment contraindicates use of steroids for these patients.

Sex hormones exert influence on hair growth, sebaceous glands, and water retention in the connective tissues. Testosterone has a peripheral influence on the hair follicle and a high testosterone production can induce hirsutism and acne vulgaris. The control of this phenomenon has been obtained by a blocking action of certain gestagens, most convincingly by cyproterone. Estrogens increase the hyaluronic acid content of the dermis and augment the water-binding capacity.

ANTIHISTAMINES

Systemic administration of antihistamines (H_1-antagonists) has been tried with moderate success for several skin diseases. The main indication is urticaria, erythema multiforme, eczematous eruptions, and drug eruptions. Each medication must be regarded as a trial, and if the patient is not relieved after 2 or 3 days on a substantial standard dose, the drug must be changed. Until now it has not been possible to classify the antihistaminic drugs according to efficacy because individual variations are extremely wide and side effects vary equally without correlation with the clinically positive effect. Many dermatologists give preference to drugs that combine antihistaminic and antiserotonin effect, even though the importance of serotonin in humans has questionable evidence. Most antihistamines have some sedative and hypnotic action. In the treatment of pruritic diseases, the sedative effect cannot be completely distinguished from the soothing of the itch, when psychosomatic etiology is suspected. Sedation, which is the most important side effect of antihistamines, will impair the patient's abilities in working and operating machinery.

ANTIMALARIALS

Primarily chloroquine and its congeners were first introduced in dermatology for protection against photosensitivity in patients with lupus erythematosus and polymorphous light eruption. They are also used for porphyria cutanea tarda. However, in porphyria cutanea tarda, chloroquine treatment may precipitate serious side effects. These are reduced when the patient is pretreated with repeated phlebotomies to reduce circulating amounts of porphyrins (14). Chloroquine has also been recommended for sarcoidosis. Chloroquine can cause pigmentary changes. It may cause achromotrichia of scalp hair, eyebrows, and lashes, and some patients develop pigmentations of face, hands, and nail beds. For systemic lupus erythematosus, chloroquine can be used in a synergistic combination with systemic corticosteroids.

CYTOTOXIC AGENTS

METHOTREXATE

Methotrexate is discussed in Chapter 27. Its indication in dermatological therapy is for severe, recalcitrant psoriasis that does not respond to standard treatment regimens, especially disabling psoriasis complicated by arthropathy and the pustular variant of psoriasis. Methotrexate is also effective in such dermatological disorders as pityriasis rubra pilaris, pemphigus vulgaris, bullous pemphigoid, and mycosis fungoides.

The use of methotrexate in psoriasis is based on epidermal cell proliferation kinetics. A psoriatic cell completes its mitotic cycle in 37 hr once a week. Therefore methotrexate is given once weekly. Two regimens are currently used (21). The first employs a dose given once a week orally, intravenously ("push"), or intramuscularly. The other gives the same dosage orally in three equally divided doses every 12 hr during a 36-hr period each week. Both work equally well; however, it is felt that one large dose gives fewer toxic side effects than divided doses.

An initial test dose of 5-10 mg should be used to detect any idiosyncratic reaction. The dosage employed with either regimen ranges from 7.5 to 25 mg/week, and is increased gradually by 2.5 mg/week. Patients' blood counts should be monitored closely as outlined in Chapter 27. Also, a liver biopsy is indicated prior to starting methotrexate for psoriasis. Complete cleaning of psoriasis is not necessary with methotrexate; however, the goal is adequate control so that conventional modalities can be used.

PSORALENS (FUROCOUMARINS)

METHOXSALEN

Methoxsalen (8-methoxypsoralen, OXSORALEN) is a naturally occurring photoactive substance found in seeds of the *Ammi majus* (Umbelliferae) plant. Chemically, it is 9-methoxy-7H-furo[3,2-g][1]-benzopyran-7-one. It is available for oral ingestion in a capsule form or a solution for topical use. When psoralens are combined with ultraviolet A (UVA) light which is of the 320-400 nm spectrum, it is termed PUVA therapy.

Reactivity of skin to UVA is enhanced by ingestion or topical application of oxsoralen. Maximum bioavailability is 2 hr after oral ingestion and 30-60 min after topical application. Ingested oxsoralen is reversibly bound to serum albumin and is preferentially taken up by epidermal cells. The mechanism of action with epidermal melanocytes and keratinocytes is unknown. However, with photoactivation oxsoralen conjugates and forms covalent bonds with DNA, leading to formation of monofunctional and bifunctional adducts to DNA (17).

Orally administered oxsoralen reaches skin via blood; topically applied it reaches transcutaneously. Orally administered oxsoralen reaches the lens of the eye in concentrations proportional to serum levels. If the lens is exposed to UVA during the time that oxsoralen is present, photochemical action may lead to irreversible binding to lens protein and DNA. This may lead to premature lens aging and cataract formation, unless the patient is protected with special filtering eye glasses.

Oxsoralen acts as a photosensitizer. Administration and subsequent exposure to UVA can lead to cell injury. Sufficient cell injury would cause inflammatory reactions. The most obvious manifestation is delayed erythema that peaks at 48-72 hr. Inflammation is followed over days to weeks by repair that is manifested by increased melanization of epidermis and thickening of stratum corneum.

Psoralens-UVA light (PUVA) therapy is used mainly for vitiligo and psoriasis. In vitiligo, a pigmentary disorder in which there is an acquired loss of epidermal melanocytes in the affected skin, it is thought that PUVA therapy stimulates melanocytes in hair follicles to move up the follicle and repopulate the epidermis. In psoriasis, a hyperproliferative disorder of epidermal cells, PUVA therapy is considered to cause DNA photodamage resulting in decreased epidermal cell proliferation.

Orally administered oxsoralen is usually used for psoriasis and extensive vitiligo. Because of the increased potency of the topically administered form (solution) of oxsoralen to induce photosensitization, it is reserved mainly for vitiligo of less than 20% skin surface involvement. Orally administered oxsoralen undergoes biotransformation in the liver prior to urinary excretion. Therefore, it should be used with caution in patients with hepatic insufficiency. Patients undergoing long-term PUVA therapy of 18-24 months' duration for psoriasis have been found to have an increased susceptibility for developing squamous cell carcinoma of the skin, particularly those individuals with fair skin or previous radiation therapy (24).

TRIOXSALEN

Trioxsalen was the first synthetic psoralen made available for medical use. Although it has greater activity than oxsoralen, the LD_{50} is six times greater. Mechanisms of action are the same as oxsoralen; however, it is only used as an orally administered drug in PUVA therapy. Indication for usage is vitiligo. Trioxsalen is rarely used in psoriasis.

PSYCHOTROPICS

A distinct dermatological problem is delusions of parasitosis (parasitophobia, acarophobia), which is commonly an isolated symptom of mental aberration. Such patients do not seek psychiatric assistance and often get offended when so advised. While complete courses of the best antiparasitic procedures will only consolidate their conviction, moderate doses of perphenazine and pimozide (11) can ordinarily distract the patient from a belief that can ruin life.

VITAMINS

Vitamin A has been tried for several skin symptoms, particularly where hair follicles are involved (acne and keratosis pilaris). The risk of intoxication is greater where a dosage over 50,000 IU/day is used. Retinoic acid derivatives are used in some skin disorders, but toxic symptoms are common and severe (see section on acne vulgaris).

TRACE METALS

Ionized zinc is required for the delayed-hypersensitivity competence of the organism, and malnourished children get thymic atrophy, which is reversed by zinc supplementation (5). In patients with acrodermatitis enteropathica, 150-300 mg/day restores all the combined defects without side effect, whereas therapeutic trials with acne vulgaris patients and for chronic ulcers have given contrasting results.

DERMATOLOGICAL SIDE EFFECTS OF SYSTEMIC DRUGS

Drug-induced skin reactions may imitate many known dermatological disorders, and any drug may cause a skin eruption. Table 20-3 correlates certain important skin changes with administration of some selected drugs. Drug-induced skin eruptions usually occur symmetrically, and often a generalized rash will follow systemic administration. The most important exceptions are the fixed drug eruption and erythema nodosum presenting as solitary lesions. The etiology is usually allergic in nature

Table 20-3
Dermatological Side Effects of Systemic Drugs

Drug	Acneiform Eruption	Alopecia	Erythema Multiforme	Erythema Nodosum	Exanthema	Fixed Drug Eruption	Lichenoid Eruption	Lupuslike Eruption	Photosensitivity	Pigmentary Changes	Porphyria Cutanea Tarda	Toxic Epidermal Necrolysis	Urticaria	Vasculitis
Adrenocorticosteroids	•													
Phenylbutazone			•		•								•	
Salicylates				•		•								
Oral contraceptives	•			•						•				
Estrogens											•			
Arsenicals							•			•				
Gold					•		•			•				•
Halogens	•			•										
Lithium	•													
Ampicillin					•									
Nalidixic acid									•					
Penicillin			•	•	•			•				•	•	
Sulfonamides			•	•				•	•			•	•	
Tetracycline									•					
Griseofulvin									•					
PAS					•		•	•						
INH								•						
Barbiturates			•		•	•						•	•	
Chlordiazepoxide						•								
Phenothiazines							•							
Anticoagulants	•													
Cytostatics	•													
Thiazides							•		•					•
Sulfonylureas									•					
Hydantoins			•		•			•		•		•		•
Hydralazine								•						
Procainamide								•						
Psoralens														
Methyldopa							•							
Allopurinol												•		
Benzoates													•	•
Chloroquine							•							
Phenolphthalein						•								
Ethyl alcohol											•			

although the type of allergy involved is difficult to determine. Because sensitization has to take place, eruptions do not start until some time after the initial dose. Laboratory investigations to support the diagnosis of allergy are often negative, and provocative tests have some risk for the patient, particularly where penicillin is concerned. The definitive establishment of a diagnosis can therefore often not be reached. The subsequent development of the lesions holds no definite proof since skin changes can disappear even when medication is continued; however, lichenoid eruptions and pigmentary changes can last for weeks or months, and the pigmentary changes may even become permanent.

Some drugs, however, cause specific skin changes that are almost pathognomonic. Carbromal provokes an itching eruption of purpuric and pigmented patches on the front of the legs followed by scaling. Meprobamate may lead to a similar reaction. Ampicillin in a large proportion of patients causes a severe morbilliform erythema on the extensor surface of the extremities. In patients with infectious mononucleosis, the incidence is about 50%. This specific rash does not indicate ampicillin allergy, whereas urticaria following ampicillin is regarded as ampicillin intolerance.

The side effects in the skin will often be isolated phenomenon, but purpuric reactions and vasculitis may often occur simultaneously in skin and internal organs. Lupus erythematosus (LE) has developed with several medications. The clinical condition has been stationary or progressive in a few patients, but most drug-induced cases of LE have shown reversibility.

In psoriatic patients, ingestion of lithium may cause severe exacerbation. In other patients, the manifestations of psoriasis start after lithium and vary in intensity with lithium dosage. Chloroquine may also cause severe psoriatic flares and complications, including exfoliative erythrodermia.

Side effects to systemic treatment rarely include contact allergy, but several systemic drugs are potential contact allergens. A contact allergy sometimes develops from handling tablets or injection fluids, but such a contact sensitivity is more often seen in nurses and pharmaceutical workers than in patients.

COSMETICS: SAFETY ASPECTS

Physically, cosmetics are similar to drugs for use on the skin; they are used as creams, lotions, ointments, powders etc. for skin conditioning, cleaning, and nutrition and may contain detergents, astringents (zinc or aluminum salts), hormones, vitamins, artificial coloring matters, among other ingredients.

Hair dyes derive from several sources (metal salts, vegetable extracts, and synthetic dyes). They are mostly small-molecular products that can diffuse into the hair shaft keratin and get evenly distributed. Many of the permanent dyes involve oxidation process on and in the hair (e.g., by peroxides). The heavy chemical processes involved in a quick (to ensure a uniform color) change of color are damaging to the surface of the hair shaft.

Thioglycolic alkali salts are used for temporary softening of keratin of hair in the waving process. Some thioglycolic salts are also used as depilatories.

Strongly active chemicals contained in many cosmetics would be toxic if they were applied in stronger concentration at higher temperature or for longer time. Some of the active chemicals as well as the additives including antioxidants, antimicrobials, emulsion stabilizers, dyes, and perfumes may be allergenic. In particular, preservatives such as parabens, sorbic acid, and ethylenediamine often cause allergic reactions to cosmetics. Outdated preservatives may also cause problems by allowing microbial growth in cosmetic preparations. When these are applied to areas such as around the eyes and eyelashes, bacterial infection may occur. A number of oxidizing hair dyes have been found positive in tests for mutagenic properties and also in long-term carcinogenicity test in rodents.

REFERENCES

1. Allen, H.B., Honig, P.J., Leyden, J.J. and McGinley, K.J. Selenium sulfide: Adjunctive therapy for tinea capitis. *Pediatrics* 69:81, 1982.
2. Bhargava, H.N., Oza, B.J. and Rojanaskul, Y. Transdermal drug delivery systems. *Drug and Cosmetic Industry* 134:52, 1984.
3. Cassidy, D.E., Drewry, J. and Fanning, J.P. Podophyllum toxicity: Report of fatal case and review of literature. *J. Toxicol. Clin. Toxicol.* 19:35, 1982.
4. Derse, D. Acyclovir. *J. Biol. Chem.* 256:11447, 1981.
5. Engasser, P.G. and Maibach, H.I. Cosmetics and dermatology: Bleaching creams. *J. Am. Acad. Dermatol.* 5:143, 1981.
6. Epstein, W.L. and Kligman, A.M. Treatment of warts with cantharidin. *Arch. Dermatol.* 77:508, 1958.
7. Goldsmith, L.A. Propylene glycol. *Int. J. Dermatol.* 17:703, 1979.
8. Kaidbey, K.H. and Kligman, A.M. Appraisal of efficacy and substantivity of new high-potency sunscreens. *J. Am. Acad. Dermatol.* 4:566, 1981.
9. Konstantinou, D., Stanoeva, L. and Yawalkar, S.J. Crotamiton cream and lotion in the treatment of infants and young children with scabies. *J. Int. Med. Res.* 7:443, 1979.
10. Leyden, J.J. and Kligman, A.M. Rationale for topical antibiotics. *Cutis* 22:515, 1978 A.
11. Lowe, N.J. and Breeding, J. Anthralin: Different concentration effects on epidermal cell DNA synthesis rates in mice and clinical responses in human psoriasis. *Arch. Dermatol.* 117:698, 1981.
12. Lowe, N.J., Breeding, J.H. and Wortzman, M.S. New coal tar extract and coal tar shampoos: Evaluation by epidermal cell DNA synthesis suppression assay. *Arch. Dermatol.* 118:487, 1982.
13. Miller, J.A. and Munro, D.D. Topical corticosteroids: Clinical pharmacology and therapeutic use. *Drugs* 19:119, 1980.
14. Milstone, E.M., McDonald, A.J. and Scholhamer, C.F. Pseudomembranous colitis after topical application of clindamycin.
15. Mosher, D.B., Parrish, J.A. and Fitzpatrick, T.B. Monobenzylether of hydroquinone: A retrospective study of treatment of 18 vitiligo patients and a review of the literature. *Br. J. Dermatol.* 97:669, 1977.
16. Nacht, S., Yeung, D., Beaslly, J.N. et al. Benzoyl peroxide: Percutaneous penetration and metabolic disposition. *J. Am. Acad. Dermatol.* 4:31, 1981.
17. Pathak, M.A., Kramer, D.M. and Fitzpatrick, T.B. Photobiology and photochemistry of furocoumarins (psoralens). In: *Sunlight and Man: Normal and Abnormal Photobiologic Responses.* Tokyo: Tokyo University Press, 1974.

18. Peck, G.L., Olsen, T.G., Yoder, F.W. et al. Prolonged remissions of cystic and conglobate acne with 13-cis-retinoic acid. *N. Engl. J. Med.* 300:329, 1979.
19. Rasmussen, J.E. The problem of lindane. *J. Am. Acad. Dermatol.* 5:507, 1981.
20. Robertson, D.B. and Maibach, H.I. Topical corticosteroids: A review. *Int. J. Dermatol.* 21:59, 1982.
21. Roenigk, H.H. Jr., Auerbach, R. and Maibach, H.I. Methotrexate guidelines: Revised. *J. Am. Acad. Dermatol.* 6:145, 1982.
22. Schacter, B. Treatment of scabies and pediculosis with lindane preparation: An evaluation. *J. Am. Acad. Dermatol.* 5:517, 1981.
23. Shelley, W.B. and Hurley, H.J. Studies on topical antiperspirant control of axillary hyperhidrosis. *JAMA* 233:1257, 1975.
24. Stern, R.S. and Melski, J.W. Long-term continuation of psoralen and ultraviolet-A treatment of psoriasis. *Arch. Dermatol.* 118:400, 1982.
25. Stoughton, R.B. Topical antibiotics for acne vulgaris: Current usage. *Arch. Dermatol.* 115:486, 1979.
26. Taylor, J.R. and Halprin, K.M. Percutaneous absorption of salicylic acid. *Arch. Dermatol.* 111:740, 1975.

GENERAL READING

AMA Drug Evaluations, 5th ed. Dermatologic Preparations. Chicago: American Medical Association, 1983, p. 1339.

Arndt, K.A. *Manual of Dermatologic Therapeutics with Essentials of Diagnosis, 3rd ed.* Boston: Little, Brown, 1983.

Maddin, S. *Current Dermatologic Therapy.* Philadelphia: W.B. Saunders, 1982.

CHAPTER 21.1

OCULAR PHARMACOLOGY

Freddy W. Chang

Ophthalmology uses a relatively small number of drugs and many routes of specialized drug administration, such as topical, subconjunctival, retrobulbar, and intraocular as well as oral, subcutaneous, intramuscular, and intravenous. Local application, the most common route of drug administration in the management of ocular disease, may be in the form of drops, cotton packs, ointment, membrane-controlled drug delivery systems, corneal baths, or subconjunctival injections. A drug in solution must have both significant lipid solubility and significant water solubility to penetrate the cornea. The corneal epithelium and endothelium contain a great amount of lipids and permit only lipid-soluble substances to pass through readily, whereas the corneal stroma tends to allow the ready penetration of water-soluble substances.

Attempts to increase drug penetration through the intact cornea have emphasized increasing the contact time between the medication and the corneal surface. Increasing the viscosity of drug vehicles (by addition of methyl cellulose, hydroxyethyl cellulose, and polyvinyl alcohol), use of pledgets or hydrophilic contact lenses saturated with the drug, or development of membrane drug delivery systems and micropump systems have been attempted.

Basically, the drugs used in ophthalmic medicine can be divided into groups, depending on their usage. Because many of them have been discussed elsewhere in this text, the material presented in this chapter will reflect that primarily relevant to ophthalmic pharmacology.

MIOTICS

Ocular administration of parasympathomimetic drugs produces *miosis* (pupillary constriction), ciliary muscle contraction, dilatation of the conjunctival and iris blood vessels, and an increase in aqueous outflow (2).

The parasympathomimetic drugs can be divided into (1) *direct acting:* carbachol, methacholine, pilocarpine; and (2) *indirect acting* (anticholinesterases): (a) *short acting:* edrophonium, neostigmine, physostigmine; (b) *Long acting/irreversible:* demecarium, diisopropylphosphorofluoridate, echothiophate.

PARASYMPATHOMIMETICS

DIRECT ACTING

Acetylcholine. The clinical usefulness of acetylcholine, is limited because it is rapidly destroyed by cholinesterases, which makes it preferable for use in ophthalmic surgery in keratoplasty, iridectomy, or cyclodialysis, where the anterior chamber is irrigated. Instillation of a 1% acetylcholine solution in the anterior chamber after cataract extraction will produce a marked miosis (of short duration) which is helpful in keeping the iris temporarily clear of the incision (6, 15).

Methacholine. Methacholine has been used for the diagnosis of Adie's tonic pupil and familial dysautonomia (Riley-Day syndrome). Although concentrations of 10% or more are necessary to produce miosis in the normal pupil when applied topically, miosis will occur in Adie's syndrome and in familial dysautonomia with 2.5% methacholine within 30 min.

Pilocarpine. Pilocarpine, the drug of choice in therapy of both open- and closed-angle glaucoma, may also be useful for counteracting mydriasis, and for treatment of hyphema and accommodative strabismus.

In glaucoma, the minimum concentration of pilocarpine that will control intraocular pressure should be used (in most patients, 2%). The frequency of instillation may range from two or three times daily to as often as every 2 hr. The major limitation to pilocarpine therapy is its duration of action (6-8 hr). A pilocarpine polymer salt, Piloplex, effectively maintains a significantly low mean intraocular pressure with less variation in diurnal values when administered twice a day (16).

Carbachol. This synthetic derivative of choline has longer duration of action than pilocarpine and is also a more potent miotic. In a 0.75% solution, it is more effective in controlling the intraocular pressure than 2% pilocarpine in chronic simple glaucoma. A 1.5% solution produces miosis that may last more than 2 days. Carbachol causes more severe headaches and accommodative spasms than pilocarpine. Because carbachol is not lipid-soluble at any pH, it penetrates the intact cornea poorly and must be dispensed with a wetting agent (usually 0.03% benzalkonium chloride) to increase corneal penetration.

INDIRECT, SHORT ACTING

An indirect, short-acting parasympathomimetic such as physostigmine is used in the management of open-angle glaucoma in patients resistant to weaker miotics and is also useful in the treatment of accommodative esotropia and in parasitic infection of the lids by *Pediculus pubis.*

Physostigmine. Topical administration of 0.5% physostigmine produces intense miosis within 30 min, lasting for 12-36 hr, with an accompanying increase in outflow facility. It is administered in 1 to 2 drops four times a day.

Physostigmine is unstable in aqueous solutions and may decompose with exposure to light and pH changes. It gradually oxidizes to rubeserine with the development of pink or rusty color.

INDIRECT, LONG ACTING/IRREVERSIBLE

Echothiophate Iodide. Echothiophate iodide is very stable in the powdered form in tightly sealed containers. In aqueous solution, it is stable for a month at room temperature, and when refrigerated remains stable for 1 year. In the treatment of open-angle glaucoma, one drop of 0.03-0.25% solution topically every 12-48 hr will produce miosis within 10-15 min; maximum miotic effect (occurring within 10-20 hr) may last as long as 96 hr.

For accommodative esotropia, a 0.125% solution is used once a day for 2-3 weeks, although 0.06% has also been found effective (12).

Diisopropylphosphorofluoridate (DFP, isoflurophate). Diisopropylphosphorofluoridate has been used in the management of primary open-angle glaucoma resistant to the shorter-acting miotics, in management of accommodative esotropia, and in the treatment of parasitic infection of the eyebrows and eyelashes from *Pediculus pubis.* Instillation of 0.05% DFP produces miosis within 5-10 min that is maximal within 15-20 min and lasts 2-4 weeks. Anhydrous peanut oil vehicle must be used to maintain its potency for more than 3 months; in aqueous solutions, the drug deteriorates so rapidly that within a week there is no miotic effect.

Demecarium Bromide. Demecarium bromide, extremely potent and the most toxic of the agents available, is water-soluble and stable in solution. It is used to treat open-angle glaucoma and accommodative esotropia. A single instillation of 0.125-0.25% solution produces miosis with an onset of 45-60 min, a maximum effect in 2-4 hr and a duration of 3-10 days. A slight miosis may be present for as long as 3-4 weeks.

ADVERSE EFFECTS

The most serious complication of anticholinesterase therapy is the formation of cataracts, although the formation of iris cysts may also result from the use of these agents. Such formation can be reversed by withdrawal of the drug or simultaneous administration of 2.5% phenylephrine (14).

THERAPY OF GLAUCOMA

In glaucoma, intraocular pressure is increased; if sufficiently high and persistent, it may produce extensive loss of visual field by damaging the optic nerve fibers. Increased pressure results from blockade of normal outflow or excessive production of the aqueous humor of the eye. The aqueous humor produced at the surface of vascular ciliary processes and the posterior aspect of the iris flows through the pupillary aperture into the anterior chamber, then passes mostly to the angle of the anterior chamber (filtration angle at the junction of the sclera with cornea). On the deep aspect of the sclera in front of the angle of the anterior chamber lies an annular venous sinus, Schlemm's canal. The thinner posterior wall of the canal is separated from the anterior chamber by a zone of trabecular tissue; intervals between the trabecular meshwork are termed Fontana's spaces. The aqueous humor percolates into Fontana's spaces where it is absorbed across the posterior wall of Schlemm's canal.

Glaucoma can be *primary* (without any known disease of the eye), *secondary* (to some obvious disease of the eye), or *congenital.* The type of primary glaucoma depends on the configuration of the angle of the anterior chamber. Narrow-angle (angle-closure, acute congestive) glaucoma is caused by a relative pupillary block between the iris and the lens due to inflammation or other causes when aqueous humor is unable to enter into the anterior chamber through the pupil and intraocular pressure is raised, causing bulging of the iris and narrowing of the filtration angle. In wide-angle (open-angle, chronic simple) glaucoma the intraocular pressure rises slowly in absence of any obstruction to the flow of the fluid through the pupil, so that the anterior chamber is bulged and the angle is widened.

The objective of therapy in both types of glaucoma is to reduce the intraocular pressure by using drugs such as miotics and agents that reduce the production of aqueous humor; the therapeutic approaches are different in two types of the disease. Narrow-angle glaucoma is almost always a medical emergency; drugs are used to control the acute attack pending removal of obstruction by surgery. The lowering of the intraocular pressure should be made 12 hr before surgery. In wide-angle glaucoma, the trabeculae are rather relaxed and lose their patency. Use of miotics to contract the iris sphincter and ciliary muscles enhances the tone of the trabecular network and improves the passage of the aqueous humor for absorption in the canal. Treatment is directed to decrease the intraocular pressure to prevent deterioration of the optic nerve and further loss of the visual field. Surgery is usually of no benefit and treatment involves drug therapy, on a permanent basis, using drugs of greater potency and of longer duration. Fig. 21.1-1 illustrates the mechanisms involved in these two types of glaucoma.

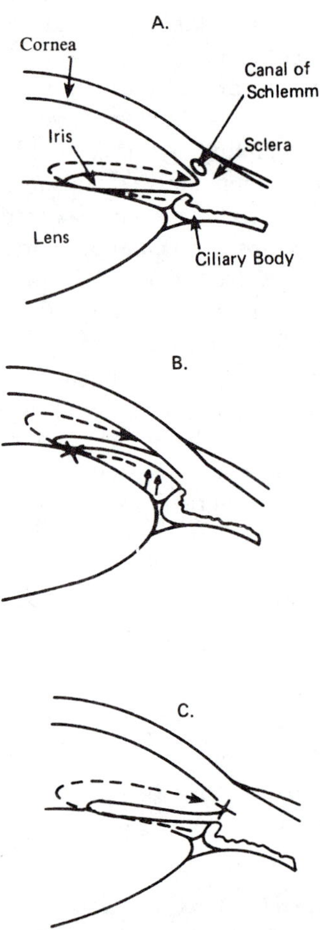

Fig. 21.1-1. *Mechanisms of glaucoma.*

(A) Normal eye; (B) angle-closure glaucoma; (C) open-angle glaucoma. Interrupted line with arrow shows the direction of flow of aqueous humor. X indicates the site of obstruction in respective type of glaucoma. (Modified from Bangier, T. *Berichte Deutch. Ophthal. Ges.*, 43:43, 1922).

ACUTE ANGLE-CLOSURE GLAUCOMA

The intraocular pressure in acute angle-closure glaucoma is usually decreased by the topical administration of a miotic together with the systemic administration of an analgesic, a carbonic anhydrase inhibitor (at frequent intervals), and osmotic agents such as urea, mannitol, and glycerol. If the patient is vomiting, mannitol, urea, or a carbonic anhydrase inhibitor may be administered intravenously.

MIOTICS

Pilocarpine 2% may be instilled topically every 10-15 min for 1-2 hr and repeated every hour for the next 4-6 hr and repeated every 3 hr for the next 12 hr. It is usually advisable to abort an attack in the fellow eye. Anticholinesterase agents more potent than physostigmine and neostigmine should be avoided because of the congestion produced in the iris and conjunctiva. Systemic symptoms of nausea, diarrhea, muscular twitching, sweating, vomiting, and urinary incontinence may follow the use of either large amounts of and/or highly concentrated solutions of miotics.

Thymoxamine, an α-adrenergic blocker, has also been used successfully in the treatment of angle-closure glaucoma, administered in a 0.5% solution and instilled every minute for five doses and then every 15 min for 2-3 hr.

CARBONIC ANHYDRASE INHIBITORS

Acetazolamide (DIAMOX) may be given orally, in an initial dose of 500 mg and 250 mg every 6 hr thereafter; if the patient is vomiting, 500 mg is administered intravenously or 250 mg may be given i.v. and 250 mg i.m. as the initial dose.

OSMOTIC AGENTS

Oral glycerin or glycerol is administered as a 50% solution with 0.9% NaCl or with orange or lime juice in a dose of 1-1.5 g/kg body weight. Commercial preparations of 50% glycerol (OSMOGLYN) and 75% glycerol (GLYROL) are also available.

Urea is administered intravenously as a 30% solution. The usual dose (1 g/kg body weight) is administered at a rate of 60 drops/min. Because this agent is a diuretic, it is considered prudent to introduce a catheter if the patient is to undergo surgery.

Mannitol is administered i.v. as a 20% solution in adults and as a 10% solution in children, over a period of 30-40 min. The adult dose is 1.5-2 g/kg body weight and the dose for children is 1.5 g/kg of body weight.

OPEN-ANGLE GLAUCOMA

MIOTICS

Pilocarpine (available in concentrations of 1-6%) is still the most important and widely used miotic for the treatment of simple open-angle glaucoma. If the intraocular pressure is high (20s to low 30s), the starting concentration is usually 1%; 2% is indicated if the intraocular pressure is in the high 30s, and 4% is used if it is higher. Because the duration of action is between 6 and 8 hr, it is normally used three to four times per day.

Carbachol chloride (available in concentrations of 0.75, 1.5, and 3%) is used to replace pilocarpine if hypersensitivity or resistance develops.

Physostigmine, available in 0.25 and 0.5% concentrations with a duration of action of about 12 hr is often substituted for pilocarpine in the medical management of chronic simple glaucoma.

Phospholine iodide (available in concentrations from 0.03 to 0.25%) needs to be instilled only once or twice a day. The advantage of increased potency is balanced by the disadvantage of increased systemic and ocular side effects. It is indicated in patients whose intraocular pressure cannot be controlled by any other means.

Demecarium bromide, comparable with phospholine iodide, is available in strengths from 0.12 to 0.25%.

SYMPATHOMIMETICS

When epinephrine is instilled in the eye, it decreases intraocular pressure by reducing aqueous formation; continued use of epinephrine will produce an increase in outflow facility. It is available in concentrations of 0.5, 1, and 2%, and is administered once to twice daily. Epinephrine can be used in the management of chronic simple glaucoma alone or as an adjunct to miotic therapy; the effects of these two drug classes are additive.

Epinephrine is the drug of choice in glaucoma therapy of patients with cataracts and young myopic patients. Prolonged use of epinephrine drops can produce local side effects such as conjunctival hyperemia and irritation and black deposits in the conjunctiva. In some patients there has been evidence of maculopathy in aphakic eyes associated with the use of epinephrine.

CARBONIC ANHYDRASE INHIBITORS

Carbonic anhydrase inhibitors are effective ocular hypotensives irrespective of the nature or the extent of resistance to outflow because they reduce the intraocular pressure by decreasing aqueous secretion.

Acetazolamide (DIAMOX). Acetazolamide is the carbonic anhydrase inhibitor of choice for emergency use because of its rapid action; the course of treatment is so short that side effects are minimal. It is usually administered orally in a dose of 250 mg twice a day to 500mg six times a day. A longer-acting form of acetazolamide (DIAMOX SEQUELS) may be administered twice a day in 500-mg doses.

Dichlorphenamide (DARANIDE). Dichlorphenamide, a more potent carbonic anhydrase inhibitor administered in doses of 50-200 mg three to four times a day, tends to have more side effects than acetazolamide but may produce less metabolic acidosis.

Methazolamide (NEPTAZANE). Methazolamide, most frequently used in patients who are unable to tolerate acetazolamide, is administered in doses of 50-100 mg three times a day. Methazolamide possesses a longer duration of action than acetazolamide, but the onset of action is slower.

SYMPATHOLYTICS

The β-adrenoceptor blocking agent propranolol was found to have ocular hypotensive activity (13), although its local anesthetic and irritative effects after topical application have mitigated against its use in therapy. Other compounds in this pharmacological class have similar ocular hypotensive effects as well as similar adverse effects when applied topically (4). The only β-blocker currently authorized for the clinical treatment of glaucoma in the United States is timolol. Katz et al. found significant reduction in intraocular pressure when one drop of 0.5, 1.0, and 1.5% timolol was administered to normal volunteers (9).

As an ocular hypotensive agent, timolol is as effective (when administered twice a day) as pilocarpine and epinephrine administered in combination. Recently, a number of side effects have been reported including some central nervous, cardiovascular, respiratory, and ocular symptoms, as well as a corneal anesthetic effect that also manifested as a superficial punctate keratitis (10, 17).

CANNABINOIDS

Since the first published report showing a significant reduction in intraocular pressure in humans who smoked marijuana (7), a number of additional studies have confirmed and extended this action. Hepler et al. (8) found that oral dosages of Δ^9-tetrahydrocannabinol (Δ^9-THC) were inconsistently effective; Green (5) tested the use of this agent as a topical drug (in a light mineral oil base) in the treatment of chronic open-angle glaucoma. Although pharmacological efficacy was obtained, some irritation of superficial ocular structures was observed. Further studies of various cannabinoids, alone or in combination with conventional antiglaucoma medications, are currently in progress (3).

MYDRIATICS AND CYCLOPLEGICS

Anticholinergic drugs are applied topically to the eye to produce pupillary dilatation (*mydriasis*) and paralysis of accommodation (*cycloplegia*). These agents paralyze the parasympathetically innervated structures, the iris constrictor, and the ciliary muscles. α-Adrenoceptor agonists stimulate contraction of the iris dilator muscles and produce mydriasis without cycloplegia, also an increase in outflow facility and vasoconstriction. It is thus evident that whereas all cycloplegic drugs produce mydriasis, all mydriatics do not produce cycloplegia.

CYCLOPLEGICS

Cycloplegics are used in refraction to paralyze the ciliary muscle and the iris sphincter, allowing the determination of the far point of the eye with relative ease. The use of a cycloplegic is generally indicated in (1) young children, (2) patients in whom subjective responses are unreliable, (3) patients whose symptoms are not warranted by the manifest refractive error, and (4) when manifest disturbances of oculomotor coordination exist.

The cycloplegics most commonly used are atropine, scopolamine, homatropine, cyclopentolate, and tropicamide.

Atropine. Atropine produces an effect of long duration. Maximum mydriasis occurs in 30-40 min and may last 7-10 days; maximum cycloplegia occurs in about 32 hr and may last 2 weeks or longer.

Atropine is indicated for refraction in children less than 5 years of age, especially if accommodative esotropia is suspected. It is also used in the treatment of iritis and iridocyclitis to prevent the formation of posterior synechiae and has been used as an occluder in the treatment of amblyopia by fogging the better eye to force the amblyopic eye to fixate.

Atropine may produce a contact dermatitis of the lids of the eye being treated; withdrawal of the drug is the only satisfactory treatment. Side effects following the use of atropine include dryness of the skin and mouth, an increase in skin temperature because of the inability to perspire, delirium due to CNS stimulation, tachycardia, and flushing of the face.

The dosage for refraction in children under 30 months of age is 1 drop of 0.5% solution three times a day for 3 days prior to the refraction and on the morning of the refraction. For children from 30 months to 5 years, the dosage is 1 drop of 1% solution three times a day for 3 days prior to the refraction and on the morning of the refraction.

Scopolamine. With scopolamine, maximum mydriasis occurs in 40 min and may last for 3-5 days; maximum cycloplegia is attained within 30-60 min and may last 5-7 days. The incidence of contact dermatitis of the lids is less than with atropine.

The most common side effects of scopolamine are flushed skin and dryness of the mouth; however, scopolamine tends to produce more CNS effects than atropine. It is usually administered in 0.2% solution two times a day before refraction.

Homatropine. Homatropine produces maximum mydriasis in 40-60 min and maximum cycloplegia in 30-60 min. Both effects may last 1-2 days. Homatropine is indicated when a shorter-acting cycloplegic is needed (for iritis or iridocyclitis) and for breaking posterior synechiae. It may be used alone or in conjunction with 1% hydroxyamphetamine (PAREDRINE) or 10% phenylephrine (NEO-SYNEPHRINE). For refraction, 2 drops of 4% homatropine are instilled 5 min apart.

Cyclopentolate (CYCLOGYL). Cyclopentolate produces maximum mydriasis and cycloplegia in 15-30 min; both effects last for 24 hr. It is indicated for cycloplegic refraction, retinal photography, and mydriasis for diagnostic procedures.

In patients with lightly colored irises, 1 drop of 1% cyclopentolate will produce adequate cycloplegia for refraction, or 1 drop of 0.5% cyclopentolate followed by a second drop 5 min later. Individuals with heavily pigmented irises are more resistant to cyclopentolate and may require repeated administration of the drug and a longer time for dilation. Instillation of three drops of 1% cyclopentolate 5-10 min apart will produce retinoscopic values comparable with those obtained when children are atropinized with three drops.

Tropicamide. Instillation of 1% tropicamide (MYDRIACYL) produces cycloplegia and mydriasis; 0.5% tropicamide solution produces mydriasis with an ineffective cycloplegia. Maximum cycloplegia is produced in 20-25 min lasting for 6 hr. However, 2-4 hr after the instillation, most patients are able to read. The accompanying mydriasis is maximum in 20-30 min and will last up to 4 hr. The administration of one drop of 1% tropicamide repeated in 5 min will produce cycloplegia of short duration; instillation of one drop of 0.5% tropicamide repeated in 5 min will produce mydriasis with insignificant cycloplegia in most individuals with lightly colored irises (11).

Drug Selection. In the selection of a cycloplegic, one must consider the age of the patient, indication for the examination, patient's occupation, iris pigmentation, and adverse effects. The younger the patient, the more potent the cycloplegic needed. Atropine should be reserved for cycloplegic refractions in children less than 6 years of age in whom accommodative esotropia is suspected. Agents such as cyclopentolate or tropicamide are indicated for older children and adults. For examination of a muscle imbalance or an accommodative esotropia, the use of a more potent cycloplegic is necessary. Because one would like to minimize the time lost from work or studies, it may be desirable to use a cycloplegic agent with a short duration of action so that accommodation can be restored within a reasonable time.

Contraindications. Cycloplegics will produce mydriasis in addition to the cycloplegia; thus, they are contraindicated in patients with a narrow anterior chamber angle or a predisposition to angle closure because of the possibility of precipitating an acute angle-closure glaucoma.

Cycloplegics are also contraindicated in patients with chronic open-angle glaucoma, as well as in patients who have had an intraocular lens implantation, in patients with a subluxated lens (rare), and in patients who have previously exhibited hypersensitivity to the drugs.

MYDRIATICS

The primary use of a mydriatic agent is to allow more accurate examination of fundus details; minute details of diagnostic importance such as diabetic microaneurysms, hypertensive arteriolar attenuation, and traumatic retinal holes are difficult to observe through a pupil of decreased size. Mydriasis may be achieved by topical application of parasympatholytic (just discussed) or sympathomimetic agents.

Sympathomimetic Mydriatics. Sympathomimetic Mydriatics may be direct or indirect acting. The only *direct-acting* sympathomimetic agent, phenylephrine, produces maximum mydriasis in 50-80 min, lasting for 3-6 hr. When phenylephrine is instilled with local anesthetic such as 0.5 proparacaine, only 2.5% phenylephrine is necessary to produce the same amount of mydriasis as 10% phenylephrine without the use of the anesthetic. The combination of drugs produces maximum mydriasis in 35-45 minutes, lasting for 3-6 hr. To produce maximal dilatation, it may be used in conjunction with 2% homatropine or 1% tropicamide; this aids the performance of both direct and indirect ophthalmoscopy, retinal photography, and other diagnostic aids such as Hruby lens examination. In addition, it is used for the restoration of flat anterior chambers, treatment of ptosis, as an adjunctive treatment of iritis, for breaking of posterior synechiae, and in conjunction with 2.5% echothiophate to prevent the formation of miotic cysts of the iris.

Phenylephrine should be used with caution in patients with cardiovascular problems. In some individuals, it may cause a liberation of iris pigment that generally appears 30 min after instillation, becomes maximal in 1-2 hr, and disappears in 12-24 hr.

Indirect-acting Sympathomimetics. Indirect-acting sympathomimetics cause increase of norepinephrine concentration at the adrenoceptor site to produce sympathomimetic effects. Cocaine is employed in concentrations of 2-4%; onset of dilatation is 15-20 min; and maximum dilatation, attained in the first hour, will last 6 hr or more. Cocaine may be used in the differential diagnosis of a Horner's pupil, although its use is limited because of its addicting properties and the associated corneal toxic propensity.

Parahydroxyamphetamine. Parahydroxyamphetamine is an excellent drug for the differential diagnosis of pre- and postganglionic sympathetic lesions, and is useful in determining the location of the lesion in Horner's syndrome. For mydriasis, one drop of 1% hydroxyamphetamine is instilled and repeated in 5-10 min. Mydriasis begins in 20-25 min, is maximal in 30-45 minutes, and lasts for 2-3 hr.

LOCAL ANESTHETICS

The clinical use of local anesthetics in ocular diagnostic and surgical procedures, such as suture removal and removal of foreign bodies, usually involves topical application, although retrobulbar injection or local tissue infiltration may be required.

TOPICAL ANESTHETICS

Cocaine. Cocaine (topically in concentrations of 1-4%) produces excellent surface anesthesia. Grayish corneal pits due to epithelial damage with further loosening of the epithelium may result in large erosions. Because of this, cocaine has been preempted by safer agents.

Tetracaine (PONTOCAINE). When topically applied in 0.5% solution, the onset of anesthesia is less than 15 sec and may last as long as 25-30 min. Tetracaine may be used to remove corneal sutures or foreign bodies. After topical instillation, however, it is not uncommon to observe with a biomicroscope a tiny superficial punctate keratitis; with repeated instillation, this epithelial damage is intensified. Because it retards corneal healing, the frequent instillation of local anesthetics to relieve irritation of a corneal abrasion or foreign body sensation is contraindicated. Tetracaine allergy should be considered when a patient complains of itching lids and swollen, irritated, and reddened eyes that persist for some days after the administration of the drug.

Benoxinate. Benoxinate (DORSACAINE) is less irritating on instillation than tetracaine. The onset of action is less than 15 sec and it lasts for 25-30 min. Benoxinate (as a 0.4% solution) may be used for the removal of corneal sutures or foreign bodies, to perform tonometry, or for other procedures requiring anesthesia of short duration.

Proparacaine. Proparacaine (OPHTHAINE) (as a 0.5% solution) produces little or no irritation on instillation, has an onset of action of less than 15 sec, and lasts for 25-30 min. The drug is indicated as for benoxinate. A small number of patients have exhibited hypersensitivity, manifested as marked epithelial stippling with stromal edema, appearing within 5-10 min after administration. In addition, there was conjunctival hyperemia and slight swelling of the lids. Patients allergic to proparacaine are not necessarily allergic to tetracaine or benoxinate.

LOCALLY INJECTED ANESTHETICS

Most ophthalmic surgical procedures can be performed with local anesthesia.

Procaine. Procaine (NOVOCAIN) is used for infiltration anesthesia, with a rapid onset of action (about 2 min) and a duration of about 1 hr. It is available in concentrations of 0.5-4.0%; for ocular procedures, however, there is rarely need for a solution stronger than 1%. Because it penetrates the cornea poorly, it is not used topically. Epinephrine may be added simultaneously with procaine to retard systemic absorption.

Chloroprocaine. Chloroprocaine (NESACAINE) is used for infiltration anesthesia, with onset of action about 2 min, lasting for about 1 hr. It possesses similar pharmacological properties to procaine and is used in concentrations of 0.5-2.0%.

Lidocaine. Lidocaine (XYLOCAINE) has a rapid onset of action (30 sec) and duration of 60-90 min. It is commonly used in concentrations of 0.5-2.0%, but for retrobulbar injections a special 4% solution is available.

Prilocaine. Prilocaine (CITANEST) is used in concentrations of 0.5-2.0% for infiltration and regional blocks.

REFERENCES

1. Abrahamson, I.A., Jr. and Abrahamson, I.A., Sr. Preliminary report on 0.06% phospholine (echothiophate) iodide in the management of esotropia. *Am. J. Ophthalmol.* 57:290, 1964.
2. Armaly, I.F. Parasympathetics and the facility of outflow: Effect and mechanism. *Am. J. Ophthalmol.* 47:879, 1959.
3. Cohen, S. Therapeutic aspects. In: *Marijuana Research Findings: 1980* (Petersen, R.C., ed.). NIDA Research Monograph 31, DHHS/NIDA pub. no. ADM-80-1001. Washington, D.C.: NIDA, 1980, p. 199.
4. Garner, A. and Rahi, A.H.S. Practolol and ocular toxicity. *Br. J. Ophthalmol.* 60:684, 1976.
5. Green, K. The ocular effects of Cannabinoids. In: *Current Topics in Eye Research* (Zadunaisky, J.A. and Davison, H., eds.). New York: Academic Press, 1978, pp. 356.
6. Harley, R. and Misahler, J. Acetylcholine in cataract surgery. *Br. J. Ophthalmol.* 50:429, 1966.
7. Hepler, R.S. and Frank, I.M. Marijuana smoking and intraocular pressure. *J. Am. Med. Assoc.* 217:1392, 1971.
8. Hepler, K.S., Frank, I.M. and Petrus, R. Ocular effects of marijuana smoking. In: *Pharmacology of Marijuana* (Braude, M.C. and Szara, S., eds.). New York: Raven Press, 1976, p. 815.
9. Katz, I.M., Hubbard, W.A., Getson, A.J. and Gould, A.L. Intraocular pressure decrease in normal volunteers following timolol ophthalmic solution. *Invest. Ophthalmol.* 15:489, 1976.
10. McMahon, C.D., Shaffer, R.N., Hoskins, H.D., Jr. and Hetherington, J., Jr. Adverse effects experienced by patients taking timolol. *Am. J. Ophthalmol.* 88:736, 1979.
11. Milder, B. Tropicamide as a cycloplegic agent. *Arch. Opthalmol.* 66:70, 1961.
12. Miller, J.E. A comparison of miotics in accommodative esotropia. *Am. J. Ophthalmol.* 49:1350, 1960.
13. Phillips, C.I., Hawitt, G. and Rowlands, D.J. Propranolol as an ocular hypotensive agent. *Br. J. Ophthalmol.* 51:222, 1967.
14. Pietsch, R.L., Bob, C.B., Finklea, J.F. and Vallotton, W.W. Lens opacities and organophosphate cholinesterase inhibiting agents. *Am. J. Ophthalmol.* 73:236, 1972.
15. Rizzuti, A.B. Acetylcholine in surgery of the lens, iris, and cornea. *Am. J. Ophthalmol.* 63:484, 1967.
16. Ticho, U., Blumenthal, M. et al. Piloplex, a new long-acting pilocarpine polymer salt. A long term study. *Br. J. Ophthalmol.* 63:45, 1979.
17. Van Buskirk, E.M. Corneal anesthesia after timolol maleate therapy. *Am. J. Ophthalmol.* 88:739, 1979.

GENERAL REFERENCES

Beitel, R.S. Cycloplegic refraction. In: *Clinical Ophthalmology, Vol. 1,* (Duane, T.R., ed.). New York: Harper & Row, 1976.

Chandler, P.A. and Grant, W.M. *Glaucoma, 2nd ed.* Philadelphia: Lea & Febiger, 1979.

Greve, E.L. (ed.). *Symposium on Medical Therapy in Glaucoma.* Boston: Kluwer, 1977.

Havener, W.H. *Ocular Pharmacology, 4th ed.* St. Louis: C.V. Mosby, 1978.

Kolder, A.E. and Hetherington, J., Jr. *Becker-Shaffer's Diagnosis and Therapy of the Glaucomas, 4th ed.* St. Louis: C.V. Mosby, 1976.

Leopold, I.H. Drugs for ophthalmic use. In: *Drugs of Choice, 1980-1981, 11th ed.* (Modell, W., ed.). St. Louis: C.V. Mosby, 1980, p. 660.

O'Connor-Davies, P. *Actions and Uses of Ophthalmic Drugs.* London: Barrie & Jenkins, 1972.

Rehak, S., Krasnov, M.M. and Paterson, G.D. (eds.). *Recent Advances in Glaucoma: International Glaucoma Symposium, Prague, 1976.* Berlin: Springer-Verlag, 1977.

Richardson, K.T. *Symposium on Ocular Pharmacology and Therapeutics: Transactions of the New Orleans Academy of Ophthalmology.* St. Louis: C.V. Mosby, 1970.

CHAPTER
21.2

AUDITORY AND VESTIBULAR PHARMACOLOGY

R. Don Brown and Charles D. Wood

Two areas of auditory and vestibular pharmacology, iatrogenic ototoxicity and the pharmacology of motion sickness, presently have a significant impact on medical practice. *Iatrogenic ototoxicity* is primarily the result of drug-induced impairment in hearing and/or equilibrium caused by action of drugs on the inner ear. On the other hand, *vestibular pharmacology* is primarily concerned with drugs that prevent motion sickness by a relatively selective action on the central nervous system (CNS).

POSSIBLE SITES OF ACTION OF DRUGS

Drugs may exert an action on the inner ear by affecting one or more of the following sites: the sensory receptors (hair cells), their afferent or efferent nerve endings, the specialized secretory epithelium, and the vasculature of the inner ear. Two types of hair cells occur, each type having a different basic shape and pattern of innervation. The type I hair cell is flask-shaped, afferent fibers synapsing directly with it and efferent fibers synapsing with the afferent terminals (not with the hair cell itself). The inner hair cell of the cochlea and the vestibular hair cell with the afferent nerve chalice are *type I sensory cells.* The *type II sensory cell* is cylindrical and has direct synaptic contact with both the afferent and efferent nerve terminals. The outer hair cells of the cochlea and the vestibular sensory cell without the chalice are type II sensory cells. The hair cells appear to serve as the primary target for ototoxicity of the aminoglycoside antibiotics.

The morphology of the synapses between the hair cells and their afferent nerve terminals is similar to that of other synapses; however, none of the common neurotransmitters (acetylcholine, norepinephrine, dopamine, γ-aminobutyric acid, serotonin, glycine) appear to be involved as transmitter substances (20). On the other hand, the efferent transmitter substance is most probably acetylcholine (11). Although drugs could affect hearing and/or equilibrium by adversely altering inner ear afferent and/or efferent synaptic physiology, these have not been demonstrated as ototoxic effects.

The stria vascularis of the cochlea and the differentiated, nonsensory epithelia of the vestibular apparatus are apparently the source of endolymph (5), a potassium-rich fluid similar to intracellular fluid in ionic composition. The stria vascularis is also responsible for generation of the cochlear endolymphatic direct current (D.C.) potential. This specified secretory epithelium, especially that of the stria vascularis, is considered the site for ototoxicity of the loop diuretics, whereas the vasculature of the cochlea has been postulated as the ototoxic site for the nonsteroidal antiinflammatory agents and quinine.

FACTORS RELATED TO DRUG DISTRIBUTION IN THE INNER EAR

Several factors govern the distribution of drugs within the fluid compartments of the inner ear (6). Drugs that gain access to the perilymphatic fluid compartment could be distributed throughout that compartment and to the cochlear and vestibular hair cells and their nerve endings. In contrast, the endolymphatic fluid compartment is not continuous with the fluid surrounding either the cochlear or vestibular hair cells; in fact, this compartment is functionally divided into cochlear and vestibular divisions. However, hydrostatic pressure changes in states, such as in Ménière's disease, can be reflected through both of the systems. Drugs may also penetrate into the area of the hair cells by passive or active transport from the capillary beds of the vascular system supplying those specific areas (i.e., the arterioles of the basilar membrane of the cochlea and those supplying the ampullae, utricle, and saccule).

EVALUATION OF OTOTOXICITY

Assessment of inner ear morphology is commonly included as a part of ototoxicity studies. However, drugs such as salicylates or loop diuretics may produce electrophysiological and behavioral evidence of ototoxicity without producing any observable structural damage to the cochlea or vestibular apparatus.

Cochlear potentials are routinely used in monitoring auditory function in experimental animals, because the cochlea is readily exposed via a simple surgical procedure. On the other hand, a variety of functional audiological testing procedures are employed to test decrements in human audition. The cochlear potentials most commonly used include: a volume conductor recording of the action potentials of the primary or first-order auditory afferents (N_1); the cochlear alternating current (A.C.) receptor potential derived from cochlear hair cell activity (presumably outer hair cells) and known as cochlear microphonics (CM); and the positive endolymphatic D.C. potential (EP). Specific information related to hearing can be obtained if electrocochleography is performed using appropriate sound stimuli and evaluating N_1; this technique can even be used in conscious human adults, sedated children, and anesthetized animals. The technique for the measurement of brain stem auditory-evoked potentials in conscious, unanesthetized subjects has only recently been developed and has not been extensively used; it appears promising, however, and has the advantage of being noninvasive.

Behavioral assessment of hearing includes determination of the intensity of sound necessary to elicit Preyer's reflex (a flicking of the pinna), pure tone audiometry, and other types of audiometry in conditioned animals and in humans. Although changes in Preyer's reflex thresholds are very crude estimates of hearing, audiometry gives the best overall picture of what the subject actually hears.

OTOTOXIC DRUGS

Drugs that produce impairment in hearing and/or equilibrium include nonsteroidal antiinflammatory drugs (NSAIDs), cinchona alkaloids, loop diuretics, aminoglycoside antibiotics, and other miscellaneous agents.

NSAID AND CINCHONA ALKALOIDS

Tinnitus, vertigo, and, in some cases, temporary hearing loss have been reported to occur with the clinical use of salicylates as well as other nonsteroidal antiinflammatory agents, such as phenylbutazone, oxyphenbutazone, indomethacin, tolmetin, sulindac, naproxen, fenoprofen, and ibuprofen (7). Transient ototoxicity is sometimes observed during treatment with the cinchona alkaloids, such as quinine and quinidine. There are only a few reports regarding permanent deafness resulting from the use of salicylates and cinchona alkaloids (38). Permanent damages to cochlea or vestibular apparatus due to NSAIDs have not been reported (30).

The changes in vestibular function due to salicylate (25) or quinine (23) intoxication are indicative of a direct effect on the peripheral vestibular apparatus. However, the changes in cochlear function induced by these agents may be due to inner ear ischemia, causing anoxia and leading to initial depression of N_1 response (more susceptible to anoxia) (12) followed by reduction in the CM responses (7). Ototoxicity induced by NSAIDs or quinine could also be due to their inhibitory effect on prostaglandin synthetase (8), or alterations produced in the endolymphatic or perilymphatic fluids. The possibility of the latter effect may be supported by significant effects of indomethacin on fluid movement across intestinal mucosa (36) and on cerebrospinal fluid production (15); increases in endolymphatic and perilymphatic pressure have been demonstrated during quinine intoxication in experimental animals (18).

LOOP DIURETICS

Ethacrynic acid and furosemide are associated with occasional manifestations of ototoxicity. These effects are primarily at the cochlea; however, ethacrynic acid may also produce vestibular toxicity (27). Both drugs can produce permanent deafness even after oral administration. Bumetanide, the newest member of this class, has less ototoxic liability (3).

Ethacrynic acid appears to exert an initial effect on the stria vascularis of the cochlea (7), producing edema and resulting in a reduction of EP and a species-dependent alteration of endolymph ionic composition (24); stria vascularis adenylate cyclase is inhibited *in vitro* in concentrations that produce EP changes *in vivo* (33). These effects can cause transient deafness. Permanent deafness may be the result of actions on both the stria vascularis and the outer hair cells.

Furosemide (frusemide) also produces changes in endolymph ionic composition, reduction of EP, depression of CM and N_1, and of auditory-evoked cortical responses, loss of sharpness of tuning in individual cochlear nerve fibers having their lowest thresholds in the higher frequency ranges, and changes in endolymph ionic composition (7).

Bumetanide also produces depression of CM and N_1 and reduction of EP (7). The dose-ototoxic response (N_1 depression) curves of ethacrynic acid, furosemide, and bumetanide are parallel (4), indicating common cochlear sites and mechanisms of action of these drugs.

AMINOGLYCOSIDE ANTIBIOTICS

Of the aminoglycosides used extensively, streptomycin is predominantly vestibulotoxic, and dihydrostreptomycin possesses a severe cochlear toxicity (and hence, has been withdrawn from clinical use). Neomycin is also primarily toxic to the cochlea and is no longer used systematically; deafness occurs after topical application and other routes of administration (39). Newer aminoglycosides, such as gentamicin and tobramycin, show both cochlear and vestibular ototoxicity with the latter occurring more often (32), whereas kanamycin and its congener amikacin are toxic primarily to the cochlea (32). In a recent survey of the clinical literature, the incidence of cochlear ototoxicity with the four commonly used aminoglycosides was kanamycin > amikacin >>> gentamicin ≈ tobramycin; the incidence of overall ototoxicity (cochlear + vestibular) was kanamycin > amikacin >>> gentamicin > tobramycin (32). Changes in the therapeutic regimen based on serum level monitoring can reduce aminoglycoside ototoxicity; this has been demonstrated for amikacin (37).

Pathophysiology. The initial cochlear lesion produced by the aminoglycoside antibiotics in humans and most experimental animals is found in the outer hair cells of the basal turn (7). As a result, the higher-frequency CM responses are affected most with a concomitant reduction in N_1 followed by reduction in cochlear EP. Depending on dosage and duration of treatment, the lesion may spread to include the inner hair cells of the basal turn followed by progressive destruction of the upper cochlear turns, and degeneration of the afferent nerve endings. Damage to the stria vascularis may follow the initial damage to the outer hair cell (7). The type I hair cell appears to be the primary target with accompanying degeneration of its nerve endings (22); as the toxicity progresses, the type II cell and its nerve endings also become affected.

The vestibular cells that play an analogous role to that of the stria vascularis of the cochlea are also damaged; the ampullar cristae appear to be more susceptible to damage than the utricular macula, whereas the macula of the saccule is least susceptible. This damage is initially manifested by vertigo, often occurring only upon turning the head (22). The responses of caloric and rotational tests are reduced in rate and duration: in cases of severe intoxication, they are sometimes entirely absent. Spontaneous nystagmus is rare, but a fine nystagmus may be produced on lateral gaze. Positional nystagmus may be absent, but optokinetic nystagmus remains normal.

Possible Mechanisms of Action. Kanamycin suppresses respiratory enzyme activity in the outer hair cell; enzyme inhibition is more pronounced in the basal than in the apical turns. Furthermore, kanamycin selectively inhibits the activity of the Embden-Meyerhof pathway in the organ of Corti (and in the kidney) without altering that of the hexose monophosphate pathway, but neither pathway is affected in the stria vascularis. In a recent study, it was found that the outer hair cells of animals made diabetic with alloxan are protected from kanamycin toxicity (19), further indicating aminoglycoside interference with carbohydrate metabolism in the outer hair cell. It has also been postulated that aminoglycoside inhibition of cochlear phosphoinositide metabolism causes derangement of selective membrane permeability of the hair cells (7). Damage to the stria vascularis of the cochlea and the analogous tissue in the vestibular apparatus could be due to two factors: suppression of respiratory enzyme and/or adenosine triphosphatase (ATPase) activity (7). Inhibition of strial ATPase occurs only at doses that are higher than those that inhibit hair cell ATPase and suppress hair cell and strial respiratory enzyme activity. Because aminoglycosides, in animals, are eliminated from perilymph more slowly than from blood, accumulation could cause inhibition of cochlear phosphoinositide metabolism and/or ATPase in patients receiving prolonged therapy with aminoglycosides.

Ototoxic Interaction of Loop Diuretics with Aminoglycosides. The risk factors associated with ototoxicity of aminoglycosides include renal impairment, treatment with a high dose over an extended period of time, advanced age, heredity, exposure of high-intensity noise, and exposure to other possible ototoxic drugs (7). In particular, it has been found that hearing loss occurred when a loop diuretic and an aminoglycoside antibiotic were used concurrently in doses not expected to cause ototoxicity if either was used alone (35, 38). In experimental animals ethacrynic acid or furosemide produce both morphological and functional indications of cochlear hair cell damage when combined with kanamycin in individually nonototoxic doses (7). There also appears to be synergistic interaction of the two types of drugs on the cochlea (34) and an additive effect on the vestibular apparatus (28). Prior exposure of a patient to one of the aminoglycosides enhances the ototoxicity observed after subsequent exposure to the same or a different aminoglycoside (32).

MISCELLANEOUS OTOTOXIC AGENTS

Certain chemotherapeutic agents (such as erythromycin) and industrial and environmental pollutants (such as the alkylmercurials, ethanol, methyl alcohol and benzene) can exert an ototoxic action (7). Additionally, following administration of a single dose of 50 mg/M^2 of cisplatin, an antineoplastic agent, ototoxicity manifested by tinnitus and/or hearing loss in the high-frequency range (4000-7000 Hz) occurs in about 30% of patients. Hearing loss may be unilateral or bilateral and tends to become more severe with repeated doses and may be more pronounced in children (31). Comprehensive listings of other ototoxic agents can be found in recent reviews (1, 7, 18, 21, 22).

Attention should be called to the fact that intratympanic instillation, or application to the external auditory canal, of local anesthetics, antiseptics, polymyxin B, chloramphenicol, erythromycin, tetracycline, and chromic acid can produce ototoxicity (7). Even cornstarch glove powder can function as a toxic agent to the ear. Apparently, the toxicity of the antiseptics and antibiotics is not related to the pH of the solutions used, although the solvent in some of the antibiotic preparations may be ototoxic itself. To minimize the toxicity of the antiseptic and antibiotic preparations, "ear drops should seldom be prescribed, especially in the presence of large perforations, where there is a history of ear surgery, or for preoperative prophylaxis" (13). To minimize the ototoxicity of the local anesthetics, it is recommended that they be iontophoretically applied (14).

MOTION SICKNESS AND ANTIMOTION SICKNESS DRUGS

MOTION SICKNESS

Exposure to an unaccustomed motion will produce motion sickness if the conditions are of sufficient intensity and duration. The first sign of motion sickness is pallor, which may be preceded by a brief flush. This is usually followed by yawning, restlessness, and cold sweat appearing on the upper lip and forehead. Next, a "stomach awareness" develops, one best described as a slight upset stomach, along with malaise and drowsiness. Nausea, excessive salivation, heavy sweating, and vomiting develop in the final stage.

Motion sickness appears to be entirely a central nervous system response dependent upon a functional vestibular system. Graybiel et al. (17) have demonstrated that a group of deaf subjects with nonfunctional vestibular systems were totally immune to motion sickness during exposure to severe conditions at sea, in aerobatics, in parabolic flight, and on the human centrifuge.

Habituation to specific conditions of motion will result if the subject is exposed to motion of a constant frequency, direction, duration, and intensity. The habituated subject is immune to motion sickness unless one or more of these parameters is altered. Habituation may result from continuous exposure or from short daily exposures. Psychological factors may also have a strong influence on the development of motion sickness, especially those factors associated with a previous episode (36).

The pharmacological spectrum of effective drugs includes scopolamine (a cholinergic-blocking agent), the antihistaminics (whose action in this case depends on acetylcholine-blocking rather than histamine-blocking properties) (9), and the amphetamines (which release norepinephrine centrally); the combination of a drug having cholinergic-blocking activity with one having noradrenergic activity proves the most effective of all.

To explain these diverse actions, the theory has been advanced (42, 43) that motion sickness is a CNS response to vestibular impulses transmitted to the vestibular nuclei, older areas of the cerebellum, and the brain stem reticular system, (Fig. 21.2-1). In the vestibular nuclei and reticular system are neurons that respond only to norepinephrine and others that respond only to acetylcholine. Some of the effective drugs block acetylcholine, and others release norepinephrine. These findings, along with the observed waxing and waning of the symptoms of motion sickness, indicate that two competing neuronal systems are involved. Habituation results from a strengthening of the influence of the noradrenergic system (41). The balance between these two systems of neurons, whether influenced by drugs or habituation, would govern susceptibility to motion sickness. The antimotion sickness drugs will shift the balance in favor of the patient.

ANTIMOTION SICKNESS DRUGS

Effective antimotion sickness drugs will raise the individual's threshold for the development of motion sick-

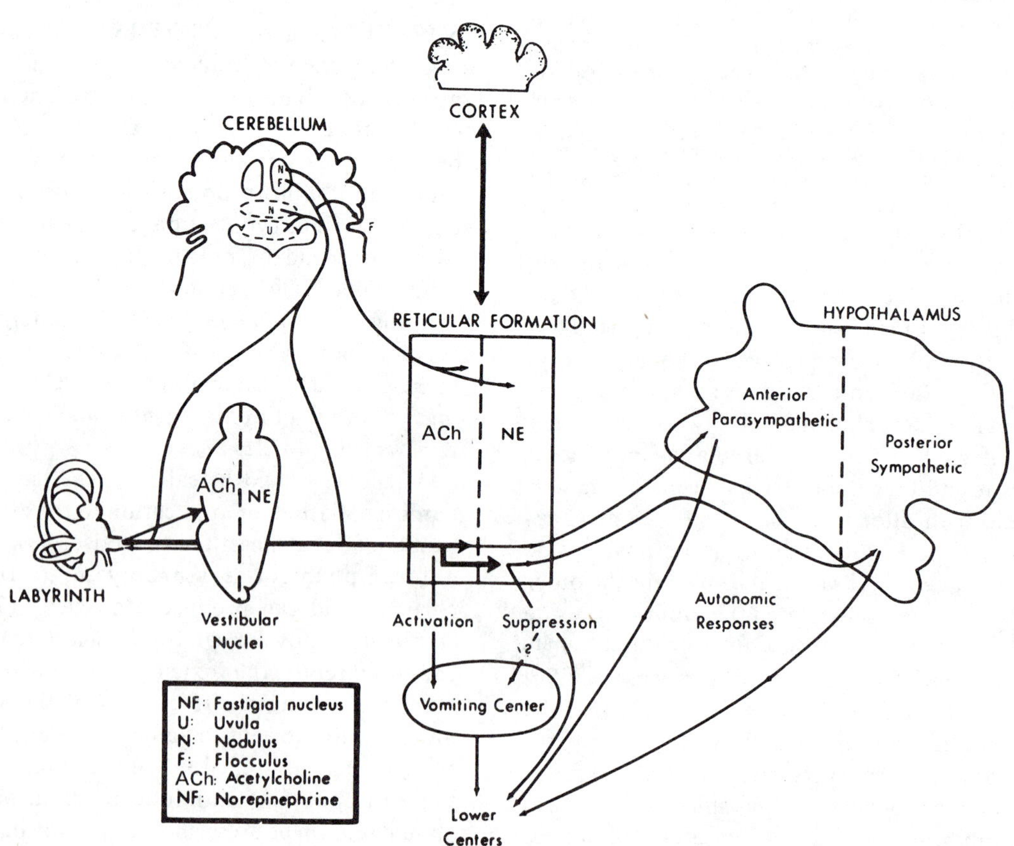

Fig. 21.2-1. *Proposed interaction of cholinergic and noradrenergic neuronal systems in the production of motion sickness* (41). Reproduced by permission.

ness and, unless the conditions are too severe or the subject is too sensitive, protect the individual from becoming frankly motion sick. During long exposures, repeated doses are required for the various antimotion sickness drugs because of their duration of action. None of the currently available preparations are ideal; all have side effects and none produce complete protection for all subjects under all conditions of motion. Table 21.2-1 summarizes the information presented on the antimotion sickness preparations.

CHOLINERGIC BLOCKERS

l-Scopolamine. The most effective single drug against motion sickness is scopolamine (hyoscine). Because it has a duration of action of 4 hours, repeated doses may be required; prolonged use for periods exceeding 24 hours is not recommended unless the dose is reduced. A transdermal applicator maintains a blood level equivalent to an oral dose of 0.2 mg given every 4 hours for a period of 60 hours. No serious side effects have been reported from this dose; with higher doses (0.5 mg or more), blurring of near vision, drowsiness, memory loss, and confusion may occur. Dryness of the mouth is reported at all dosage levels. With repetitive doses, problems have been encountered in patients with glaucoma and prostatic hypertrophy. The drug has been abused by ingesting toxic doses of 2-5 mg to produce delirium and hallucinations.

PHENOTHIAZINES

Promethazine. Promethazine is in the same range of effectiveness as scopolamine but has a duration of action of 8-12 hours. It is the only phenothiazine used as an antihistamine and the only one that is effective against motion sickness. It also has strong central anticholinergic activity. The principal side effect appears to be drowsiness, although less pronounced than that reported for scopolamine. High, prolonged dosage may evoke hypotension. Repeated doses should not be used in the presence of glaucoma or prostatic hypertrophy. Intramuscular injections of 25 mg have been reported to be effective in blocking the further buildup of symptoms after the patient has become motion sick short of vomiting. It is the only antimotion sickness drug reported to be effective as a therapeutic measure after nausea and vomiting have occurred (29). For this purpose, an i.m. injection of 25 mg is given. Some other phenothiazines and trimethobenzamide (TIGAN) are effective in the treatment of chemically induced nausea and vomiting, but are not effective in preventing motion sickness (40).

ANTIHISTAMINES

Dimenhydrinate. Dimenhydrinate is the chlorotheophylline salt of diphenhydramine (BENADRYL) and is a very effective antimotion sickness drug with a duration of action of 6 to 8 hours. It produces less drowsiness than diphenhydramine, but more than other antihistamines discussed in this chapter. Because no birth defects have been reported from animal experiments involving this drug, it is considered safe for use during pregnancy. Dimenhydrinate is one of the more effective drugs for prevention of motion sickness, ranking just below promethazine. It is satisfactory for most travel situations. A dose of 50 mg 1 to 2 hours before start of the journey may be repeated three times per day.

Cyclizine. Cyclizine is a moderately effective antihistamine of the piperazine group, with a duration of 4 hours. Little drowsiness is produced by this drug and few report dizziness while using it. It is contraindicated in the first trimester of pregnancy, as animal experiments utilizing high doses have reported birth defects. It has been included in the medical kit on the space missions as an

Table 21.2-1
Selected Antimotion Sickness Drugs[a]

Drug	Trade Name	Dose (mg)	Duration (hr)	Intensity of Motion Sickness
l-Scopolamine + d-Amphetamine	SCOPODEX (NASA)	0.3-0.6 + 5-10	6	Severe
Promethazine + Ephedrine	P_2E (NASA)	25 + 25	12	Severe
l-Scopolamine (hyoscine)		0.3-0.6	4	Severe
Promethazine	PHENERGAN	25	12 (i.m. 25-50)	Severe
Dimenhydrinate	DRAMAMINE	50	6	Moderate
Cyclizine	MAREZINE	50	4	Mild
Meclizine	BONINE	50	8	Mild

[a]All preparations are given orally, unless otherwise indicated.

alternative oral antimotion sickness preparation. This is a choice drug for civilian travel at a 50-mg dose four times per day.

Meclizine. Meclizine is also in the piperazine group, but it has a longer duration of action (6 to 12 hours) and is given twice daily. It is less effective than cyclizine, although this may be due to the long delay in reaching its peak effectiveness. Meclizine should be taken at least 2 to 3 hours before exposure to the motion environment. It is reported to cause more drowsiness and unsteadiness than cyclizine but less than dimenhydrinate. It would be best used for long exposure to moderate conditions such as encountered on a sea voyage in good weather.

SYMPATHOMIMETIC AGENTS

d-Amphetamine. Amphetamine (5-10 mg) is an effective antimotion sickness drug, alone or in combination. It ranges between dimenhydrinate and cyclizine in effectiveness, with a duration of from 6 to 12 hours depending on dosage. Side effects due to central nervous system stimulation include increased activity, increased talking, nervousness, increased blood pressure, and insomnia.

Ephedrine. Ephedrine (25 mg) is quite similar to amphetamine in effectiveness but with a shorter duration of action (about 4 hours). The side effects are similar, due to central nervous system activation.

COMBINATIONS

l-Scopolamine + d-Amphetamine. l-Scopolamine + d-amphetamine is the most effective antimotion sickness medication now available, with a duration of action from 4 to 6 hours (42, 44). Repetitive doses four times daily may produce cumulative effect of amphetamine, although the drowsiness and excitement are mutually diminished by the opposing actions of these drugs. Dry mouth is reported; in the Soviet Union, neostigmine is added to relieve this side effect (26).

Promethazine + ephedrine. Promethazine + ephedrine has similar effectiveness and appears to produce fewer side effects. Promethazine, with a >8-hour duration, would be expected to outlast ephedrine (4 hours) and produce late drowsiness. Sufficient time after administration (at least 2 hours) should be allowed before exposure to motion for an effective level of promethazine to be attained. Repetitive doses may be given every 8 to 10 hours.

PREPARATIONS OF CHOICE

The most effective preparation for prevention of motion sickness is l-scopolamine (0.6 mg) combined with d-amphetamine (10 mg), although half this dose may be sufficient under moderate conditions. This is the preparation of choice included in the medical kit on space missions. The abuse potential has limited the use of this preparation. Promethazine (25 mg) with ephedrine (25 mg) is in the same range of effectiveness. Promethazine (25 mg) can also be used alone if drowsiness is not a problem. Furthermore, it can be used in an i.m. injection (25 mg) for a therapeutic measure after motion sickness has progressed. For civilian travel, 50 mg of dimenhydrinate, (a combination of diphenhydramine and 8-chlorotheophylline), cyclizine, or meclizine two to three times a day is sufficient in most instances, if given 1 to 2 hours before exposure.

MÉNIÈRE'S DISEASE AND ITS TREATMENT

Ménière's disease is usually characterized by episodic vertigo with deafness and tinnitus (10). However, the symptoms may be localized to the cochlea or the vestibular apparatus. It is generally accepted to be caused by increased endolymphatic pressure. Therapy, aimed solely at alleviation of symptomatology, is accomplished by sedation, pharmacological and/or surgical decompression of the increased endolymphatic pressure, and if the symptoms are too disabling and the remissions short or nonexistent, by pharmacological (e.g., by streptomycin) or surgical destruction of the affected ear(s).

Efficient sedation is a mandatory component of the treatment of the acute attack to reduce anxiety and raise the threshold of response in the vestibular pathways. The neuroleptic droperidol (INAPSINE) or its combination with fentanyl citrate (INNOVAR) is sometimes used to manage the acute episode (2). In addition, atropine and epinephrine have been found to be moderately effective, presumably by altering autonomic nervous system function, improving the circulation of the inner ear, and thereby increasing the return of fluid from the endolymphatic space to the capillaries. Intravenous administration of a vasodilating cocktail (2) and local anesthetic blockade of the stellate ganglion (10) are also moderately effective and are thought to act through a similar mechanism. Although not used in management of the acute episode, furosemide and the osmotic agent, glycerin, are given as diagnostic tests for Ménière's disease (16). "Dehydration" of the endolymphatic fluid due to either type of agent produces a transient improvement in caloric response, if the patient has Ménière's disease.

The antimotion sickness drugs are employed during the acute episode and during remission. They are useful in suppressing nausea and vomiting as well as the unsteadiness that may follow an acute episode. The sedative effect of these drugs probably contributes to their therapeutic effect.

REFERENCES

1. Ajodhia, J.M. and Dix, M.R. Drug-induced deafness and its treatment. *Practitioner* 216:561, 1976.
2. Banovetz, J.D. Drugs in otolaryngology. In: *Drugs of Choice, 1978-1979* (Modell, W., ed.) St. Louis: C.V. Mosby, 1978.
3. Bourke, E. Frusemide, bumetanide, and ototoxicity. *Lancet* 1:917, 1976.
4. Brown, R.D. Cochlear N_1 depression produced by the new loop diuretic, bumetanide, in cats. *Neuropharmacology* 14:547, 1975.
5. Brown, R.D. Ethacrynic acid and furosemide: Possible cochlear sites and mechanisms of ototoxic action. *Medikon* 4:33, 1975.
6. Brown, R.D. Anatomy of the inner ear. In: *The Pharmacology of Hearing: Experimental and Clinical Bases* (Brown, R.D. and Daigneault, E.A, eds.) New York: John Wiley, 1981.
7. Brown, R.D. and Feldman, A.M. Pharmacology of hearing and ototoxicity. *Ann. Rev. Pharmacol. Toxicol.* 18:233, 1978.
8. Brune, L., Glatt, M. and Graf, P. Minireview: Mechanisms of action of antiinflammatory drugs. *Gen. Pharmacol.* 7:27, 1976.
9. Chinn, H.I. and Smith, P.K. Motion sickness. *Pharmacol. Rev.* 7:33, 1955.
10. Colman, B.H. Ménière's disease. In: Scott-Brown's Diseases of *the Ear, Nose, and Throat* (Ballantyne, J. and Grove, J., eds.) Vol. 2, 3rd ed. Philadelphia: J.B. Lippincott, 1971.

11. Daigneault, E.A. Pharmacology of the cochlear efferents. In: *The Pharmacology of Hearing: Experimental and Clinical Bases* (Brown, R.D. and Daigneault, E.A., eds.) New York: John Wiley, 1981.
12. Davis, H. Biophysics and physiology of the inner ear. *Physiol. Rev.* 37:1, 1957.
13. Ear-drops (editorial). *Lancet* 1:896, 1976.
14. Echols, D.F., Norris, C.H. and Tabb, H.G. Anesthesia of the ear by iontophoresis of lidocaine. *Arch. Otolaryngol.* 102:418, 1975.
15. Feldman, A.M., Smith, T., Epstein, M.H. and Brusilow, S.W. Effects of indomethacin on cholear toxin induced cerebrospinal fluid production. *Brain Res.* 42:379, 1978.
16. Futaki, T., Kitaharra, M. and Morimoto, M. A comparison of the furosemide and glycerol tests for Ménière's disease. *Acta Otolaryngol.* 83:272, 1977.
17. Graybiel, A., Wood, C.D. Krepton, J., Hoche, J.P. and Perkins, G.F. Human bioassay of antimotion sickness drugs. *Aerospace Med.* 46:1107, 1975.
18. Guth, P.S. and Bobbin, R.P. The pharmacology of peripheral auditory processes: Cochlear pharmacology. In: *Advances in Pharmacology and Chemotherapy,* (Gerratini, S., Goldin, A., Hawking, F. and Kopin, I.S., eds.) Vol. 9, New York: Academic Press, 1971.
19. Guth, P.S., Garcia-Quiroga, J. and Norris, C.H. Alloxan-induced diabetes confers protection against kanamycin ototoxicity. *Neurosci. Abstr.* 3:15, 1977.
20. Guth, P.S., Tachibana, M. and Sewell, W.F. Pharmacology of the cochlear afferents. In: *The Pharmacology of Hearing: Experimental and Clinical Bases* (Brown, R.D. and Diagneault, E.A., eds.) New York: John Wiley, 1981.
21. Hawkins, J.E. Drug ototoxicity. In: *Handbook of Sensory Physiology,* (Keidel, W.D. and Neff, W.D., eds.) Vol V/3, New York: Springer-Verlag, 1976.
22. Hawkins, J.E. and Preston, R.E. Vestibular ototoxicity. In: *The Vestibular System* (Nauton, R.F., ed.) New York: Academic Press, 1975.
23. Hennebert, D. and Fernandez, C. Ototoxicity of quinine in experimental animals. *Arch. Otolaryngol.* 70:321, 1959.
24. Kusakari, J. and Thalmann, R. Effects of anoxia and ethacrynic acid upon ampullar endolymphatic potential and upon high energy phosphates in ampullar wall. *Laryngoscope* 86:132, 1976.
25. Lucente, F.E. Aspirin and the otolaryngologist. *Arch. Otolaryngol.* 94:443, 1971.
26. Lukomskaya, N.Y., Nikolskay, M.I. and Mikhelson, M.Y. *Search for Drugs Against Motion Sickness.* Leningrad: Sechenov Institute of Evolutionary Physiology and Biochemistry, 1971.
27. Mathog, R.H. Vestibulotoxicity of ethacrynic acid. *Laryngoscope* 87:1791, 1977.
28. Mathog, R.H. and Capps, M.J. Ototoxic interactions of ethacrynic acid and streptomycin. *Ann. Otol.* 86:158, 1977.
29. McMurray, G.N. Evaluation of metoclopramide as an antiemetic in seasickness. *Post Grad. Med. J. (Suppl. 4)* 49:38, 1973.
30. McPherson, D.L. and Miller, J.F. Choline salicylate: Effects on cochlear function. *Arch. Otolaryngol.* 99:304, 1974.
31. Merrin, C., Beckley, S. and Takita, H. Multimodal treatment of advanced testicular tumor with radical reductive surgery and multisequential chemotherapy with cis platinum, bleomycin, vinblastine, vincristine, and actinomycin D. *J. Urol.* 120:73, 1978.
32. Neu, H.C. and Bendush, C.L. Ototoxicity of tobramycin: A clinical overview. *J. Infect. Dis. (Suppl. S206)* 134, 1976.
33. Paloheimo, S. and Thalmann, R. Tissue concentrations of ethacrynic acid and inhibition of enzymes and electrophysiological responses in cochlea. *J. Acust. Soc. Am. (Suppl. 1)* 58:S1, 1975 (abstr.)
34. Prazma, J., Browder, J.P. and Fischer, N.D. Ethacrynic acid ototoxicity potentiation by kanamycin. *Ann. Otol.* 83:111, 1974.
35. Quick, C.A. Hearing loss in patients with dialysis and renal transplants. *Ann. Otol.* 85:776, 1976.
36. Reason, J.T. and Brand, J.J. *Motion Sickness.* New York: Academic press, 1975.
37. Smith, C.R., Baughman, K.L., Edwards, C.Q., Rogers, J.F. and Lietman, P.S. Controlled comparison of amikacin and gentamicin. *N. Engl. J. Med.* 296:349, 1977.
38. Thomsen, J., Bech, P. and Szpirt, W. Otologic symptoms in chronic renal failure: The possible role of aminoglycoside-furosemide interaction. *Arch. Oto-Rhino-Laryngol.* 214:71, 1976.
39. Topical neomycin (editorial). *Med. Lett.* 15:101, 1973.
40. Wood, C.D. and Graybiel, A. Evaluation of 16 antimotion sickness drugs under controlled laboratory conditions. *Aerospace Med.* 39:1341, 1968.
41. Wood, C.D. and Graybiel, A. A theory of motion sickness based on pharmacological reactions. *Clin, Pharmacol. Ther.* 11:621, 1970.
42. Wood, C.D. and Graybiel, A. Theory of antimotion sickness drug mechanisms. *Aerospace Med.* 43:249, 1972.
43. Wood, C.D. and Graybiel, A. The antimotion sickness drugs. *Otolaryngol. Clin. North Am.* 6:301, 1973.
44. Wood, C.D., Kennedy, R.S. and Graybiel, A. Review of antimotion sickness drugs from 1954-1964. *Aerospace Med.* 36:1, 1965.

CHAPTER
21.3

DRUG EFFECTS ON TASTE AND SMELL

Robert I. Henkin

Many drugs produce unwanted effects on sensory function. Effects on visual and auditory function, resulting in nystagmus, visual perception of halos, tinnitus, egophonia, or diminution of visual or auditory acuity are commonly brought to the attention of the physician. These effects can be debilitating, the physician usually responding by terminating drug administration, which if it occurs early, is usually associated with a return of normal function. However, permanent damage to visual or auditory receptors can and does occur.

Effects of drugs on taste and smell function have not been commonly recognized until recently. Although drugs that produce anorexia, nausea, vomiting, or other signs of gastrointestinal distress are well known, drug effects that change taste and smell function have been considered to be relatively rare. With the emergence of techniques to measure taste and smell acuity (15, 18) and with the knowledge that many diseases influence taste and smell function (15, 18), drug effects have assumed increasing importance as disturbing and potentially dangerous side effects. It is the purpose of this chapter to deal with some of these relationships in order to survey the extent, magnitude, and frequency of these interactions. Because of the relatively recent emergence of this field, documentation of some of these effects may not be as systematic as similar effects on the visual and auditory systems.

Definitions

In order to describe the effects of drugs on taste and smell, it is necessary to define the manner in which taste and smell change pathologically and the manner in which these changes can be measured.

Hypogeusia is defined as a decrease in taste acuity and is a common change following drug administration. *Ageusia* is defined as a total loss of taste acuity, a total inability to detect or recognize any taste; this occurs relatively rarely. Taste acuity relates to the ability to detect and recognize tastes commonly exemplified by salt, sweet, sour, and bitter tastants (14, 15). *Detection threshold* can be measured and defined by the three-stimulus, forced-choice drop technique, in which the most dilute concentration of solute in water is detected consistently as different from two solutions of water alone (15, 28). *Recognition threshold* can be measured and defined as the most dilute concentration of solute in water recognized consistently and appropriately as either salty, bitter, sweet, or sour (15, 28). *Forced scaling* or *magnitude estimation* defines the intensity of a suprathreshold concentration of solute in water that the patient recognizes consistently and appropriately as either salty, bitter, sweet, or sour in relation to a scale from 0 to 100 with 100 considered as the most salty, bitter, sweet, or sour solution previously experienced (28).

In response to drugs, the bitter taste quality, represented by the smallest number of taste receptors in the oral cavity, is most commonly affected (15). However, most patients do not commonly seek out bitter tastants in everyday eating and drinking, except for coffee or tea to which sweeteners are commonly added. Although each taste receptor can subserve each taste quality, receptors that are most sensitive to bitter are located in taste buds on the palate (15, 21). The sweet taste quality, represented by the largest number of receptors in the oral cavity, is least commonly affected by drugs (15). Taste buds most sensitive to sweet are located over the entire lingual surface in both fungiform and circumvallate papillae. Diagnostically, changes in sweet taste are extremely useful, since these changes usually indicate severe injury to taste buds and are of great hedonic significance to the patient. Salt and sour taste qualities are intermediate in receptor sensitivity. Receptors most sensitive to salt are located in taste buds in fungiform papillae over the anterior two-third of the tongue; receptors most sensitive to sour are located in a smaller number of taste buds in palatal papillae (15).

Dysgeusia is defined as a distortion of taste function (14), a general term used to describe several aspects of distorted taste, and includes *cacogeusia*, the unpleasant, obnoxious taste associated with the intake of food and drink normally appreciated as pleasant; *parageusia*, the unusual but not necessarily unpleasant taste associated with the intake of food and drink (e.g., a normally sweet-tasting substance may taste salty); *phantogeusia*, the presence of a taste in the oral cavity without the presence of a specific food or drink stimulus; and *heterogeusia*, the uniform, usually unpleasant, taste of all food and drink. Dysgeusia usually follows the onset of hypogeusia in the initiation of taste dysfunction (15). *Taste extinction* is the rapid and complete loss of taste following the normal appreciation of the initial taste of food and drink. *Taste perseveration* is the persistence of any taste in the oral cavity for an inordinately prolonged period, dissociated from any gastrointestinal regurgitation or pulmonary stimulus, lasting for hours or days.

Hyposmia is defined as a decrease in smell acuity and is the most common smell change that occurs following drug treatment. *Detection threshold, recognition threshold,* and *forced scaling* for smell can be measured and defined (5, 18, 28) similar to taste perception except that the three-stimulus, forced-choice measurements involve two similar, relatively nonodorous stimuli, water or mineral oil, and one odorous stimulus that is commonly pyridine (pungent), nitrobenzene (bitter almond), thiophene (petrochemical), or amyl acetate (banana oil). *Magnitude estimation* is measured and defined for vapors similar to that for taste except that subjects are required to judge the intensity of suprathreshold concentrations of the vapors noted previously (5, 18, 28). Similar to taste, the decreased ability to smell perfumes, bakery, or pleasant cooking smells is commonly a sign of severe hyposmia. As in taste, increased smell thresholds indicate pathology in all smell receptors subserving a given vapor, whereas increases in forced scaling or magnitude estimation, associated with little or no change in smell thresholds, indicate a decrease in receptor number for a given vapor (18).

Abnormalities of smell acuity have been categorized clinically (14, 18). *Type I hyposmia* refers to the inability of the patient to recognize vapors at the primary olfactory area (the area of interaction between the olfactory epithelium and olfactory nerve where maximum smell sensitivity occurs), with detection preserved, albeit severely impaired. *Type II hyposmia* refers to a quantitative decrease in the ability to detect and/or recognize vapors. This defect is the most common form of hyposmia observed following drug injury to the olfactory system. *Anosmia* refers to the inability of the patient to detect or recognize vapors either at the primary or accessory (i.e., those areas innervated by cranial nerves V, VII, IX, or X) areas of olfaction (18). This type of loss is relatively rare. *Dysosmia* is defined as a distortion of smell function and includes *cacosmia*, the unpleasant, obnoxious, usually foul smells associated with the smelling of normally pleasant vapors; *parosmia*, distorted, but not unpleasant, smell sensations (e.g., flowers may smell like bananas); *phantosmia*, the presence of a smell in the nasal cavity without the presence of a specific vapor stimulus; and *heterosmia*, the uniform character, usually unpleasant, of all vapors. *Smell extinction* and *perseveration* are defined similar to that for taste perception.

Decreased flavor perception is the decreased ability to perceive flavor from food. This is commonly described by the patient as a loss of taste but, in reality, it relates more to a decrease in smell. Some patients with hyposmia may exhibit normal flavor perception whereas others may find this ability severely impaired. Similarly, some patients with hypogeusia may exhibit severe impairment of flavor perception, whereas others will exhibit very little, if any at all.

DRUG EFFECTS ON TASTE AND SMELL

The effects of several drugs on taste and smell functions are summarized in Table 21.3-1. Some agents affect taste and smell profoundly while others have only modest effects.

CARDIOVASCULAR DRUGS

Captopril has been associated with the production of hypogeusia (41) in about 20% of patients treated. Since the drug produces its antihypertensive effects through inhibition of the zinc-dependent angiotensin-converting enzyme, the mechanism of action of captopril on taste may involve chelation of zinc from other zinc metalloproteins involved in the taste process, such as gustin in saliva (25) and/or the zinc-bridge binding of

Table 21.3-1
Effects of Selected Drugs on Taste and Smell Perception[a]

Drug	Incidence %	Taste			Smell			Daily Dose: Onset Time/Recovery Time	Possible Mechanism
		Hg	Dg	Pg	Hs	Ds	Ps		
D-Penicillamine (23, 38, 43)	14-35	+	+					1-2 g/day; 2-3 weeks/variable	Cu depletion
Captopril (41)	19	+						150-450 mg; 3-4 weeks/10 days-2 weeks	Zn chelation
Amrinone (19)	40	+	+		+	+		300 mg; 2-4 weeks/unknown	Possible Zn depletion
Methimazole (10)	6	+			+			30-40 mg; 4 weeks/10 days-3 weeks	Unknown
Biguanide (50)	3	+		+				Unknown	Unknown
Oxymetazoline (19)	1-5				+			2-3 sniffs; 3-5 weeks/unknown	Local damage to olfactory receptors
L-DOPA (2, 44, 57)	20-40	+		+				1 g; 2-8 weeks/unknown	Unknown
Bromocriptine (6)	9						+	66 mg; 1-6 months/6 weeks	Unknown

[a] Abbreviations used: Dg, dysgeusia; Hg, hypogeusia; Pg, phantogeusia; Hs, hyposmia; Ds, dysosmia; Ps, phantosmia.

gustin to the family of salivary phosphoglycoproteins, lumicarmine (54, 55). Such effects could alter taste bud function directly, since gustin presumably acts as a taste bud growth factor (16). Inactivation of gustin could alter taste bud growth and development and produce hypogeusia and other symptoms of taste dysfunction (17, 56).

Amrinone, a drug used in the treatment of refractory congestive heart failure, has produced hypogeusia and dysgeusia in several patients; preliminary observations suggest that alteration in zinc metabolism, possibly by chelation, may also be a mechanism of action of this drug (19).

Oxyfedrin, a coronary vasodilator, has been reported to produce ageusia in 3% of the patients treated with this agent (48). Digitalis preparations have been associated with the production of variable phantogeusias.

DIURETICS

Several diuretics have been implicated in the production of hypogeusia or dysgeusia. *Hydrochlorothiazide* induces hyperzincuria (47), and during prolonged administration, it could induce zinc deficiency, with lower than normal levels of zinc in blood and saliva (19). Zinc deficiency per se is commonly associated with hypogeusia in several disorders (1, 11, 17, 27, 58); treatment of some patients with exogenous zinc along with continued administration of hydrochlorothiazide restored taste function to or toward normal (19).

HORMONES AND RELATED AGENTS

The production of taste dysfunction with drugs used in the treatment of hyperthyroidism such as, methylthiouracil (35, 53) and methimazole (10) (Table 21.3-1) may relate to production of a relative or absolute state of hypothyroidism or to a direct effect of these drugs on taste function. In both humans (39, 40) and experimental animals (49) hypothyroidism is associated with the production of hypogeusia, hyposmia, dysgeusia, and dysosmia. Since *thyroid hormone* appears to influence both nerve growth factor and gustin (16), these hormones could influence the taste system either indirectly or directly through inhibition of the synthesis of gustin. Thyroid hormone (34) also influences cyclic adenosine monophosphate (cAMP) phosphodiesterase (PDE) activity in isolated taste bud membranes; lack of thyroid hormone has been associated with increased cAMP PDE activity which, in turn, inhibits cAMP and taste transduction mechanisms.

Taste and smell dysfunction has been reported with use of *oral hypoglycemic agents* such as *biguanide* (50) (Table 21.3-1); however, diabetes mellitus itself has been associated with taste dysfunction (8, 12, 30). Since diabetes mellitus may influence both vascular and neural function, systems important in maintenance of normal taste and smell function, these findings are not surprising. *Chromium*, a trace metal implicated in diabetes mellitus through the action of the so-called glucose tolerance factor, has been found in human parotid saliva (46), apparently associated with proteins in fraction V (26). Oral hypoglycemic agents may interact with chromium or with other factors involved in glucose and fat metabolism, and thus may influence taste and smell at several levels of organization.

ANTIBIOTICS AND CHEMOTHERAPEUTIC AGENTS

Antibiotics of several types such as *amphotericin B*, *lincomycin*, and *metronidazole* influence both taste and smell function (50). Since these drugs commonly influence protein synthesis and since the taste buds and the olfactory receptors turn over rapidly in experimental animals, antibiotic effects on taste and smell could be mediated by alterations of receptor growth or development. *Ethambutol*, a drug used to treat tuberculosis, acts to inhibit taste perception (17) presumably by zinc depletion, since it has been shown to produce zinc depletion in the retina with resultant inhibition of the tepetum lucidum reflex in the eye of the dog (17).

The phantogeusia reported with the use of *sulfamethazine* is extremely dose dependent, with a daily dose of 2 g producing the effect, but disappearing spontaneously when the dose is decreased to 1 g/day (29, 31, 50). This drug has also been reported to produce a "sweet ageusia," a very unusual type of taste loss, since the sweet taste quality is usually the last affected by any pathological process, presumably because it is served by the largest number of taste buds in the oral cavity (15).

NASAL DECONGESTANTS

Nasal decongestants such as *oxymetazoline* (AFRIN) (19) (Table 21.3-1) can influence the smell system directly, particularly after being sprayed into the nose for prolonged periods of time to produce vasoconstriction and, hence, increased nasal air flow. This decongestant acts for 10-12 hr and, when used on a chronic basis, can produce prolonged or even permanent hyposmia. Olfactory receptors lie at the apex of the nasal airway and are in direct contact with most vapors entering the nares; chronic usage of vasoconstrictive agents that might affect either mucous secreting glands or receptors themselves may injure these sensitive structures.

ANTIINFLAMMATORY AGENTS

Acetylsalicylic acid (ASA) does not commonly produce taste dysfunction, although reports of changes in bitter taste sensation have been observed in the past (4). The effects occur well after onset of gastrointestinal symptoms and tinnitus, and symptoms have been reported to persist long after treatment was terminated. No effects on smell have been reported, although severe impairment of flavor perception has occurred. Treatment of one patient with severe hypogeusia with zinc ion (100 mg as $ZnSO_4$, orally) along with continued administration of ASA in an open trial resulted in return of normal taste acuity and flavor perception within 1 month; the patient was maintained on 50 mg of zinc ion daily with no further return of symptoms. Discontinuation of the drug was associated with a subjective return of hypogeusia and flavor loss. One possible mechanism for these effects relates to the possible interference of ASA with adenosine triphosphate (ATP)-dependent reactions, as shown in experimental animals (4, 13). Since taste buds require large amounts of high-energy phosphate bonds to carry out the various steps of taste (37), any drug that might interfere with this process could severely alter it. Effects of ASA on taste in experimental animals have been well documented for the taste of bitter (13). The possible role of prostaglandins in the taste process is also raised since several investigators have found evidence of decreased zinc absorption in rats given indomethacin, another prostaglandin inhibitor.

The influence of *colchicine* on taste function has been noted subjectively by many patients receiving this drug for attacks of acute gouty arthritis. *Gold* appears to produce taste dysfunction among some patients with rheumatoid arthritis (15). It may displace zinc from its binding site in gustin during protein synthesis, thereby inactivating gustin.

Production of hypogeusia and dysgeusia following *levamisole* (9) may relate to the action of this drug as a potent stereospecific, noncompetitive inhibitor of alkaline phosphatase (59). In studies of isolated bovine taste bud membranes, alkaline phosphatase was found to be the prevalent enzyme isolated (37). Addition of EDTA to purified taste bud membrane preparations significantly inhibited the binding of radioactive sucrose to these membranes, whereas addition of zinc to these preparations restored binding toward normal levels. These studies suggest one possible role of alkaline phosphatase, a zinc-dependent enzyme, in the taste process.

METALS AND CHELATING AGENTS

Complaints of taste dysfunction similar to those reported with gold have been observed following chronic exposure to several metals including *mercury* (36), *lead* (7), and *cadmium* (45); these metals may also replace zinc and thereby inactivate gustin. *In vitro, cobalt* competes for zinc at the primary, strong metal binding site on gustin (54), but little is known about the activities of these other metals in this system.

D-penicillamine has been observed to produce hypogeusia and dysgeusia in many patients to whom it has been administered, including patients with rheumatoid arthritis (23, 38, 43), cystinuria (20, 23), scleroderma (23), idiopathic pulmonary fibrosis (23), although rarely in those with Wilson's disease (23). It has also been shown to influence taste in experimental animals. The relatively infrequent finding of hypogeusia in patients with Wilson's disease, who have a large increase in tissue copper concentration and in whom copper depletion with D-penicillamine is infrequent, compared with the more common relative copper depletion in other patients who receive this drug and the more frequent production of taste dysfunction, suggested that the mechanism underlying this effect was that of copper depletion (23). Indeed, administration of oral exogenous copper in the face of continued D-penicillamine administration in patients with scleroderma and idiopathic pulmonary fibrosis uniformly restored taste function toward normal (23). In some patients, administration of exogenous zinc, given in large doses for prolonged periods of time along with the drug, has restored normal taste function (20). In other patients over prolonged time periods, taste function returned to normal without specific therapy. Although copper is found in human parotid saliva (46), primarily in fraction II and occasionally in fraction VI, its role in the taste process is unclear. Several metals, including copper, bind to the second or weak metal binding site on gustin (54), but only zinc seems capable of producing the physiological binding of gustin to salivary lumicarmine and, perhaps, subsequent correction of taste dysfunction (56). D-penicillamine has also been reported to produce flavor loss without production of subjective or objective hyposmia as measured by the three-stimulus, forced-choice sniff technique.

ANTITUMOR AGENTS

Decreased taste acuity following cis-platinum treatment has been observed by several investigators (19, 51). The effect of cis-platinum (19) on taste appears to be similar to that suggested for gold (i.e., replacement of zinc in gustin by a metal that produces inactivation of the protein). Its rapid onset of action may be related to its intravenous administration, with the rapid onset of several systemic effects localized to the gastrointestinal system including anorexia, nausea, and vomiting. Although nausea and vomiting may remit spontaneously within 24-28 hrs, anorexia, dysgeusia, hypogeusia, and flavor loss associated with this drug may last 3 weeks before diminishing and/or disappearing. *Adriamycin* (19) may produce hypogeusia through metal chelation or by inhibition of calmodulin secretion (33), but more work is necessary to define its mechanism of action. Indeed, several drugs which inhibit calmodulin secretion appear to induce hypogeusia also (33). *Gallium nitrate* has been reported to produce a metallic phantogeusia (3). Several other drugs used in cancer chemotherapy have been reported to be associated with the production of hypogeusia and dysgeusia; since these drugs are generally used in combinations, it is difficult to implicate specific drugs. In combination, *5-fluorouracil, CCNU, vincristine,* and other antimetabolites have produced measurable hypogeusia and dysgeusia and less frequently hyposmia. The combination of *actinomycin D, bleomycin, vindesine,* and *DTIC* has also been associated with taste changes in patients undergoing this treatment. Taste abnormalities in patients with cancer appear to be influenced by tumor burden as well as specific treatment effects.

DOPAMINE AGONISTS

Reports of effects of *L-DOPA* on taste are contradictory. *L-DOPA* has been reported to enhance taste function as well as to be associated with hypogeusia and phantogeusia (2, 44, 57). It is well known that catecholamines, metabolic products of *L-DOPA*, are localized at or near taste receptors in lower species, as demonstrated by fluorescence microscopy (22); however, their function in the taste process in humans has not been specified. *Bromocriptine* has been reported to produce phantogeusia (6) (Table 21.3-1).

MISCELLANEOUS AGENTS

Lithium, a drug used in the treatment of manic depression, has also been observed to produce taste dysfunction (19). Other drugs such as tranquilizers, including the entire class of *benzodiazepines* and their derivatives, have produced temporary or permanent hypogeusia and hyposmia (19). Some of these drugs may inhibit calmodulin secretion by the parotid gland, which may inhibit taste function since this calcium-containing protein seems to play some necessary but yet unspecified role in taste function (33). The production of hypogeusia and dysgeusia following intravenous RENOGRAFIN (*diatrizoate meglamine and diatrizoate sodium*, USP, a radiopaque contrast agent) injection was observed in one patient. In addition to an immediate allergic-type reaction with diaphoresis, skin erythema, and shortness of breath, there was an immediate loss of taste. Following administration of parenteral *diphenhydramine*, the erythema and pulmonary complaints subsided, but the hypogeusia persisted followed by the onset of dysgeusia. The patient reported recovery of near-normal taste function 2 years after the acute episode.

Some drugs just noted that influence taste function have recently been mentioned in a general review of various aspects of taste function (52).

There are profound and varied effects of drugs on taste and smell function with the number and type of drugs varying greatly as well as their possible mechanisms of action. Although patients commonly complain of taste loss following drug treatment, these complaints may indicate that they are unable to obtain the expected taste of food (i.e., a loss of flavor) that is more commonly associated with loss of smell or hyposmia than loss of taste. This must be considered when subjective complaints about drugs occur without quantitative measurement of either taste or smell function.

Although data obtained from many reports are subjective and deal with small numbers of patients, they emphasize the need to consider taste and smell dysfunction as common sequelae of drug administration. Most of these effects occur gradually, are related to drug dose, and remit spontaneously, albeit after weeks or months (in some cases) following drug discontinuation. However, some drug effects persist for long periods of time and may require therapy to restore normal function. Often, the therapy needed is unclear because the mechanisms underlying the drug effect are unknown.

MECHANISMS OF TASTE AND SMELL DYSFUNCTION

The role of zinc as one factor underlying the mechanism of drug effects appears repeatedly. At present, the roles that trace metals play in the taste process have assumed increasing significance with the increasing awareness of the importance of saliva as a fluid necessary to deliver nutrition to the taste buds and as the major proteins in human saliva, and their metal cofactors, have been isolated and characterized. Gustin, the major zinc protein in saliva, has a molecular weight of 37,000, is without subunits, contains 8% histidine, and has 1 atom of zinc per mole of protein tightly bound to the molecule, presumably to one of the histidine moieties (25): it also binds another mole of zinc less tightly, and, apparently, it is through this zinc that the lumicarmines, the family of Pro, Gly, Glx, rich, pink-violet staining phosphoproteins devoid of aromatic amino acids (55) that comprise the largest amount of protein in saliva (80% of parotid saliva) (55), are bound to gustin. This family of phosphoproteins is very unusual in that they are mainly glycoproteins, contain 6 mole of phosphate per mole of protein, have a molecular weight of 34,000, with approximately 80% of its amino acids proline, glycine, and glutamine (55). Gustin has been considered a taste bud growth factor (16), and it may be that the gustin-lumicarmine complex is the normal physiological form by which these proteins appear in the oral cavity (55). Since taste buds lack blood vessels, lymphatics, and mitotic figures, gustin has been considered to play a role in the differentiation of the surrounding epithelial cells that migrate into the taste bud and form the complex taste cells under the influence of this protein. This hypothesis is useful in the consideration of taste bud growth and development. Drugs that influence metals (e.g., zinc) by chelation, binding, or inhibition or that influence the binding of gustin to lumicarmine seem to influence taste profoundly. Obviously, the taste process is complex, involving many substances at several levels of organization, the receptor, the level of transduction of neural information at the bud, the transmission of the neural impulse along the cranial nerves, or the integration of neural information in the brain.

There is less specific information known about olfactory processes, but the physiological components of the system are basically similar to taste. There are complex chemical processes that take place at the receptor, involving binding of odorant to receptor, subsequent transduction and amplification of the initial chemical signal involving activation of cAMP (32, 34), and the subsequent cascade of events in this system including the action of specific phosphodiesterases and protein kinases. These latter events are involved in initiating depolarization of the olfactory nerve. Subsequent neural transmission and integration in the central nervous system involve many complex chemical and electrical processes that take place in the temporal lobe, the prefrontal cortex, and the limbic components of the parietal cortex.

For normal function the olfactory receptor must be bathed in mucus, as the taste receptor must be bathed in saliva. Drugs that interfere with mucus secretion in and around the olfactory epithelium can produce smell dysfunction just as those drugs that produce severe xerostomia produce taste dysfunction (24). Although the major proteins in olfactory mucus have not been isolated or characterized, some may exhibit similarities to those found in saliva, since olfactory receptors exhibit the same triad as found in taste buds (i.e., no blood vessels, no lymphatics, and few, if any, mitotic figures).

Drugs can effect any aspect of the complex processes underlying taste or olfaction and, thereby, produce dysfunction of these senses. Production of hypogeusia and dysgeusia or hyposmia and dysosmia may be related parts of the same pathological processes, based upon the common concomitant occurrence of these symptoms. When a more detailed understanding of the taste and smell processes themselves is obtained, it will be easier to understand the effects of the myriad of drugs that influence these sensory processes.

Nevertheless, it is important to realize that dysfunction of these senses, particularly if prolonged, can produce profound alteration in the function of patients. Anorexia, limitation of diet with concomitant production of vitamin and mineral deficiencies, alteration in social activities, depression, exposure to eating spoiled food, or inability to smell escaping gas or smoke cannot only affect the quality of life of patients with these disorders, but also can produce severe pathological problems and even, on rare occasions, death. The effects of drugs on taste and smell function should be considered, just as changes in visual and auditory function are considered, in order to provide effective and meaningful therapeutic practice.

REFERENCES

1. Atkin-Thor, E., Goddard, B.W., O'Nion, J., Stephen, R.L. and Kolff, W.J. Hypogeusia and zinc depletion in chronic dialysis patients. *Am. J. Clin. Nutr.* 31:1948, 1978.
2. Barbeau, A. L-Dopa therapy: Past, present, and future. *Ariz. Med.* 27:1, 1970.
3. Bedakian, A.Y., Valdivieso, M., Bodeny, G.P., Burgess, M.A., Benjamin, R.S., Hall, S. and Freireich, E.J. Phase I clinical studies with gallium nitrate. *Cancer Treat. Rep.* 62:1449, 1978.
4. Boarliere, F., Centron, H. and Rapaport, A. Action de l'acide acetysalicyclique sur la sensibilite au gout aver chez l'homme. *Rev. Franc. Etudes Clinet Biol.* 4:380, 1959.
5. Bosma, J.F., Henkin, R.I., Christianson, R.L. and Herdt, J.R. Hypoplasia of the nose and eyes, hyposmia, hypogeusia, and hypogonadotrophic hypogonadism in two males. *J. Craniofac. Genet. Develop. Biol.* 1:153, 1981.
6. Calne, D.B., Williams, A.C., Neophytides, A., Plotkin, C., Nutt, J.G. and Teychenne, P.F. Long-term treatment of parkinsonism with bromocriptine. *Lancet* 1:735, 1978.
7. Chisholm, J.J., Jr. and Kaplan, E. Lead poisoning in childhood: Comprehensive management and prevention. *J. Pediatr.* 73:942, 1968.
8. Fabbi, F. Gustatory sense modifications in diabetes. *Arch. Ohren-nasen Ukehlkopfh* 164:543, 1954.
9. Gordon, B.L. II and Yanagehara, R. Treatment of systemic lupus erythematosus with the T-cell immunopotentiator Levamisole: A follow up report of 16 patients under treatment for a minimum of four months. *Ann. Allergy* 39:227, 1977.
10. Hallman, B.L. and Hurst, J.W. Loss of taste as toxic effect of methimazole (Tapazole) therapy: Report of three cases. *JAMA* 152:322, 1953.
11. Hambidge, K.M., Hambidge, C., Jacobs, M. and Baum, J.K. Low levels of zinc in hair, anorexia, poor growth, and hypogeusia in children. *Pediatr. Res.* 6:868, 1972.
12. Harris, H., Kalmus, H. and Trotter, W.R. Taste sensitivity to phenylthiourea in goitre and diabetes. *Lancet* 2:1038, 1949.
13. Hellekant, G. and Gopal, V. Depression of taste responses by local or intravascular administration of salicylates in the rat. *Acta Physiol. Scand.* 95:286, 1973.
14. Henkin, R.I. Disorders of taste and smell. *JAMA* 218:1946, 1971.
15. Henkin, R.I. Taste in man. In: *Scientific Foundations of Otolaryngology* (Harrison, D. and Hinchcliffe, R., eds.). London: Heinemann, 1976, p. 468.
16. Henkin, R.I. Zinc, saliva, and taste: Interrelationships of gustin, nerve growth factor, saliva, and zinc. In: *Zinc and Copper in Clinical Medicine* (Hambidge, K.M. and Nichols, B.L., eds.). Jamaica, N.Y.: Spectrum, 1978, p. 35.
17. Henkin, R.I. *Zinc.* Baltimore: University Park Press, 1979.
18. Henkin, R.I. Olfaction in Human disease. In: *Looseleaf Series of Otolaryngology* (English, G.M., ed.). New York: Harper and Row, 1982, p. 1.
19. Henkin, R.I. and associates. Unpublished data.
20. Henkin, R.I. and Bradley, D.F. Hypogeusia corrected by Ni^{++} and Zn^{++}. *Life Sci.* 9:701, 1970.
21. Henkin, R.I. and Christiansen, R.L. Taste localization on the tongue, palate, and pharynx of normal man. *J. Appl. Physiol.* 22:316, 1967.

22. Henkin, R.I., Graziadei, P.P.G. and Bradley, D.F. The molecular basis of taste and its disorders. *Ann. Intern. Med.* 71:791, 1969.

23. Henkin, R.I., Keiser, H.R., Jaffe, I.A., Sternlieb, I. and Scheinberg, I.H. Decreased taste sensitivity after D-penicillamine reversed by copper administration. *Lancet* 2:1268, 1967.

24. Henkin, R.I., Talal, N., Larson, A.L. and Mattern, C.F.T. Abnormalities of taste and smell in Sjögren's syndrome. *Ann. Intern. Med.* 76:375, 1972.

25. Henkin, R.I., Lippoldt, R.E., Bilstad, J. and Edelhoch, H. A zinc containing protein isolated from human parotid saliva. *Proc. Natl. Acad. Sci.* USA 72:488, 1975.

26. Henkin, R.I., Lippoldt, R.E., Bilstad, J., Wolf, R.O., Lum, C.K.L. and Edelhoch, H. Fractionation of human parotid saliva. *J. Biol. Chem.* 253:7556, 1978.

27. Henkin, R.I., Patten, B., Re, P. and Bronzert, D.A. A syndrome of acute zinc loss. *Arch. Neurol.* 32:745, 1975.

28. Henkin, R.I., Schechter, P.J., Friedewald, W.T., De Mets, D.L. and Raff, M.S. A double blind study of the effects of zinc sulfate on taste and smell dysfunction. *Am. J. Med. Sci.* 272:285, 1976.

29. Jacobi, G.H. and Moergel, K. Azulfedine and isolierte ageusie fur de Geschmacksqualitat suss. *Internist Praxis.* 16:379, 1976.

30. Jorgensen, M.B. and Buch, N.H. Studies on the sense of smell and taste in diabetics. *Acta Otolaryngol.* 53:539, 1961.

31. Kirsner, J.B. and Henkin, R.I. Sulfamethazine-related dysgeusia. *JAMA* 241:837, 1979.

32. Kurihara, K. and Koyama, N. High activity of adenyl cyclase in olfactory and gustatory organs. *Biochim. Biophys. Acta* 291:650, 1974.

33. Law, J.S., Watanabe, K. and Henkin, R.I. Distribution of calmodulin in taste buds. *Life Sci.* 36:1189, 1985.

34. Law, J.S. and Henkin, R.I. Thyroid hormone inhibits purified taste bud membrane adenosine 3, 5-monophosphate phosphodiesterase activity. *Res. Commun. Chem. Pathol. Pharmacol.* 43:449, 1984.

35. Leys, D. Hyperthyroidism treatment with methylthiouracil. *Lancet* 1:461, 1945.

36. Louria, D.C., Joselow, M.M. and Browder, A.A. The human toxicity of certain trace elements. *Ann. Intern. Med.* 76:207, 1972.

37. Lum, C.K.L. and Henkin, R.I. Characterization of fractions from taste bud and non-taste bud enriched filtrates from and around bovine circumvallate papillae. *Biochim. Biophys. Acta* 412:362, 1976.

38. Lyle, W.H. Penicillamine and zinc. *Lancet* 2:1140, 1974.

39. McGarrison, R. *The Thyroid Gland in Health and Disease.* London: Balliere, Tindall and Cox, 1917, p. 178.

40. McConnell, R.J., Menendez, C.E., Smith, F.R., Henkin, R.I. and Rivlin, R.S. Defects of taste and smell in patients with hypothyroidism. *Am. J. Med.* 59:354, 1975.

41. McNeil, J.J. Taste loss associated with captopril treatment. *Br. Med. J.* 15:1555, 1979.

42. Mulder, N.H., Smith, M.M., Kreumer, W.M.I., Bouman, J., Sleiffer, D.T., Veeger, W. and Schraffordt Koops, H. Effect of chemotherapy on taste sensation. *Oncology* 40:36, 1983.

43. Multicenter Trial Group. Controlled trial of D-penicillamine in severe rheumatoid arthritis. *Lancet* 1:275, 1973.

44. Neundorfer, B. and Valdivieso, T. Parosmie and aromatische anosmie unter L-dopa therapie. *Nervenartz* 48:283, 1977.

45. Nilson, R. Aspects on the toxicity of cadmium and its compounds. *Proc. Natl. Sci. Ecolog. Res. Comm. Bull.* (Stockholm) 7:19, 1970.

46. Olmez, I., Gulovali, M.C., Gordon, G. and Henkin, R.I. Trace elements in human saliva. In: *Trace Substances in Environmental Health XII* (Hemphill, D.D., ed.). Columbia: University of Missouri Press, 1978.

47. Pak, C.Y., Ruskin, B. and Diller, E. Enhancement of renal excretion of zinc by hydrochlorothiazide. *Clin. Chim. Acta* 39:511, 1972.

48. Rabe, R. Isolierte Ageusie. Ein neues Symptom Als Nebenwirkung von medikamenten. *Nervenarzt* 41:23, 1970.

49. Rivlin, R.S., Osnos, M., Rosenthal, S. and Henkin, R.I. Abnormalities in taste preference in hypothyroid rats. *Am. J. Physiol.* 1:E80, 1977.

50. Rollin, H. Drug-related gustatory disorders. *Ann. Otol. Rhinol. Laryngol.* 87:37, 1978.

51. Rozencweig, M., Van Hoff, D.D., Abele, R. and Muggia, F.M. Cisplatin. *Cancer Chemother.* 1:107, 1975.

52. Schiffman, S.S. Taste and smell in disease. *N. Engl. J. Med.* 308:1275, 1337, 1983.

53. Schneeberg, N.G. Loss of sense of taste due to methylthiouracil therapy. *JAMA* 149:1091, 1952.

54. Shatzman, A. and Henkin, R.I. Metal binding characteristics of the parotid salivary protein gustin. *Biochim. Biophys. Acta* 623:107, 1980.

55. Shatzman, A.R. and Henkin, R.I. Proline, glycine, glutamic acid rich pink-violet staining proteins in human parotid saliva are phosphoproteins. *Biochem. Med.* 29:182, 1983.

56. Shatzman, A. and Henkin, R.I. Gustin concentration changes relative to salivary zinc and taste in humans. *Proc. Natl. Acad. Sci. USA* 78:3867, 1981.

57. Siegfried, J. and Zumstein, H. Changes in taste under L-dopa therapy. *J. Hematol.* 230:145, 1971.

58. Solomons, N.W., Rosenberg, I.H. and Sandstead, H.H. Zinc nutrition in celiac sprue. *Am. J. Clin. Nutr.* 29:371, 1976.

59. Van Belle, H. Kinetics and inhibition of rat and avian alkaline phosphatases. *Gen. Pharmacol.* 7:53, 1976.

Section V

DRUGS ACTING VIA CYTOTOXIC OR CHEMOTHERAPEUTIC MECHANISMS

CHAPTER
22

BASIC PRINCIPLES OF CHEMOTHERAPY

William L. West and Harold C. Neu

HISTORY AND DEFINITIONS

The term *chemotherapy* was first used to describe the type of therapy of diseases that uses synthetic chemicals acting specifically on their infective or parasitic-causative organisms. Paul Ehrlich (1854-1915), a physician and chemist, was the first to define and champion the concept of chemotherapy against much opposition. He clearly distinguished his chemical approach from the then-popular immunological approach that employed vaccines and serums for the prevention of infectious diseases. Inherent in the original definition of chemotherapy was that the term should be applied to the use of drugs/chemicals to treat infectious diseases. However, the definition of chemotherapy has been broadened to include diseases of questionable or multiple etiology (chemical, physical, or biological), such as neoplastic diseases. Currently, *chemotherapy* in its broadest sense is that branch of pharmacology that deals with drugs that may be of natural or synthetic origin and are involved in the systemic inhibition of specific causative agents of a disease.

Local actions that destroy or inhibit growth of microorganisms are best defined by the following: *antiseptics* are agents used on living tissues to kill or prevent the growth of microorganisms; *disinfectants* are agents applied to inanimate objects to kill or prevent the spread of infectious microorganisms; *germicides* kill microorganisms and may be disinfectants or antiseptics; *sanitizers* reduce the levels of microorganisms to acceptable public health standards; and *sterilization* is the complete destruction of all forms of life, including spores, by either physical or chemical means.

Although some controversy may exist, the term *antibiotic* was probably introduced with scientific meaning by the French bacteriologist, P. Vuillemin in 1899 when he reported the phenomenon of *antibiosis*, which means that certain microorganisms produce substances that are toxic to other microorganisms. *Antibiotics* are defined as natural chemical substances elaborated by microorganisms that are antagonistic toward the growth of other microorganisms in high dilutions. High dilution is a necessary part of the definition in order to distinguish antibiotics from other substances of natural origin (gastric juice, hydrogen peroxide, ethyl alcohol, etc.).

The earliest discoveries and successes in chemotherapy occurred long before Ehrlich's principles of chemotherapy and the dawn of antibacterial chemotherapy in the 1930s (see Table 22-1). The Indians in Peru had long-used bark from the cinchona tree to treat malaria, and Pelletier isolated the active substance quinine in 1820. Modern antiprotozoan chemotherapy was founded in 1904 when Ehrlich decided to search systematically for an effective remedy for trypanosomiasis and syphilis. This search culminated in the discovery of p-rosaniline for trypanocidal effects and arsphenamine for syphilis. Ehrlich postulated that he could find chemicals that were selectively toxic to parasites and not toxic to the cells of humans (the "magic bullet" concept.). He had only a limited success, and the realization of this postulate came much later with studies on the mechanism of action of sulfonamides (4).

In Table 22-1, other significant milestones in chemotherapy can be seen, namely, antimicrobial chemotherapy and the relatively newer discoveries in the treatment of viral, neoplastic, and fungal diseases.

Table 22-1
Significant Events in Chemotherapy

Date	Contributor(s)	Contributions
1623 and earlier	Indian in Peru	Used cinchona bark for malaria
1820	Pelletier	Isolated quinine from cinchona bark
1830	Pelletier	Isolated emetine from ipecac used in therapy of amebic dysentery
1854-1915	Ehrlich	"Father of chemotherapy," put forward the principles of chemotherapy and concepts of selective toxicity and receptors
1905	Thomas, Breinl	Used atoxyl in trypanosomiasis
1929	Fleming	Discovered penicillin
1932-1935	Domagk	Demonstrated protective effect of prontosil (probably first "miracle" drug) in mice infected with streptococci, published experiments on sulfonamides (1935)
1939	Florey	Isolated penicillin, cured experimental streptococcal infection
1942-1943	Goodman, Gilman, Lindskog	Used cytotoxic alkylating drugs in cancer
1944	Waksman	Discovered streptomycin, first effective antitubercular agent
1948	Farber	Used cytotoxic antimetabolites, antifolics in cancer
1956	Steinberg, Jambor, Suydam	Used systemic antifungal agents, amphotericin B
1958	Gentiles	Used broad-spectrum antifungal agent, griseofulvin
1959	Prusoff, Maxwell	Used idoxuridine in Herpes vaccinia infections and monoxydine in viral influenza
1962	Bauer	Used β-isatin thiosemicarbasone to control smallpox epidemic

Source: From Ref. 4.

The term *narrow-* or *broad-spectrum chemotherapeutic agent* is frequently used in the classification of the drugs that act on causative agents or disease. The term first used in the classification of antimicrobial drugs, describes the ability of the drug to inhibit a variety of disease-causing agents extending from viable small particles such as viruses to larger organisms such as bacteria or unicellular protozoans. The tetracycline antibiotics are examples of broad-spectrum antimicrobials.

Chemotherapeutic agents, whether broad or narrow in spectrum of activity, may either destroy the infectious agent or inhibit its growth and proliferation. *Antimetabolites* are compounds that are similar in structure to a normal endogenous substrate essential for cell growth and proliferations and that can successfully compete with these essential substrates, impairing growth. For example, sulfonamides are antimetabolites of para-aminobenzoic acid and are mainly bacteriostatic. Bacteriostatic agents do not remove the pathogens from the host directly, but indirectly they aid the defense mechanisms of the host.

NATURE OF CHEMOTHERAPY

The chemotherapy of infectious diseases differs from the therapy of many other diseases in which only the patient needs to be considered because there are three aspects to the chemotherapy that must be considered in each situation, namely, the microorganism, the chemotherapeutic agent, and the patient (Fig. 22-1). There are environmental factors that will markedly alter the therapy and make selection of a particular antibacterial agent inappropriate. In addition, the excessive use of a particular antimicrobial agent in a community may result in the selection of a population of microorganisms that are resistant to an agent.

Use of antimicrobial agents must be balanced with respect to their effect on the environment. The use of a form of an antibacterial agent that produces low tissue or serum levels, albeit adequate levels in the urine, may be satisfactory in the nonhospitalized patient, but may result in the colonization of hospital patients with bacteria resistant to a form of the agent needed in the chemotherapy of life-threatening infections. The type of microorganism will affect the choice of therapy with respect to the virulence of a particular organism, its location within the body, and the state of growth or metabolism of the microorganism. Finally, the clinical state of the patient will greatly influence the type of antimicrobial therapy that will be selected, since the patient who lacks host defenses may be unable to eradicate permanently an infecting organism that has been merely held in check by an agent that temporarily stopped the growth of the microorganism.

CAUSATIVE AGENTS OF DISEASES

Infectious diseases are produced by microbial infections or parasitic infestation. The causative agents include viruses, bacteria, protozoa, fungi, and helminths.

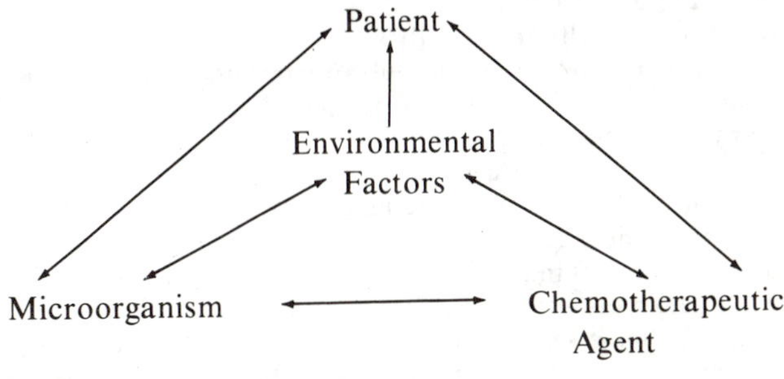

Fig. 22-1: *Factors involved in selection of a chemotherapeutic agent.*

Viruses. Viruses are a group of tiny infectious agents characterized by a lack of an independent metabolism, and by containing a nucleic acid (nucleoid) core and a protein shell (capsid). These minute submicroscopic particles that contain either ribonucleic acid (RNA) or deoxyribonucleic acid (DNA) can replicate only in living cells. The nucleic acid replication process during reproduction is similar to, yet not identical to, that occurring in the mammalian cells that they infect. Thus, subtle differences in their metabolism exist. Recently, a plethora of discoveries as to comparative biochemical differences between viruses and the mammalian cells that they infect, such as those related to the ability of the virus to penetrate and replicate in cells, have broadened the perspective for effective chemotherapeutic agents, especially since these agents exploit these subtle biochemical differences. For example, one of the first effective antiviral agents used to control a viral (pox) epidemic was the isatin 3-thiosemicarbizone, an agent that in part affects viral late-protein synthesis and assembly of viral components into a complete virus (such incomplete particles cannot infect cells); adenosine arabinoside (vidarabine), an analog of adenosine, like adenosine, is phosphorylated to the corresponding nucleotide within the cell and acts by inhibiting viral DNA polymerase; the mammalian enzyme is inhibited to a lesser extent, thus allowing for some selectivity.

Biological carcinogens such as the acute transforming retroviruses are known to insert genetic information into cells, which permits the expression of oncogenetic (*onc*) genes whose products are necessary for mammalian cell transformations (5, 15). Human dominant transforming genes isolated from certain cancers are similar to certain classes of *onc* genes derived from retroviruses. Some normal cell *onc* genes can be activated when linked to expression control elements (ECE) derived from retroviruses (3, 12, 14). ECE and *onc* genes, which appear to be linked together by chance, were shown to be causative in some animal cancers (3). Breakthroughs such as these in the isolation of genes and their products are revolutionizing viral chemotherapy.

Bacteria. Bacteria are more highly differentiated than viruses and contain genetic elements, chromosomes, and certain cytoplasmic factors that are transferable. Many reproduce by fission, but sexual fusion is possible. The unique comparative biochemistry of the firm outer wall is the target of many antimicrobial drugs. In gram-positive cocci, this outer wall consists of N-acetyl muramic acid-N-acetylglycosamine peptide complex. The final stage of cell wall synthesis is transpeptidation reaction, which cross-links the linear peptides. There are many pathogenic bacteria in which the cross-linking peptide reaction in the cell wall is not a relevant mechanism, thus limiting the therapeutic capacity of drugs that block transpeptidation (e.g., penicillins and cephalosporins). Many drugs that block the formation of the bacterial cell wall are *bactericidal* (i.e., destroy bacteria). Many drugs produce *bacteriostasis* (slow growth) of bacteria. Still others may affect membrane functions. Both bactericidal and bacteriostatic drugs appear to be the most active when the cells are rapidly dividing.

Protozoa. Protozoa are unicellular organisms, some of which are parasites in humans. Despite our early successes in chemotherapy of these diseases, as was indicated by the discovery of quinine in 1820, comparatively few advances have been made. These unicellular organisms are injured by a variety of drugs, but most of them have a low therapeutic index. Thus, these drugs are not ideal in that many are quite toxic to the host.

Malaria, trypanosomiasis, leishmaniasis, and amebiasis are perhaps the most serious of the diseases caused by protozoa. There are in our armamentarium many drugs that are selectively toxic to these parasites, but the emergence of resistant strains points out the need for a continuous search for new and effective chemotherapy. Cell-mediated immunity is active in all of these protozoan diseases.

Helminths. Worms are highly developed parasitic organisms and have in many instances highly specialized systems. Too little is known about them and the host natural defenses against these invaders. Frequently the worm is embedded in the host tissues, and the drug must act systemically to produce an effect. Immunity to these parasitic infestations is poorly understood but is probably a mixture of humoral and cell-mediated responses.

Other Agents. Whereas in the past parasitic infestations from helminths, protozoans, bacteria, and viruses have been the focus for problems in environmental health and freedom from environmental toxicity, the rapid appearance of new organic chemicals (over 700/year) in the environment from a multitude of sources such as energy production, industrial manufacturing, and agricultural use, as well as effluents from disposals of biodegradable waste of animals and humans, seems to constitute the causative agent of disease now and in the future.

The rapid introduction of new organic chemicals into the environment and their reaction with genetic materials resulting in heritable changes is now well documented (1). If increased mutations enter the genetic information pool of a given population, then deleterious effects (genetic diseases) may appear with increasing frequency. It is now possible to monitor hazardous/harmful chemicals by a number standardized or approved *in vivo* and *in vitro* methods. These bioassay methods include *gene mutation* (point mutation and small locus mutations using bacterial systems), *chromosomal mutations* (numerical changes in chromosomes, chromosomal breaks, misreplications, or misrecombinations), stimulation or recombinations, and stimulation and inhibition of chromosomal repair. Chemicals, ionizing irradiation (physical), and viruses (biological) have in common that they can induce genetic alterations leading to neoplastic or uncontrolled cancerous growth. The etiologies seem to converge in that chemicals and ionizing irradiation may also release infectious viruses and/or proviruses in the cell, which in turn may cause cancer. Regardless of the etiology, there are some fundamental differences between infectious (or parasitic) diseases and neoplastic diseases (cancer). Neoplastic diseases are more closely related to the normal cells from which they are derived. However, subtler gross and biochemical differences do exist.

CHEMOTHERAPEUTIC AGENTS

Chemotherapeutic agents are derived from both natural and synthetic products. Natural products include antibiotics and plant products. Some natural products have been the basis of, or are subjected to chemical alterations to yield, many effective semisynthetic and synthetic agents; penicillin is a good example. Although various classes of chemotherapeutic agents will be dealt in subsequent chapters, some general discussions of their mechanisms of action and drug resistance are in order here.

MECHANISMS OF ACTION

Recently, rapid advances have been made in elucidating the mechanism of action of a variety of chemotherapeutic agents. These agents exert their effects by one or more of the following mechanisms:

1. Inhibition of cell wall biosynthesis (bacteria) (e.g., cycloserine, bacitracin, vancomycin, penicillins, and cephalosporins)

2. Inhibition of cytoplasmic membrane function (bacteria or fungi) (e.g., polymyxin B, colistin)
3. Inhibition of protein and nucleic acid synthesis (bacteria, virus or cancer) (e.g., aminoglycosides, chloramphenicol, erythromycin, tetracycline, rifampin, nalidixic acid, many anticancer agents)
4. Antagonism of metabolic processes (e.g., sulfonamides, trimethoprim, many anticancer agents)

INHIBITION OF CELL WALL SYNTHESIS

The cell wall is essential for the growth and survival of bacteria. Rigid stability of the cell wall is provided by highly cross-linked latticelike structure (Fig. 22-2) composed of heteropolymeric subunits, peptidoglycans. These subunits are oligosaccharide chains of alternating pyranoside residues of two amino sugars, N-acetylglycosamine (NAG) and its 3-O-D-lactic acid derivative, N-acetylmuramic acid (NAMA). Attached to carboxyl groups of the lactic acid side chain of the NAMA moiety is a species-specific pentapeptide chain that in *Staphylococcus aureus* is L-ala-D-glu-L-lys-D-ala-D-ala. The glycan strands are crosslinked by peptide chains that are characteristic of individual microbial species. In *S. aureus* the pentaglycine chains bridge the tetrapeptide units connected to the NAMA residue of peptidoglycans.

The biosynthesis of the bacterial cell wall consists of three stages, each of which occurs at a different site in the cell (Fig. 22-3). In the first stage of biosynthesis, uridinediphospho-N-acetylmuramic acid (UDP-NAMA) is formed from uridinediphospho-N-acetylglycosamine (UDP-NAG) by soluble cytoplasmic enzymes through transfer of phosphoenolpyruvic acid to C_3-OH group of NAG, followed by its reduction to a 3-O-D-lactic acid group. The first three amino acids (AA) of the pentapeptide are then added to lactyl COOH group of UDP-NAMA in a stepwise fashion. The last two amino acids are added as a dipeptide, D-alanyl-D-alanine (D-ala-D-ala), to the tripeptide, UDP-NAMA-$(AA)_3$. Synthesis of D-ala-D-ala requires prior racemization of L-alanine by alanine racemase and condensation to the dipeptide by D-alanyl-D-alanine synthetase. The antibiotic *D-cycloserine* is a structural analog of D-alanine and competitively inhibits both alanine racemase and synthetase enzymes in this stage of cell wall synthesis. UDP-acetylmuramyl-pentapeptide UDP-NAMA-$(AA)_5$ is called *Park nucleotide* after its discoverer, who showed accumulation of this compound in the bacterial cells when subsequent synthetic stages are inhibited following treatment with penicillin.

In subsequent reactions that occur within the cell membrane, the phosphomuramyl-pentapeptide group is transferred to a membrane-bound carrier lipid, with formation of a pyrophosphate bridge and release of UMP to the OH group of muramic acid component. The second sugar (NAG) is then added from a UDP-NAG to form disaccharide-pentapeptide-pyrophospholipid. This is followed by addition to five glycine residues connected to the R_3 amino acid L-lysine residue of the heteropentapeptide.

The first half of the pentaglycine cross-link is thus formed. The completed peptidoglycan unit is then translocated from the carrier lipid to the cell wall receptor acceptor peptidoglycan under the influence of peptidoglycan synthetase, thus elongating the peptidoglycan backbone; this process also releases pyrophospho-carrier lipid, from which pyrophosphatase regenerates the mono-

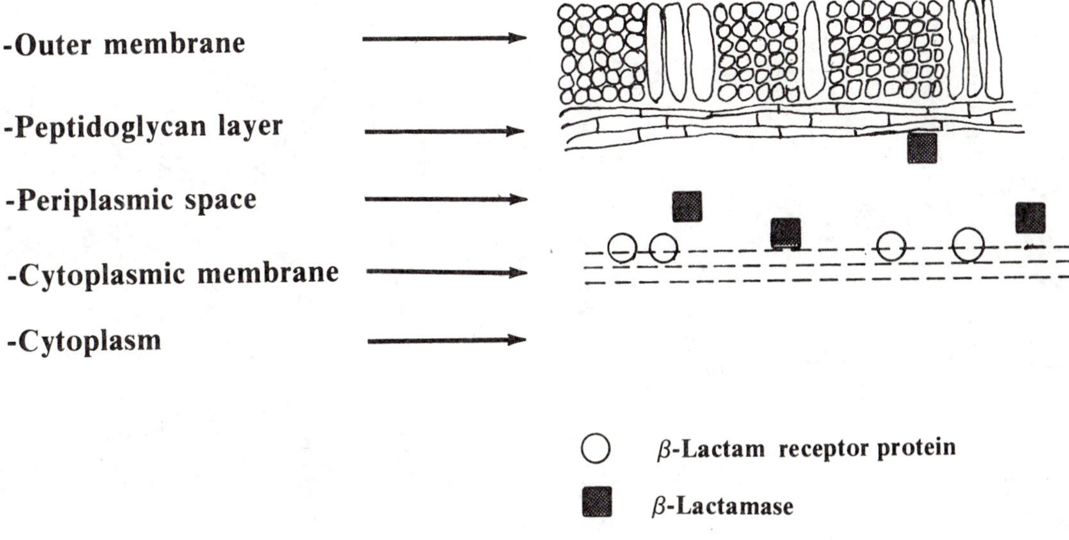

Fig. 22-2. *Structure of the bacterial cell wall.*
A penicillin or a cephalosporin must pass through the long pores of the outer membrane through the periplasmic space, wherein are located the β-lactamases, to reach the receptor proteins which make the peptidoglycan.

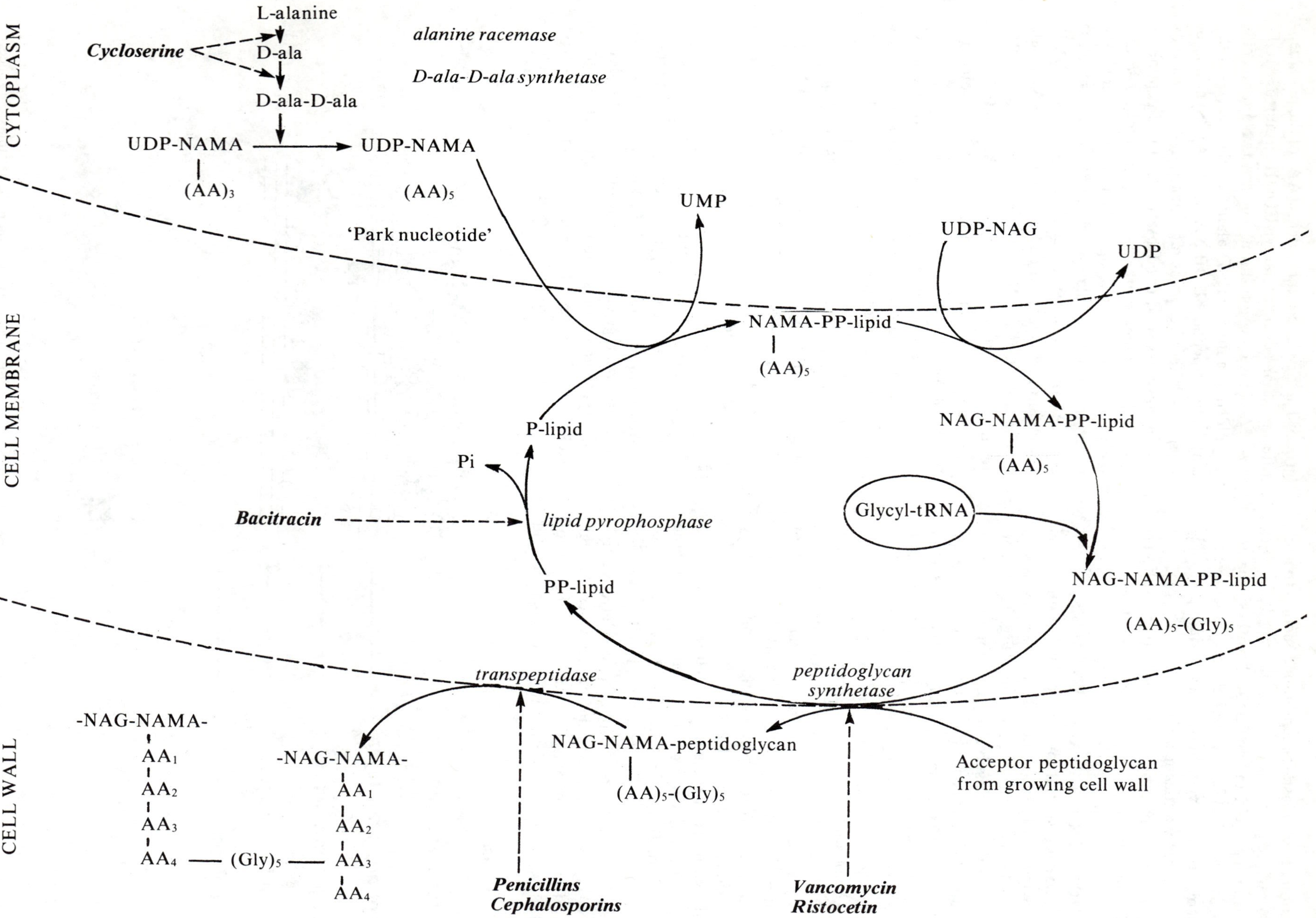

Fig. 22-3. *Sites where antibiotics interfere with bacterial cell wall synthesis.*

phospho-carrier lipid by removal of phosphate. The cell wall polymer formed in this stage is noncross-linked peptidoglycans terminating with pentapeptide units.

Several antibiotics can disrupt certain steps in this stage. *Bacitracin* is a specific inhibitor of membrane lipid pyrophosphatase probably by complexing with the lipid pyrophosphate portion of the peptidoglycan, thus preventing reentry of the lipid carrier into the reaction cycle of the cell synthesis; this antibiotic also disrupts the bacterial cell membrane. *Vancomycin* and *ristocetin* act similarly by inhibiting the activity of peptidoglycan synthetase, presumably by forming stable 1:1 complexes with acyl-D-ala-D-ala moiety and thus altering the substrate.

The final stage, which takes place outside the cell membrane, consists of completion of the cross-link between the peptidoglycan polymers. This is accomplished by a transpeptidation reaction through the influence of a membrane-bound enzyme transpeptidase and results in the cleavage of the D-alanyl-D-alanine terminus of the peptidoglycan with subsequent formation of cross-link. In *S. aureus* this reaction is completed by linking free amino group of the pentaglycine bridge of a peptidoglycan to the penultimate D-alanine carboxyl group of the pentapeptide chain of the neighboring peptidoglycan with concomitant release of D-alanine. This last stage of peptidoglycan synthesis is inhibited by β-lactam antibiotics. In bacteria grown in the presence of penicillin, uncross-linked uridine nucleotide intermediates (e.g., Park nucleotide) of cell wall synthesis accumulate.

The action of the penicillin is based on the structural analogy between penicillin and D-alanyl-D-alanine end of pentapeptide, as shown:

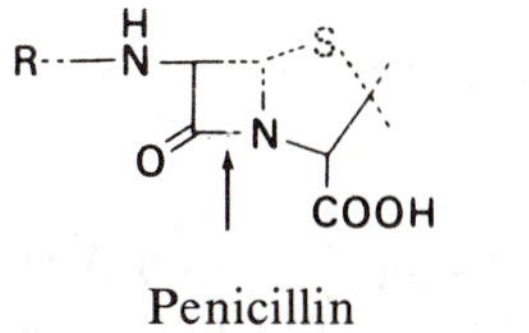

Penicillin

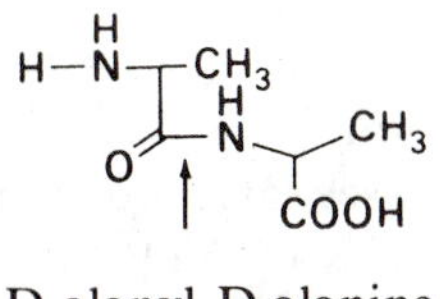

D-alanyl-D alanine

The labile CO-N bond in the β-lactam ring of penicillin lies in the same position of the peptide (marked by ↑ in the respective structures) bond involved in transpeptidation. It has been proposed that penicillin, acting as a substrate analog for normal transpeptidation, combines with the transpeptidase and thereby irreversibly inactivates it. Sites of action of the antibiotics on the bacterial cell wall synthesis (8), are illustrated in Fig. 22-3.

INHIBITION OF CYTOPLASMIC MEMBRANE FUNCTION

The cytoplasmic membrane of bacteria and fungi acts as an osmotic barrier to prevent free diffusion of substances between the external and internal environment. The polymyxins are a family of simple polypeptides, of which polymyxin B and polymyxin E are used clinically. The molecules contain both lipophilic and lipophobic groups that are able to invade the lipid protein union that makes up bacterial cell membrane. The distortion of the membrane component destroys the functional barrier of the membrane so that various ions, amino acids, and nucleosides are lost from the bacterial cell. Vancomycin and bacitracin may also damage to some extent the cytoplasmic membrane of bacterial cells. Polyene-type antifungal agents such as nystatin and amphotericin B act on a sterol component (ergosterol) of the cell membrane. Mammalian cells also contain a sterol, cholesterol. However, since certain fungi contain membranes with phospholipid/sterol ratios quite different from mammalian cells, these agents appear to be more selective for fungal cells.

INHIBITION OF PROTEIN AND NUCLEIC ACID SYNTHESIS

Many chemotherapeutic agents are known to interfere protein and nucleic acid synthesis. Protein synthesis is affected by many antimicrobial as well as anticancer agents; nuleic acid synthesis is affected mainly by anticancer agents.

Protein Synthesis. Protein synthesis may be outlined briefly as consisting of the following gross steps, namely (a) activation, (b) initiation, (c) elongation, and (d) termination (11).

Activation of Amino Acids (in cytoplasm of mammalian cell or bacteria). The activation of amino acids is catalyzed, at the expense of adenosine triphosphate (ATP), by a group of Mg^{2+}-dependent activating enzymes (aminoacyl-tRNA synthetase), each specific for one amino acid and for a corresponding tRNA. Formation of the aminoacyl complex (AA-tRNA) is necessary for their participation in the formation of proteins (see below).

$$\text{ATP} + \text{AA} \underset{\text{AA-tRNA synthetase}}{\overset{Mg^{2+}}{\rightleftharpoons}} \text{AA-AMP} + \text{PPi}$$

$$\text{AA-AMP} + \text{tRNA} \underset{\text{AA-tRNA synthetase}}{\rightleftharpoons} \text{AA-tRNA} + \text{AMP}$$

(PPi = high energy pyrophosphate)

Initiation Process (in bacteria). The first, or N-terminal amino acid for all proteins is formylmethionine. Formylmethionine (fmet) and its transfer RNA (tRNA) in the presence of an AA-tRNA-synthetase form AA-tRNA (fmet-tRNA). The messenger RNA (mRNA) attaches to the 30S subunit in the presence of a protein designated as an initiation factor, IF_3. Formylmethionine-tRNA then combines with mRNA-30S ribosomal complex with the participation of a second initiation factor, IF_2. The anticodon triplet portion of the tRNA is juxtaposed to the initiation codon in the mRNA (AUG). The presence of a third initiation factor (IF_1) is needed at this point. The combining of the 50S ribosomal subunit to the mRNA-30S-fmet-tRNA complex requires guanosine triphosphate (GTP). The GTP is then hydrolyzed and the initiation factors are released. A part of the action of aminoglycoside antibiotics is attributed to "freezing" the initiator complex.

$$\left.\begin{array}{l}\text{mRNA} + 30\text{S} + IF_2 + IF_3 \\ + \text{fmet-tRNA} + IF_1 \\ + \text{GTP} + 50\text{S}\end{array}\right\} \longrightarrow \left.\begin{array}{c}\text{enzyme} \\ \text{initiation} \\ \text{process}\end{array}\right\} \longrightarrow \begin{array}{c}\text{initiation} \\ \text{complex}\end{array}$$

The functional ribosome where assembly of amino acids takes place has a sedimentation constant of 70S. The functional ribosome moves stepwise along the mRNA gradually building a peptide chain. A polyribosome is more than one functional ribosome on a given mRNA. Tetracyclines block the reaction between the AA-tRNA and the ribosome on mRNA.

Elongation (assembly of amino acids in protein). The elongation of the polypeptide chain begins with the insertion of the second AA-tRNA in the acceptor (A) site on the 70S ribosome. This process requires the participation of GTP and two elongation factors (EF-Tu and EF-Ts). The two amino acids then become linked by a peptide bond under the direction of a peptidyl transferase enzyme. After the formation of the peptide bond, a complicated translocation takes place. In this process the dipeptidyl-tRNA is shifted from the A site to the peptidyl (P) site, the tRNA for formylmethionine is released, and the 30S subunit moves one codon along the mRNA. Elongation factor G(EF-G) and GTP hydrolysis are required for this three part process to occur. The A site is now unoccupied and ready to receive the next AA-tRNA directed by the next codon on the mRNA (11).

Chloramphenicol, macrolides, and lincomycin bind to 50S ribosomes. Chloramphenicol binds only to the 50S ribosomal subunit inhibiting the functional attachment of the aminoacyl end of AA-tRNA to the 50S subunit and thereby inhibiting transpeptidation. Chloramphenicol slightly decreases the rate of polysome (70S) breakdown, but ribosomes can slowly progress along mRNA in the absence of peptide bond formation. Chloramphenicol binding is reversible. Macrolides such as erythromycin produce conformational changes in the ribosomes so that formation of peptide bonds does not occur, although the ribosome cycle continues. These agents inhibit transpeptidation on polyribosomes and indirectly interfere with translocation when the polypeptide chain has grown to a considerable size. Lincomycin inhibits the binding of the aminoacyl end of AA-tRNA to ribosomes, either by occupying the site or by producing a conformational change in the ribosome. Lincomycin further destabilizes ribosomes so that they fall off mRNA, thus preventing polypeptide elongation.

Termination (in bacteria). Elongation is stopped on appearance of a termination code triplet such as UAA, UAG, UGA in mRNA. When one of these codons occurs, no AA-tRNA is bound to the A site. Instead this causes the hydrolysis of the peptidyl-tRNA linkage in the P site, and the ribosome then dissociates into its 30S and 50S subunits. Three releasing factors, RF_1, RF_2 and RF_3, and GTP are necessary for the completed protein to be released, and for the ribosome to be detached from the mRNA.

Nucleic Acid Synthesis. Effects of anticancer agents in protein and nucleic acid synthesis are discussed in Chapter 27. Some examples of their effects in nucleic acid synthesis are presented here. Folate reductases are important in the *de novo* synthesis of purines and in the formation pyrimidines. Methotrexate is an inhibitor of folic acid metabolism. The overall effect is the inhibition of dihydrofolate reductases and a subsequent reduction in tissue levels of N-5,10-methylene tetrahydrofolate and thymidylic acid. This leads to inhibition of DNA synthesis.

Fluorouracil is an anticancer drug mainly affecting pyrimidine metabolism and function. It is metabolically activated in tissue by uridine phosphorylase to fluorouridine and then to FUMP by uridine kinase. FUMP is further reduced to dFUMP by ribonucleotide diphosphate reductase. dFUMP formed is a specific inhibitor of thymidylate synthetase. This antagonism leads to inhibition of DNA synthesis.

ANTAGONISM OF METABOLIC PROCESSES

Sulfonamides are structural analogs of para-aminobenzoic acid (PABA), which is an essential metabolite in bacterial cell as a precursor of folic acid (Fig.22-4). Tetrahydrofolic acid is a coenzyme that is necessary for transfer and reduction of 1-carbon fragment and for the production of nucleic acid via synthesis of methionine, thymine, and other purines. Trimethoprim inhibits production of tetrahydrofolic acid by binding to the enzyme dihydrofolate reductase, which converts dihydrofolic acid to tetrahydrofolic. Microorganisms, unlike humans, are unable to utilize preformed folic acid and therefore are inhibited by these agents.

BACTERIAL RESISTANCE

Although there are many mechanisms by which bacteria can be destroyed, bacteria have developed numerous ways in which to overcome the agents developed to control them (10). The widespread use of antimicrobial agents have provided a strong selective environment that favors the appearance and maintenance of resistant bacteria (6, 9). To become resistant to antimicrobial agents, bacteria can alter a target site (binding site), alter cell permeability so that an agent does not reach a binding site, bypass a reaction blocked by an agent, reduce their requirement for a metabolite, overproduce an enzyme, or produce a metabolic antagonist. These mechanisms and the organisms in which they occur are illustrated in Table 22-2. For example, methylation of the 23 S ribosomal RNA component of the 30 S ribosome in staphylococci and streptococci results in resistance to macrolides and the lincosamide group of antibiotics. Mutations or a plasmid- (see later) coded product could interfere with the synthesis of ATP by altering electron transport or oxidative phosphorylation so that a reduction in transport of an antimicrobial agent occurred. Modification of an antibiotic, such as occurs with an aminoglycoside, reduces transport and affinity of the drug so that the agent is no longer held in the cell to bind to the ribosome (2). In this mechanism there is no reduction in extracellular concentration of drug and no modified drug would be found in the culture medium.

The best-studied mechanisms of resistance are the detoxification of antibiotics, of which β-lactamases (which hydrolyze the β-lactam ring of penicillins or cephalosporins) are an example. Bypass mechanisms are those in which a plasmid provides a cell with an enzyme that is refractory to the antimicrobial agent. Relieving an organism of the requirement for a metabolite that is usually needed allows the microorganism to ignore a blocking agent. Likewise, lack of an enzyme normally used in cell wall division such as occurs in "resistant"

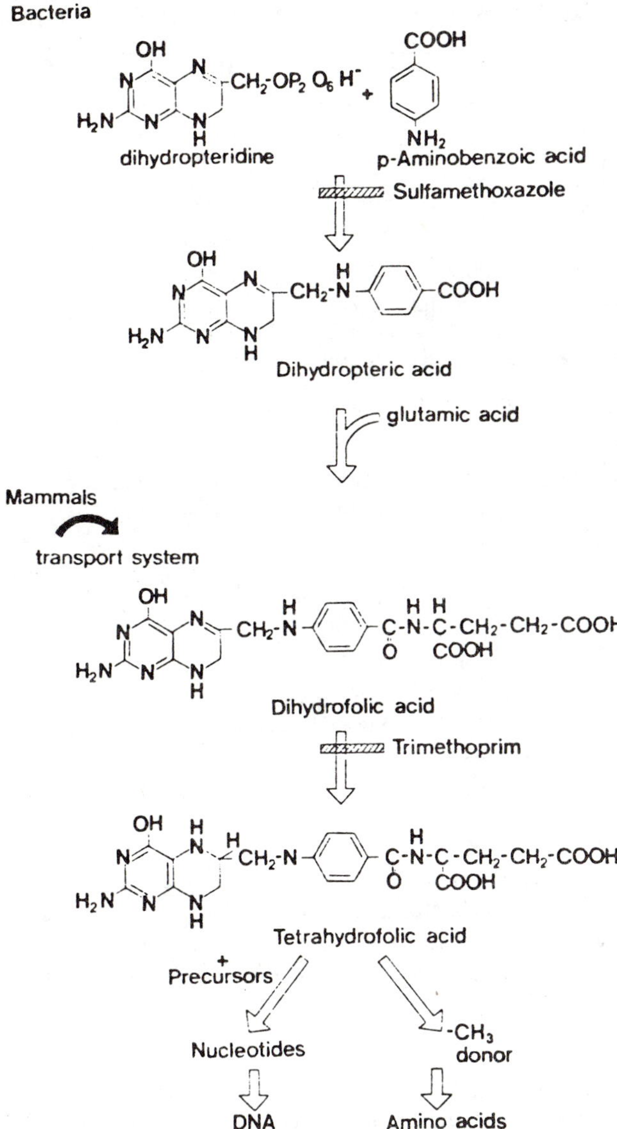

Fig. 22-4. *Sites at which sulfonamides and trimethoprim interfere with folic acid synthesis.*

staphylococci allows these bacteria to persist in the presence of penicillins. More than one mechanism of resistance for a given antibiotic can exist in a single bacterial species.

MECHANISM OF RESISTANCE

The development of resistance to an antimicrobial agent involves a stable genetic change, heritable from generation to generation. There are two major genetic mechanisms by which resistance to antibiotics and other antimicrobial agents may arise: (1) by mutation and selection, and (2) by genetic exchange.

Selection of Drug-Resistant Mutants. Drug resistance arises by a spontaneous random mutation that results in an altered susceptibility of the microorganisms to the drug, the drug serving only as a selective agent favoring the survival of resistant over sensitive organisms after the genetic alteration has occurred.

Development of resistance to antimicrobial agents may follow different temporal patterns. In some cases, a high degee of resistance may develop in a single-step mutation (e.g., resistance to streptomycin by enteric bacilli containing an altered ribosomal protein that cannot bind to the drug). The bacilli are resistant to high concentrations of the drug. In other cases, a slow stepwise development of resistance may occur (e.g., resistance of gonococcus to penicillin).

Mutations generally occur at a frequency of about 1 in 10^5-10^{10} cell divisions. The frequency of spontaneous mutation leading to resistance varies with the bacteria species and the drug; for example, the frequency of mutation of *Mycobacterium tuberculosis* in streptomycin resistance is approximately 10^{-10} and in isoniazid resistance, 10^{-6}.

This has been classically demonstrated in the laboratory by growing bacteria in the presence of subinhibitory concentration of antibiotics, but this is an inefficient approach. Bacteria produced by this technique are less virulent and are resistant to only one agent or to one member of a class of antibiotics.

Resistance Mediated by Genetic Exchange. Genetic information that controls bacterial drug resistance may occur in the chromosome as well as in the DNA of extrachromosomal genetic elements (plasmids) that replicate independently of the host chromosome. These genetic materials can be transferred from the resistant cell to a sensitive one, thus transmitting the resistant trait. Such transfer of genetic materials is an efficient mechanism of resistance and can occur in bacteria by transduction, transformation, or conjugation.

Transduction occurs by transfer of a plasmid through intervention of a bacteriophage (rather than by mating), it is particularly important in transfer of penicillinase plasmids among strains of *S. aureus*; other plasmids also transfer resistance to erythromycin, tetracycline, or chloramphenicol by this process.

Transformation involves incorporation into bacteria of DNA probably excreted by certain bacterial cells and contained in the environment. The importance of this process is uncertain.

Conjugation, which has been shown to be the major mechanism of dissemination of resistance, was first recognized in Japan in 1959 after an outbreak of bacillary dysentery caused by *Shigella flexneri* that was resistant to four different classes of antimicrobial agents, streptomycin, sulfonamides, tetracycline, and chloramphenicol. Transfer of multiple resistance is now known to occur between all genera of the *Enterobacteriaceae*. This process requires cell-to-cell contact. The genetic elements that control the process are designated *resistance factors* or *R factors* (7), which have two components, each consisting of different DNA sequences; these include the *R determinant* for drug resistance and the *resistance trans-*

Table 22-2
Mechanism of Bacterial Resistance

Drug	Target/ Mechanism	Organism
I. *Alteration of a target or binding site of a drug*		
Streptomycin	30 S ribosome	*S. faecalis*
Erythromycin and lincomycins	23 S ribosome methylated	*S. aureus*
Rifampin	DNA-directed RNA polymerase	*E. coli*
Nalidixic acid	DNA gyrase	*E. coli*
II. *Failure of a drug to enter the bacterial cell in sufficient amount or bind to receptor site*		
Tetracycline	Uptake reduced compared with that pumped out	*E. coli*
Aminoglycosides	(a) Membrane not energized	Anaerobic bacteria
	(b) Enzymatically modified drug shows reduced transport	*E. coli, Klebsiella*
Chloramphenicol	Reduced entry	*Pseudomonas*
III. *Detoxification by the Organism*		
Penicillins	β-Lactamase hydrolyzes molecule	Gram-positive, gram-negative
Cephalosporins	β-Lactamase hydrolyzes molecule	Gram-positive, gram-negative
Chloramphenicol	Chloramphenicol transacetylase	*S. aureus, E. coli*
IV. *Development of a separate pathway resistant to an agent bypassing a vulnerable metabolic step*		
Sulfonamides	Altered enzyme	*S. faecalis*
Trimethoprim	Altered dihydrofolate reductase	*E. coli*
V. *Reduced requirement for a metabolite*		
Sulfonamides	Need less thymine	*Neisseria*
Trimethoprim	Methionine	Staphylococci

fer factor (RTF) responsible for transmission of R determinant. Each of these components can exist alone, but they must act jointly for successful transfer of antibiotic resistance. When they are present in the same cell, association of the two occurs, producing an R factor. The R determinants and the RTF are independent replicons, each of which is capable of replicating and operating on its own in the bacterial cell. RTF codes for formation of specific sexual apparatus or pili through which the transfer of the resistance factors is established. Plasmids can confer resistance to 1 or even 10 antibiotics simultaneously, and have been found in most bacteria, predominantly among gram-negative bacilli (Table 22-3). The only antibacterial agents to which plasmid resistance is so far unknown are the nalidixic acid-type agents and the polymyxins. The mechanisms of resistance plasmid are given in Table 22-4.

The most alarming form of bacterial resistance is that due to transposons. Transposons are genetic elements that can move between bacterial replicons independently of the usual recombinant mechanisms of the cell. These elements facilitate transfer of genetic material between one plasmid and another, between plasmids and chromosomes, and between plasmids and bacteriophages. Transposons are not self-replicating units, but rely upon replicons for replication. Transposons mediate resistances to penicillins, aminoglycosides, and trimethoprim.

REDUCTION OF RESISTANCE

Approaches to reduce antibiotic resistance have been many. If the use of antimicrobial agents is stopped, the selective pressure exerted by the use of these agents ceases and susceptible bacteria reappear. This occurs because bacteria that are not making enzymes to overcome an agent are at an advantage in the absence of the agent in

Table 22-3
Some of the Bacteria Found to Carry Plasmid Mediating Resistance to Antibacterial Agents

Gram-Negative	Gram-Positive
Acinetobacter spp	*Bacillus* spp
Aeromonas spp	*Clostridium perfringens*
Citrobacter spp	*Staphylococcus aureus*
Enterobacter spp	*Staphylococcus epidermidis*
Escherichia coli	*Streptococcus faecalis*
Haemophilus influenzae	*Streptococcus pyogenes*
Klebsiella spp	*Streptococcus pneumoniae*
Neisseria gonorrhoeae	
Proteus spp	
Providencia spp	
Pseudomonas spp	
Salmonella spp	
Shigella spp	
Vibrio	
Yersinia	
Bacteroides	

Table 22-4
Plasmid-Mediated Resistance

Antibiotic	Mechanism	Organisms
Penicillin, ampicillin, carbenicillin, cephalosporins	β-Lactamase hydrolysis	Gram-positive, gram-negative
Oxacillin, methicillin	β-Lactamase hydrolysis	Gram-negative
Chloramphenicol	Acetylation	Gram-positive, gram-negative
Tetracycline	Permeability block	Gram-positive, gram-negative
Aminoglycosides		
Streptomycin	Acetylation	
Neomycin	Phosphorylation	Gram-positive, gram-negative
Kanamycin	Adenylation	
Gentamicin		
Tobramycin		
Amikacin		
Macrolides		
Erythromycin	Structural protein change	Gram-positive
Lincomycins	Structural protein change	Gram-negative anaerobes

terms of growth characteristics and ability to colonize human body surfaces. This approach is not practical except in special situations. Control, that is, reduction of the use of antibiotics, has in some cases resulted in less resistance by reducing selective pressure. Unfortunately, the debilitated patient who remains in the hospital for a long period is the patient most likely to need antibiotics and also to be a source of resistant strains that infect other patients. Improved hygienic practices that reduce the spread of plasmid-carrying strains have helped to reduce the proliferation of resistant bacteria. Other techniques used to reduce bacterial resistance have been the development of new antibiotics, modification of existing antibiotics, and the use of antibiotics in combination. Thus far, attempts to develop agents that will cure bacteria of resistance plasmids or prevent plasmid transfer have not been successful.

HOST

TOLERANCE

Whereas resistance is more a property of the pathogen, tolerance is more a property of the host (though not exclusive). Tolerance diminished response to a drug upon repeated administration occurs on a time scale of hours, days, or weeks and tachyphylaxis (or rapid tolerance) may occur in seconds or minutes. Drug tolerance may be due to an increased metabolism of the drug by the host (Chapter 3). During chemotherapy, both tolerance and resistance may contribute to a diminution of responsiveness.

Immunological tolerance refers to a different phenomenon (13). Using a specific antigen or haptens in high concentrations, it is possible to induce a state of unresponsiveness to an immunogen in an intact animal. Immunological tolerance is characterized by a failure of the host to synthesize antibodies or generate sensitized cells to a specific antigen while the response to all other antigens is intact and expressed in the usual way. This state of unresponsiveness is more easily induced during neonatal as compared with adult life (e.g., tolerance to tissue transplantation antigens is easily produced during neonatal life but not in the adult). The term immunological paralysis is synonymous with immunological tolerance but not with immunological suppression. The latter term denotes a state of generalized (nonspecific) suppression of immune responsiveness that occurs following the administration of cytotoxic chemotherapeutic agents such as cyclophosphamide, adriamycin, or methotrexate. Thus in immunological tolerance, there appears to be no change in the number and functions of circulation lymphocytes whereas in immunological suppression, a lymphocyte depletion (lymphopenia) occurs. Overall, immunological tolerance refers to a state whereby the individual is unable to respond immunologically to a specific antigen or hapten that it has been previously exposed to in high concentrations.

DEFENSE MECHANISM

Defense against infectious disease involves most of the host immunological capability. The immunological capability is implemented by a variety of cell types, cellular receptors, and sequential enzymatic activations, as well as resultant cellular chemical products. Many of these cellular chemical products are biologically active and are referred to as *chemical mediators*. The body responds against injury whether the causative agent is physical (heat, light, x-ray, or pressure), *biological* (bacterial, fungal, protozoal, viral, or neoplastic), or *chemical* (allergens, industrial chemicals, or biological toxins). All can gain entry and/or create matter (antigens) foreign to the body's defenses. However, the cellular and chemical mediators are quite different for each causative agent, even though they share certain common modalities. For this reason, the major components of the defense capability system are discussed in Chapters 13.5.1 and 13.5.2.

ADVERSE EFFECTS

An ideal chemotherapeutic drug would be selectively toxic to the causative agent of the disease with no adverse or toxic actions in the host. The biochemical mechanisms of toxic effects in the pathogens are different from those of their effects in the host. The predictable damage to the pathogen may vary from cell destruction to slowing of growth. On the other hand, adverse effects in the host are not always predictable.

Drugs may cause direct or indirect reactions in the host. These adverse reactions or toxicities as well as the natural defense in an individual may in part depend upon the person's age, health, and nutritional status. The manner by which adverse reactions occur may be classified as direct and indirect. If the severity of the toxic response is related to dose and the characteristic lesions are regularly produced, then the drug may act in a direct manner on the host target tissue. Such a response may be exhibited by the polyene antibiotics (i.e., amphotericin B), which possess certain specific toxic effects on mammalian cells. The immune suppressant effects of the cytotoxic anticancer drugs are the result of direct effects, and secondary bacterial infections are frequently a problem in cancer patients. The drug may act by an allergic (indirect) mechanism, as with the anaphylactic response to penicillin G. All indirect adverse reactions are not through allergic-type mechanisms. For example, certain sulfonamides may crystallize out in an acid urine, and the damage to the kidney is produced through or by mechanical (crystals) rather than chemical toxicity.

Superinfection is usually a systemic infection caused by an overgrowth of fungi inhabiting the gastrointestinal tract. Superinfection is another indirect adverse effect, which may occur as a result of long-term oral therapy and the killing off of commensal bacterial organisms.

REFERENCES

1. Auerbach, C. *Mutation Research: Problems, Results, and Perspectives.* New York: John Wiley, 1976.
2. Benveniste, R. and Davies, J. Mechanisms of antibiotic resistance in bacteria. *Ann. Rev. Biochem.* 42:471, 1973.
3. Blair, D.G., Oskarsson, M., Wood, T.G. et al. Activation of the transforming potential of a normal cell sequence: A molecular model for carcinogenesis. *Science* 212:941, 1981.
4. Busch, H. and Lane, M. (eds.). *Chemotherapy.* Chicago: Year book Medical Publishers, 1967.
5. Dalla, F.R., Gelman, E.P., Gallo, R.C. and Wong-Staal, F.O. A human *onc* gene homologous to the transforming gene (V-sis) or simian sarcoma virus. *Nature* 292:32, 1981.
6. Datta, N. Antibiotic resistance in bacteria. *Br. Med. Bull.* 40:1, 1984.
7. Foster, T.J. Plasmid-determined resistance to antimicrobial drugs and toxic metal ions in bacteria. *Microbiol. Rev.* 47:361, 1983.
8. Gale, E.F. et al. *The Molecular Basis of Antibiotic Action*, 2nd ed. London: Wiley-Interscience, 1981.
9. Neu, H.C. The emergence of bacterial resistance and its influence upon empiria therapy. *Rev. Infect. Dis.* 5:9, 1983.
10. Neu, H.C. Current mechanisms of resistance to antimicrobial agents in microorganisms causing infection in the patient at risk for infection. *Am. J. Med.* 76:11, 1984.
11. Pratt, W.B. and Fekety, R. *The Antimicrobial Drugs.* London: Oxford University Press, 1986.
12. *Pulciani, S., Santos, E., Lauver, A.V. et al. Oncogenes in human tumor cell lines: Molecular cloning of a transforming gene from human bladder carcinoma cells. Proc. Natl. Acad. Sci. USA* 79:2845, 1982.
13. Richter, M.A. *Clinical Immunology*, 2nd ed. Baltimore/London: Williams and Wilkins, 1982.
14. Wakefield, M.D., Scrace, G.T., Whittle, N. et al. Platelet derived growth factor is structurally related to putative transforming protein, p. 28 sis of Simian Sarcoma virus. *Nature* 304:35, 1983.
15. Weiss, R.A. (ed.) *RNA Tumor Viruses: Molecular Biology of Tumor Viruses,* 2nd ed. New York: Cold Spring Harbor, 1982.

CHAPTER
23

ANTISEPTICS AND DISINFECTANTS

Sven A. Kvorning

Removal or reduction of the infection potentials of intact cutaneous and mucous surfaces as well as of equipment (and air) is a prerequisite before surgery and minor technical procedures for examination and treatment. Similar procedures are necessary for rooms, furniture, instruments, and other utensils that have been used by patients with serious infections, on a smaller scale as hygienic measures before reuse of materials, and as an important practice to preserve food, and so forth.

Antiseptics are agents that kill pathogenic microbes or inhibit their multiplication or metabolic activities. Substances are usually applied topically to living tissues and are used to prevent sepsis, putrefaction, or decay. An ideal antiseptic agent should destroy all types of bacteria, fungi, viruses, and other infective agents without damaging living tissues.

Disinfectants are agents that prevent infection by destroying pathogenic microorganisms. This term commonly refers to substances applied particularly to inanimate objects (e.g., instruments, dressings, excreta). Disinfection may be accomplished by heat, irradiation, or chemicals. The reduction of bacterial flora to a level considered safe by public health requirements is usually termed *sanitization*.

Sterilization is a process that completely eliminates all microbes, including spores, fungi, and viruses. This is necessary for the laboratory instruments used for microbial culture as well as for instruments and materials needed in surgery and parenteral administrations. Sterilization demands more rigorous procedures than disinfection and can be achieved by using chemical or physical processes in greater intensity and over longer periods.

For sterilization, only compounds that are bactericidal can be used, but many bactericidals at a lower concentration have a bacteriostatic effect that will be only temporary. Sterile objects are devoid of viable germs, but toxins and pyrogens may still exist.

CHEMICAL AND PHYSICAL CHARACTERISTICS OF DISINFECTANTS

All disinfectant solutions deteriorate by storage, but they deteriorate more quickly in high dilutions than in concentrated ones. Increased temperature will also accelerate chemical breakdown (at the same time, the biological action also increases with temperature). Therefore, they should not be prepared too long before their use; old, partly inactive solutions can serve as a culture medium for microorganisms like *Pseudomonas aeruginosa*. Storing instruments in containers with antimicrobial solutions is of dubious protection and a potential danger. Most disinfectants and also detergents (such as soaps) become inactivated by contact with organic material. For this reason chemical hygiene must start with washing and cleaning. When washing and rinsing water becomes polluted (e.g., by utensils of a smallpox patient), chemical disinfection must precede the cleaning; then compounds must be chosen so that they are not inactivated by proteins. Heat sterilization of instruments is the most dependable method of killing spores and viruses.

SURFACES FOR APPLICATION

Wounds present the most delicate surface for chemicals, as they are moist and mostly composed of living cells, sometimes opening to serous cavities and often with an exudate containing catalase. For rinsing of wounds, sterile water and isotonic saline are preferable. Chlorhexidine in heat-sterilized fresh solution of 0.1% in water can be used. Suspicion of rabies demands special precautions. For treatment of contaminated wounds, chemotherapy primarily with antibiotics has almost made disinfecting chemicals obsolete. The necessary amounts are normally small, and the high cost is of little concern.

Mucous membranes are little more resistant to infection than wounds, but they are constantly contaminated by resident bacterial flora and they produce less exudate of a weaker enzymatic activity.

Skin provides a rather resistant surface against chemicals, whereas it cannot stand temperatures suitable for disinfection. The very composite character of epidermal surface, with infinite adnexal pores all containing resident and transient bacteria, requires mechanical as well as chemical treatment; if the chemical does not leave residues, the low-germ period will be very brief. The main purpose of surgical scrub with povidone-iodine in preoperative washing is to provide a long period of negative culture from the skin surface.

Inanimate objects can often be sterilized by heat and kept sterile in glass, plastic, or paper containers. For large objects, when parts or the whole cannot stand the necessary temperature, sterilization can be done by alkylating agents (e.g., ethylene oxide). When only disinfection is desired, alcohols, cationic detergents, or chlorine can be used depending on the material and nature of contamination.

When necessary, rooms can be sterilized by formaldehyde gas or disinfected by chlorine washing.

ESTIMATING THE EFFECTS

The effectiveness of a disinfectant can be rated in two different ways: (1) the number of bacteria on the treated surface can be determined before and after disinfection, and (2) the disinfectant solution can be tested during use for its ability to keep sterile or low in microbial count. The bacterial counts by the latter method will be absolutely correct, whereas those on a surface would depend much on the sampling method; a comparison therefore depends on the effectiveness of the technique. Very effective sampling is possible by washing the surface with a fast pulsating water jet. It is important that sampling be followed by a dilution that will give the surviving bacteria a chance of restitution.

MECHANISM OF DISINFECTION

The disinfectant chemicals attack microorganisms by different mechanisms: (1) denaturation of intracellular protein, (2) membrane destruction, often through extraction of membrane lipids, and (3) enzyme inhibition. The mechanism of action of all chemicals used is not known, although most have been used for years. Some effects of disinfectants are reversible; for example, the effect of mercuric ion, which acts primarily on sulfhydryl groups in enzymes, can be reversed by addition of excess of sulfhydryl groups (mercaptans). Various antiseptics and disinfectants with their mechanism of action, side effects, and uses are listed in Table 23-1.

DISINFECTING CHEMICALS

ALCOHOLS

Primary aliphatic alcohols (chain length up to C10) are germicidal, their activity increasing with chain length but simultaneously becoming less water soluble. Their bactericidal effects result from rapid coagulation of protein. Most often, ethyl or isopropyl alcohol are used in concentrations from 30 to 90%; in higher concentrations, they coagulate protoplasm of bacterial cells at the periphery and cannot penetrate into the coagulum. The 70% aqueous solution of ethyl alcohol is more effective than undiluted alcohol. Isopropyl alcohol has a slightly greater bactericidal action than ethyl alcohol due to its greater depression of surface tension. It rapidly kills vegetative forms of most bacteria in 70% (or higher) aqueous solution. Benzyl alcohol is used as a bacteriostatic agent in a number of parenteral preparations. Alcohols are lipid solvents and attack the bacterial membrane, but do not kill spores and must not be used in containers to store syringes and other instruments. The quick evaporation and, for many persons, the agreeable smell make alcohol popular for skin disinfection and for cleaning of tabletops, trays, and so forth. Ethyl and isopropyl alcohols are used also as cleansers and rubefacients for bedridden patients. Ethyl alcohol may produce allergic contact dermatitis and in high concentrations causes dehydration of the skin.

ALKYLATING AGENTS

Alkylating agents like formaldehyde and ethylene oxide replace labile H atoms in amino, carboxyl, hydroxy, and thiol groups, forming new radicals, methylene or ethylene bridges, which denature proteins. Both are active against spores in contrast to most other disinfecting compounds. They must be used as gases in closed chambers with regulated humidity and must be completely removed by careful aeration. It is most difficult to remove formaldehyde because it is sometimes condensed as paraformaldehyde, which is solid at room temperature. Ethylene oxide, which has only been used since 1940, has gained wide application for industrial sterilization of plastic equipment.

Formaldehyde is a potent, wide-spectrum germicide used as a vapor and in aqueous solution (formalin). It effectively kills microorganisms and their spores in a concentration of 1-10% in 1-6 hr, and acts by combining with and precipitating protein. It is too irritating for use as antiseptic on tissues and widely employed as a disinfectant in 2-8% concentrations. Formaldehyde has an anhidrotic action when applied to palms and soles, but not axillae.

Gluteral (glutaraldehyde) is a potent wide-spectrum dialdehyde with sporicidal and tuberculocidal activities. It kills viable microorganisms in 10 min and spores in 3-10 hr. Like formaldehyde, it has an anhidrotic action, when applied to the palms and soles, and is not generally used in the axillae for its irritant and sensitizing properties. In 2% alkaline solution in 70% isopropanol (pH 7.5-8.5), it serves as a liquid disinfectant to sterilize surgical and endoscopic instruments and plastic and rubber apparatus used for anesthesia and respiratory therapy.

Ethylene oxide is a gaseous alkylating agent that is readily diffusible, noncorrosive, and antimicrobial to all microorganisms at room temperature. It is widely used for sterilization of drugs and medical devices. It reacts with chloride and water to produce ethylene chlorohydrin and ethylene glycol, which are active germicides. For sterilization, the gas must remain in contact with the objects for several hours. For this purpose special sterilization chambers are required. It is irritant to skin and lung, and it is too toxic for topical application as antiseptic. It is mutagenic in animals and its carcinogenic potential is under investigation.

SURFACE-ACTIVE COMPOUNDS

Surface-active compounds are widely used as wetting

Table 23-1
Antiseptics and Disinfectants: Their Mechanism of Action, Side Effects, and Uses

Agents	Principal Mechanism of Action	Side Effects	Use	Preparation
Alcohols	Protein precipitation	Dehydration of skin at high concentration; contact dermatitis rare	Skin disinfection	Alcohol, USP; isopropyl alcohol, USP
Alkylating agents (aldehydes)	Protein denaturation	Irritant when inhaled	Sterilization of instruments; fumigant	Formaldehyde, USP; glutaraldehyde
Surface-active compounds (quaternary ammonium)	Alteration of cellular membrane; denaturation of lipoprotein membrane	Corrosive skin lesions in high concentration, neurotoxicity (systemic)	Disinfection of skin, mucous membrane, and abrasions	Benzalkonium chloride; benzethonium chloride, USP; cetylpyridinium chloride, USP; methylbenzethonium chloride
Halogens	Coagulation of protein and interference with enzyme action	Skin sensitivity (iodine), GI irritation following ingestion	Skin disinfection, water sterilization	Iodine solution, USP; Povidone-iodine, USP; Halazone, USP
Heavy metals	Denaturation of protein, inactivation of SH group	Acute poisoning (mercury); injury to GI mucosa	Disinfection of skin, mucous membrane, and wounds	Nitromersol, USP; phenylmercuric acetate or nitrate; hydroxyphenylmercuric chloride; thimerosal, USP; merbromin-silver nitrate, USP; zinc salts (see Chapter 14.3)
Organic dyes	Denaturation of protein; enzyme inhibition	Skin sensitization	Skin disinfection	Gentian violet, methyl violet, methylene blue
Oxidizing compounds	Oxidation of organic matter	Irritation of mucous membrane	Disinfection of wound	Hydrogen peroxide, zinc peroxide, benzoyl peroxide, USP; potassium permanganate, USP
Phenolic compounds	Protein precipitation	After ingestion and systemic absorption; GI, CV and respiratory complications; systemic neurotoxicity (hexachlorophene)	Antiseptic, caustic, antipruritic	Phenol, USP; cresol; resorcinol,USP; hexylresorcinol, USP; hexachlorophene; parachlorophenol,USP; methylparaben,NF,and analogs; thymol, NF

agents and detergents. They act by altering the energy relationship at interfaces. They emulsify sebaceous materials and remove them along with dirt and microbes. Soaps are anionic, and organic quaternary compounds are cationic surface-active agents. The latter agents are usually quaternary ammonium or pyridinium compounds. These agents have antimicrobial potentials, probably by alteration of microbial membrane permeability.

Benzalkonium chloride is the prototype of quaternary ammonium compounds. It is active against gram-positive and gram-negative bacteria, some fungi (including yeasts) and protozoa (e.g., *Trichomonas vaginalis*). Benzalkonium chloride is used to preoperatively decrease microbial flora on intact skin and mucous membrane and to reduce infection in wounds. It is used in 1:750 concentration (tincture or aqueous solution) on intact skin, minor wounds, and abrasions; in 1:2000-1:5000 (aqueous solution) for mucous membrane and diseased or broken skin; in 1:750-1:5000 (aqueous solution along with an antirust agent) for storage of instruments.

The quaternary ammonium compounds have keratolytic action and help in the removal of desquamating epithelial cells. Cationic detergents are rapidly effective at slightly alkaline pH, but can be absorbed in fabrics, cotton, cellulose sponges and other porous materials and are therefore less dependable for cold sterilization of catheters, flexible endoscopes, or other instruments. These compounds are inactivated by the presence of soaps, inorganic matter, and anionic substances. In concentrated solution, benzalkonium can cause corrosive skin lesions, and its systemic absorption may produce muscle weakness.

Methylbenzethonium chloride is effective against gram-positive and gram-negative organisms and seldom produces irritation. It is applied topically as dusting powder and used as a rinse for diapers, underclothes, and bed-linen to prevent irritant contact dermatitis.

HALOGENS

Iodine and chlorine both are antimicrobials. Bromine and fluorine are not used for this purpose.

Iodine

Iodine has been used since 1839, usually as a tincture for disinfection of skin and fresh wounds. Elemental iodine or iodophors are antiseptics with a wide spectrum of antimicrobial activity. A 1:20,000 solution of iodine kills bacteria in 1 min and spores in 15 min. Its mechanism of action is not known. Its tissue toxicity is relatively low. It is most effective disinfectant for intact skin and is used for preparation of skin before venipuncture. It can produce occasional dermatitis in hypersensitive individuals. This can be avoided by promptly removing it with alcohol.

Iodine solution, USP contains approximately 2% iodine and 2.4% sodium iodide in water and 44-50% alcohol. Iodine solution is occasionally ingested with suicidal intent. Iodine produces caustic effect on the gastrointestinal mucosa. Suspensions of protein or starch or sodium thiosulfate solution may be ingested as antidotes.

Iodophors are complexes of iodine with organic compounds serving as depots from which free iodine is slowly released. They have a broad antimicrobial spectrum. On the basis of surfactant nature of the organic compound, the iodine complexes are classified in two subtypes. Iodine can be complexed with a nonionic surfactant copolymer, Pluronic-188 to form poloxamer-iodine, or with a nonsurfactant polymer, polyvinylpyrrolidone to form povidone-iodine.

They are used as a skin disinfectant prior to surgery, injection, or aspiration and to treat minor cuts, abrasions, or burns. Povidone-iodine is available in many forms. It is used as a vaginal disinfectant for treatment of *Trichomonas* and *Gardinella* infections, although metronidazole and ampicillin are preferred, respectively, for these infections. Because it is absorbed from the vagina and may produce goiter and hypothyroidism in the fetus and newborn, its use during pregnancy should be avoided.

Chlorine

Chlorine is a potent germicidal agent. Its antimicrobial action is due to the elemental chlorine and to the hypochlorous acid that is formed when chlorine is dissolved in water at neutral or acid pH. This effect is decreased by organic matter and an alkaline pH. It is most bactericidal in acid solution because the undissociated molecule penetrates better, and it is suggested that chlorination of protein takes place even at a low concentration and temperature. Most microorganisms are killed by a concentration of $1{:}10^7$ in less than 1 min. Acid-fast bacteria, however, are more resistant; they require up to $1{:}10^4$. Because chlorine reacts with organic matter, much higher quantities are necessary with organic pollution. Excess chlorine is noticed by the acrid smell and by irritation of skin and mucous membranes, initially the eyes, but with continuous exposure (as after frequent swimming in pool water), skin manifests irritation, dryness, and scaling. Excess chlorine can be removed by sodium thiosulfate.

Chlorine is used to disinfect inanimate objects, water supplies, and swimming pools. Chlorinated lime, which forms hypochlorite solution when dissolved, is a cheap and unstable form of chlorine and mainly used for disinfection of excreta in the field.

Sodium hypochlorite solution is used to disinfect utensils. The undiluted solution containing approximately 5% sodium hypochlorite is used for root canal therapy and too irritating for use as an antiseptic. Sodium hypochlorite solution diluted (Modified Dakin's solution) containing 0.5% sodium hypochlorite can be used for irrigating suppurating wounds, but it dissolves blood clots and delays clotting.

Chloramines are amines, amides, or imides with chlorine linked to nitrogen; they are easily released to form hypochlorous acid. In solid form, chloramines are stable for transport and storage, whereas the solutions release chlorine, particularly under raised temperature. They can be used like chlorine for disinfection of drinking water and for sanitization. For disinfection of surfaces, a 0.5% solution is used, and for wounds and mucous membranes a 0.1-0.3% solution is used. The most effective chloramine is halazone. At 4-8 mg/l concentration halazone will sterilize water in 15-60 min.

Oxychlorosene is a germicidal chlorophor consisting of a mixture of hypochlorous acid and alkyl benzene sulfonates. Hypochlorous acid is slowly released from this mixture producing the germicidal activity. The sodium salt is used as a topical antiseptic for preoperative preparation of the skin and wound irrigation (0.2-0.4% solution) and urological and ophthalmological irrigations or applications (0.1-0.2% solution).

HEAVY METALS

Mercury and silver are of historical interest.

Mercury. Mercury was among the early antiseptics used by Robert Koch, and inorganic mercury had been a reputed poison for animals and humans for centuries. Inorganic mercury salts are of little importance today because they act as bacteriostatic at the concentration tolerated by living tissue and because they cause pollution of a severe degree in the environment when used for technical sanitization. Although higher concentrations precipitate proteins, their bacteriostatic effect is due to inhibition of sulfhydryl-containing enzymes. Even after a long period, the enzymes may be restored by sulfur-containing compounds (e.g., cysteine, glutathione, and so on). Highly soluble mercury salts act as depot poisons and can be used against fungi and parasites (e.g., in the anal region).

Complex organic mercury compounds (phenylmercury acetate, thimerosal, nitromersol, merbromin, etc.) are less toxic than the inorganic salts in the bacteriostatic concentrations, but they are potential contact allergens and must be critically considered when used in proprietary eyedrops, creams, and suppositories.

Silver. Silver ion precipitates protein and also interferes with the metabolism of bacteria. Inorganic salts are bactericidal in relatively low concentrations. Silver nitrate 1:1,000 rapidly destroys most bacteria upon contact; a 1:10,000 solution is considered to be bacteriostatic. Silver nitrate ophthalmic solution containing 1% of the salt is instilled into the conjunctival sac of newborns to prevent gonococcal ophthalmia. It is effective for this purpose, but may produce chemical conjunctivitis by being quite acid. Therefore, instead of this solution antibiotic ointment has been used.

Silver nitrate (0.5% aqueous solution) is sometimes applied as dressings on second- and third-degree burns to reduce infection and to induce rapid eschar formation. If it is to be applied to an extensive area over a prolonged period, it may cause depletion of sodium chloride by reacting with the salt to precipitate insoluble silver chloride. If nitrate is reduced to nitrite by bacteria in the burn, methemoglobinuria may result. Silver nitrate may stain tissue black due to deposition of reduced silver upon exposure to sunlight.

Silver sulfadiazine, 1% cream, is used in the treatment of burns and chronic pressure ulcers. It slowly releases silver and sulfadiazine and effectively suppresses microbial flora. It produces less pain than other compounds used, but it has occasionally produced leukopenia.

Colloidal silver preparations [e.g., mild silver protein (ARGYROL)] serve as depot by releasing silver ions, but in less concentrations, and hence are not effective. Prolonged use of any silver preparation may cause absorption of a small amount of silver ion, causing a permanent bluish black discoloration of skin (argyria). Silver nitrate toughened in a pencil-form application or in 10% solution soaked in a cotton pledget is used to cauterize wounds, fissures, and granulomatous tissues.

OXIDIZING AGENTS

Oxidizing agents that irreversibly alter proteins are germicidal. Their action depends on solubility, penetrability, and stability of the molecule.

Hydrogen Peroxide. Hydrogen peroxide rapidly decomposes into oxygen and water, when in contact with catalase present on wound surface and mucous membranes. The liberated oxygen can loosen and remove debris from contaminated wounds. However, the oxidation is only brief. Concentration of hydrogen peroxide should not exceed 3%. Diluted with one or more parts of water, hydrogen peroxide is used as a mouth wash, but it may irritate tongue and buccal mucosa. It is instilled in the external ear in 3% solution to loosen and remove cerumen.

Zinc peroxide (a 40% suspension) has a prolonged action, and the zinc ion is an astringent. It is mainly used against anaerobic infections of the oral cavity.

Potassium permanganate is also an oxidant and astringent. Permanganate after reduction leaves heavily brown-staining manganous oxide; even at concentrations of $1{:}10^3$, its effect against different microorganisms is rather unpredictable, and is severely hampered by presence of organic matter.

PHENOLIC COMPOUNDS

Phenols include pure phenol (C_6H_5OH) and substitution products with halogens and alkyl groups. They all denature proteins and are suited for disinfection of inorganic equipment and organic materials that are to be destroyed (e.g., polluted food and excrements from infected patients), whereas it is too toxic for disinfection even of unabraded skin. The bacteriostatic concentration of phenol is 0.5%, whereas 1.0% is bactericidal and 1.5% fungicidal. In alkaline medium, it ionizes and loses penetrability, and low temperature hampers its activity. Although phenol is not a strong disinfectant, for historical reasons it has served as a standard for comparison of antibacterial effects. The *phenol coefficient* is the ratio between the minimal sterilizing concentrations of phenol and the evaluated compound (both tested under standardized conditions against bacteria, usually *Salmonella typhi* and *Staphylococcus aureus*). Currently, phenol is seldom used as a disinfectant or an antiseptic. It is primarily used as a component of topical antipruritic preparation because of its local anesthetic and antipruritic properties. Phenol may damage skin through which it may be absorbed. Phenol should not be used in pregnant women, in infants under 6 months, or for diaper rash. Disinfectants have produced neonatal hyperbilirubinemia. Phenol has been implicated as a tumor promoter.

For halogenated phenols, the activity increases with the number of halogen atoms, while the water solubility goes down. Alkyl substitution also increases the activity of phenol. Most products contain mixtures like cresols. Some of them are insoluble in water but become miscible when mixed with soaps.

Although as a general rule soaps (because they are alkaline) impede phenol activity, hexachlorophene is extensively used as a soap additive for antimicrobial hygiene, as repeated use leaves a bacteriostatic depot on skin and hairs.

Hexachlorophene. Hexachlorophene is a chlorinated bisphenol compound that has a strong bacteriostatic action, mostly against gram-positive bacteria including staphylococci. It is used for hand washing by hospital personnel and for preoperative skin preparation. Although single application of this preparation is no more effective than soap, its regularly repeated use steadily decreases the bacterial flora of the skin. Hexachlorophene may cause irritation and burning sensation on the skin and eyes. It is absorbed through the skin, and its systemic absorption may cause cerebral irritability. When used in infants and newborns, the residues should be rinsed off thoroughly.

Cresol. *Cresol*, a mixture of three methyl isomers of phenol, is three times more bactericidal than phenol, but as toxic as the latter. Its use is limited to disinfection. Hexylresorcinol is more effective, but less toxic than phenol; it is used in mouth washes and for cleaning skin wounds. It may be irritating. *Parachlorometaxylenol* is a more effective bactericide than phenol and used for acne, seborrhea, and ear infections.

CHLORHEXIDINE

Chlorhexidine is a chlorophenyl biguanide antiseptic that disrupts the cytoplasmic membrane of bacterial cells. At pH 5-8 it is most effective against gram-positive and to a less extent gram-negative bacteria. It is rapidly acting, and its effectiveness is not significantly reduced by presence of pus or blood. High concentration of serum protein and high levels of surfactants may reduce the bacteriostatic and bactericidal effects of chlorhexidine.

On repeated application, it produces considerable residual adherence to skin and has low potential for producing contact sensitivity and photosensitivity. It is poorly absorbed even after prolonged use. It is used for preoperative preparations for surgeons and patients, treatment of superficial infections, disinfection of wound, mouth wash, and prophylaxis of dental caries. It is available as HIBICLENS SKIN CLEANSER (4% of chlorhexidine gluconate in aqueous solution), HIBITANE TINCTURE (0.5% W/V in 70% isopropanol), and HIBISTAT HAND RINSE (0.5% W/W in 70% isopropanol with emollients).

MISCELLANEOUS COMPOUNDS

Synthetic organic dyes such as gentian violet, methylene blue, and acridine dyes are bacteriostatic and fungistatic. They still are used in the treatment of acute infection not only because the staining of the surfaces keeps a record of the area treated, but also because they serve as preventives. The possibility of contact sensitization restricts their use.

Many derivatives of furan with a nitrogroup in the 5 position of the furan ring have antimicrobial properties. *Nitrofurantoin* USP (FURADANTIN) is a urinary antiseptic, and *nitrofurazone* USP (FURACIN) is a topical antimicrobial agent used (in 0.2% concentration) on superficial wounds and for surgical dressing. At the concentration used it does not interfere with wound healing. In some patients it may produce allergic pneumonitis.

GENERAL READING

AMA Drug Evaluation, 5th ed. *Antiseptics and Disinfectants.* Chicago: American Medical Association, 1983, p. 1381.

Barsam, P.C. Specific prophylaxis of gonorrheal ophthalmia neonatorum: A review. *N. Engl. J. Med.* 274:731, 1966.

Maurer, I.M. *Hospital Hygiene*, 2nd ed. London: Arnold, 1978.

Staal, E.M. and Noordzij, A.C. A new method for quantitative determination of microorganisms on human skin. *J. Soc. Cosm. Chem.* 29:607, 1978.

CHAPTER
24

THE CHEMOTHERAPY OF BACTERIAL INFECTIONS

Harold C. Neu

An ideal antimicrobial agent has a number of characteristics. The agent should have a sufficiently broad range of activity to encompass the organisms that usually would be responsible for the infection. In many situations, more than one bacterial species could be responsible for an infection. For example, in otitis media *Streptococcus pneumoniae, Haemophilus influenzae,* and *S. pyogenes* all cause the clinical syndrome. Thus, the ideal agent should inhibit all three of the species, since the species of infecting organism will not be known for 24 hours. The agent should preferably result in the death of the microorganisms, that is, be bactericidal. This is not essential in all situations and bacteriostatic agents also can be ideal agents to treat many infections. Antimicrobial agents should not produce resistance in bacteria, should not act as haptens and thereby be allergenic, nor should they be toxic to the kidney, liver, or hematopoietic or central nervous system. The ideal antimicrobial agent should be distributed to all parts of the body in which infection could occur. The administration of the agent should be simple, and the agent should be inexpensive. It is apparent that it will be impossible for any one agent to have all of these attributes, and this to a degree explains the plethora of agents available to treat infections.

DETERMINATION OF SUSCEPTIBILITY TO ANTIMICROBIAL AGENTS

Various methods to determine the susceptibility of bacteria to antimicrobial agents are available, such as growth of bacteria on agar containing the antimicrobial agent (agar dilution method), dilution of an antibiotic in broth to which bacteria are added, determination of the growth of bacteria in the presence of antibiotic by light-scattering methods, or use of antibiotic-containing filter-paper disks placed on agar plates inoculated with bacteria (2). All of the methods have potential disadvantages. The agar, broth, and light-scattering methods can reveal the precise inhibitory concentration needed but are more time-consuming than the disk method. Laboratory factors such as type of agar or broth, number of organisms used, ion concentration, and osmolality can markedly alter the results of these tests, and errors are not infrequent in actual practice due to improper attention to all of these factors.

A report of resistance or susceptibility of a bacterium to a particular agent may not always be reflected in the clinical situations (8). Because of pharmacokinetic properties of an agent, it may not be possible to achieve concentrations adequate to eradicate the particular organism. In contrast, the concentration of antibiotic in the disk method may not reflect the concentration achieved in the urine, a concentration that could be capable of eradicating a "resistant" organism, causing a urinary tract infection. Clinical experience has shown that certain agents do not cure some infections even though the bacteria are susceptible *in vitro* and even though the agent has excellent pharmacokinetic properties. For example, the cephalosporins do not eradicate infection due to *Salmonella* species even though these organisms are susceptible *in vitro* to these agents.

SELECTION OF AN ANTIBACTERIAL DRUG

Five factors should be considered in the selection of an antimicrobial agent: (1) The *clinical site of infection.* Infection of the bladder can be approached in a different manner than can infection of the humerus or of the frontal lobe of the brain. (2) The *type of infection* affects the choice of antibiotic, since bacteremia due to *Escherichia coli* or meningitis due to *S. pneumoniae* is more of a threat to life than is superficial cellulitis on the leg due to *Staphylococcus aureus.* (3) The *probable bacterial etiology* of an infection must always be considered in the selection of an antimicrobial agent, since therapy often is initiated before full bacteriological confirmation is available. An example of this is in otitis media in a child less than 3 years of age where infection usually is due to *H. influenzae, S. pneumoniae,* or *S. pyogenes.* (4) *Host factors* such as the absence of normal defense mechanisms (e.g., white cells, complement, antibody) make selection of bactericidal agent more imperative than if all of these defenses are intact. The choice of an antibiotic must reflect an understanding of host factors such as age, body size, genetic background (e.g., glucose-6-phosphate dehydrogenase deficiency), concurrent disease, allergy, pregnancy, renal function, hepatic function, and blood flow. The choice of antibiotic also must reflect what type of bacterial flora one wishes to retain. (5) The *risk/benefit ratio* of the use of a particular antimicrobial agent must be considered. In the treatment of septicemia, the use of an agent that carries a risk of ototoxicity or nephrotoxicity is justified, but such risk is not justified in the treatment of a minor wound infection.

It is essential to remember that the antibacterial activity of a drug at the site of infection is affected by *pH, presence of purulent material, decreased blood flow,* and *intracellular location of bacteria.* Any or all of these factors may exist when an abscess is treated and may thereby render an antibiotic that is potent in the test tube useless in the clinical setting.

The selection of a particular antibiotic depends upon local resistance factors. Certain agents such as ampicillin and amoxicillin, cephalexin and cephradine, carbenicillin and ticarcillin could be used interchangeably. The major common mistakes in the use of antimicrobial agents are given in Table 24-1. The antimicrobial therapy for various infectious diseases caused by pathogens is presented in Table 24-2.

Table 24-1
Major Common Mistakes in the Use of Antimicrobial Agents

1. Treatment of viral illness with antibacterial agents
2. Treatment of infection with an agent that will not reach the site of the infection
3. Treatment with an agent with known major toxic side effects when the infecting organism is susceptible to a nontoxic or less toxic agent
4. Treatment with an improper dose
5. Treatment with an improper route of administration
6. Failure to adjust a dosage program when elimination pathways are impaired
7. Treatment for too short a period
8. Failure to recognize drug interactions of antimicrobial agents with other drugs
9. Use of expensive antimicrobial agents when less expensive but effective agents could be used

COMBINATION ANTIMICROBIAL THERAPY

In general, use of a single antimicrobial agent is preferred to combination therapy, as numerous studies have demonstrated that adverse reactions increase in proportion to the number of agents used. When is combination drug use justified (4, 7)? The following situations are generally accepted as indications for combination antimicrobial therapy:

1. To treat life-threatening infection
2. To prevent emergence of bacterial resistance
3. To treat known mixed infections
4. To achieve enhanced bactericidal activity
5. To use a lower dose of one of the agents that is toxic
6. To attack an organism that exists in more than one form

Examples of each of these situations are available. Septicemia due to an unknown organism, particularly if the patient is leukopenic, requires more than one agent to cover all of the possible bacteria. Combination therapy has routinely been necessary for the treatment of tuberculosis because cavity formation provides for the ready development of resistance. Development of resistance is more difficult to demonstrate in other bacterial infections.

Infections due to the simultaneous presence of bacteria with markedly different susceptibilities, such as abscesses that follow intestinal perforation in which *E. coli, Pseudomonas,* or *Bacteroides fragilis,* all could be present and justify use of several agents. The enhancement of antibacterial activity or synergy can be shown to eradicate certain microorganisms. Examples of such synergy are:

Antibacterial Agents	Microorganisms
Penicillin + streptomycin, or ampicillin + gentamicin	*Streptococcus faecalis*
Ticarcillin + tobramycin	*Pseudomonas aeruginosa*
Trimethoprim + sulfamethoxazole	*Serratia marcescens*

These examples have clinical relevance, and the combinations have been used with success to treat serious infections (i.e., endocarditis due to *S. faecalis,* pneumonia due to *Pseudomonas,* and hospital-acquired *Serratia* infections).The basis for each combination is established. Penicillin allows the aminoglycoside to more readily enter the bacterial cell and bind to the receptor on the ribosome. In the case of trimethoprim and sulfamethoxazole, attack at two points in the same metabolic path makes it extremely difficult to bypass a pathway by a mutation. One organism in 10^6 could be resistant to either agent, but to be resistant to both is a product of the individual mutations. Two mutations in the same path would occur in 10^{12} bacterial cells, a highly unlikely concentration of microorganisms.

Other combinations of antimicrobial agents that may be used in the future are those involving compounds that

Table 24-2
Current Antimicrobial Therapy[a]

Pathogen	Clinical Illness	Drugs of Choice	
		First Choice	Alternatives
GRAM-POSITIVE COCCI			
Staphylococcus aureus	Various infections: abscesses, bacteremia, cellulitis, endocarditis, meningitis, osteomyelitis, pneumonia, others		
Nonpenicillinase-producing		Penicillin G	A cephalosporin, vancomycin
Penicillinase-producing		Penicillinase-resistant penicillin	A cephalosporin, vancomycin
Streptococcus (*viridans* group)	Bacteremia, endocarditis	Penicillin G	A cephalosporin, vancomycin
Streptococcus (anaerobic species)	Abscesses, bacteremia, endocarditis, sinusitis	Penicillin G	Erythromycin, clindamycin
Streptococcus agalactiae (group B)	Meningitis, septicemia	Ampicillin or penicillin G	Cefotaxime
Streptococcus bovis	Bacteremia, endocarditis, urinary tract infection	Penicillin G	A cephalosporin, vancomycin
Streptococcus faecalis (enterococcus)	Bacteremia, endocarditis, urinary tract infection	Ampicillin + gentamicin	Vancomycin
Streptococcus pneumoniae	Arthritis, endocarditis, meningitis, otitis media, pneumonia, sinusitis	Penicillin G	Erythromycin, a third generation cephalosporin
Streptococcus pyogenes	Bacteremia, cellulitis, erysipelas, otitis media, pharyngitis,, pneumonia, scarlet fever, sinusitis, others	Penicillin G	A cephalosporin, erythromycin, clindamycin
GRAM-POSITIVE BACILLI			
Bacillus anthracis	"Malignant pustule," pneumonia	Penicillin G	A tetracycline, erythromycin
Clostridium botulinum	Botulism	Antitoxin	
Clostridium perfringens and other species	Gas gangrene	Penicillin G	A cephalosporin, a tetracycline
Clostridium tetani	Tetanus	Antitoxin, penicillin G	A tetracycline, erythromycin
Corynebacterium diphtheriae	Diphtheria	Antitoxin, penicillin G	Erythromycin
	Carrier state	Erythromycin	Penicillin G
Listeria monocytogenes	Bacteremia, endocarditis, meningitis	Ampicillin + gentamicin	Chloramphenicol, erythromycin
Acid-Fast Bacilli			
Mycobacterium leprae	Leprosy	Dapsone + rifampin	Clofazimine, rifampin
Mycobacterium tuberculosis	Pulmonary tuberculosis	Isoniazid + rifampin	
	Miliary, renal, meningeal, and other tuberculous infections	Isoniazid + rifampin + streptomycin + pyrazinamide	
GRAM-NEGATIVE COCCI			
Neisseria gonorrhoeae (gonococcus)	Gonorrhea		
	Penicillin-sensitive	Ampicillin or amoxicillin, penicillin G	A tetracycline, cefotaxime
	Penicillinase-producing	Spectinomycin	Cefoxitin, cefotaxime
	Arthritis-dermatitis syndrome	Ampicillin or amoxicillin, penicillin G	A tetracycline

Table 24-2
Current Antimicrobial Therapy[a] (Continued)

Pathogen	Clinical Illness	Drugs of Choice	
		First Choice	Alternatives
GRAM-NEGATIVE COCCI (Contd.)			
Neisseria meningitidis (meningococcus)	Meningitis, bacteremia,	Penicillin G	Chloramphenicol
	Carrier state	Rifampin	Minocycline
GRAM-NEGATIVE BACILLI			
Acinetobacter	Various hospital infections, bacteremia	Ticarcillin + aminoglycoside	
Aeromonas hydrophila	Osteomyelitis, septicemia, wound infection	A third generation cephalosporin	Trimethoprim-sulfamethoxazole (TMP-SMX)
Arizona	Bacteremia, gastroenteritis, osteomyelitis, otitis media, pyelonephritis	Ampicillin	TMP-SMX
Bacteroides fragilis	Abscess (brain, lung, intraabdominal) bacteremia, empyema, endocarditis	Metronidazole, cefoxitin, clindamycin	Moxalactam, chloramphenicol
Bacteroides melaninogenicus	Pleuropulmonary infection	Penicillin G	Cefoxitin, clindamycin
Bacteroides bivius	Pelvic abscess and other obstetric and gynecological infection	Cefoxitin	A third generation cephalosporin
Bordetella	Pertussis	Erythromycin	Ampicillin
Brucella	Brucellosis	A tetracycline + streptomycin	TMP-SMX
Campylobacter	Bacteremia, enteritis	Erythromycin	
Citrobacter	Urinary tract and respiratory infection	A third generation cephalosporin	Aminoglycoside
Escherichia coli	Urinary tract infection,	Ampicillin	TMP-SMX
	Hospital acquired bacteremia and other infection	A third generation cephalosporin	A cephalosporin, an aminoglycoside, TMP-SMX
Eikenella corredens	Oral and pleuropulmonary infection	Penicillin G	A tetracycline
Enterobacter aerogenes	Urinary tract and other infections	A third generation cephalosporin	Aminoglycoside
Flavobacteriae	Meningitis	A third generation cephalosporin	Mezlocillin, piperacillin
Francisella tularensis	Tularemia	Streptomycin + tetracycline	Chloramphenicol
Fusobacteriae	Empyema, genital infections, gingivitis, lung abscess, ulcerative pharyngitis	Penicillin G	Chloramphenicol, clindamycin, a tetracycline, TMP-SMX
Haemophilus influenzae	Bronchitis, otitis media, sinusitis	Ampicillin	A third generation cephalosporin, TMP-SMX, chloramphenicol
	Epiglottitis, meningitis, pneumonia	Ampicillin	A third generation cephalosporin
Haemophilus parainfluenzae		Ampicillin	A third generation cephalosporin, chloramphenicol, TMP-SMX
Haemophilus ducreyi	Chancroid	TMP-SMX	A tetracycline
Haemophilus vaginalis	Vaginitis, urethritis	Metronidazole	Amoxicillin
Klebsiella pneumoniae	Pneumonia, urinary tract infection	A cephalosporin	An aminoglycoside
Pasteurella multocida	Abscesses, bacteremia, meningitis, wound infection	Penicillin G	A tetracycline
Proteus mirabilis	Urinary tract and other infections	Ampicillin	A cephalosporin, an aminoglycoside
Proteus, other species	Urinary tract and other infections	A third generation cephalosporin	Cefoxitin, an aminoglycoside

Table 24-2
Current Antimicrobial Therapy[a] (Continued)

Pathogen	Clinical Illness	Drugs of Choice: First Choice	Drugs of Choice: Alternatives
Providencia	Urinary tract and respiratory infection, wound infection	A third generation cephalosporin	Cefoxitin, ticarcillin
Pseudomonas aeruginosa	Bacteremia, pneumonia, urinary tract infection	Tobramycin + antipseudomonas penicillin	Amikacin, gentamicin
Salmonella	Acute gastroenteritis, bacteremia, paratyphoid fever, typhoid fever	Ampicillin	TMP-SMX, chloramphenicol
Serratia	Variety of nosocomial and opportunistic infections	A third generation cephalosporin	Cefoxitin, an aminoglycoside
Shigella	Acute gastroenteritis	Ampicillin	TMP-SMX, a tetracycline
Spirillum minus	Rat bite fever	Penicillin	A tetracycline
Vibrio cholerae	Cholera	Fluids + tetracycline	
Yersinia enterocolitica	Yersiniosis	A third generation cephalosporin	
Yersinia pestis	Plague	Streptomycin + a tetracycline	Chloramphenicol
SPIROCHETES			
Borrelia recurrentis	Relapsing fever	A tetracycline	Chloramphenicol
Leptospira	Meningitis, Weil's disease	Pencillin G	A tetracycline
Treponema pallidum	Syphilis	Penicillin G	Erythromycin, a tetracycline
Treponema pertenue	Yaws	Penicillin G	A tetracycline
ACTINOMYCETES			
Actinomyces israelii	Abdominal, cervicofacial, thoracic and other lesions	Penicillin G	Clindamycin, minocycline
Nocardia	Brain abscess, lesions of other organs, pulmonary lesions	A sulfonamide	Minocycline, TMP-SMX
MISCELLANEOUS AGENTS			
Chlamydia psittaci	Psittacosis (ornithosis)	A tetracycline	A sulfonamide
Chlamydia trachomatis	Inclusion conjunctivitis, lymphogranuloma venereum, nonspecific urethritis, trachoma	A tetracycline	A sulfonamide
Mycoplasma pneumoniae (Eaton agent)	"Atypical pneumonia"	Erythromycin	A tetracycline
Pneumocystis carinii	Pneumonia in impaired host	TMP-SMX	Pentamidine
Rickettsia	Brill's disease, Q fever, Rocky Mountain spotted fever, typhus fever	A tetracycline	Chloramphenicol
Ureaplasma urealyticum	Nonspecific urethritis	A tetracycline	Erythromycin

[a]Pathogens listed under a broad group and clinical illnesses due to an individual pathogen are arranged alphabetically.

inactivate enzymes that destroy a compound. For example, clavulanic acid, is a β-lactam agent with minimal antibacterial activity of its own. It inhibits many different β-lactamases so that, when combined with ampicillin, it makes ampicillin capable of destroying bacteria that would otherwise be resistant, such as *S. aureus*, *E. coli* and *Klebsiella*; these bacteria contain β-lactamases, which make these species resistant to ampicillin.

Unfortunately, combination antimicrobial therapy is not without problems, for example:

1. Enhancement of adverse reactions—"toxicity"
2. Emergence of multiple-resistant bacteria or superinfection with resistant bacteria or fungi
3. Creation of false sense of security
4. Antagonism of the activity of one agent
5. Added expense

Thus, more than one agent should be used only when laboratory and clinical studies have demonstrated unequivocably that the use of the two agents is beneficial.

USE OF PREVENTIVE ANTIMICROBIAL AGENTS

It has been estimated that more than half of the antibiotic use in the world is not to treat infection, but rather to prevent the development of infection. The preventive use of antimicrobial agents is justified when a *specific bacterial infection* will result. This implies that no infection or contamination has already occurred, that a particular species of bacteria has been shown to cause infection in the setting, that a potent antimicrobial agent is available, and that the risk of infection far outweighs the hazard of the use of the antimicrobial agent.

There are a number of areas in which the advantages of prophylactic antibiotics has been demonstrated. Healthy individuals exposed to infectious agents are protected. Examples are *M. tuberculosis, N. meningitidis,* and *N. gonorrhoeae.* Prophylactic antibiotics have prevented complications of operations in surgically traumatized areas in which contamination is probable. Examples are vaginal hysterectomy in the premenopausal woman, colon resection, and compound fractures. Antibiotics have prevented colonization of surgically implanted foreign bodies. Examples are artificial joints and heart valves. Antimicrobial agents have protected individuals susceptible to reactivation of dormant infection by virtue of other therapy. An example is the patient with a positive tuberculin reaction who is given corticosteroids to treat another disease. Prophylactic antibiotics will prevent recurrences of disease, for example, rheumatic fever. Prophylactic antibiotics will prevent infection in a patient with a biological propensity to develop a particular bacterial infection; a patient with rheumatic valvular disease will be prevented from developing bacterial endocarditis if given antibiotics prior to surgical procedures. Patients who are prone to develop infection by virtue of immunological or anatomic defects can be prevented from developing infection. Such individuals are those with asplenia, agammaglobulinemia, chronic granulomatous disease of childhood, or the woman who has recurrent urinary tract infections.

Unfortunately, there are a number of disadvantages to the prophylactic use of antimicrobial agents. First among these are toxic or hypersensitivity reactions. Superinfection, often with more resistant organisms, and alteration of the ecology of hospital flora have been noted. Improper use of prophylactic agents may temporarily mask infection, resulting in a delay in diagnosis and treatment, and it may encourage poor hygiene and surgical technique.

Understanding the basis of prophylaxis is important. The antibiotic must be delivered to the *site of probable infection* (5). The antibiotic should be bactericidal and the *duration* of use must be short to avoid toxicity and to prevent the selection of resistant bacteria.

There are various patterns of antimicrobial prophylaxis. Local methods such as irrigation of wounds, bladder, or aerosol into the respiratory tract have been of little success. However, topical silver preparations applied to burns have decreased the number of bacterial colonies in a burn eschar to a level that decreases the risk of sepsis. Systemic use of agents at the time of certain surgery, such as placement of artificial prostheses or heart valves, has reduced postoperative infection. The sporadic systemic use of antibiotics at the time of exposure to syphilis or gonorrhea, and at the time of exposure to *Neisseria* or *Haemophilus* of family contacts of a patient with meningitis, has prevented infection. Continued systemic use of antibiotics for long periods has prevented rheumatic fever or recurrence of urinary infections.

ADVERSE REACTIONS TO ANTIMICROBIAL AGENTS

All antimicrobial agents have had adverse effects associated with their use (6). Adverse reactions range from the effects on the environmental flora of the patient or of other patients in the environment, to direct toxic effects on the hematological, nervous, gastrointestinal, or renal systems (1). Table 24-3 enumerates many of these untoward effects. Fig. 24-1 shows sites of renal toxic reactions.

DRUG INTERACTIONS

Antimicrobial agents may cause a number of drug interactions that result in untoward effects (3). These are listed in Table24-4.

WHY DOES THERAPY FAIL?

Antimicrobial therapy can fail to eradicate an infection. Certain individuals have such inadequate host defenses that cure is infrequent. A patient with a hematological malignancy who is neutropenic (polymorphonuclear count $<100m^3$) who develops *Klebsiella* sepsis and pneumonia has a chance of survival even with the "best" antibiotics of less than 50%.

Many factors need to be evaluated to determine if

Adverse Reactions to Antimicrobial Agents

Agent	Mechanism	Signs
Hematological		
Chloramphenicol	Inhibit protein synthesis	Reversible anemia, leukopenia
	Damage stem cell	Aplastic anemia
Sulfonamides	G-6-PD deficiency	Hemolytic anemia
Carbenicillin	Platelet aggregation inhibited	Bleeding
Moxalactam	Prothrombin deficiency	Bleeding
Nervous system		
Aminoglycosides	Binding hair cells of organ of Corti	Deafness
	Binding vestibular cells	Vertigo
	Competitive neuromuscular blockade	Respiratory paralysis
Polymyxins	Noncompetitive neuromuscular blockade	Respiratory paralysis
Penicillins and cephalosporins	Cortical stimulation	Myoclonic seizures
Isoniazid	Vitamin B_6 deficiency	Neuropathy
Gastrointestinal		
Rifampin, isoniazid, tetracycline	Liver cell damage	Hepatitis
Neomycin	Villi damage	Malabsorption
Clindamycin, lincomycin	Pseudomembranous colitis	Diarrhea
All agents	Altered bowel flora	Diarrhea
Renal		
Penicillins	Interstitial nephritis	Fever, azotemia
Cephaloridine	Tubular necrosis	Azotemia
Aminoglycosides	Tubular necrosis	Cylinduria, azotemia
Polymyxins	Tubular necrosis	Azotemia

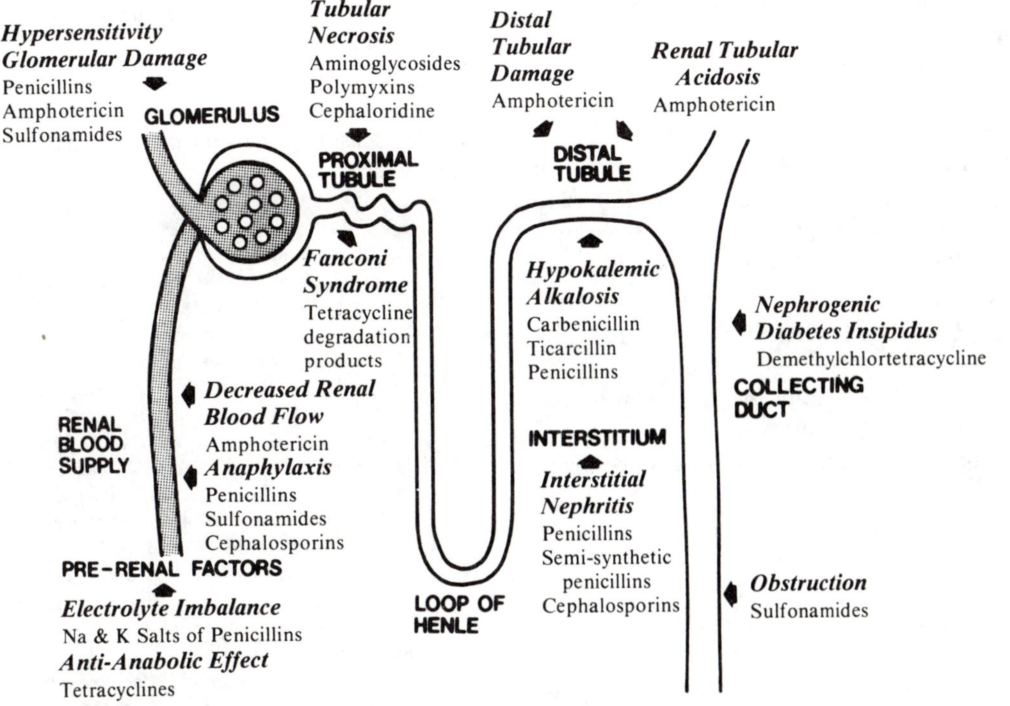

Fig. 24-1. *Sites of nephrotoxic reactions of antimicrobial agents.*
(From Appel, G.B. and Neu, H.C. The nephrotoxicity of antimicrobial agents. N. Engl. J. Med. 296:665, 1977).

Table 24-4
Drug Interactions that Occur with Antimicrobial Agents

Mechanism	Agents	Effect
Direct chemical	Carbenicillin/ticarcillin:	
	Gentamicin or tobramycin	Inactivation of aminoglycoside
	Chloramphenicol:	
	Vitamin B complex	Inactivation of antibiotic
Protein binding	Sulfonamides:	
	Tolbutamide	Hypoglycemia
	Methotrexate	Bone marrow depression
	Warfarin	Bleeding
Receptor site	Aminoglycosides:	
	Curare	Paralysis, apnea
	Methoxyflurane:	
	Tetracycline or aminoglycosides	Nephrotoxicity
	Cephaloridine:	
	Furosemide	Nephrotoxicity
	Aminoglycosides:	
	Furosemide or ethacrynic acid	Ototoxicity
	Aminoglycosides:	
	Polymyxins	Nephrotoxicity
Enhanced metabolism	Phenobarbital or phenytoin:	
	Chloramphenicol	Less antibiotic
Inhibited drug metabolism	Chloramphenicol:	
	Tolbutamide	Hypoglycemia
	Bishydroxycoumarin	Bleeding

failure of antimicrobial therapy is remedial. If fever is considered an example of failure, one must realize that all fever is not due to infection, and in some situations the antibiotic may be the cause of the fever. An improper dose of drug may have been selected. The duration of therapy may have been inadequate. Examples of this are in the treatment of osteomyelitis or bacterial endocarditis, diseases in which therapy of 4-6 weeks has been shown to be necessary. Finally, there may have been a failure to utilize measures such as drainage of abscesses, since antibiotics may not penetrate the abscess and bacteria may survive.

PRACTICAL CONSIDERATIONS IN ANTIBIOTIC USE

The following guidelines should be employed before embarking on antibiotic therapy:

1. Has infection been established by smears or gram stains?
2. Have proper cultures been obtained?
3. Do you know what organisms are expected in this type of infection?
4. Have you selected an agent with an adequate spectrum of activity?
5. Do you know the bacterial resistance patterns of your community?
6. What is the optimum effective dose, interval between doses and duration of therapy?
7. Have you selected a well-established drug?
8. Can you use the least expensive drug?
9. Have you considered the possible side effects of therapy?
10. If clinical response is not achieved, change antibiotics, but change only if *in vitro* resistance is reported or if a sufficient time has elapsed to allow the agent to work.

REFERENCES

1. Appel, G.B. and Neu, H.C. Nephrotoxicity of antimicrobial agents. *N. Engl. J. Med.* 296:663, 772, 784, 1977.
2. Bauer, A.W., Kirby, W.M.M., Sherris, J.C. and Turck, M. Antibiotic susceptibility testing by a standardized single disk method. *Am. J. Clin. Pathol.* 45:493, 1966.
3. Bint, A.J. and Reeves, D. Interactions between antibiotics and other drugs. *Antibiot. Chemother.* 25:291, 1978.
4. Klastersky, J., Cappel, R. and Daneau, D. Clinical significance of *in vitro* synergism between antibiotics and gram-negative infections. *Antimicrob. Agents Chemother.* 2:470, 1972.
5. Neu, H.C. Clinical pharmacokinetics in preventive antimicrobial therapy. *South. Med. J.* 70:13, 1977.
6. Neu, H.C. The pharmacology and toxicology of antimicrobial agents. In: *Medical Microbiology and Infectious Diseases.* (Braude, A., ed.). Philadelphia: W.B. Saunders, 1981, p. 257.
7. Rahal, J.J., Jr. Antibiotic combinations: The Clinical relevance of synergy and antagonism. *Medicine.* 57:179, 1978.
8. Sanders, W.E., Jr. and Sanders, C.C. Significance of *in vitro* antimicrobial susceptibility tests in care of the infected patient. In: *Significance of Medical Microbiology in the Care of Patients.* (Lorian, V., ed.). Baltimore: Williams and Wilkins, 1976, p. 186.

CHAPTER
24.1

SULFONAMIDES AND URINARY ANTIBACTERIAL AGENTS

Harold C. Neu

The sulfonamides were the first agents used in a systematic fashion to treat infectious diseases. Because of bacterial resistance and the development of more active agents, they have been used less frequently until the present decade, when the combination of trimethoprim and sulfamethoxazole has reawakened interest in the compounds.

THE SULFONAMIDES

History. It is ironic that the first sulfonamide, sulfanilamide, was synthesized by Gelmo in 1908, but it was not until the 1930s that the agents were used clinically. In the early 1900s, azo dyestuffs were made by the German firm of I.G. Farbenindustrie. In 1932-1935, Domagk in Germany showed that prontosil protected mice from streptococcal and other infections. He received the Nobel Prize for this work in 1939. In France, workers at the Pasteur Institute showed the prontosil split to yield paraaminobenzenesulfonamide (sulfanilamide), which was the active principal as shown in the chemical formula:

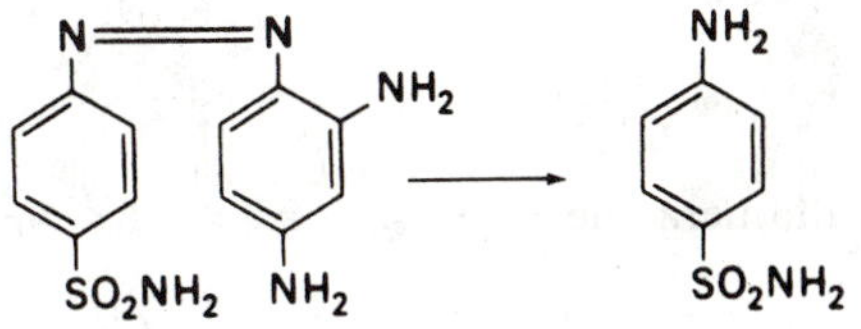

Prontosil → Sulfanilamide

Workers in Great Britain and the United States synthesized various derivatives, and by 1940 sulfadiazine was in use in the United States. More than 5000 sulfonamide substances have been synthesized, but only a small number are of use clinically.

Chemistry. All sulfonamides are white crystalline powders that are relatively soluble as sodium salts (7). The structure-activity aspects of the sulfonamides are complex, but all sulfonamides contain components that are essential for antibacterial activity (Fig. 24.1-1). The para-NH_2 group is essential and can be replaced only by groups that can be converted in the body into free amino groups. Acylated succinyl and phthalylsulfonamide derivatives are all inactive *in vitro*, but they are converted *in vivo* to active compounds. Ortho and meta amino placement results in compounds devoid of antibacterial activity. The sulfonyl group, SO_2NH_2, can be substituted, but the sulfur must be in contact with the benzene ring. Acetylation of the N′ nitrogen does not destroy activity. Substitution in the benzene ring of the sulfonamide makes inactive compounds. Structural changes in the compounds have less effect on antibacterial activity than on solubility properties. For example, sulfadiazine is 10 times as soluble at pH 7.5 as it is at pH 5.5, and sulfisoxazole is 100 times as soluble at pH 7.5 as it is at pH 5.5.

Ironically, optimal antibacterial activity was probably achieved in 1908 with sulfadiazine.

Mechanism of Action. Sulfonamides inhibit the incorporation of paraaminobenzoic acid (PABA) in dihydropteroic acid, which is a precursor of folic acid needed for the synthesis of DNA and 1-carbon fragments (20). Sulfonamides essentially are competitive inhibitors of PABA. The sulfonamides are bacteriostatic agents, but in a situation in which bacteria are exposed to amino acids and purines but no thymine, the agents can cause "thymineless death" and so are bactericidal. Sulfonamides do not interfere with mammalian cells because folate is not synthesized by mammals and is taken up by active transport (see Fig. 22-6).

NH_2 — amino group

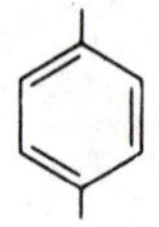

$SO_2NH - R_1$ — amide group

General Structure

Drug	R_1
Sulfanilamide	H
Sulfadiazine*	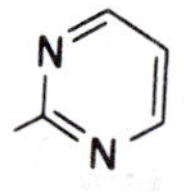 (pyrimidinyl)
Sulfamerazine	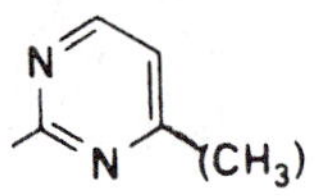 (CH_3)
Sulfamethazine	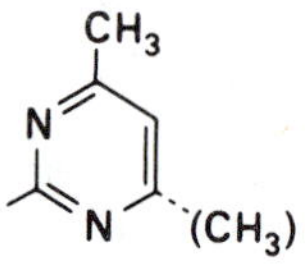 CH_3, (CH_3)
Sulfisoxazole	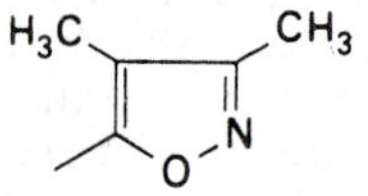 H_3C, CH_3, O, N
Sulfamethoxazole	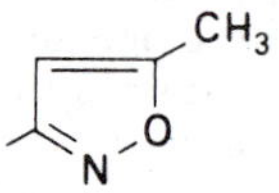 CH_3, O, N

* Silver sulfadiazine is formed by substitution of H by Ag in NH of the amide group in sulfadiazine.

Fig. 24.1-1. *Structural formulas of sulfonamide drugs.*

Resistance. It has been stated that the mutation both *in vitro* and *in vivo* results in resistance to the sulfonamides. This was postulated on the basis of animal and test tube experiments. It is more likely that in any population of bacterial cells a small number of organisms contain an altered enzyme that can bypass the sulfonamide block due to the poor affinity of the enzyme for the sulfonamide. Most clinical resistance, particularly in the gram-negative enteric bacteria, is due to the presence of plasmids that cause production of altered enzymes and thereby reduce the uptake of sulfonamides by the bacterial cell.

Whether liberation of thymine as a product of tissue breakdown will cause resistance is not well established. This would be the case only for bacteria that had a transport system for thymine.

Antibacterial Spectrum. The antibacterial spectrum of the sulfonamides varies greatly from one area of the world to another and is not predictable. Most group A streptococci are susceptible, as are many *Streptococcus pneumoniae.* Strains of *Haemophilus* are susceptible but not predictably. *Haemophilus ducreyi, Brucella, Campylobacters,* and many *Chlamydia* are inhibited. *Neisseria gonorrhoeae* today generally are resistant, as are most of group A and C *N. meningitidis*, whereas group B and Y *N. meningitidis* often are susceptible. Although *Escherichia coli* acquired in the community, which are the major cause of lower urinary tract infections, traditionally have been susceptible to sulfonamides, this is less true today. Most staphylococci, *Shigella,* anaerobic species, *Clostridia* and *Bacteroides*, and *Pseudomonas* are uniformly resistant. Most *Nocardia* are susceptible and some parasites, such as *Toxoplasma gondii*, are inhibited, as are some plasmodia. The agents are not effective against fungi.

Pharmacokinetics. ***Absorption and Distribution.*** With the exception of the sulfonamide specifically designed to exert their effect in the colon, the drugs are rapidly absorbed in the gastrointestinal tract, primarily in the small intestine. Sulfonamides are widely distributed in the body, with concentrations in tissues equivalent to those in the serum within 1-4 hours after ingestion. Sulfonamides pass readily into all body fluids—pleural, synovial, and ocular. They penetrate the CSF, producing levels 80% of the serum levels. The compounds bind to serum proteins to a varying degree, with the acetylated derivatives more highly bound. Sulfadiazine is 20% protein bound and sulfamethoxazole 65% protein bound.

The sulfonamides share the same receptor site on albumin as unconjugated bilirubin, and a number of acid drugs such as coumarins, methotrexate, phenylbutazone, and aspirin. Sulfonamides can displace all of these compounds, producing toxic effects (see later). Sulfonamides cross the placenta and are excreted in milk.

Metabolism. Sulfonamides differ in the degree to which they are metabolized. They are degraded by acetylation and oxidation, with a small amount conjugated with glucuronic acid or by sulfation. The percentage of a sulfonamide that will be acetylated is determined by the amount of time the compound remains in the body. Inactivation of sulfonamides by acetylation is genetically controlled and is similar to the acetylation of isoniazid.

Excretion. Sulfonamides are excreted primarily by glomerular filtration, with some tubular secretion and a varying degree of tubular reabsorption. Both parent and acetylated derivatives are excreted by the kidney. Several factors affect the renal excretion of sulfonamides, but degree of protein binding and pH of the urine are the most important factors (Table 24.1-1). Renal clearance of

Table 24.1-1
Usual Doses and Pharmacokinetic Properties of Sulfonamides

	Usual Adult Dosage (g/day)	Usual Pediatric Dosage (after first week of life) (mg/kg/day)	Usual Dose Frequency (doses/day)	Serum $t_{1/2}$ Normal (hr)	Serum $t_{1/2}$ Oliguria (hr)	Approximate Urine Solubility
Short Acting						
Sulfisoxazole	4	150	4-6	5-7	12	+++
Sulfacytine	0.5-1.0	Not recommended	4	4	—	++++
Sulfadiazine	4-8	90-140	4-6	2-5	12-25	+
Sulfamethizole	0.5-1.0	30-45	3-4	2-5	—	+++
Medium Long Acting						
Sulfamethoxazole	2	50-60	2	9	25	+++
Long Acting						
Sulfameter	0.5	Not recommended	1	35	—	++

sulfonamides is increased in the presence of an alkaline urine due to lowered tubular reabsorption. The solubility of sulfonamides in urine differs greatly. The presence of one sulfonamide does not affect the solubility of another. This explains the use of three agents in the triple sulfa preparations. The antibacterial activity is the sum of the three agents, but the solubility and excretion is based on the solubility of each agent alone. There is no appreciable (less than 1%) biliary excretion of sulfonamides. Sulfonamides accumulate in the presence of renal failure.

Adverse Effects. There are multiple undesirable effects associated with the use of sulfonamides (Table 24.1-2) (8, 11). The most common reactions are hypersensitivity reactions, which occur in 3-5% of patients who receive the drugs. Rash is the most frequent reaction, beginning about 10 days after use. These eruptions range from the maculopapular pruritic eruptions to petechial, severe reactions. Erythema multiforme and Stevens-Johnson syndrome have followed the use of the agents. Drug fever, serum sickness, and an arteritis syndrome can follow their use. Although blood dyscrasias are rare, hemolytic anemia can be an acute or chronic event. Sulfonamides cause individuals with glucose-6-phosphate dehydrogenase (G-6-PD) deficiency to hemolyze their red cells. Agranulocytosis, thrombocytopenia, purpura, and aplastic anemia on an allergic basis have all been reported.

Renal toxicity has been of two types. The sulfonamide crystals may precipitate in renal tubules, pelvis, or the ureters. Crystal formation is related to the solubility of the particular sulfonamide, pH, and volume of the urine. A second form of toxicity is a hypersensitivity nephritis, with changes in the glomerular membrane that are analogous to renal changes seen in other hypersensitivity nephritides. Hepatic reactions are uncommon, but there has been diffuse necrosis due to a hypersensitivity reaction. The other reactions to sulfonamides have been gastrointestinal (anorexia, nausea, or emesis), neurological (headaches, depression, tinnitus, convulsions, or peripheral neuropathy), and metabolic (hypothyroidism, goiter, or porphyria). As noted, sulfonamides compete for binding sites with drugs and bilirubin, and they have caused kernicterus in the newborn. In addition, sulfonamides can cause false-positive urine tests for glucose, albumin, urobilinogens, and porphyrins.

CLASSIFICATION

In general, sulfonamides have low aqueous solubility and form soluble salts. They vary a great deal in their solubility and absorption when given orally. On the basis of absorption and half-life, they have been classified as short-, intermediate-, long-, and ultralong-acting (Table 24.1-1). Some are poorly absorbed and used for bowel sterilization; still others are insoluble and used as topical preparations.

INDIVIDUAL SULFONAMIDES

SHORT-ACTING SULFONAMIDES

Sulfadiazine. Sulfadiazine has a relatively low solubility in acid urine, and renal crystalluria formerly was a problem. It can be used intravenously in the therapy of meningitis and as prophylaxis against meningococcal meningitis if the *Neisseria* are susceptible.

Sulfisoxazole. Sulfisoxazole is the most common agent used for treatment of lower urinary tract infections and is soluble in acid urine. It is available as a suspension, syrup, and for i.v. use.

Trisulfapyrimidine. Trisulfapyrimidine is a mixture of sulfamerazine, sulfamethazine, and sulfacetamide. Its

Table 24.1-2
Adverse Reactions to Sulfonamides

Type of Reaction	Frequency	Occurs Most Frequently With
Allergic		
Rash	3-5%	Any
Erythema multiforme	Rare	Long-acting
Fever	3-5%	Any
Arteritis	Rare	Any
Serum sickness	Rare	Any
Hematological		
Hemolytic anemia	Uncommon	G-6-PD deficient
Agranulocytosis	Rare	Any
Thrombocytopenia	Uncommon	Any
Aplastic anemia	Rare	Any
Leukopenia	Common	Any
Methemoglobinemia	Rare	Any
Renal		
Crystal precipitation	Uncommon	Sulfadiazine
Nephritis	Uncommon	Any
Hepatic		
Hepatitis	Uncommon	Any
Gastrointestinal		
Anorexia, nausea	Uncommon	Any
Pancreatitis	Uncommon	Any
Neurological		
Convulsions	Rare	Any
Peripheral neuropathy	Rare	Any
Headaches, dizziness	Uncommon	Any
Metabolic		
Hypothyroidism	Uncommon	Any
Porphyria	Uncommon	Any

advantage is that the mixture of the three agents does not result in crystalluria.

Other Agents. Other agents that are available but offer no particular benefit are sulfamethizole, sulfachlorpyridazine, sulfacetamide, sulfamerazine, sulfamethazine, and sulfisomidine.

INTERMEDIATE-ACTING SULFONAMIDES

Sulfamethoxazole. Sulfamethoxazole is similar to sulfisoxazole but is absorbed and excreted more slowly. It can be administered twice daily.

Other Agents. Other agents in this class are sulfaethidole and sulfaphenazole.

LONG-ACTING SULFONAMIDES

Long-acting sulfonamides are probably never necessary as they have a greater tendency to cause hypersensitivity reactions (3). The agents are sulfameter, sulfamethoxydiazine, sulfadimethoxine, sulfamethoxypyridazine, sulfasomizole, and sulfasymazine.

ULTRA LONG-ACTING SULFONAMIDES

Sulfadoxine has a half-life of 150 hours and has been used as a second-line agent in treatment of malaria. A similar drug is sulfametopyrazine. These agents should never be used in patients with renal insufficiency.

POORLY ABSORBED SULFONAMIDES

Conjugates of a sulfonamide with an organic acid have been developed for bowel sterilization. The drugs are of no value, and their use is to be decried. They are phthalylsulfathiazole, succinyl sulfathiazole, and phthalylsulfacetamide.

TOPICAL SULFONAMIDES

Topical sulfonamide preparations have been extremely useful in decreasing the colonization of burned skin and thereby preventing burn-wound sepsis. Mefenide (SULFAMYLON) is available as a 10% cream to treat burns. It is effective in the presence of necrotic tissue and also inhibits *Pseudomonas aeruginosa* as well as other gram-positive and gram-negative bacteria. Mefenide can be absorbed through the skin. Initially available as a hydrochloride, it caused hyperchloremic acidosis. Now it is made as an acetate, but it is a carbonic anhydrase inhibitor and can cause either alkalosis or acidosis. The major disadvantage of the drug is the severe pain that follows its topical application.

Silver Sulfadiazine (SILVADENE). Silver sulfadiazine is available as a microionized form to be applied as a cream. In this compound, a silver atom is attached to the amide nitrogen of the sulfonamide. It inhibits most bacteria, gram-positive and gram-negative species, as well as the yeast form of some fungi and also *herpes simplex.* It rarely has caused neutropenia. The compound has proved an excellent agent to control burn infections.

Sulfacetamide. Sulfacetamide is available as an ophthalmic solution for treatment of conjunctivitis.

Sulfapyridine. Sulfapyridine is a relatively toxic agent and of low antimicrobial activity, but it has been used to treat dermatitis herpetiformis. Salicylazosulfapyridine (AZULFIDINE) is used in the treatment of ulcerative colitis.

THERAPEUTIC USES OF SULFONAMIDES

The number of infections for which sulfonamides alone are the agent of first choice is small (9). Sulfonamides still are used to treat uncomplicated lower urinary tract infections (6). They are of value combined with erythromycin in treating otitis media. In most respiratory infections, other agents are preferred. Sulfonamides can be used as rheumatic fever prophylaxis, but other agents are preferred. The frequency with which *N. meningitidis* are resistant to the agents and the problems with antibacterial testing make sulfonamides still unsuitable as meningococcal prophylaxis unless the isolates are clearly known to be susceptible. Sulfonamides are no longer of value in treating intestinal infections. Various sulfonamides have been used in vaginal preparations, but most are no longer available in the United States.

They do remain the therapy of choice for nocardiosis and should be combined with pyrimethamine to treat toxoplasmosis. The topical forms are the drugs of choice in the treatment of infected burns.

TRIMETHOPRIM

Trimethoprim is available as a single agent or in combination with sulfamethoxazole. This drug is a synthetic pyrimidine first described in 1962. Its chemical structure is:

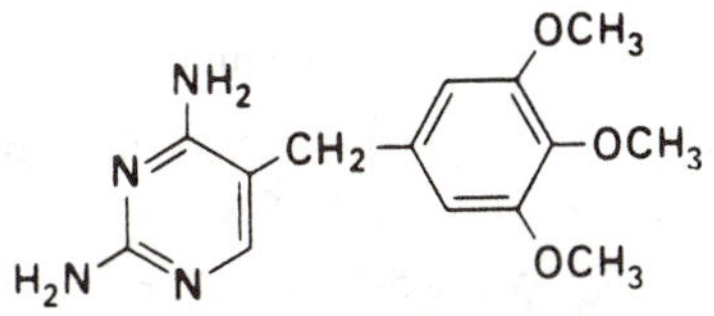

NH_2, CH_2, OCH_3, OCH_3, OCH_3, H_2N, N, N

Trimethoprim

Mechanism of Action. Trimethoprim blocks folate synthesis in bacteria by binding to the enzyme dihydrofolate reductase. This step occurs subsequent to the step at which sulfonamides block and this explains the synergistic action of trimethoprim and sulfonamides. The dihydrofolate reductase of humans has a poor affinity for trimethoprim compared with the affinity of the enzyme that is present in bacteria and certain parasites. In the absence of thymine, trimethoprim is bactericidal and in its presence bacteriostatic. When combined with a sulfonamide, the compound will usually act in a bactericidal fashion.

Resistance. Resistance is extremely uncommon but has been shown to be due to several mechanisms. Some organisms possess a dihydrofolate reductase enzyme that has a low affinity for trimethoprim. This is an intrinsic property of the organisms. Other species have a plasmid that mediates synthesis of a new enzyme that is not affected by trimethoprim. Finally, some species can utilize alternative pathways to make essential metabolites.

Antibacterial Spectrum. Trimethoprim has an extremely broad antibacterial spectrum, covering most gram-positive and gram-negative organisms with the exception of *P. aeruginosa* and *S. faecalis* (5, 18). Organisms such as *Serratia marcescens* that are resistant to all other agents are often inhibited by trimethoprim. In addition, in combination with sulfamethoxazole it inhibits *Pneumocystis carinii.*

Pharmacokinetics. Trimethoprim is well absorbed from the intestine, yielding peak serum levels about 2 hours after ingestion. The half-life of the drug is about 13-14 hours, compared with a half-life of 9-12 hours for sulfamethoxazole, with which it is combined.

Trimethoprim is distributed to all tissues, and the tissue levels often exceed those in the serum. It crosses into the CSF and also produces appreciable levels in vaginal fluid and in the normal prostate. It is bound to protein approximately 40-45%.

Trimethoprim is metabolized to inactive metabolites but is excreted primarily in the urine by glomerular filtration, with 40-75% excreted in 24 hours as active compound (4). Its renal clearance is greater in an acid urine.

Trimethoprim is available alone or in combination with sulfamethoxazole. The current formulation of trimethoprim-sulfamethoxazole (TMP/SMX) is of a 1:5 ratio. This ratio yields serum, tissue, and urine levels at a ratio of 1:10-1:20, which is the optimal concentration of the two drugs to achieve synergy.

Adverse Effects. Trimethoprim can cause gastric irritation, nausea, and anorexia (17). It will depress the bone marrow, particularly if an individual is folate depleted, such as might be the case in alcoholism or sickle-cell anemia. It will produce a megaloblastic anemia. Whether it causes actual renal damage or merely alters the kidney's ability to handle creatinine is not clear. Rash can occur with the agent but it is more common with combination product due to the sulfamethoxazole.

Therapeutic Uses. There are a number of clinical problems for which the TMP/SMX combination is indicated. It is excellent therapy for acute urinary tract infections with the exception of those due to *P. aeruginosa* and enterococci. The TMP/SMX combination effectively treats otitis media due to *H. influenzae* resistant to ampicillin. The combination is useful in the therapy of acute bacterial exacerbations of chronic bronchitis. Typhoid fever and *Salmonella* sepsis due to chloramphenicol and ampicillin-resistant isolates can be treated with TMP/SMX, and TMP/SMX is used to treat severe shigellosis since most *S. sonnei* are resistant to ampicillin. TMP/SMX has been used to treat brucellosis and endocarditis due to *Pseudomonas cepacia* occurring in narcotic addicts.

TMP/SMX is the therapeutic of choice to treat *Pneumocystis carinii* (10). It has also been used as prophylaxis against infection in the patient with leukemia or other hematological disorder who is neutropenic.

URINARY ANTIBACTERIAL AGENTS

A number of antibacterial agents have proved to be useful in the treatment of urinary tract infections even though the concentrations of the agents in serum or tissues are inadequate to treat systemic infections (15). The renal excretion of the compounds provides concentrations of the drugs in the urinary bladder that are adequate to inhibit many infecting organisms. Table 24.1-3 presents a list of urinary antibacterial agents with their doses and routes of administration.

Nitrofurantoin. There are a group of nitrofuran derivatives that have a broad spectrum of antibacterial activity, but only a few of clinical use.

Nitrofurantoin is an N-(5-nitro-2-furfurylidine)-1-aminohydantoin. The activity of the compound is related to the presence of the nitro group at the 5-position of the furan ring (Fig. 24.1-2).

The compound interferes with carbohydrate metabolism in bacteria but not in humans. It is active against most of the organisms that cause lower urinary tract infections such as *E. coli*, some strains of *Proteus, Klebsiella, Enterobacter*, and *Pseudomonas*, and some enterococci and staphylococci. It is bacteriostatic at low concentrations (5-10 μg/ml), but at high concentrations, (>100 μg/ml) it is bactericidal. Activity is increased at an acid pH. Many strains of bacteria are resistant, particularly *P. mirabilis* and *P. aeruginosa*. Resistance may developed during treatment. There is no cross-resistance with other antibacterial agents, but nitrofurantoin antagonizes the action of nalidixic acid.

Nitrofurantoin is completely absorbed from the gastrointestinal tract, but serum levels are low due to rapid breakdown in tissue. The plasma half-life of the drug is about 20 minutes. About 30-40% of a dose appears in the urine, producing levels of 15-50 μg/ml. The drug does not produce therapeutic concentrations in any tissue, and prostate levels are only one-fourth to one-half the serum levels. Levels in milk and amniotic fluid are inconsequential.

Nitrofurantoin is excreted by both glomerular filtration and tubular secretion. Clearance is linearly related to the creatinine clearance. Hence, toxic metabolites accumulate in the presence of renal failure. Urine levels in the presence of decreased renal function are too low to be therapeutically useful.

The use of nitrofurantoin has been associated with a

Table 24.1-3
Urinary Antibacterial Agents

Drug	Route	Usual Adult Dosage	Usual Pediatric Dosage (after first week of life)
Nitrofurantoin	p.o.	50-100 mg q. 6 hr	5-7 mg/kg/day divided q. 6 hr
Trimethoprim	p.o.	100 mg b.i.d.	3-6 mg/kg b.i.d.
Trimethoprim + sulfamethoxazole (TMP/SMX, cotrimoxazole)	p.o.	80 mg TMP + 400 mg SMX, b.i.d.	6-12 mg/kg TMP + 20-60 mg/kg SMX/day
Nalidixic acid	p.o.	1.0 g q. 6 hr	Do not use in infants under 3 months old, 55 mg/kg/day divided q. 6 hr
Oxolinic acid	p.o.	0.75 g q. 12 hr	Not recommended; contraindicated in infants
Cinoxacin	p.o.	500 mg q. 12 hr	Not recommended
Methenamine mandelate	p.o.	1 g after each meal and at bedtime	75-100 mg/kg/day divided q. 8 hr
Methenamine hippurate	p.o.	1 g q. 12 hr	0.5-1 g q. 12 hr

number of undesirable side effects. Gastrointestinal side effects such as nausea, emesis, and diarrhea occur in 5-10% of those who receive the drug. Skin rashes, eosinophilia, and fever develop in 4% of patients. Allergic hypersensitivity reactions including anaphylaxis have occurred, but there have been no fatalities. Hemolytic anemia occurs in some patients who are glucose-6-phosphate dehydrogenase deficient, and megaloblastic anemia occurs in some individuals. Cholestatic jaundice and hepatocellular damage also have been noted.

Nitrofurantoin can produce two types of allergic pneumonitis. The one that occurs early in therapy is heralded by chills, cough, shortness of breath, and pulmonary infiltrates. Patients usually have a skin rash and eosinophilia. The pulmonary disease rapidly resolves when the drug is withdrawn. A second form of pulmonary disease is that of chronic pulmonary interstitial pneumonitis following long-term use of the drug (14).

Peripheral neuropathy has developed after long use, particularly in patients with depressed renal function. The onset may be sudden, with pain, depressed reflexes, and muscle wasting. Neuropathy usually resolves after the drug is stopped, but the recovery is slow.

Nitrofurantoin should be used only to treat lower urinary tract infections or as prophylaxis to prevent recurrences (2, 19). When it is used in treatment, it should be given every 6 hours to provide adequate urine concentrations. As prophylaxis it can be used once nightly.

Nalidixic Acid. Nalidixic acid is one of a series of 1,8-naphthyridine derivatives (Fig. 24.1-2) synthesized in 1962. It is a pale, yellow crystalline substance with a molecular weight of 232.2.

Nalidixic acid inhibits DNA synthesis by interfering with DNA gyrase activity. It is active primarily against gram-negative organisms such as *E. coli, P. mirabilis, Klebsiella, Enterobacter*, some indole-positive *Proteus* strains, *Serratia*, and some *Shigella*. Most *P. aeruginosa* are resistant, as are gram-positive cocci and anaerobic bacteria. Resistance can develop rapidly, but there is no plasmid-mediated resistance.

The majority of an oral dose of nalidixic acid is absorbed from the intestine. Serum concentrations of 25 μg/ml are achieved, but the plasma half-life of active drug is only about 1.5 hours. Administration of the compound with alkali can increase absorption and hence urinary levels, which are also greater at an alkaline pH at which it is more soluble.

The drug is not well distributed because it is 95% protein bound and is conjugated in the liver. Only 4% of the drug appears in the feces, and it is excreted totally by the kidney. However, only 2-3% is in the unchanged form. About 13% of the drug is present in the urine as the hydroxyacid, which also is biologically active. The remainder of the drug is converted to glucuronide and dicarboxylic derivatives. In the presence of renal failure, there is accumulation of metabolites and urinary levels are inadequate.

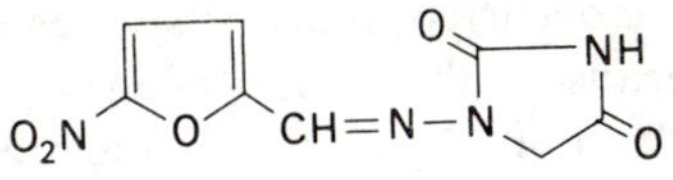

Nitrofurantoin

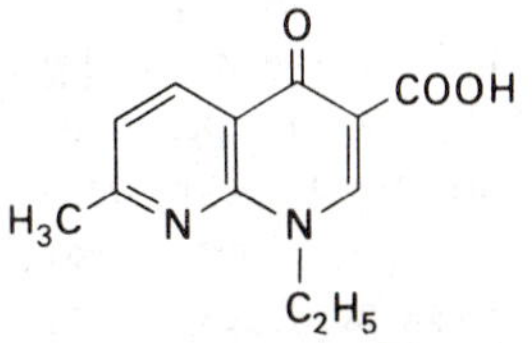

Nalidixic acid

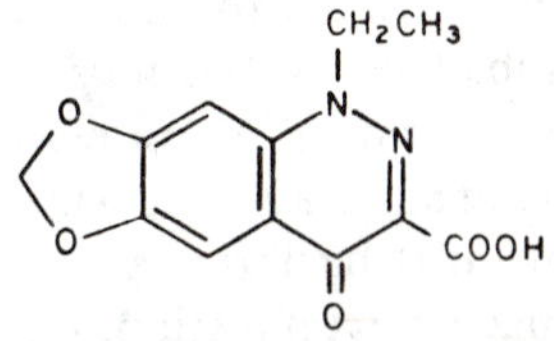

Cinoxacin

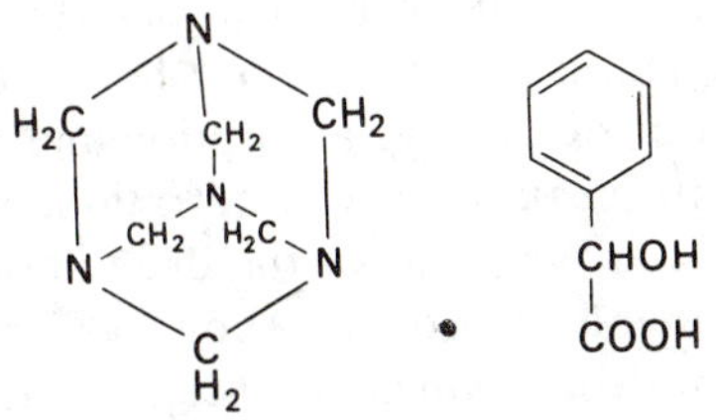

Methenamine Mandelate

Fig. 24.1-2. *Chemical structures of some urinary antibacterial agents.*

Although oral nalidixic acid is well tolerated, it produces a number of adverse side effects. Gastrointestinal complaints of nausea, emesis, and abdominal pain are the most frequent. Rashes, pruritus, urticaria, photosensitization, fever, and hepatic cholestasis have been reported. Hematological side effects have included leukopenia, hemolytic anemia, and thrombocytopenia. Neurological side effects have been seen most often in children and include benign intracranial hypertension. Headache, vertigo, and even seizures have been reported. The drug can displace warfarin from albumin, with bleeding resulting from the increased anticoagulant effect. Nalidixic acid can interfere with measurement of urinary 17-ketosteroids and can produce false-positive urine glucose tests.

Nalidixic acid is useful primarily in the treatment of uncomplicated lower urinary tract infections (16). Treatment of chronic urinary infections with the agent has been less successful and relapse rates of 50% are common. It should not be used to treat pyelonephritis. Its value in the treatment of shigellosis is questionable, and other agents would be preferred.

Oxolinic Acid. Oxolinic acid is a quinolone derivative that is analogous in activity to nalidixic acid. It inhibits gram-negative bacteria, causing urinary tract infections. *Pseudomonas* are resistant. As with nalidixic acid, resistance can develop rapidly.

Oxolinic acid is absorbed by mouth, and adequate urinary concentrations are achieved. It is metabolized in the liver, and both active drug and metabolites are renally excreted. It is excreted in milk. The compound appears to produce more neurotoxicity (restlessness, insomnia, and dizziness) than nalidixic acid, particularly in elderly subjects. Seizures have occurred. It also displaces warfarin from albumin. Because of the number of adverse effects, its use is limited. It should be avoided in the presence of decrease renal function.

Cinoxacin. Cinoxacin is a urinary antibacterial drug closely related to nalidixic acid (Fig. 24.1-2). It has an antibacterial spectrum similar to nalidixic acid covering most common gram-negative pathogens except pseudomonas. Like nalidixic acid, it inhibits DNA replication. It is bactericidal and administered orally to treat urinary tract infection. As with nalidixic acid, resistance can develop.

It is rapidly absorbed after oral administration. Following ingestion of 500 mg, mean peak serum concentration of 15 μg/ml is attained after 2 hours. Presence of food in the stomach delays absorption and causes 30% reduction in the peak serum concentration, but does not decrease the total amount of the drug absorbed. It is about 63% bound to protein. About 60% of a dose is excreted in the urine as unchanged compound and about 30-40% as inactive metabolites. More than 95% of a dose is excreted in urine within 24 hours. A mean urinary concentration of approximately 300 μg/ml is attained during the first 4 hours after a usual adult dose of 500 mg. It has a half-life of 1 to 1.5 hours in normal individuals, but elimination half-life increases to 12 hours in renal failure. The most frequent adverse effects are gastrointestinal disturbance in about 3% of patients and hypersensitivity reactions in 1 to 3% of patients. Dizziness and headaches occur in 1% of patients.

Methenamine Mandelate. Methenamine is the condensation of product of formaldehyde and ammonia. Various salts can be combined with methenamine. Mandelic acid is an aromatic acid with weak antibacterial properties. The two compounds are combined as a salt as shown in Fig. 24.1-2.

The active principle of methenamine is formaldehyde, which is liberated at an acid pH of 5.5 or lower. *E. coli* usually are susceptible to methenamine mandelate, but other organisms, particularly *Proteus* are resistant. The compound is rapidly absorbed after oral administration. Mandelic acid is excreted by glomerular filtration and tubular secretion. Urinary activity of methenamine mandelate decreases as the pH rises about 5; therefore, other acidifying agents are frequently used with it to lower the pH of the urine.

Adverse reactions are infrequent. Occasionally there is gastric irritation, and some individuals note bladder irritation with resulting urinary frequency and burning. Skin rashes are infrequent. The drug should not be used in the presence of urinary insufficiency or in individuals in whom the urine cannot be acidified. Methenamine mandelate should not be given with sulfonamides, since some sulfonamides are precipitated by formaldehyde.

Methenamine mandelate has been used primarily as an antibacterial suppressant. It is questionable whether the drug is actually useful.

Methenamine Hippurate. Methenamine hippurate is a salt of methenamine and hippuric acid. The activity is due to both the formation of formaldehyde from methenamine and the hippuric acid. The antibacterial activity is similar to that of methenamine mandelate. It is active only at pH below 5.5. The compound is well absorbed, and the hippuric acid is excreted by glomerular filtration and tubular secretion. Adverse reactions are uncommon. It should not be used in patients with renal insufficiency.

REFERENCES

1. Adam, W.R. and Dawborn, J.K. Urinary excretion and plasma levels of sulfonamides in patients with renal impairment. *Aust. Ann. Med.* 19:250, 1970.
2. Bailey, R.R., Gower, P.E. and Roberts, A.P. Prevention of urinary tract infection with lowdose nitrofurantoin. *Lancet.* 2:1112, 1971.
3. Carroll, O.M., Bryan, P.A. and Robinson, R.J. Stevens-Johnson syndrome associated with long-acting sulfonamides. *JAMA* 195:691, 1966.
4. Craig, W.A. and Kunin, C.M. Trimethoprim-sulfamethoxazole: Pharmacodynamic effects of urinary pH and impaired renal function. *Ann. Intern. Med.* 78:491, 1973.
5. Finland, M. and Kass, E.H. (eds.). Trimethoprim-sulfamethoxazole. *J. Infect Dis.* (Suppl.) 128:425, 1973.
6. Freeman, R.B., Bromer, L. and Brancato, F. Prevention of recurrent bacteriuria with continuous chemotherapy. *Ann. Intern. Med.* 69:655, 1968.
7. Hawings, R. and Lawrence, J.C. *The Sulphonamides.* New York: Grune and Stratton, 1951.
8. Koch-Wieser, J., Sidel, V.W. and Dexter, M. Adverse reactions to sulfisoxazole, sulfamethoxazole, and nitrofurantoin. *Arch. Intern. Med.* 128:399, 1971.
9. Kunin, C.M. *Detection, Prevention, and Management of Urinary Tract Infections,* 3rd ed. Philadelphia: Lea and Febiger, 1979.
10. Lau, W.K. and Young L.S. Co-trimoxazole treatment of Pneumocystis carinii pneumonia in adults. *N. Engl. J. Med.* 295:716, 1976.
11. Lehr, D. Clinical toxicity of sulfonamides, *Ann. N.Y. Acad. Sci.* 69:417, 1957.
12. Murray, M.J. and Kronenberg, R. Pulmonary reactions resembling cardiac pulmonary edema caused by nitrofurantoin. *N. Engl. J. Med.* 273:1185, 1965.
13. Pryles, C.V. The use of sulfonamides in urinary tract infections. *Med. Clin. North Am.* 54:1077, 1970.
14. Rosenow, E.G., DeRemee, R.A. and Dines, D.E. Chronic nitrofurantoin pulmonary reaction: Report of five cases. *N. Engl. j. Med.* 279:1258, 1968.
15. Stamey, T.A., Fair, W.R., Timothy, M.M., Miller, M.A., Mihara, G. and Lowery, V.C. Serum versus urinary antimicrobial concentrations in cure of urinary tract infections. *N. Engl. J. Med.* 291:1159, 1974.
16. Stamey, T.A., Nemnoy, N.J. and Higgins, M. The clinical uses of nalidixic acid: A review and some observations. *Invest. Urol.* 6:582, 1969.
17. Symposium on trimethoprim-sulfamethoxazole. *J. Infect.* 128 (Suppl.):425, 1973.
18. Trimethoprim-sulphamethoxazole. *Drugs* 1:8, 1971.
19. Vosti, K.L. Recurrent urinary tract infections: Prevention by prophylactic antibiotics after sexual intercourse. *JAMA* 231:934, 1975.
20. Weinstein, L., Madoff, M.A. and Samet, C.M. The sulfonamides. *N. Engl. J. Med.* 263:793, 842, 900, 952, 1960.

CHAPTER
24.2

β-LACTAM ANTIBIOTICS (PENICILLINS AND CEPHALOSPORINS)

Harold C. Neu

PENICILLINS

The discovery of benzylpenicillin in the 1940s made a great impact on the physician's ability to cure disease. Developments in sanitation had already reduced the incidence of many bacterial illnesses remarkably, but there was significant mortality from organisms such as the pneumococci and streptococci, which are considered minor today by hospital-based physicians. Resistance to penicillin G was quick to develop, and by the 1950s the major infectious problem was penicillin-resistant staphylococci. Developments in the technology of isolation of the penicillin nucleus made possible the production of antistaphylococcal penicillins, methicillin, and the isoxazolyl penicillins, such as oxacillin and cloxacillin (Fig. 24.2-1). Simultaneously with that development came the ability to produce a penicillin with increased gram-negative coverage, namely,

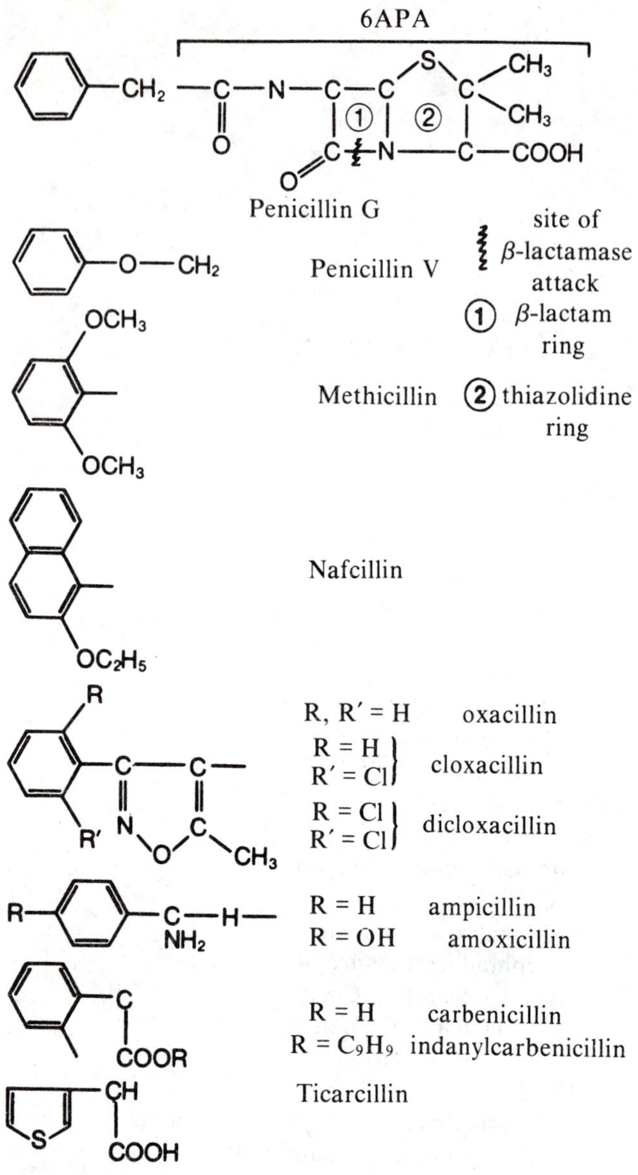

6APA

Penicillin G

Penicillin V

Methicillin

Nafcillin

R, R′ = H oxacillin

R = H, R′ = Cl cloxacillin

R = Cl, R′ = Cl dicloxacillin

R = H ampicillin

R = OH amoxicillin

R = H carbenicillin

R = C_9H_9 indanylcarbenicillin

Ticarcillin

site of β-lactamase attack

① β-lactam ring

② thiazolidine ring

Fig. 24.2-1. *Structures of commonly used penicillins.* 1 is the β-lactam ring which represents site of attack of β-lactamases and 2 is the thiazolidine ring.

ampicillin, which was effective against most isolates of *Escherichia coli, Salmonella,* and *Shigella.* Progress in hospital-support systems for care of patients with hematological malignancies, respiratory insufficiency, and burns made *Pseudomonas aeruginosa* an important organism. To attack these bacteria, new penicillins such as carbenicillin had to be developed. Recently, newer semisynthetic penicillins have been synthesized that have appreciable activity against *Klebsiella pneumoniae* and anaerobic species such as *Bacteroides fragilis.*

History. Penicillin was discovered by Alexander Fleming in 1929 in England. Fleming had been working to find human substances that would inhibit the growth of bacteria. He had already isolated lysozyme from tears. By accident he inoculated a petri dish with staphylococci that became contaminated with a mold, *Penicillium.* He went on a fishing trip and on his return noted that there was no growth of staphylococci in the area where the mold was present. He deduced that the mold elaborated a substance that subsequently he named penicillin after the species of mold. Fleming put this work aside, and it was not until the chemists Florey and Chain in 1939 began to work on the problem that the real nature of the discovery was recognized. In 1940, they showed that penicillin protected mice experimentally infected with streptococci and did not produce any toxic effect in the mice when given in large amounts. By 1941, they were able to produce enough penicillin to treat a few patients. As a result of the war, production of penicillin was undertaken in the United States, and at the end of World War II streptococcal, gonococcal, and treponemal infections were being treated. By the end of the 1940s, penicillin was available for general use in the United States. Fleming, Florey, and Chain, all received the Nobel Prize for their work on penicillin.

Chemistry. The basic structure of all penicillins consists of a thiazolidine ring, a β-lactam ring, and a side chain (Figs. 24.2-1 and 24.2-2). The penicillin nucleus is a condensation of amino acid, L-cysteinyl-D-valine. Initial production of penicillin was from a mold, *Penicillium notatum,* and subsequently from *P. chrysogenum.* A variety of natural penicillins were produced (F, X, K, etc.), but none proved more effective than benzylpenicillin, which was designated penicillin G. In 1959, Batchelor and colleagues isolated the penicillin nucleus, 6-amino-penicillanic acid (6-APA) and were able to produce semisynthetic penicillins, the first being methicillin. Basically, a semisynthetic penicillin is one in which various acyl side chains have been chemically attached to the 6-APA and produced by incorporation of specific precursors in mold cultures, by chemical alteration of wholly natural penicillins, and by synthesis from 6-APA, the last method being the most efficient. 6-APA is produced with the help of amidase from *P. chrysogenum.*

Penicillins in use are dextrorotatory compounds and usually exist as salts of alkaline earth metals, sodium, or potassium. Penicillins differ in their acid lability. Penicillin G is destroyed rapidly at pH 1, but is stable for several hours at pH 4-6. Methicillin shows a similar acid lability. Penicillin V and ampicillin, in contrast, are acid stable for several hours. All penicillins are inactivated at alkaline pH, particularly in the presence of carbohydrate.

Measurement. Penicillin G is measured in units with 1 mg of pure crystalline sodium penicillin G equal to 1667 units. All other penicillins are measured in milligrams.

Types. Penicillins can be classified on the basis of chemical structures and biological activity, as noted in Table 24.2-1. Differences within a group are usually of a pharmacological nature, although one compound of a group may have more *in vitro* activity than another. The oral absorption, distribution in the body, and renal excretion in healthy and diseased states may be remarkably different for compounds of virtually identical antibacterial activity.

Mechanism of Action. Penicillins are bactericidal antibiotics that destroy bacteria by causing lysis of the bacterial cell (14.). Penicillins act only upon bacteria that are growing.

The precise mechanism by which penicillins and cephalosporins inhibit the growth of bacteria depends on the type of cell wall present in the microorganism. Cell walls are essential for the survival of bacteria. The walls of bacteria are a complex cross-linked latticework of amino sugars and amino acids. The final stage of the cross-linking of the wall occurs outside the cell membrane. In staphylococci, this final reaction is a transpeptidation. β-Lactams, penicillins, and cephalosporins are similar in stereochemical structure to D-alanyl-D-alanine. The transpeptidase enzyme that would normally complete a linkage with alanine and the terminal glycine in the pen-

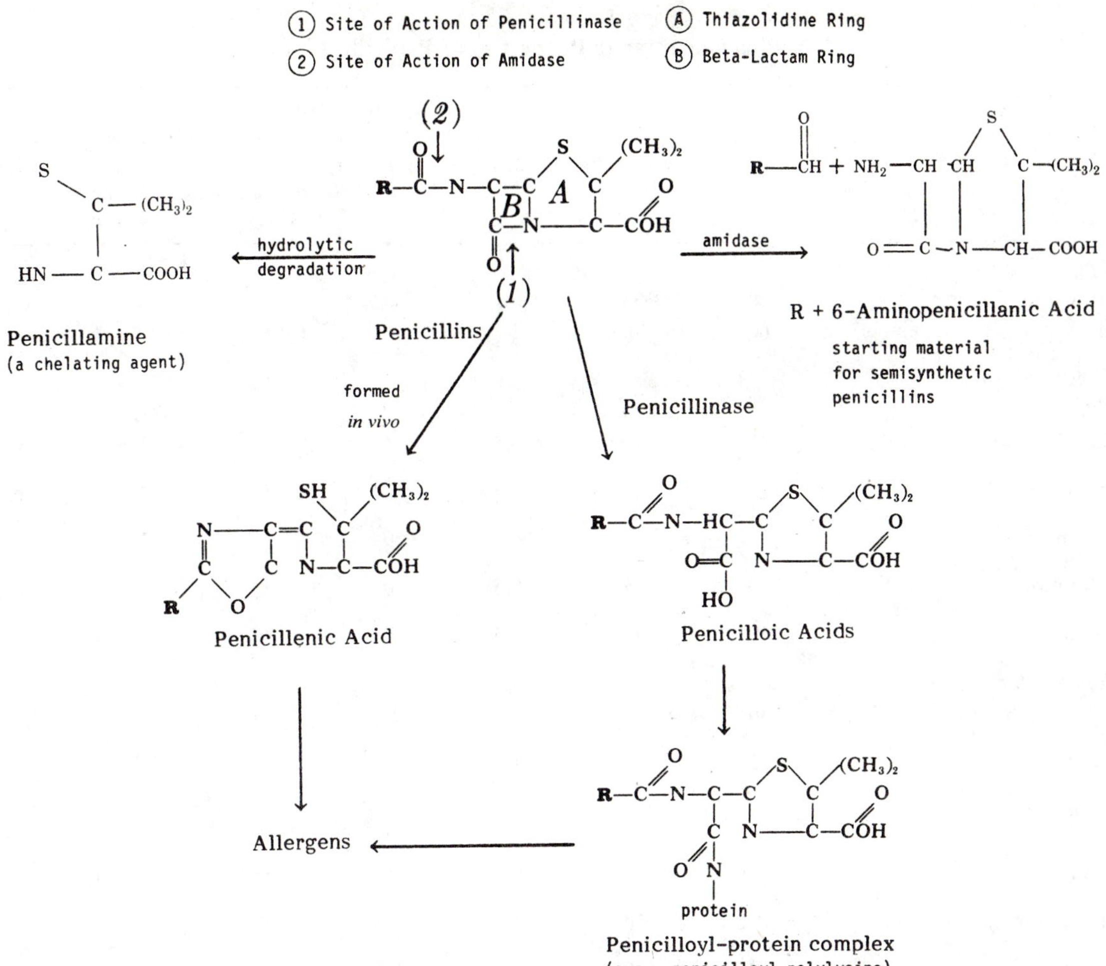

Fig. 24.2-2. *Metabolism of penicillin and formation of penicilloyl-protein complex, the cause of allergic reactions.*

taglycine bridge is acylated by penicillin and fails to complete the linkage (Fig. 22.4).

The actual lysis of the bacteria is due to bacterial enzymes, murine hydrolases, which normally cleave the wall during cell division. By disrupting normal wall synthesis, β-lactam antibiotics interfere with the inhibition of these lytic enzymes, and the cells lyse due to their increased intracellular pressure. Some penicillins cause the formation of long filamentous forms that eventually lyse but can revert to cells under certain situations. Other penicillins cause rapid bursting of the cells. These differences are related to different affinities of penicillins for the enzymes involved in elongation, septum formation, and cell shape.

It is important to realize that penicillins act only on growing bacteria and that if the environment about the bacteria is hyperosmolar, the bacteria will not be killed.

Differences in the "activity," that is, the amount of a particular penicillin needed to kill an organism, is related to three factors: (1) ability of the penicillin to go through the outer wall of the bacterium, (2) affinity for receptor proteins, and (3) resistance to β-lactamases (Fig. 24.2-2).

Bacterial Resistance. Three mechanisms of bacterial resistance to penicillins have been defined. The most important mechanism is destruction of the β-lactam nucleus, which is needed for activity. β-Lactamases are present to some extent in almost all bacteria. The enzymes may act as penicillinases or as cephalosporinases, or they may act to destroy both types of β-lactam compounds equally well. The production of β-lactamases may be plasmid-mediated as they are in *Staphylococcus aureus, E. coli, Haemophilus,* and *N. gonorrhoeae,* or chromosomally mediated as they are in *Enterobacter* and many Pseudomonas. β-Lactamases may be exoenzymes that are excreted outside the bacterium as in *S. aureus* or in the periplasmic space at the bacterial cell surface in gram-negative species. Penicillins vary in their β-lactamase stability.

The second mechanism of resistance of bacteria is failure of the penicillin or cephalosporin to reach the receptor proteins. This mechanism does not occur in gram-positive bacteria, but it is common in gram-negative species. There are proteins in the wall of gram-negative bacteria that function as channels through which mate-

Table 24.2-1
Pharmacokinetic Properties of Penicillins

Antibiotic Groups and Routes of Use	β-Lactamase Stability	Oral Absorption	Protein Binding	Serum Half-Life[a]			Dosage Reduction in Renal Failure	Effect of Dialysis
				Normal $C_{cr} > 90$/ml	Renal Failure $C_{cr} < 10$/ml	Increase in Hepatic Diseases		
I. *Natural penicillin*								
Penicillin G i.m., i.v., p.o.	–	20	55	0.5	2.5	+	Yes	+
Penicillin V p.o.	–	60	80	1		+	No	+
II. *Penicillinase-resistant penicillin*								
Methicillin i.m., i.v.	+	Nil	35	0.5	4	+	Yes	+
Nafcillin i.m., i.v.	+	Erratic	87	0.5	1.5	+++	No	No
Oxacillin i.m., i.v.	+	30	93	0.5	1	+	No	No
Cloxacillin p.o.	+	50	94	0.5	1	++	No	No
Dicloxacillin p.o.	+	50	97	0.5	1.5	++	No	No
III. *Aminopenicillin*								
Ampicillin i.v., i.m., p.o.	–	40	17	1	8	++	Yes	–
Amoxicillin i.v., i.m., p.o.	–	75	17	1	8	+	Yes	+
IV. *Antipseudomonas penicillin*								
Azlocillin i.m., i.v.	–	Nil	50	0.9	4	++	Minimal	+
Carbenicillin i.m., i.v.	–	Nil	50	1	15	++	Yes	+
Indanylcarbenicillin p.o.	–	30	50	1	15	++	Avoid	+
Mezlocillin i.m., i.v.	–	Nil	50	0.9	4	++	Minimal	+
Ticarcillin i.m., i.v.	–	Nil	50	1	15	++	Yes	+
Piperacillin i.m., i.v.	–	Nil	50	0.9	4	++	Minimal	+

[a] C_{cr}, Creatinine clearance.

rials penetrate the outer membrane. Changes in pore size will prevent molecules from reaching the penicillin binding proteins. An example of this is the ineffectiveness of methicillin (an antistaphylococcal agent) against gram-negative bacteria.

The third mechanism of resistance is failure to bind to a penicillin-binding protein. The penicillin-resistant *Streptococcus pneumoniae* and methicillin-resistant *Staphylococcus aureas* are examples of this resistance.

Antimicrobial Spectrum. The susceptibility patterns of bacteria to the various penicillins differ from community to community and hospital to hospital, but generalizations can be made. Penicillin G inhibits many clinically important bacteria such as *Streptococcus pyogenes* (group A), *S. agalactiae* (group B), *S. pneumoniae, Neisseria meningitidis, S. viridans,* nonpenicillinase producing *S. aureus, Corynebacterium diphtheriae,* anaerobic coccal species, *Clostridia, Treponema,* and a number of other species. Bacteria susceptible to natural penicillins (G, V) are usually more susceptible to these agents than to semisynthetic agents. Penicillin V can be substituted for penicillin G, except against gram-negative species, *Haemophilus* and *Neisseria.* Semisynthetic penicillinase-resistant penicillins are drugs of choice only for penicillinase-producing staphylococci. They do inhibit streptococci but not enterococci or the *Enterobacteriaceae.* The susceptibility of *Enterobacteriaceae* and *Pseudomonas* to ampicillin and carbenicillin and similar drugs is different in each community. Most anaerobic gram-positive bacteria are susceptible to most penicillins. Gram-negative anaerobic bacteria such as *Bacteroides fragilis* are susceptible only to high concentrations of penicillin G or the semisynthetic antipseudomonas penicillins.

Pharmacokinetics. Penicillins differ markedly in their oral absorption (Tabel 24.2). Some are not absorbed because of acid lability (e.g., penicillin G), some because of the ionic state (e.g., antipseudomonas penicillins). Most penicillins that are absorbed orally yield peak serum levels 1-2 hours after ingestion. Ingestion with food delays absorption and decreases the absorption of some penicillins (ampicillin), but not others (amoxicillin). Repository (long-acting due to slow release from the intramuscular tissue site) forms of penicillin G are available, but not of other agents. Penicillins are bound to protein in varying degrees, from 17% for ampicillin to 97% for dicloxacillin. *Only free drug* exerts its antibacterial activity.

The major mechanism of excretion of most penicillins is as intact molecules through the kidneys via *tubular secretion*. The rate and amount of excretion vary for each agent, but up to 4 g/h of penicillin G can be excreted. Secretion can be blocked by probenecid, which prolongs serum half-life and increases the height of the serum peak.

Penicillins accumulate in the body only in the presence of markedly decreased renal function. Dosage adjustments must be made for the newborn and for individuals whose creatinine clearance is less than 30 ml/min. In the presence of anuria, the doses of all penicillins must be reduced. Biliary excretion of all penicillins occurs but is only important for nafcillin (antistaphylococcal penicillin) and the antipseudomonas penicillins. Nafcillin is not significantly metabolized by the liver but is sequestered in the bile and undergoes enterohepatic circulation. The plasma levels are thereby maintained for a longer duration of time. In the presence of combined renal and hepatic failure, greater reduction of the dose of agents such as carbenicillin, ticarcillin, etc., must be made (4). Peritoneal dialysis and hemodialysis remove varying amounts of the different penicillins (Table 24.2-1).

Depending on the pharmacokinetic characteristics, the plasma concentration curves for different penicillin preparations show marked variations as in Fig. 24.2-3. Following administration of 300,000 U of penicillin G (i.m), penicillin V (oral), and procaine penicillin (i.m.), the peak blood levels occur at 0.5, 1, and 4 hours, and their plasma concentrations are still detectable at 5, 6, and 24 hours, respectively. After a single injection of 600,000 U of benzathine penicillin (i.m.), the peak blood level is obtained within 6 hours and can be detected in serum for 10 days.

Penicillins are well distributed to most areas of the body such as lung, liver, kidney, muscle, bone, and placenta. The levels of penicillins in abscesses, middle ear fluid, and pleural, peritoneal, and synovial fluid are sufficient to inhibit most susceptible bacteria if inflammation is present. Most penicillins are insoluble in lipid and do not penetrate mammalian cells, including white cells. Penicillins that are bound to bacteria that are ingested by white cells aid in killing the bacteria. Levels of penicillins in eye, brain, and cerebrospinal fluid are extremely low in the absence of inflammation. Penicillin and ampicillin given in high doses achieve adequate CSF levels during meningitis.

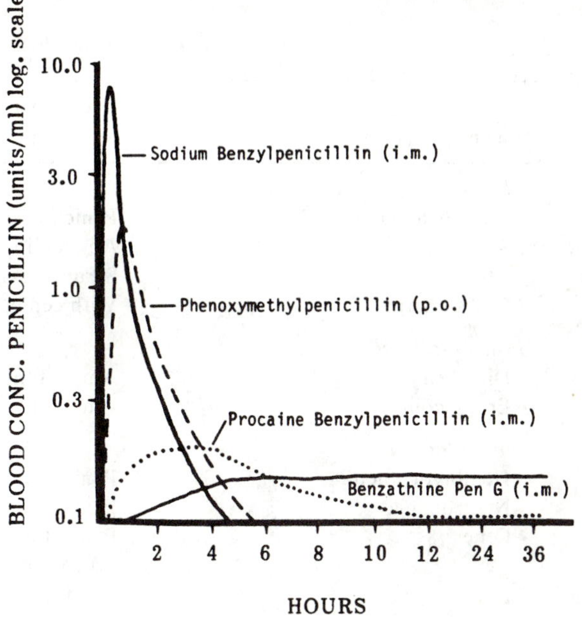

Fig. 24.2-3. *Blood concentration of various penicillin preparations.*

Urinary concentrations of all penicillins are high, even in the presence of reduced renal function, but at creatinine clearances below 10 ml/min, the urine levels will be low. Biliary levels of the penicillins exceed serum levels but are reduced in the presence of common bile duct obstruction.

Adverse Effects. The major adverse effects of penicillins are hypersensitivity reactions, which range from a minor rash to immediate anaphylaxis (Table 24.2-2). Penicillins act as haptens to combine with human proteins or proteins contaminating the solutions. There are major and minor determinants of penicillin hypersensitivity that are produced when the β-lactam ring is opened, allowing formation of amide linkage to protein (Fig. 24.2-2). Minor determinants of allergy are benzylpenicillin itself or sodium benzylpenicilloate. These minor determinants activate immunoglobulin E (IgE) antibody, causing either anaphylaxis or accelerated hypersensitivity reactions (Table 24.2-3). Anaphylactic reactions are uncommon, occurring in only 0.004-0.04% of penicillin-treated patients. Other allergic reactions, such as rash, are due to the major determinants, benzylpenicilloyl, and are probably due to IgM antibody (Table 24.2-3).

Skin testing with both major and minor determinants will detect immediate reactions to penicillin in 96% of cases. Benzylpenicilloylpolylysine (PREPEN) is available commercially, and penicillin G, broken down in an alkaline solution, can be used as the minor determinant.

Table 24.2-2
Adverse Reactions to Penicillins and Cephalosporins

Type of Reaction	Occurs Most Frequently with Penicillins	Occurs with Cephalosporins
Allergic		
Anaphylactic	Penicillin G	Rare
Skin rash	Ampicillin	Occasional
Other	Serum sickness (penicillin G)	Fever, lymphadenopathy
Cross-allergy	With cephalosporin (occurs)	With penicillin (<10%)
Gastrointestinal		
Diarrhea	Ampicillin	Uncommon
Enterocolitis	Ampicillin	Rare
Hematological		
Hemolytic anemia	Penicillin G	Rare
Neutropenia	Penicillin G, oxacillin	Rare
Other	Platelet dysfunction (carbenicillin, ticarcillin)	Eosinophilia (occasional) Prolonged prothrombin time (moxalactam)
Hepatic		
Elevated SGOT, alkaline phosphatase, SGPT	Oxacillin, nafcillin, carbenicillin	Occasional
Renal		
	Interstitial nephritis (methicillin)	Renal tubular necrosis (cephaloridine 4 g/day)
Electrolyte disturbance		
Sodium overload	Carbenicillin	—
Hypokalemia	Carbenicillin, ticarcillin	—
Neurological		
Seizures (central injection)	Penicillin G	—
Bizarre reactions	Procaine penicillin	—
Miscellaneous		
Phlebitis (on i.v. injection)	—	Common
False-positive Coombs' test	Occasional	Frequent
Urine glucose	—	Common
Disulfiram-like reactions	—	Moxalactam Cefoperazone

Development of wheal and flare reaction to the intradermal injection of the two reagents is suggestive that a patient could develop an anaphylactic reaction. A negative test does not mean that a late reaction such as rash will not occur. If an immediate allergic reaction to penicillin occurs, the treatment is epinephrine. Antihistamines and corticosteroids are of no value. Desensitization to penicillins can be accomplished by use of increasing small amounts given over many hours, but it is preferable to use another drug.

Hematological toxicity is rare. Neutropenia can follow use of high doses of any penicillin. Carbenicillin and ticarcillin bind to adenosine diphosphate (ADP) in platelets and so can alter platelet aggregation, leading to bleeding. Renal toxicity is uncommon, but interstitial nephritis has been seen with all penicillins, although most often with methicillin. The clinical syndrome is one of fever, rash, eosinophilia, proteinuria, and eosinophuria. Large doses of any penicillin, particularly carbenicillin or ticarcillin, will produce hypokalemia due to the load of nonreabsorbable ion presented to the distal tubule. Central nervous system toxicity in the form of myoclonic seizures can follow use of massive doses of any penicillin. Intramuscular injection of procaine penicillin can produce an immediate reaction manifested as CNS stimulation, resulting from too rapid release and absorption of procaine into systemic circulation. This reaction is characterized by headache, hallucination, dizziness, and sometimes seizures. Gastrointestinal disturbances such as diarrhea and abdominal pain have followed ampicillin administration but are not severe enough to require discontinuing the drug. Pseudomembranous colitis due to

Table 24.2-3
Penicillin-Induced Hypersensitivity Reactions

Type of Reaction	Responsible Antibody Class	Responsible Antigen
Immediate (2-30 min) urticaria, laryngeal edema, hypotension	IgE	Minor determinants Benzylpenicilloyl
Accelerated urticarial reaction (e.g., urticaria, pruritus, wheezing)	IgE	Benzylpenicilloyl
Late reactions (72 hr), morbiliform eruption, urticarial, Arthus-like	IgM IgG	Benzylpenicilloyl Benzylpenicilloyl
Serum sickness	IgG	Benzylpenicilloyl
Vasculitis	IgG-IgM	Minor determinants Benzylpenicilloyl

overgrowth of *Clostridium difficile* rarely occurs during ampicillin therapy. This can be quickly alleviated if the antibiotic is stopped and vancomycin is administered. Abnormalities of hepatic function tests, alkaline phosphatase, and SGOT have occurred after use of oxacillin, nafcillin, and carbenicillin. Jarisch-Herxheimer reaction occurring in syphilitic patients following administration of first dose of penicillin is described in Chapter 25.5.

INDIVIDUAL PENICILLINS

Penicillin G. Penicillin G is available in oral, parenteral, and repository preparations. It is destroyed by β-lactamases. It should be used orally only if it is taken 1 hour before or 2 hours after a meal to prevent its destruction by gastric acid. There is little reason to use oral penicillin G for acute infection at the present time.

Crystalline penicillin G in aqueous solution has been used intramuscularly, subcutaneously, intravenously, and intrathecally. Given intramuscularly as an aqueous solution, penicillin G is very rapidly cleared from the body, and it is preferable to use a repository form.

Penicillin V. Penicillin V is acid stable and administered orally. It has the same antibacterial spectrum as penicillin G and is susceptible to destruction by β-lactamase. Its distribution and excretion follow the same pattern as that of penicillin G. The drug is available in oral preparations only.

REPOSITORY FORMS

Repository penicillins are only for intramuscular use and should not be used intravenously or subcutaneously.

Procaine Penicillin. Procaine penicillin, a mixture of equal molar parts of procaine and penicillin, is a compound of low solubility and is slowly absorbed.

Benzathine Penicillin. Benzathine penicillin is a repository form of penicillin that is a combination of 2 moles of penicillin and 1 mole of dibenzylethylenediamine.

These two compounds release benzylpenicillin slowly from the region in which they were injected, thereby producing a relatively low but sustained blood level.

SEMISYNTHETIC PENICILLINS

Methicillin. Methicillin is a penicillin resistant to staphylococcal β-lactamase. There are small numbers of methicillin-resistant *S. aureus* that are resistant not because of β-lactamase activity but by virtue of altered cell wall formation. These organisms have become more common in the United States. Methicillin-resistant *S. epidermidis* are common (20-60% of isolates) in the United States and cause serious infections after cardiac surgery. Methicillin is acid unstable and must be given parenterally. Methicillin is less protein bound than the other antistaphylococcal penicillins, and although its intrinsic activity is less than that of the other antistaphylococcal penicillins, it is more active in the presence of serum than are the other agents. More allergic reactions, particularly renal toxicity in the form of interstitial nephritis, have followed the use of methicillin than have been associated with other antistaphylococcal drugs.

Nafcillin. Nafcillin has more intrinsic activity than methicillin against both staphylococci and streptococci, but it is not active against gram-negative bacteria. Absorption is erratic by mouth, and the preferred route of administration is intravenously. The antibiotic is primarily excreted by the liver and to a lesser extent by the kidney.

Isoxazolyl penicillins (oxacillin, cloxacillin, and dicloxacillin). All of these agents are stable to staphylococcal β-lactamase and inhibit both penicillin-sensitive and penicillin-resistant staphylococci. Methicillin-resistant *S. aureus* and *S. epidermidis* are resistant to these penicillins. All are absorbed after oral administration, but absorption is adversely affected by food. There are differences in serum levels among the drugs after oral ingestion, with the serum level of cloxacillin and dicloxacillin twice that of oxacillin. All the drugs are highly bound to serum proteins.

AMINOPENICILLINS

In addition to the gram-positive bacteria susceptible to penicillin G, the antibacterial spectrum of the aminopenicillins is further extended to several gram-negative cocci and bacilli. They are not stable to β-lactamase of either gram-positive or gram-negative bacteria. They are more active against group D streptococci (e.g., *S. faecalis*) than is penicillin G. Sensitivity of *N. gonorrhoeae* varies from highly sensitive to completely resistant strains. *H. influenzae* (both typable and nontypable strains) and *H. parainfluenzae* are susceptible, except for the 25% of isolates that produce β-lactamases. Although domiciliary *E. coli* are susceptible to aminopenicillins, plasmid resistance is common in hospital isolates. They inhibit *Salmonella*, but most *Shigella* now are resistant. *Klebsiella* and *Pseudomonas* are resistant.

Ampicillin. Ampicillin is moderately well absorbed after oral administration, but peak levels are delayed and lowered if it is ingested with food. Ampicillin is well distributed to body compartments and achieves therapeutic concentration in CSF and in pleural, joint, and peritoneal fluids in the presence of inflammation. It produces a rash that is not antibody mediated when given to individuals with viral illness, particularly infectious mononucleosis.

Amoxicillin. Amoxicillin is significantly better absorbed when given by mouth than is ampicillin (8). Peak blood levels are two to two and a half times those achieved with a similar dose of ampicillin, and food does not decrease absorption. Clinical studies with amoxicillin have been extensive, and it has been used in the treatment of otitis media, bronchitis, pneumonia, typhoid, gonorrhea, and urinary tract infections. It is not useful in the treatment of shigellosis. Side effects of amoxicillin are similar to those seen with ampicillin, although diarrhea may be less common than with ampicillin.

Other aminopenicillins. Hetacillin, cyclocillin, epicillin, and esters of ampicillin are available in many countries, but offer no advantage over ampicillin.

ANTIPSEUDOMONAS PENICILLINS

Carbenicillin. The principal advantage of carbenicillin is its activity against *Pseudomonas aeruginosa* and certain indole-positive *Proteus* species that are not susceptible to other penicillins. It is destroyed by β-lactamases of both gram-positive and gram-negative organisms. It inhibits some *Enterobacter* and *Serratia* strains and many *Bacteroides fragilis*, although high concentrations are required. Carbenicillin acts synergistically with amikacin, gentamicin, and tobramycin to inhibit *P. aeruginosa* (1). This antibiotic is excreted by renal tubules, but since less is converted to penicilloic acid, its half-life (72 min) is longer than that of penicillin G; it accumulates in the presence of renal failure with further accumulation if hepatic function is also depressed. Side effects due to carbenicillin are similar to those seen with other penicillins. Because it is a disodium salt and each gram contains 4.7 mEq of sodium, when administered at doses of 30-40 mg/day congestive heart failure may occur. Carbenicillin causes more hypokalemia than other penicillins due to the large load of nonreabsorbable anion delivered to the distal tubule. It has been replaced by the penicillins below.

Ticarcillin. The antibacterial spectrum of ticarcillin is identical to that of carbenicillin, except that it is two to four times more active against *P. aeruginosa*. The pharmacokinetics of ticarcillin and carbenicillin are virtually identical, as are the side effects.

Azlocillin. Azlocillin is a broad-spectrum semisynthetic penicillin that is an acyl ureido derivative of ampicillin. It is more active than carbenicillin or ticarcillin against *Pseudomonas* and against streptococcal species. It is destroyed by β-lactamases of staphylococci and some *Enterobacteriaceae*. Like carbenicillin and ticarcillin, azlocillin acts synergistically with aminoglycosides against many gram-negative bacteria. Azlocillin can only be administered by the parenteral route. Its half-life is about 1 hour in individuals with normal renal function; it is excreted primarily by tubular secretion. As with other penicillins, it is widely distributed to most body compartments. Azlocillin is used primarily to treat infections due to *Pseudomonas aeruginosa*.

Mezlocillin. Mezlocillin is an acyl ureido derivative of ampicillin that has antipseudomonas activity similar to ticarcillin and activity against streptococci similar to ampicillin. It inhibits about 50-60% of *Klebsiella*. Mezlocillin is destroyed by β-lactamases. It can only be administered by the parenteral routes. The half-life of the drug is about 1 hour, and its pharmacological properties are similar to azlocillin.

Piperacillin. Piperacillin is an acyl ureido derivative of ampicillin that contains a piperazine side chain. It has antibacterial activity against *Pseudomonas* that is eightfold greater than that of carbenicillin, and like mezlocillin it inhibits 50% of *Klebsiella*. Piperacillin has a half-life of 1 hour, is excreted by tubular secretion, and is widely distributed in the body. Adverse effects seen with its use are similar to those found with other penicillins.

ORAL ANTIPSEUDOMONAS PENICILLINS

Indanylcarbenicillin. Indanylcarbenicillin is an α-carboxy ester of carbenicillin. It has no intrinsic activity of its own, but as a sodium ester it is highly acid stable and relatively well absorbed from the gastrointestinal tract where it is hydrolyzed to yield carbenicillin as active drug. The compound does not provide adequate serum or tissue levels for systemic infections, and it is useful only for the treatment of urinary tract infections. In the presence of markedly decreased renal function, urinary levels also are inadequate.

AMDINOCILLIN (Mecillinam)

Amdinocillin acts only against gram-negative bacteria that belong to *Enterobacteriaceae, E. coli, Klebsiella,*

Enterobacter, Salmonella, etc. It does not inhibit gram-positive cocci or *Pseudomonas.* The agents binds to specific penicillin-binding protein (PBP-2) and produces osmotically fragile species. It can act synergistically with other penicillins or with cephalosporins. Amdinocillin is available as a parenteral agent or as a pivolyl ester that is orally absorbed. The pharmacokinetic properties of amdinocillin are similar to those of ampicillin, both in its oral ester form and when administered intravenously.

THERAPEUTIC USES

In the nonallergic person, a penicillin should always be the drug of choice to treat infections caused by susceptible organisms. Penicillin G remains the primary agent for treatment of *S. pyogenes* infections of the upper and lower respiratory tract. *S. pneumoniae* infections (regardless of the site of infection within the body), otitis media, pneumonia, meningitis, and arthritis still are susceptible to therapy with penicillin G. All *Neisseria meningitidis* strains are susceptible to penicillin G. *Neisseria gonorrhoeae* vary in susceptibility to penicillin G, from the highly susceptible forms that cause the disseminated forms of the disease to isolates that contain a plasmid-mediated β-lactamase. Nonetheless, in the United States penicillin G is the drug of choice to treat urogenital and disseminated forms of the illness. Similarly, penicillin G is the drug of choice for treponemal infection and syphilis, in all its forms. Puerperal infections due to anaerobic streptococci or group B streptococci (*S. agalactiae*), as well as genital clostridial infections, are best treated with penicillin G. Infections produced by anaerobic mouth flora including gram-positive and gram-negative cocci and the *Actinomyces* can be treated with penicillin G.

Staphylococcal disease should be treated with one of the semisynthetic antistaphylococcal penicillins. This includes staphylococcal pneumonia, endocarditis, osteomyelitis, and skin and soft tissue infections.

Endocarditis due to *Streptococcus viridans* group organisms should be treated with penicillin G. Endocarditis due to *S. viridans* whose penicillin-inhibitory levels are greater than 0.2 μg/ml, due to vitamin B_6-dependent streptococci or due to *S. faecalis,* would be best treated with ampicillin and gentamicin or streptomycin.

Urinary tract infections due to susceptible *E. coli, Proteus,* or enterococci are effectively treated with ampicillin.

Serious *Pseudomonas* infections such as sepsis, endocarditis, pneumonitis, or malignant otitis are best treated with carbenicillin or ticarcillin in combination with an aminoglycoside.

PROPHYLAXIS

Penicillins have been used in a number of situations for prevention of infection. Because of the problems with compliance with oral therapy, i.m. injections of 1.2 or 2.4 million U of benzathine penicillin given once each month are best to prevent recurrence of rheumatic fever.

One of the most important prophylactic uses of penicillin is for prevention of bacterial endocarditis. Patients with congenital heart disease, rheumatic or acquired valvular disease, idiopathic hypertrophic subaortic stenosis, and mitral valve prolapse syndrome with mitral insufficiency who are undergoing certain procedures that are likely to result in bacteremia should receive prophylaxis with penicillin.

Semisynthetic antistaphylococcal penicillins have been given at the time of prosthetic heart valve placement or at the time of implantation of an artificial joint. These agents should be given just before the surgery, during the procedure, and in the immediate postoperative period.

Penicillin prophylaxis has not been of benefit in prevention of meningococcal infection, bacterial infection after viral respiratory infection, or pneumonia after coma, shock, or congestive heart failure.

Dosage schedules for penicillins are given in Table 24.2-4.

CEPHALOSPORIN ANTIBIOTICS

The cephalosporins are very similar to the penicillins in antibacterial activity and pharmacology. Most cephalosporins in clinical use are derived from a fungus *Cephalosporium* whereas cefoxitin is a fermentation product of streptomyces and strictly speaking a cephamycin. Although agents in this class are considered the drug of first choice for few infections, they are the most widely used agents worldwide.

History. The story of the cephalosporins began with Professor Giuseppi Brotzu in Sardinia in July 1945. He isolated a *Cephalosporium* from seawater that had antibacterial activity against gram-positive and gram-negative bacilli. Professor Abraham and his colleagues at Oxford, workers at Glaxo in England, and others at Eli Lilly in the United States developed the cephalosporins the first of which were cephalothin and cephaloridine. Since that time, a large number of compounds have been developed and are used clinically. In 1972, the cefamycins were discovered. Structural modification of these compounds made them clinically useful.

Chemistry. Cephalosporins contain a β-lactam ring attached to a 6-membered dihydrothiazine rings, as shown in the following chemical structure. The sulfur of that ring is given position 1. Substitutions can be made at positions 3 and 7. Substitutions

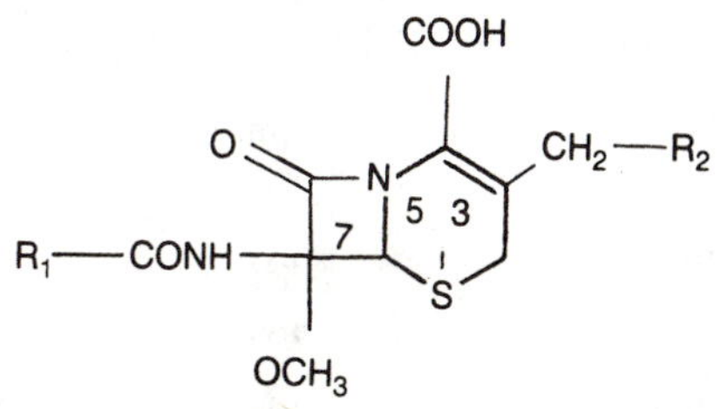

COOH
O
N
CH_2—R_2
5 3
7
R_1—CONH
S
OCH_3

Cephalosporin

at position 3 tend to affect the pharmacology of the compounds, whereas those at position 7 affect antibacterial activity, although this is not invariably so. Placement of a methoxy group at position 7 conveys resistance to β-lactamases. The structures of current cephalosporins are given in Table 24.2-5.

There are a group of cephalosporins that contain an aminothiazolyl side chain and an iminomethoxy or iminocarboxy propyl group. These agents are resistant to destruction by β-lactamases (11). Moxalactam is grouped with the cephalosporins even though it is an oxacephem, that is, oxygen replaces the sulfur in the dihydrothiazine ring.

Mechanism of Action. Cephalosporins are bactericidal-inhibiting enzymatic reactions necessary for stable bacterial cell walls. The drugs affect only growing bacteria. Their degree of antibacterial activity is dependent upon their affinity for the proteins involved in cell wall synthesis and their ability to reach the receptor sites and β-lactamase stability.

Cephalosporins mechanism to inhibit bacterial cell wall synthesis is the same as that earlier described for the penicillins. Whether they cause lysis of bacteria or produce long filamentous forms that are incapable of further replication is dependent upon the specific penicillin-binding protein for which they have great affinity.

Bacterial Resistance. Resistance of bacteria to cephalosporins is the result of three factors: (1) failure to reach a receptor site, (2) lack of affinity for important cell wall enzymes, or (3) destruction by β-lactamases (14). Cephalosporins are destroyed to varying degrees by β-lacta-

Table 24.2-4
Dosage Schedule for Penicillins

Drug	Route	Usual Adult Dosage	Usual Pediatric Dosage (after first week of life)
Penicillin G crystalline	i.m. i.v.	600,000 U q. 12 hr 1-4 million U q. 4-6 hr	50,000-300,000 U/kg/day
Procaine penicillin G (benzathine)	i.m. i.m.	600,000 U q. 12 hr 1.2 million units single injection (low, prolonged serum levels) 2.4 million U for syphilis	 300,000-1.2 million U
Penicillin V potassium	p.o.	250-500 mg q.i.d.	25,000-50,000 U/kg/day
Penicillinase Resistant			
Cloxacillin	p.o.	250-2,000 mg q. 4-6 hr	25-50 mg/kg/day
Dicloxacillin	p.o.	125-250 mg q. 6 hr before meals	25-50 mg/kg/day
Methicillin	i.m./i.v.	1-2 g q. 4-6 hr	100-200 mg/kg/day
Nafcillin	p.o. i.m. i.v.	250-500 mg q. 4-6 hr 500 mg q. 4 hr 500 mg q. 6 hr	50-100 mg/kg/day
Oxacillin	p.o., i.m./i.	0.5-2 g q. 4-6 hr	50-200 mg/kg/day
Penicillinase susceptible			
Amoxicillin	p.o. i.m. i.v.	250-500 mg q. 8 hr 0.5-1 g q. 6 hr 1-2 g q. 4-6 hr	20-100 mg/kg/day depending on indication
Ampicillin	p.o. i.m. i.v.	250-1,000 mg q. 6 hr 0.5-1 g q. 6 hr 1-2 g q. 4 hr	50-400 mg/kg/day depending on indication
Carbenicillin sodium	i.v. i.m.	4-40 g/day 500 mg/kg/day	400-600 mg/kg/day
Carbenicillin indanyl sodium	p.o.	382-764 mg q. 6 hr	Not recommended
Hetacillin	p.o.	225 mg q. 6 hr	20-40 mg/kg/day
Ticarcillin	i.m. i.v.	4-24 g/day 300 mg/kg/day	50-300 mg/kg/day
Azlocillin	i.v.	2-5 g q. 6 hr	300 mg/kg/day
Mezlocillin	i.v.	2-5 g q. 6 hr	300 mg/kg/day
Piperacillin	i.v.	2-5 g q. 6 hr	300 mg/kg/day

Table 24.2-5
Antibacterial Activity of Cephalosporins[a]

Organism	Cefazolin, Cephalothin, Cephaloridine, Cephapirin	Cefaclor, Cefadroxil, Cephalexin, Cephradine	Cefonicid, Ceforanide, Cefamandole, Cefuroxime	Cefoxitin	Ceftizoxime, Cefoperazone, Cefotaxime, Ceftriaxone, Ceftazidime	Moxalactam
	Inhibited at Achievable Concentrations (%)					
Staphylococcus aureus	95	95	95	95	95	85
S. epidermidis	95	95	95	95	95	75
Streptococcus pneumoniae	100	100	100	100	100	75
S. pyogenes	100	100	100	100	100	100
S. viridans	100	100	100	100	100	50
S. faecalis	0	0	0	0	0	0
Neisseria gonorrhoeae	100	100	100	100	100	100
Haemophilus influenzae	50	75	100	100	100	100
Escherichia coli	85	85	95	98	100	100
Klebsiella	85	85	95	98	100	100
Enterobacter	0	0	75	0	90	90
Serratia	0	0	0	70	90	90
Proteus mirabilis	95	95	95	95	100	100
Proteus, indole positive	0	0	70	80	90	95
Pseudomonas	0	0	0	0	50-95[b]	75
Clostridia	95	95	95	95	95	90
Bacteroides fragilis	10	10	20	85	50[b]	85

[a] Agents are grouped according to similarities in antibacterial activity.
[b] Ceftazidime active against Psuedomonas, but not Bacteroides.

mases, but in general they are more stable than are penicillins. Cefoxitin, cefotaxime, cefuroxime and moxalactam are β-lactamase stable.

Production of large amounts of cephalosporinases, can destroy a cephalosporin that is otherwise β-lactamase stable. This occurs with *Enterobacter* and *Citrobacter freundii.*

Antimicrobial Activity. In general, cephalosporins are excellent inhibitors of gram-positive cocci with the exception of enterococci, *S. faecalis,* and the methicillin-resistant staphylococci. The oral cephalosporins (cephalexin, cephradine) and cefoxitin are only one-tenth as active as other cephalosporins against gram-positive cocci. Among the gram-negative enteric bacilli, *E. coli, Klebsiella,* and *Proteus mirabilis* are inhibited to a degree by all of the agents, depending upon local susceptibility factors. *Enterobacter* and *Citrobacter* are inhibited by cefotaxime and moxalactam. Some *Serratia* and many indole-positive *Proteus* are inhibited by cefoxitin, most by cefotaxime and moxalactam. Cefoxitin inhibits *B. fragilis.* Cefotaxime, ceftizoxime, and moxalactam inhibit all of the aforementioned bacteria and some isolates of *P. aeruginosa* as well. Table 24.2-5 groups the agents by activity and provides their concentrations required to inhibit common organisms.

Pharmacokinetics. There are major differences in pharmacokinetic properties among the cephalosporins in oral absorption, protein binding, and renal excretion (Table 24.2-6) (9,13).

Absorption. Cephalexin, cephradine, cefadroxil, and cefaclor are all absorbed from the gastrointestinal tract. Food decreases absorption to a moderate degree. All of the other agents (Table 24.2-6) are well absorbed after intramuscular injection, but only cephaloridine, cefazolin, cefamandole, and cefuroxime are well tolerated. All of the agents are available as intravenous preparations. Serum levels differ widely among the agents after either i.m. or i.v. injection related to the degree of protein binding and to renal excretion.

Distribution. Cephalosporins do not penetrate cells, including white cells, ocular fluid, nor prostatic tissue due to their lipid-insolubility. They are, however, distributed widely and yield clinically useful levels in lung, kidney, muscle, bone, and placenta. Levels in interstitial fluid and synovial and peritoneal fluids are good. Urine levels are excellent. High concentrations are achieved in bile, particularly with cefamandole, cefoxitin, and cefazolin. Cefotaxime, moxalactam, ceftizoxime, ceftazidime, and ceftriaxone produce adequate cerebrospinal fluid concentrations to treat meningitis.

Metabolism. Compounds that possess an acetoxy side chain at position 3 of the dihydrothiazine nucleus are converted in the body by nonspecific esterases to a less active desacetyl derivative. This occurs 30-40% with cephalothin, cephapirin, and cefotaxime. The desacetyl cephalothin and cephapirin are minimally active, but desacetyl cefotaxime is more active than many other cephalosporins. Cefaclor is also metabolized in inactive fragments in serum in about 3 hours.

Elimination. Elimination of the cephalosporins occurs principally via the kidneys by a combination of glomerular filtration and active tubular secretion. Urinary concentrations of the cephalosporins are high, with most of a dose excreted in the first 2 hours after administration. Even in the presence of decreased renal function, urinary levels of cephalosporins are good until the creatinine clearance falls below 10 ml/min. Probenecid blocks excretion of most of the cephalosporins excreted by tubular secretion just as it does of penicillins. Moxalactam and ceftazidime are excreted by glomerular filtration. The renal elimination of the metabolized cephalosporins, such as cephalothin and cephapirin, is rapid; their half-life is 0.5-0.7 hr. In contrast, an agent such as cefazolin has a half-life of 1.9 hr (9). Most of the oral cephalosporins have a half-life of approximately 1 hr. Cephalosporins accumulate to varying degrees in the presence of decreased renal function (Table 24.2-6). Only minor adjustments in dosage are necessary with most cephalosporins, except cephaloridine and moxalactam, until creatinine clearances fall below 20 ml/min. Hemodialysis removes the drugs, but peritoneal dialysis has only a minimal effect.

Adverse Effects. The most common adverse effects of cephalosporin therapy are the pain on i.m. administration or phlebitis with i.v. administration, and minor gastrointestinal complaints. Allergic reactions to cephalosporins are infrequent, and cross-allergenicity with penicillin occurs in only 1% of individuals. On the other hand, rash, urticaria, eosinophilia, and fever occur in 5% of individuals who receive the drugs. Leukopenia and rarely hemolytic anemia are encountered. Dose-related nephrotoxicity due to cephaloridine has been demonstrated, and

Table 24.2-6
Pharmacokinetic Properties of Major Cephalosporins

Agent	Stability to Cephalosporinase	Route of Administration	Protein Binding (%)	Serum $t_{1/2}$ Normal (hr)	Serum $t_{1/2}$ Oliguria (hr)	Metabolized (%)	Peak Serum Levels 1 g, i.m.	Peak Serum Levels 1 g, i.v.
First-generation compounds								
Cephalothin (KEFLIN)	–	i.v.	70	0.5	3-8	30	20	70
Cefazolin (ANCEF, KEFZOL)	–	i.v., i.m.	85	1.9	25	0	60	140
Cephapirin (CEFADYL)	–	i.v.	70	0.5	3-8	30	20	70
Cephradine (ANSPOR, VELOSEF)	–	p.o.	15	1	20	0	15[a]	
Cephalexin (KEFLEX)	–	p.o.	15	1	20	0	15[a]	
Cefadroxil (DURICEF, ULTRACEF)	–	p.o.	15	1		0	10[a]	
Second-generation compounds								
Cefamandole (MANDOL)	+	i.v., i.m.	70	0.7	8	0	20	85
Cefoxitin (MEFOXIN)	++	i.v., i.m.	70	0.7	15	<5	20	70
Cefuroxime (ZINACEF)	+	i.v., i.m.	35	1.1	11	0	35	100
Cefaclor (CECLOR)	–	p.o.	15	1	30	100	12[a]	
Third-generation compounds								
Cefotaxime (CLAFORAN)	+	i.v., i.m.	30	1	2	50	20	45
Moxalactam (MOXAM)	+	i.v., i.m.	60	2	19	0	45	60
Cefoperazone (CEFOBID)	+	i.v.	85	2	3	0	30	125
Ceftizoxime (CEFIZOX)	+	i.v., i.m.	50	1.6	24	0	20	60
Ceftriaxone (ROCEPHIN)	+	i.v., i.m.	95	8	16		85	150
Ceftazidime (FORTAZ)	+	i.v., i.m.	17	1.6	16	0	35	85

[a] After 0.5 g orally.

the drug is probably no longer needed. Cephaloridine should never be used in the presence of decreased renal function. It is suggested that cephalosporins increase the toxicity of aminoglycoside antibiotics, but this is not fully established. Miscellaneous reactions that are important are false-positive chemical tests, namely Coombs', and glucose reactions if performed with Benedict's reagent. Transient increases in hepatic enzymes, SGOT, and alkaline phosphatase have been seen after use of all of the agents. Prolongation of prothrombin time occurs in some patients, particularly those with decreased renal function who receive moxalactam or cefoperazone. All drugs which contain a methylthiotetrazole ring affect vitamin K metabolism. Table 24.2-2 summarizes most of the adverse reactions.

INDIVIDUAL AGENTS

The cephalosporins and related agents have been conveniently classified as first-, second- and third-generation compounds. The first-generation or initially developed agents have a narrow spectrum of antibacterial activity compared with the later-developed compounds. The second-generation agents are generally more active against gram-negative enteric bacteria than the previous group of drugs. The third-generation compounds have a still broader *in vitro* antibacterial spectrum against gram-negative organisms, including bacteria resistant to other cephalosporins. They also show relative stability against β-lactamases. However, these compounds are less active against gram-positive bacteria compared with the first- and second-generation analogs.

Examples of compounds of these three classes currently used in the United States are given in Table 24.2-7, along with their pharmacokinetic properties. The chemical structure of these compounds are given in Fig. 24.2-4 and 24.2-5. Some of these drugs are briefly discussed next.

FIRST-GENERATION COMPOUNDS

Cephalothin, Cephapirin. Cephalothin and cephapirin are essentially identical agents microbiologically and pharmacologically. They are stable to staphylococcal β-lactamase but are destroyed by gram-negative and anaerobic β-lactamases. Both are painful if given by the intramuscular route. Their short half-lives require that doses be given at frequent intervals when treating serious infections.

Cefazolin. Cefazolin's antibacterial activity is similar to cephalothin's but is more protein bound (85%). The serum levels achieved by i.m. or i.v. routes are higher than those achieved with other available cephalosporins (3).

Cephalexin, Cephradine. Cephalexin and cephradine are oral cephalosporins that inhibit streptococci, *E. coli*, and *Klebsiella*. They are well absorbed by the oral route (6).

Cefadroxil. Cefadroxil, an oral agent, has antibacterial activity similar to that of cephalexin but has a longer half-life.

Cefaclor. Cefaclor, an oral cephalosporin, has antibacterial activity similar to cephalexin's, but is more active against *Haemophilus*. It achieves therapeutic concentrations in middle ear fluid and is useful in upper respiratory infections.

SECOND-GENERATION COMPOUNDS

Cefamandole. Cefamandole's antibacterial activity against gram-positive cocci is similar to cephalothin's, but it is more active against *Haemophilus* and inhibits some indole-positive *Proteus*, and some cephalothin-resistant *E. coli* and *Klebsiella*

Table 24.2-7
Dosages of Cephalosporins

Drug	Usual Adult Dosage	Usual Pediatric Dosage (after first week of life)
Oral	(g q. 6 hr)	(mg/kg/day)
Cephalexin	0.5-2	25-50
Cephradine	0.25-0.5	25-50
Cephaloglycin	0.25-0.5	25-50
Cefaclor	0.25-1	40-60
Cefadroxil	0.25-1	40-60
Parenteral	(g q. 4-8 hr)	
Cefazolin	0.5-1	25-100
Cephapirin	0.5-1	40-80
Cephaloridine	0.5-1	30-50
Cephalothin	0.5-2	50-150
Cephradine	0.5-2	50-100
Cefamandole	0.5-2	50-150
Cefuroxime	0.75-1.5	50-150
Cefoxitin	0.5-2	50-150
Cefotaxime	0.5-2, q. 8-12 hr	50-100
Ceftizoxime	0.5-2, q. 8-12 hr	50-100
Cefoperazone	2, q. 8-12 hr	50-100
Moxalactam	0.5-2, q. 8-12 hr	50-100
Ceftriaxone	1 q. 8-24 hr	50-100
Ceftazidime	1 q. 8 hr	50-100

(7). It does not inhibit *Bacteroides* or *Pseudomonas*. It is available for i.m. or i.v. use. Serum levels are greater than those achieved with a comparable dose of cephalothin.

Cefoxitin. Cefoxitin is less active than cephalothin against gram-positive cocci *in vitro*, but it is resistant to β-lactamases that destroy cephalothin, so it enlarges the bacterial spectrum to include *B. fragilis* and cephalothin-resistant *Enterobacteriaceae*, with the exception of *Enterobacter*. Serum levels are greater than those achieved with comparable doses of cephalothin. Cefoxitin offers a single agent to use in mixed aerobic and anaerobic infections (10).

Cefonicid. Cefonicid is similar in antibacterial activity to cefamandole. It inhibits gram-positive coccal species and most enteric gram-negative species but is inactive against *Bacteroides* and *Pseudomonas*. It has a half-life of 4-5 hours and is administered once daily by the i.m. or i.v. route.

Cefuroxime. Cefuroxime is a semisynthetic broad-spectrum cephalosporin antibiotic for parenteral administration. It is effective against a wide range of gram-positive and gram-negative organisms and highly stable in the presence of β-lactamases of certain gram-negative bacteria. After i.m. and i.v. injections of a 750-mg dose, its mean peak serum concentration is 27 μg/ml at 15 min. The serum half-life after either type of injection is approximately 80 min. About 80% of the dose is excreted by kidneys over an 8-h period, resulting in high urinary concentration. It is effective against urinary tract and lower respiratory infections caused by susceptible strains.

THIRD-GENERATION COMPOUNDS

Cefotaxime. Cefotaxime inhibits most streptococci, *Haemophilus*, and *Neisseria* at concentrations below 0.1 μg/ml. It is the most active cephalosporin, inhibiting most *Enterobacteria-*

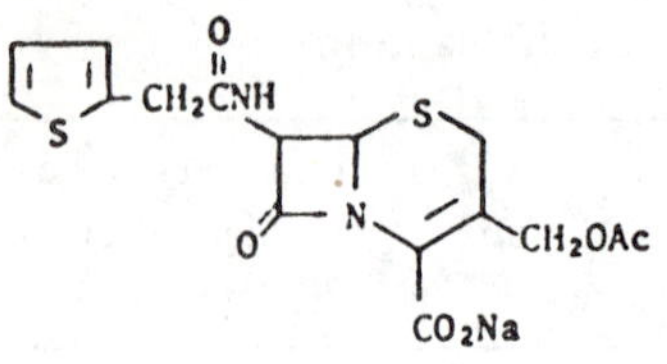

Cephalothin sodium

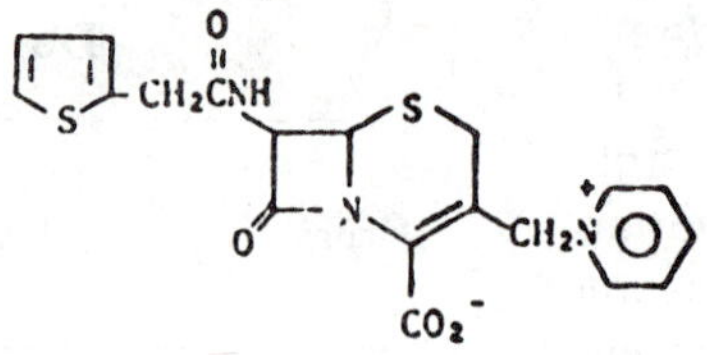

Cephaloridine

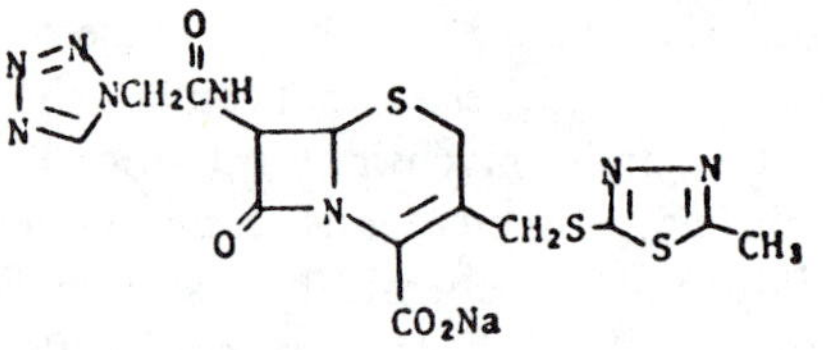

Cefazolin sodium

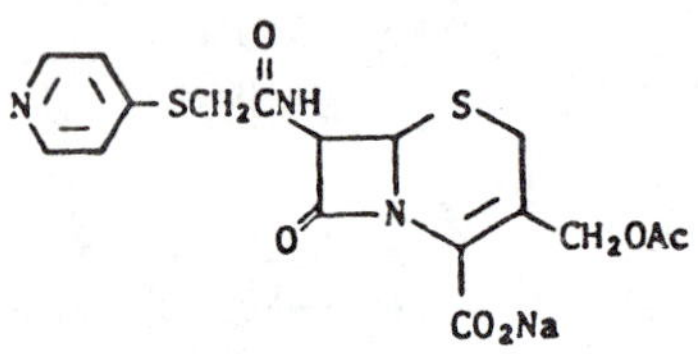

Cephapirin sodium

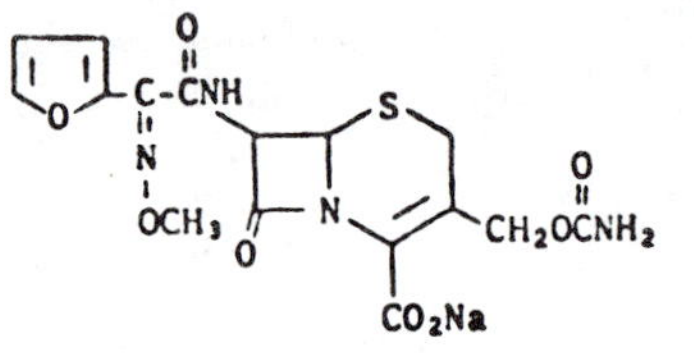

Cefuroxime sodium

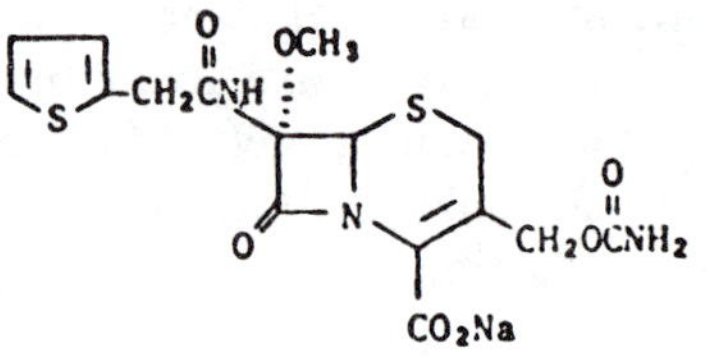

Cefoxitin sodium

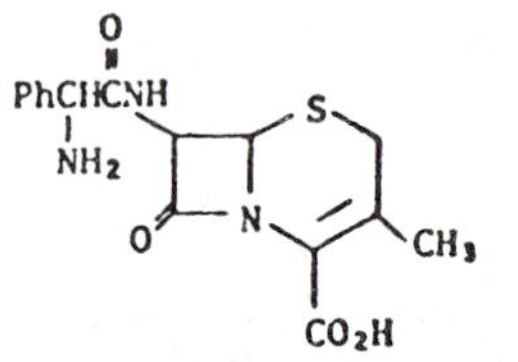

Cephalexin

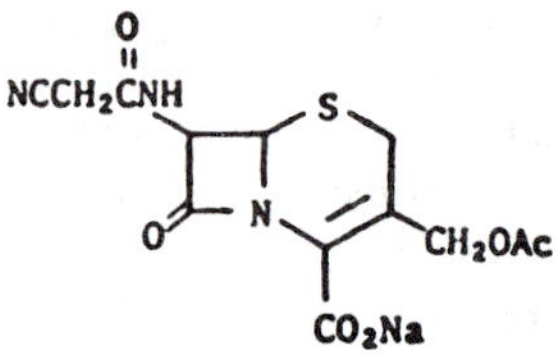

Cephacetrile sodium

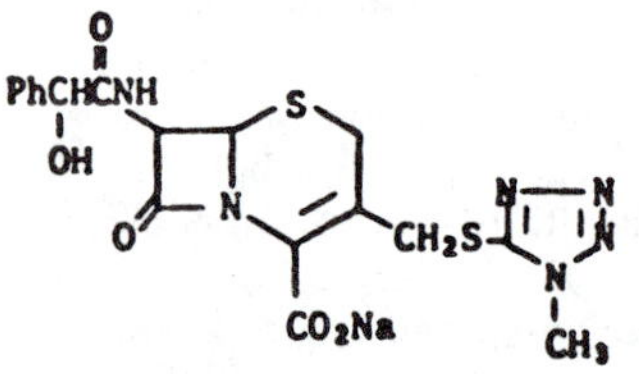

Cefamandole sodium

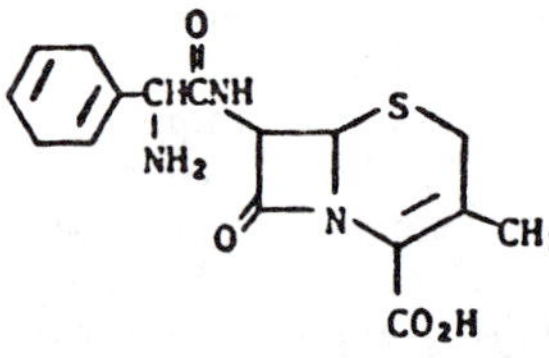

Cephradine

Fig. 24.2-4. *Structure of common cephalosporins (first and second generations).*

ceae at concentrations below 1 μg/ml. It is stable to β-lactamases. It can be used by i.m. or i.v. routes. It enters the CSF and is approved as treatment of *Haemophilus, S. pneumoniae, Neisseria* and *E. coli* meningitis.

Moxalactam. Moxalactam has less activity against staphylococci than older cephalosporins, such as cephalothin or cefazolin, and it has poor activity against *Streptococcus pneumoniae.* Moxalactam is β-lactamase stable and inhibits most *Enterobacteriaceae* at concentrations less than 1 μg/ml. It also inhibits *Bacteroides fragilis* and some *Pseudomonas aeruginosa.* It has a serum half-life of 2 h and, unlike other cephalosporins, is eliminated by glomerular filtration. It can be used by the i.m. or i.v. routes. It can cause platelet dysfunction and prolongation of prothrombin time. Vitamin K must be given when it is used.

Cefoperazone. Cefoperazone has a broad spectrum of activity inhibiting gram-positive and negative species including *Pseudomonas.* Compared with cefotaxime and moxalactam, it is only partially stable to plasmid β-lactamases. Cefoperazone is only partially excreted by renal mechanisms (25%). The majority of excretion is by the biliary tract. In the presence of major hepatic dysfunction, however, the drug is renally excreted.

Ceftizoxime. Ceftizoxime is antibacterially similar to cefotaxime. It is not destroyed by β-lactamases. It is not metabolized, and excretion is totally by renal mechanisms. It enters the CSF in therapeutic concentrations. Dosage adjustment must be made in the presence of renal failure.

Cefsulodin. Cefsulodin, a cephalosporin, inhibits only *Pseudomonas aeruginosa.* It has no appreciable activity against other bacteria. It is excreted by the kidney and has a half-life of approximately 1.5 h. It is used only to treat *Pseudomonas* infections.

Ceftriaxone. Ceftriaxone, a third-generation cephalosporin, has an antibacterial spectrum similar to that of cefotaxime. It is β-lactamase stable but not active against *Bacteroides* and poorly active against *Pseudomonas aeruginosa.* Ceftriaxone is unusual since it has half-life of 6-8 h and produces very high biliary levels of antibiotic. It enters the CSF and is effective in therapy of several forms of meningitis. Ceftriaxone can be administered once or twice daily by i.m. or i.v. routes.

Ceftazidime. Ceftazidime is an iminopropyl-carboxycephem derivative that has excellent β-lactamase stability and inhibits not only *Enterobacteriaceae* but *Pseudomonas* as well. The drug is excreted primarily by glomerular filtration, and probenecid does not alter its pharmacokinetics. It enters the CSF. It can be administered by the i.m. or i.v. routes.

Cefmenoxime. Cefmenoxime has a spectrum of *in vitro* activity similar to cefotaxime. It is stable to β-lactamases. Cefmenoxime enters the CSF. Dosage adjustment must be made in the presence of renal failure. It is not metabolized and is excreted primarily by tubular secretion.

THERAPEUTIC USES

The therapeutic indications for the cephalosporins are hard to define in spite of their broad antibacterial activ-

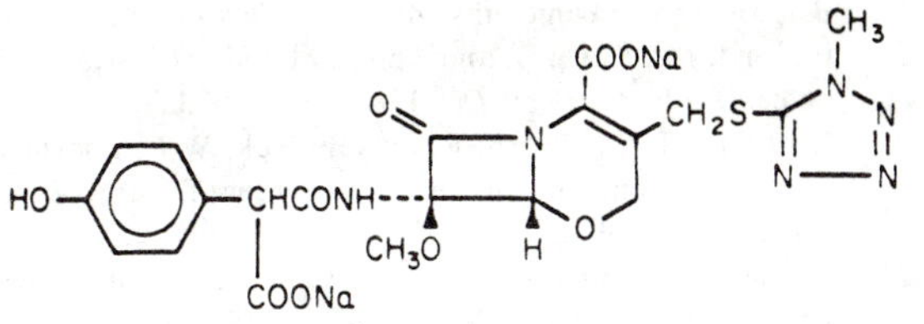

Moxalactam

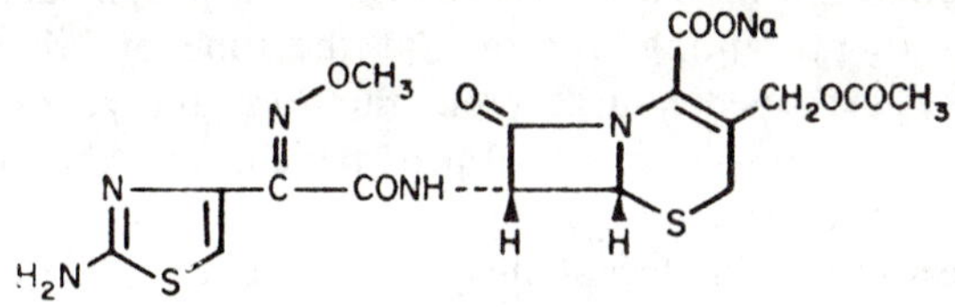

Cefotaxime sodium

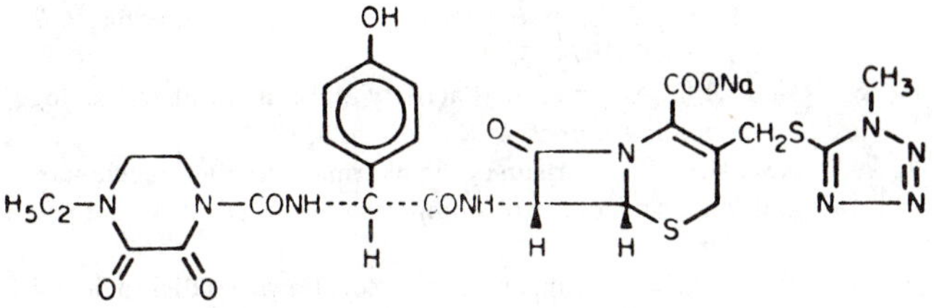

Cefoperazone

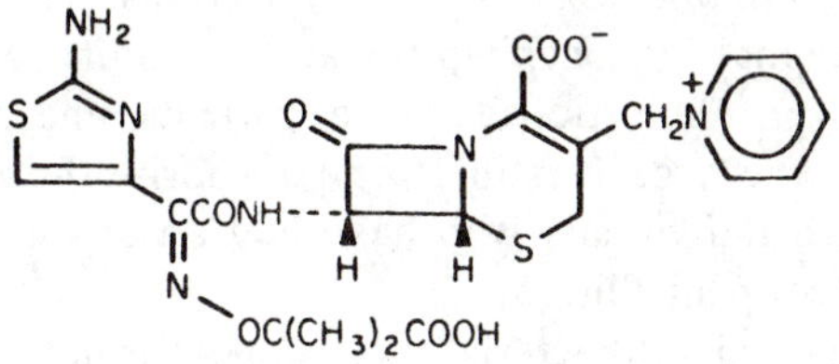

Ceftazidime

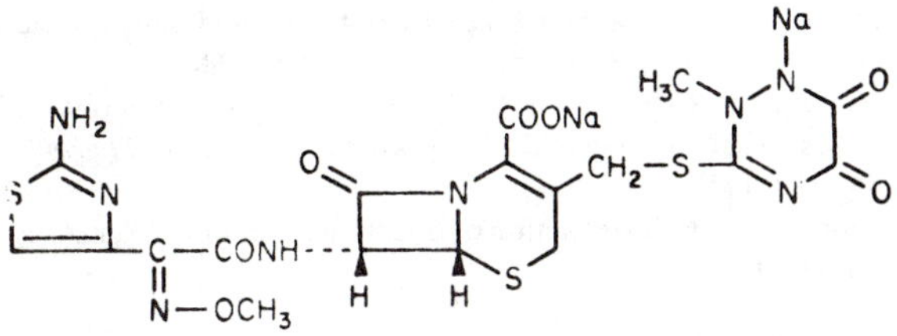

Ceftriaxone sodium

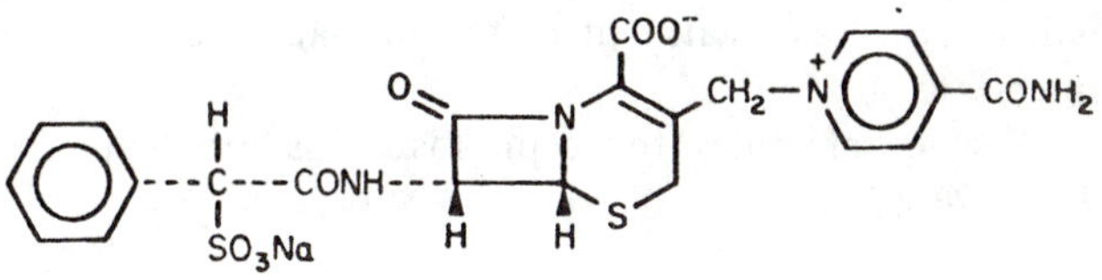

Cefsulodin sodium

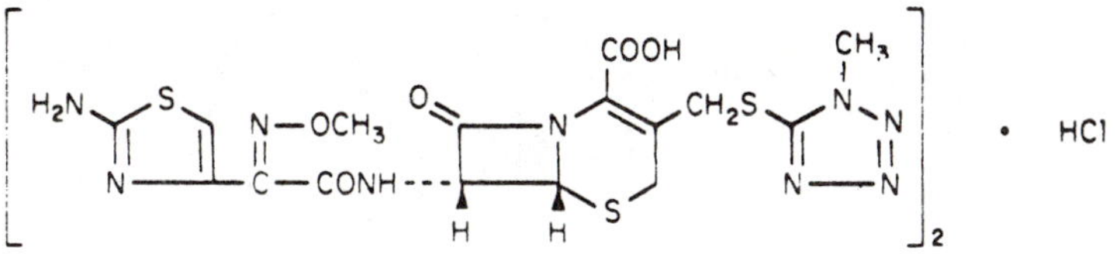

Cefmenoxime HCl

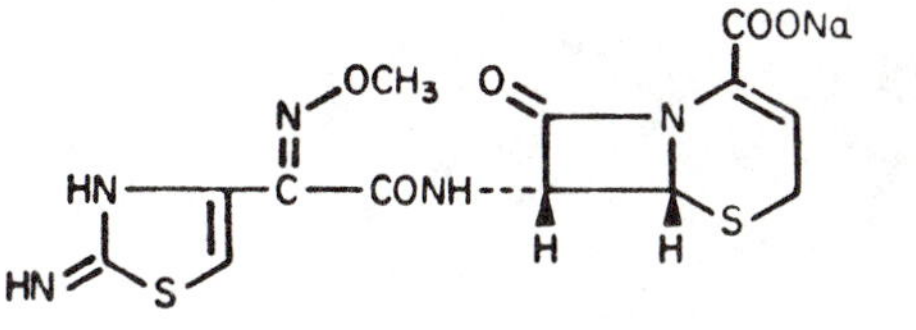

Ceftizoxime sodium (Cefizox)

Fig. 24.2-5. *Structure of common cephalosporins (third generation).*

ity. Too often these agents are used when less expensive agents would be as effective. Reasonable areas in which to use cephalosporins would be staphylococcal infections in penicillin-allergic patients and the treatment of *Klebsiella* infections. They have been used combined with aminoglycosides in the treatment of undefined bacteremia. The precise role of cephalosporins in the treatment of pneumonitis due to gram-negative species, septicemia, urinary tract infections, osteomyelitis, septic arthritis, and intraabdominal infections and gynecological infections depends upon the susceptibility of the infecting bacteria. Cefamandole, cefuroxime, cefoxitin, cefotaxime, and moxalactam may provide an alternative to use of aminoglycosides. Cefoxitin has proved useful in treatment of mixed aerobic and anaerobic infections. Cefamandole, cefuroxime, and cefaclor may be used to treat *Haemophilus* infections.

Cefotaxime, ceftizoxime, and ceftriaxone have proved useful in treatment of neonatal meningitis due to *E. coli*, and the agents have also been successfully used to treat *Haemophilus influenzae* meningitis in young children. Cefotaxime has proved useful in treatment of meningitis due to *Neisseria meningitidis* and *Streptococcus pneumoniae*. Cefotaxime would be the agent of choice to treat gram-negative meningitis due to *E. coli* or *Klebsiella* in adults.

Cephalosporins have proved useful as prophylactic agents in preventing infection at the time of biliary surgery, orthopedic surgery on fractures, and particularly during the placement of prosthetic heart valves or prosthetic joints.

The areas in which cephalosporins should not be used are much clearer. They have no role in the therapy of infections due to enterococci, *S. faecalis.* They are ineffective against methicillin-resistant *S. aureus* and will not cure *Salmonella* or *Shigella* infections. The older agents—cephalothin, cephapirin, and cefazolin—are not useful as prophylactic agents in patients undergoing surgery on the large intestine. Cephalosporins should not be given to individuals who have had an anaphylactic reaction to a penicillin (5).

The enlarged antibacterial spectrum of the new cephalosporins such as cefotaxime, ceftizoxime, ceftriaxone, ceftazidime, and related agents combined with excellent pharmacokinetic properties and retention of the safety of older agents of the class suggests that cephalosporin use will increase as treatment of hospital-acquired serious infections.

Dosage schedules for cephalosporins are given in Table 24.2-7.

REFERENCES

1. Andriole, V.T. Synergy of carbenicillin and gentamicin in experimental infection with *Pseudomonas. J. Infect. Dis.* 124(Suppl.): 46, 1971.
2. Bergan, T. The penicillins. *Antibiot. Chemother.* 25:1, 1978.
3. Finland, M., Kaye, D. and Turck, M. (eds.) Clinical symposium on cefazolin. *J. Infect. Dis.* 128(S):312, 1973.
4. Hoffman, T.A., Cestro, R. and Bullock, W.E. Pharmacodynamics of carbenicillin in hepatic and renal failure. *Ann. Intern. Med.* 73:173, 1970.
5. Levine, B.B. Antigenicity and cross-reactivity of the penicillins and cephalosporins. *J. Infect. Dis.* 128 (S):364, 1973.
6. Meyers, B.R., Kaplan, K. and Weinstein, L. Cephalexin: microbiological effects and pharmacological parameters in man. *Clin. Pharmacol. Ther.* 10:810, 1969.
7. Moellering, R.C., Jr. (ed.) Symposium on cefamandole. *J. Infect Dis.* 137(S):1, 1978.
8. Neu, H.C. Antimicrobial activity and human pharmacology of amoxicillin. *J. Infect. Dis.* 129(S):123, 1974.
9. Neu, H.C. Comparison of the pharmacokinetics of cefamandole and other cephalosporin compounds. *J. Infect. Dis.* 137(Suppl.): 80, 1978.
10. Neu. H.C. Cefoxitin: an overview of clinical studies in the United States. *Rev. Infect. Dis.* 1:233, 1979.
11. Neu, H.C. The new beta-lactamase stable cephalosporins. *Ann. Intern. Med.* 97:408, 1982.
12. Neu, H.C. Mechanisms of bacterial resistance to antimicrobial agents with particular reference to cefotaxime and other β-lactam compounds. *Rev. Infect. Dis.* 4(Suppl.):288, 1982.
13. Nightingale, C.H., Green, D.S. and Quintiliani, R. Pharmacokinetics and clinical use of cephalosporin antibiotics. *J. Pharm Sci.* 64:1899, 1975.
14. Tipper, D.J. Mode of action of β-lactam antibiotics. *Rev. Infect. Dis.* 1:39, 1979.

CHAPTER
24.3

AMINOGLYCOSIDES

Harold C. Neu

The aminoglycosides are a large group of antimicrobial compounds that share many chemical, antimicrobial, pharmacological and toxic properties. All these drugs contain amino sugars in glycosidic linkage, as shown in Fig. 24.3-1. Fig. 24.3-2 presents the chemical structures of some antibiotics of this group. They have become a major part of the clinician's armamentarium against gram-negative infections. The development of bacterial resistance and an increased awareness of their toxic properties have made it necessary to develop new agents in this class. Use of the aminoglycosides, of all the antimicrobial agents, requires an understanding of pharmacokinetic principles and a careful attention to toxicity/benefit ratios.

History. The discovery of the aminoglycosides began in 1943 with the isolation by Waksman and coworkers of an antimicrobial substance from a soil organism *Streptomyces griseus.* In 1944, it was shown that the new antibiotic, streptomycin, inhibited tubercle bacilli and a number of gram-negative bacilli. In 1949, Waksman, (who received the Nobel Prize for his work on streptomycin) and Leehevalier isolated neomycin; in 1957, Umezawa in Japan isolated kanamycin. Paromomycin was found in 1959. In 1963, gentamicin was isolated by Weinstein and coworkers in the United States as a product of *Micromonospora purpurea.* Tobramycin was isolated in 1968, and amikacin in 1972. Sisomicin, netilmicin, and dibekacin are new aminoglycosides that were developed in the late 1970s.

Nomenclature. The naming of the aminoglycosides can be confusing. All agents originating from *Streptomyces* are spelled with *mycin*; for example, kanamycin is from *S. kanamyceticus* and tobramycin from *S. tenebrarius.* Agents derived from other species are spelled with *micin*; for example, gentamicin is from *Micromonospora purpurea.*

Chemistry. The structural feature that characterizes the aminoglycosides is the presence of a six-membered aminocyclitol ring system, either streptidine or 2-deoxystreptamine. Streptidine is found in streptomycin, and 2-deoxystreptamine is found in all other agents currently in use. To this basic nucleus, various amino sugars are attached in glycosidic linkage at positions 4 and 6 of the 2-deoxystreptamine nucleus. The attached amino sugars are mono or diamino compounds at position 4. At position 6 the sugars are glucosamine, or garosamine, or gentosamine (Fig. 24.3-1).

The aminoglycosides are highly soluble in water and are stable for extended periods when in solution at pH 1-11 and at temperatures of 5-37°C. The compounds are not compatible with heparin solutions and can interact with β-lactam compounds of the penicillin and cephalosporin families; such interaction depends upon the concentration and pH of the solutions. Both agents are inactivated by this interaction; hence aminoglycosides cannot be mixed in the same infusion bottle with penicillins.

Mechanism of Action. Aminoglycosides inhibit protein synthesis by binding irreversibly to proteins in the 30S ribosome and thereby interrupting the flow of genetic information. Streptomycin sensitivity of 30S subunit has been shown to be determined by a single protein (designated P_{10} on the basis of its mobility on polyacrylamide gel electrophoresis) (3). The binding site of streptomycin is distinct from that of the other aminoglycosides. All of the aminoglycosides cause both depletion of the ribosome pool and misreading of the genetic code (Chapter

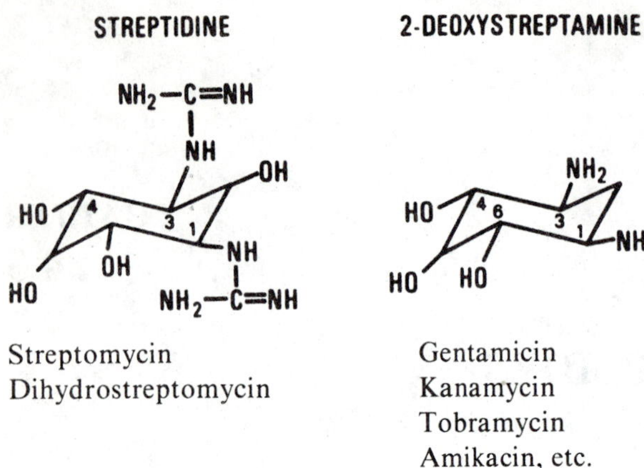

Fig. 24.3-1. *Structures of nuclei in aminoglycoside anti biotics.*

22). Antibacterial activity is markedly increased at alkaline pH, probably due to improved transport of the agents inside the bacterial cell.

Resistance. There are three mechanisms of resistance to the aminoglycosides (2, 3). The first is failure of transport of the agents inside the cell to reach the ribosome receptor site. This transport is an energy-requiring mechanism that depends on oxidative metabolism. Anaerobic bacteria are resistant to aminoglycosides by this mechanism, and facultative anaerobes (bacteria that can grow in the presence or absence of oxygen, *E. coli,* or *S. aureus)* can be relatively resistant if they are in the anaerobic environment. For example, the concentration needed to inhibit *S. aureus* is 0.1 μg in an aerobic environment but 5 μg in an anaerobic environment.

The second mechanism is the presence of altered ribosomes that do not bind well to the aminoglycosides due to absence or alteration of a protein. This mechanism is rare and is seen most frequently with streptomycin. The most common mechanism of resistance is that due to molecular modification of the aminoglycoside caused by plasmid-mediated enzymes that adenylate, phosphorylate, or acetylate the compounds. This modification of the drugs decreases the uptake of the compounds by the bacterial transport system and prevents binding to the ribosomes. The sites of which a compound can be modified are shown in Fig. 24.3-3. Substitution of side chains of two carbons or larger at position 1 of the 2-deoxystreptamine nucleus prevents inactivation at a number of these sites. This molecular modification has been utilized in amikacin and prevents its inactivation by all but a few enzymes.

Aminoglycoside-inactivating enzymes occur in many bacteria, and their presence seems to be related to local antibiotic use. Examples of common inactivating enzymes

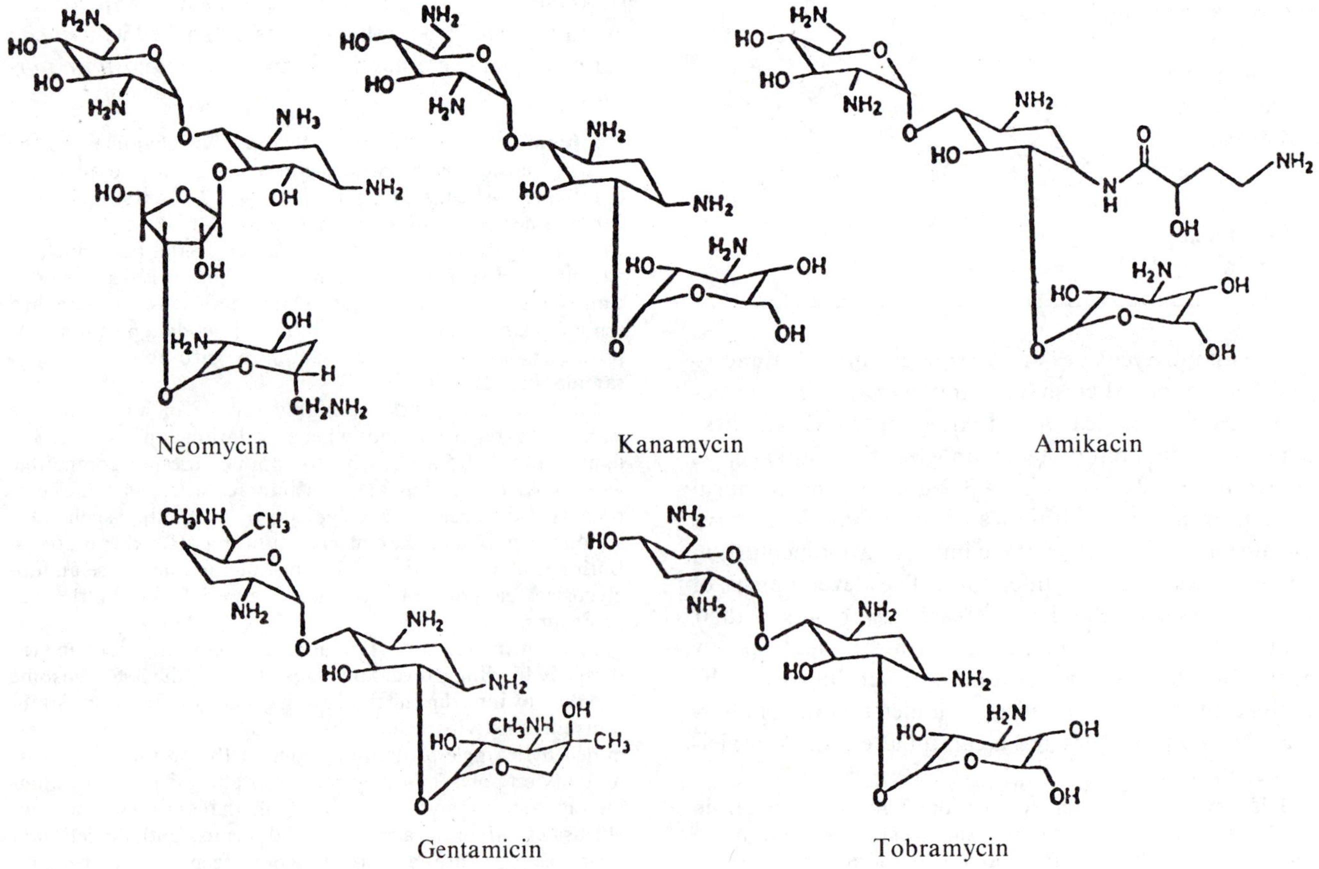

Neomycin Kanamycin Amikacin

Gentamicin Tobramycin

Fig. 24.3-2. *Structures of common aminoglycosides.*

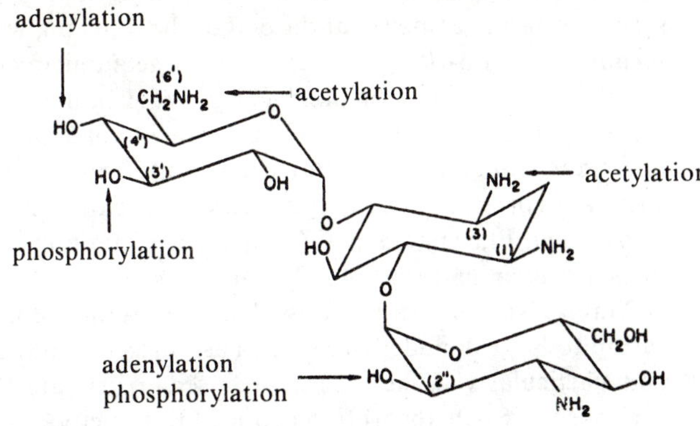

Fig.24.3-3. *Sites for inactivation in the structure of aminoglycosides.*

and the bacteria in which they occur are given in Table 24.3-1.

Antibacterial Activity. Aminoglycosides inhibit most members of the *Enterobacteriaceae* and staphylococci. They do not inhibit many of the gram-positive cocci such as *S. pneumoniae* and *S. faecalis*, and are inactive against anaerobic species, both cocci and bacilli. Activity against *Pseudomonas aeruginosa* varies. Although aminoglycosides inhibit species such as *Neisseria* and *Haemophilus*, they cannot be considered first-line compounds for treatment of infections produced by these bacteria.

Certain generalizations can be made about the antibacterial activity of these agents. Streptomycin is useful in *M. tuberculosis, Pasturella pestis, Franciella tularensis, and Brucella*, but most other bacteria causing serious infection such as *E. coli* and *Klebsiella* are resistant. Kanamycin does not inhibit *P. aeruginosa*, and many *E. coli, Klebsiella*, and *Enterobacters* are resistant. Neomycin has antibacterial activity essentially identical to that of kanamycin. Gentamicin has remained a useful agent, with most bacteria in community hospitals susceptible. However, in some hospital centers many *Serratia, Providencia, and Pseudomonas* are resistant. Tobramycin has an *in vitro* activity similar to that of gentamicin, but it is twofold more active against *P. aeruginosa.* Most *Enterobacteriaceae (i.e., E. coli, Klebsiella*, and *Proteus)* that are resistant to gentamicin are resistant to tobramycin. Some *P. aeruginosa* resistant to gentamicin are susceptible to tobramycin. Amikacin has the widest range of activity of the aminoglycosides by virtue of its resistance to inactivation. However, some *S. aureus* and *S. faecalis* are resistant to amikacin and susceptible to gentamicin. Sisomicin is similar in activity to gentamicin, but more active against *Pseudomonas.* Netilmicin is more active than gentamicin but is inactivated by some of the enzymes that do not inactivate amikacin.

Technical problems inherent in the microbiological assay of the aminoglycosides may cause differing results in bacterial susceptibility. The *in vitro* activity of the aminoglycosides is markedly affected by the cation content of agar or broth and by the pH of the medium.

Interaction with Other Antibiotics. Aminoglycosides can act synergistically with both penicillins and cepha-

Table 24.3-1
Aminoglycoside-Inactivating Enzymes

Inactivating Enzyme	Bacteria	Frequency of Occurrence	Inactivated Antibiotics	Resistant Antibiotics
3′-O-phosphotransferase	*Pseudomonas* *Klebsiella* *E. coli* *S. aureus*	Very common	Kanamycin, neomycin	Gentamicin, tobramycin, amikacin
3′-N-acetyltransferase	*Pseudomonas*	Occasional	Gentamicin	Amikacin, tobramycin
	Klebsiella *Enterobacter*	Rare	Gentamicin, tobramycin	Amikacin
2′-O-phosphotransferase	*Klebsiella*	Occasional	Gentamicin, tobramycin, kanamycin	Amikacin
6′-N-acetyltransferase	*Pseudomonas* *E. coli* *Serratia*	Uncommon	Gentamicin C_{1a} Tobramycin Kanamycin, amikacin	Gentamicin C_1
4′-O-adenyltransferase	*S. aureus*	Uncommon	Amikacin, tobramycin, kanamycin	Gentamicin
2′-N-acetyltransferase	*Proteus* *Providencia*	Occasional	Gentamicin, tobramycin	Amikacin

losporins against *viridans* streptococci, *S. faecalis*, and *S. aureus*. The mechanism of synergy is that penicillin-induced damage to the cell wall permits the entry of the aminoglycoside so that it can bind to the receptor on the ribosome. The combination of gentamicin and ampicillin also causes a more rapid killing of *Listeria monocytogenes* and *S. agalactiae* (group B). The combination of aminoglycosides (gentamicin, tobramycin, or amikacin) with the antipseudomonas penicillins – carbenicillin or ticarcillin – is synergistic both *in vitro* and *in vivo*. Combination of aminoglycosides with cephalosporins may result in synergy against some members of the *Enterobacteriaceae*, but this is less frequently seen than when effective penicillins are combined with aminoglycosides.

Pharmacokinetics. ***Absorption.*** None of the aminoglycosides when given orally produce adequate serum concentrations to treat infection. However, aminoglycosides can be absorbed when used orally or as irrigating solutions and cause toxicity. All of the compounds are well absorbed after intramuscular injection, with peak serum levels achieved in 20-90 min. Intramuscular doses of 1.5 mg/kg of gentamicin or tobramycin yield serum levels of 4 μg/ml, whereas i.m. doses of 5 mg/kg of kanamycin or amikacin yield peak serum levels of 20 μg/ml. Administered by intravenous injection, peak serum levels are achieved at the end of the infusion, with serum levels of 6-10 μg/ml achieved for gentamicin and tobramycin with infusion of 2 mg/kg over 30 min. Levels of 15 μg/ml are achieved by 30 min infusion of 5 mg/kg of amikacin or kanamycin. Bolus injection (2 min.) of the agents will produce extremely high levels, and this should be avoided. Pharmacokinetic properties of aminoglycosides are given in Table 24.3-2.

Aminoglycosides can be absorbed after topical application to large denuded areas such as burns or wounds, and particularly if the agents are used to irrigate the peritoneum. Such absorption can lead to toxicity.

Distribution. Aminoglycosides are distributed in the extracellular fluid volume. They do not enter mammalian phagocytic cells. They enter pleural, peritoneal, and synovial fluids, and can cross the placenta. Concentrations in sputum are variable. They do not enter the CSF or the eye, and intrathecal or intracisternal injection is necessary to achieve adequate concentrations in the CSF. Subconjunctival instillation will provide drug to the aqueous humor of the eye but not the vitreous. High concentrations of the drugs are achieved in renal cortical tissue, whereas their biliary concentrations are low; they

Table 24.3-2
Pharmacokinetic Properties of Aminoglycoside Antibiotics

	Gentamicin, Tobramycin, Netilmicin		Amikacin, Kanamycin	
Pharmacokinetic Properties	Dose (mg/kg), Route	Data[a]	Dose (mg/kg), Route	Data[a]
Peak serum level (μg/ml)	1, i.m. 2, i.m. 1, i.v. (2 min) 1.5, i.v.[b] 2, i.v.[b]	4 6-8 12-20 4-6 6-10	3.5, i.m. 7.5, i.m. 5-7, i.v.[b]	12 21 30-40
Serum level (μg/ml) (creatinine clearance ⩾100 mg/1.73 m^2)	i.m. i.v. (rapid)	0.5-1 (8 hr) 0.1 (8 hr)	5, i.m. 7.5, i.v.	2.1 (10 hr) 1 (10 hr)
Serum half-life (hr)				
normal		2		2
anuria		35-50		35-50
Volume distribution (%) (body weight)		25 (20-30)		25 (20-30)
Protein binding (%)		0		0
Clearance on hemodialysis (6 hr, %)		50		50
Peritoneal dialysis (removed, mg/2 l)		1		1
Urine concentrations (μg/ml)				
0-4 hr		100-300		100-800
4-8 hr		10-50		
Dose excreted (8 hr, %)		80-90		80-90

[a]Expressed in respective measure of the property.
[b]Infusion for 30 minutes.

do not enter the prostate. Aminoglycosides are not protein bound.

Excretion. Aminoglycosides are eliminated from the body by glomerular filtration. They are not metabolized and there is no major biliary excretion. The majority of the drug, 70%, is eliminated in the first 6 hours after injection, with 85% of a single dose eliminated in 24 hours. The remainder of the drug is bound to pericortical renal tissue, in the proximal tubules of the kidney. Levels of aminoglycosides in urine range from 10 to several hundred micrograms for up to 8 hours after injection in individuals with normal renal function. After a therapeutic course of aminoglycosides, drug can be detected in urine for up to a week.

The half-life of all of the aminoglycosides in normal individuals is approximately 2 hours, whether the drug is given by i.m. or i.v. injection. In the presence of decreased renal function, the serum half-life of aminoglycosides increases and urinary concentrations decrease. In anuric patients, the serum half-life of the aminoglycosides is 35-50 hours. The drugs can be removed from the body by both hemodialysis and peritoneal dialysis. Approximately 50% of a dose is removed by 6 hours of hemodialysis, and 1 mg of gentamicin or tobramycin and 3 mg of amikacin are removed per 2 liters of peritoneal dialysate. Patients with extensive burns will lose aminoglycosides through the fluid loss at the skin surface. Dosage must be adjusted in renal failure (Table 24.3-3).

Pharmacokinetics in the newborn. Aminoglycoside antibiotics are used to treat suspected sepsis in the newborn, because the organisms involved usually are gram-negative bacteria, particularly *E. coli.* The newborn differs from older children and adults in two important aspects: Renal function is not fully developed at birth, and the extracellular fluid space, which is approximately 35% of body weight, is much larger. Thus an agent such as an aminoglycoside, which is distributed primarily in the extracellular space, will produce lower levels in the premature or underweight infant but have a longer half-life.

Following an i.m. dose of 2.5 mg/kg of gentamicin or tobramycin to a neonate, mean peak serum levels of 4 μg/ml (range 2-9 μg/ml) are found at half an hour to 1 hour. Serum half-life is approximately 5 hours in neonates under /2 hours of age and may be longer in low-birth-weight infants. Concentrations of gentamicin or tobramycin in the spinal fluid reach peaks of 0.2-3.5 μg/ml 4-6 hours after a 2.5 mg/kg dose. Urinary concentrations of the drug range from 25-150 μg/ml. By 1 month of age, the pharmacokinetics of aminoglycosides in children are similar to those in adults. However, certain individuals such as children with cystic fibrosis may have lower serum levels than would be anticipated for the dose calculated on their body weight.

Adverse Effects. The most important adverse effects of aminoglycosides are toxic reactions that affect the auditory-vestibular apparatus and the kidneys. In humans, the incidence of nephrotoxicity varies from 2-10%, depending upon the agent. Streptomycin is virtually devoid of nephrotoxicity at usual doses. Neomycin has such a high rate of nephrotoxicity that it is not used parenterally. The nephrotoxicity of tobramycin appears to be slightly less than that of gentamicin and amikacin.

Nephrotoxicity appears to be dose related and is more common in elderly, debilitated patients, in those with previous renal damage, and in those who have a contracted intravascular volume.

Clinically, mild proteinuria and granular cylindruria often herald the decline in renal function. The renal failure is of a nonoliguric type with a loss of concentrating ability, presence of renal enzymuria, and β-microglobulins in the urine. Subsequently, the serum creatinine and urea nitrogen rise. The toxic reaction occurs in the proximal tubular cells with total sparing of the glomeruli and

Table 24.3-3
Reduced Dosage in Renal Failure[a]

	Creatinine Clearance (ml/min)	Percentage of Dosage 8hr	12 hr	24 hr
Gentamicin, tobramycin	80	80	90	—
Loading dose: 2 mg/kg	70	75	88	—
Maintenance dose: 1-1.5 mg/kg	60	70	85	—
	50	65	80	—
	40	55	70	95
	30	45	65	85
Amikacin, kanamycin	20	35	50	75
Loading dose: 7.5 mg/kg	15	30	40	65
Maintenance dose: 6 mg/kg	10	25	35	55

[a]Blood levels of the antibiotics should be obtained whenever renal function is changing rapidly, and for appropriate use of this table.

blood vessels. By electron microscopy myeloid bodies are seen in the tubular cells, and transport function of the proximal tubule is defective.

Toxicity usually does not appear in the first 5 days of therapy and may never occur if there is attention to serum levels of the aminoglycosides and to other factors. Toxicity can first be noted after therapy has been stopped, because a significant amount of the drug is still present in the pericortical areas of the kidney. Nephrotoxicity of aminoglycosides has often been reported in association with concomitant therapy with other drugs. It is difficult to sort out the major factors of renal damage in the critically ill patient who is septic. However, coadministration of the anesthetic methoxyflurane will increase toxicity. There is a great controversy over whether coadministration of aminoglycosides and cephalosporin antibiotics leads to increased toxicity, but the evidence does seem to point to such an association. The nephrotoxic potentiating role of loop diuretics is unclear.

Ototoxicity due to aminoglycosides is well documented (1) and is of two types, cochlear and/or vestibular. The agents differ in their damage of these functions of the eighth cranial nerve. For example, cochleotoxic reactions predominate with kanamycin, tobramycin, and amikacin, whereas gentamicin is primarily vestibulotoxic. A general estimate of overt ototoxicity is 2-3%, but in high-risk groups, such as the elderly with decreased renal function, it may reach 10-20%.

Studies in animals have shown that the aminoglycosides produce destruction of vestibular sensory cells and of cochlear hair cells. Such ototoxicity may, to a large extent, be explained by the high concentration and persistence of these antibiotics in the inner ear, their perilymph half-life being several hours (1), But the basic cellular mechanism of ototoxicity remains to be ascertained, since it cannot be predicted by daily dose, total dose, or duration of therapy. Early workers correlated excessive peak serum levels with toxicity, but this has not been substantiated. It is clear that simultaneous use of aminoglycosides and loop diuretics that are themselves ototoxic, such as furosemide and ethacrynic acid, will result in greater ototoxicity. Symptoms of vestibular toxicity include vertigo, ataxia, and nystagmus, and the symptoms may progress to the point that the patient cannot walk unaided. Auditory damage usually is manifested by high-tone hearing loss and tinnitus, but it may progress to total deafness. Damage to the vestibular and auditory apparatus may be unilateral or bilateral. It is unclear if the damage is reversible.

Neuromuscular blockade produced by the aminoglycosides appears to be due to inhibition of presynaptic release of acetylcholine, depression of motor end-plate sensitivity to acetylcholine, and interference with calcium action at the neuroreceptor. Neuromuscular blockade has rarely followed the administration of the aminoglycosides by the i.v. or i.m. route but has occurred after peritoneal lavage. It is most likely to occur in those who have recently received neuromuscular blocking agents or patients with myasthenia gravis. Neuromuscular blockade occurs with different agents in the decreasing order: neomycin > streptomycin > netilmicin > kanamycin > amikacin > gentamicin and tobramycin. It can be reversed by administration of calcium salts intravenously. Neostigmine is less effective in reversing the blockade.

Reversible dose-related malabsorption has followed the oral administration of the aminoglycosides. It is due to direct damage to villus cells and to the nonspecific binding of bile salts. It is most common with neomycin, kanamycin, and paromomycin. The absorption of fat, protein, cholesterol, iron, and digitalis is impaired.

Allergic reactions are infrequent, but rash and fever do occur in less than 1% of individuals who receive these agents. Leukopenia and elevations of liver enzyme tests have been reported.

Therapeutic Uses (5). The conditions for which aminoglycosides should be used are moderately well defined. The systemic use of aminoglycosides should be reserved for the parenteral therapy of serious infections in which other agents such as penicillins or cephalosporins would not be suitable. The drugs have no initial role in the treatment of most infections due to gram-positive cocci, although an exception would be their use in combination with penicillin or ampicillin to treat streptococcal endocarditis due to a *S. viridans* that requires penicillin-inhibitory levels above 0.2 μg/ml. They are always used to treat endocarditis due to *S. faecalis.* Gentamicin should be used in preference to streptomycin if *in vitro* studies show relative streptomycin resistance.

The major therapeutic role of the aminoglycosides is in the treatment of infections caused by members of the *Enterobacteriaceae, P. aeruginosa* and other aerobic, nonfermenting, gram-negative bacilli. In septic states, therapy often is initiated with an aminoglycoside, gentamicin, tobramycin, or amikacin, in combination with an antipseudomonas penicillin, or in combination with a cephalosporin. Such combination therapy has been recommended particularly for the neutropenic (<500 neutrophils/mm^3) febrile patient, since it has been suggested that an aminoglycoside used alone will not be effective. Source of the suspected sepsis will often mandate the choice of the other antimicrobial agent that is used with the aminoglycoside. For example, if the sepsis follows trauma or surgery to the large intestine or a gynecological source, an agent with anaerobic activity (clindamycin, ticarcillin or related penicillin, or cefoxitin) should be used until the bacterial etiology is known. If sepsis from a urinary source occurs in an immunologically intact individual, an aminoglycoside alone would be adequate therapy.

The ready colonization of the upper respiratory tract with gram-negative bacilli makes it difficult to establish how effective aminoglycoside therapy of pulmonary infections has been. The precise role of the aminoglycosides in the therapy of pulmonary infections is unclear, except perhaps in pneumonitis due to *Klebsiella* or *Pseudomonas*. All of the agents have proved effective in treating infections due to susceptible aerobic gram-negative bacilli. The agents are particularly useful in treatment of *Pseudomonas* infections in patients with cystic fibrosis.

In the treatment of urinary tract infections due to organisms resistant to the more innocuous antimicrobial agents, all of the aminoglycosides have been useful. Because of the high concentrations in the urine, cures can be achieved with lower doses with the drugs administered once or twice daily.

Various subcutaneous, postoperative, and traumatic wounds due to susceptible *Pseudomonas, Proteus*, or *Klebsiella* have been treated with aminoglycosides. Osteomyelitis due to *Pseudomonas* should be treated with an aminoglycoside and an antipseudomonas penicillin. Gram-negative meningitis in adults can be treated by intrathecal or intraventricular (via an Ommaya shunt) administration of aminoglycosides. This should not be done to treat gram-negative meningitis in the neonate, since it does not increase survival or decrease morbidity. Serious ophthalmic infections due to *Pseudomonas* can be treated by subconjunctival and even intravitreal injection of the aminoglycosides. Use of streptomycin in tuberculosis is discussed in Chapter 25.3.

Use in Patients with Renal Insufficiency. A number of different approaches to the adjustment of aminoglycoside dosage in patients has been developed. Although there are a number of nomograms based on creatinine clearance or serum creatinine that can be used to calculate doses, it is wise to utilize serum assays of the drugs to validate any program. The initial therapeutic concentrations of gentamicin, tobramycin, and netilmicin should be between 4 and 10 μg/ml, whereas the concentration of amikacin and kanamycin should be 15-30 μg/ml. Using an initial loading dose of 1.7-2 mg/kg of gentamicin, tobramycin, or netilmicin and an initial loading dose of 5-8 mg/kg of amikacin or kanamycin will achieve these concentrations. The levels produced by the initial dose will be the same for individuals with or without renal insufficiency. Subsequent adjustment of dosage can be by one of two methods: the variable-frequency method in which the interval between doses is varied, or the variable-dose method in which the dose is varied and a standard time interval is used. There is no consensus about which is a better method to achieve cure or which will better avoid toxicity. However, in the critically ill individual it is probably unwise to have long periods in which serum levels are below the inhibitory concentration. Because renal function declines with age, the serum creatinine, age of the patient, and the body mass must be utilized to calculate the actual creatinine clearance. Table 24.3-4 gives a dosage program for the aminoglycosides that will provide adequate peak levels and avoid excessively high trough levels.

Table 24.3-4
Dosage Schedule for the Aminoglycosides

Drug	Route	Usual Adult Dosage	Usual Pediatric Dosage (after first week of life)
Gentamicin	i.m./i.v.	3-7.5 mg/kg/day in 8 hourly doses; adjust dose according to renal function	<1 week 5 mg/kg/ day q. 12 hr 7.5 mg/kg/day
Kanamycin	i.m./i.v.	15 mg/kg/day in two doses; not to exceed 1.5 g/day	<1 week 15-20 mg/kg/day 20-30 mg/kg/day
Neomycin	p.o.	2-3 days; hepatic coma; 1 g q.i.d. x 2 days, then 1 g b.i.d.	Avoid
Spectinomycin	i.m.	2 g single dose	—
Streptomycin	i.m.	1-2 g/day	20 mg/kg/day, two doses
Tobramycin	i.m./i.v.	3-7.5 mg/kg q. 8 hr, adjust according to renal function	Neonate (1 week old or less) up to 4 mg/kg q. 12 hr
Amikacin	i.m./i.v.	15-25 mg/kg/day in two to three doses	15-20 mg/kg/day
Sisomicin	i.m./i.v.	3 mg/kg/day	—
Netilmicin	i.m/i.v.	3-6 mg/kg/day	3-6 mg/kg/day

INDIVIDUAL AMINOGLYCOSIDES

Streptomycin. Streptomycin was the first aminoglycoside isolated. Its use today in treatment of tuberculosis is limited to selected patients. It is useful in treatment of brucellosis, tularemia, and *Yersinia* infections (plague). Most hospital gram-negative bacteria are resistant to it. It is still used in combination with penicillin to treat streptococcal endocarditis. It should be used only by the intramuscular route.

Kanamycin. Increased resistance of *E. coli* and *Klebsiella* as well as the almost universal resistance of *Pseudomonas* to kanamycin has limited its usefulness. Auditory toxicity is more frequent with kanamycin than renal toxicity.

Neomycin. Neomycin is used as an oral or topical agent. Excessive absorption can occur causing ototoxicity and neurotoxicity. It can also cause antibiotic-associated enterocolitis, malabsorption, and hypocholesterolemia by the oral route. Organisms resistant to kanamycin are resistant to neomycin, for which susceptibility tests are not usually performed in microbiology laboratories.

Gentamicin. Gentamicin used commercially is a complex of the structurally related gentamicin C_1, C_{1a}, and C_2. Microbial susceptibility depends upon local factors of use, but many *Serratia* and *Pseudomonas* are resistant. Its use is restricted to the treatment of serious infections where other less toxic agents are ineffective. Gentamicin is ototoxic and can cause renal damage. Monitoring of serum levels will decrease nephrotoxicity.

Tobramycin. Tobramycin is more active than gentamicin against *Pseudomonas* and may have a lower nephrotoxicity potential. Pharmacologically, it is identical to gentamicin, and clinical studies have shown it to be equally efficacious clinically.

Amikacin. Amikacin is a semisynthetic derivative of kanamycin that by virtue of its side chain is resistant to inactivation by most bacteria that are resistant to other aminoglycosides. It is less active on a weight basis than gentamicin or tobramycin, but larger doses can be given without increased toxicity. Pharmacologically, it is otherwise identical to the other agents. Amikacin's use has been generally limited to treatment of serious infection due to gentamicin-resistant bacteria. It is not established that increased use will result in more bacterial resistance to the compound.

Sisomicin. Sisomicin differs chemically from gentamicin C_{1a} only by the presence of a double bond in one amino sugar. Its pharmacological properties are identical to those of gentamicin. Lower concentrations of the agent are effective against many *E. coli, Proteus* and *Klebsiella.* However, it has not been shown to have any advantage over gentamicin.

Netilmicin. Netilmicin is a semisynthetic aminoglycoside that has a spectrum similar to gentamicin but is more active than gentamicin against *E. coli* and *Enterobacter* and inhibits gentamicin-resistant *E. coli, Klebsiella,* and *Enterobacter.* It is less active against *Pseudomonas* than gentamicin. Pharmacologically it is identical to gentamicin.

REFERENCES

1. Bendush, C.L. Ototoxicity: Clinical considerations and comparative information. In: *The Aminoglycosides, Microbiology, Clinical Use and Toxicology* (Whelton, H. and Neu, H.C., eds.) New York: Marcel Dekker, 1982, p. 453.
2. Mitsuhashi, S. and Kawabe, H. Aminoglycoside antibiotic resistance in bacteria. In: *The Aminoglycosides, Microbiology, Clinical Use and Toxicology* (Whelton, H. and Neu. H.C., eds.). New York: Marcel Dekker, 1982, p. 97.
3. Moellering, R.C., Jr. Clinical microbiology and *in vitro* activity of aminoglycosides. In: *The Aminoglycosides, Microbiology, Clinical Use and Toxicology* (Whelton, H. and Neu, H.C., eds.) New York: Marcel Dekker, 1982, p. 65.
4. Neu, H.C. Pharmacology of aminoglycosides. In: *The Aminoglycosides, Microbiology, Clinical Use and Toxicology* (Whelton, H. and Neu, J.C., eds.) New York: Marcel Dekker, 1982, p. 125.
5. Neu, H.C. Clinical use of aminoglycosides. In: *The Aminoglycosides, Microbiology, Clinical Use and Toxicology* (Whelton, H. and Neu, H.C., eds.). New York: Marcel Dekker, 1982, p. 611.

ADDITIONAL READING

Ristuccia, A.M. and Cunha, B.A. The aminoglycosides. *Med. Clin. North Am.* 66:303, 1982.

CHAPTER
24.4

ANTIMICROBIAL AGENTS AFFECTING RIBOSOMAL FUNCTIONS

Harold C. Neu

The antibiotics discussed in this chapter have had wide use throughout the world. In each case, adverse reactions and the development of resistance have temporarily blunted the physician's enthusiasm for the agents. All of these compounds continue to have specific situations in which they are the preferred agents even though they are bacteriostatic compounds.

TETRACYCLINES

History. The tetracyclines were isolated in 1948 from a strain of *Streptomyces aureofaciens* by Benjamin Duggar at Lederle Laboratories in the United States. The first member of the series was called chlortetracycline. Within 2 years, oxytetracycline produced by *S. rimosus* was discovered , and by 1952, tetracycline HCl. A number of other tetracyclines—methacycline, doxycycline, and minocycline—were subsequently prepared. In contrast to the penicillins, the tetracyclines are very similar in antimicrobial activity, pharmacology, and particularly therapeutic properties. Some important differences among the drugs will be discussed.

Chemistry. The basic tetracycline structure consists of four benzene rings with various substituents on each ring (Fig. 24.4-1). The compounds are minimally soluble in water. Solutions of many of the compounds show appreciable loss of activity, although tetracycline HCl is stable for 3 weeks, and all of the compounds are stable as hydrochlorides in dry powder form.

Mechanism of Action. All tetracyclines function in the same manner. They act as bacteriostatic compounds, interfering with protein synthesis by blocking the attachment of aminoacyl tRNA to the 30 S ribosomes (Chapter 22). This binding to ribosomes is not permanent and hence they are bacteriostatic.

Resistance. The most common form of resistance in both staphylococci and the gram-negative enteric bacteria (*Escherichia coli,* etc.) is due to the presence of a plasmid that mediates the production of a protein that interferes with uptake of tetracycline by the organisms and increases removal of that tetracycline entering the bacterial cell, thereby preventing binding to the ribosomes. The same mechanism probably operates in anaerobic bacteria such as *Bacteroides,* but the precise mechanism of resistance is not established for anaerobic bacteria.

Antibacterial Spectrum. The tetracyclines have a broad range of antibacterial activity against both aerobic and anaerobic gram-positive and gram-negative organisms. In the 1950s and 1960s, many strains of *Staphylococcus aureus, S. pyogenes* (group A streptococci), and *S. pneumoniae* were resistant to the tetracyclines. Today most isolates of these species would be inhibited. Some *S. aureus* resistant to other tetracyclines are inhibited by minocycline. *Corynebacterium acnes* are inhibited by tetracyclines. Tetracyclines inhibit *Neisseria gonorrhoeae* and *N. meningitidis,* although some gonococci are resistant, particularly those from the Orient. These agents inhibit both typable and nontypable strains of *Haemophilus influenzae.* None of the tetracyclines adequately inhibit true enterococci, such as *S. faecalis*. The susceptibility of *E.coli, Klebsiella,* and *Enterobacter* to the tetracyclines is extremely variable and depends upon the local use of the drugs. All *Proteus* are resistant to tetracyclines. All tetracyclines have some activity against *P. aeruginosa,* but only at very high concentrations such as might be achieved in the urine. All of the tetracyclines inhibit *Chlamydia* and *Mycoplasma pneumoniae.* A significant number of anaerobic species, particularly *Bacteroides fragilis*, have become resistant to the tetracyclines, although some tetracycline-resistant isolates are inhibited by doxycycline. Tetracyclines also inhibit rickettsiae that cause Rocky Mountain spotted fever and *Actino-*

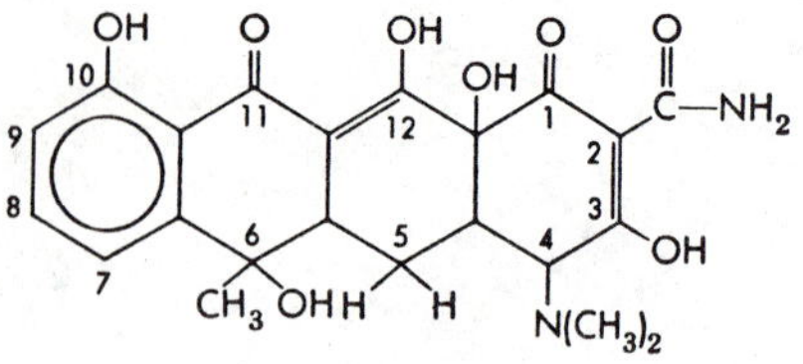

Tetracycline

Tetracyclines	Substitution at position 5	6	7
Tetracycline	-	-	-
Oxytetracycline	- OH,- H	-	-
Chlortetracycline	-	-	- Cl
Methacycline	- OH, - H	= CH_2	-
Doxycycline	- OH, - H	- CH_3, - H	-
Demeclocycline	-	- OH, - H	- Cl
Minocycline	-	- H, - H	- N $(CH_3)_2$

Rolitetracycline has a substitution only at position 2:

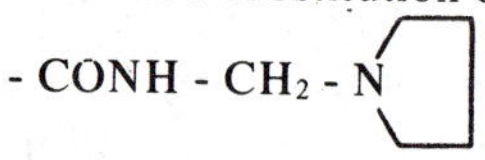

- CONH - CH_2 - N

Fig. 24.4-1. *Structural formulas of the tetracyclines.*

myces, and *Nocardia*. Table 24.4-1 shows the overall activity of these drugs.

Pharmacokinetics. ***Absorption.*** All tetracyclines are adequately absorbed from the gastrointestinal tract when taken orally except for chlortetracycline, which has poorer oral absorption (2, 5). Peak serum levels are achieved 1-2 hours after administration of an oral dose. Many substances, particularly food, markedly reduce the absorption of tetracycline hydrochloride, oxytetracycline, and chlortetracycline (Table 24.4-2). The degree to which food interferes with the absorption of doxycycline or minocycline is variable. The tetracyclines have a high affinity for divalent cations (aluminum, calcium, magnesium and also iron). The presence of calcium in the GI tract has less effect upon the absorption of doxycycline and minocycline, but iron does affect the absorption of these agents. Iron given intravenously will decrease the absorption of doxycycline by preventing enterohepatic recirculation of the drug. Tetracycline also can be administered by the intramuscular and intravenous routes, although these methods are associated with some pain due to irritation.

Distribution. All of the tetracyclines are well distributed to body tissues in humans (Table 24.4-3) (5). All of the tetracyclines are bound to protein, varying from 55 to 95%. The drugs can be demonstrated in pleural, ascitic, and synovial fluids. The biliary concentrations are high,

Table 24.4-1
Activity of Tetracyclines against Gram-Positive and Gram-Negative Bacteria

Bacteria	Mean Minimum Inhibitory Concentration (μg/ml) Tetracycline	Doxycycline	Minocycline
Gram-positive bacteria			
Staphylococcus pyogenes	3.1	1.6	0.78
Streptococcus pyogenes (group A)	0.78	0.39	0.39
Streptococcus pneumoniae (D. pneumoniae)	0.8	0.02	0.02
Streptococcus viridans ss	3.1	0.39	0.39
Streptococcus faecalis (Enterococcus, group D)	>100	50	100
Gram-negative bacteria			
Escherichia coli	12.5	12.5	6.3
Enterobacter	25	25	12.5
Klebsiella	50	50	25
Serratia	200	50	25
Proteus mirabilis	>100	>100	>100
Neisseria gonorrhoeae	0.78	0.39	0.39
Neisseria meningitidis	0.08	1.6	1.6
Haemophilus influenzae	1.6	1.6	1.6
Shigella	100	100	100
Pseudomonas aeruginosa	200	100	100
Bacteroides	100	25	100
Mycoplasma and Chlamydia			
M. pneumoniae	1.6	1.6	1.6
T. mycoplasma	0.4	0.1	
Chlamydia	2		

Table 24.4-2
Pharmacokinetic Properties of Tetracyclines

Compound	Effect upon Absorption[a] Food	Ca2+	Fe2+	Protein Binding (%)	Dose Absorbed (%)	Half-life in Serum ($t_{1/2}$, hr)	Excretion after Parenteral Injection (%)
Tetracycline[b]	++	++	++	55-65	77	10	60
Oxytetracycline	+	++	++	25-35	58	9	70
Doxycycline	+/–	+	++[c]	80-95	93	15-22	35
Minocycline	+/–	+	++	80-95	98	11-17	10
Demeclocycline	+	++	++	80-90	66	15	40

[a] +=decrease; +/– = variable.
[b] Hydrochloride.
[c] Occurs even if given i.v.

with a bile/serum ratio of 20:1 for doxycycline and 5:1 for tetracycline. The concentrations in sputum are variable, but the levels in the bronchial mucosa are appreciable. The drugs are found in salivary and lacrimal secretions. The lipid-solubility of the drugs allows them to penetrate areas such as prostatic tissue and brain. The cerebrospinal fluid levels of tetracyclines are about one-tenth the serum levels. The tetracyclines all cross the placental barrier and can accumulate in fetal bones, delaying bone growth. They are excreted in breast milk. The drugs become bound to developing teeth in children below the age of 8, codepositing with the enamel and discoloring the teeth to a brown streaked color.

Excretion. Tetracyclines differ widely in the amount excreted in the urine. Only 20% of an orally administered dose is excreted in the urine, whereas following parenteral administration, 60% of tetracycline, 70% of oxytetracycline, 40% of demeclocycline, 10% of minocycline, and 35% of doxycycline are renally excreted. The mechanism of renal excretion is glomerular filtration. All tetracyclines, except doxycycline, accumulate in the body in patients with depressed renal function.

The tetracyclines are also excreted in the bile, and a significant amount of the drugs is never absorbed and leaves via the feces, although more doxycycline is reabsorbed.

Metabolism. Only chlortetracycline undergoes metabolism. However, barbiturates and agents such as phenytoin and carbamazepine induce hepatic microsomal enzymes that inactivate doxycycline.

Adverse Effects. Tetracyclines can produce a variety of adverse effects, ranging from minor inconvenience to life-threatening (Table 24.4-4). Phototoxicity, onycholysis, and rash have followed use of all of the tetracyclines. Urticaria and rarely an anaphylactic reaction or angioneurotic edema have occurred. Demethylchlortetracycline has been associated with a lupus erythematosus type of syndrome. In children or the unborn, before the teeth are fully developed, use of tetracyclines can produce a brown, mottled staining of the teeth due to the codeposition of a tetracycline-calcium-orthophosphate complex. Gastrointestinal superinfections and hepatic side effects include glossitis and/or stomatitis, cheilosis, nausea, emesis, and diarrhea. Proctitis may be seen. Intravenous administration of tetracyclines at doses above 2 g/day has produced hepatic failure with fatty infiltration throughout the liver. Hepatic toxicity in the form of diffuse fatty metamorphosis was seen most often when tetracyclines were given to pregnant women. Although teratogenic effects due to tetracyclines have not been reported in humans, temporary depression of bone growth occurs in the fetus and young children.

Table 24.4-3
Distribution of Tetracyclines

Compound	Lung	Liver	Kidney	Brain	Sputum	Saliva	Bile	CSF[a]
Tetracycline[b]	++	++	++	+	+	+	+	10
Minocycline	++	+++	+	+++	+++	+++	+++	20
Doxycycline	++	+++	+++	+++	+++	+	+++	20

[a] Percentage of serum level.
[b] Hydrochloride.

Table 24.4-4
Major Adverse Effects of All the Tetracyclines

Site or Process Affected	Side Effects
Skin	Phototoxicity, onycholysis, rash
Allergic	Rash, urticaria, anaphylactic reaction, angioneurotic edema
Dental	Staining, dysgenesis, fluorescence
Gastrointestinal	Nausea, vomiting, diarrhea, proctitis, glossitis, stomatitis
Hepatic	Abnormal liver function tests, lethal hepatic toxicity
Superimposed infections	*Candida*, resistant staphylococci, and gram-negative bacilli
Metabolic	Catabolic effect
Renal	Azotemia, Fanconi syndrome (due to outdated tetracycline), nephrogenic diabetes insipidus (demethylchlortetracycline)
Hematological	Anemia, neutropenia, eosinophilia (rare)
Miscellaneous	Increased intracranial pressure, vertigo due to minocycline

Superinfections due to fungi such as *Candida albicans* or to gram-negative enteric species, as well as with staphylococci, were common in young women who receive tetracyclines.

The drugs are antianabolic and interfere to some extent with normal protein metabolism. When given to a patient receiving hyperalimentation, protein synthesis will be prevented. The drugs formerly caused a Fanconi-like syndrome with aminoaciduria, phosphaturia, glycosuria, etc. This was due to breakdown of tetracycline to epianhydro epimers, which no longer occurs. Nephrogenic diabetes insipidus can be produced by demethylchlortetracycline.

A number of side effects such as increased intracranial pressure, pseudotumor cerebri, and meningeal irritation are rarely seen since the drugs are no longer given to children. One important side effect, seen only with minocycline, is vertigo. This is dose related and occurs more often in females.

Therapeutic Uses. The majority of the illnesses for which tetracyclines are clearly the agents of choice are the infectious diseases, listed in Table 24.4-5. Tetracyclines should be avoided in pregnant women and in children under 8 years of age. They also should not be given to patients with severe liver disease. Tetracyclines remain the agents of choice to treat rickettsial diseases, Rocky Mountain spotted fever, typhus, Q fever, and rickettsial pox. The drugs are effective in relapsing fever. They are usually combined with streptomycin in the treatment of brucellosis and tularemia and are also used to treat plague. Pneumonitis due to psittacosis is best treated with the tetracyclines. The role of tetracyclines in the therapy of melioidosis is uncertain. They will aid in the clearing of *Vibrio cholera* from the stool of patients and carriers.

The drugs are effective therapy against *chlamydia*, particularly those of venereal origin [e.g., nongonococcal urethritis (NGU)] and are also used to treat NGU due to *Ureaplasma ureolyticum*. They should not be used to treat the chlamydial pneumonitis of the newborn, which is best treated with erythromycin. They are effective in the treatment of gonorrhea and lymphogranuloma venereum. Treatment of syphilis requires large doses, 60 g, for a prolonged period, 30 days. One common disease for which they are equal in therapy with erythromycin is pneumonitis due to *Mycoplasma pneumoniae*.

The tetracyclines offer a useful alternative to other therapies in a number of situations. They are effective in pneumococcal pneumonia and in anaerobic infection of the chest. Although tetracyclines were used to treat pulmonary infections in patients with cystic fibrosis, there is no evidence that their use was of benefit. Anaerobic infection below the diaphragm would be preferably treated with other agents, since many bacteria are resistant to tetracyclines. Tetracyclines have been used successfully to treat gas gangrene, *Haemophilus* infection, anthrax, nocardiosis, and infection due to other actinomyces.

The agents are useful to treat acute exacerbations of bronchitis, sinusitis, and acne. Tetracyclines have proved to be extremely useful in the treatment of malabsorption due to Whipple's disease or the blind-loop syndrome. The role of tetracyclines in the treatment of urinary tract infections is unclear; so many other agents are available that the drugs should rarely be used.

Misuse of tetracyclines is common. The drugs have no place as prophylaxis to prevent individuals with viral illness from developing a bacterial infection. They should not be used to treat pharyngitis and are not satisfactory therapy of staphylococcal infections. Other agents should

Table 24.4-5
Therapeutic Uses of Tetracyclines

A. *Treatment of choice*
- Rickettsial infections
  - Rocky Mountain spotted fever
  - Typhus (murine and epidemic)
  - Rickettsia pox
  - Q fever
- Chlamydial infections
  - Venereal, conjunctival
  - Psittacosis
- Brucellosis
- Tularemia
- Mycoplasma pneumonia
- Relapsing fever (*Borrelia*)
- Melioidosis
- Cholera

B. *Effective, but other agents available*
- Pneumococcal pneumonitis
- Anaerobic infections
- *Listeria* infections
- Gas gangrene
- *Haemophilus* infections
- Anthrax
- Gonorrhea
- Shigellosis
- Nocardiosis

C. *Syndromes of use*
- Bronchitis
- Sinusitis
- Acne
- Malabsorption
- Urinary infection
- Acute exacerbations of chronic bronchitis

D. *Generally ineffective or less effective than other agents*
- Pharyngitis
- Endocarditis
- Serious staphylococcal infections
- Leptospirosis
- Osteomyelitis
- Meningitis
- Gram-negative bacteremia

be used to treat endocarditis, osteomyelitis, meningitis, and gram-negative bacteremia. The one prophylactic role of a tetracycline is that of minocycline to eradicate the meningococcal carrier state. However, rifampin has replaced minocycline as the preferred agent to use because of vertigo that follows use of minocycline in many individuals.

CHLORAMPHENICOL

History. Chloramphenicol was the first broad-spectrum antimicrobial agent. It was isolated by Burkholder in 1947 from a soil sample from Venezuela from which *Streptomyces venezuelae* was discovered. Shortly thereafter, Parke-Davis Laboratories were able to synthesize the drug. Although the agent is a remarkably effective compound and often sold over the counter in many countries, its use today has been severely limited in the United States by the development of other agents. Nonetheless, its particular chemical properties make it an ideal agent to treat certain infections (1).

Chemistry. The chemical structure of chloramphenicol is as shown, consisting of propanediol moiety, a dichloroacetamide side chain, and a p-nitrophenyl group:

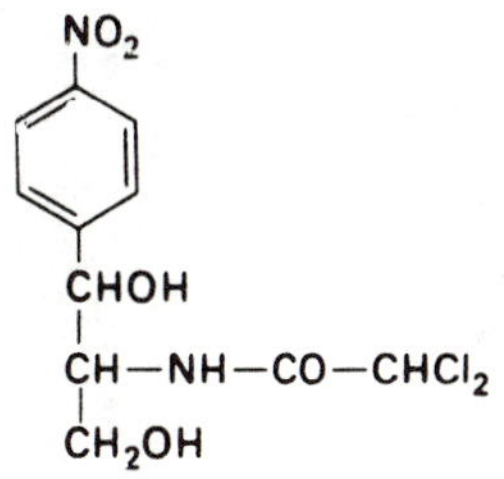

NO_2

CHOH
|
CH—NH—CO—$CHCl_2$
|
CH_2OH

Chloramphenicol

Only the D(−)threo isomer is active. Recently it has been shown that the 3′-hydroxyl group can be replaced by a fluorine atom and increased *in vitro* activity will be achieved.

Mechanism of Action. Chloramphenicol inhibits protein synthesis at the 50 S ribosomal level. Primarily it blocks the formation of the peptide bond between the amino acid on the tRNA and the peptide of the peptidyl-tRNA (Chapter 22). The drug can also inhibit protein synthesis in mammalian mitochondrial cells presumably by binding to the 70 S ribosome. Mitochondrial ribosomes are similar to bacterial ribosomes.

Resistance. The resistance of most bacteria to chloramphenicol is on the basis of a plasmid-mediated enzyme, chloramphenicol transacetylase (CAT). This enzyme is found in *S. aureus* and the various members of the *Enterobacteriaceae*. Some organisms possess a chromosomally directed CAT to account for their resistance. It appears that *P. aeruginosa* are resistant to chloramphenicol because of a failure to take up the drug. Chloramphenicol derivatives in which the 3-OH is replaced by a fluorine are not inactivated by CAT.

Antimicrobial Spectrum. Chloramphenicol has a wide range of activity that includes gram-positive, gram-negative, aerobic and anaerobic bacteria, as well as rickettsia (Table 24.4-6).

Chloramphenicol inhibits *S. aureus, S. pyogenes, S. pneumoniae, H. influenzae*, and *N. meningitidis*. Its activity against enteric gram-negative species varies from city to city and country to country. Many *E. coli, Klebsiella*, and *Proteus* are susceptible, but the resistance of hospital strains to chloramphenicol is high. *Pseudomonas* are resistant. The susceptibility of *Salmonella* and *S. typhi* depends upon the country of origin. Most strains in the United States are susceptible, whereas those from the Orient and Mexico often are resistant. *Brucella* and *Pasturella* are susceptible. *Mycoplasma, chlamydia* and rickettsia are inhibited by chloramphenicol. Bacteroides, particularly *B. fragilis* ss *fragilis*, have remained susceptible to chloramphenicol. Table 24.4-6 gives examples of the concentrations needed to inhibit important bacteria.

Table 24.4-6
Inhibitory Activity of Chloramphenicol

Organism	Minimal Inhibitory Concentrations (μg/ml)		
	Mean	Range	Percent Susceptible
Staphylococcus aureus	8	3->16	90
Staphylococcus epidermidis	4	3->16	80
Streptococcus pyogenes	4	0.3-16	100
Streptococcus pneumoniae	3	0.3-6	100
Streptococcus faecalis	6	2->16	80
Neisseria meningitidis	0.4	0.01-6	100
Neisseria gonorrhoeae	1	0.01-3	100
Listeria monocytogenes	1	0.1-3	100
Bacteroides fragilis	6	0.4-12	100
Fusobacterium	2	0.1-6	100
Clostridium	3	0.02->16	95
Haemophilus influenzae	1	0.03-8	100
Escherichia coli	4	1->16	75
Salmonella typhi	3	0.5->16	95
Klebsiella pneumoniae	8	5->16	70
Pseudomonas aeruginosa	>100		5

Pharmacokinetics. ***Absorption.*** Chloramphenicol is available as both an oral and parenteral agent. Orally it is well absorbed when given to adults as capsules containing the parent compound. If it is used as a suspension of chloramphenicol-palmitate, serum levels are less satisfactory due to variation in the rate of hydrolysis of the ester in the gastrointestinal tract that must occur to release the active compound.

As a parenteral agent in the form of chloramphenicol succinate, excellent serum levels are produced by intravenous administration, but the levels after intramuscular administration may be significantly lower, requiring larger doses if the agent is given by the i.m. route.

The blood peak levels achieved after a 1-g oral dose are reached in about 2 hours and are about 10-13 μg/ml. The half-life of the drug is 1.5-3 hours.

Distribution. Due to its solubility in lipid, chloramphenicol is extremely well distributed throughout the body. High levels are achieved in lung and liver. It readily penetrates pleural, ascitic, and synovial fluid. Unlike other antibiotics, it penetrates the eye and enters the CSF even in the absence of meningitis to a level of 50% of the serum level. Although it is bound to protein, 50%, this does not affect its distribution. Measurable levels of chloramphenicol are found in saliva and milk. There is transport across the placental barrier, so that the drug would rarely be used in the pregnant female.

Metabolism and Excretion. Chloramphenicol is conjugated in the liver with glucuronic acid to an inactive compound. About 90% of the inactive drug is excreted rapidly by the kidney. Active chloramphenicol does not accumulate in the presence of renal failure, but inactive components do. In the presence of markedly decreased renal function, the drug in the urine will not have antibacterial activity. Only a small amount of chloramphenicol is excreted in the bile.

The immature liver of the newborn or premature infant cannot conjugate chloramphenicol, and in severe liver disease in the adult this also may occur.

Adverse Effects. Bone marrow depression is the most serious side effect of the use of chloramphenicol. It occurs in some 1 in 40,000 patients who receive the drug. This is an irreversible pancytopenia that does not appear to be dose related. Mortality of the aplastic anemia exceeds 50%. This form of blood dyscrasia in the majority of patients becomes evident only weeks or months after therapy.

The more common form of hematological toxicity associated with chloramphenicol is the dose-related anemia and leukopenia. There is a reduced iron utilization for hemoglobin synthesis, vacuolation of erythroblasts, and thrombocytopenia and leukopenia. Such changes are more common when serum levels exceed 25 μg/ml. These side effects usually subside as the therapy is stopped. It is clear that frequent checks of the blood count are necessary for any patient receiving chloramphenicol.

Other hematological effects of chloramphenicol are prevention of the normal response to vitamin B_{12} and hemolysis in some patients with glucose-6-phosphate dehydrogenase deficiency.

A pediatric complication rarely seen is the Grey baby syndrome. Chloramphenicol given in doses greater than 25 mg/kg/day to premature infants produces a syndrome of abdominal distension, vomiting, pallor, cyanosis, and circulatory collapse that results in death in 60% of children. This is a result of immaturity of the hepatic glucuronyl transferase system. This enzyme immaturity coupled with the diminished glomerular and tubular function of the newborn results in elevated levels of free chloramphenicol in the circulation. Because chloramphenicol crosses the placenta, it should be used with caution in late pregnancy and avoided during lactation.

Prolonged courses of chloramphenicol therapy have produced optic neuritis in children. Gastrointestinal problems, except for overgrowth of *Candida*, are not common and hypersensitivity is rare. Chloramphenicol does interfere with the metabolism of tolbutamide, phenytoin, and bishydroxycoumarin.

Drug Interaction. Chloramphenicol has an inhibitory effect on the hepatic drug metabolizing enzymes, so that the half-life of drugs that are metabolized by this system is increased. These drugs include phenytoin, tolbutamide, chlorpropamide, and dicumarol. Drugs that can induce the hepatic microsomal enzymes will shorten the half-life of chloramphenicol.

Therapeutic Uses. The major use of chloramphenicol has been centered around its entry into the CSF on one hand and its inhibition of *Bacteroides* on the other (6). It is the drug to be used, combined with ampicillin, as initial therapy in unknown meningitis in children. This has been advocated because of the appearance of β-lactamase-producing *Haemophilus* that are resistant to ampicillin. Chloramphenicol is also the drug of choice to treat meningitis due to *Neisseria meningitidis* or *S. pneumoniae* in the patient allergic to penicillin. Although chloramphenicol enters into the CSF, it will not cure meningitis due to *E. coli* or *Klebsiella*, since it is not bactericidal for enteric bacteria. Chloramphenicol combined with penicillin was a major therapy of brain abscess, since these are frequently due to anaerobic bacteria; however, it is being replaced by metronidazole.

Chloramphenicol is excellent therapy of serious *Haemophilus* infections such as epiglottitis, osteomyelitis, and pneumonia. It is very effective in rickettsial diseases and should be used in place of tetracycline in the very ill or when renal failure is present. It also is still effective therapy of typhoid fever, but will not eradicate the carrier state and should not be used to treat *Salmonella* gastroenteritis. Chloramphenicol has been used in the treatment of abdominal wound infections due to a mixture of aerobic and anaerobic species, particularly if *Bacteroides fragilis* ss *fragilis* is involved, but it is being replaced by cefoxitin, clindamycin, and metronidazole.

Great concern has been expressed that the combined use of chloramphenicol and an aminoglycoside would result in antagonism of the normal antibacterial action of the aminoglycosides by the chloramphenicol. Animal experiments have not established that this occurs. Furthermore, clinical studies of the use of penicillin or ampicillin combined with chloramphenicol to treat experimental pneumococcal or *Haemophilus* meningitis have not shown antagonism of the action of the penicillin agent.

ERYTHROMYCIN

History. Although a number of antibiotics that belong to the macrolide family e.g., erythromycin, spiramycin, oleandomycin, and kitasamycin have been isolated, only erythromycin has been extensively used in the United States (3). Erythromycin was isolated from a strain of *Streptomyces erythreus* by McGuire and colleagues in 1952. It has been used widely in pediatric practice, and the demonstration of its activity against *Legionella pneumophila* in 1977 produced a resurgence of interest in the compound.

Chemistry. All of the macrolides contain a macrocyclic lactone ring (Fig. 24.4-2). The compounds are weak bases and exist either as a free base that is only slightly soluble in water or in the form of various esters such as the ethyl succinate, stearate, lactobionate, gluceptate, etc. The free base is acid labile and so is manufactured with an acid-resistant coating.

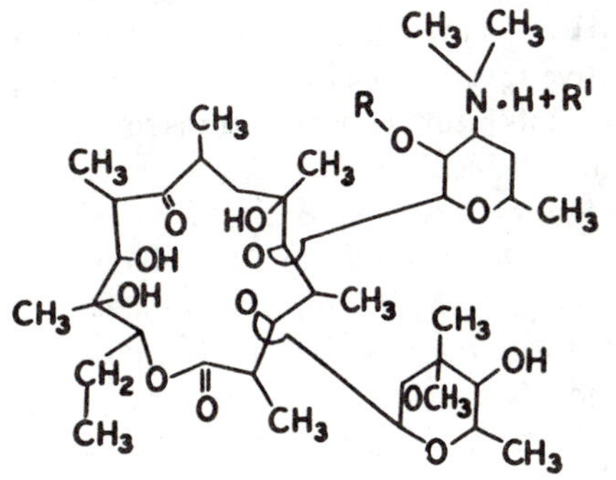

	R	R'
Erythromycin	H	
Propionyl erythromycin	CH_3CH_2CO	
Erythromycin estolate	CH_3CH_2CO	$C_{12}H_{25}OSO_3$
Erythromycin stearate	H	$C_{17}H_{35}COO$
Erythromycin ethyl succinate	$CH_3CH_2OOCCH_2CH_2COO$	

Fig. 24.4-2. *Structures of erythromycins.*

Mechanism of Action. Erythromycin inhibits protein synthesis at the 50 S ribosomal level. It is thought that erythromycin binds to the donor site on the ribosome, competing for attachment and preventing translocation of the nascent peptide from the acceptor to the donor site (Chapter 22). In the human, erythromycin probably acts in a bacteriostatic manner, although at very high concentrations it is bactericidal to some microorganisms.

Resistance. Resistance on the basis of altered ribosome can be due to the presence of plasmids or because of a mutation that alters the ribosome. Resistance is most commonly due to the presence of plasmids within the bacteria. These bacteria have an altered 23 S methylase enzyme system. Gram-negative species are resistant to erythromycin due to the inability of the compound to pass through the cell wall and hence its inability to reach its ribosome receptor site. Cross-resistance of erythromycin and clindamycin exists between many organisms, but an organism resistant to erythromycin is not necessarily resistant to clindamycin.

Antimicrobial Spectrum. Erythromycin inhibits a wide group of organisms. It inhibits *S. aureus*, both β-lactamase-producing and penicillin-susceptible isolates,

S. pyogenes, S. viridans, S. pneumoniae, and even a significant number of *S. faecalis* (true enterococci) (3). Gram-positive bacilli such as *Corynebacterium diphtheriae, Listeria monocytogenes, Bacillus anthracis* and other *Bacillus* species are inhibited. Erythromycin inhibits *N. meningitidis, N. gonorrhoeae, Haemophilus influenzae*, and *Bordetella pertussis*. It is active against *Chlamydia* and *Mycoplasma pneumoniae* and some *Ureaplasma ureolyticum*. Some *Nocardia asteroides* are inhibited.

Erythromycin at high concentrations inhibits anaerobic gram-negative species such as *B. fragilis*. In an alkaline milieu, pH 8, it can inhibit some *E. coli, Klebsiella*, and *Pseudomonas*. For example, the inhibitory concentration needed for *E. coli* is >400 μg at pH 6.3, but only 6 μg at pH 7.6. This same increase in activity is seen for gram-positive species such as *S. aureus* and *S. faecalis*. The minimal inhibitory concentrations for major bacteria are given in Table 24.4.-7.

Pharmacokinetics. ***Absorption.*** Erythromycin usually is administered by the oral route in doses given every 6 or 8 hours. It can be given by intramuscular injection in the ethyl succinate form, but it is very painful. It can also be given intravenously as the lactobionate or gluceptate. Erythromycin base that is acid coated dissolves in the duodenum, but large amounts are not absorbed and reach the large bowel. The stearate form is also only partially absorbed in the upper intestine. Although the estolate is no more readily absorbed than the other forms, its absorption is not altered by ingestion with food. Absorption varies from one individual to another, and in a life-threatening situation it may be necessary to utilize the i.v. route.

Distribution. Erythromycin is widely distributed in the body. It has a half-life ($t_{1/2}$) of 1-4 hours. Protein binding is low only 18-20%. The large difference in given half-life is due to variations in the time to reach a peak concentration. Adequate concentrations to inhibit susceptible organisms are found in liver, spleen, lungs, and pleural and ascitic fluids. It enters the CSF only in the presence of inflammation. It crosses the placenta, but the concentrations in the fetus are considerably less than in the mother. Although it enters the prostate, it is not present in an ionic state to be active. The erythromycin that is not absorbed in the intestine has local antibacterial activity in the large bowel.

Excretion. About 5% of orally administered erythromycin is excreted in active form in the urine and about 15% is excreted in urine after i.v. infusion. Urine concentrations are low in the beginning of therapy but reach levels of 30-1000 μg/ml. Erythromycin is excreted in the feces after oral administration, and levels there are 300-1000 μg/ml. The drug is also excreted in the bile.

Adverse Effects. Toxicity due to erythromycin is very uncommon; it is an unusually safe compound. Gastrointestinal irritation with nausea, emesis, and abdominal cramps are the most common toxicity of erythromycin. These reactions are infrequent in children and more common in adults, particularly females. Hepatotoxicity, which had been thought to occur only with the estolate form, can develop with any erythromycin. Hepatotoxicity is an idiosyncratic reaction that usually occurs some 10-12 days after initiation of treatment. The symptoms are fever, pruritus, and jaundice. Eosinophilia and abnormalities of liver function tests are found, increased levels of SGOT and alkaline phosphatase. A liver biopsy will show cholestasis and variable amounts of hepatic cell necrosis. The condition is reversible when the drug is stopped and neither death nor permanent hepatic dysfunction occurs.

Skin rash is rarely seen, but local irritation at the site of i.m. injection or i.v. infusion is not infrequent.

Therapeutic Uses. Erythromycin has been utilized primarily as an alternative to penicillin, particularly in the therapy of upper respiratory infections in children. It is an excellent agent to treat pneumonia, otitis media, pharyngitis caused by *S. pneumoniae*, and *S. pyogenes*. More serious infection due to *S. pneumoniae* or *Haemophilus* such as meningitis should be treated with cefotaxime or cefuroxime. Otitis media due to *Haemophilus* preferably would be treated with amoxicillin or trimethoprim-sulfamethoxazole, although erythromycin combined with a sulfonamide has been a highly effective form of therapy.

The drug can be used early in the course of pertussis, but it does not affect the course if used later. Erythromycin is the drug of choice to treat the carrier state of diphtheria. It is an excellent agent to treat chlamydial

Table 24.4-7
Antibacterial Spectrum of Erythromycin

Organism	Usual Inhibitory Concentration (μg/ml)
Streptococcus pyogenes	0.04
Streptococcus pneumoniae	0.03
Streptococcus faecalis	1.5
Streptococcus agalactiae	0.02
Staphylococcus aureus	0.5
Clostridium	0.5
Corynebacterium diphtheriae	1.6
Corynebacterium acnes	0.1
Neisseria gonorrhoeae	1
Neisseria meningitidis	0.8
Haemophilus influenzae	2.5
Bordetella pertussis	1.5
Listeria monocytogenes	0.2
Mycoplasma pneumoniae	0.01
Pasturella multocida	0.2
Chlamydia trachomatis	0.2[a]

[a] Active in *in vivo* studies.

infection of the newborn and *Mycoplasma pneumoniae* in young adults. Skin or soft tissue infections due to *S. pyogenes* or *S. aureus* respond to erythromycin therapy. More serious staphylococcal infections should be treated with other agents.

Erythromycin orally or intravenously is excellent therapy for pneumonia due to *Legionella pneumophila.* It also has been used to treat some acute exacerbations of chronic bronchitis. Although it rarely is useful in the therapy of urinary tract infections, if alkalinization of the urine above pH 7 is possible, it will eradicate some gram-negative species.

Erythromycin has been used to treat venereal disease (gonorrhea or syphilis) and nongonococcal urethritis due to *Ureaplasma ureolyticum* (see Chapter 25.5). Even though erythromycin has been used successfully to treat endocarditis due to *S. viridans* or *S. aureus,* other agents are preferred.

Erythromycin has been successfully used as a prophylactic agent in the prevention of rheumatic fever, prevention of endocarditis after dental extraction in individuals with valvular heart disease, and as an intestinal sterilizing agent given before operation on the large bowel.

OTHER MACROLIDES

Oleandomycins, although still commercially available as oleandomycin and triacetyloleandomycin, should not be used. These agents have less intrinsic antibacterial activity than erythromycin and cause more frequent hepatic toxicity. Spiramycin persists in tissues for long periods of time, and it also has activity against *Toxoplasma gondii.* It has been used to reduce the incidence of fetal toxoplasmosis.

CLINDAMYCIN AND LINCOMYCIN

History. Lincomycin was isolated from a strain of *Streptomyces lincolensis* from a soil sample near Lincoln, Nebraska by the Upjohn Research Laboratories. A variety of derivatives were prepared over the years and one of these, 7-chloro-7-deoxylincomycin (clindamycin), proved to be clinically useful. The chemical structures of lincomycin and clindamycin are:

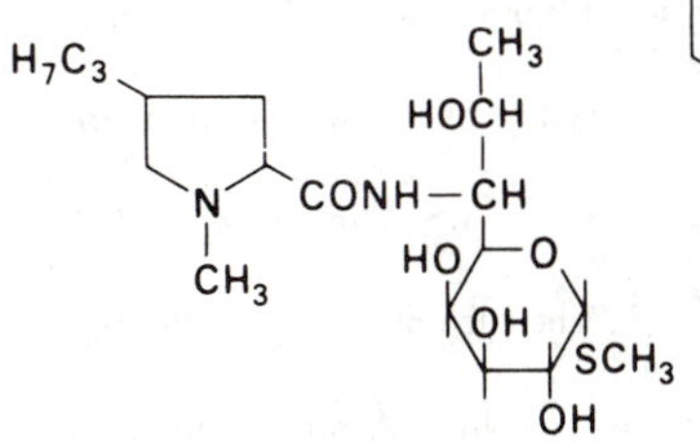

Lincomycin

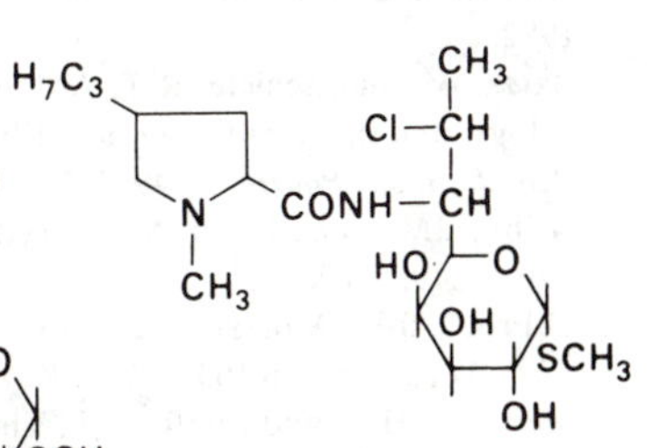

Clindamycin

Mechanism of Action. Lincomycin and clindamycin inhibit protein synthesis in a manner analogous to that of erythromycin. These agents bind to the 50 S subunit of the bacterial ribosome and interfere with peptide bond formation, perhaps via a translocation step (Chapter 22). These drugs usually act as bacteriostatic compounds, but at high concentrations they can be bactericidal.

Resistance. Resistance of bacteria to lincomycin and clindamycin can be on the basis of altered ribosomes (23 S component) or of failure to reach a receptor site in the bacteria. Plasmid resistance has been found in gram-positive cocci and in *Bacteroides.* Gram-negative bacteria are resistant due to the inability of the compounds to cross the bacterial cell wall. There is cross-resistance with erythromycin in some species.

Antimicrobial Spectrum. Lincomycin and clindamycin have a similar antibacterial spectrum of activity. They inhibit most gram-positive coccal species such as *S. aureus, S. epidermidis, S. pyogenes, S. viridans,* and *S. pneumoniae.* They are inactive against *S. faecalis,* enterococci. *Corynebacteria acnes* are inhibited. Gram-positive bacilli such as *Bacillus subtilis* and *B. cereus* and anaerobes such as *Clostridium perfringens* are in hibited; some *Clostridium,* particularly *C. difficile,* are resistant. Cross-resistance of staphylococci to lincomycin, clindamycin, and erythromycin occurs.

These drugs do not inhibit aerobic gram-negative bacteria *(Enterobacteriaceae* and *Pseudomonas).* The activity against *Haemophilus* is variable. Clindamycin in particular inhibits *Bacteroides* species, particularly *B. fragilis* ss *fragilis,* but occasional strains are resistant. The concentrations needed to inhibit mycoplasma are variable, and the agents are not drugs of choice. The *Actinomyces, A. israeli,* are inhibited but *Nocardia* are not. Inhibitory concentrations for common organisms are given in Table 24.4-8.

Pharmacokinetics. ***Absorption.*** Although both lincomycin and clindamycin are absorbed after oral ingestion, 40% of lincomycin is not absorbed and can be recovered in the feces. Clindamycin has much better absorption, and there is little need for lincomycin. The presence of food in the stomach does not impair the absorption of clindamycin. Serum half-life of clindamycin is approximately 2-3 hr.

Both agents can be given intramuscularly or intravenously. Clindamycin given parenterally is in the form of a phosphate ester. Adequate serum and tissue levels are achieved when it is given every 6-12 hr. Clindamycin has also been prepared as a suspension to be used as a topical agent in the therapy of acne.

Distribution. Adequate concentrations of lincomycin or clindamycin can be achieved in most body tissues and pleural, peritoneal, and synovial fluids, but not in the CSF. The drugs cross the placenta and also enter human milk. Extremely high concentrations are found in bone. Protein binding is approximately 80%.

Excretion. Both drugs are excreted in the urine, but only 10-15% as active drug after oral administration and about 30% when they are given parenterally. Both can accumulate to a moderate degree in the presence of renal insufficiency. A significant amount of the drugs is excreted in the bile, and biliary

Table 24.4-8
Inhibitory Concentrations of Clindamycin

Organism	Usual Inhibitory Concentration (μg/ml)
Staphylococcus aureus	0.04-0.4
Streptococcus pyogenes	0.02-0.2
S. pneumoniae	0.1-0.06
S. viridans	0.02-0.2
Actinomyces	0.03-0.3
Clostridium species	0.1-100
Peptococcus	0.1-1.6
Peptostreptococcus	0.1-0.8
Fusobacterium	0.1-1.6
Bacteroides fragilis	0.1-3.1

Table 24.4-9
Dosage Regimen

Drug	Route	Usual Adult Dosage	Usual Pediatric Dosage (after first week of life)
Tetracycline HCl	p.o., i.v.	Usual daily dose: 1-2 g in four equal doses depending on severity of infection	Not recommended for children 9 years of age and under
Chlortetracycline	p.o.., i.v.	As above	As above
Oxytetracycline	p.o., i.v.	As above	As above
Demeclocycline	p.o., i.v.	150 mg q. 6 hr, or 300 mg b.i.d.	As above
Doxycycline	p.o., i.v.	200 mg on day 1, then 100 mg/day	As above
Minocycline	p.o., i.v.	200 mg initially, then 100 mg q. 12 hr	As above
Lincomycin	i.m.,i.v. p.o.	600 mg q. 8 hr 500 mg t.i.d.	i.m./i.v.: 10 mg/kg/day in one injection p.o. 30-60 mg/kg/day divided q. 6 hr
Clindamycin	i.m., i.v. p.o.	150-600 mg q. 6 hr 150-450 mg q. 6 hr	8-20 mg/kg/day divided q. 6-8 hr
Erythromycin	i.v. p.o.	2 g day 250 mg q. 6 hr	30-50 mg/kg/day divided q. 6-8 hr
Chloramphenicol	p.o., i.v.	50 mg/kg/day q. 6 hr	50-100 mg/kg/day

levels are high. A substantial proportion of both agents is inactivated in the body. Neither drug is removed to an appreciable degree by peritoneal dialysis or hemodialysis.

Adverse Effects. The most significant toxicity that has been associated with the use of these drugs is gastrointestinal (4). Diarrhea occurs in 10-20% of individuals who receive these drugs. A more serious problem has been the development of pseudomembranous enterocolitis. It has been shown that this problem is due to the growth of *Clostridium difficile* in the intestine and the production of toxin. Thus far, there are no clinical criteria that would allow one to predict which patients will develop this problem. It can be controlled by stopping administration of the drug; if the diarrhea persists, vancomycin should be administered orally, since vancomycin inhibits *Clostridium difficile*; alternative therapy is metronidazole or bacitracin.

Hepatotoxicity with use of these drugs is poorly documented. Rashes are infrequent, but a Stevens-Johnson syndrome, generalized rash, has been reported.

Therapeutic Uses. The recognition of the syndrome of enterocolitis in the 1970s caused a reappraisal of the use of clindamycin. At the present time, use of clindamycin has been primarily to treat serious anaerobic infections. In this situation it is used in combination with an aminoglycoside. It has been used to treat staphylococcal infections such as osteomyelitis. Clindamycin is effective therapy for anaerobic pleuropulmonary disease in the penicillin-allergic patient.

Although lincomycin and clindamycin have been used to treat streptococcal infections (pharyngitis, endocarditis, soft tissue infection), their use in these situations is not encouraged and other compounds would be preferred. The oral use of clindamycin to treat acne would not seem to be wise, although the drug is quite effective and in a severe case could be temporarily used. As a topical agent, clindamycin in a suspension is useful for therapy of acne, but skin improvement will not occur until after a month or more of therapy.

DOSE SCHEDULES

Table 24.4-9 presents dose schedules for broad-spectrum antibiotics.

REFERENCES

1. Bartlett, J.G. Chloramphenicol. *Med. Clin. North Am.* 66:91, 1982.
2. Barza, M. and Schiefe, R.T. Antimicrobial spectrum, pharmacology, and therapeutic use of antibiotics. Part 1. Tetracyclines. *Am. J. Hosp. Pharm.* 34:49, 1977.
3. Gribble, M.J. and Chou, A.W. Erythromycin. *Med. Clin. North Am.* 66:79, 1982.
4. LeFrock, J.L., Molavi, A. and Prince, A.S. Clindamycin. *Med. Clin. North Am.* 66:103, 1982.
5. Meissner, H.C. and Smith, A.L. The current status of chloramphenicol. *Pediatrics* 64:348, 1979.
6. Neu, H.C. A symposium on tetracycline: A major appraisal introduction. *Bull. N.Y. Acad. Med.* 54:141, 1978.

ADDITIONAL READING

Descotes, J. et al. Pharmacokinetic drug interactions with macrolide antibiotics. *J. Antimicrob. Chemother.*, 15:659, 1985.

CHAPTER
24.5

MISCELLANEOUS ANTIMICROBIAL AGENTS

Harold C. Neu

There are a number of antibacterial agents that could be classified into groups on the basis of their effect on the bacterial cell. But it is more logical to consider the compounds individually, concentrating on the areas in which they may be particularly useful.

VANCOMYCIN

History. Vancomycin was discovered in 1956 by the Lilly Research Laboratories in a culture of *Streptomyces orientalis* found in Borneo. The agent was just beginning to be used in the early 1960s when the development of the penicillinase-resistant penicillins and subsequently the cephalosporins caused it to fall into disuse. Recent problems with organisms such as *Staphylococcus aureus* resistant to other antibiotics have caused a resurgence of interest in this agent (2).

Chemistry. Vancomycin is the only glycopeptide used clinically. It can be described as a tricyclic glycopeptide that contains three substituted phenylglycines, a glucose, a unique amino sugar (vancosamine), N-methyl leucine, and aspartic acid amide. The molecular weight is 1450. It is not related to the aminoglycosides. It forms chelates with metal ions.

Vancomycin is very soluble at pH 4, but solubility decreases rapidly as neutrality is approached. It is soluble but unstable under alkaline conditions. Vancomycin is physically incompatible with most other drugs and diluents, such as sodium bicarbonate, penicillins, and barbiturates. After dilution in sterile water for injection, it can be further diluted in 5% dextrose in water or normal saline and infused over 20-30 min.

Mechanism of Action. Vancomycin affects the cell wall synthesis by interfering with the formation of the lipid phosphodisaccharide-pentapeptide complex that is needed in the second stage of cell wall biosynthesis. It also appears to damage the cytoplasmic membrane of certain species (Fig. 22-3). It is a bactericidal antibiotic.

Spectrum of Activity. Vancomycin inhibits only gram-positive species. It is active against staphylococci, *S. aureus,* and *S. epidermidis;* streptococci such as *S. pyogenes, S. pneumoniae,* and enterococci such as *S. faecalis.* It inhibits aerobic and anaerobic gram-positive bacilli such as *B. anthrax, B. subtilis, C. diphtheriae,* and the *Clostridia, C. tetanii, C. perfringens,* and *C. difficile,* and *Actinomyces.* Staphylococci resistant to methicillin and to the cephalosporins are inhibited by vancomycin. Gram-negative bacteria, mycobacteria, and fungi are resistant. Resistance of gram-positive bacteria rarely develops.

Pharmacokinetics. ***Administration and Absorption.*** Vancomycin can only be used intravenously for treatment of systemic infections. It is not absorbed from the gastrointestinal tract, although it exerts an antibacterial action in the lumen of the intestine. There is no satisfactory intramuscular preparation. The half-life of the drug is 4-9 hr.

Distribution. Vancomycin reaches therapeutic levels in all body tissues, including lung, heart, and kidney, and in fluids such as pleural, ascitic, synovial, and pericardial, with the exception of the CSF. In the presence of severe meningeal inflammation, appreciable levels can be reached in the CSF, but this is variable. Vancomycin is only 55% bound to protein.

Excretion. Vancomycin is excreted by the kidney through glomerular filtration. There is no evidence for tubular secretion or reabsorption. There is no appreciable biliary excretion. It accumulates in the body in the presence of renal failure, and major dosage adjustments are necessary when the drug is used in individuals whose renal function is depressed. The drug is not removed by either peritoneal dialysis or hemodialysis. There is no inactivation in the body.

Adverse Effects. The true toxicity of vancomycin is not well established. Early in its use there were reports of ototoxicity and nephrotoxicity as well as severe phlebitis. With improvements in the manufacture of the compound and knowledge that the daily dose must be adjusted depending upon the patient's creatinine clearance, it has been rare to encounter ototoxicity or nephrotoxicity, but both reactions can occur. Fever, skin rashes, and eosinophilia are occasional problems. Rapid infusion causes histamine release, but it does not cause anaphylaxis.

Therapeutic Uses. Vancomycin is an excellent alternative to penicillin or cephalosporin therapy for the individual who has had a serious allergic reaction to penicillin (11). It is the drug of choice to treat staphylococcal or streptococcal (*S. viridans, S. faecalis*) infections, endocarditis, pneumonitis, or sepsis in patients who cannot receive penicillins (6). It is also the drug of choice to treat infections due to methicillin-resistant staphylococci. Vancomycin is the therapy of choice to treat antibiotic-associated diarrheal disease, whether due to *C. difficile* or *S. aureus*. It has proved to be an effective prophylactic agent to prevent endocarditis following dental extraction in individuals with valvular heart disease. It has also been used as prophylaxis in individuals undergoing cranial surgery requiring placement of shunt devices and to treat shunt infections in hemodialysis patients (1).

BACITRACIN

Bacitracin is a peptide antibiotic isolated from a strain of *Bacillus subtilis* by Johnson and colleagues at Columbia University in 1943. It was originally used systemically to treat serious staphylococcal infections, but the development of less toxic antimicrobial agents restricted its use to that of a topical agent. It is a bactericidal agent that inhibits cell wall synthesis by interfering with dephosphorylation of a lipid carrier, C_{55}-isoprenyl pyrophosphate. It is active against gram-positive cocci, staphylococci, group A streptococci, and some *Neisseria*. Resistant strains of staphylococci and streptococci have followed excessive topical use. Bacitracin is not absorbed when used topically either as an irrigating solution or as an ointment. It has caused nephrotoxicity when used systemically. The clinical use of bacitracin is in topical skin preparations and as an irrigant at the time of certain types of surgery.

GRAMICIDIN

Gramicidin is another polypeptide antibiotic that is used in eye and ear drops, creams, and ointments. It is an open-chain polypeptide that damages the lipid components of gram-positive bacteria, resulting in loss of cations. The agent is bactericidal. It cannot be used systemically.

TYROTHRICIN

Tyrothricin is a cyclic decapeptide that inhibits both gram-positive and negative bacteria. It is used only as a topical agent.

CYCLOSERINE

Cycloserine was isolated from streptomyces by several investigators in 1955. It is a D-4-amino-3-isoxazolidone. It acts as an analog of D-alanine and interferes with cell wall synthesis by inhibiting conversion of L-alanine to D-alanine and by preventing formation of D-alanyl-alanine (Fig. 22-4). Cycloserine inhibits bacteria to a variable degree. For example, *S. pyogenes* and *E. coli* are susceptible, but *Klebsiella* and *Pseudomonas* are resistant. It inhibits *Mycobacterium tuberculosis* and some strains of *Nocardia*. It is well absorbed after oral administration and is widely distributed in the body, including the CSF. Cycloserine is excreted by glomerular filtration and accumulates in the presence of renal failure. About 35% of the drug is metabolized to inactive byproducts.

Adverse Effects. These reactions have been primarily related to the nervous system. Psychic disturbance is common. Confusion, excitement, depression, and convulsions all have been reported. The drug today is rarely used to treat bacterial infections. It has been used to treat some cases of tuberculosis resistant to other agents.

POLYMYXINS

The polymyxins are a group of antibiotics that were isolated in 1947 from soil bacilli. Only two of the group—polymyxin B and polymyxin E, which is colistimethate (colistin)—have been used clinically (4).

Chemistry. The polymyxins are branched decapeptides that are available as either sulfate or methane sulfonate (Fig. 24.5-1).

Mechanism of Action. The polymyxins bind to receptor groups in the bacterial cell membrane, distorting the architecture so as to produce a loss of permeability whereby internal cations, amino acids, and nucleotides leak out of the cell.

Resistance. Gram-positive bacteria are resistant to polymyxins because the agents cannot reach the cytoplasmic membrane. *P. mirabilis* is resistant due to a similar mechanism. High concentrations of divalent cations, magnesium and calcium, antagonize the activity of the polymyxins. There is no known plasmid resistance to the polymyxins.

Antimicrobial Spectrum. Enteric gram-negative bacteria such as *E. coli, Klebsiella*, and *Pseudomonas* are inhibited, but *Proteus* and *Serratia* are resistant, as are all anaerobic species and gram-positive bacteria.

Polymyxins act synergistically with trimethoprim and sulfonamides against some isolates of *Pseudomonas, P. cepacia*, and against *Serratia marcescens*.

Pharmacokinetics. ***Administration and Absorption.*** The polymyxins are not absorbed from the gastrointestinal tract but can be administered by intramuscular injection or intravenous infusion. They have also been used by intrathecal injection, as aerosols, and as topical preparations. Polymyxins have been used orally to sterilize the intestine. Serum levels do not provide a useful guide of the amount of drug in the body. There is no appreciable absorption from the skin or mucosal or conjunctival surfaces.

Distribution. The drugs bind rapidly to a number of body tissues including liver, kidney, muscle, heart, and so on. Levels in the lung and peritoneal and pleural fluid are inadequate, although the protein binding is low, due to their binding to other tissues (8). The drugs do not enter the CSF.

Excretion. The polymyxins are excreted by the kidney, but the precise mechanism is unclear. They accumulate in the presence of renal failure. Both polymyxin B and colistin are not adequately removed from the body by either peritoneal dialysis or hemodialysis.

Adverse Effects. The most serious toxicity of the polymyxins has been nephrotoxicity with the development of renal failure (7). Proteinuria, hematuria, and casts are the first signs of toxicity, followed by a rise in the serum creatinine and blood urea nitrogen (BUN). Toxicity is related to the underlying state of renal function and the amount of the drug administered. Neurotoxicity ranges from mild paresthesias and dizziness to severe peripheral neuropathy and respiratory paralysis. This paralysis can be reversed by administration of calcium in some

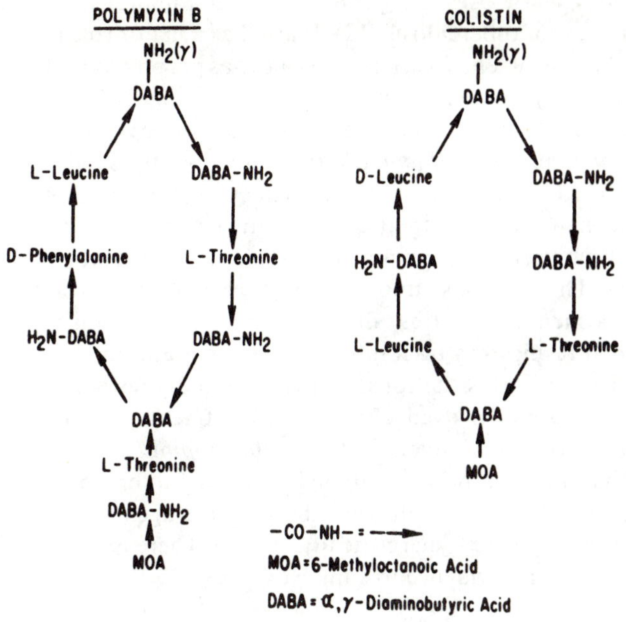

To make (SODIUM) Methanesulfonate Derivative

$$\mathrm{HC(NH)(C{=}O)-CH_2-CH_2-NH_3^+} \xrightarrow[\text{2.) NaHSO}_3]{\text{1.) HCHO}} \mathrm{HC(NH)(C{=}O)-CH_2-CH_2-NH-CH_2-SO_3^-\ Na^+}$$

Fig. 24.5-1. *Structure of polymyxin B and polymyxin E, colistin.*

cases but not by use of neostigmine. Neurotoxicity will usually resolve in 24-48 hr. Allergic reactions are uncommon. Bronchospasm has followed aerosol use. Because polymyxins liberate histamine and serotonin, this may be the mechanism of the toxicity. No serious gastrointestinal effects have followed their oral use.

Therapeutic Uses. Polymyxins have no role in the treatment of systemic infections due to the availability of more effective and less toxic agents (10). They are used as topical agents to treat surface infections due to *Pseudomonas*, such as occurs with swimmer's ear, or are applied topically to i.v. infusion sites to prevent colonization with gram-negative bacteria. Their use as an oral agent to treat *E. coli* enteritis in children is questionable.

SPECTINOMYCIN

Spectinomycin is an aminocyclitol antibiotic that has many similarities to the aminoglycosides. It binds to the 30 S ribosome and alters protein synthesis, but unlike aminoglycosides it binds to a different ribosomal protein and does not bind irreversibly. Hence, it is a bacteriostatic agent. Resistance to the agent is by plasmid-mediated enzymes or ribosomal change. It is active against a large number of gram-positive and negative bacteria, but it inhibits *Neisseria gonorrhoeae* at a level of 7-10 μg/ml. Treponema are resistant.

Spectinomycin is administered by i.m. injection at a dose of 2 g that yields serum levels of 100 μg/ml. Serum levels persist for 8 hr. The half-life in normal individuals is 2 hr. The drug is excreted by glomerular filtration. There is no metabolism of spectinomycin. Urinary levels of the drug reach 1000 μg/ml. Therapeutic concentrations are reached in urethral and cervical tissues. Concentrations in synovial fluid are adequate. Given as a single dose, toxicity is rare. Except for slight pain at the injection site, no major toxicities have been reported. Spectinomycin is used only to treat gonorrhea (9). It is the treatment of choice for β-lactamase-producing *N. gonorrhoeae* infections.

FUSIDIC ACID

Fusidic acid is produced by *Fusidium coccineum.* It has a steroid structure that is in many ways similar to some of the cephalosporins. Fusidic acid inhibits protein synthesis by interfering with the G-factor that is involved in translocation of amino acids during peptide formation on the ribosomes. Organisms resistant to fusidic acid have an altered G-factor so that GTPase is active. Gram-negative species are resistant because it cannot penetrate their cell walls. It inhibits gram-positive species such as *S. aureus*, including β-lactamase-producing isolates at very low concentrations, but it is not active against streptococci. The only gram-negative species inhibited are *Neisseria.* Gram-negative bacilli are resistant. It inhibits *Nocardia*, and most strains of *Clostridia* and *Bacteroides* are inhibited. Resistance is seen to appear during therapy when there has been a large number of infecting organisms.

Sodium fusidate is given by the oral route with good absorption. It is widely distributed in the body but does not enter the CSF. Biliary excretion occurs, but the drug is metabolized to inactive glucuronide metabolites. Essentially, no active antibiotic is excreted in the urine. It is highly protein bound, 95%, and is not removed by hemodialysis.

Adverse Effects. Toxicity to the compound has been minimal. Mild gastrointestinal upset and occasional rashes have occurred, but there has been no renal or hematological toxicity. Increased bilirubin levels have occurred, particularly after i.v. use of the drug. It is not available in the United States. It has been used with success elsewhere to treat staphylococcal infections, particularly osteomyelitis (5).

RIFAMPIN

Rifampin in the United States is generally considered an agent to be used only in the chemotherapy of tuberculosis (see Chapter 25.3). The agent, however, has a number of other uses in infectious diseases. The rifamycins are a group of antibiotics isolated from *Streptomyces mediterranei* in Italy by Lepetit Laboratories in 1957. Semisynthetic derivatives were made in the 1960s, and by the end of the 1960s large-scale studies of rifampin were begun to determine its effectiveness in the treatment of tuberculosis.

Chemistry. The compound is a zwitterion that is soluble in water at acid pH. It is soluble in nonpolar solvents.

Mechanism of Action. Rifampin prevents RNA synthesis by binding to the DNA-directed RNA polymerase in bacteria, but it does not inhibit mammalian polymerases, except at very high concentrations.

Resistance. Resistance of bacteria to rifampin can develop fairly rapidly, through production of altered DNA-directed RNA polymerases. It appears that in any large population of bacteria, particularly gram-negative bacteria, some members are resistant.

Spectrum of Activity. Rifampin inhibits gram-positive cocci such as *S. aureus* and *S. epidermidis*, including methicillin-resistant and penicillin-tolerant isolates, as well as *S. pyogenes* and *S. pneumoniae.* Enterococci often are resistant. Gram-positive bacilli—aerobic and anaerobic—are inhibited. *Neisseria meningitidis* and *N. gonorrhoeae* are very susceptible, as are many *Haemophilus influenzae*. But gram-negative bacilli such as *E. coli*, *Klebsiella*, and *Proteus* rapidly develop resistance to the drug. *Pseudomonas* are resistant. Many *Bacteroides* are susceptible. *Chlamydia* are inhibited. *Legionella pneumophila* is inhibited.

Pharmacokinetics. Rifampin is well absorbed from the gastrointestinal tract, producing peak serum levels 1.5-3 hr after ingestion. Serum levels are lowered if it is ingested with food. The drug is widely distributed in body tissues and fluids, and it enters phagocytic cells such as leukocytes and macrophages. There are good concentrations in bone and cerebrospinal fluid and in salivary and lacrimal fluids. It is about 80% bound to serum proteins.

Rifampin is metabolized in the liver by deacetylation. Both the parent compound and the deacetyl derivative are excreted in the bile. The deacetyl derivative is also biologically active. Rifampin induces the enzymes that metabolize it. Hence, its half-life is longer initially and subsequently stabilizes out at approximately 2 hr. Rifampin excreted in bile is reabsorbed from the gastrointestinal tract, but the deacetyl derivative is poorly reabsorbed. Only 10-20% of the drug is excreted in urine at usual doses, but more is excreted if the liver capacity is exceeded. Biliary obstruction impairs biliary excretion. Probenecid doubles rifampin serum levels in humans by depressing hepatic uptake and slowing deacetylation.

Adverse Effects. A number of reactions to rifampin therapy have been reported. Hypersensitivity reactions are uncommon, but intermittent use of the drug has been associated with a syndrome that resembles influenza (3). There are fever, chills, myalgias, and nausea several hours after ingestion of the drug. Hepatotoxicity is difficult to interpret because it occurs most often when the drug is administered with isoniazid. Thrombocytopenia on an immunological basis has occurred. Again, it has been seen most often with intermittent therapy. Leukopenia is rare. Interstitial nephritis is a rare side effect.

Rifampin interferes with the metabolism of a number of other drugs. It diminishes the activity of anticoagulants and of prednisone. It also reduces the efficacy of contraceptive medication. Rifampin also appears to have some immunosuppressive properties, at least in test tube systems and in animal tests. The meaning of this T-cell depression is not established.

Therapeutic Uses. The primary use of rifampin is in the treatment of tuberculosis (12). It also has a major role in the therapy of leprosy. It has been used as prophylaxis of close family contact of individuals with meningitis due to *N. meningitidis*. It is being evaluated as prophylaxis of family contacts of *Haemophilus* meningitis. It has also been used in combination with a semisynthetic penicillin or cephalosporin to treat endocarditis or osteomyelitis due to "tolerant" staphylococci, *S. aureus* or *S. epidermidis*. This use is also under study. The agent has no role in treatment of infections due to gram-negative bacilli or to treat respiratory tract infections due to gram-positive species. In both situations, resistance rapidly develops, and it has not proved effective in treatment of acute exacerbations of bronchitis due to *Haemophilus*.

Rifampin has been combined with amphotericin to treat selected fungal infections because the agents have been shown to act synergistically *in vitro*. There is so far no substantial evidence to support this use.

REFERENCES

1. Eykyn, S., Phillips, L. and Evans, J. Vancomycin for staphylococcal shunt site infections in patients on regular hemodialysis. *Br. Med. J.* 3:80, 1970.
2. Fekety, R. Vancomycin. *Med. Clin. North Am.* 66:175, 1982.
3. Grosset, J. and Leventis, S. Adverse effects of rifampin. *Rev. Infect. Dis.* (suppl. 3) 5:440, 1983.
4. Hoeprich, P.D. The polymyxins. *Med. Clin. North Am.* 54:1257, 1970.
5. Jensen, K. and Lassen, H.C.A. Fulminating staphylococcal infections treated with fucidin and penicillin or semisynthetic penicillin. *Ann. Intern. Med.* 60:790, 1964.
6. Kirby, W.M.M., Perry, D.M. and Bauer, A.W. Treatment of staphylococcal septicemia with vancomycin: Report of thirty-three cases. *N. Engl. J. Med.* 262:49, 1960.
7. Koch-Weser, J., Sidel, V.W., Federman, E.B., Kanarek, P., Finer, D.C. and Eaton, E.A. Adverse effects of sodium colistimethate: Manifestations and specific reaction rates during 317 courses of therapy. *Ann. Intern. Med.* 72:857, 1970.
8. Kunin, C.M. and Bugg, A. Binding of polymyxin antibiotics to tissues: The major determinant of distribution and persistence in the body. *J. Infect. Dis.* 124:394, 1971.
9. McCormack, W.M. and Finland, M. Drugs five years later: Spectinomycin. *Ann. Intern. Med.* 84:712, 1976.
10. Nord, M.M. and Hoeprich, P.D. Polymyxin B and colistin: A critical comparison. *N. Engl. J. Med.* 270:1030, 1964.
11. Riley, H.D., Jr. Vancomycin and novobiocin. *Med. Clin. North Am.* 54:1277, 1970.
12. Sarde, M.E. (ed.). The use of rifampin in the treatment of nontuberculosis infections. *Rev. Infect. Dis.* (suppl. 3) 5:399, 1982.

CHEMOTHERAPY OF SPECIFIC SYSTEMIC INFECTIOUS DISEASES

CHAPTER 25

CHAPTER
25.1

ANTIVIRAL AGENTS

Donald P. Levine

Although viruses are among the most common disease-causing agents and despite the fact that over 200 years have passed since Jenner introduced vaccination for the prevention of viral disease, treatment with specific antiviral chemotherapy remains an infant science. Understanding the basic nature of viruses and the mechanism of viral replication helps explain this paradox.

BIOLOGY OF VIRUS

All viruses are composed of a nucleic acid core, either deoxyribonucleic acid (DNA) or ribonucleic acid (RNA) plus nucleoproteins, enclosed by a protein coat, the capsid. Some viruses are also surrounded by an outer lipoprotein envelope. Since they are devoid of the intracellular materials for basic cellular metabolism and division, they are dependent on the host cell for survival and replication. Thus they are obligate, intracellular parasites.

Viral replication involves several sequential steps. First, the organism must come into contact with and attach itself to a living cell, a process requiring specific receptor sites. Next, penetration occurs, either by engulfment of the viral particle or by fusion of the lipid envelope with the cell membrane. Within the cell the protein coat is removed in the uncoating step, and the nucleic acid is transported to the site of replication—either the nucleus (often the case for DNA viruses) or the cytoplasm (frequently so for RNA viruses). The viral nucleic acid is then transcribed into messenger RNA (mRNA) in RNA viruses, and viral protein synthesis is initiated, either via host cell enzymes or virus-induced enzymes. During the assembly step, the newly synthesized nucleic acids and proteins are joined, thereby forming whole virus particles. These particles, called virions, are then released from the cell by budding, at which time the organism may acquire its lipoprotein envelope, the composition of which varies depending on the type of cell involved. During replication, normal cell functions generally cease while the host machinery is directed toward production of virus. In fact, cell death may occur, either during replication or at the time of virus release from the cell. Once released from the host cell, the organism is free to repeat the cycle in any other susceptible cell. In this fashion multiplication of virus and host cell injury occurs.

In the process of viral replication several steps appear potentially amenable to the action of antiviral substances: (1) adsorption; (2) penetration; (3) uncoating; (4) synthesis of viral nucleic acids and proteins; (5) assembly; and, (6) release. This chapter will consider synthetic substances designed for their specific antiviral activity.

ANTIVIRAL AGENTS

Figure 25.1-1 illustrates how the different steps of viral replication are interrupted by principal antiviral agents available at present, namely amantadine, methisazone, idoxuridine, vidarabine, acyclovir, and interferon. These drugs along with some related agents will be discussed in this chapter. The reader may also wish to refer to several recent reviews of antiviral chemotherapy (26, 31).

AMANTADINE

Amantadine hydrochloride (1-adamantanamine hydrochloride) is a synthetic salt of a primary amine possessing an unusual asymmetrical cagelike structure (18) as shown in Fig. 25.1-2.

Antiviral Activity. Amantadine is active against a variety of RNA viruses, primarily those in the orthomyxo and paramyxo groups (20). Its major activity is against influenza A viruses. Despite the sensitivity of a number of animal viruses and even some tumor viruses, there are no current, clinical applications other than prevention and treatment of influenza (5).

Mechanism of Action. Amantadine exerts its maximum inhibitory effect 5 min to 1 hr after viral exposure by interfering with the engulfment of virus into the cell (20). Trypsin removes the drug from membranes, leaving

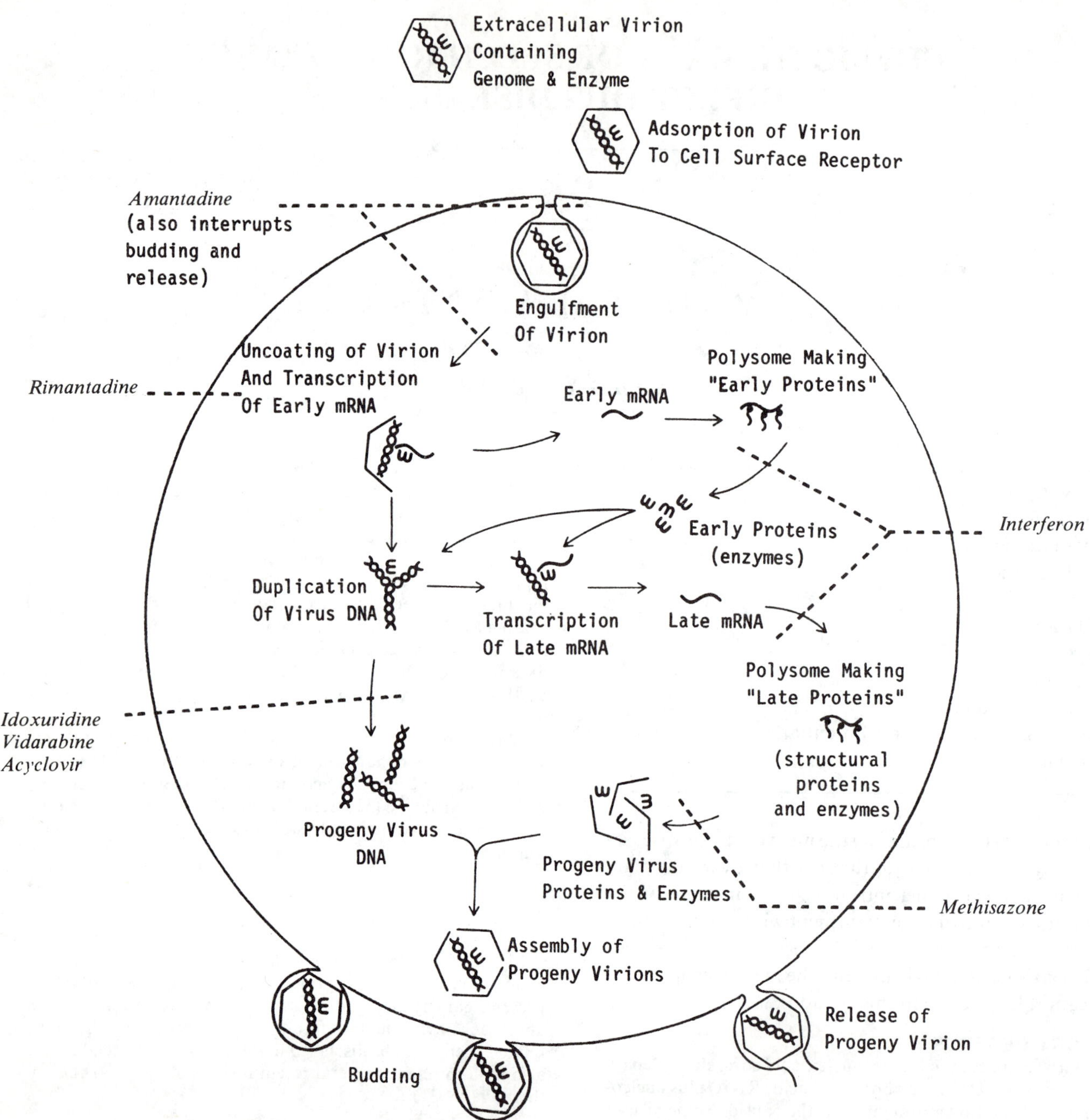

Fig. 25.1-1. *The possible interruption of steps in viral replication by various antiviral agents (---line represents interruption of a step).* (Modified from Ref. 47).

the cells more susceptible to viral infections (46). Nevertheless, inhibition of penetration may be a minor effect. Amantadine also interferes with the uncoating of viral nucleic acid (50), and may inhibit budding and release of newly formed virions by attaching to the cell's plasma membrane (35).

Pharmacokinetics. Amantadine is rapidly absorbed after oral administration and reaches peak blood levels 1-4 hr after ingestion. In human volunteers, the half-life varies between 9 and 15 hr (7). The usual dose of 100 mg orally every 12 hr leads to rapid distribution, with maximum internal organ concentration 48 hr after administration. Peak concentration occurs in the liver (12.4%) followed by kidney (5.2%), lungs (2.0%), spleen (0.7%) and heart (0.3%). Blood levels after a 200- to 300-mg daily oral dose range from 0.27 μg/ml to 1.05 μg/ml.

Metabolism and excretion vary with different species (7). Humans excrete up to 86% of a single dose unchanged in the urine according to first-order kinetics. A small amount of the drug is excreted unchanged in the feces. The rate of urinary excretion depends on urine pH. Acid urine facilitates rapid

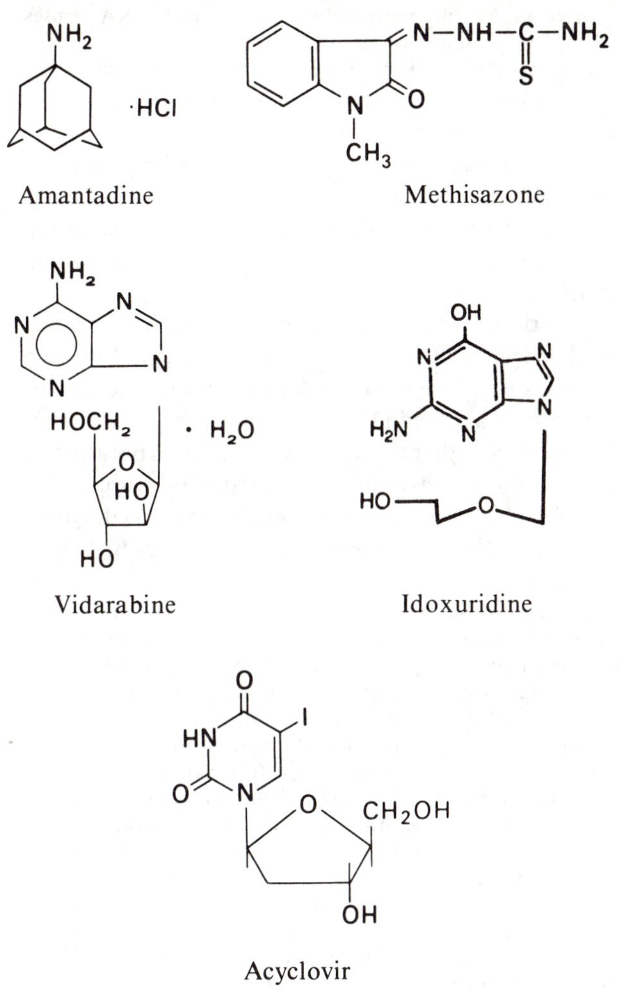

Amantadine

Methisazone

Vidarabine

Idoxuridine

Acyclovir

Fig. 25.1-2. *Chemical structures of antiviral agents.*

excretion. Thus combining the agent with bicarbonate might help maintain higher tissue concentration. Both plasma elimination and renal excretion are decreased in renal failure, necessitating a reduction in dose. Dialysis removes only a small fraction of the total body accumulation (85).

Adverse Effects. Dogs treated with a high dose (93 mg/kg) experienced central nervous system stimulation with tremor, myoclonus, and vomiting. In volunteers experiencing mild reactions after an initial 200-mg dose symptoms abated after continued use (18). When doses exceeded 400 mg/day, approximately 40% of healthy volunteers developed side effects (i.e., alteration of emotional state, depression, inability to concentrate, and anxiety). Symptoms began 3 hr after the dose and were gone by 6 hr if no additional drug was given. Insomnia has also been observed at high levels. There have also been reports of dry mouth, constipation, nausea, vomiting, diarrhea, and edema. Livedo reticularis has been noted 1 month to a year after continued use (18). All of amantadine's side effects occur more frequently in the elderly. Accordingly, the drug should be used cautiously in elderly patients, as well as patients with epilepsy, and those using central nervous system stimulants.

Therapeutic Uses. Amantadine is effective in prophylaxis and treatment of influenza A_2 strains. For prophylaxis the drug is taken before exposure or as soon as possible afterwards and is continued for as long as there is influenza present in the community. Volunteers taking 200 mg/day had 50-100% decreased incidence of disease. In addition, among amantadine users, there were fewer viral isolations and 50-70% fewer increases in serological titers. Amantadine was also shown to be preventive in family contacts and against hospital-acquired infection (18). There is an advantage of amantadine over vaccine for prophylactic purposes. Influenza undergoes antigenic drift, making a previously effective vaccine obsolete, whereas amantadine is effective against all influenza A strains. Amantadine also can be used therapeutically. It promotes more rapid disappearance of signs and symptoms, and there is faster recovery in small airways (18, 46, 53, 85). It may also be important that the drug significantly reduces the amount of viral shedding.

ANALOGS OF AMANTADINE

Rimantadine (α-methyl-1-adamantane methylamine hydrochloride), an analog of amantadine, is reported to be more active *in vitro* and *in vivo* and is better tolerated, allowing higher doses with fewer side effects. Its mechanism of action is similar to amantadine; it blocks the second step of virus uncoating that is an early stage of viral replication (9). In early clinical trials both rimantadine and the parent compound proved to have definite but similar antiviral activity with minimal side effects. In a more recent placebo-controlled, double-blind randomized trial, rimantadine was shown to be equally efficacious compared with amantadine, but was significantly less toxic ($p < 0.05$). The authors recommended rimantadine be considered the drug of choice for the prophylaxis of influenza A (25). However, it appears the major difference may be related to the pharmacokinetics of the two drugs; similar doses of the agents results in lower serum concentrations of rimantadine. Side effects have been shown to relate directly to the serum concentration (41).

METHISAZONE

Methisazone (1-methyl-1H-indole-2,3-dione 3-thiosemicarbazone) is the 1-methyl derivative of isatin 3-thiosemicarbazone and has the chemical structure as shown in Fig. 25.1-2.

Antiviral Activity. Like other ring semicarbazones, methisazone has activity against a variety of poxviruses. Unfortunately *in vitro* activity correlates poorly with *in vivo* activity (5). Derivations are effective against alastrum (a smallpox variant) and slightly less active against *variola major* (smallpox). Other DNA viruses are inhibited, but require higher concentrations than are clinically useful. Some RNA viruses are also inhibited (e.g., rhinovirus, ECHO virus, reovirus, influenza, parainfluenza, and poliovirus). Resistance to methisazone develops in pox viruses and vaccinia after several passages in tissue culture. Indeed synthesis of some strains is dependent upon the drug.

Mechanism of Action. The drug is known to adopt different steric configurations that form bi- and tridentate ligands. These ligands form complexes with metallic molecules, particularly copper, zinc, iron, and cobalt, and also sulfur and nitrogen. It is postulated that methisazone operates by interacting with metallo enzymes that are necessary for the replication of certain viruses. Sensitive organisms in direct contact with the drug are not inactivated, proving the site of action to be intracellular. It has no direct effect on viral DNA but appears to inhibit late stages in the viral growth cycle. Production of mRNA procedes normally, but translation of viral protein is blocked.

Pharmacokinetics. Methisazone is poorly absorbed from the gastrointestinal tract. Plasma levels vary after an oral dose. The maximum level is reached 4-8 hr after a dose. A peak level of 6.3 μg/ml can be obtained after a single 3-g dose in an adult. At 12 hr, most of the drug is eliminated.

Metabolism follows several paths including demethylation, replacement of S by O in the side chain and hydroxylation in the aromatic ring. Changes at the 4 and 7 positions may also occur. One of the metabolites, isatin 3-thiosemicarbazone, has approximately half the antiviral activity of the parent compound.

Interaction. In the presence of barbiturates, hydroxylated forms conjugated with glucuronic and sulfuric acids may appear. Methisazone competes with anesthetics for hepatic detoxification, and anesthesia may be prolonged. Methisazone may interfere with alcohol metabolism since it produces a marked alcohol intolerance.

Adverse Effects. Being relatively insoluble, the drug has low toxicity. In small animals LD_{50} exceeds 2000 mg/kg. Rhesus monkeys given 250 mg/kg/day orally for 1 month developed liver injury, but rats and dogs remained healthy. High doses are teratogenic in rabbits and prevent pregnancy in rats (5).

Therapeutic Uses. Primary use of methisazone is for prophylaxis of smallpox contacts and for treatment of vaccinia skin infections. It should be given on an empty stomach, since the drug delays gastric emptying. Methisazone is contraindicated in patients with liver dysfunction unless they are smallpox contacts or suffer severe complications of smallpox vaccination. Since smallpox has been eradicated, this drug appears to be of historical interest only.

IDOXURIDINE

Idoxuridine (5-iodo-2-deoxyuridine, IUdR) is a synthetic nucleoside analog containing a natural sugar, deoxyribose, with the chemical formula shown in Fig. 25.1-2.

Antiviral Activity. Initially IUdR was noted to have activity against vaccinia and herpes simplex virus, herpes simplex type 1 being more sensitive than type 2. Resistance to IUdR has developed, but its clinical significance is unknown. Other viruses found to be sensitive to IUdR are pseudorabies, B virus, myxoma virus, and some papovaviruses (5). Varicella zoster (VZ) is sensitive to IUdR, a fact that contributed to its recognition as a DNA virus. Cytomegalovirus is sensitive *in vitro*; adenoviruses are only marginally sensitive; and RNA viruses are completely insensitive.

Mechanism of Action. IUdR inhibits the replication of herpes viruses by preventing the assembly of viral components after they are synthesized, perhaps by inhibiting the synthesis of a protein required for assembly (49). An unusual aspect of IUdR is its ability to induce viral replication in certain cell hybrids. This may be an indication that the drug itself inhibits an intracellular-inhibiting protein.

In addition, IUdR, as an analog of thymidine, inhibits several enzymes important in nucleic acid and protein synthesis such as thymidine kinase, thymidine monophosphate kinase, and DNA polymerase, and is incorporated into DNA, thereby decreasing the incorporation of thymidine itself; it also produces errors in transcription and DNA-chain separation by causing increased hydrogen bonding. None of these effects entirely prevents DNA synthesis.

Pharmacokinetics. Four hours after an intravenous drip in humans, 43% of the drug appears in the urine, of which 60% is 5-iodouracil and 40% is inorganic iodide. By 24 hr 89% of the administered drug is excreted; at 48 hr approximately 95%. Nevertheless, IUdR is still detected in some tissues for as long as 70 hr after administration. The drug does not penetrate the noninflammed meninges (10), nor is it found in high concentrations in the cerebrospinal fluid (CSF) of patients with encephalitis. However, in the brain and CSF IUdR is rapidly converted to iodouracil and iodide (10). Following subconjunctival injection a therapeutic level is reached in the cornea by 30 min and a high concentration is maintained for 4 hr. Topical administration to the conjunctival sac for 3 days yields detectable levels in the cornea and conjunctiva as well as the lens and iris, but systemic levels 1000-fold below the toxic range are measured, indicating its safety when administered as an ophthalmic preparation (54).

Adverse Effects. IUdR is toxic to dividing cells. Adverse effects are dose related, occurring in all patients at a total dose exceeding 600 mg/kg, in two-thirds of the patients at 400-600 mg/kg, and in very few at doses under 400 mg/kg. When infused rapidly (50 mg/min), toxicity is minimized and the clinical effect is maximized. Adverse effects most commonly seen are thrombocytopenia, neutropenia, and stomatitis (58). Troublesome effects include anorexia, nausea, vomiting, alopecia, transient ridging of the nails, and mild iodism. Cholestatic jaundice has been reported. In animals, IUdR has a potent teratogenic effect (71).

On topical application IUdR inhibits epithelial cell DNA metabolism and causes secondary allergic responses. In the eye, the most common side effect is follicular conjunctivitis that may cause lacrimation, lymphoid follicle formation, inflammation, ptosis, and swelling of the limbus. Ultimately, scarring and corneal vascularization may occur. Corneal clouding and edema are observed, as is contact dermatitis of the eyelids. Fortunately, most of these toxic manifestations are reversible (21). When IUdR is given in solution with DMSO, most reactions to this combination are believed secondary to the vehicle.

They consist of contact dermatitis, wheals, and a garlic or metallic taste.

Therapeutic Uses. Parenteral therapy with IUdR is too toxic, and its use is limited to topical administration. IUdR in an aqueous base solution has proved effective in the treatment of varicella zoster keratitis. When combined with DMSO, which facilitates absorption, results were encouraging in both herpes simplex and varicella zoster infections (48). However, DMSO is not approved in the United States for human use. In recurrent genital herpes infection, although patients receiving the drug fared better than the controls during the initial episode, no significant difference in the recurrence rate was detected after a 2-year follow-up period (59).

ANALOGS OF IDOXURIDINE

Trifluorothymidine (5-trifluoromethyl-2′-deoxyuridine, F_3T) is a synthetic nucleoside with a natural sugar—deoxyribose.

Antiviral Effects. F_3T is active against herpes simplex virus (including IUdR-resistant strains), vaccinia, and adenovirus, and in comparative studies is effective in lower concentrations than other nucleoside analogs (61).

Mechanism of Action. After penetration of the host cell, F_3T is converted to the 5-monophosphate, the active compound, which is incorporated into replicating viral DNA, causing chain breaks and abnormal base pairing. In addition, F_3T interferes with the enzymes thymidylate synthetase and deoxythymidine kinase and mimics the feedback inhibition by deoxythymidine triphosphate. The final result is the production of abnormal progeny virus components incapable of causing further damage (61).

Pharmacokinetics. In animals, the half-life of F_3T is approximately 30 min. Urinary excretion of the parent compound and its metabolites is rapid. When applied topically to the eye, significant levels appear in the aqueous humor by 30 min. By 90 min the drug is no longer detectable. Ocular penetration is reduced in noninfected eyes. Metabolism of F_3T involves removal of the deoxyribose by nucleoside phosphorylase, with conversion to trifluorothymine. Adults metabolize the drug faster than children. F_3T is protein bound and only slightly incorporated into DNA (23).

Adverse Effects. F_3T affects rapidly metabolizing cells. Hematological findings include neutropenia, anemia, megaloblastosis, and reticulocytopenia. Hypophosphatemia and hypocalcemia occur frequently. Aside from occasional stomatitis, gastrointestinal toxicity is infrequent. In animals, F_3T is far less teratogenic than IUdR. The ophthalmic preparation may cause punctate epithelial erosions and microcysts. With continued use, epithelial edema without stromal swelling or punctate narrowing may result (61).

Therapeutic Uses. In the treatment of herpes keratitis, F_3T is significantly more effective than IUdR and vidarabine, and it is generally considered the drug of choice. However, its toxicity is intermediate between the two (61). In view of its known teratogenic effects, its use during pregnancy is contraindicated.

VIDARABINE

Vidarabine (adenine arabinoside; ARA-A, 1-β-D-arabinofuranosyladenine) is a nucleoside with an unnatural pentose sugar—arabinose. Unlike other nucleoside antiviral agents that have pyrimidine bases, ARA-A has a purine base (Fig. 25.1-2).

Antiviral Activity. ARA-A is effective against vaccinia, herpes simplex virus (HSV) (HSV-1 being more sensitive than HSV-2), cytomegalovirus (less sensitive than HSV-1), and varicella zoster. Other DNA viruses inhibited are pseudorabies, herpes virus saimiri, and myxoma virus. A single RNA virus, Rous sarcoma virus, which depends on DNA synthesis for replication, is also inhibited.

Mechanism of Action. Antiviral activity is greatest during the period corresponding to viral DNA synthesis 2-4 hr after infection. Either viral DNA polymerase or virus-induced ribonucleotide reductase is inhibited. ARA-A is not incorporated into DNA, nor does it inhibit naturally occurring nucleotides (62). Adenosine kinase is also inhibited by ARA-A, which may not be related to its antiviral activity.

Pharmacokinetics. Intramuscular injections of ARA-A are poorly absorbed. When given intravenously at 1 mg/kg, a plasma concentration of 1.4 μg/ml is obtained after 30 min; by 8 hr, none is detectable. The half-life is 30 min. After infusing 10-20 mg/kg/day for 4-10 days, the serum concentration increases rapidly to a peak of 3-6 μg/ml, but quickly falls when the infusion is stopped. This serum level reflects the concentration of ARA-A hypoxanthine (ARA-Hx, the major metabolite produced by deamination of ARA-A by xanthine oxidase) rather than the drug itself. ARA-Hx has approximately 20% as much antiviral activity as the parent compound. Further metabolism to the free base does not occur in humans.

Daily administration lengthens the half-life to 3.5 hr, but there is no accumulation (62). Continuous infusion on the other hand, results in continually increasing levels of both ARA-A and ARA-Hx. Urinary excretion of the hypoxanthine accounts for the major part of the dose and is greatest 12 hr after the infusion; 41-57.8% of the administered dose is excreted daily.

Brain levels (determined at autopsy) approximate those in plasma (which makes it useful in the treatment of encephalitis). Up to 35% of the administered dose enters the CSF (62) where approximately one-half the serum concentration is detected primarily as the hypoxanthine.

Adverse Effects. Toxicity of ARA-A includes the following (67): (1) nausea, vomiting, and anorexia, especially at higher doses; (2) weight loss; (3) weakness, which is more pronounced at higher doses; (4) megaloblastic changes in the bone marrow, primarily in the erythroid series but affecting all cell lines; (5) generalized essential tremors that occur after 5-7 days of therapy, exacerbate with activity and intention, are worse during the waking state, and rapidly improve after withdrawal of the drug; and, (6) thrombophlebitis at the site of the intravenous cannula, which is probably related to continuous infusion. Other toxic manifestations include trancelike conditions resembling akinetic mutism and chromosome breakage. The major adverse effect of ophthalmic ARA-A is transient stinging that occurs immediately.

Therapeutic Uses. Against herpetic (HSV and VZ) keratitis, ARA-A has been found to be as effective as

IUdR and F_3T. In patients with herpes simplex virus encephalitis, ARA-A at an intravenous dose of 15 mg/kg significantly decreased morbidity and mortality without evidence of acute drug toxicity (80). For these beneficial effects the drug must be given early, before neurological deficit is fixed, since the outcome is dependent on the neurological status at the onset of therapy. Also, younger patients respond better (81). Nevertheless, relapses occur, and in at least one such case virus was recovered from the brain following previous successful vidarabine treatment (24). The drug is licensed for use in biopsy-proved cases. Vidarabine also has favorable effects in neonatal herpes simplex infections (82).

In disseminated varicella zoster infection ARA-A at 5-20 mg/kg for 15 days prevented new lesion formation within 4 days; however, intact host immunity is required for successful therapy. Administration of ARA-A prior to dissemination of disease caused more rapid cessation of new lesion formation and accelerated healing, but even those receiving placebo did well. A more recent study in immunosuppressed patients demonstrated accelerated cutaneous healing and decreased cutaneous dissemination, visceral complications, and duration of post-therapeutic neuralgia, especially in patients with lymphoproliferative disease and patients over 38 years of age (79).

In cytomegalovirus (CMV) infections, there were some beneficial responses in pneumonia and urinary excretion of virus; CMV mononucleosis and disseminated CMV following renal transplantation were unaffected. Results were better in patients receiving 15-20 mg/kg/day. In hepatitis B-associated chronic active hepatitis, there were reduced titers of hepatitis B surface antigen (HB_SAG), as well as decreases in DNA polymerase activity (63). Toxicity of ARA-A may be unusually high and may limit usefulness of the drug in genital herpes infections. The use of ARA-A ointment has been disappointing.

VIDARABINE ANALOGS

Two analogs, vidarabine-5′-monophosphate and vidarabine hypoxanthine-5′-monophosphate, appear to be promising in experimental animal infections. Their major advantage appears to be greater solubility than vidarabine, which allows administration in much smaller fluid volumes. However, the efficacy of the 5′-monophosphate was equivalent to the parent compound in patients with chronic active hepatitis (44).

ACYCLOVIR (ACYCLOGUANOSINE)

The newest addition to the list of antivirals approved for clinical use is acycloguanosine (9-[2-hydroxyethoxymethyl] guanine), known as acyclovir. This agent belongs to a new class of antiviral agents with potent antiviral activity, and containing an acyclic side chain, 2-hydroxymethoxymethyl, at the 9 position. Its chemical structure is shown in Fig. 25.1-2. Current information about acyclovir has been summarized in a recent symposium (30) and a comprehensive review (66).

Antiviral Activity. Acyclovir inhibits herpes simplex virus type 1 at a concentration as low as 0.01 μM. Against HSV, it is 160 times more active than vidarabine and 10 times more active than idoxuridine. Unlike other drugs, activity is not diminished against HSV-2. It is selective for viruses of the herpes group, inhibiting multiplication of varicella zoster, and B virus, but not other DNA viruses or any RNA viruses. Since cytomegalovirus and Epstein-Barr virus do not produce virus-specific thymidine kinase, they require a different mechanism of action and are only marginally inhibited by acyclovir.

Mechanism of Action. Acyclovir is phosphorylated by HSV deoxythymidine kinase and not the corresponding host enzyme. It is then further phosphorylated to the triphosphate. This conversion occurs to only a limited extent in uninfected cells, indicating activity is related to the infecting organism. In fact, the triphosphate inhibits HSV DNA polymerase far more effectively than the normal cellular DNA polymerase. Consequently, it is extremely selective; inhibition of host cells requires a drug concentration several 1000-fold greater than necessary to inhibit the organism (33). Unfortunately, development of resistance to a acyclovir may limit its usefulness. Resistance may develop by several different mechanisms; some viruses may fail to produce thymidine kinase or may produce thymidine kinase with low affinity for the drug. Alternatively, DNA polymerase that is insensitive to the effects of phosphorylated acyclovir may be produced.

Pharmacokinetics. Gastrointestinal absorption is poor in animals. After subcutaneous injection, 94% is excreted unchanged over a 24-hr period. A minor metabolite excreted in the urine, 1% is 9-carboxymethoxymethyl guanine. Tissue distribution studies reveal rapid disappearance by 2 hr after administration, followed by slower disappearance for up to 24 hr. Blood levels are lower than in lung, liver, and intestine, but greater than in the brain. Nevertheless, brain levels are still detectable 24 hr after administration. Protein binding does not occur at low concentrations but at 88 μM/ml is 12.7%.

In humans, multiple intravenous doses (5 mg/kg every 8 hr) achieve steady-state mean peak plasma concentrations (9.7 μg/ml) that should be adequate to treat HSV-1, HSV-2, varicella zoster, and Epstein-Barr virus infections (66). The elimination half-life following i.v. infusion is approximately 2-3 hr, with most excreted through the kidneys (22, 72). In renal failure the drug accumulates, and the half-life is prolonged up to 19.5 hr. In addition, the drug is metabolized and excreted up to 44% as an inactive metabolite, carboxymethoxymethyl guanine. Acyclovir is removed by hemodialysis (52). The drug is incompletely absorbed following oral administration (73) but is not affected by food. An oral dose of 200 mg every 4 hr is associated with mean peak serum levels of 0.5 μg/ml (73). Topical administration results in little systemic absorption. Nevertheless, multiple ocular applications of a 3% ointment result in a concentration of 1.7 μg/ml in the aqueous humor (66).

Following intravenous infusion in humans, acyclovir has been found in kidney, lung, liver, heart, skin vesicles, nervous tissue, and cerebrospinal fluid, the latter in concentrations approximately 50% of serum, a fact that makes the drug theoretically attractive for central nervous system infection.

Adverse Effects. Toxicity is produced at very high doses, up to 1000 mg/kg in mice. In a mouse model of HSV-1 encephalitis, animals treated with acyclovir fared better than controls. Some survived without evidence of illness. Likewise, herpetic keratitis in rabbits and cutaneous herpes infections in guinea pigs respond well to a 1% ointment. In humans, acyclovir is well tolerated regardless of the route of administration (33). Ocular administration may be associated with transient burning or stinging and mild hypersensitivity reactions, but rarely have side effects necessitated stopping the drug. Topical application has also been associated with mild local reactions (pain, burning, stinging) that are only rarely severe enough to terminate therapy. Oral therapy is also very well tolerated; side effects have been similar to those caused by placebo. Inflammation and phlebitis are caused by extravasation of the drug. The major untoward effect of intravenous administration is transient impairment of renal function, apparently related to crystallization of the drug. This problem is alleviated by appropriate dilution and infusion rate of acyclovir and concurrent hydration of the patient.

Therapeutic Uses. Unquestionably, the high antiviral activity and low toxicity make this drug an outstanding candidate for use against the multiple manifestations of herpes virus infections in humans. Numerous studies have demonstrated its therapeutic spectrum. Topical acyclovir is comparable with other effective antiviral agents in the treatment of experimental herpetic keratitis, including infection caused by drug-resistant strains (76, 77). Efficacy has also been reported in human ocular herpetic infection (70). When compared with placebo in the treatment of primary genital herpes simplex virus infections, topical acyclovir relieved symptoms, decreased the duration of viral shedding from 7.1 to 4.1 days, and accelerated the time to lesion crusting. It did not shorten the total time to healing, prevent new lesions, or diminish the frequency or severity of recurrences. Men with recurrent disease had reduced time to crusting of lesions; a similar effect was not noted in women (16, 65). In severely immunocompromised patients, topical acyclovir resulted in significantly diminished pain and more rapid elimination of virus, but did not lead to faster healing of lesions (83). Several investigators have compared orally administered acyclovir with placebo in genital HSV infections. In initial infections treated with 200 mg orally 5 times daily, acyclovir decreased viral shedding and new lesion formation as well as the total duration of disease. Symptoms were also significantly improved (8). In patients with recurrent genital herpes infections, oral acyclovir reduced viral shedding and enhanced time to crusting and healing, or pain was not relieved. In addition, acyclovir appears to have no effect on the frequency of recurrent lesions (57). Intravenous acyclovir (5 mg/kg/day) is also effective therapy for initial genital herpes infections, in men more so than in women (17). In addition, intravenous acyclovir prevented herpetic lesions in patients undergoing bone marrow transplantation (although lesions did occur when therapy was discontinued) and prevented herpetic infections in patients undergoing therapy for acute leukemia (40, 68, 69). Other studies have also confirmed the value of intravenous acyclovir in severely immunocompromised patients (73, 78).

In nonimmunosuppressed patients with herpes zoster infections, acyclovir has been shown to ameliorate symptoms during the administration of the drug, although pain recurred in some patients posttreatment. In addition, acyclovir does not appear to prevent postherpetic neuralgia (6). Immunocompromised patients with varicella zoster infections have also been treated with acyclovir. In a double-blind randomized study in children with primary varicella, acyclovir was ineffective in terms of improvement of active lesions but did prevent visceral complications (64). In another double-blind study of patients with a variety of varicella zoster infections, acyclovir (500 mg/M^2 3 times daily for 7 days) was associated with fewer episodes of disease progression and treatment failures (3). Thus far there are no comparative trials of acyclovir for ophthalmic zoster infections.

Studies using acyclovir to treat cytomegalovirus infections are less encouraging, although in at least one instance intravenous acyclovir 500 mg/M^2 (3 times daily for 7 days) led to faster improvement and defervescence than placebo, but did not affect viral shedding or mortality (4). There are insufficient data to determine the utility of acyclovir in Epstein-Barr virus infections. Nevertheless, due to its proven efficacy in other infections, acyclovir has been approved and is available for use in topical, oral, and intravenous forms.

INTERFERON

In 1956, Isaacs and Lindemann reported the discovery of an antiviral substance produced by the very cells that were infected (45). This substance, interferon (IFN), is a heterogeneous glycoprotein. With appropriate stimulation, cells can be induced to produce IFN which, depending on the cell producer and the conditions of production, may form multimeric aggregates of smaller-molecular-weight species. These multimers possess the same activity as the monomer, which, if induced by viruses in human tissues, has a molecular weight of 12,000 (in a low-ionic environment) or 24,000 (in a high-salt environment). Other inducers stimulate interferon species with a molecular weight as high as 100,000. Although more than 20 genes code for IFN, which may explain the different molecular species, the different forms are similar enough to be inactivated by a single neutralizing serum. Standards for IFN have been set, with 1 U of interferon defined as the reciprocal of the highest dilution of a sample that reduces viral growth or effects by some appreciable amount (generally 50%) from the control (43).

Interferon is classified into types on the basis of antigenic specificities. These are alpha (α), beta (β) and gamma (γ). α-and β-IFNs are usually acid stable; γ-IFNs are usually acid labile. Currently, IFN is derived from several souces: (1) Primary human leukocytes (for IFN-α) following virus stimulation, which is impractical as a major source. (2) Human lymphoblastoid cell lines stimulated by virus: It can be reproduced in large quantities. It is stable and can undergo rigorous purification. But these are malignant cell lines, and safety of IFN so derived has not been documented. (3) Human skin fibroblast cultures: IFN-β can be produced in large quantities and does not carry the risk of viral or malignant contamination, but it possesses different biological activity. (4) Recently, cloning technology has resulted in the production of homogenous IFNs that can be produced in large quantities without the disadvantages of the other methods. The therapeutic potential of these IFNs is now being explored.

Antiviral Activity. Viruses have variable sensitivity to IFN, although in tissue cell cultures virtually all are inhibited to some extent (36). Herpes viruses are relatively resistant; among them varicella zoster (VZ) is most sensitive and HSV-1 more so than HSV-2. All strains of adenoviruses tested so far have limited sensitivity. Widely different responses are found between serotypes of rhinoviruses, although within serotypes all respond similarly, regardless of the IFN types (11). Arboviruses and myxoviruses are the most sensitive organisms, although strain variability exists. Interferon also inhibits encephalomyocarditis virus, vesicular stomatitis virus, Rous sarcoma virus, parainfluenza, cytomegalovirus, rabies, foot and mouth disease virus, Japanese encephalitis virus, influenza B and A_2, vaccinia, West Nile virus, and Newcastle disease virus. Visna virus, a retrovirus that causes a slow infection of sheep is insensitive to IFN; IFN may thus be ineffective against slow virus disease of humans (12).

Mechanism of Action. Interferon causes the synthesis of a protein that exerts an effect at the ribosomal level, interfering with the synthesis of viral coded, functional enzymes, and structural coat proteins necessary for viral replication. Among the enzymes are viral RNA replicase, viral DNA polymerase, and viral thymidine kinase. This inhibitory protein, referred to as translational-inhibitory protein, and its messenger RNA are still unidentified, and the exact site of its inhibition is unclear. It may prevent the translation of viral mRNA or possibly the transcription of viral RNA polymerase or transfer-RNA (tRNA), either of which would be manifested as inhibition at the translational level. Transcription of the viral genome may also be inhibited (43). Intracellular inhibition of viral replication caused by IFN is potentiated by the addition of 3′,5′-cyclic adenosine monophosphate (36). The nature of IFN effect on host cell function is not clear. It is of interest to note that, at least *in vitro*, combining different IFNs has been shown to produce synergistic antiviral effects (87).

Pharmacokinetics. Interferon is not absorbed orally, thus parenteral therapy is mandatory. High peak levels with rapid clearing follow intravenous infusion, although higher doses result in more sustained peaks. The half-life after intravenous infusion is approximately 20 min. Blood levels are lower after subcutaneous and intramuscular injection, but have a more sustained plateau. This may be due to passage across endothetial cells into capillaries. When applied directly to the nasal mucosa, the concentration of IFN decreases rapidly (5- to 50-fold) over the first 5 min, but is still measurable at 1 hr. Apparently it spreads quickly and binds to nasal epithelial cells. High levels are recoverable via nasal wash. The various IFN types behave differently after injection. Interferon-β given intravenously is cleared more slowly than IFN-α, whereas no differences are seen with the intramuscular route (27). Partially purified IFN enters the blood faster than purified concentrated IFN.

Tissue distribution of IFN from the blood is poor, with little diffusion into the respiratory tract, CSF, brain, aqueous or vitreous humor, fetal blood, saliva, gastrointestinal lumen, and urine. However, following induction by a potent interferon inducer, high levels in serum, brain, and CSF have been achieved (84). The metabolism of IFN is largely unknown. Approximately 10% is excreted in the urine; the fate of the rest is unknown. Interferon is concentrated in the reticuloendothelial system, particularly the liver (27). The volume of distribution in body water is lower than predicted, suggesting some form of tissue metabolism. It is interesting that cells exposed to IFN retain their antiviral activity for a long time, but the relationship, if any, between the metabolism and clinical activity of IFN is unknown.

Adverse Effects. Adverse effects of interferon include neutropenia, thrombocytopenia, fever, and interference with host serological responses to a variety of antigens. When using substances other than DNA recombinant interferon, there is the potential danger of transmitting slow viruses along with IFN since these agents are not inactivated by other methods of IFN production.

Therapeutic Uses. In a comprehensive study (56) involving three randomized double-blind, well-controlled trials, localized varicella zoster infection in cancer patients was treated with leukocyte interferon (4.2×10^4 U/kg/day to 5.1×10^5 U/kg/day). Serum levels in excess of 50 U/ml were obtained with the intermediate and highly purified preparations, and IFN accumulation occurred between the third and sixth day with the highest dose. Very early treatment prevented new lesion formation and lessened the extent of final involvement. Patients receiving the highest concentration had no distal cutaneous spread. IFN also protected against visceral involvement and postherpetic neuralgia. Fever, reticulocytopenia, and neutropenia were the only adverse effects, and IFN did not prevent the formation of complement fixation antibodies. In additional studies in immunocompromised children with zoster infection, IFN reduced the number of days of new lesion formation, prevented life-threatening dissemination, and reduced mortality (2).

Several studies using leukocyte interferon parenterally in chronic active *hepatitis B virus* infection have shown variable results. Some investigators reported diminution or elimination of laboratory indicators of active viral replication such as hepatitis B surface antigen (HB_sAG) and DNA polymerase activity, also hepatitis B core antigen (HB_cAG) and Dane particle-associated DNA (34); however, others have different findings with one or more of these parameters (34).

IFN has been used in nonrandomized fashion to treat both acquired and congenital cytomegalovirus (CMV) infections, with complete or partial clearing of viremia or viruria, but treatment adversely affects patients' immune response. However, the absence of controls prevents conclusions as to cause and effect, and in controlled therapeutic studies IFN has been disappointing in CMV infections. On the other hand, in a double-blind placebo-controlled prophylactic study, IFN was successful in reducing CMV syndromes and superinfections (42). Epstein-Barr virus shedding was diminished by α-interferon when used prophylactically in renal transplant recipients (14). Leukocyte IFN in combination with topical acyclovir significantly improved the healing time compared with acyclovir alone in patients with dendritic keratitis (15).

IFN has also been used in respiratory infections. Intranasal application prevented an influenza A_2 epidemic in the Soviet Union, where human leukocyte IFN is now available in pharmacies. In addition, freeze-dried IFN administered intranasally to a large number of children and neonates reduced the severity and duration of disease despite a relatively low dose (1). IFN nasal spray as prophylaxis against influenza B has had mixed result, although extremely high doses (14 million U/day) are effective against rhinovirus type 4 infection. Apparently, if given in adequate amounts, IFN can prevent some common respiratory infections.

In congenital rubella infections treated with IFN, viremia cleared, but viruria persisted (51). Dermal vaccinia and vaccinia keratitis respond to IFN (43). IFN may prove useful in combination with active immunization for postexposure rabies prophylaxis.

INTERFERON INDUCERS

In 1963, Isaacs deducted that cells produce interferon after exposure to chemically altered nucleic acids foreign to them or to the same host species. Although this has not been entirely correct, it has proved important in the development of a class of drugs known as interferon inducers. These agents have been classified into two types (43). Type I agents are specific IFN inducers, and type II activate lymphocytes and macrophages, inducing moderate amounts of interferon. Type I group includes class A drugs that are potent inducers (capable of stimulating > IFN 1000 U/ml in cell culture or intact animals following i.v. or i.p. injection) and are very specific. Most are a form of double-stranded RNA. Class B agents are moderate-to-poor inducers (producing < 1000 U/ml), have a narrower target spectrum, and are active only in animals, not in cell cultures.

One promising class A drug is polyriboinosinic polyribocytidilic acid polylysine (or poly rI.poly rC polylysine; poly IC-LC) and contains 2 mg of poly rI.poly rC/ml and 1.5 mg of poly-L-lysine/ml in 5% sodium carboxymethyl cellulose. Using this agent, Champney et al. (13) induced the highest levels of IFN ever recorded in humans. A daily dose of 0.2 mg/kg given over 90 min induced peak IFN concentrations at 4-8 hr, ranging from 50 to 800 U/ml. High levels persisted approximately 38 hr. Fever and lymphopenia commonly accompanied induced interferonemia, and transient, but occasionally severe, hypotension was observed on about the third day of treatment. This latter side effect necessitated alteration of the carboxymethyl cellulose molecule to develop a less toxic, lower-molecular-weight substance.

Tilorone hydrochloride (bis-diethyl-aminoethyl fluoronone) is an example of a class B inducer (43). This low-molecular-weight (412) aromatic amine is stable and soluble in water as the dihydrochloride salt. It is rapidly absorbed from the gut. A single oral dose in mice produces IFN for 24-48 hr with a peak concentration exceeding 1000 U/ml at 16 hr. It has a very low therapeutic ratio (toxic/protective dose), making it too dangerous to use. A similar drug under investigation is BL-20803 [4 (3-dimethylamino-propylamino)-1,3-dimethyl-1H-pyrazole-(3,4-b) quinolone dihydrochloride] (43). Both tilorone and BL-20803 appear to affect the same target cells (i.e., the splenic macrophages). Lymphocytes are not targets for IFN production by either drug.

Problems of Interferon Inducers. All IFN inducers (74), including virus infection, produce hyporeactivity (i.e., a diminished response upon reexposure). Characteristically, production is shut off within hours, even though the inducer is still present. The onset of hyporeactivity is inducer dependent. Hyporeactivity occurs as early as 24-48 hr with tilorone, whereas poly rI.poly rC induces IFN as long as 96 hr after injection (74). Cross-hyporeactivity also occurs (i.e., one agent causes a hyporeactive response to a different agent).

It may be hypothesized that hyporeactivity may be due to reactivation of a repressor either because of inducer breakdown or feedback by interferon itself, or both. Several mediators of hyporeactivity have been proposed. One is an antiviral protein that is induced by IFN, another a humoral substance distinguishable from IFN (36, 75). Either could act as a superrepressor, binding the operator locus previously depressed by the inducer and therefore inhibiting production. Alternatively such a substance could interfere with transcription or operate at a posttranscriptional site, such as the translation of mRNA.

Mechanism of Action. The specific mode of action of any interferon inducer is completely unknown. There is evidence, however, indicating that fixed and circulating cells of the reticuloendothelial system are good IFN producers (36). Lymphocytes, after achieving a more blastlike appearance, also produce circulating IFN. Interferon production is linked to immune recognition and apparently macrophages transfer information to leukocytes. Immunosuppressive agents affect induction, although immunosuppressed hosts are capable of IFN production.

Within any given cell, the capacity for IFN induction resides in the host genome, possibly at gene locus 21. It is postulated that more than one cistron is involved, each one coding for a different type of IFN, thus explaining the different molecular species. Most likely a repressor inactivates an operator gene adjacent to the IFN cistron, preventing continuous production. It appears that these cistrons are variably repressed, one more loosely than the other. Under the influence of an inducer, the repressor may be bound, causing the operator to switch on, resulting in the transcription of mRNA. The more loosely repressed cistron would quickly encode mRNA that could reach the ribosomes and initiate IFN synthesis. This IFN would be rapidly released, although it might confer some antiviral activity on the host cell. Although further proof of this mechanism is required, the necessity for new mRNA and protein synthesis for the production of IFN is unquestioned.

During the production of IFN, a control protein that terminates further synthesis is transcribed and translated. This protein acts at a posttranscriptional level, presumably during translation, and may be responsible for the hyporeactive state. This protein itself can be inhibited, resulting in a marked increase in IFN production (36, 43).

Adverse Effects. Nasal application of poly rI.poly rC produces irritation of the mucous membranes. On parenteral injection it produces fever, which may reach 105°F (74). Fever is dose related, occurring frequently between 1 and 10 mg/kg, and is unrelated to the amount of IFN induced. Other common effects are transient, minor changes in liver function tests, transient neutropenia, diminished *in vitro* lymphocyte DNA synthesis in response to mitogens (37, 74), and coagulation abnormalities (more common in laboratory animals than in humans). Poly IC-LC has been reported to produce an influenzalike syndrome with chills, fever, headache, and malaise for 4-12 hr after infusion, and severe hypotension (13).

Tilorone, which is used primarily as an oral agent, produces minimal gastrointestinal toxicity (74). When applied to the eye, it is deposited in the corneal epithelium. Extensive granulation in cells of the hematopoietic and reticuloendothelial systems observed in animals precludes further use of the agent in humans (74).

Another experimental inducer, BRL 5907, produces mild local irritation with coryzal symptoms following 5-10 mg/kg/day given as nasal drops. Symptoms abate with a lower dose.

Therapeutic Uses. IFN inducers have been used experimentally in rhinovirus infections and herpes simplex keratitis. Topical poly rI.poly rC compared with idoxuridine was found to be equal for prophylaxis and therapy of the acute herpes simplex virus keratitis (32), but in a placebo-controlled trial was ineffective treatment for recurrent genital herpes (19). Other experimental and clinical studies are not conclusive, and further studies are underway.

OTHER DRUGS WITH ANTIVIRAL POTENTIAL

RIBAVIRIN

Ribavirin (1-β-D-ribofuranosyl-1,2,4-carboxamide) is a broad-spectrum antiviral agent with *in vitro* activity against nearly all major virus groups, particularly influenza viruses, both A and B. Ribavirin is absorbed from the gut and can be given orally. It is phosphorylated by adenosine kinase to ribavirin 5′-monophosphate that is a competitive inhibitor of inosine 5′-monophosphate dehydrogenase. Ribavirin is virustatic, not virucidal. It probably acts by inhibiting guanine monophosphate synthesis at the step involving conversion of IMP to xanthine 5′-monophosphate, as suggested by the reversibility of the drug's activity by the addition of xanthosine, guanosine, and inosine. Ultimately, viral RNA synthesis is inhibited. In a cell-free assay influenza RNA polymerase is competitively inhibited by the phosphorylated metabolite, ribavirin triphosphate (28). Ribavirin shows low-grade toxicity in animals, but it is both a teratogen and an immunosuppressant in animals (29). It has beneficial effects in a number of animal virus infections. In humans, small-particle aerosols have produced a salutory effect against both influenza A and B (55) and respiratory syncitial virus infections (38, 39, 76). At least one study has shown oral ribavirin to be effective in the treatment of acute hepatitis A (60).

Several new antivirals are in the early stages of development. Phosphonoformic acid may prove useful as a topical agent against herpes virus infections. Bromovinyldeoxyuridine, [(E)-5-(2-bromovinyl)-2′-deoxyuridine], another antiherpes drug, also appears promising in early studies. Other new agents that may be effective against rhinoviruses or enteroviruses are arlidone (4-[b-2-chloro-4-methoxy-phenoxyl hexyl]-3,5-heptanedione) and its derivatives, 4,6-dichloroflavan and 2-(3,4-dichlorophenoxy)-5-nitrobenzenitrile.

REFERENCES

1. Arnaordova, V., Baskeva, L., Tasheva, M. et al. Treatment and prevention of acute viral respiratory infections in children with leukocyte interferon. *Arch. Immunol. Ther. Exp.* 25:731, 1977.
2. Arvin, Am., Kushner, J.H., Feldman, S. et al. Human leukocyte interferon for the treatment of varicella in children with cancer. *N. Engl. J. Med.* 306:761, 1982.
3. Balfour, H.H., Bean, B., Laskin, O.L. et al. Acyclovir halts progression of herpes zoster in immunocompromised patients. *N. Engl. J. Med.* 308:1448, 1983.
4. Balfour, H.H., Bean, B., Mitchell, C.D. et al. Acyclovir in immunocompromised patients with cytomegalovirus diseases. *Am. J. Med. (suppl.)* 73:241, 1982.
5. Bauer D.J. *The Specific Treatment of Virus Diseases.* Baltimore: University Park Press, 1977.
6. Bean, B., Braun, C. and Balfour, H.H. Acyclovir therapy for acute herpes zoster. *Lancet* 2:118, 1982.
7. Bleidner, W.F., Harmon, J.B., Hewes, W.E. et al. Absorption, distribution and excretion of amantadine hydrochloride. *J. Pharmacol. Exp. Ther.* 150:484, 1965.
8. Bryson, Y.J., Dillon, M., Lovett, M. et al. Successful treatment of initial genital herpes simplex virus infections with oral acyclovir. *N. Engl. J. Med.* 308:916, 1983.
9. Bukringkaya, N.G., Vorkunova, N.K. and Pushkarskaya, N.L. Uncoating of a rimantadine-resistant variant of influenza virus in the presence of rimantadine. *J. Gen. Virol.* 60:61, 1982.
10. Calabresi, P. Current status of clinical investigations with 6-azauridine, 5-iodo-2-deoxyuridine, and related derivatives. *Cancer Res.* 23:1260, 1963.
11. Came, P.F., Schafer, T.W. and Silver, G.H. Sensitivity of rhinoviruses to human leukocytes and fibroblast interferons. *J. Infect. Dis. (suppl.)* 133:A 136, 1976.
12. Carroll, D., Ventura, P., Hause, A. et al. Resistance of visna virus to interferon. *J. Infect. Dis.* 138:614, 1978.
13. Champney, K.J., Levine, D., Levy, H.B. and Lerner, A.M. Modified polyriboinosinic-polyribocytidilic acid complex: Sustained interferonemia and its physiological associates in humans. *Infect. Immunol.* 25:831, 1979.
14. Chessman, S.H., Henle, W., Rubin, R.H. et al. Epstein-Barr virus infection in renal transplant recipients: Effects of antithymocyte globulin and interferon. *Ann. Intern. Med.* 93:39, 1980.
15. Colin, J., Chastel, C., Renard, G. et al. Combination therapy for keratitis with human leukocyte interferon and acyclovir. *Am. Ophthalmol.* 95:346, 1983.
16. Corey, L., Nahmias, A.J., Quinon, M.E. et al. A trial of topical acyclovir in genital herpes simplex virus infections. *N. Engl. J. Med.* 306:1313, 1982.
17. Corey, L., Fife, K.H., Benedetti, J.K. et al. Intravenous acyclovir for the treatment of primary genital herpes. *Ann. Intern. Med.* 98:914, 1983.
18. Couch, R.B. and Jackson, G.G. Antiviral agents in influenza. 1976.
19. Crane, L.R., Levy, H.B. and Lerner, A.M. Topical polyriboinosinic-polyribocytidilic acid complex in the treatment of recurrent genital herpes. *Antimicrob. Agents Chemother.* 21:481, 1982.
20. Davies, W.L., Grunert, R.R., Haff, R.F. et al. Antiviral activity of 1-adamantanamine (amantadine). *Science* 144:862, 1964.
21. Dawson, C.R. and Toyin, B. Herpes simplex eye infections: clinical manifestations, pathogenesis, and management. *Surv. Ophth.* 21:121, 1976.
22. de Miranda, P., Good, S.S., Krosny, H.C., Connor, J.D., Laskin, O.L. and Lietman, P.S. Metabolic fate of radioactive acyclovir in humans. Acyclovir symposium. *Am. J. Med.* 73:215, 1982.
23. Dexter, D.L., Wolbert, W.H., Ansfield, F.J. et al. The clinical pharmacology of 5-trifluoromethyl-2′-deoxyuridine. *Cancer Res.* 32:247, 1974.
24. Dix, R.D., Baringer, J.R., Panitch, H.S. et al. Recurrent herpes simplex encephalitis: Recovery of virus after Ara-A treatment. *Ann. Neurol.* 13:196, 1983.
25. Dolin, R., Reichman, R.C., Madore, H.P. et al. A controlled trial of amantadine and rimantadine in the prophylaxis of influenza A infection. *N. Engl. J. Med.* 307:580, 1982.
26. Douglas, R.G. Antiviral drugs 1983. *Med. Clin. North Am.* 67:1163, 1983.
27. Edy, Y.G., Billiau, A. and De Somer, P. Comparison of rates of clearance of human fibroblast and leukocyte interferon from the circulatory system of rabbits. *J. Infect. Dis.* 133(Suppl.):A 18, 1976.
28. Erikson, B., Helfstrand, E., Johnson, N.G. et al. Inhibition of influenza virus ribonucleic acid polymerase by ribavirin triphosphate. *Antimicrob. Agents Chemother.* 11:946, 1977.
29. Ferm, V.H., Willhite, C. and Kilham, L. Teratogenic effects of ribavirin on hamster and rat embryo. *Teratology* 17:93, 1978.
30. Field, H.G. and Phillip, I. (eds.). Acyclovir. *J. Antimicrob. Chemother.* 12(Suppl.):1983.
31. Galasso, G.J. An assessment of antiviral drugs for the management of infectious diseases in humans. *Antiviral Res.* 1:73, 1981.
32. Galin, M.A., Chowchuvech, E. and Kronenberg, B. Therapeutic use of inducers of interferon on herpes simplex keratitis in humans. *Ann. Ophthal.* 8:72, 1976.
33. Guann, J.W., Barton, N.H. and Whitley, R.J. Acyclovir: Mechanism of action, pharmacokinetics, safety and clinical applications. *Pharmacotherapy* 3:275, 1983.
34. Greenberg, H.B., Pollard, R.B. and Lutivivk, L.I. Effects of human leukocyte interferon of hepatitis B virus infection in patients with chronic active hepatitis. *N. Engl. J. Med.* 295:517, 1976.
35. Greenhalgh, W.H. and Gaush, C.R. Localization of amantadine hydrochloride in tissue culture cells. *Bact. Proc. Absts.* 107:170, 1970.
36. Grossberg, S.E. The interferons and their inducers: Molecular and therapeutic considerations. *N. Engl. J. Med.* 287:13, 79, 122, 1972.
37. Guggenheim, M.A. and Baron, S. Clinical studies of an interferon inducer polyriboinosinic polyribocytidilic acid poly (I) poly (C) in children. *J. Infect. Dis.* 136:50, 1977.
38. Hall, C.B., Walsh, E.E., Hruska, J.F. et al. Ribavirin treatment of experimental respiratory syncitial viral infections: A controlled double-blind study in young adults. *JAMA* 249:2666, 1983.
39. Hall, C.B., McBride, J.T., Walsh, E.E. et al. Aerosolized ribavirin treatment of infants with respiratory syncitial viral infec-

tion. A randomized double-blinded study. *N. Engl. J. Med.* 308:1443, 1983.

40. Hann, I.M., Prentice, H.G., Blacklock, H.A. et al. Acyclovir prophylaxis against herpes virus infections in severly immunocompromised patients: Randomized double-blind trial. *Br. Med. J.* 287:384, 1983.

41. Hayden, F.G., Hoffman, H.E. and Spyker, D.A. Differences in side effects of amantadine hydrochloride and rimantadine hydrochloride relate to differences in pharmacokinetics. *Antimicrob. Agents Chemother.* 23:458, 1983.

42. Hirsch, M.S., Shooley, R.T., Cosimi, A.B. et al. Effects of interferon-alpha on cytomegalovirus reactivation syndromes in renal-transplant recipients. *N. Engl. J. Med.* 308:1489, 1983.

43. Ho, M. and Armstrong, J.A. Interferon. *Ann. Rev. Microbiol.* 29:131, 1975.

44. Hoffnagle, J.H., Minuk, G.Y., Dusheiko, G.M. et al. Adenine arabinoside 5'-monophosphate treatment of chronic type B hepatitis. *Hepatology* 2:784, 1982.

45. Isaacs, A. and Lindemann, J. Virus interference: I. The interferon. *Proc. R. Soc. Lond. (Biol.)* 147:258, 1957.

46. Jackson, G.G. and Stanley, E.D. Prevention and control of influenza by chemoprophylaxis and chemotherapy. *JAMA* 235:-2739, 1976.

47. Jawetz, E. Antiviral chemotherapy. In: *Viral Infections: A Clinical Approach* (Drew, W.L., ed.). Philadelphia: F.A. Davis, 1976.

48. Juel-Jensen B.E., MacCallum, F.O., Mackenzie, A.M. et al. Treatment of zoster with idoxuridine in dimethyl sulphoxide. Results of two double-blinded controlled trials. *Br. Med. J.* 2:776, 1970.

49. Kaplan, A.S. and Ben-Porat, T.L. Mode of antiviral action of 5-iodouracil deoxyriboside. *J. Mol. Biol.* 19:320, 1966.

50. Kato, N. and Eggers, H.J. Inhibition of uncoating of fowl plague virus by 1-adamantanamine hydrochloride. *Virology* 37:632, 1969.

51. Larsson, A., Forsgren, M., Hard, A.F., Segerstad, S. et al. Administration of interferon to an infant with congenital rubella syndrome involving persistant viremia and cutaneous vasculitis. *Acta Paediatr. Scand.* 65:105, 1976.

52. Laskin, O.L., Longstreth, J.A., Whelton, A. et al. Effect of renal failure on the pharmacokinetics of acyclovir. Acyclovir symposium. *Am. J. Med.* 73:197, 1982.

53. Little, J.W., Hall, W.J., Douglas, E.G. et al. Amantadine effect on peripheral airways abnormalities in influenza. *Ann. intern. Med.* 85:177, 1976.

54. Mastan, P.F. and Henderson, J.W. Penetration of idoxuridine into the anterior segment after transdermal or subconjunctival injection. *Invest. Ophthalmol.* 5:320, 1966.

55. McClung, H.W., Knight, V., Gilvert, B.E. et al. Ribavirin aerosol treatment of influenza B virus infection. *JAMA* 249:2671, 1983.

56. Merigan, T.C., Rand, H., Pollard, R.B. et al. Human leukocyte interferon for the treatment of herpes zoster in patients with cancer. *N. Engl. J. Med.* 298:981, 1978.

57. Nilsen, A.E., Aasen, T. and Haloos, A.M. Efficacy of oral acyclovir in the treatment of initial and recurrent genital herpes. *Lancet* 2:571, 1982.

58. Nolan, D.C., Lauter, C.B. and Lerner, A.M. Idoxuridine in herpes simplex virus (type I) encephalitis. Experience with 29 cases in Michigan, 1966 to 1971. *Ann. Intern. Med.* 78:243, 1973.

59. Parker, J.D. Double-blind trial of idoxuridine in recurrent genital herpes. *J. Antimicrob. Chemother.* 3(Suppl. A):131, 1977.

60. Patki, S.A. and Gupta, P. Evaluation of ribavirin in the treatment of acute hepatitis. *Chemotherapy* 28:293, 1982.

61. Pavan-Langston, D. and Foster, C.S. Trifluorothymidine and idoxuridine therapy of ocular herpes. *Am. J. Ophthalmol.* 84:818, 1977.

62. Pavan-Langston, D. and Hess, F. Ocular and systemic antiviral activity of vidarabine. *Comp. Ther.* 3:42, 1977.

63. Pollard, R.B., Smith, J.L., Neal, E. et al. Effect of vidarabine on chronic hepatitis B virus infection. *JAMA* 239:1648, 1978.

64. Prober, C.G., Kirk, L.E. and Keeney, R.E. Acyclovir therapy of chickenpox in immunosuppressed children—A collaborative study. *J. Pediatr.* 101:622, 1982.

65. Reichman, R.C., Baddger, G.H., Guinan, M.E. et al. Topically administered acyclovir in the treatment of recurrent herpes simplex genitalis: A controlled trial. *J. Infect. Dis.* 147:336, 1983.

66. Richards, D.M., Carmine, A.A., Brogden, R.N. et al. Acyclovir: A review of its pharmacodynamic properties and therapeutic efficacy. *Drugs* 26:378, 1983.

67. Ross, A.H., Julia, A. and Balakrishnan, C. Toxicity of adenine arabinoside in humans. *J. Infect. Dis.* 133(Suppl. A): 192, 1976.

68. Saral, R., Burns, W.H., Laskin, O.L. et al. Acyclovir prophylaxis of herpes-simplex-virus infections, a randomized double-blind, controlled trial in bone-marrow-transplant recipients. *N. Engl. J. Med.* 305:63, 1981.

69. Saral, R., Ambinder, R.F., Burns, W.H. et al. Acyclovir prophylaxis against herpes simplex virus infections in patients with leukemia. *Ann. Intern. Med.* 99:773, 1983.

70. Shiota, H. Clinical evaluation of acyclovir in the treatment of ulcerative herpetic keratitis. *Am. J. Med. (suppl.)* 73:307, 1982.

71. Skalko, R.G. and Packard, D.S. The teratogenic response of the mouse embryo to 5-iododeoxyuridine. *Experientia* 29:198, 1973.

72. Spector, S.A., Connor, J.D., Hintz, M. et al. Single dose pharmacokinetics of acyclovir. *Antimicrob. Agents Chemother.* 19: 608, 1981.

73. Straus, S.E., Smith, H.A., Brickman, C. et al. Acyclovir for chronic mucocutaneous herpes simplex virus infection in immunocompromised patients. *Ann. Intern. Med.* 96:270, 1982.

74. Stringfellow, D.A.' Interferon inducers as antiviral agents. *Compr. Ther.* 3:25, 1977.

75. Stringfellow, D.A., Kern, E.R., Kelsey, D.K. et al. Suppressed response to interferon induction in mice infected with encephalomyocarditis virus, semliki forest virus, influenza A2 virus herpes virus-hominis type 2 or murine cytomegalovirus. *J. Infect. Dis.* 135:540, 1977.

76. Taber, L.H., Knight, V., Gilbert, B.E. et al. Ribavirin aerosol treatment of bronchiolitis associated with respiratory syncitial virus infection in infants. *Pediatrics* 72:613, 1983.

77. Trousedale, M.D., Nesburn, A.G., Su, T. et al. Activity of 1-(2'-fluoro-2'deoxy-β-arabinofuranosyl) thymine against herpes simplex virus in cell cultures and rabbit eyes. *Antimicrob. Agents Chemother.* 23:808, 1983.

78. Wade, J.C., Newton, B., Mc Claren, C. et al. Intravenous acyclovir to treat mucocutaneous herpes simplex virus infections after marrow transplantation. *Ann. Intern. Med.* 96:265, 1982.

79. Whitley, R.J., Soong, S.J., Dolin, R. et al. Early vidarabine therapy to control the complications of herpes zoster in immunosuppressed patients. *N. Engl. J. Med.* 307:971, 1982.

80. Whitley, R.J., Soong, S., Dolin, R. et al. Adenine arabinoside therapy of biopsy-proved herpes simplex encephalitis: NIAID collaborative antiviral study group. *N. Engl. J. Med.* 297:289, 1977.

81. Whitley, R.J., Soong, S.J., Hirsch, M.S. et al. Herpes simplex encephalitis: Vidarabine therapy and diagnostic problems. *N. Engl. J. Med.* 304:313, 1981.

82. Whitley, R.J., Nahmias, A.J., Soong, S.J. et al. Vidarabine therapy of neonatal herpes simplex virus infection. *Pediatrics* 66:495, 1980.

83. Whitley, R.J., Barton, N., Collins, E. et al. Mucocutaneous herpes simplex virus infections in immunocompromised patients, a model for evaluation of topical antiviral agents. *Am. J. Med.* 73(Suppl.):236, 1982.

84. Williams, B.B., Paul, R.T. and Lerner, A.M. Pharmacokinetics of interferon in blood, cerebrospinal fluid and brain after administration of modified polyriboinosinic-polyribocytidilic acid and amphotericin B. *J. Infect. Dis.* 146:819, 1982.

85. Wu, M.J., Ing., T.S., Soung, L.S. et al. Amantadine hydrochlo-

ride pharmacokinetics in patients with impaired renal function. *Clin. Nephrol.* 17:19, 1982.

86. Younkin, S.W., Betts, R.F., Roth, F.K. et al. Reduction in fever and symptoms in young adults with influenza A/Brazil/78/H1N1 infection after treatment with aspirin or amantadine. *Antimicrob. Agents Chemother.* 23:577, 1983.

87. Zerial, A., Hovanessian, A.G., Stefanes, S. et al. Synergistic activities of type I (α,β) and type II (γ) murine interferons. *Antiviral Res.* 2:227, 1982.

ADDITIONAL READING

Douglas, R.M. et al. Prophylactic efficacy of intranasal α_2-interferon against Rhinovirus infections in the family setting. *N. Eng. J. Med.* 314:65, 1986.

Hayden, F.G. et al. Prevention of natural colds by contact prophylaxis with intranasal α_2-interferon. *N. Eng. J. Med.* 314:71, 1986.

Swallow, D.L. Antiviral agents 1978-1983. *Prog. Drug Res.* 28:127, 1984.

CHAPTER
25.2

ANTIFUNGAL AGENTS

John P. Utz

Chemotherapy of fungal infection dates back to as early as 1903, when potassium iodide was shown to be effective against sporotrichosis. Since then, effects of sulfonamides (36) (particularly sulfadiazine) (22) against *Histoplasma capsulatum* infection (1947) and of hydroxystilbamidine against *Blastomyces dermatitidis* (55) (1957) have been demonstrated. In the early 1950s, polyene antibiotics were discovered. Two important examples are nystatin (34) and amphotericin B (67), the latter being an important therapeutic agent against most systemic antifungal diseases. In 1958, the activity of griseofulvin was described in experimental dermatophytic infections (30) and that of chlorimidazole against yeast and dermatophytes (52) was shown. In 1964, flucytosine, initially developed as an antineoplastic agent, was shown to be effective against *Candida* spp. and *Cryptococcus neoformans* infections (33). Although the antifungal activity of the imidazoles was described as early as 1958 (52), members currently in use (i.e., miconazole, clotrimazole, and ketoconazole) are the most recently (1978) commercially available agents.

Despite almost 80 years of history and development of these drugs, antifungal therapy is still not adequate and has many difficulties, including the fact that the existing potent and widely used drugs such as amphotericin B are toxic and that newer and better drugs are difficult to develop.

ANTIFUNGAL DRUGS

The important antifungal agents presently used include polyene antibiotics (nystatin, amphotericin B), antimetabolite (flucytosine), imidazoles (clotrimazole, miconazole, ketoconazole), griseofulvin, and other miscellaneous agents.

MECHANISM OF ACTION

The antifungal agents produce their effects by exerting fungistatic and fungicidal actions by various mechanisms described for individual drugs. In addition to these, many agents helpful in the therapy of superficial mycoses may produce their effects by other mechanisms. Thus, keratolytic agents promote desquamation of stratum corneum, thereby removing the offending fungus and allowing penetration of drugs, and antiperspirants prevent hyperhydrosis and alter conditions for fungal growth. These agents are described in Chapter 20.

NYSTATIN

Source and Chemistry. Nystatin in a polyene antibiotic derived from *Streptomyces noursei*. It has the distinction of being the first antifungal antibiotic discovered (its name is derived from New York State). It has a general formula of $C_{46-47}H_{73-75}NO_{18}$, and contains a sequence of four to seven conjugated double bonds, four methyl groups, an amino sugar moiety, and mycosamine.

Antifungal Actions. Nystatin has extensive activity against a wide range of fungi but no antibacterial activity. *In vitro*, the minimal inhibitory concentrations (MIC) for such a range of microorganisms vary from 1.9 to 31.2 U/ml of agar. For the *Candida* spp., for which it is most commonly used, the MIC is almost uniformly 7.8 U/ml of agar. For the causative agents (*Microsporum, Trichophyton,* and *Epidermophyton* spp.) of the dermatophytoses, it is slightly less active (7.8 U/ml agar). Its activity (1.9-3.9 U/ml agar) against such systemic fungi as *B. dermatitidis, H. capsulatum,* and *C. neoformans* is in vain because serum levels cannot be obtained. In concentration of 100,000 U/ml, it is nontoxic to poliomyelitis, Coxsackie, or ECHO viruses, or the cell culture lines used in their replication; hence, nystatin is useful in such culture systems to suppress fungal growth from contaminated patient specimens. In addition, at a concentration of 1:60,000 nystatin has anti-*Trichomonas vaginalis* and anti-*Leishmania* spp. activity.

Mechanism of Action. Nystatin, like other polyenes, binds irreversibly to sterols (probably ergosterol) in fungal cell membranes. By this interaction, polyenes appear to form pores or channels in the cell membrane, thereby increasing the membrane permeability and allowing leakage of a variety of small molecules, of which potassium may be the most important.

Pharmacokinetics. Oral doses of 12 g (52,000,000 U) a day induce nausea, vomiting, and diarrhea, and produce serum levels of from 4.4 to 11 U/ml. In doses as high as 100,000 U/g of vehicle to skin or mucous membranes, no absorption or sensitization is known to occur. It may also be given as aerosol (25,000 U) or instilled onto the conjunctival sac (20,000 U/1 drop of saline solution or repeatedly into the urinary bladder), again without local or systemic effect.

Adverse Effects. Nystatin is too toxic to be given parenterally. Mild nausea or diarrhea may occur after oral administration. Irritation of skin or mucous membranes occurs even less frequently.

Therapeutic Uses. Topical use of nystatin is principally reserved for prevention or active treatment of *Candida* spp. infections of the vagina, mouth, gastrointestinal tract, skin, or nails. Such infection is manifest by inflammation of the mucous membranes (thrush) or skin, or by diarrhea. This disease is most threatening (and occasionally fatal, as a result of septicemia) in the patient immunocompromised by disease or treatment. Nystatin is inadequate for treatment of septicemia, endocarditis, or meningitis. In the dermatophytoses, topical application of the ointment does not result in penetration of the epidermis sufficient to inhibit fungi. It has also been used extensively in prophylaxis in patients immunosuppressed either naturally or deliberately in bone marrow transplant recipients (69, 72), but with disparate results.

Preparations. Nystatin, USP (MYCOSTATIN) is available as an ointment (100,000 U/g), as an oral suspension (100,000 U/ml), or as a tablet (500,000 U). The ointment is applied twice daily for purposes of convenience. The oral suspension dosage is 100,000 U for premature infants or 200,000 U for older infants four times a day. The usual dose in tablet form is one to two tablets three times a day; 1-2 weeks is customary duration of therapy.

AMPHOTERICIN B

History and Source. Amphotericins A and B were derived from a *S. nodosus* isolate recovered from a soil sample obtained from the Orinoco River region of Venezuela. Of the two compounds, amphotericin B is the more active and is clinically used.

Chemistry. Amphotericin B (Fig. 25.2-1) is a heptene but otherwise has the same mycosamine and amino sugar moiety as nystatin. It is a macrolide with both lipophilic and hydrophilic portions. Amphotericin B is insoluble in water. In a dry state, at 5°C it has virtually the same activity at the end of a year. Contrary to the package insert it is stable in suspension, at 22°C, for 24 hr, even in the presence of light (53).

Antifungal Actions. At MICs achievable in serum, amphotericin B has antifungal activity against *Aspergillus fumigatus, B. dermatitidis, Candida* spp., *C. neoformans, H. capsulatum, Coccidioides immitis, M. audouinii, Paracoccidioides brasiliensis, Rhizopus* spp., *Rhodotorula* spp., *Sporothrix schenckii, Torulopsis glabrata,* and *Trichophyton* spp. The drug inhibits some strains of *Leishmania brasiliensis, L. donovani,* and *Trypanosoma cruzi.* It also has activity against *Mycobacterium leprae* and free-living amebae of the *Naegleria* and *Hartmanella* genera that cause meningoencephalitis. Its activity was also demonstrated *in vivo* in experimentally infected animals.

Flucytosine reduced the MIC of amphotericin B necessary to inhibit *in vitro* growth of *Candida* spp. and *C. neoformans*, is additive or indifferent in *in vivo* infections with these two fungi and also *Aspergillus* spp., and reduces the dose of amphotericin B necessary and the relapse rate in cryptococcosis in humans (5, 64). Another drug, minocycline, also enhances *in vitro* activity against *Candida* spp. *T. glabrata,* and *C. neoformans.* A third drug, rifampin, reduces two to four times the MIC of amphotericin B for *Aspergillus* spp., *H. capsulatum,* and *Candida* spp. (3). It has been postulated that the synergistic effect is mediated by the amphotericin B-induced membrane defects that allow earlier entrance of the other antibiotic (e.g., flucytosine), so as to interfere with still another fungal metabolic activity (e.g., nucleic acid synthesis).

Its antifungal effects are maximal between pH 6 and 7.5 and decrease at low pH.

Mechanism of Action. Amphotericin B, like nystatin, binds irreversibly to sterols (e.g., ergosterol) in fungal cell membranes, causing a leak of potassium and other cell products.

Pharmacokinetics. Amphotericin B is poorly absorbed from the gastrointestinal tract. After intravenous administration, its plasma concentration falls rapidly (to 10% of the dose), probably due to its binding to cholesterol-containing membranes in many tissues. Details of its metabolic pathways are not known. Approximately 95% of drug in plasma is strongly bound to lipoproteins. Following administration of the therapeutic doses (e.g., 50 mg), the peak serum concentrations vary from 0.5 to 2 μg/ml. After a rapid fall, a plateau or trough level of about 0.3-0.5 μg/ml is maintained. Only about one-fourth of the amount in serum is found in the cerebrospinal fluid, bronchial or parotid gland secretions, aqueous humor, normal amniotic fluid, and hemodialysis solutions (7). In the normal patient, serum levels can be detected 7 days after a single dose. Only 5% of a single dose can be detected in urine during the following 24 hr. However, levels in urine can be measured for at least 8 weeks. About 40% of the administered dose can be accounted for in the urine during the succeeding 7 days. It has been detected in renal tissue 1 year after the last intravenous dose (48). Tissue distribution and metabolism data are not known.

Miscellaneous Actions. Amphotericin B, to a modest extent, and other members of the polyene group, notably candicidin, reduce the size of the benignly hypertrophied prostate gland of dogs and hamsters (71). Amphotericin B induces sensitivity to doxorubicin, nitrosourea, and cyclophosphamide in human neoplasia (47).

The drug has immunoadjuvant properties of enhancing the number of antibody-producing cells in the spleen and lymph node of a number of mouse strains. The immunoglobulin G (IgG) response is greater than that of IgM. In addition to enhancing serological immunity, it also augments cell-mediated immunity (54). It is not certain whether these immunological effects play a role in the chemotherapeutic effect in fungal disease patients, who have impaired cell-mediated immunity probably due to suppressor T-cell function (58).

Drug Resistance. Although some strains of *C. albicans* and *C. immitis* have been made resistant to amphotericin B by serial cultures in increasing concentrations of the drug, resistant fungi have not been encountered in patients with relapse of their infection. Some resistant

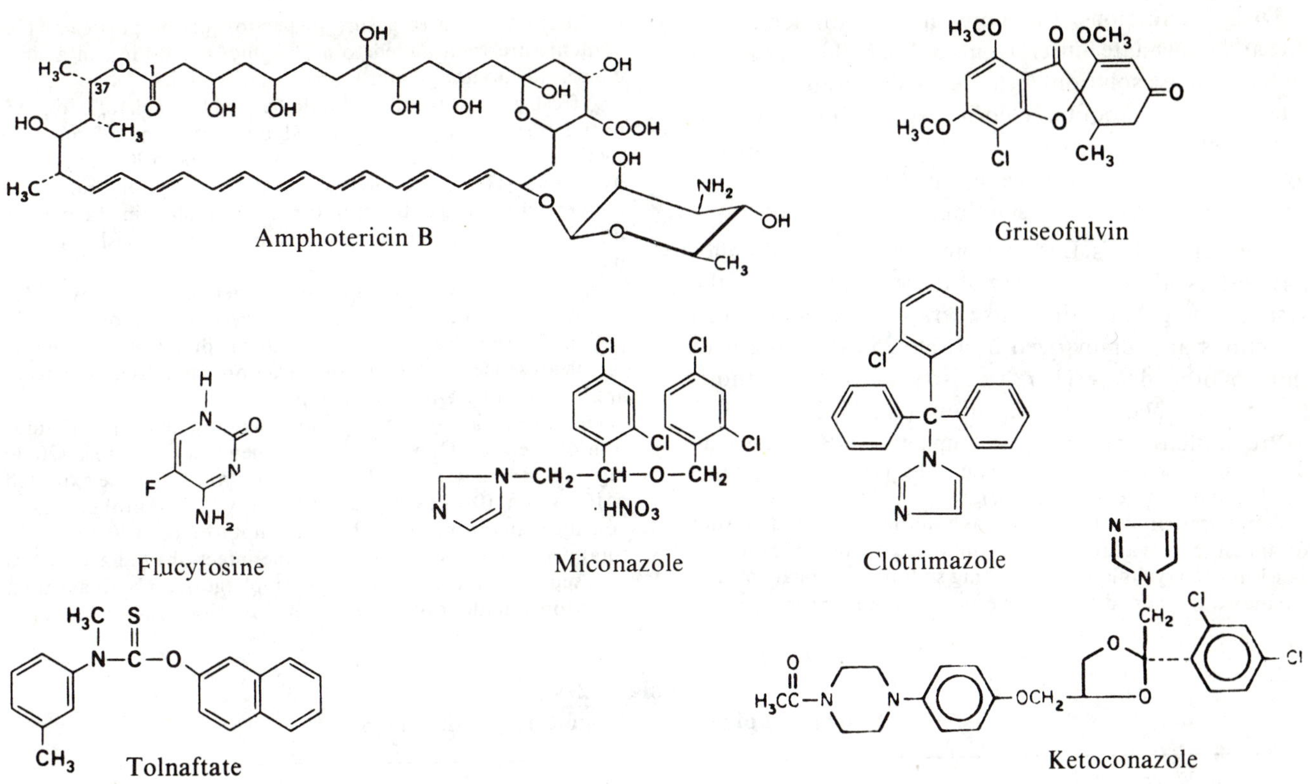

Amphotericin B

Griseofulvin

Flucytosine

Miconazole

Clotrimazole

Tolnaftate

Ketoconazole

Fig. 25.2-1: *Chemical structures of some antifungal agents.*

strains of *C. krusei, C. parakrusei,* and *C. tropicalis* have been isolated from clinical specimens (49).

Adverse Effects. Amphotericin B is the most toxic antimicrobial drug in use today, if for no other reason than daily (or alternate-day) i.v. infusions. It produces phlebitis at site of injection, chills, fever, nausea, vomiting, anorexia, diarrhea, malaise, and muscle and joint pain occur frequently, and, in the uncommon patient, with almost every infusion. Paradoxically, the most severe reactions may be with the earlier and lower doses, and diminish or disappear with later, optimal doses. Hypertension, hypotension, cardiac arrhythmias (including ventricular tachycardia and fibrillation), and cardiac arrest have been reported. Allergic or anaphylactic reactions (flushing and bronchospasm, with hypotension) have been rare, however.

Anemia develops progressively to a stable hematocrit value of from 22 to 35% during treatment. It is normocytic, normochromic, and complicates a hemolytic anemia already present from the infection (12). The drug effect is mediated via erythropoietin, rather than bone marrow depression (38). However, *in vitro* increasing amounts of drug resulted in progressive loss of potassium from erythrocytes to point of hemolysis; this effect was obviated by the presence of normal serum in the diluent. Hypokalemia may induce profound degrees of muscle weakness and electrocardiographic changes, and occurs in about 25% of patients. Distal-type renal tubular acidosis may be a major factor in pathogenesis (39).

Renal toxicity is manifest in most patients, and serum creatinine and blood urea nitrogen (BUN) values are elevated in 83-94% of patients during treatment over a prolonged period (range 4-66 months) (16). Defects in renal concentrating ability and nephrogenic diabetes insipidus have been reported (2). Uric acid clearance is increased in the proximal tubules, and there is loss of potassium, bicarbonate, and water in the distal tubules. Histological examination reveals tubular and glomerular damage (14). It shows calcification, tubular basement membrane thickening, with lumenal plugging with proteinaceous and necrotic debris, and, more recently reported, striking vacuolization in the media of small arteries and arterioles (14). The glomeruli are also affected with thickening and fragmentation of the basement membrane, hypercellularity, fibrosis, hyalinization, and calcification. Urinalysis shows hematuria, tubular cells, cylindruria, but little proteinuria. With customary total doses of 1.5-3 g, the renal toxicity is not of great importance. In two patients, however, who received 10 and 14 g, progressive renal failure and death occurred (48). In animal studies, it induces striking, dose-related decrease in renal blood flow and glomerular filtration rate as well as a marked vasoconstriction (17).

Leukopenia and thrombocytopenia are rare. Although hepatotoxicity was reported in 1960, experience during the past 20 years suggests that it occurs so infrequently as to cast doubt on its relationship to drug (4).

Drug Interactions. Amphotericin B (with deoxycholate and phosphate buffer) forms only a colloidal suspension in glucose solution or sterile distilled water. It precipitates out in sodium chloride, potassium chloride, calcium gluconate, carbenicillin, chlorpromazine, diphenhydramine, gentamicin, kanamycin, metaraminol, tetracycline, vitamins and other solutions.

Therapeutic Uses. Despite its marked toxicity, amphotericin B is still the mainstay of therapy for most of the systemic fungal infections. Its therapeutic effects in such infections are summarized in Table 25.2-1, along with those of other drugs. There are also some recent, authoritative, published recommendations (20, 35, 50, 56).

Preparations. For topical use, amphotericin B in a 3% concentration is available as a cream (20-g tube), lotion (30-ml bottle), and ointment (20-g tube).

Amphotericin B (FUNGIZONE), as a sterile lyophilized powder for infusion, is available in vials containing 50 mg amphotericin B, 41 mg deoxycholate, and 25.2 mg sodium phosphate buffer. To that vial is added 10 ml of sterile water, and the vial shaken for at least 3 min to assure dispersion of the particles. The contents are then added to a 5% glucose solution in a final concentration not greater than 10 mg/100 ml.

A fresh glucose solution should be used for each infusion. An initial dose of 1 mg is recommended by some and a 5-mg dose (with a test amount of 1 mg of that 5 over a 30- to 90-min period) by others. The blood pressure, pulse, respiratory rate, and temperature should be monitored every 30 min during the infusion. It is a common practice to give the infusion over a period of 3-6 hr.

A shorter period of 45 min has been recommended by Fields and associates (29), but fear still lingers of cardiotoxicity in patients, based on experimental studies in dogs (17). Depending on the presence and severity of a reaction, the subsequent doses are increased by 5-mg increments.

Opinion varies on optimal daily total dose of drug and duration of therapy. One school recommends a daily dose (20-30 mg) meant to give serum levels two to three times the expected MIC, and a 10-week course of therapy (27). Another school considers an optimal dose 1 mg/kg (not to exceed 50 mg) and a total dose of 1.5-3 g (37). For some infections (e.g., *Candida* spp. septicemia, mucocutaneous, esophageal, and urinary tract infection) smaller doses, 10-355 mg, over a period of 4-18 days

Table 25.2-1
Drug of Choice for Systemic Fungal Infections

Fungal Disease (causative fungus)	Form of Disease	Drug(s) of Choice and Dose Schedule[a]
Blastomycosis (*Blastomyces dermatitidis*)	All acute forms	Amph B, 1.5-2 g (TD) i.v. over 6-10 weeks
	Skin or localized	Hydroxystilbamidine isethionate, i.v.
Paracoccidioidomycosis (*Paracoccidioides brasiliensis*)	All acute forms	Sulfonamide suppressive, but not curative; amph B or ketoconazole recommended
Cryptococcosis (*Cryptococcus neoformans*)	Pulmonary or disseminated	Amph B, 1 mg/kg/day, i.v., for 6 weeks
	Meningitis	Amph B, 0.3 mg/kg/day, i.v. + FC, 150 mg/kg/day, orally, for 6 weeks
Histoplasmosis (*Histoplasma capsulatum*)	Severe progressive, chronic active, or pulmonary cavitary form	Amph B, 1.5-2 g (TD), i.v. over 10 weeks
Coccidioidomycosis (*Coccidioides immitis*)	Severe pulmonary	Amph B, 0.5-2 g (TD), i.v.
	Disseminated	Amph B, 2.5-3 g (TD), i.v.
	Meningitis	Amph B, 1 mg three times weekly intrathecally Miconazole i.v., for patients intolerant to amph B Amph B i.v., + transfer factor (a lymphocytic extract) for resistant patients. Ketoconazole, orally for months
Candidiasis (*Candida albicans* and other species)	Pharyngitis and esophagitis	Nystatin, orally or Amph B, 20 mg/day i.v. for 10 days
	Disseminated	Amph B, 0.1-2.5 g (TD) i.v.
Aspergillosis (*Aspergillus* spp.)	Invasive, nonresistant	Amph B, preferably combined with FC
Mucormycosis (*Mucor absidia and M. rhizopus*)	Systemic, especially affecting bones and joints	Amph B, 1-2 g (TD) i.v. + surgery
Sporotrichosis (*Sporothrix schenckii*)	Cutaneous and subcutaneous lymphatic form	Potassium iodide (saturated solution) up to 5 ml three times/day orally
	Severe, disseminated (e.g. pulmonary or joint)	Amph B often helpful, 2-3 g (TD), i.v.

[a] Amph B = amphotericin B; FC = flucytosine; TD = total dose.
Source: Ref. 1.

have been curative (40). When reactions are severe and repeated, 25 mg of hydrocortisone may be administered i.v. at the beginning of the infusion. Aspirin and antihistaminics, though less effective, are also useful (59). Renal function should be measured twice weekly. Although the creatinine clearance is the most sensitive measurement, serum creatinine or BUN determinations are usually preferable for reasons of ease of collection and convenience. Criteria for interrupting therapy for a day or so vary, but values of 3 for the creatinine and 50 mg/dl for BUN are frequently cited. Scalp vein needles should be used to minimize phlebitis. Similarly, heparin (1000 U/infusion) added to the bottle may be helpful. Serum potassium should also be determined twice weekly and hypokalemia corrected by oral supplementation (62). It is customary also to document the predictable fall in hemoglobin and hematocrit. However, the anemia is rarely severe, iron orally is without effect, and transfusions are unnecessary. Although nephrotoxicity has been reduced in laboratory animals by the concurrent use of mannitol i.v., it has not done so in patients. (14).

In cases of meningitis, the i.v. route may be supplemented by the intrathecal at lumbar, cisternal, or reservoir (Ommaya) sites. From 0.1 to 1 mg should be diluted in at least 5 ml of sterile water, further diluted with cerebrospinal fluid withdrawn into the syringe at time of injection, and infused slowly. Injections should be no more frequently than two to three times weekly (24). The drug may be administered directly into a pulmonary cavity via a fine catheter, or by nebulization.

Amphotericin B has also been administered into the urinary bladder via catheter, or into the renal pelvis, or in combination with the i.v. route.

It may also be given intraarticularly, especially in sporotrichosis and coccidioidomycosis. Doses by these routes vary from 5 to 50 mg.

For eye infections, it has also been injected intravitreously, subconjunctivally, and episclerally (subtenon).

FLUCYTOSINE

Chemistry and Source. Flucytosine (5-fluorocytosine) is a synthetic chemical whose structure is shown in Fig. 25.2-1.

Antifungal Action. Most isolates of *C. neoformans* and at least 50% of *Candida* spp. are inhibited by levels (up to 25 μg/ml) achievable in human serum after oral ingestion. *T. glabrata, Cladosporium trichoides,* and *Phialophora* spp. are also sensitive. Some isolates of *Aspergillus* spp. are susceptible, but not predictably so. From 7 to 8% of pretreatment isolates of *C. albicans,* other *Candida* spp., and *T. glabrata,* but only 1-2% of *C. neoformans* are resistant. Most isolates of *S. schenckii* and all of *B. dermatitidis, H. capsulatum, C. immitis,* and *Phycomyces* spp. are resistant. Marked increase in resistance has been reported and seen frequently with *C. neoformans* and *Candida* spp. isolated during treatment with otherwise optimal doses (10).

Mechanism of Action. Susceptible fungal cells convert flucytosine (5-fluorocytosine) to 5-fluorouracil by action of cytosine deaminase. 5-Fluorouracil is, thereafter, converted to deoxyuridylic acid monophosphate, an inhibitor of thymidylate synthetase, thus halting deoxyribonucleic acid (DNA) synthesis (25, 45). A second proposed mechanism is by conversion of 5-fluorouracil into ribonucleic acid with inhibition of protein synthesis (41).

Pharmacokinetics. The drug is absorbed from the gastrointestinal tract, and peak serum concentrations (30-40 μg/ml) after a usual dose (2 g) are achieved within 2-4 hr. Ninety percent of the total dose can be detected unchanged in the urine. Serum binding is estimated at 48-49% (54). In some species, but not in humans, the drug is metabolized to 5-fluorouracil. The drug is distributed widely through body tissues, and cerebrospinal fluid levels are approximately 75% of simultaneous serum levels (9). Serum half-life is approximately 4 hr. It is excreted by glomerular filtration at a rate equivalent to creatinine. With impaired renal function, serum levels are as much as 50% above those seen with normal function. Clearance by hemodialysis is also equivalent to that of creatinine.

Adverse Effects. The commonest side effects are gastrointestinal: nausea, vomiting, and diarrhea. Bowel perforation has been reported in two patients. Macular papular rashes, often requiring discontinuation of the drug, have been reported (44). Transaminase and alkaline phosphatase value elevations have been the basis for claims of hepatotoxicity (57). Thrombocytopenia, leukopenia, and anemia occur in about 5% of patients but have led to fatal complications (42). Interpretation of this bone marrow depression has frequently been difficult owing to underlying disease (e.g., leukemia), ionizing radiation, other anticancer chemotherapy, or to side effects of immunosuppression (e.g., with azathioprine). Many side effects, but especially the hematological ones, appear related to serum drug levels in excess of 100 μg/ml. This is particularly prone to occur when renal excretion of flucytosine is impaired by concurrent amphotericin B therapy. When renal function is compromised, serum levels of flucytosine should be monitored and maintained between 50 and 75 μg/ml. Less frequently encountered side effects have been confusion, headaches, hallucinations, somnolence, and vertigo.

Drug Interactions. The only known interaction is with amphotericin B as just described. *In vitro* flucytosine activity has been increased by tetracycline (41).

Therapeutic Uses. The drug can be used in *Candida* spp. infections of the urinary tract, and, when it can be established as etiological agent, in pulmonary infiltrative disease. When disease is not limited to bowel contents or mucosa, and when nystatin is not useful topically, flucytosine may be beneficial. It is usually effective for nonprogressive *C. neoformans* pulmonary disease when treatment is necessary. It may also be effective in cladosporiosis.

Flucytosine has also been effective in *T. glabrata* infections. Infections with *Phialophora* spp. and *Aspergillus* spp. have also been successfully treated. Cure of chronic cutaneous leishmaniasis has been reported with 10 days treatment (31). Cases of chromomycosis have been cured as well, but in only two cases was the oral route and a single drug used exclusively (43).

With more serious infections (i.e., *C. neoformans* meningitis), amphotericin B should be given as well (60).

Preparations. Flucytosine, USP (ANCOBON): capsules (250 or 500 mg).

Although larger doses are given in Europe, the currently recommended dosage is 150 mg/kg/day, in four equally divided doses, given at 6-hr intervals. When renal function is impaired, the interval between doses should be altered. One recent recommendation (23) is every 6 hr when the creatinine clearance is 40 mg/min or greater, every 12 hr if it is 40-20 mg/min, and every 24 hr if it is 20-10 ml/min. If the creatinine clearance is less than 10 ml/min, the interval should be determined by serum level. In patients on dialysis, 20 mg/kg dose has been recommended (19) after each dialysis.

IMIDAZOLES

Although the antifungal activities of the imidazoles were described as early as 1958 (52), members (clotrimazole, miconazole, and ketoconazole) of this group are the most recently introduced and commercially available. They have activity against a broad range of microorganisms, including both fungi and bacteria. They are related to the antithyroid agents carbimazole and methimazole, and to the antiprotozoal and antianaerobic agent, metronidazole.

Chemistry. The imidazoles, clotrimazole, miconazole, and ketoconazole, are synthesized chemicals whose structures are given in Fig. 25.2-1. They are relatively insoluble in water but can be dissolved in such organic solvents as chloroform, polyethylene glycol, and polyethoxylated castor oil (as in the preparation of miconazole for intravenous use).

Antifungal Actions. The imidazoles are active *in vitro* against the dermatophytes, the agents of the systemic mycoses, and some bacteria. Among the last, only *Staphylococcus aureus, Streptococcus faecalis,* and *Bacteroides fragilis* are sensitive. Among the systemic fungi, *B. dermatitidis* and *B. brasiliensis* are most sensitive, with MICs of 0.01-0.001 μg/ml. *C. neoformans* and *Candida* spp. have MICs of about 1 and 10 μg/ml, respectively. *Aspergillus* spp., the phycomycetes, *Torulopsis glabrata*, and *Madurella grisea* are resistant with MICs of 100 μg/ml or greater.

Mechanism of Action. The imidazoles appear to interact with cell membranes, causing leakage of cytoplasmic contents (65). Ketoconazole is a potent inhibitor of ergosterol synthesis in *C. albicans* (66). In these actions they resemble the polyenes. Low concentrations may also impede uptake of glutamines and purines.

Pharmacokinetics. Clotrimazole produces severe gastrointestinal symptoms, is poorly absorbed after oral administration, and rapidly induces liver enzymes, notably cytochrome P-450, that degrade and inactivate whatever amount is absorbed (60).

Miconazole is slightly better absorbed, with about 5-30% of the orally administered drug being detectable. After i.v. infusion of 500 mg over 15 min, peak plasma concentrations range from 2 to 9 and thereafter decline to 0.1-0.2 μg/ml at 8 hr. The volume of distribution was calculated at 14 l. It penetrates readily into infected synovial fluid and vitreous humor, but excretion in sputum is variable; CSF concentrations range from 3 to 50% of plasma levels. Ninety percent is bound to plasma proteins. It is metabolized by the liver, so that less than 1% is excreted unchanged in the urine. Neither renal impairment nor hemodialysis affects elimination, although plasma concentrations are greater in patients with azotemia owing to decreased distribution volume (11).

Ketoconazole is water soluble and readily absorbed from the gastrointestinal tract. Peak serum concentrations after doses of 10 and 160 mg/kg were 3 and 135 μg/ml, respectively. Activity decreased 10- to 1000-fold by the presence of serum. Data on metabolism, fate, and excretion are being accumulated, but it also appears to be metabolized in the liver, with inactive metabolites appearing in bile, feces, and urine. It does not penetrate into the cerebrospinal fluid.

Adverse Effects. In virtually all patients taking clotrimazole orally, side effects occur and in most are sufficiently disturbing to preclude a 6-week drug trial. These include, notably, nausea, vomiting, and diarrhea, but also abdominal cramps and even midepigastric pain. In one-fourth of patients in one study, mental disturbances have been reported. These included hallucinations and disorientation. With miconazole given intravenously, immediate reactions such as anaphylaxis, tachycardia, arrhythmias, fever, chills, and nausea were reported. Pruritus (especially with larger doses) has been sufficiently severe as to require discontinuation of the drug. Anemia and hyponatremia are common. An unusual lipoproteinemia, hyperlipidemia, hematological abnormalities, and interference of granulocyte function have been attributed to the vehicle. Data on ketoconazole are more limited, but pruritus and abnormalities of liver function tests have been reported. More recently reports of gynecomastia (26) led to demonstration of impaired adrenal (46), and testicular steroid synthesis and their displacement from serum transport proteins (32). Death (from liver disease) has also been reported (28).

Drug Interactions. Antagonism between miconazole and amphotericin B has been reported (51).

Therapeutic Uses. Clotrimazole is used locally for dermatophytic and *Candida* spp. infections. Miconazole is useful topically for the same infections. The intravenous use may be indicated when other therapy is ineffective, and sensitivity studies show activity against the isolate, in patients with candidiasis, coccidioidomycosis, cryptococcosis, and paracoccidioidomycosis. In patients with meningitis and urinary bladder infections, the intravenous route must be supplemented by the intrathecal or intrabladder irrigation routes, respectively. The dose for the former is 20 mg every 3-7 days. For the latter, the dose is 200 mg. Its eventual status is questionable, as failures, even before commercial release, were so common and striking as to merit publication of negative results (7). It is the best drug for *Pseudallescheria (Petriellidium) boydii* infections.

Ketoconazole may be a better drug for coccidioidomycosis and paracoccidioidomycosis on the basis of data that are incomplete. Animal studies suggest combined ketoconazole and flucytosine may be useful in cryptococcal meningitis (21).

Preparations. Clotrimazole is available as a 1% cream or solution (LOTRIMIN) or a 100-mg vaginal tablet (GYNELOTRIMIN), taken locally once to twice daily for from 1 to 4 weeks.

Miconazole is available as a 2% cream or lotion (MICATIN) for use on the skin and nails once or twice daily for 4 weeks, as a 2% vaginal cream (MONISTAT-7) to be applied once daily intravaginally for 14 days, and as ampule (200 mg/20 ml) for i.v. injection (MONISTAT, i.v.). The recommended i.v. dosage varies from 200- to 1200-mg infusions, which is given at 8-hr intervals, over a 30- to 60-min time period.

Ketoconazole is commercially available as a 200-mg tablet and is used at a dose of 200-400 mg/day.

GRISEOFULVIN

History. A metabolic product isolated from the yeast, *Pencillium griseofulvum* was shown to have a stunting and curling effect on hyphae of *Botrytis allii* (13). In 1958, Gentles (30) reported the use of griseofulvin orally in experimental infections with *Microsporum canis* and *Trichophyton mentagrophytes* in guinea pigs. Its first use in a patient with *T. rubrum* granuloma was reported by Blank and Roth (8).

Chemistry and Source. Griseofulvin (Fig. 25.2-1) is produced from the mycelial mat of a number of *Penicillium* spp. including, in addition to *P. griseofulvum, P. janczewskii* and *P. patulum.*

Antifungal Activity. Griseofulvin is fungistatic *in vitro* against *Microsporum, Epidermophyton, Trichophyton* spp. and dermatophytes. It is fungicidal in actively multiplying fungi, but only inhibitory in dormant cells. MIC for the dermatophytes of humans ranges narrowly from 0.20 to 0.44 μg/ml. It is ineffective in the systemic mycoses. It has no effect on bacteria, yeasts, or other fungi.

Mechanism of Action. Griseofulvin inhibits fungal mitosis. It probably causes disruption of the mitotic spindle by interacting with polymerized microtubules, as shown by its action in the mammalian cells at high concentrations. In this way, its action appears to be similar to those of colchicine and the vinca alkaloids, but its binding sites on microtubular protein are different from those of others. It slows oxidative phosphorylation and nucleic acid synthesis.

Fungal Resistance. Resistance has not been demonstrated in most of the fungal isolates from drug-treated humans. However, resistance can be made to develop *in vitro* in the dermatophytes that still can remain infectious in animals.

Pharmacological Effects. Griseofulvin has been shown to have a beneficial effect in anginal attacks, Raynaud's syndrome, and lichen planus. Of 20 patients with gout, 15 responded favorably to 2 g every 4 hr. The study was based on chemical similarity of griseofulvin to colchicine (70).

Pharmacokinetics. Peak serum levels in humans are 1.5-2 μg/ml, 4 hr following oral administration of a single dose of 1 g. Levels begin to decline at 8 hr, and only trace amounts are detected at 72 hr after dosage. The calculated half-life is 24 hr. Levels were twice as high when taken with a high-fat diet. However, from 28 to 73% of any dose is not absorbed. Within 24 hr, it can be detected in the stratum corneum, in amounts measured at 16.4, 9.7, and 4.5 ng/mg in layers 1, 2, and 3, respectively. Concentrations are higher in warmer temperatures, and concentrations fell more rapidly in skin than in serum on discontinuation. Within 72 hr, drug absorbed is excreted in the urine as the metabolite, 6-demethylgriseofulvin.

Adverse Effects. Side effects, usually mild and transient, are headache, pruritus, urticaria, dry mouth, nausea, vomiting, and diarrhea. Less frequently there is thirst, fatigue, insomnia, or irritation. There have been a few reports of lupus erythematosus syndrome. Angioneurotic edema, erythema multiforme, exfoliative dermatitis, proteinuria, and paresthesias have been reported rarely.

Griseofulvin is contraindicated in patients with porphyria and liver failure. Although it is embryotoxic and teratogenic in rats and has caused hepatic carcinomas in mice, a carcinogenic effect occurring with a latent period of less than 20 years has not been observed in humans.

Drug Interactions. Phenobarbital and phenytoin reduce serum and skin levels. Griseofulvin increases the effect of alcohol and, by increasing the rate of metabolism, diminishes the effect of anticoagulants such as warfarin.

Therapeutic Uses. Griseofulvin is indicated in patients with epidermophytosis of the skin, nails, and hair, notably in patients who have failed to respond to topical treatment. It is equally effective in infections due to *Microsporum* spp., *Trichophyton* spp. and *Epidermophyton* spp. It is less effective in palmar and plantar, and even less so in ungual, infections. For more susceptible infections, 3-6 weeks may suffice, whereas for ungual infections treatment in excess of 12 months may be necessary.

Despite its reported activity in other conditions, griseofulvin is currently not recommended for these.

Preparations. Griseofulvin, USP (GRISACTIN, GRIFULVIN V) is available as tablets (250 and 500 mg), capsules (125, 250, and 500 mg), and suspension (125 mg/5 ml). Preparations are variously microsized or ultramicrosized, and dosage is less for the latter by about one-half.

In adults, 125 mg of the ultramicrosized or 250 or 500 mg of the microsized preparation is given daily in single or divided doses. In children, 5 mg/kg of the ultramicrosized and 5 mg/lb of the microsized preparation are usual doses.

MISCELLANEOUS AGENTS

HYDROXYSTILBAMIDINE ISETHIONATE

Chemistry. Hydroxystilbamidine is a synthetic aromatic diamidine with the chemical formula, 4,4′-diamidion-2-hydroxystilbene di-(2-hydroxyethane sulfonate).

Pharmacokinetics. Hydroxystilbamidine has been administered only by the intravenous route. Nothing is known of its biotransformation or excretion. It accumulates in liver and skin.

Drug Interactions. A precipitate has been observed when hydroxystilbamidine was mixed in a 5% glucose solution with heparin.

Adverse Effects. Infrequent and late side effects include nausea, vomiting, anorexia, headache, malaise, and fever. Hepatotoxicity has been reported. Trigeminal neuropathy seen in 80% of patients given the parent drug, stilbamidine, has not been reported with hydroxystilbamidine.

Therapeutic Uses. Although once given for all forms of blastomycosis, the lack of efficacy in patients with meningitis, and to a lesser extent with pneumonias, resulted in the recommendation that use of hydroxystilbamidine be limited to patients with nonprogressive cutaneous disease (15, 68).

Preparations. The sterile vial contains 225 mg of drug, which should be diluted in sterile water and administered in at least 200 ml of normal saline or 5% glucose solution over a period of from 45 to 120 min. The vial and infusion bottle should be protected from light. Some physicians prefer a smaller initial dosage of 25-50 mg, with increments to the optimal dose. A course of treatment has usually been 8 g. A second course may be administered in relapse.

POTASSIUM IODIDE

Potassium iodide is indicated only in the cutaneous lymphatic form of sporotrichosis. It is also effective in entomophthoramycosis, a rare subcutaneous mycosis of tropical Southeast Asia,

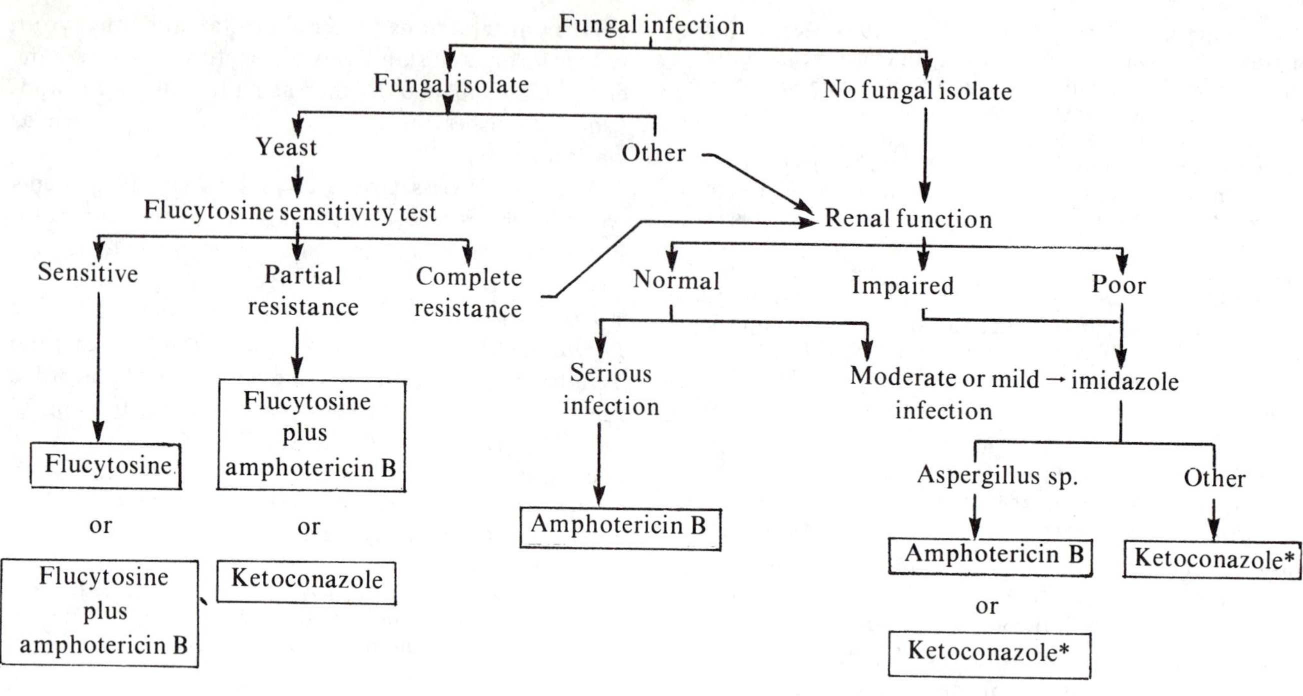

Fig. 25.2-2. *A schematic for selection of an antifungal drug for systemic mycosis* [modified from Cartwright (18)].

Indonesia, and Africa, caused by *Basidiobolus haptosporus*. However, potassium iodide is so much better tolerated than alternative drugs (e.g., amphotericin B) and the course of disease is so chronic, that one is justified in attempting therapy in other forms (e.g., pulmonary).

A saturated solution (1 g/ml) is employed and dosage is begun with 1 ml three times daily in water or other vehicle to disguise the somewhat unpleasant taste. Dosage is increased by 1 ml/day until an optimal dose of 12-15 ml is achieved. Therapy needs to be continued for a relatively prolonged period (i.e., for at least 6 weeks after disappearance of the lesions).

Iodism is frequently encountered during treatment. The earliest symptom is a brassy or otherwise unpleasant taste in the mouth. Coryza, sneezing, and tearing, all simulating a "cold," are common. Acneiform skin lesions also occur, especially in areas of heavy sweating. Nausea, heartburn, and diarrhea are evidence of gastrointestinal irritation. Parotid swelling mimics mumps. Toxic effects can usually be modulated or relieved by reducing the daily dose or ceasing therapy for a few days.

TOLNAFTATE

Tolnaftate (Fig. 25.2-1) was one of the first synthetic antifungal compounds used topically. The drug has a broad spectrum of activity against dermatophytes such as *T. mentagrophytes, T. rubrum, T. tonsurans, M. canis, M. gypseum, E. floccosum,* and *Malassezia furfur*; however, its use is primarily in the treatment of tinea pedis. It is less effective in presence of hyperkeratotic lesions that could be treated with 10% salicylic acid ointment given alternately with tolnaftate. Topical application of this agent in the just mentioned infections appears to be more effective than parenteral administration of griseofulvin but less effective than miconazole. Relapse may occur after cessation of therapy, as in the case of griseofulvin. Drug resistance and toxic or allergic reactions have not been reported.

Tolnaftate, USP (TINACTIN) is available as cream, gel, powder, aerosol powder, or topical solution in 1% concentration.

BENZOIC ACID AND SALICYLIC ACID

Benzoic and salicylic acids, USP (Whitfield's ointment containing 12% and 6% the ingredients, respectively) possesses fungistatic action of benzoate with keratolytic action of salicylate. It is used mainly in the treatment of tinea pedis.

CHOICE OF ANTIFUNGAL AGENTS

Superficial Mycoses. Griseofulvin is used for dermatophytic infections either topically or orally, depending on the site and severity of the lesion and ability of the patient to apply a cream or take a tablet. Whitfield's ointment, which is inexpensive, has also shown some effectiveness but may cause irritation.

Acute Vaginal Candidiasis. Polyenes and imidazoles are effective for acute vaginal candidiasis; the relapse rate may be lower with imidazoles.

Systemic Mycoses. The drug of choice for systemic mycoses depends on the susceptibility of the infecting fungus and the patient's renal function and ability to tolerate the drug. Table 25.2-1 presents the drug of choice for a number of systemic mycotic infections, and Fig. 25.2-2 provides a schematic for selection of a suitable antifungal drug for a patient with systemic mycosis.

REFERENCES

1. American Thoracic Society. Treatment of fungal diseases. *Am. Rev. Resp. Dis.* 120:1393, 1979.
2. Barbour, G.L., Straub, K.D., O'Neal, B.L. and Leatherman, J.W. Vasopressin-resistant nephrogenic diabetes insipidus, a

result of amphotericin B therapy. *Arch. Intern. Med.* 139:86, 1979.

3. Beggs, W.H., Sarosi, G.A. and Walker, M.I. Synergistic action of amphotericin B and rifampin against *Candida* species. *J. Infect. Dis.* 133:206, 1976.
4. Bennett, J.E. Chemotherapy of systemic mycoses. *N. Engl. J. Med.* 290:30, 1974.
5. Bennett, J.E., Dismukes, W.E., Duma, R.J. et al. Amphotericin B-flucytosine in cryptococcal meningitis. *N. Engl. J. Med.* 301:126, 1979.
6. Bhate, D.S., Hulyalkar, R.K. and Menon, S.K. Isolation of isobutyropyrrothine along with thiolutin and aureothricin from a *Streptomyces* sp. *Experientia* 16:504, 1960.
7. Bindschadler, D.D. and Bennett, J.E. A pharmacologic guide to the clinic use of amphotericin B. *J. Infect. Dis.* 120:427, 1969.
8. Blank, H. and Roth, R.J., Jr. The treatment of dermatomycosis with orally administered griseofulvin on dermatophytes. *AMA Arch. Dermatol.* 82:667, 1960.
9. Block, E.R. and Bennett, J.E. Pharmacologic studies with 5-fluorocytosine. *Antimicrob. Agents Chemother.* 1:476, 1972.
10. Block, E.R., Jennings, A.E. and Bennett, J.E. Experimental therapy of cladosporiosis and sporotrichosis with 5-fluorocytosine. *Antimicrob. Agents Chemother.* 3:95, 1973.
11. Bolaert, J., Daneels, R., Wan Landuyt, H. and Symoens, J. Miconazole plasma levels in healthy subjects and in patients with impaired renal function. *Chemotherapy* 6:165, 1976.
12. Brandriss, M.W., Wolff, S.M., Moores, R. and Stohlman, F. Anemia induced by amphotericin B. *JAMA* 189:663, 1964.
13. Brian, P.W., Curtis, P.J. and Hemming, H.G. A substance causing abnormal development of fungal hyphae produced by *Penicillium janczenskii* Zal I. Biological assay, production, and isolation of "curling factor." *Trans. Br. Mycol. Soc.* 29:173, 1946.
14. Bullock, W.E., Luke, R.G., Nutball, C.E. and Bhathena, D. Can mannitol reduce amphotericin B nephrotoxicity? Double blind study and description of a new vascular lesion in kidneys. *Antimicrob. Agents Chemother.* 10:555, 1976.
15. Busey, J.F. Blastomycosis. III. A comparative study of 2-hydroxystilbamidine and amphotericin B therapy. *Am. Rev. Resp. Dis.* 105:812, 1972.
16. Butler, W.T., Bennett, J.E., Alling, D.W., Westlake, P.T., Utz, J.P. and Hill, G.J., II. Nephrotoxicity of amphotericin B: Early and late effects in 81 patients. *Ann. Intern. Med.* 61:175, 1964.
17. Butler, W.T., Hill, G.J., II, Szwed, C.F. and Knight, V. Amphotericin B renal toxicity in the dog. *J. Pharmacol. Exp. Ther.* 143:47, 1964.
18. Cartwright, R.Y. Use of antibiotics: Antifungals. *Br. Med. J.* 2:108, 1978.
19. Christopher, T.G., Blair, A.D., Forrey, A.W. and Cutler, R.E. Hemodializer clearances of gentamicin, kanamycin, tobramycin, amikacin, ethambutol, procainamide, and flucytosine with a technique for planning therapy. *J. Pharmokinet. Biopharm.* 4:427, 1976.
20. Cohen, J. Antifungal chemotherapy. *Lancet* 2:532, 1982.
21. Craven, P.C. and Graybill, J.R. Combination of oral flucytosine and ketoconazole. *J. Infect. Dis.* 149:584, 1984.
22. Curtis, A.C. and Grekin, J.N. Histoplasmosis. *JAMA* 134:1217, 1947.
23. Cutler, R.E., Blair, A.D. and Kelly, M.R. Flucytosine kinetics in subjects with normal and impaired renal function. *Clin. Pharmacol. Ther.* 24:333, 1973.
24. Diamond, R.D. and Bennett, J.E. A subcutaneous reservoir for intrathecal therapy of fungal meningitis. *N. Engl. J. Med.* 288:186, 1973.
25. Diasio, R.B., Bennett, J.E. and Myers, C.E. Mode of action of 5-fluorocytosine. *Biochem. Pharmacol.* 27:703, 1978.
26. Dismukes, W.E., Stamm, A.M., Graybill, J.R. et al. Treatment of systemic mycoses with ketoconazole: Emphasis on toxicity and clinical response in 52 patients. *Ann. Intern. Med.* 98:13, 1983.
27. Drutz, D.J., Spickard, A., Rogers, D.E. and Koenig, M.G. Treatment of disseminated mycotic infections: A new approach to amphotericin B therapy. *Am. J. Med.* 45:405, 1968.
28. Duarte, P.A., Chow, C.C., Simmons, F. and Ruskin, J. Fatal hepatitis associated with ketoconazole therapy. *Arch Intern. Med.* 144:1069, 1984.
29. Fields, B.T., Jr., Bates, J. II and Abernathy, R.S. Effect of rapid intravenous infusions on serum concentrations of amphotericin B. *Appl. Microbiol.* 22:615, 1971.
30. Gentles, J.C. Experimental ringworm in guinea pigs: Oral treatment with griseofulvin. *Nature* 182:476, 1958.
31. Gonzalez-Ochoa, A. and Collado, C.M. Cutaneous leishmaniasis cured by 5-fluorocytosine. *Trop. Dis. Bull.* 70:732, 1973.
32. Grosso, D.S., Boyden, T.W., Pamenter, R.W. et al. Ketoconazole inhibition of testicular secretion of testosterone and displacement of steroid hormones from serum transport proteins. *Antimicrob. Agents Chemother.* 23:207, 1983.
33. Grunberg, E., Titsworth, E. and Bennett, M. Chemotherapeutic activity of 5-fluorocytosine. In: *Proceedings of the Third Interscience Conference on Antimicrobial Agents and Chemotherapy* (Sylvester, J.C., ed.). Ann Arbor, Mich: American Society for Microbiology, 1964, p. 566.
34. Hazen, E.L. and Brown, R. Fungicidin, an antibiotic produced by a soil actinomycete. *Proc. Soc. Exp. Biol. Med.* 76:93, 1951.
35. Hermans, P.E. and Keys, T.F. Antifungal agents used for deep seated mycotic infections. *Mayo Clin. Proc.* 58:223, 1983.
36. Keeny, E.L., Ajello, L. and Lankford, E. Studies on common pathogenic fungi and on *Actinomyces bovis*. *Bull. Johns Hopkins Hosp.* 75:393, 1944.
37. Kucers, A. and Bennett, N. McK. *The use of antibiotics.* Philadelphia: J.B. Lippincott, p. 575, 1975.
38. MacGregor, R.B., Bennett, J.E. and Erslev, A.J. Erythropoietin concentration in amphotericin B induced anemia. *Antimicrob. Agents Chemother.* 14:270, 1978.
39. McCurdy, D.K., Frederick, M. and Elkinton, J.R. Renal tubular acidosis due to amphotericin B. *N. Engl. J. Med.* 278:24, 1968.
40. Medoff, G., Dismukes, W.E., Meads, R.H. and Moses, J. Therapeutic program for Candida infection. *Antimicrob. Agents Chemother.* 10:286, 1970.
41. Medoff, G., Comfort, M. and Kobayashi, G.S. Synergistic action of amphotericin B and 5-fluorocytosine against yeast-like organisms. *Proc. Soc. Exp. Biol. Med.* 138:571, 1971.
42. Meyer, R. and Axelrod, J.L. Fatal aplastic anemia resulting from flucytosine. *JAMA* 228:1573, 1974.
43. Morrison, W.L., Connor, B. and Clayton, Y. Successful treatment of chromoblastomycosis with 5-fluorocytosine. *Br. J. Dermal.* 90:445, 1974.
44. Pankey, G.A., Lockwood, W.R. and Montalvo, J.M. 5-Fluorocytosine: A replacement for amphotericin B in the treatment of Candida and *Cryptococcus neoformans* infections. *J. La. St. Med. Soc.* 122:365, 1970.
45. Polak, A. Mode of action of 5-fluorocytosine and 5-fluorouracil in dematiaceous fungi. *Sabouraudia* 21:127, 1983.
46. Pont, A., Williams, P.L. and Loose, D.S. Ketoconazole inhibits adrenal steroid synthesis. *Clin. Res.* 30:99A, 1982.
47. Presant, G.A., Klahr, C. and Santala, R. Amphotericin B induction of sensitivity to adriamycin, 1,3-bis (2-chloroethyl)-1-nitrosourea (BCNU) plus cyclophosphamide in human neoplasia. *Ann. Intern. Med.* 86:47, 1977.
48. Reynolds, S.S., Tomkiewicz, I.M. and Dammin, G.J. The renal lesion related to amphotericin B treatment for coccidioidomycosis. *Med. Clin. North Am.* 47:1149, 1963.
49. Safe, L.M., Safe, S.H. and Subden, R.E. Sterol content and polyene antibiotic resistance in isolates of *Candida krusei*, *Candida porakrusei*, and *Candida tropicalis*. *Can. J. Microbiol.* 23:398, 1977.
50. Sarosi, G.A. Management of fungal diseases. *Am. Rev. Resp. Dis.* 127:250, 1983.

51. Schacter, L.P., Owellen, R.J., Rathbun, H.K. and Buchanan, B. Antagonism between miconazole and amphotericin B. *Lancet* 2:318, 1976.

52. Seeliger, H.P.R. Pilzhemmende Wirkung eines neuen Benzimidazol—Derivatives. *Mykosen* 1:162, 1958.

53. Shadomy, S., Brummer, D.L. and Ingroff, A.V. Light sensitivity of prepared solutions of amphotericin B. *Am. Rev. Resp. Dis.* 107:303, 1973.

54. Shirley, S.F. and Little, J.R. Immunopotentiating effects of amphotericin B. I. Enhanced contact sensitivity in mice. *J. Immunol.* 123:2878, 1979.

55. Snapper, I. and McVay, L.V. The treatment of North American blastomycosis with 2-hydroxystilbamidine. *Am. J. Med.* 15:603, 1957.

56. Stamm, A.M. and Dismukes, W.E. Current therapy of pulmonary and disseminated fungal diseases. *Chest* 83:911, 1983.

57. Steer, P.L., Marks, M.I., Klite, P.D. and Eickhoff, T.C. 5-Fluorocytosine: An oral antifungal compound. *Ann. Intern. Med.* 76:15, 1972.

58. Stobo, J.D., Paul, S., Van Scoy, R.E. and Hermans, P.E. Suppressor thymus derived lymphocytes in fungal infection. *J. Clin. Invest.* 57:319, 1976.

59. Tynes, B.J., Utz, J.P., Bennett, J.E. and Alling, D.W. Reduction amphotericin B reactions: A double blind study. *Am. Rev. Resp. Dis.* 87:264, 1963.

60. Utz, J.P. New drugs for systemic mycoses: Flucytosine and clotrimazole. *Bull. N.Y. Acad. Med.* 51:1103, 1975.

61. Utz, J.P., Andriole, V.T. and Emmons, C.W. Chemotherapeutic activity of X-5079C in systemic mycoses of man. *Am. Rev. Resp. Dis.* 514, 1961.

62. Utz, J.P., Bennett, J.E., Brandriss, M.W., Butler, W.T. and Hill, G.J., II. Amphotericin B toxicity. *Ann. Intern. Med.* 61:334, 1964.

63. Utz, J.P., Shadomy, J.H. and Shadomy, S. Clinical and laboratory studies of a new micronized preparation of hamycin in systemic mycoses in man. In: *Antimicrobial agents and Chemotherapy*, Ann Arbor, Mich.: American Society for Microbiology, 1968, p. 113.

64. Utz, J.P., Garriques, I.L., Sande, M.A., Warner, J.P., Mandell, G.L., Mc Gehee, R.F., Duma, R.J. and Shadomy, S. Therapy of cryptococcosis with a combination of flucytosine and amphotericin B. *J. Infect. Dis.* 132:368, 1975.

65. Van den Bossche, H. Biochemical effects of miconazole on fungi. I. Effects on the uptake and/or utilization of purines, pyrimidines, nucleosides, amino acids, and glucose by *Candida albicans. Biochem. Pharmacol.* 23:887, 1974.

66. Van den Bossche, H., Willemsens, G., Cools, W., Cornelissen, F. and VanCutsem, J.M. Effect of ketoconazole on growth and lipid synthesis of *Candida albicans. Preclinical Research Report V 1533S. New Brunswick, N.J.: Janssen Pharmaceutical Research and Development,* 1978.

67. Vandeputte, J., Wachtel, J.L. and Stiller, E.T. Amphotericins A and B, antifungal antibiotics produced by a streptomyces. II. The isolation and properties of the crystalline amphotericins. In: *Antibiotics Annual 1955.* New York: Medical Encyclopedia, 1956, p. 87.

68. Veteran's Administration Cooperative Study on Blastomycosis. A review of 198 collected cases in Veterans Administration Hospitals. *Am. Rev. Resp. Dis.* 89:659, 1964.

69. Wade, J.C., Schimpff, S.C., Hargadon, M.T., Fortner, C.L., Young, V.M. and Wiernik, P.H. A comparison of trimethoprim-sulfamethoxazole plus nystatin with gentamicin plus nystatin in the prevention of infections in acute leukemia. *N. Engl. J. Med.* 304:1057, 1981.

70. Wallace, S.J. and Nissen, A.W. Griseofulvin in acute gout. *N. Engl. J. Med.* 266:1099, 1962.

71. Wang, G.M. and Schaffner, C.P. Effect of candicidin and colestipol on the testes and prostate gland of B10 87.20 hamsters. *Invest. Urol.* 14:66, 1976.

72. Williams, C., Whitehouse, J.M.A., Lister, T.A. et al. Oral anti-Candido in patients undergoing chemotherapy for acute leukemia. *Med. Pediatr. Oncol.* 3:275, 1977.

73. Williams, T.W., Jr., Bennett, J.E. and Emmons, C.W. Chemotherapeutic and toxic activity of hamycin in experimental mycosis. In: *Antimicrobial Agents and Chemotherapy, 1964.* Ann Arbor, Mich.: American Society for Microbiology, 1965, p. 737.

CHAPTER
25.3

ANTITUBERCULOSIS AGENTS

Robert C. Hastings

Tuberculosis is an ancient infectious human disease caused by *Mycobacterium tuberculosis.* The disease has been known since at least 1000 B.C. (6). Because tuberculosis is a disease of respiratory transmission, the disease is transmitted optimally in conditions of overcrowding and poor personal and public hygiene. The development of contagious cases is associated with conditions resulting in decreased cell-mediated immunity (e.g., senescence, malnutrition, viral illnesses) and the non-availability of (e.g., poverty) or noncompliance with (e.g., alcoholism) medical care. Thus, general socioeconomic conditions have a profound influence on the incidence and prevalence of tuberculosis. Coinciding with improvements in standards of living, the incidence and prevalence of tuberculosis have declined in recent times.

In 1977, there were 30,000 new cases of tuberculosis diagnosed in the United States (29). A recent review of experience in a 525-bed private community hospital in Chicago showed approximately 5 tuberculosis patients diagnosed per 100 beds per year. Of interest, only 36% of these cases were suspected of having tuberculosis even after the chest x-ray films were available (15). Thus, tuberculosis continues to decline as a problem in the United States, but its incidence remains substantial, and circumstances have resulted in its return to the mainstream of medicine, where the index of suspicion is sometimes regrettably low.

NATURAL HISTORY

Pulmonary tuberculosis is a disease of respiratory transmission. Patients with active disease expel viable tubercle bacilli into the air in their environment by coughing, sneezing, shouting, and singing. An immunologically naive individual who inhales infectious droplet particles in the 3- to 8-μm size range has viable tubercle bacilli inoculated into his respiratory bronchioles and alveoli. The bacilli multiply for about 4-6 weeks, spread via lymphatics to regional pulmonary nodes, into the bloodstream, and disseminate throughout the body. They tend to implant and multiply in three locations: (1) the reticuloendothelial system, (2) serosal surfaces, and (3) sites with high pO_2, particularly the apices of the lungs, renal cortex, and epiphyses of growing bones. In most individuals during this time of primary dissemination, cell-mediated immunity and delayed-type hypersensitivity develop to antigens of the tubercle bacilli (tuberculoprotein) as evidenced by the development of a positive tuberculin skin test. The newly formed sensitized lymphocytes are attracted to foci of infection, and a granulomatous reaction develops. This inflammatory reaction results in objective evidence of the disease in about 10% of those infected, and about half of these individuals have symptoms (i.e., 5% of those infected) (6, 27). It should be pointed out that a full spectrum of immunological responses in tuberculosis has been described that roughly parallels that of leprosy, leishmaniasis, and syphilis (25).

In a small proportion of newly infected patients, the disease progresses uncontrollably after the time of primary dissemination, and cell-mediated immunity and delayed-type hypersensitivity do not develop. This syndrome is called *progressive primary tuberculosis* (27) and corresponds to the disseminated or lepromatous form of leprosy (Chapter 25.4). The vast majority of infected individuals heal and scar their infected foci, and the primary infection is terminated. On the other hand, a few viable bacilli remain in these scarred foci. For the rest of the individual's life these foci may break down if host defenses become impaired, and overt tuberculosis (secondary reactivation tuberculosis) results. The most common sites for this involvement are the apices of the upper and lower lobes of the lung, probably because of the high pO_2 levels maintained in these locations. From 85-90% of all cases of clinical tuberculosis are of the secondary reactivation pulmonary type (6, 27).

GENERAL PRINCIPLES OF ANTITUBERCULOSIS THERAPY

In almost all cases, chemotherapy is the only therapeutic modality necessary for the management of tuberculosis. Rest has been shown to be of no benefit (28). Because transmission is respiratory via droplets, isolation measures can be accomplished by the patient's simply covering his mouth and nose during coughing or sneezing with tissues that can be disposed of in a sanitary manner. Because the infectivity of an active tuberculosis patient virtually disappears within 1-2 weeks of starting effective chemotherapy (27), fomites are not important in transmission, and transmission, if it were to happen, would have in all likelihood already occurred in the time preceding the diagnosis; thus, there is currently no need to hospitalize tuberculosis patients in order to isolate them from contacts (22). Hospitalization is now provided only if needed by the patient because of symptoms, complications, the need for therapy of other problems, or for diagnostic problems (23).

ANTITUBERCULOSIS DRUGS

A number of available effective antituberculosis drugs are listed in Table 25.3-1 with their therapeutic doses and side effects. Depending on their efficacy and toxicity, they have been classified (3) as: *primary, or first-line,* drugs (with highest efficacy and lowest toxicity) (e.g., isoniazid, ethambutol, streptomycin, and rifampin) (23, 27), and *secondary, or second-line,* drugs (with relatively less efficacy and higher likelihood of toxicities) (e.g., pyrazinamide, p-aminosalicylic acid, and others). Recently, they have been reclassified (17) into three groups depending on their varying degree of effectiveness and potential side effects: *primary* drugs (isoniazid and rifampin are the most effective and have low toxicity);

Table 25.3-1
Treatment of Mycobacterial Disease in Adults and Children

Drugs	Dosage		Most Common Side Effects
	Daily	Twice Weekly	
Primary, or first-line			
Isoniazid	5-10 mg/kg up to 300 mg p.o. or i.m.	15 mg/kg p.o. or i.m.	Peripheral neuritis, hepatitis, hypersensitivity
Rifampin	10-20 mg/kg up to 600 mg p.o.	Not recommended	Hepatitis, febrile reaction, purpura (rare)
Ethambutol	15-25 mg/kg p.o.	50 mg/kg p.o.	Optic neuritis (reversible with discontinuation of drug; very rare at 15 mg/kg), skin rash
Streptomycin	15-20 mg/kg up to 1 g i.m.	25-30 mg/kg	Eighth cranial nerve damage, nephrotoxicity
Secondary, or second-line			
Para-aminosalicylic acid (aminosalicylic acid)	150 mg/kg up to 12 g p.o.		GI disturbance, hypersensitivity, hepatotoxicity, sodium load
Viomycin	15-30 mg/kg up to 1 g i.m.		Auditory toxicity, nephrotoxicity, vestibular toxicity (rare)
Capreomycin	15-30 mg/kg up to 1 g i.m.		Eighth cranial nerve damage, nephrotoxicity
Kanamycin	15-30 mg/kg up to 1 g i.m.		Auditory toxicity, nephrotoxicity, vestibular toxicity (rare)
Ethionamide	15-30 mg/kg up to 1 g p.o.		GI disturbance, hepatotoxicity, hypersensitivity
Pyrazinamide	15-30 mg/kg up to 2 g p.o.		Hyperuricemia, hepatotoxicity
Cycloserine	10-20 mg/kg up to 1 g p.o.		Psychosis, personality changes, convulsions, rash

Source: Modified from Ref. 3.

secondary drugs (less effective and more toxic) (e.g., ethambutol, p-aminosalicylic acid, pyrazinamide, and streptomycin), and *tertiary* drugs (least effective and most toxic) (e.g., capreomycin, cycloserine, ethionamide, and kanamycin).

PRIMARY, OR FIRST-LINE ANTITUBERCULOSIS DRUGS

ISONIAZID

History. Isoniazid (isonicotinic acid hydrazide, INH) was synthesized in 1912 and shown by three independent groups to have activity in tuberculosis in 1952. The compound was actually a chemical intermediate in the synthesis of a thiosemicarbazone that was felt more likely to be active. Routine testing of chemical intermediates for antituberculosis activity showed the remarkable activity of isoniazid (11).

Chemistry. Isoniazid (Fig. 25.3-1) is relatively water soluble and only slightly soluble in the usual organic solvents. It is a white crystalline solid. Aqueous solutions are slightly acid and relatively stable (33).

Mechanism of Action. There are a great many theories dealing with the mechanism of action of isoniazid, none of which are universally accepted. One theory states that isoniazid complexes with essential metals such as copper or iron contained in mycobacterial enzymes essential to oxidation-reduction reactions biochemically. Other theories postulate that isoniazid interacts with mycobacterial metalloporphyrin enzymes to generate toxic breakdown products or free radicals. Other proposed mechanisms involve inhibition of NAD synthesis or degradation or isoniazid conversion to isonicotinic acid and replacing nicotinamide in NAD and NADP to disturb mycobacterial oxidative and dehydrogenase systems. Interfering with mycobacterial DNA synthesis, possibly through an action on NAD, has been proposed. Still other theories involve isoniazid causing an accumulation of toxic pigments in mycobacteria, reacting with and depleting mycobacteria of pyridoxal, and inhibiting the synthesis of mycolic acids, which are unique cell wall constituents of mycobacteria (11).

Pharmacokinetics. Isoniazid is readily absorbed. Peak plasma concentrations after oral ingestion occur within 1-2 hr. Following the usual 300-mg adult doses of isoniazid, blood levels 6 hr later are 0.2-1 μg/ml. Sensitive strains of tubercle bacilli are inhibited *in vitro* by concentrations as low as 0.05 μg of isoniazid per ml. Higher concentrations are bactericidal against actively growing tubercle bacilli. Isoniazid diffuses readily into all body fluids and cells, and concentrations intracellularly are equivalent to those extracellularly. The half-life of the intact drug in blood is 1-3 hr.

Metabolism of INH is principally by acetylation in the liver. This metabolism is under genetic control. Genetically rapid acetylators show a shorter half-life of intact INH than genetically slow acetylators. Slow acetylators tend to develop neuritic side effects more frequently than rapid acetylators. On the other hand, the incidence of hepatotoxicity seems to be slightly higher in fast acetylators.

From 75-90% of a dose of isoniazid is excreted in the urine within 24 hr as metabolites, principally acetylisoniazid and isonicotinic acid. Trace amounts of isonicotinyl glycine, isonicotinyl hydrazones, and N-methyl-isoniazid are found. Unchanged drug also appears in the urine, the proportion being higher in slow acetylators, with higher proportions of acetylisoniazid being found in rapid acetylators.

Acetylator status is based on genetic differences in the activity of the enzyme, acetyl transferase, and slow acetylation is inherited as an autosomal recessive trait. Slow acetylators are thus homozygous for this trait. Rapid acetylation is inherited in a dominant fashion. Heterozygotes for the rapid trait have somewhat higher plasma isoniazid levels than individuals who are homozygotes for the rapid trait. Because peak plasma levels are the relevant factor therapeutically, antibacterial efficacy is considered to be equivalent in rapid and slow acetylators (16, 20).

Adverse Effects. Untoward effects of isoniazid are relatively rare and the drug enjoys good patient acceptability. Two types of toxicities occur with some frequency: peripheral neuritis and hepatotoxicity. The peripheral neuritis seen with isoniazid is thought to be related to the induction of a relative pyridoxine deficiency, is more common in malnourished individuals, is more common in slow acetylators, and is dose related. At adult doses of 300 mg daily, peripheral neuritis can be seen in 1-3% of patients; at 700 mg daily, in approximately 10% of patients; and at 1400 mg daily, in approximately 50%. In addition to the peripheral neuritis, other neurological side effects that have been described include insomnia, headaches, restlessness, excitement, muscle twitching, increased reflexes, paresthesias, delay in micturition, and even convulsions and psychotic episodes. Most of these side effects can be prevented or treated with supplemental pyridoxine, which does not impair the drug's antibacterial efficacy.

The incidence of isoniazid-induced hepatitis is directly proportional to age and probably alcohol intake. Estimated risks of developing hepatitis in treating individuals with reactive tuberculin skin tests are 0.13% at age 25, 0.59% at age 35, 1.09% at age 45, 1.75% at age 55, and 1.05% at age 65. Although isoniazid is 80% effective in preventing overt disease among infected individuals, by age 45 the risks of isoniazid-induced hepatitis outweigh the benefits in infected individuals with normal chest x-rays (6). Isoniazid-induced hepatitis ranges from mild to asymptomatic hepatocellular abnormalities manifested by elevations of serum transaminases to fulminant hepatic necrosis. The hepatocellular injury is attributed to toxic metabolic products of acetylisoniazid, particularly acetylhydrazine, and thus occurs more frequently in fast acetylators (19). In one large series, 22% of isoniazid-treated patients showed elevations of serum transaminases above normal. Approximately 7% had transaminase values more than five times normal, usually within

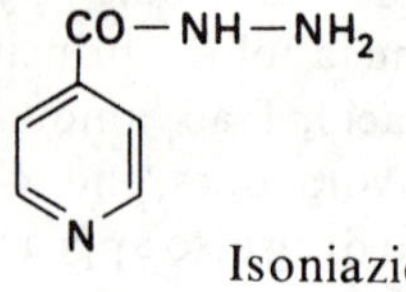

Isoniazid

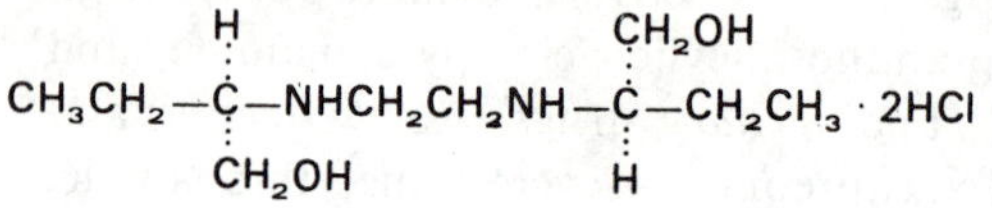

Ethambutol

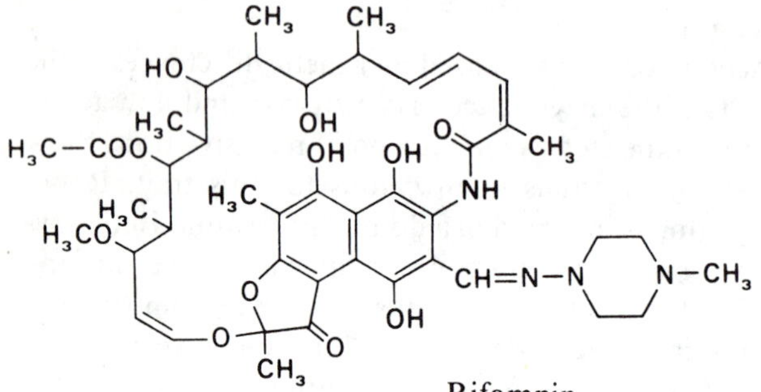

Rifampin

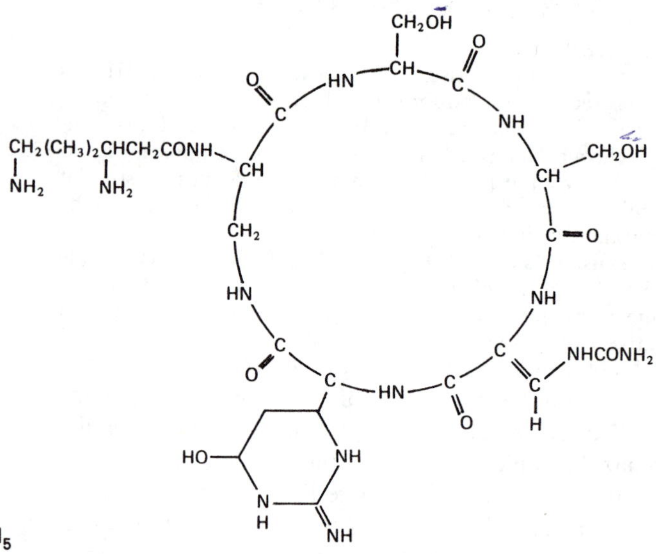

Viomycin

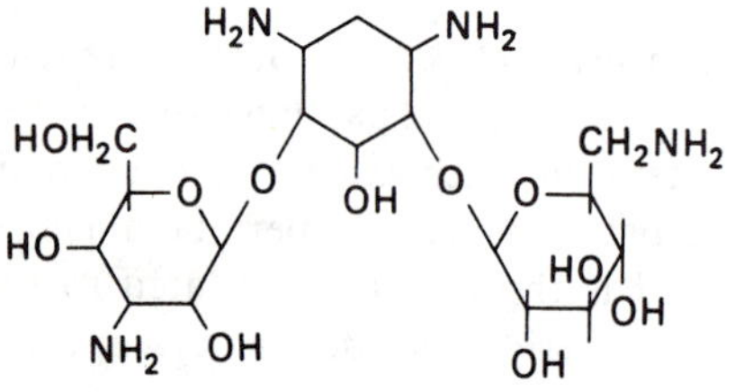

Kanamycin

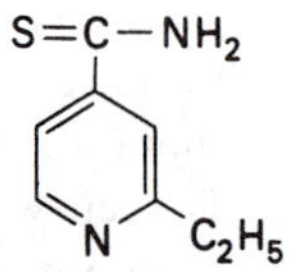

Ethionamide

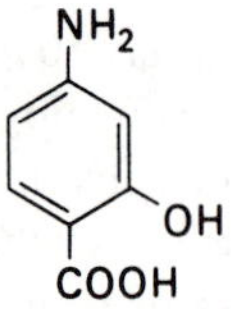

Para-aminosalicylic acid

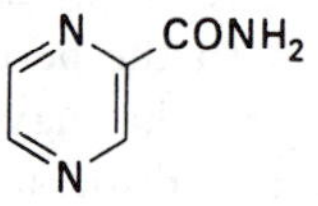

Pyrazinamide

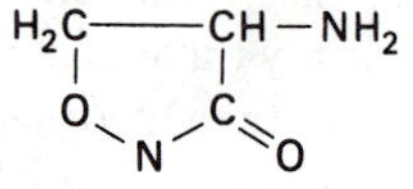

Cycloserine

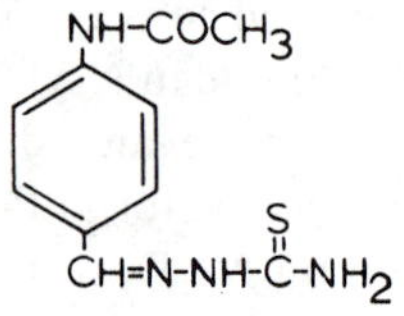

Thiacetazone

Fig. 25.3-1. *Chemical structures of some antituberculosis agents.*

the first few months of therapy, and of these, over two-thirds were asymptomatic whereas the remainder (2% of all patients) had symptoms of hepatitis (9). In other large series, the incidence of overt isoniazid hepatitis has been 0.8-1.3%, with 0.06-0.09% fatalities.

Patients with overt hepatitis have experienced mortality rates as high as 12.3% (19), but usually fatalities have occurred in patients who continued to take the drug despite symptoms and signs of toxicity such as anorexia, malaise, and jaundice. Current practice is to administer isoniazid without monitoring hepatic function in younger individuals without evidence of preexisting hepatic disease so long as they remain asymptomatic (23). In asymptomatic individuals who are monitored, many therapists recommend discontinuing isoniazid when transaminases activity is accompanied by increases in serum bilirubin or alkaline phosphatase.

A variety of allergic reactions can occur with isoniazid such as fever, skin rashes, arthralgias, and hematological reactions. These are relatively uncommon, occurring in well less than 2% of treated patients (9). In individuals with glucose-6-phosphate dehydrogenase (G-6-PD) deficiency, isoniazid can induce hemolytic anemia.

Drug Interactions. Isoniazid may interfere with the metabolism of phenytoin, decrease its excretion, or enhance its effects. To avoid phenytoin intoxication, monitoring and adjustment of the anticonvulsant dosage should be made when phenytoin is used concomitantly with isoniazid. Patients who consume alcohol daily may experience a higher incidence of isoniazid hepatotoxicity.

Therapeutic Uses. Isoniazid is the most useful of the antituberculosis drugs, having the highest efficacy and the lowest overall toxicity. Toxicities can be minimized by prophylactic pyridoxine and careful monitoring of the patient for side effects (2). The drug is extraordinarily inexpensive (6).

Preparations. *Isoniazid,* USP (isonicotinic acid hydrazide, NYDRAZID, HYZYD, etc.): tablets (100 or 300 mg), syrup (10 mg/ml), or injection (100 mg/ml). Isoniazid is administered in adult doses of 4-5 mg/kg or 300 mg daily in a single dose. For disseminated disease, doses may be as high as 10-20 mg/kg daily in adults given together with pyridoxine supplements. In infants and children, dosages of 10-20 mg/kg daily for therapy and 10 mg/kg daily for prevention are given in single doses. Intramuscular and oral doses are the same.

ETHAMBUTOL

History. The antituberculosis activity of ethambutol was established in 1961. The drug was developed in a rational synthetic program based on the knowledge that related diamines had slight antituberculosis activity. These diamines were systematically modified, based on the theory that they had activity due to their ability to chelate metal ions (11).

Chemistry. Ethambutol (Fig. 25.3-1) is a white crystalline compound that is water soluble. It is optically active. The d(+)-isomer has antituberculosis activity and is the form marketed. The l(−)-isomer exhibits 200-fold less activity.

Mechanism of Action. The biological mechanism of action of ethambutol is unknown. Theories are based on its ability to form metal chelates, together with a postulated ability of the drug or its chelate to fit a specific enzyme template. The drug may interfere with the function of polyamines (e.g., spermidine) and metal ions (e.g., magnesium) in the synthesis and stabilization of mycobacterial RNA. Ethambutol inhibits the incorporation of methionine into lipids in *M. smegmatis* (11).

Pharmacokinetics. From 75-80% of oral doses of ethambutol are absorbed from the gastrointestinal (GI) tract. Following 25-mg/kg single oral doses, peak serum concentrations of 2-5 μg/ml are attained within 2-4 hr. The minimum inhibitory concentration of ethambutol for *M. tuberculosis in vitro* is on the order of 1-5 μg/ml. The half-life of the drug in serum is approximately 8 hr. Approximately 50% of the administered dose is excreted unchanged in the urine and an additional 8-15% appears in the urine in the form of metabolites. The principal metabolic pathway appears to be an initial oxidation of the alcohol to an intermediate aldehyde, followed by conversion to a dicarboxylic acid. Approximately 20% of the initial dose is excreted in the feces as unchanged drug. Intracellular concentrations of ethambutol serve as a depot to maintain plasma concentrations. The drug does not reach to the cerebrospinal fluid normally, but can be detected in the cerebrospinal fluid of patients with tuberculous meningitis.

Adverse Effects. The most significant adverse effect of ethambutol is ocular toxicity. This is a dose-related, reversible phenomenon manifested by a gradual loss of visual acuity, decrease in visual fields, and loss of the ability to perceive the color green. These symptoms usually disappear over a period of weeks to months after the drug has been discontinued, although in rare cases recovery may be delayed for up to 1 year or more. At 15 mg/kg/day, there is a negligible incidence of this side effect. At 25 mg/kg/day, there is an incidence of approximately 2%. At a dosage of 50 mg/kg/day, approximately 33% of patients experience optic nerve toxicity. The antibacterial effectiveness of ethambutol is dose related up to at least 100 mg/kg/day.

Characteristically, ethambutol causes hyperuricemia and may precipitate acute gout. The commonly used doses of ethambutol cause hyperuricemia in approximately 50% of patients due to a decreased renal excretion of uric acid. This effect may be enhanced by isoniazid and pyridoxine.

Other side effects are rare and include the usual allergic reactions manifested by dermatitis, pruritus, arthralgias, fever, malaise, and so on. The incidence of hypersensitivity to ethambutol is relatively quite low (approximately 0.1%), and in general the reactions tend to be mild (2).

Therapeutic Uses. Ethambutol is the most commonly used companion drug with isoniazid in the conventional initial therapy with patients with pulmonary tuberculosis. It has replaced para-aminosalicylic acid in this regard because of higher patient acceptability and fewer side effects. Its optic nerve toxicity is reversible, although this has been a major drawback to its full acceptance in the past. Its antituberculosis activity is relatively modest but adequate to inhibit the appearance of isoniazid-resistant tubercle bacilli. The drug is relatively inexpensive (6).

Preparations. *Ethambutol,* USP (MYAMBUTOL): tablets (100 or 400 mg of d-isomer). The drug is administered once every 24 hr in dosages of 15-25 mg/kg for patients with normal renal function. Patients with decreased renal function require reduced dosages of ethambutol because the principal path of excretion is via the kidneys (2).

STREPTOMYCIN

Chemistry, general pharmacology, and mechanism of action of streptomycin are discussed in Chapter 24.3. Only those principles relevant to mycobacterial disease are presented here.

History. Shortly after the discovery of streptomycin in 1944, it was shown to be effective against *M. tuberculosis.* It was the first clinically effective drug available for the treatment of tuberculosis. Within several years, the problem of streptomycin resistance was noted in tubercle bacilli (20).

Pharmacokinetics. Streptomycin must be administered intramuscularly. In adults, usual doses of 1 g i.m. result in plasma concentrations of 25-30 μg/ml. The minimum inhibitory concentration of streptomycin for sensitive strains of *M. tuberculosis in vitro* are as low as 0.2-0.4 μg/ml, and most strains are inhibited by 10 μg/ml. *In vivo* in tuberculosis, the drug exerts a bacteriostatic rather than a bactericidal effect (19).

Therapeutic Uses. Streptomycin remains highly effective in the treatment of tuberculosis. Its eighth cranial nerve toxicities, the necessity for i.m. injections, the availability of oral agents of comparable safety and efficacy, and the modern outpatient management of tuberculosis have all contributed to the decline of its popularity.

Preparations. Customarily, streptomycin is administered in doses of 20 mg/kg (approximately 1 g daily for an adult) once a day for 2-3 weeks. Thereafter, the frequency can be decreased to 1 g every other day or 1 g three times weekly and then to 1 g twice each week. The dose should be reduced in older individuals and in individuals with impaired renal function. The drug is marketed generically and is available as a powder or sterile solution for injection. (2).

RIFAMPIN

History. The rifamycin antibiotics were discovered by Professor Sensi and coworkers in 1957. The chemical structures of various rifamycins were determined in 1963, and in that year rifamycin SV was first used i.m. in leprosy. In 1966, rifampin was first prepared as a synthetic modification of rifamycin B as an orally effective agent and shortly thereafter was shown to have antituberculosis activity (32).

Chemistry. Rifampin is prepared by synthetic modification of the parent compound rifamycin B, one of at least five different antibiotics produced by *Streptomyces mediterranei.* The rifamycins are ansa compounds consisting of naphthoquinone or naphthohydroquinone ring systems spanned by a long aliphatic bridge (Fig. 25.3-1). One of the substances originally produced by *S. mediterranei* is rifamycin B, which on reduction yields the naphthohydroquinone derivative, rifamycin SV. This can be modified to produce rifampin, a semisynthetic derivative of rifamycin SV.

The ansa ring is the crucial portion of the rifamycin molecule responsible for antibacterial effectiveness. The aromatic ring system can be modified to some extent without losing antibacterial effectiveness. Rifampin exists as a zwitterion. It is slightly soluble in water at pH less than 6 and is stable (33).

Mechanism of Action. Rifampin acts to inhibit transcription. It inhibits RNA synthesis by inactivating DNA-dependent RNA polymerase. One mole of rifampin is bound per mole of the enzyme. Rifampin is highly specific for bacterial RNA polymerase, with concentrations 10,000 times higher being required to inhibit the corresponding mammalian enzyme. Rifampin acts to prevent the initiation of new RNA chains. RNA chains already being constructed continue to completion in the presence of the drug. The β-subunit of bacterial DNA-dependent RNA polymerase is the site of rifampin's action. The development of rifampin resistance involves mutational change in the primary amino acid sequence of this portion of the enzyme such that rifampin no longer binds to the enzyme (11). Resistance to rifampin arises as a single-step mutation (21).

Pharmacokinetics. Blood levels of rifampin following oral administration in normal individuals vary widely. Peak levels occur between 2 and 4 hr and average 7 μg/ml, with a range from 4 to 32 μg/ml following 600-mg doses. Minimum inhibitory concentrations *in vitro* are 0.5 μg/ml or less for *M. tuberculosis* (31). The half-life of the drug in normal individuals is approximately 3 hr (2.6-6.5 hr). During the first 2 weeks of continuous therapy, there is a progressive shortening of the half-life by approximately 40% due to enhanced biliary excretion of the compound. The drug is deacetylated by the liver and excreted into the bile along with the unchanged drug. An enterohepatic circulation develops. The deacetylated metabolite is less well reabsorbed from the intestine than the parent compound; thus, metabolic deacetylation enhances eventual elimination of the drug. Rifampin competes with bilirubin and bromsulphalein (BSP) for biliary excretion. The half-life of the compound is increased in patients with hepatic dysfunction. Up to 30% of an administered dose appears in the urine, approximately half of which is unchanged drug. With high doses of rifampin, urinary excretion becomes quantitatively more significant than biliary excretion. In the usual clinical setting, however, dose adjustments are not necessary in patients with moderately impaired renal function. Despite its large molecular weight, the compound is distributed throughout the body and is present in effective concentrations in the cerebrospinal fluid. It should be noted that the deacetylated form of rifampin retains antibacterial efficacy.

Adverse Effects. Adverse reactions to rifampin are strikingly different depending on whether the drug is administered on a daily basis or whether it is administered intermittently. Side effects due to rifampin occur in 1-10% of patients when the drug is taken daily. These reactions are usually minor cutaneous, gastrointestinal, and hepatic reactions that are usually reversible and usually do not interfere with therapy. On the other hand, when intermittent regimens are used, antibodies to rifampin occur in 30% of patients and between 15 and 25% of them develop influenza-like symptoms consisting of fever, headache, dizziness, and bone pain. The two most life-threatening adverse reactions to rifampin are thrombocytopenia and renal insufficiency. These occur very rarely during continuous daily rifampin administration, but intermittent regimens either by virtue of planning or by virtue of irregular compliance by patients on prescribed daily therapy are much more likely to lead to antibody formation and the more severe reactions.

Cutaneous reactions seen with rifampin are usually mild and transient. Their frequency differs in different populations but may occur in up to 5% of treated patients. Face, scalp, neck, and conjunctival flushing with or without pruritus or rash is the usual pattern. These cutaneous reactions usually occur during the first few months of therapy and usually subside without discontinuing the drug.

Gastrointestinal reactions consist of anorexia, nausea, mild abdominal pain, and occasional nausea and vomiting. These are rarely serious. Patients should be informed that this drug imparts an orange-red color to urine, feces, sweat, tears, and saliva that is harmless.

Hepatic reactions usually consist of minor elevations in serum transaminase and occur in less than 10% of patients receiving rifampin alone. Mild degrees of transaminase elevations usually subside despite continuous drug administration. Clinical hepatitis due to rifampin occurs in less than 1% of patients. Because rifampin competes with BSP for hepatic excretion, BSP cannot be used as a test for liver function during rifampin use. A similar mechanism precludes the use of radiographic contrast media for gallbladder studies in patients taking rifampin.

Rarely, rifampin can cause thrombocytopenia, which is usually reversible within 2 days after the drug is discontinued.

The influenza syndrome, shock, shortness of breath, hemolytic anemia, and renal failure are usually seen only if rifampin is given intermittently, particularly on a regimen of once or twice each week. These adverse reactions are thought to be on the basis of an antibody to rifampin that is capable of fixing complement to red cells and platelets. Complement and immunoglobulin deposition in renal tubules and glomeruli suggest that rifampin-induced renal failure is on an immune complex basis. Characteristically, this is manifested by acute reductions in urine output. These reactions due to rifampin antibodies are best prevented by diligently instructing patients to avoid interruptions in daily drug ingestion.

Rifampin has immunosuppressive effects in humans, decreasing both cell-mediated and humoral immune responses in laboratory settings. These are of no known clinical significance, however (16, 29).

Drug Interactions. Rifampin reduces the effectiveness of warfarin-type anticoagulants. Oral contraceptives are similarly less effective. Rifampin increases the urinary excretion of methadone, resulting in a lower plasma concentration and may thus result in methadone withdrawal. Oral hypoglycemics, digitalis derivatives, dapsone, and corticosteroids may similarly show lower plasma concentrations and diminished effectiveness. There is some evidence that regular alcohol ingestion may increase the likelihood of hepatotoxicity due to rifampin. Therapeutic levels of rifampin inhibit standard assays for serum folate and vitamin B_{12}. In rodents there is some evidence that rifampin may be teratogenic.

Therapeutic Uses. Rifampin is considered to be the most significant contribution to the chemotherapy of tuberculosis since the introduction of isoniazid in 1952. It is perhaps the only other antituberculosis drug whose activity approaches that of isoniazid. Concern is in order that the indiscriminate use of rifampin for nonmycobacterial infections may favor the widespread selection of rifampin-resistant mycobacteria and thus deprive the drug of most of its usefulness. This reasoning led some authorities to be reluctant to use rifampin for the initial therapy of uncomplicated pulmonary tuberculosis, preferring to reserve its use for relapsed cases. A major drawback of the drug, particularly for underdeveloped countries, is its expense.

Preparations. *Rifampin,* USP (RIFADIN, RIMACTANE): capsules (300 mg). The usual adult dosage of rifampin is 600 mg or 10-20 mg/kg. The drug should be given as a single dose on an empty stomach because food interferes with the absorption, and reabsorption after biliary excretion, of rifampin.

SECONDARY, OR SECOND-LINE ANTITUBERCULOSIS DRUGS

Secondary antituberculosis drugs are characterized by less antimicrobial efficacy and greater clinical toxicity than the primary drugs just discussed. These compounds are usually used only in patients harboring tubercle bacilli resistant to the drugs of first choice. Considerable caution is required in the use of these secondary drugs because of the high likelihood of toxicity. The drugs are conveniently discussed as (1) alternate injectable aminoglycoside-like drugs and (2) alternate oral agents. Second-line aminoglycoside-like compounds for tuberculosis include viomycin, kanamycin, and capreomycin. Alternate oral agents include para-aminosalicylic acid, pyrazinamide, ethionamide, thiacetazone, and cycloserine.

VIOMYCIN

History. Viomycin was isolated by three independent groups in 1950 (11).

Chemistry. Viomycin is produced by fermentation from *Streptomyces pumiceus* var. *Floridae.* The compound exists as a sulfate salt and is a purple crystalline material. It is a strong base, soluble in water, but relatively insoluble in most organic solvents. Aqueous solutions adjusted to pH 5-6 are quite stable. Viomycin is a cyclic peptide antibiotic (Fig. 25.3-1), unrelated to the aminoglycosides chemically and closely related to capreomycin (see later). As will be discussed, its mode of action as well as its pattern of toxicity are quite similar to those of the aminoglycosides and this has led to widespread consideration of the compounds together (11).

Mechanism of Action. Viomycin, despite its structural differences, resembles the aminoglycosides in its mechanism of action. It inhibits protein synthesis by binding to ribosomes. Whereas streptomycin appears to bind only to the 30 S subunit of the ribosome, viomycin binds to both the 30 S and 50 S ribosome subunits. There is some degree of cross-resistance between viomycin and capreomycin. Approximately 50% of strains resistant to viomycin will also be resistant to capreomycin, although the patient has never received capreomycin.

Pharmacokinetics. After adult doses of 1-2 g, maximum plasma concentrations occur in approximately 2 hr. Most strains of tubercle bacilli are inhibited *in vitro* by 1-10 μg/ml. Excretion of viomycin is similar to that of streptomycin.

Adverse Effects. The drug is nephrotoxic, causing proteinuria, hematuria, pyuria, nitrogen retention, and electrolyte disturbances. The drug is ototoxic, resulting in deafness and less often loss of vestibular function. Nephrotoxicity appears to be reversible when the drug is discontinued; the eighth cranial nerve damage tends to be permanent. The drug is extremely painful when given intramuscularly and may cause sterile abscesses (2).

Therapeutic Uses. Viomycin has little place in the chemotherapy of tuberculosis, having been largely replaced with capreomycin, a somewhat more potent agent with somewhat less nephrotoxicity (2). It obviously cannot be given with any of the other injectable preparations because of additive toxicities.

Preparations. *Viomycin* (VIOCIN, VIOMYCIN), powder for injection. It is not available commercially in the United States at the present time. Viomycin is given in doses of 1-2 g daily for 2-4 weeks followed by the same dose two to three times a week when necessary.

CAPREOMYCIN

History. Capreomycin was isolated in 1960.

Chemistry. Capreomycin is closely related to viomycin structurally. It is produced by *Streptomyces capreolus* and is a mixture of closely related substances. It is a white solid, soluble in water, and stable in aqueous solutions at pH 4-8 (11).

Mechanism of Action. Capreomycin is thought to share the same mechanism of action as viomycin in view of the cross-resistance between the two drugs.

Pharmacokinetics. After doses of 1 g, peak blood levels of 20-40 μg/ml occur in 1-2 hr. This is five to eight times the minimum inhibitory concentration for sensitive tubercle bacilli *in vitro*. Other pharmacokinetic properties are similar to those of viomycin.

Adverse Effects. Generally capreomycin shares the pattern of toxicities of viomycin. When compared with viomycin and kanamycin, however, capreomycin is generally considered to be least toxic. Renal damage is the most consistent toxicity of capreomycin and is manifested by nitrogen retention, albuminuria, and so on. Renal abnormalities are almost always reversible when therapy is discontinued. Overall, the incidence of nephrotoxicity is less than 10% of cases (2).

Therapeutic Uses. Capreomycin has therapeutic efficacy that approaches that of streptomycin, being considerably greater than that of viomycin and somewhat greater than that of kanamycin. As mentioned earlier, capreomycin is less toxic than either viomycin or kanamycin. There is no cross-resistance between capreomycin and streptomycin. Capreomycin continues to be useful in patients with streptomycin-resistant tubercle bacilli for these reasons (2).

Preparations. *Capreomycin sulfate,* USP (CAPASTAT): ampule (1 g powder for solution in 2 ml saline or sterile water) for injection. Capreomycin is administered in adult doses of 1 g daily for 2-4 weeks followed by 1 g two or three times weekly, if necessary.

KANAMYCIN

History. Kanamycin was isolated in 1957.

Chemistry. Kanamycin is a mixture of closely related antibiotics produced by *Streptomyces kanamyceticus.* The principal component, kanamycin A, as the sulfate is a white crystalline, water-soluble solid. It is a true aminoglycoside, having two amino sugars in glycosidic linkage with 2-deoxystreptamine (30) (Fig. 25.3-1).

Mechanism of Action. Despite the fact that cross-resistance between kanamycin and streptomycin is the exception rather than the rule, it is generally considered that kanamycin has a mechanism of action similar to that of streptomycin and the other aminoglycoside antibiotics (11).

Pharmacokinetics. Intramuscular injection of 1 g of kanamycin results in a plasma concentration of 20-35 μg/ml. The drug diffuses poorly into cerebrospinal fluid. It is excreted primarily by the kidney by glomerular filtration with some secretion by renal tubules.

Adverse Effects. In daily doses of 1 g for 3 months, 39% of patients have experienced severe and permanent hearing loss. The drug is moderately nephrotoxic (2).

Therapeutic Uses. The ototoxicity of kanamycin precludes its long-term use in tuberculosis therapy. In the opinion of most authorities, kanamycin has little or no place at present in the treatment of tuberculosis (2).

Preparations. *Kanamycin sulfate,* USP (KANTREX): capsule (500 mg) or vials (500 mg/2 ml or 1 g/ml) for injection. Usual adult doses are 1 g i.m. three to five times weekly.

PARA-AMINOSALICYLIC ACID

History. Para-aminosalicylic acid (PAS) has been known chemically since 1889. In 1940, it was demonstrated that salicylates and benzoates stimulated the oxygen consumption of tubercle bacilli (5); in 1946, the tuberculostatic activity of PAS was demonstrated (24).

Chemistry. PAS (Fig. 25.3-2) and its salts are white crystalline powders. Aqueous solutions of the free acid are unstable and undergo decarboxylation. The sodium salt is relatively stable and highly soluble in water. PAS has a pK_a of 3.25 (11).

Mechanism of Action. The bulk of the evidence appears to point to a mechanism of action of PAS analogous to that of the sulfonamides in inhibiting *de novo* folate biosynthesis (11).

Pharmacokinetics. PAS is readily absorbed from the GI tract and distributed throughout total body water. The drug has a half-life of approximately 1 hr. PAS oral doses of 4 g result in plasma concentrations up to 75 μg/ml within 1-2 hr. Minimum inhibitory concentrations for sensitive tubercle bacilli *in vitro* are as little as 1 μg/ml. Over 80% of ingested doses are excreted in the urine. The drug is metabolized by acetylation in the liver. Approximately 50% of the compound in the urine is the acetylated metabolite, almost all of the remainder being the free acid.

Adverse Effects. Due to the large amount of the drug that must be ingested, the most common side effects relate to gastrointestinal intolerance. Therapy must be discontinued in approximately 19% of patients receiving PAS; in 15% of all cases, this is due to gastrointestinal intolerance in the form of nausea, vomiting, and diarrhea. Approximately 4% of patients develop hypersensitivity reactions. Hypersensitivity reactions take the form of fever, malaise, arthralgias, skin eruptions, etc. It is estimated that 20-50% of patients who tolerate PAS are, in fact, not taking the medication consistently (2).

Therapeutic Uses. The overwhelming drawback of PAS is its lack of acceptability to patients. In the past, many investigators felt that the principal cause of failure of chemotherapy of tuberculosis was the failure of patients to comply with prescribed PAS. It remains reliable and relatively safe and still may be useful in the treatment of drug-resistant tuberculosis (20).

Preparations. *Aminosalicylate sodium,* USP (PARASAL, NEO-PASALATE,): tablets (500, 690, and 1000 mg). The compound is also available as acid, aminosalicylic acid, or potassium or calcium salts, and in various other dosage forms. Adult doses of PAS are 8-12 g daily in two to three divided doses. It is also marketed generically (2).

PYRAZINAMIDE

History. Pyrazinamide was synthesized in 1936 and shown to be effective in experimental tuberculosis in 1952 (11).

Chemistry. Pyrazinamide is the synthetic pyrazine analog of nicotinamide (Fig. 25.3-2). The drug is slightly soluble in water. It is a white crystalline solid. Aqueous solutions are neutral. It has a pK_a of 0.5.

Mechanism of Action. Pyrazinamide has been postulated to interfere with the role of nicotinamide as a cofactor in mycobacterial dehydrogenase systems, similar to one of the postulated mechanisms of action of isoniazid. In view of the lack of cross-resistance between isoniazid and pyrazinamide in tubercle bacilli, this effect of pyrazinamide must differ in some detail from that of isoniazid. The enhanced antibacterial efficacy of pyrazinamide in acidic media *in vitro* suggests that pyrazinamide acts *in vivo* on tubercle bacilli in acidic loci (e.g., within phagocytic cells and caseous lesions) (11).

Pharmacokinetics. Pyrazinamide is well absorbed from the GI tract and distributed throughout the body. Oral doses of 1 g result in plasma concentrations of approximately 45 μg/ml within 2 hr. Pyrazinamide is hydrolyzed to pyrazinoic acid, which is then hydroxylated to 5-hydroxypyrazinoic acid, the major metabolite appearing in urine. The drug is excreted primarily by renal glomerular filtration. In slightly acidic media *in vitro*, 12.5 μg/ml of pyrazinamide inhibits the growth of sensitive tubercle bacilli.

Adverse Effects. Pyrazinamide produces a dose-related hepatotoxicity. In doses of 3 g/day, approximately 15% of patients have signs and symptoms of hepatic toxicity. Jaundice occurs in 2-3%. The drug routinely interferes with the excretion of urate, resulting in hyperuricemia.

Therapeutic Uses. The hepatotoxicity of pyrazinamide limits its usefulness. It is bactericidal in tuberculosis and is considered highly effective. Its use is limited to patients who can be kept under close medical supervision, and its principal use in the United States is in the retreatment of relapsing cases when less toxic drugs cannot be used (20).

Preparations. The usual adult dose is 3 g daily in divided doses. The drug is available as 500-mg tablets marketed generically (2).

ETHIONAMIDE

History. Ethionamide was synthesized in 1956, in an effort to further improve the antituberculosis activity of the thioureas and thiosemicarbazones. Its antituberculosis activity was described in 1959 (11).

Chemistry. Ethionamide (2-ethylthioisonicotinamide) (Fig. 25.3-1) is a yellow crystalline solid that is sparingly soluble in water. It is the thioamide of isonicotinic acid. Although it is related chemically to isoniazid, there is no bacterial cross-resistance between the two compounds (11).

Mechanism of Action. There is a cross-resistance between ethionamide and the thioureas and thiosemicarbazones (e.g., thiacetazone), indicating that these compounds probably share a common mechanism of action. Theories about the mechanism of action of ethionamide include inhibition of mycobacterial mycolic acid synthesis. Others suggest that it affects dehydrogenase systems in tubercle bacilli (11).

Pharmacokinetics. Ethionamide is well absorbed orally and is widely distributed, diffusing well into the cerebrospinal fluid. Following oral doses of 1 g, peak plasma concentrations in 3 hr are approximately 20 μg/ml. Minimum inhibitory concentrations of ethionamide for sensitive tubercle bacilli range from 0.6 to 2.5 μg/ml. The drug is metabolized to carbamoyl-, thiocarbamoyl-, and S-oxocarbamoyl-dihydropyridines. Less than 1% of the compound is excreted unchanged in the urine.

Adverse Effects. The principal side effects of ethionamide in doses of 1 g daily are gastrointestinal disturbances in the form of anorexia, nausea, and vomiting. These effects are thought to be mediated by a direct central nervous system action of the drug rather than direct gastric irritation. At least 30% of cases cannot tolerate ethionamide because of side effects. Approximately 9% of patients develop abnormal liver function studies. From 1 to 3% of patients develop jaundice. The drug exerts teratogenic effects in laboratory rodents (2).

Therapeutic Uses. Because of toxicity and lack of patient tolerability, ethionamide is used only in the treatment of relapsing drug-resistant tuberculosis.

Preparations. The usual adult dose is 0.5-1 g daily in one to three doses. The drug is available as TRECATOR-SC in 250 mg tablets.

THIACETAZONE

History. Thiacetazone was first synthesized in 1946 by Domagk (33). Extensive trials were conducted in leprosy in the period of 1949-1952 (1). Its antituberculosis activity was demonstrated by 1950 (8).

Chemistry. Thiacetazone (amithiozone, TB-1/698, p-acetaminobenzaldehyde thiosemicarbazone) (Fig. 25.3-1) is a pale yellow crystalline solid. It has a bitter taste and darkens on exposure to light. It is practically insoluble in water and most organic solvents except glycols.

Mechanism of Action. Thiacetazone forms a copper complex that is postulated to be the active form of the drug. Presumably, this copper complex of thiacetazone resembles actual biochemical carriers of copper and interferes with their function in mycobacteria. There is cross-resistance between thiacetazone and other antituberculosis agents containing the thioamide grouping, particularly ethionamide. This would imply that these agents share some common mechanism of action. As mentioned earlier, ethionamide has been implicated in the inhibition of mycolic acid synthesis in mycobacteria, affects dehydrogenase systems in tubercle bacilli, and may form a substituted isonicotinic acid that may interfere with NAD-dependent systems (11).

Pharmacokinetics. Thiacetazone is poorly absorbed after oral administration. After 200-mg doses, peak plasma concentrations of approximately 1 μg/ml occur 2-3 hr after dosing. The minimum inhibitory concentration for tubercle bacilli *in vitro* is 0.1-5 μg/ml (8). The estimated minimum inhibitory concentration for leprosy bacilli is approximately 0.26 μg/ml in mouse footpad infections (10).

Adverse Effects. The principal side effects of thiacetazone are hemolytic anemia, neutropenia, and renal and hepatic damage. The hepatic damage is apparently more common in doses of 200 mg daily than at doses of 150 mg daily (8). In one large series of patients taking a combination of thiacetazone plus isoniazid plus streptomycin, there was approximately a 50% incidence of side effects; approximately 20% of all patients required a change in treatment because of drug toxicities. In a group of like size receiving only isoniazid and streptomycin, some 30% of patients had side effects and approximately 6% required a change in therapy (20). Recent studies by the East African/British Medical Research Councils show 8-13% of cases experiencing drug toxicity in combinations including thiacetazone. Of interest, 2 of 242 cases on thiacetazone experienced exfoliative dermatitis (12, 13).

Therapeutic Uses. Thiacetazone is effective in delaying the emergence of isoniazid-resistant tubercle bacilli in patients under treatment. It is inexpensive and thus has a place in the management of tuberculosis in underdeveloped areas. Cross-resistance exists between thiacetazone and ethionamide, and the latter is used predominantly in developed countries. It is recommended in some combination regimens for leprosy. As monotherapy, resistance develops to thiacetazone within approximately 2 years in leprosy (8).

Preparations. Thiacetazone is not approved for use in the United States. It is available as 150-mg tablets and is given in a single dose daily in combination with other antituberculosis agents. The drug is used routinely in many developing countries of the world.

CYCLOSERINE

History. Cycloserine was isolated independently by three separate laboratories in 1955 and synthesized shortly thereafter (11).

Chemistry. Cycloserine (D-4-amino-3-isoxazolidinone) (Fig. 25.3-1) is an antibiotic produced by *Streptomyces orchidaceus.* It is a colorless crystalline compound, soluble in water, and stable at pH 10, but unstable in neutral or acid solutions. Aqueous solutions have a pH of approximately 6. The compound is amphoteric (11).

Mechanism of Action. Cycloserine is a structural analog of the amino acid D-alanine. Its antibacterial effectiveness is based on inhibition of alanine racemase and D-alanyl-D-alanyl synthetase. This deprives the cell of D-alanyl-D-alanine, which is normally incorporated as the last two peptide units of UDP-acetyl-muramyl pentapeptide. This pentapeptide is an essential cell-wall building block (11).

Pharmacokinetics. Cycloserine is rapidly and effectively absorbed after oral administration. Peak plasma levels exceed 50 μg/ml after 750-mg oral doses. Minimum inhibitory concentrations for tubercle bacilli *in vitro* are 5-20 μg/ml. The drug is freely distributed throughout body fluids and tissues with equivalent levels in the cerebrospinal fluid and plasma. Approximately 65% of the drug is excreted unchanged in the urine, and approximately 35% is metabolized by the liver.

Adverse Effects. The principal adverse reactions to cycloserine involve the central nervous system. In one series, approximately 24% of patients developed central nervous system toxicity of sufficient severity to require withdrawal of the drug. Approximately 16% of the patients developed agitated depression, 5% psychosis, 4% tremulousness and confusion, and 2% seizures. The central nervous system toxicity of cycloserine is proportional to blood levels. To minimize toxicity, dosage should be adjusted to provide blood levels below 30 μg/ml. The drug is contraindicated in individuals with epilepsy, depression, severe anxiety, psychosis, and in patients with severe renal insufficiency. Neurological reactions are said to be preventable by large doses of pyridoxine (100 mg three times daily). Therapy with cycloserine is initiated in hospitalized patients because of toxicities (2, 20).

Therapeutic Uses. Cycloserine has rather weak antituberculosis activity and formidable neurotoxicity. Although the neurological side effects are generally reversible, they severely limit the usefulness of cycloserine. Because of possible additive central nervous system toxicity, some authorities do not use cycloserine with isoniazid. The drug's usefulness is limited to the patients harboring tubercle bacilli with multiple resistance (2).

Preparations. *Cycloserine,* USP (SEROMYCIN): capsule (250 mg). Cycloserine is usually initially given in doses of 250 mg twice daily at 12-hr intervals for the first 2 weeks in adults. If well tolerated, the dose is increased by 250 mg every few days as tolerated. Dosage should be adjusted to yield plasma levels no greater than 30 μg/ml to avoid toxicities. "Trough" serum concentrations of 25-30 μg/ml can usually be attained with daily doses of 1-2 g in three divided doses. In general, a daily dose of 1 g should not be exceeded.

COMBINATION CHEMOTHERAPY OF TUBERCULOSIS

The use of combinations of antituberculosis drugs with different mechanisms of action is well established and is based on the fact that *M. tuberculosis* exhibits resistance to any one drug at a predictable rate and that the opportunities for these resistant mutants to exist in a given patient are proportional to the number of viable bacilli that patient harbors.

Drug resistance in *M. tuberculosis* is considered to be of two types, primary and secondary. Primary drug resistance refers to resistance of the bacilli that have been transmitted to a new, previously untreated patient. Obviously, this may be influenced by patterns of drug use in the individuals who were the source of the bacilli for transmission to the new patient. The frequency of primary resistance in strains of *M. tuberculosis* from previously untreated tuberculosis patients has been monitored longitudinally by the Veterans Administration since 1962 and has been shown to be stable to date. In 1973, 2.8% of strains were resistant to isoniazid, 9.7% to ethambutol, 3.2% to streptomycin, and 0.8% to rifampin (27). Thus, as an example, treating new patients with ethambutol alone would in theory be of no benefit in 9.7% of cases whereas 90.3% would at least initially show a favorable response. On the other hand, treating new patients with an ethambutol-isoniazid combination would be of no benefit in 9.7% of 2.8%, or less than 0.3% (i.e., more than 99.7% of patients would be expected to respond favorably).

Secondary drug resistance in *M. tuberculosis* refers to resistance developing during chemotherapy in a given patient. Actually, drugs do not induce the mutations that lead to drug resistance; the mutations occur naturally, and the presence of a drug merely selects for the resistant mutant because susceptible organisms are inhibited from multiplying; and, as time goes on, in the presence of the drug the predominant organisms are descended from the resistant mutant.

Resistance to any one antituberculosis drug occurs naturally in about 1 out of every 1×10^5 organisms (27). Tuberculosis cavities may contain up to 10^9 bacilli. On the other hand, noncavitary foci may contain as few as 10^2 bacilli (18). If one assumes that a contact of a tuberculosis patient who develops a positive tuberculin skin test has contracted the infection and harbors a total of 10^3 viable tubercle bacilli in his body, then the chances that one of these organisms is resistant to an antituberculosis drug (e.g., isoniazid) are $1/10^5 \times 10^3$, or $1/10^2$, or 1 chance in 100. Thus, in the absence of primary resistance, treatment of such an individual with isoniazid alone would be expected to be totally effective 99% of the time.

On the other hand, if one assumes that a patient with far-advanced cavitary pulmonary tuberculosis may harbor as many as 10^{10} viable bacilli in his body, then, in the absence of primary resistance, the most probable number of mutants in his body that are resistant to one antituberculosis drug is $1/10^5 \times 10^{10}$, or 10^5 (i.e., the chances are that the patient is harboring 100,000 bacilli that would not be affected by a single antituberculosis agent). Clearly, treating such a patient with a single drug (e.g., isoniazid) would not be effective for any length of time. The patient would be expected to improve initially, since $(10^{10} - 10^5)/10^{10}$ or 99.999% of his organisms are susceptible to isoniazid. As time went on, however, the 10^5 resistant mutants he initially harbored would be expected to multiply and the patient's disease would eventually relapse with secondary resistance despite his faithful intake of isoniazid. Obviously, such a patient's chances of long-term benefit are improved if he is treated with a combination of two antituberculosis drugs. The most probable number of mutants in his body that are resistant to both of two antituberculosis drugs at the time therapy is started is $1/10^5 \times 1/10^5 \times 10^{10}$, or 1. Thus, treating such a patient with a combination of two drugs would be beneficial, and would be beneficial longer than treating him with only one drug, but the opportunity still exists for the single mutant that is expected to be resistant to both drugs eventually to produce enough progeny to cause relapse, despite the patient's faithful intake of both drugs. To achieve statistical confidence that such a patient with far-advanced tuberculosis will not eventually relapse with resistant organisms, one must therefore utilize a combination of three drugs. The chances that the patient initially harbors an organism resistant to all three drugs becomes vanishingly small (i.e., $1/10^5 \times 1/10^5 \times 1/10^5 \times 10^{10}$, or 1 in 100,000).

Duration of Therapy. Effective chemotherapy of tuberculosis together with the patient's cell-mediated immunity reduces the bacterial population by as much as 99% in the majority of patients within 6 months after beginning therapy (6). Once this large population of bacilli has been decimated by drugs, many of the remaining organisms are in a dormant state and not multiplying, or are in an intracellular location in an acidic environment, or are sequestered in fibrotic foci, all of which may make them less susceptible to, or accessible for, the action of antituberculosis drugs. Premature cessation of chemotherapy has been empirically shown to be followed by relapse as these remaining organisms resume proliferation. Elimination of these residual persisting organisms or "sterilization" of the patient is difficult to accomplish with short-term regimens. Although such approaches have been the subject of considerable trial (6, 7, 12-14), there are many who feel that the standard approach to the chemotherapy of tuberculosis still involves 18-24 months of continuous therapy for the majority of cases, and the "cardinal signs in the therapy of tuberculosis are the failure to use multiple drugs and to maintain therapy for a sufficient period of time" (23).

Tuberculosis is a chronic disease and chronic treatment is frequently considered necessary. Most patients rapidly become asymptomatic after starting chemotherapy and within several days to 2 weeks feel well. Such an asymptomatic individual is then advised to take potentially toxic medications on a regular basis for an additional 1.5-2 years when he feels well. Quite naturally, even well-motivated patients are likely to miss doses, and all too frequently therapy becomes irregular, intermittent, or even nonexistent. The most common cause of treatment failure in tuberculosis is failure of the patient to take the prescribed medication regularly or for a sufficient duration of time.

Choice of Drugs. The number of choice of drugs to be employed in the treatment of tuberculosis must be individualized. Pertinent considerations, some of which have been already considered include:

1. The likelihood of primary resistance (community patterns, drug sensitivities in the index case if known or suspected)
2. The likelihood of developing secondary resistance (i.e., the extent of the patient's disease)
3. The likelihood of patient compliance with therapy (injections and/or drugs that can be safely used in supervised intermittent regimens might be considered in a noncompliant individual)
4. Preexisting disease (e.g., hepatic disease might make potentially hepatotoxic drugs less desirable)
5. Whether or not the patient has received previous chemotherapy for tuberculosis (the likelihood of secondary resistance already existing to specific drugs)
6. The results of *in vitro* drug sensitivities (after cultures become available)
7. Convenience of administration of the drug (e.g., injectable drugs might be convenient for a diabetic accustomed to insulin injections but impossible for a patient with rheumatoid arthritis and hand deformities)
8. Patterns of drug toxicities (e.g., three drugs all associated with hepatotoxicity might be cause for concern and additional monitoring)
9. Drug allergies
10. Cost of treatment (1 year's therapy with kanamycin, for example, costs approximately $800 for the drug

(5), plus the expense of preparing and administering the injections).

REFERENCES

1. Alonzo, A.M. The value of thiacetazone (TB-1) in leprosy. *Int. J. Lepr.* 27:321, 1959.
2. AMA Drug Evaluation. *Antimycobacterial Agents,* 5th ed. Chicago: American Medical Association, 1983, p. 1753.
3. American Thoracic Society. Treatment of mycobacterial disease. *Am. Rev. Resp. Dis.* 115:185, 1977.
4. Bates, J.H. Tuberculosis and other mycobacterial disease. In: *Current Therapy* (Conn, H.F., ed.). Philadelphia: W.B. Saunders, 1977, p. 151.
5. Bernheim, F. Effect of salicylate on oxygen uptake of tubercle bacillus. *Science* 92:204, 1940.
6. Brewin, A. The treatment of tuberculosis. In: *Rational Drug Therapy.* Philadelphia: W.B. Saunders, 1976, p. 1.
7. British Thoracic and Tuberculosis Association. Short-course chemotherapy in pulmonary tuberculosis. *Lancet* 2:1102, 1976.
8. Bushby, S.R.M. Chemotherapy. In: *Leprosy in Theory and Practice,* 2nd ed. (Cochrane, R.G., and Davey, T.F., eds.) Baltimore: Williams & Wilkins, 1964, p. 344.
9. Byrd, R.B., Horn, B.R., Solomon, D.A. and Griggs, G.A. Toxic effects of isoniazid in tuberculosis chemoprophylaxis: Role of biochemical monitoring in 1,000 patients. *JAMA* 241:1239, 1979.
10. Colston, M.J. and Hilson, G.R.F. The activity of thiacetazone, thiambutosine, and thiocarlide in the chemotherapy of experimental leprosy. *Int. J. Lepr.* 44:123, 1976.

10a. Comstock, G.W. New data on preventive treatment with isoniazid. *Ann. Intern. Med.* 98:663, 1983.

11. Doub, L. The chemical structures, properties, and mechanisms of action of the anti-tuberculosis drugs. In: *Tuberculosis* (Youmans, G.P., ed.). Philadelphia: W.B. Saunders, 1979, p. 435.
12. East African/British Medical Research Councils. Controlled clinical trial of short-course (6-month) regimens of chemotherapy for treatment of pulmonary tuberculosis. *Lancet* 1:1079, 1972.
13. East African/British Medical Research Councils. Controlled clinical trial of four short-course (6-month) regimens of chemotherapy for treatment of pulmonary tuberculosis. *Lancet* 2:1100, 1974.
14. East African/British Medical Research Councils. Controlled clinical trial of five short-course (4-month) chemotherapy regimens in pulmonary tuberculosis. *Lancet* 2:334, 1978.
15. Furey, W.W. and Stefancic, M.F. Tuberculosis in a community hospital: A five year review. *JAMA* 235:168, 1976.
16. Girling, D.J. and Hitze, K.L. Adverse reactions to rifampicin. *Bull. WHO* 57:45, 1979.
17. Glassroth, J., Robins, A.G. and Snider, D.E., Jr. Tuberculosis in the 1980s. *N. Engl. J. Med.* 302:1441, 1980.
18. Goldstein, M.S. The rational treatment of tuberculosis today. In: *American Hospital Formulary Service,* Bethesda, MD: American Society of Hospital Pharmacists; February 1977, p. 78.
19. Graham, W.G.B. and Dundas, G.R. Isoniazid-related liver disease: Occurrence with portal hypertension, hypoalbuminemia, and hypersplenism, *JAMA* 242:353, 1979.
20. Hinshaw, H.C. Treatment of tuberculosis. In: *Tuberculosis* (Youmans, G.P., ed.). Philadelphia: W.B. Saunders, 1979, p. 457.
21. Jacobson, R.R. and Hastings, R.C. Rifampin-resistant leprosy. *Lancet* 2:1304, 1976.
22. Johnston, R.F. and Wildrick, K.H. "State of the Art" review: The impact of chemotherapy on the care of patients with tuberculosis. *Am. Rev. Resp. Dis.* 109:636, 1974.
23. Kasik, J.E. Tuberculosis and other mycobacterial disease. In: *Current Therapy* (Conn, H.F., ed.). Philadelphia: W.B. Saunders, 1979, p. 155.

23a. Kuze, F., Kurasawa, T., Bando, K., Lee, Y. and Maekawa, N. *In vitro* and *in vivo* susceptibility of atypical mycobacteria to various drugs. *Rev. Infect. Dis.* 3:885, 1981.

24. Lehmann, J. Para-aminosalicylic acid in the treatment of tuberculosis. *Lancet* 250:15, 1946.
25. Lenzini, L., Rottoli, P. and Tottoli, L. The spectrum of human tuberculosis. *Clin. Exp. Immunol.* 27:230, 1977.
26. Long, E.R. *A History of the Therapy of Tuberculosis and the Case of Frederic Chopin.* Lawrence, Kans.: University of Kansas Press, 1956.
27. Mayock, R.L. and MacGregor, R.R. Diagnosis, prevention, and early therapy of tuberculosis. *Dis. Month* 22:1, 1976.
28. McConville, J.H. and Rapoport, M.I. Tuberculosis management in the mid-1970s. *JAMA* 235:172, 1976.
29. Rahal, J.J. and Simberkoff, M.S. Adverse reactions to antiinfective agents. *Dis. Month* 25:1, 1978.
30. Umezawa, H. Kanamycin: Its discovery. *Ann. N.Y. Acad. Sci.* 76:20, 1958.
31. Vall-Spinosa, A and Lester, T.W. Rifampin: Characteristics and role in the chemotherapy of tuberculosis. *Ann. Intern. Med.* 74:758, 1971.
32. Wehrli, W. and Staehelin, M. Actions of the rifamycins. *Bact. Rev.* 35:290, 1971.
33. Windholz, M. *The Merck Index,* 10th ed. Rahway, N.J.: Merck, 1983.

ADDITIONAL READING

Reed, M.D. and Blumer, J.L. Clinical pharmacology of antitubercular drugs. *Pediatr. Clin. North Am.* 30:177, 1983.

Williams, C.K.O., Aderoju, E.A., Adenle, A.D., Sekoni, G. and Esan, G.J.F. Aplastic anaemia associated with anti-tuberculosis chemotherapy. *Acta Haemat.* 68:329, 1982.

Yoshikawa, T. and Fujita, N.K. Antituberculous drugs. *Med. Clin. North Am.* 66:209, 1982.

CHAPTER
25.4

ANTILEPROSY AGENTS

Robert C. Hastings and John R. Trautman

M. LEPRAE AND HOST-PARASITE RELATIONSHIPS

Leprosy (Hansen's disease) is a chronic infectious human disease caused by *Mycobacterium leprae* that affects some 12 million persons worldwide. The principle clinical manifestations leading to diagnosis are dermatological lesions of various sorts, neurological deficits, and acute inflammatory manifestations of hypersensitivity to antigens of *M. leprae*, the so-called lepra reactions. Host-parasite relationships in leprosy are complex and dynamic. Rational therapy begins with an accurate diagnosis of both the leprosy itself and an evaluation of these host-parasite relationships that involves determining the position of a given patient within the spectrum of leprosy (i.e., that patient's classification). Well-localized leprosy with competent cell-mediated immunity and very few *M. leprae* is called tuberculoid disease. Widely disseminated, anergic disease is called lepromatous leprosy. Forms of leprosy between these two extremes are called borderline types, and the very early form of the disease before full definition of the relative balance between bacterial proliferation and cell-mediated immunity is called indeterminate leprosy.

The medical therapy of leprosy is designed to render *M. leprae* incapable of multiplication, eliminating the patient's infectivity and allowing the body to clear the bacilli. A significant and important part of the medical therapy of leprosy is the control of hypersensitivity reactions to antigens of *M. leprae* (i.e., lepra reactions). Antibacterial chemotherapy is further complicated by the ability of leprosy bacilli to persist for years in a presumably metabolically inactive condition (so-called persisters), an overall generation time of the order of 12-15 days, and the propensity of the bacilli to develop resistance to commonly used drugs.

LEPRA REACTIONS

The management of reactions in leprosy is a major portion of the overall treatment of the disease. Any effective glucocorticoid will be useful in the control of these reactions, which may occur either spontaneously or during the course of antibacterial chemotherapy for Hansen's disease. From 25 to 50% of patients with leprosy develop clinically apparent hypersensitivity reactions to antigens of *M. leprae*. These reactions are not drug allergies but are allergic responses to products of *M. leprae*. These reactions can cause considerable discomfort as well as irreversible tissue damage and must be controlled for optimal patient care. A typical initial dose of glucocorticoids for the control of these reactions would be 80 mg of prednisone. Maintenance therapy must be individualized, utilizing if possible a single dose every other day of short-acting glucocorticoids (e.g., prednisone).

DRUGS FOR THERAPY OF LEPROSY

Dapsone (4, 4′-diaminodiphenylsulfone, DDS) is a sulfone and closely related to the sulfonamides. It has the following chemical formula:

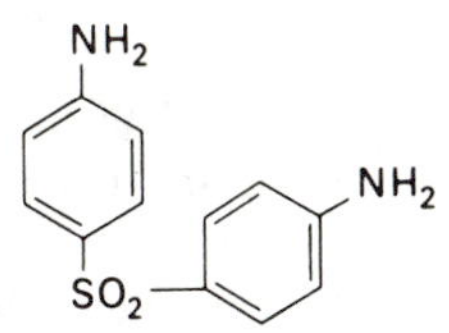

NH_2 NH_2 SO_2

Dapsone

Despite attempts to develop a better sulfone drug, dapsone remains the most effective clinically used agent in leprosy.

DAPSONE

History. Dapsone (DDS) was first synthesized in 1908. In 1937, it was demonstrated to have antibacterial activity in laboratory animals (streptococcal infections in mice) (9). That same year, it was first used clinically (for gonorrhea) (18). In 1940, it was demonstrated to offer some protection to rabbits infected with *M. avium* and to guinea pigs infected with human tubercle bacilli (8). A derivative, glucosulfone or PROMIN, was first used in the treatment of leprosy in humans in 1941 (7). The parent compound, dapsone, was first used in leprosy in 1946 (5).

Chemistry. Dapsone has a pK_b of 13 and is almost insoluble in water. The amino groups of dapsone are only very weakly basic, and at physiological pH the dapsone molecule exists almost completely as the unionized species.

Mechanism of Action. Dapsone is an analog of p-aminobenzoic acid (PABA) and acts like sulfonamide to inhibit the de novo synthesis of folic acid by *M. leprae*. The drug is bacteriostatic because of this mechanism of action.

Pharmacokinetics. Dapsone is almost completely absorbed (greater than 90%) from the GI tract, mainly from the upper part of the small bowel. Free dapsone is distributed throughout the total body water and is present in practically all tissues. High concentrations of the drug are found in kidneys (organ of excretion) and liver (organ of metabolism). DDS is 70-80% bound to plasma albumin, and its major metabolite, monoacetyl-DDS (MADDS), is 98-100% bound to albumin (30). DDS undergoes various metabolic reactions in the liver including acetylation (the major pathway), glucuronidation, sulfamation, and hydroxylation. Many of the mono- and di-substituted sulfones are broken down into the parent compound or the mono-substituted derivatives, which retain antibacterial activity. The major metabolite in human blood is MADDS. Individuals are genetically polymorphic in their capacity to acetylate dapsone. This characteristic however does not appear to have significant effects on the half-life of the drug (33). More than 85% of the drug is excreted in the urine, usually as metabolites. Smaller amounts appear in the feces, sweat, saliva, tears, milk, etc. Following 100-mg doses of dapsone orally, human blood levels of total dapsone are approximately 1.5 μg/ml. Minimal inhibitory concentrations for *M. leprae* may be as small as 0.003 μg/ml. The half-life of DDS in plasma is quite variable, 10-50 hr, with a mean of approximately 28 hr in humans (33).

Adverse Effects. On a weight basis, dapsone is more toxic than the sulfonamides. The most common side effect is gastric intolerance, which usually consists of mild nausea and occasional vomiting. Other side effects with the usual therapeutic doses include headaches, hepatitis, peripheral neuropathy, and drug sensitivity. In patients with glucose-6-phosphate dehydrogenase (G-6-PD) deficiency, normal doses of dapsone can induce a significant hemolytic anemia. In high doses, the drug may induce a hemolytic anemia, methemoglobinemia, and psychosis (36).

Therapeutic Uses. Dapsone is the drug of choice in all types of Hansen's disease except in patients with primary or secondary sulfone resistance. The existence of sulfone resistance in a given patient is diagnosed on the basis of lack of clinical response to dapsone, proof of compliance and ingestion of dapsone, and may be confirmed by the growth of *M. leprae* in the footpads of mice fed dapsone (32).

Preparations. *Dapsone*, USP (AVLOSULFON) is available in tablets (25 or 100 mg).

The dosage of dapsone in leprosy has varied widely in the past. Currently dapsone is given orally in a dosage of 100 mg daily, and considerable evidence exists that it should be administered in maximum subtoxic doses to minimize the possibility of the bacilli developing dapsone resistance (12).

THALIDOMIDE

History. Thalidomide was first synthesized in 1956 (20) and was demonstrated to be an effective sedative-hypnotic drug in animals and in humans (20, 35). It was released for use in humans as a sedative-hypnotic in 1957. In 1961, the drug was shown to be associated with congenital malformations (phocomelia) when taken by pregnant women and was withdrawn from the market (24). In 1965, the drug was demonstrated to be effective in lepra reactions of the erythema nodosum leprosum (ENL) type (13, 34). At present, it is an experimental drug.

Chemistry. Thalidomide has the following chemical structure:

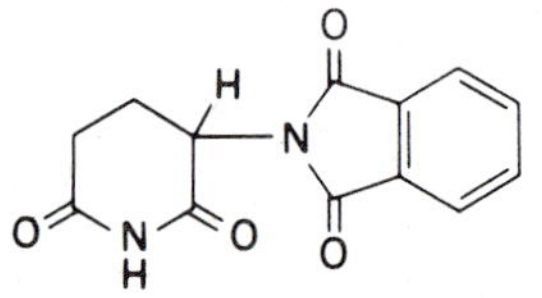

Thalidomide

The compound is practically insoluble in water. The drug is unstable in aqueous solutions and undergoes spontaneous hydrolysis at a rate that increases with pH. The α-substituted glutarimide moiety is responsible for the sedative-hypnotic action of thalidomide.

Mechanism of Action. The exact mechanism of action of thalidomide in ENL is unknown. In laboratory studies, the drug appears to inhibit the de novo synthesis of IgM-type antibodies and to inhibit the chemotaxis of human neutrophils (17). The drug has no antibacterial effect on *M. leprae* and is useful only in the control of ENL.

Pharmacokinetics. Thalidomide is well absorbed from the small intestine. The drug is distributed throughout body water with some concentration of thalidomide (mainly metabolites) intracellularly. The drug undergoes nonenzymatic hydrolysis in a pH-dependent fashion in blood. The drug and its major hydrolysis products are excreted in the urine. Trace amounts are found in feces. Peak blood levels of intact thalidomide after 100-mg oral doses of the drug are approximately 0.9 μg/ml. The half-life of the drug is approximately 3.5 hr.

Adverse Effects. Embryopathy is virtually universal if thalidomide is taken by a pregnant woman between 35-50 days after the last normal menstrual period. Thalidomide characteristically causes bony abnormalities, with phocomelia being the characteristic deformity (28). The only other side effect of significance is a peripheral neuropathy usually occurring in patients taking the drug on a regular basis for long periods of time (10).

Therapeutic Uses. Thalidomide is the drug of choice for erythema nodosum leprosum in males, and females *without* childbearing potential (13).

Preparations. The initial dosage for control of ENL is 100 mg four times daily. The drug is usually effective within 48 hr, and the dose may then be decreased to a maintenance level of between 50 and 100 mg daily, usually given at bedtime. The drug is obtained on an experimental basis only, in 100-mg tablets from Chemie Grünenthal, Stolberg, Germany. In the United States, it is available from the National Hansen's Disease Center, United States Public Health Service Hospital, Carville, Louisiana 70721.

CLOFAZIMINE

History. Clofazimine was synthesized in 1954 in an effort to find a new drug for the treatment of tuberculosis (2). In 1962, the drug was shown to be effective in murine leprosy (*M. lepraemurium*) (4) and was first used in humans (3). Shortly thereafter, the drug was shown to be both antibacterial and antiinflammatory in Hansen's disease (14, 15).

Chemistry. Clofazimine is a phenazine derivative with the following structure:

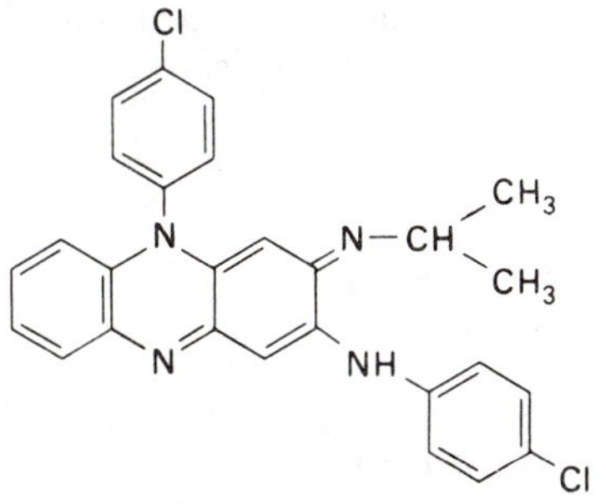

Clofazimine

It is a deep-red, stable, crystalline compound. It is insoluble in water but soluble in organic solvents.

Mechanism of Action. The mechanism of the antibacterial and antiinflammatory effects of clofazimine is not known with certainty. The drug binds to DNA and may interfere with the replication of bacterial DNA (28). The drug accumulates in cells of the reticuloendothelial system and eventually induces blockade of the reticuloendothelial system (6).

Pharmacokinetics. Clofazimine is administered orally in a micronized form and is approximately 70% absorbed from the small bowel. The drug is absorbed as a lipoprotein complex. The complex is then phagocytized by cells of the reticuloendothelial system, the lipoprotein moiety is digested intracellularly, and free drug crystallizes in phagolysosomes. The drug is soluble in fat and is stored to some extent in adipose tissues. High concentrations of the drug are found in organs of the reticuloendothelial system (e.g., liver, spleen, and lymph nodes). It is apparently not metabolized to a significant degree and appears largely in unchanged form in the urine and feces. Smaller amounts are excreted in sweat, tears, saliva, and milk. The serum concentration of clofazimine is not an accurate measure of the amount absorbed, due to its complex distribution and deposition in various organs. The half-life of the drug is complex because of the multiple compartments of its distribution. The overall half-life of elimination can be estimated to be on the order of 3 months (1).

Adverse Effects. The drug universally produces a dose-related skin pigmentation, ranging from an initial pinkish red pigmentation to a bluish black discoloration on long-term, high-dose therapy. Additionally, there is some degree of hypermelanosis, resulting in increased pigmentation of the skin due to increased melanin production in sun-exposed areas. The other major toxicity involves the GI tract and is caused by deposition of crystals of the drug in the distal small bowel wall and mesenteric lymph nodes. This results in disturbances of motility of the small bowel, with anorexia, nausea, vomiting, diarrhea, crampy abdominal pain, and weight loss. The GI toxicities are dose related and are noted in most patients after 6 months of therapy at a dose level of approximately 300 mg daily. In addition to skin pigmentation, the drug causes pigmentation of the conjunctiva and coloration of urine, stools, sputum, and sweat. Skin lesions of leprosy are selectively pigmented by the drug, sometimes resulting in a blotchy, cosmetically unacceptable pigmentation. The drug induces dryness of the skin in general, which may progress to typical ichthyosis (16).

Therapuetic Uses. Clofazimine is the drug of choice for sulfone-resistant Hansen's disease and for the long-term control of chronic reactions in all types of leprosy, including ENL, when thalidomide is contraindicated or not available (13). More recently, clofazimine has been reported as being of therapeutic benefit in pyoderma gangrenosum (25).

Preparations. To obtain antiinflammatory effects, the drug must be administered in a dosage of 100 mg three times daily or more. The antiinflammatory effect is usually apparent within 30 days. For antibacterial effects, the dose of clofazimine ranges from 50 to 100 mg daily. Clofazimine (LAMPRENE) is obtained on an experimental basis from Ciba-Geigy, Basel, Switzerland, in 100-mg capsules. In the United States, it is available from the National Hansen's Disease Center, United States Public Health Service Hospital, Carville, Louisiana 70721.

RIFAMPIN

The rifamycin antibiotics were developed in 1957 (31). A derivative, rifamycin SV, was first used in leprosy as an intramuscular preparation in 1963 (27). Rifampin was first prepared in 1966 (23) and was used as an oral preparation in Hansen's disease in 1968 (29).

The chemistry, pharmacology, and toxicity of this drug are discussed in Chapter 25.3.

Drug Interaction. Rifampin induces the metabolism of dapsone (11), but in the usual clinical setting this is of little significance.

Therapeutic Uses. Rifampin is rapidly bactericidal for *M. leprae*. Resistance to it has been described and develops in the order of 3-4 years (19). The bactericidal activity of rifampin is of marginal benefit in the usual clinical setting. Rifampin is useful when used in combination in the treatment of sulfone-resistant leprosy. The drug should not be used as monotherapy (13).

Preparations. *Rifampin*, USP (RIFADIN, RIMACTANE): capsules (300 mg). In leprosy, rifampin is administered orally in doses of 300-600 mg daily in combination with another effective antileprosy drug for the treatment of sulfone-resistant disease. Newer experimental regimens include a variety of single-dose and intermittent-dose regimens for patients with sulfone-sensitive disease in an effort to delay or prevent the emergence of sulfone-resistance.

CHEMOTHERAPY OF LEPROSY

The objectives of chemotherapy, as mentioned earlier, would be to control lepra reactions and to render *M. leprae* incapable of multiplication, in order to make the patient noninfective and allow the body to clear bacilli.

Patients with tuberculoid leprosy may manifest reversal reactions that are indicative of delayed hypersensitivity to antigens of *M.leprae*; they respond to early therapy with glucocorticoids or clofazimine. For lepra reaction of the lepromatous form (erythema nodosum leprosum), treatment with clofazimine or thalidomide is effective.

For the purpose of clearing bacilli from the patient, dapsone alone or in combination with another drug will be effective. Patients with tuberculoid or borderline tuberculoid disease having relatively few microorganisms may be treated with dapsone alone for 2-4 years. Patients with lepromatous, borderline lepromatous, and borderline diseases need more drastic and prolonged treatment; a two-drug combination, preferably including dapsone with rifampin or clofazimine, should be used. A combination of dapsone and rifampin for 3 months to 1 year followed by dapsone alone for 10 years to life has been recommended (21).

REFERENCES

1. Banerjee, D.K., Ellard, G.A., Gammond, P.T. and Waters, R.F. Some observations on the pharmacology of clofazimine (B663). *Am. J. Trop. Med. Hyg.* 23:1110, 1974.
2. Barry, V.C., Belton, J.G., Conalty, M.L., Denneny, J.M., Edward, D.W., O'Sullivan, J.F., Twomey, D. and Winder, F. A new series of phenazines (rimino-compounds) with high antituberculosis activity. *Nature* 179:1013, 1957.
3. Browne, S.G. and Hodgerzeil, L.M. B663 in the treatment of leprosy: Preliminary report of a pilot trial. *Lepr. Rev.* 33:6, 1962.
4. Chang, Y.T. Effects of B663, a rimino compound of the phenazine series, in murine leprosy. In: *Anti-Microbial Agents and Chemotherapy* (Sylvester, J.C., ed.). Ann Arbor: American Society for Microbiology, 1962, p. 294.
5. Cochrane, R.G., Ramanujam, K., Paul, H. and Russell, D. Two-and-a-half year's experimental work on the sulphone group of drugs. *Lepr. Rev.* 20:4, 1949.
6. Conalty, M.L. and Jina, A.G. The anti-leprosy agent clofazimine (B663) in macrophages: Light, electron microscope, and functional studies. In: *The Reticuloendothelial System and Immune Phenomena* (DiLuzio, N.R. and Flimming, K., eds.). New York: Plenum Press, 1971, p. 323.
7. Faget, G.H., Pogge, R.C., Johansen, F.A., Dinan, J.F., Prejean, B.M. and Eccles, C.G. The promin treatment of leprosy. *Publ. Health. Rep.* 58:1729, 1943.
8. Feldman, W.H., Hinshaw, H.C. and Moses, H.E. Effect of promin (sodium salt of p.p′-diaminodiphenylsulfone-N,N′-dextrose sulfonate) on experimental tuberculosis. Preliminary Report. *Proc. Mayo Clin.* 15:695, 1940.
9. Fourneau, E., Tréfouel, J., Nitte, F., Bovet, D. and Tréfouel, Mme. J. Action anti-streptococcique des derives sulfures organiques. *Compt. Rendu. Acad. Sci.* 204:1763, 1937.
10. Fullerton, P.M. and O'Sullivan, D.J. Thalidomide neuropathy: A clinical, electrophysiological, and histological follow-up study. *J. Neurol. Neurosurg. Psychiatry* 31:543, 1968.
11. Gelber, R.H., Gooi, H.C., Waters, M.F.R. and Rees, R.J.W. The effect of rifampin on dapsone metabolism. *Proc. West. Pharm. Soc.* 18:330, 1975.
12. Hastings, R.C. Growth of sulfone-resistant M. leprae in the foot pads of mice fed dapsone. *Proc. Soc. Exp. Biol. Med.* 156:544, 1977.
13. Hastings, R.C. Leprosy. In: *Current Therapy* (Conn, H.F., ed.). Philadelphia: Saunders, W.B. 1979, p. 32.
14. Hastings, R.C. and Trautman, J.R. B663 in lepromatous leprosy: Effect in erythema nodosum leprosum. *Lepr. Rev.* 39:3, 1968.
15. Hastings, R.C., Trautman, J.R. and Mansfield, R.E. Antibacterial effects of G 30'320 Geigy (B663) in lepromatous leprosy. *Int. J. Dermatol.* 8:21, 1969.
16. Hastings, R.C., Trautman, J.R. and Jacobson, R.R. Long-term clinical toxicity studies with clofazimine (B663) in leprosy. *Int. J. Lepr.* 44:287, 1976.
17. Hastings, R.C., Morales, M.J., Belk, S.E. and Shannon, E.J. Thalidomide analogs with potential activity in erythema nodosum leprosum. *Int. J. Lepr.* 47:672, 1979.
18. Heitz-Boyer, M. Nitti, F. and Tréfouel, J. Note preliminaire sur l'action de la paradiacetylaminodiphényl suphone (1399 F) dans la blennorrhagic. *Bull. Soc. Franç. de Dermato. Syph.* 44:1889, 1937.
19. Jacobson, R.R. and Hastings, R.C. Rifampin resistant leprosy. *Lancet* 2:1304, 1976.
20. Kunz, W., Keller, H. and Mückter, H. N-phthalyl-glutaminsaureimid (N-phthalyl-glutamic acid imide). *Arzneim. Forsch.* 6:426, 1956.
21. Languillion, J., Yawalkar, S.J. and McDougall, A.C. Therapeutic effects of adding RIMACTANE (rifampicin) 450 milligrams daily or 1200 milligrams once monthly in a single dose to dapsone 50 milligrams daily in patients with lepromatous leprosy. *Int. J. Lepr.* 47:37, 1979.
22. Lowe, J. The chemotherapy of leprosy: Late results of treatment with sulfone and with thiosemicarbazone. *Lancet* 2:1065, 1954.
23. Maggie, N., Pasqualucci, C.R., Ballota, R. and Sensi, P. Rifampicin: A new orally active rifamycin. *Chemotherapy* 11:285, 1966.
24. McBride, W.G. Congenital abnormalities and thalidomide. *Lancet* 2:1358, 1961.
25. Michaëlsson, G., Molin, L. Öhman, S., Gip, L., Lindstrom, B., Skogh, M. and Trolin, I. Clofazimine: A new agent for the treatment of pyoderma gangrenosum. *Arch. Dermatol.* 112:344, 1976.
26. Morrison, N.E. and Marley, G.M. Clofazimine binding studies with deoxyribonucleic acid. *Int. J. Lepr.* 44:475, 1976.
27. Opromolla, D.V.A. First results of the use of rifamycin SV in the treatment of lepromatous leprosy. *Proceedings of International Congress of Leprosy,* Reo de Janeiro, September 1963.
28. Pembrey, M.E., Clarke, C.A. and Frais, M.M. Normal child after maternal thalidomide ingestion in critical period of pregnancy. *Lancet* 1:275, 1970.
29. Rees, R.J.W., Pearson, J.M.H. and Waters, M.F.R. Experimen-

tal and clinical studies on rifampicin in treatment of leprosy. *Br. Med. J.* 1:89, 1970.

30. Riley, R.W. and Levy, L. Characteristics of the binding of dapsone and monoacetyldapsone by serum albumin. *Proc. Soc. Exp. Biol. Med.* 142:1168, 1973.
31. Sensi, P., Greco, A.M. and Ballotta, R. Rifamycins. I. Isolation and properties of rifamycin B and rifamycin complex. *Antibiot. Ann.* 1959-60:262, 1960.
32. Shepard, C.C. The experimental disease that follows the injection of human leprosy bacilli into foot pads of mice. *J. Exp. Med.* 112:445, 1960.
33. Shepard, C.C., Ellard, G.A., Levy, L., Opromolla, V. deAraijo, Pattyn, S.R., Peters, J.H., Rees, R.J.W. and Waters, M.F.R. Experimental chemotherapy in leprosy. *Bull. WHO* 53:425, 1976.
34. Sheskin, J. Thalidomide in the treatment of lepra reactions. *Clin. Pharmacol. Ther.* 6:303, 1965.
35. Somers, G.F. Pharmacological properties of thalidomide (alphaphthalimido glutarimide): A new sedative hypnotic drug. *Br. J. Pharmacol.* 15:111, 1960.
36. Trautman, J.R. and Enna, C.D. Leprosy. In: *Tice's Practice of Medicine*, Vol. 3. Hagerstown, MD.: Harper & Row, 1970, p. 1.

CHAPTER
25.5

SEXUALLY TRANSMITTED DISEASES

Harold C. Neu

In recent years, the changes in sexual mores and a highly mobile society have caused a major increase in sexually transmitted diseases. Gonorrhea and nongonococcal urethritis have become much more prevalent, and syphilis has also been on the increase, particularly in homosexual males. Although diseases such as chancroid, lymphogranuloma venereum, and granuloma inguinale are still uncommon, other diseases due to viruses and parasites are now known to be sexually transmissible. Table 25.5-1 lists the current diseases felt to be sexually transmitted. Table 25.5-2 gives the recommended therapies for sexually transmitted diseases.

GONORRHEA

Gonorrhea is a sexually transmitted infection caused by *Neisseria gonorrhoeae*. It can involve the urethra, endocervical, anal canal, oral pharynx, and conjunctiva by direct contact and can spread along mucosal surfaces to involve the endometrium, tubes, and peritoneum in females and epididymis in males. Systemic disease due to *Neisseria* includes arthritis, dermatitis, endocarditis, and meningitis.

Over the last several decades, the antimicrobial susceptibility patterns of *N. gonorrhoeae* have changed from susceptibility to many agents, to resistance to concentrations which heretofore were effective. In the 1970s, plasmid-mediated resistance to penicillins due to a β-lactamase similar to the one in *Escherichia coli* and *Haemophilus* was found in *N. gonorrhoeae*. The organisms that cause disseminated gonococcal infection have, however, remained susceptible to a number of antibacterial agents. The treatment of gonorrhea can be divided into types of clinical disease.

Uncomplicated Gonococcal Infections in Men and Women. Three regimens have been shown to be of equal success: (1) tetracycline hydrochloride 0.5 g by mouth four times a day for 7 days, for a total dose of 14 g; (2) amoxicillin 3 g or ampicillin 3.5 g orally, given simultaneously with 1 g of probenecid; or (3) aqueous procaine penicillin G (APPG) 4.8 million U injected i.m. divided at two sites, with 1 g of probenecid by mouth. Tetracyclines have become the drug of first choice because combined gonococcal and chlamydial infection is so common. Tetracyclines should not be given with food and should be given 1 hr before or 2 hr after meals. The tetracycline regimen should be used in patients allergic to penicillin and in those suspected of also having *Chlamydia* infection. Single-dose therapy is preferred in patients who are unlikely to complete a multiple-dose program. Some patients might be best treated with a combined regimen of oral amoxicillin 2 g with 1 g of probenecid followed by oral tetracycline 500 mg four times a day for 7 days. Doxycycline 100 mg by mouth can be substituted for tetracycline. This program provides the advantages of single-dose treatment of gonorrhea with effectiveness against chlamydial disease. Tetracycline or procaine penicillin are the preferred therapy of pharyngeal gonococcal infection. Homosexual males should be treated with procaine penicillin plus probenecid unless they are allergic to penicillin. All sexual partners should be cultured and treated with one of the programs. Patients who fail with one of these forms of therapy should be treated with 2 g of spectinomycin i.m. Oral penicillins, G or V, and repository penicillin, benzathine penicillin, have no role in the therapy of gonorrhea. Patients with β-lactamase (penicillinase) producing *N. gonorrhoeae* should be treated with 2 g of spectinomycin. If the isolate is resistant to spectinomycin, cefoxitin 2 g in 1% lidocaine given i.m. with 1 g probenecid orally will be effective, as will 1 g cefotaxime i.m. Patients who had incubating syphilis will probably be cured by any of the primary programs but not with spectinomycin. However, serological tests for syphilis should be done when the patient is next seen.

Pregnant women with gonorrhea can be treated with procaine penicillin, ampicillin, or amoxicillin. Tetracycline should not be used.

Disseminated gonococcal infection, arthritis-dermatitis syndrome, will respond to any one of the following programs: (1) ampicillin 3.5 g orally, plus 1 g probenecid orally, followed by ampicillin 0.5 g four times a day for 7 days; (2) amoxicillin 3 g orally plus 1 g probenecid followed by 0.5 g four times a day for 7 days; (3) tetracycline 0.5 g orally four times a day for 7 days; (4) cefoxitin 1 g or cefotaxime 0.5 g, either four times a day for 7 days; or (5) erythromycin 0.5 g orally four times a day for 7 days.

The precise dose of penicillin to use to treat gonococcal meningitis or endocarditis is unknown. The usual dose would be 20 million U of penicillin a day for 10 days for meningitis and the same dose for 4 weeks for endocarditis.

Infants who are born to mothers with gonorrhea are at high risk to develop infection and should receive a single i.v. or i.m. dose of 50,000 U to full-term infants and 20,000 U to low-birth-weight infants. Gonococcal ophthalmia should be treated with 50,000 U/kg/day in two i.v. doses for 7 days. Topical antimicrobial preparations are inadequate therapy. Other forms of gonorrhea in children who weigh over 45 kg should be treated with adult regimens. Tetracycline should not be used in children under 8 years of age. Uncomplicated gonorrhea in small children can be treated with a single dose of 50 mg/kg amoxicillin orally and probenecid 25 mg/kg (maximum dose 1 g).

Table 25.5-1
Sexually Transmitted Organisms and Diseases They Cause

Organism	Disease
Bacteria	
Neisseria gonorrhoeae	Gonorrhea
Chlamydia trachomatis	Non-gonococcal urethritis, proctitis
	Lymphogranuloma venereum
Ureaplasma urealyticum	Non-gonococcal urethritis
Treponema pallidum	Syphilis
Haemophilus ducreyi	Chancroid
Calymmatobacterium granulomatis	Granuloma inguinale
Salmonella	Diarrhea
Shigella	Diarrhea
Gardinella vaginalis	Vaginitis
Campylobacter foetus	Diarrhea
Virus	
HTLV-III	AIDS
Herpes virus hominis	Genital herpes
Hepatitis A, B	Hepatitis
Cytomegalovirus	Genital cytomegalovirus infection
Poxvirus group	Molluscum contagiosum
Papovavirus group	Condyloma accuminata
Fungus	
Candida albicans	Vaginitis
Protozoa	
Trichomonas vaginalis	Trichomoniasis
Entamoeba histolytica	Amebiasis
Giardia lamblia	Giardiasis
Metozoa	
Phthirus pubis	Pubic lice
Sarcoptes scabei	Scabies

NONGONOCOCCAL INFECTIONS

Nongonococcal Urethritis. Nongonococcal urethritis (NGU) is a general term that encompasses all cases of urethritis not due to *N. gonorrhoeae*, including the so-called postgonococcal urethritis, which develops several weeks after cure of gonorrhea by penicillin treatment. *Chlamydia trachomatis* accounts for 50% of the infections, and *Ureaplasma ureolyticum* for another 30%. Both of these organisms respond to treatment with tetracycline hydrochloride 0.5 g four times a day for 7 days. Failure rate is fairly high but may be due to reinfection, as the female harbors the organisms, most often asymptomatic; as with gonorrhea, the sexual partners of men with NGU should be treated in the same manner. Alternative programs have been doxycycline 0.1 g twice daily for 7 days or erythromycin 0.5 g four times a day for 7 days.

Acute Epididymoorchitis. Sexually transmitted epididymitis is usually caused by *Chlamydia* and/or *Neisseria gonorrhoeae*. Often the patient has associated urethritis. In contrast, nonsexually transmitted epididymitis is associated with urinary tract infections caused by *Enterobacteriaceae* or *Pseudomonas*. The treatment of the sexually transmitted epididymoorchitis is tetracycline 500 mg by mouth four times a day for 10 days, or doxycycline 100 mg twice daily for 10 days. Alternative therapy for nongonococcal epididymitis is erythromycin 500 mg by mouth four times daily for 10 days. If the epididymitis is gonococcal in origin, amoxicillin 500 mg three times a day orally for 10 days is useful.

Acute Pelvic Inflammatory Disease. Acute inflammatory disease of the female pelvis was formerly thought to be caused exclusively by *Neisseria gonorrhoeae*. It is now clear that other organisms such as anaerobic bacteria,

Table 25.5-2
Recommended Treatment Schedules for Gonorrhea and Pelvic Inflammatory Disease

Uncomplicated Gonococcal Infections in Men and Women

Tetracycline hydrochloride, 0.5 g, p.o., 4 times a day for 7 days, or
Aqueous procaine penicillin G, 4.8 million U i.m. plus 1 g probenecid p.o., or
Ampicillin 3.5 g or amoxicillin 3 g, either with 1 g of probenecid p.o.

Pencillinase-Producing Neisseria Gonorrhoeae (PPNG)

Spectinomycin hydrochloride, 2 g i.m., or
Cefoxitin, 2 g i.m. plus 1 g probenecid p.o., or
Cefotaxime, 1 g i.m.

Disseminated Gonococcal Infection

Aqueous crystalline penicillin G, 12 million U i.v. per day until improvement, followed by ampicillin or amoxicillin, 0.5 g p.o., 4 times a day to complete at least 7 days of treatment, or
Ampicillin 3.5 g or amoxicillin 3 g p.o., each with 1 g of probenecid p.o., followed by ampicillin or amoxicillin 0.5 g p.o. 4 times a day for at least 7 days, or
Tetracycline hydrochloride, 0.5 g p.o., 4 times a day for at least 7 days, or
Cefoxitin, 1 g, or cefotaxime, 0.5 g, i.v. 4 times a day for at least 7 days, or
Erythromycin, 0.5 g p.o., 4 times a day for at least 7 days

Neonatal Disease

Prevention of gonococcal ophthalmia
Ophthalmic ointment or drops containing tetracycline, erythromycin, or a 1% silver nitrate solution
Management of infants born to mothers with gonococcal infection
Aqueous crystalline penicillin G i.m., 50,000 U for full-term, 20,000 U for low-birth-weight infants

Neonatal infection

Gonococcal ophthalmia:
Aqueous crystalline penicillin G, 50,000 U/kg/day in 2 divided i.v. doses for 7 days plus aggressive eye irrigation
Systemic infection:
Aqueous crystalline penicillin G, 75,000-100,000 U/kg/day i.v. in 4 divided doses for at least 7 days

Childhood Disease (under 100 lb; over 100 lb treated as adult)

Uncomplicated infection
Aqueous procaine penicillin G, 100,000 U/kg i.m. plus probenecid, 25 mg/kg (maximum 1 g) p.o., or
Amoxicillin, 50 mg/kg p.o. with probenecid, as above
Systemic infection
Aqueous crystalline penicillin G, 100,000 U/kg/day i.v. in 4-6 divided doses for at least 7 days
Penicillin allergy
For uncomplicated disease: spectinomycin, 40 mg/kg i.m., or tetracycline (over 8 years of age), 40 mg/kg/day p.o. in 4 divided doses for 5 days
For systemic infection: use alternative regimens for adults in appropriate pediatric doses

Acute Salpingitis (Pelvic Inflammatory Disease)

Ambulatory patients
Cefoxitin, 2 g i.m. or amoxicillin, 3 g p.o., or ampicillin, 3.5 g p.o., or aqueous procaine penicillin G, 4.8 million U i.m., each along with probenecid, 1 g p.o., followed by doxycycline, 100 mg p.o. twice a day for 10-14 days
Hospitalized patients
Doxycycline, 100 mg i.v. twice a day, plus cefoxitin, 2 g i.v. 4 times a day for at least 4 days and 48 hr after defervescence; followed by doxycycline, 100 mg twice a day, p.o., to complete 10-14 days of therapy
Clindamycin, 600 mg i.v. 4 times a day, plus gentamicin, 2 mg/kg i.v. followed by 1.5 mg/kg i.v. every 3 hr in patients with normal renal function, for at least 4 days and 48 hr after defervescence; followed by clindamycin, 450 mg p.o., 4 times a day, to complete 10-14 days of therapy, or
Doxycycline, 100 mg i.v. twice a day, plus metronidazole, 1 g i.v. twice a day, continued for at least 4 days and 48 hr after defervescence, followed by both drugs in the same dose p.o. to complete 10-14 days of therapy

Acute Epididymitis

Tetracycline hydrochloride, 0.5 g p.o., 4 times a day, for at least 10 days or
Doxycycline, 100 mg p.o., twice a day, for at least 10 days, or
If gonococci demonstrated on smear or culture: amoxicillin, 0.5 g p.o., 3 times a day, for at least 10 days, or
If gonococci not demonstrated or cultured: erythromycin, 0.5 g p.o., 4 times a day, for at least 10 days

Modified from: Center for Disease Control. Sexually transmitted diseases treatment guidelines 1982. Morbidity and Mortality Weekly Report, 31:33S, 1982.

Bacteroides bivius, B. disiens, and occasionally *B. fragilis* as well as gram-positive cocci are important causes of this disease. Furthermore, *Chlamydia trachomatis* is particularly important in the sexually active young woman, and *E. coli, Actinomyces,* and *Mycoplasma hominis* may be involved. These organisms spread from the vagina and endocervix to the endometrium, fallopian tubes, and/or contiguous structures.

In the past, outpatient therapy with oral tetracycline, 0.5 g four times a day or with ampicillin 0.5 g four times a day for 10 days was the norm; seriously ill patients who failed to respond were given penicillin. These programs are currently felt to be unacceptable, and in 1982 the Committee for Guidelines on Sexually Transmitted Diseases recommended that patients be hospitalized and treated with doxycycline 100 mg i.v twice a day plus cefoxitin 2 g i.v. four times a day for at least 4 days, followed by doxycycline 100 mg orally twice daily to complete 10-14 days of therapy. An alternative program has been clindamycin 600 mg i.v. four times a day and gentamicin 2 mg/kg as a loading dose followed by 1.5 mg/kg every 8 hr for at least 4 days, with follow-up oral therapy with clindamycin 450 mg four times a day to complete a 10-day course. A further alternative program is doxycycline 100 mg i.v. twice daily and metronidazole 1 g twice daily for 4 days, followed by both drugs orally at the same dosage for another 10 days.

SYPHILIS

Syphilis is a chronic systemic disease due to infection by *Treponema pallidum*. It begins as a primary illness with a local lesion and regional lymphadenopathy. There is a secondary bacteremia stage with associated mucus and cutaneous lesions and general lymphadenopathy. After a latent period of years, untreated individuals may develop disease of the central nervous system, aorta, or musculoskeletal system. Latent syphilis is defined as the presence of a positive serological test for syphilis in the absence of clinical signs or symptoms of syphilis with a normal cerebrospinal fluid. Early latent syphilis is syphilis that is known to be of less than 2 years' duration.

The treatment of syphilis is based on observations that low concentrations of penicillin G will kill *T. pallidum*, but a long exposure to the drug is necessary because the organism has a generation time of 18-24 hr. Other antibiotics are much less successful.

Early Syphilis. Early syphilis (primary, secondary, or latent syphilis of less than 1 year's duration) should be treated with a single dose of 2.4 million U of benzathine penicillin G i.m. Penicillin-allergic patients should receive 15 days of tetracycline 500 mg four times a day. Syphilis of more than 1 year's duration (latent syphilis present for more than 1 year), except neurosyphilis, should be treated with benzathine penicillin G 2.4 million U i.m. once a week for 3 successive weeks. The penicillin-allergic patient should receive 30 days of oral tetracycline.

Neurosyphilis. The need to achieve adequate levels of penicillin in the cerebrospinal fluid has caused a change in therapy. The recommended program is penicillin G 12-24 million U/day i.v. for 10 days administered as 2-4 million U every 4 hr, followed by benzathine penicillin G 2.4 million U i.m. weekly for 3 weeks. An alternative outpatient program would be aqueous procaine penicillin G, 2.4 million U i.m. daily, plus probenecid 500 mg by mouth four times a day, both for 10 days, followed by three weekly i.m. doses of 2.4 million U benzathine penicillin G. The least preferred program would be 3 weeks of benzathine penicillin G.

The Jarisch-Herxheimer reaction usually develops in patients (90% or more) being treated for secondary syphilis; it may also occur in other forms of syphilis. It is manifested by headache, fever, chills, arthralgia, and myalgias, usually occurring several hours following the first administration of penicillin. The reaction is felt to be due to activation of the alternative pathway of complement. The symptoms of the reaction usually subside within 48 hr. The reaction is not noted with subsequent injections, and the drug treatment should be continued.

CHANCROID

Chancroid is caused by *Haemophilus ducreyi* and is characterized by painful genital ulcerations with suppurative inguinal lymphadenopathy. Recommended treatment is erythromycin 500 mg four times daily or trimethoprim-sulfamethoxazole 160 mg/800 mg twice daily, either program orally for at least 10 days.

LYMPHOGRANULOMA VENEREUM

Lymphogranuloma Venereum is caused by *Chlamydia trachomatis* and is characterized by multilocular suppurative inguinal lymphadinitis with late complications of rectal strictures. Tetracycline hydrochloride 0.5 g four times a day for 2 weeks is the therapy. Sulfamethoxazole 1 g by mouth twice daily or 500 mg erythromycin four times a day for 2 weeks are alternative programs.

GRANULOMA INGUINALE

Granuloma inguinale is an uncommon infection caused by *Calymmatobacterium granulomatis* that produces painless, raised red genital ulcers. Treatment with tetracycline 2 g/day for 3 weeks will prevent relapses.

VAGINITIS

Vaginitis can be caused by *Candida albicans*, *Trichomonas vaginalis*, or *Gardinella vaginalis*. The symptoms are different for each. *G. vaginalis* produces a small amount of malodorous discharge, *T. vaginalis* a profuse discharge, and *Candida* a more local pruritus. *Candida* vaginitis can be treated with topical intravaginal applications of nystatin, clotrimazole, or miconazole. *T. vaginalis* responds to a single 2 g oral dose of metronidazole; *G. vaginalis* responds to 0.5 g of metronidazole twice daily for 7 days.

VIRAL VENEREAL DISEASES

Primary herpes simplex will respond to therapy with acyclovir, 200 mg five times a day for 7 days. This treatment will reduce viral shedding and duration of disease. There is as yet no effective therapy of recurrent genital herpes, although preliminary reports of the use of oral acyclovir are encouraging. At present, there are no effective treatments for poxviruses that cause molluscum contagiosum, papovavirus that causes condyloma acuminatum, or for cytomegalovirus. External genital and perianal warts may respond to topical applications of 10-25% podophyllin in tincture of benzoin applied weekly for 4 weeks. Normal mucosa should not be exposed to podophyllin. Hepatitis B, which is common in homosexual men and can be transmitted to sexual partners of heterosexuals, can be prevented by administration of hepatitis hyperimmune globulin given twice in a 30-day period.

SCABIES

Scabies is caused by the human mite *Sacroptes scabei*. Treatment is with application of a cream or lotion containing 1% γ-benzene (KWELL), or 10% crotamiton (EURAX), or 20% benzyl benzoate. The lotion should be left on for 24 hr.

SALMONELLOSIS

Salmonellosis should not be treated, as it merely prolongs the carrier state.

SHIGELLOSIS

Most adult individuals with shigellosis will become asymptomatic without treatment, but trimethoprim-sulfamethoxazole can be used at doses of two tablets twice daily for 5 days.

CAMPYLOBACTERIOSIS

Erythromycin 0.5 g administered four times a day for 7-11 days will treat campylobacteriosis. Some strains of *Campylobacter* will respond to therapy with tetracycline.

GIARDIASIS

Metronidazole at a dose of 750 mg three times a day orally or quinacrine 100 mg orally three times a day, either for 7 days, would be effective therapy of giardiasis.

REFERENCE

1. Center for Disease Control. Sexually transmitted diseases treatment guidelines for 1982. *Morbid. Mortal. Weekly Rep.* 31:355, 1982.

CHAPTER
26

CHEMOTHERAPY OF PARASITIC DISEASES: GENERAL CONSIDERATIONS

G. Thomas Strickland and Edgar A. Steck

Human parasitic diseases have always been important to practitioners in the tropics. In fact, infections with helminths and protozoa are the most common causes of human diseases (4). The prevalence of schistosomiasis is estimated to be 200 million. More than 150 million people are believed to be infected with malaria, with approximately 1 million chidren under age 5 dying of malaria each year in Africa alone. The development of resistance by the parasites to drugs and of the mosquitoes to insecticides, and the rising cost of the latter, are leading to a resurgence of malaria in the Indian Subcontinent and other areas where it had been relatively controlled. Even greater numbers are infected with the common intestinal parasites (e.g., *Ascaris lumbricoides*, hookworm species, *Trichuris trichiura*). Parasitic diseases are increasing with the world population. Irrigation schemes to provide more food are spreading the transmission of schistosomiasis.

Parasitic diseases are becoming more prevalent in temperate climates as well as in tropical areas. Toxoplasmosis is ubiquitous, causing subclinical or clinical congenital or acquired infections in approximately one of three people worldwide. Fish tapeworm infections, echinococcosis, and trichinosis are transmitted within the Arctic Circle. Vaginal discharge and pruritus are frequently caused by *Trichomonas vaginalis*, the most common parasite infecting Americans. Diarrhea and malabsorption due to *Giardia lamblia* infection is now the most commonly reported water-borne infection in the United States. There are reports of giardiasis epidemics in ski resorts and in groups visiting Leningrad, clearly nontropical locations. Despite improvements in sanitation, more than 50 million Americans have helminth infections. The most common are pinworms (enterobiasis), roundworms (ascariasis), and whipworms (trichuriasis). Schistosomiasis is endemic in Puerto Rico and is frequently found in immigrants from there as well as from other countries.

Not only is the endemic transmission of parasitic diseases increasing in temperate climates, but also the transport of these infections is increasing in nonsuspecting hosts from the tropics to temperate areas. Subsequent to a low of 237 cases of malaria reported to the Centers for Disease Control (CDC) in 1973, there has been a progressive increase to almost 2000 in 1980. Since the end of the Vietnam war, 90% of the cases are occurring in civilians, the majority in immigrants. Therefore, due to more and faster global travel, physicians anywhere in the United States may see patients with exotic parasitic diseases. The febrile patient who was recenlty on the East African safari may have malaria or African trypanosomiasis, whereas the student from Nigeria with hematuria may have *Schistosoma haematobium* infection. The Thai wife of a former Air Force man may have opisthorchiasis, caused by eating raw freshwater fish containing the larval stage of this liver fluke. Our Mexican and Vietnamese immigrants are bringing numerous parasitic infections with them. Therefore, physicians must ask their patients, "Where have you been?"

Parasitic diseases are increasing in worldwide occurrence. Endemic parasitic diseases are increasing in the United States. Parasitic diseases are more frequently being brought into the United States by travelers and immigrants (3). It is appropriate and important that the chemotherapy of parasitic diseases be given more consideration than in the past in courses and textbooks of pharmacology.

CHOICE OF CHEMOTHERAPEUTIC AGENT

The choice of an appropriate agent to treat parasitic diseases is often complicated (2). Factors, other than efficacy, to be considered in treatment choice include availability, cost, toxicity, ease of administration, and time required to complete therapy. The ideal drug, then, is readily available, inexpensive, nontoxic, and gives excellent cure rates with one or two oral doses.

In the United States, many drugs for treatment of parasitic diseases either do not have FDA approval and so are not available (e.g., tinidazole) or have been withdrawn from the market by the manufacturer, for example iodoquinol [diiodohydroxyquin (DIODOQUIN)]. The latter drug is still available under its generic name, which was changed in 1980. Other drugs may have FDA approval for treatment of one specific disease but not another, for example, paromomycin, which is approved for ame-

Table 26-1
Drugs For Treating Parasitic Diseases

Generic Name (Trade Name)	Treatment for:[a]
A. *Drugs marketed in the United States*	
Amodiaquine (CAMOQUIN)	A: malar., malar. (proph.)
Amphotericin B (FUNGIZONE)	R: primary amebic meningoencephalitis; A: leish.
Bephenium (ALCOPAR)	A: hook., trichostrong., ternid., ascar.
Chlorguanide (PALUDRINE)	A: malar. (proph.), malar.
Chloroquine (ARALEN, RESOCHIN)	R: malar., malar. (proph.); A: ameb., clonor., parag., opisth.
Diethylcarbamazine (BANOCIDE, HETRAZAN)	R: filar., loia., oncho., tropical eosinophilia, streptocerc.; A: toxocar.
Emetine	A: ameb., clonorch., fasciol., opisth.
Iodoquinol, diiodohydroxyquin	R: ameb.
Mebendazole (VERMOX)	R: enterob., ascar., hook., trichur., capil., echin.; A: taeni., strongy.
Metronidazole (FLAGYL)	R: ameb., trichomon., giard.; A: drac., balant.
Niclosamide (YOMESAN, CESTOCIDE)	R: taeni., tape (d, f), heterop.; A: fasciolop.
Oxamniquine (MANSIL)	R: schisto. (man.)
Paromomycin (HUMATIN)	A: tape (b, d, f), ameb., balant.
Piperazine (ANTEPAR)	R: ascar.; A: enterob.
Primaquine	R: malar. (viv. & ov), proph. and treatment
Praziquantel (BILTRICIDE)	R: schist., clonor., opisth.; metag.; A: tape., parag.
Pyrantel pamoate (ANTIMINTH, COMBANTRIN)	R: enterob., ascar., hook., trichostrongy., ternid.
Pyrimethamine (DARAPRIM)	R: malar. (fal.), toxopla., cocc.; A: pneumo., malar (proph.)
Pyrimethamine-sulfadoxine (FANSIDAR)	R: malar. (fal.), proph. and treatment
Pyrvinium pamoate (POVAN, VANQUIN)	A: strongy., enterob.
Quinacrine (mepacrine, ATABRINE)	R: giard,; A: taeni.
Quinine	R: malar. (fal.)
Sulfadiazine	R: malar. (fal.), toxopl., cocc.; A: pneumo.
Sulfisoxazole (GANTRISIN)	A: malar. (fal.), toxopl., cocc., pneumo.
Tetrachloroethylene	R: fasciolop.; A: hook.
Tetracycline	A: ameb., balant., malar.
Thiabendazole (MINTEZOL)	R: strongy., trichino., cutaneous larva migrans, toxicar., drac.; A: trichur., capil., trichostrongy., enterob., ascar., hook.
Trimethoprim-sulfamethoxazole (BACTRIM, SEPTRA)	R: pneumo., cocc.; A: malar. (fal.)
B. *Drugs not marketed in the United States, available through CDC*[b]	
Bithionol (BITIN, ACTAMER)	R: parag., fasciol., A: clonor.
Dehydroemetine	A: ameb., clonor., fasciol., opisth.
Diloxanide furoate (FURAMIDE)	R: ameb.
Melarsoprol (MEL B, ARSORBAL)	R: Af. trypan. (neurological stage)
Metrifonate (BILARCIL)	R: schist. (haem.)
Nifurtimox (BAYERS 2502, LAMPIT)	R: Am. trypan.
Niridazole (AMBILHAR)	A: schist., drac.
Pentamidine (LOMIDINE)	R: babes.; A: leish., Af. trypan. (blood stage), pneumo.
Sodium stibogluconate (PENTOSTAM)	R: leish.
Sodium stibocaptate (ASTIBAN)	R: schist. (jap.); A: schist., (man., haem.)
Suramin sodium (AMTRYPOL, GERMANIN)	R: Af. trypan. (blood stage), oncho.
C. *Useful drugs not available in the United States*	
Cycloguanil pamoate (CAMOLAR)	A: Am. cutaneous leish., malar. (proph.)
Diminazene aceturate (BERENIL)	A: Af. trypan.
Levamisole	R: ascar., hook.; A: strongy., trichur., filar., oncho.
Meglumine antimoniate (GLUCANTIME)	R: leish.
Nimorazole (NAXOCIN, NULOGYL)	A: trichomon., giard., ameb.
Tinidazole (FASIGYN)	R: trichomon., giard., ameb.

Table 26-1(continued)
Drugs For treating Parasitic Diseases

Footnotes to the table.

[a]R = recommended drug
A = alternate drug.
ameb., amebiasis
ascar., ascariasis
balant., balantidiasis
babes., babesiosis
capil., capillariasis
clonor., clonorchiasis
cocc., coccidiosis
drac., dracontiasis
echin., echinococcosis
enterob., enterobiasis
filar., filariasis
fasciol., fascioliasis
fasciolop., fasciolopsiasis
giard., giardiasis
heterop., heterophysis
hook., hookworm
leish., leishmaniasis
loia., loiasis
malar., malaria
(*proph.*, prophylaxis
fal., falciparum
viv., vivax
ov., ovale)
metag., metagonimiasis
oncho., onchocerciasis
opisth., opisthorchiasis
parag., paragonimiasis
pneumo., pneumocystosis
schist., schistosomiasis
(*haem.*, haematobium
man., mansoni
jap., japonicum)
streptocerc., streptocerciasis
strongy., strongyloidiasis
taeni., taeniasis
tape., tapeworm (b, beef, d, dwarf, f, fish)
ternid., ternideniasis
toxocar., toxocariasis
toxopl., toxoplasmosis
trichomon., trichomoniasis
trichostrong., trichostrongyliasis
trichin., trichinosis
trichur., trichuriasis
trypan., trypanosomiasis
(Af, African;
Am., American).

[b]Available in the United States from Parasitic Diseases Division. Center for Disease Control, Atlanta, Georgia 30333; telephone 404-329-3311.

biasis but not for treatment of tapeworms. Several recommended and alternate drugs are made available on a limited basis in the United States by the Parasitic Diseases Division at the CDC in Atlanta (3) (Table 26-1).

The economically deprived suffer the greatest incidence of parasitic infections. In most tropical countries, treatment with the less expensive older drugs will continue despite introduction of more efficacious agents that are more costly. Piperazine, which costs roughly $ 0.25 per adult therapeutic course for ascariasis, will not be replaced readily by mebendazole, which is considerably more costly. Oxamniquine, a very efficacious and safe drug for treating schistosomiasis mansoni, is costly to produce and is expensive. The cost for treating individual patients is reasonable. It is too much, however, to be practical for treating the 10-12 million Egyptians infected with this parasite.

Some drugs used to treat parasitic diseases can cause severe toxic reactions. For instance, hycanthone, a drug with a good cure rate and reduction in egg excretion for *S. haematobium* and *S. mansoni* infections following a single intramuscular injection, has been shown to be mutagenic, teratogenic, and carcinogenic in experimental animals, may induce parasite strains to become resistant to antischistosomal agents, and occasionally causes death in humans from acute hepatic necrosis. As a consequence, drugs that require more prolonged administration, either orally (niridazole) or intramuscularly (the antimony compounds), are often used. In the United States, this usually causes no major problems. In tropical villages, however, medication is frequently not taken and physician's follow-up is often impossible.

Viruses, bacteria, fungi, and protozoa multiply in the host, and so the goal for chemotherapy in diseases caused by these agents is complete cure. Helminths, with a few exceptions (e.g., *Strongyloides stercoralis* and *Capillaria philippinensis*) do not multiply in the body, and the clinical manifestations and transmission rates are related to intensity of infection. Thus, the goal for chemotherapy of most helminth infections need not be cure, and in some cases (e.g., enterobiasis, trichuriasis) treatment may not be necessary. Even in schistosomiasis, a disease in which severe pathophysiology frequently occurs, eradication of all worms in all patients may not be a necessity. By using lower doses of chemotherapeutic agents, drug toxicity may be controlled while still reducing transmission rate and clinical manifestations to acceptable levels. In those patients who are not cured by this regimen, a marked decrease in the excretion rate of viable ova is the rule.

The toxicity of the drug must be weighed against the need for treatment. When the first drug is initially ineffective and the alternate is more toxic, it is generally advisable to retreat with the less hazardous drug before using the alternate one. Also, the nutritional state of the patient must be taken into consideration prior to prescribing potentially toxic drugs.

ADVERSE EFFECTS OF ANTIPARASITIC DRUGS

Several drugs do not have FDA approval for treating pregnant women or children. The safety of bithionol, dehydroemetine, melarsoprol, metronidazole, pentamidine, sodium stibogluconate, and suramin sodium has not been established in pregnant women or young children. The experience with pyrantel pamoate, metrifonate, and oxamniquine is still limited. Other drugs (i.e., trimethoprim, pyrimethamine, mebendazole, and tetracycline) are potentially toxic to the fetus and should not be given to pregnant women if alternative drugs are available. Quinacrine should not be given to pregnant women, to patients with a history of psychosis, or to those with psoriasis. Niridazole is not recommended in the presence of hepatocellular disease, portal hypertension, or a history of mental disorders or seizures. No antimony-containing compound should be given to patients with severe hepatic, renal, or cardiac disease. Other drugs should be substituted for emetine or dehydroemetine in the presence of cardiac disease. Melarsoprol is very toxic and should be used with extreme care in patients with liver and renal impairment, and preferably used only on hospitalized patients who are well nourished. Arsenic sensitivity is a contraindication, and a fatal reactive encephalopathy has been reported. Renal or hepatic disease and intolerance to the test dose are contraindications to the use of suramin sodium. The urine should be examined before each injection and treatment reconsidered if albuminuria is present. Primaquine can cause acute hemolytic anemia in patients with glucose-6-phosphate dehydrogenase deficiency. Severe allergic reactions frequently occur in patients with filarial infections or tropical eosinophilia who are treated with diethylcarbamazine and suramin. Concomitant corticosteroids are sometimes useful.

The multiple potential and actual complications of hycanthone are mentioned elsewhere. This drug is not recommended for treating schistosomiasis when other medications are available because of the potential toxicity, as noted in experimental animals and bacterial models, and also because of occasional fatalities associated with its use. Other excellent drugs are available, including praziquantel, a new agent with activity against all species of schistosomes infecting humans as well as against other trematodes and tapeworms, will be marketed soon.

Niridazole, metronidazole, and other nitro compounds are mutagens in bacterial culture systems. Metronidazole has also been shown to be a carcinogen in mice. Bueding believes that mutagenic and therapeutic effects of antischistosomal agents can be dissociated (1). Analogs of hycanthone and niridazole can be produced that have therapeutic efficacy and that are not mutagenic.

No patient should be denied effective treatment of a symptomatic or potentially serious parasitic disease solely on information obtained from experimental animal and bacterial culture studies. Because of the possible long-term effects of some of these agents, however, the practitioner must weigh the benefits of therapy against the dangers from administration of the drug.

REFERENCES

1. Bueding, E. Dissociation of mutagenic and other toxic properties from schistosomicides. *J. Toxicol. Environ. Health* 1:329, 1975.
2. Gilles, H.M. The search for new drugs for tropical diseases. *Trans. R. Soc. Trop. Med. Hyg.* 73:144, 1979.
3. Most, H. Current concepts. Treatment of parasitic infections of travelers and immigrants. *N. Engl. J. Med.* 310:298, 1984.
4. Schultz, M.G. Current concepts in parasitology: Parasitic diseases. *N. Engl. J. Med.* 297:1259, 1977.

ADDITIONAL READINGS

Drugs for parasitic infections. *Med. Lett. Drugs Ther.* 24:5, 1982.

Goodwin, L.G. New drugs for old diseases. *Trans. R. Soc. Trop. Med. Hyg.* 74:1, 1980.

Maegraith, B.G., and Gilles, H.M. *Management and Treatment of Tropical Diseases.* Oxford: Blackwell Scientific Publications, 1971.

Strickland, G.T. *Hunter's Tropical Medicine, 6th ed.* Philadelphia: W.B. Saunders Co., 1984.

CHAPTER
26.1

CHEMOTHERAPY OF INTESTINAL AND GENITAL PROTOZOA

G. Thomas Strickland and Edgar A. Steck

Intestinal and genital protozoan infections are among the most common infectious diseases today in both tropical and temperate climates. The estimated prevalence of amebiasis is 400 million people worldwide. Incidence in the United States has been slowly decreasing, from 5-10% of the population 40 years ago to about 0.5-1% at present.

Amebiasis is a protozoan infection caused by *Entamoeba histolytica*. The organisms occur in the intestines in two forms: trophozoite and cyst. Trophozoites, which normally live as commensals, under an unknown stimulus, will invade the intestinal mucosa, causing tissue lysis and producing diarrhea or dysentery with blood and mucus in the stool. They may be carried to the liver, lung, or brain, where they can give rise to amebic abscess. The motile trophozoites in the large bowel may encyst under adverse conditions. Although both the cysts and trophozoites are excreted in the feces, only the cysts are infective and are transmitted by the fecal-oral route via flies, fingers, food, or water. Ingested cysts liberate trophozoites in the intestine, thus continuing the life cycle in the host (Fig. 26.1-1). The majority of patients infected with *E. histolytica* are asymptomatic cyst passers. Only a minority develops invasive disease, such as dysentery and hepatic abscess. It is not known why some develop invasive disease and others do not.

Giardiasis is now the most frequently reported cause of water-borne epidemics in the United States. It occurs both in the tropics and temperate climates, and there is no longer any question of the pathogenicity of *Giardia lamblia*. The potential for visitors to Leningrad of developing the disease is well known, as is the frequent occurrence of epidemics at ski resorts. Recently, infections with either, or both, *G. lamblia* and *E. histolytica* have been reported in male homosexuals and individuals with the acquired immunodeficiency syndrome (AIDS).

Trichomoniasis is the most common parasitic disease occurring in the United States. Treatment is particularly difficult because asymptomatic males can reinfect their female sex partners if all are not treated. Vaginitis caused by *Trichomonas vaginalis* is not a life-threatening illness but can be a protracted source of discomfort.

The other pathogenic intestinal protozoan infections are rare in both the United States and the tropics: balantidiasis, isosporiasis, and *E. polecki* infection. Other protozoa found in human feces (e.g., *Entamoeba coli, E. hartmanni, Endolimax nana, Iodamoeba buetschlii, Trichomonas hominis,* and *Chilomastix mesnili)* are not associated with disease, and treatment is not believed to be indicated.

DRUGS USED IN INTESTINAL AND GENITAL PROTOZOAN INFECTIONS

DEHYDROEMETINE AND EMETINE

Following the observation in 1912 that confirmed emetine to have amebicidal activity, various derivatives and synthetic analogs were investigated extensively in both the laboratory and in clinical trials. These studies have shown that dehydroemetine retains the amebicidal properties with less toxicity than emetine.

Source and Chemistry. Dehydroemetine is a synthetic analog of emetine, an alkaloid obtained from ipecac, differing only in the lack of hydrogen atoms at positions 2 and 3 (Fig. 26.1-2). Both compounds are white crystalline powders soluble in water and alcohol.

Antiprotozoal Effect. Both drugs have a direct lethal action on *E. histolytica* and are more effective against motile trophozoites than cysts. They are thought to interfere with the multiplication of the parasite and, *in vitro*, emetine kills trophozoites at therapeutic concentrations.

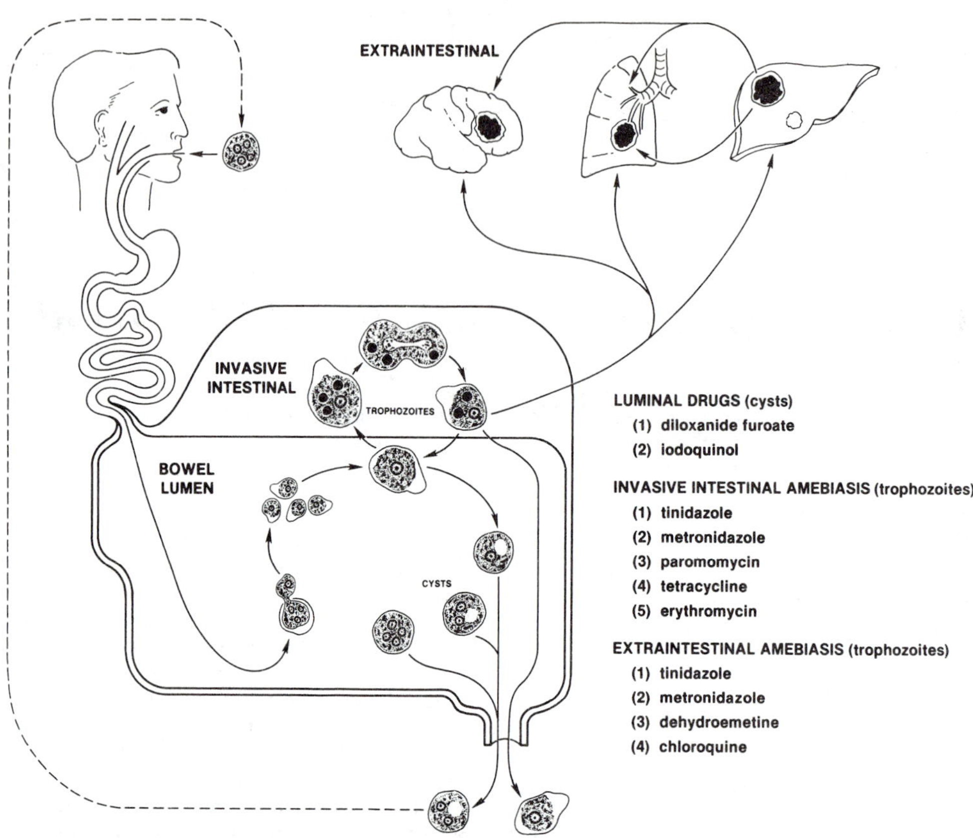

LUMINAL DRUGS (cysts)
(1) diloxanide furoate
(2) iodoquinol

INVASIVE INTESTINAL AMEBIASIS (trophozoites)
(1) tinidazole
(2) metronidazole
(3) paromomycin
(4) tetracycline
(5) erythromycin

EXTRAINTESTINAL AMEBIASIS (trophozoites)
(1) tinidazole
(2) metronidazole
(3) dehydroemetine
(4) chloroquine

Fig. 26-1. *Life cycle of Entamoeba histolytica, showing transmission and sites of infection and actions of chemotherapeutic agents.* (Redrawn from The Ciba Collection of Medical Illustrations Vol. 3, page 155)

However, these concentrations are not reached in the gut lumen, thus explaining its limited efficacy against the luminal phase of amebiasis. The selective toxicity for *E. histolytica* is probably related to the more rapid uptake of the drug by the parasite than by host cells. Studies have also shown that emetine irreversibly blocks protein synthesis in all eukaryocytes by inhibiting the translocation of peptidyl-tRNA from acceptor site to donor site on the ribosome, DNA synthesis being secondarily blocked.

Pharmacokinetics. Emetine has been studied in greater detail than dehydroemetine. It is readily absorbed following parenteral administration and is slowly excreted and detoxified. The principal route of excretion is via the kidneys. Although the drug appears in the urine within an hour of injection, cumulative toxicity is a danger, since it is still present in tissues up to 2 months after injection. Highest concentrations are found in the liver, heart, and other viscera, accounting for its cardiac toxicity and therapeutic efficacy in treating hepatic abscess. Dehydroemetine is released and excreted more rapidly than emetine from most body organs, in particular the heart. This explains its reduced toxicity.

Adverse Effects. Local reactions to either emetine or dehydroemetine are common. Following i.m. or s.c. injection, there is localized pain, stiffness, and weakness. Skin necrosis and rashes can also occur. Gastrointestinal symptoms often follow oral ingestion.

Systemic effects of the drugs involve the gastrointestinal, neuromuscular, and cardiovascular systems. Diarrhea due to increased peristalsis from direct action upon the intestinal musculature can be mistaken for an exacerbation of amebic dysentery. However, improvement frequently precedes the drug-induced diarrhea. Other gastrointestinal manifestations include nausea and vomiting. These symptoms sometimes resolve despite continuation of therapy. Dizziness, faintness, fatigue, listlessness, and headache are frequent complications.

Stiffness, weakness, aching, and tenderness of the skeletal muscles occur, particularly those of the neck and extremities. The weakness and pain generally appear before more serious symptoms and thus are guides to preventing overdosages. They usually persist until the drug is discontinued. The mechanism may be a blocking action on the neuromuscular junction. Mild sensory disturbances and tremor have been reported.

Cardiovascular toxicity is the major complication with emetine. Dehydroemetine is the preferred drug because toxicities occur less frequently, are less severe, and are shorter in duration. Some degree of cardiac toxicity occurs in the majority of patients. ECG changes are found in up to half of the patients receiving emetine, providing a sensitive and early index of toxicity. The major changes are flattening and inversion of the T wave and prolongation of the Q-T interval, which persist for varying periods after the drug is discontinued. Other

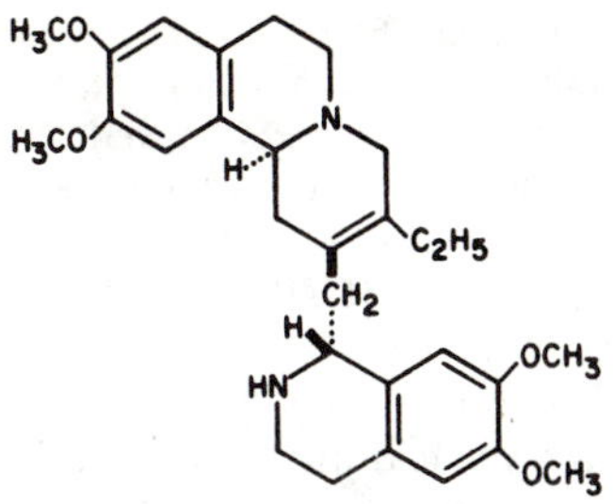

Diiodohydroxyquin

Dehydroemetine

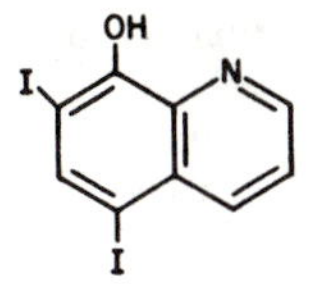

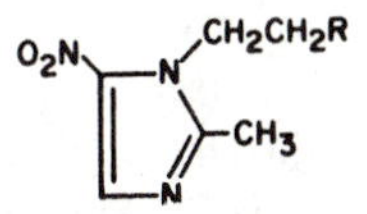

R = OH Metronidazole
R = $-CH_2CH(OH)CH_2Cl$ Ornidazole
R = $-SO_2CH_2CH_3$ Tinidazole

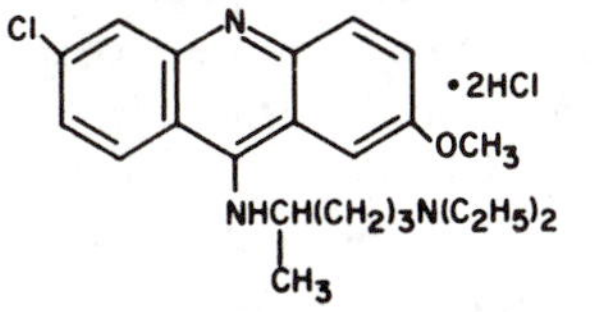

Quinacrine dihydrochloride
(Mepacrine dihydrochloride)

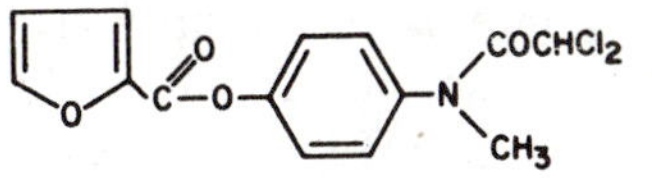

Diloxanide furoate

Fig. 26.1-2: *Drugs used in treating intestinal and genital protozoal infections.*

more serious cardiac toxicities include hypotension, precordial pain, tachycardia, and dyspnea. These may be due to a direct depressant action of the drug on the myocardium. The dyspnea is often associated with generalized weakness. The patient should be at absolute bed rest during dehydroemetine or emetine therapy and remain at partial rest for several weeks thereafter. The patient should be monitored daily by history, physical examination, and ECG. There should be a delay of at least 6 weeks between courses of therapy. Patients with heart disease should not be treated with these drugs unless the disease cannot be controlled with less toxic drugs.

Preparations. *Dehydroemetine* is available from the Parasitic Diseases Division, Centers for Disease Control, Atlanta, Georgia, in single-dose, 2 ml ampules, each containing 70 mg of the dihydrochloride in aqueous solution. The recommended dose is 1- 1.5 mg/kg/day (maximum 90 mg/day) given i.m. for up to 5 days. It is recommended that the doses be divided into two injections for children. Debilitated patients should be given reduced doses. The dose of emetine is 1 mg/kg/day given i.m. in a single or divided injection each day for up to 5 days. The maximum daily dose is 60 mg. Ten-day courses of dehydroemetine or emetine have been recommended by some, but the patient must be carefully observed for cardiac and other toxicities.

DILOXANIDE FUROATE

Diloxanide furoate is the preferred luminal amebicide because of its almost complete absence of toxicity and shorter therapeutic course than iodoquinol.

Source and Chemistry. Diloxanide furoate, a synthetic product, is a white crystalline powder almost insoluble in water. Of the acetanilide derivatives tested for antiamebic activity, the furoate ester was found to be the most active (Fig. 26.1-2).

Antiprotozoal Effect. The only pharmacological effects are those upon ameba. Diloxanide is amebicidal *in vitro*. The mechanism of action appears to involve inhibition of protein synthesis in *E. histolytica*, much as do other N-dichloroacetyl compounds such as chloramphenicol.

Pharmacokinetics. The ester undergoes hydrolysis in the upper intestinal tract and is rapidly absorbed as diloxanide. This portion of the dose is inactive systemically and is excreted in the urine as diloxanide glucuronide within 2 days. The remaining 5-10% passes to the lower intestinal tract, where it exerts its activity as a luminal amebicide before voiding in the feces.

Adverse Effects. Diloxanide has almost no toxic side effects. Flatulence is common, and occasional patients have nausea and anorexia.

Preparations. *Diloxanide furoate* is available in the United States from the CDC Parasitic Diseases Division as tablets containing 500 mg of the drug. The adult dose is 500 mg three times daily for 10 days. The course may be repeated if follow-up stool examinations contain amebic cysts. Children should be given the drug at 20 mg/kg daily in three divided doses or at a reduced dosage (i.e., 500 mg twice daily).

IODOQUINOL (Diiodohydroxyquin)

Iodoquinol is an amebicide that acts upon *E. histolytica* in the bowel lumen and is used for treating asymptomatic cyst passers and to clear the cyst stage in patients with symptomatic amebiasis.

Source and Chemistry. Iodoquinol, a tasteless, brownish yellow powder that is nearly insoluble in water, is a synthetically produced dihalogenated 8-quinolinol (Fig. 26.1-2). It is the only member of this group still used in human medicine, although many have found application in the past as antiseptics, amebicides, and trichomonacides. Iodochlorhydroxyquin has been extensively used in the treatment and prophylaxis of traveler's diarrhea and other nonspecific diarrheas but is no longer used because of its association with subacute myelooptic neuropathy (19).

Antiprotozoal Effect. The only significant pharmacological action at the recommended dose is upon amebic cysts and trophozoites in the intestinal tract. Iodoquinol is believed to act upon amebas by chelating ferrous ions, which are essential for metabolism.

Pharmacokinetics. Relatively little of the drug is absorbed from the gastrointestinal tract, explaining its therapeutic efficacy for treating the intestinal lumen stages of *E. histolytica* and its low incidence of toxicity. As expected, there is little rise in plasma iodine levels after oral therapy. The small amount of drug absorbed is mostly bound to serum lipoproteins, and the main excretory pathway is in the urine as a glucuronide.

Adverse Effects. Unlike iodochlorhydroxyquin, iodoquinol has very few side effects. The severe myelitis associated with the former drug, principally in Japanese patients being treated for nonspecific diarrhea, prohibits its use (19). The administration of iodoquinol to children in excessive doses for prolonged periods for chronic diarrhea has been associated with optic atrophy and permanent loss of vision. Minor side effects that occasionally complicate iodoquinol therapy are nausea, diarrhea, abdominal pain, headache, skin rash, thyroid enlargement, furunculosis, and chills and fever. The drug must be used with care in patients with hepatic abnormalities and is contraindicated in those with iodine intolerance.

Preparations. *Iodoquinol* is available as tablets containing 210 or 650 mg of the drug. DIODOQUIN is no longer marketed, and the drug must be ordered under its generic name, which was changed from diiodohydroxyquin in 1980. The adult dosage for the luminal amebicide is 650 mg three times daily, after meals, for 20 days. Children can be treated with 30-40 mg/kg (maximum dose of 1.95 g/day). If cysts persist in the stool after the initial course of therapy, it can be repeated.

Iodoquinol has been used at the same dosage to treat other intestinal protozoal infections: *Entamoeba polecki* (23), *Dientamoeba fragilis*, and *Balantidium coli.*

METRONIDAZOLE and TINIDAZOLE

Metronidazole is a synthetic nitroimidazole derivative that was introduced in 1959 for the systemic treatment of trichomonal infections of the urogenital tract. Subsequent synthesis and trials have shown other 5-nitroimidazoles, including tinidazole and nimorazole, to have excellent activity against some protozoa. The development of these drugs has been the most significant advance in the treatment of intestinal protozoal infections. They are active in treating trichomoniasis, systemic and intestinal amebiasis, and giardiasis. They have also been used to treat and prevent anaerobic bacterial infections, for prophylaxis during appendectomy, colon surgery, and hysterectomy (11), and to treat acute diverticulitis, nonspecific vaginitis, balantidiasis, and dracunculiasis (Chapter 26.5).

Source and Chemistry. Metronidazole is a chemically synthesized yellow crystalline 5-nitroimidazole that is only slightly soluble in water and alcohol (Fig. 26.1-2). Tinidazole is a 5-nitroimidazole, having a different substitution on the side chain at position 1 from metronidazole (Fig. 26.1-2). The nitro group is critical for antiparasitic effects of the 5-nitroimidazoles. However, various units of at least two carbons in length, may be present in position 1 (where a 2-hydroxyethyl grouping is present in metronidazole), and either a hydrogen or methyl group (as in metronidazole) may be at position 2 on the imidazole ring.

Antiprotozoal Effect. Metronidazole and the other 5-nitroimidazoles destroy *T. vaginalis* and *E. histolytica* both *in vitro* (at readily available therapeutic levels) and *in vivo*. The mechanism of action is related to reduction of its nitro group. Both carbohydrate metabolism and nucleic acid synthesis are impaired by these compounds and their congeners. They have specific anaerobicidal action, having no direct action on aerobes or facultative anaerobes. The biological properties of 5-nitroimidazoles may be mediated by a partially reduced intermediate that binds to critical sites in susceptible cells (11).

Pharmacokinetics. The 5-nitroimidazoles are rapidly absorbed following oral administration. Metronidazole is only weakly bound to serum proteins and is distributed throughout the total body water, including the cerebrospinal fluid and breast milk. It has a plasma half-life of approximately 7 hr (11). The drug has been found in amebic liver abscess pus. It is excreted in the bile and through the colonic wall into the gut lumen. Metronidazole undergoes metabolic transformation, presumably in the liver, to give four identified imidazole derivatives. Either of the two side chains can be oxidized to form either an alcohol or acid metabolite. Only the alcohol metabolite is found in the serum when renal function is normal. All metabolites are excreted in the urine, which is dark colored as a consequence. Tinidazole is metabolically more stable and has higher and more prolonged blood levels, explaining its greater efficacy than metronidazole following single daily doses (2, 3).

Adverse Effects. The most common side effects associated with 5-nitroimidazoles are self-limited and readily tolerated at the doses necessary to treat protozoal infections. They have a bitter or metallic taste and can cause anorexia, nausea, vomiting, abdominal discomfort and cramps, diarrhea, constipation, headache, dizziness, vertigo, incoordination and ataxia, insomnia, and skin rashes. Leukopenia, a peripheral neuropathy, and other rarer symptoms have been reported, but side effects severe enough to discontinue therapy are rare. Paresthesias are generally reversible if treatment is stopped when symptoms first occur. A disulfiram-like response necessitates that all patients be informed not to drink alcohol while receiving these drugs.

Metronidazole has been shown to be mutagenic to bacteria and carcinogenic in rodents. These associations have not as yet been proven in humans. Nevertheless, these drugs should not be indiscriminately prescribed and should not be used during pregnancy or be given to lactating mothers unless no alternate therapy is available (11).

Preparations. *Metronidazole* is available as 250-mg tablets. *Tinidazole* is not available in the United States but is marketed elsewhere as 200-mg tablets. The recommended adult doses are as follows: amebiasis - metronidazole, 750 mg three times daily for 5-10 days, or tinidazole, 2 g once daily for 2 or 3 days; giardiasis - metronidazole, 2 g once daily for 2 or 3 days, or tinidazole, 2 g once daily for 1-3 days; trichomoniasis - metronidazole, 2 g once, or tinidazole, 2 g once. The male sex partner(s) should also receive therapy when a woman is treated for vaginitis (14). A luminal amebicide (e.g., diloxanide furoate or iodoquinol) should also be used in treating patients with amebiasis. The pediatric dosage of these drugs is slightly reduced and depends upon body weight.

QUINACRINE

Quinacrine is an acridine derivative that was introduced as a clinically valuable antimalarial agent in 1932 and was extensively used during World War II as a suppressive and therapeutic antimalarial drug. It is no longer used in the prophylaxis and treatment of malaria but still has a place in the treatment of giardiasis.

Source and Chemistry. Quinacrine is a bright yellow crystalline powder with a bitter taste. Some 2000 acridine derivatives were synthesized and tested in the course of developing quinacrine as an antimalarial agent (Fig. 26.1-2). Chloroquine resulted as an extension of these efforts and has superceded quinacrine in the treatment of malaria.

Antiprotozoal Effect. Considerable attention has been given to the mode of antimalarial action of quinacrine. It is an effective blood schizonticidal agent. It binds to duplex DNA by intercalation and strongly inhibits DNA replication. It also inhibits RNA transcription and intrudes upon protein synthesis. This latter action explains its antigiardial effects. Lysosomal accumulation may enhance its ability to enter the parasite.

Pharmacological Effects. Quinacrine has properties other than its effects against protozoan and helminthic parasites. It has been employed as an anticonvulsant. It has inhibitory effects on various enzyme systems, including cholinesterases, accounting for some of its toxicity. Quinacrine has quinidine-like effects on cardiac arrhythmias.

Pharmacokinetics. Quinacrine is rapidly absorbed after either oral ingestion or intramuscular injection. It is widely distributed in the tissues and slowly released. The principal storage sites are the liver, spleen, kidneys, and lungs. Significant quantities of the drug can be detected in the urine 2 months after a single dose. Metabolic transformations lead to urinary excretion of two phenolic products. Other excretion products have been identified.

Adverse Effects. Quinacrine's marked staining of the skin and clothing is a nuisance. Irritant effects upon the gastrointestinal tract may cause anorexia, nausea, vomiting, abdominal pain, and diarrhea. Some individuals may have headaches, dizziness, restlessness, and, rarely, convulsions. The relatively large doses used in the treatment of tapeworm infections may cause a transitory toxic psychosis. Caution should be exercised in administering quinacrine to patients with psoriasis because the drug may cause an exacerbation and exfoliation. Because quinacrine can potentiate the hemolytic effects of primaquine, two drugs should not be administered together. Quinacrine crosses the placenta and therefore should not be given to pregnant women if other less toxic agents are available.

Preparations. *Quinacrine* is available as the dihydrochloride in 100-mg tablets. In treating giardiasis, 100 mg three times daily for 5-7 days usually gives excellent results. The pediatric dose is 7 mg/kg divided into three daily doses given over the same time frame. Although niclosamide has generally replaced quinacrine in the treatment of tapeworm infections, some practitioners still use quinacrine, particularly to treat pork tapeworm infections. The dosage and method of administration are covered in Chapter 26.6.

CHEMOTHERAPY OF AMEBIASIS

E. histolytica may remain as a commensal in the lumen of the bowel or it may invade the tissues leading to dysentery, and hepatic and other abscesses (Fig. 26.1-1). In the former situation, the patient is asymptomatic and passes cysts in the stool. With invasive disease, the patient usually has symptoms, and in the case of dysentery, erythrophagous trophozoites are present in the stool. Amebic abscess of the liver usually causes fever, hepatomegaly, right upper-quadrant abdominal pain, anorexia, and weight loss. Treatment of the two situations, cyst passers and invasive disease, differs.

Amebic dysentery has sometimes been confused with ulcerative colitis. Corticosteroids can be hazardous in this situation, and also when they are inadvertently used in patients with amebic abscess of the liver (9, 26).

TREATMENT OF THE ASYMPTOMATIC CARRIER

The asymptomatic cyst passer is not only at risk of developing invasive disease but is also a potential source of infection to others, particularly if he is a food handler. Asymptomatic carriers should usually be treated, except in some populations with poor sanitation and very high prevalence of cyst passers, where the patient will probably be reinfected. Either of two drugs is recommended for clearing cysts: diloxanide furoate (31) or iodoquinol (15) (Table 26.1-1). Therapeutic efficacy for both drugs is in the 75-85% range. The pediatric dose of diloxanide furoate is 20 mg/kg/day in three divided doses for 10 days and of iodoquinol is 30-40 mg/kg/day in three divided doses for 20 days. Neither metronidazole nor tinidazole alone is recommended for treating mild or asymptomatic intestinal amebiasis because of cost, side effects, and reduced efficacy in eliminating cysts (15, 25).

TREATMENT OF INTESTINAL AMEBIASIS

Invasive intestinal amebiasis may vary from a mild illness to severe amebic dysentery. Metronidazole or tinidazole have replaced the drugs formerly used (2, 3, 11, 15, 20) (Table 26.1-1). A luminal amebicide is also needed. The 5-nitroimidazole drugs usually eliminate trophozoites, not only in the intestine but also in extraintestinal foci. The pediatric dose of metronidazole is 35-50 mg/kg/day in three divided doses for 10 days.

Tinidazole may be slightly superior to metronidazole. In studies mostly performed on the Indian subcontinent, it had no more toxicity and better cure rates (1, 3, 7, 24, 30) in intestinal amebiasis when given as a single dose of 2 g on three consecutive days (1, 3). At a single daily dose of 60 mg/kg of body weight for 3 consecutive days, tinidazole cured 24 of 25 children with acute amebic dysentery (24).

Unlike tetracycline and erythromycin, which act by interfering with the enteric bacterial flora necessary for amebic proliferation, an aminoglycoside antibiotic, paromomycin, has a direct effect upon the ameba. The adult and pediatric dose is 25-30 mg/kg/day in divided doses at mealtimes for 5 days (Table 26.1-1). A luminal amebicide is also recommended, and the drug has no effect against extraintestinal forms of the parasite (Fig. 26.1-1). Tetracycline, 250 mg four times per day for 10-15 days, in combination with a luminal amebicide, can be used as an alternate regimen. Because this combination has no activity against extraintestinal infection, chloroquine, in a regimen of 150 mg of base twice daily for 20 days, should be added. This three-drug regimen has approximately the same efficacy as a nitroimidazole and luminal amebicide.

Dehydroemetine may be used for rapid relief of symptoms in patients with severe amebic dysentery. The drug is injected daily for no more than 4 or 5 days, and as a rule a nitroimidazole can be substituted in 3 or 4 days.

TREATMENT OF EXTRAINTESTINAL AMEBIASIS

Metronidazole (2, 8, 11, 20-22) and tinidazole (1) have replaced the older drugs in the treatment of extraintestinal amebiasis (Table 26.1-1). The latter drug is more effective than metronidazole at a single daily dose of 2 g given on 2 or 3 consecutive days because of higher blood levels (3). Metronidazole is recommended at doses of 750 mg three times daily for 5-10 days (adults) and 35-50

Table 26.1-1
Chemotherapy of Intestinal and Genital Protozoa

Disease	Recommended Drug	Adult Dose[a]	Alternate Drug	Adult Dose[a]
Amebiasis				
asymptomatic cyst passer	diloxanide furoate[b]	500 mg t.i.d. x 10 days	iodoquinol	650 mg t.i.d. x 20 days
intestinal amebiasis	metronidazole[c]	750 mg t.i.d. x 5-10 days	paromomycin	25-30 mg/kg/day t.i.d. x 5-10 days
	and		and	
	diloxanide furoate[b]	500 mg t.i.d. x 10 days	diloxanide furoate	500 mg t.i.d. x 10 days
	or		or	
	iodoquinol	650 mg t.i.d. x 20 days	iodoquinol	650 mg t.i.d. x 20 days
hepatic abscess	metronidazole[c]	750 mg t.i.d. x 5-10 days	dehydroemetine	1-1.5 mg/kg/day (max 90 mg) x 5 days
	and		and	
	diloxanide fuorate[b]	500 mg t.i.d. x 10 days	diloxanide furoate	500 mg t.i.d. x 10 days
	or		or	
	iodoquinol	650 mg t.i.d. x 20 days	iodoquinol	650 mg t.i.d. x 20 days
Giardiasis	metronidazole[c]	2 g q.d. x 3 days	quinacrine	100 mg t.i.d. x 5 days
Trichomoniasis	tinidazole	2 g once	metronidazole	2 g once

[a] All drugs are given p.o. except for dehydroemetine (given i.m.)
[b] For availability of these (from CDC) and other drugs in the United States, see Table 26-1.
[c] Tinidazole can be substituted at dose of 2 g once daily for 3 days.

mg/kg/day three times daily for 5-10 days (children). Because metronidazole does not always eradicate the intestinal phase, a luminal amebicide such as diloxanide furoate or iodoquinol should also be given to prevent recurrence.

Therapeutic failures have been reported with metronidazole treatment of hepatic abscess. In this situation, a nitroimidazole may be used for a second course, or dehydroemetine or emetine may be substituted (Table 26.1-1). Because of potential cardiac toxicity, patients receiving emetine or dehydroemetine should have electrocardiographic monitoring and should remain sedentary during therapy. Dehydroemetine is favored over emetine as it appears to have a better chemotherapeutic margin. The dosage of emetine is 1 mg/kg/day (maximum dose 60 mg/day) for 5 days. The pediatric dose is 0.5 mg/kg given twice daily. The dose of dehydroemetine is greater, 1-1.5 mg/kg/day (maximum dose 90 mg/day) for 5 days.

When suspecting amebic abscess of the liver, needle aspiration may be indicated for diagnostic purposes. Repeat aspirations may relieve pain, reduce risk of extension or rupture, and/or shorten resolution time in large hepatic abscesses (20). There is considerable controversy concerning the indications for and complications of needle aspiration of hepatic abscesses. A South African group with extensive experience in the treatment of amebic abscess of the liver gave specific criteria and outlined the advantages of needle aspiration. The reluctance to aspirate large abscesses may partially explain a reported reduced cure rate with metronidazole (20).

Treatment of nonhepatic extraintestinal amebiasis should follow the same principles as for hepatic abscess (8). Patients with ruptured abscesses and peritonitis, pulmonary infections, and pericardial involvement have poorer prognoses. With rapid diagnosis and appropriate therapy, the mortality from uncomplicated amebic abscess of the liver is approximately 1%.

CHEMOTHERAPY OF GIARDIASIS

Giardia lamblia infections are relatively common in both the tropics and nontropical areas, having a greater prevalence in places with poor sanitation. The diagnosis is suspected on clinical and epidemiological grounds and confirmed by demonstrating characteristic trophozoites or cysts in the stool or duodenal aspirates.

Quinacrine is preferred by some for treating giardiasis (4, 32) (Table 26.1-1). Metronidazole, 250 mg t.i.d. for 7-10 days, cures 65-80% (4, 13) and has equal efficacy to quinacrine when used at a higher dose (2, 11, 18) (Table 26.1-1). Tinidazole is a good alternative to metronidazole (1, 3, 12, 16, 18, 30), and other nitroimidazole derivatives (nimorazole and ornidazole) have undergone therapeutic trials outside the United States for treating giardiasis (16) as well as amebiasis (7, 21) and trichomoniasis (17). Tinidazole had an excellent cure rate in treating children with giardiasis at either a single dose of 1000-1500 mg (80-95% cures) or that dose given on 3 consecutive days (95-100% cures) (1, 3, 12, 30). The recommended dose is 50-60 mg/kg, given once only. Single-dosage therapy with metronidazole, in comparison, cures only 40-60% (3, 13). However, when the drug was given as a single dose of 2 g over three consecutive days, 91% had parasitological cures. These results compared well with a cure rate of 63% in patients treated with quinacrine, 100 mg three times daily for 10 days (33).

CHEMOTHERAPY OF TRICHOMONIASIS

Trichomonas vaginalis is a frequent cause of vaginitis. Females can be reinfected by asymptomatic males, and it is therefore recommended that both sexual partners be treated (14). A single dose of 2 g of either metronidazole (10, 11, 14, 17, 29) or tinidazole (1, 14) has been shown to be 90-95% effective, if the patient is not reinfected (2, 14). Patients should abstain from alcohol for 24 hr after administration of the drug because of its disulfiram-like effect, and pregnant women should not be given metronidazole (11).

CHEMOTHERAPY OF BALANTIDIASIS

Balantidium coli , normally a parasite of pigs, is a rare cause of diarrhea and dysentery similar to amebiasis. Tetracycline, 500 mg four times daily for 10 days, is efficacious. The pediatric dose is 10 mg/ kg four times daily (maximum dose, 2 g/ day) for 10 days. There is some controversy as to whether metronidazole is effective in human balantidiasis (5,6). At any rate, it has no apparent advantage over tetracycline. An alternate drug is iodoquinol 650 mg three times daily (pediatric dose 40 mg/ kg/ day in 3 doses, maximum 1.95 g daily) for 20 days.

CHEMOTHERAPY OF ISOSPORIASIS

Isosporiasis, caused by *Isospora belli* and *I. hominis,* is a rare cause of diarrhea and malabsorption. Long-term therapy with pyrimethamine and sulfonamides (28) or trimethoprim-sulfamethoxazole (27) with folinic acid to prevent folic acid deficiency has been successful in limited trials.

CHEMOTHERAPY OF OTHER INTESTINAL PROTOZOAN INFECTIONS

A course of tetracycline or iodoquinol, as recommended for treating amebiasis, may be tried in patients with gastrointestinal symptoms and *Dientamoeba fragilis* in their stools. A patient with intermittent episodes of abdominal cramps, diarrhea, nausea, and malaise associated with large number of *E. polecki* cysts in his stool finally responded to treatment with diloxanide furoate and metronidazole (23). Both his symptoms and stool parasites cleared, confirming that the protozoa can be pathogenic and will respond to therapy.

REFERENCES

1. Apte, V.V., and Packard, R.S. Tinidazole in the treatment of trichomoniasis, giardiasis, and amoebiasis: Report of a multicentre study. *Drugs* 15(Suppl. 1):43, 1978.
2. Baines, E.J. Metronidazole: Its past, present, and future. *J. Antimicrob. Chemother.* 4:97, 1978.
3. Bakshi, J.S., Ghiara, J.M., and Navivadekar, A.S. How does tinidazole compare with metronidazole? A summary report of Indian trials in amoebiasis and giardiasis. *Drugs* 15(Suppl. 1):33, 1978.
4. Bassily, S., Farid, Z., Mikhail, J.W. et al. The treatment of *Giardia lamblia* infection with mepacrine, metronidazole, and furazolidone. *J. Trop. Med. Hyg.* 73:15, 1970.
5. Beasley, J.W., and Walzer, P.D. Ineffectiveness of metronidazole in treatment of *Balantidium coli* infections. *Trans. R. Soc. Trop. Med. Hyg.* 66:519, 1972.
6. Botero, R.D. Effectiveness of nitroimidazine in treatment of *Balantidium coli* infections. *Trans. R. Soc. Trop. Med. Hyg.* 67:145, 1973.
7. Botero, R.D. Double-blind study with a new nitroimidazole derivative, RO-7-0207, versus metronidazole in symptomatic intestinal amebiasis. *Am. J. Trop. Med. Hyg.* 23:1000, 1974.
8. Cameron, E.W.J. The treatment of pleuropulmonary amebiasis with metronidazole. *Chest* 73:647, 1978.
9. El-Hennawy, M., and Abd-Rabbo, M. Hazards of cortisone therapy in hepatic amoebiasis. *J. Trop. Med. Hyg.* 81:71, 1978.
10. Fleury, F.J., Van Bergen, W.S., Prentice, R.L. et al. Single dose of two grams of metronidazole for *Trichomonas vaginalis* infection. *Am. J. Obstet. Gynecol.* 128:320, 1977.
11. Goldman, P. Metronidazole. *N. Engl. J. Med.* 303:1212, 1980.
12. Jokipii, A.M.M., and Jokipii, L. Comparative evaluation of two dosages of tinidazole in the treatment of giardiasis. *Am. J. Trop. Med. Hyg.* 27:758, 1978.
13. Jokipii, L., and Jokipii, A.M.M. Comparison of four dosage schedules in the treatment of giardiasis with metronidazole. *Infection* 6:92, 1978.
14. Kawamura, N. Metronidazole and tinidazole in a single large dose for treating urogenital infections with *Trichomonas vaginalis* in men. *Br. J. Vener. Dis.* 54:81, 1978.
15. Kean, B.H. The treatment of amebiasis: A recurrent agony. *JAMA* 235:501, 1976.
16. Levi, G.C., de Avila, C.A., and Neto, V.A. Efficacy of various drugs for treatment of giardiasis: A comparative study. *Am. J. Trop. Med. Hyg.* 26:564, 1977.
17. Mahony, J.D.H., Harris, J.R.W., and Farrer, C.J. Nimorazole and metronidazole in the treatment of trichomonal vaginitis. *Br. J. Clin. Pract.* 29:71, 1975.
18. Mendelson, R.M. The treatment of giardiasis. *Trans. R. Soc. Trop. Med. Hyg.* 74:438, 1980.
19. Oakley, G.P. The neurotoxicity of halogenated hydroxyquinolines. *JAMA* 225:395, 1973.
20. Powell, S.J. Therapy of amebiasis. *Bull. N.Y. Acad. Med.* 47:469, 1971.
21. Powell, S.J., and Elsdon-Dew, R. Some new nitroimidazole derivatives: Clinical trials in amebic liver abscess. *Am. J. Trop. Med. Hyg.* 21:518, 1972.
22. Powell, S.J., Stewart-Wynne, E.J., and Elsdon-Dew, R. Metronidazole combined with diloxanide furoate in amoebic liver abscess. *Ann. Trop. Med. Parasitol.* 67:367, 1973.
23. Salaki, J.S., Strickland, G.T., and Shirey, J.L. Successful treatment of symptomatic *Entamoeba polecki* infection. *Am. J. Trop. Med. Hyg.* 28:190, 1979.
24. Scragg, J.N., and Proctor, E.M. Tinidazole treatment of acute amebic dysentery in children. *Am. J. Trop. Med. Hyg.* 26:824, 1977.
25. Spillmann, R., Ayala, S.C., and DeSanchez, C.E. Double-blind test of metronidazole and tinidazole in the treatment of asymptomatic *Entamoeba histolytica* and *Entamoeba hartmanni* carriers. *Am. J. Trop. Med. Hyg.* 25:549, 1976.
26. Stuiver, P.C., and Goud, T.J.L.M. Corticosteroids and liver amoebiasis. *Br. Med. J.* 2:394, 1978.
27. Syrkis, I., Fried, M., Elian, I., Pietrushka, D., and Lengy, J. A case of severe human coccidiosis in Israel. *Isr. J. Med. Sci.* 11:373, 1975.
28. Trier, J.S., Moxery, P.C., Schimmel, E.M. et al. Chronic intestinal coccidiosis in man: Intestinal morphology and response to treatment. *Gastroenterology* 66:923, 1974.
29. Underhill, R.A., and Peck, J.E. Causes of therapeutic failure after treatment of trichomonal vaginitis with metronidazole: comparison of single-dose treatment with a standard regimen. *Br. J. Clin. Pract.* 28:134, 1974.
30. Welch, J.S., Roswell, B.J., and Freeman, C. Treatment of intestinal amoebiasis and giardiasis: Efficacy of metronidazole and tinidazole compared. *Med. J. Aust.* 1:469, 1978.

31. Wolfe, M.S. Nondysenteric intestinal amebiasis: Treatment with diloxanide furoate. *JAMA* 224:1601, 1973.
32. Wolfe, M.S. Giardiasis. *JAMA* 233:1362, 1975.
33. Wright, S.G., Tomkins, A.M., and Ridley, D.S. Giardiasis: Clinical and therapeutic aspects. *Gut* 18:343, 1977.

ADDITIONAL READING

Adams, E.B., and MacLeod, I.N. Invasive amebiasis. 1. Amebic dysentery and its complications. *Medicine* 56:315, 1977.

Adams, E.B., and MacLeod, I.N. Invasive amebiasis. 2. Amebic liver abscess and its complications. *Medicine* 56:325, 1977.

Botero, R.D. Chemotherapy of human intestinal parasitic diseases. *Ann. Rev. Pharmacol. Toxicol.* 18:1, 1978.

Drugs for parasitic infections. *Med. Lett. Drugs Ther.* 24:5, 1982.

Knight, R. The chemotherapy of amoebiasis. *J. Antimicrob. Chemother.* 6:577, 1980.

Knight, R., and Wright, S.G. Progress report. Intestinal protozoa. *Gut* 19:940, 1978.

CHAPTER
26.2

CHEMOTHERAPY OF BLOOD AND TISSUE PROTOZOA

G. Thomas Strickland and Edgar A. Steck

Protozoa commonly cause systemic infections in both tropical and temperate climates. Many of the drugs employed for treating systemic protozoan infections are not readily available in the United States and are toxic. Because blood and tissue protozoal infections are frequently fatal if not treated, some drug toxicity may need to be accepted to cure the infections.

Toxoplasma gondii infects all mammals and birds and is worldwide in distribution, occurring wherever the primary hosts, cats, are present. Transmission to humans is by several routes. The most common are by the ingestion of undercooked meat containing the cyst or trophozoite stage of the parasite or the accidental ingestion of cat feces contaminated with the highly contagious oocyst stage. Prevalence, as detected by positive serological tests, is greater in tropical countries where sanitary practices are inadequate. Nonetheless, toxoplasmosis is common in the United States and in Europe, where it has been estimated that 1% of the population between the ages of 15 and 50 are infected yearly, usually by ingesting infected undercooked meat. Rare, and potentially more serious, are transplacental infection of the fetus and infection from transfusions of blood and blood products. Congenital toxoplasmosis may be asymptomatic or only be manifested as a chorioretinitis. It may, however, cause a severe fatal illness in the newborn. Disseminated toxoplasmosis in an immunocompromised individual is also a serious life-threatening illness (21). The majority of acquired infections in older children and adults are either asymptomatic or mild self-limiting infections.

Pneumocystosis is an acute pulmonary disease characterized by fever, tachypnea, dyspnea, and cyanosis, almost always occurring in either immunocompromised individuals or in malnourished or premature infants. Infections in immunocompromised hosts occur in patients with the acquired immunodeficiency syndrome and in medical facilities where patients with malignancy, particularly lymphomas, are receiving chemotherapy. The use of corticosteroids predisposes to pneumocystosis. Lung biopsy or aspiration is usually required to make the diagnosis. Transmission is probably by the respiratory route, and activation of latent infection is believed to occur in immunocompromised patients (10, 28).

A rare protozoan infection in humans, babesiosis,has been reported with greater frequency in the United States than elsewhere. Originally described as a fatal infection in previously splenectomized individuals, *Babesia* infections have recently occurred in New England, principally on Nantucket Island, in individuals with normal splenic function. This disease, which has clinical similarities to malaria, is transmitted by the bite of infected ticks. The infection is endemic in rodents, and humans are exposed, but rarely infected, when they encroach upon the rodent habitat (19).

Primary amebic meningoencephalitis has been reported infrequently from several areas in the United States, as well as from Australia, Europe, and Africa (15). Clinically, patients have a meningitis due to infection with free-living limax amebae. The difficulty in making a rapid diagnosis has hampered the evaluation of chemotherapy (3, 6).

Human infections with *Leishmania* and trypanosomes are,in general, limited to the tropics and subtropics. However, distribution is extensive, and there are major clinical problems in many areas of the world. American physicians must constantly be alert for imported cases.

Leishmaniasis occurs in both the Eastern and Western hemispheres and has wide variations in ecological and transmission patterns, as well as clinical characteristics. The patient with Oriental sore, cutaneous leishmaniasis of the Old World, may present considerable clinical differences and show different responses to therapy than patients with either visceral leishmaniasis or New World mucocutaneous leishmaniasis. Clinical characteristics of the leishmanial infection and information regarding the geographical origin of the infection may be of some use to the physician in selecting an appropriate chemotherapeutic regimen. The drugs used for chemotherapy of the leishmaniasis are toxic and must be used with caution.

African trypanosomiasis is caused by infections with *Trypanosoma gambiense* and *T. rhodesiense* and, as its name indicates, is endemic to Africa. It presents as two different patterns of disease. A chronic, indolent infection, Gambian sleeping sickness, is more common in West and Central Africa. The more acute form, Rhodesian sleeping sickness, is more common in East and Southern Africa (25). The treatment and management of the two forms have subtle differences. The drugs used for treating African trypanosomiasis are quite toxic and great care must be taken in their use (5, 29).

American trypanosomiasis,or Chagas' disease, is a major medical problem in many parts of South and Central America. It may be present as an acute febrile illness, which is frequently not diagnosed, or as a chronic form with cardiac or gastrointestinal manifestations (8).

DRUGS USED FOR TREATING BLOOD AND TISSUE PROTOZOA

MELARSOPROL AND TRYPARSAMIDE

Melarsoprol and tryparsamide are trivalent and pentavalent arsenical compounds used to treat the central nervous system manifestations of African trypanosomiasis.

Friedheim described trypanocidal activity in an organic compound of arsenic containing a melamine nucleus in 1940. In 1949 he demonstrated that the product of reaction of dimercaprol with melarsen oxide (MEL B) or melarsoprol, had good trypanocidal efficacy and less toxicity than other arsenicals used for treating patients with central nervous system involvement. Thirty years following this observation and sixty years following the discovery that arsenical compounds had efficacy in treating African trypanosomiasis, there is no replacement for melarsoprol or tryparsamide.

Source and Chemistry. Tryparsamide, synthesized by the interaction of arsanilic acid with chloroacetamide in the presence of caustic, contains 25% pentavalent arsenic (Fig. 26.2- 1). Melarsoprol is a complex trivalent arsenical (Fig. 26.2-1) developed by Friedheim. The heterocyclic arsenical has a triazine ring attachment to melamine and is only slightly soluble in water but readily soluble in propylene glycol.

Antiprotozoal Effect. The mechanism of action of melarsoprol and tryparsamide upon trypanosomes is unknown, except that they both inactivate a great number of enzymes. Both drugs are able to penetrate the blood-brain barrier. The transport of arsenic across the blood-brain barrier appears to be facilitated by the structural features present in melarsoprol. The pentavalent arsenic of tryparsamide must be reduced to the trivalent form before it becomes active. The particular combination of arsenic and heavy metal chelator (dimercaprol) in melarsoprol provides a safer and more effective drug than tryparsamide. It is considered that this combination reduces toxicity from arsenic in the infected human yet does not reduce the level of arsenic that enters the parasite.

Pharmacokinetics. Both drugs are administered intravenously, melarsoprol giving peak blood levels within 15-20 min,

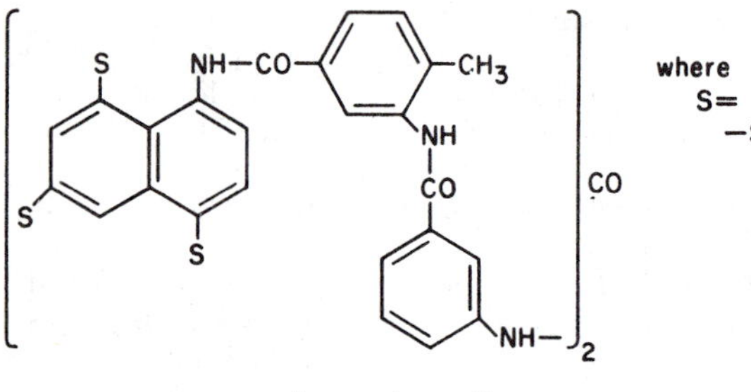

Suramin sodium

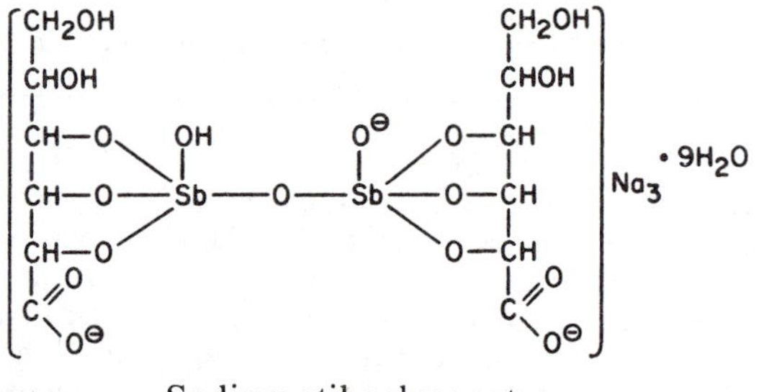

Sodium stibogluconate

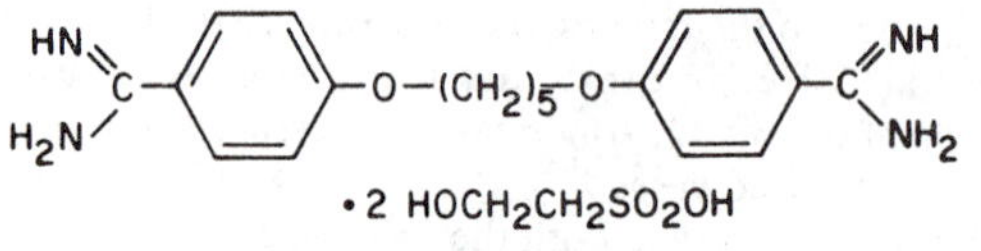

Pentamidine diisethionate

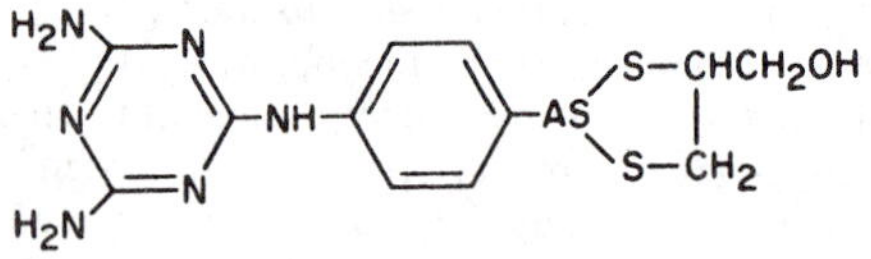

Melarsoprol

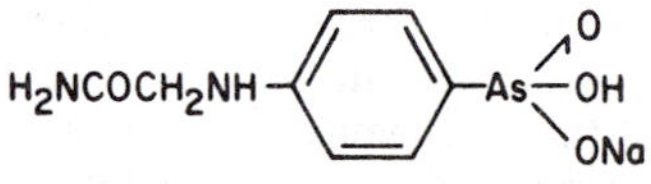

Tryparsamide

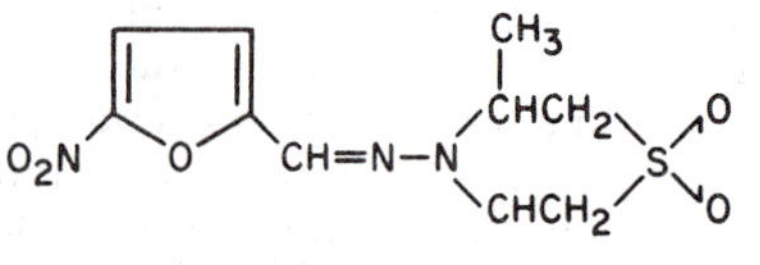

Nifurtimox

Fig. 26.2-1. *Drugs used in treating blood and tissue protozoal infections.*

falling rapidly within 2 or 3 hr. Tryparsamide has peak trypanocidal effectiveness in human blood after 24 hr disappearing within 4 days. Peak levels in the cerebrospinal fluid occur about 20 hr following injection, falling to negligible levels after 80-120 hr. Within 24 hr following the injection, 70% of tryparsamide is excreted in the urine, the majority as unchanged drug. There are no data on the tissue distribution of melarsoprol. The principal excretory route of melarsoprol is via the feces within the first 3 days following injection. About 10% of the administered drug is found in the urine.

Adverse Effects. Both tryparsamide and melarsoprol are exceeding toxic, and fatal drug reactions occur. Relatively minor reactions include nausea, vomiting, abdominal colic, skin rash, fever, albuminuria, and peripheral neuritis. More serious problems include agranulocytosis, exfoliative dermatitis, convulsions, alterations in the electrocardiogram, hypertension, cardiac arrhythmias, and shock. Reactive encephalopathy is the most common serious complication, appearing after the first 3-day course. Most of the deaths associated with arsenical therapy occur at that time. An optic neuritis that can lead to blindness has been particularly associated with tryparsamide. Dimercaprol and/or corticosteroids have been used to treat the reactive encephalopathy and optic neuritis.

Both melarsoprol and tryparsamide should be used only under the most carefully controlled hospital situations. Despite the toxicity of these drugs, the practitioner has no other choice but to use them. African trypanosomiasis with CNS involvement is always fatal if untreated.

Preparations. Melarsoprol (MEL B, ARSOBAL) is available from the Parasitic Diseases Division at the Center for Disease Control, Atlanta, Georgia for injections in the form of a 3.6% solution in aqueous propylene glycol. It is given slowly and care should be taken to avoid leakage into the surrounding tissues. Prior to administration of melarsoprol, the patient is usually treated with suramin sodium or pentamidine to reduce the blood stages of the parasite, a procedure that is believed to reduce the incidence of toxicity. Different dose schedules of melarsoprol have been used in East Africa and West Africa, all employing the drug in concentrations of 36mg/ml to a maximum dose of 200 mg. In one schedule, doses of 0.5, 1.0, and 1.5 ml are given on days 1, 3, and 5, followed by a 5 to 7 days rest. Then 2.5 ml is administered for 3 successive days, followed by another rest of 7 days. This is followed by doses of 3.0, 3.5, and 4.0 ml given on 3 consecutive days. Finally, after another 7 days rest, the patient receives 5 ml of the drug i.v. on 3 successive days. Another regimen calls for melarsoprol to be given i.v. as 1.5, 2.0, and 2.2 mg/kg at 48-hr intervals (maximum single dose 200 mg). After 7 days of rest, that is followed by doses of 2.5, 3.0, and 3.6 mg/kg at 48-hr intervals; and finally, after another 7 days respite, the patient receives three doses of 3.6 mg/kg 48-hr apart. Following these regimens, about 80-90% of patients are cured. Those relapsing may be retreated with melarsoprol but may be drug resistant. The most serious side effects generally occur after the first week of treatment.

Tryparsamide is not available in the United States; it is marketed elsewhere as a crystalline powder. Solutions should be prepared freshly by adding 10 ml of sterile distilled water to each bottle containing 2 g of the drug. It is given i.v. to patients with Gambian infections at a dose of 30 mg/kg (maximum dose is 2g) with 5 to 7 days intervals between injections, to a total of 10-12 injections. Toxicity is so common and great in children that the drugs is not recommended for treating them. Adults may be retreated after a 1-month interval if necessary.

NIFURTIMOX

Nifurtimox is a nitrofuran derivative that has been shown to have definite therapeutic efficacy in *Trypanosoma cruzi* infections. Clearance of parasitemias in both acute and chronic stages of the disease borders on 80% with use of this drug.

Source and Chemistry. Nifurtimox was developed almost 20 years ago following the observations that derivatives of 5-nitrofuran-2-aldehyde were effective in treating experimental *T. cruzi* infections (Fig. 26.2-1).

Antiprotozoal Effect. Nifurtimox has antitrypanosomal effects against both the amastigote and trypanomastigote forms of *T. cruzi.* The mechanism of action is unknown. Antileishmanial efficacy has also been reported from Brazil and Columbia.

Pharmacokinetics. Peak blood levels occur within 1-3 hr following oral administration of nifurtimox. In pharmacological studies using radioactive-labeled nifurtimox in dogs and rats, it has been demonstrated that the drug was entirely eliminated within 48 hr with 30-40% excreted in the feces and 50-60% in the urine. About 80% of the drug is absorbed after oral ingestion. Studies in pregnant rats showed that the drug crosses the placenta.

Adverse Effects. Nifurtimox has a relatively mild profile of toxic effects when it is compared with other nitrofurans. Side effects include: anorexia, nausea, vomiting, weight loss, weakness, arthralgias, peripheral neuritis, loss of memory, sleep disorders, tremor, and convulsions. Hemolytic anemia can occur in subjects with glucose-6-phosphate dehydrogenase(G-6-PD) deficiency. Depression of spermatogenesis has been noted in experimental animals. Side effects are common but usually have not required discontinuation of the drug. Children tolerate nifurtimox better than adults. Alcohol consumption increases the incidence of side effects.

Preparations. Nifurtimox is supplied as 120-mg scored tablets containing 30 mg of the active substance and is available in the United States from the CDC Parasitic Diseases Division, from whom the most current dosage schedule should be obtained. A dosage regimen frequently used requires that the tablets be taken three times daily with meals. For children up to 10 years of age, the dose is 15-20 mg/kg/day; adolescents (11-16 years of age), 12.5-15 mg/kg/day; and adults (17 years of age or older), 8-10 mg/kg/day. The duration of therapy for treating acute Chagas' disease is 90 days, and patients with chronic Chagas' disease are treated for 120 days.

PENTAMIDINE

Pentamidine has a range of antiprotozoal effects and is clinically useful in treating African trypanosomiasis, visceral leishmaniasis, pneumocystosis, and babesiosis. It was developed in the late 1930's when the diamidine group of drugs was shown to have trypanocidal activity. Pentamidine was the least toxic and most stable of these compounds.

Source and Chemistry. Pentamidine is a synthesized diamidine (Fig. 26.2-1). Of the diamidines investigated for their antitrypanosomal effects, the compounds having guanyl (amidine) functions on aromatic groupings separated by nonaromatic units were the most active. Pentamidine is an odorless white hygroscopic powder that is 10% soluble in water.

Antibiological Effect. Pentamidine is toxic to a number of different protozoa as well as to fungi. It has *in vitro* activity against *Blastomyces dermatitidis* and has been used to treat systemic blastomycosis. The mechanism of action of pentamidine is unknown. Its effects, however, may relate to its binding to the DNA of the trypanosomal kinetoplast.

Pharmacological Effects. Pentamidine and the other diamidines interact and bind strongly with DNA and polynucleotides. Pentamidine also causes diverse enzyme inhibition, such as thymidylate synthetase, which might alter cell growth patterns. Furthermore, it inhibits DNA-dependent DNA polymerase, serine proteases, and components of complement. It also causes some derangement of lipid metabolism of trypanosomes.

Pharmacokinetics. Following i.m. injection, pentamidine is excreted slowly. Blood levels of drug are low, and it remains in tissues, particularly the liver and kidneys, for months.

Adverse Effects. A multitude of toxicities have been associated with pentamidine. Immediate reactions to the drug include dizziness, breathlessness, fainting, headache, nausea, vomiting, facial flush, salivation, sweating, a rapid and thin pulse, and hypotensive shock. Pain, sterile abscess, and necrosis at the injection site are usually severe. Systemic toxicities due to pentamidine include renal function impairment, alterations in liver function, neuropathies, and blood dyscrasias. Both hypoglycemia and hyperglycemia have been associated with pentamidine therapy, and diabetes mellitus has occurred in a patient treated for visceral leishmaniasis with pentamidine.

Preparations. Pentamidine (LOMIDINE) is slowly administered parenterally as its diisethionate salt. It is available in the United States from the CDC Parasitic Diseases Division in ampules containing 200 mg of the drug. It should not be exposed to light prior to use and should be used immediately upon preparation.

For the treatment of the early stages (no cerebral involvement) of African trypanosomiasis, pentamidine is administered i.m. at a daily dose of 4 mg/kg/day for 10 days. For prophylaxis against African trypanosomiasis (which should be considered only in special situations), pentamidine has been given at a dose of 3-5 mg/kg every 3 or 4 months.

Pentamidine has been used to treat visceral leishmaniasis at a dose of 4 mg/kg/day for 10-14 days. It is particularly useful in treating patients who have been unresponsive to antimonial drugs.

Trimethoprim-sulfamethoxazole is favored for the treatment of pneumocystosis because of reduced toxicity. Pentamidine, however, at a dosage of 4 mg/kg daily for 12-14 days, is equally as effective.

In comparison with several other drugs, pentamidine was shown to be the most effective agent in treating *B. micron* infection in hamsters (16) and cured humans when used at a dose of 4 mg/kg for 14 days (7).

SODIUM STIBOGLUCONATE AND STIBOCAPTATE

Antimony compounds have been used to treat leishmaniasis since 1912 and schistosomiasis since 1918. Sodium stibogluconate (sodium antimony gluconate), a pentavalent antimony compound, is used in the treatment of visceral, cutaneous, and mucocutaneous leishmaniasis; and sodium stibocaptate (antimony sodium dimercaptosuccinate), a trivalent antimonial, is used to treat infections from all three species of schistosomes. Despite their toxicity, the antimonial compounds are still extensively used to treat both leishmaniasis and schistosomiasis. The use of antimonials to treat the later disease is due to their relatively low cost and ready availability. Another complex pentavalent antimonial, meglumine antimoniate, which has been used extensively to treat mucocutaneous leishmaniasis, contains about 30% of antimony.

Source and Chemistry. Both drugs were developed following the successful use of tartar emetic to treat leishmaniasis and schistosomiasis. Sodium stibogluconate is a colorless, amorphous powder, readily soluble in water, containing 30-34% pentavalent antimony complexed with a carbohydrate-derived acid (Fig. 26.2-1). Sodium stibocaptate is a white crystalline substance that is also soluble in water, but it is unstable and should be kept refrigerated and used within 24 hr (Fig. 26.2-1).

Antiparasitic Effect. The mechanism of action of antimonials on parasites is unknown. Trivalent antimonials readily inhibit sulfhydryl enzymes. Sodium stibogluconate's antileishmanial activity may result from action on parasite ribosomes and/or enzymes, stimulation of the host reticuloendothelial system, or alterations in host lysosomes.

Pharmacokinetics. Antimony compounds are given parenterally because of poor absorption from the gastrointestinal tract and irritation to the gastrointestinal mucosa. The trivalent and pentavalent antimonials differ in their distribution and excretion. The trivalent compounds have an increased affinity for cells. Therefore, they rapidly leave the plasma but remain circulating bound to erythrocytes. These compounds are found in high concentrations in the liver and thyroid. The majority are slowly excreted in the urine. Therefore, the patient accumulates the drug during a course of therapy, and antimony may be detected in the urine 3 months after therapy has been discontinued.

The pentavalent antimonials attain much higher plasma concentrations because they do not have as much affinity for cells as trivalent antimonials. Excretion is therefore much quicker (up to 50% of a dose excreted in the urine within 24 hr), and tissue accumulation during a course of therapy is not as great as with the trivalent antimonials. The drugs accumulate to high concentrations in the liver and spleen, partially explaining the success that sodium stibogluconate has in treating visceral leishmaniasis.

Adverse Effects. Acute and chronic toxicity is more common with the trivalent than with the pentavalent antimonials. Because the trivalent antimonials are locally toxic, sodium stibocaptate must be given intravenously, whereas sodium stibogluconate is usually given intramuscularly. Acute symptoms, more common with the administration of tartar emetic than with either stibogluconate or stibocaptate, are severe coughing, vomiting, headache, syncope, dyspnea, apnea, facial edema abdominal pain, diarrhea, vascular collapse, pruritus, and rashes. Other sequelae include pneumonia (only with use of the trivalent compounds), arthralgias, myalgias, and arthritis. Sometimes hemolytic anemia or renal damage occurs. Hepatotoxicity includes a form of hepatitis. The most serious toxicities of the antimonial compounds are cardiac abnormalities: ECG changes, cardiac arrhythmias, bradycardia, cardiac shock, and sudden death.

Preparations. Sodium stibogluconate (PENTOSTAM) is available in the United States from the CDC Parasitic Diseases Division in a sterile aqueous solution that contains 100 mg of antimony in each ml. In treating leishmaniasis, the daily dose for adults is 6 ml (600 mg of pentavalent antimony) administered either i.m. (preferred) or i.v. This is given for 6-10 days. Following rest periods of 7-10 days, the course may be repeated twice if necessary. Most patients are cured by a single course of therapy. Children under 14 years of age are treated with 4 ml doses, and infants under 1 year can be treated with daily doses of 2 ml. Cutaneous leishmaniasis has responded to infiltration of the drug solution around the edge of the lesions.

Sodium stibocaptate (ASTIBAN) is supplied in ampules containing 500 mg of the drug and is no longer available in the United States. It is administered i.m. following dilution to a 10% solution by the addition of 5 ml of water. It may be given in courses of five injections once or twice weekly to treat schistosomiasis when one of the newer agents is not available. The total dose in adults should be between 30 and 50 mg/kg, with a maximum of 2.5 g. In children, total doses of 40-60 mg/kg may be given. Because *S. mansoni* and *S. japonicum* infections are less responsive than *S. haematobium* infections, patients infected with these species generally receive the higher doses.

SURAMIN

Research in Germany during World War I, showed that the dyestuffs trypan red, trypan blue, and afridol violet were trypanocidal, led to the development of suramin sodium as a trypanocide in 1920. Suramin sodium is used in the treatment of the adult worms of *Onchocerca volvulus* and for treating the early stages of African sleeping sickness.

Source and Chemistry. Suramin sodium is a sulfonated naphthylamine derivative (Fig. 26.2-1). It is a white, cream-colored, or faintly pink crystalline powder that is readily soluble in water. All 27 isomers of the compound were synthesized and tested. The positions of the two methyl groupings on the large molecule were crucial for maximal trypanocidal activity.

Antiparasitic Effect. Suramin sodium strongly anionic, forms colloidal aggregates in solution, combines with proteins, and has enzyme-inhibitory effects. Inhibition of RNA and DNA polymerases might interfere with cell multiplication on *Onchocerca volvulus.* Because the antifilarial effects of suramin are slow, the actual mechanisms of action might include an interaction between the parasite and host.

Suramin has marked and selective effects upon the trypanosome enzyme system involving glycerol-3-phosphate dehydrogenase and NAD^+-linked glycerol-3-phosphate dehydrogenase. By accumulating in lysosomes, the drug could be localized to parasite structures.

Pharmacological Effects. Suramin sodium inhibits complement activity. However, the influence this drug has upon the host's immune response to filarial worms and to trypanosomes is unknown.

Pharmacokinetics. Following i.v. administration, suramin is firmly bound to plasma proteins, thus accounting for prolonged blood levels and retention in the body. None is detected in erythrocytes, and tissue concentrations are lower than plasma concentrations. This characteristic makes suramin useful for the prophylaxis of trypanosomiasis. The drug is not metabolically degraded to any extent, and the main excretory pathway is by the kidneys, which have higher levels of the drug than any other organ. Suramin does not penetrate into the cerebrospinal fluid to any extent.

Adverse Effects. Suramin sodium is frequently very toxic. A febrile reaction to the first one or two injections almost always occurs. Immediate reactions following injection include nausea, vomiting, abdominal pain, and hypotension that is rarely accompanied by syncope, shock, or death. During the first 24 hr following injection, other adverse effects may include pruritus, urticaria, a papular eruption, peripheral neuritis, conjunctivitis, photophobia, lacrimation, and edema. Other later complications include renal abnormalities (e.g., albuminuria and hematuria), agranulocytosis, hemolytic anemia, arthralgias, optic atrophy, and diarrhea. Albuminuria in itself is not an indication for discontinuing treatment. If the drug is administered i.m. or s.c. rather than i.v., severe local reactions and necrosis can occur.

When the drug is used to treat onchocerciasis, allergic reactions to suramin include fever, chills, myalgia, pruritus, and urticaria, which are usually associated with the death of the parasites. Therefore, it is best to treat with diethylcarbamazine first, to clear the microfilariae, and to withhold suramin therapy from the debilitated, pregnant women, and young children. Signs of nephrotoxicity must be carefully monitored and, if they do occur, the drug should be discontinued.

Preparations. Suramin sodium (GERMANIN) is available in the United States from the CDC Parasitic Diseases Division in ampules that can be made up with distilled water to a 10% solution (1.0 g drug in 10 ml). The drug must be freshly used since it is unstable.

Following a test dose of 200 mg, adult patients with African trypanosomiasis are treated with 20 mg/kg body weight (maximum 1 g) of the drug given slowly i.v. on days 1, 3, 7, 14, and 21. If necessary, the weekly doses may be extended for 5 weeks. Repeat courses should not be given prior to 3 months after the first course. Patients with central nervous system abnormalities (e.g., an abnormal cerebrospinal fluid) must also be treated with melarsoprol, as suramin does not cross the blood-brain barrier. Suramin is seldom recommended for prophylaxis of African trypanosomiasis because of the low intensity of infectivity. A single 1 g dose is believed to give protection for 3 months.

Suramin sodium is used to kill adult worms in patients with onchocerciasis. It is best to treat microfilariae with diethylcarbamazine first. If the reaction following a test dose of 200 mg is not too severe, the patient may be treated with weekly i.v. doses of 1 g of suramin for 4-6 weeks. The pediatric dosage for treating onchocerciasis is weekly i.v. injections of 20 mg/kg of suramin sodium for 4-6 weeks after a 20-mg test dose.

CHEMOTHERAPY OF TOXOPLASMOSIS

In acute toxoplasmosis, the proliferative forms, trophozoites, are rapidly multiplying. This developmental stage of the parasite is inhibited by pyrimethamine and a sulfonamide (21, 27) (Table 26.2-1). However, there may be little response to these drugs in chronic toxoplasmosis. To prevent hematological toxicity from pyrimethamine, it is recommended that folinic acid (leucovorin) be given concomitantly. In treating ocular toxoplasmosis, corticosteroids should also be employed at a

Table 26.2-1
Chemotherapy of Blood and Tissue Protozoa

Disease	Recommended Drug	Adult Dose	Route	Alternate Drug	Adult Dose	Route
Toxoplasmosis	Pyrimethamine + sulfadiazine + folinic acid	25 mg q.d. 1 g q.i.d. 5-10 mg q.d. } for 1-3 months	p.o. p.o. i.m.	see text		
Pneumocystosis	Trimethoprim-sulfamethoxazole	20 mg/kg/day 100 mg/kg/day } q.i.d. x 14 days	p.o.	Pentamidine[a]	4 mg/kg/day x 14 days	i.m.
Visceral leishmaniasis Asian cutaneous leishmaniasis American cutaneous leishmaniasis	Sodium stibogluconate[a]	10 mg/kg/day x 6-10 days (maximum dose 600 mg); may repeat after 10 days interval if necessary	i.m.	Pentamidine[a] Topical therapy Cycloguanil pamoate	2-4 mg/kg/day for up to 15 days 5 mg/kg once (maximum 350 mg base)	i.m. i.m.
American trypanosomiasis	Nifurtimox[a]	8-15 mg/kg/day given t.i.d. for 3-4 months	p.o.	None		
African trypanosomiasis, hematological stage (normal CSF)	Suramin sodium[a]	200 mg (test done), then 1 g/day on days 1, 3, 7, 14 and 21; may repeat after 1 week	i.v.	Pentamidine[a]	4 mg/kg/day for 10 days	i.m.
African trypanosomiasis, neurological stage (abnormal CSF)	Melarsoprol[a]	Three daily doses of 0.5, 1, and 1.5 ml; next week, three daily doses of 2, 2.5, and 3 ml; third week, 3.5- 5 ml daily for 3 days; continue until cured or 40 ml total dose given	i.v.	Tryparsamide	One injection of 30 mg/kg every 5 days to total of 12 injections; may be repeated after 1 month	i.v.

[a] For availability of these (the Center for Disease Control) and other drugs in the United States, see Table 26-1.

dose similar to that recommended for treating toxocariasis (Table 26.2-1) to reduce the inflammatory reaction on the eyes (18, 22). It is reported that trimethoprim-sulfamethoxazole is also effective in treating acute toxoplasmosis (17). However, the value of trimethoprim is questioned, due to negative results in animal models (24, 27). Other antibiotics used for treating toxoplasmosis, particularly during pregnancy, are clindamycin (26, 27) and spiramycin (27). Prolonged courses are required to prevent relapses.

It is difficult to evaluate the efficacy of therapy for *Toxoplasma gondii* infections; relapses have been reported. Furthermore, pyrimethamine has been shown to be teratogenic in animals. However, congenital toxoplasmosis can be devastating to the fetus, and treatment should not be withheld from a pregnant woman with acute infection. Because treatment theoretically should reduce the number of tissue cysts in the body, chemotherapy should be considered for all patients with acute toxoplasmosis.

CHEMOTHERAPY OF PNEUMOCYSTOSIS

Early diagnosis and prompt institution of chemotherapy are necessary in *Pneumocystis carinii* infections. With early treatment and no serious complications from underlying disease, 75% of patients can be cured with either pentamidine (9, 10, 28) or trimethoprim-sulfamethoxazole (9, 10) (Table 26-2-1). The experience with pentamidine has been greater. However, the combination drug, trimethoprim-sulfamethoxazole, is commercially available and FDA approved, can be given orally, and is less toxic (10). The dosage is considerably greater than that used for treating bacterial infections and is the same for both adults and pediatric patients.

CHEMOTHERAPY OF LEISHMANIASIS

Although morphologically the *Leishmania* species are indistinguishable, the spectrum of disease they cause is considerable. Some disease patterns in some areas are sensitive to antimony compounds, whereas elsewhere infections may be resistant to these drugs. Most drugs used for treating the leishmaniasis are potentially toxic, but since visceral leishmaniasis is fatal if untreated, it may be necessary to accept a certain amount of drug toxicity to cure the patient.

Newer, more potent therapeutic modalities are currently being tested in animal models. Kinnamon and colleagues (13) testing 274 different 8-aminoquinoline compounds in a hamster *Leishmania donovani* model found several to have activity manyfold that of their standard antimonial drug. By using liposomes containing antimonial compounds trapped in the aqueous phase, the drug was concentrated in the reticuloendothelial system of *L. donovani*-infected hamsters, increasing the activity of the two antimonials, sodium stibogluconate and meglumine antimoniate (GLUCANTIME), 700 times (1). Extensive laboratory studies are being conducted to determine if drugs incorporated in liposomes warrant clinical trials.

Treatment of Visceral Leishmaniasis. The recommended drug for treating visceral leishmaniasis is sodium stibogluconate (Table 26.2-1). Cure rates range from 70 to 95%, but repeat courses may be necessary, particularly in treating the Mediterranean and East African varieties. To reduce toxicity, it is recommended that repeat courses be separated by 10-day intervals. Another antimonial is meglumine antimoniate, which is not available in the United States. The alternate drug, pentamidine, is more toxic and is given i.m. 4 mg/kg/day for up to 15 doses (Table 26.2-1). The pediatric dosage is the same as the adult for both drugs. On some occasions, mucocutaneous or visceral leishmaniasis has responded to treatment with amphotericin B when it was unresponsive to treatment with either sodium stibogluconate or pentamidine.

Treatment of Cutaneous Leishmaniasis. Cutaneous leishmaniasis of the Eastern Hemisphere is often a self-limiting infection, and chemotherapy may not be indicated. Topical therapy of a few or single lesions has given good results. Sodium stibogluconate may be the best drug to initially treat cutaneous leishmaniasis. In a recent uncontrolled trial, only two relapses and no treatment failures were reported in 70 subjects treated for American cutaneous leishmaniasis with amphotericin B (23). This toxic drug is useful for treating patients with mucocutaneous lesions who fail to respond or relapse following therapy with sodium stibogluconate or cycloguanil pamoate in oil (4). The latter has been used for treating American cutaneous leishmaniasis (*L. mexicana* infections) (12).

Ethiopian diffuse cutaneous leishmaniasis has generally been unresponsive to any therapy. Treatment must be individualized, and several of the drugs may need to be tried in separate courses before an effective one may be found (2). Responsiveness of mucocutaneous leishmaniasis to therapy varies widely and is dependent upon numerous factors, including the strain of parasite, the immune status of the host, the duration of infection, and the extent and nature of prior therapy.

CHEMOTHERAPY OF TRYPANOSOMIASIS

The treatment of either African or American trypanosomiasis is currently inadequate. Drugs used for treating these infections are potentially very toxic, and efficacy is variable.

Treatment of American Trypanosomiasis. Nifurtimox (LAMPIT) is effective against both the extracellular and the intracellular amastigote stages of *T. cruzi.* The dosage schedule is complicated and lengthy (Table 26.2-1). Parasitological cures can be obtained in 90% of acute cases, but most diagnoses are made during the chronic stages after irreversible secondary changes have occurred. Cures should be supported by xenodiagnosis in which uninfected reduviid bugs (the vectors) feed on the patient and then are later examined for the presence *T. cruzi.* There is no good alternate drug for nifurtimox, although a 2-nitroimidazole, benzimidazole (RADANIL) is undergoing clinical trials (8, 14).

Treatment of African Trypanosomiasis. Pentamidine and suramin sodium (best for *T. gambiense* infections prior to evidence of central nervous system involvement), toxic drugs used for treating earlier stages of African trypanosomiasis, are not effective against the neurological stage of the disease (Table 26.2-1). The pediatric dose of pentamidine is the same as the adult dose, but it is recommended that children be treated with 20 mg/kg of suramin sodium on days 1, 4, 7, 14, and 21 following a 2 mg/kg test dose. Patients with neurological symptoms or an abnormal cerebrospinal fluid finding should receive melarsoprol, a more toxic drug (25, 29). If the patient with *T. rhodesiense* should be presumed and melarsoprol should be given, despite the absence of CNS symptoms and a normal CSF.

A brief initial course of suramin sodium may reduce some toxic manifestations. Therapeutic failures are infrequent, with 95% cure rates; more than one course of therapy may be required, however. Toxicity to the drug is especially common and severe in patients with poor nutritional status. All patients must be hospitalized during the course of treatment. Most deaths occur in patients who are in the terminal stages of the disease at the initiation of therapy, by a reactive encephalopathy, which usually occurs at the end of the first 3-day course of therapy (5).

An alternate drug for treating the neurological stage is tryparsamide (Table 26.2-1). Diminazene aceturate (BERENIL), which is used in treating cattle babesiosis, has shown promise in the treatment of early African trypanosomiasis (29). Neither drug, however, is available in the United States. In very limited trials, nifurtimox was effective in treating patients with abnormal cerebrospinal fluid examinations (11). It was given in a prolonged course, such as is used for treating American trypanosomiasis, after a single 1.5 g dose of suramin.

CHEMOTHERAPY OF BABESIOSIS

Treatment of babesiosis with relatively prolonged courses of chloroquine may give symptomatic improvement but does not clear parasitemia. Exchange transfusion has been used to reduce parasitemia. Pentamidine is effective in treating *Babesia* infections in experimental animals (16), as well as a few patients, at a dose of 4 mg/kg once daily for 14 days (7). Another aromatic diamidine, diminazene aceturate, rapidly cured a Nantucket man following failure to respond to chloroquine (20). Complications, however, were striking; albuminuria, abnormal ECG changes, and a delirious amnestic state associated with a Landry-Guillain-Barre syndrome. More recently, the combination of clindamycin and quinine has been found to be efficacious in treating babesiosis

CHEMOTHERAPY OF PRIMARY AMEBIC MENINGOENCEPHALITIS

Usually, primary amebic meningoencephalitis is diagnosed at postmortem examinations (3, 6). It presents as two distinct clinical syndromes. The first is an acute, fulminant, rapidly fatal illness usually affecting children and young adults exposed to water containing free-living amebae of the genus Naegleria. The organism is believed to gain access to the brain via the olfactory nerve. The second syndrome is caused by amebae of the genus *Acanthamoeba.* It has more insidious neurological changes, is not associated with freshwater exposure, and usually occurs in debilitated or immunosuppressed patients. Patients have had prolonged survival (15) and have survived following treatment with intravenous and intrathecal amphotericin B, sometimes in combination with miconazole and rifampin. Tetracycline also potentiates the effects of amphotericin B. The CDC's Parasitic Diseases Division should be contacted regarding the appropriate drugs and dosage to be used.

REFERENCES

1. Alving, C.R., Steck, E.A., Chapman, W.L. et al. Therapy of leishmaniasis: Superior efficacies of liposome-encapsulated drugs. *Proc. Natl. Acad. Sci. USA* 75:2959, 1978.
2. Bryceson, A.D.M. Diffuse cutaneous leishmaniasis in Ethiopia. 2. Treatment. *Trans. R. Soc. Trop. Med. Hyg.* 64:369, 1970.
3. Carter, R. F. Primary amoebic meningoencephalitis: An appraisal of present knowledge. *Trans. R. Soc. Trop. Med. Hyg.* 66:193, 1972.
4. Crofts, M.A.J. Use of amphotericin B in mucocutaneous leishmaniasis. *J. Trop. Med. Hyg.* 79:111, 1976.

5. Dugan, A.J. The treatment of African trypanosomiasis. *Trop. Doct.* 3:162, 1973.
6. Duma, R.J. Primary amoebic meningoencephalitis. *CRC Crit. Rev. Clin. Lab. Sci.* 3:163, 1972.
7. Francioli, P.B., Keithly, J.S., Jones, T.C. et al. Respone of babesiosis to pentamidine therapy. *Ann. Intern. Med.* 94:326, 1981.
8. Gutteridge, W.E. Chemotherapy of Chagas' disease. *Trans. R. Soc. Trop. Med. Hyg.* 70:123,1976.
9. Hughes, W.T. Pneumocystic pneumonia: A plague of the immuno-suppressed. *Johns Hopkins Med. J.* 143:184, 1978.
10. Hughes, W.T., Feldman, S. Chaudhary, S.C. et al. Comparison of pentamidine isethionate and trimethoprim-sulfamethoxazole in the treatment of *Pneumocystis carinii* pneumonia. *J. Pediatr.* 92:285, 1978.
11. Janssens, P.G., and DeMuynck, A. Clinical trials with "nifurtimox" in African trypanosomiasis. *Ann. Soc. Belg. Med. Trop.* 54:475, 1977.
12. Johnson, C.M. Cycloguanil pamoate in the treatment of cutaneous leishmaniasis: Initial trials in Panama. *Am. J. Trop. Med. Hyg.* 17:819, 1968.
13. Kinnamon, K.E., Steck, E.A., Loizeaux, P.S. et al. The anti-leishmanial activity of lepidines. *Am. J. Trop. Med. Hyg.* 27:751, 1978.
14. Lampit (nifurtimox) *Arzneim-Forsch.* 22:1563, 1972.
15. Lawande, R.V., Dugan, M.B., Constantinidou, M., and Tubbs, D.B. Primary amoebic meningoencephalitis in Nigeria (report of two cases in children). *J. Trop. Med. Hyg.* 82:84, 1979.
16. Miller, L.H., Neva, F.A., and Gill, F. Failure of chloroquine in human babesiosis *(Babesia microti):* Case report and chemotherapeutic trials in hamsters. *Ann. Intern. Med.* 88:200, 1978.
17. Norrby, R., Eilard, T., Svedham, A. et al. Treatment of toxoplasmosis with trimethoprim-sulphamethoxazole. *Scand. J. Infect. Dis.* 7:72, 1975.
18. O'Connor, G.R., and Frenkel, J.K. Dangers of steroid treatment in toxoplasmosis. *Arch. Ophthalmol.* 94:213, 1976.
19. Ruebush, T.K., Cassaday, P.B., March, H.J. et al. Human babesiosis on Nantucket Island: Clinical features. *Ann. Intern. Med.* 86:6, 1977.
20. Ruebush, R.K., Rubin, R.H., Wolpow, E.R. et al. Neurologic complications following the treatment of humans *Babesia microti* infection with diminazene aceturate. *Am. J. Trop. Med. Hyg.* 28:184, 1979.
21. Ruskin, J., and Remington, J.S. Toxoplasmosis in the compromised host. *Ann. Intern. Med.* 84:194, 1976.
22. Saari, M., Vuorre, I., Neiminen, H., and Raisanen, S. Acquired toxoplasmosis chorioretinitis. *Arch. Ophthalmol.* 94:1485, 1976.
23. Sampaio, S.A.P., Castro, R.M., Dillion, N.L. et al. Treatment of mucocutaneous (American) leishmaniasis with amphotericin B: Report of 70 cases. *Int. J. Dermatol.* 10:179, 1971.
24. Seah, S.K.K. Chemotherapy in experimental toxoplasmosis: Comparison of the efficacy of trimethoprim-sulfa and pyrimethamine-sulfa combinations. *J. Trop. Med. Hyg.* 78:150, 1975.
25. Spencer, H.C., Gibson, J.J., Brodsky, R.E. et al. Imported African trypanosomiasis in the United States. *Ann. Intern. Med.* 82:633, 1975.
26. Tate, G.W., and Martin, R.G. Clindamycin in treatment of human ocular toxoplasmosis. *Can. J. Ophthalmol.* 12:188, 1977.
27. Thiermann, E., Apt. W., Atias, A. et al. A comparative study of some combined treatment regimens in acute toxoplasmosis in mice. *Am. J. Trop. Med. Hyg.* 27:747, 1978.
28. Walzer, P.D., Perl, D.P., Krogstad, D.J. et al. *Pneumocystis carinii* pneumonia in the United States. *Ann. Intern. Med.* 80:83, 1974.
29. Williamson, J. Chemotherapy of African trypanosomiasis. *Trop. Dis. Bull.* 73:531, 1976.

ADDITIONAL READING

Apted, F.I. Present status of chemotherapy and chemoprophylaxis of human trypanosomiasis in the Eastern Hemisphere. *Pharmacol. Therapeutics* 11:391, 1980.

Drugs for parasitic infections. *Med. Lett. Drugs Ther.* 24:5, 1982.

Steck, E.A. *The Chemotherapy of Protozoan Diseases.* Vols. 3, 4. Washington, D.C.: Walter Reed Army Institute of Research, 1972.

Van den Bossche, H. Chemotherapy of parasitic infections. *Nature* 273:626, 1978.

CHAPTER
26.3

CHEMOTHERAPY AND CHEMOPROPHYLAXIS OF MALARIA

G. Thomas Strickland and Edgar A. Steck

MALARIAL INFECTION AND ITS TYPES

Malaria, the most widespread and lethal parasitic disease, is caused by protozoa of the genus *Plasmodium* and is transmitted by the bite of the infected female *Anopheles* mosquito. Its acute attack is characterized by febrile paroxysms proceeded by shivering and followed by sweating occurring usually at regular intervals. Humans are infected by four species of plasmodium:

1. *P. falciparum*: causing *malignant tertian malaria* (clinical attacks are severe and, if untreated, may be fatal; if treated with appropriate drugs, relapses do not occur).
2. *P. vivax* : causing *benign tertian malaria* (clinical attacks are usually milder than the malignant variety, and characterized by relapse).
3. *P. malariae* : causing *quartan malaria* (parasitemias are usually low and clinical symptoms are less than for vivax infection).
4. *P. ovale* : causing infections most commonly in West Africa.

LIFE CYCLE OF MALARIAL PARASITE

Humans are infected by sporozoites injected at the time of bite (Fig. 26.3-1). The sporozoites rapidly invade parenchymatous cells of the liver. During the following 1-2 weeks, intrahepatic schizont grows, forming thousands of merozoites. At the end of this preerythrocytic stage, as it is called, the tissue cells rupture liberating the merozoites into the bloodstream. The merozoites enter the red blood cells and start the erythrocytic stage of the asexual phase; young parasites in the erythrocytes, known as trophozoites, grow, segment, and form mature schizonts containing merozoites. Infected erythrocytes containing mature schizonts rupture, pouring merozoites into the bloodstream, along with cell debris and foreign proteins, and producing a clinical attack of malaria. Some merozoites enter new erythrocytes and repeat again and again the asexual phase of the life cycle, whereas others, after entering the red cells, develop into male and female cells (gametocytes). Another female *Anopheles* mosquito is infected during a blood meal containing both male and female gametocytes. Fertilization occurs in the gut of the mosquito with the formation of a zygote and then an ookinete. Sporogony continues and, when the mature oocyst ruptures, sporozoites migrate to the mosquito's salivary gland, from which they may be injected during a subsequent blood meal (Fig. 26.3-1).

LOCI OF ACTION OF ANTIMALARIAL DRUGS AND THEIR SIGNIFICANCE

A number of antimalarial drugs of various chemical classes are available for prophylaxis and therapy of malaria (Figs. 26.3-1 and 26.3-2). These classes of drugs have different loci of action in the life cycle of the malarial parasite and as such may be useful in different phases of prophylaxis and treatment of clinical illness (Fig. 26.3-1). Such actions of antimalarial drugs may be considered under the following categories:

Clinical Cure. Drugs that act by interrupting the erythrocytic schizogony of the malarial parasite can terminate the clinical illness and are termed schizontocides. Chloroquine, amodiaquine, mefloquine, pyrimethamine, and quinine are examples.

Suppressive Therapy. Drugs such as chloroquine, chloroguanide, and pyrimethamine can suppress the erythrocytic stage of the life cycle, preventing development of mature schizonts so that clinical disease is not produced. Such suppressive therapy may cure most falciparum malaria infections. In vivax malaria, however, the exo-erythrocytic stage may persist, and clinical attack may

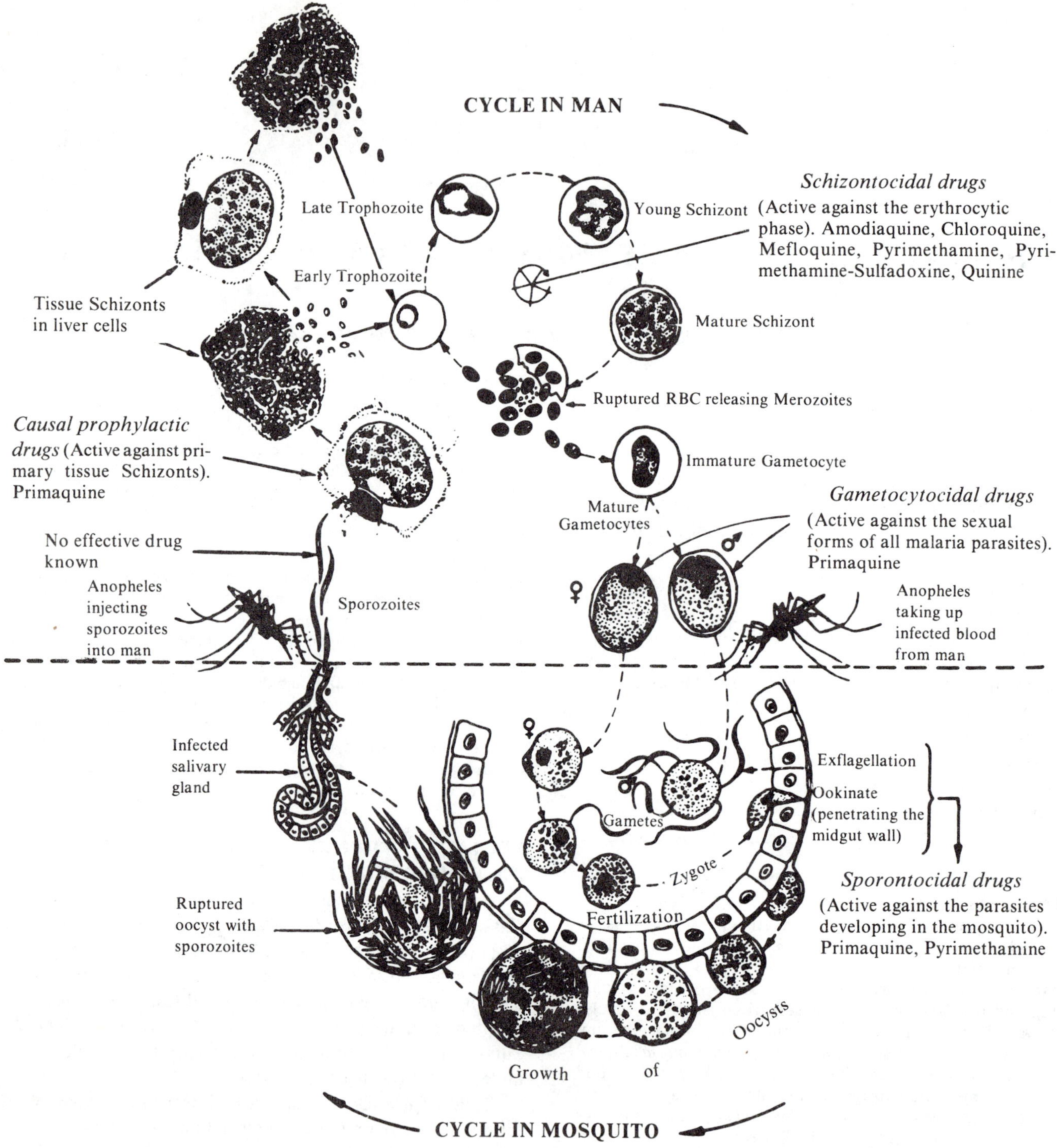

Fig. 26.3-1. *Classification of antimalarial drugs in relation to the different stages of the life cycle of the parasite.* (From Bruce-Chwatt, L.J., Bull. WHO 27:287, 1962; modified and reproduced by permission of the author and Technical Publications Division of World Health Organization).

occur after cessation of suppressive therapy. Suppressive therapy, if continued longer than the life span of the infection, can result in complete elimination of malarial parasites or suppressive cure.

Radical Cure. A drug or a drug combination can cause radical cure, if it can eradicate the erythrocytic as well as the exoerythrocytic parasites of an infection. In case of falciparum malaria, proper treatment of clinical attack or continuation of suppressive therapy as already mentioned is adequate for this purpose. For radical cure of vivax or ovale malaria, primaquine is effective in curing the exoerythrocytic stage of the parasite.

Gametocytocidal Therapy. Drugs such as primaquine can eradicate both vivax and falciparum gametocytes

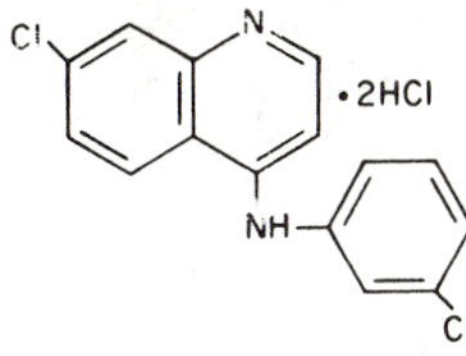

Amodiaquine dihydrochloride 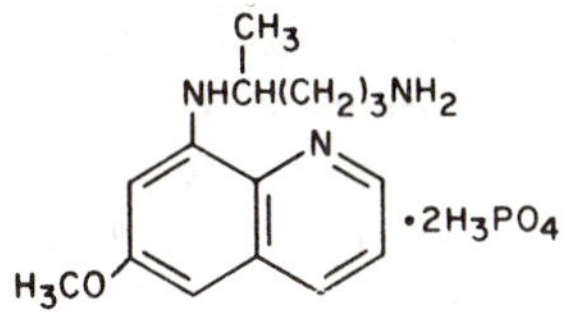 Primaquine diphosphate

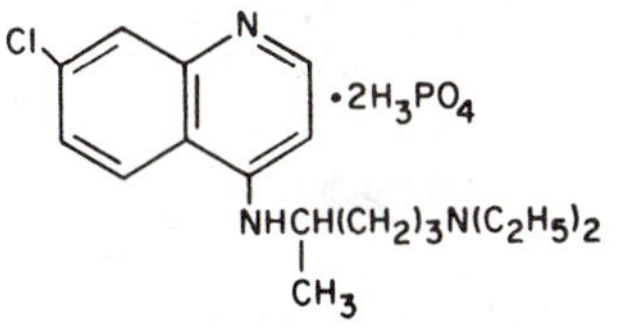

Chloroquine diphosphate 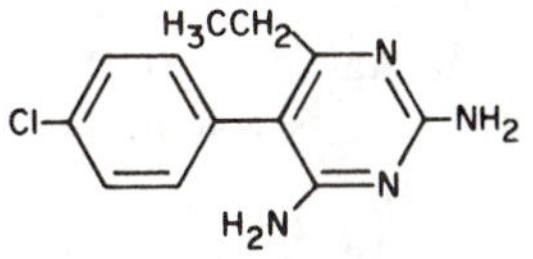 Pyrimethamine

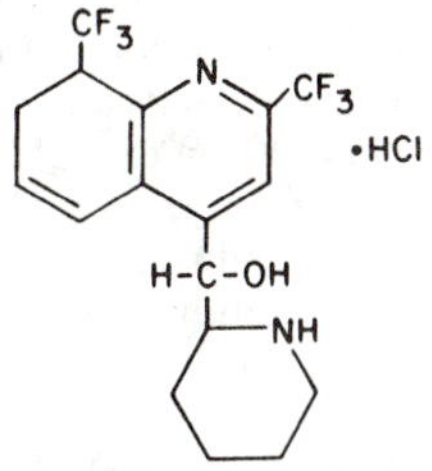

Mefloquine hydrochloride 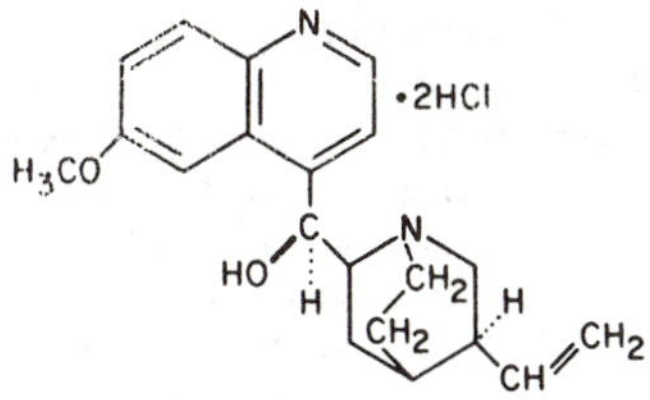 Quinine dihydrochloride

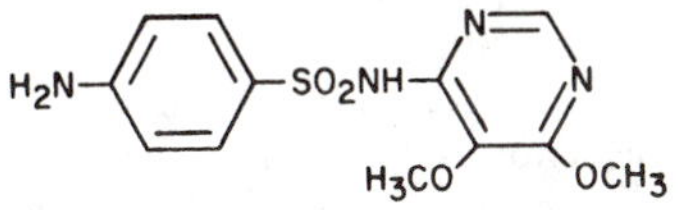

Sulfadoxine

Fig. 26.3-2. *Drugs used in treating malaria.*

within 3 days. Other antimalarial drugs are effective against vivax gametocytes, but they are ineffective against falciparum gametocytes. Gametocytocidal therapy eradicates the sexual form of the malarial parasites in human blood and eliminates the reservoir for infection of mosquitoes.

Sporontocidal Drugs. Drugs such as primaquine and pyrimethamine are active against the parasites developing in the mosquito, and thus indirectly helpful in prevention of infection in humans.

Prophylaxis. If any drug would be effective in killing sporozoites before they infect the hepatocytes, it would serve as a true causal prophylactic . Unfortunately, no such drug is clinically available. Primaquine can prevent development of malarial infection by acting on the pre-erythrocytic stage of the parasites. In practice, chloroquine and the other schizontocidal drugs are given over a prolonged period for prophylaxis.

DRUGS FOR THE PREVENTION AND TREATMENT OF MALARIA

CHLOROQUINE AND AMODIAQUINE

Chloroquine and amodiaquine are both 4-aminoquinoline derivatives with marked blood schizonticidal effects as long as the infecting strains of parasites remain susceptible (Fig. 26.3-2). They have no effect upon the exoerythrocytic forms in the liver. These drugs have been widely used in suppressive prophylaxis and treatment of malaria. Chloroquine has been subjected to greater investigation and use than amodiaquine and has also been used more frequently to treat other parasitic infections as well as other conditions. Chloroquine was first synthesized in Germany in 1934; however, it was set aside, in favor of the related 3-methyl compounds and was 'rediscovered' during the American World War II antimalarial research program. Amodiaquine was a result of detailed studies of the 4-aminoquinolines.

Source and Chemistry. Both chloroquine and amodiaquine are products of multistep syntheses. The compounds differ in the nature of the basic side chain attached to the quinoline moiety.

Chloroquine diphosphate is a white bitter powder that is stable in solution and soluble in water. Chloroquine has an asymmetric center in the basic side chain and exists in two optical isomers. The mixed isomers are used because there is no advantage in using an optically active form. The basically substituted side chain at position 4 has considerable influence upon the antimalarial potency of 4-aminoquinolines. Chloroquine is ordinarily used as the diphosphate salt 7-chloro-4-(4-diethylamino-1-methylbutylamino)-quinoline diphosphate (Fig. 26.3-2) and in France and in French-speaking African and Caribbean countries as the sulfate salt. Amodiaquine is available both as the base and the dihydrochloride, 7-chloro-4-(3-diethylamino-4-hydroxyanilino)-quinoline dihydrochloride (Fig. 26.3-2).

Antimalarial Effects. Chloroquine and amodiaquine are rapidly active against the asexual erythrocytic forms of all four human malarial species except for resistant strains of *P. falciparum*. In acute malarial attacks from susceptible strains, they rapidly control parasitemia and clinical symptoms. Most patients become afebrile within 24-48 hr and have negative malaria smears within 48-72 hr following the initiation of drug.

The 4-aminoquinoline antimalarials accumulate in parasite lysosomes and there induce breakdown of plasmodial RNA. Chloroquine combines strongly with double-stranded DNA and inhibits DNA polymerase. They alter intralysosomal pH and also cause clumping of hemozoin pigment through a decrease in digestion of hemoglobin by the parasite. Erythrocytes infected with *Plasmodia* have greater uptake of chloroquine or amodiaquine than uninfected erythrocytes. In infections with *P. falciparum* strains resistant to chloroquine, that drug is accumulated much less readily and to a lesser extent in parasitized erythrocytes. On the other hand, uptake of amodiaquine by parasitized erythrocytes remains almost the same in either chloroquine- resistant or chloroquine-sensitive *P. falciparum* strains.

Pharmacological Effects. The pharmacological profiles of chloroquine and amodiaquine are similar. Each has relaxant effects on smooth muscle and may diminish cardiac arrhythmia with minimal influence on conduction velocity. The 4-aminoquinolines prevent histamine-induced muscular contractions and block anaphylactic contractions of the tracheal muscles. Both increase the excitability of papillary muscle. Chloroquine and amodiaquine have antiinflammatory effects, partially explaining their value in treating rheumatoid arthritis and other collagen diseases. Treatment of these conditions requires much larger doses of the drug than are employed in the prophylaxis and treatment of malaria, increasing the propensity for toxicity. Chloroquine accumulates in the skin to a greater extent than amodiaquine and has caused photoallergic dermatitis. Both chloroquine and amodiaquine have some depressant effects on the bone marrow.

Pharmacokinetics. Both chloroquine and amodiaquine are rapidly and almost completely absorbed in the gastrointestinal tract. Most degradation occurs in the liver. Amodiaquine undergoes metabolic transformation more slowly than chloroquine. Effective concentrations of each drug appear readily in the plasma and tissues. About half of the drug is bound in plasma. The prolonged half-life (about 3 days following single or weekly doses) is due to prolonged high drug levels in the organs. Necropsies on suicide victims ingesting lethal amounts of chloroquine have confirmed the presence of high concentrations of the compound and its metabolites in the liver, spleen, kidneys, lung, eyes, and heart. The drug also concentrates in the brain and spinal cord, but much less so than in these other organs. The metabolism and distribution of chloroquine varies somewhat with various ethnic groups; the patterns of tissue distribution, however, are proportionately the same. Excretion of the drug is slow; half of the administered dose of chloroquine is excreted in the urine with 80% of that unmetabolized and either in free or bound form; about 10% appears in the feces. The remainder is metabolized.

The major products of the chloroquine metabolism shows removal of an ethyl grouping at the end of the side chain; other transformation products in the urine and feces are the consequence of further metabolic attack on this side chain. In common with chloroquine, amodiaquine undergoes metabolic transformations of the diethylamino moiety, one or both of the ethyl groupings are removed.

Adverse Effects. Adverse effects of chloroquine and amodiaquine are similar. At lower doses, as used for the suppression and treatment of malaria, serious adverse reactions are rare. The 4-aminoquinolines may cause minor side effects such as nausea, vomiting, diarrhea, fatigue, pruritus, skin rash and discoloration, peripheral neuropathy, vertigo, blurred vision, headache, dizziness, and confusion. Movement disorders and other transient extrapyramidal symptoms occasionally are associated with chloroquine and amodiaquine therapy. The gastrointestinal symptoms may be reduced by taking the drug after meals. Hemolysis has occurred in patients with glucose-6-phosphate dehydrogenase (G-6-PD) deficiency. More serious skin rashes (e.g., eczema, exfoliative dermatitis) and exacerbation of psoriasis rarely occur. When chloroquine is used in prolonged high doses, such as in the treatment of rheumatoid arthritis, it may cause irreversible retinopathy, characterized by a loss of central visual acuity, pigmentation of the macula, and retinal artery constriction. Retinopathy has seldom been reported following malarial suppressive doses of chloroquine as recommended in this chapter (2). Lethal doses of either drug may cause convulsions, acute circulatory failure, and respiratory and cardiac arrest. The latter has been reported following the intravenous administration of undiluted chloroquine in therapeutic doses. When parenteral administration is required, the intramuscular route is preferred. Because of high hepatic concentrations of the drug, chloroquine should be administered with caution to patients with liver disease. The same limitations hold for patients with gastrointestinal, neurological, or blood disorders. Chloroquine should not be administered during pregnancy except in the prophylaxis and treatment of malaria. For patients receiving prolonged high-dose therapy, an ophthalmological examination is recommended before and periodically during treatment.

Preparations. It is customary to express dosages of chloroquine and amodiaquine in terms of base content. Chloroquine is available in tablets containing either 250 or 500 mg of the diphosphate and for injection as the hydrochloride containing 40 mg of base per milliliter. For adults, the prophylactic antimalarial dose of chloroquine is 300 mg base (as 500 mg of diphosphate) starting 1 week prior to exposure, continuing at weekly intervals during exposure in malarious areas, and weekly for 6 weeks after return to a nonmalarious area. Children should be given 5 mg/kg chloroquine base on the same regimen for chemoprophylaxis. Treatment of chloroquine-susceptible malaria in adults should be: 600 mg chloroquine base (1000 mg diphosphate) at once, then 300 mg after 6 hr, and 300 mg daily on the next 2 days. Under similar circumstances, children should be treated with 10 mg/kg chloroquine base, followed by 5 mg/kg after 6 hr, and then 5 mg/kg daily for the next 2 days. In cases where chloroquine is not well tolerated orally, or in very severe infections, chloroquine dihydrochloride should be administered intramuscularly at a dose of 200 mg of chloroquine base. This may be repeated at intervals of 6 hr; the total dose in 24 hr should not exceed 800 mg of the base. Oral therapy should be substituted as soon as possible.

Dosage regimens of amodiaquine are similar to those described for chloroquine. For chemoprophylaxis in adults, a weekly dose of 400 mg amodiaquine base (520 mg amodiaquine dihydrochloride) is used. Children should be given amodiaquine on a weight basis, whether the dihydrochloride or base is used. Using the same weekly schedule as recommended for adults, children under 1 year, up to 150 mg base; 7-10 years, up to 200 mg base; and 11-16 years, up to 300 mg base. Treatment of susceptible malaria in adults with amodiaquine ordinarily proceeds from a loading dose of 600 mg base, followed with 400 mg at 6 hr, and again at 24 and 48 hr. In children, the respective doses are 10 mg/kg of amodiaquine base initially and 5-mg/kg doses thereafter.

The dose of chloroquine used in the past to treat *Clonorchis sinensis* infection is 300 mg of base three times daily for 6 weeks. Chloroquine has also been used in treating extraintestinal amebiasis. The availability of nitroimidazoles, however, makes chloroquine therapy for amebiasis obsolete. Chloroquine is also used to treat rheumatoid arthritis.

MEFLOQUINE

Mefloquine is a 4-quinoline-carbinolamine allied to quinine. It is an effective suppressive and curative antimalarial drug (Fig. 26.3-1) developed by the U.S. Army malarial chemotherapy program and is an advance in the management of multidrug resistant strains of falciparum malaria (11). Mefloquine is currently (1986) only available in Switzerland (where it is made) and in Thailand (where it is needed).

Source and Chemistry. Mefloquine is prepared by a complex synthetic process, and therefore is very costly. Mefloquine has structural features similar to quinine (Fig. 26.3-2). The racemic mixture of mefloquine isomers has good activity, with the erythro form showing a therapeutic advantage over the threo isomer. The drug is the purified erythro compound. Presence of the trifluoromethyl function at position 2 on the quinoline ring renders mefloquine less sensitive to metabolic inactivation and precludes phototoxic effects common among most other 2-substituted quinoline-carbinol-amines.

Antimalarial Effects. The similarity in structure of mefloquine to quinine suggests that they have similar modes of action. Mefloquine, however, does not bind significantly to DNA, whereas quinine forms an intercalation complex with DNA. The mechanism of antimalarial action therefore remains unknown.

Pharmacological Effects. Mefloquine has few effects upon the cardiovascular or pulmonary system. In animal studies, the speed of infusion influences the magnitude of effects greater than the total dose of the drug. There have been no indications of phototoxicity despite the long-term binding of mefloquine to melanin in the skin. High doses of the agent caused reduced growth and a diminished fertility index in rats and mice.

Pharmacokinetics. Mefloquine has a longer whole blood half-life than quinine, averaging 13.9 days, apparently a consequence of the functional group that bars ready metabolic degradation at position 2 of the quinoline nucleus. The drug binds extensively to plasma proteins but gives high concentrations in the lungs, gallbladder, liver, spleen, and kidneys. It undergoes extensive biliary and gastric secretion, followed by reabsorption. Most of the drug and its metabolites are accounted for in the feces of humans and experimental animals.

Adverse Effects. Preclinical toxicological studies showing that mefloquine produces minimal toxicity in animals were confirmed by tolerance trials in humans. Single oral doses of up to 1500 mg are well tolerated, but larger amounts produce transient dizziness and nausea. Long-term studies in males confirmed mefloquine to be safe for prolonged administration, with no evidence of phototoxicity. Repeated high doses of mefloquine have caused histological abnormalities in the retina of experimental animals.

Preparations. Mefloquine is formulated as tablets that contain 250 mg of the hydrochloride. Suppressive prophylaxis in areas where chloroquine-resistant strains of *P. falciparum* are prevalent was achieved by weekly administration of 250 mg of the drug, or by fortnightly doses of 500 mg. In the treatment of established cases of falciparum malaria, a single 1000-mg dose of mefloquine cured 95% (8). In treating *P. vivax* infections, primaquine is also required to achieve radical cure. The long half-life of mefloquine in the blood makes it especially suitable for chemoprophylaxis. Mefloquine is effective as a prophylactic agent against both vivax and chloroquine-resistant falciparum malaria (11). The recommended dose for malaria prophylaxis is 250 mg/ week for an adult weighing 70 kg.

PRIMAQUINE

Primaquine is an 8-aminoquinoline derivative that is a radical curative antimalarial agent. It was developed during the World War II antimalarial research in the United States, but did not receive extensive trials until the Korean war. The compound exerts causal prophylactic and gametocytocidal action against all malaria parasites (Fig. 26.3-1). Primaquine is used to prevent relapses in *P. vivax* and *P. ovale* infections. Although primaquine does have some activity against other protozoal infections, toxicity limits its use in these other conditions. Despite extensive studies, the 8-aminoquinolines remain the only class of drugs with practical utility as radical-curative and causal prophylactic agents. Pamaquine, another 8-aminoquinoline, was the first synthetic antimalarial drug marketed in 1926.

Source and Chemistry. Primaquine is a fully synthetic drug, prepared by a multistep process (Fig. 26.3-2). The basic side chain has a marked influence upon potency and toxicity in this series, with primaquine having the best chemotherapeutic index of all 8-aminoquinolines. Both d- and l-primaquine have been isolated and studied in some detail. However, no practical advantage is gained by using separated isomers, and the mixed isomers are routinely used in the form of the diphosphate, which is soluble in water and stable.

Antimalarial Effects. Primaquine has relatively few pharmacological effects other than those exerted upon malarial parasites and upon the central nervous system and blood. It is highly active against both exoerythrocytic parasites and gametocytes; it has a minimal, but erratic, action against asexual blood forms of *P. vivax*.

Despite long and successful clinical use of 8-aminoquinolines as radical-curative antimalarial, their mode of action has not been established with certainty. Included among effects reported have been interference with protein synthesis, with enzymes, and with erythrocyte phospholipid metabolism.

Pharmacological Effects. Primaquine has antiarrhythmic effects and depresses myocardial contractility. It has relatively little action on either the parasympathetic or sympathetic nervous system. Depressant effects of primaquine on the central nervous system are less marked than those of congener 8- aminoquinolines, having shorter basic side chains.

Pharmacokinetics. Difficulties in the isolation and characterization of metabolic products have left most features relating to the distribution and absorption of primaquine unsolved. Following oral administration, the drug is rapidly absorbed, with only a small proportion of the dose excreted unchanged. Peak plasma concentrations occur in 6 hr, fall rapidly, and are barely detectable after 24 hr. Metabolic attack at position 5 occurs with the 8-aminoquinolines, proceeding from the 5-hydroxy derivative to form a 5, 6-quinoline-quinone, followed by further complex degradations. Primaquine and allied compounds are degraded primarily in the liver, with transformations also in the blood.

Adverse Effects. Primaquine causes a considerable range of toxic side effects, of which the most important is intravascular hemolysis in individuals with an erythrocyte glucose-6-phosphate dehydrogenase (G-6-PD) deficiency. Therefore, it is generally recommended that a test for G-6-PD deficiency be performed in blacks and individuals of Mediterranean area and Southern Asian ancestry before administering the drug. The severity of the hemolysis is dependent upon the primaquine dose, with older erythrocytes more susceptible to hemolysis.

Therefore, lower doses of the drug often cause minimal hemolysis following an acute hemolytic episode (i.e., the remaining younger erythrocytes and reticulocytes have higher levels of G-6-PD and are more resistant to the hemolytic effects of the drug). Other untoward effects from primaquine include methemoglobinemia, hemoglobinuria, cyanosis, and, rarely, agranulocytosis, granulocytopenia, and leukopenia. The acute hemolytic anemia is usually dose related and occurs suddenly. The drug should be discontinued immediately if the patient has noticeable darkening of the urine and a drop in hemoglobin or hematocrit. Less serious toxicities include headache and gastrointestinal disturbances. Primaquine prophylaxis should be withheld until after delivery of the fetus in pregnant women, if possible.

Preparations. Primaquine diphosphate is the salt generally used. The dosage is specified in terms of the base. Tablets of diphosphate (26.3 mg of salt, equivalent to 15 mg of base) are given orally. When used for terminal suppression after leaving malarious areas, or to prevent relapses of *vivax* or *ovale* malaria due to persistent hepatic schizonts, primaquine may be administered once daily as 26.3 mg of the salt (15 mg base) for a period of 14 days, or, to diminish side effects, 79 mg (45 mg base), once weekly for 8 weeks. This is best started following or during the last 2 weeks of chloroquine suppression therapy. The foregoing dosage regimens are all for adults not having G-6-PD deficiency. In treatment of children, caution must be exercised, even in giving the recommended dosage of 0.3 mg/kg base per day for 14 days or 0.9 mg/kg base weekly for 8 weeks. Combinations of primaquine with chloroquine are not recommended.

PYRIMETHAMINE AND PYRIMETHAMINE-SULFADOXINE

Pyrimethamine and trimethoprim are 2,4-diaminopyrimidines with excellent antimicrobial activity. The former is primarily used in treating malaria and toxoplasmosis and is covered in this chapter. The latter, although used in treating pneumocystosis, is principally an antibacterial agent. Pyrimethamine's use in malaria prophylaxis and therapy has been hampered by the fact that drug resistance develops rapidly. The combination of pyrimethamine with other agents that block dihydropteroate synthetase (e.g., sulfones and sulfonamides) (Fig. 26.3-3) gives a sequential intrusion upon the plasmodial folic acid cycle, markedly decreases the liability for development of drug resistance, and potentiates the therapeutic effects. Of particular value is the combination with long-acting sulfa drugs, among which sulfadoxine has been the most satisfactory. A formulation (FANSIDAR) of pyrimethamine with sulfadoxine has become very useful in The chemoprophylaxis and treatment of chloroquine-resistant falciparum malaria and has been used in the treatment of toxoplasmosis and pneumocystosis.

Source and Chemistry. Pyrimethamine is a fully synthetic pyrimidine derivative, prepared in several steps. It is a white crystalline powder and is insoluble in water. It is a 2, 4-diaminopyrimidine which, as a consequence of investigation of nucleic acid synthesis of bacteria, was developed as an antimalarial agent (Fig. 26.3-2). It is the representative with the best antimalarial effectiveness and least toxicity of a large series of compounds.

Antimalarial Effects. Pyrimethamine is a selective inhibitor of the plasmodial enzyme, dihydrofolate reductase, and thereby interferes with nucleic acid metabolism of the parasites (Fig. 26.3-3). Dihydrofolate reductase catalyzes the reduction of dihydrofolate to tetrahydrofolate. Mammalian cells are permeable to folates, whereas bacteria and protozoa are unable to transport preformed folate. Therefore, the host cells can utilize preformed folate, whereas the protozoa, like bacteria, must synthesize their own. The biosynthesis by the parasite of purine, pyrimidine, and certain amino acids is interfered with by the drug. Pyrimethamine has a selective effect upon plasmodia, and trimethoprim is more effective against the enzymes from certain bacteria. The onset of action of the drug is delayed, and, by using alternate metabolic pathways, the parasites sometimes develop drug resistance. The combination of pyrimethamine with sulfadoxine causes a sequential blocking of essential metabolic transformation, reduces the chances for developing drug resistance, and gives a supraadditive therapeutic effect.

Pyrimethamine is active against several stages of the malaria parasite. It has effects upon the asexual blood stages (schizontocidal), possibly some against the hepatic schizonts of *P. vivax*, and some upon the sexual stages developing in the mosquito (sporontocidal) (Fig. 26.3-1).

Pharmacological Effects. Pyrimethamine has pharmacological effects and toxicity related to its inhibition of dihydrofolate reductase. Even though selective in its effects on the parasite enzyme, some inhibition of the mammalian enzyme system also occurs. Consequences sometimes include muscular weakness, convulsive seizures, emesis, diarrhea, and dehydration. These effects can be generally alleviated by the concomitant administration of folinic acid.

Pharmacokinetics. Pyrimethamine has a prolonged biological half-life of 96-hr. It is absorbed slowly and rather completely from the gastrointestinal tract. Pyrimethamine localizes in the liver, spleen, kidney, and lungs. Metabolites of the drug have not been well characterized. Both sulfadoxine and pyrimethamine are eliminated slowly in the urine and give stable and prolonged plasma levels following single doses. Pyrimethamine is excreted in the milk of nursing mothers. Sulfadoxine is a sulfonamide with a long half-life, 7-9 days.

Adverse Effects. Administration of pyrimethamine over long intervals for suppressive antimalarial effects or for the treatment of toxoplasmosis may give rise to a range of toxic effects, most ascribable to its action as a dihydrofolate reductase inhibitor. This includes bone marrow depression with leukopenia, thrombocytopenia, and megaloblastic anemia. These can be minimized by the concomitant administration of folic or folinic acid. Milder toxic effects include anorexia, nausea, vomiting, diarrhea, headache, lethargy, weakness, dizziness, and dermatitis. Neither pyrimethamine nor pyrimethamine-sulfadoxine should be given during pregnancy because of teratogenicity reported in experimental animals. Therapy of pregnant women for acute toxoplasmosis to prevent congenital toxoplasmosis in the fetus is a dilemma.

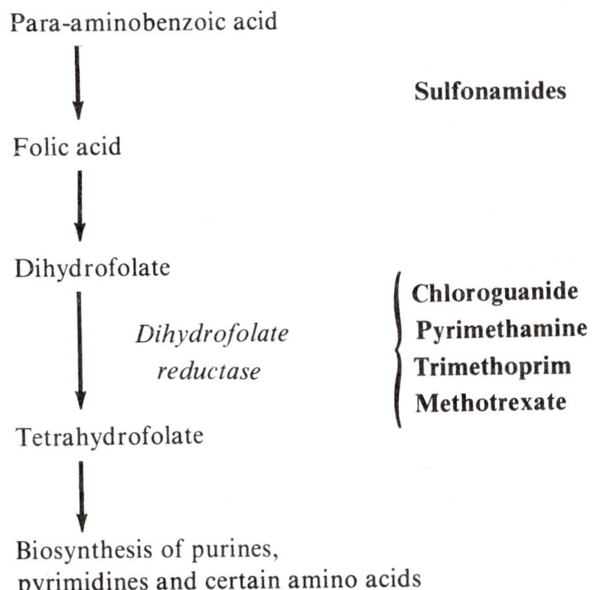

Fig. 26.3-3. *Simplified folic acid pathway to show where some of the drugs used in treating protozoa have effects.*

Some physicians only withhold treatment with pyrimethamine during the first trimester. Because it is secreted with breast milk, pyrimethamine should not be given to lactating women.

Pyrimethamine-sulfadoxine contains a long-acting sulfonamide and should not be given to patients with known allergies to the sulfonamides or pregnant women (unless essential). A reduction in the white blood cell count has been reported (11), and crystalluria occurs even in patients with normal renal function. Although rare, Stevens-Johnson syndrome, exfoliative dermatitis, and erythema multiforme have been reported in patients given this compound for malaria prophylaxis. As of this time (1986), 8 Americans have died of drug toxicity.

Preparations. Pyrimethamine (DARAPRIM) may be administered in the form of the base, which is supplied as 25-mg tablets for oral administration. Pyrimethamine is used in combination with quinine and a sulfonamide to treat chloroquine-resistant falciparum malaria (Table 26.3-1). The dosage is 25 mg twice daily for 3 days. A suitable regimen for children would be: less than 3 years, one-half tablet once daily for 3 days; from 3 to 8 years, one tablet once daily for 3 days.

A fixed combination of pyrimethamine (25 mg) with sulfadoxine (500 mg) (FANSIDAR) offers definite advantages over pyrimethamine alone in the chemoprophylaxis and treatment of chloroquine- resistant falciparum malaria. However, strains of *P. falciparum* resistant to this drug have recently been reported from Southeast Asia. When used for prophylaxis, a single FANSIDAR tablet may be given once weekly starting 1 week before exposure and continued until 6 weeks after the last exposure. Infants under 3 years old may be given one-quarter tablet and children between the ages of 3 and 8 may be given one-half tablet. However, because of recent information regarding toxic drug rashes, very careful guidelines have been set by the Centers for Disease Control (CDC), Atlanta regarding the use of this drug in malaria prophylaxis. Pyrimethamine-sulfadoxine is used to treat chloroquine-resistant falciparum malaria, with or without quinine, at a single dose of three tablets (75 mg pyrimethamine and 1500 mg sulfadoxine) (5,6,8). The pediatric dosage would be: one-half tablet for infants up to 1 year old; one tablet for children between 1 and 3; 1.5 tablets for children between the ages of 3 and 8; and two tablets for children over 8 years old.

Pyrimethamine in combination with a sulfonamide and folinic acid is used to treat toxoplasmosis (Table 26.3-1). If available, pyrimethamine-sulfadoxine can be used to treat *Toxoplasma gondii* infections. After a loading dose of three tablets, one tablet daily for 3-4 weeks is recommended. Concomitant folinic acid (leucovorin), up to 10 mg/day, should be given to prevent hematological complications. The recommended pediatric dose is: less than 3 years old, one-half tablet for 1 day, followed by one-quarter tablet daily for 4 weeks; between ages 3 and 8, one tablet for 1 day, followed by one-half tablet daily for 4 weeks; over 8 years old, the adult dosage.

Trimethoprim is superior to pyrimethamine in the treatment of pneumocystosis; FANSIDAR should not be used for this purpose if SEPTRA or BACTRIM is available.

QUININE

Quinine has been a traditional antimalarial for centuries. Its use was markedly affected by the newer synthetic drugs (e.g., quinacrine, chloroquine, pyrimethamine) that were introduced as a consequence of difficulties in obtaining quinine. The spreading prevalence of strains of falciparum malaria resistant to the synthetic antimalarials has caused renewed interest in the use of quinine.

Source and Chemistry. Quinine is a complex alkaloid that has been synthesized through multistep procedures. Because of the expense involved in synthesis, it is customarily isolated from the bark of the cinchona tree. Quinine, a natural product, is a quinoline derivative having a complex basic side chain attached to position 4 through an intermediate carbinolamine unit (Fig. 26.3-2).

Antimalarial Effects. Quinine binds strongly to both DNA and nucleic acids. Those actions have been viewed as fundamental to its antimalarial effects. Recent investigation, however, place doubt on the extent to which DNA binding may account for the antimalarial activity of quinine, as in the instance of mefloquine.

Quinine is schizontocidal (Fig. 26.3-1) and is gametocytocidal for *P. vivax* and *P. malariae* , but not for *P. falciparum*.

Pharmacological Effects. Quinine has a complex profile of pharmacological effects that include actions on the cardiovascular system qualitatively similar to those exhibited by its diastereoisomer, quinidine. It depresses the myocardium, as well as smooth muscles, and has a curare-like effect on skeletal muscle. Quinine causes vasodilatation by direct action on smooth muscle wall and may cause hypotension. It is both a local irritant and local anesthetic. It has analgesic and antipyretic effects. Other central nervous system actions are evident in toxic side effects of quinine.

Pharmacokinetics. Quinine undergoes absorption readily and is quickly transformed metabolically to at least five compounds. It is concentrated in the liver, spleen, and kidneys. Peak

Table 26.3-1
Chemotherapy of Malaria

Disease	Recommended Drug	Adult Dose	Route	Alternate Drug	Adult Dose	Route
Treatment: acute disease						
chloroquine-susceptible *falciparum, vivax, malariae,* and *ovale* malaria	chloroquine phosphate	1 g (600 mg base), then 300 mg base at 6, 24, and 48 hr	p.o. or i.m.	amodiaquine[a] dihydro-chloride	780 mg (600 mg base), then 400 mg base at 6, 24, and 48 hr	p.o. or i.m.
chloroquine-resistant *falciparum* malaria	quinine sulfate,	650 mg t.i.d. x 10-14 days	p.o./i.v.[b]	see text		
	pyrimethamine	25 mg b.i.d. x 3 days	p.o.			
	sulfadiazine, or sulfisoxazole	500 mg q.i.d. x 5 days	p.o.			
Treatment: prevention of relapse due to persistent hepatic schizonts;[c]						
vivax and *ovale* malaria	primaquine	26.3 mg (15 mg base)/day x 14 days or 79 mg (45 mg base)/week x 8 weeks	p.o.	none		
Prophylaxis: suppression of disease while in malarious area						
Geographic areas:						
Southeast Asia, Western Pacific, South America, Panama & East Africa	pyrimethamine and sulfadoxine[d]	25 mg, 500 mg } once weekly	p.o.	see text		
All other areas including West Africa	chloroquine phosphate	500 mg (300 mg base) once weekly; continue for 6 weeks, after last exposure	p.o.	amodiaquine[a] dihydro-chloride	520 mg (400 mg base) once weekly, continue for 6 weeks after last exposure	p.o.
Prophylaxis: radical cure after leaving malarious area						
Areas endemic for only *P. falciparum*	chloroquine	500 mg (300 mg base) once weekly for 6 weeks after last exposure	p.o.	amodiaquine[a] dihydro-chloride	520 mg (400 mg base) once weekly for 6 weeks after last exposure	p.o.
Areas endemic for *P. vivax, P. ovale*	chloroquine and	500 mg (300 mg base) once weekly for 6 weeks after last exposure	p.o.	amodiaquine[a] dihydro-chloride	520 mg (400 mg base) once weekly 6 weeks after last exposure	p.o.
	primaquine	15 mg base daily for 14 days or 45 mg weekly for 8 weeks	p.o.	none		

[a] Not available in the United States.
[b] Severely ill patients should be treated with intermittent slow i.v. infusions of 5-10 mg/kg (maximum dose of 600 mg) every 12 hr (see text).
[c] Primaquine is not necessary in patients with proven *P. falciparum* or *P. malariae* infections, since persistence of hepatic schizonts has not been demonstrated with these parasites.
[d] It is generally recommended that chloroquine be given in addition to pyrimethamine and sulfadoxine combination (FANSIDAR) in areas with high endemicity of *P. vivax* infections. See text regarding management of FANSIDAR-resistant strains of *P. falciparum.*

plasma concentrations occur within 2-3 hr after a single oral dose. Most is bound to plasma proteins. With continued administration, there is no accumulation in the tissues, and the metabolic degradation products are excreted in the urine, most of which have been identified as hydroxy derivatives. Acidification of the urine increases renal excretion.

Quinine readily crosses the placenta, but cerebrospinal fluid levels are 1/20 to 1/50 of those in the plasma. Recent, detailed investigation of the pharmacokinetics of quinine has improved dosage regimens. Impaired liver function associated with malaria infection results in decreased metabolic transformations of the drug. The three chief metabolites of quinine result from hydroxylation at position 2 of the quinoline ring, at position 2 of the quinuclidine moiety, and at both of those positions. The others are derived from more deep-seated oxidation (i.e., conversion of the vinyl grouping to a carboxylic acid function and complete disruption of the quinuclidine structure to give 6-methyloxyquinoline-4-carboxylic acid). Synthesis of numerous subsituted quinoline-4-carbinolamines has produced compounds with marked antimalarial potency and enhanced duration of effectiveness. Mefloquine resulted from this approach.

Adverse Effects. Quinine is bitter in taste. Cinchonism produced by high doses of the alkaloid denotes tinnitus, headache, nausea, abdominal pain, and minor visual disturbances. In severe cases, quinine may cause deafness, blindness, diverse and severe gastrointestinal disturbances, plus other problems involving the cardiovascular and nervous systems and the skin. Rashes frequently occur in patients receiving quinine, including angioedema of the face. Susceptible individuals may suffer asthma attacks, and various hematological effects, including hemolytic anemia and agranulocytosis. Under certain circumstances, very high doses of quinine may cause convulsions, delirium, coma, or death. Quinine is a local irritant. When given orally, it causes gastric pain, nausea, and vomiting. Intramuscular use is limited by severe local pain and sterile abscesses. When given intravenously, it can cause thrombophlebitis with sclerosis of veins. It can also cause damage to the renal tubules and has been associated with blackwater fever (severe hemolysis and renal failure in malaria). Quinine can cause hypoprothrombinemia, which is prevented by administration of vitamin K.

Preparations. Quinine is customarily administered orally as the hemisulfate, and intravenously as the dihydrochloride. The former is supplied as tablets containing 325 mg of the hydrated salt, or in capsules containing 130, 200, or 325 mg of the hydrated salt. In oral treatment of malaria in adults, 650 mg of the hemisulfate is given every 8 hr for 10-14 days; children are treated with 25-30 mg/kg/day, given three times daily for the same interval. In severe cases of malaria, especially falciparum infections, intravenous infusion of quinine dihydrochloride in physiological saline is given slowly. The dose for adults is 600 mg of drug in 300 ml saline infused over a 3- to 4-hr period every 12 hr (6,7). In the treatment of children with severe falciparum malaria, quinine should be administered by infusion at a level of 5-10 mg/kg of body weight during 4 hr, repeated twice daily for 2 days, or until 2 g of quinine base has been given. In those who might have chloroquine resistant infections, that course is followed by the oral administration of 1.5 g of mefloquine or the pyrimethamine-sulfadoxine combination, if these drugs are available.

Quinine is generally more toxic and less effective than the other antimalarials. Its use should be reserved for treating only those strains of falciparum malaria that might be chloroquine resistant, and it should be used in combination with other antimalarial drugs. Hall recommends an initial short course of i.v. quinine to treat patients with severe infections of chloroquine-sensitive malaria (6,7).

TREATMENT OF PATIENTS WITH SYMPTOMATIC MALARIA

The first steps in the treatment of patients with symptomatic malaria are to establish the species diagnosis, the parasite density, the immune status of the patient, and the most likely geographical location where infection occurred. The species diagnosis is best made with a Giemsa-stained thin blood smear. The parasite density and immune status are important because they correlate with severity of illness. An American tourist with a high parasitemia will usually be considerably sicker than an African student with rare trophozoites on his thick blood film. The geographical location of acquiring infection may help in establishing the parasite species (e.g., a recent visitor to India probably has a *P. vivax* infection) and helps in selecting appropriate therapy for falciparum malaria.

Treatment of *P. vivax, P. malariae,* and *P. ovale* Infections. Patients infected with *P. vivax, P. malariae,* or *P. ovale* can be treated with chloroquine, and if no complications or other contraindications are present, can be treated as outpatients. Response in the adult is rapid to 1.5 g of chloroquine base given over 2 days with relatively less for children under 12 years of age (12) (Table 26.3-1). There are several alternate drugs, of which amodiaquine has been recommended (3).

Patients with *P. vivax* and *P. ovale* infections should also be treated with primaquine to eradicate any possible remaining hepatic stages of the parasite (Table 26.3-1).

Treatment of *P. falciparum* Infections. The chemotherapy of falciparum malaria is complicated. Patients believed to have been infected in areas where chloroquine-resistant strains of *P. falciparum* are rare can be treated with chloroquine in the same dosage as that used to treat the other three species of human malaria (Table 26.3-1). These areas, as of 1984, include Central America north of the Panama Canal, west Africa, the Mediterranean basin, western Asia to Iran. There is very little chloroquine resistance reported from central and western India (2). Cases of chloroquine-resistant falciparum malaria acquired in East Africa have been confirmed since 1978 and have become more frequent since 1982.

The best alternate drug for treating chloroquine-sensitive strains is amodiaquine (3) (Table 26.3-1). Chloroquine or amodiaquine can cause death following injections, particularly in children. If parenteral therapy is indicated, the intramuscular route is preferred. The recommended dose for children (20 mg/kg/total dose) is less per kilogram than that prescribed for adults (30 mg/kg/total dose) because of increased toxicity in children (6).

Chloroquine-resistant falciparum malaria has been frequently reported from Southeast Asia, Bangladesh, Nepal and eastern India, Indonesia and Papua-New Guinea, and northern South America. Patients suspected of having been exposed in these areas should be treated for chloroquine-resistant infection.

The recommended treatment for uncomplicated chloroquine-resistant falciparum malaria is quinine, pyrimethamine, and sulfadiazine (Table 26.3-1). The pediatric dose is: quinine, 25 mg/kg/day in three doses for 10-14 days; pyrimethamine, body weight less than 10 kg - 6.25 mg/day, body weight 10-20 kg - 12.5 mg/day, body weight 20-40 kg - 25 mg/day; and sulfadiazine, 100 mg/kg/day in four doses for 5 days (maximum 2 g/day). The combination of pyrimethamine and a sulfonamide has synergism (13), and the quinine/pyrimethamine/sulfadiazine regimen has been successful in 92-98% of cases. In patients with complicated malaria, the quinine should be given slowly by intravenous infusion. Hall recommends that severely ill patients be treated with intermittent, 4-hr infusions of quinine given every 12 hr (6,7). The dose is inversely related to the severity of the disease, since the half-life is prolonged due to hepatic involvement. No more than 20 mg/kg should be administered daily in the early stages of infection, and in severely ill patients with renal and/or hepatic failure 5 or 10 mg/kg may be the maximum tolerated dose. Careful monitoring of the pulse and blood pressure is necessary to detect arrhythmia and hypotension. A practical way of giving i.v. quinine is to mix the 12-hr dosage in 300 ml of normal saline and give it over a 3- to 4-hr period at a steady rate. The course of quinine may be completed by oral administration after the patient improves, and pyrimethamine and sulfadiazine can be started at that time. Hall believes that quinine is the most rapidly acting drug in patients severely ill with chloroquine-resistant falciparum malaria (6,7).

There are several alternatives to the previously described regimen. Pyrimethamine-sulfadoxine can be substituted for the pyrimethamine and sulfadiazine. A short 2-day course of quinine followed by a single dose of three FANSIDAR tablets cured 96% of patients in Thailand infected with chloroquine-resistant falciparum malaria (6,8). Almost as good results (85% radical cure) have been reported in treating partially immune patients with a single dose of the pyrimethamine-sulfadoxine combination alone (5). Mefloquine, a quinoline methanol under development by the U.S. Army malaria research program, cured 94% of patients in Thailand with a single dose (6). The combination of a 2-day course of quinine and a single dose of mefloquine was even more effective, curing all 35 patients tested (8). Mefloquine, however, is available only in Thailand and Switzerland at this time (1986) (6).

To further complicate matters, there has been clear documentation since 1980 of strains of *P. falciparum* from Southeast Asia that are not only resistant to chloroquine but also to FANSIDAR. Individuals with falciparum malaria contracted in Thailand, Cambodia, Laos, Vietnam, the Philippines, and Indonesia who relapse after treament with a drug combination containing FANSIDAR should probably be retreated with a 3-to 10- day course of quinine, and with tetracycline, 250 or 500 mg four times daily for 7-10 days. If mefloquine is available, it could be substituted for the latter drug.

Quinine, 540 mg every 8 hr for 1 day, and concurrently, BACTRIM or SEPTRA [sulfamethoxazole (800 mg); trimethoprim (160 mg)] every 12 hr for 5 days initially cleared fever and asexual parasitemia in all patients treated, with presumptive radical cures in 85% (4). The trimethoprim-sulfonamide combination is inferior to the pyrimethamine-sulfonamide combinations for treating malaria and is not recommended for this purpose.

If pyrimethamine and a sulfonamide are not available, tetracycline can be substituted. A regimen of quinine, 540 mg every 8 hr for 1 day only, and tetracycline, 500 mg four times daily for 7 days, gave presumptive radical cures in 85% (4). Amodiaquine, another drug not always available, may be a better substitute for quinine than chloroquine, since it is more effective against chloroquine-resistant strains of *P. falciparum* (3).

Most of the studies evaluating chemotherapy of chloroquine-resistant falciparum malaria had natives from malarious areas as the infected subjects. These individuals had various levels of malarial immunity, and their responses to the infection and the therapy could be different from those of nonimmune patients seen in the United States. Therefore, conservative management is recommended, giving the longer courses of the more potent drugs to nonimmune persons infected with chloroquine-resistant falciparum malaria.

Eradication of Hepatic Stages of Malaria. In infections with *P. vivax* and *P. ovale*, there is frequently a persistence of the exoerythrocytic phase in the liver following cure of the clinically symptomatic blood stages. Additional treatment with primaquine is necessary to prevent relapses and generally should be given to those leaving or living outside of areas endemic for malaria (3,10) (Table 26.3-1). The short course of primaquine for adults is 26.3 mg (15 mg of base) daily for 14 days. A less toxic but longer course is 79 mg (45 mg of base) weekly for 8 weeks. The pediatric dose is 0.03 mg/kg of base daily for 14 days or 0.09 mg/kg once weekly for 8 weeks. Late relapses following the daily schedule should be treated using the weekly schedule. In an area where seasonal vivax malaria occurs, the combination of a single dose of amodiaquine, 600 mg base, and a short 5-day course of primaquine, 15 mg base daily, cut the incidence of malaria in half when compared with amodiaquine therapy alone (1). A single dose of 45 mg of primaquine also reduced the number with subsequent parasitemia, but it was not as effective as the 5-day course.

Because primaquine causes hemolysis in persons with a G-6-PD deficiency, appropriate tests may be performed to detect this defect before initial primaquine therapy. At the standard daily or once-weekly dosage, hemolysis is usually subclinical in blacks with G-6-PD deficiency.

CHEMOPROPHYLAXIS OF MALARIA

Chloroquine, at a once-weekly dosage of 500 mg (300 mg base), started 1 week prior to arrival in the malaria endemic area, continued while in the area and for 6 weeks after return, will prevent almost all infections except those caused by chloroquine- resistant falciparum strains (2) (Table 26.3-1). Alternate drugs include amodiaquine,

520 mg (400 mg base) on a similar once-weekly schedule, and chloroguanide (PROGUANIL, PALUDRINE), 100 mg daily, continued for 6 weeks after leaving the malarious area. Pyrimethamine, 25-50 mg once weekly, has also been used for prophylaxis. Other regimens are preferred, however, because of the high incidence of parasite resistance to pyrimethamine or chloroguanide when used alone.

Chloroquine alone is inadequate prophylaxis for chloroquine-resistant falciparum malaria. One may elect, however, to use this drug for those without heavy malarial exposure and treat all breakthrough cases of falciparum malaria as chloroquine resistant. FANSIDAR has been shown to be highly successful in preventing falciparum malaria when administered every week (11), every 2 weeks (10,11), and even every 4 weeks (9) in Thailand. The weekly dosage is recommended. This combination drug contains 25 mg of pyrimethamine (half-life about 96 hr) and 500 mg of sulfadoxine (half-life about 200 hr). It is not as effective as chloroquine in preventing vivax malaria.

Recently there have been reports of falciparum malaria occurring in individuals in eastern Thailand who had received prophylaxis with chloroquine and FANSIDAR or a quinine-sulfadiazine-pyrimethamine combination. It is difficult to make a recommendation regarding an appropriate prophylactic regimen to use in this area. There would be a reluctance to recommend daily quinine because of potential drug toxicity. Chloroquine and FANSIDAR prophylaxis is probably the better choice, followed by the treatment of any cases of falciparum malaria as being resistant to these drugs. Mefloquine was shown to be even more effective for chemoprophylaxis of resistant falciparum malaria and vivax malaria in semi-immune inhabitants of eastern Thailand (11).

If exposure to vivax or ovale malaria is suspected, the 8-aminoquinoline, primaquine, is recommended to prevent blood stage infection from persistent exoerythrocytic stages (Table 26.3-1).

REFERENCES

1. Cedillos, R.A., Warren, M.W., and Jeffery, G.M. Field evaluation of primaquine in the control of *Plasmodium vivax*. *Am. J. Trop. Med. Hyg.* 27:466, 1978.
2. Center for Disease Control. Chemoprophylaxis of malaria. *Morbid. Mortal. Weekly Rep.* 27 (Suppl.):81, 1978.
3. Clyde, D.F. Treatment of drug-resistant malaria in man. *Bull. WHO* 50:243, 1974.
4. Colwell, E.J., Hickman, R.L., and Kosakal, S. Quinine-tetracycline and quinine-bactrim treatment of acute falciparum malaria in Thailand. *Ann. Trop. Med. Parasitol.* 67:125, 1973.
5. Doberstyn, E.B., Hall, A.P., Vetvutanapilrul, K., and Sonkom, P. Single-dose therapy of falciparum malaria using pyrimethamine in combination with diformyldapsone or sulfadoxine. *Am. J. Trop. Med. Hyg.* 25:14, 1976.
6. Hall, A.P. The treatment of malaria. *Br. Med. J.* 1:323, 1976.
7. Hall, A.P. The treatment of severe falciparum malaria. *Trans. R. Soc. Trop. Med. Hyg.* 71:367, 1977.
8. Hall, A.P., Doberstyn, E.B., Karnchanachetanee, C. et al. Sequential treatment with quinine and mefloquine or quinine and pyrimethamine-sulfadoxine for falciparum malaria. *Br. Med. J.* 1:1626, 1977.
9. Lewis, A.M., and Ponnampalam, J.T. Suppression of malaria with monthly administration of combined sulphadoxine and pyrimethamine. *Ann. Trop. Med. Parasitol.* 69:1, 1975.
10. Pearlman, E.J., Lampe, R.M., Thiemanun, W., and Kennedy, R.S. Chemosuppressive field trials in Thailand. 3. The suppression of *Plasmodium falciparum* and *Plasmodium vivax* parasitemias by a sulfadoxine-pyrimethamine combination. *Am. J. Trop. Med. Hyg.* 26:1108, 1977.
11. Pearlman, E.J., Doberstyn, E.B., Sudsok, S. et al. Chemosuppressive field trials in Thailand. 4. The suppression of *Plasmodium falciparum* and *Plasmodium vivax* parasitemias by mefloquine (WR 142,490), a 4-quinolinemethanol. *Am. J. Trop. Med. Hyg.* 29:1131, 1980.
12. Peters, W. Malaria: Chemoprophylaxis and chemotherapy. *Br. Med. J.* 2:95, 1971.
13. Schmidt, L.H., Harrison, J., Rossan, R.N., et al. Quantitative aspects of pyrimethamine-sulfonamide synergism. *Am. J. Trop. Med. Hyg.* 26:837, 1977.

ADDITIONAL READING

Drugs for parasitic infections. *Med. Lett. Drugs Ther.* 24:5, 1982.

Peters, W. *Chemotherapy and Drug Resistance in Malaria.* New York: Academic Press, 1970.

Richards, W.H.G. Some promising leads in experimental malarial drugs. *Adv. Pharmacol. Ther.* 10:71, 1979.

Rozman, R.S., and Canfield, C.J. New experimental antimalarial drugs. *Adv. Pharmacol. Chemother.* 16:1, 1979.

WHO Scientific Group. Chemotherapy of malaria and resistance to antimalarials. *WHO Tech. Rep. Ser.*, no. 529, 1973.

CHAPTER
26.4

CHEMOTHERAPY OF INTESTINAL NEMATODE INFECTIONS

G. Thomas Strickland and Edgar A. Steck

Intestinal nematode infections are the most common medical condition in the world. In *This Wormy World*, published in 1947, Stoll estimated that there were many more worm infections than people between the Tropics of Cancer and Capricorn (28). If anything, there has been an increase in human intestinal nematode infections in the years since Stoll's publication. Many people, both in the tropics and the United States, are infected with the 'big three,' *Ascaris, Trichuris, and hookworm.* The prevalence of intestinal nematode infections in the United States has only been estimated. Warren, referring to Stoll's earlier figures, estimated that in 1972, 42 million Americans had enterobiasis, 4 million had ascariasis, 2.2 million had trichuriasis, 700,000 had hookworm, and 400,000 had strongyloidiasis (34).

There are several general points worth mentioning pertinent to intestinal nematode infections: (a) Many infections are not serious (i.e., enterobiasis or trichuriasis), and reinfection following treatment is frequent. Therefore, therapy may not always be indicated. (b) More important than drug therapy in the control of transmission is improvement in education and sanitation. (c) Many patients have multiple infections; therefore, the introduction of the new broad-spectrum anthelmintics (e.g., mebendazole, levamisole, pyrantel pamoate) has been very useful (Tables 26.4-1 and 26.4-2). Single-drug therapy for multiple intestinal nematode infections is cost effective, improves patient compliance, and decreases the potential for drug toxicities. (d) Many people infected with intestinal nematodes are very poor and the expense of the newer broad-spectrum anthelmintics at the personal, village, or national level may be prohibitive. Therefore, the older, less efficacious, but cheaper drugs, are still used. (e) Patients with heavy infections of intestinal nematodes, particularly with *T. trichiura,* are less likely to be cured than those having light infections (17,25).

DRUGS USED IN TREATING INTESTINAL NEMATODE INFECTIONS

BEPHENIUM HYDROXYNAPHTHOATE

Bephenium hydroxynaphthoate is a quaternary ammonium salt that has been used to treat hookworm infections, ascariasis, trichostrongyliasis, and ternideniasis.

Source and Chemistry. Bephenium is used as the hydroxynaphthoate salt, which is bitter in taste, has a low solubility in water, and is pale yellow in color (Fig. 26.4-1).

Anthelmintic Action. Bephenium hydroxynaphthoate produces irreversible paralysis in ascarid musculature. The drug causes muscular excitation followed by paralysis associated with loss of reactivity to acetylcholine. No anticholinergic effects have been noted in humans. Bephenium causes hookworms to lose their attachment to the gastrointestinal mucosa, following which they are expelled.

Pharmacokinetics. The drug is poorly absorbed when given by mouth and less than 0.5% is excreted in the urine.

Adverse Effects. The bitter taste sometimes causes nausea and vomiting. Less common side effects include mild headache, abdominal pain, and diarrhea.

Preparations. Bephenium hydroxynaphthoate (ALCOPAR) is available in packets containing 5 g of granules that contain 2.5 g of the bephenium base. The drug is given orally on an empty stomach, preferably with flavored syrups, juices, or milk to render it more palatable. The adult dosage for treating hookworm (more efficacious against *Ancylostoma duodenale), Trichostrongylus orientalis,* and *Ternidens diminutus* infections is 5 g, twice daily, for 1 (*A. duodenale*) or 2 (other parasites) days. Food should be withheld following ingestion of the packet for at least 2 hr. The drug also has some anthelmintic effects upon *Ascaris lumbricoides.*

Table 26.4-1
Efficacy of Broad-spectrum Anthelmintics[a]

Infection	Mebendazole	Pyrantel Pamoate	Levamisole	Thiabendazole	Pyrvinium Pamoate	Piperazine Citrate	Bephenium Hydroxy-naphthoate
Enterobiasis	+++	+++	–	+++	+++	+++	–
Ascariasis	+++	+++	+++	++	–	–	+
Hookworm	+++	++	++	++	–	–	++
Strongyloidiasis	–	–	+	+++	++	–	–
Trichuriasis	++	–	–	+	–	–	–
Trichostrongyliasis	+++	++	++	++	–	–	+

[a] – = less than 30% cured; + = 30-60% cured; ++ = 60-85% cured; +++ = greater than 85% cured.

LEVAMISOLE

Levamisole is the l-isomer of an imidazothiazole derivative, tetramisole, which was, and is, extensively used to treat gastrointestinal nematode infections in veterinary practice. Levamisole is widely used outside of the United States as a broad-spectrum anthelmintic (8,30,31) and has also been shown to modulate the immune response (11,29).

Source and Chemistry. Levamisole, the levo-rotatory isomer of tetramisole, is white, stable, and water soluble. It was identified as the component responsible for the fast, short- acting anthelmintic effects of tetramisole and is marketed as levamisole HCl (Fig. 26.4-1).

Anthelmintic Action. Levamisole undergoes metabolic cleavage into an imidazolone derivative that is responsible for some of its anthelmintic effects. The parent compound, however, has both *in vitro* and *in vivo* activity. Ascarids immersed in levamisole solutions have spastic contractions followed by paralysis. Levamisole causes stimulation and then contraction of ganglion-like structures in ascarids, and thereafter neuromuscular inhibition of a depolarizing type. The worms are then passively eliminated. Levamisole is a potent and stereospecific inhibitor, both *in vitro* and *in vivo* , of fumarate reductase in several groups of immature and adult nematodes. This enzyme system is species specific, and the drug must penetrate the cuticle of the worm to exert its effects. Therefore, the anthelmintic spectrum of levamisole is limited to various nematode species.

Pharmacological Effects. Both tetramisole and levamisole stimulate parasympathetic and sympathetic ganglia of mammals. This is accompanied by inhibition of norepinephrine reuptake. They have positive inotropic and chronotropic actions and are convulsants at high doses.

Levamisole is also a nonspecific stimulator of the

Table 26.4-2
Chemotherapy of Intestinal Nematodes (Roundworms)

Parasite	Disease	Recommended Drug	Adult Dose[a]	Alternate Drug	Adult Dose[a]
Enterobius vermicularis	enterobiasis (pinworm)	mebendazole	100 mg once	pyrantel pamoate	11 mg/kg once (maximum 1 g)
Ascaris lumbricoides	ascariasis (roundworm)	pyrantel pamoate	11 mg/kg once (maximum 1 g)	mebendazole	100 mg b.i.d. for 3 days
Necator amerricanus and *Ancylostoma duodenale*	ancylostomiasis (hookworm)	pyrantel pamoate	11 mg/kg/day (maximum 1 g) for 3 days		100 mg b.i.d. for 3 days
Strongyloides stercoralis	strongyloidiasis (threadworm)	thiabendazole	25 mg/kg/day b.i.d. for 2 days	pyrvinium	5 mg/kg/day for 7 days (maximum 2.5 g)
Trichuris trichura	trichuriasis (whipworm)	mebendazole	100 mg b.i.d. for 3 days	thiabendazole	25 mg/kg/day b.i.d. for 4 or 5 days

[a] Administered p.o.

immune response (29) and has been used for this purpose in the chemotherapy of malignancies (11) and to treat patients with immunodeficiencies.

Pharmacokinetics. Tetramisole and levamisole are water soluble and readily absorbed following oral administration. They are widely distributed in the tissues. Peak plasma levels are achieved within 2 hr following oral administration. Plasma half-life is about 4 hr with essentially all of the drug eliminated within 2 days. Levamisole and tetramisole are metabolized extensively in the liver, and the metabolites are primarily eliminated in the urine and feces within 24 hr.

Adverse Effects. Levamisole has a low incidence of side effects. Anorexia, nausea, vomiting, abdominal pain, dizziness, and headache have been reported (18). The more serious side effects (e.g., granulocytopenia, transient optic neuritis) have occurred in individuals receiving levamisole for modulation of the immune response. The drug has been used extensively and for prolonged periods in veterinary medicine with a low incidence of untoward toxicities.

Preparations. The drug is marketed outside the United States in tablets containing 40, 50, 80, or 150 mg of the hydrochloride. The dosage for treating ascariasis, hookworm infection, strongyloidiasis, and trichuriasis is 2.5 mg/kg given orally in a single dose (8,30,31). Clinical evaluation of its effects upon *Filariae* and the immune response is undergoing broad study.

MEBENDAZOLE

Mebendazole is a broad-spectrum anthelmintic that was introduced in the treatment of *Ascaris* infections, but also has excellent efficacy in the treatment of *Enterobius vermicularis*, hookworm, and *T. trichiura*. It has also been shown to act upon cestode infections, including *Echinococcus granulosus* and *E. multilocularis* (14) and the larvae of *Trichinella spiralis* in mice.

Source and Chemistry. Mebendazole is a yellowish amorphous powder, slightly soluble in water; it is a member of the benzimidazole family and related to thiabendazole (Fig. 26.4-1).

Anthelmintic Action. Mebendazole is effective against adult intestinal-dwelling nematodes and cestodes and their tissue-stage larvae due to its ability to inhibit glucose uptake irreversibly. This leads to endogenous depletion of glycogen stored within the parasite which itself results in a decreased formation of adenosine triphosphate, required for survival and reproduction of the helminth. Ultrastructural studies have shown that the primary effect of mebendazole is degeneration of cytoplasmic microtubules resulting in blockage of transport secretory granules from within the Golgi apparatus of the cytoplasm. The death of the helminth is believed to occur secondary to autolysis from release of hydrolytic or proteolytic enzymes from within the secretory granules, or to impaired feeding because of the inability of enzymes required for absorption or digestion to reach the absorptive site, or from reduced cell-coat protection due to blocked transport of cell-coat materials from the secretory granules (14). Following treatment, immobilization and death of the parasites occur slowly. Hookworm and *Trichuris* ova fail to develop to the larval stage following therapy.

Pharmacokinetics. Following oral administration, only a small amount of the drug is absorbed and only 5-10% may be

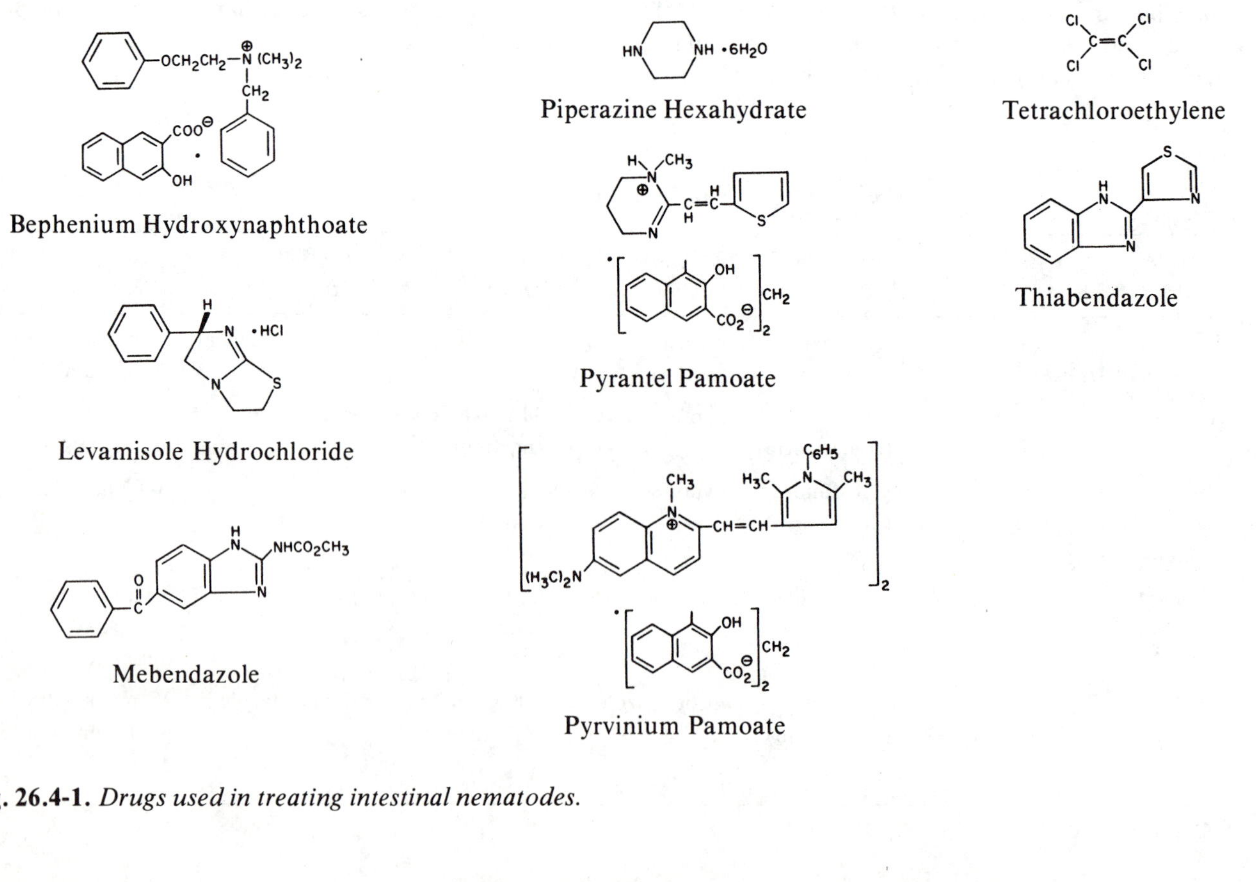

Bephenium Hydroxynaphthoate

Piperazine Hexahydrate

Tetrachloroethylene

Levamisole Hydrochloride

Pyrantel Pamoate

Thiabendazole

Mebendazole

Pyrvinium Pamoate

Fig. 26.4-1. *Drugs used in treating intestinal nematodes.*

detected in the urine within 2 days. Peak plasma levels occur about 2 hr following oral ingestion and represent 0.5% or less of the oral dose (3). The poor absorption of the drug is an advantage in treating intestinal-dwelling helminths but is a disadvantage for treating tissue-invasive parasites.

Adverse Effects. A single case of reversible leukopenia has been reported in a patient on prolonged high dosage. These same doses may also cause nausea and vomiting. Rats treated with prolonged high doses have developed testicular atrophy, and the drug has teratogenic effects in pregnant female rats.

Preparations. Mebendazole (VERMOX) is available as 100 mg tablets. The same dose schedule is used for children as adults. A single 100-mg tablet is given for 1 day to treat enterobiasis or twice daily for 3 days to treat ascariasis, trichuriasis, and hookworm infection. The dosage may be repeated if the patient is not cured. Mebendazole is also used in the treatment of *Capillaria philippinensis* (200 mg twice daily for 20 days); *Taenia saginata* and *T. solium* (200-300 mg twice daily for 3 days); *Echinococcus granulosus* and *E. multilocularis* (40 mg/kg/day for 2-12 months); *Hymenolepis nana* (200-300 mg twice daily for 5-7 days); and *Strongyloides stercoralis* and *Trichinella spiralis* (dose unspecified). Because the drug is teratogenic and embryotoxic in pregnant rats, it is contraindicated in pregnancy (14).

PIPERAZINE

Piperazine in the form of the hydrated base or a salt has been used to treat ascariasis and enterobiasis for some 30 years. Because it is inexpensive, it still is used to treat these parasites even though it is less effective and has more side effects than the newer broad-spectrum anthelmintics.

Source and Chemistry. Piperazine citrate (Fig. 26.4-1) and adipate are common commercial forms of the drug. These salts are soluble in water and are stable white crystals.

Anthelmintic Action. Piperazine acts as a parasympathetic blocking agent causing paralysis of ascarids. They are then expelled alive and active in the stools.

Pharmacokinetics. Piperazine is readily absorbed from the gastrointestinal tract, and both it and its metabolites are excreted in the urine. The appearance of side effects varies inversely with the rate of excretion of the drug and is more frequent in patients with renal dysfunction.

Adverse Effects. High doses cause depression of the central nervous system, whereas lethal doses cause convulsions. Toxicities from lower doses include headache, vertigo, blurred vision, incoordination, tremors, and somnolence. When given intravenously, piperazine may cause a transient hypotension. Other occasional, and mild, side effects include anorexia, nausea, vomiting, abdominal cramps, diarrhea, muscle weakness, and urticaria. Piperazine has been used without ill effects during pregnancy. It should not, however, be used in patients with renal dysfunction or a history of epilepsy.

Preparations. Piperazine preparations (ANTEPAR, MULTIFUGE) contain the hexahydrate of the base or salts, but dosage is expressed in terms of the base. Tablets ordinarily contain 500 mg equivalent of the base, and syrups have a concentration of 500 mg in 5 ml. In treatment of ascariasis in children, piperazine, 75 mg/kg, is given as a single dose on each of 2 consecutive days (maximum dose, 3.5 g/day). Adults are given the 3.5-g dose on the same schedule. In the treatment of pinworm infections, the dosage for both adults and children is 65 mg/kg (maximum dose 2.5 g/day) once daily for 7 days. These regimens cure nearly 100% of those treated.

PYRANTEL PAMOATE

Pyrantel pamoate has a broad spectrum of anthelmintic activity and is used extensively in both human and veterinary medicine. It has excellent activity in the treatment of ascariasis, enterobiasis, hookworm infection, and other rarer intestinal nematode infections. Oxantel, an m-phenol analog of pyrantel, has been evaluated as a single-dose treatment for trichuriasis.

Anthelmintic Action. Pyrantel is a depolarizing neuromuscular blocking agent, both in worms and invertebrates. As a consequence, spastic paralysis occurs in the worms which are subsequently expelled from the gastrointestinal tract. The effects upon *Ascaris* muscle are slow in onset and difficult to reverse by washing.

Adverse Effects. Side effects are mild and unusual. They include anorexia, nausea, vomiting, abdominal pain, diarrhea, headache, dizziness, and skin rashes.

Preparations. Pyrantel pamoate (ANTIMINTH, COMBANTRIN) contains 34% of base as the salt and is ordinarily supplied as a sweetened suspension containing 50 mg of base per milliliter and as tablets containing 125 mg of the base. To treat *Enterobius* or *Ascaris* infections, the dose for both adults and children is 11 mg/kg, to a maximum of 1 g given once. Hookworm and *Trichostrongylus* respond better to the same dose on 3 consecutive days.

PYRVINIUM PAMOATE

Pyrvinium pamoate is a poorly soluble salt of a cyanine dye with therapeutic efficacy in treating pinworms and strongyloidiasis. It resulted from experiments in the late 1940s showing that cyanine dyes possess marked antifilarial activity.

Source and Chemistry. Pyrvinium pamoate is a salt of a cyanine dye (Fig. 26.4-1) that is insoluble in water and deep red in color.

Anthelmintic Action. As a cyanine dye, pyrvinium pamoate exerts a range of selective effects upon nematodes, including interference with respiratory enzyme systems and with the absorption of exogenous glucose.

Pharmacokinetics. The drug is almost nonabsorbable when given orally.

Adverse Effects. Side effects are usually minimal. Occasional patients have mild anorexia, nausea, vomiting, and abdominal pain. Objects that come into contact with the drug or posttreatment stools are stained red.

Preparations. Pyrvinium pamoate (POVAN, VANQUIN) is available as 50 mg base in tablets and as a flavored pediatric suspension containing 50 mg of base per 5 ml. In treating pinworm infections, the adult and pediatric dose is 5 mg/kg, up to a maximum dose of 350 mg, given once prior to mealtime. A second dose can be given after 1 or 2 weeks to eliminate worms developed from ova ingested after the first dose. In the treatment of strongyloidiasis, the same dose is given over 7 successive days.

TETRACHLOROETHYLENE

Tetrachloroethylene has been used as an anthelmintic for longer than four decades and still has value in treating *Necator americanus* infections and is used in treating infections caused by *Fasciolopsis buski*, *Heterophyes heterophyes* , and *Metagonimus yokogawi*, although newer drugs are more effective and less toxic. It is also widely used in veterinary medicine.

Source and Chemistry. Tetrachloroethylene was first prepared by Michael Faraday in 1821 and was introduced about a century later as a replacement for carbon tetrachloride in the treatment of hookworm infections. It is an unsaturated halogenated hydrocarbon (Fig. 26.4-1). Its odor is similar to ether and it is highly insoluble in water.

Anthelmintic Action. The drug is believed to cause a reversible paralysis of hookworms. It also gradually releases lysosomal enzymes from the worms and interferes with digestion of nutrients by the helminths.

Pharmacokinetics. In the absence of fat or ethanol, tetrachloroethylene is absorbed to a negligible extent from the gastrointestinal tract.

Adverse Effects. Tetrachloroethylene causes side effects due to irritation of the gastrointestinal tract and depression of the central nervous system. It can cause nausea, vomiting, a burning sensation in the stomach, abdominal pain, diarrhea, headache, dizziness, vertigo, giddiness, inebriation, and occasionally loss of consciousness. Severely anemic patients may collapse during therapy, especially following purging.

Preparations. Tetrachloroethylene is supplied in soft gelatin capsules containing 0.2, 1.0, or 2.5 ml of the compound. The patient avoids fats or ethanol the night before and takes the drug on an empty stomach. He abstains from food another 4-6 hr. The adult dose is 5 ml, and children are given 0.12 ml/kg (maximum 5 ml) for the treatment of *Necator americanus* infections. Because therapeutic efficacy is not as good for *Ancylostoma duodenale* , tetrachloroethylene is not recommended for treating infections with that parasite. Repeat courses may be given if necessary. Tetrachloroethylene may cause a dangerous migration of ascarids. If the patient has a concomitant *Ascaris* infection, this should be treated first.

THIABENDAZOLE

Thiabendazole resulted from studies on the therapeutic effects of substituted benzimidazole compounds and is one of the earliest broad-spectrum anthelmintics. It has efficacy against intestinal nematode infections (i.e., strongyloidiasis, trichuriasis, hookworm, ascariasis, enterobiasis, trichostrongyliasis, and capillariasis) and tissue nematode infections (i.e., trichinosis, toxocariasis, cutaneous larva migrans, and dracontiasis). Some of its beneficial effects are believed to be related to its antiinflammatory properties, which reduce tissue reaction to the infection.

Source and Chemistry. Thiabendazole is a stable white crystalline powder almost insoluble in water but readily soluble in either weak alkali or acids. It is a substituted benzimidazole (Fig. 26.4-1).

Anthelmintic Action. Thiabendazole has considerable activity against intestinal nematodes and probable activity against tissue-invasive nematodes. The latter action may be due to its antiinflammatory, antipyretic, and analgesic properties (5), although it has been shown to be larvicidal *in vitro* at low concentrations. The mechanism of action is unknown. Like some other anthelmintics, it inhibits the helminth-specific enzyme fumarate reductase.

Pharmacokinetics. Absorption is rapid after oral administration with peak plasma levels occurring within 1 hr. The majority of thiabendazole is excreted in the urine within 24 hr as the conjugated glucuronide or sulfate or 5-hydroxythiabendazole.

Adverse Effects. Gastrointestinal side effects, such as anorexia, nausea, vomiting, and epigastric discomfort, and dizziness frequently occur at therapeutic doses. Less frequent side effects include diarrhea, drowsiness, giddiness, headache, pruritus, and skin rash. Other, rarer side effects have also been reported. Few, however, are life threatening. Thiabendazole can be hepatotoxic and sometimes has central nervous system side effects.

Preparations. Thiabendazole (MINTEZOL) is available in 500-mg chewable tablets, as an oral suspension containing 500 mg/5 ml, or as a topical suspension. It is best given after meals to reduce side effects. The usual dose is 25 mg/kg/day (maximum dose, 3 g), given in two divided doses. This is given for 1 day to treat enterobiasis and for 2 days to treat strongyloidiasis, ascariasis, hookworm infection, trichostrongyliasis, and trichuriasis (although a longer course may be more effective in treating the last-mentioned). A 30-day course was used to treat intestinal capillariasis (34). The drug is best used topically to treat cutaneous larva migrans (creeping eruption) (Chapter 26.5). Seven-day courses have generally been used to treat systemic nematode infections [e.g., visceral larva migrans (toxocariasis), trichinosis, or dracontiasis (guinea worm infection)]. Dracontiasis has been treated with 3-day courses as well. Cutaneous larva migrans, when treated orally, is usually treated for only 2 days.

TREATMENT OF ENTEROBIASIS

The adult female pinworm emerges through the anus at night to lay eggs in the perineal area, causing pruritus. When the host scratches, eggs are transferred to his fingers where they can reinfect him or some other person when swallowed. Ingested eggs hatch in the small intestine to release larvae, which pass directly to the large intestine where they mature.

Enterobiasis is the most common helminth infection in the United States and is found throughout the country in all socioeconomic classes. Prevalence in some institutions may be particularly high. When a child is found to be infected, it is worthwhile performing a Scotch-tape test on other family members. Some treat all family members, assuming that all are infected.

There are several excellent drugs for treating pinworm (Tables 26.4-1 and 26.4-2). Pyrantel pamoate is effective at a single dose of 11 mg/kg (1 tsp/25 kg) (25). Mebendazole, given at a single dose of 100 mg, cures almost everyone (3,16,25). A third drug, pyrvinium pamoate, at a single dose of 5 mg/kg (maximum dose, 250 mg) is nearly as effective with a 70-90% cure rate reported (4). Piperazine citrate, at a dose of 65 mg/kg/day (maximum 2.5 g) for 7 days, cures about 95% of those infected. It is recommended that the patient be treated a second time after 2 weeks to cure any subsequent infections from eggs in the environment.

TREATMENT OF ASCARIASIS

Ascaris ova are passed in the stool and require 2 weeks' incubation in the soil before they become infective. After ingestion, the eggs hatch in the duodenum and the larvae enter the venous circulation and pass to the lungs, where they migrate across the pulmonary-capillary beds before traveling up the respiratory tree. They are then swallowed and pass to the jejunum, where they mature and mate. Ascariasis is frequently contracted by eating contaminated salads and raw vegetables and is more common in areas where human feces are used for fertilization. Passing an adult ascarid from the anus or nose can be unpleasant. Heavy infections, particularly in children, have been associated with intestinal obstruction. *Ascaris* infection also has an adverse effect on nutritional status.

For these reasons, it is recommended that all *Ascaris* infections be treated unless the patient has a light infection and the physician is certain the patient will not be reinfected. Mebendazole given twice daily for 3 days cures almost everyone (Tables 26.4-1 and 26.4-2) (13,25, 36). Pyrantel pamoate given at a single dose is nearly as effective (12,20). Piperazine citrate is cheaper than either of the other two drugs and gives a cure rate of 65-70% when given as a single dose of 75-150 mg/kg (maximum dose 3.5 g) (17,18), and 70-90% when given at a dose of 50-75 mg/kg/day (maximum dose 3.5 g) for 2 days (12). Levamisole cures 90-95% when given at a single dose of 2.5 mg/kg (8,17,18,30,31).

TREATMENT OF HOOKWORM INFECTIONS

Hookworm is caused by infection with either *Necator americanus* or *Ancylostoma duodenale*. The later is not endemic to the United States but may be found in immigrants. Ova of the two species are indistinguishable, the disease is similar, and the treatment is usually the same, except the *N. americanus* may require higher and longer-acting doses of drugs to cure heavy infections compared with *A. duodenale*.

Hookworm eggs hatch in the soil, and the resulting larvae penetrate the bare skin of the host, then migrate through the body similar to *Ascaris* before settling in the large intestine as adult worms. Hookworm disease associated with heavy infections is caused by gastrointestinal blood loss, resulting in anemia and hypoproteinemia. A pruritic cutaneous eruption, *ground itch*, sometimes occur with skin penetration, and eosinophilic pneumonia has been described when the larvae migrate through the lung. Improvements in education and sanitation, including indoor toilets, have reduced the incidence of hookworm infection in the United States from 1.8 million to 700,000 during the past 30 years (34). However, hookworm remains a worldwide medical problem, with an estimated 300 million people infected.

It is recommended that all patients with hookworm infections be treated. Mebendazole has a 90-100% efficacy at a dose of 100 mg twice daily for 3 days, curing almost all light infections (13,14,25) (Tables 26.4-1 and 26.4-2). Shorter courses of the drug, as recommended for treating other nematodes, reduce the worm burden and give reasonable cure rates. Pyrantel pamoate is almost as efficacious as mebendazole when given as a single dose (11 mg/kg/day) for 3 consecutive days (1,2,7,26). Both drugs have very little toxicity, which is primarily gastrointestinal. Another broad-spectrum anthelmintic, levamisole, is extensively used outside of the United States for treating hookworm infection. Levamisole, at a single oral dose of 2.5 mg/kg, is reported to cure about 70-75% of those infected (8,30,31). Thiabendazole has good efficacy in treating hookworm infections at a dosage of 25 mg/kg for 3 days (6). Hookworm can also be treated with either tetrachloroethylene (better for *N. americanus*) 0.10- 0.12 ml/kg (maximum dose 5 ml) once (2,26), or with bephenium hydroxynaphthoate (better for *A. duodenale*) 5 g twice daily for 1 or 2 days (2,7,26).

TREATMENT OF STRONGYLOIDIASIS

Strongyloides worms have a complicated life cycle. The major mode of infection is similar to hookworm, with infective filariform larvae penetrating the skin and migrating through the lungs prior to reaching the upper small intestine where the adult worms are found. As in hookworm, a skin-penetrating rash and migratory pneumonia rarely occur. *S. stercoralis*, however, also has the capability of internal autoinfection, with noninfectious rhabdiform larvae metaphasing to filariform larvae while still within the intestinal tract. The larvae penetrate the intestinal mucosa or perianal skin and repeat the cycle of infection. A hyperinfection syndrome has been reported in immunosuppressed or malnourished hosts (9,22). An overwhelming systemic infection results with fever, abdominal pain, shock, and often gram- negative sepsis. For this reason, all patients with strongyloidiasis should be treated.

Threadworm infection is less common than enterobiasis, ascariasis, and hookworm infections. Because of relatively increased diagnostic difficulty, it is probably underreported, with a recently estimated prevalence of 400,000 in the United States (34).

It is also more difficult to treat than some of the other intestinal nematode infections. Thiabendazole remains the best drug (6,15,22). Cure rates of 80-90% can be obtained following a dose of 25 mg/kg/day twice daily for 2 days. Patients with systemic disease should be treated longer, perhaps for 5-7 days (22). Pyrvinium pamoate gives nearly as good results but requires a 7-day course (5 mg/kg/day, maximum 2.5 g) (32,33). Levamisole cured 55% and reduced *S. stercoralis* larvae output by 55% following single-dose therapy (8).

TREATMENT OF TRICHURIASIS

Whipworm infections are acquired by the ingestion of ova that have incubated in the soil. The larvae do not migrate through the tissues, and adult worms inhabit the large intestine. *T. trichiura* seldom causes symptoms. Heavy infections, however, particularly in children, can cause diarrhea, abdominal pain, rectal prolapse, and intestinal blood loss. Worldwide prevalence of trichuriasis is in the hundreds of millions with an estimated 2.2 million infections in the United States (34). It is not necessary to treat patients with mild trichuriasis.

Mebendazole is effective at a dose of 100 mg twice daily for 3 days (13,14,16,21,23-25,36). Cure rates range between 60 and 80% and are inversely related to worm burden (16,36). Another useful drug is thiabendazole. A dose of 25 mg/kg/day twice daily for 4 or 5 days has been reported to give cure rates of only 30-40% (6).

TREATMENT OF OTHER INTESTINAL NEMATODES

The less common human nematode infections generally respond to one of the broad-spectrum anthelmintics.

INTESTINAL CAPILLARIASIS

A rare but potentially fatal infection with *Capillaria philippinensis* was reported in epidemic form in the Philippines. Intestinal capillariasis initially only responded to long-term treatment with thiabendazole, 25 mg/kg/day twice daily for 30 days (35). Subsequently, it was shown that mebendazole at a dose of 100 mg four times daily for 20 days caused less gastrointestinal toxicity and cured all of 33 receiving initial treatment (27). Retreatment at the same dosage for 30 days cured 29 of 32 who had relapsed following earlier therapy. Intestinal capillariasis is an unusual intestinal nematode infection requiring long-term chemotherapy, as autoinfection occurs and unhatched eggs present in the small intestinal tissues are not destroyed by the drug.

TRICHOSTRONGYLIASIS

Stoll estimated that more than 5 million people, primarily in Asia, were infected with one of the *Trichostrongylus* species (28). Humans are usually infected by ingestion of infective larvae, and the adult worms live with their heads embedded in the small intestinal mucosa. As in hookworm disease, heavy infections can cause an iron-deficiency anemia from chronic blood loss. Drugs shown to be effective in treating trichostrongyliasis are levamisole, thiabendazole (6,15), mebendazole, and pyrantel pamoate (1,7,20). These drugs are used at the same dose as used to treat hookworm and have the same efficacy (Table 26.4- 1).

TERNIDENIASIS

Infection with *Ternidens diminutus* is relatively common in certain localities in Africa. The parasite inhabits the wall of the large bowel where it can cause either cystic nodules or anemia from chronic blood loss. Drugs evaluated for therapy include bephenium hydroxynaphthoate (9) and pyrantel pamoate (10).

REFERENCES

1. Bell, W.J., and Nassif, S. Field study of pyrantel pamoate in the treatment of mixed roundworm, hookworm, and *Trichostrongylus* infections. *J. Egypt Med. Assoc.* 55:111, 1972.
2. Botero, D., and Castano, A. Comparative study of pyrantel pamoate, bephenium hydroxynaphthoate, and tetrachloroethylene in the treatment of *Necator americanus* infections. *Am. J. Trop. Med. Hyg.* 22:45, 1973.
3. Brugmans, J.P., Thienpont, D.C., van-Wijgaarden, I., et al. Mebendazole in enterobiasis: Radiochemical and pilot clinical study in 1278 subjects. *JAMA* 217:313, 1971.
4. Buchanan, R.A., Barrow, W.B., Heffelfinger, J., et al. Pyrvinium pamoate. *Clin. Pharmacol. Ther.* 61:716, 1974.
5. Campbell, W.C. Anti-inflammatory and analgesic properties of thiabendazole. *JAMA* 216:2143, 1971.
6. Campbell, W.C., and Cuckler, A.C. Thiabendazole in the treatment and control of parasitic infections in man. *Tex. Rep. Biol. Med.* 27 (Suppl. 2):665, 1969.
7. Farahmandian, I., Sahba, G.H., Arfaa, F., and Jalali, H. A comparative evaluation of the therapeutic effect of pyrantel pamoate and bephenium hydroxynaphthoate of *Ancylostoma duodenale* and other intestinal helminths. *J. Trop. Med. Hyg.* 75:205, 1972.
8. Gatti, F., Vanderick, M., Parent, S., et al. Treatment of roundworm infection in African children with a single dose of tetramisole (R8299). *Ann.Soc. Belg. Med. Trop.* 49:51, 1969.
9. Goldsmid, J.M. The use of bephenium hydroxynaphthoate for the treatment of human infections with *Ternidens diminutus*. Railliet and Henry, 1909. *J. Trop. Med. Hyg.* 74:19, 1971.
10. Goldsmid, J.M., and Saunders, C.R. Preliminary trial using pyrantel pamoate for the treatment of human infections with *Ternidens diminutus. Trans. R. Soc. Trop. Med. Hyg.* 66:375, 1972.
11. Hadden, J.W. Levamisole: A synthetic immunopotentiator under evaluation. *Clin. Bull. Mem. Sloan-Kettering Cancer Ctr.* 5:32, 1975.
12. Hatchuel, W., Isaacson, M., and DeVilliers, D.J. Pyrantel pamoate in roundworm infestations: A comparative trial with piperazine citrate given in a single dose. *S. Afr. Med. J.* 47:91, 1973.
13. Hutchinson, J.G.P., Johnston, N.M., Plevey, M.V.P., et al. Clinical trial of mebendazole, a broad-spectrum anthelmintic. *Br. Med. J.* 2:309, 1975.
14. Keystone, J.S., and Murdoch, J.K. Mebendazole. *Ann. Intern. Med.* 91:582, 1979.
15. Markell, E.K. Pseudohookworm infection-trichostrongyliasis: Treatment with thiabendazole. *N. Engl. J. Med.* 278:831, 1968.
16. Miller, M.J., Krup, I.M., Little, M.D., and Santos, C. Mebendazole: An effective anthelmintic for trichuriasis and enterobiasis. *JAMA* 230:1412, 1974.
17. Miller, M.J., Farahmandian, I., Arfaa, F., et al. An evaluation of levamisole for treatment of ascariasis. *South. Med. J.* 71:137, 1978.
18. Moens, M., Dom, J., Burke, W.E. et al. Levamisole in ascariasis: A multicenter controlled evaluation. *Am. J. Trop. Med. Hyg.* 27:897, 1978.
19. Purtilo, D.T., Meyers, W.M., and Connor, D.H. Fatal strongyloidiasis in immunosuppressed patients. *Am. J. Med.* 56:488, 1974.
20. Rim, H.J., and Lim, J.K. Treatment of enterobiasis and ascariasis with Combantrin (pyrantel pamoate). *Trans. R. Soc. Trop. Med. Hyg.* 66:170, 1972.
21. Sargent, R.G., Savory, A.M., Mina, A., and Lee, P.R. A clinical evaluation of mebendazole in the treatment of trichuriasis. *Am. J. Trop. Med. Hyg.* 23:375, 1974.
22. Scowden, E.B., Schaffner, W., and Stone, W.J. Overwhelming strongyloidiasis: An unappreciated opportunistic infection. *Medicine* 57:527, 1978.
23. Scragg, J.N., and Proctor, E.M. Mebendazole in the treatment of severe symptomatic trichuriasis in children. *Am. J. Trop. Med. Hyg.* 26:198, 1977.
24. Scragg, J.N., and Proctor, E.M. Further experience with mebendazole in the treatment of symptomatic trichuriasis in children. *Am. J. Trop. Med. Hyg.* 27:255, 1978.
25. Seah, S.K.K. Mebendazole in the treatment of helminthiasis. *Can. Med. Assoc. J.* 115:777, 1976.
26. Senewiratne, B., Hettiarachchi, J., and Senewiratne, K. A com-

parative study of the relative efficacy of pyrantel pamoate, bephenium hydroxynaphthoate, and tetrachloroethylene in the treatment of *Necator americanus* infection in Ceylon. *Ann. Trop. Med. Parasitol.* 69:233, 1975.

27. Singson, C.N., Banzon, T.C., and Cross, J.H. Mebendazole in the treatment of intestinal capillariasis. *Am. J. Trop. Med. Hyg.* 24:932, 1975.
28. Stoll, N.R. This wormy world. *J. Parasitol.* 33:1, 1947.
29. Symoens, J., and Rosenthal, M. Levamisole in the modulation of the immune response: The current experimental and clinical state. *J. Reticuloendothel. Soc.* 21:175, 1977.
30. Thienpont, D., Brugmans, J., Abadi, K., and Tanamal, S. Tetramisole in the treatment of nematode infections in man. *Am. J. Trop. Med. Hyg.* 18:520, 1969.
31. Vakil, B.J., Dalal, N.J., Gangrade, R.R., and Bhise, K.B. Clinical trial with l-tetramisole in roundworm and hookworm infections. *Trans. R. Soc. Trop. Med. Hyg.* 66:250, 1972.
32. Wagner, E.D. Pyrvinium pamoate in the treatment of strongyloidiasis. *Am. J. Trop. Med. Hyg.* 12:60, 1963.
33. Wang, C.C., and Galli, G.A. Strongyloidiasis treated with pyrvinium pamoate. *JAMA* 193:847, 1965.
34. Warren, K.S. Helminthic diseases endemic in the United States. *Am. J. Trop. Med. Hyg.* 23:723, 1974.
35. Whalen, G.E., Rosenberg, E.B., Gutman, R.A., et al. Treatment of intestinal capillariasis with thiabendazole, bithionol, and bephenium. *Am. J. Trop. Med. Hyg.* 20:95, 1971.
36. Wolfe, M.S., and Wershin, J.M. Mebendazole: Treatment of trichuriasis and ascariasis in Bahamian children. *JAMA* 230:1408, 1974.

ADDITIONAL READING

Botero, D.R. Chemotherapy of human intestinal parasitic diseases. *Ann. Rev. Pharmacol. Toxicol.* 18:1, 1978.

Drugs for parasitic infections. *Med. Lett. Drug Ther.* 24:5, 1982.

Gilles, H.M. Clinical features and treatment of intestinal nematodes. *Trop. Doc.* 8:62, 1978.

CHAPTER
26.5

CHEMOTHERAPY OF TISSUE NEMATODES

G. Thomas Strickland and Edgar A. Steck

Nematodes inhabiting extraintestinal tissues of humans include the *Filariae* , the Guinea worm, *Trichinella*,and larvae of several other species normally parasitic in animals, such as the dog and cat hookworms and ascarides.

Filariasis is widespread, affecting in its various forms about 300 million people throughout the world. *Wuchereria bancrofti, Brugia malayi* , and *B. timori* , transmitted by mosquitoes, infect 250 million people, mainly in West, Central, and East Africa, Egypt, the Malagasy Republic, the Indian subcontinent, Southeast Asia, China, the Philippines, Indonesia, and some other Pacific islands and South America. The adult worms live in the lymphatic vessels and lymph nodes, obstructing the flow of lymph, causing inflammation and swelling (elephantiasis) of the arms, legs, and genitals.

Loa loa , another filarial parasite, is transmitted by the bite of the *Tabanid* fly (a horsefly). Loiasis is prevalent in Cameroon, the Congo, southern Nigeria, and Zaire. Adult worms move about in the subcutaneous tissues, producing characteristic Calabar swellings, and sometimes cross the cornea.

Onchocerciasis, or river blindness, is transmitted by the bite of the blackfly (*Simulium* species). This is the most important human filarial disease, with an estimated 30 or 40 million people infected in West, Central, and East Africa, and Yemen as well as Mexico, Central America, and northern South America. Because the blackfly breeds only in fast-flowing water and the parasite develops in the fly only at a temperature of 18°C or above, transmission occurs only in hot tropical regions with fast-flowing rivers. Onchocerciasis is manifested by various skin and eye lesions, the latter frequently progressing to blindness. In some African villages, over half of the adult males are blind. The adult worms produce characteristic nodules in the subcutaneous tissues. Each female produces thousands of microfilariae that are believed to cause the majority of the skin and eye pathology by direct invasion.

Other tissue-invasive human nematode infections are not as prevalent as the filariae. Dracunculiasis, Guinea worm infection, is highly endemic in some areas of tropical Africa and India and sporadic in Arabia and central Asia. Humans become infected from drinking water containing infected copepods, *cyclops* sp, the intermediate host.

Trichinosis, although rare now in the United States, is worldwide in distribution, occurring wherever pork is eaten. Undercooked meat contaminated with viable infectious larvae is the means of transmission. The most significant reservoir of human infection is the hog, although infections have occurred following the ingestion of wildlife (e.g., bush pig and bear).

Cutaneous larva migrans caused by infection with dog and cat hookworms is worldwide in distribution and relatively common in the southeastern United States. Toxocariasis, the most common form of visceral larva migrans, caused by human infection with dog and cat ascarides, is also worldwide in distribution. Many infections are either asymptomatic or not diagnosed. Other animal nematode infections occasionally occurring in humans are gnathostomiasis and angiostrongyliasis.

The treatment of tissue nematode infections is generally unsatisfactory. In some situations, therapeutic efficacy is uncertain (e.g., treatment of ocular onchocerciasis and toxocariasis). In others, such as Bancroftian filariasis, only the microfilariae can be effectively and safely treated because adult worms are relatively resistant to chemotherapy. In tissue nematode infections, the pathophysiological changes are caused more by the immune response to the parasite than by the parasite itself. Therefore, therapeutic principles should include methods of reducing inflammation (e.g., the use of corticosteroids). This is most important when specific therapy kills the parasite. The response to antigens released by dying parasites can cause severe immune reactions, which can be serious, especially when occurring in the eyes. Several of the drugs used to treat human tissue nematode infections (i.e., niridazole and thiabendazole) are partially effective because of their immunosuppressive properties. With the exception of diethylcarbamazine, these drugs are covered in other chapters.

DRUGS USED FOR TREATING TISSUE NEMATODES

DIETHYLCARBAMAZINE

Diethylcarbamazine resulted from detailed investigations of piperazine derivatives for anthelmintic activity. It has been extensively used to treat filariae and other tissue-invasive nematodes in both human and veterinary medicine.

Source and Chemistry. Diethylcarbamazine, a piperazine derivative (4-diethylcarbamyl-1-methylpiperazine), has the following chemical structure and is available as a dicitrate salt:

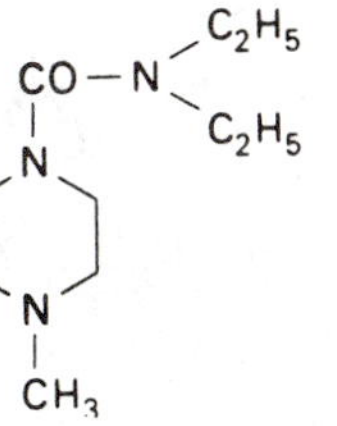

Diethylcarbamazine

It is soluble in water, colorless, and has an unpleasant sweet taste.

Anthelmintic Action. Diethylcarbamazine is inactive against microfilariae *in vitro*. *In vivo*, however, it causes the microfilariae of *W. bancrofti, B. malayi*, and *L. loa* to rapidly disappear from the circulation. It kills microfilariae of *O. volvulus* in the skin but not in nodules. The drug is believed to make the parasites more susceptible to the host's humoral and cellular immunological responses. It has considerable action against adult worms of *W. bancrofti, B. malayi*, and *L. loa*, but has little effect upon adult *O. volvulus*. Its macrofilaricidal action is believed to be greater against *Brugia* than against *Wuchereria* .

Pharmacological Effects . High doses in animals have caused convulsions, increased respiration rate and vomiting secondary to central nervous system stimulation, and increased blood pressure associated with tachycardia and peripheral vasoconstriction. Diethylcarbamazine also has some antiinflammatory effects.

Pharmacokinetics. Diethylcarbamazine is absorbed readily from the gastrointestinal tract, with peak blood levels occurring about 3 hr after ingestion. Most of the drug and its metabolites are excreted in the urine within 24 hr. Approximately 15% is recovered unchanged, 50% is excreted as the 4-oxide, and 25% as 1-ethylcarbamyl-4-methylpiperazine.

Detailed studies of the distribution of the drug have been performed for guidance in selecting the most appropriate treatment schedule. It has been shown to accumulate in the kidneys and liver and penetrate readily into hydrocele fluid. Otherwise, it is distributed almost uniformly throughout the body and has minimal accumulation following repeated doses.

Adverse Effects . Toxic effects are more frequent and greater in infected than in noninfected individuals. Side effects to the drug itself are occasional anorexia, nausea, vomiting, headache, drowsiness, malaise, weakness, and arthralgias. Reactions due to its filaricidal action are greatest in patients being treated for onchocerciasis: pruritus of skin and eyes, eye pain, photophobia, lacrimation, conjunctival and cutaneous edema, chills, restlessness, sweating, cough, syncope, fever, malaise, headache, joint and muscle pains, tachycardia, hypotension, tachypnea, increased skin temperature, enlargement and tenderness of lymph nodes and along the course of lymphatics, and, rarely, pneumonia and death (5). There is usually an initial leukocytosis with an increase in the eosinophilia that occurs in these infections. These symptoms usually occur within 24 hr of treatment and last for 3-7 days. The nodules are sites of alive and dead worms with resulting surrounding tissue reaction. Particular difficulties occur with patients having ocular onchocercal lesions. The concomitant use of corticosteroids usually reduces the worst reactions associated with diethylcarbamazine therapy. In some cases of loiasis, an allergic encephalitis occurs with treatment, whereas patients with Bancroftian and Malayan filariasis generally have similar but less severe reactions than patients with onchocerciasis. They have fewer eye symptoms, and they almost invariably have lymphangitis, lymphadenitis, and/or lymph node abscesses due to death of immature or adult worms in the lymphatics. The presence of the reaction following diethylcarbamazine has been used as presumptive evidence of infection.

Preparations. Diethylcarbamazine citrate (HETRAZAN, BANOCIDE) is available as 50-mg tablets. In the treatment of *W. bancrofti, B. malayi, B. timori, L. loa*, and tropical eosinophilia, a frequently used dosage regimen is following: a 50-mg test dose on day 1, 50 mg three times daily on day 2, 100 mg three times daily on day 3, and 4-6 mg/kg/day given in three divided doses from day 4 for up to 21 days.

The course of diethylcarbamazine is generally considered to be 36 mg/kg in Brugian filariasis and 72 mg/kg in Bancroftian filariasis. This can also be given as 6 mg/kg/day over 6 consecutive days (for the former) or over 12 consecutive days (for the latter). It is best to give a 50- or 100-mg test dose initially. Courses of 7 days are generally given for treating onchocerciasis (Table 26.5-1), although some use the same dosage schedule as is used for treating Bancroftian filariasis. If the patient has a severe reaction to the drug, subsequent doses are withheld temporarily. It is used with care in treating patients with ocular onchocerciasis, often initially given at half dosage and with local and/or systemic corticosteroid coverage. Suramin sodium (Chapter 26.2) is often also used to kill adult *Onchocerca*.

TREATMENT OF FILARIASIS

Diethylcarbamazine is the only approved effective drug for treating infections with *W. bancrofti* (25), *B. malayi* (25), *B. timori* (22), *L.loa* (25), and tropical eosinophilia (Table 26.5- 1). The latter symptom complex (i.e., cough, wheezing, dyspnea, pulmonary infiltration on chest x-ray, and hypereosinophilia) is believed to be caused by occult infections with human or animal filariae.

Diethylcarbamazine is active against microfilariae and may kill or sterilize some adult worms. Repeat courses may be necessary (25). *B. malayi* appears to be more susceptible to the drug than *W. bancrofti*. Patients having tropical eosinophilia who are successfully treated with diethylcarbamazine have reductions in their peripheral blood eosinophilia, a reduced cough, and an improved chest x-ray.

Diethylcarbamazine treatment usually leads to a flare-up in symptoms, probably due to the immunological response to increased parasite antigens released by dying microfilariae and macrofilariae. Special caution should

Table 26.5-1
Chemotherapy of Tissue Nematodes

Disease	Recommended Drug	Adult Dose	Route	Alternative Drug	Adult Dose	Route
Bancroftian filariasis	diethylcarbamazine[a,b]	day 1, 50 mg day 2, 50 mg t.i.d.	p.o.	none		
Malayan filariasis		day 3, 100 mg t.i.d. days 4-21, 2 mg/kg t.i.d.		none		
Tropical eosinophilia		[some prefer shorter course (e.g., 7-14 days)		none		
Loiasis		particularly for Malayan filariasis, tropical eosinophilia, and loiasis]		none		
Onchocerciasis (river blindness)	diethylcarbamazine[a,b] (kills microfilariae) and	day 1, 50 mg day 2, 100 mg, b.i.d. day 3-7, 200 mg, b.i.d.	p.o.	surgical removal of nodules		
	suramin sodium[a,c] (kills adult worms)	100-200 mg (test dose) then 1 g weekly for 6 weeks	i.v.			
Dracunculiasis (Guinea worm)	metronidazole[d]	250-500 mg t.i.d. x 5-10 days	p.o.	niridazole[a,d]	25 mg/kg b.i.d. (max. 1.5 g) 7 - 10 days	p.o.
Trichinosis	thiabendazole	25 mg/kg b.i.d. x 5-7 days	p.o.	salicylates or corticosteroids	600 mg q. 4 hr p.r.n. 30-40 mg prednisone q.d. x 3-5 days, then reduce dose	p.o.
Cutaneous larva migrans (creeping eruption)	thiabendazole	applied topically		thiabendazole	25 mg/kg b.i.d. x 2 days	p.o.
Toxocariasis (visceral larva migrans)	thiabendazole	25 mg/kg b.i.d. x 5 days	p.o.	corticosteroids	30-40 mg prednisone q.d. x 3-5 days, then reduce dose	p.o.

[a]For availability of these drugs from the Center for Disease Control, see Table 26 -1.
[b]Severe skin and eye reactions frequently occur. Therefore, the initial lower dosage is recommended. With severe reactions, corticosteroids may be indicated (ophthalmic corticosteroids for eye reactions).
[c]Preferable to treat only patients with skin disease or eye involvement, and after diethylcarbamazine has been used.
[d]Protruding worms should be removed by slowly rolling them onto a small stick.

be taken in treating *L. loa*, as an encephalopathy may be provoked. Corticosteroids may be required to reduce the allergic response.

Levamisole (Chapter 26.4) also has microfilaricidal and macrofilaricidal actions (16). It has been evaluated at different dose schedules in Malayan aborigines infected with *W. bancrofti, B. malayi*, or both parasites. The most effective dosage was 100 mg initially, followed by 100 mg twice daily for 10 days. All six treated with this dosage became amicrofilaremic. Drug toxicity was common, with fever occurring in 60% of those treated with levamisole.

The therapeutic end point should be a 90-95% reduction in microfilaremia and a relief from symptoms if they were present before treatment. Treatment is not usually recommended for individuals positive for blood microfilariae of *Dipetalonema perstans* and *Mansonella ozzardi*, as pathogenicity has not been confirmed and no effective therapy is known (4). However, *Dipetalonema streptocerca* infections cause dermatitis and respond to diethylcarbamazine at the dosage used for treating filariasis or onchocerciasis (18).

TREATMENT OF ONCHOCERCIASIS

Diethylcarbamazine kills the microfilariae of *O. volvulus* but has little effect on the adult worms (1,24) (Table 26.5-1). A few hours following the first dose, a sharp febrile reaction, rash, and pruritus frequently occur. This is believed to be caused by mass destruction of microfilariae and is used as a provocative test (1,2,5). Because of this reaction, smaller initial test doses of diethylcarbamazine are recommended for patients with onchocerciasis, as well as filariasis and loiasis. When microfilariae can be seen or are thought to be in the eye, concurrent corticosteroids are recommended during the first few days of diethylcarbamazine therapy. This is to reduce the inflammatory reaction around dying larvae (1,2).

When treating onchocerciasis, diethylcarbamazine should be used, and in most mild infections no other therapy may be necessary. This drug can be repeated if subsequent skin snips become positive or if surgical removal of nodules (containing adult worms) does not relieve symptoms. In heavily infected cases prone to visual complications, suramin sodium may be given following diethylcarbamazine to destroy the adult worms (1,6,12,24). Severe onchocerciasis should be treated with diethylcarbamazine under steroid cover to eliminate the microfilariae. The adult worms can then be treated with suramin (1,2,12,14). Suramin sodium is a very toxic drug, and it must be used with the patient under close medical supervision (Chapter 26.2). Both immediate and delayed adverse reactions occur. The more common immediate reaction includes nausea and vomiting, collapse, and abdominal colic. Later reactions during the first 24 hrs include fever, photophobia, abdominal distension and constipation, and cutaneous hyperesthesia of the soles or palms. Of the reactions occurring after several days, renal toxicity is the most common. Exfoliative dermatitis, stomatitis, and jaundice rarely occur, whereas generalized weakness is rather common. Allergic reactions associated with parasite death also occur rather frequently. The urine should be checked for albumin before each course of suramin (12). The long-term effects of suramin on the eye lesions are still uncertain; optic atrophy may be more frequent in infected patients treated with suramin.

Diethylcarbamazine has been applied to the skin in the treatment of onchocerciasis in an attempt to reduce toxicity. However, when compared with orally administered drug, not only is topically administered diethylcarbamazine less effective, it is also more toxic (23). The microfilaricidal effects of topically applied diethylcarbamazine (13) and levamisole (14) in the cornea look promising. Metrifonate (Chapter 26.6) also causes toxic allergic reactions and reduces microfilarial counts in skin snips from patients with onchocerciasis (3). It is not, however, as effective as diethylcarbamazine.

TREATMENT OF DRACONTIASIS

Niridazole (15), metronidazole (15,20,21), and thiabendazole (19) have all been reported to accelerate relief from pain, the healing of ulcers, and the expulsion of Guinea worms (Table 26.5- 1). The ancient method of wrapping the worm around a stick and removing it slowly over several days is still very popular.

TREATMENT OF TRICHINOSIS

Specific treatment for the tissue stage of *T. spiralis* infection is still unproved. Thiabendazole will eliminate adult worms in the intestine but has little effect on the larvae in muscle (7) that cause most of the clinical symptoms (i.e., fever, headache, myositis, periorbital edema, rash, myocarditis, convulsions, and hypereosinophilia) (Table 26.5-1). It has an antiinflammatory effect (7). Salicylates are also recommended, whereas corticosteroids can be given to treat more severe infections (8). Mebendazole (Chapter 26.4) reduced the number of larvae developing in experimentally infected mice and should be evaluated in human infections (17).

TREATMENT OF CUTANEOUS LARVA MIGRANS AND VISCERAL LARVA MIGRANS

Thiabendazole has some value in the therapy of both cutaneous larva migrans (9) and toxocariasis (9,26), partially due to its antiinflammatory activity (7) (Table 26.5-1). It is effective in treating creeping eruption when applied topically to the skin as a suspension three to six times daily for up to 3 weeks (10,11). Ethyl chloride spray or locally applied carbon dioxide snow is not as efficacious. Diethylcarbamazine has also been recommended for treatment of toxocariasis at a dosage of 2 mg/kg three times daily for 30 days. In severe infections, and when treating eye lesions, the antiinflammatory action of corticosteroids is helpful.

TREATMENT OF ANGIOSTRONGYLIASIS AND GNATHOSTOMIASIS

Angiostrongyliasis is an eosinophilic meningoencephalitis in the Far East and Eastern Pacific and an acute abdominal infection with eosinophilia in Costa Rica and Honduras. Gnathostomiasis is one of the larva migrans infections, principally occurring in the Far East. It has been frequently reported as an eosinophilic myeloencephalitis in Thailand, with involvement of the spinal cord. Little is known about the therapeutic efficacy of drugs for treating these two infections. Salicylates and corticosteroids may be used to reduce inflammation and headache. Thiabendazole (9) and diethylcarbamazine have been used as well.

REFERENCES

1. Anderson, J., and Fuglsang, H. Ocular onchocerciasis. *Trop. Dis. Bull.* 74:257, 1977.
2. Anderson, J., and Fuglsang, H. Further studies on the treatment of ocular onchocerciasis with diethylcarbamazine and suramin. *Br. J. Ophthalmol.* 62:450, 1978.
3. Awadzi, K., and Gilles, H.M. The chemotherapy of onchocerciasis: Further trials with metrifonate. *Ann. Trop. Med. Parasitol.* 74:355, 1980.
4. Bartholomew, C.F., Nathan, M.B., and Tikasingh, E.S. The failure of diethylcarbamazine in the treatment of *Mansonella ozzardi* infections. *Trans. R. Soc. Trop. Med. Hyg.* 72:423, 1978.
5. Bryceson, A.D.M., Warrell, D.A., and Pope, H.M. Dangerous reactions to treatment of onchocerciasis with diethylcarbamazine. *Br. Med. J.* 1:742, 1977.
6. Budden, F.H. The natural history of ocular onchocerciasis over a period of 14-15 years and the effect of this on a single course of suramin therapy. *Trans. R. Soc. Trop. Med. Hyg.* 70:484, 1976.
7. Campbell, W.C. Anti-inflammatory and analgesic properties of thiabendazole. *JAMA* 216:2143, 1971.
8. Campbell, W.C., and Blair, L.S. Chemotherapy of *Trichinella spiralis* infections (a review). *Exp. Parasitol.* 35:304, 1974.
9. Campbell, W.C., and Cuckler, A.C. Thiabendazole in the treatment and control of parasitic infections in man. *Tex. Rep. Biol. Med.* 27 (Suppl. 2):665, 1969.

10. Davis, C.M., and Israel, R.M. Treatment of creeping eruption with topical thiabendazole. *Arch. Dermatol.* 97:325, 1968.
11. Goldsmith, J.M., and Froese, E.H. A note on cutaneous larva migrans and its treatment with topical thiabendazole. *Cent. Afr. J. Med.* 23:250, 1977.
12. Hawking, F. Suramin: With special reference to onchocerciasis. *Adv. Pharmacol. Chemother.* 15:289, 1978.
13. Jones, B.R., Anderson, J., and Fuglsang, H. Effects of various concentrations of diethylcarbamazine citrate applied as eye drops in ocular onchocerciasis, and the possibilities of improved therapy from continuous non-pulsed delivery. *Br. J. Ophthalmol.* 62:428, 1978.
14. Jones, B.R., Anderson, J., and Fuglsang, H. Evaluation of microfilaricidal effects in the corneas from topically applied drugs in ocular onchocerciasis: Trials with levamisole and mebendazole. *Br. J. Ophthalmol.* 62:440, 1978.
15. Kale, O.O. A controlled field trial of the treatment of dracontiasis with metronidazole and niridazole. *Ann. Trop. Med. Parasitol.* 68:91, 1974.
16. Mak, J.W., and Zaman, V. Drug trials with levamisole hydrochloride and diethylcarbamazine citrate in Bancroftian and Malayan filariasis. *Trans. R. Soc. Trop. Med. Hyg.* 74:286, 1980.
17. McCracken, R.O., and Taylor, D.D. Mebendazole therapy of parenteral trichinellosis. *Science* 207:1220, 1980.
18. Meyers, W.M., Moris, R., Neafie, R.C., Connor, D.H., and Bourland, J. Streptocerciasis: Degeneration of adult *Dipetalonema streptocerca* in man following diethylcarbamazine therapy. *Am. J. Trop. Med. Hyg.* 27:1137, 1978.
19. Muller, R. The possible mode of action of some chemotherapeutic agents in Guinea worm diseases. *Trans. R. Soc. Trop. Med. Hyg.*65:843, 1971.
20. Padonu, K.O. A controlled trial of metronidazole in the treatment of dracontiasis in Nigeria. *Am. J. Trop. Med. Hyg.* 22:42, 1973.
21. Pardanani, D.S., Trivedi, V.D., Joshi, L.G., et al. Metronidazole (Flagyl) in dracunculiasis: A double blind study. *Ann. Trop. Med. Parasitol.* 71:45, 1977.
22. Partono, F., Purnomo, and Soewarta, A. A simple method to control *Brugia timori* by diethylcarbamazine administration. *Trans. R. Soc. Trop. Med. Hyg.* 73:536, 1979.
23. Taylor, H.R., Greene, B.M., and Langham, M.E. Controlled clinical trial of oral and topical diethylcarbamazine in treatment of onchocerciasis. *Lancet* 1:943, 1980.
24. Thylfors, B. Ocular onchocerciasis. *Bull. WHO* 56:63, 1978.
25. WHO Expert Committee on Filariasis. Third report. *WHO Tech. Rep. Ser. no.* 542, 1974.
26. Wiseman, R.A., Woodruff, A.W., and Pettitt, L.E. The treatment of toxocarial infection: Some experimental and clinical observations. *Trans. R. Soc. Trop. Med. Hyg.* 65:591, 1971.

CHAPTER
26.6

CHEMOTHERAPY OF CESTODE AND TREMATODE INFECTIONS

G. Thomas Strickland and Edgar A. Steck

Greater than 300 million people are infected with tapeworms or flukes. The distribution of these diseases in humans is worldwide, and the pathophysiology associated with the infections ranges from minimal or no symptoms to severe debilitating disease. Some infections (e.g., clonorchiasis, opisthorchiasis, and paragonimiasis) are geographically localized, being limited by eating habits. Others (e.g., schistosomiasis), being transmitted by contact with water, have a wider distribution. Infections with these agents range from minor importance [e.g., *Hymenolepis nana* (dwarf tapeworm) infection] to one of the five most important human medical problems, schistosomiasis.

DRUGS USED FOR TREATING CESTODES AND TREMATODES

BITHIONOL

Bithionol is used more in veterinary medicine for treatment of animal tapeworm infections than in human medicine. More recently developed compounds have greater chemotherapeutic efficacy with less toxicity for treating human cestode infections. Bithionol, however, is still used for the treatment of the trematode infections, paragonimiasis and fascioliasis.

Source and Chemistry. Bithionol is a member of a phenolic compound series (Fig. 26.6-1), used as antimicrobial agents, soaps, and sanitary chemicals.

Anthelmintic Action. Bithionol acts against cestodes and trematodes in a complex manner to damage the epithelium and interfere with biochemical processes of the worms. With cestodes, especially, it interferes with production of adenosine triphosphatases. The flukes are dependent upon succinate dehydrogenase, the enzyme responsible for conversion of fumarate into succinate. Bithionol both inhibits that enzyme system and intrudes upon oxidative phosphorylation of the trematodes. Bithionol has prompt destructive effects upon the cuticle and intestinal epithelium of young *Fasciola hepatica* worms.

Pharmacokinetics. Bithionol undergoes metabolic transformation, especially in the liver, to give the corresponding sulfoxide and some of the sulfone. The sulfoxide has greater anthelmintic effects than the parent sulfide and has been marketed itself. Unchanged bithionol is excreted chiefly in the bile in the form of the glucuronide, and excretion of the drug and its transformation products occurs principally in the feces.

Adverse Effects. Bithionol is ordinarily administered after fasting, thereby accentuating some of its gastrointestinal side effects. It frequently causes anorexia, nausea, vomiting, diarrhea, and abdominal pain. Other less common side effects include headache, dizziness, and skin rashes (e.g., urticaria and photosensitivity). Extremely high doses lead to symptoms similar to those of phenol poisoning, including central nervous system stimulation with tremors, hypotensive shock due to direct myocardial depression, and hepatic toxicity.

Preparations. *Bithionol* (BITIN) is available in the United States from the Centers for Disease Control in Atlanta, Geor-

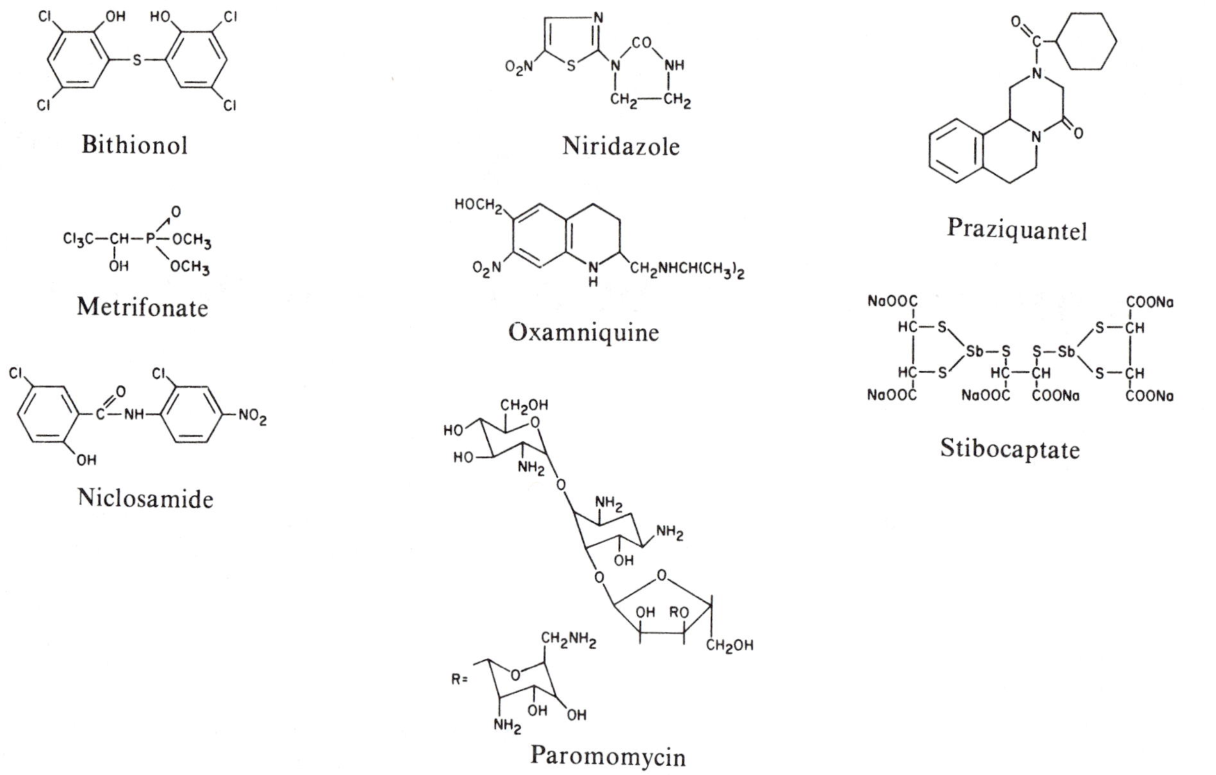

Bithionol

Niridazole

Praziquantel

Metrifonate

Oxamniquine

Stibocaptate

Niclosamide

Paromomycin

Fig. 26.6-1. *Drugs used in treating cestode and trematode infections.*

gia, as 250 mg tablets. In treating *Paragonimus* and *Fasciola* fluke infections, the oral dose of bithionol is 30-50 mg/kg, given on alternate days, for a course of 10-15 doses (Table 26.6-1).

METRIFONATE

Metrifonate is an organophosphorus compound, introduced in 1969, that has antischistosomal effects only against *Schistosoma haematobium* infections. It is an unusual example of an insecticidal compound that has been found to be safe for human use despite the fact that it is a cholinesterase inhibitor. Metrifonate has therapeutic effects against other helminth infections, including hookworm, ascariasis, trichuriasis, filariasis, onchocerciasis, and cutaneous larva migrans. It is an orally effective, inexpensive drug that causes few side effects, even in children.

Source and Chemistry. The insecticidal effectiveness of organophosphorus compounds is dependent upon inhibition of cholinesterase. The structural characteristics of these compounds' selectivity inhibits enzymes. Among the compounds investigated, the most satisfactory balance between host and parasite toxicity was a compound used to protect plants from insects (Fig. 26.6-1), first given the generic name trichlophone, but later changed to metrifonate.

Anthelmintic Action. It is presumed that the anthelmintic effects of metrifonate are based upon its action as an organophosphorus-type cholinesterase inhibitor. The compound has an inhibitory action *in vitro* on the cholinesterases of both *S. haematobium* and *S. mansoni* There is no therapeutic efficacy in treating *S. mansoni* infections, however. Immature parasites are minimally affected by doses of the drug having marked schistosomicidal effects on adults. The host immune response may play a role in destruction of the parasites.

Pharmacological Effects. Metrifonate is relatively free of toxicity from increasing acetylcholine in the body. Therapeutic doses of the drug cause inhibition of both plasma and erythrocyte cholinesterase. Although there is greater inhibition in the former enzyme, recovery of activity to normal levels is more prompt than with erythrocyte cholinesterase. Metrifonate has minimal parasympathetic effects.

Pharmacokinetics. Metrifonate is readily taken up in lipids and may be better absorbed if taken with food. It and its active components' (dichlorvos) plasma levels peak at 1-1.5 hr following the oral administration of a therapeutic dose. The drop in erythrocyte and plasma cholinesterase activity occurs early and persists for several days.

Adverse Effects. At therapeutic doses, toxic effects of metrifonate rarely appear as more than minimal gastrointestinal intolerance (i.e., nausea, vomiting, abdominal pain, diarrhea). It may also cause weakness, headache, dizziness, vertigo, and dyspnea from bronchospasm. Extensive trials on infected children have revealed little toxicity, even among populations having a high incidence of hereditary enzyme deficiencies. Metrifonate may cause minimal, transient alterations in the electrocardiogram and a rise in serum bilirubin. Effects on plasma and erythrocyte cholinesterase have been noted. It appears to transiently alter sperm counts, decreasing numbers and increasing abnormal forms. However, metrifonate has not been shown to cause testicular damage. Toxic doses may require administration of cholinesterase reactivators to prevent metabolites or the drug itself from causing a dangerous decrease in cholinesterase levels.

Preparations. Metrifonate (BILARCIL) is available in the form of scored 100-mg tablets outside of the United States. The usual regimen for treatment of *S. haematobium* infections is administration of 7.5-10 mg/kg at fortnightly to monthly intervals for a maximum of three doses (Table 26.6-1). Metrifonate should not be given at shorter intervals, as problems related to prolonged depression of cholinesterase might occur. It has efficacy as a chemoprophylactic against *S. haematobium* infections and also has minimal activity against the microfilariae of *Onchocerca volvulus*.

NICLOSAMIDE

Niclosamide is a salicylamide derivative that has a broad profile of effectiveness against cestodes. Included among tapeworm infections for which its use has been recommended are: *Taenia saginata* (beef tapeworm); *T. solium* (pork tapeworm); *Diphyllobothrium latum* (fish tapeworm); and the dwarf tapeworm (*H. nana*). Niclosamide is also an alternate drug for treatment of the intestinal fluke infections, fasciolopsiasis and heterophyiasis, which are caused by *Fasciolopsis buski* and *H. heterophyes*.

Source and Chemistry. Niclosamide, a salicylamide (Fig. 26.6-1), is a yellowish white tasteless and odorless powder that is insoluble in water.

Anthelmintic Action. Niclosamide inhibits oxidative phosphorylation in cestode mitochondria. It stimulates oxygen uptake by *H. diminuta* at low concentrations, but respiration is inhibited and glucose uptake is blocked at higher concentrations. The scolex and proximal segments of the tapeworm are killed and digested.

Table 26.6-1
Chemotherapy of Cestodes (Tapeworms) and Trematodes (Flukes)

Parasite	Recommended Drug	Adult Dose	Route	Alternative Drug	Adult Dose	Route
Diphyllobothrium latum, *Taenia saginata*, *Taenia solium*	niclosamide[a,b]	Four tablets (2 g) chewed thoroughly in single dose	p.o.	paromomycin	1 g q. 15 min x four doses	p.o.
Hymenolepis nana	niclosamide[a,b]	Four tablets (2 g) chewed in single dose q.d. x 5 days	p.o.	paromomycin	40-50 mg/kg once/day x 5-7 days	p.o.
Echinococcus granulosus	mebendazole	40-50 mg/kg/day t.i.d. x 30 days, may repeat if necessary	p.o.	surgical removal		
Schistosoma mansoni	oxamniquine[b,c]	15 mg/kg once	p.o.	niridazole[a]	25 mg/kg/day (maximum 1.5 g) x 6-8 days	p.o.
Schistosoma haematobium	metrifonate[a,b]	10 mg/kg q. 2-4 weeks (maximum 3 doses)	p.o.	niridazole[a]	25 mg/kg/day (maximum 1.5 g) x 5-7 days	p.o.
Schistosoma japonicum	praziquantel[b]	30 mg/kg twice in one day	p.o.	niridazole[a]	25 mg/kg/day (maximum 1.5 g) x 8-10 days	p.o.
Clonorchis sinensis	praziquantel[b]	25 mg/kg t.i.d. for one day	p.o.	see text		
Paragonimus sp	bithionol[a,b]	30-50 mg/kg/day b.i.d. on alternate days x 10-15 doses	p.o.	see text		
Fasciola hepatica				dehydro-emetine[a] or emetine[a]	1 mg/kg (maximum 65 mg) every other day x 12-15 doses	i.m.
Fasciolopsis buski	tetrachloro-ethylene[b]	0.1 mg/kg (maximum 5 mg) in single dose on empty stomach	p.o.	niclosamide[a]	four tablets (2 g) chewed thoroughly in single dose after a light meal	p.o.

[a] For availability of these drugs from the Center for Disease Control, see Table 26-1.

[b] Praziquantel will be the recommended drug when it is available.

[c] In children, a larger dose (20 mg/kg) has been suggested. In patients contracting their disease in Egypt, Sudan, and East and South Africa, a larger dose of 20 mg/kg given once daily on three successive days is recommended.

Pharmacokinetics. Almost no niclosamide is absorbed following oral administration.

Adverse Effects. Niclosamide has almost no side effects, only occasional minimal malaise, anorexia, nausea, and abdominal discomfort.

Preparations. Niclosamide (NICLOCIDE) is available as 500-mg chewable tablets. For adults having taeniasis, the dose is four tablets (2 g) chewed thoroughly (Table 26.6-1). For treating dwarf tapeworm infections, the same regimen is repeated on 5 consecutive days. Children weighing 10-35 kg are treated with two tablets (1 g), and those greater than 35 kg are given three tablets (1.5 g).

NIRIDAZOLE

Niridazole a heterocyclic nitro compound with therapeutic action against all three human schistosomal species, the Guinea worm, and ameba, was developed following the observation that nitrothiazole derivatives have antiparasitic effects.

Source and Chemistry. Niridazole is a synthesized nitrothiazole derivative having both an imidazole and urea structure in a fused ring (Fig. 26.6-1). Studies on the nitroimidazoles have shown this combination to have structure activity relationships. It is a yellow crystalline powder that is odorless and tasteless and nearly insoluble in water.

Anthelmintic Action. Niridazole is selectively taken up by the schistosome worms and their ova. The female worm is most sensitive to effects of the drug; eggshell formation is inhibited by small doses, and the ovary is decreased in size. Spermatogenesis is halted and the testes of male worms are affected only by high doses. Female worms are destroyed by leukocytic infiltration and autolysis in the host's liver, whereas male worms are immobilized by tissue reaction and eventually undergo autolysis. The actual mechanism by which niridazole adversely affects schistosomes is unknown.

Pharmacological Effects. Niridazole has both *in vitro* and *in vivo* amebicidal activity. Its other pharmacological actions are all toxicities, with the exception of its immunosuppressive effects that may account for some of its therapeutic efficacy, particularly in the treatment of Guinea worm infection. It is a potent and long-acting suppressor of cell-mediated immune responses.

Pharmacokinetics. Niridazole is slowly, but almost completely, absorbed from the gastrointestinal tract following oral administration. Metabolic transformations occur in the liver with the reduction products including the nitroso, hydroxylamino, and amino compounds. The parent compound and breakdown products are bound to plasma proteins, accounting for high blood levels. They are also uniformly distributed throughout the body. The antischistosomal and antiamebic activities of niridazole are not shared by its metabolites. Therefore, the therapeutic efficacy and side effects of the drug are not dependent upon the functional integrity of the liver. The drug is eliminated equally in the urine and feces (by way of the bile). urine becomes dark in color and there is an unpleasant body odor.

Adverse Effects. Niridazole is a relatively toxic drug. Anorexia, nausea, vomiting, abdominal cramps, dizziness, and headache occur frequently. Occasional complications include diarrhea, rash, insomnia, paresthesias, and changes in the electrocardiogram. Rarer and more serious toxicities include changes in the electroencephalogram, psychosis, convulsions, and hemolytic anemia in patients with glucose-6-phosphate dehydrogenase (G-6-PD) deficiencies. Niridazole transiently reduces spermatogenesis and has been shown to be mutagenic and carcinogenic in laboratory animals. EEG changes, agitation, confusion and auditory hallucinations, and convulsions are more common in patients with portal hypertension and/or hepatic dysfunction and occur more frequently in adults than in children.

Preparations. Niridazole (AMBILHAR) is not available in the United States. It is supplied as 500-mg scored tablets. For treating schistosomiasis, it is used orally for both adults and children at a dosage of 25 mg/kg (maximum 1.5 g) for 5-10 days in either one or two daily doses (Table 26.6-1). It is more effective in children than in adults and is more effective in treating *S. haematobium* than *S. mansoni* or *S. japonicum* infections. Therefore, the shorter course would be recommended for treating children with *S. haematobium* infections, whereas the longer course would be needed in treating adults with *S. japonicum* infections. Because portacaval shunting due to schistosomal hepatic fibrosis leads to increased central nervous system toxicity, it is often difficult to use niridazole to treat adults with *S. mansoni* and *S. japonicum* infections. Niridazole is contraindicated in the presence of hepatocellular disease, portal hypertension, or in patients with a history of mental disorders or seizures. Because of its mutagenic effects, niridazole should not be given to pregnant women.

Niridazole has been replaced by more effective and less toxic drugs for treating amebiasis. For the treatment of dracunculiasis, niridazole has been given at the same daily dose as used in treating schistosomiasis for a 7- to 15-day course.

OXAMNIQUINE

Oxamniquine is an antischistosomal drug that has excellent therapeutic efficacy and almost no toxicity in treating *S. mansoni* infections. It is ineffective for treating either *S. haematobium* or *S. japonicum* infections.

Source and Chemistry. Oxamniquine (Fig. 26.6-1) is the active metabolite among a series of tetrahydroquinolines screened for antischistosomal activity in experimental animals infected with *S. mansoni*. It is a yellow-orange crystalline solid that is almost insoluble in water. It is produced by an oxidative fermentation process carried out on an intermediate compound made by a complicated synthesis.

Anthelmintic Action. Oxamniquine is active against *S. mansoni*, both *in vitro* and *in vivo*. Studies in animals have shown that following treatment, the adult worm population shifts from the mesenteric veins into the liver. This occurs as early as 2 days after treatment, but the majority of worms shifted between the fourth and fifth day. The shift was irreversible for the male worms. Some female worms survived treatment and shifted back to the mesentery during the second week. Oviposition ceased within 48 hr after treatment. Male worms were more susceptible to oxamniquine, and the surviving females did not lay eggs. There were strain differences in dose responses; an East African strain required 50% greater dose to eradicate 99% of the males than a Puerto Rican strain of *S. mansoni*. Oxamniquine has some activity against immature *S. mansoni* larvae, since treatment during the prepatent period reduced eventual worm loads as well as tissue egg loads.

Pharmacological Effects. Oxamniquine has almost no pharmacological actions other than its effects upon *S. mansoni* worms. Intravenous doses of 50 mg/kg in humans have caused behavioral changes, respiratory depression, akinesia, and increased irritability.

Pharmacokinetics. Studies in both experimental animals and humans have shown that the drug is well absorbed after either oral or intramuscular administration. Human plasma concentrations reach a peak at 1-1.5 hr following oral administration of therapeutic doses. The plasma half-life is 1.5-2.5 hr. The drug is best administered in a fasting state, since prior food delays and reduces serum concentrations. It is rapidly and extensively metabolized by the liver into inactive acidic metabolites, which are largely excreted in the urine within the first 12 hr. There are no apparent racial differences in the metabolism of oxamniquine.

Adverse Effects. The most frequent side effects associated with oxamniquine therapy are dizziness and drowsiness, both of which are usually mild and transient. Other side effects include headache, anorexia, nausea, vomiting, abdominal pain, diarrhea, and urticaria. The drug colors the urine orange. Rare complications are hallucinations, psychic excitement, and convulsions. A 1-to 4-day episode of fever, eosinophilia, pulmonary infiltrates, and transient elevations in serum enzymes, sometimes occurring 4-7 days after initiating therapy, is probably the host's response to dying worms (20).

Preparations. Oxamniquine (VANSIL) is marketed as 250-mg capsules and a syrup containing 50 mg/ml. The recommended adult dosage for treating *S. mansoni* infections contracted in the Western Hemisphere and West Africa is 12-15 mg/kg in a single oral dose (Table 26.6-1). Children usually require a higher dose (i.e., 20 mg/kg) to obtain an 80% cure rate and 95% reduction in ova excretion. In *S. mansoni* infections acquired in Egypt, the Sudan, and East and South Africa, a dose of 60 mg/kg is usually required for the same therapeutic response. This can be given as single 20-mg/kg doses on 3 consecutive days or as 15 mg/kg given twice daily for 2 days.

In high doses, oxamniquine has embryocidal effects in rabbits and mice and should be used with caution in pregnancy.

PAROMOMYCIN

Paromomycin was first isolated from cultures of *Streptomyces rimosus* and is currently used only to treat tapeworm infections and the intestinal phase of *Entamoeba histolytica* infections. Like neomycin, it also has activity against intestinal bacteria.

Source and Chemistry. Paromomycin is a natural product of a specific soil organism. It is an aminoglycoside antibiotic, with structural similarities to neomycin (Fig. 26.6-1).

Anthelmintic Action. Aminoglycoside antibiotics inhibit bacterial protein synthesis. The specific modes of antiparasitic actions are unknown. Paromomycin is not only directly amebicidal but also acts by interfering with the enteric bacterial flora that is essential for the pathogenic amebae. Other antibiotics (e.g., erythromycin and tetracyclines) are believed to be amebicidal by this latter mechanism. Paromomycin may be effective in treating tapeworm infections due to its inhibitory effect upon oxidative phosphorylation in mitochondria and/or due to changes in the basal membrane of the parasite.

Pharmacokinetics. The small proportion of the drug absorbed following oral ingestion is metabolized in the liver, and the metabolites are excreted in the urine. Toxic levels may accumulate in patients with impaired renal function.

Adverse Effects. Nephrotoxicity is the major adverse effect from paromomycin. Ototoxicity is less common than with some other aminoglycosides. Because toxic levels may accumulate in patients with reduced renal function, this is a contraindication to its use. Other toxic effects include anorexia, nausea, vomiting, abdominal pain, and diarrhea. Albuminuria is evidence for impending renal toxicity. Rarely, patients complain of skin rash, headache, and vertigo.

Preparations. Paromomycin sulfate (HUMATIN) is available as 250-mg capsules and a flavored syrup for pediatric use containing 125 mg/5 ml. In treating tapeworm infections, a single dose of 75 mg/kg (maximum dose 4 g) ordinarily suffices (Table 26.6-1). In *H. nana* infections, it is recommended that the patient be treated for 5-7 days with single daily 40 to 50 mg/kg doses. The dosage for treating intestinal amebiasis is 25-30 mg/kg/day in three divided doses for 5-10 days.

PRAZIQUANTEL

Praziquantel is a broad-spectrum anthelmintic that should be effective against all *Schistosoma* species that infect humans, certain liver flukes (*Clonorchis* and *Opisthorchis*), and the lung flukes(*Paragonimus*), as well as some extraintestinal (particularly in the skin and central nervous system) cestode infections, and cysticercosis, due to *T. solium*. It is relatively nontoxic, well tolerated by patients, and can be given orally in one dose or several doses in a single day. Its use has recently been approved in the United States (41).

Source and Chemistry. Praziquantel is a heterocyclic isoquinoline pyrazine derivative (Fig. 26.6-1) that is an entirely new chemical group to be developed as an antiparasitic agent. It is a colorless, almost odorless, crystalline powder with a bitter taste. It is stable under normal conditions and soluble in many organic solvents, sparingly soluble in ethanol, and insoluble in water. It is used as a micronized preparation.

Anthelmintic Action. *In vivo* studies in mice have shown that for up to 7 days or later than 28 days after *S. mansoni* infection, treatment with praziquantel kills between 70 and 95% of worms. Concentrations as low as 1 μg/ml of the drug are toxic to schistosoma, juvenile worms, and adult worms *in vitro*. Concentrations as low as 0.004 μg/ml cause an immediate contraction and subsequent immobilization of the parasites. Intensive vacuolization of the tegument occurs without destroying the surface coat. These are the sites for cellular attack by the immune system.

Praziquantel interferes with the parasite's carbohydrate metabolism; the absorption of glucose is reduced, the excretion of lactate is increased, and endogenous glucogen is decreased. It also stimulates the parasite's cellular uptake of sodium and calcium whereas it inhibits the uptake of potassium.

It also has considerable effects upon cestodes *in vitro*, stimulates motility, impairs function of suckers, and causes strong contractions of the entire strobila. Concentrations of the drug as low as 1 ng/ml stimulate movement in hymenolepid cestodes and preadult *Echinococcus*. Praziquantel has other metabolic blocking effects. It diffuses into *Ascaris* muscle mitochondria, where it inhibits the various mitochondrial activities including $NADH^+$ (reduced form of nicotinamide adenine dinucleotide) oxidase and NADH fumarate reductase systems. This inhibitory effect would result in a decreased adenosine triphosphate (ATP) synthesis.

Pharmacokinetics. The drug is readily and almost completely absorbed after oral administration, with maximum serum concentrations occurring within 1-3 hr. The plasma half-life is short (1 to 1.5 hr) due to rapid and complete metabolism in the liver. Over 80% of the drug metabolites are excreted in the urine within 4 days, with almost all of that excreted during the first 24 hr. The highest concentrations of the drug are present in the liver and kidneys. Praziquantel is excreted in the milk of lactating women at a concentration of about one-quarter that of the plasma concentration (36).

Adverse Effects. Side effects reported from the clinical trials performed are greater with single higher doses than with lower multiple doses, and more common in individuals with heavy infections. These include malaise, fatigue, anorexia, nausea, abdominal pain, backache, headache, dizziness, drowsiness, fever, sweating, and urticaria. The reported symptoms occur frequently, are usually mild or moderate, and last only a few hours. It is recommended that the drug not be used during the first 3 months of pregnancy.

Preparations. Praziquantel (BILTRICIDE) is marketed as 600-mg tablets. Results of therapeutic trials have shown it to be effective in treating the following trematode and cestode infections: (a) *Schistosoma haematobium* or *S. intercalatum*, better than 95% cured with a single 40-mg/kg dose; (b) *S. mansoni*, greater than 80% cured following a single dose of 40 mg/kg; (c) *S. japonicum*, 80% cured following two 30-mg/kg doses on the same day; in some studies treatment with three doses of 20 mg/kg body weight given in 1 day produced high degree of parasitological cure and was superior to results with a single dose of 50 mg/kg (41); (d) *Clonorchis sinensis*, better than 95% cured following three 25-mg/kg doses on a single day; (e) *P. westermani*, 90% cured following three doses of 25 mg/kg for 2 days; (f) *Opisthorchis viverrini*, 100% cured with three 25-mg/kg doses per day for either 1 or 2 days; (g) *Taenia saginata* or *T. solium*, better than 95% cured with single 5-mg/kg or 10-mg/kg doses; (h) *H. nana*, better than 85% cured with a single dose of 15 mg/kg; (i) *D. latum*, 96% cured with single 25 mg/kg dose; (j) *D. pacificum*, 100% cured with a single 10-mg/kg dose; (k) praziquantel has also been evaluated and shown to be effective for treating *S. mekongi* and *Metagonimus yokogawai* infections, as well as for treating cerebral cysticercosis.

CHEMOTHERAPY OF CESTODES

Adult tapeworms are hermaphroditic and are flat and ribbonlike. The larval forms may require more than one secondary host and develop in the tissues. Adult tapeworms live free in the digestive tract of the primary host, attached to the intestinal mucosa by means of suckers, hooks, or grooves in the head and absorb food directly through the cuticle. Eggs are passed in the stool, usually still within gravid segments. When the eggs are ingested by the appropriate secondary host, the larvae develop into various encystic forms. The clinical pattern of disease in humans reflects these various methods of development; the cysticercoid of *H. nana* presents as intestinal irritation, the cysticercus of *T. solium* leads to multiple small lesions, often in the brain, causing seizure disorders, and the *Echinococcus* produces large space-occupying lesions, with preference in the liver.

The most common tapeworms infecting humans are listed in Table 26.6-2. *Taenia saginata* is the most common in the United States, as well as worldwide (estimated 40 million infected). Humans are infected by eating rare or raw beef containing the larval stage. Beef tapeworm infection is less common in the United States now than in the past, since American cattle have a reduced infectivity rate and most commercial beef is frozen for prolonged periods, a practice that inactivates the larval cysticerci.

T. solium (pork tapeworm) infection is rare in the United States and Western Europe. The estimated world incidence in 3 million. Humans are usually infected by eating pork containing cysticerci. Pigs, wild boars, and bear are the usual intermediate hosts. Contaminated sausage has been the source for several epidemics. In

Table 26.6-2
Tapeworms Infecting Humans

Parasite	Common Name	Primary Host(s)	Intermediate Host(s)
Taenia saginata	beef tapeworm	human	cattle
Taenia solium	pork tapeworm	human	pig, human
Diphyllobothrium latum	fish tapeworm	human	water flea, fish
Echinococcus granulosus	hydatid disease	dog, other canines	human, sheep, cattle, deer
Echinococcus multilocularis	alveolar hydatid disease	fox, dog, cat	mice, other field rodents, human
Hymenolepis nana	dwarf tapeworm	human	human, mouse
Hymenolepis diminuta	rat tapeworm	rat, mouse, human	flea, cockroach, mealworm
Dipylidium caninum	dog tapeworm	dog, cat, human	dog or cat flea

contrast to *T. saginata*, both larval and adult forms of *T. solium*, can develop in humans.

Diphyllobothrium latum (fish tapeworm) infection is most common is temperate areas such as Scandinavia, the Baltic area, Central Europe, Canada, and the Northern United States. Humans are infected by the ingestion of raw or undercooked freshwater fish. The adult, the longest tapeworm of humans (reaching 10 m and having 4000 segments), causes no pathophysiology other than occasional megaloblastic anemia. This is due to a competitive absorption of vitamin B_{12} by the parasite. More than 10 million people are estimated to be infected with the fish tapeworm.

Echinococcus granulosis (hydatid disease) is the only common tapeworm infection in which humans are a secondary, and not the primary, host. Humans are one of several secondary hosts, including sheep, cattle, and deer (Table 26.6-2). Canines are the definitive hosts, and human infection usually follows ingestion of the eggs excreted by infected dogs. This disease is focal in nature, occurring principally in areas where sheep and cattle raising and infected dogs are all present. The larval form develops into a cyst that produces symptoms as it enlarges. The most frequent organs involved are the liver and lung. A related species, *E. multilocularis*, is more malignant, producing numerous small cysts that become confluent and may even metastasize.

H. nana (dwarf tapeworm) infection is spread by fecal-oral exposure and occurs frequently in mental hospitals and schools for young children.

Treatment of Adult Tapeworms

Niclosamide has markedly simplified the treatment of tapeworm infections (Table 26.6-1). It is well tolerated, simple to administer, and has an excellent cure rate in treating fish, beef, pork, and dwarf tapeworm infestations (16, 38, 42). Mebendazole has excellent activity against tapeworms but requires a dosage three times that recommended for treating intestinal nematode infections (300 mg, either two or three times daily, for 3 days) to cure *T. solium* and *T. saginata* infections (2, 42). Praziquantel, a new drug that may replace others in the therapy of schistosomiasis, also has excellent activity against mature cestodes (10, 21) in single doses of 5-25 mg/kg.

A 5-day course of niclosamide, as opposed to a single dose, has been recommended for treating dwarf tapeworm infections because of an increased propensity for relapses (16, 38, 43) (Table 26.6-1). Praziquantel may prove to be the superior drug for treating *H. nana* infections. Single well-tolerated doses of 15 and 25 mg/kg body weight cured 94-98% of infected children (21,51). Niclosamide gives a 90-95% cure rate when used to treat human tapeworm infections, and the results with paromomycin are similar (7, 54, 61). The latter drug can be given at a dosage of 40 mg/kg/day for 5 days or as a 75-mg/kg single dose, with a maximum of 4 g (7). The pediatric dose of niclosamide is one-half (two tablets) the adult dose for children up to a weight of 35 kg. Three tablets (1.5 g) can be given in a single dose, or in five daily doses for *H. nana* infections, to children weighing more than 35 kg.

Tapeworms Rarely Infecting Humans. *H. diminuta* and *Dipylidium caninum*, also respond to niclosamide (28). Of 19 patients, 17 with *H. diminuta* were cured with a once daily 2-g dose of the drug given for 5-7 days, and 13 of 13 with *D. caninum* infection responded to a single 2-g dose of niclosamide.

In the past, the standard and unpleasant regimen for treating tapeworms was with quinacrine, 1 g in 40-50 ml of water by duodenal tube following a 36- to 48-hr liquid diet. This was followed with a saline purge 30-60 min later. Others have continued to recommend quinacrine for the treatment of *T. solium* infections, since niclosamide separates proglottids from the tapeworm's scolex and cervical region. Niclosamide and praziquantel in the doses needed to treat *T. solium* infection only rarely cause mild nausea, whereas quinacrine often causes severe gastrointestinal symptoms. Also, duodenal intubation frequently causes vomiting. Therefore, it is recommended that *T. solium* infections also be treated with niclosamide or praziquantel.

Treatment of Cysticercosis

There is currently no specific therapy for the larval stage of pork tapeworm infection, although praziquantel with concomitant corticosteroids is being evaluated. Palliative surgery and anticonvulsants may be indicated. Short courses of corticosteroids have been used to reduce the inflammatory response during the acute invasive period.

Treatment of Echinococcosis

Surgical resection has been the standard therapy for hydatid disease. Mebendazole has been shown to have activity against the larval stages of *E. granulosis*, and high-dose therapy (40-50 mg/kg/day) for at least a 30-day course has given considerable clinical improvement in human cases of hydatid disease. Repeated courses may be necessary (6,33). Wilson and colleagues treated patients with more malignant *E. multilocularis* infections, at a dosage of 40 mg/kg of body weight per day indefinitely (59). There is need for a more soluble form of mebendazole or related drug.

CHEMOTHERAPY OF TREMATODES

Schistosomiasis is the most important human fluke infection, with an estimated prevalence of 200 million infected. There are three species frequently infecting humans: *S. japonicum* infections occur in the Orient; *S. haematobium* is endemic to Africa and the Middle East; while *S. mansoni* is present in South America and the Caribbean, as well as in Africa and the Middle East. Other species infecting humans are *S. intercalatum and S. mekongi*, occurring only in limited regions of West Africa and Kampuchea (Cambodia) respectively. *S. matheei*, usually infecting sheep, may rarely also infect humans. Although schistosomiasis is not transmitted within the United States, many infected immigrants or visitors are seen in tropical medicine clinics.

Humans are infected by exposure to water containing the infectious larval stage of the parasite, the cercariae, which penetrates the skin (Table 26.6-3). They are shed from the snail intermediate host, which had been infected by a free-swimming ciliated miracidium. Humans start the cycle by excreting egg-containing feces or urine into fresh water. The miracidia then hatch from the egg in the fresh water and swim about until they find a susceptible snail.

Two species of schistosomes, *S. mansoni* and *S. japonicum*, principally involve the gastrointestinal tract, causing diarrhea and other gastrointestinal complications, fibrosis of the liver, and splenomegaly. The third species, *S. haematobium*, principally involves the urinary tract leading to hematuria, bacterial urinary tract infections, and obstructive uropathy. Treatment for the three species differs.

Hermaphroditic flukes infecting humans are listed in Table 26.6-3. All are transmitted by the ingestion of metacercariae that have encysted in fish, in crabs or crayfish, or on water nuts or water plants. Cooking inactivates the infectious stage. Therefore, transmission of infection requires that these intermediate hosts be eaten raw or undercooked.

Clonorchiasis occurs principally in the Far East. The prevalence rate is approximately 10 million infected worldwide. It is not unusual for Chinese immigrants to the United States to have *Clonorchis* ova in their stools. Opisthorchiasis is another liver fluke. Immigrants from northeast Thailand and Laos are frequently infected with *O. viverrini*. It is estimated that 4 million people in Thailand are infected with this species. *F. hepatica* is also a biliary fluke. It is a common parasite of sheep and is worldwide in distribution, being prevalent in low, wet pastures. Humans are infected as a result of eating wild watercress and other plants that harbor the encysted metacercariae.

F. buski is an intestinal fluke that is normally a parasite of pigs. It is found mainly in the Far East. Humans are infected by ingestion of metacercarial-contaminated water caltrop or water chestnuts. The lung fluke, *Paragonimus sp*, is endemic to the Far East, West Africa, and northern South America. It causes a chronic lung infection that is frequently mistaken for tuberculosis. Humans are infected by eating raw or undercooked crabs and crayfish that contain the infectious metacercariae. Paragonimiasis is a major medical problem in Korea.

Treatment of Schistosomiasis

Metrifonate, an organophosphorus compound, has reduced the mean egg counts by 95% in children infected with *S. haematobium* following three oral doses of 7.5 mg/kg given at 4-week intervals (27, 46). The recommended dose is 7.5-10 mg/kg every 2-4 weeks with a maximum of three doses (Table 26.6-1). With this dose schedule, cure rates ranging from 45 to 93% have been reported with very few side effects (26, 27, 58). Metrifonate is also cost effective and safe when used to prevent infection in children living in endemic areas (26, 27). A single-dose regimen of metrifonate, 12.5 mg/kg, and niridazole, 25 mg/kg, was recommended (45). However, a single 10-mg/kg dose of metrifonate alone reduced egg output by 96.5% and cured 22% of Kenyan school children (3).

In Brazilian patients infected with *S. mansoni*, oxamniquine is reported to have cure rates of 65-85% with one oral dose of 15 mg/kg (12, 32). Children have fewer side effects from the drug but require a higher dose (20 mg/kg) to get similar results (75% cure and 95% reduction in ova excretion) (32). In Egypt, Sudan, and South and East Africa, the dose that cures 70-90% of patients is four times that of the dose in Brazil and West Africa (e.g., 60 mg/kg body weight) (1, 4, 20, 40, 44, 47). This is best given as a single dose of 20 mg/kg on 3 successive days (1, 4, 20), or two divided doses of 15 mg/kg over 2 successive days (40, 44). Toxicity is minimal even at this higher dose and usually consists of transient dizziness, drowsiness, headache, and gastrointestinal symptoms. Patients with

Table 26.6-3
Flukes Infecting Man

Parasite	Disease	Intermediate Host(s)	Source of Infection
Schistosoma mansoni	schistosomiasis mansoni	snail	water, through skin (cercariae)
Schistosoma japonicum	schistosomiasis japonicum	snail	water, through skin (cercariae)
Schistosoma haematobium	urinary schistosomiasis	snail	water, through skin (cercariae)
Clonorchis sinensis	chinese liver fluke	fish	ingestion of raw fish
Opisthorchis sp		fish	ingestion of raw fish
Paragonimus sp	lung fluke	crab, crayfish	ingestion of raw intermediary host
Fasciolopsis buski	intestinal fluke	snail	ingestion of raw contaminated water nuts
Fasciola hepatica	sheep liver fluke	snail	ingestion of raw contaminated plants

advanced lesions, including ascites, who could not be treated with other drugs tolerated and improved with oxamniquine therapy (4). A lower dose of 40 mg/kg cured 60-80% of patients treated and reduced egg excretion to 40-80% of pretreatment levels (1,40).

It is important to remember that oxamniquine is effective in treating only *S. mansoni* infections, whereas metrifonate is only useful for treating schistosomiasis haematobium. Cure rates with antimonial compounds are generally good, but repeated parenteral doses are required, and untoward reactions, including cardiotoxicity, are not infrequent (18,58). There is an extensive report of treating World War II American servicemen with mild schistosomiasis japonicum with antimony potassium tartrate (Tartar emetic) (37). They reported better results (84% cure) with tartar emetic than with stibophen (FUADIN) (47% cure), and others (60) had a relapse rate of at least 42% in 165 patients treated with stibophen. Persistence of active infection can occur without symptoms. Of 30 asymptomatic Swedish patients, 7 still had viable ova found on rectal-snip biopsy on an average of 13 years following treatment with stibocaptate (24). However, the newer drugs including praziquantel, have generally made the antimonials obsolete for treating schistosomiasis.

Niridazole has activity against all schistosome species (Table 26.6-1). Cure rates range from 75 to 95% in treating schistosomiasis haematobium (13, 29) and 50-80% in treating *S. mansoni* infections (17, 18, 29, 30). The cure rates for patients in Japan and the Philippines with schistosomiasis japonicum ranged from 40 to 70% (49). Caution is necessary in patients with hepatosplenic manifestations, as individuals with portal hypertension frequently have acute psychotic episodes or epileptic seizures during niridazole chemotherapy (13, 17, 30, 49, 58). Reducing the dose of niridazole does not decrease the incidence or severity of toxicity (17). Niridazole has also been reported to be mutagenic (5) and carcinogenic in animals.

Hycanthone is a drug with an excellent cure rate and/or reduction in egg excretion following a single intramuscular injection of 2.5 or 3.0 mg/kg in patients infected with either *Schistosoma haematobium* (57, 58) or *S. mansoni* (11, 30, 47, 57, 58). It causes a high incidence of nausea, vomiting, and abdominal pain in treated patients, however, and has been criticized as being mutagenic, teratogenic, and carcinogenic in experimental animals (5, 8). It can cause acute toxic hepatitis (19) and death from acute hepatic necrosis in humans (57). In the field, it is difficult to comply with the longer courses of therapy required with either niridazole or the antimonial compounds (30, 58). It has been suggested that lower doses of hycanthone (e.g., 0.75-2.0 mg/kg) are less toxic and, although less likely to produce a radical cure, may reduce the transmission of schistosomiasis by decreasing worms and eggs (47, 55). Recent animal studies indicate that the liver is more susceptible to hycanthone than is the parasite. At dosages too small for chemotherapeutic effect, hepatocellular carcinomas, precancerous nodules, and micronodular hepatocellular lesions were found in the livers of schistosome-infected mice treated with hycanthone (22).

Praziquantel, a broad-spectrum antischistosomal and anticestodal compound, is active against all three schistosome species in rodents and monkeys. Clinical studies indicate that the drug is well tolerated and gives 80-100% cure rates with one or two doses in humans, infected with any of five species (14, 15, 25, 31, 36, 50, 62). Praziquantel is the closest to the ideal drug for treating schistosomiasis.

Treatment of Other Fluke Infections

Bithionol replaced some of the older drugs in the treatment of paragonimiasis (34) and fascioliasis (23) (Table 26.6-1). Cure rates are in the 80-95% range after a single course of treatment for either infection. A dihydroxy biphenyl compound, menichlopholan, gave a 90% cure rate when used for treating paragonimiasis with a single dose of 2 mg/kg body weight in a clinical trial in Nigeria (39). Tetrachloroethylene can still be used for treating fasciolopsiasis (53). Hexachloroparaxylol (HETOL) has given cure rates of 82 and 87% at dosages of 60 and 70 mg/kg given twice daily for 5 days to patients with *C. sinensis* infections (62). However, this drug, which has also been useful for treating *O. felineus* infections, was withdrawn by the manufacturer because of excessive toxicity in experimental animals. Niclosamide, at a dosage of 2 g after breakfast daily for 2 or 3 successive days, has been reported to cure 72-79% of patients with heterophyiasis, a rare infection caused by infection with the intestinal fluke, *H. heterophyes* (52).

Praziquantel has been reported to be very effective in treating most human trematode infections and has replaced the other less effective drugs. Three 25-mg/kg doses in a single day cured 95% of patients infected with *C. sinensis* (48). Cure rates for treating *P. westermani* infections when the drug was given at a dose of 25 mg/kg three times daily for 1, 2, and 3 days were 80, 90, and 100%. *O. viverrina* infections were all cured with 1-day treatment at a dose of 25 mg/kg given three times after meals (9). Praziquantel has also been effective in treating *Metagonimus yokogawai* infections.

REFERENCES

1. Abdel-Wahab, M.F., Oldfield, E.C., Strickland, G.T. and El-Sahly, A. Oxamniquine therapy of schistosomiasis in an Egyptian village. In: *Current Chemotherapy of Infectious Diseases*, Vol. 2 (Nelson, J.D. and Grassi, C., eds.). Washington, D.C.: American Society of Microbiology, 1980, p. 1108.
2. Arambulo, P.V., Cabrera, B.D. and Cabrera, M.G. The use of mebendazole in the treatment of *Taenia saginata* taeniasis in an endemic area in the Philippines. *Acta Trop.* 35:281, 1978.
3. Arap Siongok, T.K., Ouma, J.H., Houser, H.B. and Warren, K.S. Quantification of infection with *Schistosoma haematobium* in relation to epidemiology and selective population chemotherapy. 2. Mass treatment with a single oral dose of metrifonate. *J. Infect. Dis.* 138:856, 1978.
4. Bassily, S., Farid, Z., Higashi, G.I. and Watten, R.H. Treatment of complicated schistosomiasis mansoni with oxamniquine. *Am. J. Trop. Med. Hyg.* 27:1284, 1978.
5. Batzinger, R.P. and Bueding, E. Mutagenic activities *in vitro* and *in vivo* of five antischistosomal compounds. *J. Pharmacol. Exp. Ther.* 200:1, 1977.

6. Bekhti, A., Schaaps, J.P., Capron, M. et al. Treatment of hepatic hydatid disease with mebendazole: Preliminary results in four cases. *Br. Med. J.* 2:1047, 1977.
7. Botero, D.R. Paromomycin an effective treatment of *Taenia* infections. *Am. J. Trop. Med. Hyg.* 19:234, 1970.
8. Bueding, E. Dissociation of mutagenic and other toxic properties from schistosomicides. *J. Toxicol. Environ. Health* 1:329, 1975.
9. Bunnag, D. and Harinasuta, T. Studies on the chemotherapy of human opisthorchiasis in Thailand. 1. Clinical trial of praziquantel. *Southeast Asian J. Trop. Med. Publ. Health* 11:4, 1980.
10. Bylund, G., Bang, B. and Wikgren, K. Tests with a new compound (Praziquantel) against *Diphyllobothrium latum*. *J. Helmintho.* 51:115, 1977.
11. Cook, J.A., Jordan, P., Woodstock, L. and Pilgrim, V. A controlled trial of hycanthone and placebo in schistosomiasis mansoni in St. Lucia. *Ann. Trop. Med. Parasitol.* 71:197, 1977.
12. daSilva, L.C., Sette, H., Chamone, D.A.F. et al. Clinical trials with oxamniquine in the treatment of human Mansonian schistosomiasis. *Trans. R. Soc. Trop. Med. Hyg.* 69:288, 1975.
13. Davis, A. Field trials of Ambilhar in the treatment of urinary bilharziasis in school children. *Bull. WHO* 35:827, 1966.
14. Davis, A. and Wegner, D.H.G. Multicentre trials of praziquantel in human schistosomiasis: Design and techniques. *Bull. WHO* 57:767, 1979.
15. Davis, A., Biles, J.E. and Ulrich, A.M. Initial experiences with praziquantel in the treatment of human infections due to *Schistosoma haematobium*. *Bull. WHO* 57:773, 1979.
16. El-Masry, N.A., Farid, Z. and Bassily, S. Treatment of *Hymenolepis nana* with niclosamide, mepacrine, and thiabendazole. *East Afr. Med. J.* 51:532, 1974.
17. Faigle, J.W., Coutinho, A.D., Koeberle, H. et al. The metabolism of niridazole (Ambilhar) in man. 2. Investigations on patients suffering from clinically advanced forms of *Schistosoma mansoni* infection. *Ann. Trop. Med. Parasitol.* 64:383, 1970.
18. Farid, Z., Bassily, S. Lehman, J.S. et al. A comparative evaluation of the treatment of *Schistosoma mansoni* with niridazole and potassium antimony tartrate. *Trans. R. Soc. Trop. Med. Hyg.* 66:119, 1972.
19. Farid, Z., Smith, J.H., Bassily, S. et al. Hepatotoxicity after treatment of schistosomiasis with hycanthone. *Br. Med. J.* 1:88, 1972.
20. Farid, Z., Bassily, S., Higashi, G.I. et al. Further experience on the use of oxamniquine in the treatment of advanced schistosomiasis. *Ann. Trop. Med. Parasitol.* 73:502, 1979.
21. Groll, E. Praziquantel for cestode infections in man. *Acta Trop.* 37:293, 1980.
22. Haes, W.M. and Bueding, E. Long-term hepatocellular effects of hycanthone and of two other antischistosomal drugs in mice infected with *Schistosoma mansoni. J. Pharmacol. Exp. Ther.* 197:703, 1976.
23. Hardman, E.W., Jones, R.L.H. and Davis, A.H. Fascioliasis: A large outbreak. *Br. Med. J.* 3:502, 1970.
24. Hedman, P. and Bengtsson, E. A 13-year follow-up of antimony-treated *Schistosoma mansoni*-infected patients. *Am. J. Trop. Med. Hyg.* 26:693, 1977.
25. Ishizaki, T., Kamo, E. and Boehme, K. Double blind studies of tolerance to praziquantel in Japanese patients with *Schistosoma japonicum* infections. *Bull. WHO* 57:787, 1979.
26. Jewsbury, J.M. and Cooke, M.J. Prophylaxis of schistosomiasis: Field trial of metrifonate for the prevention of human infection. *Ann. Trop. Med. Parasitol.* 70:361, 1976.
27. Jewsbury, J.M., Cooke, M.J. and Weber, M.C. Field trial of metrifonate in the treatment and prevention of schistosomiasis infection in man. *Ann. Trop. Med. Parasitol.* 71:67, 1977.
28. Jones, W.E. Niclosamide as a treatment for *Hymenolepis diminuta* and *Dipylidium caninum* infection in man. *Am. J. Trop. Med. Hyg.* 28:300, 1979.
29. Kanani, S.R., Knight, R. and Woodruff, A.W. The treatment of schistosomiasis with niridazole in Britain. *J. Trop. Med. Hyg.* 73:162, 1970.
30. Katz, N. Clinical evaluation of niridazole and hycanthone in schistosomiasis mansoni endemic areas. *J. Toxicol. Environ. Health* 1:203, 1975.
31. Katz, N., Rocha, R.S. and Chaves. A. Preliminary trials with praziquantel in human infections due to *Schistosoma mansoni. Bull. WHO* 57:781, 1979.
32. Katz, N., Zicker, F. and Pereira, J.P. Field trials with oxamniquine in a schistosomiasis mansoni endemic area. *Am. J. Trop. Med. Hyg.* 26:234, 1977.
33. Kern, P., Dietrich, M. and Volkmer, K.J. Chemotherapy of echinococcosis with mebendazole: Clinical observations of 7 patients. *Z. Tropenmed. Parasitol.* 30:65, 1979.
34. Kim, J.S. Treatment of *Paragonimus westermani* infections with bithionol. *Am. J. Trop. Med. Hyg.* 19:940, 1970.
35. Leopold, G., Lingethum, W., Groll, E., Dickmann, H.W., Nowak, H. and Wegner, D.H.G. Clinical pharmacology of normal volunteers of praziquantel, a new drug against schistosomes and cestodes. *Eur. J. Clin. Pharmacol.* 14:281, 1978.
36. McMahon, J.E. and Kolstrup, N. Praziquantel: A new schistosomicide against *Schistosoma haematobium*. *Br. Med. J.* 2:1396, 1979.
37. Most, H., Kane, C.A., Lavietes, P.H. et al. Schistosomiasis japonica in American military personnel: Clinical studies of 600 cases during the first year after infections. *Am. J. Trop. Med.* 30:239, 1950.
38. Most, H., Yoeli, M., Hammond, J. et al. Yomesan (niclosamide) therapy of *Hymenolepis nana* infections. *Am. J. Trop. Med. Hyg.* 20:206, 1971.
39. Nwokoli, C. and Volkmer, K.J. Single dose therapy of paragonimiasis with menichlopholan. *Am. J. Trop. Med. Hyg.* 26:688, 1977.
40. Omer, A.H.S. Oxamniquine for treating *Schistosoma mansoni* infection in Sudan. *Br. Med. J.* 2:163, 1978.
41. Pearson, R.D. and Guerant, R.L. Praziquantel: A major advance in anthelmintic therapy. *Ann. Int. Med.* 99:195, 1983.
42. Pena-Chavarria, A., Villarejos, V.M. and Zeledon, R. Mebendazole in the treatment of taeniasis solium and taeniasis saginata. *Am. J. Trop. Med. Hyg.* 26:118, 1977.
43. Perera, D.R., Western, K.A. and Schultz, M.G. Niclosamide treatment of cestodiasis: Clinical trials in the United States. *Am. J. Trop. Med. Hyg.* 19:610, 1970.
44. Pitchford, R.J. and Leewis, M. Oxamniquine in the treatment of various schistosome infections in South Africa. *S. Afr. Med. J.* 53:677, 1978.
45. Pugh, R.N.H. Malumfashi endemic disease research project. V. Concurrent single dose metrifonate and niridazole in urinary schistosomiasis. *Ann. Trop. Med. Parasitol.* 72:495, 1978.
46. Reddy, S., Oomen, J.M.V. and Bell, D.R. Metrifonate in urinary schistosomiasis: A field trial in northern Nigeria. *Ann. Trop. Med. Parasitol.* 69:73, 1975.
47. Rees, P.H., Bowry, H.N., Roberts, J.M.D. et al. The treatment of schistosomiasis mansoni in Murang'a district, Kenya: A double blind controlled trial of three hycanthone regimens and oxamniquine. *Am. J. Trop. Med. Hyg.* 24:823, 1975.
48. Rim, H.J., Lyn, K.S., Lee, J.S. and Joo, K.H. Clinical evaluation of the therapeutic efficacy of praziquantel (Embay 8440) against *Clonorchis sinensis* infection in man. *Ann. Trop. Med. Parasitol.* 75:27, 1981.
49. Santos, A.T., Blas, B.L., Nosenas, J.S. et al. Niridazole in the treatment of schistosomiasis japonica. *J. Philippine Med. Assoc.* 47:203, 1971.
50. Santos, A.T., Blas, B.L., Nosenas, J.S. et al. Preliminary clinical trials with praziquantel in *Schistosoma japonicum* infections in the Philippines. *Bull. WHO* 57:793, 1979.

51. Schenone, H. Praziquantel in the treatment of *Hymenolepis nana* in children. *Am. J. Trop. Med. Hyg.* 29:320, 1980.

52. Sheir, Z.M. and Aboul-Enein, M.E-S. Demographic, clinical, and therapeutic appraisal of heterophyiasis. *J. Trop. Med. Hyg.* 73:148, 1970.

53. Suntharasamai, P., Bunnag, D., Tejavanij, S. et al. Comparative clinical trials of niclosamide and tetrachloroethylene in the treatment of *Fasciolopsis buski* infection. *Southeast Asian J. Trop. Med. Publ. Health* 5:556, 1974.

54. Tanowitz, H.B. and Wittner,M. Paromomycin in the treatment of *Diphyllobothrium latum* infection. *J. Trop. Med. Hyg.* 76:151, 1973.

55. Warren, K.S., Arap Siongok, T.K., Ouma, J.H. and Houser, H.B. Hycanthone dose response in *Schistosoma mansoni* infection in Kenya. *Lancet* 1:352, 1978.

56. Webbe, G. The hatching and activation of taeniid ova in relation to the development of cysticercosis in man. *Z. Tropenmed. Parasitol.* 18:354, 1967.

57. WHO reports on schistosomal drugs. 1. Report of WHO consultant group on hycanthone. *Bol. Of. Sanit. Panam.* 6:82, 1972.

58. WHO reports on schistosomal drugs. 2. Report of a WHO consultant group on the comparative evaluation of new schistosomicidal drugs for use in treatment campaigns. *Bol. Of. Sanit. Panam.* 6:89, 1972.

59. Wilson, J.F., Davidson, M. and Rausch, R.L. A clinical trial of mebendazole in the treatment of alveolar hydatid disease. *Am. Rev. Respir. Dis.* 118:747, 1978.

60. Winkenwerder, W.L., Hunningen, A.V., Harrison, T. et al. Studies on schistosomiasis japonica. 2. Analysis of 364 cases of acute schistosomiasis with report of results of treatment with Fuadin in 184 cases. *Bull. Johns Hopkins Hosp.* 79:406, 1946.

61. Wittner, M. and Tanowitz, H. Paromomycin therapy of human cestodiasis with special reference to hymenolepiasis. *Am. J. Trop. Med. Hyg.* 20:433, 1971.

62. Yokogawa, M., Koyama, H., Araki, K. et al. Mass treatment of clonorchiasis sinensis with 1,4-bistrichloromethylbenzole. 2. Minimal effective dose. *Z. Tropenmed. Parasitol.* 20:494, 1969.

63. Zhejiang Clinical Cooperative Research Group for Praziquantel. Clinical evaluation of praziquantel in treatment of schistosomiasis japonica: A report of 181 cases. *Chin. Med. J.* 93:375, 1980.

ADDITIONAL READING

Botero, D.R. Chemotherapy of human intestinal parasitic diseases. *Ann. Rev. Pharmacol. Toxicol.* 18:1, 1978.

Drugs for parasitic infections. *Med. Lett. Drugs Ther.* 24:5, 1982.

Katz, N. Chemotherapy of Schistosomiasis mansoni. *Adv. Pharmacol. Chemother.* 14:1, 1977.

Woolhouse, N.B. Biochemical and pharmacological effects in relation to the mode of action of antischistosomal drugs. *Biochem. Pharmacol.* 28:2413, 1979.

CHAPTER
27

CHEMOTHERAPY OF NEOPLASTIC DISEASES

Rose J. Papac

The use of drugs in the treatment of malignant disease is a fairly recent development. The rationale for their use is based upon the concept that effective treatment will result in the destruction of tumor cells. This may be accomplished by direct cytotoxicity to proliferating cells, by interference with cell division, or by growth inhibition.

Most of the drugs useful in cancer chemotherapy exert their effects upon metabolic or replicative processes by the following mechanisms: inhibition of reactions providing nucleotide precursors of DNA and/or RNA; direct damage to nucleic acids; combination with or incorporation into DNA; functioning as a template for RNA synthesis; inhibition of DNA polymerase; or, combination with specific cellular protein receptors.

As a result of specific biochemical mechanisms, some drugs are effective only against cells involved in the synthesis of DNA (cell cycle-dependent drug), whereas others destroy nonreplicating cells. Cell cycle-dependent drugs are linked to a specific phase of the cell cycle, with its characteristic activity, such as S phase (DNA synthesis), M phase (mitosis), G_1 phase (the postmitotic rest), or G_2 phase (the postsynthetic rest). Some cells are in a nonproliferating phase (G_0 phase). The growing fraction of a tumor represents the proportion of cells in the cycle as compared with the total cell population.

The degree to which drugs influence a tumor may depend upon the growth fraction, the phase of the cell cycle most vulnerable to the drug, inherent cytotoxicity of the agents, and many other factors in the host. With few exceptions, almost all antineoplastic agents lack specificity with regard to the site of their actions, so that some normal tissues are almost invariably affected as well as tumor tissue. Rapidly replicating normal tissues, namely bone marrow, mucosa of the oral cavity and gastrointestinal tract, germinal tissues, lymphoid tissues, and hair follicles are often affected by cytotoxic drugs. The consequences are granulocytopenia with increased risk of infection, thrombopenia, anemia, oral and gastrointestinal lesions, impaired spermatogenesis and oogenesis, lymphopenia, immunosuppression, and alopecia.

Extensive experimental screening for new compounds has yielded compounds that are clinically useful at acceptable levels of toxicity, and these have been selected for inclusion in this report. In this rapidly changing field, the current status of compounds is subject to frequent change so that the clinical importance of new compounds may not withstand the test of time.

The use of tumor chemotherapy is primarily considered to be palliative (i.e., to diminish the morbidity due to neoplastic disease in its advanced stages). In recent years, however, chemotherapy has been described as curative for several neoplasms. It is being employed as an adjunctive treatment in earlier stages of malignant disease, to increase the cure rate or to increase the disease-free interval. Additionally, the simultaneous use of drugs with different mechanisms of action is a widespread practice aimed at improving therapeutic benefits.

Although the judicious application of tumor chemotherapy provides palliation for increased numbers of patients with neoplastic diseases, the commonest types of malignant disease are not substantially affected by its use, so that for many patients with malignant disease it offers primarily hope and attentive medical care.

CLASSES OF ANTITUMOR AGENTS

Currently available chemotherapeutic agents for treatment of neoplastic diseases are listed in Table 27-1 in several arbitrary groups based partly on their chemical and partly on their pharmacological characteristics. Sites of their action in the cell cycle are shown in Figure 27-1, and their mechanism of action in Figure 27-2.

ALKYLATING AGENTS

The basis for the pharmacological action of alkylating agents as antineoplastic agents is their ability to exert destructive effects upon proliferating tissue. Because they are among the first chemotherapeutic agents to be of clinical value, they have led to the understanding and development of many other compounds.

History. The initial clinical use of alkylating agents is a result of investigation with chemical warfare agents. The sulfur mustards, used during World War I as mustard gas, were noted to have local vesicant actions. Krumbhaar and Krumbhaar (61) observed, in autopsy studies of victims exposed to sulfur mustard, that lymphoid tissue showed evidence of cytotoxicity. In 1929, Berenblum (7) found these agents to be 'anticarcinogenic'. In 1933, Adair and Bagg (1) applied sulfur mustards topically to cutaneous metastases and observed vesicant effects, and concluded the toxicity was excessive. During World War II, Gilman and Phillips (44) studied the biological and pharmacological effects of the nitrogen mustards. The initial clinical trial was in 1942 in a patient with lymphosarcoma who manifested a dramatic response and severe reversible toxicity.

Many modifications of the basic chemical structure have been developed. The concept that the use of special prosthetic groups would contribute specificity of action for certain tumors stimulated this development. The general spectrum of effects has not been altered, but reduction of certain toxic effects and ease of administration have made some agents more useful.

Cytotoxic Effect. Although the alkylating agents usually affect cells in the late G_1 or S phase more than those in G_2 phase, they may also destroy nonproliferating cells in G_0 Phase. Accordingly, these agents are considered to be cell-cycle nonspecific and can be used clinically in tumors with small growth fractions (with low percentage of dividing cells).

Mechanism of Action. Alkylating agents are compounds that are either electrophiles or generate electrophiles, producing active species that may be carbonium ions or polarized molecules with positively charged regions (74,85). Most of these agents possess a reactive bis -(2-chlorethyl) group that in aqueous solution generates highly reactive ethyleneimmonium intermediates that act readily through formation of carbonium ions. One of the two 2-chlorethyl side chains undergoes a first order substitution nucleophilic (S_N 1) cyclization, with release of a chloride ion and formation of highly reactive ethyleneimmonium ion intermediate as shown in the following reaction:

$$H_3C-N(CH_2CH_2Cl)_2 \longrightarrow CH_3-\overset{+}{N}(R')<(CH_2-CH_2) \longrightarrow >CH_2$$

Nitrogen mustard Ethyleneimmonium intermediate

They are capable of reacting with substances containing various nucleophilic groups, such as phosphate, amino, sulfhydryl, hydroxyl, carboxyl, and imidazole. Purine and pyrimidines of DNA are believed to be the most sensitive target of alkylation, resulting in the destruction of the cell. The primary site of action is the 7-nitrogen of the purine base, guanine, which is strongly nucleophilic, and its alkylation may lead to chain scission, depurination, and miscoding. This reaction can result in cross-linking of nucleic acid chains of three types: linking of two twin helices (cross-linking between two guanine moieties); interhelical cross-linking (abnormal base pair between guanine and thymine); and reaction between adjacent groups on the same chain.

Adverse Effects. Adverse effects of the nitrogen mustards include mutagenicity, bone marrow depression, suppression of gonadal function, suppression of the immune response, involution of lymphoid tissue, and carcinogenicity (44). Because of the similarities of these effects to those of ionizing radiation, these compounds are called radiomimetic. Important differences exist, however.

Variability exists within this class of agents with regard to certain toxic effects. Certain agents induce less severe thrombopenia, and the sequence of marrow depression may vary. Some agents cause damage to hair follicles, and there may be variable stimulation of the CNS vomiting center.

Resistance. It is noteworthy that resistance to an agent does not imply resistance to the entire class of compounds. In several diseases (e.g., myeloma, lymphoma) (77), failure to respond to one alkylating agent may be associated with response to another.

Table 27-1
Dosage and Route of Administration of Antineoplastic Agents

Drug	Usual Dose[a]
Alkylating Agents[b]	
Mechlorethamine (nitrogen mustard, HN_2, MUSTARGEN)	0.4 mg/kg or 10 mg/M^2 (singly), i.v.; in combination, 6 mg/M^2, i.v., 0.2-0.4 mg/kg, intracavitary
Cyclophosphamide (CYTOXAN)	40-50 mg/kg, i.v. → 10-15 mg/kg., i.v. q. 7-10 days or 1-5 mg/kg p.o. q.d.
Melphalan	6 mg/day or 0.15 mg/kg/day, p.o. → 2 mg/day or 0.05 mg/kg/day, p.o.
Chlorambucil (LEUKERAN)	0.1-0.2 mg/kg/day, p.o. → 2 mg/day, p.o.
Uracil mustard	1-2 mg/day, p.o.
Busulfan (MYLERAN)	66 μg/kg/day, p.o. → 33 μg/kg/day., p.o.
Nitrosoureas	100-200 mg/M^2
carmustine (BCNU, BICNU)	i.v. infusion q. 6 weeks
lomustine (CCNU, CEENU)	50-200 mg/M^2, p.o. q. 6 weeks
semustine (METHY-CCNU, methyl-lomustine)	50-200 mg/M^2, p.o. q. 6 weeks
Antimetabolites	
Folic acid analogs	
Methotrexate (amethopterin)	0.4 mg/kg i.v., twice weekly; 2.5-5 mg/day, p.o. 15-30 mg/day, p.o.; i.m. for 5 day, q. 1-2 weeks (choriocarcinoma) 10-25 mg/day, p.o. for 4-8 days, q. 7-10 days (Burkitt's tumors) 12 mg/M^2 q. 2-5 days intrathecal (prophylaxis in meningeal leukemia)
Pyrimidine analogs	
Fluorouracil (5-fluorouracil, 5-FU, ADRUCIL)	12 mg/kg/day, i.v. for 4 days → 10-15 mg/kg/week, i.v.
Cytarabine (cytosine arabinoside, Ara-C, CYTOSAR-U)	100-200 mg/M^2, i.v., b.d. for 5-7 days → 1 mg/kg, s.c., q. 1 or 2 weeks
5-Azacytidine	50-200 mg/M^2, i.v., q.d. for 5 days , q. 2-3 weeks
Purine analogs	
Mercaptopurine (6-mercaptopurine, 6-MP, PURINETHOL)	2.5 mg/kg or 100-200 mg/day, p.o. → 50-100 mg/day, p.o.
Thioguanine (6-thioguanine, 6-TG)	2-3 mg/kg/day, p.o.
Antitumor antibiotics	
Dactinomycin (actinomycin D, COSMEGEN)	15 μg/kg or 500 μg (adult) i.v., q.d. for 5 days
Bleomycin sulfate (BLENOXANE)	10-20 U/M^2, i.v., i.m., s.c. once or twice weekly → 1 U/day or 5 U/week i.v. or i.m.
Daunorubicin (daunomycin, rubidomycin, CERUBIDINE)	60 mg/M^2 (singly) or 45 mg/M^2/day (in combination), i.v., q. d. for 2-3 day, q. 3-4 weeks
Doxorubicin hydrochloride (ADRIAMYCIN)	60-75 mg/M^2, i.v. q. 3 weeks
Streptozocin (streptozotocin)	0.5-1.5 g/M^2, i.v. q. week for 4 weeks
Vinca Alkaloids	
Vincristine sulfate (VCR, ONCOVIN)	1-2 mg/M^2, i.v. (total dose not to exceed 2 mg) weekly
Vinblastine sulfate (VBL, VELBAN)	0.1-0.15 mg/kg, i.v. weekly
Hormones	
Adrenocorticosteroids (PREDNISONE)	20-100 mg, p.o. q.d. or q.i.d.
Progestin (hydroxyprogesterone caproate, DELALUTIN)	1 g, i.m. twice weekly
Medroxyprogesterone acetate (PROVERA)	400-1000 mg, i.m. week → 400 mg, i.m. monthly
Megestrol acetate (MEGACE)	40-320 mg/day, p.o. (endometrial carcinoma) 160 mg/day, p.o. (breast carcinoma)
Estrogen	
diethylstilbestrol	5-15 mg/day, p.o. (breast carcinoma); 1-3 mg/day, p.o. (prostate carcinoma)

[a] U = unit: → = followed by maintenance dose.

[b] All these agents require careful monitoring of peripheral blood counts, generally weekly, with reduction of dosage appropriate to the level of blood counts.

Table 27-1(continued)
Dosage and Route of Administration of Antineoplastic Agents

Drug	Usual Dose[a]
Androgen	
testosterone propionate	100 mg, i.m. three times weekly (breast carcinoma)
	100 mg, i.m. five times weekly (renal cell carcinoma)
2-α-methyl-dihydrotestosterone propionate (DROLBAN)	100 mg three times weekly (breast carcinoma)
Miscellaneous Agents	
Procarbazine hydrochloride (MATULANE)	100-300 mg/M^2 q.d., p.o.
Dacarbazine (DTIC, DTIC-DOME)	250 mg/M^2/day, i.v. for 5 days, q. 3 weeks
Hydroxyurea (HYDREA)	20-30 mg/kg q.d., or 80 mg/kg q. 3rd day, p.o.
Cisplatin (DDP, PLATINOL)	50-120 mg/M^2/ i.v. q. 3-4 weeks (ovarian tumor), or 15-20 mg/M^2/day, i.v. for 5 days (testicular tumor)
L-Asparaginase (asparaginae, ELSPAR)	200 IU/kg/day, i.v. for 28 days or 1000 IU/kg/day for 10 days
Mitotane (o, p′-DDD, LYSODREN)	2-16 g/day, p.o. (divided doses)

[a] U = unit: → = followed by maintenance dose.

[b] All these agents require careful monitoring of peripheral blood counts, generally weekly, with reduction of dosage appropriate to the level of blood counts.

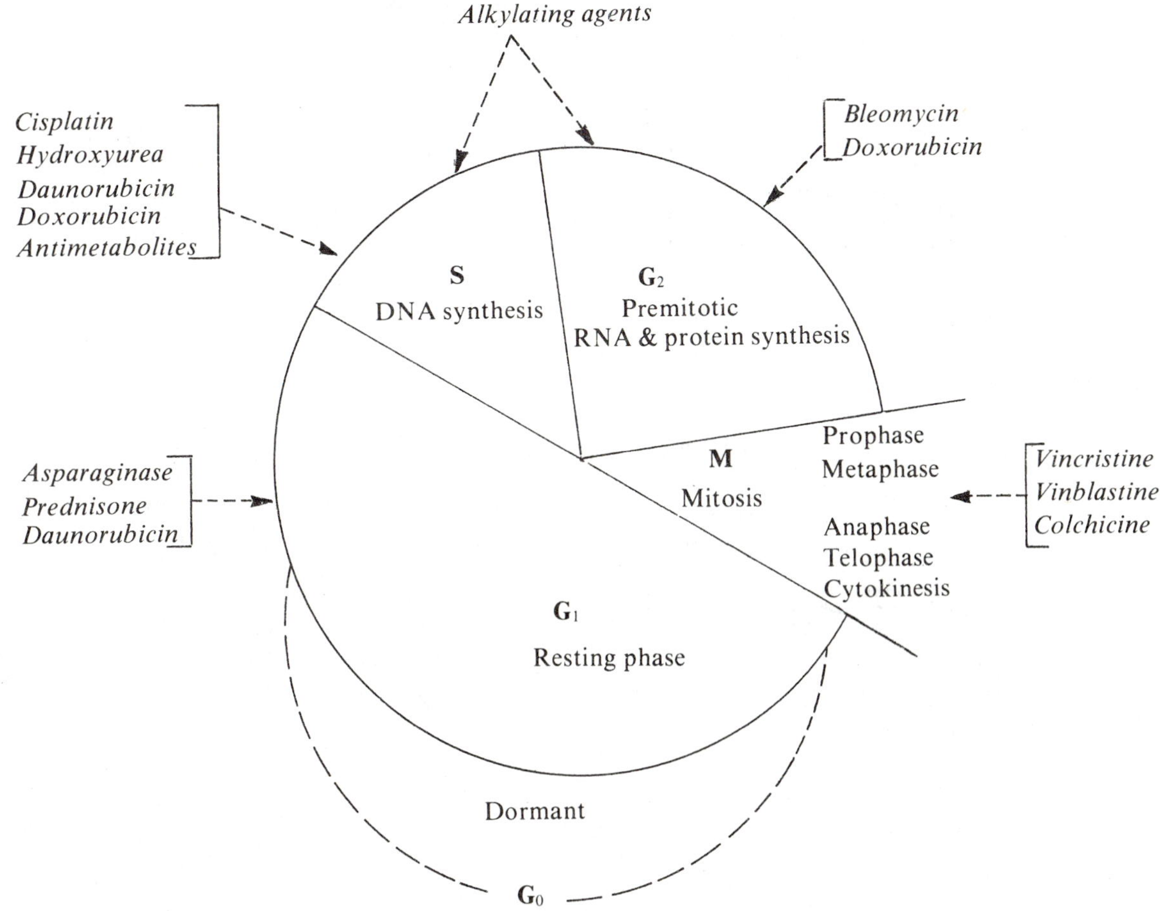

Fig. 27-1. *Effects of antineoplastic agents on cell cycle.*

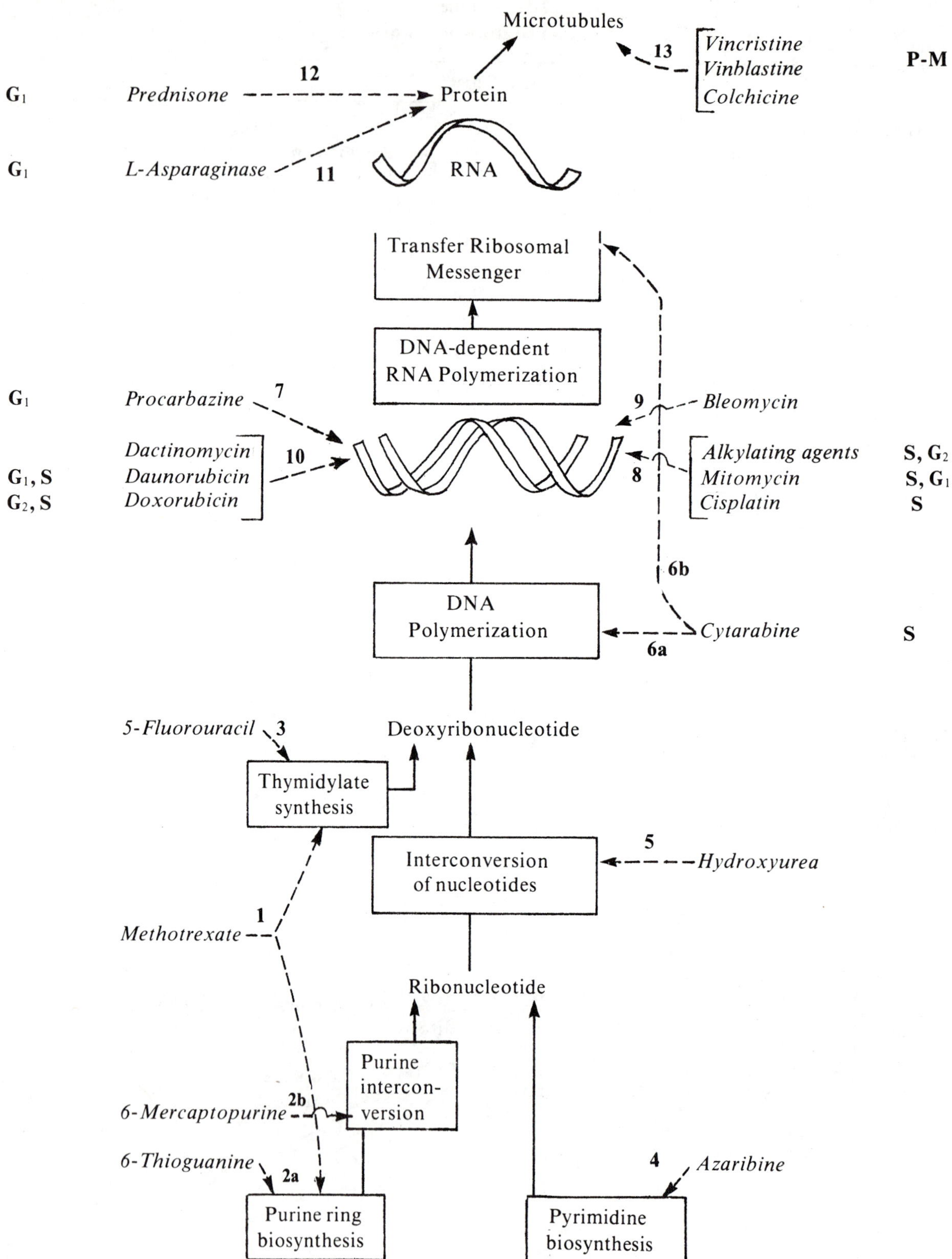

Fig. 27-2. *Sites and mechanisms of action of antineoplastic agents.*

Footnotes to Fig. 27-2:
1a. inhibition of thymidylate synthesis, and
1b. inhibition of purine ring biosynthesis.
2a. Inhibition of purine ring biosynthesis, and
2b. inhibition of interconversion of purines.
3. 5-FdUMP, an active metabolite of 5-FU (5-fluorouracil), inhibits thymidylate synthetase.
4. Inhibition of *de novo* pathway of pyrimidine biosynthesis.
5. Inhibition of conversion of ribonucleotides to deoxyribonucleotides.
6a. Inhibition of DNA polymerization, and
6b. RNA dysfunction.
7. Degradation of DNA.
8. Alkylation of biologically active moieties of nucleic acids and protein.
9. DNA scission.
10. Intercalation between base pairs in DNA.
11. Asparagine deprivation and inhibition of protein synthesis.
12. Inhibition of protein synthesis (?).
13. Inhibition of polymerization and disruption of microtubules.

Of the many nitrogen mustards that have been synthesized, mechlorethamine has had the widest clinical application, and therefore it is used as a standard of reference. Representative agents are shown in Figure 27-3. The biological activity is based upon the presence of the bis-(2-chlorethyl) groups. These groups have been linked to: amino acids [e.g., phenylalanine (melphalan)]; phenyl groups, as with aminophenylbutyric acid (chlorambucil); pyrimidine base (uracil mustard); sugar (mannitol mustard); and a cyclic phosphamide ester (cyclophosphamide). A series of methanesulfonic acid esters are also presumed to be alkylating agents, busulfan being the most notable example. Ethyleneimines (such as thio-TEPA, and so on) resemble the active form of the nitrogen mustards. There are several active compounds, although they are less widely used.

It is noteworthy that compounds structurally related to the nitrogen mustards but possessing only a single chlorethyl group, known as monofunctional agents, possess some biological activity but have shown little clinical effectiveness on tumors. The haloalkylamine adrenoceptor blocking agents such as dibenamine and phenoxybenzamine are examples (Chapter 7.2).

MECHLORETHAMINE

The chemical structure of mechlorethamine is shown in Figure 27-3. The compound is biologically active for only a few minutes when put into solution; therefore, prompt use is essential. It rapidly undergoes chemical transformation, combining with water or reactive compounds, and cannot be identified in either blood or tissues after a few minutes.

Adverse Effects. Severe nausea and vomiting are an almost invariable occurrence, resulting from gastrointestinal irritation and direct central nervous system effects. These reactions can usually be controlled by premedication with antiemetics and narcotic analgesics. This effect generally subsides within 8 hr but may persist as long as 48 hr.

Mechlorethamine may produce reversible menstrual irregularities as a result of arrest of maturation of graafian follicles and may produce fetal abnormalities when given to pregnant mothers, as evidenced in experimental

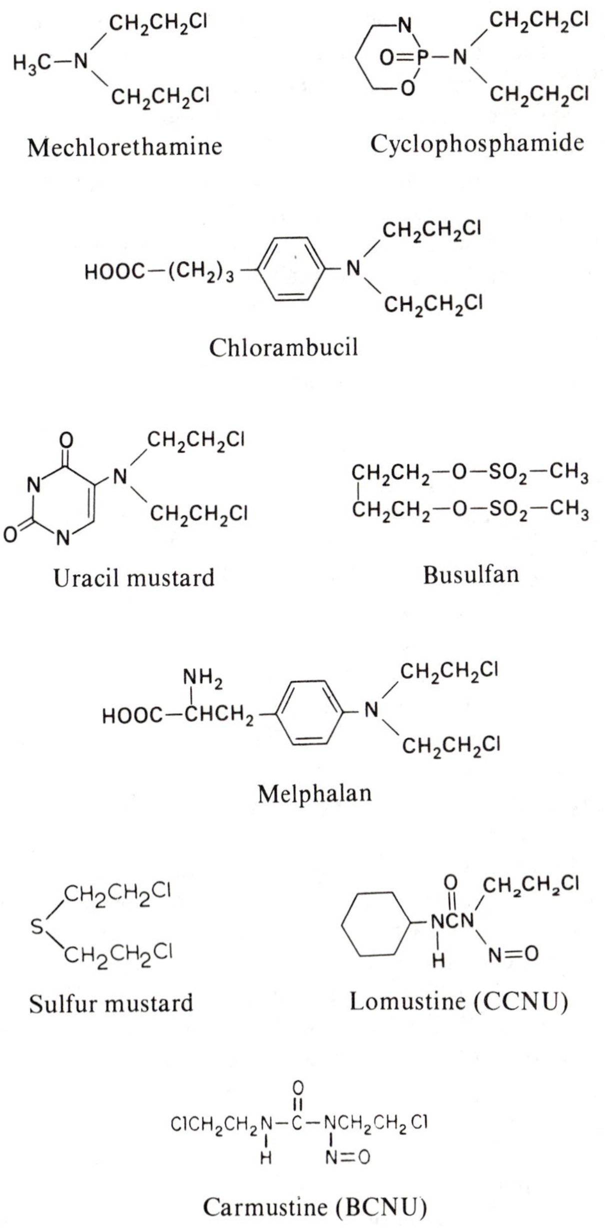

$H_3C-N(CH_2CH_2Cl)_2$

Mechlorethamine

Cyclophosphamide

$HOOC-(CH_2)_3-C_6H_4-N(CH_2CH_2Cl)_2$

Chlorambucil

Uracil mustard

$CH_2CH_2-O-SO_2-CH_3$
$CH_2CH_2-O-SO_2-CH_3$

Busulfan

$HOOC-CH(NH_2)CH_2-C_6H_4-N(CH_2CH_2Cl)_2$

Melphalan

$S(CH_2CH_2Cl)_2$

Sulfur mustard

Lomustine (CCNU)

$ClCH_2CH_2NH-C(=O)-N(N{=}O)CH_2CH_2Cl$

Carmustine (BCNU)

Fig. 27-3. *Chemical structures of alkylating agents.*

animals. Bone marrow depression develops from 5 to 21 days following nitrogen mustard treatment, the usual nadir of values occurring at about 14 days after treatment. There is reticulocytopenia, moderate fall in hemoglobin, then leukopenia and thrombopenia. Lymphopenia occurs within a few days, followed by granulocytopenia. Infection may occur during granulocytopenia if severe, and bleeding may develop if thrombopenia is marked. Thrombophlebitis and thrombosis can occur following injection; hence, it is advisable to administer the drug into the tubing of an intravenous infusion.

Therapeutic Uses. The most striking clinical benefit of mechlorethamine, when used singly, occurs in Hodgkin's disease. Present use, however, is almost always in combination with other agents for treatment of this disease. Tumor regression occurs, with lesser degrees of tumor reduction and for generally lesser periods, in patients with other types of malignant lymphoma; chronic leukemia; polycythemia vera; mycosis fungoides; carcinoma of ovary, breast, and bronchus; Wilms' tumor, seminoma; neuroblastoma; anaplastic carcinoma of lung; and, epidermoid carcinoma of lung. Rarely, tumor regression occurs in cases of adenocarcinoma of the lung, colon, soft tissue sarcoma, and malignant melanoma. Direct intracavitary use for control of malignant effusion provides effective palliation (at systemic doses).

CYCLOPHOSPHAMIDE

It was originally postulated that cyclophosphamide compound could be selectively activated in neoplastic tissues by phosphatase and phosphamidase, which are known to be present in high concentration in tumor cells. No evidence for this selective activity has been demonstrated, however, and its metabolism to an active compound occurs apparently in the liver through the microsomal cytochrome P-450 mixed-function oxidase system (26). Cyclophosphamide is converted to 4-hydroxycyclophosphamide, which is in a steady state with the acyclic tautomer, aldophosphamide. The aldophosphamide undergoes a nonenzymatic cleavage to yield phosphoramide mustard (27) and acrolein (3), both highly cytotoxic (Figure 27-4).

Because cyclophosphamide is activated by mixed-function enzyme system in the liver, corticosteroids and sex hormones, which appear to inhibit this enzyme, would decrease the action and toxicity of this antitumor compound, whereas barbiturates, which stimulate the enzyme system, would produce opposite effects.

Adverse Effects. The predominant side effects are bone marrow depression, alopecia, and gastrointestinal toxicity. Significant thrombopenia occurs in only 20% of patients; the nadir of marrow depression occurs 7-10 days following treatment but may be 21 days. Nausea and vomiting are common but not generally as severe as with nitrogen mustard. Extravasation of the drug does not yield severe local reaction. Scalp alopecia is frequent but reversible.

Sterility and testicular atrophy are common in males, and suppression of ovarian function develops at low doses in females. Hemorrhagic cystitis with hyperplastic changes is noted on bladder biopsy. This is related to high concentration of metabolites in the urine and can be avoided with good hydration. Long-continued use has rarely been associated with bladder carcinoma (24).

High doses have resulted in a few cases of cardiac toxicity; pulmonary toxicity has also been reported (75). Impaired water excretion with hyponatremia and inappropriately concentrated urine has developed at high dose levels (32); a direct effect on the distal renal tubule is postulated. Hyperpigmentation of skin and transverse ridging of the nails have been noted.

Therapeutic Uses. The clinical spectrum of therapeutic activity is similar to that of nitrogen mustard. Indeed, in the few controlled comparative studies in which either compound seems superior, the comparability of dosage may be questioned (77). Nevertheless, cyclophosphamide offers certain advantages because of oral administration in addition to its i.v. injection, such as lesser gastrointestinal side effects, and differing marrow toxicity (reduced incidence of thrombopenia).

Therapeutic applications include Hodgkin's disease, non-Hodgkin's lymphoma, multiple myeloma, small cell cancer of the lung, cancer of the breast and ovary, neuroblastoma, and Burkitt's lymphoma. Rarely, cyclophosphamide is effective in cases of acute lymphocytic leukemia and cancer of stomach, pancreas, lung, and nasopharynx. Its general use is in drug combinations, except for nodular lymphomas and Burkitt's lymphoma, in which it is highly effective as a single agent.

In recent years, more attention has been focused on cyclophosphamide due to its marked immunosuppressive action. It has been used in nonneoplastic disorders, such as nephrotic syndrome in children, rheumatoid arthritis, Wegener's granulomatosis, and in the control of organ rejection after transplantation (Chapter 13.5-3).

MELPHALAN

The phenylalanine derivative of nitrogen mustard, melphalan, or its isomer, l-sarcolysin, is shown in Figure 27-3. The spectrum of activity is similar to that of other alkylating agents, although the commonest use is in multiple myeloma and polycythemia vera.

Melphalan produces dose-dependent bone marrow depression. Pulmonary toxicity, characterized as diffuse infiltrates, has been described. The potential carcinogenicity is of concern because of the development of leukemia in patients with myeloma treated with this agent. Nausea and vomiting occur after large doses.

URACIL MUSTARD

The primary use of uracil mustard (Figure 27-3) has been thrombocythemic states (essential thrombocythemia, polycythemia vera, and chronic granulocytic leukemia), since it tends to produce thrombopenia of greater

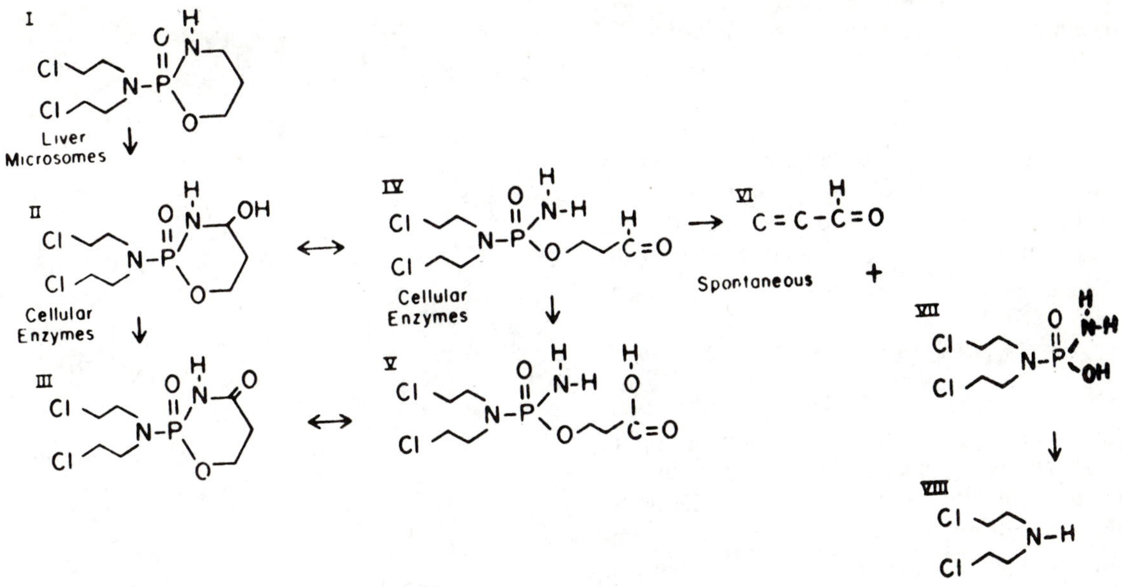

Fig. 27-4. *Metabolic transformation of (I) cyclophosphamide, (II) hydroxycyclophosphamide, (IV) aldophosphamide, and (V) phosphoramide mustard (65).*

degree at therapeutic doses, as compared with other oral alkylating agents.

CHLORAMBUCIL

Chlorambucil (Figure 27-3), one of the earliest oral alkylating agents developed, is the slowest acting and least toxic nitrogen mustard and therefore has had extensive clinical use. In large doses, it will induce nausea and emesis due to CNS stimulation. Occasionally skin reactions occur, and very rarely pulmonary toxicity has been noted. As with other alkylating agents, amenorrhea and azoospermia may develop. The most important toxicity is bone marrow depression, which can be averted by carefully monitoring peripheral blood counts of patients on therapy. The drug is used predominantly in chronic lymphocytic leukemia but is useful in Hodgkin's disease, other lymphomas, and primary macroglobulinemia. Its use in solid tumors is not common, although its effectiveness is best documented in carcinomas of ovarian and testicular origin.

BUSULFAN

Busulfan was developed because of research interest in the properties of alkanesulfonic acid esters (Figure 27-3). It was found to induce granulocytopenia in humans. In screening systems for antitumor agents, it was an inactive compound.

Adverse Effects. Myelosuppression is the most important and frequent pharmacological effect of this drug. The hematopoietic effects include granulocytopenia (dose related) and thrombopenia. Unusual complications include generalized increase in skin pigmentation, gynecomastia, cheilosis, glossitis, pulmonary fibrosis, porphyria cutanea tarda, erythema multiforme, amenorrhea, and a wasting syndrome analogous to Addison's disease.

Therapeutic Uses. Busulfan is the most effective agent available for the management of chronic granulocytic leukemia, producing benefit in 85-90% of patients. It is also used in other myeloproliferative diseases polycythemia vera, myelofibrosis, and essential thrombocytosis.

NITROSOUREAS

Several nitrosoureas, particularly carmustine [BCNU, 1,3- bis-(chloroethyl)-1-nitrosourea)], lomustine [CCNU, 1-(2- chloroethyl)-3-cyclohexyl-3-(4-methylcyclohexyl)-1-nitrosourea], and semustine [methyl CCNU, 1-(2-chloroethyl)-3-(4- methylcyclohexyl)-1-nitrosourea] are clinically useful, and the subjects of extensive biochemical pharmacological study (Figure 27-3). Although they react with DNA in several ways, including alkylation involving the chloroethyl end of the molecule, carbamoylation (48) of cellular proteins with the formation of an isocyanate was thought to inhibit DNA repair. Recent studies suggest, however, that the alkylating activity is the principal mediator of cytotoxicity (48).

Adverse Effects. Nausea and vomiting are frequent, occurring in 2-6 hr and subsiding rapidly. The most significant and serious side effect of nitrosoureas is bone marrow suppression, which is delayed and sometimes prolonged. Leukopenia and thrombopenia tend to develop 6-8 weeks after administration of therapeutic doses. In patients who have had previous treatment with myelotoxic agents, severe marrow depression is usually observed. Alopecia and gynecomastia are reported with BCNU (88). Pulmonary toxicity also occurs with nitrosoureas (6). Metabolic encephalopathy has been reported with methyl CCNU. Following prolonged therapy with nitrosoureas, interstitial nephritis associated with renal failure has been documented (87).

Therapeutic Uses. The greatest clinical use has been in Hodgkin's disease, gastrointestinal carcinoma, carcinoma of the lung, malignant melanoma, and primary brain tumors. The lipid- solubility of the nitrosoureas (62) is the pharmacological basis for their usefulness in primary brain tumors because it enables them to cross the blood-brain barrier.

ANTIMETABOLITES

Antimetabolites are chemically similar to endogenous metabolites in that they enter the same metabolic system but differ enough to disrupt normal metabolic pathways. The antimetabolites disrupt normal biosynthesis by competing for important enzymatic reactions in the synthesis of nucleic acids. Further, they can be incorporated into DNA and RNA in place of the normal nucleotides, leading to error in coding, transcription, or translation. Antimetabolites with clinical value are analogs of folic acid, pyrimidines, and purines. These compounds are most effective during the DNA synthetic phase of the cell cycle (S phase).

FOLIC ACID ANALOGS

METHOTREXATE

The most clinically important folic acid analog is methotrexate, whose structure and that of folic acid are shown in Figure 27-5. The first clinically successful folate antagonist, aminopterin (39), yielded the first instance of successful treatment of acute leukemia with cytotoxic agents. Methotrexate has supplanted aminopterin because it has less toxicity at therapeutic doses thar aminopterin.

Methotrexate

5-Fluorouracil (5-FU)

Mercaptopurine

6-Thioguanine

Cytarabine (Cytosine arabinoside)

5-Azacytidine (Aza-CR)

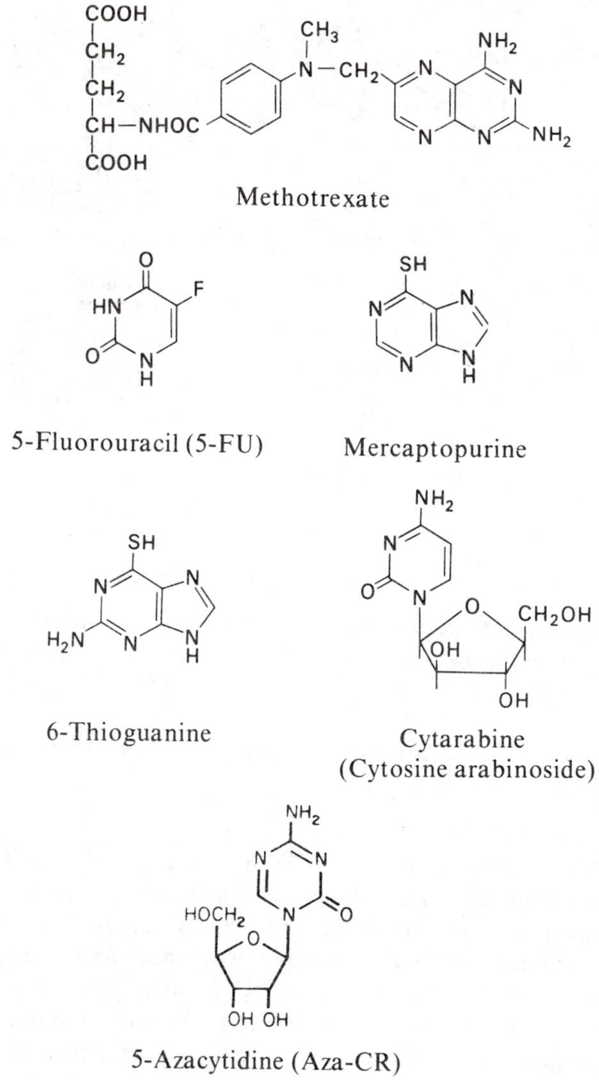

Fig. 27-5. *Chemical structures of antimetabolites.*

Tetrahydrofolic acid (THF), which is derived from folic acid, is a coenzyme responsible for metabolic transfer of 1- carbon units. Methotrexate is a potent competitive inhibitor of dihydrofolate reductase, the enzyme that converts dihydrofolate to tetrahydrofolate. The drug causes a major interference in cellular metabolism, thus resulting in an acute intracellular deficiency of folate coenzymes. In humans cells, the reaction most sensitive to depletion of tetrahydrofolate is thymidylate biosynthesis(8).

Pharmacokinetics. Following administration, there is an initial rapid phase of drug distribution. Single doses reach peak concentrations in the range of 0.1-1 μM in plasma. Bone marrow appears to withstand concentrations above the cytotoxic threshold of 1 μM for up to 42 hr with acceptable toxicity. Pharmacokinetic studies indicate a triphasic plasma disappearance with an initial mean half-life of 0.8 hr, followed by a secondary phase with a mean half-life of 3.5 hr, and a terminal phase with a mean half- life of 27 hr (9,24). The variability in plasma disappearance seems to be due to extensive enterohepatic circulation and probably enteric bacterial metabolism. Excretion of greater than 90% of the drug as intact compound occurs in urine.

A derivative of tetrahydrofolate, leucovorin, or folinic acid can protect against the inhibition of dihydrofolate reductase. This has been used extensively in the clinical treatment of cancer to prevent toxicity of high-dose methotrexate to normal cells while destroying malignant cells (63).

Adverse Effects. The major toxicity of methotrexate, noted with conventional doses, is myelosuppression consisting of granulocytopenia, anemia with megaloblastic bone marrow, and thrombopenia. In some patients, marrow recovery is accompanied by a brief leukemoid picture with thrombocytosis. Mucositis and gastrointestinal symptoms can occur. Toxicity to the intestinal epithelium is evident within 6 hr as swelling and cytoplasmic vacuolization, followed by desquamation of epithelial cells and extrusion of plasma into the lumen of the bowel.

Because most of the usual dose is excreted in the urine, impaired renal function is a cause of concern with the use of methotrexate. With reduced creatinine clearance, dosage should be decreased; with severe renal impairment, methotrexate is contraindicated.

Renal dysfunction occurs with high-dose regimens and may be related to the presence of a metabolite, 7-OH-methotrexate, in the kidneys and urine (24). Because the solubility of methotrexate rises in less acid solution, alkalinization of urine and diuresis are used during high-dose therapy to avoid renal toxicity.

During high-dose therapy, hepatic enzymes are elevated. In psoriasis, for which low doses are administered, there is a high incidence of cirrhosis (31). Neurotoxicity occurs with intrathecal use and may be in the form of an acute arachnoiditis, neuropathies, seizures, and even a fatal necrotizing encephalopathy.

Unusual forms of toxicity include pulmonary infiltrates with fever (presumed to be lung hypersensitivity), increased skin pigmentation, and rarely alopecia.

Therapeutic Uses. In choriocarcinoma and related trophoblastic tumor in women, methotrexate produces complete and lasting regression in 75% of cases. It is an unquestionable example of cure with cytotoxic treatment.

Although methotrexate is useful in acute lymphocytic leukemia, it is seldom used as primary treatment, although it is still utilized in the management of this disease (43). Complete remission occurred in about half the children in whom it has the initial treatment. In adult acute nonlymphocytic leukemia, its effectiveness is very limited. Large doses in combination with leucovorin can cause rapid reduction of elevated blood counts in acute leukemia.

In solid tumors, methotrexate is the most effective form of cytotoxic therapy for head and neck carcinomas; it has also shown benefit in cases of mycosis fungoides, osteogenic sarcoma, carcinoma of ovary, breast, and testis, and aggressive lymphoma.

The drug has proved particularly useful in the management of meningeal malignancies given intrathecally, particularly leukemia and lymphomas; and occasionally in solid tumors metastatic to meninges.

PYRIMIDINE ANALOGS

5-FLUOROURACIL (5-FU)

The development of therapeutic pyrimidine analogs was stimulated by the synthesis of 5-fluorouracil (Figure 27-5) in 1957 by Heidelberger and Ansfield (49). The clinical use of the drug is based largely upon empiric consideration, although recent developments are still expanding knowledge of the molecular and cellular mechanisms of its action.

5-FU is an antimetabolite of uracil, the normal pyrimidine base involved in the biosynthesis of RNA. 5-FU is initially converted to 5-fluorouridine monophosphate (5-FUMP), then to 5- FdUMP (5-fluoro-2′-deoxyuridine-5′-monophosphate), which inhibits thymidylate synthetase, an enzyme that catalyzes methylation of deoxyuridylic acid to thymidylic acid (73). Inhibition of thymidylate synthetase blocks the synthesis of DNA. Further, fluorouracil may be incorporated in RNA, thus depressing RNA synthesis directly by blocking incorporation of uracil and orotic acid into RNA (58).

Pharmacokinetics. A single intravenous dose of fluorouracil is rapidly distributed into the total body water with peak blood levels of 0.2-2 mM occurring immediately. The drug is rapidly cleared with a half-life of 10-20 min. The catabolism of fluorouracil occurs in the liver. The drug is reduced by dihydrouracil dehydrogenase and then nonenzymatically cleared with the formation of 2-fluoro-β-alanine, urea, ammonia, and CO_2.

Adverse Effects. When the drug is used by prolonged continuous infusion, myelosuppression is allegedly reduced. The relative efficacy of oral administration is controversial. Hepatic artery or portal vein infusion is of interest in patients with tumors confined primarily to the liver, since the liver is the main site of metabolic degradation (4). The response rate is reputed to be higher than those obtained with systemic administration. Randomized comparison of hepatic artery infusion versus i.v. administration of 5-fluorouracil does not indicate significant difference in terms of response rate or survival, however (45).

The major side effects of 5-fluorouracil are on the bone marrow, lining of the gastrointestinal tract, and oral mucosa. When the drug is administered weekly, bone marrow effects may be limited to leukopenia, although megaloblastic change occurs in the marrow. When it is given daily until toxicity occurs, more profound marrow depression develops, resulting in anemia and thrombopenia. Stomatitis is a frequent sign of early toxicity. Diarrhea occurs occasionally, as well as skin eruptions. Central nervous system toxicity, notably cerebellar ataxia, may be noted in a very small number of patients.

Therapeutic Uses. 5-Fluorouracil is clinically important as the initial drug with effectiveness in adenocarcinoma of the gastrointestinal tract. Though the response rate is low (15-20%) and the duration of benefits brief (median 3 months), it is relatively free of serious toxicity in therapeutic doses.

The drug has shown activity in adenocarcinoma of breast, ovary, and prostate, and in some cases of carcinoma arising in the head and neck, lung, and urinary bladder. It is effective for intracavitary use in controlling malignant effusion.

Its major use is in combination with other agents for adenocarcinomas of the gastrointestinal tract and breast. In gastrointestinal tumors found to be locally incurable, 5-fluorouracil is used in combination with radiotherapy, as this combination yielded improved survival when compared with radiotherapy used singly. Although improved survival is an important determinant of benefit, the reduced morbidity due to the tumor (i.e., gastrointestinal bleeding or relief of obstruction) is often a more important clinical result of this approach.

CYTARABINE

Cytarabine (cytosine arabinoside, Ara-C), an analog of the naturally occurring nucleosides, cytidine and deoxycytidine (Figure 27-5), was synthesized in 1959 and found to have profound effects on the growth of experimental tumors.

Cytosine arabinoside is enzymatically converted to the monophosphate and diphosphate form, and then to the active cytosine arabinoside triphosphate. This compound is incorporated into DNA and to a limited extent into RNA. The bases of polyarabinonucleotide cannot stack normally due to steric hindrance produced by the 2′-hydroxyl being in the trans position to the 3′-hydroxyl. This can lead to nucleic acid dysfunction and inhibition of DNA and RNA polymerase activity. Its effects are primarily exerted during the S phase of the cell cycle.

Pharmacokinetics. The drug is rapidly distributed to all body compartments following intravenous administration. When it is given orally, however, there is poor and unpredictable absorption, with less than 20% of the drug reaching the general circulation. Most of the drug is destroyed by deaminase, which is found in the gastrointestinal tract. Cytarabine's elimination is biphasic, with a rapid excretion half-life of 7-17 min and a slower elimination half-life to 110 min. An important factor determining response is the metabolic competition for the compound by two opposing systems: deamination by cytidine deaminase to an inactive compound, uracil arabinoside, and activation by deoxycytidine kinase to the nucleotide form (84).

Adverse Effects. The most serious toxicity is hematopoietic, with anemia, leukopenia, and thrombopenia developing from 3 to 21 days after its use. A striking observation is marked megaloblastosis of the marrow developing in 48 hours. At large doses, mucositis and alopecia occur. Transient elevation of liver enzymes is common.

Therapeutic Uses. Cytarabine is one of the most clinically effective agents in the treatment of acute myelogenous leukemia. As a single agent, it induces significant benefit, although superior results are reported with its use in combinations. Recent interest has focused on the use of large doses by infusion for relapsed cases of leukemia. In leukemic patients, a high blood level of the nucleotide, with its greater cellular retention, is associated with greater therapeutic effectiveness. Interestingly, low doses of cytarabine also have proved useful in the treatment of acute leukemia and myelodysplastic syndromes, the presumed mechanism being induction of differentiation rather than cytotoxicity.

Though it does not have widespread use in other tumors, cytarabine has shown antitumor activity in patients with carcinoma of head and neck, melanomas, and carcinomas arising in the gastrointestinal tract. It has been included in combinations of drugs used for treatment of diffuse histiocytic lymphoma. Intrathecal use for meningeal leukemia has been successful.

5-AZACYTIDINE

5-Azacytidine is of interest because of its effectiveness in acute myelogenous leukemia (92) and lack of cross-resistance with cytarabine. Like cytarabine it is subject to deamination and requires phosphorylation for activity. It is incorporated into both RNA and DNA and causes profound inhibition of protein synthesis (Figure 27-5) (24).

Because the clinical toxicity is severe at therapeutic levels-particularly nausea, diarrhea, leukopenia, and hepatotoxicity its major usefulness is in relapsed cases of acute myelogenous leukemia (92). Rhabdomyolysis (60) as a complication of azacytidine, is also reported.

PURINE ANALOGS

6-MERCAPTOPURINE

6-Mercaptopurine (6-MP), synthesized by Hitchings and Elion in 1954 (50), was the first clinically useful purine analog and the first useful agent for treatment of adult nonlymphocytic leukemia (Figure 27-5). Mercaptopurine was established as a chemical analog of the natural purine, hypoxanthine, which is an intermediate in the biosynthetic pathway of adenine and guanine.

Although the drug has been studied for over 20 years, its precise mechanism of action as a cytotoxic agent is not definitely established. Mercaptopurine is a substrate for hypoxanthine-guanine phosphoribosyl transferase (HGPRT) and is converted to 6-thioinosine-5-monophosphate (T-IMP). T-IMP accumulates in the cell and interferes with several metabolic functions as such, inhibition of the conversion of guanosine monophosphate (GMP) to guanosine diphosphate (GDP) by guanylate kinase, oxidation of IMP to xanthylate by inosinate dehydrogenase, and inosinate to adenosine-5-phosphate. These reactions are necessary in the interconversion of IMP to guanine and adenine. In addition, T-IMP causes a pseudofeedback inhibition in the first step in the *de novo* pathway of purine synthesis and is cell-cycle specific for the S phase.

Pharmacokinetics. Mercaptopurine can be given orally and causes little damage to the intestinal epithelium. Elimination is such that half of the dose can be recovered as metabolites in the urine in 24 hr. Metabolism follows two main pathways: (a) methylation of the sulfhydryl group followed by oxidation of the derivatives, and (b) oxidation to 6-thiouric acid by xanthine oxidase.

Adverse Effects. The major toxic effect includes bone marrow depression; this, however, is delayed and develops gradually, it is quickly reversed when therapy is stopped. Other effects include hepatic damage, nausea, vomiting, leukopenia, thrombocytopenia, hemorrhage, and cholestatic jaundice.

Therapeutic Uses. 6-Mercaptopurine is useful in the treatment of adult nonlymphocytic leukemia. It is also effective in therapy of acute lymphocytic leukemia and chronic granulocytic leukemia.

6-THIOGUANINE (6-TG)

6-Thioguanine was synthesized by Elion and Hitchings in 1955 and appeared in early studies to have the same metabolic effects as 6-mercaptopurine. Thioguanine is an analog of the natural purine, guanine (Figure 27-5), and seems to exert its cytotoxic effect by competing for guanine in nucleic acid synthesis.

Thioguanine, like 6-mercaptopurine, is a substrate for HGPRT and is converted to 6-thioguanosine-5-monophosphate (6-thio- GMP). 6-Thio-GMP competitively inhibits guanylate kinase and is an irreversible inhibitor of inosinate dehydrogenase, thereby producing a disruption in polynucleotide synthesis. Like 6- mercaptopurine, it causes a pseudofeedback inhibition of *de novo* synthesis of purines.

Pharmacokinetics. The compound can be given orally, with peak plasma concentration achieved in 8 hr. It is metabolized in the liver to yield a 5-methylation product, 2-amino-6-methylthiopurine, which is excreted into the urine.

Adverse Effects. Its major toxic effect is bone marrow depression, but unlike 6-mercaptopurine, thioguanine was found to have cumulative toxicity with repeated doses.

Therapeutic Uses. In 1969, TG was found when used with Ara-C to make one of the most effective drug combinations for treatment of adult acute nonlymphocytic leukemia. Its predominant use is in various combinations for induction or maintenance of remission in acute leukemia.

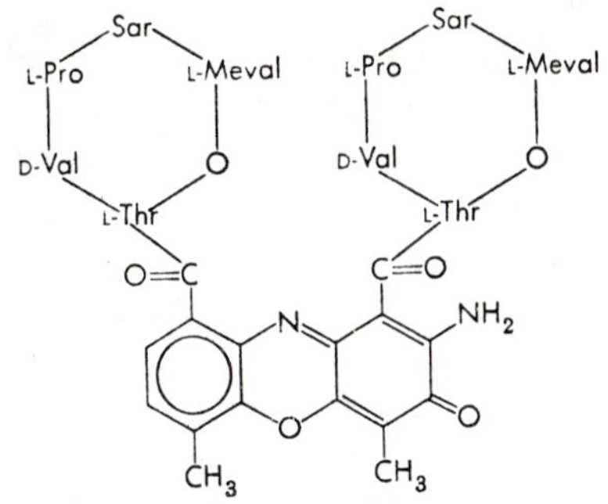

Dactinomycin
Sar = sarcosine
Meval = N-methylvaline

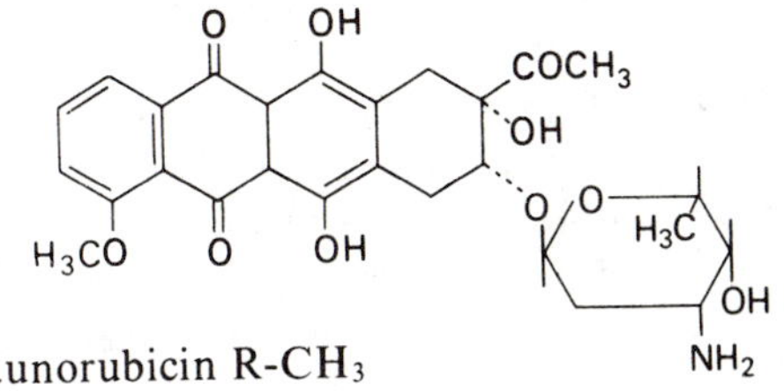

Daunorubicin R-CH_3
Adriamycin R-CH_2OH

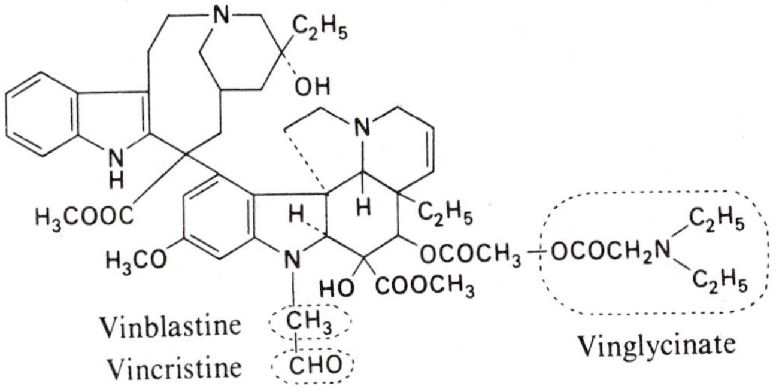

Vinblastine (CH_3)
Vincristine (CHO)
Vinglycinate

Fig. 27-6. *Chemical structure of some antineoplastic antibiotics and plant alkaloids.*

ANTIBIOTICS

Antibiotics that are clinically useful as antitumor agents affect nucleic acid functions or synthesis, although it is not certain that the cytotoxic effects are a consequence of their effect on DNA.

DACTINOMYCIN (ACTINOMYCIN D)

Dactinomycin is a peptide-containing antibiotic (Figure 27-6) derived from a species of *Streptomyces* . It forms stable complexes with DNA and is known to intercalate between adjacent guanine and cytosine base pairs of DNA with resultant unwinding of the double-helical structure. This effect causes the inhibition of DNA-dependent RNA polymerases, and thus the transcription of DNA is blocked (82). The drug is cell-cycle specific for late G_1 and S phase, and primarily affects those cells with a large growth fraction.

Adverse Effects. The drug has a wide spectrum of toxicity: nausea and vomiting occurring a few hours after administration, marrow depression with early thrombopenia and later pancytopenia, glossitis, alopecia, diarrhea, cheilitis, and oral ulceration. In areas of prior irradiation, erythema and increased pigmentation may develop (78).

Therapeutic Uses. In adults, use of dactinomycin is rather limited. Its application is mainly confined to resistant tumors choriocarcinoma that has failed methotrexate therapy, relapsed cases of Hodgkin's disease, and lymphoma. In pediatric oncology, it plays an important role in treatment of Wilms' tumor in conjunction with surgery and radiotherapy (67). As a single agent, it is very effective for embryonal cell carcinoma of the testis. It is useful in cases of advanced rhabdomyosarcoma (67).

BLEOMYCIN

Bleomycin, discovered by Umezawa, is a mixture of copper-chelating glycopeptides from *Streptomyces verticulus* and has both antibacterial and antitumor effects. This mixture includes the low-molecular-weight (1500 daltons) peptides, bleomycin A_2 and bleomycin B_2, with the A_2 species possessing the most antitumor activity.

It produces strand scissions in DNA, involving both double-stranded and heat-denatured single strands. Bleomycin is presumed to cause scission of DNA by chelating Fe^{2+} and binding DNA with its bithiazole group to form a DNA-Fe^{2+}-bleomycin complex. This complex is then oxidized to DNA-Fe^{3+}-bleomycin, which can again be reduced to Fe^{2+}-bleomycin by dissociating DNA. Each cycle of oxidation and reduction generates free radicals, possibly superoxide or hydroxyl, which attacks the glycosidic linkage in DNA, causing release of one purine or pyrimidine base (DNA scission). Fe^{2+}-bleomycin can later combine with a fresh molecule of DNA, and the process is repeated. Bleomycin inhibits progression of cells through the premitotic and mitotic phases of the cell cycle (24).

Bleomycin appears in high concentration in the lung and skin following parenteral administration. These tissues contain a low concentration of bleomycin hydrolase, an enzyme responsible for deactivation of the drug. Elimination of bleomycin is biphasic, with a half-life of 1.5 hr in the first phase and 9 hr in the second phase. The majority of the drug is excreted in the urine unchanged.

Adverse Effects. The early development of skin toxicity with bleomycin led to the present dose schedule of administration, once or twice weekly. Induration and erythema of the fingers and hands may develop. Sclerodactylia and increased pigmentation have been noted. Fever is a frequent occurrence several hours following administration but can often be prevented by premedication with antihistamines.

A major hazard of bleomycin treatment is pulmonary fibrosis, generally but not invariably dose related, occurring in about 10% of cases (91). The development of pulmonary toxicity is rare at total doses below 300 mg but has developed at lesser doses.

Clinically, pulmonary toxicity is characterized by dyspnea, cough, low-grade fever, dry basilar rales, and an interstitial infiltrate on chest x-ray. Pulmonary function studies show decreased diffusion capacity, vital capacity, and oxygen saturation.

Therapeutic Uses. Bleomycin has antitumor activity in squamous cell carcinomas, particularly those of the head and neck. Minimal effects are observed in squamous cell malignancies of esophagus and lung. It is effective in malignant lymphoma, for which it is used most frequently in combination chemotherapy. It also has demonstrated activity, singly and in combination, in cases of testicular carcinoma.It is capable of controlling malignant effusions when instilled intracavitarily. It is of particular interest that in humans the drug is not myelosuppressive so that it is particularly useful in combination chemotherapy.

ANTHRACYCLINE ANTIBIOTICS

Daunorubicin and Doxorubicin. Daunorubicin (daunomycin) and doxorubicin derived from fungal fermentation of *Streptomyces peucetius* var. *caesius* were introduced into clinical use in the past decade and constitute an important new class of agents. Structurally, both have a tetracyclic ring attached to the sugar daunosamine and differ only in the hydroxyl radical on the 14-carbon of doxorubicin (Figure 27-6).

Both agents are known to interfere with DNA function by intercalation. The anthracyclines intercalate between adjacent base pairs on the DNA strand and cause an uncoiling of the double-helix structure. This uncoiling prevents transcription of DNA by the DNA-directed RNA polymerase. Another possible mechanism includes the anthracycline's ability to cause DNA chain scission through the production of reactive free radical. DNA polymerase is also affected, but to a lesser degree.

The anthracyclines are distributed to all tissues following intravenous administration and appear in high concentration in the heart, lung, liver, and kidney. Elimination is triphasic, with half-lives in 12 min, 3 hr, and 30 hr.

The metabolism of doxorubicin in humans is known to be hepatic followed by biliary excretion. In patients with impaired hepatic function, delayed elimination may lead to severe clinical toxicity, so that dose modification is necessary if hyperbilirubinemia is present. Recent studies of the pharmacology of doxorubicin suggest that administration by continuous infusion or at frequent intervals using small doses may yield less toxicity and greater therapeutic efficacy (15,36).

Adverse Effects. The anthracyclines produce marrow depression, predominantly leukopenia and thrombopenia. Nausea and vomiting develop in about half the cases, mucositis in 10%, and alopecia in virtually 100% of patients. Hyperpigmentation, fever, skin rash, and local tissue necrosis are infrequent complications.

A serious complication of anthracycline treatment is cardiac toxicity. Refractory heart failure was noted with the use of these drugs in early trials. Pathological changes consistent with cardiomyopathy-decreased myocardial myofibrils, fragmentation, mitochondrial swelling, and intracellular inclusions were noted.

Several clinical patterns of cardiac toxicity are reported, the most striking being the abrupt onset of congestive heart failure, which is dose related and occurs in over 20% of cases receiving over a total cumulative dose of 550 mg/M^2. A report of toxicity at low cumulative doses (16) has described pericarditis, myocarditis, and heart failure, occurring 10 to 12 days after drug administration. Transient ECG abnormalities may develop early. If mediastinal or pulmonary irradiation (adjacent to the heart) has been given, however, toxicity develops at lower dose levels. Patients receiving doxorubicin must be carefully monitored for alteration of cardiac function. Measurement of systolic time interval and ejection fraction have been found to be parameters useful in detecting subclinical evidence of cardiac toxicity.

Therapeutic Uses. In acute leukemia, daunorubicin has shown clinical activity that is comparable to the best available agents. Its use is primarily in that disease. In acute promyelocytic leukemia, it is the most effective single agent. Doxorubicin, also effective in acute leukemia, has shown significant antitumor response in cases of malignant lymphoma, myeloma, carcinoma of breast, ovary, stomach, soft tissue sarcoma, thyroid carcinoma, Ewing's tumor, and Wilms' tumor.

MITOMYCIN C

Mitomycin C is an antitumor antibiotic isolated from *Streptomyces caespitosus.* It is a potent alkylating agent, when activated, and may degrade DNA, as well (53). Although it has been studied for 20 years, recent investigations indicate that at low dose levels, below those considered cytotoxic, in cell cultures it functions as a hypoxic cell sensitizer (40).

Adverse Effects. The principal toxicity of mitomycin C is delayed cumulative marrow suppression. The usual interval for nadir of peripheral count values to develop is about 30 days. Other side effects include alopecia, nausea, vomiting, diarrhea, and rarely nephrotoxicity and pulmonary fibrosis (30).

Therapeutic Uses. Mitomycin C is useful for adenocarcinomas of various sites, particularly those arising in the gastrointestinal tract. Squamous cell tumors have also shown response to mitomycin C. It has demonstrable effectiveness when instilled into the urinary bladder for superficial bladder tumors (72).

Over several years, mitomycin C has been incorporated into several drug combinations that are fairly commonly used. These include fluorouracil, adriamycin, and mitomycin (FAM) for tumors of the gastrointestinal tract; and fluorouracil, cisplatin, and mitomycin for squamous cell carcinomas of the esophagus and anorectal region (41,67).

Studies using low-dose mitomycin as a biological modifier to sensitize hypoxic cells are also in progress (94).

STREPTOZOCIN

Streptozocin, an antibiotic obtained from the fermentation of *Streptomyces acromogenes*, is known to inhibit DNA synthesis. Animal toxicity studies indicating a diabetogenic effect led to its evaluation in insulinoma. In this specific tumor, about 25- 30% of patients respond to therapy (85).

Additionally, it has some effect on malignant carcinoid tumors and malignant lymphomas. Nephrotoxicity consisting of renal tubular damage is a serious side effect that has limited its usefulness.

PLANT ALKALOIDS

Originally studied for possible hypoglycemic activity, these agents, derived from the periwinkle plant, were shown to induce bone marrow suppression in rodents. There are six alkaloids demonstrating tumor-inhibiting properties, but only two have had extensive clinical trials, vinblastine and vincristine (56) (Figure 27-6).

Vinca alkaloids are cell-cycle specific, producing metaphase arrest of cultured human cells, an observation that has suggested that this is the mechanism of their biological effect (24). Microtubular interaction involving binding to a subunit protein, tubulin, leads to disruption of a functionally intact microtubular system; therefore the chromosomes disperse throughout the cytoplasm (exploded mitosis) and ultimately the cell dies. Both vinca alkaloids inhibit DNA biosynthesis; vincristine inhibits isolated RNA polymerase preparations and vinblastine prevents the activity of cytoplasmic DNA polymerase in nucleated erythrocytes.

Pharmacokinetics. Both vinblastine and vincristine are rapidly distributed to tissue following parenteral administration and are barely detectable in plasma in an hour. Vinblastine is eliminated in a biphasic fashion, with half-lives of 5 min and 190 min, and 21% of the drug is excreted in the urine unchanged. Vincristine is characterized by a triphasic elimination, with half-lives of 1,7, and 169 min; 12% of the drug appears in the urine unchanged, and 69% is excreted in the feces, of this 40% as metabolites.

Adverse Effects. The clinical toxicity of these agents is mainly neurological (23), with paresthesia, loss of deep tendon reflexes, muscle weakness, foot drop, and less commonly ptosis, ataxia, athetosis, and hoarseness. Generally, but not always, the findings are reversible with cessation of treatment. Severe constipation and colicky abdominal pain also may occur. Alopecia develops in 10-20% of cases. Marrow depression, mainly leukopenia, is much more frequent with vinblastine at therapeutic doses. Vincristine has a lesser myelosuppressive effect and is often used with other agents, as there is less possibility of cumulative marrow toxicity. Pain at the site of the tumor has been noted rarely following drug injection.

Therapeutic Uses. Although only minor differences in structure are noted in comparing these compounds, notable differences exist in this therapeutic spectrum and toxicity.

Vinblastine as a single agent is one of the most effective agents for treatment of Hodgkin's disease. It is also useful in choriocarcinoma, cancer of breast, and testicular carcinoma. Its present use is in combination, primarily for testicular tumors. Vincristine is a very active agent in the management of acute lymphocytic leukemia and is one of the conventional drugs used to induce remission. It is also effective in Hodgkin's disease (less so than vinblastine), non-Hodgkin's lymphoma, neuroblastoma, soft tissue sarcoma, and Wilms' tumor. It is frequently used in combination for treatment of carcinoma of breast, gastrointestinal tract, rhabdomyosarcoma, and malignant melanoma.

HORMONES

The application of hormones to the therapy of malignant disease includes two general indications: (a) to induce regression of tumors that seem to possess specific hormonal- mediated growth dependency, and (b) to provide useful palliation by virtue of their effects in reducing inflammation or altering the immune state. Hormone antagonists have also recently been found to possess antineoplastic effects.

ADRENOCORTICOSTEROIDS

The greatest value of adrenocorticosteroids is in the treatment of acute lymphoblastic leukemia, in which, when combined with vincristine, a complete remission develops in about 90% of cases. This lympholytic effect and the ability to suppress mitosis have long been appreciated. Recently, the presence of receptors on leukemia cells have been investigated to examine the mechanism of effectiveness. Variations in clinical sensitivity do not appear to be related to the presence or absence of eceptors.

Occasionally, acute nonlymphocytic leukemia responds to adrenocorticosteroids. Malignant lymphomas also show significant tumor regression of brief duration. Because marrow depression is not a significant side effect, corticosteroids are useful in drug combinations, as in therapy for malignant lymphomas.

A useful contribution of corticosteroids, particularly in the hematological neoplasms, is in the management of immune hemolytic anemia and thrombopenia. In solid tumors, corticosteroids are used to reduce edema associated with radiation, notably in the management of intracranial metastases, spinal cord compression (19), superior caval obstruction (79), and esophageal carcinoma with severe obstruction. In the hypercalcemia (68) of malignant lymphomas, myeloma, leukemia, and carcinomas of breast and prostate, steroids are also useful.

Adverse Effects. Steroid administration is associated with many iatrogenic complications including immunosuppression, Cushing's syndrome, diabetes mellitus, poor wound healing, peptic ulcer disease, psychosis, and other side effects.

ESTROGENS

The use of estrogen in neoplastic disease is confined to those tumors dependent, in some instances, on the presence of sex hormones for their growth, notably, carcinoma of the breast and prostate.

In mammary carcinoma, estrogen therapy is used infrequently. In premenopausal women, estrogen is seldom used because it is thought to accelerate the disease. In postmenopausal women, estrogens are useful in patients whose dominant disease is local soft tissue metastasis (22). The presence of receptors for estrogens in the tissue seems to be predictive for the effect of therapy because some patients who are receptor-negative do respond to estrogens, although they are small number. The effects of the drugs may not be evident for 8-12 weeks.

Estrogen is also used in advanced carcinoma of the male breast, generally after orchiectomy. It has provided useful palliation in a significant number of cases.

The use of estrogens in prostatic carcinoma is a consequence of early studies demonstrating shrinkage of the prostate following castration, with reversal of castration effects by androgen. Estrogen was found to inhibit the effect of androgen. In 1941, Huggins et al (51) tried bilateral orchiectomy in patients with advanced prostatic carcinoma. Later, estrogen administration was found to yield comparable results.

The precise mechanism by which estrogens induce tumor regression is unknown. Examination of tumor tissue for steroid receptors suggests that the presence of receptors may predict response to estrogen therapy (59,69).

The indication for the use of estrogen in prostatic carcinoma is limited to advanced disease. In early stages of disease and at high doses, estrogen therapy is associated with increased risk of cardiovascular complications (10).

In patients who are refractory to diethylstilbestrol (DES), useful palliation has developed with other estrogenic substances, notably diethylstilbestrol diphosphate and estramustine phosphate (72).

Adverse Effects. Major side effects include fluid retention, anorexia, nausea, breast tenderness, decrease in libido, dizziness, abdominal cramps, and irritability. Hypercalcemia rarely develops but constitutes a medical emergency manifested as profound physiological disturbances and ectopic calcification.

ANDROGENS

The administration of androgens for mammary carcinoma in the female followed the demonstration of benefit from castration. Extensive clinical trials in patients with advanced disease indicate that androgens are preferred treatment for patients whose dominant site of metastatic disease is skeletal. Regressions occur in about 20% of cases (22). The presence of estrogen receptor in the tumor and metastases is a useful method of predicting response to hormonal therapy (59,69).

Androgen in high doses can cause regression in a small number of patients with advanced renal cell carcinoma (77). The mechanism is unknown, although recent studies demonstrated the presence of steroid receptors in tumor tissues in some cases.

The adverse effects and low response rate have led to extremely infrequent use of androgens in management of carcinoma of the female breast.

Adverse Effects. Adverse effects include fluid retention and virilization with deepening of the voice, hirsutism, clitoral enlargement, and increased libido. As with the estrogens, hypercalcemia can occur but is rare.

PROGESTATIONAL AGENTS

Progestational agents are used predominantly in the management of patients with advanced endometrial carcinoma. About one-third of patients will show tumor regression. Progestational agents are also useful in some instances of renal cell carcinoma; and carcinoma of female breast.

ANTIESTROGEN

A recent development in the hormonal management of disseminated breast carcinoma is the use of antiestrogen. Tamoxifen, a compound shown to inhibit uterine uptake of estrogen and to inhibit estrogen effects on the uterus and vaginal epithelium of rodents, is the most widely used.

Adverse Effects. Nausea and vomiting occur in some patients, and hot flashes are also noted. Hypercalcemia has been reported; and very rarely, after prolonged periods, at high dose levels, ophthalmological toxicity is observed.

Therapeutic Uses. Tamoxifen is shown to be of greatest benefit in postmenopausal women with advanced mammary cancer (22). About one-third of patients develop tumor regression, predominantly those with soft tissue metastases, those with estrogen receptor-positive tissue, and possibly those with low serum estrone levels.

MISCELLANEOUS AGENTS

PROCARBAZINE

In the search for monoamine oxidase inhibitors, a group of substituted hydrazines that exhibited antineoplastic properties were discovered. Of these, one of special potency and interest 1-methyl-2-p-(isopropylcarbamoyl) benzyl hydrazine hydrochloride (MATULANE,procarbazine) is clinically useful (Figure 27-7).

It is well established that this compound produces free-reacting CH_3 radicals, resulting in methylation of DNA and RNA. The metabolic pathways involved are complex. An exponential drop of DNA viscosity *in vitro* is noted with exposure to this agent in the presence of molecular oxygen; this can be reduced by the addition of catalase or peroxidase. Hydrogen peroxide is a byproduct of autooxidation of procarbazine at 37° C, an observation leading to the concept of hydrogen peroxide-induced DNA degradation. This is not, however, considered to be the major mechanism for procarbazine action.

Chromatid breaks have been observed in Ehrlich ascites cells. Procarbazine acts as a powerful carcinogen in rodents and also induces teratogenesis (2).

Adverse Effects. The major toxicity is bone marrow depression with leukopenia, thrombopenia, and anemia. Nausea and emesis are frequent. Rare side effects are

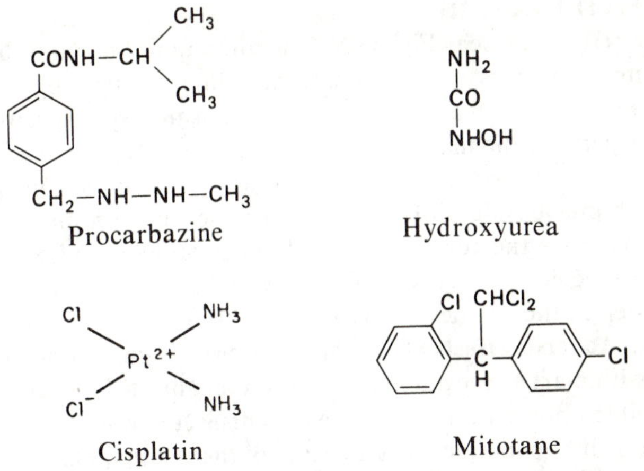

Procarbazine

Hydroxyurea

Cisplatin

Mitotane

Fig. 27-7. *Chemical structure of miscellaneous antineoplastic agents.*

stomatitis, diarrhea, fever, myalgia, and CNS effects including lethargy, ataxia, hyperexcitability, and euphoria. Pulmonary toxicity (57) consisting of infiltrates with fever and eosinophilia is also reported.

The carcinogenic potential of procarbazine is a consideration in regard to the reported cases of second malignancies following successful treatment of Hodgkin's disease with combination chemotherapy that has included procarbazine.

Therapeutic Uses. The greatest therapeutic efficacy of procarbazine is in Hodgkin's disease, in which it ranks as one of the most effective agents, used singly (19). Present use, however, is in combination therapy. It is active, to a lesser extent, in other malignant lymphomas. Responses are reported in cases of carcinoma of the lung, malignant melanoma, and myeloma.

DACARBAZINE (DTIC)

Analogs of the intermediate compound of purine biosynthesis, 5-aminoimidazole-4-carboxamide ribonucleotide, were synthesized by Shealy. On the basis of effectiveness in tumor-screening system, DTIC [5-(3,3-dimethyl-1-triazeno-imidazole-4- carboxamide)] had extensive clinical study.

DTIC is considered, on the basis of its structural relationship to nitrogen mustard, to produce alkylation after activation by the hepatic microsomal enzymes. Interference with purine and protein synthesis seems likely as well. Because it is lethal to proliferating cells, however, it is not a cell-cycle specific agent.

Adverse Effects. The most significant toxicities are myelosuppression, consisting of leukopenia and thrombopenia as well as nausea and vomiting. Fever and hepatotoxicity are also reported.

Therapeutic Uses. As a single agent, DTIC provides to be active in malignant melanoma, for which it is now used in combination with other agents. Some activity, however, has been reported in cases of Hodgkin's disease, malignant lymphoma, carcinoma of lung, and soft tissue sarcoma (42).

HYDROXYUREA

Hydroxyurea (Figure 27-7) a compound known to be myelosuppressive in animals, has shown antineoplastic activity in animal tumors. It is useful primarily in specific aspects of the management of leukemia (89).

The mechanism of cytotoxic action is inhibition of ribonucleoside diphosphate reductase, the enzyme that catalyzes the conversion of ribonucleotides to deoxyribonucleotides. This step appears to be the rate-limiting step in the synthesis of DNA.

Adverse Effects. The major toxicity is hematopoietic, with marked megaloblastic marrow change that is reversible upon discontinuance of the drug. Leukopenia and thrombopenia occur. Occasionally nausea, emesis, dermatitis, alopecia, stomatitis, or neuritis may develop.

Therapeutic Uses. Hydroxyurea is a useful agent in the management of chronic granulocytic leukemia and polycythemia vera. It also is used in acute leukemia, often with cranial irradiation, in patients with high blast counts (over 50,000 mm^3) to induce rapid decrease in count and prevent leukostasis in cerebral vessels. It has some activity in solid tumors, notably epidermoid tumors of the head and neck and malignant melanoma.

CISPLATIN

Cisplatin (*Cis*-dichlorodiammineplatinum II, DDP) is a complex formed by a central atom of platinum surrounded by chlorine and ammonia atoms in the *cis* position in the horizontal plane (Figure 27-7). The antitumor activity was first noted in 1969. The precise mechanism of antitumor mechanism is unknown, although it inhibits DNA synthesis and apparently induces intrastrand cross-linking of DNA (24). There is no cell-cycle specificity. Intraarterial administration does not yield significantly higher drug levels to the tumor (20).

Adverse Effects. The most serious toxicity is renal, with cumulative dose-related renal tubular impairment (38). Hydration and infusion of mannitol or furosemide are used to decrease nephrotoxicity, as well as to prolong the duration of the infusion. Ototoxicity, manifested as tinnitus or hearing loss, also occurs (Chapter 21.2). Nausea and vomiting are also common and troublesome. Myelosuppression may occur. A few instances of anaphylaxis after earlier cisplatin therapy have been reported. Neuropathy and elevated SGOT are reported.

Therapeutic Uses. Cisplatin is a very effective agent in nonseminomatous testicular tumors and in ovarian tumors. In clinical practice, it is generally included in combination chemotherapy of these diseases (37). It has shown activity in epidermoid tumors of the head and neck, and lung, and carcinoma of the urinary bladder (38).

L-ASPARAGINASE

The enzyme l-asparaginase is of particular interest because it represents an instance of specificity of action for neoplastic tissue (28). The lymphoblast of acute leukemia requires the amino acid l-asparagine for growth, whereas most normal tissues synthesize their own l-asparagine. The enzyme is capable of depriving malignant cells of an essential constituent. The development of mutant sublines has limited effectiveness of the drug.

Adverse Effects. Allergic reactions are the most serious complications of treatment, and anaphylactic reactions develop in about 10% of cases. Hypoglycemia and coagulation disorders can also occur.

Therapeutic Uses. Primary use has been in the induction of remission in acute lymphocytic leukemia. Capizzi et al (21) have shown that with appropriate scheduling, asparaginase can reduce toxicity and improve therapeutic effects of methotrexate.

MITOTANE (*o,p′*-DDD)

Mitotane (*o,p′*-DDD) also exerts selective antineoplastic activity, related to its toxic effects on the adrenal cortex. It is an isomer of the insecticide DDT (Figure 27-7). It causes a rapid reduction of adrenocorticosteroids in the blood and urine.

Adverse Effects. Anemia and nausea are the most frequent side effects, but lethargy and occasional dermatitis may develop.

Therapeutic Uses. Mitotane is used for palliative treatment in both functioning and nonfunctioning adrenal cortical carcinomas, with lesser benefit in the latter type of tumor.

ETOPOSIDE (VP 16-213)

Since its introduction into clinical trials in 1973, etoposide has shown effective antineoplastic activity in a wide spectrum of human malignant diseases. VP 16-213 (4′-demethyl-epipodophyllotoxin-β-D-ethylidene-glucoside) is a derivative of podophyllin, an extract of the mandrake root (52).

Its mechanism of action is as a cell-cycle dependent and phase-specific agent (35). It causes metaphase arrest in cultured cells and prevents cells from entering metaphase, a G_2 or late S phase effect. In HeLa cells single-strand DNA breaks occur and G_2 dependency for cell kill is demonstrable in human lymphoblastoid cells (64).

Pharmacokinetics. Etoposide is generally given intravenously since oral absorption is variable (18). The drug has a mean serum half-life of 11.5 hours and about 45% is recoverable in urine after 72 hours (29). Spinal fluid levels are very low. The drug is administered over 30 minutes to avoid hypotension and bronchospasm.

Adverse Effects. Commonly, nausea, vomiting, alopecia and marrow suppression, predominantly manifested as a leukopenia, are toxic effects of VP 16-213. The leukopenia is maximal from 10 to 14 days after treatment with recovery from 6 to 10 days later. Thrombopenia is relatively infrequent. Two cases of toxic hepatitis following high-dose VP 16-213 are reported. Liver biopsy was consistent with a drug-induced toxic hepatitis (55). A cause of Stevens-Johnson syndrome presumed related to VP 16-213 is also described (54).

Therapeutic Uses. As a single agent, VP 16-213 has therapeutic activity in small cell carcinoma of the lung, germ cell tumors, Hodgkin's disease, non-Hodgkin's lymphoma, and acute nonlymphocytic leukemia (93). The highest response rates are observed in previously untreated patients. For small cell carcinoma of the lung, it ranks among the most effective agents studied. Its clinical use generally involves incorporation into combination chemotherapy programs for small cell carcinoma of the lung, germ cell malignancies, and lymphomas.

INTERFERON

Interferon is a naturally occurring protein that has antiviral, antiproliferative, and immunological properties (Chapter 25.1). Interferon is species specific, with differing biological, antigenic, physical, and chemical properties. Clinical experience with human leukocyte interferon is limited to investigational use at this time. Antitumor response is documented in some patients with advanced breast cancer (13), multiple myeloma, and malignant melanoma (14,47), and renal cell carcinoma.

COMBINATION CHEMOTHERAPY

The use of drugs in combination for the treatment of cancer is a consequence of limited success obtained with the agents used singly. Many combinations in clinical use are selected empirically. As the numbers of single agents have increased, the dimensions of combination chemotherapy have expanded enormously. Scientific bases for drug combinations have been devised and are based upon kinetic, biochemical, toxicological, and pharmacological consideration. Several excellent reviews of the rationale and results are available (33,86).

With regard to the kinetic basis for combination chemotherapy, it is of importance that in cell destruction mechanism, a given dose of drug destroys a constant fraction of cells, which constitutes first-order kinetics. Therefore to increase therapeutic potential and eradicate the tumor, combination chemotherapy is a logical approach.

Conceptually, the biochemical approach to combined drug programs is aimed at decreasing the production and availability of essential products for cell growth and replication, which may occur according to three basic schemes: (a) sequential inhibition of different enzymatic pathways leading to production of an essential metabolite; (b) simultaneous inhibition of parallel pathways, termed concurrent inhibition ; and, (c) production of biochemical lesions at different loci in the biosynthesis of macromolecules, known as complementary inhibition.

The use of most drug combinations in clinical practice is still based upon empirical rather than pharmacological considerations. In fact, although the use of drug combinations far exceeds the use of single agents, controlled trials comparing single agents with drug combinations are relatively few in number (25). In some controlled trials, the number of cases is too small for the results to be conclusive in view of the variability in disease pattern.

In some diseases, however, uncontrolled trials offer convincing evidence of therapeutic superiority, as historical controls suggest limited efficacy with less intensive therapy [e.g., Hodgkin's disease (34)and cancer of breast with liver metastases (22)].

The definition of therapeutic benefit with combined chemotherapy in combination with radiotherapy is exceedingly important. The risks and morbidity of combined modality treatment may be such that they do not warrant this approach.

It is noteworthy that the best results of combined therapy are in diseases that show responsiveness to single agents (5,11,37,43,46,67). Those diseases that show few responses to single agents are not generally greatly benefited by drug combinations. Nevertheless, combination chemotherapy has become the norm for most neoplastic diseases. As shown in Table 27-3, the use of MOPP and ABVD in patients in Hodgkin's disease is standard therapy; for non-Hodgkin's lymphomas, recent therapeutic strategies include multiple aggressive regimens of which PROMACE and COMLA are 2 examples. CHOP represents a standard regimen. PAC and CHAD are examples of combinations in current use in ovarian carcinoma. PVB is an example of a combination of efficacy in germ cell tumors.

Table 27-2 lists some diseases in which combined modality therapy is commonly used, and Table 27-3 lists some commonly used drug combinations.

ADJUNCTIVE CHEMOTHERAPY

Because of the limited efficacy of antineoplastic agents in reducing bulky tumor masses, the concept of treatment when the tumor mass is relatively small has emerged (90). Micrometastatic disease should be more susceptible to control than bulk disease. Support for this view is obtained from drug response data in rodent tumors.

From this concept, the clinical use of adjuvant chemotherapy in the management of cancer has emerged. Following surgical removal of bulk disease or radiotherapy to the primary tumor, and when wound healing is considered adequate, chemotherapy is administered. Maximal tolerated doses are given, intermittently, to diminish immunosuppression. A duration of 6 months to 2 years of such treatment seems to be a reasonable interval.

There is now a considerable experience with adjunctive chemotherapy in many diseases (12,46,61,67). The most convincing evidence of benefit is in Wilms' tumor and rhabdomyosarcoma (67). In premenopausal patients with operable carcinoma of the breast, disease-free survival is prolonged in women receiving adjunctive chemotherapy (12). Benefit is most frequent in patients whose ovarian function is suppressed, although this may not be the only mechanism of effectiveness.

The use of adjunctive chemotherapy is an attractive concept and its use is widespread in clinical trials at this time. In patients with osteogenic sarcoma and ovarian and testicular malignancies, the data suggest benefits. The long term risks of such treatment have not been assessed, however, nor have there been adequate confirmatory data to conclude that such treatment is indicated in all patients with these diseases.

Immunotherapy as an adjunct to primary forms of tumor treatment is still an investigative procedure. It appears that some benefit occurs in patients with acute leukemia (80), in complete remission, who receive immunotherapy, and in patients with epidermoid lung cancer (70) at early stages.

A major thrust of present-day tumor immunotherapy research is directed toward development of improved types of immunotherapy, since trials with presently available agents, though not indicative of success, still suggest a probability of benefit.

TABLE 27-2
Disease in which Combined Modality Therapy is Commonly Used

Hodgkin's disease, stages IIIB and IV
Diffuse lymphocytic and histiocytic lymphoma, stages III and IV
Ovarian carcinoma, advanced
Embryonal carcinoma, advanced
Small cell carcinoma of lung
Acute leukemia
Carcinoma of breast
Soft tissue sarcoma
Neuroblastoma

Table 27-3
Commonly Used Drug Combinations

MOPP or COPP

	Dosage	
Cyclophosphamide (CYTOXAN)	650 mg/M^2	i.v.
Mechlorethamine (MUSTARGEN)	6 mg/M^2	i.v.
Vincristine (ONCOVIN)	1.4 mg/M^2	total is not to exceed 2 mg i.v.
Procarbazine	100 mg/M^2	p.o.
Prednisone	40 mg/M^2	p.o.

A course of MOPP or COPP is given monthly for a total of six drug cycles, each consisting of 28 days. Of this period, treatment is given for 14 days, and 14 days involve no treatment wih the cytotoxic agents. Of the six drug cycles, only three include prednisone—the first, third and fifth.

In MOPP, MUSTARGEN and in COPP, CYTOXAN are used with other drugs.

MUSTARGEN and ONCOVIN are given on days 1 and 8 of each cycle. Procarbazine and prednisone are given from days 1-14 of each cycle.

Dose modification for blood count depression is as follows:

Total granulocyte count (TGC, in mm^3); platelet count (PC, in mm^3)				Dose of Mechlorethamine, Procarbazine (%)
TGC	4-5000;	PC	>100,000	100
TGC	3-4000;	PC	75-100,000	75
TGC	2-3000;	PC	50-75,000	50
TGC	1-2000;	PC	25-50,000	25
TGC	1000:	PC	< 25,000	No therapy

CVP

	Dosage		
Cyclophosphamide (CYTOXAN)	400 mg/M^2	p.o.	
Vincristine	1.4 mg/M^2	total dose not to exceed 2 mg	i.v.
Prednisone	100 mg/M^2	p.o.	

CYTOXAN is given for 5 days with prednisone, and vincristine only on day 1 of a 21-day cycle. Six drugs are administered.

CMF

	Dosage	
Cyclophosphamide (CYTOXAN)	100 mg/M^2	p.o.
Methotrexate	40 mg/M^2	i.v.
Fluorouracil	500 mg/M^2	i.v.

CYTOXAN is given for days 1-14 of a 28-day cycle; methotrexate and FU are administered on days 1 and 8 of the cycle. A total of 12 cycles is given.

Table 27-3 (continued)
Commonly Used Drug Combinations

	Dosage	
ABVD		
Doxorubicin (Adriamycin)	25 mg/ M^2, days 1 and 15	i.v.
Bleomycin	10 U/ M^2, days 1 and 15	i.v.
Vinblastine	7 mg/ M^2, days 1 and 15	i.v.
Dacarbazine	375 mg/ M^2, days 1 and 15	i.v.
Repeat every 28 days		
[Ref.: Santoro A., and Bonadonna, G.: Prolonged disease-free survival in MOPP resistant Hodgkin's disease after treatment with adriamycin, bleomycin, vinblastine and dacarbazine (ABVD). *Cancer Chemother Pharmacol* 2:101, 1979.]		
CHOP	Dosage	
Cyclophosphamide	650 mg/ M^2, day 1	i.v.
Doxorubicin	60 mg/ M^2, day 1	i.v.
Vincristine	1.4 mg/ M^2, day 1	i.v.
Prednisone	45 mg/ M^2, days 1 to 14	p.o.
Repeat every 28 days		
[Ref.: McKelvey E.M., Gottlieb J.A., Wilson H.E. et al. Hydroxyldaunomycin (adriamycin) combination chemotherapy in malignant lymphoma. *Cancer* 38:1484, 1976.]		
PROMACE	Dosage	
Etoposide	120 mg/ M^2, days 1 and 8	i.v.
Cyclophosphamide	650 mg/ M^2, days 1 and 8	i.v.
Doxorubicin	25 mg/ M^2, days 1 and 8	i.v.
Methotrexate	1.5 gm/ M^2, day 14 followed by	i.v.
Leucovorin after 24 hr,	50 mg/ M^2 q 6 hr for 5 doses	p.o.
Prednisone	60 mg/ M^2, days 1 to 14	p.o.
Repeat every 28 days		
(Ref.: Fischer, R.I., DeVita, V.T., Jr., Hubbard, S.M., et al. Diffuse aggressive lymphomas: Increases survival after alternating flexible schedules of PROMACE and MOPP chemotherapy. *Ann Intern Med* 98:304, 1983.)		
COMLA	Dosage	
Cyclophosphamide	1.5 gm/ M^2, day 1	
Vincristine	1.4 mg/ M^2, days 1 and 8	
Methotrexate	120 mg/ M^2, days 22, 29, 36, 43, 50, 57, 64, 71	i.v.
Cytosine arabinoside	300 mg/ M^2, days 22, 29, 36, 43, 50, 57, 64, 71	i.v.
followed by Leucovorin	25 mg/ M^2 every 6 hours for 4 doses	p.o.
Repeat every 28 days		
[Ref.: Sweet, D.L., Golomb, H.M., Ultman, J.E., et al: Cyclophosphamide, vincristine, methotrexate and leucovorin rescue, and cytarabine (COMLA) combination sequential chemotherapy for advanced diffuse histiocytic lymphoma. *Ann Intern Med* 92:875, 1980.]		
PVB	Dosage	
Cisplatin	20 mg/ M^2 for 5 days	i.v.
Vinblastine	0.2 mg/kg for 2 days	i.v.
Bleomycin	30 U weekly	i.v.
Repeat every 3 weeks except for bleomycin given for 12 weeks		
(Ref.: Einhorn, L., Donahue, J.P.: Cis-diammine-dichloroplatinum, vinblastine, and bleomycin combination chemotherapy in disseminated testicular cancer. *Ann Intern Med* 87:293, 1977.)		
PAC	Dosage	
Cisplatin	20 mg/ M^2 for 5 days	i.v.
Adriamycin	50 mg/ M^2, day 1	i.v.
Cyclophosphamide	750 mg/ M^2, day 1	i.v.
Repeat every 28 days		
(Ref.: Ehrlich, E.C., Einhorn, L., Williams, S.D., et al. Chemotherapy for Stage III-IV epithelial ovarian cancer with cisplatin, adriamycin, and cyclophosphamide: A preliminary report. *Cancer Treat Rep* 63:281, 1979.)		

Table 27-3 (continued)
Commonly Used Drug Combinations

CHAD	Dosage	
Cyclophosphamdie	600 mg/ M^2, day 1	i.v.
Hexamethylmelamine	200 mg/ M^2, days 8 to 22	p.o.
Adriamycin	25 mg/ M^2, day 1	i.v.
Cisplatin	50 mg/ M^2, day 1	i.v.
Repeat every 28 days		

[Ref.: Smith, J.P.: Treatment of ovarian cancer. In: *Advances in Cancer Chemotherapy,* (Carter, S.K., Goldin A., Kuretroi, K., et al, Eds.) Baltimore, University Park Press, 1978, p. 493.]

REFERENCES

1. Adair, F.E. and Bagg, H.J. Experimental and clinical studies in the treatment of cancer by dichlorosulphide (mustard gas). *Ann. Surg.* 93:190, 1931.
2. Adamson, R.H. Carcinogenicity studies with procarbazine. In: *Proceedings of the Chemotherapy Conference on Procarbazine (Matulane: NSC-77213): Development and Application* (Carter, S.K., ed.). U.S. Government Printing Office: Washington, D.C., 1970, p. 29.
3. Alarcon, R.A., and Meienhofer, J. Formation of the cytotoxic aldehyde acrolein during the *in vitro* degradation of cyclophosphamide. *Nature (New Biol.)* 233:250, 1971.
4. Ansfield, F.J., Ramirez, G., Davis, H.L., Jr. et al. Further clinical studies with intrahepatic arterial infusion with 5-fluorouracil. *Cancer* 36:2413, 1975.
5. Bagley, C.M., Jr., DeVita, V.T., Jr., Berard, C.W., and Canellos, G.P. Advanced lymphosarcoma: Intensive cyclical combination chemotherapy with cyclophosphamide, vincristine, and prednisone. *Ann. Intern. Med.* 76:227, 1972.
6. Beelot, P.A., and Valdiserri, R.O. Multiple pulmonary lesions in a patient treated with BCNU [1,3-bis-(2-chlorethyl)-1-nitrosourea)] for glioblastoma multiforme. *Cancer* 43:46, 1979.
7. Berenblum, I. The modifying influence of dichlorethyl sulphide in the induction of tumors in mice by tar. *J. Path. Bact.* 32:425, 1929.
8. Bertino, J.R. The mechanism of action of the folate antagonists in man. *Cancer Res.* 23:1286, 1963.
9. Bischoff, K.B., Dedrick, R.L., Zaharko, D.S. et al. Methotrexate pharmacokinetics. *J. Pharm. Sci.* 60:1128, 1971.
10. Blackard, C.E. The Veterans Administration cooperative urological research group studies of carcinoma of the prostate: A review. *Cancer Treat. Rep.* 59:225, 1975.
11. Bodey, G.P., and Rodriguez, V. Approaches to the treatment of acute leukemia and lymphoma in adults. *Semin. Hemat.* 15:221, 1978.
12. Bonnadonna, G. et al. Are surgical adjuvant trials altering the course of breast cancer? *Semin. Oncol.* 5:450, 1978.
13. Borden, E.C., Holland, J.F., Dao, T.L. et al. Leucocyte-derived interferon (alpha) in human breast carcinoma. *Ann. Intern. Med.* 97:1, 1982.
14. Borgstrom, S., von Eyben, F.E., Flodgren, P. et al. Human leukocyte interferon and cimetidine for metastatic melanoma. *N. Engl. J. Med.* 307:1080, 1982.
15. Boston, R.C., and Phillips, D.A. Evidence of a possible dose-dependent doxorubicin plasma kinetics in man. *Cancer Treat. Rep.* 67:63, 1983.
16. Bristow, M.R., Thompson, P.D. et al. Early anthracycline cardiotoxicity. *Am. J. Med.* 65:823, 1978.
17. Bruckman, J.E., and Bloomer, W.D. Management of spinal cord compression. *Semin. Oncol.* 5:135, 1978.
18. Brunner, K.W., Sonntag, R.W., Ryssel, H.J., and Cavalli, F. Comparison of the biologic activity of VP 16-213 given intravenously and orally in capsules or drink ampules. *Cancer Treat. Rep.* 60:1377, 1976.
19. Brunner, K.W., and Young, C.W. A methylhydrazine derivative in Hodgkin's disease and other malignant neoplasms: Therapeutic and toxic effects studies in 51 patients. *Ann. Intern. Med.* 63:69, 1965.
20. Campbell, T.N., Howell, S.B., Pfeifle, C.E. et al. Clinical pharmacokinetics of intra-arterial cisplatin in humans. *J. Clin. Oncol.* 1:763, 1983.
21. Capizzi, R.L., Bertino, J.R., and Handschumacher, R.E. L-asparaginase. *Ann. Rev. Med.* 21:433, 1970.
22. Carbone, P.P., and Davis, T.E. Medical treatment for advanced breast cancer. *Semin. Oncol.* 5:417, 1978.
23. Carpentieri, V., and Lockhart, L.H. Ataxia and athetosis as side effects of chemotherapy with vincristine in non-Hodgkin's lymphoma. *Cancer Treat. Rep.* 62:561, 1978.
24. Chabner, B.A., Myers, C.E., Coleman, C.N., and Johns, D.G. The clinical pharmacology of antineoplastic agents. *N. Engl. J. Med.* 292:1107, 1975.
25. Chlebowski, R., Irwin, L., Pugh, A. et al. Survival of patients with metastatic breast cancer treatment with either combination or sequential chemotherapy. *Clin. Res.* 27:53-A, 1979.
26. Cohen, J.L., and Jao, J.Y. Enzymatic basis of cyclophosphamide activation by hepatic microsomes of the rat. *J. Pharmacol. Exp. Ther.* 174:206, 1970.
27. Colvin, M., Brundrett, R.B., Kan, M.N. et al. Alkylating properties of phosphoramide mustard. *Cancer Res.* 36:1121, 1976.
28. Cooney, D.A., and Handschumacher, R.E. L-asparaginase and l-asparagine metabolism. *Ann. Rev. Pharmacol.* 10:421, 1970.
29. Creaven, P.J., and Allen, L.M. EPEG (VP 16-213) a new antineoplastic epipodophyllotoxin. *Clin. Pharmacol. Ther.* 18:221, 1975.
30. Crooke, S.T., and Bradner, W.T. Mitomycin C: A review. *Cancer Treat. Rev.* 3:121, 1976.

31. Dahl, M.G., Greogory, M.M., and Scheuer, P.J. Liver damage due to methotrexate in patients with psoriasis. *Br. Med. J.* 1:625, 1971.

32. DeFronzo, R.A., Braine, H., Colvin, O.M. et al. Water intoxication in man after cyclophosphamide therapy; Time course and relation to drug activation. *Ann. Intern. Med.* 78:861, 1973.

33. DeVita, V.T., and Schein, P.S. Use of drugs in combination for the treatment of cancer. *N. Engl. J. Med.* 288:998, 1973.

34. DeVita, V.T., Jr., Serpick, A.A., and Carbone, P.P. Combination chemotherapy in the treatment of advanced Hodgkin's disease. *Ann. Intern. Med.* 73:881, 1970.

35. Drewinko, B., and Barlogie, B. Survival and cycle-progression delay of human lymphoma cells *in vitro* exposed to VP 16-213. *Cancer Treat. Rep.* 60:1295, 1976.

36. Drewinko, B., Yang, L., Barlogie, B., and Trujillo, J.M. Comparative cytotoxicity of bisantrene, mitroxantrone, ametantrone, dihydroxyanthracenedione diacetate, and doxorubicin on human cells *in vitro* . *Cancer Res.* 43:2648, 1983.

37. Einhorn, L.H., and Donohue, J. Cis-diammine dichloroplatinum, vinblastine, and bleomycin combination chemotherapy in disseminated testicular cancer. *Ann. Intern. Med.* 87:293, 1977.

38. Einhorn, L.H., and Williams, L.D. The role of cis-platinum in solid tumor therapy. *N. Engl. J. Med.* 300:289, 1979.

39. Farber, S., Diamond, L.K., Mercer, R.D. et al. Temporary remissions in acute leukemia in children produced by folic acid antagonist, 4-aminopteroylglutamic acid (aminopterin). *N. Engl. J. Med.* 238:787, 1948.

40. Fracasso, P.M., Keyes, S.R., Rockwell, S., and Sartorelli, A.C. Biotransformation of mitomycin C by NADPH-cytochrome P-450 reductase and DT-diaphorase in cultured cell lines. *Proc. Am. Assoc. Cancer Res.* 24:249, 1983.

41. Franklin, R., Steiger, Z., Gangadhar, V. et al. Combined modality therapy for esophageal squamous cell carcinoma. *Cancer* 51:1062, 1983.

42. Frei, E. III., Luce, J.K., Talley, R.W. et al. 5-(3,3- Dimethyl-l-triazeno) imidazole-4-carboxamide (NSC 45388) in the treatment of lymphoma. *Cancer Chemother. Rep.* 56:667, 1972.

43. Frei, E. III., and Sallan, S.E. Acute lymphoblastic leukemia: Treatment. *Cancer* 42:828, 1978.

44. Gilman, A., and Phillips, F.S. The biological actions and therapeutic applications of the B-chloroethyl amines and sulfides. *Science* 103:409, 1946.

45. Grage, T.B. et al. Results of a prospective randomized study of hepatic artery infusion with 5-fluorouracil versus intravenous 5-fluorouracil in patients with hepatic metastases from colorectal cancer: A central oncology group study. *Surgery* 86:550, 1979.

46. Greco, F.A., Einhorn, L.H., Richardson, R.L. et al. Small cell cancer: Progress and perspective. *Semin. Oncol.* 5:323, 1978.

47. Gutterman, J.U., Blumenschein, G.R., Alexanian, R. et al. Leucocyte interferon induced tumor regression in human metastatic breast cancer, multiple myeloma and malignant lymphoma. *Ann. Intern. Med.* 93:399, 1980.

48. Heal, J.M., Fox, P.A., and Schein, P.S. Effect of carbamoylation on the repair of nitrosourea-induced DNA alkylation damage in L1210 cells. *Cancer Res.* 39:82, 1979.

49. Heidelberger, C., and Ansfield, J.F. Experimental and clinical uses of fluorinated pyrimidines in cancer chemotherapy. *Cancer Res.* 23:1226, 1963.

50. Hitchings, G.H., and Elion, G.B. The chemistry and biochemistry of purine analogs. *Ann. N.Y. Acad. Sci.* 60:195, 1954.

51. Huggins, C., Stevens, R.E., Jr., and Hodgens, C.V. Studies on prostate cancer: Effects of castration on advanced carcinoma of prostate gland. *Arch. Surg.* 43:209, 1941.

52. Isell, B.E., and Crooke, S.T. Etoposide (VP 16-213). *Cancer Treat. Rev.* 6:107, 1979.

53. Iyer, V., and Szybalski, W. Mitomycins and porfiromycin: Chemical mechanisms of activation and crosslinking of DNA. *Science* 145:55, 1964.

54. Jameson, C.H., and Solanki, D.L. Stevens-Johnson syndrome associated with etoposide therapy. *Cancer Treat. Rep.* 67:1050, 1983.

55. Johnson, D.H., Greco, F.A., and Wolff, S.N. Etoposide-induced hepatic injury. A potential complication of high-dose therapy. *Cancer Treat. Rep.* 67:1023, 1983.

56. Johnson, I.S., Armstrong, J.G., Gorman, M., and Burnett, J.P., Jr. The vinca alkaloids: A new class of oncolytic agents. *Cancer Res.* 23:1390, 1963.

57. Jones, S.E., Moore, M., Blank, N., and Castellino, R.A. Hypersensitivity to procarbazine manifested by fever and pleuropulmonary reaction. *Cancer* 29:498, 1972.

58. Kent, R.J., adn Heidelberger, C. Fluorinated pyrimidines. XL. The reduction of 5-fluorouridine 5′-diphosphate by ribonucleotide reductase. *Mol. Pharmacol.* 8:465, 1972.

59. Kiang, D.T., Frenning, D.H., Goldman, O.I. et al. Estrogen receptors and responses to chemotherapy and hormonal therapy in advanced breast cancer. *N. Engl. J. Med.* 299:1330, 1978.

60. Koeffler, H.P., and Haskell, C.M. Rhabdomyolysis as a complication of 5-azacytidine. *Cancer Treat. Rep.* 62:573, 1978.

61. Krumbhaar, E.B., and Krumbhaar, H.D. The blood and bone marrow in yellow cross gas (mustard gas) poisoning: Changes produced in the bone marrow of fatal cases. *J. Med. Res.* 40:497, 1919.

62. Levin, V.A., and Wilson, C.B. Chemotherapy: The agents in current use. *Semin. Oncol.* 2:63, 1975.

63. Levitt, M., Mosher, M.B., DeConti, R.C. et al. Improved therapeutic index of methotrexate with 'leucovor in rescue'. *Cancer Res.* 33:1729, 1973.

64. Loike, J.D., and Horowitz, S.B. Effects of VP 16-213 on the intracellular degradation of DNA in HeLa cells. *Biochemistry* 15:5443, 1976.

65. Ludlum, D.B. Alkylating agents and the nitrosoureas. In: *Cancer: A Comprehensive Treatise, Vol. 5. Chemotherapy* (Becker, F.F., ed.). Plenum Press: New York, 1977.

66. Macdonald, J.S., Schein, P.S., Woolley, P.V. et al. 5-Fluorouracil, mitomycin C and adriamycin (FAM): A new combination chemotherapy program for advanced gastric carcinoma. *Ann. Intern. Med.* 39:533, 1980.

67. Maurer, H.M. Solid tumors in children. *N. Engl. J. Med.* 299:1345, 1978.

68. Mazzaferri, E.L., O'Dorisio, T.M., and LoBaglio, A.F. Treatment of hypercalcemia associated with malignancy. *Semin. Oncol.* 5:141, 1978.

69. McGuire, W.L. Hormone receptors: Their role in predicting prognosis and response to endocrine therapy. *Semin. Oncol.* 5:428, 1978.

70. McKneally, M.F., Maver, C., Kausel, H.E., and Alley, R.D. Regional immunotherapy with intrapleural BCG for lung cancer. *J. Thorac. Cardiovasc. Surg.* 72:333, 1976.

71. Mishina, T., Oda, K. Murata, S. et al. Mitomycin C: Bladder instillation therapy for bladder tumors. *J. Urol.* 114:217, 1975.

72. Mittelman, A., Catane, R., and Murphy, G. New steroidal alkylating agents in advanced stage D carcinoma of the prostate. *Cancer Treat. Rep.* 61:307, 1977.

73. Myers, C.E., Young, R.C., Johns, D.G. et al. Assay of 5-fluorodeoxyuridine 5′-monophosphate and deoxyuridine 5′-monophosphate pools following 5-fluorouracil. *Cancer Res.* 34:2682, 1974.

74. Ochoa, M., Jr., and Hirschberg, E. Alkylating agents. In: *Experimental Chemotherapy of Neoplastic Diseases* (Schnitzer, R.J., and Hawking, F., eds.). Academic Press: New York, 1967, p. 1.

75. O'Connell, T.X., and Berenbaum, M.C. Cardiac and pulmonary effects of high doses of cyclophosphamide and isophosphamide. *Cancer Res.* 34:1586, 1974.

76. Papac, R.J., Ross, S.A., and Levy, A. Renal cell carcinoma: Analysis of 31 cases with assessment of endocrine therapy. *Am. J. Med. Sci.* 274:281, 1977.

77. Papac, R.J., and Wood, D.A. Long term results achieved with the use of alkylating agents in malignant lymphoma and Hodgkin's disease. *Acta Unio. Int. Contra. Cancer* 20:377, 1964.
78. Pearson, D., Deakins, D.B., Hendry, J.H., and Moore, J.V. Interaction of actinomycin D and radiation. *Int. J. Radiat. Oncol. Biol. Phys.* 4:71, 1978.
79. Perez, C.A., Present, C.A., and Van Amburg III, A.L. Management of superior vena cava syndrome. *Semin. Oncol.* 5:123, 1978.
80. Powles, R.L., Russel, J. et al. Immunotherapy for acute myelogenous leukemia: A controlled clinical trial 2.5 years after entry of the last patients. *Br. J. Cancer* 35:273, 1977.
81. Price, C.C., Gaucher, G.M., Koneru, P. et al. Mechanism of action of alkylating agents. *Ann. N.Y. Acad. Sci.* 163:593, 1969.
82. Reich, E. Biochemistry of actinomycin. *Cancer Res.* 23:1428, 1963.
83. Rose, D.P., and Davis, T.E. Ovarian function in patients receiving adjuvant chemotherapy for breast cancer. *Lancet* 1:1174, 1977.
84. Rustum, Y.M., and Preisler, H.D. Correlation between leukemic cell retention of 1-β-d-arabinosfuranosylcytosine 5′-triphosphate and response to therapy. *Cancer Res.* 39:42, 1979.
85. Sadoff, L. Patterns of intravenous glucose tolerance and insulin response before and after treatment with streptozotocin (NSC-85998) in patients with cancer. *Cancer Treat. Rep.* 56:61, 1972.
86. Sartorelli, A.C. Some approaches to the therapeutic exploitation of metabolic sites of vulnerability of neoplastic cells. *Cancer Res.* 29:2292, 1969.
87. Schacht, R.C., and Baldwin, D.C. Chronic interstitial nephritis and renal failure due to nitrosourea therapy. *Kidney Int.* 14:661, 1978.
88. Schorer, A.E., Oken, M.M., and Johnson, G.A. Gynecomastia with nitrosourea therapy. *Cancer Treat. Rep.* 62:574, 1978.
89. Schwartz, J.H., and Canellos, G.P. Hydroxyurea in the management of hematologic complications of chronic granulocytic leukemia. *Blood* 46:11, 1975.
90. Skipper, H.E. Adjuvant chemotherapy. *Cancer* 41:936, 1978.
91. Sostman, H.D., Matthay, R.A., and Putman, C.E. Cytotoxic drug-induced lung disease. *Am. J. Med.* 62:608, 1977.
92. Van Hoff, D.D., Slavik, M., and Muggia, F.M. 5-Azacytidine: A new anticancer drug with effectiveness in acute myelogenous leukemia. *Ann. Intern. Med.* 85:237, 1976.
93. Vogelzang, N.J., Raghavan, D., and Kennedy, B.J. VP 16-213 (Etoposide). The mandrake root from Issyk-Kul. *Am. J. Med.* 72:136, 1982.
94. Weissberg, J. Personal communication.

ADDITIONAL READING

Ho, M. Recent advances in the study of interferon. *Pharmacol. Rev.* 34:119, 1982.

Ozols, R.F. et al. Antineoplastic agents: Chemotherapy of ovarian cancer. *Semin. Oncol. 11:251, 1984.*

CHAPTER
27.1

INTERACTIVE EFFECTS OF RADIATIONS AND DRUGS

Gerald H. Sokol and Paul Berger

RADIOTHERAPY AND CHEMOTHERAPY

Chemotherapy provides essentially a systemic means for treating disseminated spread of cancer and may control micrometastatic disease (4). Radiation may react locally with chemical agents *additively* to increase damage or *interactively* to create more than an additive effect (*sensitization*). Alternatively, they may act separately with no interaction or negatively in that a resistive effect may occur. The interactions may occur by changing the distribution of cells in the cycle or number of cells surviving (and hence sensitivity), or they may sensitize the cells by altering protein or nucleic acid synthesis. Radiation may sterilize tumor in areas not amenable to chemotherapy. Preradiation chemotherapy may induce tumor regression to allow for smaller fields of irradiation and increase tumor control, whereas chemotherapy applied during radiation may sensitize cells to radiation while sterilizing distant subclinical disease. Chemotherapy after radiation may control subclinical disease while allowing for maximal local surgical or radiotherapeutic treatment with less host toxicity during a vulnerable period of debility secondary to radiation or surgery.

RADIOTHERAPY AND IMMUNOTHERAPY

Whereas radiation and drugs normally kill cells by first-order kinetics (a fixed *fraction* of cells are destroyed per given dose), immunotherapy kills by zero-order kinetics (i.e., a fixed *number* of cells are destroyed per given dose). Hence, the 'last' cancer cell becomes vulnerable to killing. Immunotherapy may counteract immunosuppression induced by radiation, drugs, or tumor effects and enhance host immunity. In addition, by reducing tumor burden, immunological mechanisms that eliminate antibodies that 'block' a successful immunological assault on tumors may become operational. Last, radiation may alter cells in such a way that they are not viable but may still induce an immunological host response.

New modalities of cancer treatment (including new physical modalities such as hyperthermia; new particles of radiation including protons, neutrons, and π-mesons; radiosensitizers; hypoxic cell sensitizers; and new chemotherapeutic agents) add complexity to the combined modality treatment of cancer.

RADIOBIOLOGY

THERAPEUTICALLY USEFUL RADIATION

Many forms of radiation can produce biological effects, but radiotherapy is principally concerned with ionizing types. Therapeutically useful radiation can be divided into particulate and electromagnetic types. X-rays and γ-rays are both electromagnetic radiations commonly used in therapy. Their high speed and lack of mass or charge allow excellent penetration into target tissue to reach deep-seated malignancies. Electrons (β-particles) are negatively charged (-1) and have a small mass (0.00055), they have limited penetrating ability and a well-defined depth of penetration, making them useful for irradiation of surfaces to a high dose while sparing deeper structures. Neutrons are uncharged particles (mass 1; charge 0) that can penetrate deeply with theoretical benefits. Negative π-mesons (mass 0.15; charge 1) deposit the bulk of their energy at depth rather than on the surface, making them ideally suited for irradiating deep tumors while sparing overlying normal structures.

A common denominator shared by all therapeutically useful radiations is the production of an energetic charged particle to mediate the tissue ionization that initiate biological changes. Some radiations (electrons and protons) can ionize target tissue directly, whereas others (neutrons and x-rays) must produce a charged particle to cause target ionization (indirectly ionizing).

The radiations used for treatment with isotopes, implants, and external therapy using ^{60}Co or ^{137}Ce derive their energy from radioactive decay; the clinically important emissions are β-particles and γ-rays.

MOLECULAR, CELLULAR, AND TISSUE EFFECTS

It is assumed that a critical target molecule(s) exists in tissue, injury to which is critical in establishing the eventual effect of the radiation exposure. Although this target may be ionized directly, this is uncommon. Water, being by far the most abundant molecule, is the one most commonly hit. Thus, most often, radiation exposure produces a charged particle that in turn ionizes water, producing unstable products with a half-life of 10^{-10} sec. These products then react to create free radicals, unionized substances that are highly reactive because of an unpaired electron in the outer shell. These free radicals, whose brief life span (10^{-5} sec) is nevertheless much longer than that of the ions, are thought to be the intermediaries between ionization and react with the target molecule:

$$H_2O \xrightarrow{\text{irradiation}}$$

$$H_2O^+ + H_2O \rightarrow H_3O^+ + OH^\cdot \text{ (free radical)}$$
$$e^{\pm} + H_2O \rightarrow H_2O^- \rightarrow OH^- + H^\cdot \text{ (free radical)}$$

Free radicals may recombine or react. In the latter case, the results may be innocuous, produce toxic molecules (e.g., OH+ H_2O_2), or cause significant changes in critical target molecules.

At the cellular level, radiation damage is of three types: interphase death, delay in division, and reproductive failure. *Interphase death* , occurs before the cell enters mitosis. This is uncommon and clinically relevant only concerning the oocyte and lymphocyte. *Division delay* is reflected in the mitotic index, defined as the fraction of cells in mitosis, which remains constant under steady-state conditions. After exposure to radiation, there is a delay in a cell's progression through mitosis, resulting in a fall in the index; the extent of recovery is dose dependent. *Reproductive failure* represents a decrease in the number of cells capable of reproducing indefinitely. Radiation causes effects in many subcellular structures, including chain breakage in fatty acids, structural changes in proteins, functional changes in enzymes, and alterations in membrane permeability. The nucleus of the cell contains the critical target for radiation, as shown by Munro using polonium- tipped microneedles to demonstrate the increased radiosensitivity of the nucleus as compared with the cytoplasm (26). Tritium- labeled compounds similarly implicate chromosomal exposure as instrumental in producing observed effects. Damage to the critical target in the nucleus would produce heritable defects.

The radiosensitivity of a cell is greatly dependent upon its place in the cell cycle. In general, sensitivity is greatest in M and G_2 phases, with late S being the most resistant time. Those cells with a long G phase have an early resistant period followed by a late sensitive one.

Chemical compounds (to be described in detail later) can act as either sensitizers (e.g., oxygen, pyrimidines) or radioprotectors (e.g., sulfhydryl compounds) with respect to these various cellular effects of radiation.

When a tissue is irradiated, death occurs in the stem cell population destined to replace the mature functioning cells after the latter has had a completed life span. Mature cells themselves are, as a rule, radioresistant. Thus, radiation-induced effects consist of the initial lesion and the late manifestation of that lesion. The organ may initially appear functionally intact, but the defect will become apparent when the metabolically active population dies off and no replacements are available to maintain function.

Rubin and Casarett have proposed the following classification of cell radiosensitivity (36): *group I cells* (e.g., erythroblasts, intestinal crypt cells, germinal cells of epidermis) are stem cells that are immature, mitotically active, and therefore radiosensitive; *group II cells* (e.g., myeloblasts) are those that mature while dividing; *group III cells* (e.g., liver cells) are more differentiated and more radioresistant and, though they do not normally divide, can be made to do so under conditions of stress; *group IV cells* (e.g., nerve and muscle cells), mature and nondividing, are the most radioresistant. Between Groups II and III are the connective tissue cells that form the supporting structure for the organs. Observed organ effects depend upon both dose of radiation and type of parenchymal cells irradiated.

WHOLE BODY EFFECTS

Acute Effects. The clinical syndromes observed after acute whole body radiation exposure have prodromal, latent, and manifest phases. The severity of the prodromal phase correlates with exposure dose, larger doses giving harsher symptoms with shorter intervals to expression. There are gastrointestinal and neuromuscular symptoms; diarrhea, fever, or hypertension usually indicates a supralethal dose. The following latent period (during which there is no apparent defect because the lack of stem cell replacements has not yet become of significance) has a duration that is also dose dependent; at high exposure levels, the prodromal and latent stages may merge imperceptibly.

At doses below 1000 rads (the LD_{50} is about 300 rads), the *hematopoietic syndrome*, caused by obliteration of the bone marrow precursors, is seen. Although all cell lines are affected, the relatively long life of the mature red blood cells prevents a deficit in that population. This syndrome, which can cause death in humans up to 60 days after exposure, is manifested by symptoms of sepsis due to leukopenia and/or bleeding due to thrombocytopenia. Anemia, if it occurs, is due to bleeding.

At doses between 1000 and 10,000 rads, the stem cells of both the gastrointestinal and hematopoietic systems are destroyed; the deficit, first observed in the former, causes the *gastrointestinal syndrome*. The death of the basal cells in the crypts of Lieberkühn prevents replacement of mature epithelium as it sloughs. The denuded epithelium results in the loss of both electrolyte homeostasis and protection against intraluminal microorganisms. Death due to sepsis, dehydration, or electrolyte imbalance occurs in 3-10 days.

At doses above 10,000 rads, death occurs within hours so that the gastrointestinal and hematopoietic syndromes are never given a chance to become manifest. The victim undergoes progressive neurological degeneration, leading inevitably to coma and death. Though the mechanism is uncertain, cerebral edema with herniation of the brain through the basilar foramina is thought to contribute.

Late Effects. Late radiation effects are seen after a longer latency period and at lower doses and dose rates than acute effects;they include life shortening, carcinogenesis, and mutagenesis. When small animals are exposed to low doses of radiation, their lives are shortened although they show no evidence of acute radiation syndromes and maintain normal weight. Histological findings include a decrease in the parenchymal components of tissues and increase in the connective tissue part, findings compatible with accelerated aging. Originally, the life shortening was thought to reflect increases in all morbidities as part of aging, but recent data suggest that increasing incidence of neoplasia is the cause.

Evidence for carcinogenesis in humans includes skin cancers in physicians working with radiation, lung cancer in pitchblende miners who inhale radioactive ore, bone sarcoma in radium dial painters, cancer of the liver in patients after use of THOROTRAST as a contrast agent, carcinoma of the thyroid in children irradiated for benign disorders such as enlarged thymus, and increased leukemia in Japanese survivors of the atomic bomb blasts at Hiroshima and Nagasaki, in patients irradiated for ankylosing spondylitis, and in American radiologist. All types of leukemia except the chronic lymphatic variety may be seen.

Mutagenesis is of great importance because of its heritable nature. Somatic sequelae affect only the victim, whereas mutations may create an indefinite burden. In radiation mutagenesis, the mutations that occur are not unique but an increased incidence of those that occur naturally. There appears to be no threshold dose beneath which mutations will not occur. Any exposure increases the incidence of mutations to some extent, with the incidence increasing proportionately over certain dose ranges. Finally, this effect is independent of fractionation, with the effect cumulative. Data in humans are sparse because the mutations are recessive and may not be observed for several generations. For example, no mutagenic effects have yet been observed in the Japanese atomic survivors.

Observations on effects on the embryo and fetus in mice and humans (27) reveal that large (above 250 R) exposures within 3 weeks of conception produce resorption or abortion, whereas exposure in weeks 3-6 produces severe structural abnormalities. Specific defects are associated with the precise time of exposure, an organ being most susceptible at the time of earliest appearance of differentiation. Later in pregnancy, retarded development, both intellectual and physical, and microcephaly are seen. After 30 weeks, structural defects are not usually seen, although there may be functional ones. Because *in utero* exposure may increase the incidence of subsequent neoplasia, especially leukemia, diagnostic x-rays should be obtained within the first 10 days of the menstrual cycle, if possible.

CLINICAL APPLICATIONS OF RADIATION AND RADIATION-DRUG COMBINATIONS

THERAPEUTIC USES OF RADIONUCLIDES

Though therapeutic uses stimulated the early developments of nuclear medicine, most uses of radionuclides have been diagnostic, and advances in therapeutic applications lag somewhat because of the great achievements of external beam radiotherapy and chemotherapy. Their diagnostic uses are thoroughly reviewed in other sources (13).

Radiotherapeutic uses of nuclides are summarized in Table 27.1-1. The use of therapeutic nuclides started in 1939 with the use of ^{32}P in the treatment of leukemia. Later, ^{32}P was used to treat polycythemia vera (15), and ^{131}I was used for inducing myxedema in patients with refractory cardiac failure (4) and, later, for treating hyperthyroidism.

Currently, radionuclides may be classified into three categories: *electron emitters* (β-particles, positrons, conversion electrons, and Auger electrons), *photon emitters* (γ -rays, x-rays, and annihilation radiation), and *α-particle emitters*.β-Particles dissipate their energy in a small volume of tissue, whereas photons have a much greater depth of penetration. α-Particles with their sharp localization of radiation, high radiation density, and high radiation level per particle have little current role in therapeutic nuclear medicine.

The pharmacological considerations for radionuclides, as for drugs, depend on the kinetics and metabolism of the agent under a given pathophysiological condition (chemical nature of the compound, rate of administration, biokinetics, transport mechanisms, half-life, etc.). Specificity of localization, however, is far more important in therapeutic nuclear medicine than in diagnostic nuclear medicine because of the high radiation doses involved.

As radiation may affect disposition of drugs (see later), so may chemotherapeutic agents affect the distribution of radionuclides. Adriamycin, bleomycin, cisplatin, vincristine, and methotrexate have been reported (in animals) to alter the distribution of certain radioactive materials, as have nonchemotherapeutic agents such as clindamycin, acetazolamide, phenothiazines, sex hormones, and glucocorticoids (21).

Future applications of therapeutic radionuclides lie in greater specificity of localization with intralymphatic (2) or intravenous administration of a β-emitter bound to an immunoglobulin with specificity for tumor antigens (24). Radiolabeled antimetabolites such as ^{131}I-labeled iododeoxyuridine provide potential for nuclear uptake and specific destruction of DNA. More specific chemical coupling providing more specific localization of α-emitters such as ^{211}At, and the uses of liposomes as carriers of therapeutic radioactive nuclides, are currently under investigation (3).

COMBINATIONS OF RADIATION AND DRUGS

Radiation therapy alone may result in the cure of many types of tumors, whereas chemotherapy alone is generally not considered curative, although specific chemotherapy holds promise for the cure of testicular cancers, ovarian carcinomas, and choriocarcinomas (8). The combination of two modalities is expected to enhance cure rate over either alone, but toxicity as well may also be enhanced.

Nitrosoureas added to surgery and radiotherapy seem to have had a significant effect on the course of glioblastoma, increasing survival by approximately 25% (44). Trials in head and neck cancer are equivocal. Bleomycin and 5-fluorouracil (5-FU) may have effectiveness in improving survival (7). There is good evidence that prolonged disease-free survival can be obtained with the combination of nitrogen mustard, vincristine, prednisone, and procarbazine in conjunction with radiation therapy for Hodgkin's disease (35). Excellent long-term survival in Hodgkin's disease using a five-drug combination and low dose radiation to sites of bulky disease have been obtained by Prosnitz et al (32). There is an early suggestion of potential benefit of combining cyclophosphamide, 5-FU, and prednisone with radiation in management of postmenopausal breast cancer (1). In a recent review (33) usefulness of radiation as an adjuvant to chemotherapy of Hodgkin's disease, breast carcinoma, and gastrointestinal cancer has been further reiterated.

Combination modality treatment in lung cancer remains unproductive, except in oat cell cancers where radiation to 'sanctuary' sites (brain) combined with treatment to the primary tumor and chemotherapy with cyclophosphamide, adriamycin, and vincristine seems promising for improved survival (19). Early studies by Moertel et al. suggest a potentiation of radiation by 5-FU in the treatment of rectal, pancreatic, and gastric carcinomas, but additional information is needed (25). Piver et al. suggest that the combination of hydroxyurea and radiation therapy improves disease-free survival in advanced carcinomas of the uterine cervix (30). The survival rates of children with Wilm's tumor have improved from 30% to over 85% with the combined use of surgery, chemotherapy with actinomycin D and/or vincristine, combined with local or regional abdominal irradiation (9). Survival rates have been markedly improved in rhabdomyosarcoma with radiotherapy to the "bed of the tumor", following complete surgical excision, combined with cyclophosphamide, actinomycin D, vincristine, and adriamycin (23, 42). By combining radiation and drugs improvement of survival has been made in childhood leukemia (11, 34), with up to 50% survival at 5 years, and in Ewing's sarcoma.

INTERACTIVE EFFECTS OF RADIATION AND DRUGS

TOXIC INTERACTIONS

The progress in survival and enhanced tumor control by combination therapy has led to an increased incidence of normal tissue toxicity, both acute and late. Acute toxicity primarily involves rapidly proliferating cell systems (e.g., bone marrow, oral or gastrointestinal mucosa, and skin); the effects are usually short lived and spontaneously resolve.

Late complications, noted months or years following treat-

Table 27.1-1
Radiation Doses for Certain Radiopharmaceuticals Used for Therapy

Radiopharmaceutical	Therapy Procedure	Organ	Radiation Dose/Administered Activity
			Dose(rad/mCi)
cholesterol ^{3}H	adrenals	whole body	0.23
		adrenals	833.0
cholesterol ^{14}C	adrenals	whole body	3.5
		adrenals	7,142.0
colloid (chromic phosphate) ^{32}P	liver (injected through superior mesenteric and celiac arteries)	liver	439.0
colloid (chromic phosphate) ^{32}P	intracavitary	retroperitoneal lymph nodes	517.0
		omentum	450.0
		peritoneal serosa	317.0
		liver	61.0
		spleen	60.0
		kidneys	52.0
colloid ^{198}Au	intracavitary	retroperitoneal lymph nodes	51.7
		omentum	45.0
		peritoneal serosa	31.7
		liver	6.1
		spleen	6.0
		kidneys	5.2
sodium phosphate ^{32}P	polycythemia vera	marrow	13.0
		trabecular bone	10.0
		cortical bone	1.0
etiodol ^{32}P	endolymphatic (injected into lymphatic vessel)	lymph nodes	10,000-20,000
etiodol ^{131}I	endolymphatic (injected into lymphatic vessel)	lymph nodes	1,250-2,500
microspheres ^{90}Y	liver (injected into hepatic artery)	liver	100.0
polyphosphate ^{32}P	bone (injected i.v.)	bone marrow	56.8
			76.6
polyphosphate ^{33}P	bone (injected i.v.)	bone marrow	15.3
			15.5
sodium iodide ^{125}I	thyroid (oral)	whole body	0.34
		thyroid (10% uptake)	622.0
		thyroid (30% uptake)	1,250.0
		thyroid (50% uptake)	2,300.0
sodium iodide ^{131}I	thyroid (oral)	whole body	0.45
		thyroid (10% uptake)	600.0
		thyroid (30% uptake)	1,310.0
		thyroid (50% uptake)	2,370.0
sodium sulfate ^{35}S	chondrosarcoma chordoma (injected i.v.)	chondrosarcoma	4,650.0[a]
		normal cartilage	4,050.0[a]
		bone marrow	990.0[a]
		chordoma	1,470.0[a]

[a] Average tissues doses for an administered activity of 30 mCi/kg of body weight.
Source: From Ref. 36.

ment, are governed primarily by vascular and connective tissue changes in slow proliferating tissues and include hepatitis, fibrosis, brain necrosis, myelitis, and meningitis.

Phillips and Fu have classified critical organs into categories: (1) organs essential to life that must be critically protected (spinal cord, brain, liver, kidney, stomach, intestines); and (2) organs that would not produce life-threatening difficulties should injury occur (oral mucosa, skin, esophagus, salivary glands, gonads, cartilage, endocrine glands) (28).

Clinically significant radiation-drug toxicity enhancement has been reviewed by Phillips and Fu (29), as well as Dritschilo and Piro (10). Two types of reactions have been described: enhanced acute reaction and "recall" reactions, where a flare-up of previous radiation injury may occur weeks to months after radiation when chemotherapy is administered (Table 27.1-2).

Second tumors, an additional hazard of combined modality treatment, have been reviewed with respect to pediatric tumors (22). Canellos has described an increased risk of secondary malignant neoplasms in patients with Hodgkin's disease who have been treated with radiation and chemotherapy (6).

Table 27.1-2
Radiation-Drug Toxic Interactions

Interaction	Organ
Enhancement of Radiation Effect	
ActinomycinD	Skin, esophagus, lung, GI, GU, liver, bone, soft tissues.
Adriamycin	Skin, esophagus, lung, heart, GI, GU, bone, soft tissues
Bleomycin	Skin, esophagus, GI, lung
Cyclophosphamide	Lung, bladder
Hydroxyurea	Skin, esophagus, lung
5-Fluorouracil	Skin, GI, liver, eye
Methotrexate	Skin, CNS
Vincristine, vinblastine	Esophagus, lung
BCNU	GI
Cytosine arabinoside	Optic nerve
Recall of Radiation Effect	
ActinomycinD	Skin, esophagus, lung
Adriamycin	Skin
Bleomycin	Skin, lung
Methotrexate	Skin
Steroids (withdrawal)	Lung, heart

Source: From Ref. 10.

RADIOPROTECTORS

Radioprotectors are drugs that, when delivered shortly before exposure to radiation, increase the resistance of normal tissues to radiation injury; the drugs might preferentially increase tumor sensitivity to radiation or preferentially protect normal tissues from radiation injury. They are thought to act as scavengers for radiation-induced free radicals, thus reducing the number of free radicals available to interact with critical target molecules. These compounds, like the oxygen sensitizers, are effective in the presence of sparsely ionizing radiation but not high-density ionizing types. Additional potential mechanisms of radioprotection might include agents that promote recovery of specific tissues and/or expand the size of the critical target cell population, postirradiation tissue transplantation, and supportive therapy (45).

Preclinical research (*in vitro* and animal systems) suggested efficacy of multiple sulfhydryl-containing agents including cysteine,β-mercaptoethylamine (MEA), aminoethylisothiuronium (AET), and their phosphorylated derivatives. This soon grew to include induced hypoxia, hypothermia, "biochemical shock", cyanide, ethyl alcohol, vitamins, chlorophyll, extracts of tea leaves, cabbage, and broccoli. These nonsulfhydryl agents appear to be only marginally effective, however.

To provide a therapeutic advantage (i.e., protecting normal tissue while injuring tumor tissue) four mechanisms may be involved: (1) taking advantage of quantitative and qualitative differences in enzymatic machinery, (2) differing rates of activation or rates of catabolism, (3) differing rates of absorption by the various cell types (e.g., enhanced electronegativity of tumor cells or membrane alteration), and (4) differing vasculature and hence oxygenation, with tumor cells frequently outgrowing their blood supply, resulting in a hypoxic core of tumor cells less responsive to sulfhydryl radioprotective drugs (5, 18).

Significant toxicity is associated with the most efficacious radioprotectors, although the phosphorothioate derivative of MEA (MEA-PO_4) appears to be less toxic. Alkylaminoalkylphosphorothioate toxicity increases with the length of the aminoalkyl substitution (N-position of MEA); the protective efficacy increases as per unit of sulfur increases. WR-2721 [S-2-(3-aminopropyl-amino)ethylphosphorothioic acid], which is not active *in vitro* but must be dephosphorylated to free sulfhydryl, appears to represent the optimal combination, the most effective radioprotectant yet developed.

As yet, there are no studies that test directly whether radioprotective drugs increase the effectiveness of therapy in solid tumor radiotherapy. There are human studies, however, that suggest that normal tissue protection is possible. Topical application of sulfhydryl agents has been shown to enhance the radiation resistance of skin (20), oral mucosa (14), and rectum (44). Freibel has indicated that the p.o. administration of N-acetylhomocysteine thiolactone can diminish the development of intestinal injury in patients undergoing radiotherapy for gynecological malignancies (12). Additionally, mercaptopropionylglycine (MPG) seems to increase radiation resistance by 10-20% with relatively small doses (38).

RADIOSENSITIZERS AND HYPOXIC CELL SENSITIZERS

A *radiosensitizer* is by definition any agent that enhances the amount of injury induced by radiation. This definition could include "true" radiosensitizers (agents that must be present at the time of radiation application), agents that inhibit the ability of tissue to repair radiation damage, and agents that alter radiation tolerance of a nontarget tissue (reducing oxygen consumption of well-oxygenated tumor tissues, allowing better oxygen penetration to previously hypoxic cells). The interaction of anticancer cytotoxic agents with radiation is discussed elsewhere in this chapter.

Factors contributing to tumor resistance to radiation and potential chemical approaches to their abolition include (46): (1) inherent cellular resistance (most likely), (2) greater ability to repair radiation injury (possible), (3) a greater rate of proliferation (occasionally), (4) a hypoxic subpopulation resistant to radiation (often), and (5) noncycling of cells (possible).

Attempts at clinical radiosensitization have made use of analogs of DNA, including the halogenated pyrimidine 5-chlorodeoxyuridine (5-CUDR), 5-bromodeoxyuridine (5-BUDR), and 5- iododeoxyuridine (5-IUDR). The agents are incorporated into DNA while 5-fluorodeoxyuridine (5-FUDR) inhibits *de novo* DNA synthesis by interfering with the action of thymidylate synthetase. The presence of these weakened backbone structures may make DNA more sensitive to radiation damage, or these agents may interfere with repair mechanisms. Analogs of purine such as 6-mercaptopurine (6-MP) or 6-thioguanine may also sensitize cells to radiation but are not as selective as pyrimidine analogs. Additionally, their sensitization seems to be oxygen dependent, and the compounds are toxic. Actinomycin D inhibits RNA synthesis and, as noted previously, can potentiate radiation effect, whereas hydroxyurea kills cells at the end of the G_1 or S phase. Partially synchronized cells in G_1 may be relatively more radiosensitive (31). Chloroquine was felt to increase net tumor injury but laboratory and clinical studies have failed to indicate any tumor selectivity (46).

Hypoxic cells are known to be more resistant to x-rays than well-oxygenated cells, and oxygen, particularly at low pressure, sensitizes the effects of radiation on cells; some trials of hyperbaric oxygenation during radiation therapy, however, have failed to suggest an improved therapeutic ratio (16).

Chemical agents may mimic the presence of oxygen and thereby radiosensitize hypoxic cells, as demonstrated by Bridges in 1960 with N-ethylmaleimide. There appeared to be a direct correlation between electronegativity of an agent and the ability of an agent to sensitize anoxic cells. More recently, imidazoles such as metronidazole (FLAGYL) and misonidazole have shown promising clinical activity in hypoxic cell sensitization (43, 46). Nitrofurantoins, vitamin K analogs, and hyperthermia have also been suggested as radiosensitizers.

RADIATION EFFECTS ON PHARMACOKINETICS OF DRUGS

As radiation may alter the function of any organ system (e.g., induce hepatitis, nephritis, myocardial injury, pneumonitis, gastritis, and enteritis), either on a clinical or subclinical level, it is not surprising that the pharmacokinetics of drugs are altered in irradiated organisms. Table 27.1-2 reviews sites of radiation effects and potential sources of altered drug biodynamics. Radiation may alter drugs or chemicals by radiolysis if doses and conditions are correct, although this is rarely a clinical problem. More clinically relevant are radiation effects on drug absorption and bioavailability because of altered gastric acidity, gastric or intestinal motility, mucosal barriers, or intestinal blood flow. Altered absorption of nutrients, vitamin B_{12}, digoxin, and clorazepate have been demonstrated (40).

Radiation may affect vascular permeability, blood flow, or skin fibrosis, thereby altering the distribution of parenterally administered drugs, as has been demonstrated with subcutaneous implants of γ-globulin in irradiated skin, and the subcutaneous absorption of diazepam from irradiated skin (41).

Radiation may also affect drug metabolism; modified catabolism of nicotinic acid, impaired demethylation of meperidine, and N-demethylation of chlordiazepoxide (39) have been demonstrated. Radiation may alter the blood-brain barrier and hence change the permeability of drugs into the central nervous system, and alter the function of multiple endocrine organs changing the metabolic conversion of drugs (38).

REFERENCES

1. Ahmann, D.L., Payne, W.S., Scanlon, P.W., et al. Repeated adjuvant chemotherapy with phenylalanine mustard or 5-fluorouracil cyclophosphamide and prednisone with or without radiation, after mastectomy for breast cancer. *Lancet* 1:893, 1978.
2. Ariel, I.M. Lymphography in the endolymphatic administration of radioactive isotopes for the treatment of certain cancers. In: *Therapy in Nuclear Medicine* (Spencer, R.P., ed.). New York: Grune and Stratton, 1978, p. 313.
3. Atkins, H.L. Potential future applications with therapeutic agents. *Semin. Nucl. Med.* 9:121, 1979.
4. Blumgart, H.L., Freedberg, A.S., and Kurland, G.S. Treatment of incapacitated euthyroid cardiac patients with iodine. *JAMA* 157:1, 1955.
5. Brenk, H.A.S. Vanden, and Jamieson, D. Studies of mechanisms of chemical radioprotection *in vivo* II. *Int. J. Radiol. Biol.* 4:379, 1962.
6. Canellos, G.P. Second malignancies complicating Hodgkin's disease in remission. *Lancet* 1:1294, 1975.
7. Carter, S.K. The chemotherapy of head and neck cancer. *Semin. Oncol.* 4:413, 1977.
8. Carter, S.K., and Soper, W.T. Integration of chemotherapy into combined modality treatment of solid tumors: I. The overall strategy. *Cancer Treatment Rev.* 1:1, 1974.
9. D'Angio, G.J., Evans, A., Breslow, N. et al. The treatment of Wilm's tumor: Results of the national Wilm's tumor study. *Cancer* 38:633, 1976.
10. Dritschilo, A., and Piro, A. Clinical combinations of radiation and drugs in the management of adult tumors. In: *Radiation Drug Interactions in Cancer Management* (Sokol, G.H., and Maickel, R.P., eds.). New York: John Wiley, 1980.
11. Fernbach, D.J., George, S.L., Sutow, W.N. et al. Long-term results of reinforcement therapy in children with acute leukemia. *Cancer* 36:1552, 1975.
12. Freibel, H.G. Clinical experiences on the effect of the oral application of N-acetylhomocysteine thiolactone on the intestinal reaction in the radiotherapy of gynecological malignancies. *Strahlenther.* 124:540, 1964.
13. Gopal, S.,Buck, R., Cooper, J. et al. *Radiopharmaceuticals.* New York: The Society of Nuclear Medicine, 1975.
14. Grasser, H., Muller-Fassbender, H., Prechtel, K. et al. Tier experimentelle und klinische ergebrisse mit oxyphenbutazon bei bestrahlungen in mundhohenlen und keiferbereich. *Med. Monatsschr.* 26:430, 1972.
15. Hamilton, J.G., and Lawrence, J.H. Recent clinical developments in the therapeutic application of radiophosphorus and radioiodine. *J. Clin. Invest.* 21:624, 1942.
16. Henk, J.M., Kunther, P.B., and Smith, C.W. Radiotherapy and hyperbaric oxygen in head and neck cancer: Fincal report of the first controlled trial. *Lancet* 2:101, 1977.
17. Hertz, S., and Roberts, A. Application of radioactive iodine in the therapy of Graves' disease. *J. Clin. Invest.* 21:624, 1942.
18. Irie, H., and Yoshihara, H. Influence of radiation protective agents on the therapeutic effects of radiation for malignant tissues. *Chemotherapia* 3:176, 1961.
19. Johnson, R.E., Brereton, H.G., and Kent, C.H. Small cell cancer of the lung: Attempt to remedy cause of past therapeutic failure. *Lancet* 2:289, 1976.
20. Kastratovic, M. Prevention and therapy of radiodermatitis in postoperative radiotherapy following mastectomy. *Fortschr. Med.* 89:889, 1971.
21. Lentle, B.C., Scott, J.R., Noujaim, A.A. et al. Iatrogenic alterations in radionuclide biodistributions. *Nucl. Med.* 9:131, 1979.
22. Li, L.P., and Stone, R. Survivors of cancer in childhood. *Ann. Intern. Med.* 84:551, 1976.
23. Mauer, H.M., Donaldson, M., Fernandez, C. et al. The intergroup rhabdomyosarcoma study: A preliminary report. *Cancer* 40:2015, 1977.
24. McGaughey, C. Feasibility of tumor immunoradiotherapy using radioiodinated antibodies to tumor-specific cell membrane antigens with emphasis on leukemias and early metastases. *Oncology* 29:302, 1974.
25. Moertel, C.G., Childs, D.S., Reitmeier, R.J. et al. Combined 5-fluorouracil and supervoltage radiation therapy of locally unresectable gastrointestinal cancer. *Lancet* 2:865, 1969.
26. Munro, T.R. The relative radiosensitivity of the nucleus and cytoplasm of Chinese hamster fibroblasts. *Radiat. Res.* 42:451, 1970.
27. Murphy, D.P *Congenital Malformations.* Philadelphia: J.B. Lippincott, 1947.
28. Phillips, T.L., and Fu, K. Acute and latent effects of multi-modal therapy on normal tissues. *Cancer* 40:489, 1977.
29. Phillips, T.L., and Fu, K. Quantification of combined radiotherapy and chemotherapy effects on critical and normal tissues. *Cancer* 37:1186, 1976.
30. Piver, M.S., Barlow, W., Vongtoma, N. et al. Hydroxyurea and radiation therapy in advanced cervical cancer. *Am. J. Obstet. Gynecol.* 120:969, 1974.
31. Prasad, K.N. *Cellular Radiation Biology in Human Radiation Biology.* Hagerstown, MD: Harper & Row, 1974, p. 82.
32. Prosnitz, L.R., Farber, L.R., Fischer, J.J. et al. Long-term remissions with combined modality therapy for advanced Hodgkin's disease. *Cancer* 37:2826, 1976.
33. Prosnitz, L.R., Kapp, D.S., and Weissberg, J.B. Medical Progress. *Radiotherapy* 309:771, 1983.
34. Rosen, G. Management of malignant bone tumors in children and adolescents. *Pediatr. Clin. North Am.* 23:183, 1976.
35. Rosenberg, S.A., and Kaplan, H.S. Management of I, II, and III Hodgkin's disease with combined radiotherapy and chemotherapy. *Cancer* 35:55, 1975.

36. Rubin, P., and Casarett, G.W. *Clinical Radiation Pathology.* Philadelphia: W.B. Saunder, 1968.
37. Saenger, E.L., Kereiakes, J.G., Sodd, V.J. et al. Radio-therapeutic agents: properties, dosimetry, and radiobiological considerations. *Semin. Nucl. Med.* 9:72, 1979.
38. Sokol, G.H., Greenblatt, D.J., and Kaufman, S.D. Radiation effects on normal tissues: Pharmacokinetic and therapeutic implications. In: *Radiation-Drug Interactions in Cancer Management* (Sokol, G.H., and Maickel, R.P., eds.). New York: John Wiley, 1980, p. 79.
39. Sokol, G.H., Greenblatt, D.J., Littman, P. et al. Chlordiazepoxide metabolism in mice following hepatic irradiation. *Pharmacology* 13:248, 1975.
40. Sokol, G.H., Greenblatt, D.J., Lloyd, B.L. et al. Effects of abdominal radiation therapy on drug absorption in humans. *J. Clin. Pharmacol.* 18:388, 1978.
41. Sokol, G.H. Unpublished data.
42. Sugahara, T., Horikawa, M., Hitika, M. et al. Studies on a Sulfhydryl radioprotector of low toxicity. *Experientia* 27(Suppl.): 53, 1977.
43. Urtasun, R.C., Band, P., and Champna, J.D. Radiation and high-dose metronidazole in supratentorial glioblastoma. *N. Engl. J. Med.* 294:1364, 1976.
44. Walker, M.D., and Horowitz, B.S. BCNU in the treatment of malignant brain tumors: A preliminary report. *Cancer Chemother. Rep.* 541:263, 1970.
45. Yarmoneuko, S.P. Analysis of the action mechanism of radioprotective agents in light of their practical use on the protective effects of agents introduced into the rectum. *Med. Radiol.* (Moscow) 9:66, 1964.
46. Yuhas, J.M. Chemical radiosensitization as a means of improving solid tumor radiotherapy. In: *Radiation-Drug Interactions in Cancer Management* (Sokol, G.H., and Maickel, R.P., eds.). New York: John Wiley, 1980, p. 137.
47. Yuhas, J.M. On the potential application of radioprotective drugs in solid tumor radiotherapy. In: *Radiation-Drug Interactions in Cancer Management* (Sokol, G.H., and Maickel, R.P., eds.). New York: John Wiley, 1980, p. 113.

Section VI

ENVIRONMENTAL PHARMACOLOGY AND TOXICOLOGY

CHAPTER

28

INTERACTION OF ORGANISM (HUMANS) WITH CHEMICAL ENVIRONMENT

This section deals with the pharmacological and toxicological effects of chemicals that pollute the environment of living organisms, particularly humans. The pollution of the atmosphere began presumably when fire was first lit by cavemen. However, at the present time urbanization and industrialization have rapidly increased the magnitude of pollution by occupational and industrial chemicals. Their effects have been variable from mild to severe and from acute to chronic, depending on the dose and duration of exposure to the chemicals. Very special types of chronic toxicological reaction have been the production of tumor (carcinogenic effect) and alteration of some hereditary character or mutation (mutagenic effect). These effects of industrial and environmental chemicals are discussed in the following chapters.

CHAPTER
28.1

HEAVY METALS AND CHELATING AGENTS

Samar N. Dutta and Sachin N. Pradhan

A mysterious nervous illness characterized by numbness of mouth and extremities, slurring speech, unsteady gait, and tunnel vision was reported in 1953 among the population of Minamata, a small town at the southern-most part of the main island of Japan. Extensive investigation led to conclusions in 1956 that the epidemic outbreak of the disease resulted from an unknown toxic substance in fish, and finally by 1961 the causative agent was identified as methyl mercury. The latter was traced to the effluent of a chemical plant emptied directly into Minamata Bay. A total of 121 Minamata cases have been recorded in the literature. During the period from 1965 through 1970, another outbreak of methyl mercury poisoning occurred in Niigata, Japan, which affected an additional 47 cases. A more extensive episode, involving 6000 cases and causing 500 deaths, resulted from mercury-contaminated bread made from cereal grains treated with alkyl mercury fungicides in Iraq in 1971-1972.

Although heavy metals were previously used in therapeutics, current interest lies primarily with their adverse effects, which can occur through air and water pollution and food contamination in humans, as well as in domestic and wild animals. A number of heavy metals, including mercury, lead, arsenic, cadmium, thallium, antimony, copper, zinc, and selenium have been of specific toxicological interest.

Study of pharmacokinetics of heavy metal compounds is important for understanding their short- and long-term toxicities. Metals in their elemental form are poorly absorbed from the body surface; when suspended in lipid media, however, their chances of absorption from skin are markedly increased. Inorganic metals in circulation are capable of reacting with a variety of binding sites, forming complexes, and hence their excretion is slow. For a particular toxic effect, their reaction with ligands of a biological system is a prerequisite. Metal complexes are formed primarily with sulfhydryl groups and to lesser degrees with amino, carboxylate, imidazole, and hydroxyl radicals of essential enzymes. Complexes with sulfur and nitrogen atoms are more stable than with oxygen. Clinical toxicities of various heavy metals such as arsenic, lead, and mercury depend upon the sensitivity of the tissues affected and the extent of interference of normal function caused by metal complexes.

Metallothionein (MT), a low molecular weight protein, rich in cysteine and contained in various organs of different mammalian species, has a high affinity for certain metals such as zinc, mercury, copper, and cadmium. Synthesis of MT can be induced by these metals, and the protein may serve as a scavenging agent by binding with them (7).

There are a few chemicals [e.g., the sodium and calcium salts of ethylenediaminetetra-acetic acid (EDTA), deferoxamine, dimercaprol, and D-penicillamine] known as chelating agents (*chela* means "prehensile claw of a crab"), which possess some reactive electrophilic groups or ligands that can compete with the endogenous ligands in the body for heavy metal ions and form stable heterocyclic ring complexes (chelates) that are then excreted. Thus, they can prevent or reverse heavy metal binding in the body. These heavy metal chelators are water soluble, nonionic, and chemically stable, and they are excreted by the kidney. Efficacy of chelating agents depends largely on their affinity to metal ions (Table 28.1-1). Stability of a chelate depends on the ligand atom. Thus, lead and mercury have greater affinity for S and N ligands (e.g., -SH, -S-S-, $-NH_2$, =NH) than for O ligands (e.g., -OH, -COO-); the opposite is the case with calcium. Chelates are generally less stable at low pH.

HEAVY METALS

LEAD

Sources. Common sources of lead are soil, dust, old paints, putty or plaster, gasoline combustion engines, ceramic glazes, solder in tin cans, old lead water pipes, certain inks (colored), battery casings, and lead smelters. Lead is present in its various sources in inorganic (e.g., oxides and salts) and organic (e.g., alkyls) forms. Lead oxide is used in red lead paints and dry

Table 28.1-1
Net Affinity Constants for Some Metal Ions and Chelating Agents

Metal Ion	Net Affinity Constants[a]			
	EDTA	DTPA	PA	DFOA
Pb^{2+}	6.3	7.2	4.8	
Hg^{2+}	10.1	14.8	9.9	
Cu^{2+}	7.1	9.6	8.9	4.2
Fe^{3+}	13.4	15.6		20.7
Zn^{2+}	4.6	6.5	2.4	1.2

[a] EDTA, ethylenediaminetetra-acetate; DTPA, diethylenetriaminepentaacetate; PA, D-penicillamine; DFOA, deferoxamine.

The affinity constant K_{ML}^{M} for a metal (M) and a ligand donor chelating agent (L) is defined by:

$$K_{ML}^{M} = \frac{[KM]}{[K][M]}$$

The net affinity of the chelator (K'_M) for the metal M is approximated by:

$$K'_M = \frac{K_{ML}^{M}[L]}{\alpha_L + K_{CaL}^{Ca}[Ca^{2+}]}$$

in which α_L is calculated from the affinity of the ligand groups for hydrogen ions at the biological pH.
Source. Ref.5.

batteries and dominantly occurs in smelters and storage battery plants, which are some of the sources of its industrial exposures. Ambient air contains a complex mixture of halides, carbamates, oxides, phosphates, and sulfates. Sources of lead in air range from large particle size dusts to chemical forms comprising aerosols. Lead alkyls (tetramethyl, tetraethyl, etc.) are added to gasoline as antiknock agents. There are instances where lead poisoning results from ingestion of lead- contaminated health foods and Chinese herbal medicines. The use of lead is decreasing, resulting in somewhat reduced levels in the the environment.

Absorption, Distribution, and Elimination. Lead reaches the bloodstream via the gastrointestinal and respiratory tracts, and to a lesser extent through the skin and mucous membrane. In adults, about 5-10% of ingested lead is absorbed, compared with 30-40% in a preschool child (35). Iron deficiency and calcium have been suggested to increase intestinal absorption of lead (3). About 5% of the ingested lead binds to soft tissues in the adult and the rest goes to bone, where it is relatively inert. In contrast, in children roughly 33% of absorbed lead reaches bone marrow, kidney, and brain (19). Lead is also bound to plasma proteins and erythrocytes. Metabolically active diffusible plasma lead constitutes about 2% of the total body burden (total amount of chemical in the body at steady state following repeated exposure), and a dynamic interchange of lead occurs between this pool and bound lead in various soft and hard tissues. Distribution of lead through the body is relatively slow.

Lead is excreted into the bile, feces,and urine. In humans, urinary excretion of lead bears a direct relationship to its plasma levels. The plasma half-life of lead has been reported to be about 30 days.

Effects on Organ Systems. Lead mainly affects the hemopoietic system, CNS, kidneys, and liver. It interferes with heme synthesis (Fig. 28.1-1). The enzyme δ-aminolevulinic acid dehydratase (ALAD), which is required to synthesize porphobilinogen from two molecules of δ-aminolevulinic acid (ALA), is inhibited by lead. The ALAD activity needs to be sufficiently inhibited by lead for the ALA level to build up in the red blood cells and to be excreted in greater amounts in the urine. Lead also interferes specifically with the conversion of protoporphyrin and nonheme iron into heme, resulting in accumulation of free protoporphyrin and zinc protoporphyrin in the red blood cells. It also leads to accumulation of coproporphyrin, which is excreted in the urine. The osmotic and mechanical fragility of the red blood cell membrane has been reported to increase as a result of coating the cell membrane with lead salts.

Varying degrees of demyelination of axons and nerve cell bodies may occur with increased body burden of lead. In the kidney, it causes swollen proximal tubular lining cells, mitochondrial changes, nuclear inclusion bodies, and proximal tubular dysfunction (15). Lead-induced renal tumors in rats have been reported (23). It has been suggested that lead at relatively low concentrations inhibits microsomal formation of cortisol metabolites in lead-toxic children (32).

Lead Poisoning. Massive exposure to lead may cause acute poisoning. Prolonged exposure causes an insidious poisoning that is the most common form. In children, regular ingestion of dried lead paint for 3-6 months is necessary before manifestation of clinical symptoms. Concentration of lead in blood is the only index of exposure to the external dose (e.g., concentration of lead in the environment) as well as being an internal index linked to various biological effects of lead. Traditionally, lead concentrations of 70 μg/100 ml in blood and 200 μg/100 ml in urine have served as biological threshold limit values in considering the "safe" levels of occupational exposure. Lead poisoning, however, can occur among lead-exposed workers with a blood level equal to or less than 70 μg/100 ml. The concentration of lead in various tissues (e.g., blood, urine, hair,nail, and bone) does not correlate with the tissue responses. A significant correlation, however, has been demonstrated between blood lead, erythrocytic protoporphyrin, urinary lead, and urinary lead EDTA complex (1).

In adults, the common symptoms of inorganic lead poisoning are abdominal pain, constipation, diarrhea, vomiting, asthenia, paresthesia,and mental symptoms. Organic lead poisoning results in sleep disturbances, nausea,anorexia, vomiting, diarrhea, abdominal pain, vertigo, headache, muscular weakness, tremor, weight loss, irritability, arthralgia, and a metallic taste in the mouth.

In children, symptoms of organic lead poisoning are the same as in adults. Symptoms of inorganic lead poisoning include drowsiness, gastrointestinal symptoms, ataxia, and stupor. In severe cases, wrist drop and encephalopathy may develop. Anemia is common with the inorganic form but not with organic lead. In 80% of all chronic lead poisonings, a gingival blue "lead line" is formed. This blue line is caused by the action of hydrogen sulfide (a product of bacterial degradation) on the lead compound. Hematological indices of lead poisoning are blood ALA, erythrocytic ALAD activity (decreased), erythrocytic protoporphyrin (increased), bone marrow sideroblasts, reticulocytes, punctate basophils (stippled red cells), and increased red blood cell fragility. Large amounts of ALA and coproporphyrin are excreted in the urine in patients with lead intoxication. In some children symptoms of lead poisoning are not recognizable until several years after the exposure. Impairment of cognitive functions and behavioral delay are mainly seen in these children during the developmental years (24).

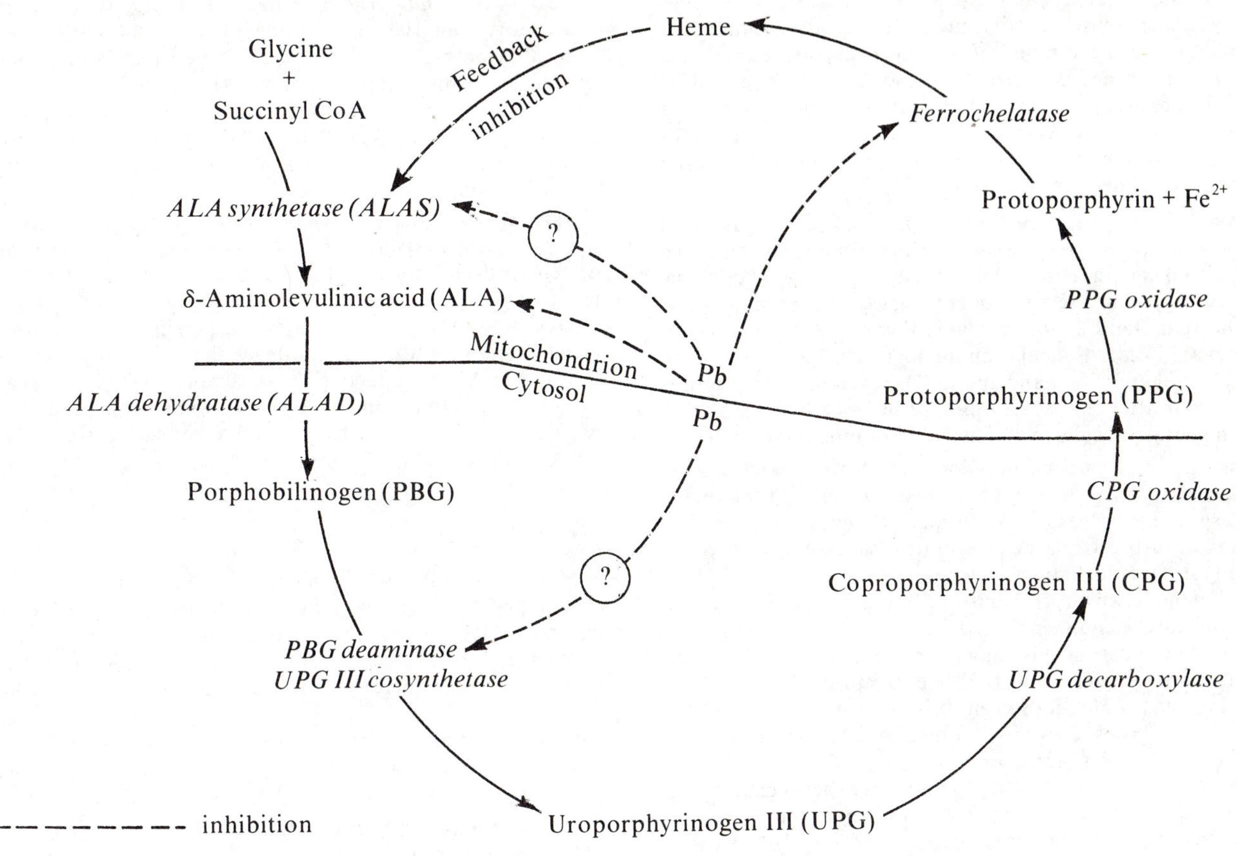

Fig. 28.1-1. *Sites of action of lead in heme synthesis.*

Criteria for Diagnosis of Lead Poisoning. Several parameters should be taken into consideration in establishing a diagnosis of lead poisoning. It has been suggested that the following criteria be satisfied: (a) presence of signs and symptoms of lead poisoning, (b) a positive history of exposure to lead, and (c) at least one parameter of both increased absorption and lead poisoning must show significant change from the standard reference values (33). An erythrocytic ALAD level less than 21 units of activity has been suggested to indicate an exposure to lead that has been excessive as well as potentially hazardous to individual health (30). All children with pica, anemia, hyperkinetic behavior, or neurological disease including seizures should be tested for lead by determination of blood lead and erythrocyte protoporphyrin determinations (13).

Treatment of Lead Poisoning. For organic lead poisoning there is no specific therapy. The mortality rate is about 20% (14). Prolonged sedation is usually instituted, and chelating agents such as calcium disodium edetate ($CaNa_2$ EDTA), dimercaprol, and D-penicillamine are the principal drugs of therapy in chronic lead poisoning. Lead binds to all ligand sites (O,N,S) of these chelating agents.

The chelating agent $CaNa_2$ EDTA is the drug of choice; it forms a stable complex with lead by displacement of the calcium. Chelating agents, however, do not displace lead in bone, and once abnormal absorption is terminated, practically all the lead in the body is shifted to bone. The recommended dose of calcium EDTA in children is 50 mg/kg/day for 5 days by i.v. or i.m. route. The lead chelate formed is excreted in the urine, 50% in the first 4 hr posttherapy. Adequate urine flow must be established prior to initiation of drug therapy, and renal damage is a contraindication for this drug therapy. In children, some clinicians recommend a calcium EDTA mobilization test to determine the body burden of lead (9). For adults a daily dose of 2 g (in 5% glucose solution i.v.) is given for 5 days. In more severe poisoning, dimercaprol should be given initially at doses of 4 mg/kg and 2.5 mg/kg, i.m., for children and adults, respectively. Subsequently, calcium EDTA may be given at doses of 8-12.5 mg/kg every 4 hr concurrently with BAL for 5 days. In lead encephalopathy, therapy may be extended to 7 days.

For moderate toxicity, penicillamine, which not only chelates lead but also provides sulfhydryl groups, may be considered as the agent of choice. It is also useful as a follow-up treatment after initial calcium disodium EDTA. The recommended dose of penicillamine is 30 mg/kg (p.o.) up to a daily total of 2 g in divided doses. To relieve increased intracranial pressure in lead encephalopathy urea, mannitol or dexamethasone may be needed.

Besides specific antidotal therapy, other measures employed in the management of lead toxicity include cessation of exposure, saline purgation to promote fecal excretion of unabsorbed lead, intravenous calcium to control colic and to maintain adequate fluid and electrolyte balance.

ARSENIC

Chemistry. Arsenic was known to medical alchemists for more than 2400 years in Greece and Rome as both a medicinal agent and a poison. Arsenic preparations were mentioned in the writings of Paracelsus in the sixteenth century. The element is found to a small extent as an arsenide of true metals. Arsenic preparations are used for hardening copper, lead alloys, and in the manufacture of certain types of glass. In organic arsenical preparations, arsenic is bound to a carbon atom by a covalent bond. Arsenic exists in trivalent (arsenite) and pentavalent (arsenate) forms. Examples of tri- and pentavalent arsenicals are: arsphenamine, oxophenersine, and carbarsone, glycobiarosol, respectively. Trivalent compounds are more toxic and presumably are converted to "arsenoxide" to act as a protoplasmic poison. Pentavalent arsenicals penetrate more readily from the intestine than the trivalents.

Arsine. Arsine (or arsenic trihydride) is a colorless gas with a garlic odor. It is very toxic and the principal source of industrial aresenic poisoning today. Arsine poisoning is of great concern, because it produces severe Coombs'-negative anemia, hemolysis,and renal failure, and available therapy is inadequate. Its toxic manifestations include anorexia, headache, nausea, vomiting, hemoglobinemia,and anuria. Dark red urine is generally seen 4-6 hr after exposure, followed in 24-48 hr by jaundice. Death geneally results from renal and/or pulmonary failure.

Absorption, Distribution, Biotransformation, and Excretion. Inorganic arsenic is readily absorbed through the intact skin, especially in a lipid-base ointment. Soluble salts of arsenic are well absorbed from the gastrointestinal tract and through mucous surfaces including the lung.

Following its absorption into the circulation 95-99% of the inorganic form is found in the red blood cells bound to globin of hemoglobin. In serum, it is bound to protein. In about 24 hr, the metal leaves the blood and is distributed to the liver, kidney, lung, intestinal wall, and spleen. It is also found in the muscle and nervous tissues. Chronic administration leads to accumulation in the skin, hair, and bones.

Following chronic arsenic poisoning in experimental animals, the metal is concentrated in the hair in amounts four to six times (per unit of weight) as great as in the liver (25). In various tissues it is firmly bound to —SH groups of the protein fraction and released slowly. In the hair and bone, it remains for years. Inorganic arsenic crosses the placental barrier and may cause neonatal death (20).

The thioarsenic compounds that result from reacting with various cellular metabolism are fairly stable but ultimately undergo further oxidations to active aresenoxides, and then to additional oxidation products: $RAs = AsR \rightarrow RAsO \rightarrow RAs$.

Following administration of a single large dose, arsenic is excreted in the urine within the first 4 days. Excretion begins as early as 2-8 hr postadministration and continues up to 10 days. Complete excretion may take as long as 70 days after repeated dosings. Small amounts are excreted in the feces and sweat.

Effects on Organ Systems. Sulfhydryl enzyme systems, especially pyruvate oxidase, are inhibited as a result of combination of arsenic with sulfhydryl groups of proteins. Arsenic also uncouples oxidative phosphorylation in the liver mitochondria.

A variety of hematological abnormalities (leukopenia, relative lymphocytosis, eosinophilia, and anemia) has been reported (11). Studies have shown that inorganic arsenic interferes with DNA synthesis in human lymphocyte cultures (29). There is evidence to indicate that arsenic may be carcinogenic in the skin and lung in humans(17,27).

Arsenic Toxicity. Chronic toxicity leads to loss of weight, skin pigmentation, hyperkeratosis of palms and soles, eczema and peripheral neuropathy (sensory type), hematological effects, garlic odor of breath and perspiration.

The U.S. Environmental Protection Agency's (EPA) recommended maximum allowable concentration of arsenic in drinking water is 50 $\mu g/l$.

The minimum lethal dose of arsenic trioxide is about 60-180 mg. Acute intoxication with smaller doses causes vomiting, diarrhea, abdominal pain, muscle cramp, and hemoglobinuria. Severe poisoning may lead to shock and death within 20-48 hr.

Laboratory Diagnosis of Arsenic Toxicity. Blood arsenic level above 7 $\mu g/100$ ml is considered abnormal. Patients with clinical symptoms of arsenic poisoning excrete more than 0.1 mg/24 hr. Urinary coproporphyrin III excretion is markedly increased. Analysis of hair and nail samples for arsenic is also helpful (normal values are 0.025-0.088 mg/100 g of hair), but it should be carried out as part of an epidemiological investigation of a group of patients.

Treatment of Acute Arsenic Poisoning. In addition to supportive measures such as induction of emesis or gastric lavage, dimercaprol (2,3-dimercaptopropanol, BAL) is the drug of choice in acute intoxication. For severe cases, the initial dose of BAL is 5 mg/kg, i.m., followed by 2.5 mg/kg every 4 hr for six doses, with an additional six doses thereafter at 6- to 12-hr intervals. BAL is ineffective in arsine poisoning (12). It is also not of any use in chronic arsenic poisoning probably because the damage has already occurred. Exchange transfusion and hemodialysis are the treatment of choice in acute arsine poisoning.

MERCURY

Mercury is a silver-white, heavy liquid metal, slightly volatile at ordinary temperatures. It is present in three forms: elemental, inorganic (Hg^{+}, Hg^{++}), and organic. Organic mercury compounds (e.g., methyl mercury) vary widely in molecular structure and contain mercury forming a bond with one carbon atom.

Both elemental mercury vapor and short-chain alkyl mercury produce consistent toxic effects on the CNS, whereas the inorganic mercury primarily shows renal toxicity.

Absorption, Distribution, Biotransformation, and Excretion. Absorption of mercury varies with its chemical form. For elemental mercury, the most important route of absorption is the respiratory tract. In a suitable vehicle, elemental mercury may be absorbed through the skin, especially if oxidation occurs. Otherwise, elemental mercury is probably not absorbed as such. Inhaled mercury vapor is oxidized to mercuric oxide within the body rapidly enough to cause intoxication (18). Orally ingested mercury is absorbed from the gastrointestinal tract if oxides or sulfides are formed. The soluble inorganic mercurials in food are absorbed up to about 7%, although much remains localized in the intestinal mucosa and its contents. Organic mercury compounds are highly absorbed from the gastrointestinal tract because of their lipid solubility.

Concentration of mercury in blood is a biological indicator of its exposure. In the blood, one-half of absorbed mercury is firmly bound to the albumin (in combination with sulfhydryl groups), and the other half is associated with the red blood cells, resulting in rapid distribution to the tissues. Within a few hours, highest concentration occurs in the kidneys; in decreasing amounts it is found in liver, blood, spleen, respiratory mucosa, intestine, skin, salivary glands, heart, skeletal muscle, brain, and lung. It is stored in the bone and bone marrow for only a short period (about 24 hr); 8-85% of total mercury in the body is stored in the kidney at the end of 7-8 days, virtually localized in the proximal tubules (31). Further increase in absorbed mercury raises the concentration in other body tissues without affecting the kidney levels.

Minute amounts of inorganic mercury compounds cross blood-brain and placental barriers. In contrast, organomercurials pass both these barriers in large amounts.

Ionic metal preferentially forms covalent bonds with sulfur of sulfhydryl groups. Mercury also complexes with other ligands such as carboxyl, phosphoryl, amide, and amine groups. The major route of excretion of mercury is the kidney, but sufficient amounts are excreted in the feces, bile, and saliva. Excretion of mercury starts almost immediately after its absorption, and tissue concentration declines at different rates; brain levels decrease slowly, kidney retains 60-80% of the mercury about 1 week after exposure, and mercury levels in the kidney and urine generally indicate the severity of exposure. Of the mercuric ions, 60-70% are excreted through the kidney as sulfhydryl-mercury complex (cysteine and n-acetylcysteine) of the type RHg-SR. Methyl mercury is primarily excreted through the feces and to a lesser degree through the urine.

Effects on Organ Systems. Elemental mercury volatilizes rapidly at room temperature and enters the body by inhalation. After reaching the bloodstream it acts on two major target organs, the CNS and kidney. The CNS effects produced by the mercury vapor are neuropsychiatric in nature, whereas those from exposure to alkyl mercury (e.g., methyl mercury) are predominantly sensorimotor.Tremor seems to occur in both types of mercury poisoning, increasing progressively in mercury vapor exposure. Neuropsychiatric manifestations include marked shyness,insomnia, and emotional instability with periods of depression and irritability. The latter manifestations are generally seen at relatively low levels of exposure and are collectively known as *erethism*. Fits of crying and laughing along with intellectual deterioration are characteristics of methyl mercury poisoning. Neurological effects of methyl mercury poisoning include motor incoordination, paralysis, and altered reflexes. The early signs of sensory disturbances include paresthesias and narrowing of visual fields.

Regardless of the chemical form of mercury, maximum concentration of the metal occurs in the kidney. Acute severe intoxication with inorganic mercury, although relatively rare, leads to initial anuria (which may last for several days) followed by polyuria. Chronic occupational exposure to mercury compounds results in proteinuria, and in severe intoxication it may cause nephrotic syndrome. In methyl mercury poisoning, the renal function is not affected. Several other toxic effects of mercury are known to occur, including stomatitis, gingivitis, excessive salivation, and a metallic taste in the mouth with mercury vapor inhalation. Discoloration of anterior surface of the lens (*mercurialentis*) and pneumonitis have also been known to occur as a result of exposure to mercury vapor. Inflammation of the mouth, esophagus, stomach, and small intestine results from poisoning with inorganic mercury salts. Inorganic mercury seems to play a role in an infant disease known as acrodynia, or "pink disease" (4).

Mechanism of Action. Biochemical, neurophysiological, and pharmacological mechanisms of action of methyl mercury have been reviewed by Chang (6). The integrity of the blood-brain barrier is disrupted by both inorganic and alkyl mercury compounds. Both types of mercury compounds are widely distributed in the brain and cause degenerative changes. Sensory neurons are more severely affected than the motor neurons. Nerve fibers are also affected with degeneration of axoplasm and myelin sheath. Mercury compounds are known to inhibit enzymes of both glycolytic pathways and protein synthesis. Mercury also blocks synaptic and neuromuscular transmission.

Treatment of Mercury Poisoning. Although blood levels of mercury are not always reliable, in most instances blood levels above 20 µg/100 ml are generally considered abnormal. High urine level of mercury, or a significant increase following a challenge with BAL or penicillamine, often helps in establishing the diagnosis of mercury poisoning and decision about chelation therapy (Table 28.1-2).

In acute inorganic mercury poisoning, death occurs usually from uremia. The treatment is primarily directed to prevent the shock of dehydration and to remove mercury from the body. Dimercaprol (BAL) is known to promote excretion of mercury. The recommended dose of BAL in mercury poisoning is 5 mg/kg, i.m., initially; thereafter, 2.5 mg/kg once or twice daily for about 10 days (2). N-Acetyl-D,L-penicillamine has been reported to enhance excretion of methyl mercury. However, clinical efficacy of penicillamines in the treatment of methyl mercury poisoning is unsatisfactory.

In an attempt to interfere with the reabsorption of mercury secreted in the bile, a polythiol nonabsorbable resin (8 g/day) was tested in acute or chronic mercury poisoning. Such a ther-

Table 28.1-2
Laboratory Assessment of Toxicity of Lead and Mercury and Requirement of Chelation Therapy

Heavy Metal	Blood/Urine/Hair Levels	Challenging Test [a] With Chelating Agent	Requirement of Chelation Therapy[b]
Lead	Patient symptomatic:		
	b.l.[c], >70	Not needed	++
	b.l., >60; ery. prot.[c], >250	Not needed	++
	b.l., 30-60; ery. prot., 100-250	Needed: urine Pb increases to >500 µg/l during the test	+
	Patient asymptomatic:		
	b.l., 50-70; ery. prot., 110-250	Needed	++
	b.l., <30; ery. prot., <50	Not needed	-
Mercury	Blood level >4 µg/ ml and urine level >20 µg/ ml	Confirmed by a BAL or penicillamine provocative test	+
	Hair concentration of methyl mercury >400 µg/g and red blood cell to plasma level ratio about 10:1		+

[a] A simplified 8-hour $CaNa_2EDTA$ provocative test for lead has been found useful (22).

[b] +, ++ indicate requirement of therapy; ++ signify patient considered as "urgent risk."

[c] b.l., blood level µg/100 ml; ery. prot., erythrocyte protoporphyrin, µg/100 ml of blood.

apy results in increased fecal excretion of mercury and lowering of its blood level (34).

RELATIVE TOXICITIES OF HEAVY METALS

Toxicities of several heavy metals and their treatment are summarized in Table 28.1-3.

CHELATING AGENTS

DISODIUM EDETATE

Disodium edetate (disodium salt of ethylenediaminetetra-acetic acid, Na_2 EDTA, edathamil disodium) (Fig. 28.1-2) has characteristics of a weak acid and is soluble in water.

Pharmacological Effects. Compared with EDTA, disodium edetate chelates calcium ions with greater affinity. Most of its pharmacological effects are attributed to this chelation of calcium ions, which results in altered physiological response. Chelation of other trace metals (e.g., zinc, cadmium, magnesium, lead, and vanadium) may also occur, generally without any clinical consequences. Rapid injection of concentrated solution of Na_2 EDTA may lead to hypocalcemia, tetany, convulsions, cardiac arrhythmias, and respiratory arrest. Although a transient decrease in prothrombin time may occur, blood coagulation returns to normal within 12 hr after administration. Hypotension, hypokalemia, hypomagnesemia, reduced plasma glucose, and reduced insulin requirements have also been reported due to this drug.

Pharmacokinetics. Na_2 EDTA is poorly absorbed from the gastrointestinal tract. Its biological half-life in humans is about 60 min. It is mainly distributed in the extracellular fluid; only a trace is oxidized in the liver. Within 24 hr after administration, more than 90% of the dose is eliminated through the kidney; glomerular filtration is the principal mechanism involved in renal excretion.

Adverse Effects. Common adverse reactions to Na_2 EDTA include chills, fever, pain at the site of injection,- hypotension, muscle cramp, urinary frequency, skin eruptions, nausea, vomiting, and anorexia. There are rare reports of acute renal tubular necrosis during Na_2 EDTA therapy.

Contraindications and Precautions. Na_2 EDTA is usually contraindicated in patients with healed calcified tuberculous lesions,as there is a possibility of decalcification following its use. It is also contraindicated in patients with renal disease. The Na_2 EDTA preparation contains about 1 g of sodium per 5 g; this fact should be taken into consideration in patients on restricted sodium intake.

Therapeutic Uses. Na_2 EDTA is used in the emergency treatment of refractory hypercalcemic patients in whom rapid substantial lowering of serum calcium is indicated. Suggested dosage ranges from 15 to 50 mg/kg, administered intravenously in 500 ml of sodium chloride or 5% dextrose solution over 3-4 hr. Frequency of administration depends on the degree of hypercalcemia. Serum electrolytes, electrocardiogram, and blood pressure should be monitored during therapy.

Preparations. *Disodium edetate*, USP injection (150 mg/ml in 20 ml ampules or 200 mg/ml in 15-ml ampules).

CALCIUM DISODIUM EDETATE

Calcium disodium edetate, $CaNa_2EDTA$ (Fig. 28.1-2) is a neutral compound, soluble in water, but practically insoluble in organic solvents.

Pharmacological Effects. $CaNa_2$ EDTA does not cause hypocalcemia. It is primarily used in the treatment of lead poisoning. It combines with lead within a wide range of physiological pH. The chelate with lead is water soluble, stable, and readily excreted through the kidney. Chelation with copper, cadmium, nickel, chromium, manganese, and gold is clinically insignificant. $CaNa_2$ EDTA is ineffective in mercury and arsenic poisoning.

Pharmacokinetics. $CaNa_2$ EDTA is poorly absorbed from the gastrointestinal tract; hence, it is given intravenously and not orally. In addition, it promotes intestinal absorption of lead, since the lead chelate is more soluble than lead salts themselves. The drug is not metabolized in the body, but over 95% is eliminated in 24 hr.

Adverse Effects. $CaNa_2$ EDTA has a relatively low toxicity. Pain at the site of injection is a common reaction. Other side effects include hypotension, chills, fever, and allergic reactions. Rare fatal cases of acute renal necrosis have been reported after therapy with high doses. Because lead displaces calcium from the agent, hypercalcemia may be produced in some patients.

Contraindications. Calcium disodium edetate is contraindicated in patients with severe renal impairments.

Therapeutic Uses. $CaNa_2$ EDTA is indicated in the treatment of lead poisoning. In adults, it is given intravenously for 3-5 days, allowing adequate time for optimal chelation and excretion of lead in the urine. Renal elimination of lead begins to occur within 24-48 hr. The average daily dose in adults is 2-3 g in divided doses. In children with lead poisoning, therapy should be started when serum levels of lead are between 50 and 79 mg/100 ml and there are evidences of deranged heme synthesis. The average dose is 50 mg/kg in divided doses. The i.v. dose is diluted in 500 ml normal saline or 5% dextrose solution and is given over a period of 6-8 hr. The severity of lead poisoning, age, response to initial therapy, and side effects determine the frequency of administration and the number of courses necessary.

$CaNa_2$ EDTA is also used as a diagnostic agent. If lead blood levels are between 30 and 70 μg/dl and disorders of heme synthesis are suspected, a 24 hr diagnostic $CaNa_2$ EDTA mobilization test may be performed to determine the body burden of lead. In this test about 50 mg/kg of $CaNa_2$ EDTA is administered to a patient and a 24-hr

Table 28.1-3
Toxicities of Heavy Metals and Their Treatment

Metals	Common Source of Poisoning	Biological Effects	Clinical Features of Poisoning	Treatment
Lead	Occupational: lead smelters, lead-containing paint	Cerebral vascular damage, demyelination and axonal damage in neurons, inhibition of cholinergic and adrenergic synaptic evoked transmitter release; proximal renal tubular damage and glomerular atrophy; increased mechanical fragility of red blood cells and decreased Hb synthesis	Nonhemolytic anemia, nausea, abdominal colic, constipation, weakness, aminoaciduria, glycosuria, nephritis, ataxia, tremor, coma, and convulsions	$CaNa_2EDTA$, dimercaprol (BAL), D-penicillamine
Mercury	Occupational exposure to mercury vapors in chloralkali industry	Disruption of blood-brain barrier, altered brain metabolism; neuronal damage; protein synthesis and glycolytic pathways affected; glomerular and tubular damage; local corrosive action	Salivation, nausea, vomiting, diarrhea, anuria, polyuria, stomatitis, gingivitis, insomnia, nervousness, psychic symptoms, paresthesia, ataxia, constriction of visual field, motor weakness, and slurring speech	$CaNa_2EDTA$, BAL, D-penicillamine, N-acetyl D,L-penicillamine
Arsenic	Occupational exposure to dusts from the smelting of copper, zinc, lead, etc.; rodenticides, herbicides, insecticides	Binds to tissue proteins (-SH groups), teratogenic, chromosomal damage	Diarrhea, vomiting, abdominal pain; cardiomyopathy, respiratory inflammation, vesicular skin rash, renal impairments, hematological disturbances, muscle spasm, vertigo, delirium, coma; peripheral neuropathy, hyperpigmentation *Arsine gas:* vertigo, headache, nausea, vomiting, hematuria, jaundice, stupor, psychomotor disturbances, severe kidney damage	BAL, hemodialysis in arsine poisoning
Cadmium	Occupational: inhalation of cadmium oxide fumes	*In vitro*, inhibition of multiple enzymatic activity; hepatic, pulmonary, and renal tubular damage; hemolytic, carcinogenic	Acute gastroenteritis, pneumonitis, pulmonary edema, emphysema, proteinuria, glycosuria; aminoaciduria, anemia; osteomalacia (itai itai disease)	No known effective therapeutic agent
Iron	Therapeutic preparations (iatrogenic)	Corrosive; hepatic damage; coagulation defects; hemochromatosis	Vomiting, diarrhea, lethargy, circulatory collapse, hepatic damage, coagulation defects, hyperpyrexia, coma, convulsions; hemochromatosis; skin pigmentation, diabetes mellitus, hepatomegaly, cardiac failure, hypogonadism	Deferoxamine
Thallium	Rodenticides, pesticides	Accumulation in nervous tissues; hepatic and renal damage	Alopecia, ataxia, choreiform movements, vomiting, delirium, hallucinations, coma; blindness, paresthesia, facial paralysis, liver necrosis, and renal impairments	Prussian blue, activated charcoal; KCl (enhances urinary excretion)

Table 28.1-3 (continued)
Toxicities of Heavy Metals and Their Treatment

Metals	Common Source of Poisoning	Biological Effects	Clinical Features of Poisoning	Treatment
Antimony	Therapeutic preparation (emetics, in schistosomiasis, filaria)	Trivalent compounds combine with SH groups of enzymes	Vomiting, diarrhea, abdominal pain; dermatitis, conjunctivitis (exposure to dust) *Stibine* (SbH_3): acute hemolysis, CNS effects	BAL
Copper	Drinking of copper contaminated beverages	Proximal renal tubular damage, excessive tissue deposition; hemolysis	Wilson's disease: aminoaciduria, glycosuria, phosphaturia, uricosuria; acute overdose; hemolytic anemia, hepatic necrosis with jaundice.	D-penicillamine
Zinc	Occupational: inhalation of zinc oxide or zinc chloride fumes	Oral zinc chloride: tissue necrosis; inflammatory reactions from inhalation	*Oral overdose:* nausea, vomiting, diarrhea, fever; *fumes:* fever, chills, pneumonitis	

Source: From Refs. 15-17, 26, 28.

urine sample is collected. The results are expressed as μg of lead/mg of $CaNa_2$ EDTA administered. A 24-hr lead/$CaNa_2$ EDTA ratio greater than 1 indicates high lead concentration.

Preparations. *Calcium disodium edetate,* USP (CALCIUM DISODIUM VERSENATE); tablets (500 mg); injection (20% solution) in 5-ml container.

TRISODIUM CALCIUM PENTATE

Trisodium calcium pentate (diethylenetriaminepentaacetate, DTPA; pentathamil) is an investigational drug that facilitates excretion of radioactive or other isotopes of heavy metals such as lanthanum, yttrium, americium, scandium, and plutonium. It does not promote excretion of strontium, polonium, or uranium. It is structurally related to $CaNa_2$ EDTA and is sometimes used in lead-poisoning patients not responding to $CaNa_2$-EDTA.

DEFEROXAMINE

Ferrioxamine B is a siderochrome isolated from *Streptomyces griseus*; it is an octahedral complex containing iron. Removal of iron produces deferoxamine (Fig. 28.1-2).

Pharmacological Effects. Deferoxamine has a high affinity for ferric ion, with which it readily combines to form a stable, water-soluble colored chelate, ferrioxamine. Its affinity for ferrous ion is considerably less. It can also form complexes with the iron component of ferritin, hemosiderin, and less so with transferritin, without affecting any other metal ions or trace elements. It does not affect the iron component of hemoglobin or myoglobin.

Pharmacokinetics. Deferoxamine is poorly (only about 15%) absorbed from the gastrointestinal tract. In the intestinal lumen it combines with iron and renders it nonabsorbable. Although its metabolic pathways have not been determined, it is known to be metabolized by circulating enzymes. The Fe^{3+} chelate is excreted in the urine, imparting a reddish-brown color. Stoichiometrically, 100 mg of deferoxamine sequesters 8.5 mg of ferric iron.

Adverse Effects. Generally, deferoxamine is well tolerated by most patients. Reactions attributable to deferoxamine include hypotension, tachycardia, urticaria, skin rash, and pruritus following rapid i.v. administration, and histaminelike local cutaneous manifestation after s.c. injection. Long-term administration has been reported to cause allergic reactions, blurred vision, diarrhea, abdominal pain, leg cramps, fever, and cataracts. Rarely, loss of vision as a toxic effect of deferoxamine has been reported (8).

Therapeutic Uses. Deferoxamine is used as an adjunct in the treatment of acute iron intoxication. The usual dose is 1 g i.m. initially, followed by 500 mg every 4 hr for two doses. Thereafter, depending upon the degree of poisoning (using serum iron level as a measure) and response of the patient, an additional 500 mg may be administered every 4-12 hr. The total daily dose should not exceed 6 g. When the patient is in shock or in cardiovascular collapse, the drug should be administered slowly by the i.v. route, 1 g (15 mg/kg/hr) initially, followed by additional doses i.m. as indicated. It should not be given in patients with severe renal impairment. It is also used in the treatment of secondary hemochromatosis and to promote iron excretion in cases of iron overloading resulting from repeated blood transfusions. Intensive chelation therapy with deferoxamine at a dose of 100-200 μg/day has been suggested by some investigators in the management of thalassemia to reduce the rate of iron

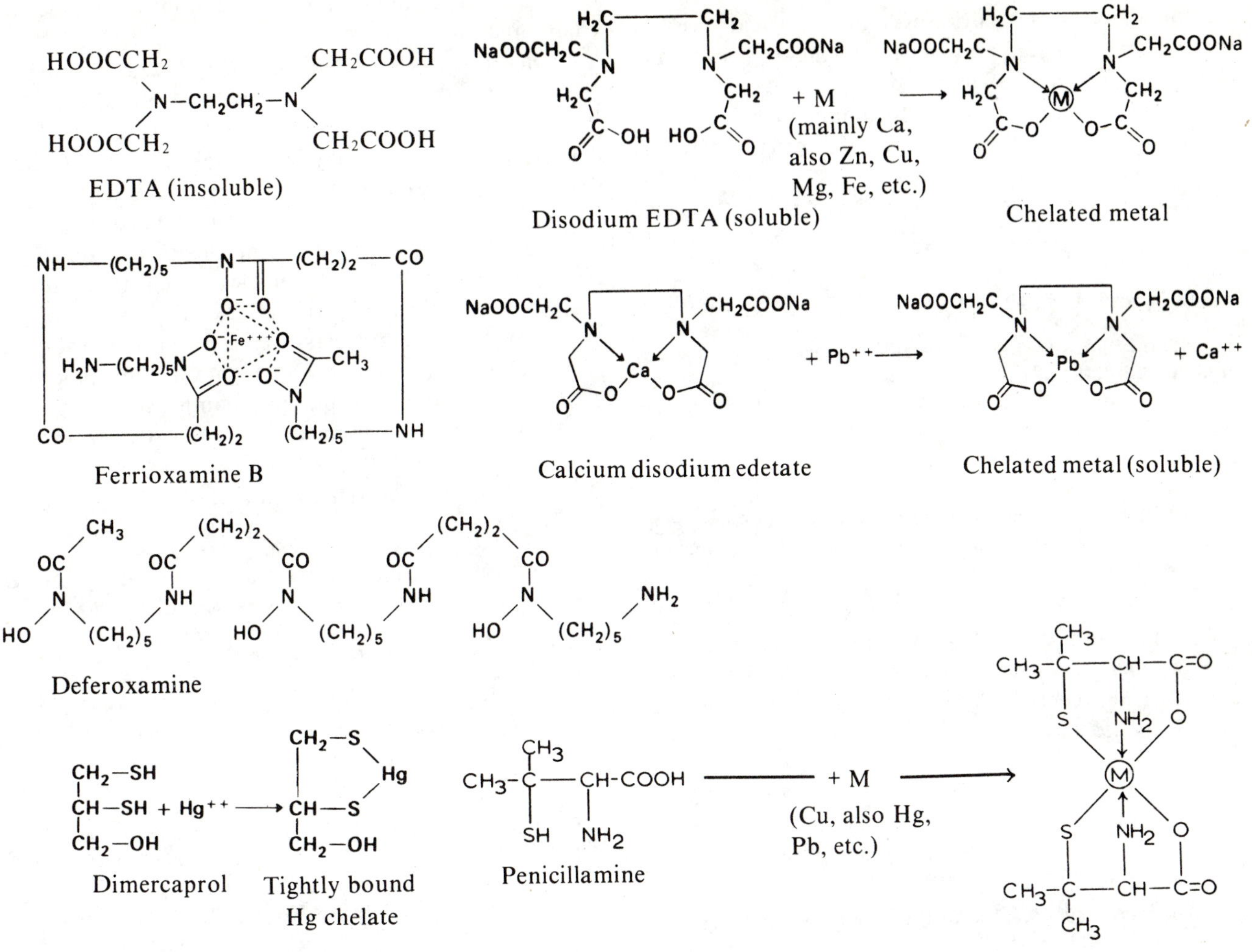

EDTA (insoluble)

Disodium EDTA (soluble) + M (mainly Ca, also Zn, Cu, Mg, Fe, etc.) ⟶ Chelated metal

Ferrioxamine B

Calcium disodium edetate + Pb^{++} ⟶ Chelated metal (soluble) + Ca^{++}

Deferoxamine

Dimercaprol + Hg^{++} ⟶ Tightly bound Hg chelate

Penicillamine + M (Cu, also Hg, Pb, etc.) ⟶

Fig. 28.1-2. *Chemical structures of some chelating agents.*

loading from recurrent transfusion (10, 21). In secondary hemochromatosis, concomitant administration of ascorbic acid seems to enhance the chelating effect of deferoxamine. Ascorbic acid is discontinued if cardiac decompensation results from combined therapy.

Preparations. *Deferoxamine mesylate,* USP (DESFERAL MESYLATE): 500-mg lyophilized powder in ampule.

DIMERCAPROL (BAL)

The chemical structure of dimercaprol (British anti-Lewisite, BAL) is given in Fig. 28.1-2. BAL is a colorless liquid with an offensive, mercaptan-like odor. It is soluble in water (1 g in about 20 ml), alcohol, and vegetable oil.

Pharmacological Effects. Dimercaprol forms complexes with arsenic, mercury, and gold. It hastens excretion of lead when combined with calcium disodium edetate in severe lead poisoning in children. To a lesser extent, it also increases excretion of copper in Wilson's disease. Clinically, it has no beneficial effect in arsine (AsH_3), antimony, and bismuth poisoning. Dimercaprol complexes of iron, cadmium, or selenium are more nephrotoxic than the metal alone. In low doses, it has no other significant pharmacological properties.

Pharmacokinetics. Dimercaprol is administered exclusively by i.m. injection, circulates in the extracellular fluid, and has a short half-life. The drug is rapidly metabolized and excreted through the kidney within 4 hr of administration. Some dimercaprol is excreted in the urine as a glucuronic acid conjugate.

Adverse Effects. At therapeutic doses, the side effects of dimercaprol or BAL are generally mild and short lasting. They include tachycardia, increased blood pressure, weakness, headache, burning sensation in the lips, mouth, and throat, a feeling of constriction in the chest or throat, lacrimation, blepharospasm, diaphoresis, salivation, nausea, and vomiting. The drug imparts an unpleasant odor to breath. Large doses of dimercaprol may cause hypertension, metabolic acidosis, coma, or convulsions. It is potentially nephrotoxic and should not be used in acute renal failure.

Therapeutic Uses. BAL is the drug of choice in the treatment of acute mercury poisoning. The usual dose for mild arsenic and gold poisoning is 2.5 mg/kg (i.m.) four times daily for 2 days, two times on day 3, and then 2.5 mg daily for 10 days. For mercury poisoning, the initial dose is 5 mg/kg followed by 2.5 mg/kg once or twice daily for 10 days.

Preparations. *Dimercaprol*, USP (2,3-dimercaptopropanol, BAL): injection (BAL 10%, w/v, and benzyl benzoate in peanut oil in 3-ml containers).

2,3-DIMERCAPTOSUCCINIC ACID

2,3-Dimercaptosuccinic acid is an investigational congener of dimercaprol that is orally effective against mercury, arsenic, and lead poisoning,and about 30 times less toxic than dimercaprol.

PENICILLAMINE

Chemically, penicillamine is D-β-β-dimethylcysteine (Fig. 28.1-2). This drug is obtained by acid hydrolysis of penicillin and is also made synthetically. It is a crystalline powder freely soluble in water with a characteristic odor and bitter taste.

Pharmacological Effects. Penicillamine chelates copper, mercury, zinc, and lead, and probably other metals. It can react with cysteine to form a more soluble mixed disulfide. In addition to chelation of excess copper from the liver in both primary biliary cirrhosis and Wilson's disease, it has also been suggested that the drug reduces immune complexes and immunoglobins in primary biliary cirrhosis. Chelation of lead with this drug is less than satisfactory.

Pharmacokinetics. Unlike other chelating agents, penicillamine is well absorbed from the gastrointestinal tract. It is partly oxidized to a disulfide and excreted in the urine.Chelates of penicillamine with copper, lead,iron, and arsenic are soluble and readily excreted by the kidneys. Compared with cysteine, penicillamine is somewhat resistant to actions of cysteine desulfhydrase or L-amino acid oxidase and hence relatively stable *in vivo*.

Adverse Effects. Common side effects associated with short-term therapy with penicillamine include maculopapular skin rash (possibly hypersensitivity reactions), transient impairment of taste, ecchymoses, pruritus, fever, lymphadenopathy, leukopenia, thrombocytopenia, and arthralgia. Rare cases of cholestatic jaundice and pancreatitis have been reported during penicillamine therapy.

Long-term administration of penicillamine may result in severe adverse reactions such as bone marrow depression and immune complex abnormalities. Nephrotic syndrome, Goodpasture's syndrome, proteinuria, and optic neuropathy (with D and DL form) have been reported. There is no cross-sensitivity between penicillin and penicillamine.

Contraindications and Precautions. Penicillamine is contraindicated in pregnancy because it may be teratogenic. Skin rashes seen after long-term therapy may resemble pemphigus, and medication should be discontinued.

Therapeutic Uses. Penicillamine is used in removing copper in primary biliary cirrhosis and Wilson's disease. The usual daily dose in adults is 125-250 mg initially for 4-8 weeks, thereafter 500-750 mg daily as a maintenance dose. It is also used in mercury, zinc, and lead poisoning, as well as in cysteinuria and rheumatoid arthritis.

The drug is also used in asymptomatic lead poisoning with moderately elevated blood lead levels. In severe lead poisoning, it may be given after initial $CaNa_2$ EDTA therapy. Penicillamine has also been reported to be effective in arsenic poisoning. The efficacy of penicillamine in mercury poisoning has not been confirmed.

Preparations. *Penicillamine*, USP (CUPRIMINE): capsules (125, 250 mg) or tablets (250 mg).

REFERENCES

1. Alessio, L., Bertazzi, P.A., Tofoletto, F., and Foa, V. Free erythrocyte protoporphyrin as an indicator of the biological effects of lead in adult males. *Int. Arch. Occup. Environ. Health* 37:73, 1976.
2. *AMA Drug Evaluations*, 5th ed. Chicago: American Medical Association, 1983, p. 1869.
3. Aronow, R., Brege, B., Chen, H.Y. et al. The influence of oral penicillamine and diet on lead poisoning in rats. *Clin. Toxicol.* 11:221, 1977.
4. Bidstrup, P.L. *Toxicity of Mercury and Its Compounds.* London: Elsevier, 1964.
5. Catsch, A., and Harmuth-Hoene, A. New developments in metal antidotal properties of chelating agents. *Biochem. Pharmacol.* 24:1557, 1975.
6. Chang, L.W. Neurotoxic effects of mercury: A review. *Environ. Res.* 14:329, 1977.
7. Cherian, M.G., and Nordberg, M. Cellular adaptation in metal toxicology and metallothionein. *Toxicology* 28:1, 1983.
8. Davies, S.C., Hungerford, J.L., Arden, G.B. et al. Ocular toxicity of high dose intravenous desferrioxamine. *Lancet* 2:181, 1983.
9. Dillard, R.A. Detection, evaluation, and management of children exposed to lead. *Texas Med.* 74:65, 1978.
10. Editorial. High-dose chelation therapy in thalassemia. *Lancet* 1:373, 1984.
11. Feussner, J.R., Shelburne, J.D., Bredehoft, S., and Cohen, H.J. Arsenic induced bone marrow toxicity: Ultrastructural and electron-probe analysis. *Blood* 53:820, 1979.
12. Flowler, B.A., and Weissberg, J.F. Arsine poisoning. *N. Engl. J. Med.* 291:1171, 1974.
13. Garrettson, L.K. Lead. In: *Clinical Management of Poisoning and Drug Overdose* (Haddad, L.M., and Winchester, J.F., eds.). Philadelphia: W.B. Saunders, 1983, p. 649.
14. Gordon, N.C., Brown, S., Khosla, V.M., and Hansen, L.S. Lead poisoning. *Oral Surg.* 47:500, 1979.
15. Goyer, R.A. Toxicology of lead on kidney and other organs. In: *A Symposium on Health Effects of Occupational Lead and Arsenic Exposure* (Carnow, B.W., ed.). HEW Publication No. (NIOSH) 76-134. U.S. Government Printing Office, Washington, D.C., 1976, p. 86.
16. Hammond, P.B. Metals. In: *Quick Reference to Clinical Toxicology* (Hanenson, I.B., ed.). Philadelphia: J.P. Lippincott, 1980, p. 163.
17. Hammond, P.B., and Beliles, R.P. Metals. In: *Casarett and Doull's Toxicology* (Doull, J., Klaassen, C.D., and Amdur, M.D., eds.). New York: MacMillan, 1980, p. 409.
18. Hughes, W.L. A physiochemical rationale for the biological

activity of mercury and its compounds. *Ann. N.Y. Acad. Sci.* 65:454, 1957.

19. Lin-Fu, J.S. Vulnerability of children to lead exposure and toxicity. *N. Engl. J. Med.* 289:1229, 1973.
20. Lugo, G., Cassady, G., and Palmisano, P. Acute maternal arsenic intoxication with neonatal death. *Am. J. Dis. Child.* 117:328, 1969.
21. Marcus, R.E., Davies, S.C., Bantock, H.M. et al. Desferrioxamine to improve cardiac function in iron-overloaded patients with thalassemia major. *Lancet* 1:392, 1984.
22. Markowitz, M.E., and Rosen, J.F. Assessment of lead stores in children: Validation of an 8-hour $CaNa_2$ EDTA provocative test. *J. Pediatr.* 104:337, 1984.
23. Moore, M.R., and Meredeth, P.A. The carcinogenicity of lead. *Arch. Toxicol.* 42:87, 1979.
24. Needleman, A.L., Gunnoe, C., Leuiton, A., et al. Deficits in psychological and classroom performance of children with elevated dentine lead. *N. Engl. J. Med.* 300:689, 1979.
25. Oehme, F.W. Mechanisms of heavy metal toxicities. *Clin. Toxicol.* 5:151, 1972.
26. Osterberg, R. Physiology and pharmacology of copper. *Pharmacol. Ther.* 9:121, 1980.
27. Ott, M.G., Holder, B.B., and Gordon, H.L. Respiratory cancer and occupational exposure to arsenicals. *Arch. Environ. Health.* 29:250, 1974.
28. Perry, H.M., Jr., Thind, G.S., and Perry, E.F. The biology of cadmium. *Med. Clin. North Am.* 60:759, 1976.
29. Peters, J., and Berger, A. Zür Einfluss anorganischen Arsens auf die DNA-synthese menschlicher Lymphozyten *in vitro. Arch. Dermatol. Forsch.* 242:343, 1972.
30. Repko, J. Behavioral toxicology of inorganic lead exposure. In: *A Symposium on Health Effects of Occupational Lead and Arsenic Exposure* (Carnow, B.W., ed.). HEW Publication No. (NIOSH)76-134. U.S. Government Printing Office, Washington, D.C., 1976, p. 59.
31. Rothstein, A., and Hayes, A.D. The metabolism of mercury in the rat studied by isotope techniques. *J. Pharmacol. Exp. Ther.* 130:166, 1960.
32. Saenger, P., Markowitz, M.E., and Rosen, J.F. Depressed excretion of 6β-hydroxycortisol in lead-toxic children. *J. Clin. Endocrinol. Metabol.* 58:363, 1984.
33. Waldron, H.A., and Stofen, D. *Subclinical Lead Poisoning.* New York: Academic Press, 1974.
34. Winek, C.L., Fochtman, F.W., Bricker, J.D., and Wecht, C.H. Fatal mercuric chloride ingestion. *Clin. Toxicol.* 18:261, 1981.
35. Ziegler, E.E., Edwards, B.B., Genson, R.L. et al. Absorption and retention of lead by infants. *Pediatr. Res.* 12:29, 1978.

CHAPTER
28.2

NONMETALLIC OCCUPATIONAL AND ENVIRONMENTAL POLLUTANTS

Michael A. Evans and Mahin D. Maines

ATMOSPHERIC POLLUTANTS

It was not until 1952, when over 4000 persons died in London within a span of a few days due to air pollution, that the quality of the atmosphere became universally recognized as an important variable of the environment. Similar incidents of smaller magnitude have occurred in the United States associated with the use of high-sulfur coal, local atmospheric conditions, and geographical terrain. Almost all of the air pollutants today are a result of transportational and industrial activity such as electric power generation and burning of refuse and fuel. The atmosphere then acts as a medium for transport, dilution, and physical and chemical transformation of individual pollutants.

In an effort to classify air pollutants, two general groups are considered: (a) *primary pollutants*, which are emitted directly into the atmosphere from identifiable sources; and (b) *secondary pollutants*, which are produced in the air by interaction among one or more primary pollutants and normal atmospheric components. The five major primary pollutants that account for 98% of air pollution are listed in Table 28.2-1.

The chemical nature of air pollutants and their subsequent effects on health vary in different localities, based on the climatic conditions and the source of pollutants. The term *smog* was first used to denote a mixture of smoke (suspended particles) and fog associated with the London type of pollution, chemically characterized by high concentrations of sulfur dioxide and smoke produced by combustion of high-sulfur coal in a cool, humid atmosphere (46). Because of its chemical nature, this type of smog is sometimes referred to as the *reducing type* of pollution; under certain meteorological conditions, it is capable of producing adverse effects on health, mainly among the elderly and those suffering from cardiac and/or respiratory disorders. A second type of air pollution, characterized by a high content of hydrocarbons, oxides of nitrogen, and photochemical oxidants produced by automobile exhaust and sunlight, occurs with particular frequency and intensity in areas such as the Los Angeles basin. Because of its chemical nature, this is sometimes referred to as an *oxidizing* type of pollution (46). In the Los Angeles type of smog, the primary photochemical event involves dissociation of NO_2 to NO and oxygen radicals, which can initiate secondary free radical events. The types of free radicals and semistable compounds formed commonly include ozone, aldehydes, organic hydroperoxides, and peroxyacetal nitrate (PAN). In the presence of ozone and energy, NO_2 can also be oxidized to NO_3 and eventually to nitric acid. The acute health effects of the oxidizing type of air pollution are associated with eye irritation, impairment of athletic performance, and increased incidence of bronchitis and upper respiratory infections. Chronic exposure may con-

Table 28.2-1
Major Atmospheric Pollutants and Their Sources

Class	Primary Pollutants	Secondary Pollutants	Sources
Oxides of carbon	CO, CO_2	None	Combustion of organic material
Sulfur compounds	SO_2, H_2S	SO_3, H_2SO_3, H_2SO_4	Combustion of sulfur-containing fuels
Nitrogen compounds	N_2, NO	NO_2, NO_3, N_2O_5, HNO_3+O_3	Combination of N_2 and O_2 during high-temperature combustion
Hydrocarbons	C_1-C_5 compounds	Aldehydes, ketones, acids	Combustion of fuel, petroleum refining, solvent use
Particulate matter			

tribute to and/or aggravate diseases associated with respiratory illness, including: (a) chronic bronchitis, (b) pulmonary emphysema, (c) bronchial asthma, (d) chronic obstructive ventilatory disease, (e) nonspecific upper respiratory disease (infections), and (f) lung cancer.

OXIDES OF CARBON

Carbon monoxide. Carbon monoxide (CO) is a colorless, odorless, and nonirritant gas slightly lighter than air. It is a product of incomplete combustion of carbonaceous material. CO acts as a chemical asphyxiant at tissue level by preventing transport of oxygen to the cells. The background or natural concentration of CO is estimated to be approximately 0.1 ppm in the atmosphere of the Pacific Ocean compared with that of large urban areas, where the average value is between 20 and 60 ppm. Concentrations as high as 90 ppm have been measured in underground garages, tunnels, and buildings over highways. The main sources of CO in the environment are automobile exhaust (where it is present in a concentration of 4-7%), and combustion of coal (where it ranges from 10 to 40% of the gaseous effluent). CO is also encountered as a health problem in poorly ventilated rooms with flame space heaters and with charcoal burners.

The mechanism of CO toxicity is based on its affinity for hemoglobin (Hb). Carbon monoxide combines with Hb at a rate approximately one-tenth of that of O_2, but it dissociates from Hb at a rate of 2100 times slower than O_2. Thus, the affinity of CO for Hb is about 210 times greater than the affinity of O_2. Equilibrium for ambient CO with Hb is dependent on body size, blood volume, and physical activity. For a resting adult male, half-saturation value is reached in about 4 hr. The association of CO with Hb to form carboxyhemoglobin decreases the amount of hemoglobin available for O_2 transport and decreases the ease with which O_2 dissociates from the remaining sites of the Hb molecule.

The *toxic reactions* that follow inhalation of CO are primarily the result of tissue hypoxia produced by insufficient oxygen transport. The reduction of oxygen-carrying transport is proportional to the amount of COHb present. Because of the CO- induced shift in the oxyhemoglobin dissociation curve, the amount of oxygen available to the tissue is further reduced in CO poisoning. This secondary effect of CO on Hb transport of O_2 is best illustrated by comparing the tissue O_2 perfusion capability of blood in an anemic individual having a 7% Hb with another individual having a hemoglobin value of 14% but with half of it in the form of COHb. In both individuals, the oxygen-carrying capacity of blood is the same (7%), but because of the interference of COHb with the release of oxygen carried as O_2 Hb, the anemic individual demonstrates few symptoms whereas the person with COHb poisoning will be near collapse.

The normal concentration of COHb in the blood of nonsmokers ranges from 0.3 to 1% and is attributed to endogenous production of CO from heme catabolism. Cigarette smoking can temporarily increase COHb to a level between 5 and 10%. These levels can produce impairment in psychomotor function and increase coronary blood flow and cardiac output in normal individuals. In patients with coronary heart diseases, decreased coronary sinus blood pO_2 and impaired oxidative metabolism are observed (23). Factors that govern the toxicity of CO include: (a) concentrations of the gas in inspired air, (b) rate of respiration, (c) duration of exposure, (d) hemoglobin concentration, and (e) oxygen demand of the tissues. Thus, anemic individuals and those with coronary insufficiency or arteriosclerosis are more susceptible to CO than normal individuals. The elevated metabolic rate of children and small animals compared with that of adults and large animals renders them more susceptible to CO poisoning. Because the effect of CO is an impairment of transport of oxygen to the tissue, under conditions of reduced O_2 tension, such as in high altitude, the effects of a given concentration of CO will be correspondingly more severe. This is reflected in air-quality standards for CO, which are more stringent for high-altitude areas compared with those at normal elevations (23). Effects of chronic or subchronic exposure to low levels of CO in healthy individuals appears to be entirely reversible. Although there is no conclusive evidence of tissue pathology associated with chronic exposure to moderate levels of CO, chronic exposure to low levels of CO has been implicated as a contributory factor for the rise in the number of various types of accidents and cardiovascular disease (23).

CO Poisoning. The spectrum of CO levels that produce toxicity and the associated range of COHb is given in Table 28.2-2 (46). Not all symptoms are experienced by every individual poisoned with CO; many of the symptoms may be lacking, particularly with rapid inhalation of high concentrations of CO. In the heart, severe CO poisoning can produce sinus tachycardia, atrial fibrillation, ST segment depression, along with ischemic changes and subendocardial infarction. Other clinical symptoms commonly found in patients with CO poisoning include skin lesions (blisters), excessive sweating, pyrexia, leukocytosis, and albuminuria (38). An important consideration is that less than a factor of 10 separates concentrations that are nontoxic for 1-hr exposure and those at which fatality occurs. The relative toxicity of CO to an organ is a function of its sensitivity to O_2 depletion. Both the brain and heart are particulary sensitive to changes in tissue pO_2 . The heart has a particularly high oxygen extraction ratio, and the supply of oxygen to the organ can be increased only by an increased blood flow. In persons with coronary heart disease, low levels of CO have been shown to aggravate existing circulatory conditions, particularly angina pectoris and peripheral arteriosclerosis. In the brain, the sensitivity of the higher centers to oxygen deprivation by far exceeds that of the lower centers. Studies on neurological parameters have demonstrated dose-dependent impairment of vigilance, reaction time, coordination, and tracking sensory process and complex intellectual behavior at 50-100 ppm of CO.

Pathology of Acute CO Poisoning. Pathological lesions from CO exposure result from tissue hypoxia. In the CNS, the progression from severe headaches to coma is believed to be due to cerebral edema and increased intracranial pressure resulting from transudation of extravascular fluids across hypoxic capillaries. Extensive demyelination and symmetrical bilateral necrosis of globus pallidus are characteristic findings in cases of delayed death involving CO poisoning.

Diagnosis and Treatment. Diagnosis of acute CO poisoning is based on circumstances surrounding the victim, hypoxia associated with a bright red color of the skin, and elevated COHb levels in the blood (18). Treatment of CO poisoning consists of removing the person from the CO environment, application of adequate oxygen supply, plus supportive measures. If respiration has failed, artificial respiration with O_2 must be immediately instituted. At high tension, oxygen can accelerate CO displacement from the Hb molecule and also dissolve as a gas in the plasma to provide additional O_2 to the tissue. Metabolic acidosis due to tissue hypoxia is often observed with CO poisoning, and appropriate supportive therapy must be instituted. Tissue demands for O_2 are minimized by keeping the patient quiet. Hypothermia has been shown to be a valuable adjunct in minimizing residual neurological sequelae (13). Delayed recovery from severe CO poisoning often results in cerebral damage and permanent functional impairment.

Carbon Dioxide. Although not generally considered an air pollutant, carbon dioxide (CO_2) contributes to what is called the greenhouse effect in the atmosphere. The concentration of

Table 28.2-2
Symptoms and Treatment of COHb Poisoning

CO Concentration and Duration	Blood Concentration COHb (%)	Signs and Symptoms	Treatment
	0-2	No human health effects	
<30 ppm	2-5	Impairment of time-interval discrimination	Fresh air, patent airways, rest
30 ppm, 8 hr	5-10	Impairment of select psychomotor facilities	Same
100 ppm, 8 hr	10-20	Slight headache, dilation of cutaneous vessel	Same
200 ppm, 8 hr	20-30	Nausea, throbbing headache abdominal discomfort, vomiting, flushing of skin	100% O_2, symptomatic therapy, rest
300 ppm, 8 hr	30-40	Dimness of vision, cherry red mucosal membranes, weakness, collapse, vomiting	Same
500 ppm, 4 hr	40-50	Syncope, collapse, coma, mental confusion, tachycardia, possible convulsions	Hyperbaric O_2 (2-2.5 atm), exchange transfusion, hypothermia, symptomatic therapy
1500 ppm, 1 hr 5000 ppm, 10 min	50+	Cheyne-Stokes respiration, intermittent convulsions, depressed respiration and cardiac function, coma	Same

CO_2 in air is variable and depends on the rate of production and elimination. The combustion of fossil fuel is the main source of CO_2 production, and photosynthesis is the major route of elimination of CO_2. Systemically, the physiological effects of carbon dioxide are of importance in the regulation of respiration, circulation, and CNS functions.

SULFUR COMPOUNDS

Sulfur compounds in the atmosphere principally occur as hydrogen sulfide, sulfur dioxides, sulfuric acid, and various types of sulfates such as ammonium sulfate. Other types of sulfur compounds, such as mercaptans, are present regionally in trace amounts, generally as a result of emission by local industry.

Hydrogen Sulfide. The two general sources for hydrogen sulfide (H_2S) are biological decay and industrial processes. High local concentrations of H_2S produced by industry have resulted in episodes of acute toxicity in humans (33). Hydrogen sulfide is commonly formed in the course of production of rubber, rayon, and glue, as well as in well caissons and tunnels. Fortunately, because of its characteristic rotten-egg odor, concentrations as low as 0.025 ppm can be detected and poisonings are fairly infrequent (23,53).

The mechanism of H_2S toxicity is similar to that of cyanide, which involves the inhibition of the cytochrome oxidase system, thereby causing severe tissue hypoxia. In addition, H_2S exerts direct effects on the chemoreceptors of the carotid bodies and CNS, causing hyperpnea and paralysis of the respiratory center.

Because of its high irritancy, acute exposure to low levels of H_2S can cause painful conjunctivitis, rhinitis, cough, and pulmonary edema. Continued exposure to high concentrations (above 700 ppm) produces sudden collapse, unconsciousness, respiratory paralysis, and death within 30-60 min. Acute intoxication with H_2S is treated by administering nitrites to produce methemoglobin, which in turn competes with ferric iron in cytochrome oxidase for the hydrosulfide anion (HS^-). The sulfmethemoglobin formed by the HS^- is then excreted through the kidney or gradually metabolized to sufate and other sulfur oxides.

Sulfur Dioxide and Sulfuric Acid. Sulfur dioxide (SO_2) is a colorless gas with a pungent, irritating odor. It is readily soluble in water (11 g/100 ml) and forms sulfurous acid (H_2SO_3). SO_2 is also oxidized to sulfur trioxide (SO_3). This reaction may be catalyzed by heavy metals, oxides of nitrogen, hydrocarbons, and particulate matter found in polluted air. Sulfur trioxide immediately interacts with water vapor to form sulfuric acid (H_2SO_4). H_2SO_4 is 4-20 times more irritating to the respiratory tract than SO_2 and 3-4 times more than SO_3.

The major source of SO_2 in the atmosphere is combustion of fuels (coal and petroleum products) containing sulfur. Sulfur trioxide readily combines with moisture in air to form sulfuric acid (H_2SO_4).

Absorption and Distribution. Although highly soluble in water, SO_2, at levels pertinent to air pollution, is not removed during passage through the upper respiratory tract. Absorption of SO_2 in the upper respiratory tract is inversely related to the flow rate and concentrations; thus, at higher respiration rates and lower concentrations, proportionately greater amounts of SO_2 reach the bronchioles of the lung (52). Once inhaled, SO_2 is readily distributed throughout the body, even if exposure is limited to the upper respiratory tract. Moreover, inhaled SO_2 is very slowly removed from the respiratory tract. Studies utilizing $^{35}SO_2$ have shown that trace amounts of radioactivity can be detected in the respiratory system 3 weeks following exposure to labeled SO_2. Binding of the labeled sulfur moiety to tissue proteins is in part responsible for the retention of the compound (4).

Mechanism of Toxicity. The degree of irritation of sulfur dioxide, sulfuric acid, and sulfates to the respiratory tract is dependent largely on their concentration in the atmosphere and the size of the particles. As noted earlier, SO_2 under conditions of high humidity and in the presence of particulate matter is converted to H_2SO_4, which causes irritation to the respiratory tract and acute respiratory illness.

The acute exposure to SO_2 causes an increase in flow resistance in the nasal cavity and respiratory tract. This increased resistance is a concentration-dependent phenomenon (4). Flow resistance returns to normal within 1 hr after termination of exposure to the gas. This reaction is a nonspecific reflex response of the bronchial tree to an irritant.

Pathophysiology. Exposure to SO_2, H_2SO_4 mist, or acid sulfates is associated with acute irritation of the upper respiratory tract and conjunctiva, aggravation of cardiopulmonary disease, and exacerbation of asthmatic attacks and chronic obstructive pulmonary disorders. Moreover, exposure to SO_2-polluted atmosphere causes excessive mucus production and hyperplasia of the bronchial mucosa, which in turn promotes bacterial infection of the respiratory tract. On the basis of morbidity and mortality, smokers appear to be a high-risk population when compared with nonsmokers (10). Some individuals display a heightened sensitivity to SO_2 such that their exposure to 5-10 ppm SO_2 in polluted air can cause severe bronchospasm.

The rapidity of the onset of SO_2-induced increase in flow resistance and its reversal by atropine or cooling of the vagosympathetic nerve tract indicate that changes in smooth muscle tone are the cause of the bronchoconstriction. SO_2 in the upper airway produces an increased resistance in the lungs via the vagal reflexes (11). Exposure to SO_2 also acts to reduce ciliary action and mucus flow in the respiratory tract (11). Decreased activity and ultimately the cessation of ciliary beat is directly related to the concentration of SO_2 and the duration of exposure. Long exposure periods exceeding 10 min result in a marked slowing or complete cessation of mucus flow. The slowing of mucus transport is also accompanied by an increased mucus secretion, leading to as much as a five-fold increase in thickness of the mucus blanket. The increased mucus flow may persist for as long as 1 month after cessation of exposure to SO_2. Histamine release from lung slices can be promoted by exposure to combined sulfuric acid mist and SO_2, but not by exposure to sulfuric acid mist alone. Sulfate salts are most effective in promoting histamine release.

In humans, acute exposures to concentrations as low as 1 ppm are associated with an increase in respiratory frequency, secondary to the increase in flow resistance and decreased tidal volume. These changes are dose related and occur within 1 min of exposure (20). At a concentration of 20 ppm, the damage to the respiratory organ is reversible when exposure ceases. Concentrations above 20 ppm cause waterlogging to the lungs and larynx and eventually respiratory paralysis. The recurring episodes of excessive mucus production and productive cough which accompany chronic exposure to SO_2 cause hyperplasia of the bronchial mucous gland and thickening of the mucosa of the bronchial tract (11).

GASEOUS NITROGEN COMPOUNDS

Nitrogen in the environment forms compounds such as ammonia, amides, amines, amino acids, and nitrates in the reduced states, as well as a large number of nitro, nitroso, nitrite, and nitrate derivatives in the oxidized state.

Ammonia. The most prevalent form of reduced nitrogen in the atmosphere is ammonia, which has a background concentration of 1-20 ppm. The major source of ammonia is bacterial breakdown of amino acids in organic waste material.

Ammonia gas is highly irritating and, when inhaled in dilute form, produces an alkaline caustic action on the upper respiratory tract. Additionally, the medullary and vasomotor centers are reflexly stimulated through irritation of the trigeminal nerve to promote bronchoconstriction, coughing, and respiratory arrest. High concentrations of ammonia vapor produce pulmonary edema, uvulitis, opacification of the eye, and death. Solutions containing ammonia in the hydroxide form are local irritants and produce a rubefacient and vesicant action when applied to the skin. The ammonium ion formed by the dissociation of ammonium hydroxide is also a systemic poison and can produce convulsions and coma (8).

Treatment for poisoning with ammonia gas involves removal of the patient to an uncontaminated atmosphere and symptomatic care for eye, nose, and throat irritations and respiratory difficulties. If readily available, a 5% boric acid solution may be used instead of water for eye irrigation. If liquid ammonia is taken internally, the patient should drink large amounts of water to dilute the chemical. If the patient is in shock, extreme pain, or unconscious, do not induce vomiting.

Oxides of Nitrogen. The three principal oxides of nitrogen in the atmosphere are nitrous oxide (N_2O), nitrogen oxide (NO), and nitrogen dioxide (NO_2). The latter two are usually collectively referred to as *nitrogen oxides* (NO_x). Nitrous oxide is used as an anesthetic in minor surgery and is commonly called laughing gas. Nitrogen oxide is a colorless, odorless, and tasteless gas produced by both biological activities and pollution sources. In polluted atmospheres, it is rapidly oxidized to nitrogen dioxide (NO_2) through secondary photochemical reactions involving ozone (O_3) or hydroxyl radicals (OH). Nitrogen dioxide is a reddish brown gas with pungent odor. With moisture, NO_2 can also be converted to nitrous (HNO_2) and nitric acid (HNO_3), which can eventually form both inorganic and organic nitrates. Both acids are irritating and corrosive to the mucous lining of the lungs.

Acute nitrogen dioxide poisoning leading to instant pulmonary edema and death has been recognized in a number of occupational syndromes and pathological entities such as Silo-filler's Disease. Nitrogen oxides are formed in silage made from forage (usually corn) of high nitrate concentration. Due to the heavier density, the oxides accumulate around the base of the silo, where even acute exposure can cause severe irreversible pulmonary emphysema. The high concentration of NO in tobacco smoke allows conjecturing the conversion of NO to NO_2 in the airways as a possible etiology in certain respiratory diseases associated with cigarette smoking (i.e., emphysema). The NO in tobacco smoke results from combustion of nitrate. The atmospheric concentrations for nitrogen dioxide and nitric oxide in urban areas ranges from 0.06 to 0.6 ppm. Much higher levels of nitrogen oxides, sufficient to produce pathological changes following acute exposure, are reached in closed silos and other selected occupations, including manufacturing of nitrogen explosives and nitric acid. The greatest hazard of exposure to nitrogen oxides is that their serious effects are not felt for several hours, despite the fact that dangerous amounts may be inhaled before any real discomfort occurs. Pulmonary edema may not develop up to 72 hr after exposure.

Cellular Damage with NO_2. Nitrogen dioxide is a direct cellular irritant. Because of its low water solubility, however, it produces extensive damage in the peripheral areas of the lung. The initial pulmonary lesions from NO_2 exposure appear within 24 hr after exposure, and the symptoms consist of detection of fibrin in the airway, increased numbers of macrophages, and loss of type I alveolar cells (squamous bronchiolar alveolar epithelial cells) with replacement by type II cells (granular pneumonocytes). Similar lesions are observed with ozone and oxygen toxicity, indicating the nonspecific nature of their irritant action. The loss of type I cells can be observed within a few hours after exposure to NO_2, and replacement by type II cells occurs within 1 day, with almost complete replication of epithelium by 6-9 days following exposure. If exposure continues, other cellular changes, including loss of cilia in the bronchioles, loss of the normal contour of the cuboidal cells in the terminal airway, and large crystaloid deposits within the cuboidal cells appear at a higher level of the airway (21). In acute exposure to sublethal amounts of NO_2, the lungs of rats show ruptured and disoriented mast cells. This occurrence may be interpreted as the potential onset of an acute inflammatory response. At higher concentrations of NO_2, lymphocyte infiltration, septal breaks, vesicular dilatation, and total collapse of the alveoli with frank edema become evident. Chronic intermittent exposure of NO_2 in rats leads to swelling of collagen fibrils and thickening of the basement membranes, and the ensuing weakening of the connective tissue framework of the lung. The weakening of the connective tissue is associated with a decreased lung recoil or contractility. The development of sporadic narrowing and fibrosis of the terminal bronchioles coincides with gross enlargement of the lung and dilatation of the air spaces. The gross enlargement of the lung, however, is accompanied by a 50% reduction in the number of air spaces and a 25% reduction in alveolar surface area (11). This process is initially reversible if exposure is promptly discontinued; under continued exposure, the connective tissue becomes irreversibly hyperplastic, leading to the loss of alveoli and enlarged air sacs. Emphysema-like damage in the alveoli is often accompanied by narrowing of the terminal bronchial lumen due to hypertrophy of the epithelium and the accumulation of amorphous proteinaceous material. Frequently, fibrin strands and alveolar macrophages accumulate at the junctions of the terminal ducts.

Prior exposure to low concentrations of NO_2 and other edemagenic agents can produce a tolerance to subsequent acute exposure of irritant gases. Unfortunately, the tolerance does not extend to chronic effects.

Biological Effects. The biological effects of NO_2 resemble those of other oxidizing agents. Lipid peroxidation, as evidenced from both *in vivo* and *in vitro* studies, is a prominent feature of NO_2 toxicity. It is speculated that NO_2-catalyzed lipid peroxidation involves formulation of nitroso free radicals (NO), which initiates auto-oxidation by methylene hydrogen abstraction. Unlike ozone-induced lipid peroxidation, which involves initial reaction with ethylene groups and leads directly to peroxidation, NO_2-induced lipid peroxidation is mediated by peroxyl free radical production. Thus, phenolic antioxidants like vitamin E that react with peroxyl free radicals are effective inhibitors of NO_2-catalyzed peroxidation but not that of ozone. Exposure to NO_2 also leads to alteration in the molecular structure of collagen and elastin. The efficiency of NO_2 uptake in the respiratory tract is about 90% and reflects its conversion of nitrate (NO_3^-) and nitrite (NO_2^-) ions. After acute exposure to NO_2, these ions appear immediately in the blood and are found within 15 min in the urine. The formation *in vivo* of methemoglobin, however, has not been linked to the nitrite. Acute exposure to NO_2 produces a dose-related increase in respiratory frequency and decrease in lung compliance. The overall minute volume remains the same, whereas tidal volume is decreased due to compliance changes. Clinical studies have also revealed a 92% increase in airway resistance in five subjects exposured for 10 min to 5 ppm NO_2. Often, the change in resistance is not apparent until 30 min after the termination of exposure, suggesting the involvement of a secondary factor, possibly histamine, in the resistance change (3). The toxicity of NO_2 in air pollution is complicated by a number of modifying factors. Gray and coworkers (26) have demonstrated that short exposures at high concentrations of NO_2 are considerably more toxic than lower concentrations applied over a longer interval of time.

Occupational exposure associated with NO_2, including nitric acid manufacturing, electric arc welding, silo workers, and nitrogen-containing explosives (e.g., TNT), has been shown to lead to gradual production of respiratory tract irritation and pulmonary fibrosis. In these reports, however, concentrations of NO_2 range from 25 to 30 times higher than concentrations associated with air pollution. In humans, exposure to as little as 25 ppm of nitrogen oxide for an 8 hr period can cause pulmonary symptoms after a virtually asymptomatic period of from 5 to as much as 48 hr. Higher concentrations of 50-100 ppm result in delayed pulmonary edema after only a 30-60 min exposure period, whereas a few breaths of nitrogen oxide at about 200 ppm will cause severe pulmonary damage. Physical signs and symptoms associated with nitrogen oxide toxicity are time related and include respiratory discomfort, headache, and dizziness during the immediate period after exposure; 5-8 hr after exposure, the victim can become cyanotic, experiencing irregular respiration, choking, dizziness, and tightness in the chest. Untreated cases frequently terminate in death caused by pulmonary edema (8).

The main objective in treatment of exposure to NO_2 is to provide an adequate supply of oxygen to the tissues. Oxygen therapy (100% O_2) at 1 hr intervals, combined with a small dose of morphine to diminish anxiety and dyspnea, should be instituted. Antibiotics and steroid therapy are recommended to minimize the likelihood of development of respiratory infection, inflammatory reactions, and pulmonary fibrosis.

HYDROCARBONS

The hydrocarbons, primary ingredients of photochemical smog, consist of saturated hydrocarbons or paraffins ranging from methane to aromatics and olefins (55). In themselves, the hydrocarbons have a relatively low toxicity, but because of their reactivity with sunlight, ozone, and nitrogen oxides, they can be oxidized to alcohols, ethers, aldehydes, ketones, peroxides, and organic acids, which are significantly more toxic. Many of these compounds, particularly formaldehyde and acrolein, are primary skin irritants and account for the odor and eye irritation of photochemical smog.

Among the various hydrocarbons present in the polluted air, two aliphatic complexes, formaldehyde (CH_2O) and acrolein ($CH_2{=}CHCHO$), are most problematic. They exert a direct irritant effect on the eyes and mucous membranes and give rise to lacrimation, sneezing, cough, dyspnea, rapid pulse, and allergic skin reactions. Concentrations of formaldehyde in Los Angeles in 1962 ranged from 0.02 to 0.19 ppm. In clinical studies, eye irritation was shown to begin at levels of 0.01-1 ppm. Acrolein produces symptoms similar to those caused by formaldehyde but is considered more toxic to humans. The threshold for odor perception of acrolein, however, is 0.3 ppm as compared with 0.06 ppm for formaldehyde (57). Vapors of aromatic hydrocarbons, which include benzene, toluene, styrene, and xylene, are more irritating than equivalent concentrations of aliphatic hydrocarbons. The aromatic complexes, however, unlike the aliphatic hydrocarbons, constitute more of a serious occupational hazard than an environmental hazard.

The major sources of polycyclic aromatic hydrocarbon (PAH) compounds in the atmosphere are: (a) heat and power generators, (b) refuse burning, (c) coke production, and (d) motor vehicle emissions. Various PAH compounds have known carcinogenic activity, and several studies have correlated lung cancer with the concentration of these compounds, especially benzo(a)-pyrene (BP), in the polluted air (31). Among some 40 PAHs known to occur in polluted atmospheres, those complexes with less than three-, or more than six-membered rings, do not as a rule exhibit carcinogenic activity.

PARTICULATES

Particulate is a term used to describe all small solid particles and liquid droplets in the air. The main sources of man-made particulates in the atmosphere are domestic or industrial burning of coal and other fuels and the automobile exhaust. Many of the particles found in the atmosphere exhibit a high order of toxicity to plant and animal species; they are grouped into several broad categories based on molecular dimension and chemical composition. (a) Dust particles are solid pollutants dispersed in the atmosphere by mechanical disintegration of material. Their size may vary from angstrom size to 100-nm diameter. (b) Fumes are particles formed by condensation. The majority of particles have a diameter less than 0.1 nm. Most common fumes of toxicological interest are oxides of metal. (c) Smokes are extrafine particulate matter that, unlike fumes, do not readily settle. Smoke particles are generally less than 0.5 nm in diameter. (d) Mists are liquid particles formed by either condensation on solid particulates or uptake of liquid by hygroscopic particles in the air. (e) Soot is finely divided adherent carbon particles formed by incomplete combustion of coal. (f) Haze is formed by suspension of dust or salt particles in water droplets. In addition to these nonviable particulates, viable particulates (e.g., bacteria, fungi molds, and their spores and pollen) can be also present in the atmosphere and pose special health related problems that are beyond the scope of this chapter.

The particulates vary greatly in their chemical composition, and numerous interactions can occur among the particulates of the various air pollutants. The major health hazard associated with particulates in the atmosphere is due to interaction of particulate matter with gaseous pollutants. Formaldehyde, for example, attaches to particulate matter and can be carried into the alveolar spaces to produce inflammation. By virtue of their comparatively large external surface area, particles may absorb chemicals such as carcinogens. This interaction may increase the penetration of the latter compounds into the lung, prolonging their residence in the lung tissue and enhancing their carcinogenic effect. Particles also provide surface area for condensation nuclei for water vapor to produce droplets in which hygroscopic gases such as SO_2 may be converted to acids. Some particulate matters, when inhaled, can directly cause lung damage and promote fibrotic proliferation of the lung tissue. The lesions are characterized by the size, hygroscopicity, shape, and charge density, and the disposition site of the particulate matter (36). This type of lung damage, which is referred to as *pneumoconiosis*, is primarily associated with industrial exposure to particulate matter rather than air pollution.

The site of deposition for particulate matter in the pulmonary tract is dependent on particle size. The size of most particles deposited in the nasopharyngeal region is in the range of 5-30 μm, and therefore present little health hazard to the individual. As the airway narrows from trachea to bronchial and bronchiolar region, smaller particles ranging in size from 1 to 5 μm are deposited according to size. Particles ranging from 0.5 to 1 μm are distributed throughout the alveolar segment of the respiratory tract; smaller particles can diffuse in tracheobronchial region and become deposited in appreciable numbers in this area of the respiratory tract. Clearance of particles is dependent on the relative amount deposited in the respiratory tract and the tissue site of deposition. Solubility of the particles also affects the relative clearance; if a particle passes through the membrane with relative ease, the systemic dose will be high. Particles that are deposited in the conducting airways and the bronchiolar region are removed by ciliary conduction of mucus toward the trachea and pharynx, where they are swallowed or expectorated. Removal of particles deposited in the alveolar region is conducted by either mechanical alveolar movement during respiration or by a shearing effect from layers of mucus fluids to transport the particles to the terminal bronchiole. Alveolar macrophages also facilitate the transfer of particles to the level of the ciliated respiratory epithelium, where they are cleared by either ciliary clearance or by entering the lymphatic system. Clearance rate is dependent on the tissue site of particle deposition and ranges from a half-life of 12-24 hr for the upper respiratory tract to several months for particles deposited in the lung parenchyma. Particles that are soluble within the lung tissue may have a half-life of several years. Some particular matters that pose serious health hazards to humans are discussed in detail in the following sections.

Silica Dust. Chronic inhalation of silica dust produces irreversible lung damage characterized by fibrogenic nodules, enlarged tracheobronchial lymph nodes, and increased susceptibility to tuberculosis and other bacterial infections. Silica exists in several forms but produces silicosis only in crystalline forms, such as quartz. Following inhalation, the smaller particles are phagocytized by alveolar macrophages and are eventually destroyed by the silica particles, releasing lysosomal enzymes as well as substances that stimulate collagen formation and lipid factors that increase macrophage proliferation. Proliferation and migration of the macrophages to the site of injury initiate the process of nodular development, which in turn involves increased localized synthesis of collagen. The development of the fibrogenic nodule in silicosis is often associated with increased susceptibility to pulmonary infections. The combination of infection and nodular development leads to the conglomerate form of silicosis. The nodules are usually located in the upper half of the lung and can be readily detected in chest x-rays. Right heart failure is a common finding at this stage of the disease. Other silicates including talc, mica, kaolin, and Fuller's earth are also associated with development of pulmonary fibrosis, particularly in industrial settings associated with mining and milling of these materials.

Asbestos. Asbestos consists of a group of chain silicates that occur as filaments. The most important commercial variety of asbestos is chrysotile, a hydrated magnesium silicate containing small amounts of aluminum and iron. Chrysotile constitutes over 90% of the asbestos used in industry. Chronic deposition of asbestos fibers in the lung leads to production of a fibrotic reaction termed *asbestosis* that produces a loss of elasticity of the lung, resulting in shortness of breath. Usually 5-10 years of exposure to asbestos is required before asbestosis becomes apparent. The incidence of lung cancer is also particularly high in asbestos insulation workers (60). Bronchial cancer is usually detected some 20-30 years subsequent to exposure and is particularly prevelant among cigarette smokers. In addition, asbestos produces mesothelioma , an otherwise rare type of tumor in the lining of the pleura and peritoneal cavities. Among asbestos workers, 1 out of 10 deaths occurring some 25-40 years after the initial exposure is caused by mesothelioma. An increased incidence of mesothelioma has also been observed in residence of areas surrounding asbestos-using industries and among household members of asbestos workers (11).

Clinical diagnosis of asbestosis is confirmed by fine basal rales, pleural thickening, with eventual calcification that can be detected by x-ray and a history of asbestos exposure. Bronchitis is uncommon in the early development of the disease but may appear in response to the continuing pleural thickening. The fibrotic lesions in asbestosis, as opposed to silicosis, tend to be more diffuse predominate in the lower portions of the lung. The development of fibrosis has a rather short period of latency and is usually related to exposure to high concentrations of asbestos. Frequently, fibrosis develops at the bronchioles, where there is a preferential disposition of the asbestos fibers. Total capacity and compliance of the lung are decreased in asbestosis without any evidence of airway constriction. As fibrosis further develops, alteration in pulmonary vasculature and impaired transfer of oxygen from the alveolus to blood are also observed. As shown by increased incidence of cancer of gastrointestinal tract in asbestos-exposed workers and among people residing in areas with asbestos-contaminated drinking water, the site of asbestos toxicity may be a function of the route of absorption (36).

Organic Fiber. Organic fibers and dust represent occupational hazards in select industrial settings and are associated with pulmonary disorders. Concentrations of dust in air and duration of exposure are important factors in determining the onset and severity of disorders. Other factors, including respiratory infections and smoking, significantly also contribute to the expression of the pulmonary disfunctions. *Bagassosis* is a pulmonary disease resulting from chronic inhalation of dried cellulose fiber (bagasse) from dried stalks of sugar. Signs and symptoms include shortness of breath, fever, chills, and loss of weight. The causative agents in bagassosis are molds and fungi stored in bagasse that promote an immune response. Subsequent exposure of the patient is therefore contraindicated since attenuation of the immune system after the first attack is inevitably experienced. *Byssinosis* is a respiratory disease associated with chronic inhalation of cotton, flax, or hemp fiber in industrial exposure. The symptoms include tightness in the chest and breathing difficulties. The bronchoconstriction caused by the dust appears to be due to agents in the material that are antigenic in nature, having histamine and 5-hydroxytryptamine-releasing effects. Other symptoms associated with byssinosis include chronic bronchitis and febrile syndromes.

SECONDARY POLLUTANTS

The secondary pollutants produced during photochemical reactions are among the most hazardous of all atmospheric chemicals. They include: ozone, aldehydes, peroxyacyl nitrates (PANs), organic hydroperoxides, and other free radicals formed by photoactivation of primary air pollutants. These gaseous compounds exert their toxic effects upon surface contact, and their effects can range from health-impairing physiological impairments to anatomical lesions and death. Collectively, their presence in the atmosphere increases the oxidizing properties of ozone and nitrogen dioxide and adds to the health hazards of photochemical smog.

Ozone. Ozone is a natural constituent of the stratosphere, where it is formed by the conversion of O_2 to O_3. It is a bluish gas about 1.6 times as heavy as air and highly reactive. Its concentration varies from 0.02 ppm in the atmosphere of rural areas to 0.2 ppm in the stratosphere. In urban areas, the concentration of ozone in the atmosphere is about 0.1 ppm. The concentration of ozone in polluted air is highly dependent on nitrogen oxide production and availability of sunlight. Brief exposure to high concentration of ozone elicits edema and inflammatory response. Studies conducted by Alpert et al (3) in rats suggest that the ozone threshold for leakage of plasma into lungs lies between 0.25 to 0.50 ppm. Other species may exhibit even a higher degree of sensitivity. Acute pulmonary inflammatory response is a regular feature of ozone exposure and entails a significant increase in polymorphonuclear leukocytes, engorged blood vessels, thickening of the respiratory bronchioles, and an inflammatory exudate in the alveolar spaces. The inflammatory response occurs at levels below those identified with pulmonary edema. Ozone at levels of 0.26-1 ppm can cause loss of ciliated cells throughout the airway passages and promote cytoplasmic vacuolization of the ciliated cells. Loss of type I cells and breakage of capillary endothelium due to the deep lung irritation of ozone are also observed. Exposure to higher levels of ozone (5 ppm) can produce focal lesions in the lung tissue, with necrosis and internal bleeding of the capillary endothelium. Chronic exposure to ozone at 1-ppm concentration produces chronic bronchitis as well as bronchiolytic, emphysematous, and fibrotic changes in the lung (51). These changes are dose- and time-dependent and appear to follow a course similar to NO_2 in producing lung damage. In response to type I cell death initially, the epithelium becomes hyperplastic; thereafter, fibroblasts and connective tissue elements increase to replace the damaged respiratory epithelium. The increase in connective tissue disrupts the symmetry of the small airways and proximal alveoli and restricts the lumen of the smaller airways. Factors such as age, temperature, and increased ventilation (exercise) have been shown to alter the toxicity of ozone (51). Several mechanisms of action have been proposed to account for biological damage produced by ozone and include the following:

1. ***Nonspecific cellular irritation and release of histamine.*** Acute ozone exposure produces an almost immediate, and persistent (17), release of histamine. Although pretreatment with antihistamines reduces the edemagenic response due to ozone exposure, ozone-exposed animals react more severely to parenterally administered histamines; thus, release of histamine cannot fully explain all of the cellular changes produced by ozone.

2. ***Oxidation of sulfhydryl (-SH) groups.*** Oxidation of -SH groups by ozone and protection against ozone-induced tissue damage by GSH precursors have been demonstrated (51). The oxidation of -SH groups may be a result of, rather than a cause of, ozone injury because the cycle of lung GSH level mimics the cellular death cycle induced by ozone exposure. The cellular cycle consists of a decrease in type I cells, with subsequent cellular hyperplasia of type II cells that have a particularly high concentration of -SH compounds.

3. ***Lipid peroxidation.*** It has been demonstrated that the interaction of ozone with unsaturated fatty acids leads to the formation to free radicals and peroxidation of the unsaturated lipids (24). Ozonides are stable intermediates formed upon the direct addition of ozone to the double bond of fatty acids. The formation of ozonides can increase vascular permeability and initiate peroxidation of cellular membrane. The so-called Heinz bodies are produced by incubation of erythrocytes with fatty acid ozonides. This treatment also lyses red blood cells, reflecting oxidation of cellular membrane.

4. ***Formation of toxic free radicals*** . The pathological alterations produced by ozone resemble those caused by ionizing radiation and involve production of free radical species. Protection against ozone toxicity and ionizing radiation by free radical scavenger suggest similarity of the mechanism of toxicity for both agents; moreover, detection of free radical signals in the electron paramagnetic resonance (EPR) spectrum of ozone further indicates a similarity of the mechanism of action. Exposure of ozone produces changes in protein structure that are similar to those observed with radiation damage. Ozone promotes intra- and inter-molecular cross-linking of proteins and alters normal lung tissue structure. These effects most likely contribute to ozone-induced decrease in lung elasticity. Breakdown of hyaluronic acid in ground substances also facilitates penetration of bacteria into the lung tissue and may be the underlying reason for the increased sensitivity of ozone-exposed animals to bacterial infection.

5. ***Neurohormonal mechanisms*** . The likelihood of the involvement of neurohormonal reactions in the expression of ozone toxicity is supported by experimental evidence demonstrating an increased resistance to ozone-induced pulmonary edema in rats following ablation of the thyroid gland. Similar protection is afforded by selected lesions of the spinal cord. Moreover, thyroid-stimulating agents have been shown to increase the edemagenic response of lung tissue to ozone.

HOUSEHOLD PRODUCTS

In 1972, 44,515 cases of accidental ingestions of household agents were reported to the National Clearinghouse for Poison Control Centers. Children under 5 years were responsible for 85-90% of all cases. The toxic potential of household agents is greatly variable. The importance of some agents lies mainly in the number of people involved; with others, there is a disproportionate morbidity that is reflected in the hospitalization rate (29).

SOAPS AND DETERGENTS

Most household cleaning agents (soaps) and detergents are ingested with a relatively high frequency by children; it is noted, however, that relatively mild consequences are associated with most of the agents in this group. The toxicity of these agents is most often related to the local damage produced as a result of their irritant or caustic properties related to irritant properties of fatty acid salts. Rarely are systemic toxic effects noted from the ingestion of these agents.

Classes of Household Cleaning Agents and Their Ingredients. Household cleaning agents can be grouped into the following four classes with their ingredients:

1. *Soaps*: Sodium, potassium, or ammonium salts of fatty acids.
2. *Nonionic detergents* : Medium- to long-chain polyether sulfates, alcohols or sulfonates (e.g., alkyl aryl polyether sulfates, alcohols, or sulfonates; alkyl phenol polyglycol ethers, polyethylene glycol alkyl aryl ethers, and sorbitan monostearate, spans, and tweens).
3. *Anionic detergents* : sulfonated hydrocarbons or phosphorylated hydrocarbons (e.g., alkyl sodium sulfate, sodium lauryl sulfate, sodium aryl alkyl sulfonate, dioctyl sodium sulfosuccinate, and sodium oleate). Laundry compounds have added water softeners such as sodium phosphate.
4. *Electric dishwasher detergents* : organic phosphate and carbonate salts (e.g., sodium tripolyphosphate, tetrasodium pyrophosphate, and hexametaphosphates).

Toxic Effects. Class I and II agents, when ingested, may cause mild gastrointestinal irritations and vomiting, and diarrhea may ensue. Nonionic detergents are only slightly irritating to the skin.

Acute oral toxicities of the anionic detergents (class III agents) vary considerably with their formulations and additives; irritation with vomiting, intestinal distention, and diarrhea are the usual symptoms, however. These agents irritate the skin by removing the natural oils, causing redness, soreness, and papular dermatitis.

Most of the organic phosphates of class IV agents possess a much higher pH than other household detergents. They also bind calcium and, after ingestion, are capable of seriously reducing the serum calcium levels. Hydrolysis of the polymeric phosphates will produce acidosis. They are quite capable of producing severe local corrosive effects as well as systemic toxicity. Ingestion is followed by intense oral mucosal irritation and corrosion manifested by severe pain, vomiting, and diarrhea. The vomitus may contain blood. Subsequent absorption of the phosphates produces a shock-like state, hypotension, bradycardia, cyanosis, and may culminate in hypocalcemic tetany.

Treatment. No treatment is indicated except when large quantities are consumed. Then dilution with water and demulcent therapy such as milk will reduce the gastric irritation. Ingestions of large amounts often produce spontaneous emesis.

For anionic detergents, emesis by dilution with water is indicated if a moderate amount (greater than 100 mg/kg) has been ingested without any spontaneous emesis. For organic phosphate detergents of group IV, immediate dilution is recommended, and emesis induced otherwise is contraindicated.

Ammonia

Household ammonia products contain varying concentrations (5-30%) of ammonium hydroxide, which produces cell injury as a direct result of its causticity. The ingestion by a child of about 30 ml of a 25% solution will prove fatal. Its contact with eyes is usually followed by permanent injury and blindness; when it is ingested, acute irritation and corrosion of the mouth, throat, and stomach ensue. Treatment for ingestion of ammonia involves dilution and demulcent therapy. Neutralization is often unnecessary, as this will be accomplished by the stomach acids. In addition, blood pH should be monitored due to possible systemic absorption of the alkaline ammonia. The ammonium ion, in contrast to sodium and potassium ions, is a systemic poison producing convulsions and coma.

Bleaches

Household bleaches usually contain varying concentrations of either sodium perborate, sodium peroxide, or sodium or calcium hypochlorite. The potential toxicity of the household preparations should not be equated with those of the highly caustic pure preparations of the listed chemicals. Toxicity for the liquid bleaches is related to concentration of active ingredients in the preparation rather than the volume ingested. The concentrated nature of granular bleaches renders these preparations more toxic.

Symptoms associated with the systemic intake of bleaches include mucous membrane and gastrointestinal irritation, nausea, and vomiting. In addition, one or more of the following disorders, including hypotension, fever, contracted abdominal musculature, and possible perforation of the esophagus and stomach, may be present. Treatment for ingestion of bleach is symptomatic and is focused on the dilution of the acid with large quantities of water or milk and neutralization/demulcent therapy with milk of magnesia.

Select bleaches may contain sodium perborate, which decomposes to form peroxide and borate. Borate is strongly alkaline and irritating, and displays the spectrum of the toxic systemic effects of boric acid. The symptoms of borate toxicity include gastrointestinal irritation with hemorrhage, shock, vascular collapse, and convulsions, followed by CNS depression. Treatment for sodium perborate includes gastric lavage, parenteral administration of fluids to counterbalance losses by vomiting and diarrhea, and treatment for shock. Borate is concentrated and excreted by the kidney; accordingly, renal failure is a possible consequence of borate ingestion and thus dialysis may also be required. A few commercial bleaches, as well as some disinfectants, metal cleaning agents, and rust inhibitors, also contain oxalic acid, which is corrosive in nature. When this is ingested, the mucous membranes display a whitish discoloration; the lips and the face are usually not affected. The acute symptoms include gastric pain, bloody vomiting, and cardiovascular collapse. The latter is associated with hypocalcemia and can be treated by immediate ingestion of a calcium-rich solution such as milk or chalk in water. Oxalic acid is absorbed by activated charcoal; therefore, a charcoal slurry preparation may be administered by mouth or gastric tube. Shock should be anticipated. Renal damage from calcium oxalic crystals may be a later-onset development.

Household Caustics

Drain cleaners, oven cleaners, and other similar household products contain heterogenous alkaline or acidic preparations that are caustic to the upper digestive tract. Usually these agents contain concentrated solutions of strong acids or alkalis such as sodium or potassium hydroxide, sodium or potassium carbonates, sodium bisulfate, sodium bioxalate, or oxalic acid. The principle difference between the caustic effects of acids and alkalis is that acids tend to produce a coagulation type of necrosis that protects the deeper layers of the esophagus from destruction, although complete destruction of the tissue can occur with acids. Alkaline caustics are usually much more likely to produce total destruction of the esophageal musculature, resulting in either perforation or late stricture. After ingestion, burns usually appear about the lips, face and buccal mucosa. Burns rarely occur in the esophagus in the absence of burns on the lips or the mouth. Long-term treatment with high doses of corticosteroids is often required. This type of therapy, however, can potentially be dangerous in itself.

The toxicity of caustics is associated with their ability to combine with proteins to form proteinates and with fats to form soap, thus producing penetrating burns on contact with tissue. The degree of causticity is related to concentration of the agent and the length of time it is in contact with the tissue. Caustics, when they come in contact with the skin, may produce first-, second-, or even third-degree burns, depending on concentration and duration of contact. Contact with the eyes may cause severe conjunctivitis as well as corneal destruction. Symptoms of caustic ingestion include a burning pain from mouth to stomach. Swallowing is usually difficult at first and may then become impossible. Mucous membranes are soapy and white but subsequently become brown, edematous, and ulcerated; vomitus is bloody and may contain shreds of mucous membrane. The pulse is feeble and rapid; respiration is increased and collapse may ensue. In the cases of severe poisoning, death due to shock, asphyxia from glottic edema, intercurrent infection, pneumonia, or mediastinitis may occur in 48-72 hr. Within weeks, esophageal stricture develops. Corrosive acid ingestion produces fewer permanent effects on the esophagus than do the alkalis, and it is not unusual for individuals so affected to develop pyloric stenosis instead of esophageal strictures.

Treatment for ingestion of household caustics consists of immediate dilution with water or milk followed by neutralizing substances and demulcents. Because of their corrosive action, gastric lavage or emesis should be avoided, and the airway should be maintained clear to prevent asphyxia secondary to glottal edema. Antiinflammatory steroid therapy and antibiotics should be initiated within 24 hr after ingestion to reduce esophageal stricture formation and infection. If esophageal perforation is suspected, endoscopic examination should be performed. Approximately 25% of those who ingest strong caustics die from the immediate effects. Damage to the esophagus and stomach after ingestion, however, may progress for 2-3 weeks. A high percentage of those who ingest strong caustics and recover from the immediate effects have persistent esophageal strictures. In addition, the corneal damage from eye contact is almost always permanent.

PETROLEUM DISTILLATES

Petroleum distillates are usually found in solvents, fuel, as additives in household cleaners, polishes, cements, paint thinner, and waxes. The majority of petroleum distillates contain a mixture of straight and branched chain aliphatic hydrocarbons (e.g., kerosene, naphtha, gasoline, mineral spirits) and because of their low surface tension tend to spread over a large surface area such as the lungs. This physical effect accounts for the major hazard from ingestion of these compounds.

The systemic toxicity of petroleum distillates is relatively low, and the estimated lethal adult dose for gasoline is approximately 90-120 ml. Without aspiration, ingesting of petroleum distillates produce CNS depression and possibly other systemic side-effects, usually related to their direct irritant properties. Severe CNS symptoms are seen in less than 3% of the cases, with initial euphoria and mania that later progress to headache, depression, coma, and convulsions. The effects are of a narcotic type depression. The pathogenesis of the CNS effects has not been clearly elucidated. No permanent sequelae of a neurological nature have ever been reported with petroleum distillate poisoning. The exact dose known to produce CNS effects has not been determined; it appears to be fairly large, however. With chlorinated solvents, myocardial sensitization to epinephrine with fatal cardiac arrhythmias also develops.

The major hazard from ingestion of petroleum distillates is due to aspiration and development of chemical pneumonitis. The aspiration hazard of petroleum distillates is primarily related to the viscosity of the hydrocarbons. The low-viscosity petroleum distillates spread rapidly over mucosal surfaces and are easily aspirated. This is especially significant in children, whose tracheobronchial tree has a relatively small total surface area. In comparison with the oral lethal dose (90-120 ml), there is general agreement that the lethal intratracheal dose is as little as 3-5 ml. Even without vomiting and subsequent aspiration, the mere presence of petroleum distillates in the hypopharynx can cause chemical pneumonitis. Pulmonary involvement has been noted to be as high as 87% of those ingesting petroleum distillates. The pulmonary involvement may be initially asymptomatic, or the child may exhibit symptoms of respiratory distress such as coughing, choking, breath holding, cyanosis, and even massive pulmonary edema. The natural history of the pulmonary involvement is steady radiographic and clinical deterioration over the first 24-72 hr, with subsequent resolution in 3-6 days. Death in fatal cases is due to hemorrhagic pulmonary edema and usually occurs in the first 6-18 hr. Unfortunately, there appears to be no way to determine in advance which cases will develop to such severity. Histopathological examination reveals the presence of alveoli filled with proteinaceous material, interstitial edema, and occasionally frank hemorrhage. The weakened alveolar wall may lead to emphysema and development of pneumothorax. Bacterial pneumonia may complicate the original chemical pneumonitis. Generally, pulmonary signs are the most important both from the point of prognosis and treatment. Gastrointestinal irritation is manifested by severe abdominal pain, nausea, and vomiting, and often the odor of hydrocarbon can be detected on the patient's breath. Because of the need to balance between possible systemic toxicity from absorption and chemical pneumonitis related to aspiration, treatment for oral ingestion of petroleum distillates is based on the dose taken and the toxicity of the solvent. In general, the stomach should be emptied if the distillates ingested

(a) are suspected to be greater than 1 mg/kg,

(b) are toxic (i.e., trichloroethane), and

(c) contain heavy metals, pesticides, or other toxic substances.

If a sufficient quantity has been ingested to warrant emptying of the stomach, vomiting should be induced only in patients with an intact gag reflex. In patients without a gag reflex, a cuffed endotracheal tube should be inserted before gastric lavage is performed. In children under 6 years of age, a cuffed endotracheal tube is not used because the cricoid ring provides the necessary seal at this age. In addition to the treatment listed, general supportive care should be maintained. The use of epinephrine should be avoided due to the possible solvent-induced sensitization of the myocardium.

Aromatic hydrocarbons (benzene, xylene, toluene) are commonly found in paint and varnish removers, lacquers, and cements. Because of their high volatility and CNS effects, this class of solvents is found not only in cases of accidental ingestion but also in cases of voluntary and purposive solvent inhalation. The symptoms derived from acute inhalation of these solvents include a number of immediate and transient effects including euphoria, dizziness, violent behavior, hallucinations, and delusions; these immediate CNS effects usually last for the duration of active sniffing and for 15-60 min afterwards. The users then experience 1 or 2 hr of drowsiness and stupor, with all of the dependent effects gradually wearing off in several hours. Habitual repeated abuse of solvents leads to psychological dependence, a gradual pulmonary fibrosis, and possible neuropathy. A number of unpleasant side effects are also experienced from inhalation of these solvents. These include photophobia, rhinitis, coughing, nausea, chest pain, and anorexia. Systemic damage of the liver, kidney, and the hematopoietic system may also be present after chronic exposure to select solvents such as benzene or chlorinated hydrocarbons (see the following).

Benzene. Benzene is an aromatic hydrocarbon and a constituent of auto fuel. It is also an industrial solvent and widely used for chemical synthesis. Acute exposure to a large amount of benzene by inhalation or ingestion causes varying degrees of CNS depression. On chronic exposure, benzene produces CNS and gastrointestinal disorders such as headache, drowsiness, nervousness, anorexia, and pallor. The more serious toxic effects or chronic benzene poisoning include fatty degeneration of the heart, liver, and adrenal glands, aplastic anemia, and leukemia. The effects on bone marrow cells are suspected to be caused by covalent binding of a reactive intermediate of benzene oxidation to nucleophilic sites on protein and nucleic acids. Benzene is rapidly converted to phenol and is excreted in the urine as a sulfate ester of phenol. The urinary levels of the ester reflect the level of exposure to benzene.

Toluene. Toluene is also an aromatic hydrocarbon widely used as an industrial solvent, in glues, varnishes, paints, and lacquers, and as a chemical intermediate in organic synthesis. It is a CNS depressant, it does not, however share the toxic effects of benzene on bone marrow.

Carbon Tetrachloride. Carbon tetrachloride (CCl_4) is a halogenated hydrocarbon previously used as an anthelmintic, spot remover, and carpet cleaner. Brief exposure to CCl_4 causes mild irritation to eyes, nose, and throat, and nausea and vomiting. Continued exposure or absorption of CCl_4 in large quantities causes varying degrees of CNS depression leading to coma and death. Sudden death may occur due to ventricular fibrillation or medullary depression. The most serious systemic effect from CCl_4 exposure is hepatic and renal necrosis. Biochemical manifestations of hepatic injury in the form of a marked increase in the activities of serum transaminase and some cellular enzymes may appear after several hours or 2-3 days after exposure. The histopathology includes hepatic steatosis and hepatic centrolobular necrosis. CCl_4-induced hepatic injury appears to be mediated through an active metabolite, trichloromethyl free radical (CCl_3). This active metabolite is formed by the homolytic cleavage of the parent compound by the drug-metabolizing enzymes in the endoplasmic reticulum membranes. The hepatotoxic effects of CCl_4 are enhanced by enzyme inducers such as phenobarbital and DDT, and are also potentiated by ethanol and to even a greater extent by isopropanol (43, 63). Renal damage is signaled by an early reversible lesion of proximal tubules and a reversible oliguria. In severe cases, oliguria may progress to near anuria within a week.

Like CCl_4, other members of this group [e.g., chloroform, dichloromethane (methylene chloride), and 1,1,2-trichloroethane] are also CNS depressants, and some, such as chloroform, have been used as anesthetic agents. They also sensitize the myocardium to catecholamine-induced arrhythmia. Hepatotoxic and nephrotoxic effects may also be evident with chloroform due to production of the active metabolite, phosgene. Dichloromethane (a paint remover) 1,1,1-trichloroethane and trichloroethylene are dry- cleaning agents that appear to be comparatively less toxic than chloroform.

Treatment for ingestion of aromatic and chlorinated hydrocarbons is the same as for petroleum distillates.

ALIPHATIC HYDROCARBONS

The straight short-chain (C_1 - C_4) aliphatic hydrocarbons include methane, ethane (present in natural gas), and also propane and butane (in bottled gas). Methane and ethane do not have general systemic effects but can produce asphyxia by lowering the partial pressure of oxygen. Higher chain length (C_5 - C_8) aliphatic hydrocarbons, like most organic solvents, are CNS depressants and produce dizziness and incoordination. n-Hexane and methyl n-butyl ketone also produce slowly reversible polyneuropathy. This toxic effect is suggested to be due to metabolite, 2,5-hexanedione.

ALCOHOLS

Aliphatic alcohols are straight- or branched-chained alcohols that, because of their general low toxicity and chemical properties, have a wide application in industrial and household products. Because of its appropriate physiological effect, metabolic pathway, and relative low order of toxicity, ethanol is considered the prototype of aliphatic alcohols and has been extensively studied in humans and animals. Other monohydroxy and dihydroxy (glycols) alcohols are in general qualitatively similar to ethanol in their systemic effects but may carry additional hazards due to select metabolite pathways.

Isopropanol is used in rubbing alcohol, hand lotion, antifreeze, and deicing preparations. During acute poisoning, isopropanol produces CNS depression like ethanol, but with more marked gastritis, nausea, vomiting, pain, hemorrhage, and possibility of aspiration into respiratory tract during vomiting. The acute toxicity of isopropanol is about twice that of ethanol and lasts significantly longer because it is oxidized more slowly. Blood levels of 150 mg% are associated with deep coma. Acetone, also a CNS depressant, is a major metabolite of isopropanol. A common effect with isopropanol toxicity is the presence of a severe acetonuria without acidosis. Symptoms of acute intoxication with isopropanol include dizziness and headaches progressing to stupor and coma. Hypothermia, hypotension and circulatory collapse, and respiratory failure constitute other symptoms of isopropanol toxicity. Treatment for the intoxication is similar to that for ethanol and includes supportive therapy for respiratory depression, lowering of body temperature, and gastric lavage. Hemodialysis may be beneficial for treatment of acute poisoning with isopropanol.

The glycols are heavy, colorless, odorless, water-soluble liquids with a sweet pungent taste that contributes to their occasional use as a substitute for ethanol and as a suicide agent. These chemicals are used as heat exchangers in antifreeze, hydraulic fluids, as a plasticizer, and solvents for drugs, cosmetics, lotions, ointments, and food additives. The major glycols used in industry are ethylene, diethylene, hexylene, and propylene glycol. Aside from acute CNS depression associated with all the glycols and shared by propylene glycol, the latter is essentially nontoxic and undergoes metabolic transformation.

Ethylene and diethylene glycol can produce severe renal damage leading to acute renal failure. Ethylene glycol is oxidized by alcohol dehydrogenase to the dialdehyde (glyoxal) and then to glyoxylic acid. The latter, on decarboxylation, yields carbon dioxide and formic acid that contribute to metabolic acidosis during poisoning. Glyoxylic acid is also oxidized to oxalic acid. In turn, the chelation of serum calcium by oxalic acid brings about muscle spasms and renal damage due to precipitation of calcium oxalate in renal tubules. The CNS effects of glycols include intoxication, nausea, vomiting, depressed reflexes, seizures, and tetany. Metabolic effects include acidosis, hyperkalemia, and hypocalcemia. Other signs and symptoms following ingestion of glycols include tachycardia, pulmonary edema, tachypnea, cardiac enlargement, and congestive failure. Renal toxicity (oliguria) can occur within 12 hr of ingestion and can last as long as 5-7 weeks.

Treatment for ethylene glycol poisoning is similar to that for methanol toxicity and includes use of a base such as sodium bicarbonate for acidosis, use of ethanol to prevent oxidation of the glycol to oxalic acid by competing for alcohol dehydrogenase, intravenous administration of mannitol to produce an osmotic diuresis (contraindicated if oliguria is present), dialysis for increased elimination, and calcium preparation to treat muscle spasm.

INDUSTRIAL AGENTS

In recent years, increasing concern has focused on the widespread environmental contamination of select industrial chemicals and waste products (28), with major emphasis given to the polyhalogenated biphenyls, chlorinated dioxins, and phthalate esters. These compounds are characterized by hydrophobicity, slow rate of environmental degradation, bioaccumulation, and production of long-term systemic toxicity.

Polychlorinated biphenyls (PCBs) were introduced to U.S. industry in 1930, and became popular for their noninflammability, high-plasticizing ability, and high-dielective constant properties. They are used in the production of transformer, capacitor, hydraulic, and heat-transfer fluids, as plasticizers in waxes, and as solvents, adhesives, and sealants. It is estimated that annually about 4000 tons of PCBs gain entry to the waterways in the United States (27). The two major sources for human exposure to PCBs are food materials namely, PCB stored in fish and other aquatic food sources and industrial accidents that contaminate food ingredients and animal feed.

The polybrominated biphenyls (PBBs) are closely related to PCBs in structure and toxicological properties. Exposure to these compounds can produce a wide variety of adverse health effects. Chronic exposure to these polyhalogenated biphenyls produces porphyria, liver damage, and nervous disorders. Many, but not all, polyhalogenated aromatic chemicals are potent inducers (25) of delta-aminolevulinic acid (ALA) synthetase, the initial and rate- limiting enzyme in heme biosynthetic pathway, and can also alter the activities of other enzymes of the pathway, such as ALA dehydratase (35). In addition, both PCBs and PBBs interfere with reproduction in phytoplanktons, animals, and humans.

The PCBs and PBBs are mixtures of high and low halogen-containing isomers. The high halogen-containing isomers are particularly resistant to degradation. Long-term exposure to those agents causes liver hypertrophy, induction of the microsomal mixed-function oxidase system, and increased metabolism of endogenous steroids and increased estrogenic activities. The PCBs and PBBs have a unique ability of inducing both the cytochrome P-450 as well as the cytochrome P-448 types. Various polycyclic hydrocarbon carcinogens are activated as a consequence of oxidation by cytochrome P-448 types. Chronic exposure to polyhalogenated aliphatic compounds such as methylchloride (a solvent) and vinylchloride (a precursor for various synthetic products) also causes hepatic porphyria, liver damage, thrombocytopenia, and sclerodermal-like cutaneous changes. Other major effects that have been noted in patients exposed to

PCBs and PBBs include severe acne, numbness, neuralgic pains, jaundice, and long-term immunosuppression. A major contributing factor to the toxicity of PCBs and PBBs is their extremely long half-life and lipophilicity, which can lead to accumulation with tissue in the body fat. A major route for excretion of these compounds is via the breast milk, which can pose a serious health hazard to nursing infants.

The term *chlorinated-dibenzo-p-dioxins* or, more simply, *chlorinated dioxins* refers to a series of 75 compounds that are byproducts in the synthesis of trichlorophenols or trichlorophenoxyacetic acid. Only a few of the 75 compounds have been extensively studied for their chemical and biological properties. However, sufficient data have been gathered to indicate that 2,3,7,8-tetrachloro-dibenzo-p-dioxin (TCDD) is up to 1000 times more toxic than other chlorinated dioxins and is believed to be the most toxic synthetic substance known. At nonlethal doses, it produces loss of body weight, hepatic porphyria, and degenerative changes in thymus and liver,

The term *chlorinated-dibenzo-p-dioxins* or, more simply, *chlorinated dioxins* refers to a series of 75 compounds that are byproducts in the synthesis of trichlorophenols or trichlorophenoxyacetic acid. Only a few of the 75 compounds have been extensively studied for their chemical and biological properties. However, sufficient data have been gathered to indicate that 2,3,7,8-tetrachloro-dibenzo-p-dioxin (TCDD) is up to 1000 times more toxic than other chlorinated dioxins and is believed to be the most toxic synthetic substance known. At nonlethal doses, it produces loss of body weight, hepatic porphyria, and degenerative changes in thymus and liver, with thymic atrophy being a highly sensitive index of TCDD exposure. This agent is also a potent fetotoxin and teratogen. Symptoms of acute toxicity with TCDD include nausea, vomiting, fatigue, polyneuritis, and sensory impairment. Laboratory findings show that lipids and prothrombin times are elevated. The major sources of TCDD in the environment is the manufacturing of 2,4,5- trichloro-phenoxy acetic acid (2,4,5-T), an important herbicide used widely in weed control programs. TCDD is a trace byproduct of 2,4,5-T synthesis. Agent Orange, a mixture containing 2,4,5-T, was extensively used by the U.S. Armed Forces in Vietnam, and concern has been expressed that individuals exposed to the herbicide may suffer long-term health complications. Several major industrial accidents have also produced involuntary exposures to TCDD. Accumulation of TCDD in the environment primarily occurs in the soil, where it tends to persist for more than 1 year after application. Degradation of the chemical in the soil takes place largely by photochemical procedures. The concentration of chlorodioxins in 2,4,5-T has decreased significantly with public awareness of their toxicity.

Phthalate ester plasticizers are extensively used in automotive, construction, household packing, apparel, toy, and medicinal products. Approximately 1 billion pounds of 20 different compounds are produced each year (37). The two most abundantly used chemicals of this group are di-2- ethylhexylphthalate (DEHP) and di-n-butyl phthalate (DBP). When incorporated into polyvinyl chloride as a plasticizer, phthalic acid esters impart flexibility and may account for as much as 40% of the final weight of the plastic. Because they are not chemically bonded in the matrix, phthalic acid esters can escape from the plastic into air and water, where they become significant environmental pollutants. In general, phthalate esters have a low order of acute toxicity. Both DEHP and DBP at low concentrations, however, may be detrimental to reproduction of some aquatic organisms. Several studies also indicate that DEHP has a much greater toxicity to poliferating cells in comparison with nonproliferating cells. DEHP is rapidly metabolized and eliminated from the body. In humans, its half- life following i.v. administration is approximately 28 min. In the body, it is initially hydrolyzed to mono-ethylhexylphthalate, an extremely toxic agent, which is further metabolized and excreted in the urine (57).

PESTICIDES

Pesticides are chemical agents intended for killing or injuring specific undesirable life forms; many pesticides, however, are generally toxic to many other organisms, including humans. Chemicals are selected as pesticides on the basis of their predicted selective toxicity to an organism, which in turn is based on the presence of biological differences between the target organism and humans. As the target organism ascends the evolutionary scale, however, the biological differences between the organism and humans are diminished. A number of herbicides used in control of weeds are, therefore, fairly nontoxic in humans. On the other hand, agents that are used for control of rodents (rodenticides) have relatively the same degree of toxicity to humans as to animals.

Acute poisoning with pesticides usually occurs in humans as a result of occupational exposure or careless use of the toxic agents. The mortality rate for pesticides in the United States is estimated at 0.65/1 million population, but there are an estimated 100 nonfatal poisonings for each fatal case (30). Additionally, new and more sensitive methods of detection suggest the possibility of persistent and subtle changes in the state of health due to low-level chronic exposure to pesticides.

Within each class of pesticides there are chemicals that have a diversity of actions in an organism and display varied toxicological spectra. The three major classes of pesticides, classified on the basis of their target organisms, are: (a) insecticides, (b) herbicides, and (c) rodenticides.

INSECTICIDES

Insecticides are the most widely used of all the classes of pesticides and account for the majority of cases of acute human poisoning with pesticides. Most insecticides are lipophilic in nature and are designed to penetrate the chitin exoskeleton of the insects. Because skin, like chitin, is readily penetrated by lipophilic substances, insecticides constitute an important class of environmental toxicants. The mechanism of toxicity for most insecticides is based on their effects on the nervous tissue. Because of the commonalities of the target organs, toxicity of these chemicals, when assessed on the basis of dosage per unit of body weight, does not greatly differ among various species, including humans. Because most insecticides are absorbed from the skin, however, the large surface area to body weight ratio of the insects greatly increases the effective dosage for these animals. This anatomical property also contributes to the species- selective toxicity of insecticides. Insecticides are classified into three major chemical categories: the chlorinated hydrocarbons, the organophosphates, and the carbamates. The last class includes the various substituted ureas and amides, which can act as herbicides and fungicides as well as insecticides.

ORGANOPHOSPHATES AND CARBAMATES

The organophosphorus and carbamate insecticides are widely used in the United States and have frequently been implicatd in human poisonings. Organophosphates were developed during the 1930's and 1940's in Germany as substitutes of nicotine-based insecticides. Later they were used as nerve gases in chemical warfare. The originally synthesized organophosphates are rapidly hydrolyzed and were of little practical use in agriculture. The substitution of sulfur for oxygen in the phosphate moiety of the complex conferred stability and increased the potential selective toxicity of the compounds. The organophosphates act by inhibiting acetylcholinesterase activity that is critical to the transmission of cholinergic nerve impulses. Systemically, the sulfur containing organophosphates are readily converted, by oxidative enzymes, to the oxygen analogs, which can rapidly and irreversibly inhibit acetylcholinesterase activity. The carbamate insecticides are relatively rapid-acting, reversible inhibitors of cholinesterase enzymes and directly inhibit acetylcholinesterase in a mechanism similar to oxygen containing organophosphates. All carbamates contain a carbamic acid ester linkage and, depending on the nature of the secondary group of the molecule, display a wide acute toxicity dose range (0.8-850 mg/kg LD_{50} in rats)(22). Table 28.2-3 lists several carbamate insecticides with their oral and dermal toxicities. Compared with organophosphates, most of the aromatic carbamates have low-dermal toxicities, except for TEMIK (aldicarb), and are not broad-spectrum insecticides. The members of this class of insecticides react slowly with water, and rapidly with strong alkali, to yield hydrolysis products that are usually either nontoxic or less toxic than the parent compound. The anticholinesterase insecticides may be absorbed across any cell barrier and are readily absorbed

Table 28.2-3
Some Carbamate Insecticides and Their Acute Lethal Toxicities

Compound	LD_{50} in Male Rats (mg/kg)	
	Oral	Dermal
BAYGON (PROPOXUR)	83	2400
CARBARYL	850	4000
MOBAM	150	2000
TEMIK (ALDICARB)	0.8	3

Source: Values obtained in standardized tests in the same laboratory; from Ref. 22.

through the respiratory tract or the eyes, resulting in local effects on these tissues. Absorption of sufficient quantities of the chemical, regardless of the route, results in generalized systemic effects.

Activation and Inactivation. The enzyme systems that catalyze the conversion of the organophosphate insecticides to their respective oxygen analogs belong to the microsomal mixed-function oxidase system. Although the liver has the greatest capacity to catalyze the reaction, other tissue including brain and lung also demonstrate activity. The organophosphates are inactivated by ester hydrolysis and by an NADPH-requiring microsomal enzyme that cleaves the aryl phosphorus bonds. Plasma and tissue carboxylesterases can also hydrolyze select organophosphates (e.g., malathion). In several species of insects, the amount of this enzyme is relatively low, providing an increase in selective toxicity of these agents. Hydrolysis of the carbamic acid ester linkage also produces metabolites that lack anticholinesterase activity. Several carbamates can undergo oxidative metabolism, forming products more toxic than the parent compound. TEMIK, a very potent carbamate (oral LD_{50}, 0.8 mg/kg, rat), is metabolized to a sulfoxide and sulfone, both of which exhibit greater anticholinesterase activity than the parent compound (15).

Mechanism of Action. As noted earlier, both the organophosphate and carbamate insecticides produce their acute toxic actions by inhibiting acetylcholinesterase. The toxicity that occurs in the course of poisoning with these agents can be accounted, for the most part, by the resulting excess accumulation of acetylcholine at the neuroeffector junctions and autonomic ganglia. Insecticides impair the enzyme activity by binding to the esteratic site, which is normally occupied by acetylcholine. Organophosphates and carbamates phosphorylate and carbamylate, respectively, occupy the esteratic site and form a relatively stable bond with the enzyme (1). In general, the carbamates are considered reversible inhibitors of cholinesterase enzymes, with a relatively short duration of action, whereas organophosphates are considered irreversible inhibitors and may even undergo an aging process in which dealkylation of the organophosphate occurs to further strengthen the phosphorylated bond with the enzyme. In this case, the rate of regeneration of cholinesterase activity coincides with the rate of synthesis of new enzyme.

Adverse Effects. The inhibition of acetylcholinesterase and the accumulation of endogenous acetylcholine produce 'cholinergic crisis' in the patient (Table 28.2-4). Because most organophosphates must be activated by metabolism to their respective oxygen analog before binding to the enzyme, the onset of toxic symptoms is usually not observed until about 1 hr after exposure. This is in contrast to the rapid appearance of symptoms of toxicity with carbamates, which are apparent 15-30 min after exposure. Respiratory failure is the common cause of death from organophosphate and carbamate poisoning. Breathing is impaired because of bronchoconstriction, excessive bronchial secretion, muscular weakness, and depression of the medullary centers that control respiration. Other major signs and symptoms include profuse sweating and salivation, abdominal pain and diarrhea, constriction of pupils (miosis), and muscular weakness. Symptoms of poisoning begin promptly and progress rapidly. Respiratory symptoms are usually the first to appear after inhalation of vapor or aerosol; gastrointestinal symptoms usually appear first after ingestion. Localized sweating and muscle fasciculation are usually the first signs observed after cutaneous exposure. If untreated, the duration of toxic symptoms for organophosphates generally lasts from 1 to 5 days. In comparison, acute respiratory symptoms from the carbamates last from 1 to 2 hr and no chronic sequelae develop. Delayed neurotoxic effects leading to functional disturbance in sensory and motor nerves with polyneuritis, sensory disturbance, and muscular weakness have also been reported for several of the organophosphates; these effcts are believed to be due to binding of the toxins to a specific protein fraction in the nerve tissue and are related to axonal degeneration followed by myelin degeneration (2). Some carbamate and organophosphates, when given intravenously, produce pronounced anesthetic effect and respiratory failure that appear unrelated to their anticholinesterase effects (56). One of the carbamates, carbaryl, produces teratogenic effects in experimental animals, particularly in beagle dogs. This may be related to the fact that beagle dogs do not metabolize carbaryl to L-naphthol, a major metabolite in most other species, including human (59). Exposure to carbamate compound can produce in the rat, dog, and human cloudy swelling of cells in proximal convoluted tubules of kidney (61).

Treatment. Treatment for poisoning by acetylcholinesterase inhibitors is focused on four principles: a) preventing further absorption of the compound; b) providing assistance of life-support systems; c) inhibiting excess accumulation of acetylcholine; and d) in the case of organophosphate poisoning, regeneration of acetylcholinesterase enzyme. Death often results from a lack of proper diagnosis, improper or ineffective method of resuscitation, and use of improper and/or inadequate therapeutic agents. Essential features of proper treatment include the removal of the victim from the toxic environment and immediate disposal of clothing and any liquid contamination of the patient. Washing of the contaminated skin and hair with soap or detergent and water followed by an alcohol wash is recommended. If ingestion or inhalation has occurred, gastric lavage may be considered. Inhaled material may be deposited in the upper respiratory tract and subsequently carried to the pharynx and swallowed. Levin tube may be used to empty a distended stomach. Supportive therapy for respiratory depression and respiratory distress include the removal of secretion in the bronchial tree and applying positive-pressure method of artificial respiration until cyanosis is overcome. Thereafter, 2-4 mg of atropine should be administered i.v. This dose of atropine may be repeated at 5 to 10 min intervals until signs of atropinization appear (dry, flushed skin and tachycardia). A mild degree of atropinization should be maintained for at least 48 hr. In cyanotic patients, atropine may promote ventricular fibrillation. Atropine is very effective in reducing tracheobronchial secretions and bronchial constriction, and is moderately effective in decreasing central respiratory depression. It is ineffective against action of insecticides on peripheral neuromuscular junction and paralysis.

Oximes are given as specific therapy for poisoning by organophosphorus compounds. They react directly with the alkylphosphorylated enzyme to free the active unit. Pralidoxime (2-PAM chloride; PROTOPAM), the prototype of oximes used in therapy, is very effective at the skeletal neuromuscular junctions to reduce paralysis. Because of the polar quaternary structure and limited distribution of oximes in the body, however, they are not very effective at the autonomic effector site or the CNS (41). In adults, 2-PAM is given at an initial dose of 1 g, preferably by infusion as a 5% solution in sterile water over a 15 to 30 min period. If this is not practicable, the dose may be given slowly by i.v. injection as a 5% solution in saline. After about 1 hr, a second dose of 1 g may be administered if muscular weakness persists. For children, the dose is reduced 20-50 mg/kg. Additional doses may be given cautiously if muscle weakness persists. Pralidoxime is a weak anticholinesterase; therefore, when used in excess amounts, it may provoke respiratory depression. Because of 'aging' phenomenon, treatment with 2-PAM is most effective if given within a few hours after poisoning by an anticholinesterase. The drug has few beneficial effects if given more than 48 hr after exposure, though occasionally patients may respond after such an interval. In the cases of toxicity, the possibility of heart block by anticholinesterase should be considered. Where the poison has been ingested, the likelihood of continuing absorption from the lower bowel should be taken into

Table 28.2-4
Signs and Symptoms Associated with Acute and Subacute Exposures to Cholinesterase-Inhibiting Insecticides

Muscarinic Manifestations	
Gastrointestinal	Anorexia, nausea, vomiting, abdominal cramps, diarrhea, tenesmus, involuntary defecation, "heartburn," substernal pressure
Sweat glands	Increased sweating
Salivary glands	Increased salivation
Lacrimal (tear) glands	Increased lacrimation
Cardiovascular system	Bradycardia, fall in blood pressure
Bronchial tree	Tightness in chest, wheezing suggestive of bronchoconstriction, dyspnea, cough, increased bronchial secretion, pulmonary edema
Pupils	Pinpoint (miosis) and nonreactive
Ciliary body	Blurring of vision
Bladder	Increased urinary frequency, involuntary urination
Nicotinic Manifestations	
Striated muscle	Muscular twitching, fasciculation, cramping, weakness (including muscles of respiration)
Sympathetic ganglia and adrenals	Pallor, tachycardia, elevation of blood pressure
CNS Manifestations	Uneasiness, restlessness, anxiety, tremulousness, tension, apathy, giddiness, withdrawal and depression, headache, sensation of "floating," insomnia with excessive dreaming (nightmares), ataxia, slurred, slow speech with repetition, drowsiness, difficulty in concentrating, confusion, emotional lability, coma with absence of reflexes, Cheyne-Stokes respirations, convulsions, hyperpyrexia, depression of respiratory and circulatory centers (with dyspnea and fall in blood pressure)

account. In such cases, additional doses of PROTOPAM may be administered at 6 to 8 hr intervals.

The severity of poisoning with organophosphates can be determined by measuring the cholinesterase activity in the red blood cells (62). Plasma (pseudo) cholinesterase level is subject to variations by factors such as dietary habits, liver damage, and others. In addition, the activity of plasma cholinesterase fluctuates more readily than that of the red cells upon exposure to organophosphates. Red cell cholinesterase, unless reactivated by oximes, recovers only as fast as new erythrocytes are formed. Treatment of poisoning by carbamates is the same as that for organic phosphorus compounds, except that PROTOPAM and other oximes are not recommended for routine use (40). Severe intoxication is usually treated with atropine and recovery is rapid. Due to the relatively short duration of action of carbamates, the measurement of cholinesterase activity usually aids only in the confirmation of the poisoning.

CHLORINATED HYDROCARBONS

The chlorinated hydrocarbons, characterized by DDT (chlorophenoethane or dichlorodiphenyltrichloroethane), were originally synthesized in 1875. The extensive use of DDT was encouraged because of its wide range of insecticidal activity, ease of synthesis, stability to light and air, and relatively low level of mammalian toxicity. The chlorinated hydrocarbons, as a class, are no longer favored for uses as pesticides because of their persistence in the environment.

CLASSIFICATION

The chlorinated hydrocarbon insecticides can be chemically classified into several groups as listed in Table 28.2-5 along with their acute lethal toxicity. Because all the chlorinated hydrocarbon insecticides have similar biological properties, the discussion of toxicity will focus primarily on DDT, followed by mention of distinctive features of each class of compounds.

DDT. ***Adverse effects.*** Acute nonfatal poisoning with DDT is rare, occurring mainly as a result of suicide attempts. The average adult would probably have to ingest 10-20 g of DDT (in an oily solution) to be severely poisoned. DDT and other chlorobenzene derivatives in large doses induce prompt nausea and vomiting due to a local effect on the stomach. Because petroleum distillates are used as solvents for insecticides, the possibility of aspiration of the distillates poses a potential health hazard. Other symptoms include fatigue, heaviness and

Table 28.2-5
Some Chlorinated Hydrocarbon Insecticides and Their Acute Lethal Toxicity

Chemical Classes and Compounds	LD_{50} in Male Rats (mg/kg) Oral	Dermal
Chlorobenzene derivatives		
DDT	113 (p,p'DDT)	—
	217 (technical)	2510
DDE	880	—
DDA	740	—
Methoxychlor	5000-7000	—
Benzene hexachloride		
Lindane	88	1000
Polycyclic chlorinated compounds		
Aldrin	39	98
Dieldrin	46	90
Endrin	18	18
Heptachlor	100	195
Chlordane	335	840
Chlorinated camphenes		
Toxaphene	40	600
Strobane	200	—
Other chlorinated hydrocarbons		
Mirex	740	>2000
Chlordecone (KEPONE)	95	345 (rabbit)

Source: Values for most of the compounds except for toxaphene, strobane, and chlordecone are obtained in standardized tests in the same laboratory; from Ref. 22.

aching of limbs, paresthesia of lips, tongue, and face, impaired vision, nervous irritability, apprehension, disorientation, and mental sluggishness. Sympathetic discharge from the CNS sensitizes the cardiac myocardium, and arrhythmias, including ventricular fibrillation, may occur. Chronic exposure to high, but nonfatal, doses of DDT in experimental animals can produce centrolobular necrosis of the liver. In the case of exposure to larger doses or lack of treatment, twitching of the eyelids is observed. This develops into coarse tremors, first in the head and neck, then progressing to the extremities. Convulsions, coma, and death ensue.

Chronic exposure to DDT results in accumulation of residues in humans and other animals, but the health significance of these residues is not readily apparent. For example, in one study the intake of DDT in food by lactating women was estimated to be 0.0005 mg/kg body weight/day; their milk contained 0.08 ppm of DDT, which results in the intake of 0.01 mg/kg/day of DDT by the infants, or about a 20-fold increase compared with that of the mothers (45). No evidence was found suggesting that infants had been harmed by the insecticide.

Mechanism of toxicity. The mechanism of DDT toxicity is associated with blockage of potassium flow across the nerve membrane, resulting in an increased negative afterpotential in the nerve cells and thus disrupting nerve functions (39). In animals, the most prominent action of DDT is direct CNS stimulation, which resembles pentylenetetrazol-induced stimulation. The severity of the convulsions parallels the concentration of DDT in the brain. Clinically, the CNS stimulation is observed in a sequence of symptoms that directly reflect the progressive increase in the amount of insecticide in the brain. The sequence is composed of tremors, increased reflex excitability, generalized spasms, and clonic-tonic convulsions. The frequency of convulsions increases until respiration is depressed and death ensues. Chlorinated hydrocarbons, including DDT, sensitize the heart to catecholamines. Thus, injection of epinephrine, even in small amounts, can cause cardiac arrhythmias and ventricular fibrillation.

Disposition. DDT is slowly and incompletely absorbed from the gastrointestinal tract. Appreciable percutaneous absorption occurs when DDT is dissolved in organic solvents. The chlorinated cyclodiene insecticides such as endrin, aldrin, and heptachlor differ significantly from DDT in that they are readily absorbed from the intact skin. Following absorption, DDT tends to accumulate in adipose tissues, and elimination from adipose stores is estimated at a rate of approximately 1% of the total body storage per day. An important aspect of toxicity is the time interval during which the pesticide is absorbed into the body. If moderate amounts are absorbed over a period of days or weeks, redistribution in the body fat may prevent accumulation in the brain and overt CNS toxicity. The same total amount given as a single dose, however, may be fatal. The slow release of DDT from the storage depots apparently accounts for the prolonged induction of mixed-function oxidase system observed in a number of animal studies (44). A hazard of unknown magnitude with chlorinated hydrocarbons is represented by their transplacental passage. DDT is slowly metabolized to dichlorophenylacetic acid (DDA); less than 20% of the total dose, however, is excreted as DDA.

Methoxychlor. Methoxychlor, a chlorinated ethane derivative, is increasingly being used to replace DDT. It is much less toxic than DDT in mammals, and its half-life is only about 2 weeks compared with 6 months for DDT. It is rapidly metabolized by O-methylation and then conjugation before its excretion in urine.

Benzene Hexachloride (BHC). Benzene hexachloride (BHC), also called benzene hexachlorocyclohexane, is a mixture of eight isomers. The γ-isomer, known as lindane, is most toxic and mostly responsible for the insecticidal activity. The α- and γ-isomers of BHC are CNS stimulants, while the β- and γ-isomers are CNS depressants. Lindane induces hepatic mixed-function oxidase activity and has been implicated in several cases of aplastic anemia. The α- and β-isomers of BHC are known to produce hepatoma in rodents. Lindane, in comparison with DDT, is relatively less persistent in the environment. Benzene hexachloride (γ-isomer, lindane) has symptoms similar to those of DDT and the chlorobenzene compounds. There are some definite differences, however. One such difference is that this compound is absorbed through the skin. Also, there is more hyperirritability seen with this compound than with chlorobenzene compounds. Lindane is more acutely toxic than DDT but is not considered to be a cumulative poison.

Other Chlorinated Hydrocarbons. The polycyclic and other chlorinated hydrocarbon complexes such as aldrin, heptachlor, toxaphene, mirex, and chlordecone are somewhat more toxic than the chlorobenzene derivatives. Poisoning with these compounds can occur from ingestion, inhalation, or skin contact. In the case of poisoning with these agents, symptoms of both sympathetic and parasympathetic stimulations are observed; thus, neurological symptoms are of little diagnostic value. They have also been shown to cause liver and kidney damage. As with chlorobenzene derivatives, this class of compounds is readily absorbed from the intact skin and manifests symptoms of toxicity (Table 28.2-3). Polycyclic chlorinated hydrocarbon complexes may produce convulsions without manifestation of less serious warning signs such as headache, dizziness, nausea, vomiting, and mild jerking. This rather unusual mode of action contributes to a number of fatalities from acute poisoning with these compounds. Aldrin and heptachlor are metabolized to their corresponding epoxides, which are, when administered acutely, equally or more toxic than the parent compounds (41).

The symptoms of poisoning with chlorinated camphenes such as toxaphene differ somewhat from those of other chlorinated hydrocarbon insecticides in that nausea and vomiting can occur prior to convulsions and the chlorinated camphenes show an abrupt onset of toxicity. Toxaphene is the major insecticide in this class of chlorinated hydrocarbons and during recent years has ranked first in quantity used in the United States. It consists of mixed isomers of chlorinated camphene containing more than 170 C_{10} compounds, including isomers of hexa-, hepta-, and nano-chloroboranes and chloroborenes (48). Like other chlorinated hydrocarbons, toxaphene causes CNS toxicity and has been reported to be a carcinogen. It is readily metabolized, which probably accounts for its relatively low persistence in the environment (48).

Similar to other chlorinated hydrocarbon insecticides, mirex and chlordecone (KEPONE) produce CNS stimulation, hepatic injury, microsomal enzyme induction, and carcinogenicity in rodents (14,32,58). They are extremely persistent in the environment and are concentrated several 1000-fold in the food chain. Mirex is probably oxidized to chlordecone; the latter complex, however, does not appear to be biodegradable. Exposed industrial workers show various symptoms of toxicity including tremors, ocular flutter, widened gait, mental deterioration, liver injury, and reduced fertility (54). Oral administration of an anion-exchange resin, cholestyramine, interrupts enterohepatic circulation of chlordecone and enhances its fecal excretion by 3 to 18-fold (12).

HERBICIDES

The use of several herbicides can pose a significant health hazard due to either contamination with synthetic byproducts and/or metabolism to toxic molecular species. The herbicides can be divided into five major categories based on their mechanism of herbicidal action. These are the photosynthetic inhibitors, the inhibitors of chloroplast development, growth regulators, phototoxic herbicides, and respiratory uncouplers (Table 28.2-6). About 45% of all herbicides are photosynthetic inhibitors and therefore have a rather slow course of action in plants. Inhibitors of either chloroplast development or growth regulators are used to hinder growth, whereas phototoxic herbicides and uncouplers of respiration are used to block mitochondrial electron transfer processes and production of adenosine triphosphate (ATP) by oxidative phosphorylation. These types of herbicides are toxic to all cells with intact mitochondrial functions. In addition to these five classes of chemical herbicides, arsenic-containing compounds are available and are commonly used as both household and agricultural herbicides. The toxicity of these compounds to humans is related to their content of arsenic, and poisoning with these compounds manifests symptoms of arsenic toxicity.

ORGANONITROGENS

Adverse effects with organonitrogen herbicides such as trazines, acetanilides, and acetamides are rarely observed in animals or humans (16). At exceedingly high doses (500-1000 mg/kg), certain organonitrogens are capable of causing injury to the nervous system, liver, kidney, and capillary membranes. Large doses of trazine compounds can produce anemia and impaired renal function. Many organonitrogens, however, are irritating to the skin and mucous membranes and some, such as acetanilides and acetamides, may produce sensitization. Clinical features observed with toxicity of these compounds include skin rashes, nausea, vomiting, and diarrhea. Protracted dermatitis is observed in cases of poisoning with acetanilides and acetamides. Herbicides are generally dissolved in organic solvents such as petroleum distillates, and the major hazard of toxicity for this class of herbicides is related to the toxicity of the solvent (49).

BIPYRIDYLS

The bipyridyls (e.g., paraquat, diaquat) are highly polar, water-soluble compounds that act as contact herbicide against a broad spectrum of plant life.

Paraquat. Paraquat is used worldwide as a defoliant and weed killer. At low concentration, it is also used in household products for lawn and garden weed control. Diaquat is used for the control of water weeds. Due to their strong adsorption to plant tissue and soil particles, their herbicidal action is limited to the area of application.

Table 28.2-6
Major Classes of Chemical Herbicides

Class	Mechanism of Action	Example
Photosynthesis inhibitors	Prevent electron transfer between photosystems I and II	Organonitrogen: Substituted ureas, Triazines Uracils carbamates
Phototoxic herbicides	Compete for electrons from photosystem I	Bipyridyls: Paraquat Diaquat
Inhibitors of chloroplast development	Inhibit formation of chloroplast	Amitrole, dichlormate, pyrichlor
Uncouplers of respiration and oxidative phosphorylation	Block synthesis of ATP	Pentachlorophenol, dinitrophenols hydroxybenzonitriles
Growth regulators	Suppress cell division, abnormal cell division	Chlorophenoxy compounds: 2,4-D; 2,4,5-T

The toxic action of paraquat in humans is mediated through free radical generated reactions via a cyclic single reduction-oxidation of the bipyridyl, using NADPH as the reducing agent (6). The loss of cellular NADPH is considered to be one aspect of the cellular toxicity of paraquat. Reoxidation of the reduced bipyridyl by molecular oxygen leads to formation of superoxide radical (O_2^-) that dismutes, nonenzymatically, to singlet oxygen (O_2). Both oxygen radicals can lead to lipid peroxidation and loss of cellular glutathione (9). The pattern of organ toxicity produced by diaquat markedly differs from that of paraquat. Paraquat is particularly toxic to the lung. This has been attributed to an energy-dependent system in the lung that selectively concentrates paraquat but not diaquat (47).

Because of their high polarity and water solubility, dermal absorption of bipyridyls is minimal. Direct pulmonary absorption is also minimal with exposure to commonly used bipyridyl-containing sprays. In concentrated form, paraquat is an irritant and can produce skin irritation, nose bleeding, and a protracted keratitis in the eyes. Paraquat has been used in recent years for eradication of marijuana plants. High residues of paraquat have been found in marijuana cigarettes, and it has been reported that a slow accumulation of scar tissue in the lung may occur in chronic smokers of marijuana contaminated with paraquat.

Oral ingestion of paraquat concentrate accounts for nearly all incidences of serious morbidity and mortality with bipyridyls and produces a unique sequence of toxicological events. The initial toxicity of paraquat may persist for several days and is limited to irritation of the gastrointestinal tract and damage to the kidney, liver, and lung. Damage to the kidney and liver are associated with metabolism and renal excretion of paraquat and are generally reversible. Selective uptake of paraquat by the lung tissues, however, results in a diffuse tissue reaction that can eventually lead to fatal lung injury. Appearance of the respiratory distress associated with the lung injury is delayed for 3-14 days, and its progression is irreversible. The diffuse lung injury consists initially of intra-alveolar edema and hemorrhage related to the destruction of lipid membranes, a reactive proliferation of bronchiolar epithelium,and local atelectasis. Eventually, a rapid proliferation of fibroblasts and increase in fibrous connective tissue in the alveoli. The progressive impairment of gas exchange accompanied by cough, dyspnea, and tachypnea goes beyond the magnitude of response observed with general inflammatory reactions and has led to death in a number of cases.

On the basis of pharmacokinetic studies in humans and dogs, Davies et al. (15) have suggested that plasma concentrations of more than 0.2 $\mu g/ml$ paraquat, when accompanied by impaired renal function will usually result during the initial 24 hr after exposure in fatal pulmonary toxicity. Thus, treatment of paraquat poisoning must be instituted within 10 hr after exposure and prior to appearance of pulmonary symptoms. Treatment consists primarily of removal of paraquat by decontamination of skin, gastric lavage, and cathartics and hemodialysis. In animals, superoxide dismutase, administered i.v. or as an aerosol, has been successfully used as antidote for paraquat poisoning. The applicability of this enzyme in treatment of human poisoning is not known. Corticosteroids are of questionable value in treatment of paraquat poisoning, and supplemental oxygen, to overcome the progressive impairment in gas exchange, is contraindicated unless pO_2 drops below 60-70 mmHg. Increased levels of alveolar oxygen attenuate the pathological process. Based on a review of 96 published cases of paraquat poisoning, it is estimated that consumption of 10-15 ml of commercially prepared concentrates of paraquat constitutes the lethal dose for adults.

Diaquat in comparison with paraquat is relatively free of pulmonary toxicity. In large doses, diaquat produces irritation of the gastrointestinal tract with severe dehydration. As with paraquat, large doses of diaquat, once absorbed, can also produce acute renal and liver injury.

CHLOROPHENOXY COMPOUNDS

The compounds 2,4-dichlorophenoxyacetic acid (2,4-T) and 2,4,5-trichlorophenoxyacetic acid (2,4,5-T) exert herbicidal effects by stimulating growth hormone in plants. This effect is selective for plants and has no counterpart action in animals. Toxic doses of chlorophenoxy compounds in animals produce a variety of symptoms including stiffness of extremities, muscular atrophy, paralysis, and eventually coma. Pathological changes associated with 2,4,5-T toxicity are nonspecific and confined to irritations of the stomach with some liver and kidney damage. In humans, an oral dose of 3-4 g produces symptoms of toxicity; in some patients, peripheral neuritis and muscular weakness following heavy occupational exposure have been reported. The chlorophenoxy compounds are rapidly excreted as conjugates in the urine and have a half-life of approximately 20 hr. Recent concern over the toxicity of 2,4,5-T is focused on a contaminant, 2,3,7,8-tetrachlorodibenzo-p-dioxin (TCDD), produced in the industrial manufacturing of 2,4,5-T. The molecular basis for toxicity and teratogenicity of TCDD is not clearly established, although interactions with DNA/RNA function are apparently involved in the manifestations of the adverse effects.

NITROPHENOLS AND CHLOROPHENOLS

These substances have long been used as contact herbicides and are toxic to all aerobic cells. Their mechanism of action involves uncoupling of carbohydrate oxidation with oxidative phosphorylation. The uncoupling leads to the depletion of body carbohydrates and fat stores and to increased cellular oxygen consumption and heat production. Severe poisoning by these compounds generally occurs in hot environments that accentuate the adverse effects of increased heat production. In addition to their metabolic effect, the phenols also have a specific toxic effect on the CNS, liver, and kidney. Recently, the use of pentachlorophenol as a germicide in diaper rinse was linked to the death of two infants (5). In children, the important features of poisoning with chlorophenols are dehydration and metabolic acidosis.

Nitrophenols and nitrocresols are efficiently absorbed through the skin as well as the gastrointestinal tract and are highly toxic to humans. The major clinical features of acute poisoning with these compounds are associated with the increased heat production and include profuse sweating, headache, weakness, malaise, and fever. Tachycardia and tachypnea are also usually present. Cerebral effects are characterized by apprehension, restlessness, anxiety, and manic behavior. Contact with nitro-containing herbicides produces an intense yellow staining of skin and hair and staining of urine. Those observations indicate absorption of sizable amounts of nitro-containing herbicide through the skin. Chronic low-level exposure to this class of herbicides produces weight loss due to increased cellular metabolism.

Treatment for poisoning with the nitro and chlorophenol herbicides is focused on decreasing the body burden of the herbicide and reducing the severity of fever and CNS symptoms. If poisoning involves dermal exposure, the skin should be washed thoroughly with soap and water. Emesis with syrup of ipecac or intubation is used when poisoning from ingestion of the herbicides is suspected. Caution must be taken because of the possible aspiration of petroleum distillates used to dissolve the herbicides. Intravenous fluids should be administered to increase urinary excretion of the agents and to support physiological mechanism for heat loss. The increased body temperature and tissue anoxia should be treated with sponge baths, cooling blankets, and oxygen therapy. Aspirin and other antipyretics are contraindicated for control of body temperature. In animal studies, these chemicals have been shown to enhance the toxicity of nitro and chlorophenol herbicides (50). During convalescence, a high-calorie, high-vitamin diet should be maintained to facilitate the repletion of body fat and carbohydrate stores.

RODENTICIDES

A wide variety of chemicals has been used in the past for the control of rodents. In most cases, the actual toxicity of these compounds in humans is very similar to that of the rodent, and species selectivity is imposed by placement of the chemical agent in selected areas. Thus in most cases, human poisoning with this class of pesticides is a result of acute accidental or intentional (suicidal) ingestion of the chemical. The major rodenticides include the anticoagulants, red squill, sodium fluoroacetate, and strychnine sulfate.

ANTICOAGULANTS

The most successful and widely used class of rodenticides are the anticoagulants. The coumarin anticoagulants consist of warfarin or warfarin analogs. These agents act to inhibit the synthesis of prothrombin and factors VII, IX, and X involved with blood clotting, resulting in hemorrhage throughout the entire body. The 1,3-indandione type of anticoagulants has a similar mode of action but also produces neurological disorders and cardiopulmonary injury that may result in death before hemorrhage occurs. In rodents, the symptoms of poisoning with the anticoagulants generally require several days before they are fully expressed.

Ingestion of sufficient amounts of anticoagulant rodenticide to produce generalized hemorrhagic condition in humans only occurs in cases of suicide attempts, chronic low-level consumption, and ingestion of large amounts of grain contaminated with the agents by malnourished individuals. In most cases of poisoning with anticoagulants, the individual remains asymptomatic or exhibits hypoprothrombinemia. Larger doses can produce hematuria, nose bleeding, bleeding gums, and generalized weakness as a result of anemia. Anticoagulants are efficiently absorbed from the gastrointestinal tract, and this usually continues for several days after ingestion. Thus, in cases of poisoning, emesis with syrup of ipecac and the administration of activated charcoal to reduce the absorption are recommended. Vitamin K (phytonadione) is given to reverse the depression in synthesis of clotting factor. Vitamin K_3 (menadione) and Vitamine K_4 (menadiol) have little or no therapeutic efficacy. In some cases, irrespective of the vitamin K_1 dosage, reversal of increased prothrombin time requires as long as 3 days. In severe cases of poisoning, the antidotal therapy is supplemented with transfusion of fresh blood or fresh frozen plasma. Prothrombin time is a sensitive and reliable diagnostic indicator of anticoagulant poisoning and is useful in determining the course of recovery.

RED SQUILL

Red squill is an extract derived from the bulbs of a cabbage-like plant (*Urginen maritima*) and contains glycosides similar to those in foxglove (digitalis). The toxicity of red squill is similar to that of digitalis and acts by impairing cardiac function. The glycosides in red squill also have a centrally acting emetic effect that contributes to the safety of red squill to large mammals and humans (34). Rodents are not capable of vomiting. Symptoms associated with poisoning with red squill include vomiting, cardiac irregularity, convulsions, and death from ventricular fibrillation. Quinine sulfate reduces the cardiac toxicity of red squill and is used in treatment of the toxicity.

SODIUM FLUOROACETATE

This compound, commonly known as Compound 1080 or Compound 1081 (fluoroacetamide), is largely used by licensed pest control operators, especially in poisoning of large predatory mammals such as coyotes. At the cellular level, fluoroacetate is incorporated as the acetate into the citric acid cycle and converted into fluoroacetyl coenzyme A, which then condenses with oxaloacetate to form fluorocitrate. Normal conversion of citrate to isocitrate is based on the abstraction of hydrogen by the enzyme aconitase. The fluoride-carbon bond in fluorocitrate is much stronger than the hydrogen-carbon bond in acetate, and thus the aconitase activity is effectively inhibited. As a result, large quantities of citrate accumulate and the citric acid cycle is blocked (42). The symptoms from acute poisoning with fluoroacetate are related to the organs most sensitive to interruption of the energy supply from the citric acid cycle. These include the central nervous systems (convulsions) and the heart muscles (arrhythmic contraction, ventricular fibrillations, and cardiac failure). Death in humans from fluoroacetate poisoning is usually due to cardiac failure. The LD_{50} of fluoroacetate ranges from 2 to 10 mg/kg. Large quantities of acetate given as glycerol monoacetate can antagonize fluoroacetate poisoning and have been used successfully in selected cases.

STRYCHNINE SULFATE

The alkaloid from the Nux vomica plant is a potent convulsant with a lethal dose of 1-5 mg/kg. It blocks the inhibitory pathway of the Renshaw cell over the motor cells in the spinal cord and results in increased stimulation by spinal reflexes of motor nerves. Toxicity resembles tetanus convulsions in response to sensory stimuli, and treatment is based on sedation and deprivation of sensory stimuli until the compound is eliminated by urinary excretion.

REFERENCES

1. Aldridge, W.N. The nature of the reaction of organophosphorus compounds and carbamates with esterases. *Bull. WHO* 44:25, 1971.
2. Aldridge, W.N., Barnes, J.M., and Johnson, M.K. Studies on delayed neurotoxicity produced by some organophosphorus compounds. *Ann. N.Y. Acad. Sci.* 180:314, 1969.
3. Alpert, S.M., Gardner, D.E., Hurst, D., Lewis, T.R., and Coffin, D.L. Effect of exposure to ozone on defensive mechanisms of the lung. *J. Appl. Physiol.* 31:247, 1971.
4. Amdur, M.O. Air pollutants. In: *Casarett and Doull's Toxicology* (Doull, J., Klaassen, C.D., and Amdur, M.O., eds.). New York: Macmillan, 1980, p. 608.
5. Armstrong, R.W., Eichner, E.R., and Klein, D.E. *J. Pediatr.* 75:317, 1969.
6. Autor, A.P. (ed.). *Biochemical Mechanisms of Paraquat Toxicity.* New York: Academic Press, 1977.
7. Bates, P.V., Bell, G.M., Burnam, C.P. et al. Short-term effects of ozone on the human lung. *J. Appl. Physiol.* 32:176, 1972.
8. Broker, W., Mossman, A.L., and Siegel, D. *Effects of Exposure to Toxic Gases - First Aid and Medical Treatment.* Lyndhurst, N.J.: Matheson, 1977.
9. Bus, J.S., Aust, S.D., and Gibson, J.E. Paraquat toxicity. *Environ. Health Perspect.* 18:139, 1976.
10. Carnow, P.W. Relationship of SO_2 levels to morbidity and mortality in high-risk populations. *Proceedings of Air Pollution Medical Research Conference,* New Orleans, Oct. 5, 1970.
11. Coffin, D.L., and Stokinger, H.E. Biological effects of air pollutants. In: *Air Pollution,* Vol.2 (Stern, A.C., ed.). New York: Academic Press, 1926, p. 232.
12. Cohn, W.J., Boylan, J.J., Blanke, R.V. et al. Treatment of chlordecone (Kepone) toxicity with cholestyramine. *N. Engl. J. Med.* 298:243, 1978.
13. Craig, T.V., Hunt, W., and Atkinson, B. Hypothermia - its use in severe carbon monoxide poisoning. *N. Engl. J. Med.* 261:854, 1959.
14. Cueto, C., Page, N., and Saffiotti, U. *Report of Carcinogenesis Bioassay of Technical Grade Chlordecone (Kepone R).* Bethesda, MD: National Cancer Institute, 1976.
15. Davies, D.S., Hawksworth, G.M., and Bennett, P.N. Paraquat poisoning. *Proc. Eur. Soc. Toxicol.* 18:21, 1977.
16. Dolgaard-Mikkelson, S., and Paulsen, E. Toxicology of herbicides. *Pharmacol. Rev.* 14:225, 1962.
17. Easton, R.E., and Murphy, S.D. Experimental ozone pre-exposure and histamine. *Arch. Environ. Health* 15:160, 1967.
18. Elo, T. Carbon monoxide, cyanides and sulfides. In: *Quick Reference to Clinical Toxicology* (Hanenson, I.B., ed.). Philadelphia: Lippincott, 1980, p. 177.
19. Fairshter, R.D., and Wilson, A.F. Paraquat poisoning: manifestations and therapy. *Am. J. Med.* 59:751, 1975.
20. Frank, N.R., Amdur, M.O., Worchester, J., and Whittenberger, J.L. Effects of acute controlled exposure to SO_2 on respiratory mechanics in healthy male adults. *J. Appl. Physiol.* 17:252, 1962.
21. Freeman, G., Crane, S.C., Stephens, R.J., and Furiose, N.J. The subacute nitrogen dioxide induced lesion of the rat lung. *Arch. Environ. Health* 18:609, 1969.
22. Gaines, T.B. Acute toxicity of pesticides. *Toxicol. Appl. Pharmacol.* 14:515, 1969.
23. Goldsmith, J.R., and Friberg, L.T. Effects of air pollution on human health in air pollution. In: *Air Pollution* (Sterns, A.C., ed.). New York: Academic Press, 1976, p. 458.
24. Goldstein, B.D., Lodi, C., Callinson, C., and Balchum, O.J. Ozone and lipid peroxidations. *Arch. Environ. Health* 18:631, 1969.
25. Goldstein, J.A., Hickman, P., and Jue, D.L. Experimental hepatic porphyria induced by polychlorinated biphenyls. *Toxicol. Appl. Pharmacol.* 27:437, 1974.
26. Gray, E.L., Patton, F.M., Goldberg, S.B., and Kaplan, E. Toxicity of the oxides of nitrogen. *Arch. Ind. Hyg. Ox. Med.* 10:418, 1954.
27. Hammond, A.L. Chemical pollution: polychlorinated biphenyls. *Science* 175:155, 1972.
28. Hammond, E.C., and Selikoff, I.J. Public control of environmental health hazards. *Ann. N.Y. Acad. Sci.* 329:10, 1979.
29. Hanenson, I.B. (ed.). *Quick Reference to Clinical Toxicology.* Philadelphia: J.B. Lippincott, 1980.
30. Hayes, W.J., Jr. *Toxicology of Pesticides.* Baltimore: Williams & Wilkins, 1975.

31. Hoffmann, D., and Wynder, E.L. Organic particulate pollutants in air pollution. In: *Air Pollution*, Vol. 2. (Sterns, A.C., ed.). New York: Academic Press, 1977, p. 362.
32. IARC. *Monographs on the Evaluation of the Carcinogenic Risk of Chemicals to Man, Vol. 5. Some Organochlorine Pesticides.* Lyon, France: International Agency for Research on Cancer, 1974.
33. Kellogg, W.W., Cadle, R.D., Allen, E.R., et al. The sulfur cycle. *Science* 175:587, 1972.
34. Lisella, F.S., Long, K.R., and Scott, H.G. Toxicology of rodenticides and their relation to human health. *J. Environ. Health* 33:231, 1971.
35. Maines, M.D. Evidence for the catabolism of polychlorinated biphenyl-induced cytochrome P-448 by microsomal heme oxygenase, and the inhibition of delta - aminolevulinate dehydratase by polychlorinated biphenyls. *J. Exp. Med.* 144:1509, 1976.
36. Manzel, D.B., and McClellan, R.O. Toxicology responses of the respiratory system. In: *Casarett and Doull's Toxicology* (Doull, J., Klaassen, C.D., and Amdur, M.O., eds.). New York: Macmillan, 1980, p. 246.
37. Marx, J.L. Phthalic acid esters, biological impact uncertain. *Science* 173:46, 1972.
38. Meigs, J.W., and Hughes, J.P.W. Acute carbon monoxide poisoning. An analysis of one hundred five cases. *A.M.A. Arch. Ind. Hyg.* 6:344, 1952.
39. Narahashi, T. Mode of action of DDT and allethrin on nerve: Cellular and molecular mechanisms. *Residue Rev.* 25:275, 1969.
40. Natoff, I.L., and Reiff, B. Effect of oximes on the acute toxicity of anticholinesterase carbamates. *Toxicol. Appl. Pharmacol.* 25:569, 1973.
41. O'Brien, R.D. *Insecticides, action and metabolism.* New York: Academic Press, 1967.
42. Peters, R.A. *Biochemical Lesions and Lethal Synthesis.* New York: Macmillan, 1963.
43. Plaa, G.L. Toxic responses of the liver. In: *Casarett and Doull's Toxicology*, 2nd ed. (Doull, J., Klaassen, C.D., and Amdur, M.O., eds.). New York: Macmillan, 1980, p. 206.
44. Polland, A.P., Smith, D., Kuntzman, R., et al. Effect of extensive occupational exposure to DDT on phenylbutazone and cortisol metabolism in human beings. *Clin. Pharmacol. Ther.* 11:724, 1970.
45. Quimbey, G.E., Armstrong, J.F., and Durham, W.F. DDT in human milk. *Nature* (London) 207:726, 1965.
46. Robinson, E., and Robbins, R.L. *Air Pollutants in Air Pollution Control, Part II* (Strauss, W., ed.). New York: Wiley, 1972, p. 1.
47. Rose, M.S., and Smith, L.L. Tissue uptake of paraquat and diaquat. *Gen. Pharmacol.* 8:173, 1977.
48. Saleh, M.A., Turner, W.V., and Casida, J.E. Polychlorobornane components of toxaphene: structure-toxicity relations and metabolic reductive dechlorination. *Science* 198:1256, 1977.
49. Smith, R.J. Poisoned pot becomes burning issue in high places. *Science* 200:417, 1978.
50. Sproull, D.H. A comparison of sodium salicylates and 2:4-dinitro-phenol as metabolic stimulants *in vitro* . *Biochem. J.* 66:527, 1957.
51. Stokinger, H.E. Ozone toxicology. A review of research and industrial experience 1954-1964. *Arch. Environ.Health* 10:719, 1965.
52. Strandberg, L.G. SO_2 absorption in the respiratory tract. *Arch. Environ. Health* 9:160, 1964.
53. Subcommittee on Hydrogen Sulfide. *Hydrogen Sulfide*, Baltimore: University Park Press, 1979.
54. Taylor, J.R., Selhorst, J.B., Houff, S.A., and Martinez, A.J. Chlordecone intoxication in man. 1. Clinical observations. *Neurology* 28L:626, 1978.
55. Urone, P. The primary air pollutants - gaseous. In: *Air Pollution*, Vol. 1 (Sterns, A.C., ed.). New York: Academic Press, 1976, p. 24.
56. Vandekar, M., Plestina, R., and Wilhelm, K. Toxicity of carbamates of mammals. *Bull. WHO* 44:241, 1971.
57. Waldbott, G.L. *Health Effects of Environmental Pollutants.* St. Louis: C.V. Mosby, 1978.
58. Waters, E.M., Huff, J.E., and Gerstner, H.B. Mirex. An overview. *Environ. Res.* 14:212, 1977.
59. Weil, C.S., Woodside, M.D., Carpenter, C.P., and Smyth, H.F., Jr. Current status of tests of carbaryl for reproductive and teratogenic effects. *Toxicol. Appl. Pharmacol.* 21:390, 1972.
60. Whipple, H.E. Biologic effects of asbestosis. *Ann. N.Y. Acad. Sci.* 132:1, 1965.
61. Wills, J.H., Jameson, E., and Coulston, F. Effects of oral doses of carbaryl on man. *Clin. Toxicol.* 1:265, 1968.
62. Wills, J.H. The measurement and significance of changes in the cholinesterase of erythrocyte and plasma in man and animals *CRC, Crit. Rev. Toxicol.* (March):153, 1972.
63. Zimmerman, H.J. *Hepatotoxicity: The Adverse Effects of Drugs and Other Chemicals on the Liver.* New York: Appleton-Century-Crofts, 1978.

CHAPTER
28.3

CARCINOGENIC AGENTS

Elizabeth K. Weisburger

History. From the numerous reports carried by the newspapers and magazines on carcinogens in the environment, one would surmise that cancer is a modern disease. This is not the case, for examinations of dinosaur bones, Egyptian mummies, and archaeological discoveries have shown evidence of cancer in such specimens (32).

Toward the end of the Middle Ages, the introduction of technical and industrial processes resulted in occupational cancer. For example, it is surmised that a disease of the cobalt miners of Schneeberg, Germany, in the early sixteenth century was lung cancer, caused by uranium, radium, and their volatile decay products in the ores. In 1775, the surgeon Percivall Pott deduced that scrotal cancer in English chimney sweeps was due to their occupational exposure to soot. One hundred and fifty years later, Passey induced tumors in mice from painting them with extracts of soot; this evidence that carcinogenic materials were present in soot substantiated Pott's hypothesis (44).

Various other cases of cancer in humans, traced to long-term exposure to chemicals, have been discovered (Table 28.3-1; Fig. 28.3-1). A sizable proportion of these carcinogens are industrial materials. These include such substances as the dyestuff intermediates 2-naphthylamine and benzidine, and the synthetic intermediates vinyl chloride, *bis*-2-chloromethyl ether, and acrylonitrile (7, 46). Carcinogens, however, are not limited to organic synthetic intermediates. Not only are some metals or their salts carcinogens, but also numerous compounds formed by plants, fungi, or bacteria are carcinogens in animals. The presence of one such product, aflatoxin B_1, in foodstuffs is associated with excess liver cancer in males in certain areas of the world (47). Finally, the continued use or misuse of certain drugs is likewise correlated with the appearance of neoplasms in a higher than normally expected incidence of the users (17). These situations include: excessive use of phenacetin, diphenylhydantoin, certain oral contraceptives, diethylstilbestrol, some anabolic steroids, 2-naphthylamine mustard (Chlornaphazine), immunosuppressive drugs (17, 31) and several other drugs such as melphalan, busulfan, and methyl-CCNU (4) used in the chemotherapy of neoplastic diseases (Table 28.3-2). In such cases the risk-benefit ratio to the patient must always be considered. An overwhelming deficiency of the immune system, acquired immunodeficiency syndrome (AIDS), perhaps facilitated by the use of certain drugs, has also been implicated in the development of the neoplasm known as Kaposi's sarcoma (11, 14, 26).

Definitions (21, 32). *Cancer* is usually defined as the uncontrolled growth of cells or tissues. Some tumors are benign, meaning that they grow slowly, are fairly well delineated, and affect surrounding tissues by compression. Cells in benign tumors often have normal chromosomes and rarely divide. *Malignant* tumors often grow rapidly, may not be well defined, and often actively invade surrounding tissues, while cells of these tumors may metastasize or move to another organ, either through the circulatory or lymphatic system.

Benign tumors are generally named with reference to the tissue in which they arise. Thus a benign tumor of cartilage is a chondroma (chondro + oma); of fibrous tissue a fibroma; of glandular tissue an adenoma.

Tumors are also divided into classes depending on the embryological origin of the tissues in which they arise. In the early embryo, cells are arranged in three layers: ectodermal, mesodermal, and endodermal. As the embryo develops, ectodermal cells form skin, its appendages, and nerve tissue. Mesodermal cells form bone, muscle, cartilage, and related tissues - the structures that hold the organism together. Endodermal cells yield the intestinal system and associated organs. Thus, cancers originating in mesodermal tissue are called *sarcomas*, and those from ectodermal or endodermal tissues are *carcinomas*. Carcinomas comprise the majority of the cancers seen in the general population.

In analogous fashion, a malignant tumor of the cartilage

would be a chondrosarcoma; of fibrous tissue, a fibrosarcoma; of glandular tissue, an adenocarcinoma. There are also tumors that do not fit neatly into these descriptions for which other classifications, based on their apparent origin, are needed.

METABOLISM AND MECHANISM OF ACTION OF CARCINOGENS

The exact mechanisms by which carcinogens react are still unknown, although many processes have been examined and delineated to some extent. *Primary carcinogens* are compounds that are active as constituted without the need for activation. Examples are alkylating agents such as the nitrogen mustards, β-propiolactone, ethylenimine, methyl methanesulfonate, and propane sultone. *Procarcinogens* require activation, usually by metabolic processes, to show a carcinogenic effect; these constitute the great majority of chemical carcinogens. Still other compounds can show a combination of these actions (24).

Furthermore, certain substances may have an extremely weak effect alone but enhance the action of other carcinogens when applied together. Such compounds are called *cocarcinogens. Promoters* are other compounds that enhance the action of chemical carcinogens. Usually animals are given a single treatment with a known carcinogen, followed by repeated treatments with the promoter to obtain tumors. Although the most frequently used promoters in laboratory research are terpene-like (phorbol) esters of long-chain fatty acids isolated from the seeds of the plant *Croton tiglium* , other compounds also have promoting effects (39). The most potent of these, teleocidin and its analogs, are derived from fungi or algae (12).

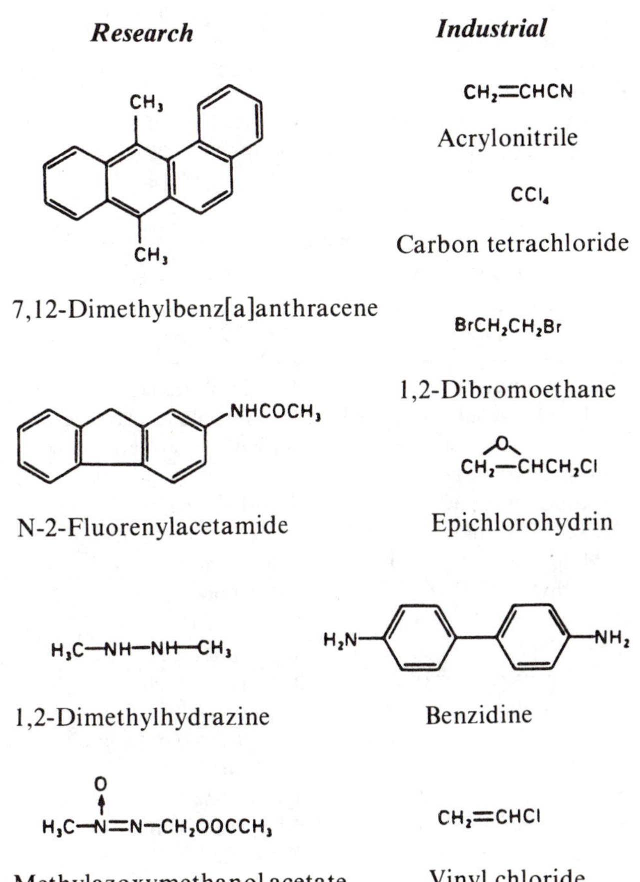

Fig. 28.3-1. *Structures of representative chemical carcinogens.*

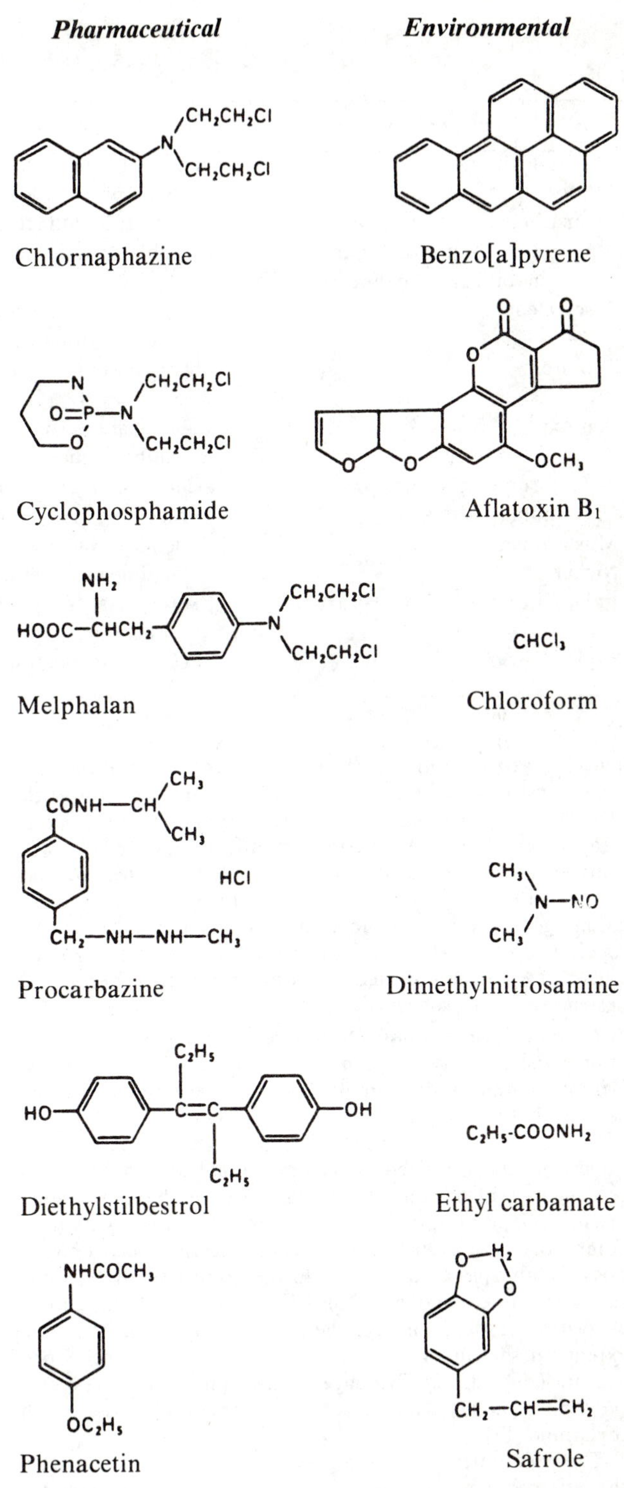

Fig. 28.3-1. *Structures of representative chemical carcinogens* (Continued).

At present, it is presumed that the crucial reaction of an activated carcinogen is with the genetic material of the cell -namely, the nucleic acids. Deoxyribonucleic acid (DNA) carries the genetic information of the cell, and ribonucleic acids (RNA) transfer this information into the making of proteins. Different types of carcinogens are activated in various fashions; in turn, these activated intermediates attach to different positions on the nucleic acids (45). The attachment to the nucleic

Table 28.3-1
Substances Associated with Carcinogenic Risk in Humans

Type of Compound	Products or Process	Type of Cancer or Organs Affected
Acrylonitrile	Polymer production	Lung, intestine
Aflatoxin	Oilseed processing or food use	Liver
Aromatic amines (auramine, benzidine, 2-naphthylamine, 4-aminobiphenyl, magneta)	Dyestuff manufacture, rubber manufacture	Urinary bladder
Arsenic compounds	Smelting, chemical or insecticide manufacture	Skin, liver, lung
Asbestos	Insulation production and installation	Mesothelioma or pleural and peritoneal cavity
Benzene	Chemical intermediate, shoemaking, rubber cement	Leukemia
Bis(chloromethyl) ether	Chemical intermediates	Lung
Chromium (chromates)	Processing of chromite ores	Nasal cavity, lung
Mustard gas	Chemical warfare	Respiratory tract
Nickel	Smelting, electrolysis	Nasal cavity, lung
Polycyclic aromatic hydrocarbons	Soots, tars, creosotes, shale, and mineral oils	Respiratory tract, skin
Vinyl chloride	Polymer production	Liver

acids leads to disruption of their normal functions and weakens their physical structure, making it more susceptible to breakage. On the other hand, there are various enzyme systems ("repair" enzymes) that recognize modified or faulty DNA and remove or excise these altered sections,allowing other enzymes to rebuild the DNA (6). Thus, isolated small exposures to a carcinogen may lead to no overt neoplasms because of the repair processes. However, when the repair process is overwhelmed by large repeated doses of carcinogens, permanent destructive changes occur.

Aromatic Amines and Derivatives. Carcinogenic aromatic amines such as 2-naphthylamine, benzidine, 4-aminobiphenyl, 2-fluorenamine, and its amide, 2-fluorenylacetamide, are activated to N-hydroxy derivatives by enzymes of the P-450 family (22). The P-450 enzyme has several forms that have been separated and characterized (23); monoclonal antibodies to the enzyme have also been prepared (29). Although other schemes are possible, it appears most likely that in turn the N-hydroxy compounds are esterified by acetic, sulfuric, glucuronic, or possibly phosphoric acid to form the respective esters. These esters are quite reactive and mostly attach to the carbon in the 8-position of the guanine in the DNA or RNA, and to a lesser extent on the nitrogen in the 2-position (24) or the N-6 of adenine (Fig. 28.3-2). Evidence for attachment to the oxygen in the 6-position has also been obtained for N-hydroxy-1- naphthylamine (18).

The moiety attached to the C-8 is relatively easily removed by the repair enzymes; that at the N-2 seems less accessible to this process because it is in the minor groove of the DNA. The consequence of attachment to the O-6 position is not yet known. There have been various physicochemical studies on the effects of aromatic amines on nucleic acids that substantiate the displacement of the normal nucleic acid functions such as base pairing, and the weakening of the structure (43).

With improvements in separation of aromatic amine-nucleic acid adducts, the multiplicity of the adducts has become apparent as well as the variation in their persistence (2, 19, 30, 37).

Aromatic nitro compounds are reduced by nitro reductases to the N-hydroxy derivatives, which then proceed by the same process as those from the aromatic amines. The extent of the various steps may vary, depending on the exact nitro compound. Thus, although the nitro compounds corresponding to many aromatic amines are carcinogenic, in most cases they are less potent carcinogens than the amines, or they may affect different sites. An exception is 4-nitroquinoline-N-oxide, which is reduced to a hydroxylamine but is active by itself without metabolic activation.

The N-hydroxylamines, however, account for only a small fraction of the metabolic products of aromatic amines. Hydroxy-

Table 28.3-2
Drugs Associated with Increased Cancer Risk (4, 17)

Drug	Cancer Type
Amphetamines[a]	Hodgkin's disease
Androgenic-anabolic steroids	Hepatocellular carcinoma
Antilymphocyte serum	Reticulum cell sarcoma
Antineoplastic agents	
Chlornaphazine	Bladder cancer
Cyclophosphamide } Melphalan }	Acute myelomonocytic leukemia
Methyl-CCNU	Leukemia
Arsenic	Skin cancer
Chloramphenicol[a]	Leukemia
Contraceptives (oral)	Hepatic adenoma
Diethylstilbestrol	Vaginal and cervical adenoma (in female offspring)
Phenytoin[a]	Lymphoma
Phenacetin	Renal carcinoma
Reserpine[a]	Breast cancer
Thorotrast	Hemangioendothelioma of liver

[a] Epidemiologic evidence suggestive but inadequate.

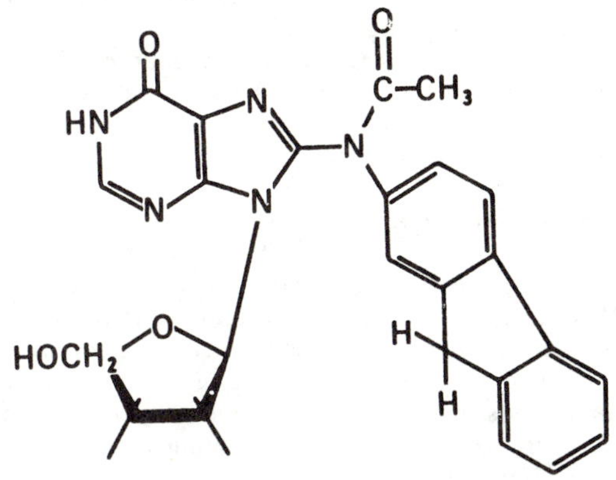

Fig. 28.3-2. *Major product from reaction of 2-fluorenylacetamide with deoxyribonucleic acid, N-(deoxyguanosin-8-yl)-2-fluorenylacetimide.*

lation on ring positions, also mediated by the P-450 enzymes, followed by conjugation to form water-soluble glucuronides or sulfates generally is more prominent, yielding detoxified products. Acetylation of amino groups or conjugation with glutathione leading to mercapturic acids may also occur. On an overall basis, therefore, metabolism of aromatic amines mainly affords detoxification products. The active carcinogenic N-hydroxy intermediates are usually formed in appreciable amounts only after repeated administration of the aromatic amines.

Halogenated Hydrocarbons. Carcinogenic halogenated hydrocarbons include chloroform, carbon tetrachloride, the industrial intermediate vinyl chloride, 1,2-dibromoethane, 1,2-dichloroethane, 1,2-dibromo-3-chloropropane, and trichloroethylene, plus others of more complex structure. There has been much effort recently on the metabolic activation and interactions of these compounds (20, 28). Although the pathway of activation of carbon tetrachloride involves formation of the carbonium ion, CCl_3^+, there has been little definitive work on the position of attachment to nucleic acids.

Due to its large industrial production, much effort has been expended on vinyl chloride. There is divided opinion whether vinyl chloride is activated by metabolism to an epoxide or whether some other pathway operates, such as formation of chloroacetaldehyde. With respect to reaction with nucleic acids, vinyl chloride attaches to the N-1 and the 6-amino positions of adenine, and at the N-3 and N-4 positions of cytosine (3), forming new rings that may lead to a disruption in nucleic acid function. In addition, a 7-hydroxyethylguanine has been identified, evidence for a chloroethylene oxide intermediate (5).

The halogenated hydrocarbons are also detoxified by conjugation with glutathione through glutathione transferase and therefore may deplete liver glutathione levels in the animal. However, 1,2-dibromoethane may also be activated by glutathione conjugation to yield a sulfur mustard analog (38).

Chloroform, carbon tetrachloride, and trichloroethylene all were once used as drugs or anesthetics. Environmentally, chloroform is found at low levels in water supplies due to reaction of organic constituents of the water with chlorine during the disinfection process.

Nitrosamines, Nitrosamides, and Nitrosoureas. Dialkylnitrosamines such as the dimethyl analog $(CH_3)_2N\text{-}NO$ are oxidized enzymatically to several intermediates. One of these, methyl(hydroxymethyl)nitrosamine, is too unstable to exist as such, but the acetyl ester has been synthesized. Another presumed intermediate is monomethylnitrosamine, formed by oxidative removal of one methyl group. This compound, however, is also unstable and decomposes to a carbonium ion, assumed to be the intermediate that attacks proteins and nucleic acids. Initially it was noted that dialkylnitrosamines led to alkylation of the 7-position of the guanine of nucleic acids. At present, the degree of alkylation and dealkylation on the oxygen at position O-6 of guanosine is considered of more interest in the process of carcinogenesis. However, alkylation of several other positions on the nucleic acid bases also occurs (33).

Nitrosamides and nitrosoureas decompose spontaneously at higher pH levels to release carbonium ions, which attach to many sites of nucleic acids or proteins. Nitrosoureas have facilitated the development of animal tumor models rarely seen with other types of laboratory carcinogens. For example, injection of nitrosomethylurea into pregnant rats affords tumors of the nervous system, not in the mother, but in the offspring.

Nitrosamines and nitrosamides are of environmental interest due to their possible endogenous formation from secondary or tertiary amines or amides and nitrite (25, 36). Such amines may occur in certain foods; in addition, many drugs have such structures. Nitrite is present to a limited extent in cured meats. The major portion, however, is formed largely through reduction of nitrate, present in vegetable foods, by bacteria in the salivary plaque or intestinal tract (36).

Ascorbic acid inhibits endogenous nitrosation by competing for the nitrite, thus reducing the risk of carcinogenicity. Unfortunately, ascorbate cannot inhibit the carcinogenicity of preformed dialkylnitrosamines.

Polycyclic Aromatic Hydrocarbons. The polycyclic aromatic hydrocarbons such as benzo[a]pyrene are ubiquitous in the environment because they are formed by combustion processes or even synthesized by algae (10). Benzo[a]pyrene is a weaker carcinogen than some other polycyclic aromatic hydrocarbons used as laboratory models. The metabolism of benzo[a]pyrene proceeds through oxidation by an inducible monooxygenase of the P-450 family to the 7,8-epoxide, which is a substrate for glutathione-S-transferase or epoxide hydratase, leading either to mercapturic acids and precursors or dihydrodiols, respectively (Fig. 28.3-3). By a second step, the 7,8-dihydrodiol affords a 7,8-dihydrodiol-9,10-epoxide, which is a transient but important intermediate that reacts with DNA (13). In this case, the hydrocarbon nucleus attaches to the amino group on the 2-position of guanosine (24, 45). Metabolism of the polycyclic hydrocarbons usually is a regio- and stereospecific process (27, 40).

Besides this covalent type of binding, polycyclic aromatic hydrocarbons are capable of attaching to nucleic acids through physicochemical means. They may be tucked into the DNA helix or intercalated (stacked) between the base pairs of the DNA, causing some uncoiling of the DNA (21).

As with the aromatic amines, polycyclic aromatic hydrocarbons are detoxified by hydroxylation and conjugation to form soluble glucuronides or sulfates or by oxidation to quinones. The glutathione-mercapturic pathway is also a viable detoxification mechanism for aromatic hydrocarbons.

Other Organic Compounds. Many other organic compounds besides those mentioned previously are carcinogens. Ethyl carbamate, 1,2-dimethylhydrazine, cycasin, acrylonitrile, and bis-(chloro-methyl)ether are examples.The latter two compounds are industrial intermediates that have been associated with excess cancers in exposed personnel.

The exact mechanism of action is not known for each of the compounds mentioned. Ethyl carbamate, which affects mice and infant rats, is presumed to be activated through an N-hydroxy intermediate because the latter compound acylates cytosine. A hypothesis that vinyl carbamate is an activated intermediate remains unproven (9).

1,2-Dimethylhydrazine, often used as a model to cause colon

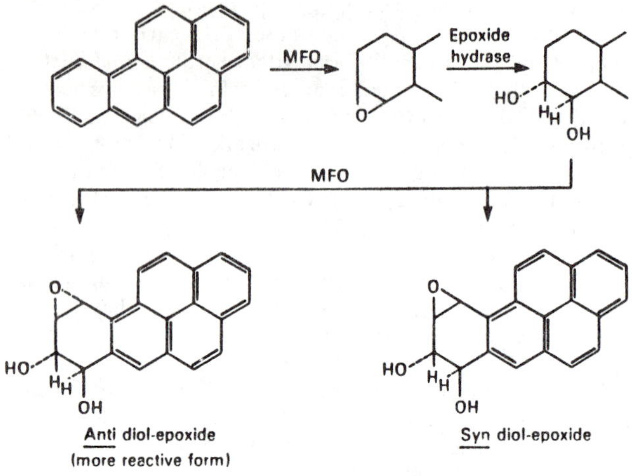

Fig. 28.3-3. *Benzo*[a]pyrene activation.

carcinogenesis in animals, is oxidized through azomethane and azoxymethane to methylazoxymethanol, a compound that decomposes spontaneously, yielding a methyl carbonium ion as the activated intermediate, which in turn alkylates nucleic acids. A glycoside of methylazoxymethanol is cycasin, a carcinogen that occurs in the nuts of the cycad plant which grows in tropical or subtropical areas of the world.

Bis-(chloromethyl)ether and *bis*-(chloroethyl)sulfide are active alkylating agents without the need for metabolic activation. Acrylonitrile or vinyl cyanide is metabolized through an epoxide and by glutathione conjugation, but its effect on the genetic material of the cell has not been investigated.

Aflatoxin B_1 is activated by oxidation to an epoxide, similar to polycyclic aromatic hydrocarbons. The major product from reaction of the aflatoxin epoxide with DNA *in vitro* has been identified as 2,3-dihydro-2-(N^7-guanyl)-3-hydroxyaflatoxin B_1 in which the aflatoxin moiety attached to the 7-position of guanine, analogous to the situation with dimethylnitrosamine or β-propiolactone. However, by high-performance liquid chromatography, 11 peaks, indicating adducts, could be separated (8); by use of monoclonal antibodies, 5 adducts were recognized (15). The imidazole ring opened forms have also been characterized (16).

Metals. Although many metals or their salts are essential micronutrients for the mammalian organism, in certain cases they act as carcinogens (35). Those usually considered in this category are arsenic or its salts, beryllium salts, cadmium salts, chromium compounds (hexavalent), nickel compounds, and lead salts. In addition, asbestos exposure is associated with an excess of mesotheliomas in exposed persons who smoke.

Arsenic salts, at various oxidation states, did not induce tumors when tested in animals. However, persons exposed to arsenic through medicinal preparations, in the drinking water, or industrially have a higher-than-normal incidence of skin and/or liver cancer.

Exposure to chromates or nickel compounds is associated with an increased incidence of cancers of the respiratory tract in industrial workers. Despite this, trivalent chromium is an essential micronutrient involved in sugar metabolism. Cadmium salts have induced tumors in experimental animals when given by very specific routes, but there is only suggestive evidence for cancer in exposed workers. Hypertension, another damaging disease, is associated with exposure to cadmium. Beryllium and lead salts have led to cancer in several species of laboratory animals, but the evidence that they are carcinogens in humans is less substantial.

Exposure to various other metallic elements such as uranium, radium, and thorium (diagnostically as THOROTRAST) is associated with increased cancer because of their radioactivity. As is the case with asbestos, smoking has a synergistic effect in the development of neoplasms of the respiratory tract in people exposed to uranium and its radioactive daughters.

STRUCTURAL CORRELATIONS

The structure of a compound can furnish some clues to its possible activity, based on comparisons with known carcinogens. However, reliance on structure alone as a criterion of carcinogenicity is unwise, since many intrinsic factors influence the response of animals to any compound. Furthermore, as more compounds are tested, the guidelines may change. Despite these uncertainties, a few leads can be summarized for various classes of compounds (1).

Aromatic Amines and Aminoazo Dyes. An amino group in the most reactive or most readily substituted position of the aromatic nucleus is more likely to result in a carcinogen than if the amino group is in another position. Amino groups adjacent to a ring annulation are more likely to be noncarcinogens. A methyl group adjacent to an aromatic amino group may increase the carcinogenicity compared with the unmethylated compound. In many cases, the substitution of polar groups such as hydroxyl, sulfonic, or carboxylic on the ring may decrease any carcinogenic effect. Blocking positions usually involved in metabolic hydroxylation by fluorine, methoxy, or methyl often increases the effect, relative to the unsubstituted compound.

Polycyclic Aromatic Hydrocarbons. Linear condensed hydrocarbons are generally noncarcinogenic, as are those of three or fewer rings or those greater than 120 Å in size. Similar guidelines generally hold with respect to substituents as with the aromatic amines. As an example, chrysene itself has minimal carcinogenic activity, but that of certain methylchrysenes is considerably greater.

N-Nitroso Compounds. Most symmetrical and unsymmetrical dialkylnitrosamines are active unless the substituent alkyl groups are very bulky, as tert-butyl. Usually activity decreases as the length of the alkyl chain increases. Many heterocyclic N-nitroso compounds are potent carcinogens. Nitroso-alkyl or -arylureas and amides are generally active carcinogens. An exception is p-tolylsulfonyl-N-methyl-N-nitrosamide, a compound employed as a laboratory reagent to generate diazomethane.

Some nitroso compounds, however, are not carcinogenic. For example, nitrosoproline, dicyclohexyl- and dibenzylnitrosamines are not effective under conditions where other nitrosamines are. Among the nitroso heterocyclics, changing the position of a substituent such as a methyl group can dramatically alter the carcinogenic potency for unknown reasons. There is much research currently on nitroso componds that may lead to new structure-activity concepts for this area.

Other Compounds. Several compounds with strained rings are fairly active carcinogens. Examples are simple aziridines, alkyl diepoxides, β-propiolactone or 1,3-propane sultone. Unstrained lactones such as butyrolactone have minimal or no activity.

Diarylthioureas are inactive, but alkylthioureas often cause liver or thyroid neoplasms. Thioacetamide, which may be considered as similar to a thiourea, is also a hepatocarcinogen in mice.

INHIBITION OR SUPPRESSION OF CHEMICAL CARCINOGENS

In view of all the carcinogens that are present in the environment or that can be formed endogenously, it is evident that there must be environmental factors that modify the action of such carcinogens; otherwise, cancer rates in most populations would be higher than they are now. Laboratory studies have shown that many factors influence the response to fairly potent carcinogens in experimental animals. Whether these hold in humans is still a question. A new area in research is the chemoprevention of cancer by proper administration of antioxidants, vitamin A analogs, naturally occurring plant constituents, or other relatively nontoxic substances. This concept contrasts with the philosophy of much current effort, where the aim is to cure an existing neoplastic state. The adage, "An ounce of prevention is worth a pound of cure," certainly applies to this situation. The first step in prevention, however, should be to limit exposure to carcinogens to as low a level as feasible. Industrially, the use of closed systems in manufacturing, respirators, proper clothing and gloves, showering at the end of the workday, and working neatly to avoid contaminating the workplace are essential. For the general population, avoiding smoking, certain moldy or other harmful foods, and eating a moderate but varied diet may be useful.

Factors Modifying Response to Carcinogens. There have been many discussions on this topic, mostly in treatises on the conduct of long-term toxicity or carcinogenicity studies (46). The most important factors are delineated briefly here.

In animal experiments with carcinogens, it was discovered that great differences existed in *species* response to the same carcinogen. Mice and rabbits responded when polycyclic aromatic hydrocarbons were painted on their skins, whereas rats and monkeys did not. Guinea pigs and monkeys were resistant to most aromatic amines, but rats, mice, hamsters, and dogs developed tumors after being fed such compounds. Of interest, *all* species tested, including monkeys, had tumors when challenged with N-nitrosodiethylamine.

Likewise, within a given species there were appreciable *strain* differences in response, both in the incidence of tumors and in the organs affected by the neoplastic agents. In many cases, neonatal animals were more sensitive to carcinogens than adult animals. Recent studies indicate, however, that older animals are affected somewhat more by vinyl chloride. Thus *age* is an important consideration. Because the enzymes metabolizing carcinogens to the active intermediates are often mediated through hormones, *sex* also determines the response. Males may be highly affected by one carcinogen, females very little, and vice versa. The *immune* status of the animals is another important but often overlooked factor.

Diets restricted in calories may suppress the action of certain carcinogens, but a deficiency in certain vitamins or other nutritional factors may increase their action. The relative proportion of carbohydrates, proteins, or fats in the diet may influence carcinogenesis. Diets high in fat often enhance carcinogenic effects because the resulting increase in bile acids has a promoting action for some carcinogens. However, diets high in certain vegetable materials, may have a protective action because some of the plant constituents induce enzymes that aid the detoxification of the carcinogens. Other *enzyme inducers* such as phenobarbital, phenothiazines, naphthoflavones, DDT, some other pesticides, a polychlorinated biphenyl, the antioxidants BHT (butylated hydroxytoluene) and BHA (butylated hydroxyanisole) and some polycyclic aromatic hydrocarbons have thus depressed the action of various chemical carcinogens (41).

Chemoprevention. There are no simple means to prevent cancer in many populations since it is a complex disease or series of diseases. Furthermore, everyone is exposed to many factors that may either enhance or suppress the progression of cancer. Although model experiments in animals have afforded leads on the factors that affect chemical carcinogens, extrapolation to humans is not always possible.

A new development has been the use of derivatives of vitamin A, the retinoids, to prevent or suppress the development of tumors in experimental animals from some potent carcinogens (34). In tissue culture experiments, the retinoids have reversed preneoplastic conditions and caused cells to assume a normal appearance. However, it will require additional research and development, before these results can be applied to inhibit or suppress precancerous conditions in humans from progressing to overt cancers. Additionally, the benefits of such intervention must outweigh the risks (42).

REFERENCES

1. Arcos, J.C., and Argus, M.F. *Chemical Induction of Cancer, Vol. IIA.* New York: Academic Press, 1974.
2. Beland, F.A., Dooley, K.L., and Jackson, C.D. Persistence of DNA adducts in rat liver and kidney after multiple doses of the carcinogen N-hydroxy-2-acetylaminofluorene. *Cancer Res.* 42: 1348, 1982.
3. Bergman, K. Reactions of vinyl chloride with RNA and DNA of various mouse tissues *in vivo* . *Arch. Toxicol.* 49:117, 1982.
4. Boice, J.D., Jr., Greene, M.H., Killen, J.Y., Jr. et al. Leukemia and preleukemia after adjuvant treatment of gastrointestinal cancer with semustine (methyl-CCNU). *N. Engl. J. Med.* 309: 1079, 1983.
5. Bolt, H.M., and Filser, J.G. Irreversible binding of chlorinated ethylenes to macromolecules. *Environ. Health Perspect.* 21:107, 1977.
6. Cerutti, P.A. In: *DNA Repair Mechanisms, ICN-UCLA Symposia in Molecular and Cellular Biology, Vol. IX.* New York: Academic Press, 1978, p. 1.
7. Cole, P., and Goldman, M.B. In: *Persons at High Risk of Cancer. An Approach to Cancer Etiology and Control.* New York: Academic Press, 1975, p. 167.
8. Croy, R.G., and Wogan, G.N. Quantitative comparison of covalent aflatoxin-DNA adducts formed in rat and mouse livers and kidneys. *J. Natl. Cancer Inst.* 66:761, 1981.
9. Dahl, G.A., Miller, J.A., and Miller, E.C. Vinyl carbamate as a promutagen and a more carcinogenic analog of ethyl carbamate. *Cancer Res.* 38:3793, 1978.
10. Dipple, A. In: *Chemical Carcinogens, ACS Monograph 173.* Washington, D.C.: American Chemical Society, 1976, p. 245.
11. Durack, D.T. Opportunistic infections and Kaposi's sarcoma in homosexual men. *N. Engl. J. Med.* 305:1465, 1981.
12. Fisher, P.B., Miranda, A.F., Mufson, R.A. et al. Effects of teleocidin and the phorbol ester tumor promoters on cell transformation, differentiation, and phospholipid metabolism. *Cancer Res.* 42:2829, 1982.
13. Gelboin, H.V. Benzo[a]pyrene metabolism, activation, and carcinogenesis: Role and regulation of mixed-function oxidases and related enzymes. *Physiol. Rev.* 60:1107, 1980.
14. Gold, K.D., Thomas, L., and Garrett, T.J. Aggressive Kaposi's sarcoma in a heterosexual drug addict. *N. Engl. J. Med.* 307:498, 1982.
15. Groopman, J.D., Haugen, A., Goodrich, G.R. et al. Quantitation of aflatoxin B_1 -modified DNA using monoclonal antibodies. *Cancer Res.* 42:3120, 1982.
16. Hertzog, P.J., Smith, J.R.L., and Garner, R.C. Characterization of the imidazole ring-opened forms of *trans*-8,9-dihydro-8-(7-guanyl)-9-hydroxy aflatoxin B_1. *Carcinogenesis* 3:723, 1982.
17. Hoover, R., and Fraumeni, J.F., Jr. Drugs. In: *Persons at High Risk of Cancer: An Approach to Cancer Etiology and Control.* New York: Academic Press, 1975, p. 185.
18. Kadlubar, F.F., Miller, J.A., and Miller, E.C. Guanyl O^6-arylamination and O^6-arylation of DNA by the carcinogen N-hydroxy-1-naphthylamine. *Cancer Res.* 38:3628, 1978.

19. Kadlubar, F.F., Unruh, L.E., Beland, F.A., et al. *In vitro* reaction of the carcinogen, N-hydroxy-2-naphthylamine, with DNA at the C-8 and N^2 atoms of guanine and at the N^6 atom of adenine. *Carcinogenesis* 1:139, 1980.

20. Kluwe, W.M., and Hook, J.B. Potentiation of acute chloroform nephrotoxicity by the glutathione depletor diethyl maleate and protection by the microsomal enzyme inhibitor piperonyl butoxide. *Toxicol. Appl. Pharmacol.* 59:457, 1981.

21. LaFond, R.E. *Cancer, The Outlaw Cell.* Washington, D.C.: American Chemical Society, 1978.

22. Lotlikar, P.D., and Hong, Y.S. Microsomal N- and C-oxidations of carcinogenic aromatic amines and amides. *Natl. Cancer Inst. Monogr.* 58:101, 1981.

23. Lu, A.Y.H., and West, S.B. Multiplicity of mammalian microsomal cytochrome P-450. *Pharmacol. Rev.* 31:277, 1980.

24. Miller, E.C., and Miller, J.A. The metabolism of chemical carcinogens to reactive electrophiles and their possible mechanisms of action in carcinogenesis. In: *Chemical Carcinogens ACS Monograph 173.* (Searle, C.E., ed.). Washington, D.C.: American Chemical Society, 1976, p. 737.

25. Mirvish, S.S. N-Nitroso compounds: Their chemical and *in vivo* formation and possible importance as environmental carcinogens. *J. Toxic Environ. Health* 2:1267, 1977.

26. Nahas, G.G. Opportunistic infections and Kaposi's sarcoma in homosexual men. *New Engl. J. Med.* 306:932, 1982.

27. Neidle, S., Subbiah, A., Kuroda, R., and Cooper, C.S. Molecular structure of(±)-7,8,9,10-tetrahydroxy-7,8,9,10-tetrahydrobenzo[a]pyrene determined by x-ray crystallography. *Cancer Res.* 42:3766, 1982.

28. Parchman, L.G., and Magee, P.N. Metabolism of [^{14}C] trichloroethylene to $^{14}CO_2$ and interaction of a metabolite with liver DNA in rats and mice. *J. Toxicol. Environ. Health* 9:797, 1982.

29. Park, S.S., Fujino, T., West, D., Guengerich, F.P., and Gelboin, H.V. Monoclonal antibodies that inhibit enzyme activity of 3-methylcholanthrene-induced cytochrome P-450. *Cancer Res.* 42:1798, 1982.

30. Poirier, M.C., True, B.A., and Laishes, B.A. Formation and removal of (guan-8-yl)-DNA-2-acetylaminofluorene adducts in liver and kidney of male rats given dietary 2-acetylaminofluorene. *Cancer Res.* 42:1317, 1982.

31. Rosenthal, J.T., Iwatsuki, S., Starzl, T.E., Taylor, R.J., and Hakala, T.R. Histiocytic lymphoma in renal transplant patients receiving cyclosporine. *Transplant Proc.* 15:2805, 1983.

32. Shimkin, M.B. *Contrary to Nature.* DHEW Publication No. (NIH) 76-720, Washington, D.C.: US Department of Health, Education and Welfare, 1977.

33. Singer, B. N-Nitroso alkylating agents. Formation and persistence of alkyl derivatives in mammalian nucleic acids as contributing factors in carcinogenesis. *J. Natl. Cancer Inst.* 62:1329, 1979.

34. Sporn, M.B., Squire, R.A., Brown, C.C., Smith, J.M., Wenk, M.L., and Springer, S. 13-*cis*-Retinoic acid: Inhibition of bladder carcinogenesis in the rat. *Science* 195:487, 1977.

35. Sunderman, F.W., Jr. Carcinogenic effects of metals. *Fed. Proc.* 37:40, 1978.

36. Tannenbaum, S.R., Sinskey, A.J., Weisman, M., and Bishop, W. Nitrite in human saliva. Its possible relationship to nitrosamine formation. *J. Natl. Cancer Inst.* 53:79, 1974.

37. Tarpley, W.G., Miller, J.A., and Miller, E.C. Rapid release of carcinogen-guanine adducts from DNA after reaction with N-acetoxy-2-acetylaminofluorene or N-benzoyloxy-N-methyl-4-aminoazobenzene. *Carcinogenesis* 3:81, 1982.

38. van Bladeren, P.J., Breimer, D.D., Rotteveel-Smijs, G.M.T., et al. The relation between the structure of vicinal dihalogen compounds and their mutagenic activation via conjugation to glutathione. *Carcinogenesis* 2:499, 1981.

39. Van Duuren, B.L. Tumor-promoting and cocarcinogenic agents in chemical carcinogenesis. In: *Chemical Carcinogens ACS Monograph 173.*(Searle, C.E., ed.). Washington, D.C.: American Chemical Society, 1976, p. 24.

40. Vyas, K.P., Levin, W., Yagi, H., et al. Stereoselective metabolism of the (+)- and (-)- enantiomers of *trans*-1,2-dihydroxy-1,2-dihydrochrysene to bay-region 1,2-diol-3,4-epoxide diastereomers by rat liver enzymes. *Mol. Pharmacol.* 22:182, 1982.

41. Wattenberg, L.W. Guest editorial: Inhibition of chemical carcinogenesis. *J. Natl. Cancer Inst.* 60:11, 1978.

42. Wattenberg, L.W. Inhibitors of chemical carcinogenesis. *Adv. Cancer Res.* 26:197, 1978.

43. Weinstein, I.B., and Grunberger, D. Structural and functional changes in nucleic acids modified by chemical carcinogens. In: *Chemical Carcinogenesis, Part A.* New York: Marcel Dekker, Inc., 1974, p. 217.

44. Weisburger, E.K. Cancer-causing chemicals. In: *Cancer, the Outlaw Cell.* Washington, D.C.: American Chemical Society, 1978, p. 73.

45. Weisburger, E.K. Mechanisms of chemical carcinogenesis. *Ann. Rev. Pharmac. Toxicol.* 18:395, 1978.

46. Weisburger, E.K. Industrial and environmental cancer risks. In: *Dangerous Properties of Industrial Materials*, 5th ed., New York: Reinhold, 1979, p. 259.

47. Wogan, G.N. Naturally occurring carcinogens. In: *The Physiopathology of Cancer, Vol. 1*, Basel: Karger, 1974, p. 64.

ADDITIONAL READING

Harris, C.C. The carcinogenicity of anticancer drugs: A hazard in man. *Cancer* 37:1014, 1976.

Harris, C.C. Guest editorial: A delayed complication of cancer therapy - cancer. *J. Natl. Cancer Inst.* 63:275, 1979.

Sieber, S.M., and Adamson, R.H. Toxicity of antineoplastic agents in man - Chromosomal aberrations, antifertility effects, congenital malformations, and carcinogenic potential. *Adv. Cancer Res.* 22:57, 1975.

CHAPTER
28.4

MUTAGENIC AGENTS

Sidney Green and K.S. Lavappa

Definition of Mutation. Mutations are heritable alterations in the genetic material, deoxyribonucleic acid (DNA), of an organism and may occur in both somatic and germinal cells. Somatic mutations may lead to various diseases in the organism, whereas germinal mutations are transmitted from generation to generation. Heritable gonadal mutations are far more serious than somatic mutations. Mutations can be dominant or recessive in nature. They can occur spontaneously or can be induced by chemicals, radiation, and viruses. There are two types: point mutations and chromosomal aberrations. A variety of environmental insults have been known to cause both point mutations and chromosomal aberrations. The mutagenic effects of some antineoplastic agents, phenothiazine derivatives, industrial chemicals, as well as several other agents, are presented as examples. The carcinogenic and teratogenic effects of some of these agents are briefly discussed. Inasmuch as the carcinogenicity and teratogenicity may originate via mutation, a discussion of the evidence supporting this view is also provided.

TYPES OF MUTATIONS

Point Mutations. Point mutations, or gene mutations, involve one or a few base pairs of the DNA of an organism. They can be classified as (a) base pair substitutions, or (b) frameshift, also known as addition and deletion.

Base Pair Substitution. Two types of base pair substitution occur: transitions and transversions. If the substitution involves purine for purine, or pyrimidine for pyrimidine, then the mutation is called a *transition*. On the other hand, if the substitution involves purine for pyrimidine, or a pyrimidine for purine, then the mutation is called a *transversion*.

Frameshift, or Addition and Deletion. Frameshift mutations, involve deletion or addition of base pairs in the DNA. These involve large and small macrolesions. Frameshift mutations are readily reverted by many mutagens.

Chromosomal Aberrations. Chromosomal aberrations can be classified into structural aberrations and numerical aberrations. *Structural aberrations* result from breakage of chromosomes and reunion of broken ends. *Numerical aberrations* are changes in the number of chromosomes resulting from errors in the movement of chromosomes during meiosis or mitosis, mainly as a consequence of spindle malfunction.

Structural Aberrations. There are two major types of structural aberrations, namely, chromosome type and chromatid type. The *chromosome type* is produced when mutagens act in the G_1 phase of the cell cycle where the sites of breakage and reunion involve the entire chromosome. The *chromatid type* is produced when mutagens exert their effect in the S or G_2 phase of the cell cycle in which each chromosome has already divided into two chromatids. Some alkylating chemicals produce only chromatid-type aberrations regardless of the stage of the mitotic cycle at which the cell is exposed.

Structural aberrations include the following: *chromosome break*, a discontinuity in both chromatids of the chromosome; *chromatid break*, a discontinuity in one chromatid of the chromosome; *deletion*, paired acentric fragments resulting from a single chromosome break; *minutes*, small acentric fragments of chromosomes or chromatids; *acentric rings*, chromosome with a ring-like configuration lacking a centromere; *centric rings*, chromosome with a ringlike configuration and a centromere; *asymmetrical interchange*, exchange of material between chromosomes resulting in dicentric chromosomes (chromosomes with two centromeres); and *symmetrical interchange*, exchange of material between chromosomes, resulting in a quadriradial configuration.

Numerical Aberrations. Numerical aberrations include trisomics, monosomics, and polyploidy. Trisomics and monosomics result when both chromosomes of a pair undergo nondisjunction during gametogenesis. The gamete containing an extra chromosome, when fertilized by a normal gamete from the opposite sex, will lead to a trisomic zygote. On the other hand, the gamete lacking a chromosome, when fertilized by a normal gamete from the opposite sex, will lead to the formation of a monosomic zygote, which rarely survives. Continued duplication of chromosomes without accompanying cell division leads to polyploidy.

EFFECTS THAT MAY ORIGINATE VIA MUTATION

Carcinogenicity. The process of carcinogenesis may involve mutations as primary or multistage events. There is a great deal of evidence indicating that carcinogens such as chemicals, radiation, and viruses are also mutagens causing genetic changes (60). Studies of chemical carcinogenesis (4), radiation carcinogenesis (41), and dominantly inherited tumors (37) have suggested that mutations are involved in cancer at possibly two stages. Altered patterns of chromosomes, both structural and numerical, and mitotic anomalies have been noted in many malignant cells. There are some tumors, however, that do not show altered patterns of chromosomes. Consequently, it is not clear whether chromosome alteration in tumor cells is a cause or a consequence of cancer.

Teratogenicity. Some chemical agents are teratogenic in nature and induce congenital abnormalities in experimental animals. They are also mutagenic in nature and produce gene mutations and chromosomal aberrations. Chemical agents that produce both teratogenic and mutagenic effects include cyclophosphamide (CP), methylmethanesulfonate (MMS), and ethylmethanesulfonate (EMS) (31). When administered to pregnant mice, 6-aminonicotinamide, a vitamin antagonists, induces both cleft palate and chromosomal aberrations in the cleft palate tissue of the fetus (38). Some teratogenic agents, such as chlorambucil and griseofulvin, however, do not induce mutations (31). The relationship between teratogenicity and mutagenicity is still not clearly understood.

In the human population, some congenital abnormalities are inherited as Mendelian genes (40). Some other types of congenital abnormalities, such as Down's syndrome, cri-du-chat syndrome, Turner's syndrome, and Kleinfelter's syndrome, are associated with specific chromosomal alterations (63).

MUTAGENIC AGENTS

Mutagenic agents are defined as those physical or chemical agents capable of significantly increasing mutational events in experimental animals, thereby posing a possible danger to humans.

Antineoplastic Agents. Antineoplastic agents are used clinically in the treatment of many forms of cancer. The rationale for their use is that they exert their effects on various cellular processes, particularly those controlling the division of cancerous cells. Antineoplastic agents have been found to be mutagenic, carcinogenic, and teratogenic in experimental animals.

Triethylenemelamine (TEM). Triethylenemelamine is an alkylating agent that produces its effects by cross-linking with DNA. It is mutagenic in a variety of systems. Chromosomal aberrations have been demonstrated in cultured human lymphocytes treated with TEM. Translocations and chromosome fragmentation in spermatocytes of mice treated with TEM have also been observed. TEM induces dominant-lethal mutations in rats and mice, and heritable translocations in the F_1 progeny of treated male mice. The mutagenic activity of TEM has been reviewed by Fishbein et al. (16). Intraperitoneal and subcutaneous administration of TEM to mice results in the development of pulmonary tumors. Similarly, rats treated with TEM develop a high incidence of sarcomas (17).

TEM is also a potent teratogen and is embryolethal in the rat. Intraperitoneal injection of TEM at 0.3-0.6 mg/kg to the rat on days 11-12 of pregnancy produces defects in the central nervous system, palate, and skeleton. Growth retardation, enlargement of the myocele, and somite degeneration have also been reported in mouse embryos (30).

Cyclophosphamide. Cyclophosphamide is an antitumor agent widely used in cancer chemotherapy (39). It is also effective in the treatment of rheumatoid arthritis and Wegener's granulomatosis.

Cyclophosphamide has been shown to be mutagenic in a variety of systems, requiring metabolic activation before producing mutagenic byproducts. Chromatid aberrations in treated laboratory mammals and in human lymphocyte cultures following cyclophosphamide (CYTOXAN) therapy have been detected (17). Dominant-lethal mutations and heritable translocations are also induced by cyclophosphamide. Induction of micronuclei in the bone marrow cells of laboratory rodents and the induction of univalents during meiosis have also been attributed to the action of cyclophosphamide. Intraperitoneal administration of cyclophosphamide to mice and rats produces pulmonary tumors, reticular cell sarcoma, and lymphomas. Weisburger et al. have recently reviewed the carcinogenic properties of some drugs used in clinical cancer chemotherapy, including cyclophosphamide (67).

Cyclophosphamide is a potent teratogen, inducing skeletal defects, cleft palate, and exencephaly in rats treated with 7-10 mg/kg of the drug on days 11-12 of pregnancy (7). It has also been shown to be teratogenic in mice and in humans.

6-Mercaptopurine. 6-Mercaptopurine induces dominant-lethal mutations in mice. Increases in the frequency of chromatid and isochromatid deletions on days 14 and 15 after treatment with 150 or 250 mg/kg in cells analyzed at the diakinesis-metaphase I stage of spermatogenesis of mice have also been noted (19). A high incidence of lymphomas was found in mice treated intraperitoneally with 6-mercaptopurine (13).

This SH-containing purine analog and its derivatives are teratogenic in the chick and the rat. An intraperitoneal injection of 31-125 mg/kg of 6-mercaptopurine to rats on day 11 or 12 of pregnancy produced defects in the extremities and in the tail of the fetuses (8). In the chick, the compound produced facial defects.

Vincristine. Vincristine, an alkaloid derived from the plant *Vinca rosea*, is a spindle poison producing a colchicine-like effect. It is used in cancer chemotherapy. It induces micronuclei and polyploidy in bone marrow cells (51). At lower doses the spindle disruption is partial, but at higher doses the disruption is drastic and leads to polypoid cells. Patients treated with vincristine for Hodgkin's disease develop malignancies such as acute leukemia (1).

This antineoplastic agent is teratogenic in hamsters, rats, and monkeys. Intravenous injection of 0.1 mg/kg of vincristine to Syrian hamsters on the eighth gestational day produces skeletal and eye defects (14). Similar effects have been found in rats. Teratogenic effects of vincristine have also been demonstrated in the rhesus monkey.

Mitomycin C. Mitomycin C, an antineoplastic antibiotic used in cancer chemotherapy, has been found to be mutagenic. Human lymphocyte cultures treated with mitomycin C exhibited chromatid aberrations and chromosome rearrangements (18).

Subcutaneous administration of mitomycin C to mice (23) and intraperitoneal administration of mitomycin C to rats (67) induced a high incidence of sarcomas. This growth inhibitor isolated from *Streptomyces caespitosus* produced effects in mouse fetuses, such as skeletal defects of the palate and brain (59).

Actinomycin D. Actinomycin D, a chromopeptide antibiotic, has been used as an antineoplastic agent. Biochemically, it is known to suppress DNA-dependent RNA synthesis and binds to DNA as revealed by tritium-labeled autoradiography (49). Actinomycin D also induces inhibition of mitosis and chromosome breakage in Chinese hamster cells *in vitro*. Chromosome damage (such as chromatid breakages and rearrangements) has also been detected in human lymphocytes and skin and HeLa cell cultures (44). Chromatid aberrations were also detected in human embryonic cells. Breakage of chromosomes appears to be preferentially in the centromeric areas.

Induction of sarcomas in two strains of mice by subcutaneous injection of actinomycin D has been demonstrated (33). The drug has also been shown to induce mammary carcinomas, hepatomas, and squamous cell carcinomas in DBA and Swiss albino mice when administered either subcutaneously or intraperitoneally (12). Similarly, fibrosarcomas in Fisher rats were induced by the intraperitoneal or intravenous injection of actinomycin D.

Actinomycin D is teratogenic in rats when administered daily for the first 10 days of pregnancy. Teratogenic effects include defects of the nervous system and bronchial arch malformations (61). Similar effects have been noted in rabbits. Rumplessness in chicks following injection at 48 hr of incubation has also been produced by actinomycin D.

Phenothiazines. Phenothiazine derivatives are widely used in the treatment of psychiatric diseases. Studies in animals and humans have indicated that these tranquilizing drugs are also mutagenic in nature.

Chlorpromazine. Chlorpromazine forms stable free radicals when photoactivated by ultraviolet light; these free radicals intercalate with DNA (5). Studies on the frequencies of chromosome aberrations in patients treated with chlorpromazine showed variations beginning from no change (9) to increases (43). Recently, Kelly-Gavert and Legator have clearly demonstrated that chromosome aberrations and point mutations can be induced in Chinese hamster cells following treatment of cultures with ultraviolet-irradiated chlorpromazine (34). Induction of sister chromatid exchanges (SCE) following treatment of Chinese hamster cells with chlorpromazine and visible light has also been demonstrated. The general consensus is that chlorpromazine is nonteratogenic (32).

Triflupromazine. Induction of chromosome breakage and rearrangements in cultured rat kangaroo cells treated with triflupromazine has been demonstrated. Inhibition of mitosis was also noted in rat kangaroo cells treated with 20 μg/ml of the drug for 3 days (20). Dose-dependent increases in dominant-lethal mutations are also induced by triflupromazine (47).

Miscellaneous Agents. In addition to the antineoplastic agents and phenothiazine tranquilizers, there are a variety of chemicals that are able to produce mutations, carcinogenicity, and teratogenicity. Table 28.4-1 provides a list of some of these drugs and industrial chemicals with their reported mechanism of mutagenic effect. It appears that the correlation among an agent's ability to produce mutagenicity, carcinogenicity, and teratogenicity is extremely good for the antineoplastic agents. This is generally true for the agents that have a clearly defined site of action in DNA. Very little definitive information about this correlation can be gleaned from the small number of chemicals selected in this table, however. It is certainly evident that a chemical may share more than one of these properties.

Table 28.4-1
Mutagenicity and Its Correlation with Teratogenicity and Carcinogenicity[a]

Chemical	Mechanism of Action	Mutagenicity	Teratogenicity	Carcinogenicity
Antineoplastic agents				
Triethylenemelamine	Alkylating agent	+ (16)	+ (30)	+ (62)
Cyclophosphamide	Alkylating agent	+ (17)	+ (7)	+ (66)
6-Mercaptopurine	Base analog	+ (18)	+ (8)	+ (13)
Vincristine	c-Mitotic agent	+ (51)	+ (14)	+ (2)
Mitomycin C	Alkylating agent	+ (18)	+ (59)	+ (23, 67)
Actinomycin D	Intercalating agent	+ (44)	+ (61)	+ (12, 33)
Phenothiazines				
Chlorpromazine	Arylating agent	+ (34)	- (32)	0
Triflupromazine	Arylating agent	+ (20, 47)	0	0
Miscellaneous agents				
Antiepileptics				
Phenytoin	Not certain	+ (50)	+ (15)	+ (28)
Schistosomacides				
Hycanthone	Intercalating agent	+ (21)	+ (42)	+ (27)
CNS stimulant, alkaloid				
Caffeine	Base analog	+ (36)	+ (10)	+ (58)
Industrial chemicals				
Benzene	Not certain	+ (48)	+ (65)	± (26)
DDT, pp′	Not certain	+ (46)	- (45)	+ (25)
Formaldehyde	Alkylating agent	+ (55)	- (52)	+ (57)
TCDD-2,3,7,8-tetrachloro-dibenzo-p-dioxin	Intercalating agent	± (22)	+ (11)	? (29)
Methyl mercury	Not certain	+ (54)	+ (35)	0
Cadmium compounds	Not certain	+ (5, 53, 64)	+ (3)	+ (24)
Ethyl alcohol	Not certain	+ (3)	+ (56)	0

[a] Numbers in parentheses denote references: +, significant activity; -, nonsignificant activity; ±, ambiguous results; 0, information lacking; and ?, questionable results.

REFERENCES

1. Adamson, R.H., and Sieber, S.M. Antineoplastic agents as potential carcinogens. In: *Origins of Human Cancer* (Hiatt, H.H., Watson, J.D., and Winsten, J.A., eds.). Cold Spring Harbor Laboratory, 1977, p. 429.
2. Badr, F.M., and Badr, R.S. Induction of dominant lethal mutation in male mice by ethyl alcohol. *Nature* 253:134, 1975.
3. Barr, M. The teratogenicity of cadmium chloride in two stocks of wistar rats. *Teratology* 7:237, 1973.
4. Berenblum, I. The mechanism of carcinogenesis: A study of the significance of cocarcinogenic action and related phenomena. *Cancer Res.* 1:807, 1941.
5. Carr, C.R. The relevance of phenothiazine during metabolism to pharmacologic and toxic effects. *Aggressologie* 9:249, 1968.
6. Cea, G.C., Alarcon, M.A., and Weigert, G.T. Induction of chromosome aberration and sister chromatid exchange (SCE) in human lymphocytes by cadmium chloride. *IRCS Med. Sci.: Libr. Compend.* 11:997, 1983.
7. Chaube, S., Kury, G., and Murphy, M.L. Teratogenic effects of cyclophosphamide (NCA-26271) in the rat. *Arzneim-Forsch.* 15:1222, 1967.
8. Chaube, S., and Murphy, M.L. *Advances in Teratology*, Vol. 3. New York: Academic Press, 1968.
9. Cohen, M.M., Hirschhorn, K., and Frosch, W.A. Cytogenic effects of tranquilizing drugs *in vivo* and *in vitro* . *JAMA* 207:2425, 1969.
10. Collins, T.F.X., Welsh, J.J., Black, T.N., and Collins, E.V. A comprehensive study of the teratogenic potential of caffeine in rats when given by oral intubation. *Regulatory Toxicol. Pharmacol.* 1:355, 1981.
11. Courtney, K.D., and Moore, J. Teratology studies with 2,4,5-trichlorophenoxyacetic acid and 2,3,7,8- tetrachlorodibenzo-p-dioxin.*Toxicol. Appl. Pharmacol.* 20:396, 1971.
12. DiPaolo, J.A. Experimental evaluation of actinomycin-D. *Ann. NY Acad. Sci.* 89:408, 1960.
13. Doell, R.G., Cyr, C., deV. St., and Grabar, P. Immune reactivity prior to development of thymic lymphoma in C_{57} B_1 mice. *Int. J. Cancer* 2:103, 1967.
14. Ferm, V.H. Congenital malformations in hamster embryos after treatment with vinblastine and vincristine. *Science* 141:426, 1963.
15. Finnel, R.H. Phenytoin-induced teratogenesis: A mouse model. *Science* 211:483, 1981.
16. Fishbein, L., Flamm, W.G., and Falk, H.L. (eds.). *Chemical Mutagens.* New York: Academic Press, 1970, p. 145.
17. Fishbein, L., Flamm, W.G., and Falk, H.L. (eds.). *Chemical Mutagens.* New York: Academic Press, 1970, p. 149.
18. Fishbein, L., Flamm, W.G., and Falk, H.L. (eds.). *Chemical Mutagens.* New York: Academic Press, 1970, p. 236.
19. Generoso, W.M., Preston, J., and Brewen, J.G. 6-Mercaptopurine: An inducer of cytogenetic and dominant- lethal effects in premeiotic and early meiotic germ cells of male mice. *Mutat. Res.* 28:437, 1975.
20. Green, S., Palmer, K.A., and Legator, M.S. *In vitro* cytogenetic investigation of calcium cyclamate, cyclohexalamine, and triflupromazine. *Food Cosmet. Toxicol.* 8:617, 1970.
21. Green, S., Sauro, F.M., and Legator, M.S. Cytogenetic effects of hycanthone in rats. *Mutat. Res.* 17:239, 1973.
22. Green, S., Moreland, F., and Sheu, C. Cytogenetic effects of 2,3,7,8-tetrachlorodibenzo-p-dioxin on rat bone marrow cells. *FDA-Bylines* No. 6, 292, 1977.
23. Ikegami, R., Akamatsu, Y., and Haruta, M. Subcutaneous sarcomas induced by mitomycin-C in mice. *Acta Pathol. Japan* 17:495, 1967.
24. International Agency for *Research on Cancer. Monograph* 2:74, 1973.
25. International Agency for *Research on Cancer. Monograph* 5:83, 1974.
26. International Agency for *Research on Cancer. Monograph* 7:203, 1974.
27. International Agency for *Research on Cancer. Monograph* 13:91, 1977.
28. International Agency for *Research on Cancer. Monograph* 13:201, 1977.
29. International Agency for *Research on Cancer. Monograph* 15:87, 1977.
30. Jurand, A. Action of triethylenemelamine (TEM) on early and late stages of mouse embryos. *J. Embryol. Exp. Morphol.* 7:526, 1959.
31. Kalter, H. Correlation between teratogenic and mutagenic effects of chemicals in mammals. In: *Chemical Mutagens: Principles and Methods for Their Detection,* Vol. 1. (Hollaender, A., ed.). New York: Plenum Press, 1971, p. 57.
32. Kalter, H. *Toxicology of the Central Nervous System.* Chicago: University of Chicago Press, 1968, p. 164.
33. Kawamata, J., Nakabayashi, N., Kawai, A., and Ushida, T. Experimental production of sarcomas in mice with actinomycin. *Med. J. Osaka Univ.* 8:753, 1958.
34. Kelly-Gavert, F., and Legator, M.S. Photoactivation of chlorpromazine; Cytogenetic and mutagenic effects. *Mutat. Res.* 21:101, 1973.
35. Khera, K.S. Teratogenic effects of methyl mercury in the cat: Note on the use of this species as a model for teratogenicity studies. *Teratology* 8:293, 1973.
36. Kuhlman, W., Fromme, H.G., Heege, E.M., and Ostertag, W. The mutagenic action of caffeine in higher organisms. *Cancer Res.* 28:237, 1968.
37. Kundson, A.G. Mutation and cancer: Statistical study of retinoblastoma. *Proc. Natl. Acad. Sci.* USA 68:820, 1971.
38. Lavappa, K.S. Teratogenic and cytogenetic effects of 6-aminonicotinamide in mice. *Genetics* 80:S50, 1975.
39. Livingston, R.B., and Carter, S.K. *Single Agents in Cancer Chemotherapy.* New York: Plenum Press, 1970.
40. McKusick, V.A. *Mendelian Inheritance in Man: Catalogs of Autosomal Dominants, Autosomal Recessives, and X-linked Phenotypes.* Baltimore: Johns Hopkins Press, 1966.
41. Mole, R.H. Cancer production by chronic exposure to penetrating gamma irradiation. *Natl. Cancer Inst. Monogr.* 14:217, 1964.
42. Moore, J.A. Teratogenicity of hycanthone in mice. *Nature* (Lond.) 239:107, 1972.
43. Neilsen, J., Friedrich, U., and Tsuboi, T. Chromosome abnormalities in patients treated with chlorpromazine, perphenazine, and lysergide. *Br. Med. J.* 3:634, 1969.
44. Ostertag, W., and Kersten, W. The action of proflavin and actinomycin D in causing chromatid breakage in human cells. *Exp. Cell Res.* 39:296, 1965.
45. Ottobani, A. Effect of DDT on the reproductive life-span in the female rat. *Toxicol. Appl. Pharmacol.* 22:497, 1972.
46. Palmer, K.A., Green, S., and Legator, M.S. Cytogenetic effects of DDT and derivatives of DDT in a cultured mammalian cell line. *Toxicol. Appl. Pharmacol.* 22:355, 1972.
47. Petersen, K.W., and Legator, M.S. Dominant lethal effects of triflupromazine in hybrid C_3 D_2 F_1/J mice. *Mutat. Res.* 17:87, 1973.
48. Picianno,D. Cytogenetic study of workers exposed to benzene. *Environ. Res.* 19:33, 1979.
49. Reich, E., Franklin, R.M., Shatkin, A.J., and Tatum, E.L. Action of actinomycin-D on animal cells and viruses. *Proc. Natl. Acad. Sci.* USA 48:1238, 1962.
50. Roman, I.C., and Caratzali, A. Effects of anticonvulsant drugs chromosomes. *Br. Med. J.* 4:234, 1971.
51. Schmid, W. The micronucleus test for cytogenetic analysis. In: *Chemical Mutagens: Principles and Methods for Their Detection,* Vol. 4. (Hollaender, A., ed.). New York: Plenum Press, 1976, p. 31.

52. Sheveleva, G.A. Investigation of the specific effect of formaldehyde on the embryogenesis and progeny of white rats. *Toksikal. Novykh. Promysh. Khim. Veshchestv.* 12:78, 1971.

53. Shirarashi, Y., Kvrahashi, H., and Yosida, T.H. Chromosomal aberrations in cultures of human leucocytes induced by cadmium sulfide. *Phoc. Japan Acad.* 48:133, 1972.

54. Skerfving, S., Hansson, K., and Lindsten, J. Chromosome breakage in humans exposed to methyl mercury through fish consumption. *Arch. Environ. Health* 21:133, 1970.

55. Slizynska, H. Cytological analysis of formaldehyde-induced chromosomal changes in Drosophila Melanogaster. *Proc. R. Soc. Edin.* 66:288, 1957.

56. Streissguth, A.P., Landesman-Dwyer, S., Martin, J.C., and Smith, D.W. Teratogenic effects of alcohol in humans and laboratory animals. *Science* 209:353, 1980.

57. Swerberg, J.A., Kerns, W.D., Mitchell, R.J., Gralla, E.J., and Pavkov, K.L. Induction of squamous cell carcinoma of the rat nasal cavity by inhalation exposure to formaldehyde vapor. *Cancer Res.* 40:3398, 1980.

58. Takayma, S., Kuwabara, N., and Sugimura, T. Induction by caffeine of various tumors in Wistar rats. Presented at the International Life Sciences Institute *Caffeine Workshop,* Kona, Hawaii, November 8-11, 1978.

59. Tanimura, T. Effects of mitomycin-C administered at various stages of pregnancy upon mouse fetuses. *Okajimas Folia Anat. Jap.* 44:337, 1968.

60. Temin, H.M. On the origin of the genes for neoplasia: G.H.A. Clowes Memorial Lecture. *Cancer Res.* 34:2835, 1974.

61. Tuchmann-Duplessis, H., and Mercier-Parot, L. Ciba Foundation *Symposium on Congenital Malformations.* Boston: Little, Brown, 1960.

62. Walpole, A.L. Carcinogenic action of alkylating agents. *Ann. NY Acad. Sci.* 68:750, 1958.

63. Warkany, J. *Congenital Malformations.* Chicago: Year Book Medical Publisher, 1971.

64. Watanabe, T., Shimada, T., and Eendo, A. Mutagenic effects of calcium on mammalian oocyte chromosomes. *Mutation Res.* 67:349, 1979.

65. Watanabe, G., and Yoshida, S. The teratogenic effect of benzenes in pregnant mice. *Acta Med. Biol.* 17:285, 1970.

66. Weisburger, E.K. *Carcinogenicity of alkylating agents.* Public Health Rep. 81:772, 1966.

67. Weisburger, J.H., Griswold, D.P., Prejean, J. et al. The carcinogenic properties of some of the principal drugs used in clinical cancer chemotherapy: Recent results. *Cancer Res.* 52:1, 1975.

Section VII
SPECIAL AREAS IN PHARMACOLOGY

CHAPTER
29

PEDIATRIC PHARMACOLOGY

John T. Wilson

Many prescription drugs have not been adequately evaluated in children, particularly in infants, in terms of their dose, adverse effects, or other label requirements (135). The physician must often depend on empirical or adult-derived information on dose and adverse effects when a drug is to be used for the child. However, for many drugs, extrapolation of pediatric dose from the adult dose has been difficult, and adverse reactions in the child have been markedly different from those seen in adults. Pediatric drug data, not readily available in the package insert or Physicians Desk Reference (PDR), must be sought from recent literature or from practitioners who have experience with a particular drug. These situations impose an additional burden on those who take care of children. In some countries, such as the United States, children are denied the use of many potentially valuable drugs that are not adequately evaluated in infants and children; such sick children in need of unevaluated drugs have been categorized as "therapeutic orphans" (105,106). This chapter highlights child versus adult differences in pharmacotherapy.

CONSEQUENCES OF IMMATURITY

Maturity is the final expression of biological and psychological development that proceeds through a chain of closely interlinked events. The child has many organs and systems that are undergoing overall growth in specific qualitative or quantitative aspects, and such changes continue through puberty. Developmental changes are also responsible for differences in drug disposition seen throughout childhood. Therefore, the weight-adjusted drug dose may not be the same for a preschool child as for a 10-year-old.

Furthermore, during a period of latent or rapid growth, some drugs that may cause severe or protracted toxicity can alter the final mature expression of a system. Drug toxicity may remain covert until full performance is demanded at maturity. These concepts of drug effects on host and host effects on drug (134) need to be appreciated for appropriate use of drugs in children.

AGE-INDIVIDUALIZED DOSAGE

Individualization of drug therapy is the *sine qua non* of rational therapeutics. Pragmatically, however, this is attainable for very few patients. Average or recommended doses continue to be used until plasma level monitoring and pharmacokinetic applications become more widespread. Although many physiological parameters (e.g., total body water, creatinine clearance) are related to body surface area, there are genetic, environmental, and other influences that impact on drug disposition to obviate acceptance of a single principle for pediatric dose calculations. A successive approximation to the calculation of a child's dose is thus in order. Age-related differences in pharmacokinetics, in addition to those of body size, can be used to guide calculations. Altered absorption, distribution, and elimination are most marked in the newborn, especially in prematures, but for many drugs, disposition processes may equal or exceed the adult capacity by late infancy and/or childhood. Relevant pharmacodynamics, toxicity, and disease effects on drug disposition can be used to modulate the age-adjusted dose.

PHARMACOKINETICS

Bioavailability. Absorption and the hepatic first-pass effect (hepatic extraction ratio, presystemic clearance) are the primary determinants of oral bioavailability for a drug. Absorption is dependent on dissolution characteristics and physicochemical properties of the drug, gastric and intestinal contents, anatomical and metabolic factors at the site of absorption, intestinal transit time, and mesenteric blood flow. Blood flow is also important for age-related differences in rate of absorption from parenteral routes. An influence on rate of absorption (i.e., to slow the absorption process) may lower plasma levels with or without affecting total bioavailability of a drug.

As shown in Table 29-1, age-related estimates of bioavailability are not similar for all drugs. They can be influenced by absorption as well as by volume of distribution and elimination rate; hence, drug plasma level comparisons between adults and children per se may not be an accurate index of bioavailability. Differences in rate of oral absorption in the neonate may be due to several factors: (a) rapid changes in gastric acidity and gastric emptying time play important roles; (b) the newborn infant has a relative achlorhydria, and gastric emptying time is somewhat longer in the newborn; and (c) in the infant a high intestinal level of β-glucuronidase activity (56) may enhance enterohepatic recirculation of parent drugs that undergo glucuronidation and thus may influence assessment of the absorption rate.

Table 29-1
Change in Bioavailability of Various Drugs in the Neonate in Comparison with Older Children and Adults

Drug	Bioavailability[a]	
	Oral Route	Intramuscular Route
Penicillin G	+	
Ampicillin	+	
Nafcillin	+	
Rifampin	–	
Gentamicin	–	–
Phenytoin	–	0
Phenobarbital	–	
Nalidixic acid	–	
Acetaminophen (paracetamol)	–	
Phenylbutazone	0	
Co-trimoxazole	0	
Sulfonamides[b]	0	
Digoxin	0	–
Diazepam	0	0

[a] Change: +, increase; –, decrease; 0, normal.
[b] Sulfafurazole (sulfisoxazole), sulfadiazine, sulfasomidine, sulfamethoxypyrazine.
Source: Adopted from Ref. 84.

Furthermore, irregularity of peristalsis (with transit time of upper intestine delayed and that of colon being rapid) as well as variable permeability of GI mucosa are also factors. Selective effects (e.g., diminished gastric acidity in the neonate) have been used to explain an increased bioavailability of orally administered penicillin (51). Phenobarbital absorption in newborns is decreased in infants up to 15 days of age, as is also time for the oral absorption of phenytoin and rifampin (Table 29-1).

Hepatic first-pass elimination, a phenomenon not evaluated in children for most xenobiotics, can also influence bioavailability of orally administered drugs. Propranolol and dextropropoxyphene show wide interindividual variability of plasma levels in children, as in adults. This is consistent with their high hepatic first-pass elimination (136). The newborn and older infants have pathways of hepatic drug metabolism that may be involved with hepatic first-pass elimination, and these show variation in their maturation. This may explain much of the interage and interindividual variations.

Gastrointestinal disorders can also influence absorption of orally administered drugs in infants and children. Generally, any disorder that can increase the gastric emptying rate and peristalsis (i.e., diarrhea, steatorrhea, gluten enteropathy, and so on) can decrease the oral absorption of drugs. Conversely, disease-induced increase in intestinal permeability (i.e., as seen with celiac disease and Crohn's disease) can facilitate the absorption of specific agents in infants and children so affected (94). Thus, absorption of ampicillin can be impaired in children with diarrhea and that of cephalexin in infants with celiac disease.

Protein Binding and Volume of Distribution. A decrease in total body water and extracellular water and an increase in intracellular water occur during postnatal development (100). These changes, in addition to qualitative as well as quantitative protein binding differences for certain substrates, may alter the apparent volume of distribution for a variety of drugs. Of clinical note is the influence of this alteration on the total drug in plasma and concentration of free drug, both of which have an impact on estimation of a "therapeutic" plasma level. The effect of these binding and distribution differences on drug elimination by glomerular filtration has been summarized (125) (Table 29-2). A marked decrease (from 45 to 17%) in extracellular water in the newborn versus the adult accounts for a fall in the $t_{1/2}$ ratio (newborn/adult) relationship to plasma protein binding for drugs excreted by glomerular filtration (100,125). It is important to note that total serum albumin (3.3-3.5 g/100 ml) is similar for full-term newborns and adults (41,52). Selective distribution is conceivably dependent on disparate growth rates and age-dependent proportions of cell constituents for certain organs (Table 29-3), concomitant blood flow changes, and also on the different proportion of extracellular volume of water in a certain tissue as influenced by

Table 29-2
Relationships Between Protein-Binding, Volume of Distribution, and Half-Life of Elimination for Drugs Excreted by Glomerular Filtration in the Newborn Infant and Adult[a]

	Drug Distributed In								
	Plasma Water			Extracellular Water			Total Body Water		
Protein Binding (% bound)	V_D (ml)	$t_{1/2}$ (min)	F	V_D (ml)	$t_{1/2}$ (min)	F	V_D (ml)	$t_{1/2}$ (min)	F
Newborn infant (3400 g)									
0	140	32	—	1530	354	—	2650	612	—
50	280	64	2	1670	387	1.10	2790	645	1.05
95	2800	640	20	4190	970	2.74	5310	1220	2
Adult (70,000 g)									
0	3000	16	—	12,000	64	—	41,000	218	—
50	6000	32	2	15,000	80	1.25	44,000	234	1.07
95	60,000	320	20	69,000	368	5.75	98,000	521	2.38

[a] Calculated from equations (5) and (12) of Keen (Ref. 58). F is the factor by which plasma binding increases the length of time for which the free-drug concentration exceeds any given value, assuming the initial free-drug concentration is the same in each case.
Source: From Ref. 125.

growth (17). The effect of these developmental changes, separate or combined, on volume of drug distribution has largely not been defined in children. Most data remain of an observational nature, although competing effects of endogenous substances present at particular ages have been shown for drug protein binding. In general, concern about volume of distribution and protein binding has focused on the neonate infant clearly at risk for bilirubin encephalopathy and respiratory depression, each of which may ensue from alterations in these pharmacokinetic parameters.

The apparent volume of distribution for several drugs is shown in Table 29-4. It is evident that more data are available for older children than for infants. Additionally, no unidirectional trend is discernible for all drugs, although most show differences of various magnitudes between children and adults. Sulfonamides, for example, show a consistent decrease in volume of distribution with age. An interindividual variation in apparent volume of distribution is found for some drugs in both children and adults (see sulfonamides, Table 29-4).

Table 29-3
Contribution of Organs and Tissues to Body Weight in the Newborn and Adult

Organs/ Tissues	Percent of body weight	
	Newborn	Adult
Skeletal muscle	25	40
Skin	4	6
Skeleton	18	14
Heart	0.5	0.4
Liver	5	2
Kidneys	1	0.5
Brain	12	2

Source: Adopted from Ref. 132.

Newborns and infants generally show a decrease in plasma protein binding as compared with adults. For some drugs, this decrease is a consequence of endogenous competitors or a variable physicochemical environment prevalent at a certain age. Thus, the binding sites may be occupied by high concentrations of bilirubin, free fatty acids, or maternal hormones during the first few days of life. Sick neonates may also show metabolic disturbances (such as acidosis) due to a disease, and use of multiple drugs, both of which can alter drug protein binding. Phenytoin binding to plasma protein is decreased 25-48% in neonates with hyperbilirubinemia (29,99), and sulfaphenazole has a lower affinity for neonatal albumin because of a tightly bound endogenous ligand such as bilirubin (18). It is important to recognize that binding is also a function of both affinity for the drug and amount of binding protein in plasma. Plasma protein (particularly albumin) is quantitatively reduced, and there is also some qualitative change both for albumin and γ-globulin in their binding capacity. A decrease in plasma protein binding generally produces a higher tissue level of free drug, which, depending on the extent of binding and intrinsic plasma clearance, may occur with or without a discernible fall in plasma level of total drug. For a highly bound drug such as phenytoin, a marked decrease in binding can produce an increase in the free-drug fraction

Table 29-4
Age Dependency in Apparent Volume of Distribution (V_d)

Drugs	V_d (l/kg)			
	Newborn (term-1 month)	Infant (2-12 months)	Child (2-18 years)	Adult
Antimicrobials				
Ampicillin (27, 84)	0.48	—	—	0.4-07
Clindamycin (24)	—	—	12[a]	34[a]
Gentamicin (24, 117)	0.52-0.56	0.51	0.22-0.35	0.28-0.31
Kanamycin (24, 27, 117)	0.37-0.81	—	—	0.17-0.29
Sulfisoxazole (24, 84, 117)	0.35-0.43	0.33-0.43	0.29-0.38	0.16
Sulfamethopyrazine (117)	0.36-0.47	0.25-0.47	0.21	0.22-0.25
Ticarcillin (89)	0.66	—	0.35	—
Anticonvulsants				
Diazepam (24, 84, 86)	1.4-1.82	1.3	2.6	0.7-2.6
Dipropylacetate (24)	—	—	0.25	0.15
Ethosuximide (24)	—	—	0.69	0.9
Phenobarbital (48, 53, 84, 86)	0.59-1.54	0.41-1.31	0.5-0.61	0.5-0.78
Phenytoin (25, 84, 93)	1.2-1.4	—	0.78	0.60-0.78
Cardiovascular and Diuretics				
Digoxin (24, 84, 100)	4.9-10.2	15.4-16.3	16.1	5.17-7.35
Furosemide (2, 5)	0.83	—	—	0.1
Antiinflammatory agents				
Phenylbutazone (24, 84)	0.20-0.25	0.16	0.11-0.15	0.02-0.15
Salicylate (84)	0.15-0.35	—	—	0.13-0.20
Bronchodilator				
Theophylline (3, 24, 30)	0.43-1.07	—	0.3-0.5	0.3-0.6
Miscellaneous				
Bromosulphthalein (BSP) (54, 131)	0.056-0.061	0.068-0.070	0.068	—

[a] $V_d = l/m^2$

such that the therapeutic and toxic effects are seen at lower plasma levels of total drug. Age-related plasma protein binding for selected drugs is shown in Table 29-5. Use and interpretation of these values must consider both the drug and plasma protein concentrations in infants for whom binding was determined. Also to be considered is the influence of disease (e.g., renal failure, hyperbilirubinemia) as well as the number of drug binding sites with differential affinity constants and capacity. Protein binding as a function of initial and/or total body burden (total amount of the drug in the body at a steady-state level following its repeated administration) of a drug at a given time is being recognized more frequently (61,139), so that extent of binding must be interpreted in relation to the plasma concentration.

Elimination: Metabolism and Excretion. Any reduction in elimination processes in the young increases the risk for drug toxicity and vitiates simple weight-adjusted dose calculation. Rapid developmental changes of drug elimination rates necessitate frequent monitoring of steady-state plasma levels so that either very low or high dosing, and hence toxicity, can be avoided. Functional immaturity of metabolic and renal systems underlies many observed changes in drug disposition.

In contrast to results from many animal species, human newborn and older infants have some capacity for oxidative drug biotransformation, as demonstrated by studies of plasma drug decay (82, 111), urinary metabolite excretion (111), and analysis of hepatic mixed-function oxidase system (112). A decreased first-order elimination rate is seen for most drugs in newborn infants, but thereafter the rate for some drugs [e.g., phenobarbital (115), phenytoin (37), and theophylline (30)] increases to that similar to or higher than that in adults.

Table 29-5
Plasma Potein Binding of Various Drugs in Neonates and Adults

Drug	Bound (%)	
	Newborns	Adults
Ampicillin	9-11	15-29
Nafcillin	68-69	87-90
Sulfafurazole (sulfisoxazole)	65-70	~84
Sulfamethoxypyrazine	~57	65-70
Salicylate	63-84	80-85
Phenylbutazone	85-90	96-98
Digoxin	14-26	23-40
Diazepam	~84	94-98
Phenytoin	75-84	89-92
Phenobarbital	28-36	46-48
Pentobarbital	37-40	39-45
Imipramine	~74	85-92
Desmethylimipramine	64-71	80-94

Source: From Ref. 84.

Zero-order kinetics for drug elimination are also found in children and include phenytoin (55), salicylate (74), phenobarbital (53, 135), and theophylline (126). Because many drug-metabolizing pathways are of low capacity in the newborn, changes from first-order to zero-order, or mixed first-order/zero-order kinetics may occur at a lower total body burden of drug as compared with children and adults.

Drug conjugation by glucuronidation and sulfation appears to be decreased more than drug oxidation in the newborn and young infant. A typical example is that of chloramphenicol; a decrease in glucuronide conjugation of this drug contributes to the "gray baby" syndrome and death in premature infants. A marked reduction in chloramphenicol dose and prolongation of the dosing interval are needed to avert this toxicity (128). Sulfation is more active in the infant and child until about 12 years of age, as has recently been shown for the metabolism of acetaminophen (1, 73, 81). It is important to note, however, that though sulfation is a high-affinity pathway in infants and children, it has a limited capacity. The urinary profiles of chlorpromazine, meperidine, and promazine conjugates in the newborn are dissimilar to those in the adult (92). Quantitative differences in the urinary profile of salicylate in newborns probably reflect a low rate of glucuronidation (71). Quantitative differences in metabolite profile (i.e., dependency on one route more than another) may predispose the child to toxicity when saturation kinetics are operative for primary routes of elimination (137). Other conjugations with glutathione or amino acids are low in the newborn, as shown for bromsulphthalein (BSP) (131). Acetylation of p-aminobenzoic acid is high in the newborn compared with later in life, but this may be a function of the drug per se since sulfonamide acetylation is low in the newborn (36). A simplified, conceptually useful summary of the development of these various drug biotransformation processes is seen in Figure 29-1.

Drug conjugation and oxidation by liver microsomes in children and adults can be induced by a wide variety of drugs and certain chemicals in foods. The onset and extent of induction are often unpredictable and require reassessment of drug dose when the child is exposed to an inducing agent (e.g., phenobarbital, carbamazepine, phenytoin, rifampin) (84, 97, 98, 103, 119). Enzyme induction per se was first shown for bilirubin conjugation by administration of phenobarbital (22, 141). This was later confirmed and noted for other inducing agents (119). Enzyme induction in the newborn may pose potential risks (133). Enhanced conjugation of salicylamide after phenobarbital treatment of newborn infants demonstrated enzyme induction for exogenous substrates (141). It is important to recognize that enzyme induction may increase the elimination rate of many drugs similar to that found for adults (50). Placental transfer of enzyme inducers can in utero markedly increase the drug metabolic capacity of the newborn [e.g., for diazepam (103)]. A history of prepartum drug administration is important for dose calculation in newborn infants if the elimination or disposition of the drug to be given is governed by biotransformation processes. An often overlooked effect of enzyme induction in children is the increase in plasma levels of active metabolite(s) as shown for carbamazepine epoxide (98, 100).

Maturation of drug biotransformation processes is not limited to the liver. As seen in Table 29-6, plasma esterases important for drug hydrolysis are lower in the infant as compared with the adult.

Maturation of existing nephrons, including tubule elongation, occurs postnatally (77). Renal function in the newborn and young infant is deficient with regard to glomerular filtration rate and tubular secretion (about one-third of the function in the adult), both of which rapidly develop in the first 2-3 weeks of life and then more slowly to about 1 year of age (129). A decrease in renal blood flow and anatomical immaturity compound these excretion deficiencies. Other immature functions contributing to alterations in renal function include base excretion, concentration, and reabsorption ability; the extent of their influence on renal drug elimination in the newborn remains to be assessed completely. Two classes of antibiotics (penicillins and aminoglycosides) frequently used in the neonate depend on active tubular secretion and glomerular filtration for their elimination. Because their rate of elimination is decreased in the neonate (as for the aminoglycosides) a decrease in dose and/or increase in dosing interval must be made to avoid accumulation to toxic levels. As seen in Table 29-7, the half-life of a hypothetical drug is increased as a consequence of immature glomerular filtration and tubular secretion mechanisms (100, 125).

The net effect of an immature renal or metabolic process for the elimination of some drugs can be illustrated by changes in plasma drug half-lives, as summarized in Table 29-8. The utilization of this information for pediatric drug dosing is exemplified by theophylline (7, 30, 40, 100). Marked developmental changes in theophylline half-life are seen in the preschool child. A high plasma clearance of theophylline, with a concomitant decrease in elimination half-life, necessitates frequent dosing if a desired steady-state level is to be achieved without the risk of high, potentially toxic levels soon after a dose is given (Table 29-9). Recognition of this dilemma has led to the development of

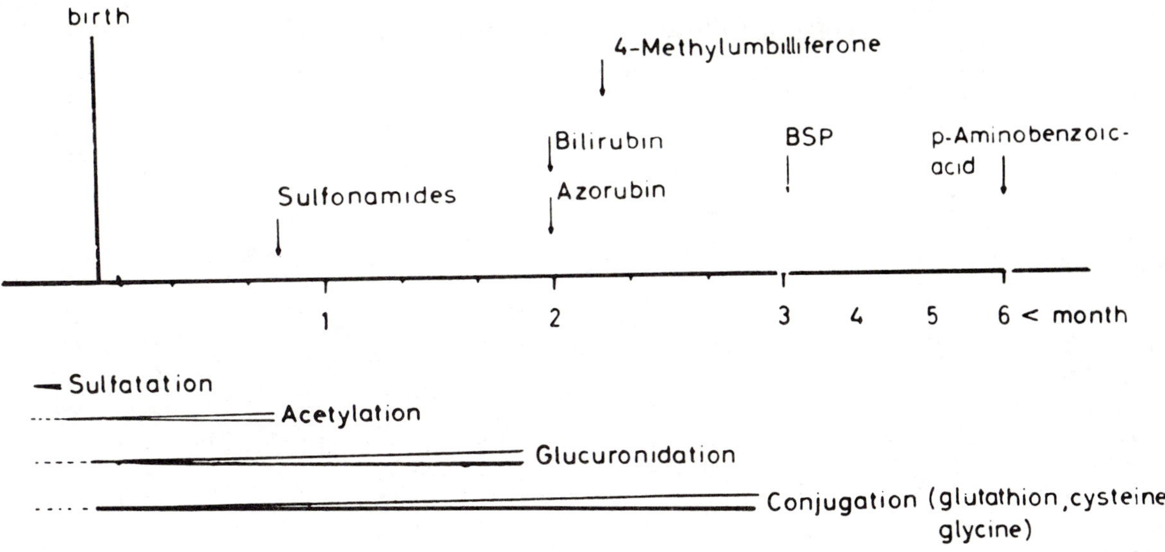

Fig. 29-1. *The sequence of maturation of different metabolic liver functions* (From Ref. 42).

prolonged-release preparations of theophylline for children (7, 127). It is of interest that the half-life of prednisolone, another drug used in pedriatric asthma therapy, is shorter in children as compared with adults (44). A relatively rapid rate of drug elimination is found for many drugs given to prepubertal children. Age-dependent and interindividual variation in the clearance of many drugs emphasizes the need for plasma-level monitoring after about five to seven half-lives have elapsed from the

Table 29-6
Blood or Tissue Enzyme Assays in the Young Child and Adult

Drug	Process	Units	Amount Metabolized per Minute				
			Premature	Term	Infants	Children	Adults
Aspirin	Esterase	nM/ml	8	11	13	14	13
Acetylcholine	Esterase (RBC)	μM/ml	4.6-5.8	5.3	7-9	9-10	10
Butyrylcholine	Esterase (plasma)	μM/ml	0.3-1.1	1.2	2-2.3	2.1-2.5	2.0
Phenylacetate	Arylesterase (plasma)	μM/ml	6.5	8.4	19.5	24.2	27.8
Paroxon	Esterase (plasma)	nM/ml	3.6	3.4		6.1	7.3
Procaine	Esterase (plasma)	nM/ml	1.7	7	8-9	10-11	10

Source: From Ref. 24.

Table 29-7
Calculation of Half-Life for a Proposed Drug with the Same Clearance as Inulin (Glomerular Filtration) or Para-Aminohippuric Acid (Tubular Secretion)[a]

	Weight (kg)	Inulin Clearance (ml/min)	Inulin $t_{1/2}$ (min)	PAH Clearance (ml/min)	PAH $t_{1/2}$ (min)
Infant	4.5	About 10	100	About 25	40
Adult	70	130	67	650	13

[a]The example is shown for an infant (1.5 months old) and an adult. The drug is supposed to distribute in the extracellular water space. $t_{1/2} = 0.693 \times V_d/\text{clearance}$.

Source: From Ref. 100.

Table 29-8
Age Dependency of Plasma Drug Half-Lives [a]

Drugs	Newborn (term-1 month)	Infant (2-12 months)	Child (2-16 years)	Adult
Acetaminophen (24, 84)	2.2-5	—	3.1-4.5	2-3.6
Aminopyrine (84)	30-40	—	—	2-4
Antipyrine (24)	—	—	6.6	12-15
Amobarbital (24, 84)	17-60	—	—	12-27
Ampicillin (24, 27, 54, 117)	0.67-4.9	1.6-2.3	—	1-1.8
BSP (30)	7.7-9.6	6.1-7 min	5.5 min	—
Caffeine (3, 24)	32-149	—	—	4-5
Carbamazepine (24)	8-28	—	14-19	18-55
Carbenicillin (24, 117)	1.5-4.7	1.6	—	1
Cephaloridine (24)	2.1-5.4	1.1	—	1-1.5
Cephalothin (24)	2.4	0.3	0.2-0.3	0.5-0.9
Chloramphenicol (24)	8-15	—	4	2.3
Clindamycin (24)	—	—	1.5-3.4	3.2-4.8
Clonazepam (24, 26, 88)	—	—	22-38	20-60
Diazepem (24, 88)	25-100	—	18	15-42
Diazoxide (24)	—	24	10-19	24-36
Digoxin (24, 88)	26-107	19-25	36-37	31-60
Dipropylacetate (24)	—	—	9.4	15.3
Doxycycline (24)	6.9	3.7	3.2-3.7	12-22
Ethosuximide (15, 24)	—	—	23-68	56
Gentamicin (24, 78, 84 108)	2.3-3.5	1.7-5.4	1-1.6	—
Indomethacin (84)	14-20	—	—	4-11
Kanamycin (24, 27, 78, 117)	1.5-7.5	—	—	2-2.2
Lidocaine (24)	3	—	—	1.2-2.2
Mepivacaine (24)	9	—	—	0.12
Methicillin (25, 117)	0.8-3.3	0.8-0.9	—	0.4
Nalidixic acid (84)	2.4-5.7	—	1.2-2.5	—
Nortriptyline (24, 84, 111)	56	—	—	17-27
Oxacillin (24)	1.2-1.5	1.1	—	0.4-0.7
Penicillin (24)	1.4-9.7	0.9-2.2	—	0.6-0.7
Phenobarbital (24, 48, 53, 84, 93)	40-500	37-133	53-64	53-140
Phenytoin (24, 84, 93)	17-104	—	5	12-29
Phenylbutazone (24, 84)	21-34	17	20-40	12-82
Prednisolone (44)	—	—	84-210 min	175-246 min
Salicylate (24, 84)	4.5-11.5	—	2-3.1	2-4
Sulfamethopyrazine (117)	135-280	53-68	44-50	62-63
Sulfisoxazole (24, 117)	7.8-12.4	7-11	4-5.8	5.7-6
Theophylline (3, 24, 30)	—	—	1.4-7.9	3.5-12
Ticarcillin (89)	5.6	—	0.9	—
Tobramycin (24, 117)	3.9-6.1	—	—	2-2.2
Tolbutamide (24, 84)	10-40	—	—	4.4-9

[a] Adapted from Ref. 24 which has the original citations in addition to those shown. Their data for term—perinatal and "newborn" have been combined under the "newborn" category for this table, because some articles did not give information sufficient to distinguish "newborns" from "neonates" 1-28 days old. Individual values or ranges are used in most cases. The original work should be consulted for details about the statistical variation between subjects and the conditions used for collection of data. Values for $t_{1/2}$ are in hours unless otherwise indicated.

Table 29-9
Pitfalls in Theophylline Dosing As a Function of Differences in Clearance[a]

	$K_{el(\beta)}$ /hr	V_d (ml/kg)	V_{pl} (ml/kg/hr)	Dose (mg)	Interval (hr)	Estimated plasma level (μg/ml) 0 hr	2 hr	4 hr	6 hr	8 hr
Low clearance	0.2	422	84	96	6	9.5	6.37		2.86	
				240	6	23.7	15.88		7.13	
				480	6	47.4	31.77		14.27	
High clearance	0.6	422	253	96	6	9.5	2.86		0.26	
				240	6	23.7	7.13		0.65	
				480	6	47.4	14.27		1.29	
				96	2	9.5	12.36	13.22	13.48	13.56

Assume 6-year-old child, weight 24 kg: $C_o = \text{dose}/V_d$
$C_t = C_oe^{-kt}$ or $C_t = C_oe^{-kt} + (C_ie^{-kt})_i + \ldots (\ )_n$ for multiple dosing.

[a] $K_{el(\beta)}$ = the apparent first-order rate constant for elimination; V_d = apparent volume of distribution; C_o, C_t = concentration at o, t time;
Source: Adopted from Ref. 100.

onset of dosing. More frequent monitoring is required for those drugs that show nonlinear kinetics of elimination or have a narrow therapeutic index.

PHARMACODYNAMICS

Mechanism of Drug Action. A fundamentally similar mechanism of drug action in children as compared with that in adults is usually assumed unless evidence has been accumulated to the contrary. Known exceptions include drug toxicity or adverse effects that result from circumstances peculiar to immaturity, such as stunting of growth from administration of tetracyclines or steroids, tetracycline staining of teeth, bilirubin encephalopathy secondary to a drug interaction at the level of bilirubin-albumin binding, and aspirin hepatotoxicity or metabolic acidosis. Similar mechanism of action in adults and children may prevail for these effects, but the final consequences are determined by the immature status of the organism.

A quantitative and possibly qualitative difference with regard to mechanism of action may exist for digoxin. A wide range exists for digoxin doses, 7.5-12.5 μg/kg, for premature neonates; 15-20 μg/kg for infants; 10-15 μg/kg for children (100). The newborn infant apparently requires a higher weight-adjusted dose as compared with older children or adults to achieve comparable plasma levels. Some infants tolerate high plasma levels of digoxin without toxicity (113, 130), even though it has been shown that plasma levels correlate with higher myocardium levels found in infants (43, 60, 65). Volume of distribution or clearance differences have been postulated to explain digoxin dose requirements for young infants, but a developmental change in cardiac sensitivity, sodium-potassium-dependent adenosine triphosphatase, or other reaction has not been ruled out for the human newborn (49, 70, 100, 113, 120).

The apparent need for higher doses, increased plasma levels, and even a digitalizing dose in newborn infants has been questioned (113). Toxicity manifested by poor feeding, emesis, and ECG changes (AV nodal block and atrial conduction abnormalities in contrast to ventricular arrhythmias in adults) is often overlooked. Serum levels above 3 ng/ml are more frequently associated with toxicity in young infants as compared with levels above 2 ng/ml in adults (113). Both serum level and clinical status must be repeatedly assessed for selection of the appropriate dose until more precise data are available on the pharmacodynamics of digoxin in children.

Receptor or transmitter development contributes to age-dependent differences in drug responses and their mechanisms. α-Adrenoceptors and their response to phenylephrine have been demonstrated in the eye of premature and full-term infants by studying the mydriatic response. Underdevelopment of sympathomimetic amine storage mechanism for prematures, however, was indicated by use of tyramine (75). Enhanced response of newborns to reserpine indicates an increased sensitivity of storage site receptors (87). Infusion of norepinephrine in term newborns resulted in nonshivering thermogenesis. Premature infants apparently have a requirement for higher doses of epinephrine to increase blood pressure. Enhanced myocardial sensitivity to fluorothane has also been found for newborns (79). Relative resistance to succinylcholine (weight-adjusted dose) and sensitivity to tubocurarine have been found for newborns and are indicative of a decreased response to depolarizing drugs in newborns compared with adults (19,90). When doses of succinylcholine were adjusted for body surface area, however, the duration of neuromuscular blockade was similar for most infants as compared with adults (124).

As previously noted, newborn infants and children respond to enzyme-inducing agents. The quantitative response may be larger in those young infants who have low levels of a given enzyme, especially that contained in the hepatic microsomal mixed-function oxidase system.

Biological responses of prednisolone have been correlated with its dose and pharmacokinetics (44). Single doses (0.5 mg/kg or greater) of prednisolone inhibited somatomedin activity and cell-mediated immunity. Peak plasma levels greater than 19 μg/dl were associated with a 73% and 96% effect on these biological factors, respectively. These factors are conceivably related to the adverse effects and efficacy of this drug, so that such plasma level correlates will enable pharmacodynamic assessment of clinical effect.

A shift to the right in phenobarbital plasma levels was seen with regard to lowering of serum bilirubin concentration (123). A relationship between phenobarbital exposure time and decrease in serum bilirubin was apparent and indicative of enzyme induction as a mechanism for lowering serum bilirubin levels (11, 114). These data are of interest even though phenobarbital is not a drug of choice for hyperbilirubinemia of the newborn (133).

The net effect of furosemide to promote fluid and electrolyte loss has recently been substantiated for the newborn (102), and efficacy demonstrated (31). Duration of action (6 hr) correlated with the observed half-life (7.7 hr), which was about eightfold that of the adult (2). Antagonism by indomethacin suggests that prostaglandin E is involved in the mechanism of action of furosemide (37).

Efficacy and Tolerance. The apparent age-dependent increase in tolerance (and possible decreased response) to digoxin in the young infant has been discussed. Improvement in pulmonary function (forced expiratory volume in the first second) by theophylline is seen in adults and children with plasma levels of 10-20 μg/ml. Risk of toxicity and little improvement in efficacy are expected when plasma levels of theophylline exceed 20 μg/ml (100). Specific clinical toxicity in premature infants with inadvertent high theophylline plasma levels needs to be studied in order to define tolerance (3, 67).

Longitudinal changes in airway resistance following salbutamol administration were found in children 7 months to 3.5 years of age, significant changes in resistance not being detected until 2 years of age (68). Asthmatic children 5-14 years old showed a dose- and time-course-dependent response to terbutaline, a β_2-adrenergic amine. An improvement in maximum midexpiratory flow rate was found for doses of 50-140 μg/kg, whereas a dose of 100 μg/kg seemed to be the most efficient dose with a maximal effect at 180 min (4).

A dose and plasma-level relationship as well as an age-dependent response has been described for some anticonvulsants. Adult plasma level-efficacy relationships are frequently used in the absence of data for children (36, 100). Effective plasma level of phenytoin for control of epilepsy in the majority of children was found to be above 5 μg/ml and below 20 μg/ml. However, toxicity has been demonstrated over a wide range (13.8-40 μg/ml) of plasma levels at dosages ranging from 5.6 to 9.5 mg/kg/day; toxicity was common at plasma levels exceeding 20 μg/ml (Figure 29-2). A wide range of plasma levels was seen for ethosuximide when used to control absence seizures; about 93% of the controlled patients had plasma levels of 40 μg/ml (15, 104). Use of plasma-level information for efficacy purposes requires knowledge of drug binding and also of relationship of free-drug fraction to total drug. The free (unbound) plasma concentration of drug is responsible for efficacy as well as toxicity (10), and disease or other drugs can change the free fraction of drug. Meaningful plasma level-dose correlates are obtained when midpoint, or preferably nadir, measurements are made under steady-state conditions. Age *per se* is known to increase the plasma level dose ratio for some drugs (e.g., phenobarbital, carbamazepine, valproic acid) (86). This plasma level/dose ratio may be influenced by other drugs, environmental factors, and renal or hepatic diseases. Compliance is an additional caveat to be considered when dose alterations are made on the basis of such data. Active metabolites also influence the interpretation of an "effective" plasma level. Thus, consideration should be given to the serum concentrations of active metabolites like phenobarbital and phenylethylmalonamide (PEMA) for primidone (35), dimethadione for trimethadione (9), and carbamazepine-10-11-epoxide for carbamazepine (98). Given these considerations, it is more appropriate, where possible, to depict "accepted therapeutic" plasma levels in relation to a weight-adjusted dose for certain age-defined groups of children who are also characterized with regard to single- or combined-drug treatment.

It is apparent that the literature on pediatric clinical pharmacology is largely replete with drug disposition data for children. Of equal importance and meaning for therapeutics are data on

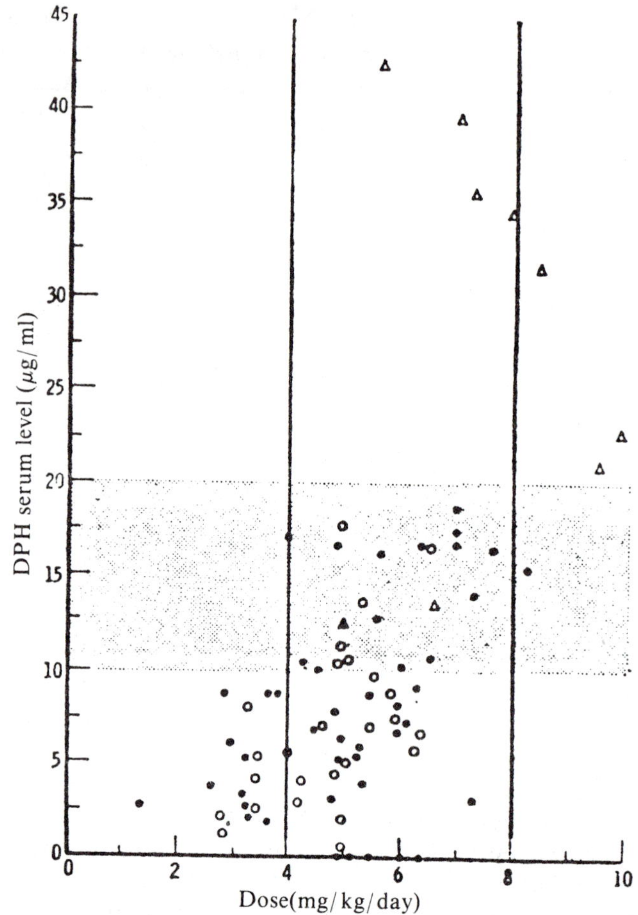

Fig. 29-2. *Diphenylhydantoin (DPH): efficacy, toxicity, and dose-serum level relationships in children.*

DPH dosage (mg/kg/day) plotted against serum levels (*μg/ml*): O, clinically controlled; •, uncontrolled epilepsy; △, patients with signs of drug toxicity. Shaded area indicates levels usually considered safe and clinically effective (From Ref. 12).

pharmacokinetic-clinical effect correlates (i.e., pharmacodynamics); the final link needed for accurate dose estimates. Efficacy data, some in relation to dose and drug disposition, are being obtained more frequently in children, as illustrated by recent investigations summarized in Table 29-10. Aspirin, a drug used for over half a century for the treatment of arthritis, has recently been evaluated for efficacy-disposition correlates. Interindividual variation in response was minimized by adjustment of salicylate plasma levels to an acceptable range for children with juvenile rheumatoid arthritis (6).

ADVERSE EFFECTS

Physical and Biochemical Effects. Most unwanted effects peculiar to pediatric pharmacotherapy are a result of immaturity or a childhood disease that predisposes to drug risks. An example that encompasses both is the jaundiced infant with sepsis. Hyperbilirubinemia results from an immature bilirubin conjugation system in the liver. Sepsis, often accompanied by acidosis, requires antimicrobial therapy. Treatment of premature infants with a sulfonamide produced a higher incidence of bili-

Table 29-10
Efficacy of Some Drugs in Children's Diseases As Shown in Recent Studies

Drug	Condition
Propranolol	Cardiac dysrhythmias, idiopathic hypertrophic subaortic stenosis, paroxysmal hypoxemic episodes associated with ventricular infundibular stenosis (41), hypertension (45)
Methylprednisolone	Status asthmaticus (47)
Phenobarbital	Febrile seizures (96), familial cholestasis (30)
Methylphenidate	Hyperkinesis (69, 107)
Lithium	Behavioral disorder (hostility, aggressiveness, manic excitement) (23)
Dopamine	Shock (28)
Minoxidil	Hypertension (110)
Diazepam	Tetanus (59)
Imipramine	Enuresis (59)
Beclomethasone dipropionate aerosol	Asthma (62)
Furosemide	Salt and water retention (31)
Nitroprusside	Hypertension with normal renal function (76)
Salbutamol	Asthma (68)
Theophylline	Apnea of prematurity (3, 67, 95)

rubin encephalopathy (109). Another example is the high concentration of tetracycline in bones and decidual teeth of the child given tetracycline prior to 7 years of age, with consequent adverse effects (63). These or other associated effects could be more prevalent in children with cystic fibrosis because of the frequent and long-term administration of antimicrobial agents. On a more positive note, a limited follow-up study of aminoglycoside therapy in neonates revealed no substantial ototoxicity.

A list of selected childhood diseases, drugs administered, and the associated adverse or toxic effects, is given in Table 29-11.

Psychological Effects. Impairment of psychosocial and intellectual development secondary to drugs is difficult to substantiate. Only recently have investigations been undertaken in this area, as stimulated by the prolonged effects of narcotic withdrawal in the neonate and from studies of maternal-infant bonding. The anesthetics and analgesics used during delivery have been shown to adversely affect psychophysiological functioning in the newborn; effects were seen for 1 month, with coping ability affected most severely (13). Sucking behavior also is abnormal in infants of addicted mothers (66). Coppolillo (21) has recently reviewed the long-term psychiatric implications of drug impediments to mothering behavior, including relationships to child abuse, materialistic orientations, and barriers to mother-child cross-stimulation.

DISEASE EFFECTS

The effects of childhood disease on drug disposition and action appear to be fundamentally similar to those found for certain categorical diseases (e.g., liver, renal) in adults. The reader is referred to studies with adults as summarized by Benet (8) and by Tillement et al (116). Childhood diseases such as systemic lupus erythematosus prolonged the half-life of prednisolone (44), whereas renal clearance of dicloxacillin was increased in children with cystic fibrosis (55). Acetaminophen clearance is decreased in those children with Gilbert's syndrome (25). Renal disease decreases the clearance of many drugs, notably the aminoglycoside antibiotics. A nomogram for adjustment of gentamicin half-life according to the creatinine clearance has been developed for children (142); however, its utility remains to be prospectively evaluated in a large population of children. Use of this and other nomograms (5) can facilitate dosing and interval adjustments to avoid drug toxicity, if disease effects on nomogram relationships are considered. Hypoalbuminemia associated with nephrotic syndrome can produce a significant increase in the free fraction of highly bound drugs (116). Enhanced toxicity related to low serum albumin has been shown for diazepam, phenytoin, and prednisolone (46).

DRUG INTERACTIONS

A carefully compiled list of drug interactions (5), as well as a review of pharmacokinetic approaches (72), has been published. Differences of a quantitative nature from those interactions described for adults are expected for the newborn who shows a decreased plasma protein binding for many drugs (Table 29-5) and a decrease in oxidative and conjugation activity with consequent decrease in their clearance (Table 29-8). The latter may exaggerate a drug interaction that occurs through competitive metabolic mechanisms. Dependence on one biotransformation pathway (e.g., sulfation) may enhance risks from administration of two drugs that utilize the same pathway.

An enzyme-inducing interaction has been demonstrated for phenytoin, phenobarbital, and carbamazepine given to children (36, 100). Premature and full-term newborns show an induction of diazepam metabolism such that an elimination half-life similar to older children is seen (Table 29-12) (103). An interesting age-specific interaction has been found for furosemide and indomethacin (34). Furosemide increased prostaglandin E excretion whereas indomethacin decreased it in infants with patent ductus arteriosus. Thus, furosemide may be less effective when used in customary doses in those receiving indomethacin.

Table 29-11
Drug Toxicity and Adverse Effects Found in Children

Drug	Effect
Hereditary conditions (21)	
Sulfonamides, primaquine, nitrofuran derivatives, acetophenetidin, chloramphenicol	Hemolysis in those with an erythrocyte enzyme deficiency
Sulfonamides, acetanilid, nitrites, amines	Methemoglobinemia in those with erythrocyte diaphorase deficiency
Sulfonamides, nitrites, primaquine	Hemolysis in those with hemoglobin variants (H and Zurich)
Salicylates, menthol, tetrahydrocortisone	Prolonged elimination by glucuronide conjugation in those with Crigler-Najjar syndrome
Allopurinol, azathioprine, 6-mercaptopurine, 8-azaguanine	Active drug metabolites not formed in those with Lesch-Nyhan syndrome
Barbiturates	Crisis in hepatic porphyria
Warfarin, dicumarol	Decreased effectiveness in those with genetic predisposition to a need for a higher dose
Digitalis	Decreased cardiac output in those with muscular subaortic stenosis
Norepinephrine, intradermal histamine	Respective increase in pressor response and lack of a flare response in those with familial dysautonomia
Atropine	Increased response in those with mongolism
General anesthetics and succinylcholine	Hyperpyrexia, acidosis, muscle rigidity in those with malignant hyperpyrexia
Isoniazid (14, 122)	Behavioral deterioration, irritability, hyperkinesis and sleep difficulties in child with probable block in kynurenine pathway of tryptophan metabolism
	Hepatotoxicity in a child with rapid acetylator phenotype
Inadvertant dosing in utero (83)	
Analgesics, barbiturates	Neonatal depression
Salicylates, barbiturates, phenytoin	Coagulation defects in the newborn
Local anesthetics	Bradycardia and neonatal depression
Propylthiouracil, carbimazole	Goiter
Coumarin (oral anticoagulants)	Neonatal hemorrhage
Tetracyclines	Discoloration of teeth
β-Adrenoceptor blockers	Neonatal depression and bradycardia
Reserpine	Nasal stuffiness, lethargy
Magnesium sulfate	Neuromuscular weakness, lethargy
Ethanol	Floppy infant, withdrawal symptoms (121)
Administration as a result of therapeutic indication	
Barbiturates	Drug metabolism increased
Benzodiazepine	Neonatal depression (59)
Aminoglycosides	Ototoxicity (33)
Tetracyclines	Tooth discoloration and delayed bone growth
Chloramphenicol	Cardiovascular collapse
Sulfonamides	Kernicterus in newborn
Hexachlorophene	CNS toxicity (118)
Hydroxyzine	Caused wheezing in a child with asthma (80)
Phenobarbital	Behavior disorder in children with febrile seizures (16, 64, 140)
Phenytoin	Exanthema related to body burden of the drug soon after onset of therapy
Acetaminophen	Hepatic necrosis after high single or repeated dose (91, 134)
Aspirin	Hepatotoxicity (101)

In general, the type, mechanism, and locus of drug interactions are similar for adults and children. In the absence of data, however, extrapolations from adult information must be cautiously applied to those drugs used frequently in combination for treatment of childhood disease.

Table 29-12
Drug Interaction: Induction of Diazepam Metabolism by Barbiturates

Age Group	Type of Treatment	Apparent Half-Life (hr)
Newborns		
Premature	a	75 ± 35
	b	11
Full term	a	31 ± 2
	b	18 ± 1
Infants	a	10 ± 2
Children	a	17 ± 3

a = no exposure to barbiturates; single dose of diazepam either directly to the child or to the mother.
b = previous exposure to barbiturates either during intrauterine life or during first days of extrauterine life.

Source: From Ref. 85.

REFERENCES

1. Alam, S.N., Roberts, R.J., and Fischer, L.J. Age-related differences in salicylamide and acetaminophen conjugation in man. *J. Pediatr.* 90:130, 1977.
2. Aranda, J.V., Perez, J., Sitar, D.S. et al. Pharmacokinetic disposition and protein binding of furosemide in newborn infants. *J. Pediatr.* 90:507, 1978.
3. Aranda, J.V., Sitar, D.S., Parsons, W.D., Loughnan, P.M., and Neims, A.H. Pharmacokinetic aspects of theophylline in premature newborns. *N. Engl. J. Med.* 295:413, 1976.
4. Ardal, B., Beaudry, P., and Eisen, A.H. Terbutaline in asthmatic children: A dose-response study. *J. Pediatr.* 93:305, 1978.
5. Avery, G.S. *Drug Treatment.* Sydney: ADIS Press, 1976.
6. Bardare, M., Cislaghi, G.U., Mandelli, M., and Sereni, F. Value of monitoring plasma salicylate levels in treating juvenile rheumatoid arthritis. *Arch. Dis. Childhood* 53:381, 1978.
7. Bell, T., and Bigley, J. Sustained-release theophylline therapy for chronic childhood asthma. *Pediatrics* 62:352, 1978.
8. Benet, L.Z. (ed.). *The Effect of Disease States on Drug Pharmacokinetics.* Washington, D.C.: American Pharmaceutical Association and Academy of Pharmaceutical Sciences, 1976.
9. Booker, H.E. Trimethadione and other oxazolidinediones: Relation of plasma levels to clinical control. In: *Antiepileptic Drugs* (Woodbury, D.M., Penry, J.K., and Schmidt, R.P., eds.). New York: Raven Press, 1972, p. 403.
10. Booker, H.E., and Darcey, B. Serum concentrations of free diphenylhydantoin and their relationship to clinical intoxication. *Epilepsia* (Amst.) 14:177, 1973.
11. Boreus, L.O., Jalling, B., and Wallin, A. Plasma concentrations of phenobarbital in mother and child after combined prenatal and postnatal administration for prophylaxis of hyperbilirubinemia. *J. Pediatr.* 93:695, 1978.
12. Borofsky, L.G., Louis, S., Kutt, H., and Roginsky, M. Diphenylhydantoin: Efficacy, toxicity, and dose-serum level relationships in children. *J. Pediatr.* 81:995, 1972.
13. Brackbill, Y. Psychophysiological measures of pharmacological toxicity in infants: Perinatal and postnatal effect. In: *Basic and Therapeutic Aspects of Perinatal Pharmacology* (Morselli, P.L., et al., eds.). New York: Raven Press, 1975, p. 21.
14. Brenner, A., and Wapnir, R.A. A pyridoxine-dependent behavioral disorder unmasked by isoniazid. *Am. J. Dis. Child.* 132:773, 1978.
15. Browne, T.R., Dreifuss, F.E. et al. Ethosuximide in the treatment of absence (petit mal) seizures. *Neurology* 25:515, 1975.
16. Buchtal, F., and Lennox-Buchtal, M.A. Phenobarbital: Relation of serum concentration to control of seizures. In: *Antiepileptic Drugs* (Woodbury, D.M., Penry, J.K., and Schmidt, R.P., eds.). New York: Raven Press, 1972, p. 335.
17. Cheek, D.B. Extracellular volume: Its structure and measurement and the influence of age and disease. *J. Pediatr.* 58:103, 1961.
18. Chignell, C.F., Vesell, E.S., Starkweather, D.K., and Berlin, C.M. The binding of sulfaphenazole to fetal, neonatal, and adult human plasma albumin. *Clin. Pharmacol. Ther.* 12:897, 1971.
19. Churchill-Davidson, H.C., and Wise, R.P. Neuromuscular transmission in the newborn infant. *Anesthesiology* 24:271, 1963.
20. Cohen, S.N., and Weber, W.W. Pharmacogenetics. *Pediatr. Clin. North Am.* 19:21, 1972.
21. Coppolillo, H.P. Drug impediments to mothering behavior. *Addictive Dis.* 2:201, 1975.
22. Crigler, J., and Gold, N.I. Sodium phenobarbital-induced decrease in serum bilirubin in an infant with congenital nonhemolytic jaundice and kernicterus. *J. Clin. Invest.* 45:998, 1966.
23. DeLong, G.R. Lithium carbonate treatment of select behavior disorders in children suggesting manic-depressive illness. *J. Pediatr.* 93:689, 1978.
24. Done, A.K., Cohen, S.N., and Strebel, L. Pediatric clinical pharmacology and the therapeutic orphan. *Ann. Rev. Pharmacol. Toxicol.* 17:564, 1977.
25. Douglas, A.P., Savage, R.L., and Rawlins, M.D. Paracetamol (acetaminophen) kinetics in patients with Gilbert's syndrome. *Eur. J. Clin. Pharmacol.* 13:209, 1978.
26. Dreifuss, F.E., Penry, J.K. et al. Serum clonazepam concentrations in children with absence seizures. *Neurology* 25:255, 1975.
27. Driessen, O.M.J., Sorgedrager, N., Michel, M.F. et al. Pharmacokinetic aspects of therapy with ampicillin and kanamycin in newborn infants. *Eur. J. Clin. Pharmacol.* 13:449, 1978.
28. Driscoll, D.J., Gillette, P.C. et al. The use of dopamine in children. *J. Pediatr.* 92:309, 1978.
29. Ehrnebo, M., Agurell, S. et al. Age differences in drug binding by plasma proteins: Studies on human foetuses, neonates, and adults. *Eur. J. Clin. Pharmacol.* 3:189, 1971.
30. Ellis, E.F., Koysooko, R., and Levy, G. Pharmacokinetics of theophylline in children with asthma. *Pediatrics* 58:542, 1976.
31. Engle, M.A., Leury, J.E. et al. The use of furosemide in the treatment of edema in infants and children. *Pediatrics* 62:811, 1978.
32. Fichter, E.G., and Curtis, J.A. Sulfonamide administration in newborn and premature infants. *AMA Am. J. Dis. Child* 90:596, 1955.
33. Finitzo-Hieber, T., McCracken, G.H., Jr., Roeser, R.J. et al. Ototoxicity in neonates treated with gentamicin and kanamycin: Results of a four-year controlled follow-up study. *Pediatrics* 63:443, 1979.
34. Friedman, Z., Demers, L.M. et al. Urinary excretion of prostaglandin E following the administration of furosemide and indomethacin to sick low-birth-weight infants. *J. Pediatr.* 93:512, 1978.
35. Gallagher, B.B., and Baumel, I.P. Primidone: Biotransformation. In: *Antiepileptic Drugs* (Woodbury, D.M., Penry, J.K., and Schmidt, R.P., eds.). New York: Raven Press, 1972, p. 361.
36. Garrettson, L.K. Pharmacology of anticonvulsants. *Pediatr. Clin. North Am.* 19:179, 1972.
37. Garrettson, L.K., and Jusko, W.J. Diphenylhydantoin kinetics in overdosed children. *Clin. Pharmacol. Ther.* 17: 481, 1975.
38. Garrettson, L.K., and Kim, O.K. Apparent saturation of diphenylhydantoin metabolism in children. *Pediatr. Res.* 4:455, 1970.

39. Ghent, C.N., Bloomer, J.R., and Hsia, Y.E. Efficacy and safety of long-term phenobarbital therapy of familial cholestasis. *J. Pediatr.* 93:127, 1978.

40. Ginchansky, E., and Weinberger, M. Relationship of theophylline clearance to oral doses in children with chronic asthma. *J. Pediatr.* 91:655, 1977.

41. Gitlin, D., and Boesman, M. Serum alpha -fetoprotein, albumin, and gamma G-globulin in the human conceptus. *J. Clin. Invest.* 45:1826, 1966.

42. Gladtke, E., and Heimann, G. The rate of development of elimination functions in kidney and liver of young infants. In: *Basic and Therapeutic Aspects of Perinatal Pharmacology* (Morselli, P.L. et al., eds.). New York: Raven Press, 1975, p. 393.

43. Gorodischer, R., Jusko, W.J., and Yaffe, S.J. Tissue and erythrocyte distribution of digoxin in infants. *Clin. Pharmacol. Ther.* 19:256, 1976.

44. Green, O.C., Winter, R.J. et al. Pharmacokinetic studies of prednisolone in children. *J. Pediatr.* 93:299, 1978.

45. Griswold, W.R., McNeal, R., Mendoza, S.A., Sellers, B.B., and Higgins, S. Propranolol as an antihypertensive agent in children. *Arch. Dis. Child.* 53:594, 1978.

46. Gugler, R., and Azarnoff, D.L. Drug protein binding and the nephrotic syndrome. *Clin. Pharmacokinet.* 1:25, 1976.

47. Harfi, H., Hanissian, A.S. et al. Treatment of status asthmaticus in children with high doses and conventional doses of methylprednisolone. *Pediatrics* 61:829, 1978.

48. Heinze, E., and Kampffmeyer, H. Biological half-life of phenobarbital in human babies. *Klin. Wocherschr.* 49:1146, 1971.

49. Hernandez, A., Kouchoukos, N., Burton, R.M., and Golding, D. The effect of extracorporeal circulation upon the tissue concentration of digoxin H. *Pediatrics* 31:952, 1968.

50. Hoppel, C., Rane, A., and Sjoqvist, F. Kinetics of phenytoin and carbamazepine in the newborn. In: *Basic and Therapeutic Aspects of Perinatal Pharmacology* (Morselli, P.L. et al., eds.). New York: Raven Press, 1975, p. 341.

51. Huang, N.N., and High, R.H. Comparison of serum levels following the administration of oral and parenteral preparations of penicillin to infants and children of various age groups. *J. Pediatr.* 42:657, 1953.

52. Hyvarinen, M., Zelter, P., Oh, W. et al. Influence of gestational age on serum levels of α-l-fetoprotein, IgG globulin, and albumin in newborn infants. *J. Pediatr.* 82:430, 1973.

53. Jalling, B. Plasma and cerebrospinal fluid concentrations of phenobarbital in infants given single doses. *Dev. Med. Child. Neurol.* 16:781, 1974.

54. Jusko, W.J. Pharmacokinetic principles in pediatric pharmacology. *Pediatr. Clin. North Am.* 19:81, 1972.

55. Jusko, W.J., Mosovich, L.L., Gerbracht, L.M., Matter, M.E., and Yaffe, S.J. Enhanced renal excretion of dicloxacillin in patients with cystic fibrosis. *Pediatrics* 56:1038, 1975.

56. Kandall, S.R., Thaler, M.M., and Erickson, R.P. Intestinal development of lysosomal and microsomal beta glucuronidase and bilirubin uridine diphosphoglucuronyl transferase in normal and jaundiced rats. *J. Pediatr.* 82:1013, 1973.

57. Karlberg, P., Moore, R.E., and Oliver, T.K., Jr. Thermogenic and cardiovascular responses of the newborn baby to noradrenaline. *Acta Pediatr. Scand.* 54:225, 1965.

58. Keen, P. Effect of building to plasma proteins on the distribution, activity, and elimination of drugs. In: *Handbook of Pharmacology*, Vol. 28 (Brodie, B.B., and Gillette, J.R., eds.). Berlin: Springer, 1971, p. 213.

59. Khoo, B.H., Lee, E.L., and Lam, K.L. Neonatal tetanus treated with high dosage diazepam. *Arch Dis. Child.* 53:737, 1978.

60. Kim, P.W., Yanagi, R., Krasula, R.W., Soyka, L.F. et al. Postmortem tissue digoxin concentration in infants and children. *Circulation* 52:1128, 1975.

61. Kiosz, D., Simon, C., and Malerczyk, V. Die plasmaeiweibbindung von clindamycin, cephazolin and cephradin bei neugeborenen and erwachsenen. *Klin. Padiatrie* 187:71, 1975.

62. Klein, R., Waldman, D. et al. Treatment of chronic childhood asthma with beclomethasone dipropionate aerosol: A double-blind crossover trial in non-steroid dependent patients. *Pediatrics* 60:7, 1977.

63. Kline, A.H., Blattner, R.J., and Lunin, M. Transplacental effect of tetracyclines on teeth. *JAMA* 188:178, 1964.

64. Knudsen, F.U., and Vestermark, S. Prophylactic diazepam or phenobarbitone in febrile convulsions: A prospective, controlled study. *Arch. Dis. Child.* 53:660, 1978.

65. Krasula, R.W., Hastreiter, A.R., Levitsky, S. et al. Serum, atrial, and urinary digoxin levels during cardiopulmonary bypass in children. *Circulation* 49:1047, 1974.

66. Kron, R.E., Finnegan, L.P. et al. The assessment of behavioral change in infants undergoing narcotic withdrawal: Comparative data from clinical and objective methods. *Addictive Dis.* 2:257, 1975.

67. Latini, R., Assael, B.M. et al. Kinetics and efficacy of theophylline in the treatment of apnea in the premature newborn. *Eur. J. Clin. Pharmacol.* 13:203, 1978.

68. Lenney, W., and Milner, A.D. At what age do bronchodilator drugs work? *Arch. Dis. Child.* 53:532, 1978.

69. Lerer, R.J., Lerer, M.P., and Artner, J. The effects of methylphenidate on the handwriting of children with minimal brain dysfunction. *J. Pediatr.* 91:127, 1977.

70. Levy, A.M., Leaman, D.M., and Henson, J.S. Effects of digoxin on systolic time intervals of neonates and infants. *Circulation* 46:816, 1972.

71. Levy, G. Salicylate pharmacokinetics in the human neonate. In: *Basic and Therapeutic Aspects of Perinatal Pharmacology* (Morselli, P.L. et al., eds.). New York: Raven Press, 1975, p. 319.

72. Levy, G. Pharmacokinetic approaches to the study of drug interactions. *Ann. N.Y. Acad. Sci.* 281:24, 1976.

73. Levy, G., Khanna, N.N., Soda, D.M., Tsuzuki, O., and Stern, L. Pharmacokinetics of acetaminophen in the human neonate: Formation of acetaminophen glucuronide and sulfate in relation to plasma bilirubin concentration and d-glucaric acid excretion. *Pediatrics* 55:818, 1975.

74. Levy, G., and Yaffee, S.J. The study of salicylate pharmacokinetics in intoxicated infants and children. *Clin. Toxicol.* 1:409, 1968.

75. Lind, N., Shinebourne, E., Turner, P., and Cottom, D. Adrenergic neurone and receptor activity in the iris of the neonate. *Pediatrics* 47:105, 1971.

76. Luderer, J.R., Hayes, A.H. et al. Long-term administration of sodium nitroprusside in childhood. *J. Pediatr.* 91:490, 1977.

77. MacDonald, M.S., and Emery, J.L. The late intrauterine and postnatal development of human renal glomeruli. *J. Anat.* 93:331, 1959.

78 McCracken, G.H., Threlkeld, N. et al. Intravenous administration of kanamycin and gentamicin in newborn infants. *Pediatrics* 60:463, 1977.

79. Marini, A., Zuccoli, G. et al. Farmaci ed apparato cardiovascolare nel neonato II anestetici volatili. *Minerva Pediatr.* (Suppl.) 16:1056, 1964.

80. Massoud, N. Hypersensitivity to vistaril in a child with asthma. *J. Pediatr.* 93:308, 1978.

81. Miller, R.P., Roberts, R.J., and Fischer, L.F. Acetaminophen elimination kinetics in neonates, children, and adults. *Clin. Pharmacol. Ther.* 19:284, 1976.

82. Mirkin, B.L. Diphenylhydantoin: Placental transport, fetal localization, neonatal metabolism, and possible teratogenic effects. *J. Pediatr.* 78:329, 1971.

83. Mirkin, B.L. Pharmacodynamics and drug disposition in pregnant women, in neonates, and in children. In: *Clinical Pharmacology*, 2nd ed. (Melmon, K.L., and Morrelli, H.F., eds.). New York: Macmillan, 1978, p. 127.

84. Morselli, P.L. Clinical pharmacokinetics in neonates. *Clin.*

Pharmacokinet. 1:81, 1976.

85. Morselli, P.L. Antiepileptic drugs. In: *Drug Disposition During Development* (Morselli, P.L., ed.). New York: Spectrum, 1977.

86. Morselli, P.L. Psychotropic drugs. In: *Drug Disposition During Development* (Morselli, P.L., ed.). New York: Spectrum, 1977.

87. Mueller, R.A., and Shideman, F.E. A comparison of the absorption, distribution, and metabolism of reserpine in infant and adult rats. *J. Pharmacol. Exp. Ther.* 163:91, 1968.

88. Nalstoff, J., Lund, M., and Larsen, N.E. Assay and pharmacokinetics of clonazepam in humans. *Acta Neurol. Scand.* (Suppl.) 53:49, 1973.

89. Nelson, J.D., Kusmiesz, H. et al. Clinical pharmacology and efficacy of ticarcillin in infants and children. *Pediatrics* 61:853, 1978.

90. Nightingale, D.A., Glass, A.G. et al. Neuromuscular blockade by succinylcholine in children. *Anesthesiology* 27:736, 1966.

91. Nogen, A.G., and Bommer, J.E. Fatal acetaminophen overdosage in a young child. *J. Pediatr.* 92:832, 1978.

92. O'Donoghue, L.E.J. Distribution of pethidine and chlorpromazine in maternal, foetal, and neonatal biological fluids. *Nature* 229:124, 1971.

93. Painter, M.J., MacDonald, H. et al. Phenobarbital and diphenylhydantoin levels in neonates with seizures. *J. Pediatr.* 92:315, 1978.

94. Parsons, R.L. Drug absorption in gastrointestinal disease with particular reference to malabsorption syndromes. *Clin. Pharmacokinet.* 2:45, 1977.

95. Peabody, J.L., Neese, A.L. et al. Transcutaneous oxygen monitoring in aminophylline treated apneic infants. *Pediatrics* 62:698, 1978.

96. Pollack, M.A. Continuous phenobarbital treatment after a 'simple febrile convulsion'. *Am. J. Dis. Child.* 132:87, 1978.

97. Rane, A., Bertilsson, L., and Palmer, L. Disposition of placentally transferred carbamazepine (Tegretol) in the newborn. *Eur. J. Clin. Pharmacol.* 8:283, 1975.

98. Rane, A., Hojer, B., and Wilson, J.T. Kinetics of carbamazepine and its 10,11 epoxide metabolite in children. *Clin. Pharmacol. Ther.* 19:276, 1976.

99. Rane, A., Lunde, K.M. et al. Plasma protein binding of diphenylhydantoin in normal and hyperbilirubinemic infants. *Pediatr. Pharm. Ther.* 78:877, 1971.

100. Rane, A., and Wilson, J.R. Clinical pharmacokinetics in infants and children. *Clin. Pharmacokinet.* 1:2, 1976.

101. Rich, R.R., and Johnson, J.S., Salicylate hepatotoxicity in patients with juvenile rheumatoid arthritis. *Arthrit. Rheumat.* 16:1, 1973.

102. Ross, B.S., Pollak, A.,and Oh, W. The pharmacologic effects of furosemide therapy in the low-birth-weight infant. *J. Pediatr.* 92:149, 1978.

103. Sereni, F., Mandelli, M., Principi, N. et al. Induction of drug metabolizing enzyme activities in the human fetus and in the newborn infant. *Enzyme* 15:318, 1973.

104. Sherwin, A.L., and Robb, J.P. Ethosuximide: Relation of plasma levels to clinical control. In: *Antiepileptic Drugs* (Woodbury, D.M. et al., eds.). New York: Raven Press, 1972, p. 443.

105. Shirkey, H.C. (ed.). *Pediatric Therapy,* 5th ed. St. Louis: C.V. Mosby, 1975.

106. Shirkey, H.C. Editorial comment: Therapeutic orphans. *J. Pediatr.* 72:119, 1968.

107. Shouse, M.N., and Lubar, J.F. Physiological basis of hyperkinesis treated with methylphenidate. *Pediatrics* 62:343, 1978.

108. Siber, G.R., Smith, A.L., and Levin, M.J. Predictability of peak serum gentamicin concentration with dosage based on body surface area. *J. Pediatr.* 94:135, 1979.

109. Silverman, W.A., Anderson, D.H., Blanc, W.A., and Crozier, D.N. A difference in mortality rate and incidence of kernicterus among premature infants allotted to two prophylactic antibacterial regimens. *Pediatrics* 18:614, 1956.

110. Sinaiko, A.R., and Mirkin, B.L. Management of severe childhood hypertension with minoxidil: A controlled clinical study. *J. Pediatr.* 91:138, 1977.

111. Sjoqvist, F., Bergfors, P.G., Borga, O., Lind, M., and Ygge, H. Plasma disappearance of nortriptyline in a newborn infant following placental transfer from an intoxicated mother: Evidence for drug metabolism. *J. Pediatr.* 80:496, 1972.

112. Soyka, L.F. Isolation and characterization of reduced nicotinamide adenine dinucleotide phosphate: Ferri cytochrome c oxidoreductase and identification of cytochrome b5 in the liver of human infants. *Biochem. Pharmacol.* 19:945, 1970.

113. Soyka, L.F. Digoxin: Placental transfer, effects on the fetus, and therapeutic use in the newborn. In: *Clinics in Perinatology*, Vol. 2 (1) (Yaffe, S.J., ed.). Philadelphia: W.B. Saunders, 1975, p. 23.

114. Stern, L., Khanna, N.N. et al. Effect of phenobarbital on hyperbilirubinemia and glucuronide formation in newborns. *Am. J. Dis. Child.* 120:26, 1970.

115. Svensmark, O., and Buchtal, F. Diphenylhydantoin and phenobarbital: Serum levels in children. *Am. J. Dis. Child.* 108:82, 1964.

116. Tillement, J.P., Lhoste, F., and Giudicelli, J.F. Diseases and drug protein binding. *Clin. Pharmacokinet.* 3:144, 1978.

117. Tognoni, G. Antibiotics. In: *Drug Disposition During Development* (Morselli, P.L., ed.). New York: Spectrum, 1977, p. 123.

118. Tyrala, E.E., Hillman, L.S. et al. Clinical pharmacology of hexachlorophene in newborn infants. *J. Pediatr.* 91:481, 1977.

119. Vaisman, S.L., and Gartner, L.M. Pharmacologic treatment of neonatal hyperbilirubinemia. In: *Clinics in Perinatology,* Vol. 2(1) (Yaffe, S.J., ed.). Philadelphia: W.B. Saunders, 1975, p. 37.

120. Vargo, T., Lewis, R., Burdine, J., and Schwartz, A. Comparison between puppies and adult dogs following infusion of digoxin. *Pediatr. Res.* 8:355, 1974.

121. Vogelstein, B., Kowarski, A.A., and Lietman, P.S. The pharmacokinetics of amikacin in children. *J. Pediatr.* 91:333, 1977.

122. Walker, S.H., and Park-Hah, J.O. Possible isoniazid-induced hepatotoxicity in a two-year-old child. *J. Pediatr.* 91:344, 1977.

123. Wallin, A., Jalling, B., and Boreus, L.O. Plasma concentrations of phenobarbital in the neonate during prophylaxis for neonatal hyperbilirubinemia. *J. Pediatr.* 85:392, 1974.

124. Walts, L.F., and Dillon, J.B. The response of newborns to succinylcholine and d-tubocurarine. *Anesthesiology* 31:35, 1969.

125. Weber, W.W., and Cohen, S.N. Aging effects and drugs in man. In: *Handbook of Experimental Pharmacology,* Vol. 28(3) (Gillette, J.R., and Mitchell, J.R., eds.). Berlin: Springer-Verlag, 1975, p. 213.

126. Weinberger, M., and Ginchansky, E. Dose-dependent kinetics of theophylline disposition in asthmatic children. *J. Pediatr.* 91:820, 1977.

127. Weinberger, M., Hendeles, L., and Bighley, L. The relation of product formulation to absorption of oral theophylline. *N. Engl. J. Med.* 299:852, 1978.

128. Weiss, C.F., Glazko, A.J., and Weston, J. Chloramphenicol in the newborn infant. *N. Engl. J. Med.* 262:787, 1960.

129. West, J.R., Smith, H.W., and Chasis, H. Glomerular filtration rate, effective renal blood flow, and maximal tubular excretory capacity in infancy. *J. Pediatr.* 32:10, 1948.

130. Wettrell, G., Andersson, K.E., Bertler, A., and Lundstrom, N.R. Concentrations of digoxin in plasma and urine in neonates, infants, and children with heart disease. *Acta Paediatr. Scand.* 63:705, 1974.

131. Wichman, H.M., Rind, H., and Gladtke, E. Die Elimination von Bromsulphalein beim Kind. *Z. Kinderheilk.* 103:263, 1968.

132. Widdowson, E.M. Changes in body proportions and composition during growth. In: *Scientific Foundations of Paediatrics* (Davis, J.A., and Dobbing, J., eds.). Philadelphia: W.B. Saunders, 1974, p. 158.

133. Wilson, J.T. Phenobarbital in the perinatal period. *Pediatrics* 43:324, 1969.

134. Wilson, J.T. Developmental pharmacology: A review of its application to clinical and basic science. *Ann. Rev. Pharmacol.* 12:423, 1972.

135. Wilson, J.T. Pragmatic assessment of medicines available for young children and pregnant or breast-feeding women. In: *Basic and Therapeutic Aspects of Perinatal Pharmacology* (Morselli, P.L. et al., eds.). New York: Raven Press, 1975, p. 411.

136. Wilson, J.T., Atwood, G.F., and Shand, D. Disposition of propoxyphene and propranolol in children. *Clin. Pharmacol. Ther.* 19:264, 1976.

137. Wilson, J.T., Kasantikul, V., Harbison, R., and Martin, D. Death in an adolescent following an overdose of acetaminophen and phenobarbital. *Am. J. Dis. Child.* 132:466, 1978.

138. Wilson, J.T., and Wilkinson, G.R. Chronic and severe phenobarbital intoxication in a child treated with primidone and diphenylhydantoin. *J. Pediatr.* 83:484, 1973.

139. Windofer, A., Jr., Kuenzer, W., and Urbanek, R. The influence of age on the activity of acetylsalicylic acid-esterase and protein-salicylate binding. *Eur. J. Clin. Pharmacol.* 7:227, 1974.

140. Wolf, S.M., and Forsythe, A. Behavior disturbance, phenobarbital, and febrile seizures. *Pediatrics* 61:728, 1978.

141. Yaffe, S.J., Levy, G., Matsuzawa, T., and Baliah, T. Enhancement of glucuronide-conjugating capacity in a hyperbilirubinemic infant due to apparent enzyme induction by phenobarbital. *N. Engl. J. Med.* 275:1461, 1966.

142. Yoshioka, H., Takimoto, M., Matsuda, I., and Hattori, S. Dosage schedule of gentamicin for chronic renal insufficiency in children. *Arch. Dis. Childhood* 53:334, 1978.

ADDITIONAL READING

Blumer, J.L., and Reed, M.D. Clinical pharmacology of aminoglycoside antibiotics in pediatric. *Pediatr. Clin. North Am.* 30:195, 1983.

Jaffe, S. (ed). *Pediatric Pharmacology: Therapeutic Principles in Practice.* New York: Grunne and Stratton, 1980.

MacLeod, S.M., and Radde, J.C. *Textbook of Pediatric Clinical Pharmacology.* Littleton, Mass.: Wright-PSG, 1984.

Maxwell, G.M. *Principles of Pediatric Pharmacology.* New York: Oxford University Press, 1984.

Reed, M.D., and Blumer, J.L. Clinical pharmacology of antitubercular drugs. *Pediatr. Clin. North Am.* 30:177, 1983.

Smith, A.L., and Weber, A. Pharmacology of chloramphenicol. *Pediatr. Clin. North Am.* 30:209, 1983.

CHAPTER
30

GERIATRIC PHARMACOLOGY

Saradindu Dutta and Samar N. Dutta

This is a new branch of pharmacology that deals with actions and interactions of drugs in elderly patients (age 60-65 years or older). For sometime, various clinical studies have shown that many drugs act differently in senescent subjects than they do in young adults. Since such information has been acquired from a group of persons who are not only old, but also suffer from more than one disease, and therefore consume many drugs, it has been difficult to accept that such drug super-or under-sensitivity is a specifically age-related phenomenon.

However, studies with animals, in which one can conduct clearly defined longitudinal studies, have revealed that there is indeed an age-dependent prolongation of effect of drugs such as pentobarbital, secobarbital, and presumably other drugs that are metabolized by hepatic cytochrome P-450 enzymes (30). In addition to prolongation of drug action as affected by age-related change in pharmacokinetic parameters, there is also evidence of general decrease or increase in responsiveness to drugs in the aging target organs (18, 21, 42, 43).

By extrapolating experimental results from age-related studies it is possible to deduce that some of the super- or under-sensitivity as noted in the elderly patients is perhaps caused by alteration in pharmacokinetic and/or pharmacodynamic profiles of the elderly patients. Thus, when a particular drug manifests unusual effect in the elderly, the physician should take into consideration all possible factors that can play a role in causing this change in drug action. In an attempt to provide such insight to physicians, this chapter will deal with various pharmacokinetic and pharmacodynamic processes that may be altered, resulting in modification of drug action in the elderly.

AGE-RELATED CHANGES IN PHARMACOKINETIC FACTORS

Available data from clinical studies have shown that the plasma concentration of drugs in elderly patients are higher than those in the young adult (34). Figure 30-1 shows a typical age-related increase in serum concentration of digoxin as noted in patients following administration of a fixed dose of β-acetyldigoxin (5).

As in the case of digoxin, a similar effect of age on plasma concentrations has been observed with drugs such as penicillin, dihydrostreptomycin, and tetracycline (34). The reactions for this age-related increase in plasma level are not easily understood. When higher concentrations are associated with a prolonged half-life, it is reasonable to conclude that the drugs that are eliminated by the kidney and/or liver may have stayed longer in blood and caused a higher plasma level in older patients because of their age-related change in kidney or liver functions. There are instances in which certain drugs may show longer half-life and higher blood levels in older patients

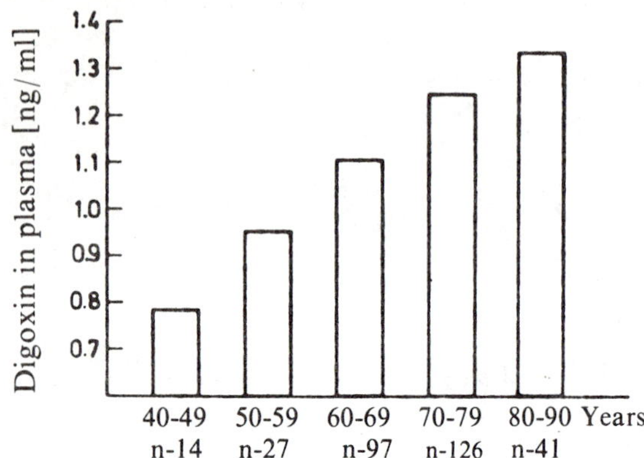

Fig. 30-1. *Mean serum digoxin concentrations in relation to age among a series of patients receiving a fixed dose of β-acetyldigoxin (0.4 mg/day)* (From Ref. 5).

without obvious dysfunctions of kidney and liver. Therefore, one has to take into consideration of all the possible factors that may be affected by senescence and may be involved in changing pharmacokinetic properties of many drugs in elderly patients. The following section deals with these factors individually.

Absorption. The entire gastrointestinal tract undergoes changes caused by the effects of aging. With advancing age there is frequent loss of teeth, and such loss of teeth seems to cause a reduction in salivary flow. It has been reported that in very advanced old age one may observe a complete lack of salivary flow (39, 50). There is also a significant reduction in salivary ptyalin (2) content and the absorbing capacity of the oral mucosa with advancing age. It can be postulated that because of these changes in the salivary secretion and oral mucosa, elderly people would not be able to easily absorb sublingual or buccal tablets resulting in varying degrees of ineffectiveness of those drugs that are absorbed mainly from the oral cavity (34).

Additionally, the passage of tablets may be delayed by the aging esophagus. It has been pointed out that with aging changes such as "deglutition, relaxation of the lower esophageal sphincter, delayed esophageal emptying, dilation of esophagus" are occasionally observed in elderly patients (34). These defects may interfere with the passage of tablets into the stomach. Tablets were reported to be retained in the esophagus for longer than 10 min because of the earlier mentioned defects (9, 13). Therefore, it should be realized that many solid drugs administered orally, if not taken with meals and with an adequate amount of fluids, may not be processed appropriately by the aging esophagus, and this may contribute to unpredictable drug effect.

On theoretical grounds unpredictable absorption of drugs may be caused also by age-related change in the pH condition of the stomach. Since most drugs are weak acids or bases, their absorption in stomach depends greatly on what proportions of these drugs remain in unionized moiety in gastric contents (Chapter 2). Because with advancing age there is a decrease in basal and histamine-stimulated acid secretion in the stomach causing achlorhydria or hypochlorhydria, it has been postulated that weakly acidic drugs may not be well absorbed in the elderly subjects. However, actual studies in the elderly with weakly acidic drugs have not substantiated such a postulate. Similarly, because of aging there is a general decrease in the volume of fluids in the gastrointestinal tract, it is concievable that elderly patients will also have difficulty in absorbing poorly soluble drugs, such as ampicillin, digoxin, and griseofulvin. Finally, it has been suggested that the drug absorption from the stomach can also be significantly affected by such age-related diseases as atrophic gastritis and emotional stress, because these conditions significantly reduce gastric emptying of the ingested drugs. With advancing age, the stomach appears to empty slowly as indicated by slow and incomplete absorption of drugs such as diazepam (20).

After the stomach, the next site of drug absorption is the upper small intestine which with advancing age may lose a large fraction of absorptive cells, and thus, becomes inefficient to absorb drugs rapidly (4). Drug absorption from the intestine can also be decreased by an age-related reduction in the mesenteric blood flow. It has been suggested that since the mesenteric and splanchnic blood carries the absorbed drug from the intestine to the general circulation for its ultimate effect on target organs, any reduction of blood flow would cause lower drug absorption and reduce its effective blood levels. Therefore, these kinetic factors explain in some way why certain drugs may reach lower blood levels in elderly patients. However, the common problem with most drugs, as shown in Figure 30-1, is that they reach higher blood levels with advancing age. In order to explain such an observation, it has been proposed that with advancing age intestinal peristaltic activity diminishes, resulting longer retention of a drug in close contact with the absorbing surface and, thus, enhancing its absorption. However, this does not seem to be a satisfactory explanation, because increased retention time for drugs in close contact with the absorbing cells also may lead to their fast intraluminal and/or intramucosal degradation. Although in a recent report it has been clearly demonstrated that calcium absorption from the intestine is reduced in elderly women, resulting in low plasma 25-hydroxyvitamin D and 1,25-dihydroxyvitamin D (16) with an element such as calcium, one cannot invoke intraluminal degradation as the cause of slow absorption in the elderly.

Distribution. With advancing age cardiac output diminishes, which alters blood distribution to various organs. For example, it has been stated that in order to distribute blood effectively in the presence of diminishing cardiac output, the brain and heart as well as skeletal muscle preferentially receive more of the diminished cardiac output than do the liver and the kidneys (34). Thus such altered distribution of blood favors decreased hepatic metabolism and renal excretion of some drugs, which results in increased supply of drugs to target organs such as the CNS or heart.

Body Weight and Body Compartments. It has been reported that between age 25 and 65 total body water can decrease by 15-20%, and so can the extracellular fluid by approximately 35-40% (34). On the other hand, fat weight to body weight ratio increases by 25-45%. These changes in body compartments with advancing age can affect pharmacokinetic parameters of various drugs in several ways: for example, (a) water-soluble agents that distribute in body water would reach higher concentration and show exaggerated action in the elderly because their volume of distribution is reduced, and (b) lipid-soluble drugs, on the other hand, that deposit in body fat would find a larger volume of distribution and consequently might show longer plasma half-life and prolonged drug action. For many drugs, elderly people do indeed exhibit prolonged half-life as shown in Table 30-1.

Plasma Protein Content. With advancing age a fall in mean serum albumin levels is noted. The serum albumin level changes from 4 g/100 ml at age 40 or under to approximately 3.58 g/100 ml in those aged 80 years or above (23, 52). Such an age-related reduction in the serum albumin can affect pharmacokinetic properties of drugs in two ways. First, since less plasma albumin leads to an increase in the concentration of free drug and since drug effect is directly related to the concentration of a given drug as available in free state, one can expect to see an exaggerated drug effect in the elderly because of increased availability of free drug. Thus, a drug such as warfarin, which remains 97% bound to plasma albumin in young adults, may show adverse effects in the elderly, supposedly due to a reduction of plasma protein (28). On the other hand, when there is less binding of a drug due to hypoalbuminemia, many drugs would be rapidly eliminated by the metabolic and excretory actions of the liver and kidney. With phenytoin, a faster elimination leading to shorter or unpredictable drug action was observed (27). Contrary to these findings, another clinical study (6) reported that in the presence of a reduction of serum albumin concentration of less than 3 g/100 ml, phenytoin caused adverse effects in about 11% of patients, compared with 3.8% of patients with normal albumin levels. Thus, it appears that the age-related hypoalbuminemia can influence drug action in the elderly by a number of conflicting factors.

Plasma Protein Binding. It has been suggested that certain age-related renal disease can cause a change in the molecular structure of albumin that may result in a decreased binding of acidic drugs such as aspirin, phenylbutazone, phenytoin, sulfadiazine, and thiopental. Renal disease seems also to affect binding of neutral molecules such as digoxin (12).

Binding to Red Blood Cells. With advancing age, binding of certain drugs (e.g., meperidine, acetazolamide, chlorthalidone) to red blood cells has been reported to be reduced, thereby causing higher blood levels of these drugs in the elderly (20).

Hepatic Elimination. Both structure and function of the liver are affected by the aging process. Since the liver has the highest capacity to metabolize drugs for their elimination from the body, any dysfunction of this vital organ during the aging process is expected to prolong their plasma half-life. The drugs are metabolized by the liver primarily by the enzymatic activities of mixed-function oxidases, N-acetyltransferase, and nitro-reductase. Therefore, one may speculate that the activities of these enzymes may fall during the aging process, because of gradual death of hepatocytes, reduced blood flow to this organ, and/or loss of catalytic activity of drug-metabolizing enzymes. With increasing age, functioning hepatocytes have been shown to be gradually reduced (29, 30). However, experimentally or otherwise there is no evidence that this age-related change in hepatic mass can cause a reduction in hepatic drug metabolism (46). It is possible that age-induced loss of hepatocytes is compensated for by an increased activity of the surviving cells.

Between 30 and 70 years of age, cardiac output decreases about 40% in humans (22), and any decrease in cardiac ouput would directly reduce the amount of blood flowing through the liver and less amount of a drug would be delivered to the drug-metabolizing site. It can be inferred that during the aging process there would be a reduction of drug metabolism by the liver. However, there is no experimental evidence supporting such a cause and an effect relationship between an age-related reduc-

Table 30-1
Age-Related Increase in Half-Life of Some Commonly Used Drugs

Drug	Half-Life β (hr)	
	Young (<50 Years)	Old (>50 Years)
Diazepam	38-44	86-94
Chlordiazepoxide	10	18
Imipramine	19	24
Phenylbutazone	81	105
Quinidine	7	9
Warfarin	37	44
Acetaminophen	1.75	2.17
Cimetidine	1.8	2.3
Digoxin	51	73
Dihydrostreptomycin	6.5	8
Indomethacin	1.53	1.73
Morphine	3	4.5
Penicillin G	0.4	0.93
Theophylline	4.4	7.68

Source: Refs. 19 and 41.

tion in cardiac output and decreased hepatic drug metabolism. Nevertheless, drugs with high extraction ratios such as isoproterenol, nitroglycerin, etc., which are dependent on liver blood flow and removed during the first-pass through this organ, must be used with great caution in the elderly.

With regard to age-dependent loss of enzyme catalytic activity, although direct evidence from animal and clinical studies is lacking, Salem et al. (45) reported a reduced induction of drug metabolism in the elderly. This indicates that elderly patients may not be able to easily synthesize new enzymes when provoked and to develop tolerance to a drug. Therefore, in this group of patients any upward adjustment of drug dosage may be harmful.

Renal Elimination. An age-related deterioration of renal function occurs because the kidney loses 20% of its weight between the fourth and eighth decades (36). The weight loss involves a gradual reduction in the number of nephrons. These changes are primarily caused by the process of aging itself and perhaps affected by an age-related decline in mean renal blood flow per unit tissue mass (11). As in the case of the liver, the age-dependent reduction in cardiac output causes renal blood flow to decline by about 50% between the fourth and eighth decades. Thus, with advancing age glomerular filtration rate (GFR) as well as tubular excretory function declines. The impairment of GFR affects the elimination of polar drugs such as the penicillins, aminoglycosides, digoxin, procainamide, etc., and thereby prolongs their half-life in the elderly. On the other hand, certain drugs such as the tetracyclines, cephalothin, and carbenicillin do not manifest their therapeutic effect in urinary tract infection when GFR goes down to less than 20 ml/min (34). The peak plasma levels and half-life of drugs (e.g., penicillin, dihydrostreptomycin, tetracycline, and kanamycin) that are predominantly excreted by the kidney are altered by age-related changes in renal hemodynamics and in the nephrons (51).

It is essential to point out that of all the age-related changes that affect prolongation of drug effect in the elderly the decrease of GFR can be assessed ahead of time, and an appropriate dosage can be prescribed to avoid adverse drug reaction. For example, by measuring the urinary and serum creatinine levels, one can accurately calculate creatinine clearance and determine the degree of renal impairment of the elderly patient under study and prescribe a drug accordingly.

Table 30-2 summarizes various pharmacokinetic parameters that are affected by the aging process.

AGE-RELATED CHANGES IN PHARMACODYNAMIC FACTORS

In contrast to the much emphasized roles of pharmacokinetic factors in age-related change in drug action, relatively little attention has been paid to pharmacodynamic factors. In recent years, a limited but an interesting body of information has emerged characterizing drug responsiveness of various isolated organs per se in relation to aging (10, 18, 21, 42, 43). Although many contradictory findings exist, in general these studies have documented that during the period ranging from adulthood to senescence, in contrast to maturational development, an end-organ super- or under-sensitivity develops toward various drugs.

Changes in Organ System Function. The functional capacity of many organ systems (kidney, heart, lung) is diminished with old age. Since cardiac drugs are most commonly used by the elderly, the problems associated with these drugs will be discussed. Although it is generally recognized that pharmacokinetic factors are prima-

Table 30-2
Cause and Effect of Age-Related Changes in Physiological Processes

Process Affected	Probable Causes	Possible Effects
A. Absorption		
1. Mouth	Reduced salivary secretion and oral mucosal-absorbing surface	Reduced sublingual and buccal drug absorption
2. Esophagus	Slow peristalsis and longer tablet retention	Reduced drug absorption
3. Stomach	Reduced pH and gastric emptying	Reduced acidic drug absorption
4. Intestine	Reduced mesenteric blood flow,	Decreased absorption,
	Decreased peristalsis,	Decreased absorption,
	Longer contact with mucosa	Increased absorption
B. Body composition	Decreased water compartment	Increased concentration of polar drugs
	Increased fat weight	Half-life of lipid-soluble drugs increased
C. Plasma protein	Decreased concentration	Increased drug action and elimination
D. Elimination		
1. Liver	Decreased blood flow and organ weight	Decreased drug metabolism
2. Kidney	Decreased blood flow and organ weight	Decreased drug excretion and increased half-life

rily responsible for increased incidence of quinidine and digitalis toxicity in the aged, there is suggestive evidence that pharmacodynamic factors may also be involved. Studies in cats have demonstrated that long-term administration of "toxic" doses of digitalis glycoside results in development of severe degenerative (ventricular) histological lesions, including scar tissue, more frequently in older animals than in young animals (10). The presence of scar tissue in tbe heart of aged subjects has been suggested as the focus of increased irritability resulting in ectopic beats during digitalis therapy (14).

Alteration of End-Organ Receptors. The effect of aging on adrenoceptor function has been most widely studied among the pharmacodynamic factors affecting drug response in the elderly. Norepinephrine has been shown to have less effect on the contractile activity of cardiac muscle prepared from senescent (25-month-old) versus young (12-month-old) rats. Similar age-related difference in responsiveness has been noted with isoproterenol (26). By contrast, calcium-induced positive inotropic effect was found to be similar in both old and adult age groups. It appears that with advancing age under *in vivo* conditions adrenergic agonists for some reason lose their ability to interact with receptors, whereas the mechanism to mobilize calcium from the extracellular pool and its subsequent interaction with the contractile proteins remain unaltered by aging. Interestingly, it has been observed by *in vitro* measurements that density and/or affinity of β-adrenoceptors, cyclic adenosine monophosphate (cAMP), or protein kinase activation of cardiac tissue are not affected by senescence (25).

Evidence also exists which shows that with increasing age β-adrenergic activities of various tissues such as strips of thoracic aortae of rats, rabbits, and guinea pigs (15), iris (32), and tracheal smooth muscle (1) are also decreased. In regard to vascular smooth muscle, old rabbit thoracic aorta was shown to relax very poorly to isoproterenol in comparison with the aortic strips obtained from young animals, whereas nitroglycerin demonstrated no such age-dependent difference in relaxation (15). It becomes evident that like that of cardiac tissue adrenergic receptors of smooth muscle cells are perhaps also affected by senescence whereas contractile mechanisms remain unaffected.

Metabolic responses (β-adrenoreceptor mediated) to sympathomimetic agents are also decreased in old age; lipolytic response to norepinephrine in isolated human fat cells is inhibited. The data relating alteration in α-adrenoceptor functions with aging are conflicting, and it appears that there is no change in those receptors sensitivity (31). Age-related alterations in receptor sensitivity also occur in several hormone receptors (see Chapter 12).

The clinical implication of this loss of β-adrenergic activity with advancing age is that direct- or indirect-acting adrenergic agents are apt to produce less effect in the elderly, whereas β-receptor-blocking drugs are expected to show an exaggerated action. Indeed, with propranolol such as enhanced effect has been observed by Conway (8). This drug caused a marked fall in blood pressure and decreased cardiac function in old people (50-65 years) in contrast to what it did in young subjects (18-35 years).

Increased receptor sensitivity to sedative effects has also been reported in the elderly to diazepam (38) and nitrazepam (7). In aged subjects a lower blood level of warfarin has been shown to induce marked depression of clotting factor synthesis (49).

Alteration of Ion Channels. By studying the effects of lidocaine, quinidine, phenytoin, and verapamil on the electrical properties of rat atrial and ventricular tissues obtained from various age groups, Roberts and Goldberg (18, 21, 43) demonstrated that the electrophysiological effects shown by these ion channel-blocking agents were affected by the age of the animal. The decrease in action potential amplitude by lidocaine was reported to remain unaltered in atrial muscle prepared from 1-, 6-, and 24-month age groups, whereas this drug produced the highest effect on muscle prepared from the 28-month-old group.

When the effect of lidocaine was evaluated on the isolated rat heart prepared from similar age groups, this drug seemed to show more depressant effect on atrial rate, but a lesser effect on ventricular rate with increasing age. These results imply that with advancing age the sodium channels of rat atrial muscle are more susceptible to blockade by lidocaine than ventricular tissue. The clinical implication of this finding is that the effect of lidocaine in suppressing atrial arrhythmia could increase with increasing age whereas the opposite would happen in case of ventricular arrhythmia. However, human studies have revealed no evidence of any difference in antiarrhythmic potential of lidocaine in elderly patients (44).

The study of quinidine on the atrial muscle prepared from different age groups revealed no particular age-dependent effects on action potential amplitude. In the isolated heart, quinidine showed less depressant effect with increasing age both on atria as well as on ventricle. Furthermore, a study on the papillary muscle obtained from 7 patients, aged 7-60 years, revealed no differences in quinidine action on such electrophysiological parameters as rate of depolarization and amplitude and duration of action potential (37). These results indicate that there may not be much change in the antiarrhythmic action of quinidine in elderly patients.

Verapamil, a calcium channel-blocking agent, has also been studied in the rat atrial muscle and isolated hearts obtained from different age groups. As was noted with the sodium channel-blocking drug, lidocaine, the study with verapamil also showed more depressant effect on action potential amplitude of atrial muscle with increasing age. It appears that senescence perhaps affects both sodium and calcium channels equally and brings about certain change in their molecular makeup, so that they become more sensitive to blocking action.

Adverse Drug Reactions in the Elderly. Several surveys indicate that with increasing age use of both prescription and nonprescription drugs increase (35). Thereby, incidence of adverse reactions to drugs seem to increase three to seven times in elderly patients compared with young people (47).

An estimated 3-5% of hospital admissions are attributed to drug reactions, and about 15-30% of all admissions are complicated by drug reactions beginning in the hospital (24). About 11-21% of patients over 60 years develop adverse reactions to drugs (56). Table 30-3 shows some common drug-induced adverse reactions in elderly patients.

GENERAL PRINCIPLES REGARDING THE USE OF DRUGS IN THE ELDERLY

Patients Condition and Diagnosis. As with any therapeutic program, it is important to match the desired and undesired actions of a drug or drugs to the therapeutic needs of a particular patient. The best match will be based on the patient's presenting condition, symptoms, and history. This is of particular importance in treating older patients, since the incidence of multiple pathology is higher, there is greater biological variability, and the therapeutic goal is more demanding. It is important to clearly identify the goals of a proposed therapeutic program to help in decisions regarding drug selection and dose. No therapeutic program, to particularly in the elderly, will achieve maximum benefit and reduced risk if it is not developed within this context.

Dose. More and more evidence has accumulated that suggests a lower initial dose of most drugs should be considered for elderly patients. This is particularly true when multiple drug programs are implemented (40). Various dosage guidelines have been suggested (33); for example, a 10% reduction in dose at age 65 years, a 20% reduction at age 75, and 30% reduction by age 85 has been suggested (51). Others have proposed that drug dose should be reduced by 20% by age 65 and 30% by age 80. One should realize that those guidelines are simple in nature and have been proposed in this manner because one does not know what to expect by way of adverse reaction in various elderly age groups. Current prescribing information for drugs should take into consideration physiopathological factors on an individual basis.

Simplicity of Dosage Regimens. Dosage regimens for the elderly should be made as simple as possible and drugs should be clearly labeled. It is also important that adherence to the drug program be monitored. Older individuals tend to be forgetful, and therefore the physician or pharmacist should encourage daily recording of medications taken.

Concomitant Use. Concomitant use of drugs in the elderly is of particular concern, first because the elderly may be more sensitive to the drugs themselves, and second, they may interact in such a way as to promote the actions of one of the drugs which in the elderly can precipitate an undesirable or unwanted response.

The guidelines and principles described here are more

Table 30-3
Adverse Reactions Caused by Drugs Commonly Used by the Elderly

Drugs	Adverse Reactions
Barbiturates	Mental confusion, paradoxical excitement, hypoglycemia, hallucinations, liver dysfunction, porphyria
Anticholinergics	Hallucinations, disorientation, acute attack of glaucoma (narrow-angle), constipation
Antipsychotics	Extrapyramidal reactions, galactorrhea, postural hypotension, liver dysfunction
Benzodiazepines	Mental confusion, psychomotor impairment, diarrhea, vertigo
L-DOPA	Involuntary movements, psychic depression, cardiac arrhythmias, hallucinations
Methyldopa	Depression, drowsiness, paranoia, extrapyramidal syndrome, galactorrhea, liver dysfunction
Reserpine	Depression, mental confusion, hypotension, extrapyramidal syndrome
Digitalis	Confusional state, diarrhea, cardiac arrhythmias, gynecomastia, visual dysfunctions
Diuretics	
Thiazides	Dehydration, aplastic anemia
Furosemide	Deafness, hyperuricemia, hyperglycemia
Spironolactone	Diarrhea, gynecomastia, hirsutism
Antiarrhythmics	Blood dyscrasias, systemic lupus erythematosus (procainamide), visual dysfunction (quinidine)
Antihypertensives	Hemolytic anemia (methyldopa), edema, postural hypotension, peripheral neuropathy (hydralazine)
Cimetidine	Constipation, galactorrhea, gynecomastia
Sulfonylureas	Blood dyscrasias, hypoglycemia, liver dysfunction
Antiarthritics	Adrenal insufficiency, cataracts, Cushing's disease, edema, glaucoma, hirsutism, hyperglycemia, osteoporosis, peptic ulcer and psychosis (corticosteroids), neutropenia (indomethacin)

Source: Refs. 3 and 17.

or less obvious; yet they are not consistently applied. A recent report noted that "polypharmacy and a lack of current concepts of clinical pharmacology in the elderly can lead to increased morbidity and mortality in this group of patients" (48). In this study concerning the patterns of drug use in a geriatric nursing facility, 50 patients over 60 years of age were being cared for by seven physicians. The average number of drugs received per patient was seven with a range of four and one-half to nine. Of particular interest was the finding of a direct relationship between the lack of a specific indication for drug use and an adverse reaction. There was a 70% chance of an adverse reaction when no indication or diagnosis was recorded for drug use. There was also a lack of consistency by individual physicians in their approach to therapy of a similar disease. Thus, there is a need for teaching a rational approach to therapeutics based on clinical pharmacology as applied to the elderly.

REFERENCES

1. Aberg, G., Adler, G., and Ericsson, E. The effect of age on β-adrenoceptor activity in tracheal smooth muscle. *Br. J. Pharmacol.* 147:181, 1973.
2. Bayless, T.M. Malabsorption in the elderly. *Hosp. Pract.* 14:57, 1979.
3. Berlinger, W.G., and Spector, R. Adverse drug reactions in the elderly. *Geriatrics* 39:45, 1984.
4. Berman, P.M., and Kirsher, J.B. The aging gut. II. Disease of the colon, pancreas, liver and gallbladder, functional bowel disease and iatrogenic disease. *Geriatrics* 27:117, 1972.
5. Bodem, G., Ochs, H.R., and Dengler, H.J. The effect of disease on cardiac glycoside pharmacokinetics. In: *Cardiac Glycosides. II. Pharmacokinetics and Clinical Pharmacology* (Greeff, K., ed.). New York: Springer-Verlag, 1981, p. 219.
6. Boston Collaborative Drug Surveillance Program. Diphenylhydantoin side effects and serum albumin levels. *Clin. Pharmacol. Ther.* 14:529, 1973.
7. Castelden, C.M., George, C.F., Mercer, D. et al. Increased sensitivity to nitrazepam in old age. *Br. Med. J.* 1:10, 1977.
8. Conway, J. Effect of age on the response to propranolol. *Int. Z. Klin. Pharmacol. Ther. Toxikol.* 4:148, 1970.
9. Crowson, T.D., Head, L.H., and Ferrante, W.A. Esophageal ulcers associated with tetracycline therapy. *JAMA* 235:2747, 1976.
10. Dearing, W.H., Barnes, A.R., and Essex, H.E. Experiments with calculated therapeutic and toxic doses of digitalis; effects on the myocardial cellular structure. *Am. Heart J.* 25:648, 1943.
11. Epstein, M. Effects of aging on the kidney. *Fed. Proc.* 38:168, 1979.
12. Erill, S., Calvo, R., and Carolos, R. Plasma protein carbamylation and decreased acidic drug protein binding in uremia. *Clin. Pharmacol. Ther.* 27:612, 1980.
13. Evans, K.T., and Roberts, G.M. Where do all the tablets go? *Lancet* 2:1237, 1976.
14. Fine, W. The effects of drugs on old people. *Med. Press* (London) 242:4, 1959.
15. Fleisch, J.H., and Hooker, C.S. The relationship between age and relaxation of vascular smooth muscle in the rabbit and rat. *Circ. Res.* 38:243, 1976.
16. Francis, R.M., Peacock, M., Taylor, G.A. et al. Calcium malabsorption in elderly women with vertebral fractures: evidence for resistance to the action of vitamin D metabolites on the bowel. *Clin. Sci.* 66:103, 1984.
17. Frieser, A.J.D. Adverse drug reactions in the geriatric client. In: *Pharmacologic Aspects of Aging* (Pagliaro, L.A., and Pagliaro, A.M., eds.). St. Louis: C.V. Mosby, 1983, p. 257.
18. Goldberg, P.B., and Roberts, J. Age-related changes in rat atrial sensitivity to lidocaine. *J. Gerontol.* 36:520, 1981.
19. Goldberg, P.B., and Roberts, J. (eds.). *Handbook of Pharmacology of Aging.* Boca Raton: CRC Press, 1983.
20. Goldberg, P.B., and Roberts, J. Pharmacologic basis for developing rational drug regimens for elderly patients. *Med. Clin. North Am.* 67:315, 1983.
21. Goldberg, P.B., Stoner, S.A., and Roberts, J. Influence of age on activity of antiarrhythmic drugs in rat heart. *Adv. Exp. Med. Biol.* 97:309, 1978.
22. Goldman, R. Decline in organ function with aging. In: *Clinical Geriatrics,* 2nd ed. (Rossman, I., ed.). Philadelphia: Lippincott, 1979.
23. Greenblatt, D.J. Reduced albumin concentration in the elderly. *J. Am. Geriatr. Soc.* 27:20, 1979.
24. Gryfe, C.I., and Gryfe, B.M. Drug therapy of the aged. *J. Am. Geriatr. Soc.* 32:301, 1984.
25. Guarnieri, T., Filburn, C.R., Zitnik, G. et al. Diminished contractile response to catecholamines in senescent myocardium, but unaltered β-receptors, cyclic AMP, or kinase activation. *Clin. Res.* 27:127A, 1979.
26. Guarnieri, T., Filburn, C.R., Zitnik, G. et al. Contractile and biochemical correlates of β-adrenergic stimulation of the aged heart. *Am. J. Physiol.* 239:H507, 1980.
27. Hayes, M.J., Langman, M.J.S., and Short, A.H. Changes in drug metabolism with increasing age. 2. Phenytoin clearance and protein binding. *Br. J. Clin. Pharmacol.* 2:73, 1975.
28. Hayes, M.J., Longman, M.J.S., and Short, A.H. Changes in drug metabolism with increasing age. 1. Warfarin binding and plasma protein. *Br. J. Clin. Pharmacol.* 2:69, 1975.
29. Kato, R., Chiesara, E., and Frontino, G. Induced increase of meprobamate metabolism in rats pretreated with phenobarbital or phenaglycodol in relation to age. *Experientia* 17:520, 1961.
30. Kato, R., Takanaka, A., and Onoda, K.G. Studies on age difference in mice for the activity of drug-metabolizing enzyme of liver microsomes. *Jap. J. Pharmacol.* 20:572, 1970.
31. Kelly, J., and O'Malley, K. Adrenoceptor functioning and ageing. *Clin. Sci.* 66:509, 1984.
32. Koyczyn, A.D. Sympathetic pupillary tone in old age. *Arch Ophthalmol.* 94:1905, 1976.
33. Lamy, P.P. Therapeutics and the elderly. *Addict. Dis.* 3:311, 1978.
34. Lamy, P.P. Modifying drug dosage in elderly patients. In: *Current Geriatric Therapy* (Covington, T.R., and Walker, J.I., eds.). Philadelphia: W.B. Saunders, 1984, p. 35.
35. Lamy, P.P. *Prescribing for the elderly.* Littleton, Mass.: PSG Publishing, 1980.
36. McLachlan, M.S.F. The ageing kidney. *Lancet* 2:143, 1978.
37. Nawrath, H., and Eckel, L. Electrophysiological study of human ventricular heart muscle treated with quinidine: Interaction with isoprenaline. *J. Cardiovasc. Pharmacol.* 1:415, 1979.
38. Reidenberg, M.M., Levy, M., Warner, H. et al. Relationship between diazepam dose, plasma level, age, and central nervous system depression. *Clin. Pharmacol. Ther.* 23:371, 1978.
39. Richey, D.P., and Bender, A.D. Effects of human aging on drug absorption and metabolism. In: *The Physiology and Pathology of Human Aging* (Goldman, R., and Rockstein, M., eds.). New York: Academic Press, 1975, p. 59.
40. Ritschel, W.A. Pharmacokinetic approach to drug dosing in the aged. *J. Am. Geriatr. Soc.* 24:344, 1976.
41. Ritschel, W.A. Pharmacokinetics in the aged. In: *Pharmacologic Aspects of Aging* (Pagliaro, L.A., and Pagliaro, A.M., eds.). St. Louis: C.V. Mosby, 1983, p. 219.

42. Roberts, J. Autonomic drugs. In: *Handbook on Pharmacology of Aging* (Goldberg, P.B., and Roberts, J., eds.). Boca Raton: CRC Press, 1983, p. 155,
43. Roberts, J., and Goldberg, P.B. Changes in responsiveness of the heart to drugs during aging. *Fed. Proc.* 38:1927, 1979.
44. Rossen, K.M., Lau, S.H., Weiss, M.B., and Damato, A.N. The effect of lidocaine on atrioventricular and intraventricular conduction in man. *Am. J. Cardiol.* 25:1, 1970.
45. Salem, S.A., Rajjayabun, P. Shepherd, A.M., and Stevenson, I.H. Reduced induction of drug metabolism in the elderly. *Age Ageing* 7:68, 1978.
46. Sata, T., Miwa, T., and Tauchi, H. Age changes in human liver of different races. *Gerontologia* 16:368, 1970.
47. Schmucker, D.L. Age-related changes in drug disposition. *Pharmacol. Rev.* 30:445, 1978.
48. Segal, J.L., Thompson, J.F., and Floyd, R.A. Drug utilization and prescribing patterns in a skilled nursing facility: The need for a rational approach to therapeutics. *J. Am. Geriatr. Soc.* 27:117, 1979.
49. Shepherd, A.M., Hewick, D.S., Moreland, T.A. et al. Age as a determinant of sensitivity to warfarin. *Br. J. Clin. Pharmacol.* 4:315, 1977.
50. Stare, P.J. Three scores and ten plus more. *J. Am. Geriatr. Soc.* 25:529, 1977.
51. Vestal, R.E. Drug use in the elderly: A review of problems and special considerations. *Drugs* 16:358, 1978.
52. Wallace, S., and Whiting, B. Factors affecting drug binding in plasma in elderly patients. *J. Clin. Pharmacol.* 3:327, 1976.
53. Williamson, J., and Clopin, J.M. Adverse reactions to prescribed drugs in the elderly: A multicenter investigation. *Age Ageing* 9:73, 1980.

ADDITIONAL READING

Anderson, S., and Brenner, B.N. Effects of aging on the renal glomerulus. *Am. J. Med.* 80:435, 1986.

Meier, D.E. Cardiovascular drugs. In: *Geriatric Medicine* (Cassel, C.K., and Walsh, J.R., eds.). New York: Springer-Verlag, 1984, p. 618.

Stilwell, J.E. Psychotherapeutic drugs. In: *Geriatric Medicine* (Cassel, C.K., and Walsh, J.R., eds.). New York: Springer-Verlag, 1984, p. 637.

CHAPTER
31

ADVERSE DRUG REACTIONS

M.G. Bogaert and A.F. De Schaepdryver

Adverse drug reactions have been recognized ever since drugs have been used, but awareness of their importance by the medical world, the public, and official bodies has mainly come with the sulfanilamide-diethylene glycol problems in the United States in 1937 and with the thalidomide disaster in Europe in the early 1960s.

Since then detection and prevention of drug-induced diseases have become a major field of research. Although large efforts are being made, it is a utopic hope to expect that this will lead to a happy world with only perfectly safe drugs. We continue to hope for more specific drugs (i.e., drugs that would act only to restore the disturbed functions to normal), but for the time being the available drugs will have unwanted side effects; it is the role of the physician prescribing a drug to evaluate its benefits and risks in each particular situation. Also the patient should share this responsibility (11).

In order to play the role of advisor to the patient about the benefit/risk ratio of a drug, the physician needs to know more about drug-induced illnesses than what is written in the package insert. It is certainly helpful to read on the package insert of a new anti-inflammatory agent that the drug is less likely to give problems in the patient with a history of peptic ulcer than other anti-inflammatory drugs; that its chemical relationship to another drug makes hematological reactions theoretically possible; that interference with the protein binding of coumarin-anticoagulants has not been seen but is not excluded. However, in order to use this information fruitfully the physician has to be aware of the limited predictive value of toxicity studies in animals and of the difficulty in assessing drug-induced illness in humans. The physician should know that, for uncommon reactions, studies in a few hundreds or even a few thousands of patients do not allow an accurate assessment of their frequency. This has been amply demonstrated by the problems encountered with newer nonsteroidal anti-inflammatory drugs soon after their introduction on the market (2). The physician should, on the other hand, know the factors that predispose to some adverse drug reactions.

This chapter will provide some background information on drug-induced illnessess that may help in evaluating the benefit/risk ratio in a particular situation and in making the correct therapeutic decisions. A brief description of the possible mechanisms of adverse drug reactions will be followed by a discussion of predisposing factors and of the situations in which adverse reactions are more likely to occur. After that, the problem of detection of adverse effects is surveyed.

MECHANISMS OF ADVERSE DRUG REACTION

An adverse reaction is often only the extension of one of the drug's known pharmacological effects, an effect that may not be related to the therapeutic response. For most pharmacological effects, the doses needed to obtain the same effect, or alternatively, the response seen with the same dose, show wide variations from species to species as well as from one individual to another. So, with the dose needed to obtain a beneficial pharmacological effect in most patients, a grossly exaggerated response may be seen in a few patients. These interindividual differences arise from pharmacokinetic or from pharmacodynamic variations. Pharmacokinetic factors such as increased absorption and decreased biotransformation or excretion can lead to increased concentrations of the drug in the organism. Pharmacodynamic factors, on the other hand, can alter the sensitivity of the target organ for the pharmacological effects of the drug.

However, other side effects cannot be explained as an exaggeration of a drug's pharmacological effects. For these unexpected reactions, the term *idiosyncratic reactions* has often been used without clear definition. Enzymatic abnormalities are probably responsible for many of these reactions, and for some of them a pharmacokinetic cause has been detected. In the group of unexpected reactions to a drug, drug allergy (or hypersensitivity) is important. Allergy depends on the formation of an antibody in response to an antigenic stimulus from the drug. As for other allergic reactions, types 1, 2, 3, and 4 reactions can be distinguished (see Chapter 13.5.2). The most dramatic manifestation of drug allergy is the anaphylactic reaction, other manifestations being skin rash, drug fever, serum sickness, liver disease, nephropathy, hematological disorders, and so forth. A definite diagnosis of the immunological nature of reactions is often difficult (e.g., for the hematological reactions), and it should not be assumed that all effects of a drug that cannot be produced in animals are necessarily due to allergy. *In vivo* tests (mainly skin tests) and *in vitro* tests (lymphocyte transformation, detection of antibodies, and so on) for detecting drug allergy have been developed but are at present of limited value.

It is important to point out that adverse reactions are sometimes related to the manufacturing, storage, labeling, or delivery of a drug. An example is the increased risk of toxicity with digoxin when changes in the manufacturing process led to a sudden, unrecognized increase in bioavailability. Adverse reactions resulting from prescription errors are also frequent. Finally, problems of compliance from the part of the patient may play a role.

PREDISPOSING FACTORS

Although many adverse reactions are unexpected, some predisposing factors exist that may lead to the recognition of the patients more at risk, or at least provide an explanation of the adverse reaction.

Pharmacokinetic Factors

Interactions with other drugs or with food in the gastrointestinal tract can occasionally lead to increased *absorption*. The increased absorption of monoamines after blockade of the monoamine oxidase in the intestinal mucosa by inhibitory drugs is well known. Some drugs (e.g., lidocaine and propranolol), although well absorbed from the gut or the stomach, are extensively metabolized by the liver enzymes so that only a fraction of the dose given reaches the systemic circulation in unchanged form. This first-pass phenomenon is unpredictable and for some drugs saturable, so that chronic administration, or administration of a higher dose, causes unexpectedly high levels in the organism as compared with the levels reached after single administration of a low dose. Moreover, interactions with other drugs,food and disease states can influence the first-pass phenomena, due to changes in drug-metabolizing enzyme activity or in splanchnic blood flow.

Drug interactions or pathological conditions can alter the *distribution* of a drug. Altered distribution of digoxin in renal failure could be an important cause of increased risk of adverse reactions to the drug; however, it is difficult to incorporate this factor into nomograms for adaptation of posology in relation to the degree of renal failure.

A decreased *serum protein-binding* with an increased free fraction of the drug in plasma has been found for many drugs in situations such as renal failure, nephrotic syndrome, hepatic disease, etc. For most drugs the elimination (excretion by the kidney or biotransformation by the liver) and the pharmacological activity are related to the free fraction of drug in the plasma, so that an increase in free fraction will increase the pharmacological effect but accelerate the elimination of the drug. In most cases it is not known to what extent these changes in protein-binding lead to changes in pharmacological effect or to side effects. Drug interactions at the serum protein-binding level have been much studied and discussed as possible causes of side effects. The consequences of those interactions are often less dramatic than would be implied from the *in vitro* studies. Indeed, for drugs with a large distribution volume, the increase in free concentration resulting from a given decrease in percentage of protein-binding is often negligible. Moreover, the increase in free concentration often tends to wane in time, as for many drugs the rate of biotransformation and of renal excretion increases with higher free concentrations (10). Finally, an increase in free drug concentration will only influence the effect for those drugs that have a steep concentration-response curve.

Urinary excretion is the main pathway of elimination for some drugs, and renal failure is an important cause of exaggerated reactions for such drugs if they have a narrow therapeutic-toxic range. For digoxin and aminoglycoside antibiotics, for example, renal failure is probably the most important single cause of toxicity (e.g., in the elderly). Guidelines for adaptation of the dose in relation to the decrease in renal function have been proposed. Even when doses are adapted according to those guidelines, careful observation of the patient and occasional determination of plasma levels are mandatory. Indeed, even the more sophisticated guidelines do not take into account all factors: for example, for digoxin, changes in distribution could alter profoundly the disposition of the drug in patients with renal failure; for the aminoglycoside antibiotics, the concentrations in the target organs are probably not adequately reflected by the plasma level profile.

Urinary excretion of drugs can be modified by variations in tubular reabsorption, dependent upon the urine flow and the degree of ionization of the drug. However, for drugs for which urinary excretion is only a small part of their overall elimination, even a profound change in tubular reabsorption does not lead to clinically relevant changes in concentration in the organism.

For many drugs, *biotransformation* in the liver is the main pathway of elimination. The rate of hepatic biotransformation shows wide interindividual variations, even in the absence of hepatic dysfunction. This variability explains in many cases why for same dose of drugs, such as tricyclic antidepressants, antiarrhythmics, anticonvulsants, and so forth, some patients do not show any effect, whereas others have very serious overdosage problems. There is no way of predicting the rate of biotransformation of a particular drug, and toxicity (or on the other hand, undertreatment) can only be avoided by individual dose titration. When the diagnosis of overdosage symptoms is difficult, plasma level determination can be of help.

The interindividual differences in rate of biotransformation are in part due to genetic factors. In most cases these influences are multifactorial, leading to a continuous distribution of rate of biotransformation and of drug response. In some cases, a discontinuous variation is found and the population can be divided into two or more distinct groups: this is called *pharmacogenetic* variation in biotransformation. Lack of normal cholinesterase, for example, leads to an exaggerated and long-lasting response to succinylcholine. For drugs such as sulfonamides, isoniazide, hydralazine, and procainamide, genetically determined rapid and slow acetylators can be distinguished. Whereas it is usually said that slow acetylators have a higher risk of developing side effects with these drugs, the reverse could be true for isoniazide and procainamide, and it has been suggested that the acetylated metabolites may be responsible for the isoniazide liver damage and for the procainamide lupus syndrome. A genetic defect can lead to an unusual pathway of biotransformation of a drug, resulting in an unusually high concentration of a metabolite and in toxic effects. There is much interest in the existence of extensive and of poor metabolizers for substances such as debrisoquin, etc.

Variability in biotransformation rate is, however, in part also due to environmental factors. Enzymes can be induced or inhibited by administration of other drugs, by food, or by pollutants, and this can lead to toxicity. For example, for coumarin anticoagulants bleeding is sometimes seen in a patient on concomitant treatment with barbiturates when administration of the enzyme-inducing barbiturate is inadvertently stopped, so that the rate of biotransformation of coumarin slows down to its normal rate.

Apart from the problem of variability, there is the difficulty that for some drugs (e.g., phenytoin) biotransformation proceeds according to zero-order kinetics (saturation kinetics, dose-dependent kinetics), even for therapeutic doses. In that case, a small increase in dose can lead to a disproportionate increase in concentrations in the organism, and ensuing toxicity. No clear-cut rules can be given for the effect of liver disease on the fate of drugs; for many drugs, impaired metabolism has been described, but there is no parameter of endogenous hepatic function that can be correlated with the slowing of drug metabolism. For a few drugs (e.g., lidocaine and propranolol) biotransformation does not depend so much on the activity of the enzyme system as on the rate of their delivery to the liver (i.e., on the hepatic blood flow). In those cases, the decrease in blood flow to the liver, as seen in some situations, leads to a much higher concentration of the drug in the organism; the toxicity of lidocaine due to high and persisting plasma levels in patients with cardiac and hepatic insufficiency has been amply demonstrated.

Pharmacodynamic Factors

Altered sensitivity of the target organs is important in determining the effect of a given dose of a drug. There is, as for the pharmacokinetic factors, a wide interindividual variability in organ sensitivity. The sensitivity of the target organs moreover can be increased by disease states, e.g., cardiac failure or bronchospasm in individuals with underlying cardiac or bronchial disease treated with a β-adrenolytic drug. Interactions can likewise increase the response toward a given concentration of the drug in the organism.

Idiosyncratic reactions are often due to changed sensitivity of the target organs. A few of those reactions have been recognized as belonging to the pharmacogenetic group. Glucose-6-phosphate dehydrogenase deficiency predisposes to hemolysis by a number of antimalaria drugs and also by analgesics, chloramphenicol, etc. Malignant hyperpyrexia after a general anesthetic or a curarizing agent, and glaucoma after administration of glucocorticoids etc., also belong to this group. For many other unexpected reactions to drugs, genetic or other biochemical deficiencies will probably be detected.

There is a tendency to overemphasize pharmacokinetic factors as the cause of adverse reactions and to forget the importance of pharmacodynamic factors. This is mainly so for drugs such as the digitalis glycosides, antiarrhythmics, antiepileptics, aminoglycoside antibiotics, psychotropic drugs etc., for which plasma levels are monitored. Toxicity is not unusual in patients with so-called therapeutic plasma levels of these drugs, and this is the consequence of pharmacodynamic variability.

SITUATIONS WITH INCREASED RISK OF ADVERSE REACTIONS

Race. Cholestatic jaundice by oral contraceptives appears to be more common in Scandinavian women. For several known pharmacokinetic phenomena, such as glucose-6-phosphate dehydrogenase deficiency and fast or slow acetylation of drugs, important differences exist among people of different origins.

Sex. Women present more adverse reactions to drugs than men; moreover, women are more likely to develop hematological complications upon administration of drugs such as chloramphenicol.

Age. The neonate, and especially the premature baby, has an insufficient renal excretory capacity, and the enzymes responsible for biotransformation (in particular the glucuronyltransferase system) are still immature. Many drugs are therefore eliminated much more slowly than in older children: for chloramphenicol, the grey syndrome characterized by cyanosis, vascular collapse etc., is well known (see Chapters 24.4 and 29). The fact that the body composition of the neonate is completely different from that of the adult is also responsible for marked changes in drug effects. Drugs such as sulfonamides and salicylates displace bilirubin from plasma albumin, with increased chances of development of kernicterus. Much less is known about the possible differences in sensitivity of the target organs of the drug in the very young children compared with older children or adults.

For children, adaptation of dosage to the age of the patient is of course important mainly for drugs with a large potential for producing side effects, but no general rules can be given. For example, theophylline is transformed more rapidly by children than by adults; for digoxin, at a certain period of childhood, the doses needed per kilogram are much higher than in adults. Problems specific for childhood are tetracycline-induced changes in dentition and in ossification, and growth stunning by androgens.

Elderly patients develop more adverse drug reactions than the younger population. Drug prescription is more frequent in this age group, and the number of drugs taken per patient is high. Elderly patients often have difficulties in understanding and following the prescribed regimen, and overdosage by mistake is frequent (see Chapter 30). Moreover, for a given dose, concentrations reached in the organism are often much higher: the lean body mass is decreased, biotransformation of drugs in the liver tends to slow down, and renal function as a rule is diminished. There are also changes in target organ sensitivity, predisposing, for example, to postural hypotension with antihypertensive drugs, to micturition problems with anticholinergic agents, to arrhythmias with digitalis products, and to confusion with hypnosedative drugs.

Disease States. In renal failure urinary excretion of drugs is decreased proportionate to the decrease in creatinine clearance. There are, moreover, changes in the distribution of drugs (e.g., for digoxin); protein binding can be altered; biotransformation is affected in an unpredictable way. There is also a change in the sensitivity of the target organs toward the therapeutic and toxic effects of many drugs.

The results obtained in hepatic disease are less clear-cut, probably due to the heterogeneity of the patient groups studied. Biotransformation as a rule tends to slow down. Here, too, one should not only think of pharmacokinetic factors; patients with ascites and edema, for example, are much more sensitive to drugs that change the water and electrolyte balance. Other disease states (e.g., cardiac failure, thyroid dysfunction, bronchial asthma, etc.) can predispose to side effects for certain categories of drugs. Atopic patients have a higher incidence of allergic drug reactions. Finally, one should realize that there are a number of unknown factors that increase the risk of adverse reactions. For example, it is difficult to see why the adverse reactions to nitrofurantoin in the United Kingdom, Sweden, and Holland are so different, although in this particular case differences in reporting rather than differences in incidence could be implicated (14).

DETECTION OF SIDE EFFECTS

Studies in animals can detect only some of the adverse reactions that will occur in humans. Even if an adverse reaction is due to an exaggerated pharmacological effect, only the study in humans will lead to an exact definition of the risk, taking into account factors such as the typical pattern of drug metabolism, the interactions with other drugs, and pathological conditions. This is even more true for the so-called unexpected reactions, allergic and others.

A major problem in assessing the adverse reactions to drugs in humans is that most if not all side effects of drugs, trivial or severe, can also be seen in patients not in contact with any drug. Finding an unwanted effect after administration of a drug does therefore not necessarily imply a causal relationship, and the number of subjective symptoms that are found in placebo-treated patients is quite impressive. Moreover, some serious drug-induced effects only become manifest after a long period of exposure and also sometimes long after treatment has been stopped.

It is therefore necessary to discuss the problem of assessment of adverse drug reactions with respect to the magnitude of the added risk of illness caused by the use of a drug compared with the magnitude of the baseline risk without the drugs. Jick (8) defines arbitrarily as a 'low risk', a rate of newly occurring illness of less than 1/10,000 per year; as a 'high risk', a rate of more than 1/200 per year; and in between the risk is said to be 'intermediate'. Jick distinguishes five categories of adverse reactions.

Category 1: Side effects with a high drug-induced risk and a low baseline risk. Thalidomide-induced phocomelia is an example. Adverse effects in this category will probably always be detected quite soon.

Category 2: Side effects with a low drug-induced risk rate and a high baseline risk rate. A large number of unknown side effects of drugs belong probably in this category, but detection is almost impossible, even if very marked efforts would be done.

Category 3: Side effects with a low drug-induced risk and a low baseline risk. Here, we can mention aplastic anemia by chloramphenicol, sclerosizing peritonitis after practolol, and vaginal cancer in the offspring of mothers who have taken diethylstilbestrol.

Category 4: Side effects with a high drug-induced risk and a high baseline risk. The possibility of tolbutamide-induced cardiovascular mortality as seen in the University Group Diabetes Program is an example.

Category 5: Side effects with an intermediate drug-induced risk and an intermediate baseline risk.

For side effects for which the drug-induced risk is low compared with the baseline risk, in particular when they develop only after a certain period of time, careful observation of the patient by the physician will clearly not be sufficient, and a more systematic approach will be required.

A number of strategies for detecting side effects of drugs have been applied. Before marketing of a drug, randomized controlled clinical trials are usually done, even though on limited numbers of patients. Thereby common, acute side effects are easily detected, but infrequent and delayed side effects will probably not be recognized. For the latter, long-term clinical trials on large numbers of patients are more appropriate, but those are not frequently done before marketing of the drug. It is often not possible to carry these trials out on a randomized basis. Even then, considerable discussion often arises about the validity of the results. This is well illustrated by the ongoing debate about possible cardiovascular complications of tolbutamide in the University Group Diabetes Project, and by the more recent controversy about the suspicion of carcinogenicity of clofibrate in the WHO cooperative trial in the primary prevention of ischemic heart disease using clofibrate (15).

For late and infrequent adverse effects, spontaneous reporting by the physician is certainly still the most valuable tool; reporting the suspicion, for example in letters to clinical journals, is one way of disseminating the information, but there has been criticism about the uncritical publishing of such observations; attempts to improve this reporting have been published (9). Spontaneous reporting systems have been set up in different countries, and in certain cases valuable information has been gained.

A more systematic approach to the discovery of side effects for drugs already on the market is the postmarketing surveillance. A well-known system is the Boston Collaborative Drug Surveillance Program. In this particular program, undesirable unexpected effects that the physician attributes to the intake of a drug, old or new, are reported. Lately there has been much interest in the problem of postmarketing surveillance for new drugs on large numbers of patients; for example, in Great Britain several proposals about such a system have been made (12), but there is still discussion about the best way to perform these surveillance studies. Results of procedures such as the 'prescription-event monitoring' at the University of Southampton are awaited by a wide audience (7).

In the different systems discussed hitherto, one proceeds from cause to effect (i.e., from drug to possible side effect). For rare drug-related events, proceeding from effect to cause is probably more appropriate. This approach is also called *case control study* but the names *trohoc* and *retrospective* are also used (4). Patients with the possible drug related illness are compared with a group without this illness, and the proportion of people in the two groups who have and who have not used a particular drug is compared. For diseases with a low drug-induced risk or with a long incubation period, case control studies are probably the best and perhaps the only way of detection. As in all nonrandomized studies, there is a considerable methodological difficulty in selecting the appropriate controls. This is well illustrated by the differences in the estimation of the magnitude of the association between estrogens and endometrial cancer in different case control studies (5).

Summarizing the problem of detection of drug-induced illness, one could say that careful observation of the patient by the physician is more than ever necessary. However, as many drug-related events are rare and occur also not infrequently without drugs, more systematic approaches such as the clinical trial and postmarketing surveillance are necessary. It should not be expected, however, that those methods will always give clear-cut and indisputable answers.

A special problem is that of detecting drug-induced teratogenicity. Although the thalidomide catastrophy has stimulated animal research in this field, preclinical data are probably only of very limited value. Whereas teratogenicity in humans has been proven for thalidomide, antineoplastic drugs, and some hormones, for a number of agents (e.g., anticonvulsant drugs) there is only a strong suggestion of teratogenicity in humans. For many other drugs, teratogenicity is suspected, but no clear evidence exists. One can hope that spontaneous reporting to central agencies will help to detect drug-induced teratogenicity early; another approach is the registration of all birth defects in the hope of recognizing certain trends. The possibility of neural tube defect in infants born to mothers treated during the pregnancy with the anticonvulsant valproate has again elicited discussions about the best way to detect such effects (3). The fact that in 4% of live-born infants major morphological anomalies are present is a major hindrance when one tries to evaluate the danger or safety of a drug during pregnancy. The value of these systems remains to be shown, but one can expect that detection of these rather low drug-induced risks in patients with high baseline risks will be difficult.

Drug treatment of a pregnant woman is mandatory in some situations, but recent surveys suggest an overconsumption of drugs by those women and a lack of awareness of the problem from her and from the physician. It is disappointing that the warning about possible teratogenicity by hormonal pregnancy tests, in the presence of much better alternatives of diagnosis of early pregnancy, seem not to have influenced a number of physicians (1, 13).

CONCLUSION

When a subjective adverse reaction occurs that is annoying for the patient, the decision to stop the drug will often be taken by the patient. However, for serious drug-induced illnesses it is often the physician who will have to make the decision whether or not to prescribe, for a given indication, a drug for which an adverse reaction has been described. If for that condition no other efficacious drug is available and if treatment of the disease is mandatory, the decision is relatively easy. If alternative drugs are available, one often tends to avoid the drug for which a serious adverse reaction is known, but comparative studies of adverse reactions with different drugs of the same class are often lacking. In some countries clofibrate was withdrawn after the WHO trial in 1978, but other lipid-lowering drugs that are less studied carry perhaps an even greater risk of adverse reactions.

In fact the physician is expected to base the therapeutic decision on an evaluation of the benefit/risk ratio of a drug, but in many cases has only very rough estimates or no estimates at all of the magnitude of benefit and of risk. However, we should not think that if good estimates of benefit/risk ratios were available, decision making would always be very easy. If we had an exact estimate of the risk of sudden death in a patient with ventricular dysrhythmias, of the prophylactic effect of an antiarrhythmic thereupon, and of the risk of agranulocytosis induced by the antiarrhythmic, what would we do? Would we consider that the drug-induced risk is acceptable as long as the number of patients who die from the drug does not exceed the number of patients one saves by administering the drug?

In conclusion, it can be said that the drugs we are using do carry a certain risk of adverse reactions, and that exact figures for that risk are often not available. Knowledge of certain predisposing factors will certainly diminish the frequency of adverse reactions to drugs. Finally, it is important to realize that a serious adverse reaction to a drug used in a situation in which the drug was not really needed should be distinguished from a reaction from a drug given as a last resource to a terminally ill patient (6).

REFERENCES

1. Brewer, C.L. Continued use of hormonal pregnancy tests. *Br. Med. J.* 1:437, 1978.
2. Dukes, M.N.G. The seven pillars of foolishness. In: *Side Effects of Drugs, Annual 8* (Dukes, M.N.G., ed.). New York: Elsevier, 1984, pp. XVII.
3. Editorial. Valproate and malformations. *Lancet* 2:1313, 1982.
4. Feinstein, A.R. The epidemiologic trohoc, the ablative risk ratio, and 'retrospective' research. *Clin. Pharmacol. Ther.* 14:291, 1973.
5. Horwitz, R.I. and Feinstein, A.R. Alternative analytic methods for case-control studies of estrogens and endometrial cancer. *N. Engl. J. Med.* 299:1089, 1978.
6. Ingelfinger, F.J. Counting adverse drug reactions that count. *N. Engl. J. Med.* 294:1003, 1976.
7. Inman, W.H.W. Postmarketing surveillance of adverse drug reactions in general practice. II: Prescription-event monitoring at the University of Southampton. *Br. Med. J.* 282:1216, 1981.
8. Jick, H. The discovery of drug-induced illness. *N. Engl. J. Med.* 296:481, 1977.
9. Jones, J.K. Criteria for journal reports of suspected adverse drug reactions. *Clin. Pharmacol.* 1:554, 1982.
10. Koch-Weser, J. and Sellers, E.M. Binding of drug to serum albumin. *N. Engl. J. Med.* 294:526, 1976.
11. Laurence, D.R. and Black, J.W. *The Medicine You Take.* Glasgow: W. Collins Sons, 1978.
12. Lawson, D.H. Detection of drug-induced disease. *Br. J. Pharmacol.* 7:13, 1979.
13. Meire, F., Vuylsteek, K., Buylaert, W. and Bogaert, M. Continued use of hormonal pregnancy tests. *Br. Med. J.* 1:856, 1978.
14. Penn, R.G. and Griffin, J.P. Adverse reactions to nitrofurantoin in the United Kingdom, Sweden and Holland. *Br. Med. J.* 284:1440, 1982.
15. WHO-Cooperative trial in the primary prevention of ischaemic heart disease using clofibrate. Report from the Committee of Principal Investigators. *Br. Heart J.* 40:1069, 1978.

ADDITIONAL READING

Davies, D.M. *Textbook of Adverse Drug Reactions*, 2nd ed. Oxford: Oxford University Press, 1981.

CHAPTER 32

ACUTE POISONING AND THERAPY

Daniel A. Spyker and George D. Armstrong

ACUTE POISONING: FUNDAMENTALS

All substances are poisons
The right dose differentiates a poison and remedy
— Paracelsus

Pharmacology might well be considered the science and art of using specific effects of poisons. The truth of Paracelsus' sixteenth century observation cannot be overemphasized. Most health professionals recognize the toxicity of barbiturates or aspirin, but the lethal potential of excessive oral sodium chloride or even water is less appreciated. Yet, saline emetics have caused pediatric deaths and water intoxication in compulsive water drinkers in well known.

Clinical toxicology is a new medical discipline, first specialty boards in 1975, that seeks to understand, manage, and prevent the toxic effects of drugs, chemicals, and naturally occurring substances.

In this chapter the endeavor is to:

- Provide an epidemiological perspective on acute poisoning exposures, morbidity, and mortality;
- Outline the basic strategy in the management of acute poisoning;
- Examine the toxicology and treatment of commonly encountered acute poisonings.

EPIDEMIOLOGY

There are an estimated 5 million accidental poisonings each year in the United States, of which 5000 are fatal; these numbers are steadily increasing (41). Poisoning is the fourth most frequent cause of accidental death, after automobile accidents, drownings, and burns. Acute poisoning is one of the most common pediatric medical emergencies, representing approximately 10% of emergency admissions and 5% of all hospital admissions. Ninety percent of all reported poisonings are accidental and involve children less than 10 years old. The U.S. Consumer Product Safety Commission estimated that, in 1983, over 130,000 children under 5 were treated in hospital emergency departments (EDs) for potentially toxic substances, and 13.9% were hospitalized (48). However, most hospital admissions for poisoning involve adult suicide attempts (Table 32-1). There is a third group at high risk, adolescents and young adults, wherein the poisoning is frequently labeled *drug abuse* . In a study of 255 drug-overdose patients, Stern et al (65) noted that 1-2% of all emergency ward visits and 5% of all admissions to an intensive care unit were for drug-overdose patients. In a

Table 32-1
Annual Morbidity (Principally Pediatric) and Mortality (Principally Adult Suicides) for Acute Poisoning

	Accidental	Intentional
Typical age range (years)	2-10	20-40
Poisoning incident cases	5,000,000	500,000
Hospital admissions	10,000	100,000
Mortality	150	5000
Recurrence Rate (%)	60	25

follow-up study, 5% died of drug overdose within a year of the index visit, and 42% had been readmitted for overdose or psychiatric illness. A history of drug abuse was present in 26%, regular alcohol use 70%, and 75% had received psychiatric treatment.

Approximately half of all ingestions involve medications with prescription drugs being slightly more common than non-prescription drugs. The usual drugs of abuse, or street drugs, collectively account for less than 1% of poisonings reported to poison centers. Tables 32-2 and 32-3 represent reports submitted by poison control centers to the Poisoning Surveillance and Epidemiology Branch formerly the National Clearinghouse for Poison Control Centers.

The toxic principle most often involved in poisonings is ethanol, either alone or in multiingredient products. Salicylates are the second most common, and petroleum distillates are third.

Mortality from acute poisoning based on death certificates is reported in Tables 32-4 and 32-5.

A poisoning mortality rate of 8 per million child-years for children under 19 was determined by Gallagher et al. in a Massachusetts study (27). Further demographics for poisonings were covered in an article by Armstrong et al. (7).

POISON CONTROL CENTERS

Recognition of acute poisoning as a major source of morbidity and mortality, particularly in the pediatric age group, gave rise to the concept of the poison control center (PCC) in 1953. The number of local PCCs officially designated by state health departments increased until 1970 but has steadily decreased since. For many of these centers the volume of calls is low and the quality of responses variable at best (61). Over the past 10 years centers with full-time, specially trained poison information specialists answering a large number of calls regional centers have gradually been replacing local PCCs, consolidating resources, and concentrating expertise to maximize service to the public. This evolution represents a major advance in the standardization and quality of PCC service (45).

Regional poison centers reduce severity of poisoning and emergency health care costs. By providing early, effective care, regional centers reduce morbidity and mortality from poisoning. Since approximately 85% of poison calls can be managed at home with telephoned directions and guidance, the need for transport to emergency facilities is usually obviated (40).

FUNDAMENTALS OF TREATMENT

"Acute poisoning is often mismanaged. It is impossible at times to determine whether recovery occurred because of or in spite of the treatment employed" (5).

Poisoning is a medical emergency. There are five principal elements to the management of a severely poisoned patient. The first is support. Many people who die of poisoning die simply because they stop breathing. The primary concern must be to secure an airway, making

Table 32-2
Top Nine Poisoning Categories
Poison Center Reports to the Poisoning Surveillance and Epidemiology Branch

	Number	Percent	All Ages Number	Combined Percent
Medications	29,310	40	49,621	41
Cleaning and polishing agents	10,508	14	14,889	12
Plants	9,402	13	11,723	10
Others and unknowns	7,637	10	20,172	17
Cosmetics	7,296	10	8,297	7
Pesticides	4,064	6	7,220	6
Paints and solvents	2,899	4	4,660	4
Petroleum products	2,026	3	3,696	3
Gases and fumes	140	<1	1,220	1

Source: Poisoning Surveillance and Epidemiology Branch Division of Drug Experience, National Center for Drugs and Biologics, 1981; n = 121,498.

Table 32-3
Poisoning Demographics

Age (Year)	All Ages (%)	Sex		Age Group Female (%)
		Male	Female	
<6	52[a]	13,112	10,950	45
6-12	4	1,166	823	41
13-17	3	572	743	56
>17	21	4,327	5,414	55

[a] Of the 52% <6, 39%, were ages 1 or 2.

Source: AAPCC/FDA Cooperative Poison Control Center Pilot Study, 1983.

Table 32-4
Poisoning Deaths, 1980

Category	Number	Percent		Modal Age Group
		Category	Total	
Accidental	4,331	100	40	
Drugs	2,492	58	23	25-29
Nondrug liquids and solids	597	14	5	50-54
Gases and vapors	1,242	29	11	20-24
Suicide	5,453	100	50	
Drugs	2,761	51	25	25-29
Nondrug liquids and solids	274	5	3	25-29
Gases and vapors	2,418	44	22	25-29
Undetermined	1,140	100	10	25-29
Total number of deaths	10,924			

Source: National Center for Health Statistics.

Table 32-5
Total Poisoning Deaths by Substances and Motivations, 1980

Category	Accidental		Suicidal		Undetermined Manner	
	Number	%	Number	%	Number	%
Analgesics/antipyretics/antirheumatics	636	15	310	6	202	18
Barbiturates	155	4	498	9	65	6
Other sedatives	59	1	99	2	28	2
Psychotropics	271	6	754	14	140	12
Other drugs	1,371	32	1,100	20	391	34
Nondrug liquids and solids	597	14	274	5	67	6
Gases and vapors	1,242	29	2,418	44	247	22
Totals	4,331		5,453		1,140	

Total number of poisoning deaths — 10,924.
Source: National Center for Health Statistics.

sure the patient is in fact breathing and that circulation is established. As always, the primary strategy is to consider treatable problems. Hypoglycemia occurs in alcoholics and in diabetes mellitus as well as in drug overdoses. Therefore, patients in a coma of unknown etiology should be suspected of hypoglycemia and treated accordingly.

Identification is a critical element that can proceed simultaneously with the other three parts of our strategy, which are to minimize absorption of the poison, to increase elimination wherever possible, and last (and probably least) to use specific antidotes.

Support. The major element of treatment is basic life support of the patient's airway, breathing, and circulation (A-B-C). Even recently, cardiac compression was taught as a quick, sharp compression of the sternum, but cardiac compression should comprise at least half of the compression relaxation cycle. Shorter compression results in substantial decrease of cardiac output (30-40%) (66).

The appropriate uses of electrical defibrillation (advanced life support) and drug therapy have been well summarized by Goldberg (28). Sodium bicarbonate should not be used routinely in cardiac arrest unless the patient has been apneic for more than 5 minutes (10). The "1 amp every 5 minutes" rule of thumb is probably excessive. Arterial blood gas determinations should be available and can provide guidance for acid-base manipulations. Patients whose blood is kept slightly alkaline (e.g., pH 7.45) are less likely to develop fatal arrhythmias.

Convulsions should be controlled with specific treatment where possible (e.g., ventilation, buffers for acidosis). Intravenous diazepam is the drug of choice for treating most seizures.

Minimize Absorption. Routine application of the principles of decreasing absorption of a toxin can significantly impact the morbidity and mortality associated with acute poisoning. The fundamentals of minimizing absorption include dilution, emesis or lavage, activated charcoal, and saline cathartics.

Dilution. Although currently recommended in at least one toxicology textbook (6), no clinical or experimental evidence supports the use of water in the treatment of ingested systemic poisons. Dilution with water may, in fact, increase the plasma concentration of certain drugs, such as sodium salicylate and quinine (32). Thus, although water is generally valuable when used with ipecac, water alone may be potentially harmful as a first-aid measure (15).

We recommend oral administration of water when the toxin ingested produces tissue irritation or corrosion. Milk is generally preferable if immediately available. The use of neutralizing substances, such as vinegar for alkaline ingestions, may cause more harm than benefit due to the heat of neutralization. Thus two large glasses (500 cc) of milk or water should be the first therapeutic measure.

Emesis. There are only two contraindications to inducing emesis. One is the ingestion of a caustic such as a strong acid or strong base, where the risk to patient from emesis may exceed the risk of leaving the poison in the stomach. The second is inability to protect the airway (absence of gag reflex, convulsions, or coma). The agent of choice for inducing emesis in the absence of these situations is syrup of ipecac (21). Table 32-6 shows that the gag reflex may be present in comatose patients and absent in 22% of emergency department staff.

The dose is 30 ml (2 tablespoons) for an adult, and 15 ml (1 tablespoon) for a child over 1 year old. Water should be given with ipecac (3 or 4 glasses for adults, 8-10 oz for children). Fluids are essential and may be given before or after ipecac with equal efficacy (13). The dose may be repeated once, if vomiting does not occur within 30 minutes. Success of this method is between 95 and 99%. Although failure of ipecac in the past was indication for lavage, the toxicity was probably overestimated, and the decision to lavage if ipecac fails to induce vomiting should be made on an individual basis (55).

Apomorphine effectively induces vomiting, but is available only in injectable form, as a hypodermic tablet that must be reconstituted. CNS or respiratory depression, toxicity, and excessive vomiting are not infrequent. Naloxone reverses the depression due to apomorphine and should always be readily available if apomorphine is administered.

In 776 cases where ipecac was recommended by telephone, 89% vomited after the first dose (within 30 min) and 98% after the second dose (60 min). Zero complications were noted in that group, and 93% were asymptomatic by the time of the 4-hr follow- up (6).

Even in patients overdosing on antiemetics, 81% vomited after the first dose and 95% by the second dose (32).

Table 32-6
Clinical Use of the Gag Reflex in Assessing Level of Consciousness

Level of Consciousness	Gag Reflex	
	Present	Absent
Comatose	9	2
Lethargic	14	0
Awake	12	1
All patients	35	4 (8%)
ED staff	14	4 (22%)

Gastric Lavage. When the contraindications to emesis are present as previously outlined, gastric lavage with a large-bore tube is the treatment of choice. A cuffed endotracheal tube should be protecting the airway prior to lavage. The only contraindication to lavage would be the ingestion of a caustic. In this case, endoscopy (ideally in the operating room) should be carried out within the first 24 hr of exposure. Fifteen percent of patients with esophageal burns have no readily visible oral or pharyngeal burns. Therefore, esophagoscopy must be considered based on history and symptoms.

If gastric lavage is used, a large-bore tube (37 French for adults) is essential. The patient should be in the left-side, head-down position. Each wash should be approximately 100-300 ml of either half normal saline or tap water. The patient should be lavaged until the aspirate is clear, the tube and/or the patient readjusted, and lavaged with additional lavage fluid.

Lavage or ipecac must be considered in any medically serious overdose, no matter how long since ingestion. Many drugs such as narcotics and those with anticholinergic activity (including tricyclics, phenothiazines, and antihistamines) suppress peristalsis and keep drugs in the stomach many hours after ingestion.

A 45-year-old patient who ingested 38 g of meprobamate was admitted to the hospital in a coma and recovered to the point of ambulation following appropriate treatment, but suffered a cardiopulmonary arrest 25 hr after admission. Autopsy revealed 25 g of meprobamate in a stomach concretion (35).

Intact LOMOTIL tablets (diphenoxylate HCl with atropine) were recovered from a pediatric patient 27 hr after overdose (58). Even protracted active vomiting does not guarantee emptying the stomach, as evidenced by autopsy following a colchicine overdose (25).

Ipecac or lavage removes 50% of stomach contents at most. One human study comparing lavage with emesis showed more aspirin was removed by ipecac-induced emesis than gastric lavage, even when ipecac was administered after lavage (1).

Activated Charcoal. The fine, black, fluffy powder used as an antidote since the nineteenth century results from the destructive distillation of organic materials, usually wood pulp. Following activation with steam or strong acid, activated charcoal's surface area (1000 m^2/ml) and electrostatic properties favor binding with most poisons.

N-acetyl cysteine (NAC) effectively reduces acetaminophen hepatotoxicity when given within 24 hr. Clinical toxicologists disagree as to whether syrup of ipecac and/or activated charcoal should be used in the treatment of acetaminophen overdose. *In vitro*, activated charcoal binds NAC (14). Serum levels of NAC, however, remain unaffected by concomitant charcoal (51). In the presence of conflicting data, our approach to acetaminophen overdoses has been to use ipecac and charcoal if less than 4 hr have elapsed since ingestion, and follow with NAC.

In France and Belgium, activated charcoal serves as first-line treatment for overdose in home and hospital. Activated charcoal is widely available in homes and pharmacies and generally enjoys the wide use and availability that ipecac does in this country. In those countries, ipecac is much less known or used for acute poisoning.

Clearly, activated charcoal decreases absorption of many orally administered drugs, and now we find evidence that it doubles elimination of methylxanthines (9) and barbiturates (8) given intravenously. In a simulated study of aspirin overdose, patients treated with syrup of ipecac alone had absorption reduced by 27%, activated charcoal + cathartic by 41%, and the combination (syrup of ipecac + activated charcoal + cathartic) by 25% (18).

We are beginning a gradual but major change in our initial approach to the treatment of the poisoned patient (both oral and parenteral). Based on experimental and clinical data, and extensive experience in Europe, we are beginning to recommend activated charcoal as a first-line treatment for most acute poisonings. The editorial board for Poisindex(C), the most widely used primary poison information system, has decided to make this change in many of the 291 treatment protocols.

Although scientific evidence supports the advantages of charcoal in many situations, we face a major marketing barrier with both professionals and the conscious patient before the full benefits of this black, messy powder can be realized in the treatment of the poisoned patient.

The appropriate dose of charcoal is 5-10 times the weight of the ingested substance, or 1 g/kg of body weight. The dose is generally given in water but other vehicles have also been used. Some vehicles (such as milk) reduce the effectiveness of charcoal. Black, heme-negative stools provide an indication of transit time.

A sorbitol-charcoal suspension has also demonstrated efficacy, may be prepared in advance, and offers improved palatability for the awake patient (53); 1 g/kg of charcoal in a 70% sorbitol solution would be a reasonable dose. Sorbitol has seen wide use as an osmotic cathartic, often used with sodium polystyrene sulfonate (KAYEXALATE) given rectally, and has occasionally been used intravenously as a calorie source. Sorbitol is thought to be absorbed slowly when taken orally, and to cause a slight increase in serum glucose (69).

The "universal antidote" - burnt toast, tea, and milk of magnesia - comprises charcoal, tannic acid, and magnesium oxide and has no place in the modern management of acute poisoning (19).

Cathartics. Cathartics are substances that enhance the elimination of bowel contents. Oil-based cathartics should be avoided due to the risk of aspiration pneumonia. Sodium sulfate, magnesium sulfate, and magnesium citrate are all useful cathartics. The recommended dose of sodium sulfate and magnesium sulfate is 250 mg/kg. In the event of contraindication to sodium absorption, such as congestive heart failure, magnesium sulfate (Epsom salts) should be used. Two tablespoons of Epsom salts in two glasses of water provide effective catharsis. Magnesium sulfate is contraindicated in renal failure. Saline cathartics do not interfere with charcoal adsorption (68).

Decontamination. Topical exposure to pesticides, caustics, and hydrocarbons poses an easily overlooked risk. Successive washings alternating soap and water with alcohol are recommended. Tincture of green soap is useful because it combines soap and alcohol. Care must be taken so that washers do not become contaminated themselves.

Identify Poison. History taking and identification preferably should proceed simultaneously with the medical management of the severely poisoned patient.

Toxicology screens provide qualitative evaluations of blood, gastric contents, and urine for toxins that commonly cause acute poisoning. It takes 2-6 hr to complete a drug screen. Most drugs have enough differential solubility (e.g., chloroform solubility much greater than water solubility) to permit separation and quantitation by many methods such as gas chromatography (11). The separation provided by gas chromatography and the identification permitted by mass spectrophotometry are combined in the gas chromatograph/mass spectrophotometer. This approach can provide drug quantitation and identification in most cases of unknown intoxication (34).

Increase Elimination. Efforts aimed at enhancing the elimination of a drug will be successful only if the agent or its active metabolites are excreted unchanged by the kidneys. Drugs that are lipid-soluble have a large volume of distribution; only a small fraction of the drug will be accessible (i.e., in the bloodstream) at any given time, and the best efforts to enhance elimination through forced diuresis or even dialysis will be minimally successful. Drugs in this category include phenothiazines and tricyclic antidepressants.

Various procedures (e.g., hemoperfusion, hemodialysis, and peritoneal dialysis) are being used in treatment of drug overdose. Continuous circulation of blood outside the body through various adsorbent materials such as charcoal or resin defines hemoperfusion. Hemodialysis involves extracorporeal perfusion of blood across a semipermeable membrane removing elements from blood based on their diffusion. Hemoperfusion is more effective in removing substances that are lipid-soluble, highly protein bound, and poorly distributed in plasma water. Such substances are poorly removed by hemodialysis or peritoneal dialysis. In animal experiments as well as in humans, hemoperfusion has been shown to enhance the rate of drug elimination and to reduce coma time, which may improve survival (52).

Dialysis or charcoal hemoperfusion is indicated: (a) when maximal supportive measures fail to maintain adequate cardiorespiratory function; (b) if the presence of hepatic, renal, or pulmonary diseases compromises toxin elimination; (c) for intoxication with drugs whose metabolites are equally or more toxic than the parent compounds (e.g., methanol, ethylene glycol); and, (d) for intoxication with dialyzable drugs such as ethchlorvynol, ethanol, and meprobamate. Hemodialysis is generally two to three times more effective than peritoneal dialysis. Dialysis or hemoperfusion should be considered early for heavy metals and lithium (22).

Specific Measures or Antidotes. There are five key elements in the management of acute poisoning. *Support* is essential for all poisonings. *Identification* needs to proceed simultaneously. A major impact on morbidity and mortality can be made with the routine steps to *minimize* absorption , including emesis or lavage, activated charcoal, and saline catharsis. Measures increasing the rate of elimination should be taken cautiously and then only to support vital functions. *Antidotes* are an infrequent part of managing the acutely poisoned patient and should be used only with specific indications. There are few "antidotes" in the sense of specific pharmacological antagonists. Some need to be used on suspicion of exposure and suggestive clinical state without awaiting confirmatory laboratory tests.

Specific measures and/or antidotes for some drugs and chemicals are discussed in the following section. Specific antidotes for some drug overdosages and poisonings and their mechanisms of action are presented in Table 32-7.

ACUTE POISONINGS: SPECIFIC AGENTS

BARBITURATES

Sedative-hypnotic drug use declined in the 1970s, experienced a resurgence, and has been declining once again. This class of medication accounted for 27 million prescriptions (1 billion doses) in the United States in 1976 and 29 million in 1983 (3). The 1983 data represent a decline of 3% when compared with 1982 (47). Sedative-hypnotics were implicated in 12% of 1906 drug-related accidental poisoning deaths. Barbiturates alone accounted for 7% of these.

Historical Perspective. Barbiturates have been a leading cause of death from drug overdose since the 1920s. During the 1930s, when gastric lavage and activated charcoal was the principal treatment, mortality was about 20%. During the 1940s, stimulation of respiration via CNS stimulants (analeptics) came into vogue. No appreciable reduction in mortality was realized until intensive life support supplanted analeptics in the 1960s. This method of basic cardiorespiratory support was reported as reducing the mortality to 1.5% in a series of 18,600 barbiturate poisonings at a Copenhagen hospital and became known as the *Scandinavian method* (16).

Clinical Effects. Central nervous system depression is the primary effect of barbiturates. The Glasgow Coma Scale (Table 32-8) provides a reproducible measure of CNS depression based on motor response, verbal response, and eye opening. The score appears to be a useful predictor of outcome; a score of less than 8 is defined as coma (67).

In addition to coma grade, the laboratory parameters of greatest predictive value (increased likelihood of mortality) include low arterial blood pH, low pO_2, and high central venous pressure (1). These parameters probably reflect the degree of hypoxia and shock prior to treatment.

Clinical effects in addition to CNS depression include suppression of peristalsis, stimulation of antidiuretic hormone, dilation of venules, and hypothermia. Bullous skin lesions of the hands, buttocks, and between the knees are found in 6% of patients (29). These blisters are not specific for barbiturates and should be managed as a burn. Severe barbiturate intoxication is likely to cause fatal pulmonary (atelectasis, bronchopneumonia, edema) and renal complications.

Treatment. The primary concern is the support of vital functions and basic measures to minimize absorption and increase elimination. Repeated doses of activated charcoal have demonstrated reduction of phenobarbital half-life from 110 to 45 hr even following intravenous administration (8). The importance of adequate fluid replacement in treating neurogenic shock cannot be overemphasized (62). Physiological fluids to raise the central venous pressure to 13 cm H_2O or, preferably, a pulmonary capillary wedge pressure of 18 mmHg should precede the use of pressor agents in the treatment of hypotension.

Short-acting barbiturates are less water-soluble and more lipid-soluble and therefore more subject to metabolism. The long-acting barbiturates such as phenobarbital are principally eliminated by glomerular filtration, and are thus amenable to alkalinization and diuresis.

Since the mortality associated with phenobarbital overdosage is relatively low, alkalinization alone may be prudent considering the dangers of high-volume forced diuresis.

Hemodialysis or charcoal hemoperfusion are indicated for poisoning with long-acting barbiturates when vital functions cannot be maintained (22). These short-acting agents have a large apparent volume of distribution and thus are not significantly removed (less than 5%) by urinary manipulations or hemodialysis. It may be neces-

Table 32-7
Specific Antidotal Therapy for Some Drug Overdosage and Poisoning

Drug or Poison	Specific Therapy	Mechanism
Centrally acting drugs		
Narcotic analgesics (including methadone, meperidine, heroin, morphine, pentazocine, dextropropoxyphene)	Naloxone	Opiate receptor antagonist
Acetaminophen (paracetamol)	N-acetylcysteine, cysteamine	Sulfhydryl donors, inactivation of toxic metabolite, protection of liver glutathione level
Antipsychotics (e.g., phenothiazines, butyrophenones) causing extrapyramidal reactions	Anticholinergics (e.g., benztropine, diphenhydramine, procyclidine, orphenadrine)	Restoration of balance between dopaminergic and cholinergic activity in CNS
Autonomic agents		
Sympathomimetics	β-Adrenoceptor blockers	Pharmacological antagonist
β-Adrenoceptor blockers	Atropine	Inhibition of vagal activity
	Isoproterenol	Pharmacological antagonist
	Glucagon	Direct stimulation of myocardial adenylate cyclase
Cholinesterase inhibitors: (e.g., organophosphates, neostigmine, physostigmine, pyridostigmine)	Atropine	Pharmacological antagonism
	Pralidoxime	Regeneration of cholinesterase
Anticholinergic agents	Physostigmine	Cholinesterase inhibition and pharmacological antagonism
Chemotherapeutic agents		
Isoniazid	Pyridoxine	Inhibits neurotoxicity
Methotrexate	Tetrahydrofolic acid	Bypass of inhibited enzyme reaction
Miscellaneous agents		
Insulin and oral hypoglycemics	Dextrose	Normalization of plasma glucose
Fluorides	Calcium salts	Decreased intestinal absorption of fluoride
Iron salts	Deferoxamine	Chelation
Heavy metals	Calcium disodium edetate, penicillamine, dimercaprol	Chelation
Cyanide	Cobalt edetate	Chelation
	Nitrite	Methemoglobinemia
	Thiosulfate	Provision of sulfur for metabolism to thiocyanate
Nitro compounds causing methemoglobinemia	Methylene blue	Reduction of Fe^{+++} to Fe^{++} and conversion of methemoglobin to hemoglobin
Coumarin anticoagulants	Clotting factors	Replacement of clotting factors
	Vitamin K_1	Pharmacological antagonist
Methanol, ethylene glycol	Ethanol	Inhibition of conversion to toxic metabolites

sary to manage abstinence syndrome after management of acute toxicity.

ETHANOL

Epidemiology. Alcohol is the most frequently encountered toxic constituent in poisonings. Alcohol includes methyl, wood, industrial, grain, ethyl, denatured, Columbia Spirit, all fusal oil, and methylated spirits, with ethanol predominating. As with the other sedative-hypnotics, the brain is the target organ. Ethanol exhibits a narrow therapeutic index. The level of 100 mg/dl represents "legally drunk" in most states; in a naive

Table 32-8
Glasgow Coma Scale

Observation		Score
Best motor response	Follows simple commands	6
	Pulls examiner's hand away when pinched	5
	Pulls part of body away when pinched	4
	Flexion to pain (decorticate)	3
	Rigid extension to pain (decerebrate)	2
	No motor response to pain	1
Best verbal response (arouse patient with pain if required)	Oriented and converses	5
	Confused or disoriented	4
	Inappropriate words	3
	Incomprehensible sounds	2
	No response	1
Eye opening	Spontaneous	4
	On verbal command	3
	To pain	2
	No response	1
	Total	3-15

drinker, respiratory arrest would be expected to occur at a level of 450 mg/dl. A level of 500 mg/dl corresponding to a dose of 3 g/kg of body weight distributed throughout the total body water will be lethal in about 50% of subjects. However, levels in excess of 780 mg/dl have been reported in tolerant individuals (38).

Pharmacology. Ethanol is rapidly and completely absorbed from the gastrointestinal tract and is distributed in the total body water (V_d 0.6 l/kg). The potentially lethal dose for an average (70 kg) man is 240 ml of absolute ethanol or 490 ml (about one pint) of 100-proof liquor (20). A quart or even a fifth ingested rapidly exceeds the estimated LD_{50}.

Ethanol is metabolized almost entirely by the liver. This process is half-saturated at a serum level of 10 mg/dl, and kinetics are thus described by the V_{max}, which is 7 mg/dl/hr. Thus, the rate of elimination is independent of drug level (zero-order process).

Treatment. Treatment is primarily supportive. Emesis (or lavage), activated charcoal, and saline cathartics should be used. The latter two substances are of value in preventing deeper intoxication if they are administered within 2 hr after ingestion of large amounts of alcohol. Contrary to popular belief, breathing oxygen-enriched air has no effect on ethanol kinetics. Intravenous fructose has reportedly increased ethanol metabolism by up to 25%, but because fructose induces nausea, vomiting, and possibly lactic acidosis, its use is not recommended (37). However, glucose must frequently be used to correct the resultant hypoglycemia.

BENZODIAZEPINES

VALIUM was the largest selling prescription drug, until recently supplanted by DYAZIDE, INDERAL, and TYLENOL - Codeine. It ranked fourth in the total number of prescriptions dispensed by retail pharmacies in 1983 (4). There is no known documented fatal overdose from oral diazepam or chlordiazepoxide alone, since the benzodiazepines have a large therapeutic index compared with other sedative-hypnotics.

A patient with an overdose of diazepam alone will almost always be arousable. Complications arising from benzodiazepines taken with other sedative-hypnotics are similar in frequency and severity to those for the other drug alone (31).

Management of pure benzodiazepine overdose consists of removal and support. More severe coma or other problems suggest another drug (e.g., alcohol) may be involved, and management should be directed at that agent.

SALICYLATES

Analgesics and antipyretics represent the medication category most frequently ingested as well as the most common drug-induced lethal poisoning. Lethal poisonings are most often associated with analgesics other than aspirin and acetaminophen. Aspirin is still the most common single agent ingested, but acetaminophen accounts for an increasing proportion of sales and poisonings. Many combination drugs contain salicylates. Oil of wintergreen (methylsalicylate) contains 1 g/ml of salicylate. Salicylism is not infrequent in the elderly and goes unrecognized in as many as 25% of the patients (38).

Aspirin is rapidly and completely absorbed from the gastrointestinal tract and is rapidly hydrolyzed to salicylic acid (half-life 16 minutes). Salicylate half-life is 15-30 hr in overdose, but urinary elimination may be increased 20-fold by raising the urine pH by one unit.

Clinical Effects. Tinnitus and impaired hearing are usually the earliest symptoms, followed by severe vomiting, hyperthermia, hypoglycemia (rarely hyperglycemia), convulsions, and coma. Salicylate is a direct respiratory stimulant, and respiratory alkalosis usually precedes the metabolic acidosis associated with salicylism. The major complications at high doses are pulmonary edema, hemorrhage, and renal failure.

Treatment. Treatment is based on dose. Some general guidelines:

<100 mg/kg: No treatment

>100 mg/kg: Ipecac, charcoal, and cathartic

>240 mg/kg: Ipecac, charcoal, and bring to emergency room

>360 mg/kg: Median lethal dose (LD_{50}), vigorous support, consider hemoperfusion.

Support of vital functions and minimization of absorption are the central strategy. Large doses may result in prolonged absorption (up to 8 hr). Comparison of blood levels (standard thresholds) with blood-level curves (the Done nomogram) provides an assessment of severity (45).

Alkalinization of urine to enhance elimination has been the stated objective of bicarbonate administration. Evidence now suggests the principal value of alkalinization is extracellular ion trapping (23). Sodium bicarbonate is an extracellular buffer and the drug of choice. Concomitant potassium administration (even though plasma K^+ may be near-normal value) is usually necessary to alkalinize the urine. Likewise, a urine to plasma pH gradient will favor salicylate excretion, but difficulty is often encountered in alkalinizing the urine in severely poisoned patients.

ACETAMINOPHEN

Acetaminophen has been widely advertised as safer than aspirin. It has long been popular in the United Kingdom (where it is known as paracetamol) and accounted for 1000 hospitalizations and 30 deaths per month in the late 1970s (24).

At normal doses, acetaminophen causes less gastrointestinal irritation and blood loss than an equivalent dose of aspirin. In overdose (42), or in patients with hepatic sensitization (2), hepatic injury ranging from transient enzyme elevation to fatal hepatic necrosis may occur.

Pharmacology. Most acetaminophen is conjugated in the liver to glucuronide (50%), or sulfate (40%), or excreted unchanged (6%). A small amount is metabolized via the P-450 mixed-function oxidase system to a reactive compound that is normally scavenged by hepatic glutathione stores. When these scavenging systems are overwhelmed, the reactive metabolite binds to sulfhydryl-rich macromolecules and causes centrilobular necrosis. Thus, acetaminophen toxicity will be increased in overdose, glutathione depletion, or increased P-450 activity. P-450 blockers and sodium sulfate (which enhances the sulfation process) have been shown to decrease toxicity in experimental animals. Acetaminophen represents a class of hepatotoxins for which the initial severity of symptoms (nausea, vomiting, abdominal pain) bears no relation to the ultimate severity of the poisoning (hepatocellular necrosis).

Treatment. Introduction of a sulfhydryl-rich, glutathione alternative to bind the active metabolite (since glutathione does not penetrate cells) is needed for treatment. N-acetylcysteine (NAC, MUCOMYST) appears to be an effective substitute for glutathione. Oral treatment with NAC has been tested in a multicenter study. Approximately 1800 patients have been followed in an evaluation of oral NAC. Its value seems clearly established if given within 10 hr of acetaminophen ingestion. Parenteral NAC also appears to be effective (54).

Serum acetaminophen levels in excess of 200 μg/ml at 4 hr postingestion often result in hepatotoxicity (57) and should be treated with NAC. If serum levels are not readily available, NAC treatment should be initiated for ingestions of more than 140 mg/kg and discontinued if levels rule out severe poisoning.

NARCOTICS

Narcotics include naturally occurring opiates (such as codeine and morphine) as well as synthetic and semisynthetic derivatives (such as propoxyphene and pentazocine). All of these compounds cause CNS depression and are antagonized by naloxone.

Epidemiology. Products containing codeine and propoxyphene are most often reported to poison control centers, although heroin and propoxyphene account for more emergency room visits and are involved most often in medical examiners' cases.

The toxicity of these compounds is an extension of their pharmacological effect. Toxic and lethal doses are highly variable due to individual differences (e.g., age) and tolerance. Methadone is considered to be lethal at a dose of 100 mg, but a fraction of that dose is potentially lethal to children, whereas a tolerant individual might survive 1000 mg.

Clinical Effects. Central nervous system depression, including respiratory depression, cyanosis, and any degree of coma may be present. Although a hallmark of narcotism is pinpoint pupils, the pupils may be dilated if meperidine has been taken, or if concomitant hypoxia is severe. Convulsions and pulmonary edema are not uncommon complications (26).

Treatment. Narcotics reduce the motility of the gastrointestinal tract; therefore, lavage (with airway protected), activated charcoal, and cathartics should be considered in a comatose patient, no matter how long since the exposure.

Naloxone, the antidote of choice, is a narcotic antagonist with virtually no contraindications. Due to the short half-life (1-1.5 hr), repeated doses may be required (50).

A therapeutic trial in an adult consists of 2 mg (5 ampules) naloxone i.v. with evaluation after 5 minutes and a repeat dose if response is absent or questionable. Propoxyphene and pentazocine may require doses of naloxone up to 4 or 5 mg (59).

ANTICHOLINERGICS

Although they differ in therapeutic indication and in toxicity, the tricyclic antidepressants (amitriptyline, imipramine), the phenothiazine tranquilizers (chlorpromazine), antihistamines (chlorpheniramine, diphenhydramine), the belladonna alkaloids (atropine, scopolamine), and antiparkinson drugs (trihexyphenidyl, benztropine), all share cholinergic-blocking activity. Poisoning with such agents can be life-threatening.

Epidemiology. In 1974, 24 million prescriptions were written for tricyclic antidepressants. Studies showed many patients failed to take the medication as instructed (40%), whereas others abused it seeking a euphoric state (25%) (17). The National Poison Center Network, received 1626 tricyclics reports in 1978 (1% of all reports), of which amitriptyline accounted for over one-half. A common cause of poisoning from belladonna alkaloids is from abuse of plants (jimson weed) and drugs to achieve a "high" (39).

Clinical Effects. Most untoward effects associated with cholinergic-blocking agents are manifestations of their pharmacological actions and generally dose related. They can be divided into central and peripheral effects. Central effects include hyperactivity, disorientation, anxiety, delirium, hallucinations, convulsions, nausea, vomiting, coma, medullary paralysis, and death. Peripheral effects may include mydriasis, xerostomia, dysphagia, thirst, tachycardia, vasodilatation, hyperpyrexia, hypotension or hypertension, urinary retention, decreased gastrointestinal motility, decreased secretions, leukocytosis, rash (face and upper trunk), and respiratory arrest.

The anticholinergic syndrome has been characterized as:

> "Hot as a fire, Red as a beet,
> Dry as a bone, Blind as a bat,
> and Mad as a hatter"

Treatment. Treatment can be successful if the diagnosis is correct and the patient has not suffered anoxia or other adverse effects. The peripheral and central nervous system effects can be reversed by judicious use of sodium bicarbonate in life-threatening cases and physostigmine in addition to aggressive measures to support life and prevent or treat shock. Specific indications for physostigmine are convulsions, severe hallucinations, hypertension, and cardiac arrhythmias. Although coma can be reversed by physostigmine, it should not be used merely to keep the patient awake. For adolescents and adults a therapeutic trial consists of 2 mg given slowly (over 2 minutes). A second dose of 1-2 mg may be given in 20 minutes if no reversal has occurred. A therapeutic dose is the smallest dose that produces reversal and should be repeated as often as life-threatening symptoms recur. Physostigmine is metabolized within 30-60 minutes, and repeated doses may be necessary; however, a continuous drip should not be used.

Contraindications to the use of full doses of physostigmine include asthma, gangrene, cardiovascular disease, and mechanical obstruction of the gastrointestinal or urogenital tracts. Under these conditions one-fourth to one-half the usual dose should be used, with caution. Cardiac monitoring is essential. Tricyclics exert a quinidine-like cardiac toxicity that may require intervention with antiarrhythmic drugs (lidocaine or phenytoin), electrical cardioversion, or both. However, alkalinization of blood (pH 7.5) and physostigmine frequently lead to spontaneous conversion.

INSECTICIDES

Insecticides comprise about 3.5% of poisonings reported to the NCPCC. Insecticides may be grouped according to toxicity and treatment into:

1. Organophosphates (e.g., malathion, parathion)
2. Carbamates (e.g., SEVIN)
3. Pyrethrums and related compounds
4. Halogenated hydrocarbons (e.g., DDT)

Pyrethrine compounds are generally present in such small amounts that except for possible irritation and dermatological reactions, they are relatively innocuous. The halogenated compounds have lost favor as insecticides due to their persistence in the soil and carcinogenic potential. From an acute toxicity perspective, they are much safer than the organophosphates. Largely due to the banning of DDT and similar compounds, the use of more toxic and less persistent organophosphates has increased.

Organophosphate poisoning produces cholinergic overdrive or the SLUDE syndrome (salivation, lacrimation, urination, defecation, and emesis); respiratory paralysis represents the major complication. Red blood cell cholinesterase is decreased in acute or chronic poisoning. Atropine, the antidote of choice, reverses most parasympathetic symptoms, but is not effective in overcoming block at the myoneural junction. Pralidoxime (2-PAM) is a useful adjunct to atropine but is ineffective for carbamates. Pralidoxime should not be used alone.

HYDROCARBONS

Hydrocarbons include petroleum distillates (kerosene, gasoline, and so on), alkylbenzenes (benzene, toluene, xylene, and so on), and others.

For many years the treatment of hydrocarbon ingestions consisted of gastric lavage and symptomatic and supportive care. Steroids and antibiotics were employed prophylactically. Induced emesis was contraindicated. More recently, there has been a trend toward induced emesis when evacuation of the stomach is deemed necessary.

Green (30) studied 116 cases of hydrocarbon ingestion (1969-1974) and found 68% incidence of clinical pneumonia. He found no statistical difference between those that did and did not vomit, and no difference in complications between the lavaged and nonlavaged groups.

Ng et al. (49) compared pretreatment and posttreatment radiographs in 255 hydrocarbon ingestions over a 5 year period. Persistent or worsened pneumonitis occurred in 19% of the ipecac-induced emesis group versus 39% for a lavage group. Thus, available objective data seem to favor ipecac over cautious gastric lavage in the treatment of uncomplicated hydrocarbon ingestion.

The target organ of hydrocarbons is the lung. Aspiration from gagging and choking may cause coughing, cyanosis, and other signs of respiratory distress. Pneumonitis, pulmonary edema, pneumatocele, and pneumothorax are potential consequences. Radiographs are useful in the diagnosis but are not foolproof.

Some of the individual hydrocarbons, as well as the hydrocarbons mixed with toxic substances (e.g., solvent for pesticides), have significant systemic toxicity and affect other organs. However, for most hydrocarbon ingestions, the prevailing opinion is to empty the stomach only if systemic toxicity is anticipated (1 ml/kg for gasoline or kerosene). Prophylactic antibiotics and steroids have no place in the treatment of hydrocarbon ingestions.

PLANTS

Epidemiology. The increasing popularity of house plants has been followed by an increase in the number of contacts reported. Plants account for about 10% of reports from poison control centers (see Table 32-2). Most exposures occur among 1- and 2-year-old children (64). Mushrooms comprise only 1% of all reports from poison centers, but are associated with significant morbidity and mortality. The deadly amanita (*Amanita phalloides*) accounts for about 95% of all fatal mushrooms poisonings.

Symptoms. If present, symptoms are usually gastrointestinal. The possibility for foreign-body blockage of the airway is ever present. Any plant, especially those with fibrous leaves, has the potential for moderate-to-severe intoxications. The raphide (needle-like) structure of calcium oxalate crystals appears to be the cause of local irritation, swelling, and edema from plants such as dieffenbachia (dumb cane) and rhubarb (36).

A useful (but not foolproof) rule of thumb for mushroom poisoning is that if the patient begins vomiting within 6 hr after ingestion, complete recovery with no sequelae is likely. If the vomiting begins after 6 hr, one should suspect a severe poisoning. It should be obvious that treatment should not be based on a rule of thumb, but on a careful history, identification of the mushroom by mycologists whenever possible, and symptoms. "There are old mushroom eaters; there are bold mushroom eaters; but there are no old, bold mushroom eaters".

Treatment. Home treatment with syrup of ipecac and observation for ingesting and irrigation or washing for contact can be employed in most plant exposures. Severe intoxications should be referred to a hospital emergency department. The beliefs that boiling mushrooms renders them nontoxic or that atropine is the antidote for mushroom poisoning have both been discounted. Atropine is useful when indicated to counteract cholinergic symptoms. Symptomatic and supportive treatment is the therapeutic mainstay. Hemodialysis is employed for some intoxications (e.g., *Amanita phalloides*).

CYANIDE/LAETRILE

Epidemiology. Cyanide is discussed here since it is an uncommon, but none-the-less important source of morbidity and mortality in humans and because it represents a severe and treatable poisoning. Commercial uses of cyanide include fumigation, metal polishes, electroplating solutions, and in photographic processes. It occurs in plants including the cassava bean, twigs and especially seeds from wild cherries, plums, peaches, apples, pears, and apricots.

Laetrile. Laetrile is a common name for amygdalin, which is particularly common in almonds, apricot pits, yew, and appleseeds. Amygdalin has been employed medically for centuries as a treatment for drunkenness and hemorrhoids. It was first marketed as laetrile in 1950 as a cure for cancer. The astounding public acceptance of this compound has resulted in its legalization in about half of the 50 states and use in 50,000 patients per year (33).

A multicenter clinical trial of amygdalin (laetrile) involving 178 patients revealed NO SUBSTANTIVE BENEFIT that could be attributed to the treatment. Several patients with symptoms of cyanide toxicity or blood cyanide levels approaching the lethal range attested to the hazards of amygdalin therapy (44). Although scientifically sound, such results have not closed the book on the laetrile story.

Amygdalin, itself practically nontoxic, is converted to cyanide via β-glucosidase. This enzyme, present in almonds, fruits, and vegetables, exibits greater activity in an alkaline medium. Thus, the cyanide production from the activity of β- glucosidase on amygdalin represents much more of a risk to the patient taking amygdalin orally.

Nitroprusside. Use of the direct-acting vasodilator, nitroprusside, carries the risk of cyanide toxicity, particularly when used in high doses in patients with compromised renal function. The nitroprusside molecules (not the metabolites) account for the hypotensive action, and each molecule contains 5 cyanide (CN) groups. The nitroprusside molecule rapidly breaks down releasing all 5 CN^- ions via nonenzymatic reaction with free and intracellular hemoglobin producing (a) methemoglobin from oxidation of hemoglobin iron (Fe^{2+} to Fe^{3+}) and (b) an unstable nitroprusside free radical. One of the CN^- ions reacting with the methemoglobin forms a less toxic metabolite, cyanmethemoglobin. The four remaining CN^- ions are formed into thiocyanates (SCN^-), which are also less toxic metabolites.

Mechanism of Toxicity. Cyanide inhibits hematin compounds, most importantly cytochrome oxidase. Catalase, peroxidase, and methemoglobin are also inhibited as well as the nonhematin compounds tyrosinase, xanthine oxidase, and lactic dehydrogenase.

Cyanide is extremely well absorbed via the skin, inhalation, or gastrointestinal tract. Cyanide metabolism involves vitamin B_{12} via several pathways, but the major route is via thiocyanate involving rhodanase with thiosulfate as the substrate.

The oft-cited bitter almond odor associated with cyanide cannot be appreciated by 20-40% of the population due to a sex- linked recessive genetic defect. Laboratory tests are available for determination of cyanide or thiocyanate, but treatment must not be delayed for laboratory evaluation.

Clinical effects of this cellular asphyxiation include dryness of the mouth, burning of the throat, and air hunger leading to hyperpnea. Apnea, seizures, and cardiovascular collapse will follow quickly in severe cyanide poisoning.

Treatment. Basic life-support measures, and in particular oxygen, represent the first line of treatment for cyanide overdose. A cyanotic patient who does not 'pink up' with adequate oxygenation should be considered cyanide poisoned until proven otherwise. The differential between the methemoglobinemia of nitrite or nitrate poisoning and cyanmethemoglobin of cyanide intoxication must usually be determined based on history. Otherwise, a simple rapid examination of a spot of blood for the chocolate brown color of methemoglobinemia may be adequate.

Cobalt salts have been used for more than 75 years as chelators of cyanide. They are still not routinely available for treatment of cyanide intoxication, but nitrates and thiosulfate (Lilly cyanide antidote kit) are usually effective for those who reach the emergency department (ED) alive. Every emergency department should stock two or more cyanide treatment kits. Amyl nitrite should be started with oxygen therapy, and patient should inhale for 30 seconds out of each minute. As soon as available, sodium nitrate 0.35 ml/kg should be given i.v., followed by sodium thiosulfate 1.6 ml/kg i.v. This regimen should be repeated in 20 minutes if symptoms persist. Diazepam represents the first-line drug for treatment of persistent seizures. An exchange transfusion may be considered for persistent excessive methemoglobinemia.

REFERENCES

1. Afifi, A.A., Sacks, S.T., Liu, V.Y. et al. A cumulative prognostic index for patients with barbiturate, glutethimide and meprobamate intoxication. *N. Engl. J. Med.* 285:1497, 1971.
2. Anonymous: Acetaminophen hepatotoxicity. *Med. Lett.* 20:61, 1978.
3. Anonymous: Total number of Rx's slumps again for the 4th year in a row. *Pharm. Times* 44:41, 1978.
4. Anonymous: Top 200 drug products account for 68.1% of all Rxs. *Pharm. Times* 27:34, 1984.
5. Arena, J.M. Poisoning. *Emergency Med.* 8:171, 1976.
6. Arena, J.M. First treatment for poisoning. In: *Poisoning Toxicology, Symptoms, Treatment,* 4th ed. Springfiled, Ill.:Charles C Thomas, 1979.
7. Armstrong, G., Fow, M. and Veltri, J. Poisoning: Epidemiology and prevention. *Family Commun. Health* 6(3):41, 1983.
8. Berg, M.J., Berlinger, W.G., Goldberg, M.J. et al. Acceleration of the body clearance of phenobarbital by oral activated charcoal. *N. Engl. J. Med.* 307:642, 1982.
9. Berlinger, W.G., Spector, R., Goldberg, M.T. et al. Enhancement of theophylline clearance by oral activated charcoal. *Clin. Pharmacol. Ther.* 33:351, 1983.
10. Bishop, R.L. and Weisfeldt, M.L. Sodium bicarbonate administration during cardiac arrest. *JAMA* 235:506, 1976.
11. Boxer, L., Anderson, F.P. and Rowe, D.S. Comparison of ipecac-induced emesis with gastric lavage in the treatment of acute salicylate ingestion. *Pediatrics* 74:800, 1969.
12. Braico, K.T., Humbeert, J.R., Terplan, K.L. and Lehotay, J.M. Laetrile intoxication: Report of a fatal case. *N. Eng. J. Med.* 300:236, 1979.
13. Bukis, D. and Kuwahara, L. Results of forcing fluids: Pre-versus post-ipecac. *Vet. Hum. Toxicol.* 20:90, 1978.
14. Chenouth, R.W. and Czajka, P.A. N-acetylcysteine adsorption by activated charcoal. *Vet. Hum. Toxicol.* 22:392, 1980.
15. Chin, L. Gastrointestinal dilution of poisons with water - an irrational and potentially harmful procedure. *Am. J. Hosp. Pharm.* 28:712, 1971.
16. Clemmesen, C. and Nilsson, E. Therapeutic trends in the treatment of barbiturate poisoning - the Scandinavian method. *Clin. Pharmacol. Ther.* 2:220, 1961.
17. Cohen, M.J., Handbury, R. and Handbury, S. Abuse of amitriptyline. *JAMA* 240:1372, 1978.
18. Curtis, R.A., Barone, J. and Giacona, N. Efficacy of ipecac and activated charcoal/cathartic: Prevention of salicylate absorption in a simulated overdose. *Arch. Intern. Med.* 144:48, 1984.
19. Daly, J.S. and Cooney, D.O. Interference by tannic acid with the effectiveness of activated charcoal in 'universal antidote'. *Clin. Toxicol.* 12:515, 1978.
20. David, D.J., and Spyker, D.A. The acute toxicity of ethanol -dosage and kinetic nomograms. *Vet. Hum. Toxicol.* 21:272, 1979.
21. Decker, W.J. In quest of emesis: fact, fable, and fancy. *Clin. Toxicol.* 4:383, 1971.
22. Doffler, A., Bernstein, M., LaSette, A. et al. Fixed- bed charcoal hemoperfusion treatment of drug overdose. *Arch. Intern. Med.* 138:1691, 1978.
23. Done, A.K. Aspirin revisited. *Emergency Med.* 9:151, 1977.
24. Douglas, A.P., Hamlyn, A.N. and James, O. Controlled trial of cysteamine in treatment of acute paracetamol (acetaminophen) poisoning. *Lancet* 1:111, 1976.
25. Ellwood, M.G. and Robb, G.H. Self-poisoning with colchicine. *Postgrad. Med. J.* 47:129, 1971.
26. Frand, et al. Methadone-induced pulmonary edema. *Ann. Intern. Med.* 76:975, 1972.
27. Gallagher, S., Guyer, B., Kotelchuck, M. et al. A strategy for the reduction of childhood injuries in Massachusetts: SCIPP. *N. Engl. J. Med.* 307:1015, 1982.
28. Goldberg, A.H. Current concepts - cardiopulmonary arrest. *N. Eng. J. Med.* 290:381, 1974.
29. Goldfrank, L. and Osborn, H. The barbiturate overdose. *Hosp. Phys.* Sept. 30, 1977.
30. Green, V.A. *Petroleum distillates. Bulletin.* Bethesda, MD: National Clearinghouse for Poison Control Centers, May-June, 1976.
31. Greenblatt, D.J., Allen, M.D., Noel, B.J. et al. Acute overdosage with benzodiazepine derivatives. *Clin. Pharmacol. Ther.* 21:497, 1977.
32. Henderson, J.L., Picchioni, A.L. and Chin, L. Evaluation of oral dilution as a first aid measure in poisoning. *J. Pharmacol. Sci.* 55:1311, 1966.
33. Herbert, V. Laetrile: The cult of cyanide promoting poison for profit. *Am. J. Clin. Nutr.* 32:1121, 1979.
34. Horwitz, J.P., Hills, E.B., Andrezejewski, D. et al. Adjunct hospital emergency toxicology service - a model for a metropolitan area. *JAMA* 235:1708, 1976.
35. Jenis, E.H., Payne, R.J. and Goldbaum, L.R. Acute meprobamate poisoning a fatal case followed by a lucid interval. *JAMA* 201:361, 1969.

36. Lampe, K. *Plant dermatitis. Symposium of Poisonous Plants in Urban and Suburban Environment*. New York: Albert Einstein School of Medicine and N.Y. Botanical Gardens, April, 1978.
37. Levy, R., Elo, T. and Hanenson, I.B. Intravenous fructose treatment of acute alcohol intoxication. *Arch. Intern. Med.* 137:1175, 1977.
38. Lindbald, B. and Olsson, R. Unusually high levels of blood alcohol. *JAMA* 236:1600, 1976.
39. Mahler, D.A. Anticholinergic poisoning from jimson weed. *JACEP* 5:440, 1976.
40. Micik, S. Establishment of a regional poison center. *Clin. Toxicol.* 13:587, 1978.
41. Micik, S. *Developing Regional Poison Systems*. Washington, D.C.: Health, Education Welfare, HRA 232- 78-0173, 1979.
42. Mitchell, J.R., Jollow, D.J., Potter, W.Z. et al. Acetaminophen induced hapatic necrosis. I. Role of drug metabolism. *J. Pharmacol. Exp. Ther.* 187:185, 1973.
43. Moertel, C.G., Ames, M.M., Kovach, J.S. et al. A pharmacologic and toxicological study of amygdalin. *JAMA* 245:591, 1981.
44. Moertel, C.G., Fleming, T.R., Rubin, J.R. et al. A clinical trial of amygdalin (laetrile) in the treatment of human cancer. *N. Engl. J. Med.* 306:201, 1982.
45. Moriarty, R.W. Regionalization: The Pittsburgh experience. *Clin. Toxicol.* 12:271, 1978.
46. Morse, D.L., Boros, L. and Findley, P.A. More on cyanide poisoning from laetrile. *N. Engl. J. Med.* 301:892, 1979.
47. *National Prescription Audit*. IMS America Ltd., 1983.
48. Nelson, R., Fow, M., Brancato, D. et al. Poisoning among children - United States. *MMWR* 33(10):129, 1984.
49. Ng, R.C., Darwish, H. and Steward, D.A. Emergency treatment of petroleum distillate and turpentine ingestion. *Can. Med. Assoc. J.* 111:537, 1974.
50. Ngai, S.H. et al. Pharmacokinetics of naloxone in rats and in man. *Anesthesiology* 44:398, 1976.
51. North, D.S., Peterson, R.G. and Drezelok, E.P. Effect of activated charcoal administration on acetylcysteine serum levels in humans. *Am. J. Hosp. Pharm.* 38:1022, 1981.
52. Papadopoulou, Z.L. and Novello, A.C. The use of hemoperfusion in children past, present, and future. *Pediatr. Clin. North Am.* 29:1039, 1982.
53. Picchoni, A.L., Chin, A. and Gillespie, T. Evaluation of activated charcoal-sorbitol suspension as an antidote. *J. Clin. Toxicol.* 19:433, 1982.
54. Prescott, L.F., Illingworth, R.N., Critchley, J.A. et al. Intravenous n-acetylcysteine: the treatment of choice for paracetamol poisoning. *Br. Med. J.* 2:1097, 1979.
55. Rauber, A. The cardiac safety of ipecac used as a therapeutic emetic. *Vet. Hum. Toxicol.* 20:166, 1978.
56. Rubino, M.J., Davidoff, F., Baselt, R. and Fletterick, C. Cyanide poisoning from apricot seeds: Case report and review of the literature. *Ann. Meeting Prog. AACTAAPCC,* Louisiana, 1978.
57. Rumack, B.H., and Matthew, H. Acetaminophen poisoning and toxicity. *Pediatrics* 55:871, 1975.
58. Rumack, B.H. and Temple, A.R. Lomotil poisoning. *Pediatrics* 53:495, 1974.
59. Rumack, B.H., Temple, A., Becker, C.H. et al. *Poisindex.* Denver, Col.:Micromedex, 1979.
60. Sadoff, L., Fuchs, K. and Hollander, J. Rapid death associated with laetrile ingestion. *JAMA.* 239:1532, 1978.
61. Scherz, R.G., and Robertson, W.O. The history of poison control centers in the United States. *Clin. Toxicol.* 12:291, 1978.
62. Shubin, H. and Weil, M.H. The mechanism of shock following suicidal doses of barbiturates, narcotics and tranquilizer drugs, with observations on the effects of treatment. *Am. J. Med.* 38:853, 1965.
63. Smith, F.P., Butler, T.P.,Cohan, S. and Schein, P.S. Laetrile toxicity: A report of two cases. *JAMA* 238:1361, 1977.
64. Spoerke, D.G., and Temple, A.R. One year's experience with potential plant poisonings reported to the intermountain regional poison control center. *Vet. Hum. Toxicol.* 20:85, 1978.
65. Stern, T., Mulley, A., and Tibault, G. Life-threatening drug overdose. *JAMA* 251(15):1983, 1984.
66. Taylor, G.J., Tucker, W.M., Greene, H.L. et al. Importance of prolonged compression during cardiopulmonary resuscitation in man. *N. Engl. J. Med.* 296:1515, 1977.
67. Teasdale, G. and Jennett, B. Assessment of coma and impaired consciousness: A practical scale. *Lancet* 2:81, 1974.
68. Thompson, W.L., Dayton, H.E. and Sunshine, I. Adsorbent and cathartic interactions with drugs *in vitro* and *in vivo*. In: *Pharmacology-Toxicology Symposium.* Bethesda, MD:National Institutes of Health, 1977, p. 57.
69. Wick, A.N., Almen, M.C. and Joseph, L. The metabolism of sorbitol. *J. Am. Pharm. Assoc.* 40:542, 1951.

CHAPTER
33

MEDICAL DIAGNOSTIC AGENTS

Roger P. Maickel

The use of diagnostic agents is of great importance in clinical medicine and requires an extensive presentation of materials and technology far beyond the scope of this textbook. Accordingly, this chapter combines an introduction to the knowledge of such agents with an overview of their pharmacology and uses. The reader who wishes detailed information should consult the general references listed at the end of the chapter.

Basically, the term *diagnostic agents* refers to specific chemicals used to aid the physician in making a rational and accurate diagnosis of an abnormal or pathological state of an organism. For practical considerations, all of the agents so used can be divided into five categories, each of which can be generally described as presented in Table 33-1.

RADIOISOTOPES I

These agents are used to determine body function(s) by virtue of their ability to act as tracers, i.e., to permit knowledge to be gained of body functions or malfunctions through procedures involving quantitative measurements of specific chemical entities. The types of studies using these agents can be subdivided into two categories: dilution and kinetics. The first category, *dilution* studies, involves procedures in which a known amount of radiolabeled material is administered and, after sufficient time has elapsed for equilibrium to be achieved, the degree of dilution of the radioisotope in the total compartmental volume is determined. Procedures of this type can be useful in determining compartments such as total blood volume, plasma volume, or extracellular fluid volume; variations on this technique can be useful in determining the survival or turnover time of erythrocytes.

The second type of studies is often referred to as *kinetic* or *excretion* studies because measurements made are of the relative amount of a radiolabeled substance that is absorbed by or excreted from the body over a standardized time period. The basic procedure involves administration of a known dose of a radiolabeled material, followed by the determination of the levels of the substance and/or metabolites (over time) in blood and excreting routes such as expired air, bile, feces, and urine. Studies

Table 33-1
Categories of Agents Used in Diagnostic Medicine

Radioisotopes I	agents used in dilution or kinetic studies
Radioisotopes II	agents used in localization or scanning studies
Radiopaque agents	agents used to facilitate X-ray examinations
Diagnostic chemicals	agents used to determine organ function
Diagnostic drugs	agents used to test for specific disease states by virtue of pharmacological actions

of this type are useful in the determination of renal and hepatic function, iron absorption and distribution, vitamin B_{12} absorption, and intestinal absorption processes in general. In addition, this type of study can be used, in a quasidiagnostic maneuver, to examine the rate(s) and/or route(s) of metabolism of drugs or endogenous compounds *in vivo* as a possible indication of some abnormal or pathological state.

RADIOISOTOPES II

These are agents that permit the measurement of the radionuclide to be made by direct determination of the radiation it emits from the body, i.e., without the necessity for removing blood or collecting samples of excretory materials. By using an external, noninvasive measuring device (such as an appropriate γ-counting system) it is possible to determine the localization or uptake of a selected ion or compound into a particular site, tissue, or organ. Supplementation of the actual measuring device with appropriate computerized systems for quantitation and/or imaging permits visual characterization of the structure or function of organs, systems, or tumors. Examples of such procedures include scanning of bone, brain, liver, lung, kidney, spleen, and thyroid, as well as examination of iodine uptake by the thyroid gland. In some cases, whole body counting is used to measure the radioactivity present in the entire body; through these procedures make for a minimal resolution of spatial localization, they can be used to determine the overall retention of substances in the body and find applications in the characterization of genetic abnormalities such as potassium content in muscular dystrophy as well as iron absorption and retention.

A summary of specific isotopes used as diagnostic tools and some examples of their applications is presented in Table 33-2.

RADIOPAQUE AGENTS

The largest single use of diagnostic agents is in the area of substances that facilitate X-ray diagnosis by visualizing specific body organs or systems through an ability to absorb X-radiation. These agents, also known as *contrast media*, may be subdivided into two classes: barium salts and iodine-containing compounds.

Barium Salts. The use of one specific barium salt, namely $BaSO_4$, dates back at least 70 years. The extremely low water solubility of this compound ($<$ 3 mg/l at 25°C), its low systemic toxicity on oral administration (probably due to poor absorption), and its lack of osmotic activity even when given as a thick suspension, make it the agent of choice for X-ray studies of the gastrointestinal tract. Depending on the area to be examined, the barium sulfate preparation can be given p.o. as a paste or thick cream (esophageal studies) or as a suspension of the consistency of milk (gastric or small intestine studies). Alternatively, the latter formulation can be given as a retention enema to visualize the colon. The opacity of the material permits study of gastrointestinal tract contours; time-delay radiograms can demonstrate motility phenomena; after passage from the stomach or colon, a residual "coating" may remain that is sufficient to permit further studies.

Barium sulfate, USP, is generally given in a total dosage of $\leq$ 300 g, p.o. or $\leq$ 360 g by rectal enema. The USP preparation has a maximum particle size limitation and virtually no toxicity. Although a possible hazard exists from respiratory aspiration or leakage through an esophageal fistula or gastrointestinal perforation, the relatively innocuous nature of the substance gives a high safety potential.

Iodine-Containing Compounds. Iodine-containing organic compounds, with a diversity of chemical structures, are the most widely used radiopaque agents for X-ray diagnostic efforts. A selected number of these agents, as presented in Figure 33-1, provides examples of structural diversity rather than an all-inclusive listing. Depending on the physicochemical and pharmacokinetic properties unique to a particular structure, the diagnostic application is often relatively specific. Table 33-3 presents a summary listing of the currently accepted uses for iodinated diagnostic agents.

Urinary System. The urinary system may be examined by intravenous or retrograde pyelography. In the former, the radiopaque agent is given by i.v. administration and, after excretion by the kidneys, can be seen in those organs, the ureters, and the urinary bladder within a relatively short time. In retrograde studies, the agent is instilled through catheters placed in a ureter or into the urinary bladder. Compounds useful for urinary tract diagnostic procedures should be readily soluble in water, should not be bound to plasma proteins, and should be res-

Table 33-2
Examples of Use of Radioisotopes in Diagnostic Medical Procedures

Isotope	Form	Application(s)
^{22}Na	sodium chloride	studies of electrolytes
^{42}K	potassium chloride	potassium space determination
^{51}Cr	sodium chromate	blood volume, RBC survival time
^{59}Co	cyanocobalamin	absorption of vitamin B_{12}
^{99m}Tc	sodium pertechnetate	scanning of brain
^{125}I	various forms	total body water, lung and thyroid scanning, liver and renal function
^{197}Hg	chloromerodrin	scanning of kidney and brain
^{3}H	drugs	metabolism/disposition/kinetics
^{14}C	drugs	metabolism/disposition/kinetics
^{35}S	drugs	metabolism/disposition/kinetics

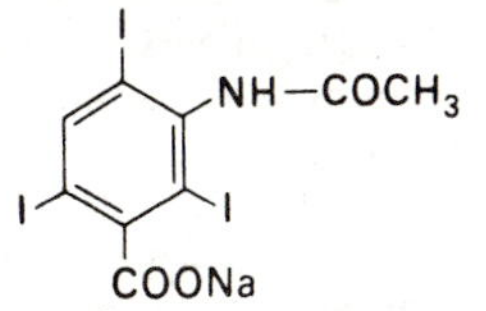

Sodium acetrizoate

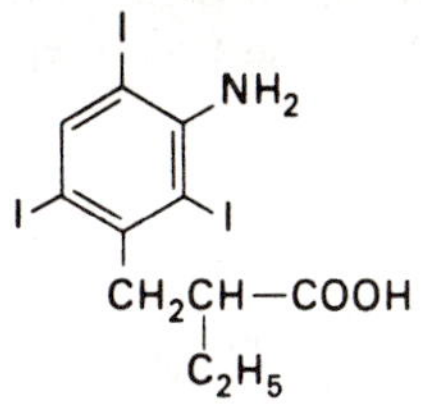

Iopanoic acid

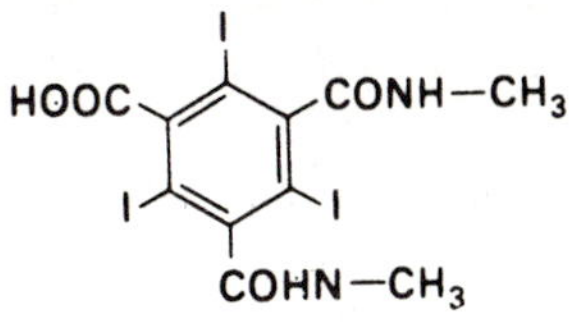

Iothalamic acid

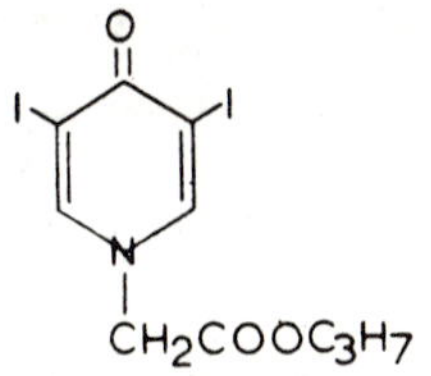

Propyliodone

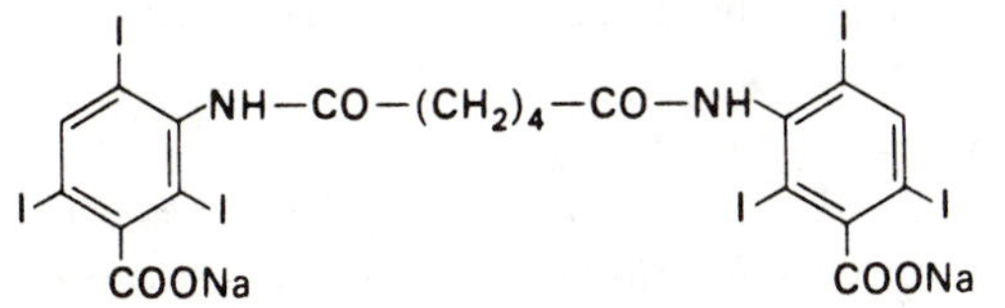

Sodium iodipamide; iodipamide meglumine

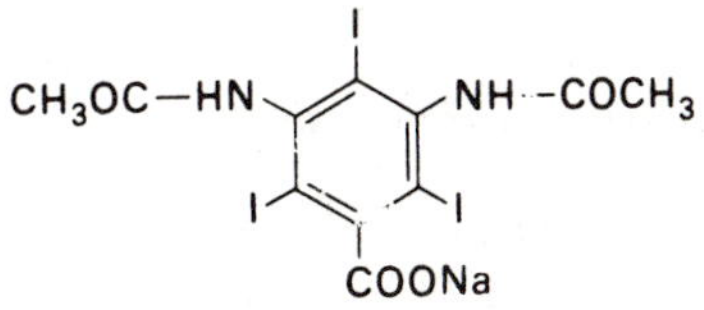

Sodium diatrizoate

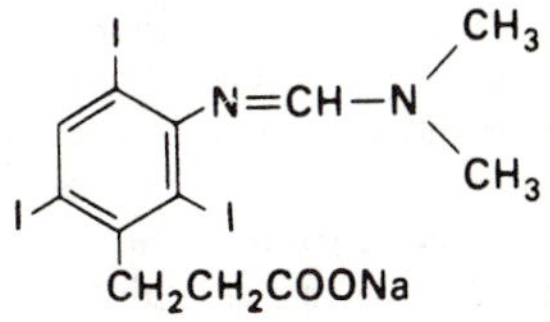

Sodium ipodate

Fig. 33-1: *Structures of common iodinated radiopaque agents.*

Table 33-3
Examples of Iodinated Radiopaque Agents and Their Uses

Substance	Use(s)	Formulation/Dosage
Acetrizoate sodium		
(CYSTOKLON)	cystography	30% sol.
(PYRELOKON-R)	retrograde pyelography	20% sol.
Diatrizoate		
(CARDIOGRAFIN)	angiocardiography	85% sol., 40-50 ml
	thoracic angiography	85% sol., 15-20 ml
(GASTROGRAFIN)	alimentary tract	76% sol., 30-90 ml
(RENOGRAFIN-60)	excretory urography	60% sol., 25 ml
(RENOVIST)	excretory urography	69% sol., 25 ml
(RENOGRAFIN-30)	retrograde pyelography	30% sol.
Iodipamide		
(CHOLOGRAFIN)	cholangiography	20-50% sol., 20-40 ml, i.v.
	cholecystography	20-50% sol., 20-40 ml, i.v.
Iopanoic acid		
(TELEPAQUET)	cholecystography	2-6 g, p.o.
Iothalamate		
(CONRAY-400)	excretory urography	66.8% sol., 25 ml
	angiography	66.8% sol., 1 ml/kg
	angiocardiography	66.8% sol., 40-50 ml
(ANGIO-CONRAY)	angiography	80% sol., 1 ml/kg
	angiocardiography	80% sol., 40-50 ml
(CONRAY)	excretory urography	60% sol., 25-30 ml
	direct cerebral angiography	60% sol., 35-50 ml
	retrograde brachial cerebral angiography	60% sol., 35-50 ml
	other angiography	60% sol., 20-40 ml
Ipodate		
(ORAGRAFIN)	cholangiography	
	cholecystography	3 g, p.o.
Propyliodone		
(DIONOSIL)	bronchiography	suspension in peanut oil by intratracheal injection at a dose of 0.75 ml/year of age to a maximum of 18 ml

tricted in distribution to the extracellular fluid space. They should have maximal tubular secretion and minimal tubular reabsorption as well as minimal osmotic activity.

Biliary System. The biliary system, on the other hand, requires a different set of characteristics if it is to be satisfactorily examined. The route of passage of these agents, from blood to liver to bile, is of necessity a slow process. Therefore, the desirable agent for cholecystography is one that is highly bound to plasma proteins, poorly filtered by the glomerulus, reabsorbed and not actively secreted in the tubules, and biotransformed to compounds such as glucuronides that will be excreted largely through biliary secretory pathways. The agents may be given i.v. or, if well absorbed from the gastrointestinal tract, p.o.

Circulatory System. The circulatory system may be examined by using angiography with intravenous or, in carefully selected cases because of the high risk involved, intra-arterial administration of iodinated radiopaque agents. The agents and procedures involved are highly technologically specific.

Respiratory Tract. The respiratory tract can be visualized with suitable iodinated radiopaque agents. The agent of choice is propyliodone administered as a suspension in olive oil. Although not completely without hazard, this preparation has largely supplanted the iodized oils first used in bronchography.

Several other highly specialized diagnostic procedures also make use of iodine-containing radiopaque agents; these are specialty uses that belong to the province of radiological medicine. As with all medical procedures and with administration of any foreign organic compound into the body, there is a significant risk associated with the use of the iodine-containing radiopaque agents. The problems associated with these agents may be divided into three categories:

1. Interference with diagnostic laboratory tests for thyroid function is not a direct risk, although the long half-life of the radiopaque agents in the body makes valid use of thyroid function tests impossible for as long as six to nine months. The radiopaque agents are highly bound to plasma proteins; they also interfere with inorganic-organic iodine exchange processes.
2. A second and more serious problem of these agents is their ability to produce, in some individuals, an idiosyncratic allergic reaction. The magnitude of the allergic response ranges from a modest hay fever type syndrome to one of full-blown anaphylactic shock. The response may be induced by radiopaque agents given by any route (i.v. or p.o.), and may or may not require a prior sensitization episode. In fact, patients responsive on their first exposure to iodine-containing radiopaque agents may not respond to subsequent exposures.
3. The most severe adverse effect of these agents is that observed in a very few patients who respond to a single exposure with major toxic symptoms: dizziness, nausea and vomiting, cyclic changes in blood pressure, mental confusion, cyanosis, and even loss of consciousness and death. This type of toxic reaction has been considered to involve damage, expressed in both function and morphology, of parenchymal cells in a variety of organs.

DIAGNOSTIC CHEMICALS

More than 40 years ago, the *Quick test* was established as a procedure to determine the functional status of the liver. The procedure was a simple one: The patient was given a dose of benzoic acid and the rate of urinary excretion of hippuric acid (benzoylglycine) was determined. This type of procedure, one that does not involve a pharmacological agent and a consequent pharmacological response, is the model for the class of diagnostic agents to be discussed in this section; they are listed in Table 33-4.

Cardiac Function. Agents for the study of cardiac function include those for determination of parameters such as blood volume and cardiac output. The first of these to be put to successful clinical use (more than 40 years ago) was Evans blue. This compound, a highly water-soluble, high-molecular-weight (961), relatively stable compound, is virtually completely bound to plasma albumin (> 40 μg/ml of plasma). In humans, the rate of plasma decline is less than 10% per hour initially; the later exponential phase has a half-life of greater than 15 days. Although it can be readily measured in plasma by visible absorption (620-625 nm), the accuracy of the measurement is influenced by the degree of oxygen saturation of the blood. The only side effect reported in humans, in any significant number of instances, is that of a blue-green tinge to the skin.

Table 33-4
Examples of Diagnostic Chemicals and Their Uses

Substance	Use(s)	Formulation/Dosage
p-Aminohippurate (PAH)	Renal function	Sterile sol. 2g/10 ml at alkaline pH; dose to plasma concentrations of 10-20 mg/l (renal plasma flow) or 400-600 mg/l (tubular secretion rate)
Evans Blue	Blood volume	Single-dose ampules containing 25 mg (5.0 ml of 0.5% sol.) for i.v. injection
Indocyanine Green (CARDIO-GREEN)	Cardiac, hepatic function	Sterile powder (25 or 50 mg vials) to be freshly dissolved in sterile coater; i.v. administration at 0.15 mg/kg (hepatic function) or 5 mg/kg(cardiac output)
Inulin	Renal function	Sterile ampules containing 5.0 g in 50 ml at slightly alkaline pH; i.v. injection of 100 ml (10 ml/min)
Sulfobromophthalein (BROMSULPHALEIN, BSP)	Hepatic function	Sterile ampules (3.0, 7.5, 10.0 ml) containing 50 mg/ml in aqueous sol., i.v. dose is 0.5-2.0 mg/kg
Phenolsulfonphthalein (PHENOL RED)	Renal function	Sterile solution (6 mg/ml) in physiological saline; i.v. dose is 6 mg

More recently, the use of Evans blue has been supplanted by radioisotope tracer technology and by the use of indocyanine green. Both of these utilize noninvasive techniques of measurement, the former by external γ-monitoring and the latter by use of the CAT densitometer.

Liver Function. Liver function can be assessed by the use of indocyanine green and sulfobromophthalein. Their major applications are for the assessment of hepatic blood flow and hepatic (biliary) secretory function. Indocyanine green is taken up (after i.v. injection) almost exclusively by the liver and excreted unchanged in the bile. The rate of plasma decay is a measure, in the first (rapid) phase, of hepatic uptake and, in the second (slow) phase, of biliary secretion. Indocyanine green is devoid of toxicity.

Sulfobromophthalein is taken up (after i.v. dosage) by kidney (< 5%) and skeletal muscle (25 – 30%), the remainder is taken up by the liver, where it is conjugated with reduced glutathione and excreted in the bile. Thus, estimation of liver uptake, conjugation function, and biliary excretion can be made with a single compound. Unfortunately, the popularity of sulfobromophthalein has been compromised by toxic side effects, including fatal initial hypersensitivity reactions in asthmatics, delayed hypersensitivity after paravascular injection, and localized acute thrombophlebitis.

Renal Function. Renal function tests are used, primarily in concert with other measurements, to facilitate the estimation of kidney impairment. Three compounds are used: *p*-aminohippuric acid (PAH), inulin, and phenolsulfonphthalein.

p-Aminohippuric acid (PAH) is administered i.v. as the sodium salt. It is not bound to plasma proteins to any significant extent, is not metabolized, and distributes primarily in extracellular space, although a small amount does enter the intracellular compartment. Small amounts are excreted by glomerular filtration, but the major excretory route is via the active secretory processes of the proximal convoluted tubules; the PAH clearance rate exceeds 600 ml/min. This active secretory process can create drug-drug interactive situations; concomitant presence of some diuretics, penicillin, or salicylates when PAH is administered can result in competitive interactions at the secretory sites.

Inulin is a plant starch with molecular weight of approximately 5000 and significant water solubility. After i.v. administration to humans, the distribution of inulin is restricted to the extracellular space; it can be used as a determinant of that compartment. Inulin is not metabolized, nor does it bind to plasma proteins. Excretion takes place only in Bowman's capsule, where inulin is filtered by the glomerular system; no significant excretion or reabsorption occurs in the tubules. The renal clearance in normal humans is equal to the glomerular filtration rate (125 ml/min); any deviation (beyond that of experimental error) is suggestive of a renal malfunction.

Phenolsulfonphthalein (phenol red) is only slightly soluble in water unless the pH is greater than 9.0. Following i.v. injection, the compound is highly bound to plasma proteins and is distributed largely into the intravascular compartment. Although it is not metabolized, a significant fraction (15-25%) of the dose is removed by the liver and secreted in the bile; thus, the presence of liver disease may be a confounding variable in the use of phenol red to determine renal function. In the kidney, a modest amount (< 10% of single-pass excretion) is filtered out by the glomerulus, whereas the remainder is secreted in the proximal convoluted tubules.

The toxic effects of these three agents are minimal. Hypersensitivity for phenolsulfonphthalein, and feelings of warmth and nausea from PAH, have been reported. In early work, a few pyrogenic reactions to unsatisfactory inulin preparations have been observed.

DIAGNOSTIC DRUGS

A number of therapeutic agents, or related compounds, are also used as diagnostic tools. The details of the specific agents, their mechanism(s) of action, pharmacodynamic and pharmacokinetic aspects of their action, and other details such as side effects and toxicities are presented elsewhere in this book. Table 33-5, however, presents a collective summary of some commonly used agents and their applications in diagnostic medicine. As pharmacological research continues to discover more information regarding mechanism of action of drugs, applications such as these should become more numerous.

Table 33-5
Examples of Diagnostic Drugs and Their Uses

Drugs	Use/Application
L-Arginine	A solution of arginine HCl (10 g/100 ml) for i.v. administrations as a diagnostic test for growth hormone secretion response
Dexamethasone	Suppression of adrenocortical and/or anterior pituitary secretory functions to test for endocrine malfunctions
Epinephrine	Conjunctival instillation with observation of pupillary dilatation to test for denervation of post-ganglionic sympathetic pathways
Histamine	Pressor response to i.v dosage as a test for pheochromocytoma; also can be used to test for gastric acid secretion
Mannitol	Available as 5-20% sterile solutions for i.v. use in testing renal function
Metyrapone	Tablets (250 mg) for test of pituitary function
Norepinephrine	Pressor response to i.v. infusion may be decreased (amyloidosis) or increased (denervation hypersensitivity)
Pentagastrin	Test of functionality of gastric secretion by parietal cells; has largely replaced histamine in such tests
Phentolamine	Depressor response after i.v. administration, concomitant decrease in blood glucose and rise in plasma insulin in pheochromocytoma
Tyramine	Pressor response to i.v. dosage is enhanced in pheochromocytoma

GENERAL READING

Henry, J.B. (ed.). *Todd-Sanford-Davidson Clinical Diagnosis and Management by Laboratory Methods,* 16th ed. Philadelphia: W.B. Saunders, 1979.

Herfindal, E.T., and Hirschman, J.L. (eds.). *Clinical Pharmacology and Therapeutics,* 2nd ed. Baltimore: Williams & Wilkins, 1979, p. 719.

Melmon, K.L., and Morrelli, H.F. (eds.). *Clinical Pharmacology, Basic Principles in Therapeutics,* 2nd ed. New York: Macmillan, 1978, p. 1146.

Modell, W. (ed.). *Drugs of Choice,* 1982-1983. St. Louis: C.V. Mosby, 1982, p. 356.

Robertson, D., and Smith, C.R. *Manual of Clinical Pharmacology.* Baltimore: Williams & Wilkins, 1981, p. 320.

Wagner, H.N., Jr. (ed.). *Nuclear Medicine.* New York: HP Publishing, 1975, p. 255.

CHAPTER
34

OVER-THE-COUNTER DRUGS

George R. Spratto and Nicholas G. Popovich

Self-medication, already an integral form of health care within the United States, will become even more important in the next decade. It is estimated that there are more than 350,000 nonprescription products available within the United States with more than 8 billion dollars spent for their purchase in 1980. Self-medication with these products will continue to escalate because of spiraling health care costs, as well as a greater awareness and emphasis on the need for persons to become involved in their own health maintenance.

It is predicted that Americans will be handling their health care problems more knowledgeably, more confidently, and more effectively in the future. Further, future over-the-counter (OTC) products will be improved through the application of science, through the exercise of uniform and appropriate regulation, and by the competitiveness of the proprietary drug industry. The Food and Drug Administration (FDA) OTC Review Process has been a comprehensive and thorough process, which when completed in the late 1980s will provide OTC products that are effective for intended use and provide suitable information for the consuming public.

The use of over-the-counter medications has increased in recent years, in part, due to intensive advertising campaigns in the mass media. Such advertising currently reaches a largely uninformed laity who are, in general, oblivious to safety and effectiveness as well as the proper use of such products. In addition, many people who regard pain or discomfort as situations that should not be tolerated, seek relief through the avenue of self-medication. Thus, people attempt to treat themselves for some real or perceived medical problem while not under the care of a physician.

The purpose of this chapter will be to identify problems associated with the use and misuse of those drugs that are available without a prescription to the consuming public. Central to the presentation will be ways in which OTC medications can interact with prescription and other medication(s). For information, several over-the-counter category examples with active ingredient(s) are listed in Tables 34-1 and 34-2.

PROBLEMS OF SELF-MEDICATION

Humans have an insatiable desire to self-medicate. If an individual achieves relief from an OTC product, not only has the condition been treated, but the person has also enjoyed the emotional satisfaction of producing relief by his or her own efforts and judgment. This is a significant factor in the treatment of many minor medical problems that involve a strong psychogenic or placebo component.

If the right to self-medicate were curtailed, physicians would be inundated by patients who previously had treated themselves successfully for a variety of medical problems. It is incomprehensible, for example, to imagine what hardships would ensue if aspirin were made available only by prescription.

On the other hand, although self-medication is part of the American life style, it is the responsibility of the physician, the pharmacist, and other members of the health care team to ensure that self-medication is properly performed. Patients must be educated to recognize the limitations of their own therapeutic competence and the inherent dangers associated with exceeding these limitations.

Table 34-1
Ingredients of Selected Internal Over-The-Counter (OTC) Categories

OTC Category	Ingredients	Product Examples
Antacids	Aluminum hydroxide gel	ALUDROX, ALTERNAGEL
	Calcium carbonate	ALKA-2, TUMS
	Calcium carbonate-magnesium hydroxide combination	LO-SAL
	Dihydroxyaluminum sodium	ROLAIDS
	Magaldrate	RIPOAN
	Sodium bicarbonate	ALKA-SELTZER ANTACID
Antidiarrheals	Bismuth subsalicylate	PEPTO-BISMOL
	Calcium polycarbophil	MITROLAN
	Electrolyte replacement	INFALYTE, LYTREN, PEDIALYTE-RS
	Kaolin-pectin combination	KAOPECTATE, KAOPECTATE CONCENTRATE
	Kaolin-pectin-belladonna alkaloid combination	DONNAGEL
	Psyllium mucilloid	KONSYL, METAMUCIL
Cold/allergy	Phenylpropanolamine HCl/chlorpheniramine maleate combination	A.R.M., ALLEREST, CORSYM, TRIAMINIC
	Pseudoephedrine HCl	AFRINOL, NOVAFED, SUDAFED
	Pseudoephedrine HCl/brompheniramine maleate combination	DISOPHROL, DRIXORAL
	Pseudoephedrine HCl/chlorpheniramine maleate combination	CHLOR-TRIMETON DECONGESTANT, SUDAFED PLUS
	Pseudoephedrine HCl/triprolidine HCl combination	ACTIFED
Internal analgesics	Acetaminophen	ANACIN-3, DATRIL, PANADOL, TYLENOL
	Aspirin	BAYER, ECOTRIN
	Aspirin, buffered	ASCRIPTIN, ALKA-SELTZER, BUFFERIN
	Ibuprofen	ADVIL, NUPRIN
Sleep aids	Diphenhydramine HCl	COMPOZ, NYTOL W/DPH, SLEEP-EZE 3
	Doxylamine succinate	UNISOM NIGHTTIME SLEEP-AID
	Pyrilamine maleate	NERVINE NIGHTTIME SLEEP-AID, SOMINEX
Stimulants	Caffeine	NODOZ, CAFFEDRINE, VIVARIN
Weight control	Stimulant	
	Phenylpropanolamine HCl	ACUTRIM, DEXATRIM (Caffeine free)
	Phenylpropanolamine HCl/caffeine combination	DEXATRIM, PROLAMINE, RESOLUTION I
	Decreased taste sensation	
	Benzocaine	AYDS, SLIM-LINE
	Bulk producer	
	Alginic acid combination	PRETTS
	Psyllium mucilloid	KONSYL, METAMUCIL

PURPOSE OF OTC DRUG THERAPY

The intent of self-medication is to produce temporary relief of minor ailments and discomfort for those conditions that are safe for self-treatment. There are some products, however, that are used for cure or control of minor disease conditions such as athlete's foot and acne. OTC products are generally not indicated for prolonged or continual use except on the advice of the physician.

PROBLEMS AND DANGER OF OTC DRUG THERAPY

Generally, consumers perceive OTC products as entirely safe and effective. Mistakenly, many believe advertising is rigidly controlled so that ineffective and/or potentially dangerous products cannot be sold. Thus, the consumer has little awareness of, and often overlooks, the possible dangers or shortcomings of OTC medication. However, there are a number of potential problems associated with the use of OTC products. Problems frequently arise simply because the patient disregards (or does not even read) the product label, which provides essential information about directions for use, cautions, and warnings. There is also the widespread belief that if a little medication helps a particular problem, a little more will be even better. This notion has been nurtured in the past by the proprietary industry which compounded pro-

Table 34-2
Ingredients of Selected External Over-The-Counter (OTC) Categories

OTC Category	Ingredients	Product Examples
Acne	Gel, lotion, cream	
	Benzoyl peroxide, 5%; 10%	BUF-OXAL 10, CLEARASIL, OXY-5
	Sulfur, 2%; 4%	FINAC, POSTACNE, TRANSACT, XERAC
	Sulfur/resorcinol combination	ACNOMEL (8%/2%), EXZIT (4%/2%), REZAMID (5%/2%), SULFORCIN (4%/1%)
	Medicated cleansers	
	Benzoyl peroxide, 5%, 10%	FOSTEX 10% BP WASH, PANOXYL BAR
	Sulfur, 10%	SULFUR SOAP
	Sulfur, 2%/salicylic acid, 2% combination	ACNOMEL CAKE, FOXTEX CAKE
Antifungals	Miconazole nitrate, 2%	MICATIN
	Tolnaftate, 1%	AFTATE, TINACTIN
	Undecylenic acid derivatives	CRUEX, DESENEX, NP-27 (LIQUID)
Corns/Calluses	Salicylic acid disks/Pads	DR. SCHOLL'S ZINC PADS
	Salicylic acid, 13.6%/Zinc chloride, 2.2% combination	FREEZONE
Dandruff	Coal tar derivatives	DENOREX, PENTRAX, TEGRIN
	Selenium sulfide, 1%	SELSUN BLUE
	Sulfur, 2%/Salicylic acid, 2% combination	FOSTEX, SEBAVEEN, SEBULEX
	Zinc pyrithione, 1%	DANEX, ZINCON
	Zinc pyrithione, 2%	HEAD AND SHOULDERS
Decongestants	Topical, nasal	
	Naphazoline HCl, 0.05%	PRIVINE
	Oxymetazoline HCl, 0.05%	AFRIN, DURATION, NEO-SYNEPHRINE 12 HOUR
	Phenylephrine HCl, 0.125-1%	DURATION MILD, SINEX, SUPER ANAHIST
	Xylometazoline HCl, 0.1%	4-WAY LONG-ACTING, SINUTAB LONG-LASTING
	Topical, ophthalmic	
	Naphazoline HCl, 0.012%	ALLEREST, CLEAR EYES, DEGEST-2, NAPHCON
	Phenylephrine HCl, 0.12%	ISOPTO-FRIN, PRE-FRIN
	Tetrahydrozoline HCl, 0.05%	MURINE PLUS, OPT-EASE, VISINE
Dermatitis	Hydrocortisone, 0.5%	CALDECORT, CORTAID, DERMOLATE, LANACORT
Dry skin	Lactic acid, 5%	LACTICARE
	Mineral oil combinations	EUCERIN, KERI, LUBRIDERM, NIVEA
	Petrolatum combinations	ECLIPSE AFTER SUN, pH-STABIL, PURPOSE
	Urea, 2%; 10%	AQUACARE, AQUACARE-HP, CARMOL
Otic	Swimmer's ear	
	Boric acid, 2.75%	DRI-EAR, EAR DRY, SWIM EAR
	Ear wax removal	
	Carbamide peroxide, 6.5%	DEBROX, MURINE EAR
Pediculocides	Pyrethrins, 0.3%/Piperonyl butoxide, 3% combination	R&C, RID, TRIPLE X
	Pyrethrins, 0.33%/Piperonyl butoxide, 4% combination	A-200 PYRINATE
Psoriasis	Coal tar derivatives	ESTAR, TARBONIS, TEGRIN
	Hydrocortisone, 0.5%	CALDECORT, CORTAID, DERMOLATE, LANACORT
	Moisturizing bath oils	ALPHA KERI, LUBATH
	Moisturizing cream combinations	LUBRIDERM, NIVEA
	Urea, 2%, 10%	AQUACARE, AQUACARE-HP, CARMOL
Wart	Calcium pantothenate/ascorbic acid/starch combination	VERGO, WART-AID
	Salicylic acid, 17%/Flexible collodion combination	COMPOUND-W, OFF-EZY, WART-OFF
	Salicylic acid, 40% plaster	MEDIPLAST

ducts containing half the amount needed for a therapeutic response. It was not uncommon for a patient merely to double the dose. Further, the anticipation of beneficial effects may be influenced by the recommendations of friends, relatives, and/or advertising. In addition, many people believe that prior experience with a drug or drug product, or the fact that it is advertised in the mass media, is sufficient for their purpose. A brief description of potential problems associated with the use of OTC products is in the following sections.

Adverse Effects. Even if the medication is used according to the instructions on the label, it is possible for a person to develop adverse drug reactions. For example, magnesium hydroxide used in antacids can cause diarrhea.

Overdose. Drug toxicity may be manifested as a result of excessive use (overdose) of the medication. Such toxic effects may be intentional or accidental. Children are often the victims of accidental poisoning, especially with oral analgesics (e.g., aspirin) and chewable vitamin-iron combinations. Even a relatively innocuous OTC product (e.g., mouthwash/rinse) has been implicated in several childhood poisonings from over ingestion. Adult education is a necessary prerequisite to the correct storage and use of OTC products. In addition, the development of products that are less esthetically attractive to children (e.g., physical appearance, taste, and odor) and with child-resistant containers (particularly those prone to misuse by children) may offer a partial solution to this dilemma.

Inappropriate Therapeutic Use. The classic example of inappropriate therapeutic use is the administration of a drug for canker sore relief for an oral ulcer that is persistent and nagging. If the sore within the mouth lasts for longer than 3 weeks, it may be an early warning sign of cancer.

With the recent availability of 0.5% topical hydrocortisone products for mild itching and inflammation, it is apparent that persons are misusing these. For example, these products are being used for acne vulgaris, nasal polyps, internal hemorrhoids, and diaper rash. Further, these products are even being used to treat styes. This latter use has far-reaching implications if conditions are such to encourage the development of an ophthalmological infection.

Masking of Serious Symptoms of an Illness. The masking of serious symptoms may cause patients to delay seeking appropriate medical care. The use of aspirin in pyrogenic infections or the use of cough suppressants for unsuspected tuberculosis or lung cancer are two notable examples.

Drug-Drug Interactions. With the availability of OTC drug products in numerous retail outlets, often without any pharmacist to consult, there is a greater risk for drug interactions to occur with either routinely administered prescription or nonprescription medications. In the recent past, a tremendous interest has been generated toward the understanding of how one drug can influence another drug's action in the body. Much of this research effort has been directed toward an understanding of prescription medication. Nonprescription drugs, however, are active entities, and thus, it is entirely possible that these drugs will interact with prescription medication. Table 34-3 illustrates some of the more common drug interaction mechanisms that are possible with drugs in nonprescription products and prescription products.

Multidrug OTC Products. The combination of two or more ingredients in a single OTC product leads to great confusion in evaluating the effectiveness of such combinations. Are two or more ingredients as effective or more effective than a single component? Often, the reason given for combining two or more drugs in a single poduct is to increase the beneficial effect while decreasing the chance for adverse effects (i.e., the ingredients can be present in lower doses). Each ingredient, however, should make a contribution to the therapeutic effectiveness of the medication, and no ingredient should decrease the safety or efficacy of any of the active ingredients. One of the goals of the FDA OTC Advisory Panels was to establish combinations of drugs for a product based upon rational need of the drugs in the product. The achievement of this objective is readily apparent by observation of rational combination cough-cold products that are marketed.

Patient Compliance. A dramatic reversal of a medical problem is not always possible. For example, to attain a cure from athlete's foot not complicated by an infected toenail, an antifungal product might have to be applied daily for 4-6 weeks. Similarly, to attain control of acne, the continual daily application of a product for 2-3 weeks might be necessary. The unsuspecting, poorly informed person might judge the product to be ineffective when the product is used an insufficient period of time.

Patient Misunderstanding. Nonprescription medications, even if used correctly, might not be efficacious unless the patient removes predisposing factors to the problem. For example, the treatment of acne is enhanced and promoted by a thorough, daily cleansing program, and the usc of oil-based cosmetics or soaps must be curtailed before the acne process can be reversed.

It is apparent that the consumer must be better educated to the use of OTC products. In addition, the patient should have the benefit of consultation with a member of the health profession (e.g., a pharmacist) who can monitor and counsel the patient and thus avoid potential problems. This will become even more crucial in future years as more potent legend medication (e.g., ibuprofen and pyrantel pamoate) become available on an OTC basis.

Table 34-3
Common Mechanisms for Drug-Drug Interactions with Representative Examples

OTC Drug	Interactant	Effect
A. OTC drugs that act additively or synergistically when administered with other drugs		
Aspirin	Coumarin anticoagulants	Increased prothrombin time (bleeding)
	Nonsteroidal antiinflammatory agents (e.g., MOTRIN, NAPROSYN, CLINORIL)	Increased potential for gastric upset; possible diminished activity of the NSAIAs
Atropine alkaloids (antidiarrheals, e.g., DONNAGEL, DONNAGEL-PG)	Anticholinergics (e.g., PROBANTHINE), tricyclic antidepressants (e.g., ELAVIL), and phenothiazines (e.g., THORAZINE)	Additive anticholinergic effects (e.g., dry mouth, blurred vision)
Benzoyl peroxide (Antiacne products, e.g., OXY-5)	Tretinoin (RETIN-A), Isotretinoin (ACCUTANE)	Additive peeling and skin irritation; dry skin
Bismuth subsalicylate (in PEPTO-BISMOL)	Aspirin	Salicylate toxicity (e.g., ringing, buzzing, or fullness in ears) if taken in high doses
Diphenhydramine (sleep-aid products, e.g., COMPOZ, NYTOL with DPH)	Alcohol (as a beverage or a vehicle in medicinal products)	Additive CNS depression
Epinephrine HCl (antiasthmatic products, e.g., MEDIHALER-EPI)	Tricyclic antidepressants (e.g., ELAVIL)	Increased pressor response to epinephrine
Phenylpropanolamine HCl (cold-decongestant products, e.g., CONTAC, SINE-OFF)	Phenylpropanolamine HCl (diet aid products, e.g., DEXATRIM, DIETAC)	Overdose; restlessness, insomnia, irritability
Potassium chloride (salt substitutes, e.g., NO-SALT)	Potassium supplements (e.g., K-LYTE, SLOW-K)	Possible hyperkalemia
B. OTC drugs that enhance or diminish the absorption of another drug from the GI tract		
Bismuth subsalicylate (in PEPTO-BISMOL)	Tetracycline HCl and other tetracyclines	Decreased tetracycline absorption
Docusate sodium (e.g., COLACE) Docusate calcium (e.g., SURFAK) Docusate potassium (e.g., DIALOSE)	Danthron (an irritant cathartic)	Suspected hepatitis due to enhanced danthron absorption
	Mineral oil	Increased systemic absorption of mineral oil
Iron supplements (e.g., FEOSOL, MOL-IRON, FERGON)	Tetracycline HCl and other tetracyclines	Decreased tetracycline absorption
Kaolin-pectin (e.g., KAOPECTATE, DONNAGEL)	Digoxin, chlordiazepoxide	Decreased absorption and bioavailability for these drugs
Magnesium-aluminum hydroxide gel (e.g., MAALOX, KOLANTYL, MYLANTA)	Tetracyclines, digoxin, phenytoin	Decreased tetracycline absorption, as well as decreased digoxin and phenytoin absorption
Mineral oil	Fat-soluble vitamins	Chronic mineral oil use can decrease the absorption of fat-soluble vitamins
C. OTC drugs that alter the distribution (e.g., plasma protein binding) of other drugs		
Aspirin (e.g., BAYER, ANACIN)	Coumadin, DIABINESE, methotrexate	Displacement of drug from plasma protein-binding sites resulting in an increased pharmacological response.

Table 34-3
Common Mechanisms for Drug-Drug Interactions with Representative Examples(Continued)

OTC Drug	Interactant	Effect
D. OTC drugs that alter the renal excretion or effectiveness of another drug		
Ammonium chloride (menstrual products, e.g., AQUA-BAN)	Weakly basic drugs dependent upon urinary excretion (e.g., TCADs, amphetamines)	Urinary acidification would enhance excretion of these drugs
Sodium bicarbonate (antacid products, e.g., ALKA-SELTZER ANTACID)	Weakly basic drugs dependent upon urinary excretion (e.g., quinidine, amphetamine)	Urinary alkalinization would diminish excretion of these drugs, possibly leading to toxicity
	Methenamine mandelate	Urinary alkalinization prevents conversion of methenamine to the active formaldehyde in the urine
	Nitrofurantoin	Urinary alkalinization decreases the bactericidal effect of nitrofurantoin
E. Drugs that decrease the biotransformation of another drug resulting in increased toxicity		
Phenylephrine, phenylpropanolamine, ephedrine, (decongestant products, e.g., CONTAC, CORICIDIN-D)	Monoamine oxidase (MAO) inhibitors	MAO inhibitors decrease biotransformation with possible hypertensive crisis
F. OTC drugs that interfere with or affect the desired effect of another drug		
Alcohol (vehicle, e.g., NYQUIL NIGHT-TIME COLDS LIQUID MEDICINE)	Metronidazole (FLAGYL) Chlopropamide (DIABINESE) Disulfiram (ANTABUSE)	Antabuse-like effect
Aspirin	Probenecid (BENEMID) Sulfinpyrazone (ANTURANE)	Inhibition of the uricosuric effect of probenecid or sulfinpyrazone
Epinephrine HCl (antiasthmatic aerosols)	Digitalis	Possible cardiac arrhythmias
Ephedrine SO_4 (antiasthmatic oral products, TEDRAL)	Guanethidine	Blockade of guanethidine's entrance to the site of action, thus decreased antihypertensive effect
Milk of magnesia (laxative or antacid)	Aspirin (ECOTRIN), Bisacodyl (DULCOLAX) Methenamine mandelate (MANDELAMINE)	Premature release of these drugs from their enteric-coated tablet in stomach; could result in stomach distress on patient's part
Sodium lauryl sulfate (a soap)	Benzalkonium chloride (a germicide)	Germicidal activity is decreased by chemical reaction with the soap if the soap is not thoroughly rinsed from the skin prior to application of germicide

CHAPTER
35

PRESCRIPTION WRITING

Nicholas G. Popovich and George R. Spratto

The *prescription* represents a mechanism through which a treatment modality is provided to the patient. A prescription order may be written and issued by a physician, dentist, veterinarian, or other properly licensed medical practitioner. The prescription for each patient is a unique entity, designating a specific medication or medications for a specific patient at a specific time. The prescription may be written and signed by a physician or it may be verbally communicated to the pharmacist (except for a few controlled substances) via a telephone or other communication system. The pharmacist is obliged to transcribe the verbally transmitted prescription into a written form and, if necessary according to statute, obtain the prescriber's signature on the prescription at a later time.

According to Smith, there are several manifest functions of the prescription, as listed in Table 35-1 (7).

The *Ebers Papyrus*, which dates from the eighteenth dynasty (written about the sixteenth century B.C.), is considered to be an unofficial formulary or recipe book of medicines. Some of the formulas in the *Ebers Papyrus* included as many as 35 ingredients. Often the quantity of drug is stated accurately in the formula; details of preparation and administration are also given at times. The late historian Dr. George Urdang pointed out, however, that these formulas that have come from Assyrian-Babylonian and Egyptian antiquity are not prescriptions as such but merely recipes or formulas to be used as a guide to mixing medicines (6). The Arabians, credited with the preservation of the art of pharmacy and medicine, as early as the seventh century A.D., after their conquest in Europe, brought with them a revival of science and learning. While in Syria, the Arabians translated Greek manuscripts into their own language and continued this tradition while in Persia. The Arabians are credited with founding hospitals to teach practical medicine. Christian and Jewish authors translated the works of ancient civilization into Arabic, and in this way knowledge filtered through Syria to Persia, and finally to the Arabs (4). In 1240, Frederick II of Hohenstaufen brought about legislation that separated medicine and pharmacy in the Two Sicilies. To this date, pharmacists in some European countries must swear conscientiously to fill the prescriptions of physicians (6). In the fourteenth century, specialization in the two professions emerged in England (3); the Stonor Letters in the Public Record Office include four prescriptions by a physician addressed to an apothecary in 1480. From the prescription form and symbols, it becomes obvious that the manner and art of prescription writing have changed very little over the centuries (3).

DESCRIPTION OF THE PRESCRIPTION

The prescription is usually written upon a printed form that possesses blank spaces for the necessary information. Such blanks are often supplied to the physician in the form of a pad containing approximately 100 blank forms. There is no set form required for a prescription order, since any type of paper or other material may be used by a physician.

Table 35-1
Manifest Functions of the Prescription

1. Legal documentation
2. Record source
3. Means of communication
4. Therapy modality
5. Means of medical control of therapy
6. Means of clinical trial
7. Mechanism sample

Depending upon a physician's prescribed request, the prescription can be classified as *compounded, noncompounded* (i.e., dispensed), *generic, trade name, controlled, new,* or *refill.* Table 35-2 lists a glossary of these types and their definition.

COMPONENT PARTS OF THE PRESCRIPTION

The pharmacist has the responsibility to interpret the intent of the prescriber from the prescription. For the purpose of discussion, a prescription may be subdivided according to the following headings:

1. The name and address of the patient
2. The date prescribed
3. The superscription
4. The inscription and subscription
5. The signatura
6. The renewal instructions
7. The name of the prescriber

With the exception of the inscription and the name of the prescriber, some or all of these parts of a prescription may be missing in an actual situation, whereupon it becomes the responsibility of the pharmacist to obtain the missing information from the patient and/or the prescribing physician. The component parts of a prescription are illustrated in Figure 35-1.

The *name and address* serve to identify for whom the prescription is intended. Placement of the correct name on the prescription label serves to prevent a mix-up of medication within a household. The full name and the address are required by federal law on all prescriptions for controlled substances (2). Although it is not included here, the age of the patient is a good additional piece of information, especially with pediatric patients where dosage calculations may have to be double-checked for safety. Preferably, the name and address of the patient should be placed upon the prescription by the prescriber. Unfortunately, however, it is not uncommon for the prescription to reach the pharmacist's hands with the name and address of the patient omitted.

The *date* prescribed is important from the standpoint of ascertaining the life of the prescription. This is especially so with records of narcotics and controlled substances that are governed by special laws and regulations. For instance, federal law states that "no prescription for a controlled substance listed in Schedule III or IV shall be filled or refilled more than 6 months after the date on which such prescription was issued and no such prescription authorized to be refilled may be refilled more than five times" (2).

The *superscription* consists of the symbol R_x. It is generally understood to be a contraction of the Latin verb *recipe* ("take thou"). This is the representative symbol of the prescription and the profession of pharmacy. Its origin dates back to the Egyptian era, when it was the sign of Isis and an invocation to the goddess for health.

The *inscription* is the principal portion of the prescription. It contains the name and quantity of the prescribed medicament(s). This is the most critical portion of the prescription. With the advent of manufactured trade names and dosage forms, there has been a movement toward the use of the English language instead of Latin. Latin is used occasionally, primarily in those prescriptions that need compounding. The prescription in Fig. 35-2 directs that a total suspension volume of 60 ml be prepared and dispensed to the patient.

The quantities of the ingredients are written in either the apothecary or metric system of weights and measures, although the use of the apothecary system is gradually diminishing. The official compendium and pharmaceutical manufacturers have advocated the use of the metric system for some time.

Pharmacists must be familiar with the symbols and abbreviations of both systems and be able to convert from one to the other. It is not uncommon for both systems to be found in the same prescription. When prepared dosage forms such as tablets, capsules, sustained-release capsules, and so on, are prescribed in the metric system, the pharmacist may dispense the corresponding approximate equivalent in the apothecary system and vice versa. To calculate quantities required in a compounded prescription or a pharmaceutical formulation, however, exact equivalents rounded to three significant figures must be used.

When the metric system is used, the decimal may be replaced by a vertical line that may be imprinted on the prescription blank or written in by the physician (Fig. 35-2). The symbol g (for grams) or ml (for milliliter) are often eliminated. It is understood that solids are dispensed by weight (i.e., g) and liquids by volume (i.e., ml). As a general rule, Arabic figures are used to designate quantities in the metric system. In the apothecary system, quantities are designated by a symbol followed by a Roman numeral. Custom also indicates that fractions be used with the apothecary system. Table 35-3 lists the more typical symbols or abbreviations for units of measure found within a prescription.

The *subscription* indicates to the pharmacist directions from the physician to prepare the prescription. This portion of the prescription is generally omitted because many of today's prescriptions require little, if any, compounding. In a vast majority of prescriptions, the sub-

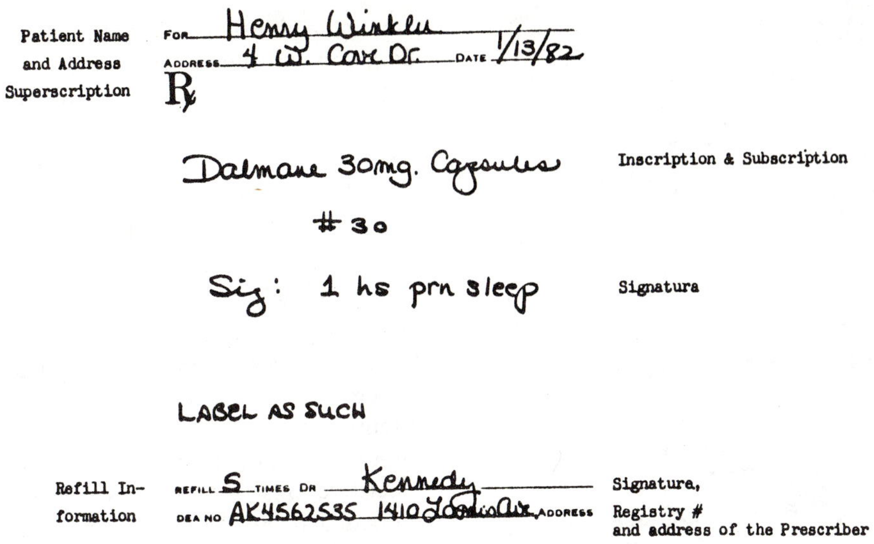

Patient Name and Address	For Henry Winkler Address 4 W. Cave Dr. Date 1/13/82	
Superscription	℞	
	Dalmane 30mg. Capsules #30	Inscription & Subscription
	Sig: 1 hs prn sleep	Signatura
	LABEL AS SUCH	
Refill Information	Refill 5 times Dr Kennedy DEA No AK4562535 1410 [illegible] Address	Signature, Registry # and address of the Prescriber

Fig. 35-1. *Component parts of the prescription.*

scription serves to designate the dosage form requested and number of doses to be supplied to the patient.

The *signatura* (i.e., signa, sig., S.) is the intended direction to the patient. The pharmacist has the responsibility to place this information on the prescription label of the container. This information must be sufficient to allow the patient to understand fully the amount of drug product to be taken and the frequency and manner of administration. The use of the phrase "as directed" is not satisfactory for the signatura. It should not be used unless absolutely necessary. In these instances it is important that the physician supply the patient with separate oral or written instructions. It is known, however, that oral instructions to the patient can often be forgotten or misinterpreted. This only leads to confusion and misunderstandings on the patient's part on how to use the prescribed product correctly. Hence correct patient compliance with the prescribed medication can be severely handicapped.

Because erroneous interpretations have occurred when the patient endeavored to read the directions when written in English, most physicians continue to write the signa in Latin abbreviations. For the average prescription, comparatively few abbreviations are necessary. Table 35-4 lists the more common Latin abbreviations and their meanings.

For informational purposes, some physicians include the name and strength of the prescribed product within the signatura. In some states, this information is required on the prescription label. The physician may imply that the prescription label contains the name of the product by either including the name and strength of the drug actually in the signa (e.g., Sig: Tabs 1 q 6 h, q.i.d., Sumycin 250 mg) or by indicating on the prescription (i.e., label contents) that the prescription label contains the name and strength of the medication (Fig. 35-3).

Table 35-2
Glossary of Prescription Types

Compounded	Prescription order requires mixing of one or more ingredients (i.e., active medicaments) with one or more pharmaceutical necessities (e.g., vehicle, suspending agent) to obtain a finished product
Noncompounded	Prescription order does not require mixing of two or more ingredients to obtain a finished product; prefabricated drug products (e.g., DARVON Compound-65 Pulvules) including simple products (e.g., PENTID "400" for syrup) that are reconstituted by adding a diluent or solvent are in this category
Generic	Prescription order for a drug by its official name (e.g., tetracycline HCl)
Trade name	Prescription order for a drug by its registered trademarked or brand name (e.g., ACHROMYCIN V)
Controlled	Prescription order that requests a Schedule II, III, IV, or V drug
New	Original prescription order filled for the first time
Refill	A repeat filling of the original prescription order

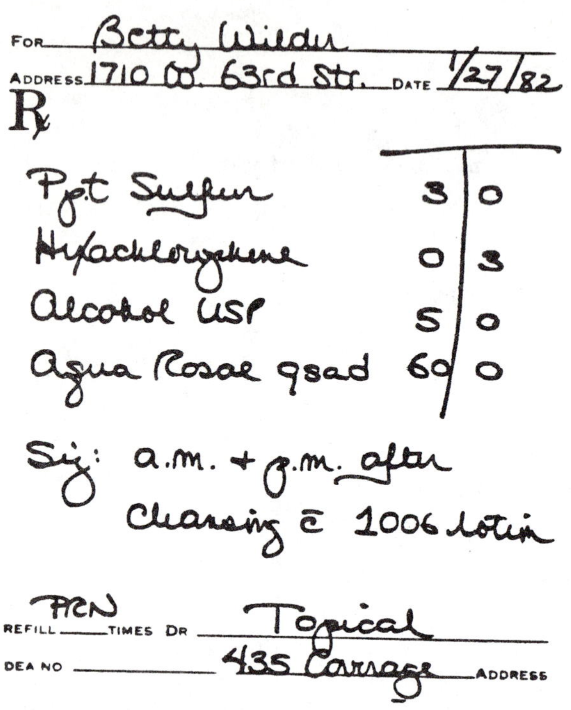

FOR Betty Wilder

ADDRESS 1710 W. 63rd Str. DATE 1/27/82

℞

Ppt Sulfur 3 | 0

Hexachlorophene 0 | 3

Alcohol USP 5 | 0

Aqua Rosae qsad 60 | 0

Sig: a.m. + p.m. after cleansing c̄ 1006 lotion

REFILL PRN TIMES DR Topical

DEA NO 435 Carriage ADDRESS

Fig. 35-2. *An example of a compounded presription.*

The practice of labeling the prescription label with the name of the product and quantity has several useful purposes. It serves to make the identity of the prescription medication readily ascertainable when there is (a) an accidental or intended overdose, (b) a desire to adjust a dosage regimen, (c) a need to identify previously prescribed medication, and (d) a situation where a knowledge of the medication is required but it is not practical to contact the pharmacy where it was dispensed (e.g., a telephone conversation with the patient).

Snipes has proposed a signatura code intended to offer speed, versatility, simplicity, and accuracy for the prescribing physician (8). It is a convenient code for the physician and would seem to offer less confusion about the intended administration of the medication for the nurse, the pharmacist, and the patient. Snipes proposed that the signatura of the prescription be written as a four-digit code in Arabic numerals. The first digit represents the dose to be taken *after breakfast*, the second gives the *after lunch* dose , the third the *after dinner* dose , and the fourth the *bedtime* dose. When a medication is to be taken before meals, the signatura is written with the "a.c." dose(s) underlined. An "O" indicates that no dose is to be taken at the specified time.

Table 35-5 compares Snipes' proposed method of writing instructions versus the conventional method. It becomes apparent that Snipes' method does offer simplicity and time saved in writing. The examples are intended to illustrate how this system can convey a high variety of instructions. The limitation of this system is in those medications that necessitate irregular schedules, *pro re nata*, or specific time schedules (i.e., around the clock). In these instances, the conventional method of direction writing is necessary.

In some cases, the prescription order may be conveyed orally to the pharmacist. Here the pharmacist must commit the physician's verbal communication to writing (Fig. 35-4); the transcribed order must contain all necessary information.

LEGAL CONSIDERATIONS

Ownership of the Prescription. The pharmacist has the general right to keep the written prescription once he/she has filled and delivered the prescription to the patient. Federal and state drug control laws are in agreement that retention of the prescription constitutes proof of dispensing the drug or drug product to the patient. If the pharmacist refuses to fill a prescription, the pharmacist is obligated to return the prescription to the patient. In general, the pharmacist has the legal right to refuse to fill a prescription, although this right may be modified by a state pharmacy board. For example, West Virginia prohibits the pharmacist from refusing to fill a prescription without a good reason. This prohibition is mainly directed at those pharmacists who decline to fill a compounded prescription because of the time involved in its preparation.

Prescription Copies. A copy of any prescription is *not* a prescription and can only be used for informational purposes. A pharmacist presented with a copy of a prescription cannot legally dispense the medication. It is the responsibility of the pharmacist to contact the prescribing physician and receive a new prescription either in written or verbal form.

A copy of a prescription should be marked as such. In some states, the pharmacy board rules specify that a prescription copy be marked in red ink with the words "Copy - For Informational Purposes Only."

Table 35-3
Typical Symbols or Abbreviations of Measure Used in Prescription

Unit of Measure, Term	Symbol or Abbreviation
Drop, drops	gtt
Fluid	f or fl
Fluid dram	f ʒ
Fluid ounce	f ℥
Grain	gr
Gram	g
Kilogram	kg
Milligram	mg
Milliliter	ml[a]

[a] A milliliter (ml) is the approximate equivalent of a cubic centimeter (cc). It is the recognized symbol for fluid measure.

Table 35-4
Some Common Latin Abbreviations and Their Meanings

Word or Phrase	Contraction	Meaning
Ad	Ad	To, up to
Ad Libitum	Ad lib	At pleasure
Ana	aa.	Of each
Ante cibos	a.c.	Before meals
Aqua	aq.	Water
Aures utrae	a.u.	Each ear, both ears
Aurio dextra	a.d.	Right ear
Aurio laeva	a.l.	Left ear
Bis-in-die	b.i.d.	Twice daily
Capsula	caps	Capsule
Charta	chart	Paper
Collyrium	collyr.	An eye wash
Cum	c	With
Da, detur	d., det.	Give, let be given
Dentur-tales doses	d.t.d.	Let such doses be given
Emulsum	emuls.	Emulsion
Et fac, fiat, fiant	F.	And make
Gutta, guttae	gtt.	A drop, drops
Hora somni	h.s.	At bedtime
Non repetatur	non rep.	Do not repeat
Noct, nox, noctis	noct.	Night
Numerus	no.	Number
Oculo utro	o.u.	Each eye, both eyes
Oculus dexter	o.d.	Right eye
Oculus laevus	o.l.	Left eye
Oculus sinister	o.s.	Left eye
Per os	p.o.	By mouth
Post cibos	p.c.	After eating
Pro re nata	p.r.n.	When necessary
Quaque	q	Each, every
Quantum sufficiat	q.s.	As much as is sufficient
Quater-in-die	q.i.d.	Four times a day
Repetatur	rept.	Let it be repeated
Semis	ss	A half
Signa	sig, S.	Mark thou
Sine	s	Without
Statim	stat	Immediately, first dose
Ter-in-die	t.i.d.	Three times daily
Unguentum	ung	Ointment
Ut dictum	ut dict	As directed

Prescription Refills. It is at the discretion of the prescribing physician whether any prescription will be refillable. When the physician writes or verbally transmits the prescription to the pharmacist, refill information should be given. The physician (Fig. 35-1) or pharmacist (Fig. 35-4) indicates this within the space provided on the prescription blank for refill information. In the absence of refill instructions, the prescription, by law, is considered to be nonrefillable. This situation may be terribly inconvenient, especially to those patients maintained on daily maintenance medications (e.g., LANOXIN, ALDOMET, DIABINESE). The pharmacist has no alternative but to contact the physician for refill directions when the need arises after the original filling of the prescription.

In general, antibiotic medications should not be refillable unless the physician is of the opinion that a second

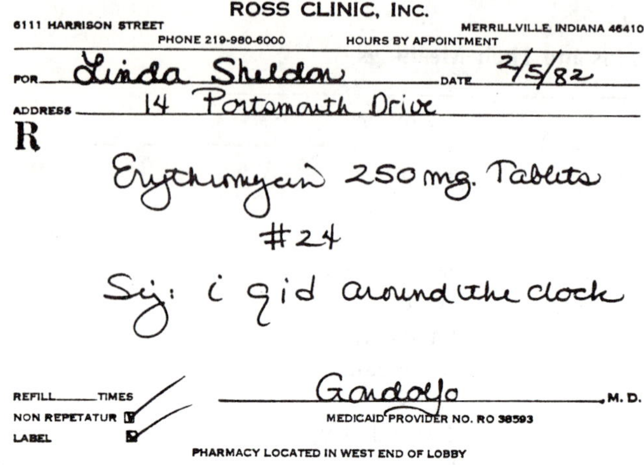

ROSS CLINIC, INC.
6111 HARRISON STREET MERRILLVILLE, INDIANA 46410
PHONE 219-980-6000 HOURS BY APPOINTMENT
FOR Linda Sheldon DATE 2/5/82
ADDRESS 14 Portsmouth Drive
R
Erythromycin 250 mg. Tablets
#24
Sig: i qid around the clock

REFILL ___ TIMES
NON REPETATUR
LABEL
Gandolfo M. D.
MEDICAID PROVIDER NO. RO 38593
PHARMACY LOCATED IN WEST END OF LOBBY

Fig. 35-3. *Representative prescription illustrating the prescribing physician's directions to list the product prescribed on the container label.*

or third course of therapy may be beneficial. In this case, the physician may indicate the refill instructions as indicated in Fig. 35-5 (i.e., refill two times in 1 month). Otherwise it is conceivable that the patient may attempt to use antibiotic refills to self- medicate at a later time, a practice that of course can be dangerous.

A specific number of refills should be indicated to obviate interpretation of *prn (pro re nata)* refills, which, according to a strict definition of the law, are refillable only once. State law will indicate the length of time for prescription validity. In the state of Indiana, for example, a prescription is valid for a period of not more than 1 year after the original date of filling. If a medication is continued for more than 1 year, the patient must either secure a new prescription from the physician, or the pharmacist must contact the physician for approval of the new prescription. At this time, a new prescription number is assigned to the medication and the process repeated as need be.

There are limitations on the types of medications that may or may not be refilled. Federal law dictates that prescriptions for controlled substances in Schedule II are nonrefillable. Controlled substances in Schedules III and IV are, however, refillable, for a period of 6 months, a maximum of five times.

Controlled Substance Prescriptions. All prescriptions for controlled substances must be dated and signed by the physician on the date of issuance. In addition, the prescription must contain the full name and the address of the patient and the Drug Enforcement Administration (DEA) registration number of the physician. The physician should sign his/her name as he/she would a legal document or a check (e.g., William H. Jennings or W.H. Jennings). Prescriptions must be written with ink, indelible pencil, or typewritten, and must be manually signed by the physician. It is permissible for a nurse or a secretary to prepare the prescription for signature by the physician. It is, however, the responsibility of the prescribing physician to ensure that the prescription conforms in all essential respects to the laws and regulations. Similar liability rests upon the pharmacist who endeavors to fill a prescription not prepared in accordance with law and regulations.

In those instances where an intern, resident, foreign-trained physician, or physician on the staff of a Veteran Administration facility are exempted from registration under Code of Federal Regulations (CFR) 1301.24 and such a person writes a prescription for a controlled substance, the registration number of the hospital and the special internal code number assigned to him/her by the institution should appear on the prescription. An official

Table 35-5
Comparison of Snipes' Method of Prescription Writing Versus Conventional Method

Example	Medication Prescribed	New Method	Old Method	Prescription Label
1	MACRODANTIN 50 mg	1 1 1 1	i p.c. and h.s. q.i.d.	Take one capsule after meals and at bedtime four times daily
2	PRELUDIN ENDURET 75 mg	1 0 0 0	i q a.m.	Take one tablet after breakfast
3	VALIUM 5 mg	1 0 1 0	1 b.i.d.	Take one tablet after breakfast and after supper
4	GANTRISIN 500 mg	2 2 2 2	ii q.i.d.	Take two tablets after meals and at bedtime, four times daily
5	ORNADE SPANSULES	1 0 0 1	i b.i.d.	Take one capsule after breakfast and at bedtime
6	DIMETANE-DC EXPT.	10 cc: 1 1 1 1	2 dr. q.i.d.	Take two teaspoonfuls after meals and at bedtime
7	DONNATAL TABLETS	1 1 1 1	1 q.i.d. a.c. and h.s.	Take one tablet before each meal and at bedtime

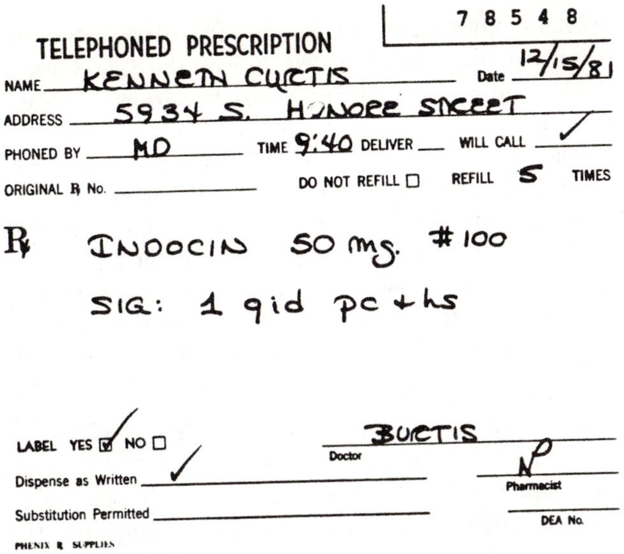

TELEPHONED PRESCRIPTION 78548

NAME KENNETH CURTIS Date 12/15/81

ADDRESS 5934 S. HONORE STREET

PHONED BY MD TIME 9:40 DELIVER ___ WILL CALL ✓

ORIGINAL ℞ No. ___ DO NOT REFILL ☐ REFILL 5 TIMES

℞ INDOCIN 50 mg. #100

SIG: 1 qid pc + hs

LABEL YES ☑ NO ☐ BURTIS Doctor

Dispense as Written ✓ Pharmacist

Substitution Permitted ___ DEA No.

PHENIX ℞ SUPPLIES

Fig. 35-4. *Example of a telephoned prescription by the pharmacist.*

exempted from registration under CFR 1301.25 shall include on all prescriptions issued by him/her the branch of service or agency (e.g., "U.S. Air Force" or "Public Health Service") to which he/she belongs and his/her service identification number, in lieu of the registration number of the practitioner required for control drugs. The service identification number for a public health service employee is his/her social security identification number. Each prescription must have the name of the officer stamped, typed, or handprinted on it, as well as the signature of the officer.

The law allows a pharmacist to dispense a controlled substance (Schedule II) only pursuant to a written prescription signed by a prescribing individual practitioner, except in an emergency situation. In this latter instance, a pharmacist may dispense a controlled substance listed in Schedule II upon receiving an oral authorization of a prescribing individual practitioner, provided that:

1. The quantity prescribed and dispensed is limited to the amount adequate to treat the patient during an emergency period.
2. The verbal prescription is reduced immediately to writing by the pharmacist. The pharmacist must ensure that the prescription is complete in all respect exclusive of the signature of the prescribing physician.
3. If the prescribing physician is unknown to the pharmacist, the pharmacist must make a reasonable effort to determine that the oral authorization came from a registered individual practitioner. This process may include a callback to the prescribing physician using his/her telephone number as listed in the telephone directory and/or other good-faith methods to ensure his/her identity.
4. Within 72 hr after autherization of an emergency prescription, the prescribing physician must effect a written prescription for the emergency quantity prescribed and ensure its delivery to the dispensing pharmacist. On the face of the prescription "Authorization for Emergency Dispensing" and the date of the oral order must appear. This written prescription may be delivered to the pharmacy in person or by mail. However, if mailed it must have been postmarked within the 72-hr period. If the prescribing physician fails to provide the prescription in the required time of 72 hr, the pharmacist must notify the DEA regional office or the oral prescription is void and the pharmacist is liable.

It is conceivable that in the course of writing a prescription for a controlled substance, the physician may inadvertently make an error in the quantity requested for the patient. In this case, an alteration of the prescription is required. Unless state laws dictate otherwise, it is suggested that the prescribing physician sign his/her name adjacent to the error or initial the error. Initials could be easy to duplicate illegally in the future, whereas a signature would be somewhat more difficult; the signature of the prescribing physician also seems to be the best approach because it would then appear twice on the prescription face (Fig. 35-6). The easiest and best solution to this problem is merely to rewrite an entirely new prescription with the correct quantity on another blank.

Beyond federal laws, each individual state may have further regulations with respect to prescribing controlled substances. For instance, in the state of Illinois prescriptions written for Schedule II drugs can only be written upon Official Triplicate Prescription forms provided to practitioners by the Department of Registration and Education. When issuing a prescription on a triplicate

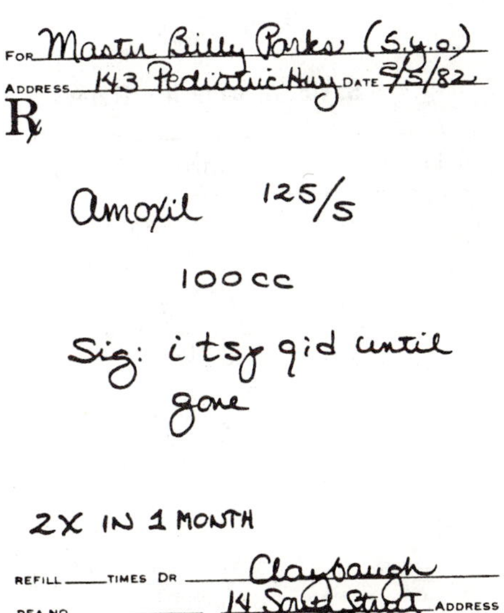

FOR Master Billy Parks (5 y.o.)

ADDRESS 143 Pediatric Hwy DATE 5/5/82

℞

Amoxil 125/5

100 cc

Sig: i tsp qid until gone

2X IN 1 MONTH

REFILL ___ TIMES DR Claybaugh

DEA NO ___ 14 South Street ADDRESS

Fig. 35-5. *Representative prescription illustrating the time length for refilling the prescription.*

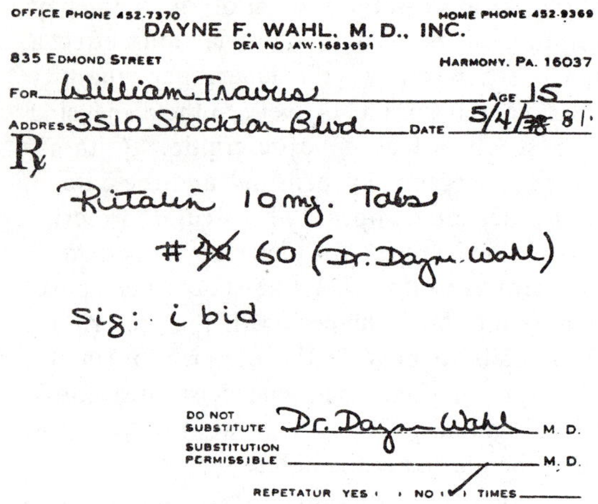

OFFICE PHONE 452-7370 HOME PHONE 452-9369
DAYNE F. WAHL, M. D., INC.
DEA NO AW-1683691
835 EDMOND STREET HARMONY, PA. 16037
FOR William Travers AGE 15
ADDRESS 3510 Stockton Blvd. DATE 5/4/81
℞
Ritalin 10 mg. Tabs
60 (Dr. Dayne Wahl)
Sig: i bid

DO NOT SUBSTITUTE Dr. Dayne Wahl M. D.
SUBSTITUTION PERMISSIBLE ______ M. D.
REPETATUR YES ( ) NO (✓) TIMES ______

Fig. 35-6. *A legally altered Schedule II prescription (where permissible by law).*

form, the prescribing physician keeps one copy; the original and the second copy go to the patient, who presents both to the pharmacist for filling. Subsequently, the pharmacist keeps one copy for the pharmacy files and forwards the other copy to the Department of Education and Registration by the fifteenth day of the following month.

Table 5-3 lists representative examples of controlled substances according to schedule, and Table 35-6 offers some general information about prescribing controlled drugs and/or drug products.

It is not legal for a prescribing physician to predate or postdate a prescription for a controlled substance. This circumstance is presented when the prescribing physician desires to leave a narcotic controlled substance prescription (e.g., DEMEROL) with the patient for future use (e.g., terminal patient with severe pain). This problem is magnified in those states where the law dictates that the narcotic prescription be filled *only* on the date it bears. There is no prohibition in federal law from filling the controlled substances prescription several days after its issuance or from filling a controlled substance prescription for a large amount of drug—provided no issue of bad faith is present. In the case of a prescription for a large amount of narcotic controlled substance, the pharmacist may be required to ascertain from the prescribing physician whether a legitimate medical purpose exists to support good faith in filling the prescription.

WRITING THE PRESCRIPTION

Latin Versus English. Latin is considered to be the language of the medical world. In that context in years past, Latin was the official language in which a physician communicated to a pharmacist instructions for the patient. With the advent of prepackaged dosage forms and coined trade names for medicaments, however, the use of Latin has steadily diminished. As mentioned, Latin terms and abbreviations are still used to an extent in the signatura and occasionally in the subscription. It is realistic to assume that in this day and age, the prescription should be written in English whenever possible to minimize interpretation difficulties that may arise from an incorrectly used Latin term or "unofficial" Latin abbreviation of the physician's own making (e.g., *aa*, meaning *a*ffected *a*rea). As long as Latin "abbreviations" and words appear in prescriptions the pharmacist must be able to interpret them correctly.

It is a practice of some physicians to write the name of the medication or drug product in an abbreviated or shorthand form. Unless the abbreviation is readily identifiable and obvious, this practice should be discouraged. *SSKI* is the common abbreviation for saturated solution of potassium iodide. When *CPM* appears, however it

Table 35-6
Basic Information Relevant to Writing Prescriptions for Controlled Substances

Schedule of Drug	Form of Prescription	Signature of Physician	Refills
II	Written only (verbal in emergency)	Required	Nonrefillable
III	Written	Required	In accordance with physician's directions, maximum 5 x in 6 months
	Verbal	Pharmacist writes Rx	
IV	Written	Required	In accordance with physician's directions, maximum 5 x in 6 months
	Verbal	Pharmacist writes Rx	
V	Written	Required	In accordance with physician's directions, time limit dependent upon state law
	Verbal	Pharmacist writes Rx	

might not be obvious to every pharmacist that the physician has written a prescription for chlorpromazine.

Prescription Legibility. A formidable problem that confronts the pharmacist at the time the prescription is received is the deciphering and/or interpreting the physician's order. With continued experience, the pharmacist becomes accustomed to physicians' writing and becomes in essence a handwriting expert. The fact remains, however, that the clearly written prescription is preferred. It reduces greatly the time spent deciphering the prescription and may even obviate an otherwise unnecessary telephone call to the physician for prescription clarification. If a physician's signature is naturally illegible, the physician's name should appear somewhere on the blank. A growing problem that further compounds the encountered interpretation of the written prescription is that the names of many drugs and/or drug products look and/or sound like those of other drugs.

Names of pharmaceutical products have on occasion been changed to negate the possible confusion associated with the name of the other product. Several years ago, a brand name of amoxicillin was changed from LAROCIN to LAROTID. This was to decrease the possibility that the product would be confused with LANOXIN, a product with cardiac action. The need for clarification and enunciation is also evident when a prescription is telephoned to the pharmacist. A good example of this would be a telephoned prescription for KOLYUM, which could inadvertently be interpreted as VALIUM. In the Wolfer and Stevens study, similarity in drug names accounted for 16% of prescription-filling errors, ranking second only to lack of concentration (9).

Omission(s) on the Prescription. The physician should make every effort to assure that the prescription is as complete as possible. This is particularly so with respect to omission in the superscription (i.e., name and strength of the drug product prescribed). It is implicit that the strength of a medication be indicated on the prescription. Omission of the dose strength does not imply to the pharmacist that the lowest strength or the usual dose product be dispensed; the prescriber must always be consulted. For example, the decision to dispense 50-mg tablets of HYDRODIURIL when a prescription for HYDRODIURIL is received and no strength is indicated cannot be justified on the basis that this is the most frequently used dosage strength.

It is the responsibility of the pharmacist to be familiar with the available strengths and dosage forms of prefabricated medications to detect such omissions and supply the physician with the necessary information. Similarly, whenever possible, the physician should indicate the dosage form desired. An increasing number of oral products are now available in both tablet and capsule form in equal amounts. It is important that the patient receive the intended dosage form. It *cannot* be assumed that the capsule and tablet would be interchangeable in drug-release characteristics, either. For example, the capsule dosage form of COMPAZINE 10 mg is a sustained-release dosage form.

Measures to Prevent Illegal Prescription Alteration. With the advent of the drug culture, many drug abusers have become adept at writing their own prescriptions and forging the physician's name. Indeed, with the advent of consumer prescription price books from several chain-store pharmacies, instruction is clearly given on "how to read a prescription" (5). This serves as a perfect vehicle for the forger to ensure that everything is just right on the prescription blank. The key to control is *prevention on the physician's part* and *observation on the pharmacist's part.* Prescription blanks carelessly left in open view of the patient serve as an easy means for some patients to steal a few blanks; only the most observant physician would realize that several prescription blanks had been removed. Indeed, the worst practice for a physician is to presign blank prescription forms for later use and leave them unattended with the patient. Prescription blanks must be stored carefully out of sight of the patient.

The pharmacist must also be cautious about forged and/or altered prescriptions. Work experience will help familiarize the pharmacist with the local physicians' handwriting. An observant pharmacist will be able to pick out the forgery quite easily on the basis of the handwriting on the prescription. Prescriptions are also easily altered, however, by changing or increasing the amount of medication prescribed. For example, the number 4 could be changed to the number 24, or the Roman numeral XX (i.e., 20) could be changed to XXX (i.e., 30) (1). Pharmacists must be observant of these common tricks, especially for drugs with an abuse potential. Written prescriptions in different-colored ink (for one number) or one number placed too close to another may be clues to prescription alteration. Similarly, the size of the pen used on the prescription might not be consistent throughout all of the numbers.

Precautions About Polypharmacy. Whenever possible, the physician should write for the least number of prescription medications the patient will use and need. It has been shown that patient compliance with medications is adversely affected by increasing the number of patient medications. Confusion is probably the foremost problem of noncompliance in this sense. It becomes very difficult for patients to recall at what times to take certain medications or how often during the day. In the practice of medicine, however, there exist many instances when patients will require more than one medication. Frequently, physicians merely write two prescriptions on one blank to save time. This practice *should be discouraged.* It should be followed *only* if the physician, the clinic, or the hospital uses a polyprescription form. Although the polyprescription form is convenient for the physician and in general ensures that the patient will not lose any of the prescriptions, it can place a hardship on the pharmacist. This burden arises when the physician writes a prescription for a controlled substance on a polyprescription form. Legal requirements stipulate that a prescription for a controlled substance be filed separately from ordinary prescriptions. Thus, the pharmacist must take additional efforts to ensure that the letter of the law is upheld.

Size and Frequency of the Prescribed Dose. The size and frequency of the dose must be carefully considered by the physician prior to writing the prescription. It is the responsibility of the pharmacist to determine the safety of the prescribed dose prior to dispensing the medication to the patient. This determination by the pharmacist must be made for relatively toxic drugs as well as for seemingly innocuous drugs. The dosage and its frequency are intended to best befit the needs of the patient. The pharmacist must consider the patient's age, weight, surface area, and physical condition while evaluating a dosage regimen. Aside from these considerations, the dosage form requested, any possible interactions with other drugs, and the frequency of administration are all weighed by the pharmacist. Because of the number of variables, there is no steadfast rule on dosing. It is basically empirical, commensurate with the physician's experience. There are a number of references (e.g., *Pediatric Dosage Handbook, Facts and Comparisons, AMA Drug Evaluations*) that contain useful dosing information. In special instances, however, such as pediatric medicine, the experience of the physician usually dictates the dose and frequency, even though there are several empirical rules based on weight and age for estimation of doses of children and infants. In the recent past, if has been observed that a dose does not always follow a simple linear function of body weight and that its calculation as amount of drug per kilogram of body weight is inaccurate. Clinical experience has demonstrated that the doses of a number of drugs are more nearly proportional to the surface area of the body.

SELECTION OF A PRESCRIPTION BLANK TYPE

There are a multitude of prescription blank types that are available from a number of manufacturers of professional prescription packages. Vanity sometimes plays an important role in the selection of a prescription blank. Colors, style of type size, and even subdued photo imprints are considered. When selecting a prescription blank for one's practice, however, the following points are offered as a guideline in the selection process:

1. Select a prescription blank of normal size (e.g., 5 1/2 in. by 4 in.). Odd-size prescription blanks are either too small or too large. These are extremely difficult for a pharmacist to file conveniently.
2. Prescription blanks should contain the physician's name, address, city, telephone number, DEA number, and state registry number when applicable (Fig. 35-6). The mere address of "San Francisco" is sometimes inappropriate, depending upon the class of medication prescribed.
3. The place for refill directions and labeling instructions should be prominent on the face of the prescription (Fig. 35-3). If the prescribing physician does not believe in prescription refills, it is possible to have *NR* (i.e., nonrefillable) imprinted upon the blank.
4. The prescription blank should have adequate space on the reverse side for an adequate record of refills when necessary.
5. A place for instructions about generic substitution and/or its permissibility is advised. Figure 35-6 illustrates this concept according to the position of the physician's signature.

SUMMARY AND CONCLUSIONS

Prescription writing is an art, and it is imperative that the physician exercise this art in a diligent fashion. The time spent to write a prescription that is complete, correct, and legible will ensure that the patient receives the correct medication, dosage form, and dosage regimen. Communication between the physician and the pharmacist is encouraged to identify any problems (i.e., legal, nonlegal) associated with the writing of the prescription.

REFERENCES

1. Abbott, L. Battling drugstore burglary: An inmate tells how. *Am. Pharm.* 18:26, 1978.
2. Fink, J.L. III (ed.). *Pharmacy Law Digest.* Medica, PA: Harwal Publishing Co., 1984, p. CS1306.21.
3. Matthews, L.G. *History of Pharmacy in Britain.* Edinburg: E. & S. Livingstone, 1962.
4. Mez-Mangold, L. *A History of Drugs.* Basel, Switzerland: F. Hoffman-LaRoche, 1971, p. 49.
5. *Osco Prescription Price Book.* Oak Brook, Ill.: Osco Drug, 1974, p. 203.
6. Plein, E.M. The prescription. In: *Prescription Pharmacy.* Philadelphia: J.B. Lippincott, 1970, p. 1.
7. Smith, M.C. The prescription: Everything you wanted to know but didn't think to ask. *Am. Pharm.* 18:31, 1978.
8. Snipes, F.L. Putting zip in prescription writing: A proposal. *Postgrad. Med.* 63:185, 1978.
9. Wolfer, R.R., and Stevens, R.M. A 12-month study of reported dispensing errors (in patients). *Hosp. Pharm.* 6:2, 1971.

APPENDIX A

PHARMACOKINETIC PARAMETERS

W.A. Ritschel

It is generally accepted that changes in drug concentrations in the body as a function of time are related to the course of pharmacological effects. The change of drug concentration with time depends on the four main pharmacokinetic phases: (a) absorption (the systemic uptake of the drug in solution at the site of administration or absorption), (b) distribution (the process of drug penetration and permeation out from systemic circulation into tissues, different body compartments, and other body fluids), (c) metabolism (the biotransformation of the parent molecule to usually less effective or ineffective, more polar metabolites), and (d) elimination (the process of final removal of the drug independent of pathway, particularly via the kidney and liver, but also via lungs, skin, saliva, or milk).

Pharmacokinetic parameters characterize the fate of a drug in the body. Clinically most important are the following: (a) elimination half-life, $t_{1/2}$, the time required to reduce the drug plasma concentration to one-half after equilibrium is established; (b) the apparent volume of distribution, V_d, the fictitious volume of distribution, a volume that would be required to dissolve the total amount of drug at the same concentration as that found in blood or plasma: (c) the fraction of unchanged drug excreted into urine, F_u; and (d) the fraction of drugs systemically absorbed after extravascular administration, F, also called absolute bioavailability.

An additional parameter is clinically important, namely the therapeutic concentration or therapeutic range.

The elimination half-life, $t_{1/2}$, can easily be converted into the terminal elimination rate constant β:

$$\beta = 0.693/t_{1/2} \qquad \text{Eq. 1}$$

Knowing the V_d and β one can simply calculate the total clearance, Cl_{tot}:

$$Cl_{tot} = V_d \cdot \beta \qquad \text{Eq. 2}$$

Since $t_{1/2}$ is given in hours, the dimension for β is 1/hr. V_d has the dimension l/kg. Hence, the dimension for Cl_{tot} = l/kg/hr. Multiplying V_d or Cl_{tot} by the body weight one obtains the individual patient's volume of distribution or clearance of a given drug.

How can pharmacokinetic parameters clinically be used? There are numerous applications possible. But principally there are two groups for use, namely for characterization of a given drug to answer some clinically relevant questions and for dosage regimen design.

Questions belonging to the first group are, for instance:

1. How long does it take to completely eliminate the drug from the body?
   Answer: 10 x $t_{1/2}$ in hours.
2. How long does it take to reduce a drug blood level to 50, 25, and 10% of its original value?
   Answer: 1 x $t_{1/2}$, 2 x $t_{1/2}$, 4 x $t_{1/2}$ in hours, respectively.
3. Using identical dose sizes for multiple dosing how long does it take to reach steady-state concentration in blood?
   Answer: 5 x $t_{1/2}$ in hours.
4. Will renal impairment influence the $t_{1/2}$ of a drug and prolong its elimination?
   Answer: It depends on the magnitude of fraction of unchanged drug eliminated in urine. The closer F_u approaches 1 the longer will be the drug's $t_{1/2}$ with increasing renal impairment.
5. Can you predict a drug's $t_{1/2}$ in renal failure?
   Answer: An estimate is easily obtained using the drug's F_u value and the patient's observed creatinine clearance:

$$t_{1/2\ \text{renal failure}} = \frac{t_{1/2\ \text{normal}}}{\left[\left(\frac{Cl_{creatinine}}{120} - 1\right) \cdot F_u\right] + 1} \qquad \text{Eq. 3}$$

6. For which drugs may displacement from protein binding cause a clinical problem?
   Answer: Only for acidic drugs with protein binding of more than 80% and a V_d larger than 0.15 l/kg.

Questions belonging to the second group, for instance:

1. Since a patient has impaired renal function and it has been determined that $t_{1/2}$ will be prolonged (see Eq. 3), what should be the dosing interval in renal failure, $\tau_{renal\ failure}$?
   Answer:

$$\tau_{renal\ failure} = \tau_{normal} \cdot (t_{1/2\ renal\ failure}/t_{1/2\ normal}) \qquad \text{Eq. 4}$$

2. The normal maintenance dose, D_{normal}, for a drug is known. Because of a patient's renal impairment one wishes to reduce the dose size $D_{renal\ failure}$ and keep the dosing interval.

$$D_{renal\ failure} = D_{normal} \cdot (t_{1/2\ normal}/t_{1/2\ renal\ failure}) \qquad \text{Eq. 5}$$

3. Can you predict an optimal dose size, D, for an individual patient based on pharmacokinetic parameters and a described therapeutic concentration, $C_{ss\ desired}$?
   Answer: Yes, the maintenance dose size, DM, based on the mean therapeutic concentration is calculated as follows:

$$DM = \frac{C_{ss\ desired} \times V_d \times \text{body weight in kg} \times \tau}{1.44 \times t_{1/2} \cdot F} \qquad \text{Eq. 6}$$

   τ is the chosen dosing interval (i.e., every 4, 6, 8, or 12 hrs, respectively), $t_{1/2}$ is the drug's elimination half-life, and F is the bioavailability.

The pharmacokinetic parameters listed in Table A-1 have been compiled from the literature and recent reviews (1-5). The values represent mean values, usually from several studies. They may vary between individual reports and studies depending on method of assay, length of blood sampling, dose size, age of subjects, time of administration, administration of drug before, with, or after meals, disease and disease states, etc. Hence, the values do not represent absolute figures valid for all subjects and all circumstances. Not only may disease and disease state largely affect one or more pharmacokinetic parameters, but also interindividual variation may be large for some drugs. For instance, the $t_{1/2}$ of theophylline may range interindividually between 3 and 15 hours over a fivefold range, whereas the other parameters remain practically constant. In the case of phenytoin the $T_{1/2}$ of 22 hours is a rough estimate. The $t_{1/2}$ for this drug is dose-dependent.

One may ask, How useful are my pharmacokinetic parameters if their values are rather variable than absolute? Without question the pharmacokinetic parameters may be very helpful for the clinician in answering numerous questions regarding dosing and side effects and to design dosage regimens to achieve a desired therapeutic drug concentration. However, monitoring of drug concentration becomes an integral part of optimizing therapy. Drug monitoring, if indicated, should be performed to finally adjust the dosage regimen to the desired therapeutic level.

REFERENCES

1. Avery, G.S. (ed.) *Drug Treatment*, 2nd ed. Sydney: Adis Press, 1980.
2. Bochner, F., Carruthers, G., Kampmann, J., and Steiner, J. *Handbook of Clinical Pharmacology*, 2nd ed. Boston: Little, Brown, 1983.
3. Ritschel, W.A. *Handbook of Basic Pharmacokinetics*, 2nd updated ed. Hamilton, IL.: Drug Intelligence Publications, 1982.
4. Ritschel, W.A. *Graphic Approach to Clinical Pharmacokinetics*, Barcelona, Spain: J.R. Prous, 1983.
5. Sadée, W, and Beelen, G.C.M. *Drug Level Monitoring*, New York: John Wiley, 1980.

Table A-1
Pharmacokinetic Parameters of Important Drugs

Drug	$t_{1/2}$ (hr)	V_d (l/kg)	F_u	F	Therapeutic Range (μg/ml)
Acebutolol	2.9	2.9	0.4	0.4	0.5-2.0
Acetaminophen	2.5	1.1	0.05	0.85	1-10
Acetazolamide	3.5	0.2	0.9	1.0	5-100
Acetyldigoxin	53.0	4.2	0.2	0.8	
Acetylprocainamide	6	1.4	0.8	0.85	2-22
Acetylsalicylic Acid	0.25	0.21	0.01	1.0	20-300
Alprenolol	2.7	3.4	0.01	0.01	
Amikacin	2.5	0.25	0.9	1	10-25
p-Aminosalicylic Acid	0.85	0.23	0.25	0.9	230
Amitriptyline	17.1	8.8	0.05	0.65	0.3-0.9
Amobarbital	21	1.1	0	1	1-8
Amoxicillin	1.2	0.47	0.7	0.92	2-8
Amphetamine	12.2	4.0	0.65	1	0.01-0.03
Amphotericin B	20	4.0	0.05	0.03	0.2-2.0
Ampicillin	0.9	0.52	0.9	0.5	2-8
Antipyrine	11.5	0.62	0.1	1	
Azidocillin	0.8	0.28	0.6	0.3	0.01-0.8
Butobarbital	37.5	0.8	0.08	1	1-5
Carbamazepine	37.7	1.2	0.01	0.9	4-12
Carbenicillin	0.8	0.15	0.8	0.5	10-125
Carisoprodol	8.0	0.66	0.3	1	10-30
Cefamandol	0.6	0.2	1.0	1	0.5-5
Cefazolin	1.6	0.17	0.8	0	0.1-63
Cephacetrile	1.0	0.18	0.85	0	3
Cephalexin	0.9	0.33	0.9	0.9	6-50
Cephaloridine	1.2	0.23	0.85	0.05	0.1-16
Cephalothin	0.6	0.31	0.6	0	0.1-6.3
Cephapirin	0.75	0.15	0.7	0.05	1-12
Cephradine	0.76	0.32	0.9	1	0.5-12
Chloramphenicol	2.7	0.57	0.1	0.8	5-40
Chlordiazepoxide	15.0	0.3	0	1	1-3
Chlorpromazine	30	21.0	0.01	0.32	50-300
Chlorpropamide	32	0.15	0.2	1.0	50-150
Chlortetracycline	5.6	1.74	0.18	0.7	0.5-6
Cimetidine	2.0	1.8	0.7	0.7	0.25-1
Clindamycin	2.8	1.1	0.1	0.9	0.002-0.5
Clofibrate	16.7	0.12	0.3	1	80-150
Clonazepam	27	2.5	—	0.9	0.01-0.07
Clonidine	8	3.5	0.3	0.8	0.0002-0.002
Cloxacillin	0.5	0.15	0.75	0.8	7-14
Codeine	3.3	3.45	0.1	0.5	0.025
Colistin Sulfate	3	0.55	0.8	1 i.m.	1-5
Colistimethate	3	0.5	0.75	1 i.m.	1-5
Demethylchlortetracycline	13.6	1.8	0.4	0.7	0.5-3
Desipramine	17	41.9	0.1	1	0.15-0.3
Diazepam	32.9	2.0	0.005	1	0.1-1
Diazoxide	30	0.2	0.4	1.0	15-25
Dicloxacillin	0.8	0.29	0.7	0.8	15-18
Dicumarol	8.2	0.13	0.01	0.8	5-10
Digitoxin	164	0.6	0.08	0.9	0.01-0.035

Table A-1
Pharmacokinetic Parameters of Important Drugs (Continued)

Drug	$t_{1/2}$ (hr)	V_d (l/kg)	F_u	F	Therapeutic Range (μg/ml)
Digoxin	43	6.3	0.76	0.62	0.0008-0.002
Diphenhydramine	5.2	3.7	0.03	0.5	0.01-0.1
Disopyramide	7	0.5	0.6	0.8	3-6
Doxycycline	20	1.0	0.55	1	1-2
Erythromycin	1.4	0.6	0.15	0.4	0.5-2.5
Ethambutol	3.5	2.3	0.85	0.8	1-5
Ethosuximide	50	0.6	0.3	1.0	50-100
Flucloxacillin	0.8	0.12	0.55	0.5	0.4
Furosemide	1.5	0.2	0.75	0.6	0.1-0.2
Gentamicin	2	0.25	0.9	0 p.o. 1 i.v., i.m.	0.5-10
Glutethimide	8.7	2.2	0.002	1	0.2-0.8
Griseofulvin	14	1.5	0.01	0.5	0.3-1.3
Hexobarbital	4.1	1.3	0	1	2-4
Hydralazine					
Fast acetylator	5	0.5	0.02	0.22	0.5-1.5
Slow acetylator	4	0.5		0.38	0.5-1.5
Imipramine	7	30	0	1	0.15-0.5
Isoniazid					
Fast acetylator	1.1	0.6	0.3	0.9	0.5-15
Slow acetylator	3.6	0.6	0.5	0.9	0.5-15
Kanamycin	2	0.25	0.81	0 p.o. 0.7 i.m.	2-8
Lidocaine	1.8	1.5	0.1	0.35	1.5-7
Lincomycin	5.4	0.4	0.15	0.4	0.09-3
Lithium	19.2	0.8	1.0	1.0	0.6-1.4 meq/l
Lorazepam	13	0.8	0.01	1	0.02-0.05
Meperidine	3.5	4.7	0.1	0.52	0.2-0.6
Meprobamate	12	0.7	0.1	0.9	5-15
Metformin	1.5	60.0	0.8	0.32	1-10
Methacycline	13	1.8	0.4	0.7	1-10
Methadone	15	1.5	0.2	1	0.1-0.4
Methicillin	1	0.3	0.75	0 p.o.	1-6
Metronidazole	11	0.65	0.4	0.9	1-2.5
Mexiletine	10.5	9.0	0.1	0.88	0.75-2.0
Mezlocillin	0.8	0.38	0.5	0 p.o.	4-8
Miconazole	22.5	21	0.01	0.3	0.001-10
Minocycline	12	0.43	0.1	0.9	0.5-3
Morphine	2.3	1.0	0.1	0.4 p.o.	0.07-0.1
Nadolol	14.1	2.0	0.6	0.4	0.1-0.3
Nafcillin	0.5	0.3	0.38	0.5	0.03-1
Nitrazepam	31	2.1	0.01	0.8	0.03-0.06
Nortriptyline	27	20	0.02	0.6	0.05-0.8
Oxacillin	1	0.33	0.55	0.7	5-6
Oxazepam	12	1.2	0.02	1	1-2
Oxprenolol	1.9	1.2	0.05	0.45	0.06
Oxytetracycline	9.2	1.9	0.25	0.77	0.05-3
Penicillin G	0.7	0.5	0.8	0.3	1.5-3
Penicillin V	0.6	0.4	0.26	0.4	3-5
Pentazocine	2.5	4.0	0.05	0.5	0.1-0.6

Table A-1
Pharmacokinetic Parameters of Important Drugs (Continued)

Drug	$t_{1/2}$ (hr)	V_d (l/kg)	F_u	F	Therapeutic Range (μg/ml)
Pentobarbital	22.3	1.0	0.01	1	1-4
Phenobarbital	90	0.7	0.35	0.9	10-50
Phenylbutazone	72	0.25	0	1	40-150
Phenytoin	22	0.65	0.05	0.9	10-20
Pindolol	2.2	1.5	0.5	0.9	0.005-0.01
Practolol	10.5	1.6	0.9	1	1-2
Primidone	6.5	0.8	0.1	0.8	5-12
Probenecid	5	0.15	0.05	1	100-200
Procainamide	3	2	0.5	0.85	4-10
Propoxyphene	6.5	5.4	0.015	0.2	0.2-0.8
Propranolol	3.8	5.5	0.01	0.35	0.05-0.1
Quinidine	6.3	3	0.2	0.75	1-4
Ranitidine	2.3	1.2	0.8	0.6	0.1
Rifampin	3	0.6	0.15	1	0.5-10
Salicylate	4	0.14	0.15	1	20-300
Streptomycin	2.4	0.26	0.5	0 p.o.	20-25
Sulfadiazine	17	0.9	0.6	0.9	100-150
Sulfamerazine	22	0.35	—	0.9	50-200
Sulfamethazine	9	0.5	0.3	0.9	50-200
Sulfamethizole	1.5	0.35	0.75	0.9	50-200
Sulfamethoxazole	10	0.3	0.35	0.9	50-200
Sulfisoxazole	6	0.16	0.5	1	90-150
Tetracycline	6.8	1.3	0.6	0.8	0.5-2
Theophylline	5.5	0.45	0.08	1	10-20
Timolol	4.9	3.1	0.1	0.75	0.005-0.01
Tobramycin	2	0.25	0.9	1	2-10
Tocainide	12.5	2	0.4	1.0	5-10
Tolbutamide	7	0.12	0	1	50-100
Trimethoprim	8.8	2.0	0.6	1	0.5-12
Valproate	12.2	0.14	0.05	0.9	20-100
Warfarin	46	0.11	0	0.9	1-10

INDEX

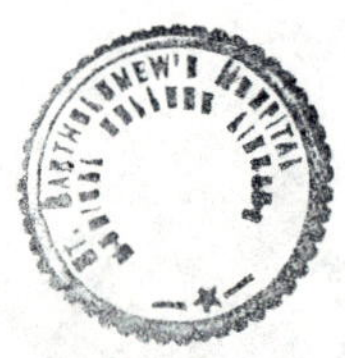

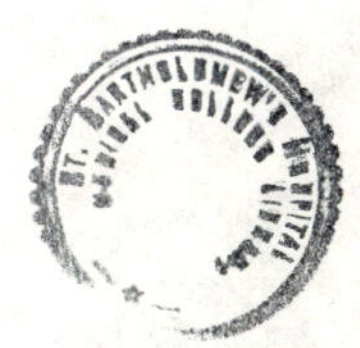

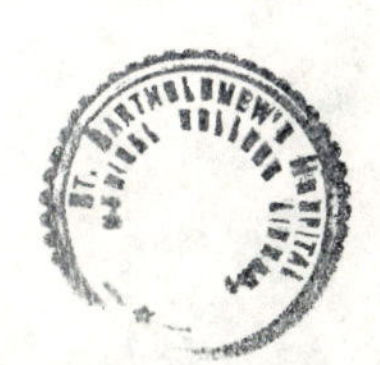